Instructor Resources—Redefined!

INTRODUCING
Pearson Nursing Class Preparation Resources

- **New and Unique! Correlation to Today's Nursing Standards!**
  - Correlation guides link book and supplement content to nursing standards such as the *2010 ANA Scope and Standards of Practice, QSEN, National Patient Safety Goals, AACN Essentials of Baccalaureate Education* and more
- **New and Unique! Pearson Nursing Lecture Series**
  - Highly visual, fully narrated and animated, these short lectures focus on topics that are traditionally difficult to teach and difficult for students to grasp
  - All lectures accompanied by case studies and classroom response questions for greater interactivity within even the largest classroom
  - Useful as lecture tools, remediation material, homework assignments and more
- **Additional instructor resources!**
  - Find assets such as **videos, animations, lecture starters, classroom and clinical activities** and more!
  - **Add selected resources** to presentations that can be shown online or exported to PowerPoint™ or HTML pages
  - Organized by topic and **fully searchable** by type and keyword
  - **Upload your own resources** to keep everything in one place
  - **Rate resources** and view other instructor ratings
- **Pearson Nursing Question Bank**
  - Even **more** accessible with both pencil and paper and online delivery options
  - Expanded question bank for each chapter
  - **All New!** Approximately 30% of questions now in alternate-item format
  - **Complete rationales** for both correct and incorrect answers mapped to learning outcomes

Book-specific resources also available to instructors including:

- Online Instructor's Manual with detailed lecture outlines and activities
- Comprehensive PowerPoint™ presentations integrating lecture notes and images
- Image library
- Classroom Response Questions
- Online course management systems complete with instructor tools and student activities

mynursinglab

- Saves instructor time by providing quality feedback, ongoing formative assessments, and customized remediation for students
- **New!** Select *Real Nursing Simulation* scenarios
- Includes select set of *Real Nursing Skill 2.0* videos
- Available with *Pearson's Interactive e-Text*
  - Integrated media and website links
  - Full search capability and note-taking functionality
  - Customizable organization

REAL NURSING SIMULATIONS

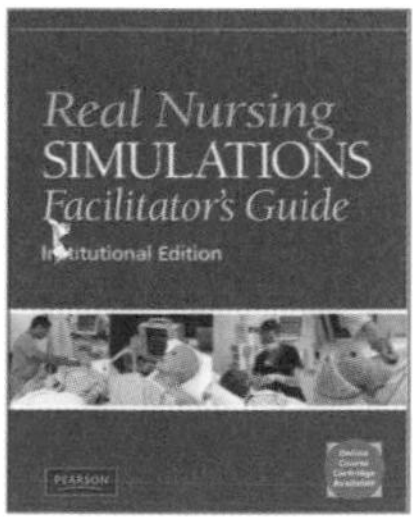

- 25 simulation scenarios that span the nursing curriculum
- Consistent format includes learning objectives, case flow, set-up instructions, debriefing questions and more!
- Companion online course cartridge with student pre- and post-simulation activities, videos, skill checklists and reflective discussion questions

Brief Contents

OLDS'

Maternal-Newborn NURSING & Women's Health

Across the Lifespan

NINTH EDITION

Michele R. Davidson, PhD, CNM, CFN, RN
Associate Professor of Nursing and Women's Studies
George Mason University
Fairfax, Virginia

Marcia L. London, RN, MSN, APRN, CNS, NNP-BC
Senior Clinical Instructor and Director of Neonatal Nurse Practitioner Program (Ret.)
Beth-El College of Nursing and Health Sciences
University of Colorado
Colorado Springs, Colorado
Staff Clinical Nurse
Urgent Care and After Hours Clinic
Colorado Springs, Colorado

Patricia A. Wieland Ladewig, PhD, RN
Vice President for Academic Affairs
Regis University
Denver, Colorado

Pearson
Boston Columbus Indianapolis New York San Francisco Upper Saddle River
Amsterdam Cape Town Dubai London Madrid Milan Munich Paris Montreal Toronto
Delhi Mexico City São Paulo Sydney Hong Kong Seoul Singapore Taipei Tokyo

Library of Congress Cataloging-in-Publication Data
Davidson, Michele R.
Olds' maternal-newborn nursing & women's health across the lifespan / Michele R. Davidson, Marcia L. London, Patricia A. Wieland Ladewig. -- 9th ed.
p. ; cm.
Olds' maternal-newborn nursing and women's health across the lifespan
Maternal-newborn nursing & women's health across the lifespan
Includes bibliographical references and index.
ISBN-13: 978-0-13-210907-9
ISBN-10: 0-13-210907-7
1. Maternity nursing--Handbooks, manuals, etc. 2. Newborn infants—Diseases—Nursing—Handbooks, manuals, etc. I. London, Marcia L. II. Ladewig, Patricia W. III. Title. IV. Title: Olds' maternal-newborn nursing and women's health across the lifespan. V. Title: Maternal-newborn nursing & women's health across the lifespan.
[DNLM: 1. Maternal-Child Nursing--methods. 2. Neonatal Nursing--methods. 3. Nursing Assessment--methods. 4. Pregnancy Complications--nursing. 5. Women's Health. WY 157.3]
RG951.O43 2012
618.2'0231--dc22
2010042912

Notice: Care has been taken to confirm the accuracy of information presented in this book. The authors, editors, and the publisher, however, cannot accept any responsibility for errors or omissions or for consequences from application of the information in this book and make no warranty, express or implied, with respect to its contents.

The authors and publisher have exerted every effort to ensure that drug selections and dosages set forth in this text are in accord with current recommendations and practice at time of publication. However, in view of ongoing research, changes in government regulations, and the constant flow of information relating to drug therapy and reactions, the reader is urged to check the package inserts of all drugs for any change in indications or dosage and for added warning and precautions. This is particularly important when the recommended agent is a new and/or infrequently employed drug.

Publisher: Julie Levin Alexander
Assistant to Publisher: Regina Bruno
Executive Acquisitions Editor: Kim Mortimer
Editorial Assistant: Marion Gottlieb
Assistant Editor for Media: Sarah Wrocklage
Director of Marketing: David Gesell
Marketing Manager: Phoenix Harvey
Marketing Specialist: Michael Sirinides
Development Editors: Elena Mauceri and Lynda Hatch
Development, Supplements: Pamela Lappies
Managing Editor, Production: Patrick Walsh
Production Editor: Heather Willison, S4Carlisle Publishing Services
Production Liaison: Anne Garcia
Media Project Managers: Rachel Collett and Leslie Brado
Manufacturing Manager: Ilene Sanford
Art Editor: Patricia Gutierrez
Media Product Manager: Travis Moses-Westphal
Senior Design Coordinator: Chris Weigand
Interior Design: Mary Siener and Christine Cantera
Cover Design: Mary Siener
Cover Image: Getty Images, Kick Images, Tsoi Hoi Fung
Composition: S4Carlisle Publishing Services
Image Specialist: Annette Linder
Manager, Cover Visual Research & Permissions: Karen Sanatar
Art Studio: Argosy Publishing
Printer/Binder: Courier Kendallville
Cover Printer: Lehigh-Phoenix Color/Hagerstown

Chapter opener credits: Page 1: Corbis/Superstock Royalty Free; Page 24: Purestock/Florian Flake/ Superstock; Page 44: Kevin Schafer/Alamy Images Royalty Free; Page 59: Glow Asia/Superstock Royalty Free; Page 80: SS Photography / FreeDigitalPhotos.net; Page 99: David Morgan/Alamy Images; Page 116: Corbis/Superstock Royalty Free; Page 145: Kablonk/Superstock Royalty Free; Page 165: djcodrin / FreeDigitalPhotos.net; Page 186: Terry Vine/Blended Images/Alamy; Page 216: Blend Images/Superstock Royalty Free; Page 242: Image Source/Superstock Royalty Free; Page 277: moodboard/Superstock Royalty Free; Page 295: Blend Images/Superstock Royalty Free; Page 317: Steve Smith/Superstock Royalty Free; Page 344: Rubberball/Superstock Royalty Free; Page 378: Hola Images/Alamy Images Royalty Free; Page 394: Exactstock/Superstock Royalty Free; Page 416: Fancy Collection/Superstock Royalty Free; Page 450: Blend Images/Superstock Royalty Free; Page 496: Galleo Images/Superstock Royalty Free; Page 528: OJO Images/Superstock Royalty Free; Page 554: Tetra Images/Superstock Royalty Free; Page 594: Rubberball/Superstock Royalty Free; Page 634: Radius/Superstock Royalty Free; Page 662: Purestock/Greer & Associates/SuperStock; Page 692: Fancy Collection/Superstock Royalty Free; Page 724: Rubberball/Superstock Royalty Free; Page 755: Exactostock/Superstock Royalty Free; Page 782: Ruberball/Superstock Royalty Free; Page 823: Blend Images/Superstock Royalty Free; Page 849: Blend Images/Superstock Royalty Free; Page 889: Courtesy of Joanna Allen / Pearson Education; Page 938: Exactostock/ Superstock Royalty Free; Page 990: Exactostock/Superstock Royalty Free; Page 1019: OJO Images/Superstock Royalty Free; Page 1054: Corbis/ Superstock Royalty Free; Page 1086: Exactostock/Superstock Royalty Free; Page 1114: Courtesy of Joanna Allen /Pearson Education.

PEARSON

www.pearsonhighered.com

10 9 8 7 6 5 4 3 2 1
ISBN-13: 978-0-13-210907-9
ISBN-10: 0-13-210907-7

Sally B. Olds is the quintessential nurse and teacher—

She sees possibilities where others see problems, abilities where others see limitations.

She cares passionately about childbearing families and has a clear vision of what excellent nursing means.

She stresses the importance of clinical skill and acumen but never loses sight of the human side of caregiving.

She is committed to students, to helping them to learn and grow, to develop their own sense of the difference a nurse can make.

She is the best of the best of nursing. . .

And so, with the deepest affection and respect we dedicate this book to Sally, our dear friend and colleague.

Thank you for the inspiration you provided, the warmth you brought, and the expertise you shared.

We hope you enjoy many days of sunshine, blessings, and joy.

And, as always, to our beloved families

To Nathan Davidson, Hayden, Chloe, Caroline, and Grant

To David London, Craig and his fiancé Jennifer, and Matthew

To Tim Ladewig, Ryan, Amanda, Reed, and Addison, and Erik, Kedri, Emma, and Camden

About the Authors

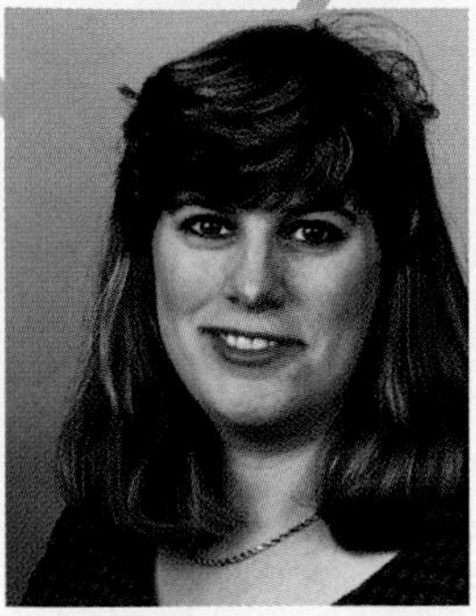

Michele Davidson

Michele Davidson received an ADN degree from Marymount University in 1990 and upon graduation began working in postpartum and the newborn nursery in Washington, DC. Because of her interest in educating expectant and new families, she began an education and consulting service providing childbirth education classes, lactation consulting services, and newborn care courses. During this time she also worked as a reproductive endocrinology/infertility nurse while she obtained a BSN from George Mason University. Dr. Davidson then attended Case Western Reserve University where she earned her MSN and a nurse-midwifery certificate. She worked as a nurse-midwife at Columbia Hospital for Women in Washington, DC, while completing her PhD in nursing administration and healthcare policy from George Mason University (GMU). Dr. Davidson began teaching at GMU in 1999. Dr. Davidson has developed an immersion clinical experience for GMU students on a remote island in the Chesapeake Bay, where she teaches community health nursing to students who reside in the community. In 2003, she founded the Smith Island Foundation, a nonprofit organization in which she serves as executive director. In her free time, Michele enjoys spending time with her mother, gardening, reading, and spending time at their home on Smith Island with her nurse practitioner husband, Nathan, and their four young children, Hayden, Chloe, Caroline, and Grant. Dr. Davidson recently received certification as a Certified Forensic Nurse. Her research interests include maternal-newborn and women's mental health issues.

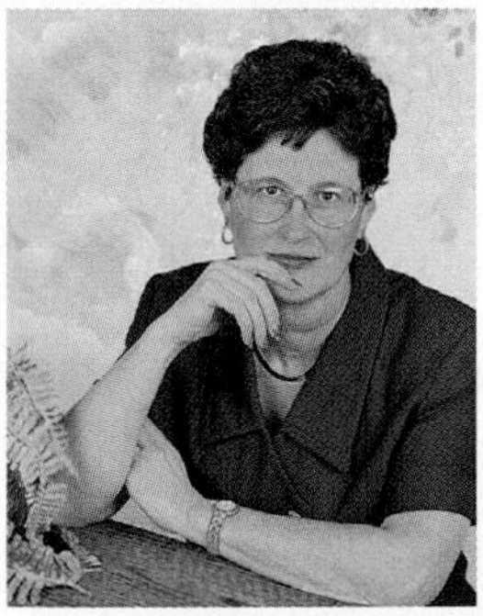

Marcia L. London

Marcia L. London has been able to combine her two greatest passions by being both a nurse caring for children and families and a teacher for almost 40 years. She received her BSN and school nurse certificate from Plattsburgh State University in Plattsburgh, New York. After graduation, she began her nursing career as a pediatric nurse at St. Luke's Hospital in New York City, then moved to Pittsburgh, where she began her teaching career. Mrs. London accepted a faculty position at Pittsburgh's Children's Hospital Affiliate Program and received her MSN in pediatrics as a clinical nurse specialist from the University of Pittsburgh. Mrs. London began teaching at Beth-El School of Nursing and Health Science in 1974 after opening the first intensive care nursery at Memorial Hospital of Colorado Springs. She has served in many administrative and faculty positions at Beth-El, including coordinator for nursing care of children for 32 years. Mrs. London maintained her clinical skills working in an urgent care and after-hours clinic, doing undergraduate pediatric clinical supervision, and teaching class. She obtained her postmaster's neonatal nurse practitioner certificate in 1983 and subsequently developed the neonatal nurse practitioner (NNP) program and the master's NNP program at Beth-El. She is active nationally in neonatal nursing and was involved in the development of the Neonatal Nurse Practitioner Educational Program Guidelines. She has contributed five chapters to various neonatal nursing texts. Mrs. London is active in nurse practitioner education in general. She was involved in the revision of the Core Competency for Nurse Practitioners and Curriculum Guidelines for Nurse Practitioner Education, as a member of the Education Committee of the National Organization of Nurse Practitioner Faculties, and participated as part of the Core Competency Validation Expert Panel. Mrs. London has also pursued her interest in college student learning by taking doctoral classes in higher education administration and adult learning at the University of Denver in Colorado. She feels fortunate to be involved in the education of her future colleagues. Her teaching philosophy is that, with support, students can achieve more than they may initially believe they are capable of achieving. She believes in lifelong learning and applying it to her nursing care of patients as part of her faculty practice. Mrs. London and her husband have two sons and one dog (Reilly, daughter by proxy). Her son, Craig is involved in computer informatics and his fiancé Jennifer a future nurse. Matthew studied media arts and animation, and both sons are more than willing to give Mom and Dad helpful hints.

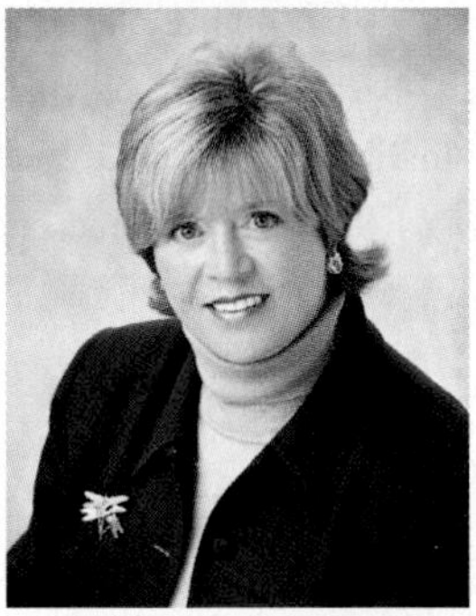

Patricia A. Wieland Ladewig

Patricia A. Wieland Ladewig received her BS from the College of Saint Teresa in Winona, Minnesota. After graduation, she worked as a pediatric nurse before joining the U.S. Air Force. After completing her tour of duty, Dr. Ladewig relocated in Florida, where she accepted a faculty position at Florida State University. There she embraced teaching as her calling. Over the years, she taught at several schools of nursing while earning her MSN in maternal-newborn nursing from Catholic University of America in Washington, DC, and her PhD in higher education administration from the University of Denver in Colorado. In addition, she became a women's health nurse practitioner and maintained a part-time clinical practice for many years. In 1988 Dr. Ladewig became the first director of the nursing program at Regis College in Denver and, in 1991, when the college became Regis University, she became dean of the Rueckert-Hartman College for Health Professions (RHCHP). Under her guidance, the Department of Nursing, now the Loretto Heights School of Nursing, added a graduate program and RHCHP added two new schools: the School of Physical Therapy and the School of Pharmacy as well as two departments: the Department of Health Services Administration and the Department of Health Care Ethics. Dr. Ladewig has now taken on a new role as Vice President for Academic Affairs at Regis University. She is excited by the opportunity this position gives her to help ensure the quality of academic programs across the entire university. When not at work or writing textbooks, Pat and her husband, Tim, enjoy skiing, Colorado Rockies baseball games, and traveling. However, their greatest pleasure comes from their family: son Ryan, his wife, Amanda, and grandchildren Reed and Addison; and son, Erik, his wife Kedri, and grandchildren Emma and Camden.

Thank You

Contributors

We are grateful to the contributors to the ninth edition of *Olds' Maternal-Newborn Nursing & Women's Health Across the Lifespan*. Thanks, also, to Pamela Lappies for editorial assistance on the supplements.

Jessica L. Anderson MSN, CNM, WHNP
University of Colorado College of Nursing
Senior Instructor
Aurora, CO
Chapter 15: Antepartum Nursing Assessment

Nancy Benner RNC, BSN
Presbyterian/St. Luke's Medical Center
Denver, CO
Chapter 31: The Normal Newborn: Needs and Care

Laura Bonazzoli MFA
Medical Writer
Chapter 3: Complementary and Alternative Therapies

Jessica Breese CNM, MS
University of Colorado
Aurora, CO
Chapter 21: Assessment of Fetal Well-Being

Jenny Clapp RN, MSN
University of North Carolina Greensboro
Greensboro, NC
Chapter 35: Postpartum Family Adaptation and Nursing Assessment

Alyssa Consigli RD, CD
University of Vermont
Burlington, VT
Chapter 18: Maternal Nutrition

Robin Webb Corbett PhD, RNC
East Carolina University
Greenville, NC
Chapter 6: Women's Health: Commonly Occurring Infections

Cathy Emeis PhD, CNM, FACCE, LCCE
Oregon Health and Science University
Portland, OR
Chapter 28: Birth-Related Procedures

Cori Feist MS, CGC
Oregon Health and Science University
Portland, OR
Chapter 12: Special Reproductive Concerns: Infertility and Genetics

Victoria Flanagan RN, MS
Dartmouth-Hitchcock Medical Center
White River Junction, VT
Chapter 19: Pregnancy at Risk: Pregestational Problems

Brigitte Hall RN, MSN, IBCLC
Georgetown University Hospital
Washington, DC
Chapter 32: Newborn Nutrition

Carol Ann Harrigan RN, MSN, NNP-BC
Cardon Children's Medical Center
Mesa, AZ
Chapter 33: The Newborn at Risk: Conditions Present at Birth

Jennifer Hensley CNM, WHNP, LCCE, EdD
University of Colorado
Denver, CO
Chapter 05: Women's Health: Family Planning

Stephanie Holaday DrPH, MSN, CNE
Trinity (Washington) University
Washington, DC
Chapter 22: Processes and Stages of Labor and Birth, and *Chapter 23:* Intrapartum Nursing Assessment

Janet L. Houser PhD, RN
Regis University
Denver, CO
Research Evidence in Practice features

Vanessa Howell RN, MSN
Memorial Health Care System – NICU
Colorado Springs, CO
Chapter 30: Nursing Assessment of the Newborn

Joanne Jonell MS, RNC-MNN
Regis University
Denver, CO
Chapter 17: Adolescent Pregnancy

Connie J. Kirkland MA, NCC
George Mason University
Fairfax, VA
Chapter 9: Violence Against Women

Cheryl Pope Kish RNC, MSN, EdD, WHNP
Georgia College & State University (retired)
Milledgeville, GA
Chapter 39: The Postpartum Family at Risk

Deborah Cooper McGee RNC, MSN, PNNP, RDMS
Obstetrix Medical Group of Colorado, Presbyterian St. Luke's Medical Center
Arvada, CO
Chapter 20: Pregnancy at Risk: Gestational Onset

Julie Nadeau RN, MS
University of the Incarnate Word
San Antonio, TX
Chapter 36: The Postpartum Family: Needs and Care, and Chapter 37: Home Care of the Postpartum Family

Patricia Posey-Goodwin RN, MS
University of West Florida
Pensacola, FL
Chapter 2: Care of the Family in a Culturally Diverse Society, *Chapter 24:* The Family in Childbirth: Needs and Care, and *Chapter 25:* Pain Management During Labor

Susan Saindon MSN, WHNP
South Denver Obstetrics and Gynecology
Littleton, CO
Chapter 4: Health Promotion of Women Across the Lifespan

Candice Schoeneberger PhD, WHCNP
Regis University
Denver, CO
Half of Chapter 16: The Expectant Family: Needs and Care

Kelly E. Shields RNC, BS, MSN, NCBF
St. David's Medical Center
Austin, TX
Chapter 38: Grief and Loss in the Childbearing Family

Patricia Shinn RN, MS
State University of New York (SUNY) at Canton
Canton, NY
Chapter 13: Preparation for Parenthood

Lisa Ann Smith-Pedersen APRN, MSN, NNP-BC
NNP, Denver Children's Hospital
Denver, CO
Chapter 34: The Newborn at Risk: Birth-Related Stressors

Donna Marie Stewart RN, MSN, NNP-BC
Memorial Health Care System-NICU
Colorado Springs, CO
Chapter 29: Physiologic Responses of the Newborn to Birth

Wendi Strauss MS, RNC-OB
Regis University
Denver, CO
Half of Chapter 16: The Expectant Family: Needs and Care

Supplement Contributors

Instructor Resources

Ann Bianchi RN, MSN
University of Alabama
Huntsville, AL

Stephanie Bronsky BSN, MSN Ed
Ashford University
Clinton, IA
Instructor's Resource Manual and PowerPoint Slides

Mary Goodrich BSN, MA
FlexEd
Las Vegas, NV
Testbank

Kathy Johnson RN, MA
University of South Dakota
Sioux Falls, SD

MyNursingLab

Kim D. Cooper RN, MSN
Ivy Tech Community College
Terre Haute, IN

Amy M. Corbitt RN, MSN
Children's Hospital of the King's Daughters
Norfolk, VA

Kelly Gosnell RN, MSN
Ivy Tech Community College
Terre Haute, IN

Christine Kuoni RN, MSN, CNE
San Antonio College
San Antonio, TX

Dawna Martich RN, MSN
Nursing Education Consultant
Pittsburgh, PA

Fawn Updike RN, MSN Ed
Ivy Tech Community College
Columbus, OH

Reviewers

We are grateful to all the nurses, both clinicians and educators, who reviewed the manuscript of this textbook. Their insights, suggestions, and eye for detail helped us prepare a more relevant and useful textbook, one that will prepare caring and competent nurses in the field of maternal-newborn and women's health nursing.

Ann Aschenrenner RN, MSN
Columbia College of Nursing

Nancy J. Cooley MSN, CAGS, FNP-BC
University of Maine at Augusta

Gail Coster RN, MSN, CWHNP
California State University Long Beach

Donna M.J. Davis RN, NP-BC, CNS, MSN
Imperial Valley College

Patricia Boyle Egland RN, MSN, CPNP-PC
The City University of New York

Jamie L. Houchins RN, MSN
Ivy Tech Community College

Linda Irle MSN, FNP, CNP
University of Illinois

Karen Jagiello MSN, RNC
James Madison University

Christine King Kuoni RN, MSN, CNE
San Antonio College

Hilda Diane Malloy RN, PhD
Saint Louis University

Sharon Y. Pompey RN, MSN
Schoolcraft College

Jane Ragozine MSN, WHNP-BC, CLC
Kent State University

Sonia Rudolph RN, MSN, ARNP, FNP-BC
Jefferson Community & Technical College

Janet Ruiz RN, MS
Front Range Community College

Linda V. Walsh CNM, MPH, PhD
University of San Francisco

Lisa Sneed RN, MSN, NCSN
Park University

Acknowledgments

Our goal with every revision is to incorporate the latest research and information from the literature of nursing and related fields to make our text as relevant and useful as possible. This would not be possible without the support and encouragement of our colleagues in nursing. The comments and suggestions we have received from nurse educators and practitioners around the country have helped us keep this text accurate and up to date. Whenever a nurse takes the time to write or to speak to one of us at a professional gathering, we recognize again the intense commitment of nurses to excellence in practice. And so we thank our colleagues.

We are grateful, too, to our students, past, present, and future. They stimulate us with their interest; they reinvigorate us with their enthusiasm; they challenge us with their questions to make each edition of this text clear and understandable. We learn so much from them.

In publishing, as in health care, quality assurance is an essential part of the process. That is the dimension our reviewers have added. Some reviewers assist us by validating the accuracy of the content, some by their attention to detail, and some by challenging us to examine our ways of thinking and to develop a new awareness about a given topic. Thus, we extend our sincere thanks to all those who reviewed the manuscript for this book. Their names and affiliations are listed on the preceding pages.

We are also grateful to the contributors to the ninth edition of ***Olds' Maternal-Newborn Nursing & Women's Health Across the Lifespan***. Their knowledge of clinical practice and current literature in their areas of expertise helps make the chapters relevant and accurate. They, too, are listed on the preceding pages.

The success of a project of this scope requires the skills and dedication of many people. We would personally like to thank the following people:

Thanks to Kim Mortimer, our new editor. Kim has been supportive and helpful throughout the project. She brings a wealth of publishing experience to challenge us, a fresh eye to refocus us, and a warmth and responsiveness that has already enabled us to bond as a team.

Julie Alexander, our publisher, has played an important role in the development of our text. Her leadership of Prentice Hall Health has resulted in the growth of a company committed to excellence, to technology, and to student support. She is a visionary in publishing.

We cannot say enough good things about our developmental editor Elena Mauceri, and her colleague and partner on this project, Lynda Hatch. We have worked with Elena on other books and deeply appreciate her creativity, organizational skill, and ability to stay calm and unflappable. Things simply go more smoothly because of all she brings to a project. Having Lynda join her has been an added benefit. Lynda, too, has a wonderful eye for detail and brings a new perspective to our work. We have enjoyed getting to know her and deeply appreciate all she has done to keep us on track. We thank you both. Our thanks to Marion Gottlieb, who managed the myriad details required in the administration of this project; Mary Siener, Maria Guglielmo, and Christopher Weigand for the stunning interior and cover design; to Anne Garcia for the production support; to Patty Gutierrez, who skillfully managed our photographs and illustrations; and to Heather Willison of S4Carlisle Publishing Services. Without support in these crucial areas, our work would not be as visually appealing and accurate as it is.

We are especially grateful to Kim Mohler, RN, and to Kaitlyn and Kyle Kersey—and their beautiful baby, Braeden—for their participation in the "Through the Eyes of a Nurse" features and videos. This edition benefits immensely because they were willing to share with nursing students this special time of their lives.

During these times of uncertainty in the healthcare environment, we are sustained by our passion for nursing and our vision of what childbirth means. Time and again, we have seen the difference a skilled nurse can make in the lives of people in need. We, like you, are committed to helping all nurses recognize and take pride in that fact. Thank you for your letters, your comments, and your suggestions. We are renewed by your support.

Michele R. Davidson
Marcia L. London
Patricia W. Ladewig

Preface

Most often, pregnancy and childbirth are times of great joy, a celebration of life, and a promise of the future. But they may also be times of deepest sorrow as families deal with illness, complications, and loss. Nurses play a central role in all aspects of the childbearing experience, from the earliest days of pregnancy, through the moments of birth, and during the early days of parenthood. Often the quality of the nursing care that a family receives profoundly influences their perceptions of the entire experience—for better or for worse. However, the changes occurring in the healthcare delivery system are altering the way we practice nursing and have staggering implications for nurses everywhere, even nurses caring for childbearing women and their families.

Now, more than ever, nurses must be flexible, creative, and open to change. They must be able to think critically and problem solve effectively. They must be able to meet the teaching needs of their patients so that their patients can, in turn, better meet their own healthcare needs. They must be open to an increasingly multicultural population. They must understand and use the healthcare technology available in their chosen area of practice. Most crucially, they must never lose sight of the importance of excellent nursing care to promote patient safety and in improving the quality of people's lives.

Important Themes in This Edition

The underlying philosophy of ***Olds' Maternal-Newborn Nursing & Women's Health Across the Lifespan*** remains unchanged. We believe that pregnancy and birth are normal life processes and that family members are partners in care. We believe that women's health care is an important aspect of nursing. We remain committed to providing a text that is accurate and readable—a text that helps students develop the skills and abilities they need now and in the future in an ever-changing healthcare environment.

Partnering with Families Through Health Promotion Education

Developing a partnership with women and their families is a pivotal aspect of maternal-newborn nursing, and one key element of that partnership is patient and family health promotion teaching. It is a crucial responsibility of the maternal-newborn nurse to find opportunities to educate patients and their families, and we continue to emphasize and highlight this in the ninth edition. Again, the focus is on the teaching that nurses do at all stages of pregnancy and the childbearing process, including the important postpartum teaching that is done before and immediately after families are discharged.

In this textbook, we also subscribe to the paradigm that women and childbearing families need health promotion and health maintenance interventions, no matter where they seek health care or what health conditions they may be experiencing. Nurses integrate health promotion and health maintenance into the care for women and childbearing families in a variety of birthing and community settings where they go to obtain health supervision care. This textbook integrates health promotion and health maintenance content throughout, most visibly in Unit 2, *Women's Health* and Chapter 37, "Home Care of the Postpartum Family." In addition, a new heading, **Health Promotion Education**, has been added that emphasizes the health promotion education that women and childbearing families need.

Because we believe that nursing excellence must include partnering with women and their families for all outcomes, we have included Chapter 38, "Grief and Loss in the Childbearing Family." It is designed to assist nurses to support families as they deal with the painful losses—maternal, fetal, and neonatal—that sometimes turn moments of great joy into times of deep sorrow. We know that it often takes time for nurses to find authentic ways to support grieving families. Our aim in having this chapter is to help you understand the dynamics of loss and to offer concrete guidance about effective nursing approaches.

We further the concept of partnering with childbearing families with a special feature called **Through the Eyes of a Nurse**. This feature helps you prepare for clinical experiences, with this unfolding story of an expecting couple and their nurse. **Through the Eyes of a Nurse** vignettes show the interaction between the nurse and the couple surrounding a typical topic of concern for expecting women and their partners. Viewing the partnership that develops will prepare you for success in clinical encounters and in practice.

The book's companion Web site features the interaction between Kaitlyn and Kyle and their nurse during four examinations at various stages throughout their childbirth experience. Author Michele Davidson introduces each segment to help you notice the important communication and patient education that takes place. View the partnership that develops and use it to help you prepare for clinical by answering the questions about what you have seen.

The companion Web site includes videos of four examinations to model nurse-patient interaction:

- ***Through the Eyes of a Nurse:*** The First Trimester
- ***Through the Eyes of a Nurse:*** The Second Trimester
- ***Through the Eyes of a Nurse:*** The Third Trimester
- ***Through the Eyes of a Nurse:*** The Postpartum Visit: *Welcoming the New Arrival*

Another special feature that focuses on the nurse's partnership with the woman and family is the full-color foldout, **A Day in the Life of a Nurse-Midwife**. This pictorially depicts the many opportunities that a nurse-midwife has throughout the course of a day to partner with women and families to optimize the nurse-patient relationship.

Women's Health Care

This edition continues to provide expanded coverage of women's health care with updated information on contraception, commonly occurring infections, health maintenance recommendations, menopause, and a variety of gynecologic conditions such as polycystic ovarian syndrome and pelvic relaxation. Special attention is given to violence against women, which is the focus of a separate chapter. Other pressing societal issues are also covered in a separate chapter, as well as throughout the women's health unit. Moreover, because of the text's focus on community-based care, gynecologic cancers are covered briefly in the text.

Nursing Excellence in Maternal-Newborn and Women's Health

Truly effective nurses have both a solid understanding of underlying nursing theory and excellent clinical skills. Perhaps equally important, they have a deep appreciation of the essential need to partner with childbearing women and their families to ensure optimum outcomes for all. But how do we help students develop this level of expertise? We believe that nursing excellence as it relates to women's health and to childbearing families starts here, in the pages of this text. This book provides essential theoretical content within a contemporary, holistic, family-centered context. Our goal is to lay a foundation that you can build on with each clinical experience you have.

You may notice a change in terminology from "postpartal" and "intrapartal" to "postpartum" and "intrapartum." The latter terms reflect the official style of the American College of Obstetricians and Gynecologists. Because the former versions are still commonly recognized and used, we have left some as-is within the text, but you'll see the change to the official –um endings in chapter titles and headings.

Evidence-Based Practice

Nursing professionals are increasingly aware of the importance of using evidence-based approaches as the foundation for planning and providing effective care and to foster patient safety and quality improvement. The approach of evidence-based practice draws on information from a variety of sources, including nursing research. To help nurses become more comfortable integrating new knowledge into their nursing practice, a brief discussion of evidence-based practice is included in Chapter 1, "Current Issues in Maternal-Newborn Nursing."

A new feature entitled **Research Evidence in Practice** further enhances the approach of using research to determine nursing actions. It describes a particular problem or clinical question and investigates the research evidence from a variety of sources including systematic reviews of research literature, recent research findings, and national organization policy that have direct application to nursing practice. The feature asks the student to use critical thinking (clinical reasoning and clinical judgment) to determine what additional information is needed, what the evidence showed best practice at this time, and invite the student to apply critical thinking skills to further identify nursing approaches to meet women's health and maternal-newborn nursing care issues.

Commitment to Diversity

As nurses and as educators, we recognize the importance of honoring diversity and of providing culturally competent care. Thus, we continually strive to make our text ever more inclusive. Chapter 1, "Current Issues in Maternal-Newborn Nursing," briefly introduces cultural issues relevant to maternity and newborn nursing care. Chapter 2, "Care of the Family in a Culturally Diverse Society," provides the theoretical basis for the consideration of cultural factors that influence a family's expectations of their healthcare providers and their experience with the healthcare system. We elaborate upon this information throughout the text in a boxed feature entitled **Developing Cultural Competence**. In addition, we have worked hard to ensure that our photos, illustrations, charts, and case scenarios are inclusive in their appearance and in the information they provide. As our society becomes more global in nature, nurses need to cultivate their awareness of these issues because they ultimately do affect how we deliver health care in this country.

Critical Thinking

The abilities needed to think critically and problem solve effectively are learned skills that you can cultivate and develop. To help students hone their critical-thinking skills, **Clinical Judgment** case studies present a brief scenario and **Critical Thinking** questions ask students to determine the appropriate response in that situation. Suggested answers to the questions are provided on the book's companion Web site so that students will have immediate feedback on their decision-making skills.

Another feature that emphasizes these skills is **Critical Thinking in Action**, found at the end of each chapter. This case study introduces a patient situation at the end of each chapter with questions to enable the student to decide which nursing actions are appropriate. Suggested answers appear on the book's companion Web site.

Nursing Professionalism

Professionalism requires that the astute professional nurse demonstrate professional standards of moral, ethical, and legal conduct and model the values of the nursing profession as he or she cares for women and childbearing families. With these expectations, a new feature called **Professionalism in Practice** has been added. This feature focuses on topics such as legal and ethical considerations, contemporary nursing practice issues, professional accountability, patient advocacy, and home and community care considerations.

Patient Education

Patient education remains a critical element of effective nursing care, one that we emphasize in this text. Nurses teach their patients during the care of women, all stages of pregnancy, the childbearing process, and while providing care for specific conditions. Throughout the book, we include **Patient Education** features that present a special healthcare issue or problem and the related key teaching points for care by the patient and family.

The tear-out **Patient/Family Teaching Cards** are also handy tools for you to use while studying or for quick pocket-size reference in the clinical setting. Furthermore, a foldout, full-color **Maternal-Fetal Growth and Development Chart** depicts maternal/fetal development month by month and provides specific teaching guidelines for each stage of pregnancy. You can use this chart as another tool for study or as a quick clinical reference.

Complementary and Alternative Therapies

Nurses and other healthcare professionals recognize that today, more than ever, complementary and alternative therapies have become a credible component of holistic care. To help nurses become more familiar with these therapies, Chapter 3, "Complementary and Alternative Therapies," provides basic information on some of the more commonly used therapies. Then throughout the text, we expanded the topic by providing a heading and an icon that highlight specific therapies your patients might be using or therapies you might suggest, keeping patient safety upmost in our thoughts. In all cases, research is cited for safe practice of these therapies.

Community-Based Nursing Care

By its very nature, maternal-newborn nursing is community-based nursing. Only a brief portion of the entire pregnancy and birth is spent in a birthing center or hospital. Moreover, because of changes in practice, even women with high-risk pregnancies are receiving more care in their homes and in the community and spending less time in hospital settings. Similarly, most aspects of women's health care are addressed in ambulatory settings.

The provision of nursing care in community-based settings is a driving force in health care today and, consequently, is a dominant theme throughout this edition. Four chapters provide a theoretical perspective and important tools in caring for childbearing families in the community setting: Chapter 15, "Antepartum Nursing Assessment;" Chapter 16, "The Expectant Family: Needs and Care;" Chapter 36, "The Postpartum Family: Needs and Care;" and Chapter 37, "Home Care of the Postpartum Family." We have addressed this topic in a variety of ways. **Community-Based Nursing Care** is a heading used throughout the text to assist you in identifying specific aspects of this content. Because we consider **Home Care** to be one form of community-based care, it is often a separate heading under Community-Based Nursing Care.

Other New or Expanded Concepts in This Edition

Nursing is a dynamic profession, which requires textbooks to reflect current practice. As such, we have added several important areas of content in the ninth edition.

- Ensuring appropriate **nutrition** during pregnancy and infancy is important to promote growth, development, and health. A growing national focus on healthy nutrition patterns underscores the importance of this information. Chapter 18, "Maternal Nutrition" and

Chapter 32, "Newborn Nutrition" address nutrition for pregnant women and newborns.

- **Pain management** is a priority in healthcare settings. All of the chapters in Unit 5, *Birth* address pain assessment and management, and it is the primary focus in Chapter 25, "Pain Management During Labor." We discuss applicable pain assessment and management when appropriate in other chapters in Unit 6, *The Newborn* and Unit 7, *Postpartum.*
- Content related to caring for **women with intellectual disabilities** has been added to Chapter 8, "Women's Care: Social Issues." Such women are more commonly choosing to live independently and even become mothers. Therefore, we have added coverage of caring for mothers with intellectual disabilities in Chapter 36, "The Postpartum Family: Needs and Care."

Organization: A Nursing Care Management Framework

Nurses today must be able to think critically and to solve problems effectively. For these reasons, we begin with an introductory unit to set the stage by providing information about maternal-newborn nursing and important related concepts. Subsequent units progress in a way that closely reflects the steps of the nursing process. We clearly delineate the nurse's role within this framework. Thus, the units related to pregnancy, labor and birth, the newborn period, and postpartum care begin with a discussion of basic theory followed by chapters on nursing assessment and nursing care for essentially healthy women or infants. Within the nursing care chapters and content areas, we use the heading **Nursing Care Management** and the subheadings **Nursing Assessment and Diagnosis, Planning and Implementation**, and **Evaluation**.

Complications of a specific period appear in the last chapter or chapters of each unit. The chapters also use the nursing process as an organizational framework. We believe that students can more clearly grasp the complicated content of the high-risk conditions once they have a good understanding of the normal processes of pregnancy, birth, and postpartum and newborn care. However, to avoid overemphasizing the prevalence of complications in such a wonderfully normal process as pregnancy and birth, we avoid including an entire unit that focuses only on complications. To aid student study, we have developed a new chapter, Chapter 26, "Childbirth at Risk: Prelabor Complications," which focuses on content that impacts both pregnancy and labor and birth. This new chapter allows more discussion of the impact of pregestational physiologic and pathophysiologic conditions so that students can apply the principles they have learned to changes experienced in pregnancy.

NURSING CARE MANAGEMENT

The *Nursing Care Management* head delineates the important care management role of the nurse within the organizing framework of the nursing process to help you understand what nursing actions are needed. Numerous special features reinforce the nursing care management role.

NURSING CARE PLAN

Nursing Care Plans address nursing care for patients who have complications, such as a woman with preeclampsia. We designed this feature to help you approach care from the nursing process perspective. These care plans use a nursing diagnosis approach in planning and providing care when pregnancy-related and newborn complications arise. We have added four care plans to this edition: Epidural Anesthesia, Hemorrhage in the Third Trimester and at Birth, A Woman with Engorgement, and Induction of Labor.

CLINICAL PATHWAY For Newborn

Clinical Pathways describe nursing actions as women are integrated into care of other health professionals. They help you organize care for healthy women and evaluate its effectiveness.

ASSESSMENT GUIDE Prenatal Assessment

Assessment Guides help you organize your questions and steps during a physical assessment, and provide normal findings, alterations, and possible causes, as well as guidelines for nursing interventions.

Features That Help You Use This Text Successfully

Instructors and students alike value the in-text learning aids that we include in our textbooks. The following guide will help you use the features and resources from ***Olds' Maternal-Newborn Nursing & Women's Health Across the Lifespan***, Ninth Edition, to be successful in the classroom, in the clinical setting, on the NCLEX-RN® examination, and in nursing practice.

Each chapter begins with a personal **vignette** and photo that sets the tone for the chapter.

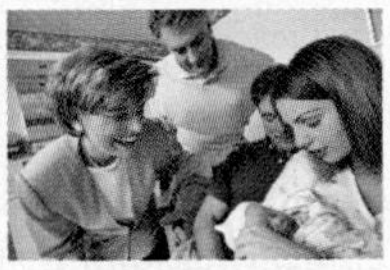

I can't imagine going through pregnancy, birth, or those initial few weeks after my daughter was born without my family. My brother called regularly throughout my pregnancy to check on me. Dad gave me pep talks on eating right and taking care of myself. My husband and my mom were both with me during my labor and my unexpected cesarean birth. After Rosario was born, my husband accompanied our new daughter to the nursery and mom stayed with me, talking and hold… ence a family can ma…

LEARNING OUTCOMES

1. Describe the significance of using the nursing process to promote health in the woman and her family during pregnancy.
2. Describe actions the nurse can take to help maintain the well-being of the expectant father and siblings during a family's pregnancy.
3. Discuss the significance of cultural considerations in managing nursing care during pregnancy.
4. Identify the common discomforts of pregnancy and their causes.

Learning Outcomes introduce you to the topics covered in each chapter. The terminology in the new Bloom's taxonomy is reflected in these learning outcomes.

KEY TERMS

Amenorrhea *64*	Menopause *67*	Premenstrual dysphoric disorder (PMDD) *66*
Climacteric *69*	Osteoporosis *70*	Premenstrual syndrome (PMS) *66*
Dysmenorrhea *65*	Perimenopause *69*	
Hormone therapy (HT) *72*		

Key Terms introduce each chapter, with page numbers showing where each term first appears in the chapter, in bold type.

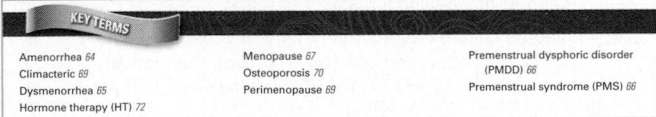

PATIENT TEACHING What to Tell the Pregnant Woman About Assessing Fetal Activity

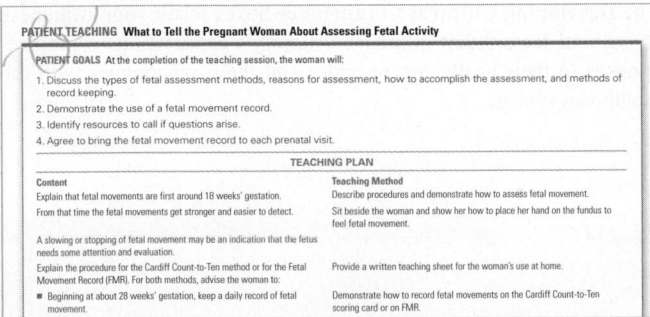

PATIENT GOALS At the completion of the teaching session, the woman will:

1. Discuss the types of fetal assessment methods, reasons for assessment, how to accomplish the assessment, and methods of record keeping.
2. Demonstrate the use of a fetal movement record.
3. Identify resources to call if questions arise.
4. Agree to bring the fetal movement record to each prenatal visit.

TEACHING PLAN

Content	Teaching Method
Explain that fetal movements are first around 18 weeks' gestation.	Describe procedures and demonstrate how to assess fetal movement.
From that time the fetal movements get stronger and easier to detect.	Sit beside the woman and show her how to place her hand on the fundus to feel fetal movement.
A slowing or stopping of fetal movement may be an indication that the fetus needs some attention and evaluation.	
Explain the procedure for the Cardiff Count-to-Ten method or for the Fetal Movement Record (FMR). For both methods, advise the woman to:	Provide a written teaching sheet for the woman's use at home.
■ Beginning at about 28 weeks' gestation, keep a daily record of fetal movement.	Demonstrate how to record fetal movements on the Cardiff Count-to-Ten scoring card or on FMR.

The teaching that nurses do at all stages of pregnancy and childbearing and throughout the life of a woman is one of the most important aspects of their work. The **Patient Teaching** boxes in the textbook help you plan and organize your patient teaching.

Health Promotion Education

In counseling the pregnant woman, the nurse needs to avoid "talking down" to her or "preaching" to her. The nurse should present information in a clear, logical way, using appropriate language but avoiding jargon. Examples are often helpful in clarifying material. The nurse should also answer all questions appropriately and clearly.

When a person requires nutritional counseling, a dietary change usually is necessary. However, change is often difficult. Counseling will be more effective if the nurse understands the woman's values and explains the needed change in a way that is meaningful to the patient. Because the pregnant woman must follow the plan, it should be developed in cooperation with her; be suitable for her financial level and background; and be based on reasonable, achievable goals.

The following example demonstrates one way a nurse can implement a plan with a patient based on the nursing diagnosis.

Diagnosis: *Imbalanced Nut… ments related to low intake…*

Patient goal: The woman wi… to the DRI level.

Patient teaching often involves empowering the patient in their own health promotion, and this content is now called out with a special icon and **Health Promotion Education** headings and icon.

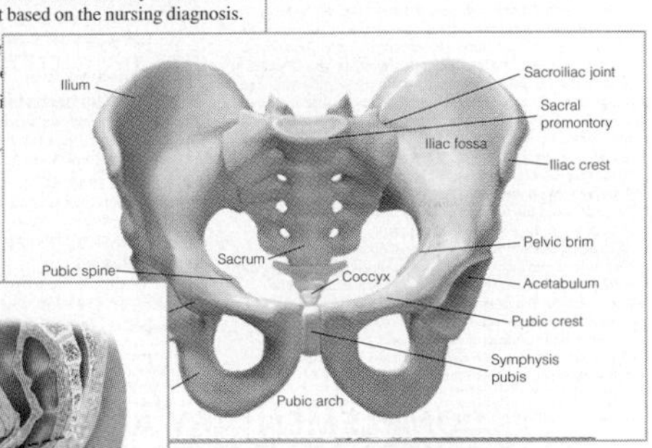

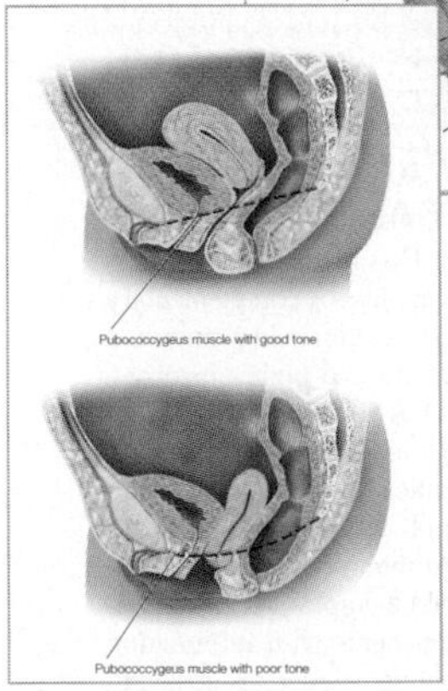

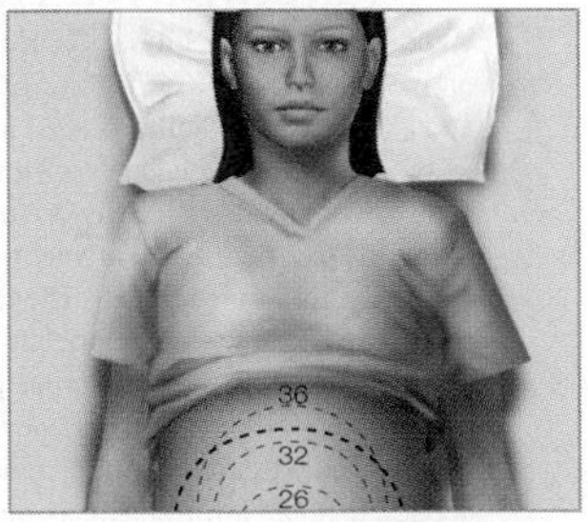

We have continued our tradition of providing top-notch visuals to enhance students' learning by including nearly **100 new lifelike obstetric illustrations**. The 9th edition continues to provide a large amount of tabular material that provides students with quick reference to high-priority information.

Application: Pelvic Structures

Bony Pelvis

The female bony pelvis has two unique functions:

- To support and protect the pelvic contents
- To form the relatively fixed axis of the birth passage

Because the pelvis is so important to childbearing, its structures should be understood clearly.

Bony Structure

The pelvis is made up of four bones: two innominate bones, the sacrum, and the coccyx (or tailbone) (Figure 10-11 ■). The pelvis resembles a bowl or basin; its sides are the innominate

The companion Web site thumbtabs in each chapter remind you to use the accompanying supplemental materials found on the text's companion Web site. These thumbtabs cross-reference additional information or specific activities related to the concepts introduced on that page in the textbook. These resources enhance learning and provide an application beyond the textbook experience.

Features

To help you understand the use of reliable information to plan and provide effective nursing care, **Research Evidence in Practice** boxes relate research evidence to women's health and maternal-newborn nursing. Each feature asks the student to use critical thinking skills to analyze the data to best meet women's health and maternal-newborn nursing care issues.

RESEARCH EVIDENCE IN PRACTICE Passive Descent Versus Immediate Pushing in Women with Epidural Analgesia

CLINICAL QUESTION

Which method of pushing—passive descent or active pushing upon full cervical dilatation—most benefits women with epidural analgesia?

RESEARCH EVIDENCE

Epidural analgesia has become a common method of pain management for laboring women, yet one of its side effects is a decrease in a woman's lower body sensations. This may inhibit the natural urge to push upon full cervical dilatation. Traditionally, active management of labor meant that women were directed to push immediately upon full cervical dilatation, whether they felt the urge or not. The chief concern leading to this practice was that an extended second stage of labor was deleterious for both mother and baby, leading to acidosis, maternal exhaustion, and neonatal morbidity.

The natural second stage of labor includes a period of rest and descent, often described as passive descent. This practice involves allowing the woman to delay pushing until she feels the urge to push, or the head is visible vaginally.

A group of obstetric and gynecologic nurse experts conducted a meta-analysis of studies comparing the effects and outcomes of immediate pushing versus passive descent in women with epidural analgesia. The results demonstrated that immediate pushing did not reduce the incidence of acidosis or shorten the second stage of labor. Indeed, prolonged active pushing was shown to increase the incidence of fetal and maternal acidosis, increased the risk of having an instrument-assisted

spontaneous vaginal birth. Pushing time was lengthened with immediate pushing as compared to passive descent.

Furthermore, passive descent had additional benefits in that it allowed for further fetal descent and rotation, better situating the fetus in the woman's pelvis. It also caused further release of oxytocin that augmented the progress of labor. These findings suggest that the duration of active pushing should be limited, not the duration of the second stage of labor.

No differences were found between immediate pushing and passive descent in terms of the rate of cesarean birth, lacerations, or episiotomies.

WHAT QUESTIONS REMAIN UNANSWERED?

Are there any conditions under which active pushing should be used? Are there differences in these findings when women do not use epidural analgesia?

WHAT IS BEST PRACTICE?

Passive descent should be used during birth to safely and effectively increase spontaneous vaginal births, decrease instrument-assisted birth, and shorten pushing time.

CRITICAL THINKING

How can the nurse help the mother recognize the urge to push at an effective time when epidural analgesia is in place?

References

Brancato, R., Church, S., & Stone, P. (2008). A meta-analysis of passive descent versus immediate pushing in nulliparous women with epidural analgesia in the second stage of labor. *Journal of Gynecological and Neonatal Nursing, 37*, 4–12. doi:10.1111/J.1552-6909.2007.00205.x

COMPLEMENTARY AND ALTERNATIVE THERAPIES

According to the National Center for Complementary & Alternative Medicine (NCCAM) (2008), the use of complementary and alternative medicine (CAM) is more common in women and in those with higher levels of education and higher incomes. Many women are electing to use CAM therapies, such as homeopathy, herbal medicine (phytomedicine), acupressure, acupuncture, biofeedback, Therapeutic Touch, massage, and chiropractic, as part of a holistic approach to their healthcare regimens. Nurses are in a unique position to bridge the gap between conventional therapies and CAM therapies. As patient advocates, nurses are able to provide patients with information needed to make informed decisions about their health and health

Complementary and Alternative Therapies have become a credible component of holistic care. To help you become familiar with this content, we have integrated this content into the chapter content to inform you about therapies your patients might be using or therapies you might safely suggest. In all cases, research is cited for safe practice of these therapies. Special icons denote the location of this content.

PROFESSIONALISM IN PRACTICE

2008 Prenatally and Postnatally Diagnosed Conditions Act

The Prenatally and Postnatally Diagnosed Conditions Act was signed into law in 2008. This law requires that medical providers give parents accurate, updated, and scientific information regarding their child's diagnosis, prognosis, treatment, and life expectancy. Nurses are often an important source of information and support when a prenatal or postnatal diagnosis of a genetic condition or birth defect is made.

Nursing professionalism is fostered in new features called Professionalism in Practice, which focuses on topics such as legal and ethical considerations, contemporary nursing practice issues, professional accountability, patient advocacy, and home and community care considerations.

CLINICAL JUDGMENT

Case Study: Jillian Rundus

Jillian Rundus is a 31-year-old G1P0 who is 35 weeks' pregnant. She presents for a routine office visit with complaints of nausea and abdominal pain rating 7/10. She has had a headache and general malaise for 2 days. She denies visual changes. Upon examination, you find her to be alert and oriented and her physical exam is unremarkable with the exception of abdominal tenderness and a blood pressure of 170/110. She has had no previous history of hypertension. Fetal heart rate ranges from 140–150 beats per minute.

Critical Thinking

What should the nurse do at this time?

See www.nursing.pearsonhighered.com for possible responses.

Clinical Judgment case studies help students hone their critical thinking and clinical reasoning skills by presenting a brief scenario and **Critical Thinking** questions to determine the appropriate response in that situation.

DEVELOPING CULTURAL COMPETENCE

Culture and Response to Fetal Loss

Remember that individual responses to fetal loss following miscarriage may vary greatly and may be influenced by ethnic or cultural norms.

- Miscarriage may be viewed in many ways. For example, it may be seen as a punishment from God, as the result of the evil eye or of a hex or curse by an enemy, or as a natural part of life.
- When grieving over a pregnancy loss, women from some cultures and ethnic groups may show their emotions freely, crying and wailing, whereas other women may hide their feelings behind a mask of stoicism.
- In some cultures the woman's partner is her primary source of support and comfort. In others, the woman turns to her mother or close female relatives for comfort.
- Avoid stereotyping women according to culture. Individual responses are influenced by many factors, including the degree of assimilation into the dominant culture.

The **Developing Cultural Competence** boxes foster your awareness of cultural factors that influence a family's expectations of and responses to their healthcare provider and their experiences with the healthcare system.

DRUG GUIDE Magnesium Sulfate

PREGNANCY RISK CATEGORY: B

OVERVIEW OF OBSTETRIC ACTION

Magnesium sulfate acts as a CNS depressant by decreasing the quantity of acetylcholine released by motor nerve impulses and thereby blocking neuromuscular transmission. This action reduces the possibility of convulsion, which is why magnesium sulfate is used in the treatment of preeclampsia. Because magnesium sulfate secondarily relaxes smooth muscle, it may decrease the blood pressure, although it is not considered an antihypertensive. Magnesium sulfate may also decrease the frequency and intensity of uterine contractions; as a result it is also used as a tocolytic in the treatment of preterm labor.

ROUTE, DOSAGE, FREQUENCY

Magnesium sulfate is generally given intravenously to control dosage more accurately and prevent overdosage. An occasional physician still prescribes intramuscular administration. However, it is painful and irritating to the tissues and does not permit the close control that IV administration does. The IV route allows for immediate onset of action. It must be given by infusion pump for accurate dosage.

large doses may cause cardiac arrest. A potential for uterine atony and postpartum hemorrhage may occur from magnesium's tocolytic effect. Magnesium can cause a rapid suppression of parathyroid hormone release which may cause a transient hypocalcemia. If symptoms of myoclonus, delirium, or EKG abnormalities are present, calcium gluconate should be administered.

EFFECTS ON FETUS/NEWBORN

The drug readily crosses the placenta. A transient decrease in fetal heart rate (FHR) baseline and variability may occur. In general, magnesium sulfate therapy does not pose a risk to the fetus. Ill effects in the newborn may actually be related to fetal growth retardation, prematurity, or perinatal asphyxia.

NURSING CONSIDERATIONS

1. Monitor the blood pressure closely during administration.
2. Monitor maternal serum magnesium levels as ordered (usually every 6–8 hours). Therapeutic levels are in the range of 4–8 mg/dl. Reflexes often disappear at serum magnesium levels of 9–12 mg/dl; respiratory depression may occur at levels

Drug Guide boxes for selected medications commonly used in maternal-newborn nursing guide you in correctly administering the medications and evaluating your actions.

CLINICAL PATHWAY For Intrapartum Stages

Category	First Stage	Second and Third Stage	Fourth Stage Birth to 1 Hour Past Birth
Referral	Review prenatal record Advise CNM/physician of admission	Labor record for first stage	Report to recovery room nurse ■ ***Expected Outcomes*** Appropriate resources identified and utilized
Assessments	Admission assessments: Ask about problems since last prenatal visit; labor status (contraction frequency and duration), membrane status (intact or ruptured); coping level; support; woman's desires during labor and birth; ability to verbalize needs; laboratory testing (blood and UA) Intrapartal assessments: Cervical assessment: from 1 to 10 cm dilatation; nullipara (1.2 cm/h), multipara (1.5 cm/h) Cervical effacement: from 0% to 100%, multiparas may not fully efface prior to birth. Fetal descent: progressive descent from −4 to +4 Membrane assessment: intact or ruptured; when ruptured, Nitrazine positive, fluid clear, no foul odor Comfort level: woman states is able to cope with contractions Behavioral characteristics: facial expressions, tone of voice, and verbal expressions are con-	Second stage assessments: • BP, P, R q5–15min • Uterine contractions palpated continuously • FHR q15min (for low-risk women) and q5min (for high-risk women) if reassuring; if nonreassuring, monitor continuously Fetal descent: descent continues to birth Comfort level: woman states is able to cope with contractions and pushing Behavioral characteristics: response to pushing, facial expressions, verbalization Third stage assessments: • BP, P, R q5min • Uterine contractions, palpate occasionally until placenta is delivered, fundus maintains tone and contraction pattern continues to birth of placenta Newborn assessments: • Assess Apgar score of newborn • Respirations: 30–60, irregular • Apical pulse: 110–160 and somewhat	Immediate postbirth assessments of mother q15min for 1h: • BP: 90–135/60–85; should return to prelabor level • Pulse: slightly lower than in labor; range is 60–90 • Respirations: 12–24/min; easy; quiet • Temperature: 36.2–37.6°C (98–99.6°F) • Fundus firm, in midline, at the umbilicus • Lochia rubra; moderate amount; less than 2 pad/h; no free flow or passage of clots with massage • Perineum: sutures intact; no bulging or marked swelling; minimal bruising may be present; no c/o severe pain nor rectal pain • Bladder nondistended; spontaneous void of greater than 100 ml clear, straw-colored urine; bladder nondistended following voiding • If hemorrhoids present, no tenseness or marked engorgement; less than 2 cm diameter

In keeping with the changing approaches to nursing care management, **Clinical Pathways** are designed to help you plan and manage care within normally anticipated time frames.

PROCEDURE 21-3 Assisting During Amniocentesis

NURSING ACTION

Preparation

- Explain the procedure and the indications for it and reassure the woman.
- Determine whether an informed consent form has been signed. If not, verify that the woman's doctor has explained the procedure and ask her to sign a consent form.

Rationale: *It is the physician's responsibility to obtain informed consent. The woman's signature indicates her awareness of the risks and gives her consent to the procedure.*

Equipment and Supplies

22-gauge spinal needle with stylet

10- and 20-ml syringes

1% lidocaine (Xylocaine)

Povidone-iodine (Betadine)

Three 10-ml test tubes with tops (amber colored or covered with tape)

Rationale: *Amniotic fluid must be protected from light to prevent breakdown of bilirubin.*

Procedure: Sterile Gloves

1. Obtain baseline vital signs including maternal blood pressure (BP), pulse, respirations, temperature, and fetal heart rate (FHR) before procedure begins.

- Palpate the woman's fundus to assess for uterine contractions.
- Monitor her using an external fetal monitor for 20 to 30 minutes after the amniocentesis.
- Determine a treatment course to counteract any supine hypotension and to increase venous return and cardiac output.

Rationale: *Monitoring maternal and fetal status postprocedure provides information about response to the procedure and helps detect any complications such as inadvertent fetal puncture.*

8. Assess the woman's blood type and determine any need for Rh immune globulin.
9. Administer Rh immune globulin if indicated (see Procedure 20.2 on page 482).

Rationale: *To prevent Rh sensitization in an Rh-negative woman, Rh immune globulin is administered prophylactically involving amniocentesis.*

10. Instruct the woman to report any of the following changes or symptoms to her primary caregiver:
   - Unusual fetal hyperactivity or, conversely, any lack of fetal movement
   - Vaginal discharge—either clear drainage or bleeding
   - Uterine contractions or abdominal pain
   - Fever or chills

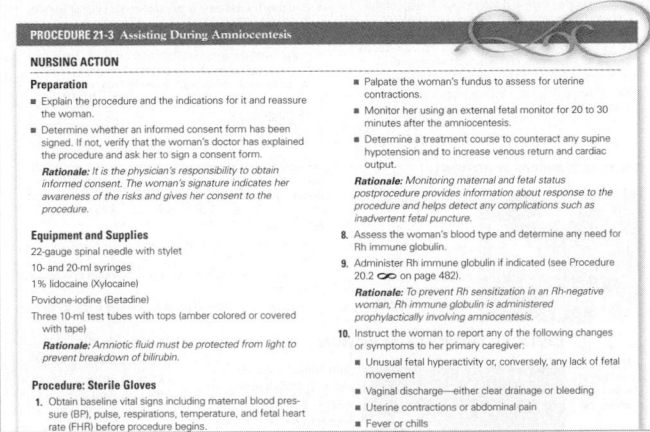

Procedure boxes offer step-by-step techniques that show you the tasks expected of a nurse in clinical situations, preparing you for your clinical experiences. Included in each box are the preparation steps with rationales, equipment and supplies needed, and steps for the procedure itself, with rationales for the nurse's actions.

ASSESSMENT GUIDE Subsequent Prenatal Assessment

Physical Assessment/Normal Findings	Alterations and Possible Causes*	Nursing Responses to Data[†]
VITAL SIGNS		
Temperature: 36.2°–37.6°C (97°–99.6°F)	Elevated temperature (infection)	Evaluate for signs of infection. Refer to healthcare provider.
Pulse: 60–90/min Rate may increase 10 beats/min during pregnancy	Increased pulse rate (anxiety, cardiac disorders)	Note irregularities. Assess for anxiety and stress.
Respiration: 12–22/min	Marked tachypnea or abnormal patterns (respiratory disease)	Refer to healthcare provider.
Blood Pressure: Less than or equal to 135/85 (falls in second trimester)	Greater than 140/90 or increase of 30 mm systolic and 15 mm diastolic (preeclampsia)	Assess for edema, proteinuria, and hyperreflexia. Refer to healthcare provider. Schedule appointments more frequently.
WEIGHT GAIN		
First Trimester: 1.6–2.3 kg (3.5–5 lb)	Inadequate weight gain (poor nutrition, nausea, intrauterine growth restriction [IUGR])	Discuss appropriate weight gain.
Second Trimester: 5.5–6.8 kg (12–15 lb)	Excessive weight gain (excessive caloric intake, edema, preeclampsia)	Provide nutritional counseling. Assess for presence of edema or anemia. Refer to dietitian as needed.
Third Trimester: 5.5–6.8 kg (12–15 lb)		
EDEMA		
Small amount of dependent edema, especially in last weeks of pregnancy	Edema in hands, face, legs, and feet (preeclampsia)	Identify any correlation between edema and activities, blood pressure, or proteinuria: Refer to healthcare provider if indicated.
UTERINE SIZE		

Assessment Guides assist you with diagnoses by incorporating physical assessment and normal findings, alterations and possible causes, and guidelines for nursing interventions.

Through the Eyes of a Nurse
Genetic Testing Options in Pregnancy

Family's Experience

"There seems like there are so many tests available, we are really confused about what to do. We don't feel like we have any risk factors, but we want to make sure our baby is healthy. What tests should we get? Which ones do we really need?"

Nurse's Response

"There are various testing options. I can explain your options and help you weigh the pros and cons of each test. Because of your age and the fact that you do not have any risk factors identified in your medical or family history, you would not be a candidate for the amniocentesis or chorionic villus sampling tests. You may want to consider the other optional tests though, such as the quadruple screen, nuchal translucency test, and cystic fibrosis testing.

"The quadruple screen is a test that screens for neural tube defects and trisomy 18 and 21. This test is only a screening tool, which means it does not tell you if your baby *definitely* has one of these problems. It could help us know if your baby is at risk though. The test is not perfect and you can get false-positives or false-negatives. If the test did come back abnormal, you have other testing options such as a more detailed sonogram or an amniocentesis.

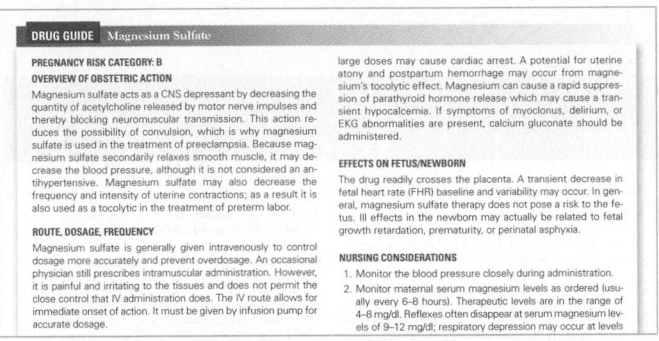

"The nuchal translucency test is a blood test and sonogram combined that screens for trisomy 18 and 21. The test is more accurate than the quadruple screen and is done earlier. Some insurance may not cover the test though, so you will need to call your insurance company to see if it is covered.

"The cystic fibrosis test screens for known gene mutations that cause cystic fibrosis. If your screen is positive, we will then have the father of the baby tested to determine if he is also a carrier. If you are both carriers, there is a 25% chance that the baby could have the disease. If only one of you is a carrier, there would be a chance the baby would also be a carrier, but the baby could not inherit the disease."

Nurse's Actions and Rationale

The nurse's role is to explain all testing options and to answer questions related to the various tests. The nurse presents the information in an objective manner without expressing a personal opinion. The couple must weigh each choice carefully and determine what tests are right for them. The nurse can also provide written resource material to the couple. The couple should be allowed to discuss the information and make an informed decision.

523

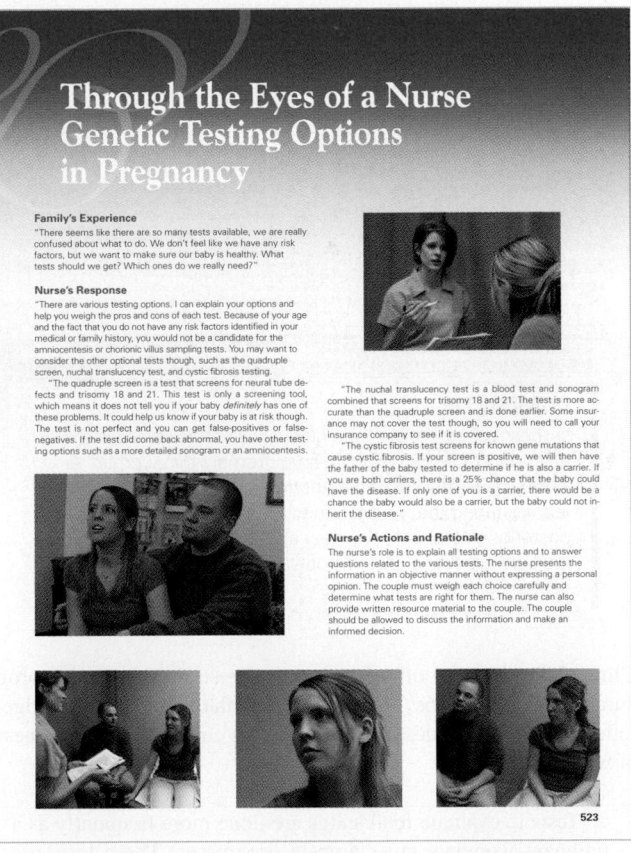

The relationship you create with your patients and their families is the most essential and rewarding part of your nursing career. You will enjoy your job and be more effective in it when you develop these bonds. **Through the Eyes of a Nurse** shows you how one nurse establishes a connection with a couple throughout the pregnancy and after the birth of their baby. We believe that seeing this partnership develop—in your textbook and on the videos on the companion Web site—will help you understand how this wonderful process works.

Features

Nursing Care Plans address nursing care for women who have complications such as preeclampsia or diabetes mellitus, as well as for high-risk newborns. We designed this information to enhance your preparation for the clinical setting.

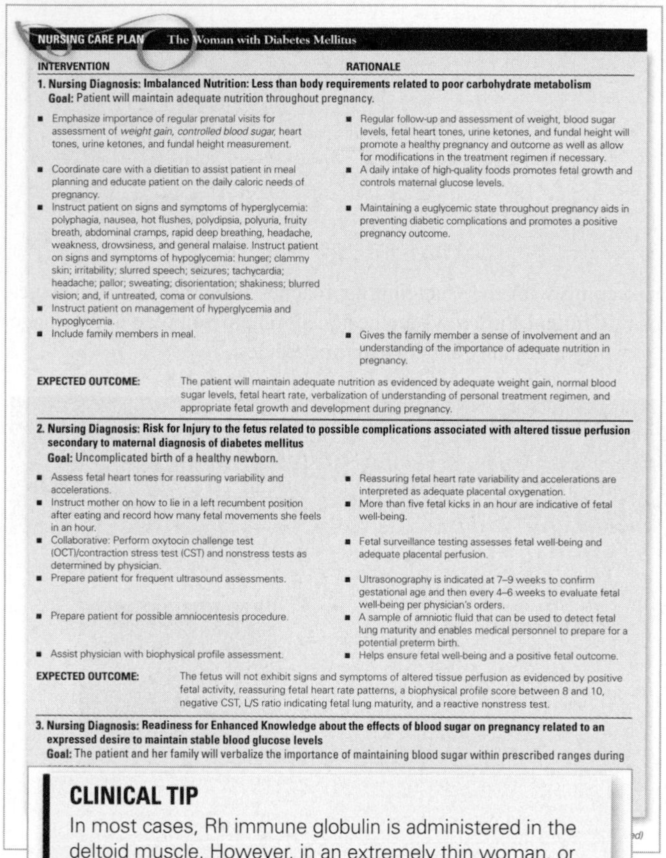

NURSING CARE PLAN The Woman with Diabetes Mellitus

INTERVENTION	RATIONALE
1. Nursing Diagnosis: Imbalanced Nutrition: Less than body requirements related to poor carbohydrate metabolism Goal: Patient will maintain adequate nutrition throughout pregnancy.	
■ Emphasize importance of regular prenatal visits for assessment of *weight gain, controlled blood sugar,* heart tones, urine ketones, and fundal height measurement.	■ Regular follow-up and assessment of weight, blood sugar levels, fetal heart tones, urine ketones, and fundal height will promote a healthy pregnancy and outcome as well as allow for modifications in the treatment regimen if necessary.
■ Coordinate care with a dietitian to assist patient in meal planning and educate patient on the daily caloric needs of pregnancy.	■ A daily intake of high-quality foods promotes fetal growth and controls maternal glucose levels.
■ Instruct patient on signs and symptoms of hyperglycemia: polyphagia, nausea, hot flushes, polydipsia, polyuria, fruity breath, abdominal cramps, rapid deep breathing, headache, weakness, drowsiness, and general malaise. Instruct patient on signs and symptoms of hypoglycemia: hunger; clammy skin; irritability; slurred speech; seizures; tachycardia; headache; pallor; sweating; disorientation; shakiness; blurred vision; and, if untreated, coma or convulsions.	■ Maintaining a euglycemic state throughout pregnancy aids in preventing diabetic complications and promotes a positive pregnancy outcome.
■ Instruct patient on management of hyperglycemia and hypoglycemia.	
■ Include family members in meal.	■ Gives the family member a sense of involvement and an understanding of the importance of adequate nutrition in pregnancy.
EXPECTED OUTCOME:	The patient will maintain adequate nutrition as evidenced by adequate weight gain, normal blood sugar levels, fetal heart rate, verbalization of understanding of personal treatment regimen, and appropriate fetal growth and development during pregnancy.
2. Nursing Diagnosis: Risk for Injury to the fetus related to possible complications associated with altered tissue perfusion secondary to maternal diagnosis of diabetes mellitus Goal: Uncomplicated birth of a healthy newborn.	
■ Assess fetal heart tones for reassuring variability and accelerations.	■ Reassuring fetal heart rate variability and accelerations are interpreted as adequate placental oxygenation.
■ Instruct mother on how to lie in a left recumbent position after eating and record how many fetal movements she feels in an hour.	■ More than five fetal kicks in an hour are indicative of fetal well-being.
■ Collaborative: Perform oxytocin challenge test (OCT)/contraction stress test (CST) and nonstress tests as determined by physician.	■ Fetal surveillance testing assesses fetal well-being and adequate placental perfusion.
■ Prepare patient for frequent ultrasound assessments.	■ Ultrasonography is indicated at 7–9 weeks to confirm gestational age and then every 4–6 weeks to evaluate fetal well-being per physician's orders.
■ Prepare patient for possible amniocentesis procedure.	■ A sample of amniotic fluid that can be used to detect fetal lung maturity and enables medical personnel to prepare for a potential preterm birth.
■ Assist physician with biophysical profile assessment.	■ Helps ensure fetal well-being and a positive fetal outcome.
EXPECTED OUTCOME:	The fetus will not exhibit signs and symptoms of altered tissue perfusion as evidenced by positive fetal activity, reassuring fetal heart rate patterns, a biophysical profile score between 8 and 10, negative CST, L/S ratio indicating fetal lung maturity, and a reactive nonstress test.
3. Nursing Diagnosis: Readiness for Enhanced Knowledge about the effects of blood sugar on pregnancy related to an expressed desire to maintain stable blood glucose levels Goal: The patient and her family will verbalize the importance of maintaining blood sugar within prescribed ranges during	

CLINICAL TIP

In most cases, Rh immune globulin is administered in the deltoid muscle. However, in an extremely thin woman, or in the cases of a larger-than-normal dose, consider administering the medication in the ventrogluteal or posterior gluteal site. You may also divide the dose into multiple injections. Both Rhophlac and WinRho-SFD may be administered intravenously.

Clinical Tip features offer hands-on suggestions for specific procedures and interventions. The authors' wealth of clinical knowledge—reflecting many decades of experience—are reflected in these pearls of wisdom.

Tests to evaluate fetal status are done more frequently as a pregnant woman's preeclampsia progresses. These tests are described in detail in chapter 21 ∞. Monitoring fetal well-being is essential to achieving a safe outcome for the fetus. The following tests are used:

Cross-reference icons (∞) help the student to easily locate related information in other chapters.

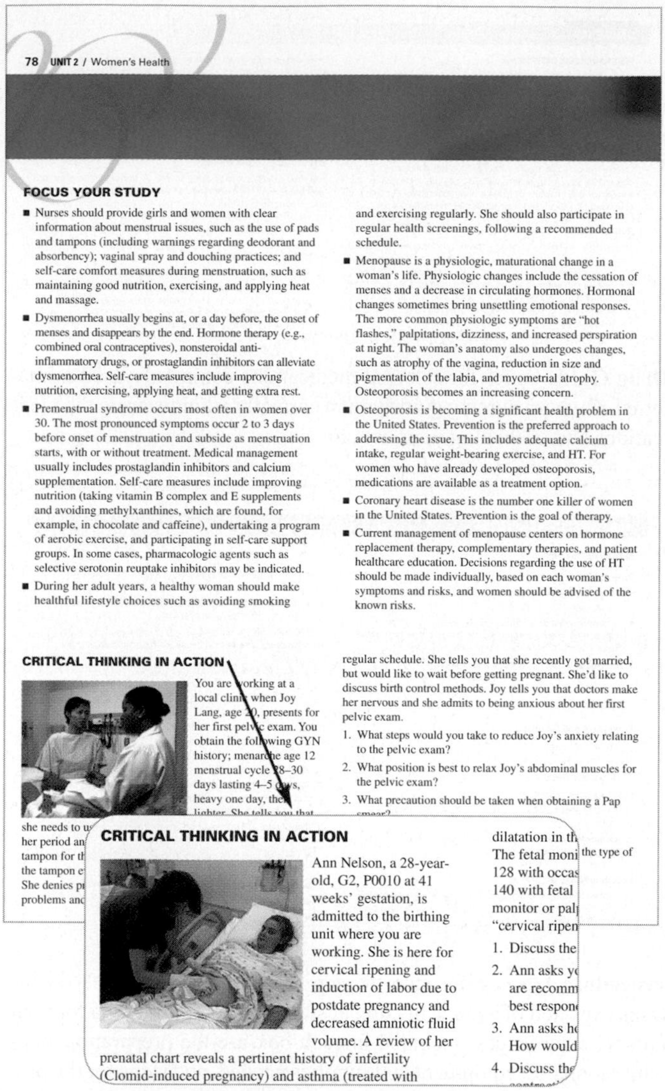

78 UNIT 2 / Women's Health

FOCUS YOUR STUDY

- Nurses should provide girls and women with clear information about menstrual issues, such as the use of pads and tampons (including warnings regarding deodorant and absorbency); vaginal spray and douching practices; and self-care comfort measures during menstruation, such as maintaining good nutrition, exercising, and applying heat and massage.
- Dysmenorrhea usually begins at, or a day before, the onset of menses and disappears by the end. Hormone therapy (e.g., combined oral contraceptives), nonsteroidal anti-inflammatory drugs, or prostaglandin inhibitors can alleviate dysmenorrhea. Self-care measures include improving nutrition, exercising, applying heat, and getting extra rest.
- Premenstrual syndrome occurs most often in women over 30. The most pronounced symptoms occur 2 to 3 days before onset of menstruation and subside as menstruation starts, with or without treatment. Medical management usually includes prostaglandin inhibitors and calcium supplementation. Self-care measures include improving nutrition (taking vitamin B complex and E supplements and avoiding methylxanthines, which are found, for example, in chocolate and caffeine), undertaking a program of aerobic exercise, and participating in self-care support groups. In some cases, pharmacologic agents such as selective serotonin reuptake inhibitors may be indicated.
- During her adult years, a healthy woman should make healthful lifestyle choices such as avoiding smoking and exercising regularly. She should also participate in regular health screenings, following a recommended schedule.
- Menopause is a physiologic, maturational change in a woman's life. Physiologic changes include the cessation of menses and a decrease in circulating hormones. Hormonal changes sometimes bring unsettling emotional responses. The more common physiologic symptoms are "hot flashes," palpitations, dizziness, and increased perspiration at night. The woman's anatomy also undergoes changes, such as atrophy of the vagina, reduction in size and pigmentation of the labia, and myometrial atrophy. Osteoporosis becomes an increasing concern.
- Osteoporosis is becoming a significant health problem in the United States. Prevention is the preferred approach to addressing the issue. This includes adequate calcium intake, regular weight-bearing exercise, and HT. For women who have already developed osteoporosis, medications are available as a treatment option.
- Coronary heart disease is the number one killer of women in the United States. Prevention is the goal of therapy.
- Current management of menopause centers on hormone replacement therapy, complementary therapies, and patient healthcare education. Decisions regarding the use of HT should be made individually, based on each woman's symptoms and risks, and women should be advised of the known risks.

CRITICAL THINKING IN ACTION

You are working at a local clinic when Joy Lang, age 20, presents for her first pelvic exam. You obtain the following GYN history; menarche age 12 menstrual cycle 28–30 days lasting 4–5 days, heavy one day, then lighter. ... regular schedule. She tells you that she recently got married, but would like to wait before getting pregnant. She'd like to discuss birth control methods. Joy tells you that doctors make her nervous and she admits to being anxious about her first pelvic exam.

1. What steps would you take to reduce Joy's anxiety relating to the pelvic exam?
2. What position is best to relax Joy's abdominal muscles for the pelvic exam?
3. What precaution should be taken when obtaining a Pap smear?

CRITICAL THINKING IN ACTION

Ann Nelson, a 28-year-old, G2, P0010 at 41 weeks' gestation, is admitted to the birthing unit where you are working. She is here for cervical ripening and induction of labor due to postdate pregnancy and decreased amniotic fluid volume. A review of her prenatal chart reveals a pertinent history of infertility (Clomid-induced pregnancy) and asthma (treated with

Each chapter ends with **Focus Your Study**, which outlines the main points of the chapter, and **Critical Thinking in Action** exercises, which present brief patient scenarios with questions that help you apply concepts learned in the chapter. Not only can you review chapter content in an easy, quick-view format, but you can also apply the concepts used in preparation for clinical work, ensuring success in partnering with your patients.

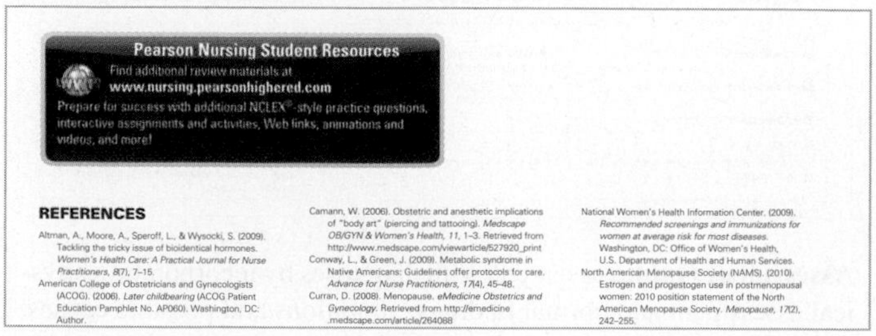

Pearson Nursing Student Resources
Find additional review materials at www.nursing.pearsonhighered.com
Prepare for success with additional NCLEX®-style practice questions, interactive assignments and activities, Web links, animations and videos, and more!

REFERENCES

Each chapter wraps up with a list of **References**, and directions to **the companion Web site** for additional resources.

Resources for Student Success

Companion Web site This Web site offers study tools to enrich your learning. Included are NCLEX-RN®-style questions with rationales, case studies, care plans, an audio glossary, animations, Through the Eyes of a Nurse videos, Newborn Reflex videos, interactive activities, and other material to prepare you for success in the classroom, in clinicals, and on the NCLEX-RN® exam.

MyNursingLab This Web site gives you an opportunity to test yourself on key concepts and skills and track your progress throughout the course. The personalized study plan is designed to help you achieve success. MyNursingLab features NCLEX-RN® practice questions and activities of all types with image- and media-based questions, and other interactive exercises. MyNursingLab also comes with an option to use Pearson's Interactive E-Text. The E-Text includes integrated, rich media; links to Web sites; organization that can be customized; search capability; and note-taking functionality.

Clinical Handbook for Olds' Maternal-Newborn Nursing & Women's Health Across the Lifespan (ISBN: 0-13-211849-1)—This pocket guide serves as a portable, quick-reference to maternal-newborn nursing care. Encompassing pregnancy through the postpartum and newborn stages, this handbook allows you to take the information you learn in class into any clinical setting.

Student Workbook (ISBN: 0-13-255778-9)—This popular study tool incorporates strategies for you to focus your study and increase comprehension of concepts of nursing care.

Resources for Faculty Success

Companion Web site—This site provides the tools faculty need for ease in classroom preparation and evaluation. Included are the testbank with peer-reviewed NCLEX-RN®-style questions, integrated PowerPoint presentations, an image library, and animations and videos.

MyNursingLab—This Web site saves instructors time by providing quality feedback, ongoing formative assessments, and customized remediation for students. It provides easy, one-stop access to a wealth of teaching resources, such as a testbank with 35 questions per chapter, PowerPoint slides, and video suggestions.

MyNursingLab is also available with Pearson Interactive E-Text, which includes integrated, rich media; links to Web sites; organization that can be customized; search capability; and note-taking functionality.

Instructor's Resource Manual—This online manual contains detailed, chapter-by-chapter lecture outlines to be used with the Lecture Summary PowerPoint slides and includes individual, small group, and large group activities.

Contents

Special Features

Assessment Guide

Clinical Judgment

Clinical Pathway

Developing Cultural Competence

Drug Guide

Nursing Care Plan

Patient Teaching

Procedure

Professionalism in Practice

Research Evidence in Practice

Through the Eyes of a Nurse

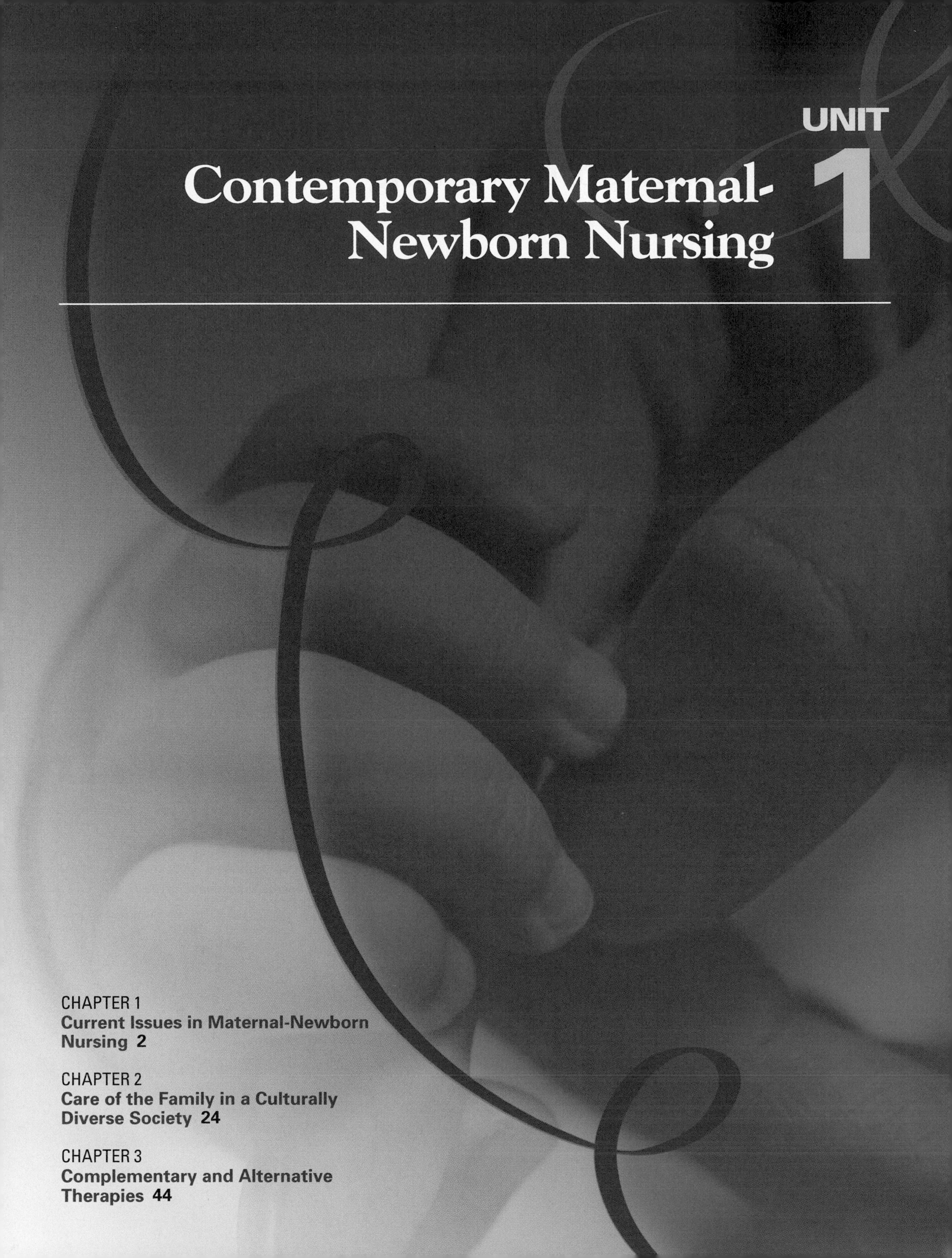

UNIT 1 Contemporary Maternal-Newborn Nursing

CHAPTER 1

Current Issues in Maternal-Newborn Nursing

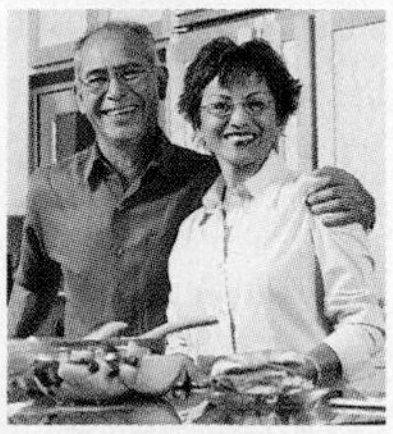

Our daughter just told us that she is 3 months pregnant with our first grandchild. As a labor and delivery nurse for 30 years, I've helped with hundreds of births, but it still seems magical to me, especially now. I'm excited for her and a little worried because I know all the risks as well as the joys. She is so happy; when I am with her I just want to laugh out loud. I already know I love being a grandmother!

LEARNING OUTCOMES

1. Discuss the impact of the self-care movement on contemporary childbirth.
2. Compare the nursing roles available to the maternal-newborn nurse.
3. Describe the use of community-based nursing care in meeting the needs of childbearing families.
4. Identify specific factors that contribute to a family's value system.
5. Delineate significant legal and ethical issues that influence the practice of nursing for childbearing families.
6. Evaluate the potential impact of some of the special situations in contemporary maternity care.
7. Contrast descriptive and inferential statistics.
8. Relate the availability of statistical data to the formulation of further research questions.
9. Identify the impact of evidence-based practice in improving the quality of nursing care for childbearing families.

KEY TERMS

Assisted reproductive technology (ART) *15*
Birth rate *17*
Certified nurse-midwife (CNM) *9*
Certified registered nurse (RNC) *9*
Clinical nurse specialist (CNS) *9*
Evidence-based practice *20*
Infant mortality rate *18*
Informed consent *12*
Intrauterine fetal surgery *14*
Maternal mortality rate *19*
Nurse practitioner (NP) *9*
Nurse researcher *9*
Professional nurse *9*
Therapeutic insemination (TI) *15*

The practice of most nurses is filled with special moments, shared experiences, times in which they know they have practiced the essence of nursing and, in doing so, have touched a life. What is the essence of nursing? Simply stated, nurses care for people, care about people, and use their expertise to help people help themselves.

> ❝ I like working with students. I enjoy the enthusiasm they bring, the questions they ask, the ways they cause me to examine my practice. I love being a nurse. I am passionate about the importance of what I do, and I feel the need to seize every chance to influence those who will be practicing beside me someday. Last week was a perfect example. I had a nursing student working with me in one of our birthing rooms. It was her first day caring for a laboring woman, and she was scared and excited at the same time. We were taking care of a healthy woman who had two boys at home and really wanted a girl.
>
> As labor progressed, the student and I worked closely together monitoring contractions, teaching the woman and her husband, doing what we could to ease her discomfort. Sometimes the student would ask how I knew when to do something, a vaginal exam, for example, and I'd have to think beyond "I just do" to give her some clues. At the birth the student stayed close to the mother, coaching and helping with breathing. The student was excited but felt she had an important role to play, and she handled it beautifully. At the moment of birth the student and the dad were leaning forward watching as the baby just slipped into the world. There wasn't a sound until the student said in a voice filled with awe, "Oh, it's a girl!" Then we all laughed and hugged each other. What a day—using my expertise to help others and helping a future nurse recognize the importance of what we do! ❞

All nurses who provide care and support to childbearing women and their families can make a difference. Expert nurses, like the nurse in the preceding situation, have a clear vision of what is possible in a given situation. This holistic perspective that expert nurses develop is based on a wealth of knowledge bred of experience and enables them to act "intuitively" to provide effective care. In reality nurses' intuition reflects their internalization of information. When faced with a clinical situation, expert nurses draw almost subconsciously on their stored knowledge and judgment. New nurses need time to develop this level of skill and can benefit greatly from mentoring and coaching by their more seasoned colleagues.

This intuitive perception is integral to the "art of nursing," especially in areas such as maternal-newborn nursing, where change occurs quickly and families look to the nurse for help and guidance. Labor nurses become attuned to a woman's progress or lack of progress; nursery nurses detect subtle changes in the infants under their care; antepartal and postpartal nurses become adept at assessing and teaching. Similarly, nurses who are cross-trained as labor, delivery, recovery, and postpartum (LDRP) nurses become skilled at caring for childbearing families during all phases of childbirth. Thus skilled nursing practice depends on a solid base of knowledge and clinical expertise delivered in a caring, holistic manner.

> ❝ My first pregnancy ended in spontaneous abortion at 8 weeks, so this time I decided not to tell anyone I was pregnant until I was 3 months along. We had just told both families the news the preceding day when it happened again. I began bleeding heavily, and we rushed to the ED. Here I was, a maternal-newborn nursing instructor, and I couldn't seem to handle a pregnancy. I was in the bathroom when I passed the fetus into the Johnny cap. My poor baby—so small, maybe 3 or 4 inches long. I began to sob uncontrollably as I rang for the nurse. I told her what happened, and she helped me to bed. My husband sat with his arm around me as I cried while the nurse took our baby out. A few minutes later, she came back and said, "I saw on your record that you are Catholic. Would you like me to baptize your baby?" I said, "Oh, yes, please," and she left. I've never forgotten how that made me feel. She saw me as a total person. I'm still teaching, and now I have two children. Whenever I teach high-risk pregnancy, I tell that story to the students. I want them to know what a difference a nurse can make. ❞

Many nurses who work with childbearing families are sensitive, intuitive, knowledgeable, critical thinkers. They are technically skilled, empowered professionals who can collaborate effectively with others and advocate for those individuals and families who need their support. Such nurses do make a difference in the quality of care that childbearing families receive.

Contemporary Childbirth

The scope of practice of maternal and newborn nurses has changed dramatically in the past 30 years. Today's maternal-newborn nurses have far broader responsibilities and focus more on the specific goals of the individual childbearing woman and her family (Figure 1-1 ■).

Contemporary childbirth is characterized by an emphasis on the family, and family-centered childbirth is accepted and encouraged. Fathers are active participants in the birth experience. Families and friends are also often included. Siblings are encouraged to visit and meet their newest family member and may even attend the birth. In addition, new definitions of family are evolving as discussed in chapter 2 ∞. For example, the family of the single mother may include her mother, sister, another relative, a close friend, or the father of the child. Many

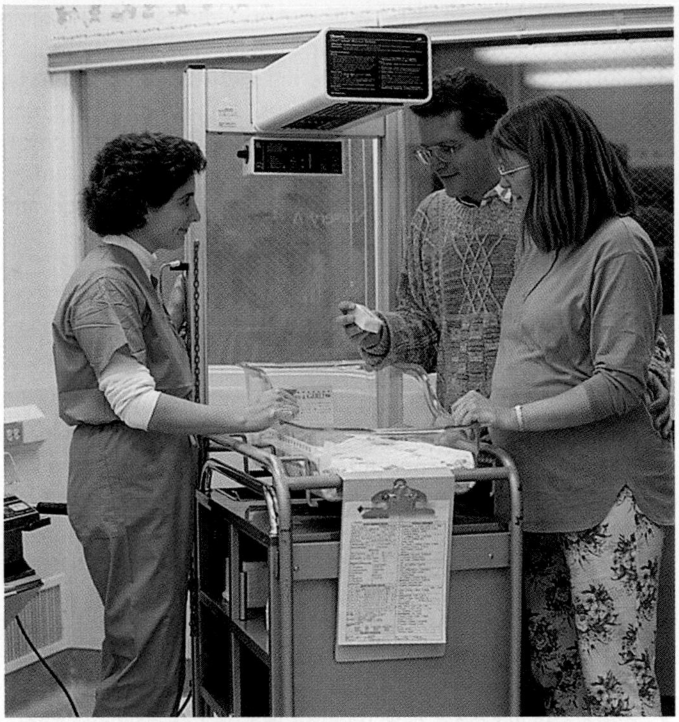

Figure 1-1 ■ Individualized education for childbearing couples is one of the prime responsibilities of the maternal-newborn nurse.

cultures also recognize the importance of extended families, where several family members often provide care and support.

Contemporary childbirth is also characterized by an increasing number of choices about many aspects of the childbirth experience, including the place of birth (hospital, free-standing birthing center, or home birth); the primary caregiver (physician, certified nurse-midwife, or certified midwife); and birth-related experiences (methods of childbirth preparation, use of analgesia and anesthesia, and position for labor and birth, for example).

In many areas of the United States there is a movement from a natural, family-focused, low-tech form of childbirth—sometimes called normal childbirth—to high-tech birthing. This movement is influenced in part by childbearing families, sometimes called generation Y or the iGeneration, who have grown up with technology and know no other way. They may view elective induction and mother-requested cesarean birth as accepted options, for example. This movement is often reinforced by caregivers who, aware of legal liability issues, practice defensive medicine. Furthermore, many hospitals now support a high-tech model of maternity care because it is "easier" to manage more patients if their pain is controlled by epidurals and their contractions are monitored by electronic fetal monitors (Zwelling, 2008). This high-tech approach can potentially interfere with family-focused care. Zwelling (2008) has identified several actions that nurses can take to promote family-focused, low-tech childbirth, including:

- Advocating vigorously within the community for normal childbirth.
- Working to ensure that childbirth preparation classes are readily available.
- Increasing personal labor support skills as well as technical skills.
- Accepting doulas as part of the labor team.
- Promoting changes in the birth environment where they work.
- Participating in interdisciplinary committees to develop and implement standardized practices for care.

It seems likely that home follow-up nursing care will continue to gain acceptance because it is a cost-effective approach with favorable long-term family outcomes. In addition, families can access a variety of community resources, from local programs focusing on specific topics such as parenting or postpartal exercise to the widely recognized support provided by national organizations such as La Leche League.

For families with access to the Internet, a wealth of information and advice is available. For example, the Department of Health and Human Services' Office on Women's Health offers a wide variety of educational resources designed to help promote women's health and well-being. Web links to a variety of other organizations and consumer publications also exist.

Interest in complementary and alternative medicine (CAM) practices is growing nationwide and is having an impact on the care of childbearing families. In response to this trend, the National Institutes of Health now has an Office of Alternative Medicine. Nurses caring for childbearing families need to recognize that a significant percentage of Americans are using some form of unconventional or alternative practice, although they may not share this information with their healthcare provider. Thus it is important for nurses to communicate a willingness to work with the women and their families to recognize and respect these alternative approaches. To assist nurses caring for these childbearing families, we have devoted chapter 3 ∞ to complementary and alternative therapies.

Many women elect to have their pregnancy and birth managed by a certified nurse-midwife (CNM), a registered nurse who is also prepared as a midwife. In 2006, for example, CNMs and CMs attended 7.4% of all births in the United States and 10.8% of all vaginal births (American College of Nurse-Midwives (ACNM), 2009a). The preparation and role of the CNM is described on page 9.

Some women choose to receive care from a direct-entry certified midwife or even a lay midwife, who is an unlicensed or uncertified midwife trained through an informal route such as apprenticeship or self-study rather than a formal educational program (Midwives Alliance of North America [MANA], 2009). Midwives who complete a direct-entry midwifery education program that meets the standards established by the American College of Nurse-Midwives (ACNM) may take a certification exam to become a *certified midwife (CM)*. ACNM has mandated that, as of 2010, a graduate degree is required for entry into clinical practice as either a CNM or CM. The ACNM Position Statement does support the continued recognition of CNMs and CMs without graduate degrees who completed their education prior to 2010 so that they can retain their licenses and become licensed in additional states (ACNM, 2009b).

The North American Registry of Midwives (NARM) is also a certification agency. Midwives certified through NARM may

RESEARCH EVIDENCE IN PRACTICE Factors Influencing Planned Home Birth and Outcomes

CLINICAL QUESTIONS

What are the factors that influence the choice to give birth at home? What are the comparable outcomes of home versus hospital births for low-risk pregnancy?

RESEARCH EVIDENCE

Home birth remains controversial, even though it is commonplace in many cultures. Healthcare providers' attitudes about maternity care options influence the advice they give to expectant mothers as to where to give birth. The mother's desire to influence the conditions under which she gives birth also has a powerful impact on the choice of birth site. Evidence integrating qualitative inquiry, surveys of provider attitudes, and quantitative research comparing birth outcomes can help determine the factors that influence the choice to give birth at home and describe the comparable outcomes of planned home birth.

In a large, multisite study of certified nurse-midwives and their attitudes toward home birth, the provider's comfort and amount of experience with planned home birth was the primary predictor of willingness to advise mothers to give birth at home. In a qualitative study of mothers who gave birth at home, women felt strongly positive about the experience. They reported feeling more relaxed during the perinatal period, felt more informed about the process, and believed they were more fully engaged in the planning of their care. These mothers had a great deal of trust in their midwives' skills and knowledge and felt a genuine sense of support throughout the process.

In a large (n = 6692) Canadian study, women with expected low-risk pregnancies who gave birth at home were compared with similar women who gave birth in the hospital. There was no difference in maternal or neonatal mortality or morbidity; both groups had low mortality rates. All measures of serious maternal morbidity were lower in the planned home birth group as were rates for all interventions, including cesarean birth.

Still, more than 12% of planned home births end up with the mother transported to the hospital to complete the birth. Nulliparas were more likely to require transport than multiparas, most commonly due to failure to progress. Women who planned a home birth also ended up giving birth in the hospital when their selected provider was unavailable to them. A pregnancy exceeding 42 weeks increased the risk of transfer for both primiparas and multiparas.

WHAT QUESTIONS REMAIN UNANSWERED?

Even though these studies were large, the women who gave birth at home were self-selected and not randomly assigned to groups. Are there characteristics of women who choose home birth that influence outcomes, such as nutritional choices or exercise? What are the mortality and morbidity rates for women who plan a home birth but are transported to the hospital to complete the birth?

WHAT IS BEST PRACTICE?

When the provider is experienced and establishes a trusting relationship with the mother, planned home birth can be a viable alternative for the mother with a low-risk pregnancy. Women who have had previous births may be able to complete a home birth more easily than those who are having their first baby. The rate of serious outcomes for low-risk birth is the same for mothers who give birth at home and in the hospital and, in some cases, may result in fewer interventions.

CRITICAL THINKING

What characteristics of a mother might make her a good candidate for a planned home birth? How can these characteristics be assessed in the prenatal period?

References

Hutton, E., Reitsma, A., & Kaufman, K. (2009). Outcomes associated with planned home and planned hospital births in low-risk women attended by midwives in Ontario, Canada, 2003–2006: A retrospective cohort study. *Birth: Issues in Perinatal Care, 36*(3), 180–189.

Janssen, P., Henderson, A., & Vedam, S. (2009). The experience of planned home birth: Views of the first 500 women. *Birth: Issues in Perinatal Care, 36*(4), 297–304.

Lindgren, H., Hildingsson, I., Christensson, K., & Radestad, I. (2008). Transfers in planned home births related to midwife availability and continuity: A nationwide population-based study. *Birth: Issues in Perinatal Care, 35*(1), 9–15.

Vedam, S., Stoll, K., White, S., Aaker, J., & Schummers, L. (2009). Nurse-midwives' experiences with planned home birth: Impact on attitudes and practice. *Birth: Issues in Perinatal Care, 36*(4), 274–282.

become midwives through a formal educational program at a college, university, or midwifery school, or through apprenticeship or self-study. They are eligible to use the credential *certified professional midwife (CPM)* (MANA, 2009).

Some women choose to give birth at home although healthcare professionals do not generally recommend this approach. The concern of the healthcare professional is that, in the event of an unanticipated complication that threatens the well-being of the mother or her infant, delay in obtaining emergency assistance might result. Some CNMs do attend home births; however, the majority of home births are attended by CMs, CPMs, or lay midwives. In fact, in 2006, just over half of 1 percent (0.59%) of births occurred at home. Of these, about 61% were attended by midwives. Of midwife-attended home births, one fourth (27%) were done by CNMs; 73%, however, were done by other midwives (MacDorman & Menacker, 2010).

The Self-Care Movement and Health Promotion Education

The *self-care* movement began to emerge in the late 1960s as consumers sought to understand technology and take an interest in their own health and basic self-care skills. More and more people have begun to exercise, control their diet, and monitor their psychologic and physiologic status. They thus assume many primary care functions. Furthermore, today's healthcare consumers are requiring greater information and accountability from their healthcare providers. These consumers recognize that knowledge, indeed, is power.

Practicing self-care—assuming responsibility for one's own health—often requires assertiveness and taking an active role in seeking necessary information. Healthcare providers can help foster self-care by focusing on *health promotion education* during every patient encounter. This may be as simple as discussing actions that foster a healthy lifestyle, such as exercising regularly or wearing a helmet when biking, skiing, or snowboarding, or it may be more involved for a person with a chronic health condition. Health promotion education can be especially effective when it is related to a specific health concern. For example, discussion about the importance of a healthy diet, weight control, and regular exercise may be particularly impactful for a woman who learns she has high cholesterol or who is diagnosed with gestational diabetes mellitus. Nurses can foster self-care by providing information readily and by acknowledging people's right to ask questions and become actively involved in their own care.

Gradually, as more and more people have come to recognize that promoting health can help decrease healthcare costs, health promotion education activities have increased significantly. Literature and handouts are available in offices, pharmacies, stores, and other public places. Television, radio, newspapers, and magazines regularly address health-related topics. Community organizations have become more active in promoting health through events such as bicycle safety camps for youngsters and by providing car seats to low-income families so that newborns are protected from the moment they leave their place of birth.

Maternal-newborn care offers a special opportunity to promote health-related activities and to foster active participation in health care because it is essentially health focused; in most cases, patients are well when they enter the system. The consumer movement that has already influenced childbirth encourages people to speak up for preferences in dealing with healthcare providers.

We believe that health promotion education and its corollary, self-care, will be vital parts of health care for years to come. Obviously, self-care is not always realistic or appropriate, especially in acute emergencies, but in many situations it is appropriate. With this in mind, throughout this book we have attempted to suggest ways in which nurses might offer health promotion education that would enable the childbearing family to meet its own healthcare needs. We see this as one of nursing's most important functions and one that nurses are especially well qualified to perform.

The nursing profession has been at the forefront in recognizing that people who are able to do so should take an active role in their own health care, and we agree. Because of that, in previous editions we used the term *client* as more descriptive of this relationship. Many of the students and faculty who use our book have expressed a preference for the term *patient*, however, because it is the norm in most clinical areas. We have returned to this more traditional language because we feel sure that the practice of nursing has evolved sufficiently so that both nurses and the people they serve understand that it is the nurse's professional expertise and skill that is sought in an equal partnership.

The Healthcare Environment

Healthcare issues are at the top of policy and legislative agendas. Cost, access, and quality of health care have become the "bywords" of the times. In 2007, healthcare expenditures in the United States were $2.2 trillion, a 6% increase over the previous year. The healthcare share of the gross domestic product (GDP) was 16%, up from 14% in 2000. This share of the GDP is greater than that of any other developed country. Switzerland is the next closest country, spending 11.3% of its GDP on health care (National Center for Health Statistics [NCHS], 2010).

Despite this increase in spending, however, not all adults and children in the United States have access to health care. In 2007, 16.6% of the population (43.3 million people) were without health insurance. For people living in poverty, Medicaid is the most prevalent form of insurance, covering almost 14% of people (36.2 million), including pregnant women who fall into specified income categories (NCHS, 2010).

Almost all adults over age 65 are covered by Medicare, so the vast majority of uninsured are under age 65. The percentage of people covered by private insurance declined from 73% in 1999 to 67% in 2007. This decrease has been offset, however, by increases in the percentage of people with Medicaid or coverage through the Children's Health Insurance Program (CHIP) (NCHS, 2010). As a result, the percentage of uninsured people under age 65 has not changed significantly. See Figure 1-2 ■.

Taken together, Medicare, Medicaid, and other federal, state, and local programs account for 45% of healthcare spending as shown in Figure 1-3A ■. Of those dollars, almost two thirds are spent on hospitalizations and physician and clinical services (Figure 1-3B ■ [NCHS, 2010]).

For women who become pregnant, early prenatal care is one of the most important approaches available to reduce adverse pregnancy outcomes. In 2006, 83.2% of pregnant women in the United States began prenatal care in the first trimester. However, these percentages vary significantly among groups, with black or African American, Hispanic or Latina, and Native American women less likely to receive early and adequate prenatal care than white and Asian women (NCHS, 2010). As mentioned previously, the United States spends more per capita than any other country in the world on health care; nevertheless, compared with other industrialized nations, the United

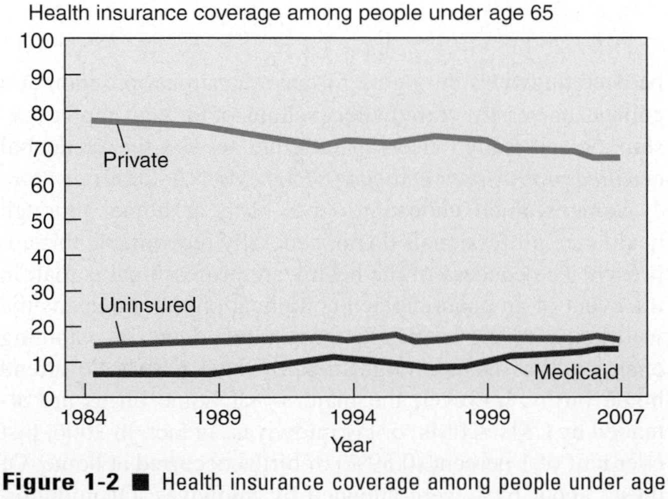

Figure 1-2 ■ Health insurance coverage among people under age 65 in the United States, 2009.

Source: Centers for Disease Control and Prevention/National Center for Health Statistics (CDC/NCHS). (2010). Health, United States, 2009. *Figure 19. Data from the National Health Interview Survey.*

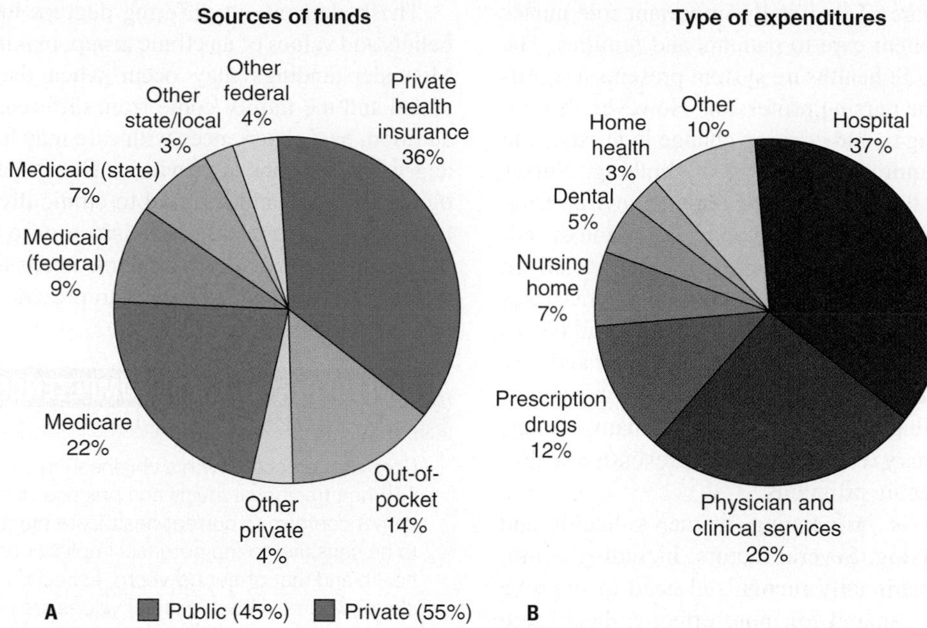

Figure 1-3 ■ Personal healthcare expenditures in 2007 totaled $1.9 trillion. Figure A demonstrates that 45% of the funding comes from public sources, while 55% comes from private health insurance or out-of-pocket dollars. Figure B demonstrates that almost two thirds of expenditures are related to hospitalizations and physician/clinical services.

Source: Centers for Disease Control and Prevention/National Center for Health Statistics (CDC/NCHS). (2010). Health, United States, 2009. *Figure 21. Data from the Centers for Medicare and Medicaid Services.*

States has higher infant mortality rates, similar life expectancy, and less access to care. Many people who have insurance fear changing or losing jobs because they may lose healthcare benefits and access to insurance. They may be denied insurance in the future because of preexisting conditions. The increase in serious, debilitating illnesses, such as AIDS and tuberculosis, and in chronic illnesses, such as diabetes and hypertension, makes this problem of "job lock" and lack of transferability of insurance benefits even more significant. For some uninsured people, the only access to the healthcare system is an emergency department. This inappropriate use of expensive services for basic primary care is both an access and a cost problem.

Among the insured, many people are enrolled in some type of managed care organization because, in an effort to curtail costs, many employers have moved from fee-for-service coverage to some form of managed care. Thus managed care is now the dominant form of healthcare delivery in the United States. The move toward managed care has sparked concerns about the quality of health care. Because a fee-for-service model allows the consumer to register dissatisfaction by choosing to seek care elsewhere, quality is a high priority among fee-for-service providers. A managed care model, in contrast, limits consumer choice and, in turn, potentially affects quality. Establishing managed care's effects on quality poses a problem because in the U.S. system, quality indicators such as outcomes of care usually have not been well determined. An outcome-based system is essential if there is to be comprehensive healthcare reform.

Changing the current system requires a new way of thinking and providing services. Primary healthcare services should be the base on which all other secondary and tertiary services are built. Today in the United States the opposite is still the case. The system emphasizes high-technology care rather than prevention. However, morbidity and mortality from disease are reduced significantly when people use preventive health services. The *Health Insurance Portability and Accountability Act (HIPAA)* of 1996, which was fully implemented in 2002, has also had an impact on health care. HIPAA has two areas of focus: It protects the health insurance coverage of employees and their family if they lose a job or change jobs. It also addresses the privacy and security of health information and requires that national standards be established for the electronic transmission of healthcare data. The *privacy rule* is the federal regulation developed to meet HIPAA requirements. It defines the policies and procedures to be followed to safeguard an individual's protected health information. It also guarantees people access to their medical records and provides recourse for them if their medical privacy is violated. HIPAA regulations have caused healthcare facilities to take a wide variety of actions to ensure client/patient privacy. It has also empowered individuals by giving them access to information about their health care. Academic programs that prepare nurses, physicians, and other healthcare professionals have had to develop tools and resources to ensure that their students understand privacy requirements and comply with them.

Providing all segments of the population with access to primary health care should be the chief criterion for meaningful reform of the U.S. healthcare system. This includes a focus on health promotion, prevention, and individual responsibility for one's own health. In this model, secondary healthcare services would use a smaller proportion of the healthcare dollar.

The current emphasis on healthcare reform has yielded an unexpected benefit: Many healthcare providers and consumers have become more aware of the vitally important role nurses play in providing excellent care to patients and families. The emerging shift in the U.S. healthcare system presents a significant opportunity for the nursing profession. However, this opportunity for responding to and creating change in nursing and healthcare delivery requires a new way of thinking. Nurses must clearly articulate their role in the changing environment. They need to define and differentiate practice roles and the educational preparation required for those new roles, especially in community-based nursing practice and advanced practice roles such as nurse practitioners (NPs) and certified nurse-midwives (CNMs). Nurses must delineate the roles of caregiver and care manager. Nurses also need to assume greater roles in promoting health and preventing disease. In reality, in many settings nurses assume the primary responsibility for preventive healthcare services and screening programs.

Healthcare reform is influencing women's health and maternal-newborn nursing. Several factors, including demographic changes, the nationally recognized need to improve access to care, public demand for more effective healthcare options, new research findings, and women's preferences for health care, are contributing to changes in the field. Changes are predicted in clinical procedures, provider roles, care settings, and financing of care. As access to health care and the need to control costs increase, so will the need for, and utilization of, nurses in advanced practice roles.

Culturally Competent Care

The U.S. population has a varied mix of cultural groups with ever-increasing diversity. Approximately 44% of all children less than 18 years of age are from families of minority populations (Forum on Child and Family Statistics, 2009). Culture develops from socially learned beliefs, lifestyles, values, and integrated patterns of behavior that are characteristic of the family, cultural group, and community. The cultural background and values of childbearing families are often quite different from those of the nurse.

Specific elements that contribute to a family's value system include the following:

- Religion and social beliefs
- Presence and influence of the extended family as well as socialization within the ethnic group
- Communication patterns
- Beliefs and understanding about the concepts of health and illness
- Permissible physical contact with strangers
- Education

Specific differences in beliefs between families and healthcare providers are common in the following areas:

- Help-seeking behaviors
- Pregnancy and childbirth practices
- Causes of diseases or illnesses
- Death and dying
- Caretaking and caregiving
- Childrearing practices

These elements in differing degrees influence the cultural beliefs and values of an ethnic group, making the group unique. Misunderstandings may occur when the healthcare professional and the family come from different cultural groups. In addition, past experiences with care may have made the family angry or suspicious of providers. Nurses need to be able to recognize, respect, and respond to ethnic diversity in a way that leads to an outcome that is satisfactory to both the patient and the healthcare provider. The nurse needs to identify culturally relevant facts about the patient to provide culturally appropriate and competent care.

DEVELOPING CULTURAL COMPETENCE
Values Conflicts

Conflicts can occur with a childbearing woman and her family when traditional rituals and practices of the family's elders do not conform to current healthcare practices. Nurses need to be sensitive to the potential implications for the woman's health and that of her newborn, especially after they are discharged home. When cultural values are not part of the nursing care plan, a woman and her family may be forced to decide whether the family's beliefs should take priority over the healthcare professional's guidance.

When the family's cultural values are incorporated into the care plan, the family is more likely to accept and comply with the needed care, especially in the home care setting. It is important for nurses to avoid imposing personal cultural values on the women and families in their care. By learning about the values of the different ethnic groups in the community—their religious beliefs that have an impact on healthcare practices, their beliefs about common illnesses, and their specific healing practices—nurses can develop an individualized nursing care plan for each childbearing woman and her family.

Because of the importance of culturally competent care, this topic is discussed in more depth in chapter 2 ∞ and throughout the book as well.

Professional Options in Maternal-Newborn Nursing Practice

"As a man, I don't always find it easy to be a labor and delivery nurse. I have three children of my own and attended all their births. It meant a lot to me to be there, and I like helping others to have good childbirth experiences, too. I don't fit some people's image of a nurse; so they refer to me as a "male nurse" as opposed to a real nurse, and they ask why I didn't go into medicine instead. Why can't they understand that I'm a nurse because it's what I really want to be—and I'm darned good at it, too. More men are choosing nursing now, and I think that will help. I hope to see the day when we don't have "female doctors" and "male nurses," but doctors and nurses, period!"

Maternal-newborn nurses are found in the maternity departments of acute care facilities, in physicians' offices, in clinics, in college health services, in school-based programs dealing with sex education or adolescent pregnancies, in community health services, and in any other setting where a patient has a need for maternity care. The depth of nursing involvement in various settings is determined by the qualifications and the role or function of the nurse employed. Many different titles have evolved to describe the professional requirements of the nurse in various maternity care roles. These titles include the following:

- A **professional nurse** is a graduate of an accredited basic program in nursing who has successfully completed the nursing examination (NCLEX-RN) and is currently licensed as a registered nurse (RN). Professional nurses are typically educated as generalists.
- A **certified registered nurse (RNC)** has shown expertise in a particular field of nursing such as labor and delivery by taking a national certification examination.
- A **nurse practitioner (NP)** is a professional nurse who has received specialized education in either a Doctor of Nursing Practice (DNP) or master's degree program and thus can function in an expanded role. (Note: Early nurse practitioner programs were sometimes certificate programs.) The area of specialization determines the NP's title, so that there are family nurse practitioners, neonatal nurse practitioners, pediatric nurse practitioners, women's health nurse practitioners, and so forth. Nurse practitioners often provide ambulatory care services to the expectant family (women's health nurse practitioner, family nurse practitioner); some NPs also function in acute care settings (neonatal nurse practitioner, perinatal nurse practitioner). NPs focus on physical and psychosocial assessment, including health history, physical examination, and certain diagnostic tests and procedures. The nurse practitioner makes clinical judgments and begins appropriate treatments, seeking physician consultation when necessary. The emerging emphasis on community-based care has greatly increased opportunities for NPs.
- A **clinical nurse specialist (CNS)** is a professional nurse with a master's degree who has additional specialized knowledge and competence in a specific clinical area. CNSs assume a leadership role within their specialty and work to improve patient care both directly and indirectly.
- A **certified nurse-midwife (CNM)** is educated in the two disciplines of nursing and midwifery and is certified by the American College of Nurse-Midwives (ACNM). The certified nurse-midwife is prepared to manage independently the care of women at low risk for complications during pregnancy and birth and the care of normal newborns (Figure 1-4 ■).

The term *advanced practice nurse* is used to describe nurses who, by education and practice, function in an expanded nursing role. The term, often used in a legal sense in state nurse practice acts, most frequently applies to NPs, CNSs, certified registered nurse anesthetists (CRNAs), and CNMs. As NPs assume a more prominent role in providing care, the distinctions between the roles of the nurse practitioner and the clinical nurse specialist are beginning to blur and these roles may ultimately merge.

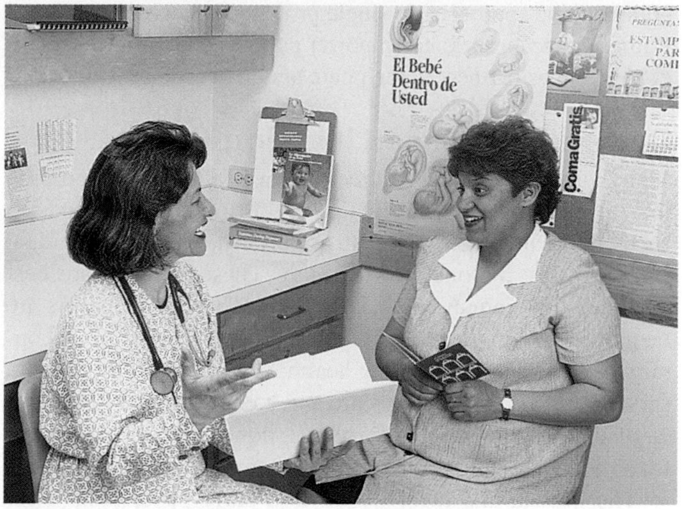

Figure 1-4 ■ A certified nurse-midwife confers with her patient.

Source: Photographer, Jenny Thomas.

The **nurse researcher** has an advanced doctoral degree, typically a Doctor of Philosophy (PhD) and assumes a leadership role in generating new research. Nurse researchers are typically found in university settings although more and more hospitals are employing them to conduct research relevant to patient care, administrative issues, and the like.

Collaborative Practice

Managed care has led to a rethinking of care delivery. One approach that is becoming increasingly popular is collaborative practice. Collaborative practice is a comprehensive model of health care that uses a multidisciplinary team of health professionals to provide cost-effective, high-quality care. In maternal-newborn settings, the team generally includes CNMs and NPs in practice with physicians (often obstetricians or family practice physicians) and may include other health professionals, such as lactation consultants, social workers, or CNSs (Figure 1-5 ■).

In a successful team, each individual has autonomy but functions within a clearly defined scope of practice. In such a

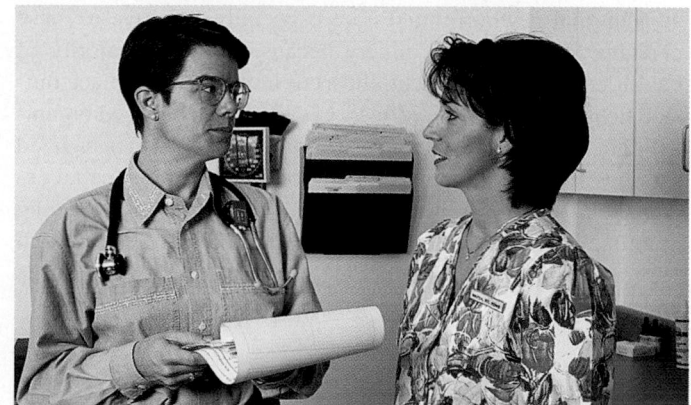

Figure 1-5 ■ A collaborative relationship between nurse and physician contributes to excellent patient care.

Source: Photographer, Elena Dorfman.

collaborative approach, no single profession "owns the patient." Rather, the team seeks to empower patients and families and include them as partners in their care and in decision making.

Community-Based Nursing Care

Many advocates of a new direction for health care support the increasing emphasis on primary care. Primary care includes a focus on health promotion, illness prevention, and individual responsibility for one's own health. These services are best provided in community-based settings. Third-party payers are beginning to recognize the importance of primary care in containing costs and maintaining health. Community-based health services providing primary care and some secondary care will be available in schools, workplaces, homes, churches, clinics, transitional care programs, and other ambulatory settings.

The growth and diversity of third-party payer plans offer both opportunities and challenges for women's health care. The potential exists for third-party payers to work with consumers to provide a model for coordinated and comprehensive well-woman care that includes improved screening and preventive services. One challenge payers will face is how to relate to essential community providers of care—organizations such as family planning clinics or women's health centers—that offer a unique service or serve groups of women with special needs (adolescents, disabled women, ethnic or racial minorities). Community-based care remains an essential element of health care for uninsured and underinsured individuals as well as for those individuals who benefit from programs such as Medicare or state-sponsored health-related programs. Some of these programs, such as those offered through public health departments, are broad based; others, such as parenting classes for adolescents, are geared to the needs of a specific population.

Community-based care is also part of a trend initiated by consumers, who are asking for a "seamless" system of family-centered, comprehensive, coordinated health care, health education, and social services. This seamless system requires coordination as patients move from primary care services to acute care facilities and then back into the community. The shortened length of hospital stays further mandates the need for coordination of services. Nurses can assume this care management role and perform an important service for individuals and families.

Application: Scope of Practice

Maternal-newborn nurses are especially sensitive to these changes in healthcare delivery because the vast majority of health care provided to childbearing families takes place outside hospitals in clinics, offices, and community-based organizations. In addition, maternal-newborn nurses offer specialized services such as childbirth preparation classes or postpartal exercise classes. In essence, we are already experts at providing community-based nursing care. However, it is important that we remain knowledgeable about current practices and trends and open to new approaches to meet the needs of women and children.

Home Care

The provision of health care in the home is emerging as an especially important dimension of community-based nursing care. The shortened length of hospital stays has resulted in the discharge of individuals who still require support, assistance, and teaching. Home care can help fill this gap. Conversely, home care also enables individuals to remain at home with conditions that formerly would have required hospitalization.

Nurses are the major providers of home care services. Home care nurses perform direct nursing care and also supervise unlicensed assistive personnel who provide less skilled levels of service. In a home setting, nurses can use their skills in assessment, therapeutics, communication, teaching, problem solving, and organization to meet the needs of childbearing families. They also play a major role in coordinating services from other providers, such as physical therapists or lactation consultants.

Postpartum and newborn home visits are becoming a recognized way of ensuring that childbearing families make a satisfactory transition from the hospital or birthing center to the home. We see this trend as positive and hope that this method of meeting the needs of childbearing families becomes standard practice. Chapter 36 ∞ discusses home care in more detail and provides guidance about making a home visit. In addition, throughout the text we have provided information on how home care can meet the needs of women with health problems such as diabetes or preterm labor, which put them at risk during pregnancy. We believe that home care offers nurses the opportunity to function in an autonomous role and make a significant difference for individuals and families.

Legal and Ethical Considerations

Professional nursing practice requires full understanding of practice standards; institutional or agency policies; and local, state, and federal laws. Professional practice also requires an understanding of the ethical implications of those standards; policies; and laws that impact care, care providers, and care recipients. Every professional nurse is responsible for obtaining and maintaining current information regarding ethics and laws related to nursing practice and health care.

Scope of Practice

State nurse practice acts protect the public by broadly defining the legal *scope of practice* within which every nurse must function and by excluding untrained or unlicensed individuals from practicing nursing. Although some state practice acts continue to limit nursing practice to the traditional responsibilities of providing patient care related to health maintenance and disease prevention, most state practice acts cover expanded practice roles that include collaboration with other professionals in planning and providing care, diagnostic and prescriptive privilege, and the delegation of patient care tasks to other specified licensed and unlicensed personnel. Specified care activities for certified nurse-midwives (CNMs) and women's health, perinatal, or neonatal nurse practitioners may include diagnosis and prenatal management of uncomplicated pregnancies (CNMs may also manage births) and prescribing and dispensing medications using protocols in specified circumstances. A nurse must function within the scope of practice or risk being accused of practicing medicine without a license.

Correctly interpreting and understanding state practice acts enables the nurse to provide safe care within the limits of nursing practice. State boards of nursing may provide official interpretation of practice acts when the limits are not clear. On occasion hospital policy may conflict with a state's nurse practice act. It is important to recognize that hospital or agency policy may restrict the scope of practice specified in a state practice act, but such policy cannot legally expand the scope of practice beyond the limits stated in the practice act.

Nurse practice acts are subject to change. One component of professional nursing practice is the responsibility of each nurse to remain up to date regarding scope of practice and even to participate actively in promoting appropriate changes.

Nursing Negligence

Negligence is defined as omitting or committing an act that a reasonably prudent person would not omit or commit under the same or similar circumstances. Negligence consists of four elements:

1. There was a duty to provide care.
2. The duty was breached.
3. Injury occurred.
4. The breach of duty caused the injury (proximate cause).

Duty may be breached by omission—failing to give a medication, failing to assess properly, failing to notify a physician of a change in a laboring woman's condition, and so on. Duty may also be breached by commission—giving the wrong medication, placing an infant in the wrong crib, and so on. The injury that results may be physical or mental (pain and suffering). In determining whether nursing negligence occurred, the care that was given is compared with the standard of care. If the standard was not met, negligence occurred.

Standards of Nursing Care

Standards of care establish minimum criteria for competent, proficient delivery of nursing care. Such standards are designed to protect the public and are used to judge the quality of care provided. Legal interpretation of actions within standards of care is based on what a reasonably prudent nurse with similar education and experience would do in similar circumstances.

Sources of Care Standards

Written standards of care are provided by a number of different sources. The American Nurses Association (ANA) has published standards of professional practice since 1950. In 1973, the ANA Congress for Nursing Practice began to write generic standards for all nurses in all settings. In addition, the ANA Divisions of Practice have published standards that include nursing practice for maternal-child health. The Council of Perinatal Nurses has published standards for perinatal nursing. Other specialty organizations, such as the Association of Women's Health, Obstetric, and Neonatal Nurses (AWHONN), the Association of Operating Room Nurses (AORN), and the National Association of Neonatal Nurses (NANN), have developed standards of specialty practice. Agency policies, procedures, and protocols also provide appropriate guidelines for care standards. The Joint Commission on Accreditation of Healthcare Organizations, referred to simply as The Joint Commission, a private, nongovernmental agency that audits the operation of hospitals and healthcare facilities, has also contributed to the development of nursing standards.

Agency policies, procedures, and protocols also provide appropriate guidelines for care standards. For example, *clinical practice guidelines* and clinical pathways are comprehensive interdisciplinary care plans for a specific condition that describe the sequence and timing of interventions that should result in expected patient outcomes. Clinical practice guidelines or clinical pathways are adopted within a healthcare setting to reduce variation in care management, to limit costs of care, and to evaluate the effectiveness of care.

Although standards do not carry the force of law, they carry important legal significance. Any nurse who fails to meet appropriate standards of care invites allegations of negligence or malpractice. (*Malpractice* is negligent action of a professional person.) However, any nurse who practices within the guidelines established by agency, local, or national standards is assured that patients are provided with competent nursing care, which, in turn, diminishes the potential for litigation.

Ethical Components of Care Standards

Standards of care are based on a legal model rather than on ethics. However, they incorporate important ethical components that extend the narrow legal interpretation of the term *standard*. Although there is a great deal of interplay between the two disciplines, each has a different perspective.

Law is based primarily on a rights model that establishes rules of conduct to define relationships among individuals. Law may also define relationships to impersonal entities like formal organizations, agencies, or hospitals.

Ethics, in contrast, is based on a responsibility or duty model that considers a wider range of factors than the rights model of law. Ethics incorporates factors such as risks, benefits, other relationships, concerns, and the needs and abilities of persons affected by and affecting decisions.

Law and ethics are interrelated; they share a similar decision process and standards. Both disciplines incorporate fact-finding, conflict negotiation, prioritization of related issues and values, and the application of resolutions of particular cases in decision making. Professional nurses must consider the ethical implications of legal decisions and the legal implications of ethical decisions.

Understanding the distinctions among medical or healthcare decisions, legal decisions, and ethical decisions is important. Consider the case in which parents from a culture unfamiliar to the nurse refuse surgery for their newborn based on a deeply held spiritual belief that intentional cutting of a body will result in spiritual death. Such a decision to forgo surgery may be viewed as negligent in the eyes of the law, unwise and inappropriate from a medical perspective, yet fully justifiable ethically. Similarly, legally sanctioned maintenance of life support for a severely damaged newborn with little hope for meaningful existence may remain a medically viable alternative, but to

Application: Standards of Care

many it is not ethically justifiable. Recognizing the type of decision to be made often helps measure the worth and outcome of a decision more appropriately.

Patients' Rights

Law and ethics impact all of nursing practice, and several topics have specific implications for maternal-child nursing practice. Patients' rights encompass such topics as informed consent, privacy, and confidentiality.

Patient Safety

The Joint Commission has identified patient safety as an important responsibility of healthcare providers. Patient safety goals, which are evaluated and updated regularly, are requirements for accreditation. The Joint Commission has also developed recommendations related to newborn identification and prevention of kidnapping. These goals and recommendations can be found on The Joint Commission Web site. (Infant identification and security are discussed in chapter 24 ∞.)

Informed Consent

Informed consent is a legal concept designed to allow patients to make intelligent decisions regarding their own health care. Informed consent means that a patient, or a legally designated decision maker, has granted permission for a specific treatment or procedure based on full information about that specific treatment or procedure as it relates to that patient under the specific circumstances of the permission. Although this policy is usually enforced for such major procedures as surgery or regional anesthesia, it pertains to any nursing, medical, or surgical intervention. To touch a person without consent (except in an emergency) constitutes battery.

Several elements must be addressed to ensure that the patient has given informed consent. The information must be clearly and concisely presented in a manner understandable to the patient and must include risks and benefits, the probability of success, and significant treatment alternatives. The patient also needs to be told the consequences of receiving no treatment or procedure. Finally, the patient must be told of the right to refuse a specific treatment or procedure. Each patient should be told that refusing the specified treatment or procedure does not result in the withdrawal of all support or care.

The individual who is ultimately responsible for the treatment or procedure should provide the information necessary to obtain informed consent. In most instances, this is a physician. In such cases, the nurse's role may be to witness the patient's signature giving consent. A nurse who knows the patient and the procedure may certainly help the physician obtain the patient's consent by clarifying the information the physician provides. It is also part of the nurse's role to determine that the patient understands the information before making a decision. Anxiety, fear, pain, and medications that alter consciousness may influence an individual's ability to give informed consent. An oral consent is legal but written consent is easier to defend in a court of law.

Society grants parents the authority and responsibility to give consent for their minor children. Parents are presumed to possess what a child lacks in maturity, experience, and capacity for judgment in life's difficult decisions. Although the age of majority is 18 years in most states, variations in certain states require that nurses be aware of the law in the state where they practice. Children under 18 or 21 years of age, depending on state law, can legally give informed consent in the following circumstances:

- When they are minor parents of the infant or child patient
- When they are *emancipated minors* (self-supporting adolescents under 18 years of age, not subject to parental control)
- When they are adolescents between 16 and 18 years of age seeking birth control, mental health counseling, or substance abuse treatment (Anderson, Schaechter, & Brosco, 2005)

Mature minors (14- and 15-year-old adolescents who are able to understand treatment risks) can give consent for treatment or refuse treatment in some states.

Special problems can occur in maternity nursing when a minor gives birth. It is possible, depending on state law, that a minor may be able to consent to treatment for her infant but not for herself. In some states, however, a pregnant teenager is considered an emancipated minor and may, therefore, give consent for herself as well.

Additionally, some states require a married woman to obtain the consent of her spouse when a procedure involves sterilization or threatens the life of a fetus. Although childbearing women sign a general consent form on admission to an agency, separate informed consent is often required for surgery, cesarean birth, the administration of anesthesia, tubal ligation, or participation in research.

Refusal of a treatment, medication, or procedure after appropriate information also requires that a patient sign a form to release the physician and agency from liability. Jehovah's Witnesses' refusal of blood transfusion or Rh immune globulin is an example of such refusal.

Nurses are responsible for educating patients about any nursing care provided. Before each nursing intervention, the maternal-child nurse lets the individual and/or family know what to expect, thus ensuring cooperation and obtaining consent. Afterward, the nurse documents the teaching and the learning outcomes in the person's record. The importance of clear, concise, and complete nursing records cannot be overemphasized. These records are evidence that the nurse obtained consent, performed prescribed treatments, reported important observations to the appropriate staff, and adhered to acceptable standards of care.

Right to Privacy

The *right to privacy* is the right of a person to keep his or her person and property free from public scrutiny. Maternity nurses need to remember that this includes avoiding unnecessary exposure of the childbearing woman's body. In the context of health care, the right to privacy dictates that only those responsible for a person's care should examine the person or discuss his or her case.

Most states have recognized the right to privacy through statutory or common law, and some states have written that right into their constitution. The ANA, the National League for Nursing (NLN), and The Joint Commission have adopted professional standards protecting patients' privacy. Healthcare agencies should also have written policies dealing with patient privacy. The Health Insurance Portability and Accountability Act (HIPAA), discussed previously, also has a provision to guarantee the security and privacy of health information.

Laws, standards, and policies about privacy specify that information about an individual's treatment, condition, and prognosis can be shared only by the health professionals responsible for his or her care. Authorization for the release of any patient information should be obtained from competent individuals or their surrogate decision makers. Although it may be legal to reveal vital statistics such as name, age, occupation, and prognosis, such information is often withheld because of ethical considerations. The patient should be consulted regarding what information may be released and to whom. When a patient is a celebrity or is considered newsworthy, inquiries may be best handled by the public relations department of the agency.

Confidentiality

Given the highly personal and intimate information requested of patients, the need for maintaining confidentiality is crucial for the development of trust in the relationship between the individual and the provider. Privileged communications exist between patient and physician, patient and attorney, husband and wife, and clergy and those who seek their counsel. In some states, laws of privilege also protect nurses. Nurses should become well informed about privileged communication laws in their state.

A patient may waive the right to confidentiality of medical records by action or words. For example, if a childbearing woman sues a physician, hospital, or other care provider, she waives the right to confidentiality of the medical record because the record becomes a source of evidence. Patients commonly consent to disclose information to insurance companies or to their employers. Computerization of medical records has created a greater concern for the integrity of records and the potential invasion of privacy.

In some instances, the public good takes precedence over an individual's right to privacy. For example, state laws require that care providers report gunshot wounds, child abuse, elder abuse, and some communicable diseases.

The Federal Patient Self-Determination Act requires all healthcare institutions that are reimbursed by Medicare or Medicaid to provide all hospitalized individuals with written information about their rights, which include expressing a preference for treatment options and making *advance directives* (writing a living will or authorizing a durable power of attorney for healthcare decisions on the individual's behalf). This often comes as a surprise to young women and couples of childbearing age who may have no experience of hospitals. However, with an advance directive in place, a childbearing woman can be certain that, even if she becomes incompetent, she can retain her autonomy about healthcare decisions. Nurses often discuss these issues with patients and their families and can help them explore their beliefs and values about treatment options and dying.

> **PROFESSIONALISM IN PRACTICE**
>
> ***Confidentiality and the Pregnant Adolescent***
> Breaching confidentiality is a potential problem for pregnant adolescents, who are just learning whom they can trust in the healthcare system. Make sure you openly discuss the limits of confidentiality for such things as mandatory reporting requirements with the patient and family. Inadvertent disclosure of personal information may lead to psychologic, social, or physical harm for some patients.

Special Ethical Situations in Maternity Care

Maternity care is fraught with unique circumstances in which an ethical dilemma may arise. These include situations of maternal-fetal conflict, issues related to termination of pregnancy, embryonic and fetal research, reproductive assistance, and cord blood banking.

Maternal-Fetal Conflict

Until fairly recently, the fetus was viewed legally as a nonperson. Mother and fetus were viewed as one complex patient—the pregnant woman—of which the fetus was an essential part. However, advances in technology have permitted the physician to treat the fetus and monitor fetal development. The fetus is increasingly viewed as a patient separate from the mother, although treatment of the fetus necessarily involves the mother. This type of approach, by nature adversarial, tends to emphasize the divergent interests of the mother and her fetus rather than focus on their shared interests. This focus on the fetus intensified in 2002 when President George W. Bush announced that "unborn children" would qualify for government healthcare benefits. The move was designed to promote prenatal care, but it represented the first time that any U.S. federal policy had defined childhood as starting at conception.

Most women are strongly motivated to protect the health and well-being of their fetuses. In some instances, however, women have refused interventions on behalf of the fetus, and forced interventions have occurred. These include forced cesarean birth, coercion of mothers who practice high-risk behaviors such as substance abuse to enter treatment, and, perhaps most controversial, mandating experimental in utero therapy or surgery in an attempt to correct a specific birth defect. These interventions infringe on the autonomy of the mother. They may also be detrimental to the baby if, as a result, maternal bonding is hindered, the mother is afraid to seek prenatal care, or the mother is herself harmed by the actions taken. Attempts have also been made to criminalize the behavior of women who fail to follow a physician's advice or who engage in behaviors that are considered harmful to the fetus. These forced interventions raise two thorny questions: (1) What practices should be monitored? and (2) Who will determine when the behaviors pose such a risk to the fetus that the courts should intervene?

The American College of Obstetricians and Gynecologists (ACOG) Committee on Ethics (2004) has affirmed the fundamental right of pregnant women to make informed, uncoerced decisions about medical interventions and has taken a direct stand against coercive and punitive approaches to the maternal-fetal relationship, citing the following "overwhelming rationale" for avoiding such approaches.

1. Coercive and punitive legal approaches to pregnant women who refuse medical advice fail to recognize that all competent adults are entitled to informed consent and bodily integrity. . . .
2. Court-ordered interventions in cases of informed refusal, as well as punishment of pregnant women for their behavior that may put a fetus at risk, neglect the fact that medical knowledge and predictions of outcomes in obstetrics have limitations. . . .
3. Coercive and punitive policies treat medical problems such as addiction and psychiatric illness as if they were moral failings. . . .
4. Coercive and punitive policies are potentially counterproductive in that they are likely to discourage prenatal care and successful treatment, adversely affect infant mortality rates, and undermine the physician-patient relationship. . . .
5. Coercive and punitive policies directed toward pregnant women unjustly single out the most vulnerable women. . . .
6. Coercive and punitive policies create the potential for criminalization of many types of otherwise legal maternal behavior" (ACOG, 2005, pp. 6–9).

ACOG and the American Academy of Pediatrics (AAP) recognize that cases of maternal-fetal conflict involve two patients, both of whom deserve respect and treatment. Such cases are best resolved by using internal hospital mechanisms including counseling, the intervention of specialists, and consultation with an institutional ethics committee. Court intervention should be considered a last resort, appropriate only in extraordinary circumstances.

Abortion

Care Plan Activity: Request for Second Trimester Abortion

Since the 1973 Supreme Court decision in *Roe v. Wade,* abortion has been legal in the United States. It can be performed until the period of viability, that is, the point at which the fetus can survive independently of the mother. After viability, abortion is permissible only when the life or health of the mother is threatened. Before viability, the mother's rights are paramount; after viability, the rights of the fetus take precedence. Abortion is often defined as a pregnancy that is terminated before 20 weeks' gestation or, if the gestation is not certain, a fetus that weighs less than 500 g. In truth, although opinion varies somewhat, it is generally accepted that "births before 26 weeks, especially those weighing less than 750 g, are at the current threshold of viability and that those preterm infants pose a variety of complex medical, social, and ethical considerations" (Cunningham et al., 2010, p. 807).

Personal beliefs, cultural norms, life experiences, and religious convictions shape people's attitudes about abortion. Ethicists have thoughtfully and thoroughly argued positions supporting both sides of the question. Nevertheless, few issues spark the intensity of response seen when the issue of abortion is raised.

At present, decisions about abortion are made by a woman and her physician. Nurses (and other caregivers) have the right to refuse to assist with the procedure if abortion is contrary to their moral and ethical beliefs. However, if a nurse works in an institution where abortions may be performed, the nurse may be dismissed for refusing. To avoid being placed in a situation contrary to their values and beliefs, nurses should determine the philosophy and practices of an institution before going to work there. A nurse who refuses to participate in an abortion because of moral or ethical beliefs does have a responsibility to ensure that someone with similar qualifications is able to provide appropriate care for the patient. Patients may never be abandoned, regardless of the nurse's beliefs.

Fetal Research

Research with fetal tissue has been responsible for remarkable advances in the care and treatment of fetuses with health problems and advances in the treatment of progressive, debilitating adult diseases such as Parkinson disease, Alzheimer disease, and DiGeorge syndrome. Therapeutic research with living fetuses has been instrumental in the treatment of infants who are Rh sensitized, the evaluation of lung maturity using the lecithin/sphingomyelin ratio, and the treatment of pulmonary immaturity in the newborn. Because it is aimed at treating a fetal condition, therapeutic fetal research raises fewer ethical questions than does nontherapeutic fetal research. To be approved, nontherapeutic research requires that the risk to the fetus be minimal, that the knowledge to be gained be important, and that the information be unobtainable by any other means. Control over research standards and attention to state and federal regulations remain foci of debate regarding fetal research.

Intrauterine fetal surgery, which began in 1981 and developed through therapeutic research, is a therapy for anatomic lesions that can be corrected surgically and are incompatible with life if not treated. Intrauterine fetal surgery involves opening the uterus during the second trimester (before viability), treating the fetal lesion, and replacing the fetus in the uterus. The risks to the fetus are substantial, and the mother is committed to cesarean births for this and subsequent pregnancies because the upper, active segment of the uterus is incised during the surgery. The parents must be informed of the experimental nature of the treatment, the risks of the surgery, the commitment to cesarean birth, and alternatives to the treatment.

As with other aspects of maternity care, caregivers must respect the pregnant woman's autonomy. The procedure does involve health risks to the woman, and she retains the right to refuse any surgical procedure.

Healthcare professionals are generally encouraged to provide a clear summary of the risks and benefits of a given approach and to follow the principle of nondirectiveness, in which only the patient's values are discussed during the decision-making process. However, it is likely that some "slippage" in approach occurs, which can result in a blurring of the boundaries between choice and coercion. This may be complicated by the reality that many women are influenced by their views about what it means to be a "good" mother, to behave responsibly. As a result some women may feel that they must opt for a risky procedure to avoid a sense of blame for failing to do their "duty" (Williams, 2006). The dilemmas associated with the consideration of fetal surgery are challenging and complex. Healthcare providers must be careful that their zeal for new technology does not lead them to focus unilaterally on the fetus at the expense of the mother.

Reproductive Assistance

The number and sophistication of reproductive assistance techniques continue to grow. Infertile couples now have available a wide range of reproductive options, from therapeutic insemination to in vitro fertilization and beyond. The ethical dimensions of such techniques are discussed here. The techniques themselves are identified and described in detail in chapter 12 ∞.

Therapeutic insemination (TI) is accomplished by depositing into a woman sperm obtained from her husband, partner, or other donor. Some women who are single are choosing TI as a childbearing option. No states prohibit therapeutic insemination using a husband's sperm because there is no question of the child's legitimacy. Legal problems may occur with TI using donor sperm, however. Because the child is the biologic child of the mother, legal concerns center on the donor. A donor must sign a form waiving all parental rights. The donor must also furnish accurate health information, particularly regarding genetic traits or diseases. Donor sperm must be tested for HIV. Husbands often are requested to sign a form to agree to the insemination and to assume parental responsibility for the child. Some men legally adopt the child so there is no question of parental rights and responsibilities. Several states have enacted legislation regarding paternity of the child conceived by insemination with donor sperm.

Assisted reproductive technology (ART) is the term used to describe any fertility treatment in which both the egg and sperm are handled. Treatments in which only the sperm are handled (e.g., therapeutic insemination) or in which a woman takes medication to stimulate egg production without subsequent egg retrieval are not included in the definition of ART. In vitro fertilization and embryo transfer (IVF-ET), a therapy offered to selected infertile couples, is perhaps the best known ART technique. Some effort has been made legislatively to address consumer concerns about ART. In the United States, the Federal Fertility Clinic Success Rate and Certification Act (FCSRCA) of 1992 addresses issues related to laboratory quality and the standardized reporting of pregnancy success rates associated with ART programs. To help ensure data accuracy, a validation process, which includes site visits to a portion of reporting clinics, is completed.

The use of ART has significantly increased multifetal pregnancies. Multifetal pregnancy occurs because the use of ovulation-inducing medications typically triggers the release of multiple eggs, which, when fertilized, produce multiple embryos, which are then implanted. Multifetal pregnancy increases the risk of miscarriage, preterm birth, and neonatal morbidity and mortality. It also increases the mother's risk of complications, including cesarean birth. To help prevent a high-level multifetal pregnancy, the American Society for Reproductive Medicine (ASRM) and the Society for Assisted Reproductive Technology (SART) have jointly issued guidelines to limit the number of embryos transferred. These guidelines are designed to decrease risk while allowing for individualized care (ASRM & SART, 2009). This practice raises ethical considerations about the handling of the unused embryos. However, when a multifetal pregnancy does occur, the physician may suggest that the woman consider fetal reduction, in which some of the embryos are aborted to give the remaining ones a better chance for survival. Clearly this procedure raises ethical concerns about the sacrifice of some so that the remainder can survive.

Prevention should be the first approach to the problem of multifetal pregnancy. It begins with careful counseling about the risks of multiple gestation and the ethical issues that relate to fetal reduction. No physician who is morally opposed to fetal reduction should be expected to perform the procedure; however, physicians should be aware of the ethical and medical issues involved and be prepared to respond to families in a professional and ethical manner (ACOG, 2007).

Surrogate childbearing is another approach to addressing the issue of infertility. Surrogate childbearing occurs when a woman agrees to become pregnant for another woman or for a couple who are usually childless. Depending on the infertile woman's or couple's needs, the surrogate may be therapeutically inseminated with the male partner's sperm or a donor's sperm, or she may receive a gamete transfer. If fertilization occurs, the woman carries the fetus to term and then releases the infant to the couple after birth.

These methods of resolving infertility raise many ethical questions, including the problem of religious objections to artificial conception, the question of who will assume financial and moral responsibility for a child born with a congenital defect, the issue of candidate selection, and the threat of genetic engineering. Other ethical questions include the following:

- What should be done with surplus fertilized oocytes?
- To whom do frozen embryos belong—parents together or separately? The hospital or infertility clinic?
- Who is liable if a woman or her offspring contracts HIV disease from donated sperm?
- Should children be told the method of their conception?

> “Our son was born after artificial insemination. Nick, my husband, was sterile because of radiation therapy, so his cousin was the donor for us. I thought that might be awkward but the whole family was so excited that there was a way to help us after Nick's battle with cancer that it has been OK. Every time we look at Vincent Joseph (he is named for his grandfathers) and see him smile, we know that we would do it again in an instant.”

Embryonic Stem Cell Research

Human stem cells can be found in embryonic tissue and in the primordial germ cells of a fetus. Research has demonstrated that in tissue cultures these cells can be made to differentiate into other types of cells such as blood, nerve, or heart cells, which might then be used to treat problems such as diabetes, Parkinson and Alzheimer diseases, spinal cord injury, or metabolic disorders. The availability of specialized tissue or even organs grown from stem cells might also decrease society's dependence on donated organs for organ transplants.

Positions about embryonic stem cell research vary dramatically, from the view that any use of human embryos for research is wrong to the view that any form of embryonic stem cell research is acceptable, with a variety of other positions that fall somewhere in between these extremes. Other questions also arise: What sources of embryonic tissue are acceptable for research? Is it ever ethical to clone embryos solely for stem cell research? Is there justification for using embryos remaining after fertility treatments?

The question of how an embryo should be viewed—with status in some way as a person or in some sense as property (and, if property, whose?)—is a key question in the debate. Ethicists recognize that it is not necessary to advocate full moral status or personhood for an embryo to have significant moral qualms about the instrumental use of a human embryo in the "interests" of society. The issue of consent, which links directly to an embryo's status, also merits consideration. In truth, the ethical questions and dilemmas associated with embryonic stem cell research are staggeringly complex and require careful analysis and thoughtful dialogue.

Case Study: Cord Blood Banking

Cord Blood Banking

Cord blood, which is taken from a newborn's umbilical cord by the physician or nurse-midwife assisting with the birth, may play a role in combating leukemia, certain other cancers, metabolic disorders, and other immune and blood system disorders such as sickle cell anemia, thalassemia, and severe aplastic anemia. This is possible because cord blood, like bone marrow and embryonic tissue, contains hematopoietic stem cells, which can replace diseased cells in the affected individual. The value of bone marrow transplants has long been recognized, and a national registry of potential bone marrow donors has been established. The process of collecting bone marrow is expensive and uncomfortable, however, and the National Marrow Donor Registry often has difficulty finding a matching bone marrow donor.

Cord blood banks that store cord blood have been established in the United States. Public banks receive cord blood given on a volunteer basis and are designed to support unrelated-donor transplant programs. Private banks are for-profit entities designed primarily for families who plan to use the cord blood for the infant who provided the blood or for another family member who might need transplantation therapy in the future because of a genetic blood condition, cancer, bone marrow failure, or inborn error of metabolism, for example (ACOG, 2008).

Ethical concerns focus on the issue of confidentiality for the mother and family throughout the process; the question of ownership of the blood (donor, parents, the blood bank, or society); the concern about fair distribution of the harvested blood; and the obligations to the family that may arise if testing of the blood reveals genetic disorders or infectious diseases.

Both ACOG and the American Academy of Pediatrics (AAP) have issued statements about umbilical cord blood banking. ACOG (2008) stresses the importance of providing balanced information about the advantages and disadvantages of public vs. private banking and the need for healthcare professionals to disclose any financial interests they have in private cord blood banks.

The AAP (Lubin & Shearer, 2007) recommendations support the ACOG opinion and address other clinical considerations too. Key recommendations include:

- Parents are encouraged to bank their newborn's cord blood privately if they have an older child who has a condition that could benefit from a cord blood transfusion.
- In general, parents are encouraged to donate their newborn's cord blood to a public bank because it might help treat someone in need.
- Private cord blood banking as "insurance" against possible future personal or family need is discouraged because often the genetic traits associated with the condition that develops are present in the cord blood.
- Collection centers should test all donated cord blood for infectious and genetic disorders and should have a protocol developed for notifying families of abnormal results.
- Written consent for cord blood donation should be obtained before labor begins.

Implications for Nursing Practice

The complex ethical issues facing maternal-newborn nurses have many social, cultural, legal, and professional ramifications. Nurses, like all healthcare professionals, need to learn to anticipate ethical dilemmas, clarify their own positions and values related to the issues, understand the legal implications of the issues, and develop appropriate strategies for ethical decision making. To accomplish these tasks, they may read about bioethical issues, participate in discussion groups, or attend courses and workshops on ethical topics pertinent to their areas of practice. Most nurses develop solid skills in logical thinking and critical analysis. These skills, coupled with theoretic knowledge about ethical decision making, can serve nurses well in dealing with the many ethical dilemmas found in health care.

Statistical Data and Maternal-Infant Care

Increasingly nurses are recognizing the value and usefulness of statistics. Health-related statistics provide an objective basis for projecting patient needs, planning use of resources, and determining the effectiveness of treatment.

There are two major types of statistics: *descriptive* and *inferential. Descriptive statistics* describe or summarize a set of data. They report the facts—what is—in a concise and easily retrievable way. How the data are compiled and presented is determined by the question being asked. An example of a descriptive statistic is the birth rate in the United States. Although no conclusion may be drawn from these statistics about why some phenomenon has occurred, they can identify certain trends and high-risk "target groups" and generate possible research questions.

Inferential statistics allow the investigator to draw conclusions or inferences about what is happening between two or more variables in a population and to suggest or refute causal relationships between them. For example, descriptive statistics reveal that the infant mortality rate in the United States has declined over the past decade. Exactly why that trend has occurred cannot be answered by simply looking at these data, however. More data and inferential statistics using smaller samples of the population of pregnant women are needed to determine whether this finding is because of earlier prenatal care, improved maternal nutrition, use of electronic fetal monitoring during labor, and/or any number of factors potentially associated with maternal-fetal survival.

Descriptive statistics are the starting point for the formation of research questions. Inferential statistics answer specific questions and generate theories to explain relationships between variables. Theory applied in nursing practice can help change the specific variables that may cause or contribute to certain health problems.

TABLE 1-1 Live Births and Birth Rates by Age, Race, and Origin of Mother: United States, 2007 (Estimated)

	2007	
AGE AND RACE AND HISPANIC ORIGIN OF MOTHER	NUMBER	RATE
All races and origins[1]		
Total[2]	4,317,119	14.3
10–14 years	6218	0.6
15–19 years	445,015	42.5
15–17 years	140,640	22.2
18–19 years	304,405	73.9
20–24 years	1,082,837	106.4
25–29 years	1,208,504	117.5
30–34 years	962,179	99.9
35–39 years	499,916	47.5
40–44 years	105,071	9.5
45–54 years[3]	7349	0.6
Non-Hispanic white[2]	2,312,473	11.5
Non-Hispanic black[2]	627,230	16.4
American Indian or Alaska Native total[4,5]	49,284	15.2
Asian or Pacific Islander total[2,5]	254,734	17.2
Hispanic[6]	1,061,970	23.3

[1]Includes origin not stated.
[2]The total number includes births to women of all ages, 10–54 years.
[3]The number of births shown is the total for women aged 45–54 years. The birth rate is computed by relating the number of births to women aged 45–54 years to women aged 45–49 years, because most of the births in this group are to women aged 45–49.
[4]Includes births to Aleuts and Eskimos.
[5]Data for persons of Hispanic origin are included in the data for each race group according to the mother's reported race.
[6]Includes all persons of Hispanic origin of any race.
Source: Hamilton, B. E., Martin, J. A., & Ventura, S. J. (2009). Births: Preliminary data for 2007. National Vital Statistics Reports, 57*(12), 1–23.*

This section discusses descriptive statistics that are particularly important to maternal-newborn health care. Inferences that may be drawn from these descriptive statistics are addressed as possible research questions that may help identify relevant variables.

Birth Rate

Birth rate refers to the number of live births per 1000 people. In 2007, the U.S. birth rate was 14.3 per 1000, a slight increase from the 2006 rate of 14.2. The actual number of live births rose by 1% to 4,317,119. In 2007, births rose for every race and Hispanic origin group, and the birth rate for teenagers rose 1% to 42.5 births per 1000, up from 40.5 in 2005 (Hamilton, Ventura, & Martin, 2009). Table 1-1 provides valuable information about births in the United States in 2007 by age and race of the mother.

Childbearing by unmarried women continued to increase in 2007, reaching record highs—over 1.7 million births—an increase of 5% over 2006. In fact, 39.7% of all births were to unmarried women. Moreover, these increases occurred in all ages, races, and Hispanic-origin subgroups (Hamilton et al., 2009). The cesarean birth rate reached record levels, increasing by 2% to 31.8% of all births in 2007 (Hamilton et al., 2009). Birth rates also vary dramatically from country to country. Table 1-2 identifies the birth rates for selected countries.

- Is there an association between birth rates and changing societal values?
- Do the differences in birth rates between various age groups reflect education? Changed attitudes toward motherhood?

TABLE 1-2 Live Birth Rates and Infant Mortality Rates for Selected Countries*

COUNTRY	BIRTH RATE	INFANT MORTALITY RATE
Afghanistan	38.4	153.1
Argentina	17.9	11.4
Australia	12.8	4.8
Cambodia	25.7	54.8
Canada	10.3	5.0
China	14	20.3
Egypt	25.4	27.3
Germany	8.2	4.0
Ghana	28.7	51.2
India	21.7	50.8
Iraq	30.1	44.7
Japan	7.6	2.8
Mexico	19.7	18.4
Russia	11.1	10.6
United Kingdom	10.7	4.9
United States	14.2**	6.69**

* Based on 2009 estimates.
** Based on final data for 2006.
Source: Data from The World Fact Book 2010. *Washington, DC: The Central Intelligence Agency. Retrieved March 7, 2010, from http://www.cia.gov/library/publications/the-world-factbook*

- Do the differences in birth rates among various countries reflect cultural differences? Do they represent availability of contraceptive information? Are there other factors at work?

Infant Mortality

The **infant mortality rate** is the number of deaths of infants under 1 year of age per 1000 live births in a given population. In 2003 the U.S. infant mortality rate was 6.85, a decrease over 2002. The infant mortality rate in 2006 was 6.68, a decrease of 3% from the 2005 rate of 6.87 (Mathews & McDorman, 2010). However, the infant mortality rate varied widely by race of the mother, from 5.57 for infants of white mothers to 12.9 for infants of black mothers (Mathews & McDormand, 2010). *Neonatal mortality* is the number of deaths of infants less than 28 days of age per 1000 live births. *Postneonatal mortality* refers to the number of deaths of infants between 28 days and 1 year of age. *Perinatal mortality* includes both neonatal deaths and fetal deaths per 1000 live births. (*Fetal death* is death in utero at 20 weeks' or more gestation.) Figure 1-6 ■ shows the changes in infant, neonatal, and postneonatal mortality since 1940. Figure 1-7 ■ shows the 10 leading causes of deaths of infants in the United States.

The U.S. infant mortality rate has continued to be of concern in the United States. In 2005, the United States ranked 30th in infant mortality among industrialized nations (Figure 1-8 ■). The very high percentage of preterm births in the United States

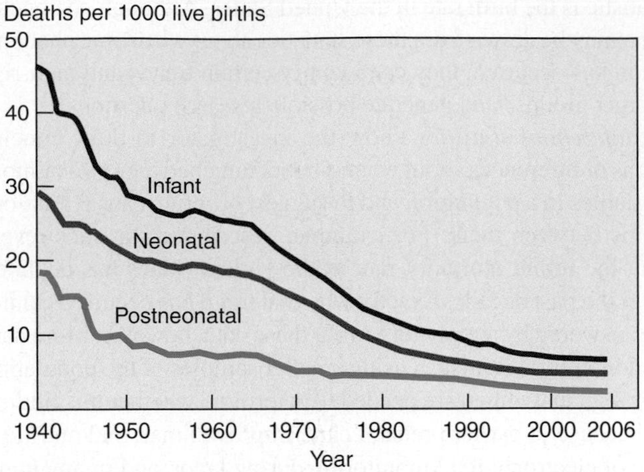

NOTE: Rates are infant (under 1 year), neonatal (under 28 days), and postneonatal (28 days–11 months) deaths per 1000 live births in specified group.

Figure 1-6 ■ Infant, neonatal, and postneonatal mortality rates in the United States from 1940 to 2006. In 2006, the infant mortality rate was 6.69, the neonatal mortality rate was 4.45, and the postneonatal mortality rate was 2.24 per 1000 live births.

Source: Heron, M., Hoyert, D. L., Murphy, S. L., Xu, J., Kochanek, K. D., & Tejada-Vera, B. (2009). Deaths: Final data for 2006. National Vital Statistic Reports, *57(14), 13.*

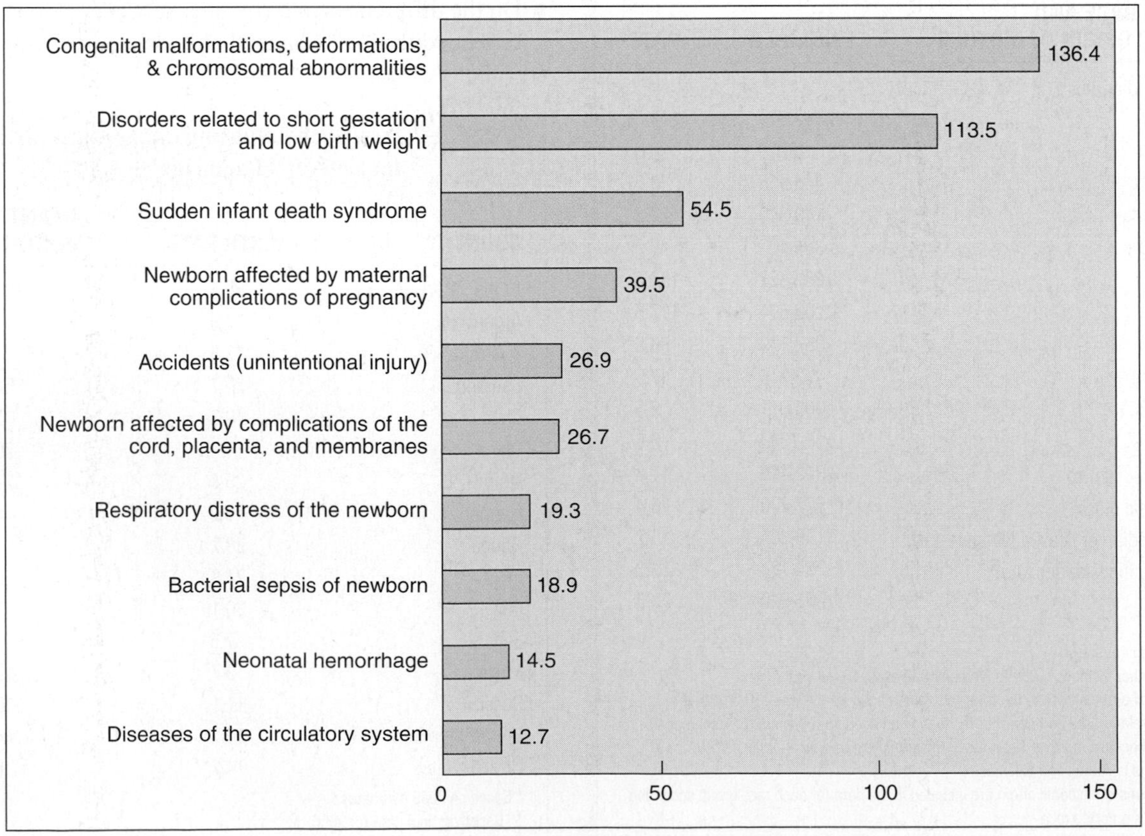

Figure 1-7 ■ Leading causes of death by mortality rate for infants in the United States, 2006.

Source: Adapted from Heron, M., Hoyert, D. L., Murphy, S. L., Xu, J., Kochanek, K. D., & Tejada-Vera, B. (2009). Deaths: Final data for 2006. National Vital Statistic Reports, *57(14), 13.*

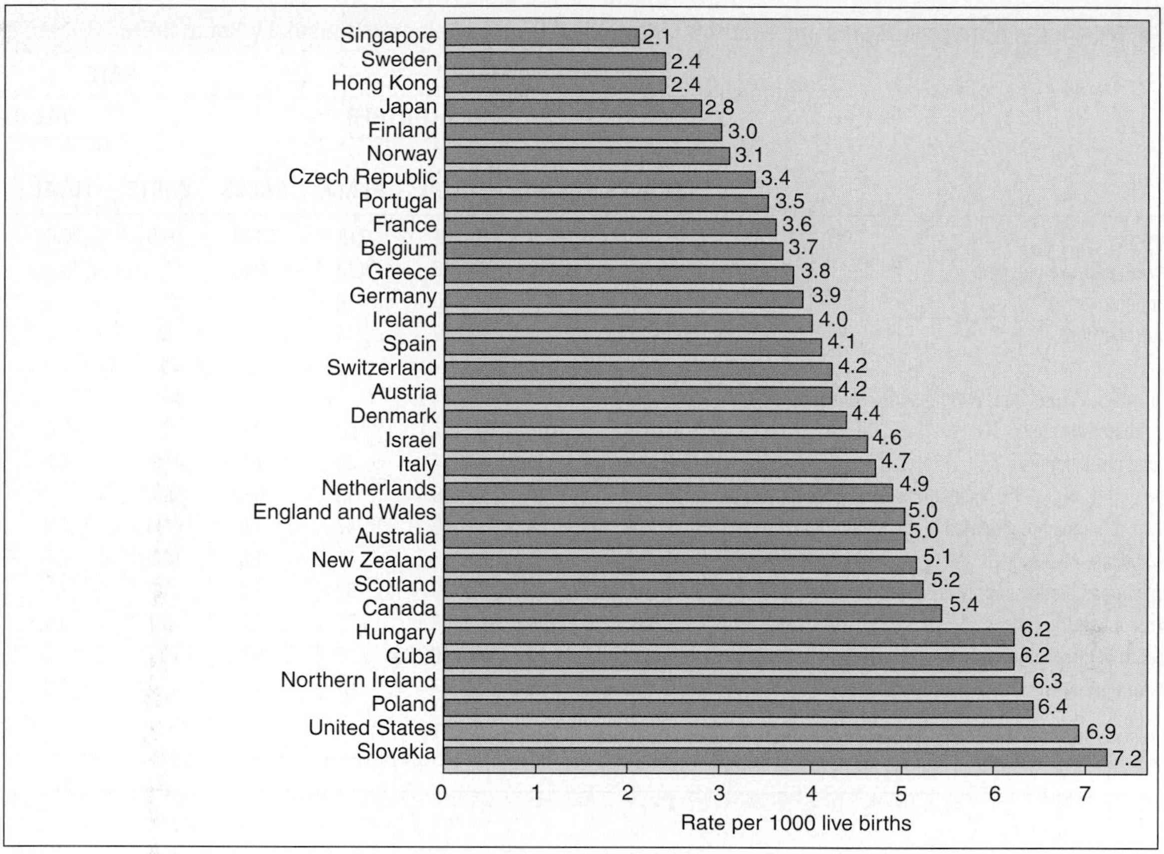

Figure 1-8 ■ Infant mortality rates for selected countries, 2005.

Source: Health, United States 2008 *in MacDorman, M. F., & Mathews, T. J. (2009). Behind international rankings of infant mortality: How the United States compares with Europe.* NCHS Data Brief, No. 23.

is the main cause of this high rate when compared to other countries (MacDorman & Mathews, 2009). While differences in reporting processes do exist, it is unlikely that these differences are the primary cause of the United States's low ranking, especially considering the fact that in 2005, 22 countries had infant mortality rates of 5.0 or less (MacDorman & Mathews, 2009). Healthcare professionals, policy makers, and the public have continued to stress the need in the United States for better prenatal care, coordination of health services, and the provision of comprehensive maternal-child services.

Table 1-2 identifies infant mortality rates for selected countries. As the data indicate, the range is dramatic among the countries listed. Unfortunately, information about birth rates and mortality rates is limited for some countries because of a lack of organized reporting mechanisms.

The information prompts questions about access to health care during pregnancy and following birth, standards of living, nutrition, sociocultural factors, and more. Additional factors affecting the infant mortality rate may be identified by considering the following research questions:

- Does infant mortality correlate with a specific maternal age?
- What are the leading causes of infant mortality in each country?
- Is there a difference in mortality rates among racial groups? If so, is it associated with the availability of prenatal care? With the educational level of the mother or father?

Maternal Mortality

The **maternal mortality rate** is the number of deaths from any cause related to or aggravated by pregnancy or its management during the pregnancy cycle (including the 42-day postpartum period) per 100,000 live births. It does not include accidental or unrelated causes. In 2006, 569 women were reported to have died from maternal cause, resulting in a maternal mortality rate of 13.3 per 100,000 live births (Heron et al., 2009).

Table 1-3 identifies the number of maternal deaths and maternal mortality rates by cause for 2006. In general, maternal mortality rates are significantly lower than they were 25 years ago. Nevertheless, worldwide, an estimated 350,000 to 500,000 women die in childbirth each year (Brooks, 2010). Six countries—India, Nigeria, Pakistan, Afghanistan, Ethiopia, and the Democratic Republic of the Congo—account for over half of these deaths (Barclay, 2010). Encouragingly, significant decreases in maternal mortality have occurred in China, Egypt, Ecuador, and Bolivia. However, in a recent study, maternal mortality rates appear to have increased in the United States, Canada, and Norway. These increases may be explained by improved determination of maternal deaths and by changes in the way late maternal deaths are included in the data (Hogan et al., 2010). Nevertheless, the U.S. maternal mortality rate of 17 per 100,000 live births in 2008 is more than double the rate in the United Kingdom, 3 times the rate in Australia, and 4 times the rate in Italy (Barclay, 2010).

TABLE 1-3 Number of Maternal Deaths and Maternal Mortality Rates for Selected Causes by Race: United States, 2006

	NUMBER				RATE			
			ALL OTHER				ALL OTHER	
	ALL RACES	WHITE	TOTAL	BLACK	ALL RACES	WHITE	TOTAL	BLACK
Maternal causes	569	313	256	218	13.31	9.5	26.8	32.7
Pregnancy with abortive outcome	26	10	16	12	0.6	*	*	*
Ectopic pregnancy	15	5	10	10	*	*	*	*
Spontaneous abortion	5	3	2	1	*	*	*	*
Medical abortion	-	-	-	-	*	*	*	*
Other and unspecified pregnancy with abortive outcome	6	2	4	1	*	*	*	*
Other direct obstetric causes	394	207	187	160	9.2	6.3	19.6	24
Eclampsia and pre-eclampsia	54	30	24	22	1.3	0.9	4.1	3.3
Hemorrhage of pregnancy and childbirth and placenta previa	39	21	18	12	0.9	0.6	*	*
Complications predominately related to the puerperium	109	54	55	47	2.6	1.6	5.8	7.1
Obstetric embolism	41	21	20	15	1.0	0.6	2.1	*
Other complications predominately related to the puerperium	68	33	35	32	1.6	1.0	3.7	4.6
All other direct obstetric causes	192	102	90	79	4.5	3.1	9.4	11.9
Obstetric death of unspecified cause	22	17	6	5	0.5	*	*	*
Indirect obstetric causes	126	79	47	41	3.0	2.4	4.9	6.2

*Figure does not meet standards of reliability followed by the National Center for Health Statistics.
Source: Heron, M., Hoyert, D. L., Murphy, S. L., Xu, J., Kochanek, K. D., & Tejada-Vera, B. (2009). Deaths: Final data for 2006. National Vital Statistics Reports, *57(14), 1–135.*

Factors influencing the decrease in maternal mortality include the increased use of hospitals and specialized healthcare personnel by antepartum, intrapartum, and postpartum maternity patients; the establishment of care centers for high-risk mothers and infants; the prevention and control of infection with antibiotics and improved techniques; the availability of blood and blood products for transfusions; and the lowered rates of anesthesia-related deaths.

Additional factors to consider may be identified by asking the following research questions:

- Is there a correlation between maternal mortality and age?
- Is there a correlation with availability of health care? Economic status?

Implications for Nursing Practice

Nurses can use statistics in a number of ways. For example, statistical data may be used to:

- Determine populations at risk.
- Assess the relationship between specific factors.
- Help establish databases for specific patient populations.
- Determine the levels of care needed by particular patient populations.
- Evaluate the success of specific nursing interventions.
- Determine priorities in caseloads.
- Estimate staffing and equipment needs of hospital units and clinics.

Statistical information is available through many sources, including professional literature; state and city health departments; vital statistics sections of private, county, state, and federal agencies; special programs or agencies (family-planning and similar agencies); and demographic profiles of specific geographic areas. Most of these sources are accessible via the Internet. Nurses who use this information will be better prepared to promote the health needs of maternal-newborn patients and their families.

Evidence-Based Practice in Maternal-Child Nursing

Evidence-based practice—that is, nursing care in which all interventions are supported by current, valid research or other forms of evidence such as committee opinions or task force recommendations—is emerging as a force in health care. It provides a useful approach to problem solving/decision making and to self-directed, patient-centered, lifelong learning. Evidence-based practice builds on the actions necessary to transform research findings into clinical practice by also considering other forms of evidence that can be useful in making clinical practice decisions. These other forms of evidence may include, for example, statistical data, quality improvement measurements, risk management measures, and information from support services such as infection control.

As clinicians, nurses need to meet three basic competencies related to evidence-based practice:

1. To recognize which clinical practices are supported by sound evidence, which practices have conflicting findings as to their effect on patient outcomes, and which practices have no evidence to support their use

2. To use data in their clinical work to evaluate outcomes of care
3. To appraise and integrate scientific bases into practice

Unfortunately, some agencies and clinical units where nurses practice still operate in the old style, which often generates conflict for nurses who recognize the need for more responsible clinical practice. In truth, market pressures are forcing nurses and other healthcare providers to evaluate routines to improve efficiencies and provide better outcomes for patients.

Nurses need to know what data are being tracked where they work and how care practices and outcomes are improved as a result of quality improvement initiatives. However, there is more to evidence-based practice than simply knowing what is being tracked and how the results are being used. Competent, effective nurses learn to question the very basis of their clinical work.

Throughout this text we have provided *snapshots* of evidence-based practice related to childbearing women, children, and families in the Research Evidence in Practice features, such as the one on page 5. We believe that these snapshots will help you understand the concept more clearly. We also expect that these examples may challenge you to question the usefulness of some of the routine care you observe in clinical practice. That is the impact of evidence-based practice—it moves clinicians beyond practices of habit and opinion to practices based on reliable, valid, current science.

Nursing Research

Research is vital to expanding the science of nursing, fostering evidence-based practice, and improving patient care. Research also plays an important role in advancing the profession of nursing. For example, nursing research can help determine the psychosocial and physical risks and benefits of both nursing and medical interventions.

The gap between research and practice is being narrowed by the publication of research findings in popular nursing journals, the establishment of departments of nursing research in hospitals, and collaborative research efforts by nurse researchers and clinical practitioners. Interdisciplinary research between nurses and other healthcare professionals is also becoming more common. This ever-increasing recognition of the value of nursing research is important because well-done research supports the goals of evidence-based practice. To make this link clear, most chapters of this text include Research Evidence in Practice.

Clinical Pathways and Nursing Care Plans

One result of nursing research into the nursing process has been the creation of clinical pathways. *Clinical pathways* specify essential nursing activities and provide basic guidelines about expected outcomes at specified time intervals. These guidelines are research based and enable the nurse to determine whether a patient's responses meet expected norms at any given time. In the text, we have provided sample clinical pathways for a woman experiencing a normal vaginal birth, for the normal newborn, and for a woman in the postpartal period.

Nursing care plans, which use the nursing process as an organizing framework, are also invaluable in planning and organizing care. Care plans are especially valuable for nursing students and novice nurses. To help organize care, this text also provides several examples of nursing care plans such as those found in chapter 19 ∞.

FOCUS YOUR STUDY

- Many nurses working with childbearing families are expert practitioners who are able to serve as role models for nurses who have not yet attained the same level of competence.
- Contemporary childbirth is family centered, offers choices about birth, and recognizes the needs of siblings and other family members.
- The self-care movement, which emerged in the late 1960s, emphasizes personal health goals, a holistic approach, and preventive care.
- The U.S. healthcare system is facing a variety of challenges including the high cost of health care and the need for cost containment while retaining quality; the large numbers of uninsured and underinsured people; high infant mortality rates as compared with other industrialized nations; and a high incidence of poverty, especially among children and women-headed households.
- The nurse who provides culturally competent care recognizes the importance of the childbearing family's

value system, acknowledges that differences occur among people, and seeks to respect and respond to ethnic diversity in a way that leads to mutually desirable outcomes.

- A nurse must practice within the scope of practice or be open to the accusation of practicing medicine without a license. The standard of care against which individual nursing practice is compared is that of a reasonably prudent nurse.
- Nursing standards provide information and guidelines for nurses in their own practice, in developing policies and protocols in healthcare settings, and in directing the development of quality nursing care.
- Informed consent—based on knowledge of a procedure and its benefits, risks, and alternatives—must be secured before providing treatment.
- State constitutions, statutes, and common law protect the right to privacy.
- Maternal-fetal conflict may arise when the fetus is viewed as a person of equal rights to those of the mother's and external agents' attempt to force the mother to accept a therapy she wishes to refuse, or similarly attempt to restrict a mother's actions to support the well-being of the fetus.
- Abortion can be performed until the age of viability. Caregivers have the right to refuse to perform an abortion or assist with the procedure.
- A variety of procedures are available to help infertile couples achieve a pregnancy. However, some of these procedures provoke serious ethical dilemmas.
- Embryonic stem cell research using human stem cells obtained from a human embryo is marked by controversy. On the one hand, it raises the possibility of treatment for a variety of major diseases such as diabetes, Parkinson disease, and Alzheimer disease. On the other hand, ethicists question the ethical implications of using embryonic tissue—especially tissue obtained specifically for stem cell research.
- Cord blood banking provides the opportunity to make stem cells available to treat a variety of cancers and blood system disorders. Its growing popularity has revealed several ethical issues, such as: Who owns the blood? How will informed consent be obtained and by whom? How will confidentiality be ensured? How can the harvested blood be distributed fairly, so that it is available to individuals from all races, ethnic groups, income levels, and so forth?
- Descriptive statistics describe or summarize a set of data. Inferential statistics allow the investigator to draw conclusions about what is happening between two or more variables in a population.
- Evidence-based practice—that is, nursing care in which all interventions are supported by current, valid research evidence—is emerging as a positive force in health care.
- Nursing research plays a vital role in adding to the nursing knowledge base, expanding clinical practice, and expanding nursing theory.

CRITICAL THINKING IN ACTION

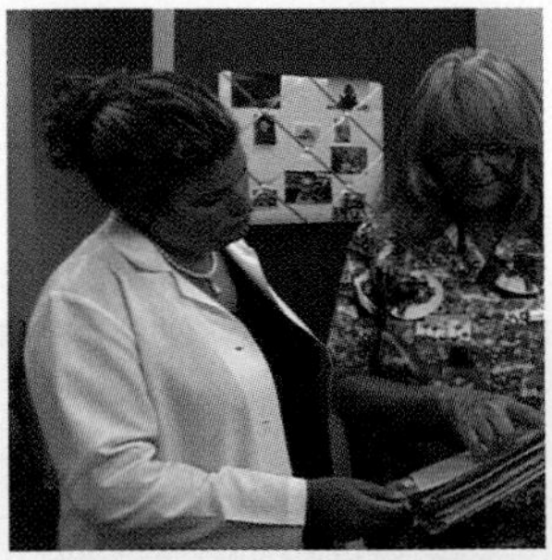

You are working as a prenatal nurse in a local clinic. Before entering a patient's room, you review the chart for pertinent information such as cultural background, significant family members, weeks of gestation, test results, birth plan, and her education for health promotion. You greet each patient and her family members by name and ask how they are coping with the pregnancy. Depending on the trimester of the pregnancy, you review the discomforts or concerns of the mother/family and what they may expect. You examine the mother, including fundal height, fetal heart rate and fetal position if appropriate, maternal blood pressure, weight gain, and urine analysis. With each patient, you discuss the community resources available such as prenatal classes, lactation consultants, and prenatal exercise/yoga classes. Based upon the information you obtain, you might refer the mother to social services or the WIC program as appropriate. At the end of the clinic session, you review the patients with the collaborating physician.

1. How would you define the terms *family* and *family-centered care?*
2. Describe how the nursing process provides the framework for the delivery of direct nursing care.
3. How would you describe the concept of community-based care?
4. How would you describe culturally competent care?

See www.nursing.pearsonhighered.com for possible responses.

REFERENCES

American College of Nurse-Midwives (ACNM). (2009a). *Fact sheet: CNM/CM-attended birth statistics.* Retrieved from http://www.midwife.org/sitefiles/news/CNM_CMAttendedBirths2006.pdf

American College of Nurse-Midwives. (2009b). *Position statement: Mandatory degree requirements for entry into midwifery practice.* Retrieved from http://www.midwife.org/siteFiles/position/Manadatory_Degree_Req_for_Entry_Midwifery_Practice_7_0.pdf

American College of Obstetricians and Gynecologists (ACOG). (2004). *Ethics in obstetrics and gynecology* (2nd ed.). Washington, DC: Author.

American College of Obstetricians and Gynecologists (ACOG). (2005). *Maternal decision making, ethics, and the law* (Committee Opinion No. 321). Washington, DC: Author.

American College of Obstetricians and Gynecologists (ACOG). (2007). *Multifetal pregnancy reduction* (Committee Opinion No. 369). Washington, DC: Author.

American College of Obstetricians and Gynecologists (ACOG). (2008). *Umbilical cord blood banking* (Committee Opinion No. 399). Washington, DC: Author.

American Society for Reproductive Medicine and the Society for Assisted Reproductive Technology. (2009). Guidelines on number of embryos transferred. *Fertility and Sterility, 92*(5), 1518–1519.

Anderson, S. L., Schaechter, J., & Brosco, J. P. (2005). Adolescent patients and their confidentiality: Staying within legal bounds. *Contemporary Pediatrics, 22*(7), 54–64.

Barclay, L. (2010). Maternal mortality increasing in US and Canada, but rapidly decreasing in other countries. *Medscape Medical News.* Retrieved from http://www.medscape.com/viewarticle/720152_print

Brooks, M. (2010). Despite progress, half a million women still die in childbirth annually. *Medscape Medical News.* Retrieved from http://www.medscape.com/viewarticle/720350_print

Cunningham, F. G., Leveno, K. J., Bloom, S. L., Hauth, J. C., Rouse, D. J., & Spong, C. Y. (2010). *Williams obstetrics* (23rd ed.). New York, NY: McGraw Hill Medical.

Forum on Child and Family Statistics. (2009). *America's children: Key national indicators of well-being, 2009.* Retrieved from http://www.childstats.gov/americaschildren/demo.asp

Hamilton, B. E., Ventura, S. J., & Martin, J. A. (2009). Births: Preliminary data for 2007. *National Vital Statistics Reports, 57*(12), 1–23.

Heron, M., Hoyert, D. L., Murphy, S. L., Xu, J., Kochanek, K. D., & Tejada-Vera, B. (2009). Deaths: Final data for 2006. *National Vital Statistics Reports, 57*(14), 1–135.

Hogan, M. C., Foreman, K. J., Naghavi, M., Ahn, S. Y., Wang, M., Makela, S. M., Lopez, A. D., . . . Murray, C. J. L. (2010). Maternal mortality for 181 countries: 1980–2008: A systematic analysis of progress toward Millenium Development Goal 5. *Lancet, 375*(9726), 1609–1623.

Lubin, B. H., & Shearer, W. T. (2007). Policy statement: Cord blood banking for potential future transplantation. *Pediatrics, 119*(1), 165–171.

MacDorman, M. F., & Mathews, T. J. (2009). *Behind international rankings of infant mortality: How the United States compares with Europe* (NCHS Data Brief No. 23). Hyattsville, MD: National Center for Health Statistics.

MacDorman, M. F., & Menacker, F. (2010). Trends and characteristics of home and other out-of-hospital births in the United States, 1990–2006. *National Vital Statisitcs Reports, 58*(11), 1–7.

Mathews, T. J., & MacDorman, M. F. (2010, April 30). Infant mortality statistics from the 2006 period linked birth/infant death data set. *National Vital Statistics Reports, 58*(17), 1–32.

Midwives Alliance of North America (MANA). (2009). *Definitions.* Retrieved from http://www.mana.org/definitions.html

National Center for Health Statistics (NCHS). (2010). *Health, United States, 2009. With Special Feature on Medical Technology.* Retrieved from www.cdc.gov/nchs/data/hus/hus09.pdf

Williams, C. (2006). Dilemmas in fetal medicine: Premature application of technology or responding to women's choice? *Sociology of Health & Illness, 28*(1), 1–20.

Zwelling, E. (2008). The emergence of high-tech birthing. *Journal of Obstetric, Gynecologic, and Neonatal Nursing, 37*(1), 85–93.

CHAPTER 2

Care of the Family in a Culturally Diverse Society

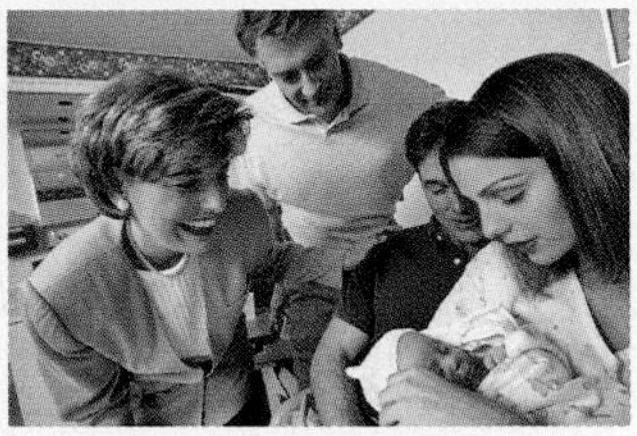

I can't imagine going through pregnancy, birth, or those initial few weeks after my daughter was born without my family. My brother called regularly throughout my pregnancy to check on me. Dad gave me pep talks on eating right and taking care of myself. My husband and my mom were both with me during my labor and my unexpected cesarean birth. After Rosario was born, my husband accompanied our new daughter to the nursery and mom stayed with me, talking and holding my hand. What a difference a family can make.

LEARNING OUTCOMES

1. Explore factors that influence the values, decision making, and roles within the family unit.
2. Discuss employment, marital, and economic trends affecting the contemporary family.
3. Distinguish among different types of families.
4. Explain major developmental tasks to be completed by the childbearing family.
5. Examine the advantages of using a family assessment tool.
6. Discuss the impact of culture in caring for the childbearing family.
7. Analyze prevalent cultural norms related to childbearing and childrearing.
8. Explain the importance of cultural competency in providing nursing care.
9. Discuss the use of a cultural assessment tool as a means of providing culturally sensitive nursing care.
10. Examine the key considerations in providing spiritually sensitive nursing care.

KEY TERMS

Although a woman may arrive for her healthcare appointment physically alone, in another sense, she is always accompanied by her family. Her parents, partner, spouse, or in-laws may accompany her in the form of internalized messages about her body, contraception, sex, or childbearing or in the form of their expectations for her behavior. In addition, her family's culture and religious beliefs will influence her healthcare practices, decisions, and needs. Thus, a nurse may provide expert teaching about condom use to an adolescent, but the teaching may not be put into practice because the patient's partner or family objects. Or a nurse may encourage a pregnant woman to increase her consumption of cow's milk, but a religious proscription against consuming animal products may prohibit this behavior. The goal of effective, holistic nursing care requires nurses to recognize that their patients' values, behaviors, decisions, and needs do not exist in a vacuum; instead, nurses must actively seek to learn about and care for the entire childbearing family.

In this chapter, we provide a perspective on the childbearing family in a culturally diverse society. We begin by discussing family values, power, and roles as well as key social changes affecting the contemporary family. We then identify a variety of different family types the nurse is likely to encounter, and explore the developmental tasks of these varied families. Because families cannot be considered in isolation from their culture, we introduce several concepts essential to culturally competent nursing care. We close the chapter with a brief look at the influence of a family's religious beliefs on health outcomes, and identify key considerations in providing spiritually sensitive nursing care.

Defining Family

There are multiple definitions of family found in the literature. For example, according to McGrath and Edwards (2009), geneticists or clinicians would base their definition of family on biology, whereas individuals might include those linked socially in their definition. The U.S. Census Bureau (2008a) defines **family** in more traditional terms as "a group of two people or more (one of whom is the householder) related by birth, marriage, adoption and residing together: all such people (including related subfamily members) are considered as members of one family."

Family Values

Family values are values that guide behavior and interactions within society and their own family units. These values are greatly influenced by external factors including cultural background, social norms, education, environmental influences, socioeconomic status, and beliefs held by peers, coworkers, political and community leaders, and other individuals outside of the family unit. Because of the influence of these external factors, a family's values may change significantly over the years.

Family Power and Decision Making

Individuals act in accordance with a set of internalized norms and values that are learned primarily through socialization (Kaakinen, Gedaly-Duff, Coehlo, et al., 2010). Within each family, there is an individual or group who possesses **family power**; that is, the potential or actual ability to change the behavior of other family members. This individual or group may affect how a patient responds to a healthcare provider, a diagnosis, treatments, or health teaching. Research has shown that many families make health-related decisions only with the aid of other family members. For example, in the Korean culture, in which elders are highly respected and play a key role in family matters, family power may rest with the grandfather. If the son wanted to make a health-related change in the family's diet, for example, he would first seek the advice and approval of his grandfather. Similarly, many Chinese identify themselves in relation to other members of the family and believe that personal independence is not as important. Thus, a Chinese patient may avoid taking action regarding a health matter unless a family leader gives permission (Galanti, 2008).

In many traditional families, the father figure is the decision maker. In traditional Cuban culture, for example, the father may be assertive and dominant and is critical to all family decisions (Galanti, 2008). In contrast, the mother typically remains at home, passive and dependent. However, Cubans in the United States have become much more egalitarian because women are usually the first ones able to find jobs and contribute to their families. Thus, among Cubans who have assimilated, one may find equal decision-making power.

In many immigrant families, the child is first to learn the new language. In families in which the father is considered the power holder, this situation can cause problems if the family perceives that the healthcare provider is relating only to the child. They may feel that their child is being placed in a superior position, which may be unacceptable to them. In most cases, children acculturate more rapidly than their parents, which can lead to stress within the family unit (Wagner et al., 2008).

Family Roles

Family roles are homogeneous sets of behaviors that are normatively defined and expected of an occupant of a given social position. Roles vary depending on age, position within the family, conflict within the family, stressors, cultural backgrounds, health status of family members, and demographic trends. However, within each family, roles commonly encountered include breadwinner, homemaker, nurturer, social planner, and peacemaker. Although roles are sometimes perceived to be gender specific, they are more accurately assigned to the family member who performs that specific function. In the majority of U.S. households in the 1950s, a male was the sole breadwinner and a female performed all homemaker functions. In contemporary society, these roles are often shared. For example, both parents may be employed and may participate equally in the care of the children. Segregated roles are more evident in certain cultures where roles are defined more sharply based on gender.

Any one individual within a family may have two or more roles. In nuclear families, roles are typically paired and consist of father-husband, wife-mother, son-brother, and so forth. In extended families the number of paired roles increases, whereas in single-parent families the numbers are less.

Increasingly important in the contemporary U.S. family is the role of the grandparent. High adolescent pregnancy rates have created a sizable population of young grandparents (as young as the 30s), and increased life expectancy rates have created a sizable population of great-grandparents. Grandparents vary in how they express their role. Role functions may include: (1) witness who is simply present for the grandchildren, (2) protector who provides care and ensures safety when needed, (3) peacemaker who helps resolve conflicts between parents and children, and (4) active participant who maintains involvement in family life in the past, present, and future.

Grandparents can offer a great deal to children and provide substantial support and advice to parents (Figure 2-1 ■). Often grandparents are able to spend more quality time with grandchildren than they did with their own children. Many grandparents are retired and use this opportunity to build lasting bonds with grandchildren. Although extended families are often geographically separated, many grandparents have identified alternative means to stay connected with grandchildren when frequent visits are not possible. These alternatives include phone calls; emails; and letters as well as sharing journals, photos, and videotapes.

> “Computers, emails, and cell phones were not the kinds of communication I grew up using; however, I decided to learn so that I could communicate with my grandchildren who don't live close by. My grandchildren send me jokes and digital photos, and it has helped me to feel like I am more a part of their lives. They think I am “cool” because I have learned to use their technology. We exchange cards electronically now for many special occasions, and we communicate much more often than we did before I knew how to use my computer. It sure doesn't replace being together face-to-face, but it does help me feel like I know them better!”

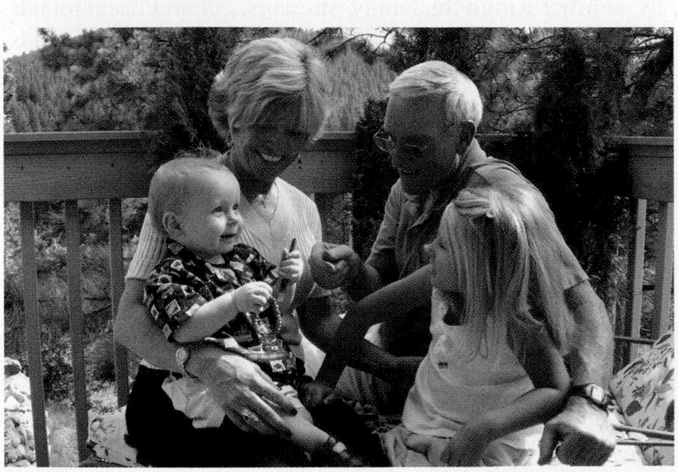

Figure 2-1 ■ Grandparents can offer nurturing and guidance to their grandchildren, not to mention lots of fun.

Source: Photographer, Paul Barton.

Changes Affecting the Contemporary Family

The contemporary family has changed dramatically from the family unit of the 1950s, which typically consisted of a working father and a stay-at-home mother who cared for the children and ran the family home (Figure 2-2 ■). Affecting the contemporary family are employment trends, changes in marriage rates, and economic trends.

Changes in the number and types of households are influenced by patterns of population growth, shifts in the age composition of the population, and the decisions individuals make about their living arrangements. Demographic trends in marriage, cohabitation, divorce, fertility, and mortality also affect family and household composition. Moreover, shifts in social norms, values, laws, and the economy and improvements in health care also influence how people organize their lives. Individual decisions produce aggregate societal changes in household and family composition (U.S. Census Bureau, 2009).

Today, the mother may be working outside the home and the father may be the stay-at-home parent. In 2007, the United States had an estimated 5.5 million “stay-at-home” parents: 5.3 million mothers and 140,000 fathers (U.S. Census Bureau News, 2009).

Employment Trends

Employment trends have changed with the shift from a male-dominated workforce to a mixed male-female workforce. Today, the majority of households consist of dual-earner families in which both parents have employment outside of the home. Dual-earner families may have different needs than traditional families. For example, when a child becomes ill in a dual-earner family, the parents must decide who will take off work to care for the child. In traditional families, the mother would care for the child and work stresses from illness-related absences would not be a concern.

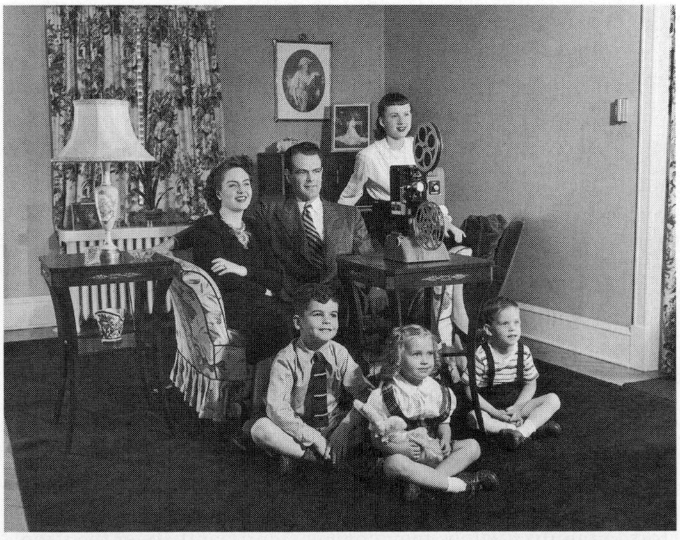

Figure 2-2 ■ The traditional family of the mid-20th century consisted of a father who worked outside of the home, a mother who performed all homemaking and childrearing functions, and one or more children.

Source: Getty Images, Inc.–Hulton Archive Photos.

Changes in Marriage Rates

Since World War II, there has been a consistent decline in marriage rates. According to the U.S. Census Bureau News (2008b), 68% of households in 2007 were family households, compared with 81% in 1970. The area with the highest percentage of single-parent households was the District of Columbia (54%), while the state with the lowest percentage of single-parent households was Utah (15%). The proportion of one-person households increased by 10%—from 17% to 27%—between 1970 and 2007. Households with children make up only one third of all U.S. households. It is interesting to note the decline in the proportion of married-couple households with their own children—from 40% of all households in 1970 to 23% in 2007. In contrast, the proportion of households that were made up of married couples without children dropped only slightly over the same time period—from 30% in 1970 to 28% in 2007. From 1950 to 2007, the proportion of family households with children that were maintained by a married couple decreased from 93% to 71%. There was a corresponding increase in the percentage of family households with children that were maintained by a mother who was a single parent (6% to 23%) and by a father who was a single parent (1% to 5%).

These changes reflect changing societal norms including a delay in the median age at first marriage. The median age for a man's first marriage was 27.7 years in 2007, up from 26.1 in 1990. The median age for a woman's first marriage was 26.0 years in 2007, up from 23.9 in 1990. According to the Centers for Disease Control and Prevention (CDC) (National Center for Health Statistics, Division of Vital Statistics, 2009), additional societal changes include an increase in the rate of nonmarital births, up 26% from 2002 to 2007, and a higher percentage of marriages that result in divorce.

Along with the high proportion of single-parent families, there is also a higher proportion of never-married individuals in the United States than ever before, and those who do marry tend to do so at a later age than in the past. A combination of factors has led to delayed childbearing (see chapter 8 ∞). There is also a growing trend for women to remain childless. The U.S. Census Bureau News report on fertility (2008) shows that 20% of women ages 40 to 44 were childless in 2006, twice as high as the level in 1980. American women spend fewer childbearing years in marriage, which increases the likelihood of nonmarital childbearing.

Other trends in the United States include increasing acceptance of single women giving birth. In 1950, 3% of births were to unmarried women. Today, the National Center for Health Statistics (2009) reported almost 30% of all births are to unmarried women. While this trend is increasing in the United States, in some cultures an unmarried woman giving birth is viewed negatively. We discuss cultural views on birth outside of marriage later in this chapter.

Economic Trends

Changes in income levels have directly affected families. Families who experienced the most economic growth had two wage earners and higher educational preparation. Although family median income levels fell slightly, between 2007 and 2008, income levels have continued to rise since 2001; unemployment statistics, however, have been on the rise since 2009.

Types of Families

Various types of families—both traditional and nontraditional—exist in contemporary society.

Traditional Nuclear Family

The *traditional nuclear family* consists of a husband provider, a wife who stays home, and children. Although the traditional nuclear family was once the norm in the United States, it is no longer the most common type of family. It has become a demographic minority as those in the United States and many cultures around the world redefine what family is.

Dual-Career/Dual-Earner Family

The *dual-career/dual-earner family* is now considered the norm in modern U.S. society. Today, two thirds of all two-parent families have both parents working. Although many women work outside the home because of financial necessity, other women work either full or part time out of personal choice. Dual-career/dual-earner families have specific challenges. Because both parents are working, child care, household chores, and spending time with other family members are priorities that need to be addressed.

Childless or Childfree Family

A growing trend exists for couples to remain childless or childfree (Figure 2-3 ■). As many as 10% of couples experience infertility problems and are considered to be childless, while another 6.5% of married couples are voluntarily without children and consider themselves to be childfree. This trend is continuing to grow with the increased opportunities available to women in the workplace, delayed marriage, availability of contraceptives to prevent unwanted pregnancy, and wider acceptance of women choosing not to become mothers.

Extended Family

Extended families consist of a couple who shares household responsibilities, chores, and expenses with parents, siblings, or other relatives. Multigenerational family living arrangements

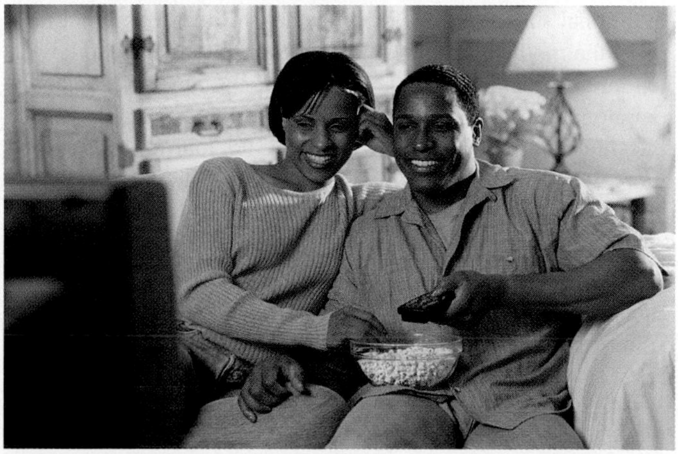

Figure 2-3 ■ Today, 5% of married couples voluntarily choose to remain childless.

Source: Michael Keller/CORBIS.

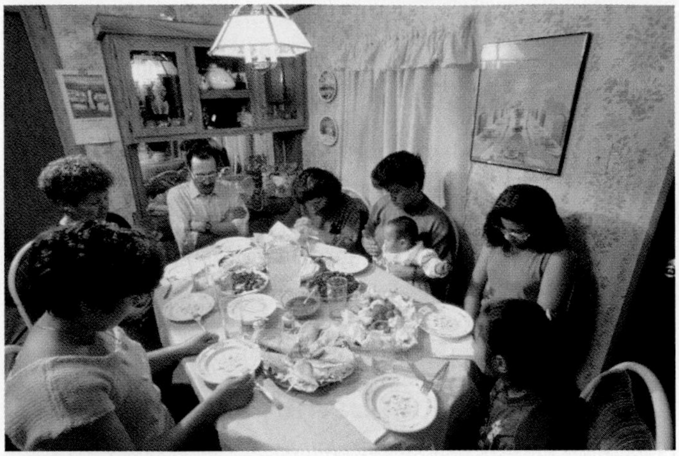

Figure 2-4 ■ In an extended kin network family, two nuclear families live in close proximity to each other and share responsibilities and resources.

Source: Zigy Kaluzny/Getty Images, Inc.—Hulton Archive photos.

are most common in non-U.S. cultures and in working-class families. Children are reared by their parents and other relatives. Extended families are also common when an elderly or ill relative requires care by the younger family members.

Extended Kin Network Family

An *extended kin network family* is a specific form of an extended family in which two nuclear families of primary or unmarried kin live in close proximity to each other. The family shares a social support network, chores, goods, and services. This type of family model is common in the Latino community (Figure 2-4 ■).

Single-Parent Family

Single-parent families are headed by only one parent (Figure 2-5 ■). While rare in the past, in the year 2006, there were 13 million one-parent families in the United States, about one third of all families. These consisted of 10.4 million single-mother families and 2.5 million single-father families (Pan, 2008).

In the traditional single-parent family the head of the household is widowed, divorced, abandoned, or separated. In the nontraditional single-parent family the head of the household, most often the mother, was never married. Single-parent families often face difficulties because the sole parent may lack social and emotional support, need assistance with childrearing issues, and face financial strain. Mothers who have not married tend to have more financial difficulties, less educational achievement, and are younger in age than those who are divorced.

Stepparent Family

Stepfamilies include a biologic parent with children and a new spouse who may or may not have children. These families are also known as *remarried families, reconstituted families,* or *blended families.* It is estimated that 75% of all divorced individuals eventually remarry. Sixty-five percent of these remarriages involve children from a prior marriage (Stewart, 2007).

Stepfamily models have both strengths and weaknesses. Although marriage is often a new opportunity for success in

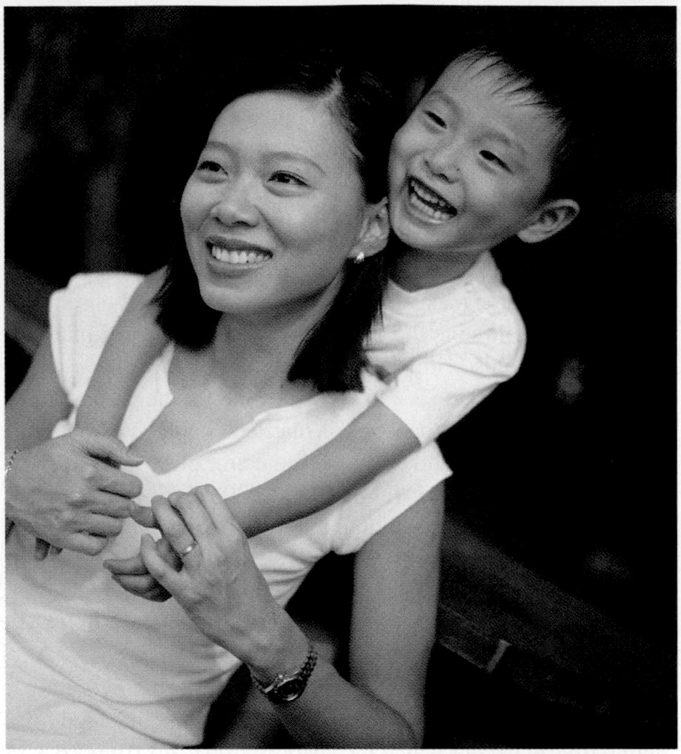

Figure 2-5 ■ Single-parent families account for nearly one third of all U.S. families.

Source: © Joyce Choo/CORBIS. All Rights Reserved.

a marital relationship for the parents, the relationship between stepparents and stepchildren can be strained. Stresses can include discipline issues, adjustment problems, role ambiguity, strain with the other biologic parent, and communication issues. Although stepfamilies may have fewer financial issues and may actually offer the child a new support person and role model, open communication is imperative to ensure a smooth transition.

Binuclear Family

A *binuclear family* is a post-divorced family in which the biologic children are members of two nuclear households, both that of the father and that of the mother. The children alternate between the two homes, typically spending a week with the father and a week with the mother. This is also called *coparenting* and involves joint custody. Legally, *joint custody* refers to situations in which both parents have equal responsibility and legal rights, regardless of where the children live. Although this type of family represents a small number as yet, there has been an increase in this type of household as fathers assume a more active role in parenting. The increased recognition of the importance of having both a maternal and paternal presence has encouraged more parents to actively raise their children together, regardless of their relationship with each other. The benefits of a binuclear family include the ability to have both the mother and father involved in the child's upbringing, a model for effective communication (in a successful family model), and additional support and role models from extended family members.

Nonmarital Heterosexual Cohabitating Family

A *nonmarital heterosexual cohabitating family* is a heterosexual couple who may or may not have children and live together outside of marriage. This may include never-married individuals as well as divorced or widowed persons. Some individuals prefer this family model for personal reasons, whereas others do so for financial reasons or to seek companionship. For example, a widow may fear losing her pension if she remarries, or an individual who owns significant assets may fear losing these assets to a spouse, especially if residing in a community-property state.

CLINICAL TIP

It is important to establish which parent has legal custody, current visitation policies, and other legal variables (restraining orders, supervised visitation, etc.) when communicating information to parents about their children. Certain legal issues may prohibit the nurse from sharing some information with the noncustodial parent.

Gay and Lesbian Families

Gay and *lesbian families* include those in which two or more people who share a same-sex orientation live together (with or without children) as well as families consisting of a gay or lesbian single parent rearing a child (Figure 2-6 ■). The number of gay and lesbian families is underreported. The 2000 census was the first census to record unmarried same sex partners living together. There were a recorded 601,209 lesbian and gay families, but it is unknown how many of those households had minor children living with them. These numbers are said to be underreported also (Smith & Gates, 2009).

Small studies have evaluated children raised by gay and lesbian couples and have found that they show no significant differences from children raised in other types of families. These children get along with their parents and peers the same as children raised in heterosexual households. Children raised in gay or lesbian families may face unique issues in interacting with peers and in revealing their parents' sexual orientation.

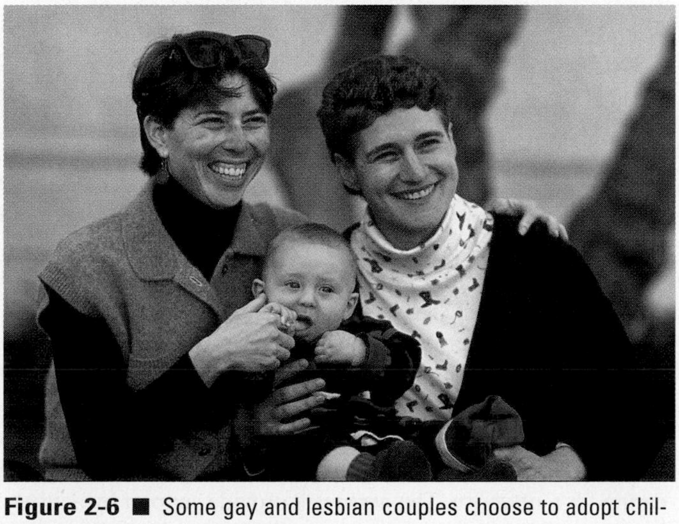

Figure 2-6 ■ Some gay and lesbian couples choose to adopt children in need of loving homes.

Source: Dana White/PhotoEdit.

Contemporary Family Development Frameworks

Family development refers to the dynamics or changes that families experience over time. It includes relationships, communication patterns, roles, and changes in interactions. Although each family is unique, the members must go through a set of fairly predictable changes. The amount of time in each stage and the duration between stages vary within each family unit.

Multiple family models and frameworks have been proposed over the years to facilitate an understanding of the complexities of family development. These developmental frameworks observe a family's progression over time by identifying specific stages in family life. Models, primarily based on the classic traditional work of Duvall (1977) and Duvall and Miller (1985), have embraced the trends and changes of contemporary society and family life. Duvall developed an eight-stage family life cycle that describes the developmental process that each family encounters. This model is based on a nuclear family (Table 2-1). The oldest child serves as a marker for the family's developmental stage except in the last two stages when the children are no longer present. Couples with more than one child may be in overlapping stages with developmental advances occurring simultaneously.

Model of the Childbearing Family

Multiple tasks exist for the childbearing family. The couple must first arrange the home to meet the needs of the newborn. This entails preparing for the infant by providing a safe environment; a safe, clean place to sleep; and appropriate clothing and supplies.

At the time of birth of the first child, the childbearing family will engage in behaviors aimed at identifying responsibility and accountability for the newborn. Couples are rapidly faced with the realization that infants require 24-hour care. Although fathers are taking a more active role in childrearing, the mother is frequently the primary care provider, especially if she is breastfeeding. Although a breast pump can be used and milk can be given by bottle, the breastfeeding mother still assumes the majority of the feeding responsibilities. The father may assume other household tasks or other baby care activities, such as changing, bathing, and putting the infant down to sleep. Many facilities are now offering special classes just for fathers that help them learn to care for their infants. During the early stages, new roles will be identified as couples strive to establish a daily routine that includes the new family member.

Another task of the couple in a childbearing family is reestablishing a satisfying sexual relationship. Nurses can play an active role in teaching couples about normal changes during this period of family life. For example, in the postpartum period, sexual activity typically declines or ceases. The parents are transitioning to new roles, especially the mother. Fatigue is common. Women may also feel discomfort because of the birth and may fear pain with resumption of sexual intercourse. Reduced desire and vaginal

TABLE 2-1 The Traditional Family Life-Cycle Stages and Developmental Tasks

Stage I	Married couple	Establishing relationship as a married couple: blending of individual needs, developing conflict-and-resolution approaches, communication patterns, and intimacy patterns.
Stage II	Childbearing families with infants	Adjusting to pregnancy and then infant; adjusting to new roles as mother and father; maintaining couple bond and intimacy.
Stage III	Families with preschool children	Understanding normal growth and development; adjusting to different temperaments and styles of children if more than one child in family; coping with energy depletion; maintaining couple bond and intimacy.
Stage IV	Families with school-age children	Working out authority and socialization roles with school; supporting children in outside interests and needs; determining disciplinary actions and family rules and roles.
Stage V	Families with adolescents	Allowing adolescents to establish their own identities and still be part of family; thinking about the future, education, jobs, working; increasing roles of adolescents in family, cooking, repairs, and power base.
Stage VI	Families launching young adults	After member moves out, reallocating roles, space, power, and communication; maintaining supportive home base; maintaining parental couple intimacy and relationship.
Stage VII	Middle-aged parents	Refocusing on marriage relationship; ensuring security after retirement; maintaining kinship ties.
Stage VIII	Aging families	Adjusting to retirement, grandparent roles, death of spouse, and living alone.

Source: Duvall, Marriage & Family Development, *Table "The Traditional Family Life-Cycle Stages and Development Tasks," © 1984 Harper & Row Publishing, Inc. Reproduced by permission of Pearson Education, Inc.*

dryness due to low estrogen levels are especially common in breastfeeding women. Counseling can provide the couple with reassurance that these changes are a common part of this developmental stage.

Couples need to communicate effectively and share thoughts and feelings as they adjust to their new roles. Fathers may feel isolated or "left out" as the mother embraces her new role. New mothers may feel overwhelmed with the responsibility of caring for an infant when alone. Even dual-career families typically have a transition period in which the mother is at home caring for the newborn and the father is working. For some women who previously worked full-time, being at home may cause feelings of isolation.

> "I thought I would love being at home with my beautiful new son. It wasn't that I didn't love him and want to be with him, I just felt like I was losing part of myself. I wasn't me anymore, and I missed talking with other adults and working. I felt tremendously guilty when I returned to work at 3 months; however, it made my time with him so much more special, and I regained my self-confidence and felt like a real person again."

As the new family adapts to changing roles and responsibilities, the roles of other family members also emerge. Some extended families take an active role, whereas others may be more passive. Family members frequently provide guidance, advice, and assistance with child care. Both sets of grandparents may have strong beliefs about childrearing and may attempt to promote their own beliefs and rituals. Couples must effectively communicate with each other and other family members to avoid conflict. Although both families may want their traditions followed in terms of childrearing, the couple may wish to develop new traditions and rituals within their own family unit.

Along with changes in family relationships, the childbearing family may also experience changes in personal relationships and outside activities. After the birth of an infant, couples are typically more involved with their home life, may stay home more often, and may engage in different activities. Many women, especially women who formerly worked outside of the home, may feel like they have less in common with previous coworkers or friends who do not have children. This may lead to new friendships with other families who have more in common with the new family unit.

> "Allie and I met in high school, and from then on, we were inseparable. Even after I got married, we stayed close, going out to lunch or shopping together every couple of weeks, and talking on the phone every few days. When she found out I was pregnant, she threw a surprise shower for me, but as my due date approached, we started to drift apart. Since my daughter's birth, we've gotten together just once. Allie says she feels excluded and that all I ever talk about is the baby. I guess she's right—my daughter is the center of my world now, so it's hard to talk about anything else. I haven't seen Allie for several months now. It makes me sad when I think about it."

Childbearing families face multiple changes and challenges as they embark into new parenthood. The nurse can assist the childbearing family by providing teaching about family-planning issues, infant care and appropriate development, and safety concerns. The nurse can also offer guidance to the couple as they transition into parenthood by identifying interventions that can assist in meeting the emotional and physical needs of caring for a newborn. The nurse can provide support by actively listening as the couple expresses feelings related to current role transitions and changes in personal and family relationships.

Resources can be provided to the new parents that will enable them to establish new relationships within their community.

Model Incorporating the Unattached Young Adult

Other models have been created to encompass the changes in contemporary families. For instance, Carter and McGoldrick (2005) modified the Duvall (1977) model to include the unattached young adult (Carter, 2010). This stage begins when the young adult leaves the family home and becomes financially independent, and lasts throughout young adulthood as long as the individual remains unmarried. Developmental tasks in this stage include differentiating self from the family unit, developing intimate peer relationships, and establishing a career and financial independence.

Because the median age at first marriage continues to rise (27.6 years for men and 26 years for women in 2007), it is important to include the unattached young adult in family models. Due to this increased age at first marriage, it is less common for adolescents to go directly from their parental home to a marital relationship. However, there is also a trend, perhaps due to economic factors, for young adults to reside with their parents well into their 20s. This is especially true for young men.

TABLE 2-2 Stages in Divorce and Postdivorce

STAGE	ISSUES
Divorce	
I. Decision to divorce	Accepting responsibility/part of responsibility for failed marriage.
II. Planning the breakup	Collaboratively working to resolve marital issues: financial, child care/custody; communicating dissolution of marriage to relatives and friends.
III. Separation	Adapting to loss of previously established family unit; reorganizing relationships with spouse and children; restructuring finances; adapting to living apart; addressing issues related to attachment to spouse; maintaining bonds with extended family and spouse's extended family.
IV. Divorce	Grieving related to loss of prior family unit; accepting that the marriage is over; retrieving positive aspects of marriage (hopes, memories, dreams, expectations); overcoming negative feelings (anger, guilt, hurt, disappointment); maintaining relationships with extended family members.
Postdivorce	
I. Single parent (custodial)	Dealing with issues related to visitation and custody; rebuilding social relationships; ensuring financial stability.
II. Single parent (noncustodial)	Continuing parenting role; identifying new means to relate to children; facilitating relationship between ex-spouse and children; providing support with childrearing decisions; providing financial support to ex-spouse for children; establishing new social relationships.

Source: From Carter, Betty and McGoldrick, Monica (Eds). The Changing Family Life Cycle: A Framework for Family Therapy, *2ed. 2005. Published by Allyn and Bacon, Boston, MA. Copyright © 1989 by Pearson Education. Reprinted by permission of the publisher.*

Model Incorporating Divorce and Remarriage

Carter and McGoldrick (2005) devised another developmental model to describe issues encountered in undergoing divorce and in postdivorce (Carter, 2010). See Table 2-2. Both emotional and developmental issues are encountered as families dissolve during the divorce process. Family members not only mourn the loss of a two-parent family, they also must adjust to a single-parent family model. Child visitation, financial issues, guilt, and attachment difficulties all play a major role in the changing family dynamics. Remarriage, which is becoming increasingly common, is another transitional stage in which family members must adjust to new roles and expectations (Table 2-3).

Model of the Lesbian or Gay Family

Lesbian or gay families face unique challenges in completing their developmental tasks. For example, they are frequently faced with discrimination and disapproval from mainstream society. In the past, many gay or lesbian families opt to keep their sexual orientation a secret. In most states, they do not have the option of legal marriage and, therefore, do not have many of the benefits of marriage that heterosexual couples have, such as insurance benefits, rights to property, custody issues, and family leave benefits associated with family illness or childbirth. Some states now recognize same-sex marriage and civil unions, which provide protection of rights for same-sex partners (Giger & Davidhizar, 2007). Chapter 8 ∞ provides an overview of some of the obstacles faced by lesbian families.

TABLE 2-3 Stages in Remarriage

STAGE	ISSUES
I. Establishing a new relationship	Resolve feelings from divorce; determine new marriage is desired; evaluate emotional readiness for new family; commit to new family.
II. Planning new marriage and family	Deal with personal fears and fears of new spouse and children; establish openness and open communication; determine financial obligations and coparenting roles with former spouses; plan for adjustment to new roles for parents and children: set new boundaries, resolve loyalty conflicts, maintain relationships with extended family members of ex-spouses, foster relationships between extended family and new spouse.
III. Remarriage and reconstitution of family	Include new spouse into family unit; dissolve previous attachment to former spouse and image of the "ideal family;" restructure family system to include stepparent role; incorporate both families into a system to support children; foster all family relationships with extended family (including ex-spouses); share special memories to enhance family bonding and integration.

Sources: Friedman, Marilyn M., Family Nursing: Research, Theory, and Practice, 4th ed., © 1998. Reproduced with permission of Pearson Education, Inc., Upper Saddle River, New Jersey. From Carter, Betty & Monica McGoldrick (Eds.) The Changing Family Life Cycle: A Framework for Family Therapy, *2e. Published by Allyn and Bacon, Boston, MA. Copyright © 1989 by Pearson Education. Reprinted by permission of the publisher.*

TABLE 2-4 Lesbian and Gay Family Stages

STAGE	ISSUES
I. Formation of couple	Establish themselves as a couple versus individuals: combine two lives together, develop trust, reveal details about self, respond empathetically to partner to encourage further risk taking in relationship, tell others about their relationship.
II. Ongoing couplehood	Move from a passionate physical relationship to a stable relationship that includes passion and dailiness; manage differences between partners and handle conflict; increase sense of security and belonging as a couple.
III. Middle years	Progress into a long-term relationship with commitment and a continued sense of security; make efforts to keep relationship fresh and new; rework rewards and disappointments.
IV. Generativity	Create a legacy beyond each partner's own self-identity that will endure.

Source: Friedman, Marilyn M., Family Nursing: Research, Theory, and Practice, 4th ed., © 1998. Reproduced with permission of Pearson Education, Inc., Upper Saddle River, New Jersey. Adapted with the permission of The Free Press, a Division of Simon & Schuster Adult Publishing Group, from THE LESBIAN FAMILY LIFE CYCLE *by Suzanne Slater. Copyright © 1995 by Suzanne Slater. All rights reserved.*

Slater (1995) developed a model specific to the stages of family life for lesbian and gay families (Table 2-4). The model identifies five stages in the development of the gay or lesbian family and addresses different issues and tasks in each stage.

Family Assessment

Case Study: Family Assessment

The nurse's understanding of the family structure helps provide insight into the family's support systems and needs. A **family assessment** is a collection of data regarding the family's current level of functioning, support systems, sociocultural information, environmental information, type of family, family structure, and needs.

To obtain an accurate and concise family assessment, the nurse needs to establish a trusting relationship with the woman and her family. Data are best collected in a comfortable, private environment, free from interruptions. The nurse can use therapeutic communication skills, such as active listening, reflection, and silence, to encourage the woman and family to verbalize information. Basic information should include:

- Name, age, sex, and family relationship of all family members residing in the household
- Cultural associations, including cultural norms and customs related to childbearing, childrearing, and infant feeding (discussed later in the chapter)
- Religious affiliations, including specific religious beliefs and practices related to childbearing
- Support network, including extended family, friends, and religious and community associations
- Family type, structure, roles, and values
- Communication patterns, including verbal and written language barriers

Health History

The health of individual family members can have a great impact on the health, well-being, and functioning of the family as a whole. The nurse should gather data about acute and chronic illnesses, genetic conditions, history of family violence, and mental health. A personal history beginning with pregnancies, pregnancy losses, infant health concerns, or deaths is also obtained. The nurse completes a comprehensive review of current health practices and health promotion behaviors to assess the family's ability to prevent accidents and chronic health conditions and performs a brief nutritional assessment. Families with nutritional excesses or deficits are provided with nutritional education to reduce the risk of nutrition-related illnesses.

The health history should also assess current exercise and activity patterns, sleep patterns, occupational exposures, use of prescription and nonprescription drugs, herbal remedies, alcohol consumption, smoking, and use of illegal drugs.

Environmental Considerations

A family's home environment can be assessed through home visits. Although not always possible, multiple home visits will yield more information than a single visit. A home visit enables the nurse to observe the family directly in their own environment and personal space. It also provides a more realistic view of family relationships, roles, parenting styles, and family needs. Often, the first visit serves as an introduction for the nurse to lay the foundation for a therapeutic relationship.

Observations should include the availability of personal space for all family members, including a place to sleep. The home should have basic necessities for daily living such as safe drinking water, a working waste-disposal system, electricity, and heat. The nurse can ensure that adequate cooking facilities, including a stove and refrigerator, are available for safe meal preparation. The availability of a phone is important so family members have access to healthcare providers and emergency services as needed.

The childbearing family should have resources available for the new baby, including a safe place to sleep, appropriate clothing, blankets, hygienic equipment, and age-appropriate resources for other children.

The home should also be inspected for potential hazards. Childproofing the home is a topic generally covered during the home visit. A safe place to bathe the infant should be identified. Parents should be taught never to leave the infant unattended during bathing and never to leave the infant in a location where a fall can occur. Environmental hazards such as open stairs, uncovered electrical outlets, fragile items that could harm the infant or other children if the items were broken, and unattended electrical appliances need to be discussed. Many new childbearing families may not recognize the potential environmental dangers and will benefit from a brief review.

During the home visit, the nurse can also assess the neighborhood in which the family lives. Observations should include availability of resources (drug store, grocery store, closest medical facility, child care resources, and schools), characteristics of the neighborhood (safety issues, proximity of public transportation), and community resources (new mothers' groups, breastfeeding support groups, and availability of infant development/first aid classes).

Upon completion of the home visit(s), the nurse can make recommendations and identify community resources and sources of support for the new family. Families can also be counseled on the availability of social services, such as the Special Supplemental Food Program for Women, Infants, and Children (WIC), and financial support programs. Parents without health insurance coverage should be encouraged to apply for Medicaid coverage for their infant. Community health programs, such as local health department immunization clinics, should also be discussed.

Family Assessment Tool

Multiple tools are available to assist the nurse in collecting data regarding the family. The Friedman Family Assessment tool is a comprehensive assessment of family functioning and other essential family data (Figure 2-7 ■). It can be used during the home visit to obtain pertinent information and provide a framework for the nurse when planning and implementing interventions for the family.

Cultural Influences Affecting the Family

When caring for families, it is critical to consider the influence of culture, which may affect how a family reacts and responds to health-related issues. Cultural beliefs that may seem strange to a person born and raised in Ohio might have significant meaning for an immigrant from West Africa. Developing knowledge about cultural beliefs and traditions can increase the nurse's appreciation of diversity; prevent violation of cultural norms; and, most important, improve the family's healthcare experience.

Within the United States there is tremendous cultural diversity. In 2008 the Census Bureau reported that 15.4% of Americans are Hispanic or Latino, 12.8% are of African descent, 4.5% are of Asian descent, 10% are American Indian or Alaska Native, 0.18% are of non-Hispanic Pacific Islander descent, and 1.7% are of two or more races. Thus it is important for nurses to have an understanding of how culture can influence family care.

Cultural Concepts

Culture can be defined as the beliefs, values, attitudes, and practices that are accepted by a population, a community, or an individual. Culture is learned and not ingrained in our genetic material, yet it can be passed on from generation to generation by means of *enculturation.* When a group is isolated, whether geographically or economically, culture is often reinforced.

Ethnicity is a social identity that is associated with shared behaviors and patterns. These include family structure, religious affiliation, language, dress, eating habits, and health behaviors. Many Americans define ethnicity by physical characteristics such as skin color. However, many individuals consider themselves to be "biracial" or identify with a specific ethnic group not because of skin color but because of a shared ideology or attitude. Many Americans are blends of ethnic backgrounds, and it is often difficult to assign a specific ethnic identity to someone. Although some beliefs and cultural practices are common among certain ethnic groups, one must be careful to avoid stereotyping individuals. It is important not to assume that because individuals identify themselves as a specific ethnicity, they must practice a certain custom.

Within the United States, cultures have in the past been forced to blend. When people from one culture are transported to another place with new cultural norms, many adapt to these new behaviors. This process by which people adapt to a new cultural norm is called **acculturation**. Moreover, when a group completely changes their cultural identity to become part of the majority culture, **assimilation** occurs.

Acculturation

Many immigrants acculturate, and sometimes the acculturation process has an effect on the family's health. Acculturation is frequently associated with improved health status and health behaviors; however, this does not suggest that the American lifestyle is somehow more healthful than others. Instead, it seems that many factors contribute to the improved health status of acculturated immigrants. Primary among these are socioeconomic factors. Many immigrants are financially better off in the United States than they were in their country of origin, particularly those who have emigrated from developing nations.

Despite economic resources, acculturation plays a major role in immigrants' use of preventive care services. It appears that the length of time spent in the United States is a predictor for utilization of health services. A study by the Kaiser Commission (Cunningham & Artiga, 2009) showed that the uninsured rate for recent immigrants is almost 3 times that of immigrants who have been in the United States for more than 20 years (63% vs. 22%). Cunningham and Artiga point out that among immigrants, recent immigrants are the most likely to lack a usual source of care and experience language barriers with a physician, and they have lower levels of physician visits than longer-term immigrants.

Often overlooked in debates and discussions related to immigrant issues is the great diversity among the immigrant population, and, in particular, the fact that their circumstances and situations change over time as they assimilate socially and economically within American society. "New immigrants should be recognized as a vulnerable group with regard to the impact of work on their well-being" (De Castro, Gilbert, & Takeuchi, 2008). In a study that investigated how immigrants' duration of time in the United States impacts the relationship between job-related stress and health conditions, researchers concluded that job-related stressors are associated with adverse health outcomes, and this relationship is strongest for newer immigrants.

Sometimes health declines with acculturation. A study examining patterns of substance abuse by Hispanics in the United States found acculturation to result in increased rather than decreased drug use (Akins, Mosher, Smith, et al., 2007). Obesity is another problem that is growing rapidly within the United States, particularly among immigrant populations.

Impact of Culture on Family Structure

Traditional family structure within the United States usually consists of a nuclear family with an extended family living separately.

Meeting of Physical, Emotional, and Spiritual Needs of Members

- Ability to provide food and shelter
  - Space management as regards living, sleeping, recreation, privacy
  - Crowding if over 1.5 persons per room
  - Territoriality or control of each member over lifespace
  - Access to laundry, grocery, recreation facilities
  - Sanitation including disposal methods, source of water supply, control of rodents and insects
  - Storage and refrigeration
  - Available food supply
  - Food preparation, including preserving and cooking methods (stove, hotplate, oven)
  - Use of food stamps and donated foods as well as eligibility for food stamps
  - Education of each member as to food composition, balanced menus, special preparations or diets if required for a specific member
- Access to health care
  - Regularity of health care
  - Continuity of caregivers
  - Closeness of facility and means of access such as car, bus, cab
  - Access to helpful neighbors
  - Access to phone
- Family health
  - Longevity
  - Major or chronic illnesses
  - Familial or hereditary illnesses such as rheumatic fever, gout, allergy, tuberculosis, renal disease, diabetes mellitus, cancer, emotional illness, epilepsy, migraine, other nervous disorders, hypertension, blood diseases, obesity, frequent accidents, drug intake, pica
  - Emotional or stress-related illnesses
  - Pollutants that members are chronically exposed to such as air, water, soil, noise, or chemicals that are unsafe
- Neighborhood pride and loyalty
- Job access, energy output, shift changes
- Sensitivity, warmth, understanding between family members
  - Demonstration of emotion
  - Enjoyment of sexual relations
    - Male: Impotence, premature or retarded ejaculation, hypersexuality
    - Female: Frigidity (inability to achieve orgasm), enjoyment of sexual relations, feelings of disgust, shame, self-devaluation; fear of injury, painful coitus
    - Menstrual history, including onset, duration, flow, missed periods and life situation at the time, pain, euphoria, depression, other difficulties
- Sharing of religious beliefs, values, doubts
  - Formal membership in church and organizations
  - Ethical framework and honesty
  - Adaptability, response to reality
  - Satisfaction with life
  - Self-esteem

Childrearing Practices and Discipline

- Mutual responsibility
  - Joint parenting
  - Mutual respect for decision making
  - Means of discipline and consistency
- Respect for individuality
- Fostering of self-discipline
- Attitudes toward education, reading, scholarly pursuit
- Attitudes toward imaginative play
- Attitudes toward involvement in sports
- Promotion of gender stereotypes

Communication

- Expression of a wide range of emotion and feeling
- Expression of ideas, concepts, beliefs, values, interests
- Openness
- Verbal expression and sensitive listening
- Consensual decision making

Support, Security, Encouragement

- Balance in activity
- Humor
- Dependency and dominance patterns
- Life support groups of each member
- Social relationship of couple: go out together or separately; change since marriage mutually satisfying; effect of sociability patterns on children

Growth-Producing Relationships and Experiences Within and Without the Family

- Creative play activities
- Planned growth experiences
- Focus of life and activity of each member
- Friendships

Responsible Community Relationships

- Organizations, including involvement, membership, active participation
- Knowledge of and friendship with neighbors

Growing with and Through Children

- Hope and plans for children
- Emulation of own parents and its influence on relationship with children
- Relationship patterns: authoritarian, patriarchal, matriarchal
- Necessity to relive (make up for) own childhood through children

Unity, Loyalty, and Cooperation

Positive interacting of members toward each other

Self-Help and Acceptance of Outside Help in Family Crisis

Figure 2-7 ■ Family Assessment Tool.

Source: Murray, R. B., & Zentner, J. P. (2001). Health promotion strategies through the lifespan *(7th ed., p. 200, Figure 4–2 Family Assessment Tool). Printed and electronically reproduced by permission of Pearson Education, Inc., Upper Saddle River, New Jersey.*

However, many immigrants to the United States live together with and rely on a network of grandparents and even aunts, uncles, and cousins. For example, Cuban families are often multigenerational and consider grandmothers to be part of the nuclear family. Further, godparents (or *compadrazgos*) are often considered part of the family even if they are not related by blood (Giger & Davidhizar, 2007).

Many Islamic families from West Africa practice polygamy. Although they do not often freely admit this when in the United States, sometimes women live in households with their co-wives. Sometimes the co-wives work well together and get along, and in some cases they do not. Often children view each co-wife as their own mother.

> **CLINICAL TIP**
> When caring for a family in which grandparents play a key role in family decision making, the nurse should include the grandparents in the decision-making and teaching sessions because their views are highly respected within the family unit.

Cultural Influences on Childbearing and Childrearing

A family's culture may influence its beliefs about and practices surrounding many aspects of childbearing and childrearing, including beliefs about the importance of children, beliefs and attitudes about pregnancy, health practices, and infant feeding behaviors.

Beliefs Regarding the Importance of Children

Children are generally valued all over the world, not only for the joy they bring, but also because they ensure continuation of the family and cultural values. This valuing of children may manifest in different ways, however. Families in the United States and many Western countries commonly have only one or two children, often out of a desire to provide the children with the best home and education they can afford, and to spend as much free time with them as possible. Many fear that additional children would too greatly dilute their financial and emotional resources. In contrast, in many cultures throughout the world, it is common to have as many children as possible. In Mali, West Africa, for example, the average woman has about seven children in her lifetime.

An understanding of the meaning of children in a culture may explain reactions of joy or shame to pregnancy. In the western United States, people of the Mormon faith view motherhood as the most important aspect of a woman's life, comparable with the male role of priesthood. In Mexican American society and among many other Hispanic groups, having children is evidence of the male's virility and is a sign of manliness, or *machismo,* a desired trait.

In cultures that value children only when they are born to a legally married couple, however, pregnancy is a shameful event if it occurs outside of marriage. In some Middle Eastern countries, for example, a woman who conceives outside of marriage would be permanently banned from her family. Pregnancy outside of marriage may even be dangerous. In many Muslim countries, an unmarried pregnant woman may seek a clandestine abortion because the consequences of carrying an illegitimate child can be social ostracism or even death—in some cases, even when the pregnancy has resulted from rape. It is not unheard of for women to be killed if the family discovers she engaged in sexual intercourse outside of marriage and became pregnant.

There are also many culturally influenced beliefs related to contraception. Many Muslims from the Middle East may use birth control but do not believe in sterilization because it is a permanent method. Other Muslims may not practice contraception because children are highly valued and it is believed that the traditional role of the woman is to bear children.

Beliefs and Attitudes About Pregnancy

Beliefs and attitudes about pregnancy may also be culturally influenced and may influence a woman's health behaviors. Thus certain health behaviors can be expected if a culture views pregnancy as a sickness, whereas other behaviors can be expected if pregnancy is viewed as a natural occurrence. Prenatal care may not be a priority for women who view pregnancy as a natural occurrence. Americans of African descent, for example, usually consider pregnancy as a state of wellness. Mexican Americans generally view pregnancy as a natural and desirable condition, and most Native American groups consider pregnancy a normal process. Although pregnancy is perceived as a natural occurrence in many cultures, it may also be viewed as a time of increased vulnerability. Individuals with European/Western ideas might expect the woman to be away from work before and right after childbirth. In Orthodox Judaism, it is a man's responsibility to procreate, but it is a woman's right, not her obligation, to do so.

Individuals of many cultures take certain protective precautions based on their beliefs. For example, many women of Malawi, Africa, avoid preparing clothes for the infant during the prenatal period because they believe that this action will lead to the birth of a stillborn infant. Similarly, many Southeast Asian women fear that they will have a complicated labor and birth if they sit in a doorway or on a step. Thus they tend to avoid areas near doors in waiting rooms and examining rooms. For many Vietnamese women, lifting the arms above the head is believed to increase the risk of preterm birth. Vietnamese women are also discouraged from sitting or lying down for lengthy periods because doing so might allow the baby to become too large.

In the Mexican American culture, the concept of *mal aire,* or bad air, is sometimes related to evil spirits. It is thought that air, especially night air, may enter the body and cause illness. Preventive measures, such as keeping the windows closed or covering the head, are used. Some Latinos may place a raisin on the cord stump of a newborn to prevent drafts from entering the baby's body.

For many Southeast Asians, the wind (or *vata*) is a potentially negative force that can disturb the body's internal harmony when a person is in a vulnerable state, such as during and after childbirth or during surgery. The natural forces thought to be more desirable during pregnancy include the earth, for groundedness, and water, for fluidity. Thus, in addition to avoiding wind and drafts, the pregnant woman is encouraged to eat creamy, oily, and other heavy foods; retire early and sleep until dawn; avoid stimulants and stress; and drink plenty of water.

Taboos refer to behaviors or things that are avoided. Many cultures, including those found in the United States, have taboos centered on the unborn baby that are meant to ensure that the baby will survive. Many of these beliefs stem from the fear of injuring an unborn child or the worry that a baby might die. In developing countries, mortality rates among infants and young children are extremely high; thus, certain traditions have centered on preventing early death. For example, it is common among Muslims to avoid naming babies until after birth and to ensure that the first words a baby hears are from God. In the western part of Mali, babies' faces are covered in mud and they are called ugly names to ward off evil spirits. Taboos also emanate from the fear that a pregnant woman has evil powers. For this reason, pregnant women are sometimes prohibited from taking part in certain activities with other people.

Many cultures ascribe to the *equilibrium model of health,* which is based on the concept of balance between light and dark, heat and cold. As described in chapter 3, Far Eastern philosophic belief systems focus on the notion of yin and yang. Yin represents the female, passive principle—darkness, cold, and wetness. Yang is the masculine, active principle—light, heat, and dryness. When the two are combined, they are all that can be.

The hot-cold classification is also seen in cultures in Latin America, the Near East, and Southeast Asia. The dimensions and meanings of this classification vary, however, and require further investigation. Spanish priests brought the concept of "hot" and "cold" to Mexico, where it was combined with ancient Aztec beliefs. Consequently, some Mexican Americans may consider illness to be an excess of either hot or cold (Galanti, 2008). To restore health, imbalances are often corrected by the proper use of foods, medications, or herbs. These substances are also classified as hot or cold. For example, an illness attributed to an excess of coldness will be treated only with hot foods or medications. The classification of foods is not always consistent, but it does conform to a general structure of traditional knowledge. Certain foods, spices, herbs, and medications are perceived to cool or heat the body. These perceptions do not necessarily correspond to the actual temperature; some hot dishes are said to have a cooling quality.

Southeast Asians believe it is important to keep the woman "warm" after the birth because blood, which is considered "hot," has been lost, and the woman is at risk of becoming "cold." Therefore, they avoid cold drinks and foods following birth. In addition, many women in India consider pregnancy a hot period and eat cool foods to counterbalance the hot state (Galanti, 2008). The concepts of hot and cold are not as important in Native American or African American beliefs. There are some similarities, however, in all of these groups because of the emphasis on a balance in nature.

Care Plan Activity: Effects of Hispanic Culture on Infant Feeding Practices

CLINICAL TIP

When caring for a woman of Asian descent, ask her if she would prefer hot water or ice water at her bedside. This can help ensure that proper oral hydration is maintained and cultural beliefs are supported.

Health Promotion Practices During Pregnancy

Health practices during pregnancy are influenced by numerous factors, such as the prevalence of traditional home remedies and folk beliefs, the importance of indigenous healers, and the influence of professional healthcare workers. In an urban setting the age of the family members, length of time in the city, marital status, and strength of the family may affect these patterns. Socioeconomic status is also important because modern medical services are more accessible to those who can afford them.

An awareness of alternative health sources is crucial for health professionals because these practices affect health outcomes. For example, many members of the Mexican American community utilize the *partera,* a lay midwife, as a healer who gives advice and treats illnesses during pregnancy as well as being in attendance during labor and birth.

Indigenous healers are also important in some cultures. In the Mexican American culture the healer is called a *curandero* or *curandera.* In some Native American tribes the medicine man may fulfill the healing role. Herbalists are often found in Asian cultures; and faith healers, root doctors, and spiritualists are sometimes consulted in the African American culture.

Cultural Norms Regarding Infant Feeding Practices

Culture can greatly affect new mothers' as well as experienced mothers' choices in feeding decisions. For example, in the Hispanic culture, women often believe that newborns need to be supplemented with infant formula before the milk comes in. Although colostrum provides vital antibodies for the infant, many Hispanic women refuse to nurse until their milk supply is established. It is important for the nurse to understand cultural norms and make recommendations that complement these norms, rather than conflict with them. In the preceding example, the nurse may advise the woman to first nurse her newborn at the breast and then offer the infant formula.

The majority of research on formula-feeding behavior has been conducted among Hispanic mothers and African American mothers. One common practice in these cultural groups is the addition of foods to the formula bottle, usually after 2 to 3 months, but for some, as early as 2 weeks into a baby's life. The kinds of food added vary from nonnutritive, high-calorie substances like sugar to adult foods like rice, beans, cereal, potatoes, yams, and eggs. Once the food is added, the nipple is often enlarged so that the baby can consume the food, creating a potential choking hazard.

Such supplementation may be done for a variety of reasons. Hispanic mothers report that it is important to add these foods to the formula to help the baby grow to be large. In Latin American culture, many people believe that "the bigger the baby, the better," so parents supplement the breast or formula, hoping for a big and healthy baby. Unfortunately, the parents are usually unaware of the fact that the addition of these foods can hurt the growth and health of the infant. Indeed, if a mother does not feed her child in the culturally accepted way, she may appear to be unfit or irresponsible within the community.

A second reason why foods are added to formulas lies in the belief that the addition of traditional foods at a very young age will prepare children to accept and enjoy their traditional foods when they are older. Food is an extremely important component of many Hispanic cultures; it ties people together and is usually the centerpiece of religious events and holidays. This relates to the third reason why foods are added to formula. During the holidays, it is considered important that everyone eat the same thing and participate equally; thus, infants are often included by being given the same foods the adults are eating.

African American mothers have also reported adding foods like cereal, potatoes, evaporated milk, or even extra scoops of powdered formula to thicken the formula. As with Hispanic families, the addition of these foods is thought to be necessary to help the child grow to be big and healthy, but more immediately, it is thought that this thickened formula will better satisfy a baby, so that he or she will sleep better through the night and allow the mother to do so as well. Thin formulas are associated with making a baby cry at night.

Overfeeding is a common cultural behavior as well. Hispanic mothers are reported to often overfeed their infants. Some mothers have reported to feed a child until he or she spits up. That is the indication that a child is eating in a healthful manner. Puerto Rican mothers believe overfeeding to be a protective care behavior that keeps a child healthy, well fed, and safe from illness or harm.

Many immigrants choose formula-feeding over breastfeeding. Although this choice may be partly due to their busy lives, it also can be due to cultural beliefs, particularly among immigrants from developing countries, where the ability to formula-feed is a status symbol because it is so expensive. In Mali, for example, a can of formula can cost the equivalent of $2, although the average individual only earns $200 per year. In the United States, formulas are more affordable and available to the poor; however, when additional cultural practices come into play, such as overfeeding and adding extra formula, the subsidized formulas can run out quickly, and mothers may choose to substitute cow's milk, use canned evaporated or condensed milk, dilute the formula, or purchase unsafe formulas on the "black market." Obviously, these choices have dangerous health implications for the infant.

A nurse may educate a mother in her native language about appropriate infant feeding practices, but the influences from her family and their cultural beliefs may have a greater impact than the health teaching on her feeding behavior. Understanding parents' beliefs and traditions can help nurses to educate families more effectively about healthful feeding behaviors.

Cultural Diversity in Family Nursing Care

Cultural attitudes, behaviors, and beliefs that are related to health can greatly affect how a patient will respond to and comply with health advice. Thus it is critical that nurses develop a holistic understanding of their patients' needs. (See www.nursing.pearsonhighered.com for a list of cultural resources.) Healthcare providers are often unaware of the cultural characteristics they themselves demonstrate. Without cultural awareness, caregivers tend to project their own cultural responses onto foreign-born patients; patients from different socioeconomic, religious, or educational groups; or patients from different regions of the country. This leads caregivers to assume that patients are demonstrating a specific behavior for the same reason that they themselves would. Moreover, healthcare providers frequently fail to recognize that medicine has its own culture, which has been dominated historically by traditional, middle-class values and beliefs.

Ethnocentrism is the conviction that the values and beliefs of one's own cultural group are the best ones or the only acceptable ones. It is characterized by an inability or unwillingness to understand the beliefs or worldview of another group or culture. To a certain extent, most people are guilty of ethnocentrism, at least some of the time. Thus the nurse who values stoicism during labor may be uncomfortable with the more vocal response of a Latin American woman. Another nurse may be disconcerted by the Southeast Asian woman who believes that pain is something to be endured rather than alleviated and is very intent on maintaining self-control in labor (Andrews & Boyle, 2008).

Healthcare providers sometimes believe that if members of other cultures do not share Western values, they should adopt them. This is especially difficult for a nurse caring for childbearing families if the nurse is a firm believer in the equality of the sexes and feminism. The nurse may find it difficult to remain silent if a woman from a Middle Eastern culture defers to her husband in decision making. It is important to remember that pressure to defy cultural values and beliefs can be stressful and anxiety provoking for these women.

To address issues of cultural diversity in the provision of health care, emphasis is being placed on developing **cultural competence**—that is, the skills and knowledge necessary to appreciate, understand, and work with individuals from different cultures. It requires self-awareness, awareness and understanding of cultural differences, and the ability to adapt clinical skills and practices as necessary.

The nurse can begin developing cultural competence by becoming knowledgeable about the cultural practices of local groups. For example, is it considered courteous to avoid eye contact? Should last names be used in conversation as a sign of respect? Is a female rather than male healthcare provider necessary? Do communication and language barriers exist? If so, how can they be addressed?

Application: Ethnocentrism and Health Care—Providing Culturally Sensitive Care

Giger and Davidhizar (2007) have suggested that care providers conduct a "cultural assessment" to glean information about health practices based on the patient's beliefs, values, and customs. This kind of assessment might include questions such as:

1. Who in the family must be consulted before decisions are made about a person's care?
2. Does the patient see primarily in the present or does he or she have a futuristic time orientation?
3. What type of health provider is most appropriate for the patient?
4. Does the patient have beliefs or traditions that may impact the care plan?

Several cultural assessment tools are in use to assist the nurse in obtaining cultural information. Giger and Davidhizar (2007) developed a transcultural assessment tool that identifies the cultural background, communication patterns, issues related to personal space, social organization, time, roles within the environment, biologic variations, and a nursing assessment (Figure 2-8 ■).

Culturally Influenced Responses

Cultural Resources

It is imperative when caring for families that nurses provide culturally sensitive care that supports cultural differences. The nurse who respects cultural diversity is an asset to the childbearing family as they adjust to their new role. Establishing a trusting relationship enables the nurse to assist the family in meeting educational needs. The nurse who considers the woman's personal values, beliefs, and customs will be a far more effective caregiver than the nurse who does not.

Biologic Differences

Genetic and physical differences occur among cultural groups and can lead to disparities in needs and care. African Americans are more likely to experience hypertension, strokes, obesity, diabetes, and sickle cell anemia. Thalassemia, another type of anemia, occurs primarily in individuals of Mediterranean descent. African Americans and Native Americans tend to have higher rates of tuberculosis than the general population. On the other hand, African Americans have higher bone mass than Caucasians and lower rates of osteoporosis. Caucasians have higher rates of heart disease. Caucasians from certain geographic regions have higher rates of cystic fibrosis, celiac disease, and Crohn's disease. Hispanics have higher rates of diabetes and lactose intolerance. Asians and Native Americans often do not metabolize alcohol readily and are more prone to either injury after alcohol ingestion or to alcohol abuse. Otitis media, or infection of the middle ear, is common in Native American and Alaskan Native children. Diabetes, liver disease, and injuries are common in Native American groups. Metabolism of certain drugs is also linked to genetics in certain groups.

Nurses must understand other genetic characteristics in order to provide culturally competent nursing assessments and interventions. Differences in skin color may make cyanosis, pallor, and jaundice difficult to recognize and describe. Mongolian spots are darkened skin spots on the lower back and buttocks of some babies with dark skin. Variations in texture of hair require different approaches to hygiene among various racial groups.

Communication Patterns

Communication is a method by which members of culture groups share information and preserve their beliefs, values, norms, and practices. To ensure effective nursing care, it is

A Transcultural Assessment Model

CULTURALLY UNIQUE INDIVIDUAL

1. Place of birth
2. Cultural definition
   What is . . .
3. Race
   What is . . .
4. Length of time in country

COMMUNICATION

1. Voice quality
   A. Strong, resonant
   B. Soft
   C. Average
   D. Shrill
2. Pronunciation and enunciation
   A. Clear
   B. Slurred
   C. Dialect
3. Use of silence
   A. Infrequent
   B. Often
   C. Length
      (1) Brief
      (2) Moderate
      (3) Long
      (4) Not observed
4. Use of nonverbal
   A. Hand movement
   B. Eye movement
   C. Moves entire body
   D. Kinesics (gestures, expressions, or stances)
5. Touch
   A. Startles or withdraws when touched
   B. Accepts touch without difficulty
   C. Touches others without difficulty
6. Ask these and similar questions:
   A. How do you get your point across to others?
   B. Do you like communicating with friends, family, and acquaintances?
   C. When asked a question, do you usually respond (in words or body movements, or both)?
   D. If you have something important to discuss with your family, how would you approach them?

SPACE

1. Degree of comfort
   A. Moves when space invaded
   B. Does not move when invaded
2. Distance in conversations
   A. 0 to 18 inches
   B. 18 inches to 3 feet
   C. 3 feet or more
3. Definition of space
   A. Describe degree of comfort with closeness when talking with or standing near others
   B. How do objects (e.g., furniture) in the environment affect your sense of space?
4. Ask these and similar questions:
   A. When you talk with family members, how close do you stand?
   B. When you communicate with coworkers and other acquaintances, how close do you stand?
   C. If a stranger touches you, how do you react or feel?
   D. If a loved one touches you, how do you react or feel?
   E. Are you comfortable with the distance between us now?

SOCIAL ORGANIZATION

1. Normal state of health
   A. Poor
   B. Fair
   C. Good
   D. Excellent

Figure 2-8 ■ Cultural assessment tool.

2. Ask these and similar questions:
   A. How do you define social activities?
   B. What are some activities that you enjoy?
   C. What are your hobbies, or what do you do when you have free time?
   D. Do you believe in a Supreme Being?
   E. How do you worship that Supreme Being?
   F. What is your function (what do you do) in your family unit/system?
   G. What is your role in your family unit/system (father, mother, child, advisor)?
   H. When you were a child, what or who influenced you most?
   I. What is/was your relationship with your siblings and parents?
   J. What does work mean to you?
   K. Describe your past, present, and future jobs.
   L. What are your political views?
   M. How have your political views influenced your attitude toward health and illness?

TIME

1. Orientation to time
   A. Past-oriented
   B. Present-oriented
   C. Future-oriented
2. View of time
   A. Social time
   B. Clock-oriented
3. Physiochemical reaction to time
   A. Sleeps at least 8 hours a night
   B. Goes to sleep and wakes on a consistent schedule
   C. Understands the importance of taking medication and other treatments on schedule
4. Ask these and similar questions:
   A. What kind of timepiece do you wear daily?
   B. If you have an appointment at 2 PM, what time is acceptable to arrive?
   C. If a nurse tells you that you will receive a medication in "about a half hour," realistically, how much time will you allow before calling the nurses' station?

ENVIRONMENTAL CONTROL

1. Locus-of-control
   A. Internal locus-of-control (believes that the power to affect change lies within)
   B. External locus-of-control (believes that fate, luck, and chance have a great deal to do with how things turn out)
2. Value orientation
   A. Believes in supernatural forces
   B. Relies on magic, witchcraft, and prayer to affect change
   C. Does not believe in supernatural forces
   D. Does not rely on magic, witchcraft, or prayer to affect change
3. Ask these and similar questions:
   A. How often do you have visitors at your home?
   B. Is it acceptable to you for visitors to drop in unexpectedly?
   C. Name some ways your parents or other persons treated your illnesses when you were a child.
   D. Have you or someone else in your immediate surroundings ever used a home remedy that made you sick?
   E. What home remedies have you used that worked? Will you use them in the future?
   F. What is your definition of "good health"?
   G. What is your definition of illness or "poor health"?

BIOLOGIC VARIATIONS

1. Conduct a complete physical assessment noting:
   A. Body structure
   B. Skin color
   C. Unusual skin discolorations
   D. Hair color and distribution
   E. Other visible physical characteristics (e.g., keloids, chloasma)
2. Ask these and similar questions:
   A. What diseases or illnesses are common in your family?
   B. Describe your family's typical behavior when a family member is ill.
   C. How do you respond when you are angry?
   D. Who (or what) usually helps you to cope during a difficult time?
   E. What foods do you and your family like to eat?
   F. Have you ever had any unusual cravings for:
      (1) White or red clay dirt?
      (2) Laundry starch?
   G. When you were a child what types of foods did you eat?
   H. What foods are family favorites or are considered traditional?

NURSING ASSESSMENT

1. Note whether the client has become culturally assimilated or observes own cultural practices.
2. Incorporate data into plan of nursing care:
   A. Encourage the client to discuss cultural differences; people from diverse cultures who hold different worldviews can enlighten nurses.
   B. Make efforts to accept and understand methods of communication.
   C. Respect the individual's personal need for space.
   D. Respect the rights of clients to honor and worship the Supreme Being of their choice.
   E. Identify a clerical or spiritual person to contact.
   F. Determine whether spiritual practices have implications for health, life, and well-being (e.g., Jehovah's Witnesses may refuse blood and blood derivatives; an Orthodox Jew may eat only Kosher food high in sodium and may not drink milk when meat is served).
   G. Identify hobbies, especially when devising interventions for short or extended convalescence or for rehabilitation.
   H. Honor time and value orientations and differences in these areas. Allay anxiety and apprehension if adherence to time is necessary.
   I. Provide privacy according to personal need and health status of the client (Note: the perception and reaction to pain may be culturally related).
   J. Note cultural health practices
      (1) Identify and encourage efficacious practices.
      (2) Identify and discourage dysfunctional practices.
      (3) Identify and determine whether neutral practices will have a long-term ill effect.
   K. Note food preferences
      (1) Make as many adjustments in diet as health status and long-term benefits will allow and that dietary department can provide.
      (2) Note dietary practices that may have serious implications for the client.

Figure 2-8 ■ Cultural assessment tool. continued

Source: Reprinted from Transcultural Nursing: Assessment and Intervention, *by J. N. Giger and R. E. Davidhizar, Copyright © 1991, with permission from Elsevier.*

essential for nurses to be able to communicate with the family. This becomes an issue when the family and nurse do not speak the same language. In such cases, translators should be provided. The Joint Commission of Accreditation of Hospital Organizations (JCAHO) requires that hospitals provide a mechanism for patients to communicate in their own language. This reduces medical errors and increases effective communication. The use of children and other family members to act in the role of translator is not recommended because of confidentiality issues. Written instructions, signs, and brochures should be offered in the individuals' native language.

Language can also affect health literacy skills. A large number of instructions are given in writing. Examples include prescriptions and directions on medication bottles, signs hanging in health facilities, consent forms for procedures and surgery, insurance forms, directions for techniques or procedures, future appointment dates, and health promotion materials. Nurses need to verify that the patient and family can read and whether alternate methods are needed. Nurses can verbally give the information and provide paper and pencil so that the family can write it down in their own language. Translation services should be available in all healthcare settings.

Variations in communication among cultures are reflected in their word meaning, voice inflection and quality, and verbal styles. Culture not only influences the manner in which feelings are expressed, but also which verbal and nonverbal expressions of communication are considered appropriate. An individual's willingness to discuss certain topics or to express or conceal certain thoughts and feelings are also influenced by the cultural norms. For example, Native Americans and people of Asian descent may feel it is appropriate to remain quiet when experiencing pain, whereas people of Italian, Jewish, and Latino descent may feel that it is best to express pain more vocally.

Use of names varies among cultural groups. Assuming that each person wishes to be called by a first name can be disrespectful. Address family members respectfully, usually using terms such as Mr., Mrs., and Ms. If the person has a title such as doctor, judge, or senator, it should be used. Ask what the person prefers to be called and record this in the health record for future reference. In some cultures such as Korean, Cambodian, and Filipino, the first name used is actually the family name. Asking for the "family name" rather than the "last name" may clarify this practice.

NONVERBAL COMMUNICATION Nonverbal communication patterns may hinder or help communication. For example, gestures and body language may be misunderstood or misinterpreted. Similarly, eye contact has different meanings among cultures. European Americans, for example, value eye contact with communication and interpret this as a sign of sincerity and interest. In other cultures, such as Asian and Native American, sustained eye contact may be considered rude or disrespectful.

Silence may also be considered a sign of respect in some cultures. Among those groups, offering an immediate response to a question may be viewed as being disrespectful because an instant reply could indicate that no thought was given to the matter. Nurses should watch for patterns in various cultures and alter their own approach to be more congruent. For example, many nurses commonly nod and say "yes" or "oh, I see" when a healthcare patient is speaking. This may seem disruptive to some cultures. Noting that the listener is silent and does not use such patterns of agreement alerts the nurse to alter his or her own response to match more closely the acceptable method of communication for the family. Nurses need to learn that silence and quiet listening can be perceived as positive approaches.

TOUCH The appropriateness of touch varies with each culture. For example, an Asian may consider touching an unfamiliar person of the opposite gender to be inappropriate, whereas touch between men and women may be viewed as appropriate by another culture. Adults commonly feel that it is acceptable to touch children of all ages but this may not be accurate. Nurses should look for responses from family to touch and progress accordingly.

SPACE Depending on an individual's specific culture, the use of space has different meanings. "Space," as defined in this context, refers to the relationship between the individual and other persons and objects in the environment. Cultures may have specific spatial preferences, such as personal distance and social distance. Some cultures tend to prefer close contact with less space because they use touch as a form of communication. Nurses should be alert for how close a childbearing woman or a child comes to them and other individuals and try to maintain this space in their interactions. Nursing procedures often cause the space barrier to be broken. Nurses need to touch patients to take vital signs, administer injections, change dressings, and the like. This does not mean that close touch is appropriate at all times. Telling all patients before touching them for procedures will help them understand what is happening.

Time Orientation

Time orientation can vary significantly among cultures. Cultural groups may place emphasis on the events of the past, those events that occur in the present, or those events that will occur in the future. Time is also influenced by development so that young children sometimes do not understand the use of clocks, the importance ascribed to being "on time," or other time orientations.

Cultures that are oriented predominantly to the past may want to begin healthcare encounters with lengthy descriptions of past healthcare treatments, family history of diseases, or individual past experiences with health. There may be little interest in learning methods of adapting to or maintaining a new plan of care.

For cultures that are oriented predominantly to the present, little consideration may be given to either the past or the future. For example, adolescents commonly focus on the present and may not engage in preventive health practices for long-term health. Short-term goals often provide more incentive to adolescents.

Cultures that are oriented predominantly to the future, such as European Americans, may not focus on what is important at the present time. For example, the family focusing on the future may focus on the dreams they had for a child's education or sports performance and have trouble setting present goals for treatment of a disease such as juvenile rheumatoid arthritis. One commonly hears that it was a big adjustment to learn to "take one day at a time." Not living up to the family's expectation for their future success may be difficult for a child who has developed an illness that has a chronic course.

Time also refers to punctuality about schedules and appointments. In the United States and Canada, the predominant culture respects promptness and considers time valuable and not to be wasted. Other cultures may not reflect this same concern for time. This may be manifested by a family's inability to follow timed medication schedules or treatments, or to show up as scheduled for an appointment. In these cases, it is not intended as a sign of disrespect.

Impact of Religion and Spirituality

The goal of truly holistic care of the childbearing family requires that the nurse understand the influence that religion and spirituality may have on the childbearing experience.

Diverse Meanings of Religion and Spirituality

The terms *religion* and *spirituality* mean very different things to different people. Although many people think of **religion** as an institutionalized system that shares a common set of beliefs and practices, others define it more simply as a belief in a transcendent power. The latter definition approaches most people's understanding of **spirituality** as a concern with the spirit or soul.

Philosophers and mystics have debated the meaning of religion for millennia, but within the last 200 years, technologic advances and the ascendance of rationalism and postmodernism have led many influential thinkers to condemn religion as mere wishful thinking. For example, in 1844, philosopher Karl Marx famously decried religion as "the opium of the people" (Marx, 1971), and in 1932, in his *New Introductory Lectures on Psychoanalysis,* psychologist Sigmund Freud stated: "Religion is an illusion . . . an attempt to get control over the sensory world, in which we are placed, by means of the wish-world . . . " (Freud, 1965). More recently, however, religious teachers have offered new visions of a religious life grounded in day-to-day experience.

Range of Religious Beliefs

The diverse meanings and approaches to religion and spirituality are reflected in the diversity of religious beliefs encountered in contemporary childbearing families. Some may belong to large institutionalized religious organizations; others may feel deeply religious yet have no formal affiliation or practice. Many patients are *agnostic,* or doubtful about the existence of a transcendent being, or truly *atheist,* meaning that they believe there is no higher power.

A childbearing family's religious beliefs, affiliation, and practices can influence deeply their experience and attitudes toward health care, childbearing, and childrearing. Members of certain religious groups such as Christian Scientists may attempt to avoid all medical interventions, whereas others such as Jehovah's Witnesses may refuse specific interventions, such as blood transfusions. Roman Catholics may refuse contraception. Many religions promote childbearing as a sacred right and responsibility, and some prescribe childrearing practices as well. In most cases, the woman and her family gain comfort from acknowledgment of and respect for their religious beliefs and practices in the healthcare setting. However, the agnostic or atheist family may be offended if care providers assume that references to God or a higher power will be comforting.

Provision of Spiritually Sensitive Nursing Care

For all these reasons, nurses are increasingly committed to providing spiritually sensitive nursing care to childbearing families. On admission to the clinic or labor setting, a religious or spiritual history is now included when assessing the childbearing family. Many patients specify a religious affiliation on admission to an acute care facility, but more specific information is also needed. The assessment can include questions about current spiritual beliefs and practices that will affect the mother and baby during the hospital stay or preferences for religious rituals during labor and birth.

Whenever possible, the nurse and other healthcare providers should attempt to accommodate religious rituals and practices requested by the childbearing family. Most such requests, such as for certain music, foods, or keeping a statue or picture by the bed, can be accommodated without causing danger; however, some, such as lighting candles, could present a risk in an acute care setting. In these circumstances, the family should be given a clear explanation of why the particular action cannot safely be carried out. In addition, nurses can provide patients with resources to meet their religious needs, such as consultation with on-staff chaplains. In settings where chaplains are not readily available, the nurse should be familiar with community resources in the area and offer referral as needed. In circumstances of spiritual distress, such as with severe fetal deformity or loss of a newborn, the family may prefer to meet with their personal religious adviser and the nurse can arrange for that visit.

Considering the diversity of religious beliefs, it is not unusual for nurses to encounter childbearing families whose beliefs conflict with their own. This is not problematic as long as the nurse avoids attempts to influence the patient's decision making. For example, a nurse who does not believe in baptism should avoid revealing this belief to a Catholic patient seeking baptism for her stillborn infant. Nurses should also examine their religious beliefs related to genetic screening procedures; use of assisted reproductive technology to achieve pregnancy; use of technology to support life in a severely compromised newborn; abortion; and even less dramatic issues such as methods of contraception, circumcision, and infant feeding. In many institutions, nurses can ask to be reassigned to a different patient if their religious beliefs are in conflict; however, if other personnel are not available, it is the nurse's responsibility to provide sensitive, appropriate, and nonjudgmental care to that patient.

FOCUS YOUR STUDY

- Family values, power, and roles are important to consider when attempting to provide holistic health care to contemporary families.
- Multiple trends have influenced changes in the traditional family, including employment trends, changes in marital status patterns, and economic trends.
- Nuclear families consist of a mother, father, and children.
- Dual-career/dual-earner families make up the majority of contemporary families in the United States.
- Childless families are a growing trend in American culture.
- Extended family members can play an active role in family life, decision making, and family roles.
- Single-parent families account for almost a third of all U.S. families, and stepparent and binuclear families are increasingly common.
- The developmental framework looks at a family over time as it progresses through predictable stages within the life cycle.
- A family assessment provides an in-depth tool to collect pertinent family life information that can assist the nurse in planning care.
- Culture plays a significant part in a family's development; roles; and observance of traditions, customs, and taboos.
- Cultural norms influence a family's beliefs about the importance of children, pregnancy, health practices, and infant feeding.
- A cultural assessment can assist the nurse in identifying cultural norms and providing culturally appropriate nursing care.
- A religious history is included when assessing contemporary families. Whenever possible, the nurse accommodates the family's religious-based preferences for care.

CRITICAL THINKING IN ACTION

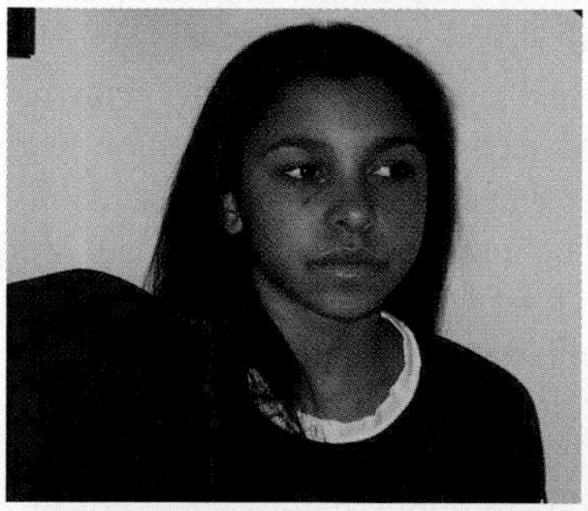

While working in an inner-city clinic for adolescents, you meet a new patient, a 14-year-old Latina girl named Juanita. She is accompanied by her parents. None of them speak English. Through an interpreter, Juanita tells you that she recently moved here with her parents. They have brought her here today because she has a sore throat. The curandero they took her to see prescribed the herbal remedy *Echinacea*, but her throat is still sore. The rapid test you perform for strep throat is positive and the nurse practitioner prescribes an antibiotic.

1. According to the national standards for culturally and linguistically appropriate services in health care set by the government, what are examples of important standards of care that you, as the nurse, can provide in the care of this adolescent?
2. How can you, as the nurse, take steps to achieve cultural competence?
3. How would you, as the nurse, be able to address some of the disparities that can exist when this patient comes to the clinic?
4. What are some examples of common food preferences in the Latino American culture?

See www.nursing.pearsonhighered.com for possible responses.

Pearson Nursing Student Resources

Find additional review materials at **www.nursing.pearsonhighered.com**

Prepare for success with additional NCLEX®-style practice questions, interactive assignments and activities, Web links, animations and videos, and more!

REFERENCES

Akins, S., Mosher, C., Smith, C., & Florence, J. (2007). *Acculturation and drug use: The effect of linguistic isolation on Hispanic substance use in Washington State.* Paper presented at the annual meeting of the American Sociological Association, August 11, 2007, New York, NY.

Andrews, M. M., & Boyle, J. S. (2008). *Transcultural concepts in nursing care* (5th ed.). Philadelphia, PA: Wolters Kluwer Health/Lippincott Williams & Wilkins.

Carter, B. (2010). *The expanded family life cycle.* New York, NY: Allyn & Bacon.

Carter, E. A., & McGoldrick, M. (Eds.). (2005). *The expanded family life cycle: Individual, family, and societal perspectives* (3rd ed.). New York, NY: Allyn & Bacon.

Cunningham, P., & Artiga, S. (2009). *Medicaid and the uninsured: How does health coverage and access to care for immigrants vary by length of time in the U.S.? The Kaiser Commission.* Retrieved from http://www.kff.org/uninsured/upload/7916_ES.pdf

De Castro, A. B., Gilbert, C. G., & Takeuchi, D. T. (2008). Job-related stress and chronic health conditions among Filipino immigrants. *Journal of Immigrant and Minority Health, 10*(6) 551–558.

Duvall, E. M. (1977). *Marriage and family development* (5th ed.). New York, NY: Harper Row.

Duvall, E. M., & Miller, B. C. (1985). *Marriage and family development.* New York, NY: Harper Collins.

Freud, S. (1965). *New introductory lectures on psychoanalysis* (lecture 35). New York, NY: W. W. Norton. (Original work published 1932)

Galanti, G. A. (2008). *Caring for patients from different cultures* (4th ed.). Philadelphia: University of Pennsylvania Press.

Giger, J. N., & Davidhizar, R. E. (2007). *Transcultural nursing: Assessment and interventions* (5th ed.). St. Louis, MO: Mosby.

Kaakinen, J., Gedaly-Duff, V., Coehlo, D., & Hanson, S. (2010). *Family health care nursing: Theory, practice and research* (4th ed.). Philadelphia, PA: F. A. Davis.

Marx, K. (1971). *Critique of the Hegelian philosophy of right.* Cambridge, England: Cambridge University Press. (Original work published 1844)

McGrath, B. B., & Edwards, K. L. (2009). When family means more (or less) than genetics. *Journal of Transcultural Nursing, 20,* 270. doi: 10.1177/1043659609334931

National Center for Health Statistics, Division of Vital Statistics. (2009, March 18). Births: Preliminary data for 2007. *National Vital Statistics Reports, 57*(12). Retrieved from http://www.cdc.gov/nchs/data/nvsr/nvsr57/nvsr57_12.pdf

Pan, W. (2008, October 3). *Single parent family statistics—Single parents a new trend?* Retrieved from http://ezinearticles.com/?Single-Parent-Family-Statistics—Single-Parents-a-New-Trend?&id=1552445

Slater, S. (1995). *The lesbian family life cycle.* New York, NY: The Free Press.

Smith, D. M., & Gates, G. (2009). *Gay and lesbian families in the United States: Same-sex unmarried partner households.* Retrieved from http://www.urban.org/publications/1000491.html

Stewart, S. D. (2007). *Brave new stepfamilies.* Thousand Oaks, CA: Sage.

U.S. Census Bureau. (2008a). *Current population survey (CPS) definitions and explanations.* Retrieved from http://www.census.gov/population/www/cps/cpsdef.html

U.S. Census Bureau, Housing and Household Economic Statistics Division, Fertility & Family Statistics Branch. (2008b). *Current population survey.* Retrieved from http://www.census.gov/population/www/cps/cpsdef.html

U.S. Census Bureau. (2009). *America's families and living arrangements: 2007.* Retrieved from http://www.census.gov/population/www/socdemo/hh-fam/p20-561.pdf

U.S. Census Bureau News. (2008). *New analysis offers state-by-state look at fertility.* Retrieved from http://www.census.gov/Press-Release/www/releases/archives/population/012510.html

U.S. Census Bureau News. (2009). *Stay-at-home moms are more likely younger, Hispanic and foreign-born than other mothers.* Retrieved from http://www.census.gov/newsroom/releases/archives/families_households/cb09-132.html

Wagner, K., Ritt-Olson, A., Soto, D., Rodriguez, Y., Baezconde-Garbanati, L., & Unger, J. (2008). The role of acculturation, parenting, and family in Hispanic/Latino adolescent substance use: Findings from a qualitative analysis. *Journal of Ethnic Substance Abuse, 7*(3), 304–327.

CHAPTER 3

Complementary and Alternative Therapies

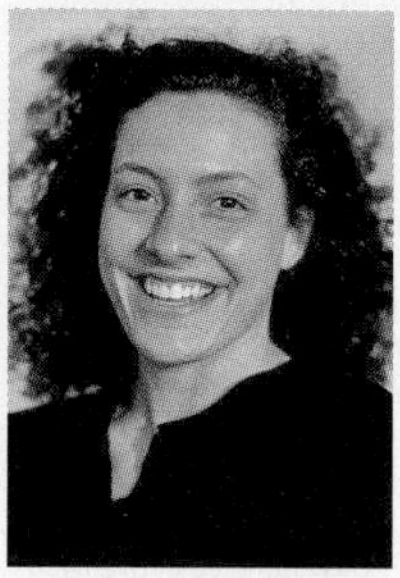

As part of a continuing education course on body-based therapies for nurses, I was giving a back massage to one of my classmates. At one point, I felt a buzz of energy shoot up my hands and arms. At that exact moment, the other student said, "Wow!" Our instructor just laughed and said, "Oh, you're just exchanging friendly energy." That experience changed forever my views as a nurse and educator. I like the fact that nursing is based in science, but I remain open to the mysteries of the human body, mind, and spirit.

LEARNING OUTCOMES

1. Distinguish between *complementary* and *alternative therapies*.
2. Identify several factors that have contributed to the rise in popularity of complementary and alternative therapies in the United States and Canada.
3. Describe the role of the National Center for Complementary and Alternative Medicine.
4. Explain the role of complementary and alternative therapies in promoting wellness, disease prevention, and holistic healing.
5. Delineate the risks of using complementary and alternative therapies.
6. Compare the basic principles and components of homeopathy, naturopathy, traditional Chinese medicine, and ayurvedic medicine.
7. Describe the use of mind-body therapies in promoting the well-being of childbearing families.
8. Contrast the different manipulative and body-based therapies.
9. Explain the advantages and disadvantages to childbearing women of therapies involving ingestion of substances such as foods, dietary supplements, herbs, and homeopathic remedies.
10. Distinguish between acupressure and acupuncture.
11. Distinguish between Reiki and Therapeutic Touch.
12. Discuss complementary therapies appropriate for the nurse to use with childbearing families.

KEY TERMS

Acupressure *54*
Acupuncture *55*
Alternative therapy *45*
Aromatherapy *54*
Ayurveda *50*
Biofeedback *50*
Chiropractic *51*
Complementary and alternative medicine (CAM) *45*
Complementary therapy *45*
Guided imagery, *51*
Hatha yoga *53*
Homeopathy *49*
Hypnosis *51*
Integrative medicine *47*
Massage therapy *52*
Naturopathy *49*
Reflexology *52*
Reiki *55*
Therapeutic Touch *55*
Traditional Chinese medicine (TCM) *49*
Visualization *51*

Until the latter part of the 20th century in the United States, it was rare for European American childbearing families to consult anyone except their obstetrician for advice about their pregnancy, birth, and postpartum. Though such patients are still encountered today, perinatal nurses are more likely to care for childbearing families who integrate other types of practitioners and therapies with traditional Western medicine. Families choosing complementary and alternative therapies may include those whose health practices are rooted in their cultural heritage, as well as European Americans who have explored one or more of the vast number of non-Western healing approaches available today. The nurse may even encounter families who consider alternative approaches superior to the diagnostics and treatments that conventional Western medicine offers, and who enter a clinic or hospital environment only reluctantly.

Because the use of complementary and alternative therapies has become so widespread, all nurses need to have at least a fundamental understanding of their benefits and risks and guidelines for their safe use. The chapter begins with an overview of the evolution of complementary and alternative therapies. A brief description of the most common therapies currently used by childbearing families is also provided.

Evolution of Complementary and Alternative Therapies

Complementary and alternative medicine (CAM) is a group of diverse medical and healthcare systems, practices, and products that are not generally considered part of conventional medicine (National Center for Complementary and Alternative Medicine [NCCAM], 2008). A **complementary therapy** may be defined as any procedure or product that is used together with conventional medical treatment. For example, a childbearing woman might request aromatherapy to help her cope with the discomfort she anticipates following a scheduled cesarean birth. Although complementary therapies were entirely absent from clinics and hospitals until the last few decades, they are now often used in conjunction with surgery, pharmaceuticals, and other conventional treatments for a variety of injuries and illnesses. They are also being more and more frequently integrated with conventional perinatal care.

In contrast, an **alternative therapy** is used in place of conventional medicine (NCCAM, 2008). For example, a woman with a postterm pregnancy may refuse medication to induce labor, and instead ingest an herb she believes will stimulate contractions. Because alternative therapies are used in place of medically prescribed treatments, people may be reluctant to discuss them with a conventional physician or registered nurse.

The very terms *complementary* and *alternative* suggest the contemporary view that herbs, homeopathy, chiropractic, and other such healing techniques are peripheral to conventional Western medicine, which is the "primary" treatment. How did we come to hold this view? And what has contributed to the resurgence in complementary and alternative therapies in the last few decades?

Historic Perspective

Five hundred years ago, a Native American woman drinking hot water steeped with chamomile to settle her stomach would never have described her beverage as a complementary or alternative therapy. She was merely following a custom handed down to her by her ancestors and practiced widely in her tribe. If her symptoms continued, she would likely have consulted a medicine woman or medicine man, who might have performed a healing ritual using other herbs, stones, chanting, and/or communion with the "animal spirits" or ancestors who had passed on. Such forms of self- and community-based treatment, though varying somewhat from one culture to another, are thought to have been the norm around the world for thousands of years.

Many therapies that are today considered complementary or alternative grew out of indigenous cultures' use of the herbs, spices, flowers, fruits, and other plants and natural materials available in the region, and reflected their health concerns. For example, it has been proposed that one rationale for the highly spiced cuisine of India is that the spices used, in addition to being widely available, have an antimicrobial effect. This would have been important for a hot region of the world where food could not be preserved without fear of spoilage. In contrast, people in colder regions of the world, such as northern Europe, developed techniques such as salting, drying, and freezing foods during long winters to preserve them from microbial decay.

Many other complementary and alternative therapies developed from cultures' spiritual beliefs. Thousands of years ago, most cultures held the belief that illnesses and injuries—as well as therapies to heal them—were spiritually based. For example, peoples from ancient China, India, and the Americas shared the belief that all animals, plants, and even minerals contain a spiritual "essence," a vibrational life force that could be employed in healing. European peoples once believed that disease was caused by supernatural forces either to punish human beings or to teach them spiritual lessons. Others, such as the people of ancient India, believed that illness demonstrated a lack of alignment of the mind and body with God. For Patanjali, who wrote the *Yoga Sutras* in the third century BCE, a healthy body was a precondition for spiritual wholeness. In some cultures, spiritual healers performed rituals to exorcise the evil spirit from the diseased body.

Around 400 BCE, Hippocrates became the first practitioner in the West known to challenge the idea that illnesses and injuries have spiritual causes and remedies. His school of medicine investigated impurities in the individual's food, water, and environment as causes of disease and attempted to base healing practices in the known laws of nature. Students began to investigate systematically the healing properties of local plants and other substances and to develop standards of practice.

Over the next millennium, indigenous peoples worldwide continued to hand down the knowledge of healing plants and practices. Shamans, alchemists, and midwives were highly respected members of their communities and were relied on for their cures. However, between the 13th and 17th centuries in Europe, church-led inquisitions sought out and killed indigenous healers, typically burning them as "witches." At the same time, the new philosophy of rationalism became popular, and community leaders began to demand empiric evidence for healing practices. During the 17th century, the scientific method gained ascendancy, single-celled organisms were discovered, and the first experiments challenging the idea of spontaneous generation of life were conducted.

From the 18th to the 19th centuries, several scientific achievements further advanced the supremacy of empirically based medical techniques. High-powered microscopes were developed that could allow detection of microorganisms such as bacteria. In 1796, the English physician Edward Jenner developed the first effective vaccine, which used material from cowpox lesions to stimulate immunity to smallpox. In the mid-1800s, the French scientist Louis Pasteur conducted experiments that led to the formulation of the *germ theory of disease,* that is, the theory that microbes can cause human disease. In the 1860s, the English surgeon Joseph Lister introduced aseptic techniques using phenol and dramatically reduced the mortality rate following surgery. His techniques were widely adopted by other surgeons and led to increased acceptance of surgery as a viable treatment. By 1875, the German scientist Robert Koch had established postulates to prove whether a certain organism was pathogenic and what disease it caused. Thus, people learned that infectious disease, which was the leading cause of death at that time, was not due to spiritual flaws.

At the same time, European colonization of countries in Asia, Africa, Australia, and the Americas brought European medical practices as well. Indigenous healers and their therapies, such as the ayurvedic system of India and the nature-based therapies of Africa, were prohibited by the colonial powers and replaced with Western procedures and pharmaceuticals. In the United States, the American Medical Association (AMA) grew in prominence, replacing female midwives with male obstetricians, and homeopathic physicians (estimated to comprise about 50% of U.S. physicians in the mid-19th century) with medical doctors who had graduated from AMA-approved schools of medicine.

National Center for Complementary and Alternative Medicine

In the early 20th century, several factors combined to ensure a virtual monopoly of conventional medicine in the United States. First, antimicrobial drugs and vaccines were developed that dramatically reduced morbidity and mortality due to infectious disease. Second, pharmaceutical companies began dominating medicine by heavily subsidizing U.S. medical schools, giving rewards and subsidies to physicians who used their drugs, and lobbying U.S. legislators for statutes and regulations favorable to their industry. Third, two world wars led to advances in both pharmaceuticals and surgical techniques that helped convince legislators of the superiority of the AMA's approach to health care.

Resurgence of Complementary and Alternative Therapies

Complementary and alternative therapies never entirely died out in the United States. Even in the 1950s, some people were able to eke out a living as chiropractors or herbalists. The social upheavals and "back to the land" movements of the 1960s and 1970s led to a renewed study of the healing therapies of indigenous cultures. Moreover, as Americans began to engage more widely in international work, study, and travel, their exposure to other healing systems and practices increased. Indeed, several American physicians, disillusioned by the limitations of conventional Western medicine, traveled to Asia and other regions to study alternative therapies.

By the final years of the 20th century, America's love affair with conventional Western medicine had begun to cool even more significantly as costs increased, health care began to be seen as more technologic and less "human," and access to healthcare professionals' time became strictly limited. Childbearing families in particular began to seek more "natural" birth experiences, without anesthesia, in homelike settings attended by female certified nurse-midwives. Americans began to recognize that many health problems, such as back pain, headaches, cancer, diabetes, heart disease, autoimmune diseases, and others, could not be cured simply by swallowing a pill or "going under the knife." Such disorders came to be seen as complex, involving lifestyle factors, cultural factors, emotional elements, and—many people believed—spiritual aspects that were ignored by conventional approaches. Increasingly, people with such diseases turned to the complementary and alternative healing community.

But perhaps the most explosive element in the resurgence of complementary and alternative therapies was—and continues to be—the Internet. With a laptop or smart phone, current information on complementary and alternative products and services is now just a click away. For example, a paper presented at a conference in Germany on the health benefits of reflexology might become available worldwide the next day. The Internet has increased not only information, but also communication among people with similar health concerns. A pregnant woman who has just begun to experience first trimester nausea can now join a chat group debating the advantages and disadvantages of ginger tea. Infertile couples can share a technique claiming to increase fertility that they learned on a trip to Asia. Suddenly, it has become easy for people to integrate complementary and alternative therapies into their own unique approach to their healthcare concerns.

Growing Integration with Conventional Western Medicine

In this new century, it seems clear that the future of American health care will see an ever increasing integration between conventional medicine and complementary therapies. Some obvious examples of this new integration in perinatal settings include the acceptance of certain herbal teas for antepartal discomforts; the use of massage, Reiki, or Therapeutic Touch during the first stage of labor; the use of music and aromatherapy during labor and childbirth; and the increased emphasis on skin-to-skin, mother-to-baby bonding in the immediate postpartum period.

Further evidence of this increased integration was the establishment in 1992 of the Office of Alternative Medicine (OAM) at the National Institutes of Health. The OAM was mandated by Congress to promote research into complementary and alternative therapies and dissemination of information to consumers. In 1998 the OAM was incorporated into a new National Center for Complementary and Alternative Medicine (NCCAM) with an expanded mission and increased funding. NCCAM is dedicated to exploring complementary and alternative healing practices in the context of rigorous science, training CAM researchers, and disseminating authoritative information to the public and professionals (NCCAM, 2008). Recently, NCCAM recognized a new domain of integrative medicine. **Integrative medicine** is an approach that combines mainstream medical therapies with complementary therapies for which there is evidence of safety and effectiveness (NCCAM, 2008). Many studies of complementary and alternative therapies are currently under way at the NCCAM, which can be accessed via the Internet.

TABLE 3-1 Concerns of the Holistic Healer

The holistic healer may be concerned with the following aspects of the patient's life:

- Exercise, breathing, and posture
- Self-care, including dental care
- Nutrition, hydration, use of dietary supplements, and method of food preparation
- Digestion and elimination
- Sleep/wake cycles
- Stress and emotional responses
- Purity of air, food, water, and environment
- Use of alcohol, tobacco, caffeine, and other substances
- Employment and unemployment
- Hobbies, sports, and other recreational activities
- Home life and relationships
- Spirituality
- Type and age of bed and bedding
- Types of clothing, cosmetics, and personal care products used
- Pets
- Exposure to and use of sound and music
- Reactions to weather and seasons
- Electromagnetic phenomena and exposure to radiation
- Exposure to sunlight and artificial light
- Travel
- Personality and temperament
- Fears (e.g., of heights, of death, etc.)

Source: Compiled from data in Lockie, P., & Geddes, N. (2000). Complete guide to homeopathy: The principles and practice of treatment. *New York, NY: DK.*

Benefits and Risks of Complementary and Alternative Therapies

Complementary and alternative therapies undisputedly have many benefits for the childbearing family and other healthcare consumers. However, many of these remedies have associated risks that must be considered thoughtfully before a decision is made to use them.

Benefits

Many complementary and alternative therapies emphasize prevention and wellness and place a higher value on holistic healing than on physical cure. In addition, many are noninvasive and have few side effects, and many are more affordable and available than conventional therapies.

Emphasis on Prevention and Wellness

The therapies of conventional Western medicine—pharmaceuticals and surgery—are typically prescribed after a disease has already manifested in symptoms. These therapies are, of course, entirely appropriate—and may be lifesaving—in certain circumstances; for example, albuterol for an acute asthma attack or an appendectomy for appendicitis. However, they may be limited in effectiveness for subacute conditions.

In contrast, most complementary and alternative therapeutic systems emphasize maintenance of wellness and prevention of illness. For example, a woman consulting a medical doctor for fatigue might be tested for iron deficiency anemia. If the lab test came back negative, the woman might be advised simply to try to get more sleep, and the physician might prescribe a sedative to help achieve a full night's rest. In contrast, a woman consulting a practitioner of complementary and alternative medicine (CAM) would likely be asked dozens of questions about every aspect of her life, including her childhood, relationships, work habits, diet, lifestyle, stressors, and even how she feels about sunny days versus rainy days (Table 3-1). These questions would attempt to unearth the underlying cause of even the most subtle complaints and to prescribe remedies in several domains (acupuncture, homeopathic treatments, herbs, nutritional modifications, lifestyle modifications, massage, color therapy, and so forth) early enough in the process of breakdown to restore wellness before significant disease manifests.

Emphasis on Healing Versus Cure

This holistic approach extends to the goal of therapy as well; that is, the goal of many complementary therapies is not curing an illness but rather healing the patient's psyche, spirit, body, and even community. The physician and author Dr. Rachel Naomi Remen describes healing as the leading forth of wholeness in people. "Sometimes people heal physically, and they don't heal emotionally, or mentally, or spiritually. And sometimes people heal emotionally, and they don't heal physically . . . People can heal and live, and people can heal and die" (Moyers, 1993, p. 344).

Noninvasive Approaches

In part because of this emphasis on healing versus cure, many of the therapeutic techniques offered by complementary systems are noninvasive and potentially enriching on many levels. For example, imagery is often used to help people with cancer enhance their immune function, but also to help increase their optimism and gain new access to feelings of love and nurturance that may have been buried by fear of their diagnosis. Meditation, hypnosis, and biofeedback are other mind-based therapies that are entirely noninvasive and can affect the patient on several levels. Massage and the other body-based therapies noninvasively promote healing of both the physical body and the patient's psyche. Music, light, colors, magnets, gems, and fragrances are also noninvasive and likely achieve their effects by subtly influencing the neurochemistry, circulation, memories, and/or emotions of the patient. Indeed, only a very few of the complementary therapies are invasive: these include acupuncture, certain techniques used in ayurveda, foods and dietary supplements, herbs, and homeopathic remedies, which are highly diluted substances.

Cost and Access

Complementary and alternative therapies may be less expensive and more readily available than conventional remedies. For example, most homeopathic remedies cost less than $15 for a vial of 100 pellets or tablets. Essential oils, herbs, and dietary supplements also tend to be far less expensive than most conventional pharmaceuticals. In fact, some complementary and alternative therapies—including meditation, prayer, visualization, dietary modifications, and regular physical exercise—are free.

Visits to complementary healers are usually somewhat less expensive than visits to medical doctors; however, most insurance carriers do not cover complementary therapies unless the primary care physician has prescribed them. On the other hand, in some cases it is far easier to access complementary healers than conventional physicians, whether in the community or via their Web sites. By searching the Internet, it is possible for a childbearing family to glean tips on everything from relieving first-trimester nausea to preventing plugged ducts during breastfeeding.

Risks

These benefits of complementary and alternative therapies notwithstanding, it is critical that all consumers—and especially childbearing families—be aware of their not-insignificant risks. These include lack of standardization, lack of regulation and research substantiating safety and effectiveness, inadequate training and certification of some healers, and financial and health risks of unproven methods.

Lack of Regulation and Standardization

Pharmaceuticals prescribed by a Western physician or nurse practitioner have been tested and approved by the Food and Drug Administration (FDA). All preparations of an FDA-approved pharmaceutical, whether a brand-name drug or a generic version, have to contain identical quantities of certain precisely regulated, purified substances.

In contrast, herbs and dietary supplements do not undergo FDA testing or need FDA approval before they are marketed. Currently, the FDA is considering adopting new regulations for products that are marketed with health claims, but no such regulations are in place at this time. This lack of regulation means that non–FDA-approved products may vary dramatically from one manufacturer to another. For example, preparations of herbs may use the flowers, leaves, or stems, all of which vary in potency, and preparations may contain various concentrations of the actual herb versus carrier materials. Additionally, some manufacturers use such harsh chemicals to process herbs that their healthful properties are reduced or lost. Some herbs lose their potency over time with different types of storage, whereas others vary in strength according to the soil in which they were grown or the season in which they were harvested. This lack of standardization means that one preparation may be highly potent, whereas another is ineffective.

Lack of Research

Claims made by manufacturers of non–FDA-approved remedies may not be backed by valid, reliable research. The National Center for Complementary and Alternative Medicine (NCCAM) cautions: "While some scientific evidence exists regarding some CAM therapies, for most there are key questions that are yet to be answered through well-designed scientific studies—questions such as whether these therapies are safe and whether they work for the diseases or medical conditions for which they are used" (NCCAM, 2007e).

Approval by the FDA guarantees that a drug has been subjected to—and passed—a rigorous process requiring, in most cases, double-blind research studies substantiating the safety and effectiveness of the drug for the purpose under investigation. For this reason, when a childbearing woman is told that a certain drug will safely relieve her nausea or induce labor, she can accept these statements with confidence.

In contrast, the claims to effectiveness and safety of some complementary therapies may be largely unsubstantiated, resting on flawed or inadequate research, testimonials, tradition, or merely the healer's say-so. Thus, the consumer choosing these therapies often has little valid and reliable evidence that they will work effectively and safely.

The current inadequacy of research into complementary and alternative therapies is often due to lack of funding. When drug manufacturers commit millions of dollars to research and development of new pharmaceuticals, they do so knowing that, if they succeed in developing a safe and effective drug, their financial gain will more than cover their investment. In contrast, no one profits financially from consumers who use meditation, prayer, visualization, dietary modifications, exercise, water therapy, music, or sunlight. Even the profits from herbs, dietary supplements, or the body-based therapies are minimal compared with the costs of research studies to substantiate their use. Fortunately, as noted earlier, NCCAM is now funding research into several of these therapies.

Research into complementary and alternative therapies is also hindered by the very nature of these therapies. It is comparatively easy to provide a control group with either the drug being studied or a placebo and then to measure reduction in symptoms, but how does one design a reliable, valid study of therapies that attempt to maintain wellness or prevent illness; that value healing rather than cure; that claim to work on subtle, vibrational levels; or that admit to the necessity of a therapeutic relationship with the healer? Currently there is so little understanding of the cultural, psychologic, emotional, and spiritual aspects of healing that investigators trained in quantitative research methodologies may be unprepared even to design valid studies. On the other hand, it is interesting to note that several qualitative nursing research studies over the past decade have studied complementary and alternative therapies with some success.

Inadequate Training and Certification

Many complementary modalities require rigorous training and testing before applicants receive certification as practitioners. For example, naturopathic, homeopathic, and chiropractic physicians usually complete a typical undergraduate premedical program before enrolling in a 4-year graduate school in their specialty. Acupuncturists, certified massage therapists, Reiki practitioners, and some other complementary therapists must complete a course of study at an approved school, achieve a certain number of hours of practice, and pass an exam before they are certified.

In contrast, many titles are unregulated. For example, many states do not require that people calling themselves "counselors," "nutritionists," "healers," "intuitives," or "consultants" have any particular education or license. Thus, consumers who purchase the services of such therapists must beware.

Financial and Health Risks of Unproven Methods

As noted earlier, complementary and alternative remedies and techniques may cost considerably less than conventional pharmaceuticals and procedures. However, consumers may make a considerable investment in unproven methods and products that may not, in the end, improve their well-being, prevent illness, or promote healing.

Although few complementary and alternative therapies actually harm consumers directly, consumers' health may indeed suffer if their belief in the therapy or healer causes them to delay or forgo conventional medical treatments. Tragically, each year in the United States, cases of fetal demise occur among childbearing families who choose to use unlicensed birth attendants in home settings.

Types of Complementary and Alternative Therapies

The following review of complementary and alternative therapies is meant as an introduction. The list is not exhaustive, and the descriptions are exceedingly brief.

The categories under which particular therapies are discussed here are somewhat arbitrary. For example, homeopathy is categorized as a complementary therapeutic system, but it could also be considered an energy therapy. Therapeutic Touch and Reiki are both energy based and body based. Massage is a sense therapy in that it employs touch, yet it is classified with the body-based therapies. In truth, the holistic nature of these therapies means that they affect the patient in many different ways.

Complementary Therapeutic Systems

The complementary therapeutic systems described here are complex and multidimensional, incorporating different techniques into a holistic approach to wellness, prevention, and healing.

Homeopathy

Homeopathy is best understood in contrast to conventional Western medicine, which is also called *allopathic medicine.* The term *allopathy* is derived from the Greek words *allos,* meaning "different," and *pathos,* meaning "suffering." Thus, allopathic medicine, which has been dominant in the United States for over 100 years, uses remedies that produce effects differing from—or in opposition to—those of the disease being treated. For example, allopathic healthcare practitioners may prescribe an anti-inflammatory to reduce swelling or a sedative to relieve insomnia.

In contrast, the term **homeopathy** is derived from the Greek word *homos,* meaning "the same." Thus, it is often described as a healing system that uses like to cure like; that is, homeopathic remedies are minute dilutions of substances that, if ingested in larger amounts, would produce effects *similar* to the symptoms of the disorder being treated. For example, *Cantharis vesicatoria* is a species of beetle (commonly called Spanish fly) whose poison causes, among other things, burning urinary tract pain and a continuous urge to urinate. Homeopathic *Cantharis* is a minute dilution of this toxin and is thus a remedy of choice for women suffering from cystitis.

Founded by the German physician Samuel Hahnemann in the late 18th century, homeopathy traces its roots to Hippocrates, who was the first physician known to have observed the principle of like curing like. Homeopathic remedies are believed to achieve their effects by stimulating the patient's immune system to mount a response against the diluted substance. Thus, it is the individual's own body, rather than the ingested remedy, that opposes the symptoms. Indeed, homeopathic physicians advise that an initial worsening of symptoms indicates that the correct remedy has been given.

It is important to note that, although homeopaths do rely on certain standard remedies such as *Cantharis* for cystitis, they believe that physical symptoms manifest disturbances on far deeper levels. Thus, they work to peel away ever-more subtle layers of disturbance, thereby effecting holistic healing.

Application: Complementary Therapies

Naturopathy

Naturopathy is commonly referred to as *natural medicine.* Its central beliefs are that nature has healing power, and that the human body has the innate power to maintain or return to a state of health—and thus to heal itself (NCCAM, 2007c). Naturopathic physicians are eclectic, employing a variety of therapies in their practice. These might include clinical nutrition, exercise, botanical medicine, homeopathy, counseling for lifestyle modification, and other therapies. Moreover, they believe that physicians should be educators as well, so they teach their patients how to nurture themselves and encourage self-responsibility (American Association of Naturopathic Physicians, 2009).

Traditional Chinese Medicine

Traditional Chinese medicine (TCM) developed more than 3000 years ago in the Chinese culture and then gradually spread with modifications to other Asian countries, including Japan, Vietnam, Tibet, and Korea. Its goal is to promote health and well-being so the underlying focus of TCM is prevention, although diagnosis and treatment of disease also play an important role.

TCM seeks to ensure the balance of energy, which is called *chi* or *qi* (pronounced "chee"). Chi is the invisible flow of energy in the body that maintains health and energy and enables the body to carry out its physiologic functions. Chi flows along certain pathways or meridians, which are discussed further in the acupressure and acupuncture section.

Another important concept in TCM is that of *yin* and *yang,* opposing internal and external forces that, together, represent the whole (Figure 3-1 ■). Yin is the female force—passive, cool, wet, and close to the earth. Yang is the masculine force—aggressive, hot, dry, and celestial. Yin and yang cannot exist independently because they are complementary and both are essential. Certain foods, behaviors, and environmental factors are believed to increase yin, whereas others increase yang. Well-being occurs when

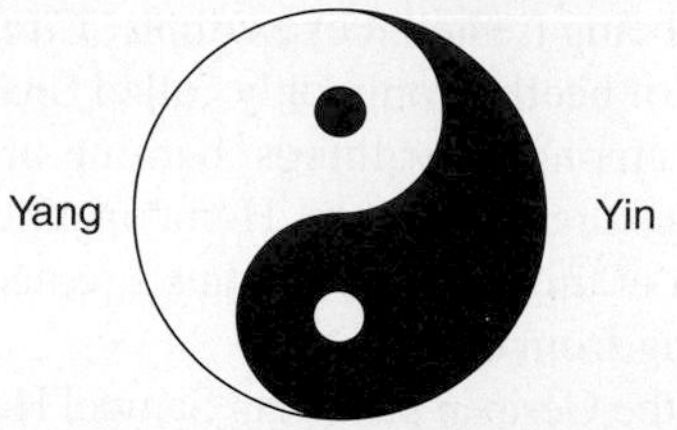

Figure 3-1 ■ Traditional Chinese symbol of the opposing forces of *yin* and *yang* in perfect balance, representing integration and wholeness.

these two opposing forces are in balance, and illness can result if this balance is disturbed over a period of time.

TCM includes the following therapeutic techniques:

- Acupuncture (discussed on p. 55)
- Herbal therapy
- Nutrition
- Acupressure (Chinese massage) (discussed on p. 54)
- *Moxibustion,* which involves the application of heat from a small piece of burning herb
- *Qigong* (pronounced "chee-goong"), which is a self-discipline that involves the use of breathing, meditation, self-massage, and movement. Typically practiced daily, the movements are nontiring and are designed to stimulate the flow of chi (Figure 3-2 ■).
- T'ai chi (pronounced "ty chee"), which is a form of martial art. It originally focused on physical fitness and self-defense but is currently used more as a health discipline. T'ai chi is helpful in improving balance.

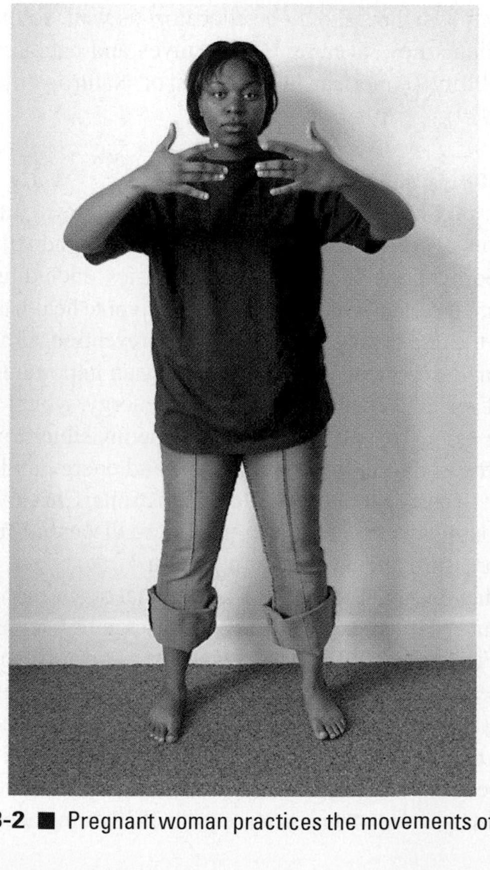

Figure 3-2 ■ Pregnant woman practices the movements of *Qigong.*

> "I am so glad that complementary therapies are becoming more accepted. I don't plan to stop going to see my doctor, but now that I am pregnant I like doing things on my own to improve my health. I used acupressure wrist bands early on and felt they really helped my nausea. I'm taking prenatal yoga classes now and I feel terrific! I think I will definitely continue doing yoga after the baby is born."

Ayurveda

The classical system of Hindu medicine is known as **ayurveda**. The term *ayurveda* is derived from the Sanskrit words *ayus,* meaning "life, health, and vitality," and *veda,* meaning "knowledge." Thus, ayurveda is the knowledge of how to live a vital, healthful life. Ayurvedic physicians believe that the five elements of ether, wind, fire, water, and earth take form in the body as three tendencies, called *doshas:* vata, pitta, and kapha. Each person's constitution is believed to reflect some combination of these three doshas. For example, vata reflects the elements of ether and wind; thus, a person in whom vata is dominant may be flighty and anxious, with dry skin, eyes, and respiratory membranes. The primary element in kapha is water, and so it is not surprising that pregnancy is considered a kapha condition.

An important part of the ayurvedic physician's job is to balance the doshas by suppressing the dosha that is dominating the patient and stimulating the dosha that is sluggish. The physician does this by addressing virtually all aspects of the patient's life. For example, a fatigued woman in whom kapha is too dominant may be prescribed hot foods and spices, certain herbs, warm colors, energizing music, pungent aromas, an earlier bed time and waking time, exercise, and other changes to stimulate her internal fire (pitta) and burn away some of her internal water (kapha). This is a simplistic example of a highly complex system, but the important thing to bear in mind about ayurveda is that, like homeopathy, naturopathy, and TCM, it approaches the patient holistically.

Mind-Body Therapies

This section discusses therapies engaging the mind in activities such as imagination, reflection, communication, and relaxation.

Biofeedback

Biofeedback is a method used to help individuals learn to control their physiologic responses based on the concept that the mind controls the body. An individual is hooked up to a system of highly sensitive instruments that relay information about the body back to that person. The effectiveness of biofeedback has been proven in countless studies, and it is now considered a conventional therapy more than a complementary one. For example, biofeedback may focus on temperature or thermal feedback, especially in treating certain vascular diseases or in promoting relaxation. It may focus on galvanic skin response, which measures sweat gland activity in the fingers or palms, in helping people learn to deal with stress. It may use electromyography (EMG) to provide feedback about muscle tension to help in the treatment of muscle spasm or tension headache, or electroencephalography (EEG) to gain feedback about brain wave activity to help with insomnia or pain.

Hypnosis

Hypnosis, whether guided by a trained hypnotherapist or induced through self-hypnosis, is a state of great mental and physical relaxation during which a person is very open to suggestions. Because hypnosis cannot make people do something against their will, it will not work unless an individual is really interested in changing. Studies have shown that self-hypnosis during invasive medical procedures such as breast biopsy can significantly reduce a patient's pain and anxiety (NCCAM, 2007a).

Meditation and Prayer

Many people think of meditation as sitting quietly with legs crossed and eyes closed, repeating a *mantra* or counting one's breaths to still the mind and bring peace. In contrast, the great spiritual teacher J. Krishnamurti (1895–1986) defined *meditation* far more simply, as something one can do every day at any moment. For Krishnamurti (2000), "Meditation is to perceive the truth each second . . ." by simply observing without judgment. When patients allow their family values, education, social conditioning, knowledge, desires, expectations, and all other "accumulations" to fade away, and listen receptively in a state of not knowing, they experience an emptiness that is itself transformative and healing (Figure 3-3 ■).

Whereas meditation is often likened to listening, *prayer* is an act of silently or vocally addressing a deity such as Allah, Jesus, Shiva, or the Great Spirit, or for those outside of a particular religious tradition, simply "talking to the Universe." Prayer specifically for health reasons is the most commonly used complementary therapy (NCCAM, 2005). The effect of prayer on healing has been studied and documented and more research is under way.

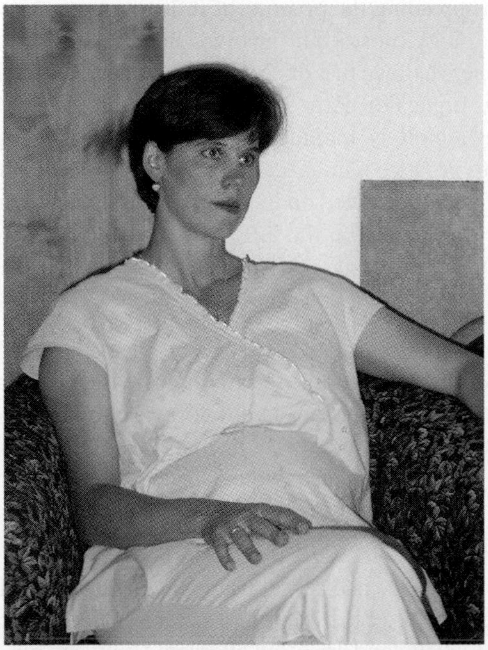

Figure 3-3 ■ Meditation does not have to be practiced in a particular pose but can be incorporated into each day. People who meditate regularly find it helpful to assume a comfortable position in a quiet area free of distractions. Eyes may be open or closed. This woman, 8 months pregnant, has chosen a comfortable position with her arms and legs supported. She is gazing into the distance, unfocused. Her goal is to open her mind and move into a receptive state.

Visualization and Guided Imagery

A complementary therapy, **visualization** has been used since ancient times. In visualization a person goes into a relaxed state and focuses on or "visualizes" soothing or positive scenes such as a beach or a mountain glade. Visualization helps reduce stress and encourage relaxation. For example, a therapist may work with a woman before childbirth to help her create positive images of labor.

Guided imagery is a state of intense, focused concentration used to create compelling mental images. It is sometimes considered a form of hypnosis. Guided imagery is useful in imagining a desired effect such as weight loss or in mentally rehearsing a new procedure or activity. Skill in using guided imagery improves with practice so people who wish to use it should set aside 5 to 20 minutes of quiet time once or twice daily and practice creating images that are personal and meaningful.

Manipulative and Body-Based Therapies

Therapies requiring practitioner manipulation of the body are discussed here, along with hydrotherapy, hatha yoga, and regular physical exercise.

Chiropractic Therapy

Chiropractic, the third largest independent health profession in the United States (behind medicine and dentistry), is based on concepts of spinal manipulation. It was developed by Daniel David Palmer, a self-taught American healer, in the late 19th century. Palmer believed that many diseases and illnesses were the result of abnormal nerve transmissions caused by misalignment of the spine (subluxation). He postulated that spinal manipulation could correct these vertebral misalignments.

To practice chiropractic in the United States, practitioners must earn a Doctor of Chiropractic (DC) degree, which typically requires 4 years of postgraduate study and clinical experience. Currently chiropractors are licensed in all 50 states and are regulated by state boards. Chiropractic has earned a higher level of insurance coverage than most other alternative therapies. Many health maintenance organizations (HMOs) and private health insurance plans, as well as Medicare, cover chiropractic treatment (NCCAM, 2007b).

Chiropractors focus on the close relationship between structure and function but also stress the importance of proper nutrition and regular exercise to good health. A number of studies have shown chiropractic to be effective in treating problems such as lower back pain. During pregnancy, chiropractic can help relieve the backache and physical stress resulting from increased body weight and a changing center of gravity.

Massage for Pregnancy

Massage Therapy

Massage has been used for centuries as a form of therapy. **Massage therapy** involves the manipulation of the soft tissues of the body to reduce stress and tension, increase circulation, diminish pain, and promote a sense of well-being. Different techniques have been developed, including, for example, Swedish massage, shiatsu massage, Rolfing, trigger point massage, Thai massage, and sports massage. Most forms of massage use approaches such as pressing, kneading, gliding, circular motion, tapping, and vibrational strokes.

Certification and/or licensure for massage therapists varies from state to state although most states require at least 500 hours of training. Massage therapists who have passed the written examination given by the National Certification Board for Therapeutic Massage and Bodywork (NCBTMB) are nationally certified. Continuing education is then required for recertification.

Certain massage therapists specialize in massage for women during pregnancy (Figure 3-4 ■). Massage is often helpful as women adapt to the discomforts of their changing bodies. In addition, certified nurse-midwives often use perineal massage before labor to stretch the muscles of the perineum around the vaginal opening and thereby prevent tearing of the tissues during childbirth. During labor, massage of the back and buttocks by the nurse, labor coach, or doula can help the woman relax and may help decrease her discomfort.

Infant massage has become increasingly popular in the United States (Figure 3-5 ■). The calm, soothing strokes of baby massage can help soothe an infant and minimize crying. In addition, research has demonstrated that massage can improve immune function, relieve pain, reduce anxiety, and promote relaxation and sleep (Sinclair, 2005).

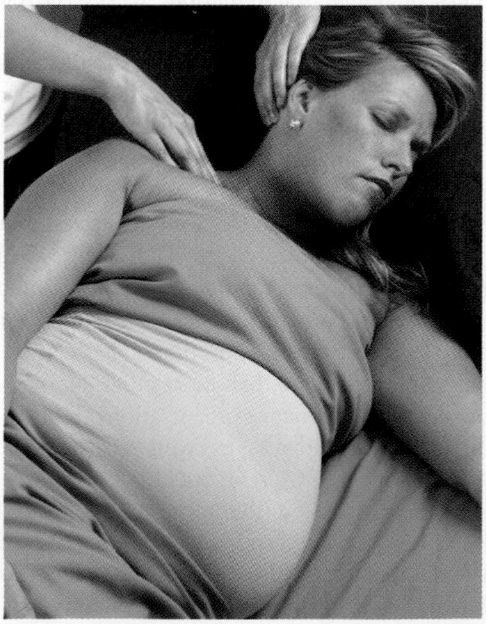

Figure 3-4 ■ Pregnant woman receiving massage. Massage is often useful in helping a pregnant woman cope with the discomforts of pregnancy.

Source: Alfred Wekelo/Shutterstock.

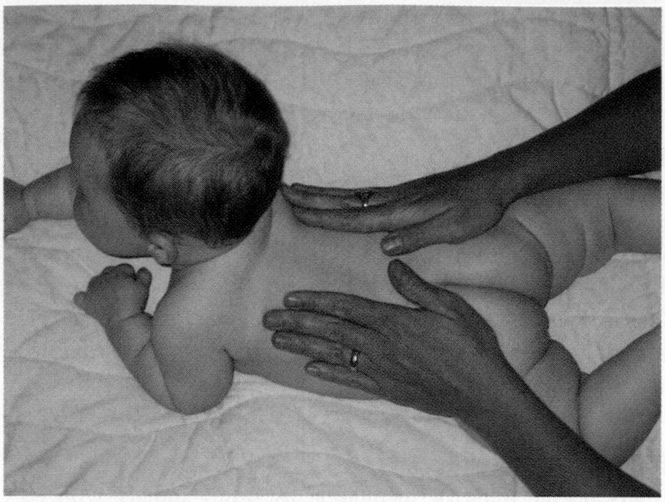

Figure 3-5 ■ Infant massage.

> “I got into infant massage when Ryan was born. I loved the time we spent together, and I am convinced it was part of the reason he was such a good baby.”

Reflexology

Reflexology is a form of massage that involves the application of pressure to designated points or reflexes on the patient's feet, hands, or ears using the thumb and fingers. Eunice Ingham, a physical therapist, mapped the specific reflex zones and is credited with spreading the practice of reflexology.

Reflexology most often involves manipulation of the feet. Practitioners believe that distinct areas of the feet correspond to particular organs or body systems. The stimulation of the appropriate region is intended to eliminate energy blockages thought to produce pain or disease. Organs on the right side of the body are represented on the right foot and organs on the left side are represented on the left foot (Figure 3-6 ■). Although they are used less frequently, the hands and ears have also been mapped.

Hydrotherapy

Hydrotherapy is the term used to describe therapy that makes use of hot or cold moisture in any form. Hydrotherapy is used to relax muscles, promote rest, decrease pain, reduce swelling, promote healing, cleanse wounds and burns, reduce fever, lessen cramps, and improve well-being. The major types of hydrotherapy include the following:

- *Compresses* (ice packs, hot water packs, towels or dressings soaked in hot or cold water and wrung out). Compresses are applied locally and are often alternated between hot and cold compresses. They are especially effective in improving circulation to a given area, thereby reducing swelling and promoting healing. They are also helpful in reducing pain or achiness in a given area.
- *Baths* (local, such as a foot bath or sitz bath, or full immersion bath). Baths serve many of the same functions as com-

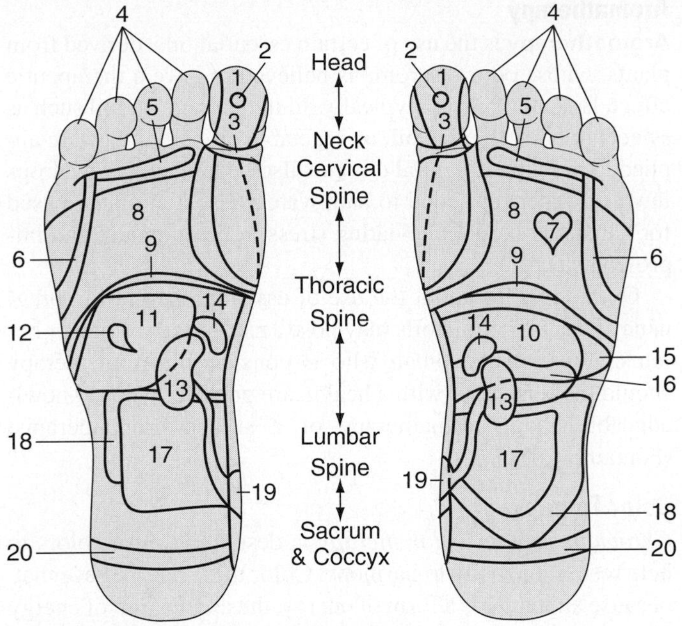

Figure 3-6 ■ Foot reflexology points.

Source: Fontaine, K. L. Complementary and Alternative Therapies for Nursing Practice, *2nd ed., 2005. p. 225. Printed and electronically reproduced by permission of Pearson Education, Upper Saddle River, NJ.*

presses but also are effective in cleansing. Warm baths are often used to promote comfort during labor.

- ***Sweat baths*** (steam bath or sauna). Sweat baths are used to open pores and induce sweating, which is thought to promote the elimination of toxins, drugs, and salts from the body. Because high heat has been associated with neural tube defects, pregnant women should not do steam baths or saunas, especially in the first trimester (Fontaine, 2011).

Hatha Yoga

When they hear the word *yoga,* most people think of people in leotards moving through a series of postures, such as the cat stretch or the salute to the sun. In reality, the term *yoga* comes from the Sanskrit word for "union," and implies a path toward union with God. **Hatha yoga** is the physical branch of yoga, and in the United States, it is commonly practiced for wellness, illness prevention, and healing. In hatha yoga, the individual moves through a series of gentle stretches and postures (called *asanas*) coordinated with deep, rhythmic breathing techniques that promote oxygenation of all body tissues.

Certain yoga positions are especially beneficial during pregnancy and can be practiced safely by most women. These techniques coordinate breathing with movement while increasing strength and suppleness, providing valuable preparation for childbirth. In many communities, yoga teachers offer classes specifically designed for pregnant women (Figure 3-7 ■).

Regular Physical Exercise

As more and more people are recognizing, regular physical exercise plays an important role in maintaining health and fitness. Exercise is important in maintaining muscle tone and strength, controlling weight, promoting cardiovascular health, improving digestion and elimination, reducing stress, promoting sleep, preventing a variety of chronic health problems, and providing an overall sense of fitness and well-being. In addition, exercise programs are an important component of ongoing therapy for a variety of health conditions.

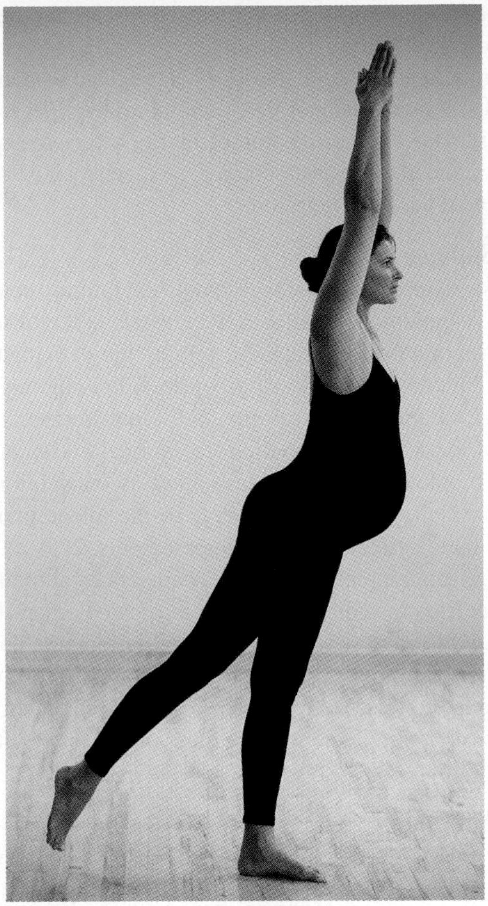

Figure 3-7 ■ Pregnant woman doing a hatha yoga stretch.

Source: Ryan McVay/Getty Images, Inc. Photodisc/Royalty Free.

For further discussion of exercise during pregnancy, please refer to chapter 16 ∞.

Nutritional and Herbal Therapies

The nutritional and herbal therapies include the use of particular foods as remedies; the use of vitamins, minerals, and other supplements; and the use of herbs.

Dietary Therapies

It has long been recognized that foods have nutrients that are necessary for health. However, the value of a nutritious diet in maintaining health is becoming more widely recognized and concerns are growing about the quality of some of the food products available today.

As part of their quest for optimum health, people make choices about their diets: whether to choose vegetarianism, a high-protein, low-carbohydrate diet, or a more balanced combination based on the U.S. Department of Agriculture's (USDA's) MyPyramid (see chapter 18 ∞); whether to consume alcohol in moderation or no alcohol at all; whether to include processed foods in the diet or not; whether to incorporate dietary supplements or not, and so forth. The literature offers a wealth of information about nutrition and diet therapy. Some of this information is grounded in data and research; other advice relies more on tradition and hearsay.

The importance of good nutrition for pregnant women and for infants and children cannot be overemphasized. Please refer to chapter 18 ∞ for a discussion of nutrition for women during pregnancy and the postpartum period and to chapter 32 ∞ for a discussion of newborn nutrition.

Use of Supplements

A *dietary supplement* is any product (excluding tobacco) intended to supplement the diet. It may be available for ingestion in the form of a powder, capsule, geltab, liquid, extract, and so forth, and it contains one or more of the following ingredients: a mineral, vitamin, herb, amino acid, other botanical supplements, or extracts and ingredients of animal and plant origin. Dietary supplements are not presented as conventional food products and they are not intended to be the sole item of a meal or of the diet (Office of Dietary Supplements, 2009).

Dietary supplements, sometimes called natural food supplements, are used to achieve a specific purpose. Perhaps the most widely used form of supplement is a multivitamin tablet or capsule. Other commonly used supplements are fish oil, flaxseed oil, ginseng, and garlic. Women who are pregnant should discuss the use of supplements with their caregiver or with a registered dietitian.

Herbal Therapies

An herb is a plant or plant part (such as leaves, flowers, or seeds) that is used for its flavor, scent, or therapeutic properties (NCCAM, 2009b). Like vitamins and minerals, herbs are a form of dietary supplement; thus, herbal formulations are not subject to Food and Drug Administration (FDA) premarket testing for safety and effectiveness. The FDA does have the authority to pull a product off the market if it is proven to be dangerous.

The use of herbs during pregnancy and breastfeeding is an especially important consideration for nurses working with childbearing families. Pregnant and lactating women interested in using herbs are best advised to consult with their healthcare provider before taking any herbs, even as teas. Lists identifying common herbs that women are advised to avoid or use with caution during pregnancy and lactation are available. For further information on specific herbs, visit the NCCAM Web site.

DEVELOPING CULTURAL COMPETENCE
Herbal Therapies

The World Health Organization estimates that 80% of the earth's population depends on plants to treat common ailments. Herbalism is an essential part of ayurvedic (Indian), traditional Asian, Native American, and naturopathic medicines. Many homeopathic remedies are also developed from herbs.

Sense Therapies

Most practitioners who use the sense therapies are trained in several. For example, to boost immunity, one healer might prescribe a varied menu of aromas, colors, and sounds.

Aromatherapy

Aromatherapy is the use of certain essential oils, derived from plants, whose odor or aroma is believed to have a therapeutic effect. Essential oils are typically diluted in a carrier oil such as sweet almond oil, olive oil, or vegetable oil before they are applied to the skin. Essential oils can also be inhaled (a few drops in warm water) or added to bath water. Essential oils are used for balancing mood, alleviating stress, relieving pain, and improving sleep.

Opinion varies about the use of essential oils during pregnancy because certain oils may pose a risk to the woman or her fetus. A pregnant woman who is considering aromatherapy should first discuss it with a healthcare provider who is knowledgeable about aromatherapy or a skilled aromatherapist (Fontaine, 2011).

Color Therapy

Chromotherapy or *color therapy* is designed to use colors to help restore the body to harmony. Color therapists believe that, because all matter is a form of energy, the application of energy to the body in the form of light can have therapeutic results. Because light can be split into colors, it is possible to deliver this energy at very precise levels and in easily controlled doses. After assessment, the color therapist exposes the patient to a particular color of light to promote healing.

Sound and Music Therapies

Sound therapy is based on the premise that when the body is exposed to the correct sound frequency (including some very low and very high frequencies that humans cannot normally hear) the body restores itself. A simple application of sound therapy is to encourage a woman in childbirth to moan on as low a pitch as possible during contractions. This opens the jaw, throat, and chest, and many women report that it promotes feelings of relaxation and power. In contrast, high-pitched squealing or screaming tightens the body and may promote feelings of fear. *Music therapy* can be considered a form of sound therapy. Music has been used during pregnancy and labor and birth to help soothe women and decrease their anxiety by stimulating endorphin release.

Energy Therapies

The energy therapies work at the most subtle level of the body to enhance immunity, reduce allergy, improve circulation, and improve neural integration.

Acupressure and Acupuncture

Both acupressure and acupuncture were originally part of traditional Chinese medicine. These practices are based on the traditional Eastern belief that the body's life energy, chi, which was discussed previously, flows along certain pathways known as meridians. The meridians—14 in number—connect all parts of the body. The places where the meridians pass close to the skin's surface are called pressure points. Stimulating specific pressure points can promote wellness, relieve pain, and contribute to healing.

Acupressure (sometimes called Chinese massage) uses pressure from the fingers and thumbs to stimulate pressure points.

Acupressure is easy to learn and is often used for self-treatment of tension-related ailments such as headaches, muscle aches, and tension due to stress. Pregnant women often use acupressure wristbands to help relieve the nausea of early pregnancy.

Acupuncture, considered the stronger technique, uses very fine (hairlike) stainless steel needles to stimulate specific points depending on the patient's medical assessment and condition. A treatment typically involves the placement of 6 to 12 needles. Acupuncture is used to treat a variety of conditions. Recent research indicates that acupuncture may improve rates of pregnancy when given with embryo transfer in women undergoing in vitro fertilization (NCCAM, 2009a).

Reiki

A Japanese technique founded in 1922 by Mikao Usui, **Reiki** is a form of hand-mediated therapy designed to promote healing, reduce stress, and encourage relaxation. Reiki practitioners place their palms on or just above specific problem areas and transfer energy to their patients to restore the balance of the patient's energy fields. Although the technique is entirely safe, the value of Reiki remains unproven (Lee, Pittler, & Ernst, 2008).

Therapeutic Touch

Therapeutic Touch is a complementary therapy designed to interface with conventional medical care. It was developed in the early 1970s by Dr. Delores Krieger, a nursing professor at New York University, and Dora Kunz, a clairvoyant healer. Therapeutic Touch is grounded in the belief that people are a system of energy with a self-healing potential. The Therapeutic Touch practitioner, often a nurse, can modulate his or her energy field with that of the patient's, directing it in a specific way to promote well-being and healing. Proponents of Therapeutic Touch believe that a strong desire to help the recipient is essential as is a conscious use of self to act as a link between the universal life energy and the other person (Fontaine, 2011). Many small studies of Therapeutic Touch have suggested its effectiveness in a wide variety of conditions, including wound healing, osteoarthritis, migraine headaches, and anxiety in patients with burns (NCCAM, 2007d). See Table 3-2 for more information about Therapeutic Touch.

Like many other conventional and complementary therapies, Therapeutic Touch should be applied cautiously to pregnant women and newborns by trained providers (Figure 3-8 ■).

TABLE 3-2 Facts About Therapeutic Touch (TT)

- Therapeutic Touch is taught in more than 100 colleges and universities worldwide and has been taught to more than 40,000 healthcare providers.
- The North American Nursing Diagnosis Association (NANDA) recognizes "energy field disturbance" as a nursing diagnosis, and professional organizations such as the American Nurses Association and the National League for Nursing have supported TT as a nursing intervention.
- TT is used as a complementary therapy for virtually all medical and nursing diagnoses as well as for surgical procedures.
- TT is best known for its ability to relieve pain and anxiety.

Source: Nurse's handbook of alternative and complementary therapies. *(1999). Springhouse, PA: Springhouse.*

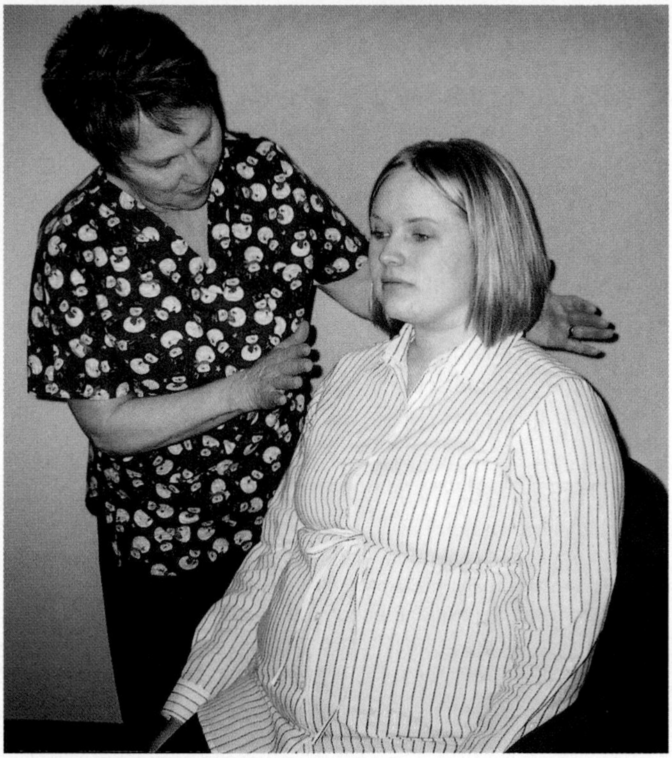

Figure 3-8 ■ During pregnancy, Therapeutic Touch is often helpful in easing pain and reducing anxiety.

Source: Nurse Healers—Professional Associates International, The official organization for Therapeutic Touch. www.therapeutic-touch.org

Application: Internet Information on Complementary Therapies.

Nursing Care of the Childbearing Family Using Complementary Therapies

Some form of complementary and alternative medicine (CAM) is currently being used by 38% of adults in the United States. Women use CAM more often than men do, as do people with higher educational levels and incomes. By race, American Indian/Alaska Natives are the greatest users of CAM, followed by whites (NCCAM, 2008).

As knowledge of complementary and alternative therapies grows, the number and type of people using one or more of them will probably increase as well. Thus, it is likely that the majority of childbearing families are using some form of CAM even though they do not share that information.

Assessing a Patient's Use of Complementary Therapies

The reality that women may use CAM and not reveal it raises some concern. Many CAM modalities are not likely to cause adverse effects during pregnancy. However, the possibility exists that there might be an adverse interaction between an herbal therapy and a medication prescribed by the caregiver. In addition, a few herbal remedies, such as cat's claw, are dangerous during pregnancy. Similarly, complications might develop from the use of certain vitamin supplements, especially if taken in megadoses.

Nurses who create a climate of respect and openness tend to be more effective in gathering information about a woman's use of complementary or alternative therapies. The following recommendations may be useful to nurses in taking a history:

- Ask questions that are direct and nonjudgmental in seeking information about the patient's use of CAM.
- Ask questions about specific therapies, including the use of herbal therapy and homeopathy. Because many people consider herbs to be natural substances and because they are often sold as dietary supplements, patients may not think to mention them.
- Avoid making negative or disparaging comments about CAM. Such comments send the message that CAM is not desirable and may discourage people from disclosing their use of CAM therapies.

Case Study: Complementary Therapies

Care Plan Activity: Use of CAM in High-Risk Adolescent Pregnancy

PROFESSIONALISM IN PRACTICE

CAM Awareness

All nurses practicing today need to have at least an awareness of complementary and alternative therapies. The NCCAM Web site is an excellent resource for healthcare providers and for childbearing women and their families.

CLINICAL JUDGMENT

Case Study: Sally Redwing

Sally Redwing is a 31-year old Native American software engineer visiting the women's health clinic for the first time. When asked the reason for her visit, she explains that she and her husband had been trying to conceive for the past year and that 2 months ago, her mother had convinced her to try her grandmother's "special herbs" to induce pregnancy. She had been taking the preparation once weekly for a few weeks when she noticed that her period was late. Yesterday she had used an over-the-counter pregnancy test kit, and the results were positive, so she was here to get "a real test" to confirm her pregnancy. When the nurse asks Sally the ingredients in her grandmother's mixture of "special herbs," Sally says she has no idea and asks whether or not the nurse thinks she should continue to use the herbs "for a while, to keep the pregnancy going."

Critical Thinking

What should the nurse advise Sally about continuing to use the herbs?

See www.nursing.pearsonhighered.com for possible responses.

Incorporating Complementary Therapies into Maternal-Newborn Nursing Care

Because the practice of nursing is holistic in nature, many nurses are open to and supportive of the use of complementary and alternative therapies. However, nurses in the United States need to know whether the nurse practice act in their state specifically addresses CAM therapies because some states do, whereas others do not. For example, in Louisiana registered nurses (RNs) may initiate and use complementary therapies for patients who seek the therapies as part of the nursing plan of care to meet goals such as relief of pain, comfort, reduction of stress, relaxation, improved coping mechanisms, and increased sense of well-being, if the individual has given informed consent. Written policies are required in all practice settings that permit the RN to perform such modalities. Nurses also need to be knowledgeable about any legal requirements that govern their use of CAM.

In working with childbearing families, or indeed with any patients, nurses who use CAM therapies should choose those methods that are within the scope of nursing practice in their state and not limited by the licensure of other providers (such as massage therapists). Nurses are also best advised to use CAM therapies that are considered somewhat mainstream and for which there is research supporting their safety and effectiveness. For example, nurses working with a pregnant woman might safely suggest acupressure wristbands for the treatment of nausea. Other therapies that nurses often employ include exercise and movement, Therapeutic Touch, visualization and guided imagery, prayer, meditation, music therapy, massage, hydrotherapy, and aromatherapy.

Nurses who use complementary modalities should document their use within the context of nursing practice. This is most effective when the modality is identified as an intervention to address a specific nursing diagnosis. Thus, music therapy might be used for a laboring woman to address the identified nursing diagnosis of pain.

Many certified nurse-midwives (CNMs) incorporate complementary and alternative therapies into their clinical practice with childbearing families. Research suggests that CNMs who prescribe CAM do so for the following reasons: nausea and vomiting, labor stimulation, perineal discomfort, lactation disorders, postpartum depression, preterm labor, postpartum hemorrhage, and labor analgesia. Research on CAM sparks great interest in the public, and momentum is increasing to design and carry out well-developed research on alternative modalities. Nurses have a role in conducting and supporting research of this type. Because of the variety of CAM therapies in use, research is needed in a host of areas.

The results of research on CAM can be found in professional journals and at the NCCAM Web site. As the evidence supporting the use of certain interventions grows, nurses and other healthcare providers are incorporating the results as part of their evidence-based practice.

FOCUS YOUR STUDY

- A complementary therapy is an adjunct to conventional medical treatment, whereas an alternative therapy is used in place of prescribed medical therapy.
- The National Center for Complementary and Alternative Medicine (NCCAM) promotes research into complementary and alternative therapies and disseminates the information to consumers and professionals.
- Integrative medicine combines mainstream medical therapies with complementary therapies for which there is some high-quality scientific evidence of safety and effectiveness.
- Use of complementary and alternative medicine (CAM) therapies may be beneficial. Many of them emphasize prevention and wellness, place a higher value on holistic healing than on physical cure, are noninvasive, and have few side effects. In addition, many are more affordable and available than conventional therapies.
- Risks of CAM include lack of regulation and standardization, lack of research substantiating safety and effectiveness, inadequate training and certification of some healers, and financial and health risks of unproven methods.
- The term *homeopathy* is derived from the Greek word *homos,* meaning "the same." It is a healing system that uses like to cure like; that is, homeopathic remedies are minute dilutions of substances that, if ingested in larger amounts, would produce effects *similar* to the symptoms of the disorder being treated.
- Traditional Chinese medicine (TCM) seeks to ensure the balance of energy, called *chi* or *qi.* Techniques of TCM include acupuncture, moxibustion, herbal therapy, nutrition, acupressure, Qigong, and t'ai chi.
- Ayurveda is the classical system of Hindu medicine. It promotes balance of the three primary forces thought to influence human health and well-being.
- Biofeedback is a method used to help individuals learn to control their physiologic responses based on the concept that the mind controls the body.
- Hypnosis, whether guided by a trained hypnotherapist or induced through self-hypnosis, is a state of great mental and physical relaxation during which a person is very open to suggestions.
- Guided imagery is a state of intense, focused concentration used to create compelling mental images.
- Chiropractic, a profession practiced by licensed chiropractors, is based on concepts of manipulation, especially spinal manipulation.
- Massage therapy involves the manipulation of the soft tissues of the body to reduce stress and tension, increase circulation, diminish pain, and promote a sense of well-being. Reflexology is a specific form of massage that involves the application of pressure to designated points on the patient's feet, hands, or ears.
- Hydrotherapy makes use of hot or cold moisture in any form to relax muscles, promote rest, decrease pain, reduce swelling, promote healing, cleanse wounds and burns, reduce fever, lessen cramps, and improve well-being.
- Hatha yoga, the physical branch of yoga, is commonly practiced to improve health and well-being, to prevent illness, and to promote healing.
- A *dietary supplement* is any product (excluding tobacco) intended to supplement the diet. It contains one or more of the following ingredients: a mineral, vitamin, herb, amino acid, other botanical supplements, or extracts and ingredients of animal and plant origin.
- Herbs, a form of dietary supplement, are used to treat the symptoms of specific ailments or to enhance overall health. Pregnant and lactating women should inform their primary care provider about any herbs they plan to take.
- Acupressure (sometimes called Chinese massage) uses pressure from the fingers and thumbs to stimulate pressure points. Acupuncture, considered the stronger technique, uses very fine needles to stimulate specific points.
- Therapeutic Touch is based on the belief that people are a system of energy with a self-healing potential. The Therapeutic Touch practitioner, often a nurse, can unite his or her energy field with that of the patient's, directing it in a specific way to promote well-being and healing.
- Many nurses are open to and supportive of complementary and alternative therapies. Nurses who incorporate such therapies into their care of patients must be certain that they are practicing within the framework of their nurse practice act and with the informed consent of their patients.

CRITICAL THINKING IN ACTION

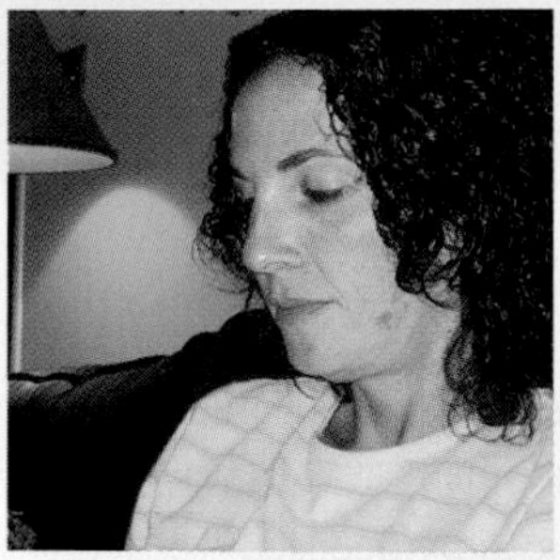

Rommy Startorius, a 34-year-old woman who has never been pregnant, is being seen for her annual gynecologic examination. As part of the health history you ask her whether she is using any forms of treatment for her health that are new since she was seen last year. Initially she reports that she has been getting massage therapy for low back pain and then, as the conversation progresses, she reports that she has been having acupuncture as well. She asks you how "regular" doctors feel about acupuncture and other forms of alternative therapy.

1. How would you describe the role of CAM in health care today?
2. What information could you provide about the use of acupuncture?
3. Mrs. Startorius asks you how she can learn about CAM therapies that have some research support for their effectiveness. How would you reply?

See www.nursing.pearsonhighered.com for possible responses.

Pearson Nursing Student Resources

Find additional review materials at **www.nursing.pearsonhighered.com**

Prepare for success with additional NCLEX®-style practice questions, interactive assignments and activities, Web links, animations and videos, and more!

REFERENCES

American Association of Naturopathic Physicians. (2009). *What is naturopathic medicine?* Retrieved from http://www.naturopathic.org/content.asp?contentid=59

Fontaine, K. L. (2011). *Complementary and alternative therapies for nursing practice* (3rd ed.). Upper Saddle River, NJ: Prentice Hall Health.

Krishnamurti, J. (2000). *To be human* (D. Skitt, Ed.). Boston, MA: Shambhala.

Lee, M. S., Pittler, M. H., & Ernst, E. (2008, April 10). Effects of Reiki in clinical practice: A systematic review of randomized clinical trials. *The International Journal of Clinical Practice, 62*(6), 947–954.

Moyers, B. D. (1993). *Healing and the mind.* New York, NY: Doubleday.

National Center for Complementary and Alternative Medicine (NCCAM). (2005, Winter). Prayer and spirituality in health: Ancient practices, modern science. *CAM at the NIH, XII*(1). Available at http://nccam.nih.gov/news/newsletter/pdf/2005winter.pdf

National Center for Complementary and Alternative Medicine (NCCAM). (2007a, Winter). *CAM at the NIH: Research Roundup, XIV*(1). Retrieved from http://nccam.nih.gov/news/newsletter/2007_winter/roundup.htm

National Center for Complementary and Alternative Medicine (NCCAM). (2007b, November). *Chiropractic: An introduction.* Retrieved from http://nccam.nih.gov/health/chiropractic

National Center for Complementary and Alternative Medicine (NCCAM). (2007c, April). *Introduction to naturopathy.* Retrieved from http://nccam.nih.gov/health/naturopathy/

National Center for Complementary and Alternative Medicine (NCCAM). (2007d, March). *NCCAM backgrounder: Energy medicine: An overview.* Retrieved from http://nccam.nih.gov/health/whatiscam/energy/D235.pdf

National Center for Complementary and Alternative Medicine (NCCAM). (2007e, February). *What is complementary and alternative medicine (CAM)?* Retrieved from http://nccam.nih.gov/health/whatiscam/overview.htm

National Center for Complementary and Alternative Medicine (NCCAM). (2008, December). *The use of complementary and alternative medicine in the United States.* Retrieved from http://nccam.nih.gov/news/camstats/2007/camsurvey_fs1.htm

National Center for Complementary and Alternative Medicine (NCCAM). (2009a, October). *Acupuncture shows promise in improving rates of pregnancy following IVF.* Retrieved from http://nccam.nih.gov/research/results/spotlight/020202.htm

National Center for Complementary and Alternative Medicine (NCCAM). (2009b, February). *Using dietary supplements wisely.* Retrieved from http://nccam.nih.gov/health/supplements/wiseuse.htm

Office of Dietary Supplements. (2009, July 9). *Dietary supplements: Background information.* Retrieved from http://www.ods.od.nih.gov/factsheets/dietarysupplements.asp

Sinclair, M. (2005). *Pediatric massage therapy* (2nd ed., p. 2). Baltimore, MD: Lippincott Williams & Wilkins.

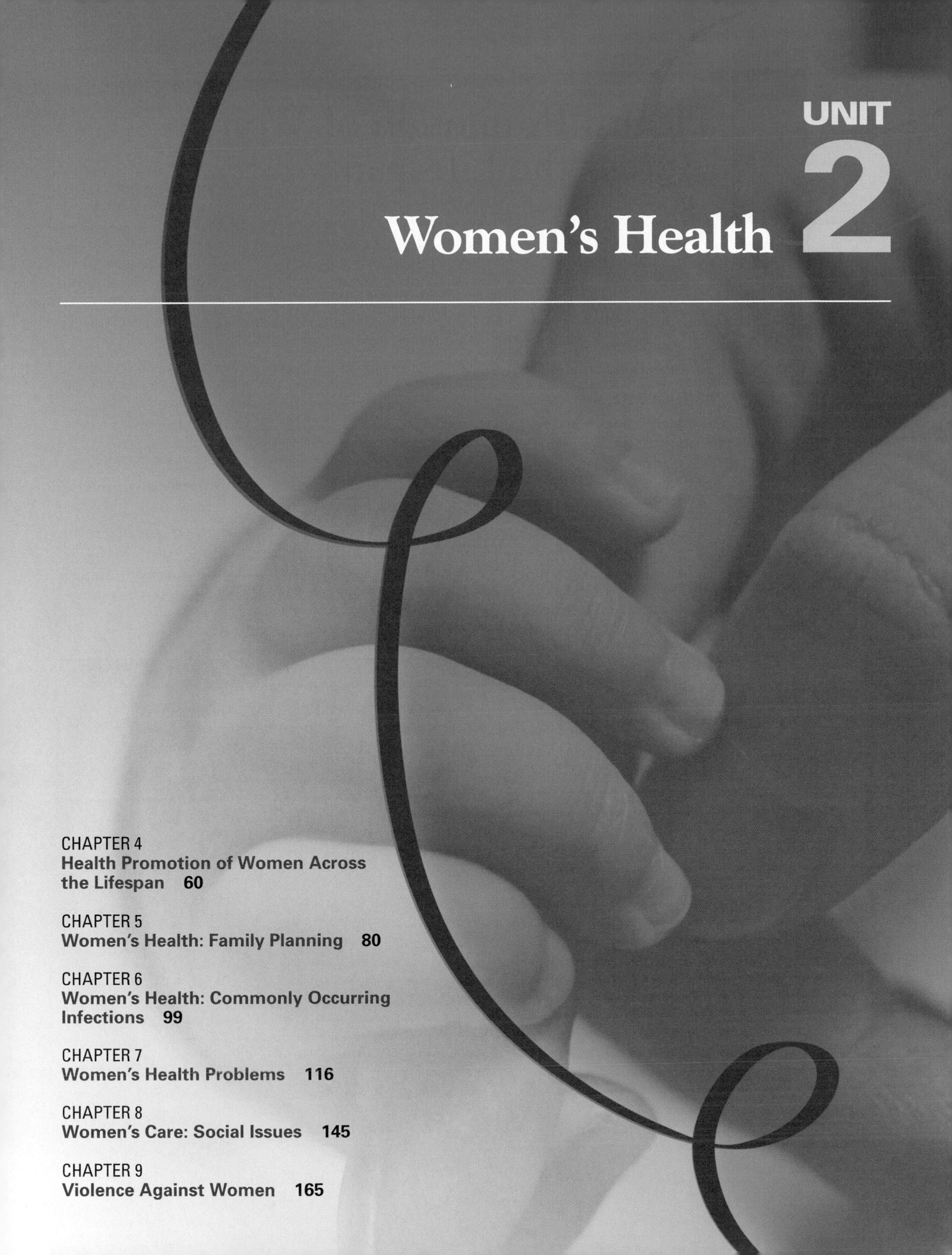

UNIT 2

Women's Health

CHAPTER 4

Health Promotion of Women Across the Lifespan

This is a great time to be a woman. I feel like I can accomplish just about whatever I put my mind to. There are more opportunities for women now in education, sports, and involvement in the community. I intend to take good care of this body and mind and strive for something great.

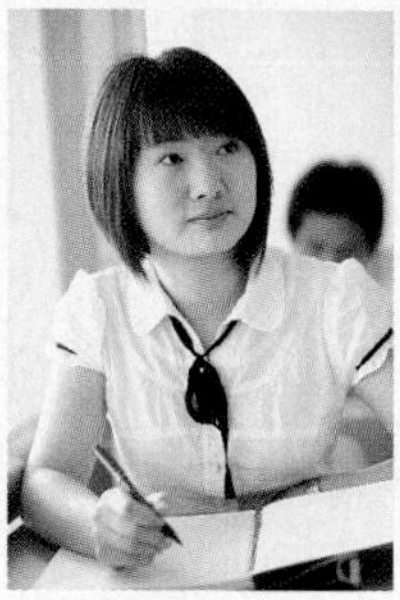

LEARNING OUTCOMES

1. Discuss the key points a nurse should consider in taking a sexual history.
2. Summarize information that women may need in order to implement appropriate self-care measures for dealing with menstruation.
3. Identify causes of amenorrhea.
4. Contrast dysmenorrhea and premenstrual syndrome.
5. Delineate the physical and psychologic aspects of menopause.
6. Explain the relationship between menopause and osteoporosis.
7. Identify medical and complementary therapies to alleviate the discomforts of menopause.

KEY TERMS

Amenorrhea *64*
Climacteric *69*
Dysmenorrhea *65*
Hormone therapy (HT) *72*
Menopause *67*
Osteoporosis *70*
Perimenopause *69*
Premenstrual dysphoric disorder (PMDD) *66*
Premenstrual syndrome (PMS) *66*

A woman's healthcare needs change throughout her lifetime. As a young girl she requires health teaching about menstruation, sexuality, and personal responsibility. As a teen she needs information about reproductive choices and safe sexual activity. During this time she should also be introduced to the importance of healthcare practices such as breast self-examination and regular Pap smears. The mature woman may need to be reminded of these self-care issues and prepared for physical changes that accompany childbirth and aging. By educating women about their bodies, their healthcare choices, and their rights and responsibilities, nurses can help women be knowledgeable consumers who assume responsibility for the health care they receive.

This chapter, the first of six devoted to women's health, focuses primarily on wellness care. Chapter 5 ∞ considers issues related to family planning. Chapter 6 ∞ focuses on infections women may encounter, and chapter 7 ∞ addresses some of the common gynecologic issues and conditions a woman may face. Chapter 8 ∞ explores some of the major social issues women face, and chapter 9 ∞ focuses on violence against women.

Community-Based Nursing Care

Women's health refers to a holistic view of women and their health-related needs within the context of their everyday lives. It is based on the awareness that a woman's physical, mental, and social statuses are interdependent and determine her state of health or illness. The woman's perception of her situation, her assessment of her needs, her values, and her beliefs are valid, important factors to be incorporated into any healthcare intervention.

CLINICAL TIP

In making decisions about effective methods for communicating with a family about healthcare issues, remember that a woman's views frequently influence the health care of her entire family because women typically coordinate the family's healthcare needs.

Nurses can provide health teaching and information about self-care practices in schools, during routine examinations in a clinic or office, at senior centers, at meetings of volunteer organizations, through classes offered by the local health department or community college, or in the home. Nurses can also help women with various forms of disability to address their unique healthcare needs and optimize their state of wellness. This community-based focus is the key to providing effective nursing care to women of all ages.

In reality, the vast majority of women's health care is provided outside of acute care settings. Nurses oriented to community-based care are especially effective in recognizing the autonomy of each individual and in dealing with patients holistically. This approach is important in addressing not only physical problems but also major health issues such as violence against women, which may go undetected unless care providers ask women specifically about violence and are alert for signs of it.

DEVELOPING CULTURAL COMPETENCE

Developing Effective Communication

The United States' population includes many ethnic and cultural groups. As a nurse you will be caring for women and families from diverse cultures. It is important to avoid ethnocentrism and to approach the childbearing woman with an openness to learning about her traditions and cultural preferences. Understanding subtle differences in various cultures will help you initiate conversation and ask questions that will allow the woman to offer information about her preferences. It is easy to misconstrue simple cultural differences. There will be times as a nurse when you say or do something that the patient or the family interprets as inappropriate and perhaps even offensive. Being sensitive to body language and facial expressions will alert you that this may have happened. Stopping what you are doing and asking questions will convey a sense of caring and can encourage communication, thus allowing the woman and her family to express concerns or misunderstandings.

The Nurse's Role in Addressing Issues of Women's Wellness and Sexuality

Women expect the nurses who care for them to be knowledgeable not only about gynecologic health, but about a wide variety of health topics. Thus it is important that nurses expand their knowledge about the issues healthy women and their families may face. These include, for example, a general knowledge of normal growth and development; recommended screening procedures for both women and men, and the ages at which these procedures are indicated; signs and symptoms of substance abuse, including alcoholism; health issues that well men face; signs of emotional stress and depression; community resources; and a variety of other topics. By keeping abreast of issues well families may face, the nurse becomes a more complete resource and acts to promote overall health.

On occasion, most women experience concern and even anxiety about some aspect of menstruation, contraception, or sexual activity. Societal standards and pressures can cause girls and adolescents to evaluate and compare with others their experiences with menstruation, sexual attractiveness, and beliefs and values about engaging in sexual activity. Young adults may be more concerned about the reproductive and health implications of sexual intercourse. The desire to achieve or avoid pregnancy and the fear of sexually transmitted infections may cause many women to modify their sexual practices and activities. Although older women share many of these same concerns, they may also experience anxiety about the onset of menopausal changes and wonder how these changes will affect their sexuality. Furthermore, throughout the lifespan women may have concerns, problems, and questions about sex roles, sexual orientation, behaviors, inhibitions, morality, and related areas such as family planning. Recently divorced or widowed women who have been in long-term marriages may need education about sexual activity and sexually transmitted infections if they are reentering the dating world.

Women frequently voice these concerns to the nurse in a clinic or ambulatory setting. Thus the nurse may need to assume the role of counselor on sexual and reproductive matters.

Nurses who assume this role must be secure about their own sexuality. They must also develop an awareness of their own feelings, values, and attitudes about sexuality so that they can be more sensitive and objective when they encounter the values and beliefs of others. Nurses also need to know about the structures and functions of the female and male reproductive systems. In addition, they should have accurate, up-to-date information about topics related to menstruation, sexuality, sexual practices, cultural differences, menopause, and common gynecologic problems.

Staying up to date on issues of sexuality and women's health requires constant vigilance: Regular journal review, attendance at reputable conferences, library and Internet searches, and diligent perusal of women's health literature are essential activities. Continuing education for the practicing nurse and appropriate courses in undergraduate and graduate nursing education programs can also help nurses achieve and maintain the requisite knowledge. These activities enhance the nurses' knowledge about these topics and improve their effectiveness in teaching and providing care for their patients.

Taking a Sexual History

Nurses today are often responsible for taking a woman's initial history, including her gynecologic and sexual history. To be effective in this role, the nurse must have good communication skills and should conduct the interview in a quiet, private place free of distractions. The sexual history is one part of a lengthier health history and covers personal and intimate topics.

> **CLINICAL TIP**
>
> When taking a history, start your interview with less intimate areas, such as medical and surgical history, and then proceed to the sexual history toward the end of the history-taking session. This approach helps the woman develop a comfort level with you before disclosing personal information.

Opening the sexual history discussion with a brief explanation of the purpose of such questions is often helpful. For example, the nurse might say, "As your nurse I'm interested in all aspects of your well-being. Often women have concerns or questions about sexual issues, especially as their life situations change. I will be asking you some questions about your sexual history as part of your general health history." This explanation will help women understand the nature of this part of the history and allow for more open, honest answers.

Case Study: Premenstrual Girl

It may be helpful to use direct eye contact as much as possible unless the nurse knows it is culturally unacceptable to the woman. The nurse should do little, if any, writing during this part of the interview. Open-ended questions are often useful in eliciting information. For example, "What, if anything, would you change about your sex life?" will elicit more information than "Are you happy with your sex life now?" The nurse should also clarify terminology to ensure accurate information is being conveyed. Proceeding from easier topics to those that are more difficult will help a natural flow of information. Throughout the interview, the nurse should be alert to the patient's body language and nonverbal cues. It is essential that the nurse listen, react in a nonjudgmental manner, and use teachable moments to educate women about their bodies. It is also important that the nurse not assume the woman is heterosexual. Nurses should be respectful of all patients when discussing their sexuality; some women will be open to this discussion, whereas others will be very reserved until a sense of trust in the caregiver is established.

After completing the sexual history, the nurse assesses the information obtained. If there is a concern that requires further medical tests and assessments, the nurse refers the woman to a nurse practitioner, certified nurse-midwife, physician, or counselor as necessary. In many instances the nurse alone will be able to develop a nursing diagnosis and then plan and implement an appropriate intervention. For example, if the nurse determines that a woman who is interested in conceiving a child does not have a clear understanding of when she ovulates, the nurse may formulate the nursing diagnosis ***Deficient Knowledge*** related to lack of information about the timing of ovulation. The nurse can implement a plan of care to evaluate the woman's knowledge, and then provide the necessary education.

The nurse must be realistic in making assessments and planning interventions. It requires insight and skill to recognize when a woman's problem requires interventions that are beyond a nurse's preparation and ability. In such cases, the nurse must make appropriate referrals.

Menstruation

Girls today begin to learn about puberty and menstruation at a young age. Unfortunately, the source of their "education" is sometimes their peers and sometimes the media; thus the information is frequently incomplete, inaccurate, and sensationalized. Nurses who work with girls and adolescents recognize this and are working hard to provide accurate health teaching and to correct misinformation about *menarche* (the onset of menses) and the menstrual cycle.

Cultural, religious, and personal attitudes about menstruation are part of the menstrual experience and often reflect negative attitudes toward women. In the past, many misconceptions surrounded menstruation. Women were often isolated or restricted to the company of other women during their monthly flow because they were considered "unclean." Currently in the Western world there are few customs associated with menstruation, although some women remain uncomfortable about discussing it. Sexual intercourse during menstruation is a common practice and is not generally contraindicated. For most couples, the decision is one of personal preference. (The physiology of menstruation is discussed in chapter 10 ∞.)

Counseling the Premenstrual Girl About Menarche

The average age of menarche is about 12.5 years for girls in the United States, but it may occur between the ages of 8 and 16. For about 2 years before menarche, a girl experiences a series of physical changes as her body develops. Maturity level and self-concept often influence a young girl's comfort in discussing these changes. However, the most critical factor in successful adaptation to menarche is the preteen's or adolescent's level of correct information and preparedness. The nurse is an excellent source of information about puberty and menarche. Information should be clear and straightforward and offered as it relates to each girl's individual situation and maturation level. The following basic information is helpful for young patients:

- *Cycle length:* Cycle length is determined from the first day of one menses to the first day of the next menses. Initially, cycle length may be irregular. It is not unusual for cycles to be unpredictable for the first year. Once established, the cycle is about 28 to 30 days, but the normal length may vary from 21 to 35 days. Cycle length often varies by a day or two from one cycle to the next, although greater normal variations may also occur.
- *Amount of flow:* The average amount of flow is approximately 25 to 60 ml per period. Usually women characterize the amount of flow in terms of the number of pads or tampons used. Flow is often heavier at first and lighter toward the end of the period.
- *Length of menses:* Menses usually lasts from 3 to 5 days, although the length may vary, and may last up to 7 days (American College of Obstetricians and Gynecologists [ACOG], 2007a).

The nurse should make it clear that variations in age at menarche, length of cycle, and duration of menses are normal, because girls are likely to be concerned if their experiences vary from those of their peers. It also is helpful to acknowledge the negative aspects of menstruation (messiness and embarrassment) while stressing its positive role as a symbol of maturity and womanhood.

Cultural factors may play an important role in menstruation for girls and women of some cultures. See Developing Cultural Competence.

Educational Topics

The nurse's primary role is to provide accurate information and assist in clarifying misconceptions so that girls will develop positive self-images and progress smoothly through this phase of maturation.

Pads and Tampons

Since early times women have made pads from cloth or rags, which required washing but were reusable. Some women made them from gauze or cotton balls. Commercial tampons were introduced in the 1930s.

Today adhesive-stripped, disposable minipads and maxipads and flushable tampons are readily available. However, the deodorants and increased absorbency that manufacturers have added to both sanitary napkins and tampons may prove harmful. The chemicals used to deodorize and increase absorbency can create irritation of the vulva and inner aspects of the vagina. This irritation may cause an external rash or internal sores from trauma to the tender mucosal lining of the vagina.

Interest is growing in the use of eco-friendly menstrual products including reusable menstrual pads made of washable cotton, menstrual cups, and menstrual sponges. These products are becoming more readily available at pharmacies and major discount stores.

Application: Teaching Adolescents How to Keep a Period Calendar

When taking a menstrual history, the nurse should attempt to determine the amount of bleeding each month. The woman can be asked what type of pad or tampon she uses, how frequently she changes, and how much blood has been absorbed. Women should be advised to change pads frequently, every 3 to 6 hours when awake, regardless of the amount of blood that is absorbed. If a woman reports that she supersaturates a maxipad every 1 to 2 hours for 2 to 3 days, she may be experiencing a gynecologic problem, requiring the need for further evaluation. Heavy menstrual flow is a leading cause of anemia in women.

The use of super absorbent tampons has been linked to the development of toxic shock syndrome (TSS). Women may prevent problems by using tampons with the minimum absorbency needed to control menstrual flow, changing them every 3 to 6 hours, and avoiding using them for vaginal discharge or abnormal bleeding. Women should be instructed on proper hygiene techniques for insertion and removal of tampons to decrease the risk of bacterial toxins being spread from hands to the vagina. Specifically, a woman should wash her hands before inserting or removing a tampon. After the tampon is unwrapped she should avoid touching the portion of the tampon to be inserted into the vagina. Most toilet systems become clogged if tampons are flushed. Thus, when a tampon is removed, it should first be wrapped in toilet tissue or placed in a disposable bag and then discarded in a trash receptacle or designated container. Finally the woman should again wash her hands.

In the absence of a heavy menstrual flow, tampons absorb moisture, leaving the vaginal walls dry and subject to injury; therefore, their use should be discouraged when the flow is too light to warrant a tampon. The absorbency of regular tampons varies. If the tampon is hard to pull out or shreds when removed, or if the vagina becomes too dry, the tampon is probably too absorbent. If a woman is worried about accidental spotting, she can check the diagrams on the packages of regular tampons. Those that expand in width are better able to prevent leakage without being too absorbent.

A woman may want to use tampons only during the day and switch to pads at night to avoid vaginal irritation. If a woman experiences vaginal irritation, itching, or soreness or notices an unusual odor while using tampons, she should stop using them and be evaluated for infection.

The choice of sanitary protection must meet the individual's needs and feel comfortable, whether it be pads or tampons. Young women should be taught to track their periods and to carry feminine hygiene products when their menses is due so that they are prepared for its onset.

Vaginal Sprays and Douching

Vaginal sprays are unnecessary and can cause itching, burning, rashes, and other problems. Healthcare providers do not generally recommend that women use them. If a woman chooses to use a spray, she needs to know that these sprays are for external use only, should be used infrequently, and should never be applied to irritated or itching skin.

Douching as a hygiene practice is unnecessary, because the vagina has numerous glands that provide a natural cleansing. Caregivers generally advise against it. The vagina has naturally occurring bacteria that aid in maintaining a pH balance to keep fungal and bacterial growth at bay. Douching upsets this vaginal flora, which can make the vagina more susceptible to infection. Douching with one of the perfumed or flavored douches can cause an allergic reaction. Propelling water up the vagina may force bacteria and germs from the vagina into the uterus. It is essential that women avoid douching during menstruation, because the cervix is dilated to permit the downward flow of menstrual fluids from the uterine lining. Douching is also contraindicated during pregnancy.

DEVELOPING CULTURAL COMPETENCE
Islamic Women and Menstruation

Islamic women who are menstruating are not allowed to enter a mosque for prayer, touch the Qur'an, or fast during Ramadan. These restrictions are based on the belief that menstruation is unclean. These women are also encouraged to limit their contact with others (Blumenthal, 2007).

Cleansing the Perineum

The secretions that continually bathe the vagina are completely odor free while they are in the vagina; only when they combine with perspiration and become exposed to the air does odor develop. Keeping one's skin clean and free of bacteria with plain soap and water is the most effective method of controlling odor. Bathing is as important (if not more so) during menses as at any other time. A long leisurely soak in a warm tub may also help to relieve cramps.

A woman can ensure herself of adequate ventilation by wearing cotton panties and clothes loose enough to allow air to circulate. After using the toilet, a woman should always wipe herself from front to back and, if necessary, follow up with a moistened paper towel or toilet paper.

The most important thing to remember is that if an unusual odor persists despite these efforts, a visit to one's healthcare provider is indicated. Certain conditions, such as vaginitis, produce a foul-smelling discharge that women often describe as having a "fishy" odor.

Associated Menstrual Conditions

A variety of menstrual irregularities have been identified. Several of them are discussed in chapter 7 ∞ in the section on dysfunctional uterine bleeding. Others are addressed in the following sections.

These terms are used to describe variations in uterine bleeding:

- *Hypomenorrhea:* short duration of menstrual flow or, in other words, uterine bleeding at normal intervals but in decreased amounts
- *Hypermenorrhea:* an abnormally long or heavy menstrual flow at normal menstrual intervals (sometimes used interchangeably with menorrhagia)
- *Oligomenorrhea:* bleeding, often irregular, occurring at intervals greater than 40 days
- *Polymenorrhea:* bleeding, either regular or irregular, occurring at intervals of less than 22 days
- *Menorrhagia:* bleeding that is excessive in amount and duration, which occurs at regular intervals (see hypermenorrhea)
- *Metrorrhagia:* bleeding, usually of a normal amount, occurring at irregular intervals
- *Menometrorrhagia:* bleeding that is excessive in amount and duration, which occurs at either regular or irregular intervals
- *Intermenstrual bleeding:* bleeding occurring between regular menstrual cycles

Amenorrhea

Amenorrhea, the absence of menses, is classified as primary or secondary. Primary amenorrhea is said to occur if menstruation has not been established by 16 years of age. Secondary amenorrhea is said to occur when an established menses (of longer than 3 months) ceases. Typically, the causes of amenorrhea are categorized into one of four groups:

1. *Hypothalamic dysfunction:* Several types of hypothalamic disorders can occur. Some are very rare disorders and may be related to a failure of the central structures of the hypothalamus to develop properly. Other disorders may be caused by a tumor. More common forms of hypothalamic dysfunction are triggered by systemic stress related to marked weight loss (anorexia, bulimia, fad dieting), excessive exercise (associated with long-distance runners, dancers, and other athletes with a low body fat ratio), and severe or prolonged stress.
2. *Pituitary dysfunction:* Pituitary disease and pituitary tumors, such as a pituitary adenoma, can cause changes in the many hormones, including prolactin, that the pituitary manufactures. A variety of medications, including several used to treat anxiety and other psychiatric disorders, can induce a mild increase in prolactin levels, resulting in amenorrhea. Amenorrhea may also be related to low prolactin levels resulting from pituitary failure. Sheehan's syndrome, head trauma, and cancer are also serious causes of hypopituitarism.
3. *Chronic anovulation or ovarian failure:* Some forms of ovarian failure are caused by genetic disorders often related to the sex chromosomes and are not treatable. Turner syndrome (see chapter 12 ∞) is one of the most common genetic disorders. Causes of chronic anovulation include polycystic ovarian syndrome or thyroid or adrenal disorders. Ovarian failure is related to exposure to radiation, chemotherapy, viral infection, and surgical removal of the ovary.
4. *Anatomic abnormalities:* This category includes a variety of structural disorders such as congenital absence of the uterus, ovaries, or vagina; congenital obstruction; or imperforate hymen.

Diagnosis begins with a thorough history and careful physical examination. For women who have had periods, this evaluation begins with a pregnancy test. For a woman who has never menstruated, the pelvic examination is a crucial assessment tool in determining that she has a normal vagina, uterus, and ovaries. Regardless of type of amenorrhea, based on initial findings, further, more specific tests are usually done. To evaluate pituitary function, a serum prolactin level is often obtained as a screening test. If serum prolactin levels are elevated, magnetic resonance imaging (MRI) will be ordered to rule out a pituitary tumor. Other pituitary hormones can be evaluated if necessary. Similarly, elevated serum follicle-stimulating hormone (FSH) levels indicate ovarian failure. A thyroid-stimulating hormone (TSH) level is assessed to rule out thyroid disease. A condition known as polycystic ovarian syndrome (PCOS) should be ruled out based on several diagnostic parameters as well (see chapter 7 ∞).

Treatment is dictated by the causative factors. Some conditions, such as imperforate hymen, are easily corrected. Other causes are not treatable. The nurse can explain that once the underlying condition has been corrected—for example, when the patient gains sufficient body weight—menses will resume. Female athletes and women who participate in strenuous exercise routines may be advised to increase their caloric intake or reduce their exercise levels for a month or two to see whether a normal cycle resumes. If it does not, medical referral is indicated.

Dysmenorrhea

Dysmenorrhea, or painful menstruation, occurs at, or a day before, the onset of menstruation and disappears by the end of menses. Dysmenorrhea is classified as primary or secondary.

Primary dysmenorrhea is defined as cramps without underlying disease. Prostaglandins F_2 and $F_{2\alpha}$, which are produced by the uterus in higher concentrations during menses, are the primary cause. They increase uterine contractility and decrease uterine artery blood flow, causing ischemia. The end result is the painful sensation of cramps. Dysmenorrhea typically disappears after a first pregnancy and may not occur if cycles are anovulatory.

Treatment of primary dysmenorrhea includes oral contraceptives (which inhibit ovulation); nonsteroidal anti-inflammatory drugs (NSAIDs) (such as ibuprofen, aspirin, and naproxen), which act as prostaglandin inhibitors; and self-care measures such as regular exercise, rest, application of heat, and good nutrition. Biofeedback has also been used with some success.

Secondary dysmenorrhea is associated with pathology of the reproductive tract and usually appears after menstruation has been established. Conditions that most frequently cause secondary dysmenorrhea include endometriosis, residual pelvic inflammatory disease (PID), cervical stenosis, uterine fibroids, ovarian cysts, benign or malignant tumors of the pelvis or abdomen, or the presence of an intrauterine device (IUD). Because primary and secondary dysmenorrhea may coexist, accurate differential diagnosis is essential for appropriate treatment.

Dysmenorrhea sometimes occurs in women who are also experiencing menometrorrhagia. In such cases, a careful examination is necessary to determine what is causing both symptoms. Testing may include transvaginal ultrasound, hysterosalpingography, and hysteroscopy. If the examination shows an endometrial polyp, treatment is removal of the polyp with a dilation and curettage (D&C) of the uterus.

For women with severe dysmenorrhea, use of continuous oral contraceptive therapy, which does not allow ovulation or menstruation to occur, may be of benefit. Hysterectomy may be the treatment of choice if there are anatomic disorders and childbearing is not desired. Presacral neurectomy may control severe dysmenorrhea caused by endometriosis.

SELF-CARE MEASURES FOR DYSMENORRHEA Some nutritionists suggest that vitamins B and E help relieve the discomforts associated with menstruation. Vitamin B_6 may help relieve the premenstrual bloating and irritability some women experience. Vitamin E, a mild prostaglandin inhibitor, may help decrease menstrual discomfort. Avoiding salt can decrease discomfort from fluid retention.

Heat is soothing and promotes increased blood flow. Any source of warmth, from sipping herbal tea to soaking in a hot tub or using a heating pad, may be helpful during painful periods. Massage can also soothe aching back muscles and promote relaxation and blood flow.

Daily exercise can ease existing menstrual discomfort and help prevent cramps and other menstrual complaints. Aerobic exercise—jogging, cycling, aerobic dancing, swimming, and fast-paced walking—is especially helpful (Figure 4-1 ■). Persistent discomfort should be medically evaluated.

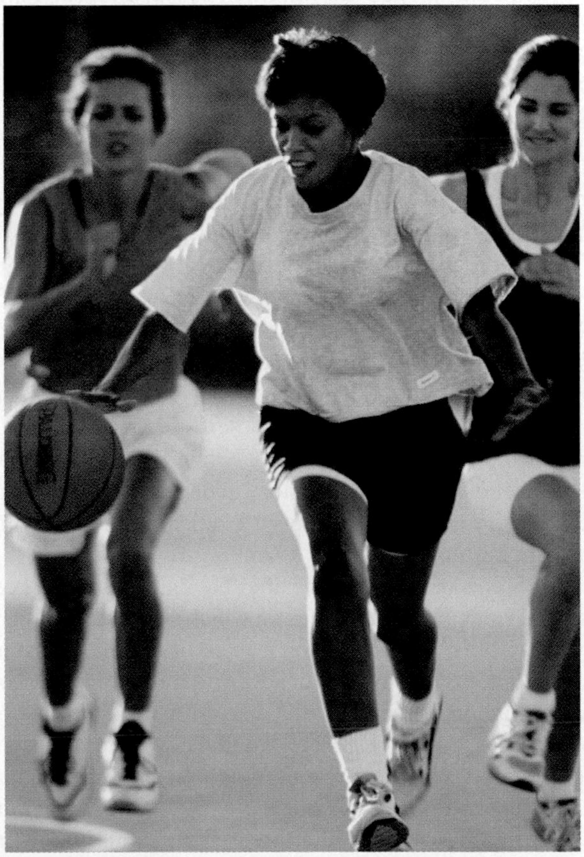

Figure 4-1 ■ Regular exercise is an important part of therapy for dysmenorrhea.

Source: Tim Pannell-CORBIS.

Premenstrual Syndrome

Premenstrual syndrome (PMS) refers to a symptom complex characterized by behavioral and physical changes that occur during the luteal phase of the menstrual cycle, anywhere from several days to 2 weeks before the onset of menstrual flow. The symptoms are relieved once the flow has started. It is estimated that clinically significant symptoms, resulting in emotional distress that impairs work, relationships, and activity levels, occur in only 12.6% to 31% of menstruating women. The majority of women seeking help with these symptoms are in their mid-20s to late 30s. A diagnosis of PMS occurs when a woman experiences one to three troublesome symptoms (Freeman, 2007).

Premenstrual dysphoric disorder (PMDD), a more serious form of PMS categorized as a depressive disorder, affects 5% to 8% of women of reproductive age (Freeman, 2007). Women with PMDD must experience at least five specific symptoms listed in the *Diagnostic and Statistical Manual,* 4th edition (DSM-IV) in the given time frame. These symptoms are relieved by menstruation and occur in most menstrual cycles.

Premenstrual symptoms include, but are not limited to, the following:

- *Psychologic:* irritability, lethargy, depression, low morale, anxiety, sleep disorders, crying spells, hostility, decreased concentration
- *Neurologic:* classic migraine, vertigo, syncope
- *Respiratory:* rhinitis, hoarseness
- *Gastrointestinal:* nausea, vomiting, constipation, abdominal bloating, increased appetite or food cravings
- *Urinary:* retention and oliguria
- *Dermatologic:* acne
- *Mammary:* swelling and tenderness
- *Musculoskeletal:* joint or muscle pain

The exact cause of PMS is unknown, although a variety of theories have been put forth to explain it. Evidence suggests that progesterone and estradiol levels are involved, although no consistent differences in these levels have been identified. Newer theories suggest that some women have an abnormal sensitivity to the normal changes of these hormones during the menstrual cycle. Central nervous system–mediated interactions between neurohormones and sex steroids may also account for the occurrence of PMS. Certain risk factors such as stress, genetics, obesity, or a history of depression or other psychiatric disorders may predispose women to these disorders (Freeman, 2007).

Diagnosis is generally made after having the woman keep a menstrual calendar for 3 months on which she carefully records daily symptoms, rating them on a scale of 0 to 4, with 0 used for no symptoms and 4 used for severe, debilitating symptoms. The information provided by the diary should be very helpful. In some cases, the diary may reveal that a woman has psychologic symptoms that are present throughout her cycle but intensify premenstrually. This is not a diagnosis of PMDD but an exacerbation of an underlying disease that should be referred for psychiatric evaluation. Except in very severe cases, treatment focuses, at least initially, on lifestyle changes and natural approaches. These are discussed in the following section. Some women will have a degree of resolution of symptoms with vitamin supplements or dietary changes, although relief will vary considerably from woman to woman.

Women with PMDD may benefit from selective serotonin reuptake inhibitors (SSRIs) such as fluoxetine hydrochloride (Prozac), sertraline hydrochloride (Zoloft), and paroxetine CR (Paxil CR) taken during the entire cycle or intermittently (half the cycle) (Endicott, 2007). The Food and Drug Administration (FDA) has also approved the use of an oral contraceptive called YAZ for PMDD. YAZ may be a good choice for women who choose an oral contraceptive as their method of contraception and who experience side effects from SSRIs or dislike the idea of taking them (Rapkin, 2008).

NURSING CARE MANAGEMENT

The nurse can help the woman identify specific symptoms and develop healthy behavior. After assessment, the nurse may advise the woman to restrict her intake of foods containing methylxanthines, such as chocolate, cola, and coffee. It is advisable for the woman to restrict her intake of alcohol, nicotine, red meat, animal fats, and foods containing salt and sugar. Concurrently, she should increase her intake of complex carbohydrates (such as whole grains, brown rice, oatmeal), protein, fruits, vegetables, and vegetable oils and increase the frequency of meals.

Supplementation with 50 to 100 mg daily of Vitamin B_6 may help women with some symptoms. A calcium supplement of 1200 mg per day is occasionally effective in reducing physical and psychologic symptoms of PMS. A magnesium supplement of 400 mg daily may help reduce fluid retention and bloating. Vitamin E taken in 400 international units daily may reduce cramping and breast tenderness. Herbal remedies such as black cohosh, ginger, red raspberry leaf, and evening primrose oil may reduce the effects of PMS. Underlying health conditions may contraindicate the use of herbal or vitamin supplements, however, and must be considered when recommending them. Natural progesterone creams derived from wild yams or soybeans may provide relief to some women; however, no scientific studies have shown this to be true (Mayo Clinic Staff, 2007).

A program of aerobic exercises such as fast walking, jogging, or aerobic dancing is generally beneficial. In fact, women who exercise regularly tend to have fewer, less severe symptoms.

An empathic relationship with a healthcare professional to whom the woman feels free to voice concerns is highly beneficial. The nurse can also encourage the woman to keep a journal to help identify life events associated with PMS. Stress reduction education, self-care groups, and self-help literature can also help women gain control over their bodies.

Health Promotion Education for Well Women

Healthcare providers are becoming increasingly aware of the value of health maintenance and disease prevention, as are many consumers of healthcare services. Women can make lifestyle choices that promote health and well-being. These choices involve a variety of factors, including:

- Eating a nutritious, balanced diet.
- Maintaining normal weight for height (no fad dieting).
- Performing regular aerobic exercise and weight training several times a week.
- Getting adequate sleep.
- Avoiding smoking and/or stopping smoking.
- Consuming alcohol in moderation.
- Managing stress effectively.
- Developing enjoyable hobbies and leisure activities.
- Developing an inner life in some form through religion, spirituality, personal reflection, yoga, and so forth.
- Fostering bonds of support and affection with family and friends.
- Obtaining regular health screenings and assessments.
- Ensuring that immunizations are up to date.

Health screening recommendations vary by age. Table 4-1 from the National Women's Health Information Center (2009) identifies general screening and immunization guidelines for low-risk women based on their ages. Nurses can share this information with well women so that they can be aware of indicated screening procedures.

Body Piercing and Tattoos

Body piercing and tattooing, often called *body art,* are rapidly becoming commonplace in today's culture among people of all ages (Figure 4-2 ■).

Tattooing is the application of minute amounts of pigments into the skin with indelible inks. The ritual of tattooing appears far back in history in most ancient cultures (Donohoe, 2006). Body piercing sites include earlobes and ear cartilage, lips, nose, tongue, eyebrow, nipples, umbilicus, and the external genitalia for the purpose of displaying some form of adornment or jewelry. Estimates suggest that in the United States as many as 50% of undergraduates have had some form of body piercing (Donohoe, 2006).

Each of these forms of body art carries with it an element of health risk. For tattooing and body piercing, risks include infections such as HIV and hepatitis B and C because of the use of inadequately sterilized equipment, as well as allergic reactions, local swelling and burns, granulomas, and keloid formation (more common in people of African descent). Tattooing has also been associated with a variety of risk-taking behaviors in adolescents (Donohoe, 2006). Oral piercing has been associated with tooth and gum damage. Among pregnant or breastfeeding women, nipple piercing has been associated with mastitis, damaged milk ducts, difficulty with breastfeeding, and galactorrhea (Camann, 2006).

Educating patients about the risks associated with these practices should include information about infection, permanent scarring, keloid formation, and care afterward. It is important for the nurse to avoid passing judgment or making generalizations about individuals who have these types of body alterations.

Menopause

Menopause, defined as the absence of menstruation for 1 full year, is a time of transition for a woman, marking the end of her reproductive abilities. Although it usually occurs between 45 and 52 years of age, the current median age of menopause in the United States is approximately 50 to 51 years of age (Curran,

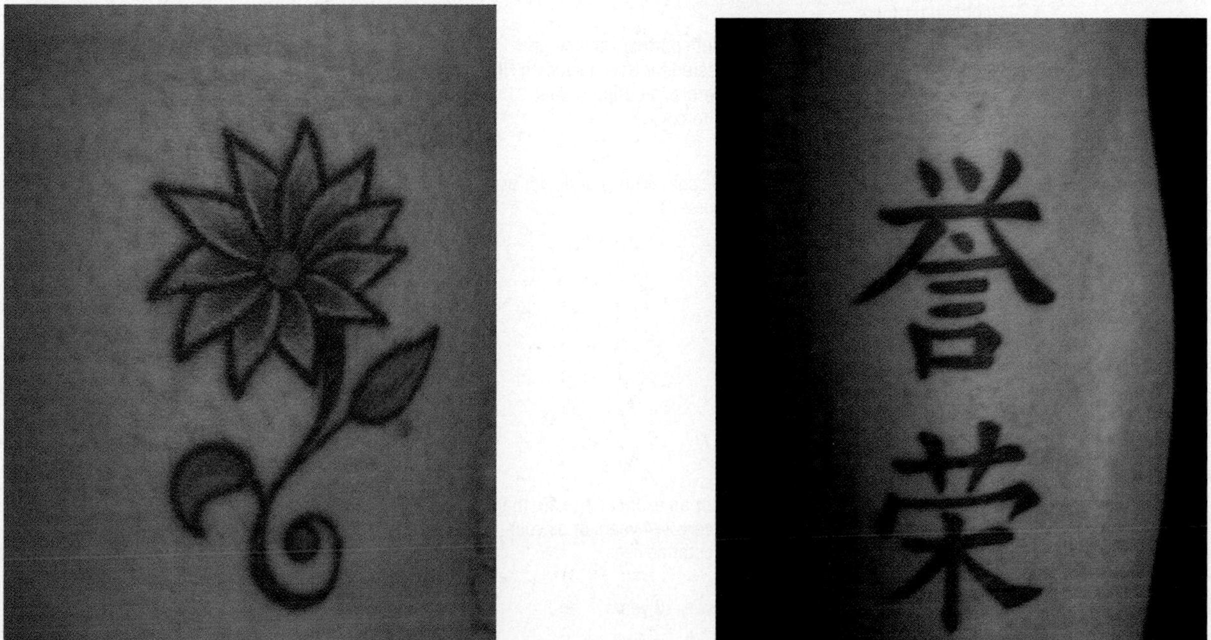

A B

Figure 4-2 ■ Tattoos vary greatly in size, complexity, and meaning to the individual. A. This tattoo, on the ankle of a young woman, is purely decorative. B. This tattoo, on the shin of a young man, is the Chinese symbol for honor. He chose it to express a personal commitment to live a life of integrity.

TABLE 4-1 Recommended Screenings and Immunizations for Women at Average Risk for Most Diseases

SCREENING TEST	AGES 18–39	AGES 40–49	AGES 50–64	AGES 65 AND OLDER
General Health				
Full checkup, including weight and height	Discuss with your doctor or nurse	Discuss with your doctor or nurse	Discuss with your doctor or nurse	Discuss with your doctor or nurse
Thyroid test	Start at age 35, then every 5 years	Every 5 years	Every 5 years	Every 5 years
HIV test	Get this at least once to find out your HIV status. Ask your doctor if and when you need the test again.	Get this at least once to find out your HIV status. Ask your doctor if and when you need the test again.	Get this at least once to find out your HIV status. Ask your doctor if and when you need the test again.	Discuss with your doctor or nurse.
Heart Health				
Blood pressure test	At least every 2 years	At least every 2 years	At least every 2 years	At least every 2 years
Cholesterol test	Start at age 20, discuss with your doctor or nurse.	Discuss with your doctor or nurse.	Discuss with your doctor or nurse.	Discuss with your doctor or nurse.
Bone Health				
Bone density screen		Discuss with your doctor or nurse.	Discuss with your doctor or nurse.	Get a bone mineral density test at least once. Talk to your doctor or nurse about repeat testing.
Diabetes				
Blood glucose test	Discuss with your doctor or nurse.	Start at age 45, then every 3 years.	Every 3 years	Every 3 years
Breast Health				
Mammogram (x-ray of breast)		Every 1–2 years. Discuss with your doctor or nurse.	Every 1–2 years. Discuss with your doctor or nurse.	Every 1–2 years. Discuss with your doctor or nurse.
Clinical breast exam	At least every 3 years starting in your 20s	Yearly	Yearly	Yearly
Reproductive Health				
PAP test	Every 1–3 years if you have been sexually active or are older than 21	Every 1–3 years	Every 1–3 years	Discuss with your doctor or nurse.
Pelvic exam	Yearly	Yearly	Yearly	Yearly
Chlamydia test	Yearly until age 25 if sexually active. Older than 26, get this test if you have new or multiple partners.	Get this test if you have new or multiple partners.	Get this test if you have new or multiple partners.	Get this test if you have new or multiple partners.
Sexually transmitted infection (STI) tests	Both partners should get tested for STIs, including HIV, before initiating sexual intercourse	Both partners should get tested for STIs, including HIV, before initiating sexual intercourse	Both partners should get tested for STIs, including HIV, before initiating sexual intercourse	Both partners should get tested for STIs, including HIV, before initiating sexual intercourse
Mental Health				
Mental health screening	Discuss with your doctor or nurse.	Discuss with your doctor or nurse.	Discuss with your doctor or nurse.	Discuss with your doctor or nurse.
Colorectal Health (use one of the following methods)				
Fecal occult blood test			Yearly	Yearly. Older than 75, discuss with your doctor.
Flexible sigmoidoscopy (with fecal occult blood test)			Every 5 years	Every 5 years. Older than 75, discuss with your doctor.
Colonoscopy			Every 10 years	Every 10 years. Older than 75, discuss with your doctor.
Eye and Ear Health				
Complete eye exam	At least once between the ages of 20–29; at least twice between the ages of 30–39; any time that you have a problem	Get an exam at age 40, then every 2–4 years or as your doctor advises	Every 2–4 years or as your doctor advises	Every 1–2 years
Hearing test	Starting at age 18, then every 10 years	Every 10 years	Every 3 years	Every 3 years
Skin Health				
Mole exam	Monthly mole self-exam; by a doctor as part of a routine full checkup starting at age 20.	Monthly mole self-exam; by a doctor as part of a routine full checkup.	Monthly mole self-exam; by a doctor as part of a routine full checkup.	Monthly mole self-exam; by a doctor as part of a routine full checkup.

TABLE 4-1 Recommended Screenings and Immunizations for Women at Average Risk for Most Diseases continued

SCREENING TEST	AGES 18–39	AGES 40–49	AGES 50–64	AGES 65 AND OLDER
Oral Health				
Dental exam	Routinely; discuss with your dentist.	Routinely; discuss with your dentist.	Routinely; discuss with your dentist.	Routinely; discuss with your dentist.
Immunizations				
Influenza vaccine	Discuss with your doctor or nurse.	Discuss with your doctor or nurse.	Yearly	Yearly
Pneumococcal vaccine				One time only
Tentanus-diptheria booster vaccine	Every 10 years	Every 10 years	Every 10 years	Every 10 years
Human papilloma virus (HPV) vaccine	Up to age 26, if not already completed vaccine series; discuss with your doctor or nurse.			
Meningococcal vaccine	Discuss with your doctor or nurse if attending college			
Herpes zoster vaccine (to prevent shingles)			Starting at age 60, one time only. Ask your doctor if it is okay for you to get it.	Starting at age 60, one time only. Ask your doctor if it is okay for you to get it.

Source: The National Women's Health Information Center. (2009). Recommended screenings and immunizations for women at average risk for most diseases. *Washington, DC: Office of Women's Health, U.S. Department of Health and Human Services.*

2008). Not all of the physiologic mechanisms initiating menopause are precisely understood; however, it is known that the onset occurs when estrogen levels drop because of cessation of ovarian function. In addition, most researchers agree that the age of onset is influenced by such factors as the woman's overall health, weight, nutrition, lifestyle, culture, and genetic factors.

Climacteric, or *change of life* (often used synonymously with *menopause*), refers to the host of psychologic and physical alterations that occur around the time of menopause. These aspects are discussed separately.

Perimenopause

Perimenopause refers to the period of time before menopause during which the woman moves from normal ovulatory cycles to cessation of menses. Women in perimenopause will generally begin having menstrual irregularities and changes in estrogen and follicle stimulating hormone (FSH). The perimenopause can last 2 to 8 years (Freeman, 2008).

Symptoms of perimenopause vary significantly in women. It is estimated that more than 80% of women in the perimenopause report some degree of vasomotor symptoms (hot flashes). It is important that women in this age group be screened thoroughly to rule out other causes of vasomotor symptoms. Mood and cognitive changes are also a common complaint, with women expressing concern over emotional instability and a decrease in memory. These may, in fact, be the more concerning symptoms women express to their healthcare providers. Changes in sexuality are common and may include decreased libido, vaginal lubrication, and comfort with sexual intercourse. Estimates indicate that nearly 75% of perimenopausal women experience these changes to some degree (Freeman, 2008).

Contraception remains a major concern for many perimenopausal women. Although a growing number of women are choosing to delay childbearing, 38% of pregnancies for women ages 40 and higher are unplanned (Speroff & Wysocki, 2009). As women age fertility decreases and the risk of spontaneous abortion increases. In women who delay pregnancy until after age 40, risks for pregnancy complications are approximately twofold to sixfold higher. These complications include hypertensive disorders, diabetes, placenta previa, and placental abruption. These complications in turn increase the rate of preterm birth, intrauterine growth restriction, and serious neonatal complications (ACOG, 2006).

In the United States, female sterilization is, in general, the most commonly used method of contraception among couples over age 35 (Sufrin & Korn, 2009). In 2002 the Food and Drug Administration approved a nonsurgical method of female sterilization known as the Essure method (see chapter 5 ∞) (Sufrin & Korn, 2009).

However, combined hormonal contraceptives (the pill, patches, and vaginal rings) continue to be popular forms of contraception during this time in a woman's reproductive life. Combined hormonal contraceptives prevent pregnancy and provide noncontraceptive benefits. Healthy nonsmokers benefit from effective contraception; regulation of menses; treatment of anovulatory bleeding; relief of symptoms of estrogen deficiency and variability such as hot flashes, sleep disturbances, menorrhagia, and vaginal dryness; and a decreased risk of endometrial and ovarian cancer. They may also experience less acne and hirsutism (abnormal hair growth, often on the face and neck) and decreased osteopenia. Thus they are considered by many to be an optimal approach to this transition, even when contraception is not a concern. Other contraceptive options for perimenopausal women include sterilization; contraceptive intrauterine devices (IUDs); progestin-only methods of contraception; and barrier methods of contraception such as male and female condoms, diaphragm, cervical cap, and spermicides (Speroff & Wysocki, 2009). (See chapter 5 ∞ for a discussion of these methods.)

Women describing problems that suggest perimenopause should be referred to their care providers. If oral contraceptives are not an option, other alternatives are available. Exercise, calcium and vitamin D, and other supplements or medications may be effective.

Psychologic Aspects of Menopause

A woman's psychologic adaptation to menopause and the climacteric is multifactorial. It is often further complicated because women of this age may be dealing with other life circumstances such as adjustment to an "empty nest" or caring for aging parents. Numerous personal factors influence a woman's ability to transition and cope with these changes, such as self-concept, physical health, marital stability, relationship with others, and cultural values. Some women express disappointment in approaching this time of their lives, whereas others may see it as a positive transition that offers freedom from menses or concern about contraception. Women who are dealing with aging, ill parents may have increased stressors that affect their emotional health and ability to deal with their symptoms. Often night sweats and insomnia affect a woman's capability to cope because of increased fatigue.

As a nurse, understanding the basic physiology of menopause offers an opportunity to provide education, supportive resources, and encouragement to women at this time in their lives. Suggesting exercises and teaching proper nutrition are critical for overall health and may help these women improve the emotional aspects associated with menopause. It is important to help women understand the changes that come with menopause and deal with their feelings during this period. Moreover, caregivers need to be alert for signs that distinguish between the mood swings that are related to hormonal changes and true clinical depression.

Today the average woman in the United States will live one third of her life after menopause (Curran, 2008). The changing perceptions of menopause and beyond are enabling menopausal women to cope more effectively and to view menopause as a time of personal growth.

> "My personal response to menopause has surprised me a little. Suddenly 52 doesn't really seem old. I look at pictures of my mother in her early 50s and she seems so much older. I imagine each generation looks back and thinks the same thing. I do wish I had known at 22 what I know now, but I still see myself as learning and growing. I know I have a lot to offer and a lot of choices in how to accomplish that. One thing I'm committed to is trying to live each day as well as I can, to stay positive, and to keep looking forward."

Physical Aspects of Menopause

Changes in the Reproductive System

The physical characteristics of menopause are linked to the shift from a cyclic to a noncyclic hormonal pattern. Beginning 2 to 8 years before menopause, women experience episodes of anovulation; reduced fertility; decreased or increased menstrual flow; menstrual cycle irregularities; and then, ultimately, amenorrhea. Generally ovulation ceases 1 to 2 years before menopause, but individual variations exist. FSH levels rise, and ovarian follicles cease to produce estrogen. As estrogen levels decline, physiologic changes occur within the reproductive organs. The uterine lining, or endometrium, thins and the uterine muscle layer, or myometrium, atrophies. The fallopian tubes and ovaries atrophy. The vaginal mucosa loses its elasticity and becomes thinner and smoother. The loss of cervical gland function leads to dryness of the mucous membranes of the vagina, which can lead to burning and itching. The vaginal pH level increases as the number of Döderlein's bacilli decreases. This change in the vaginal ecology can lead to a condition known as atrophic vaginitis and increases the woman's risk of vaginal infections.

Pubic hair thins, turns gray or white, and may ultimately disappear. The labia shrink and lose their heightened pigmentation. Menopausal women may experience a general loss of pelvic tone and support, which can lead to prolapse of reproductive and urinary tract organs and subsequent urinary incontinence (Curran, 2008). Kegel exercises and regular sexual activity help prevent this change. Breasts lose their density and are replaced by fat, which makes them more pendulous and less firm.

Sexual functioning declines with age; however, more than 75% of the middle-aged women in the Study of Women's Health Across the Nation (SWAN) cited sex as being moderately to extremely important. Contributing factors to the decline in both interest and occurrence of sexual activity are widespread. Pain during intercourse due to lack of lubrication and thinning vaginal walls is a common cause. Other factors may include a lack of partners, stress in current relationships, psychosocial factors, and a decline in general health. A positive attitude about aging and menopause as well as the overall good health of the women in the study had a highly positive effect on sexual activity and satisfaction (Avis et al., 2009). Completing a good sexual history will help the nurse to assess the woman's sexual health and allow the woman to ask questions and express concerns or frustrations.

Vasomotor Changes

Many women who are perimenopausal or menopausal experience a vasomotor disturbance commonly known as a *hot flash*. Hot flashes are typically described as a feeling of heat rising from the chest and spreading to the neck and face. Hot flashes at night are often accompanied by sleep disturbances triggered by profuse sweating (*night sweats*) in which a woman awakens with drenched night clothes and bedding. These episodes may occur as often as 20 to 30 times a day and generally last 3 to 5 minutes or less. Some women also experience dizzy spells, palpitations, and weakness. Many women find their own most effective ways to deal with the hot flashes. Some report that dressing in layers, using a fan, avoiding alcoholic beverages, or drinking a cool liquid helps relieve distress. Still others seek relief through hormone therapy or complementary therapies such as herbs or acupuncture.

Changes in the Musculoskeletal System and Skin

Osteoporosis, a decrease in bone strength related to diminished bone density and bone quality, is a major health concern for women, particularly after menopause. An estimated 10 million U.S. adults have osteoporosis; of those, 80% are women (Reiter,

2008). Women who experience menopause at a younger age and those with less bone mass when entering menopause, predicatively will have the most severe bone loss (Curran, 2008). This change is associated with lowered estrogen levels; however, the greatest influencing factor is a family history of osteoporosis. Osteoporosis puts an individual at increased risk for fractures of the hip, forearm, and vertebrae. Risk factors associated with osteoporosis are identified in Table 4-2.

As skin ages, collagen and elastin, which are what maintain firmness of the skin, weaken. The skin appears looser and thinner and wrinkles. Past sun exposure and tobacco use influence the amount of skin changes that occur. As women age, the skin becomes drier and may need increased moisturizing. Nurses, as a part of general counseling, can remind women to wear sunscreen with a sun protection factor (SPF) of at least 30 to provide 97% ultraviolet B (UVB) filter and prevent damage. Recommending annual dermatologic screening for serious skin changes is also important (Baron, Kirkland, & Santo Domingo, 2008).

Evidence suggests that estrogen regulates weight and fat metabolism in women (Kohrt, 2009), and during menopause a change in fat distribution occurs. In postmenopausal women compared to premenopausal women total body fat increases by 22%. More specifically the increase in fat accumulation occurs in the trunk region. Nurses should be especially concerned about central body obesity, which is a predictor of the development of chronic illness. This is done by calculating a waist-to-hip ratio, or dividing the woman's waist measurement by the hip measurement. Women should maintain a waist-to-hip ratio of less than 0.80 to decrease their risk for chronic disease (Grubbs, 2009).

Changes in the Cardiovascular System

An important long-range physical change of menopause is a shift in lipid and lipoprotein levels. The presence of normal estrogen levels before menopause contributes to higher levels of high-density lipoprotein cholesterol (HDL-C) or the "good" cholesterol and lower levels of low-density lipoprotein cholesterol (LDL-C) or "bad" cholesterol. Levels of HDL-C of less than 50 mg/ml are the most important predictor of coronary heart disease in women (Reiter, 2008). As estrogen levels fall during menopause, this protective mechanism ceases, which potentially places a woman at increased risk for coronary heart disease, hypertension, and strokes. During menopause women should be encouraged to have their cholesterol monitored on an annual basis if normal and every 3 to 6 months if abnormal.

TABLE 4-2 Risk Factors for Osteoporosis

- Personal history of fracture after age 50
- Current low bone mass
- History of fracture in a first-degree relative
- Being female
- Being thin (weight less than 127 lb and/or having a small frame)
- Advanced age
- Family history of osteoporosis, especially a maternal hip fracture
- Use of certain medications (e.g., corticosteroids, chemotherapy, anticonvulsants)
- Abnormal absence of menses, early onset of menopause
- Anorexia nervosa
- Low lifetime intake of calcium
- Vitamin D deficiency
- Current cigarette smoking, excessive alcohol use
- Inactive lifestyle
- Being Caucasian or Asian

TABLE 4-3 Risk Factors for CHD in Women

- Family history of heart disease
- Advancing age—over 55 or postmenopausal
- Overweight and obesity
- Cigarette smoking and/or tobacco use
- Sedentary lifestyle
- Hypertension
- Diabetes
- Elevated cholesterol
- Race (highest incidence in African American women)

Although viewed as a higher risk in men, cardiovascular disease (CVD) is still the number one killer of women in the United States. Coronary heart disease (CHD) is the major cause of heart attacks in women. In fact, approximately 50% of all deaths in women are a result of CHD. Many women perceive breast cancer as the greatest threat to their health; however 1 in 30 women will die from breast cancer, while 1 in 6 women will die from CHD (Rowe, 2007). Risk factors for CHD are identified in Table 4-3.

Metabolic syndrome is a major predisposing factor for CHD and is defined through a collection of risk factors. Clinical characteristics are waist measurement greater than 35 inches, triglycerides greater than 150 mg/dl, HDL less than 50, blood pressure over 130/85, and fasting glucose levels greater than 100 mg/dl (Conway & Green, 2009).

Changes in Cognitive Function

Memory and cognitive function change with advancing age. There is suggestion that the brain benefits from circulating estrogen and that declining estrogen levels might contribute to loss of this function as well as to the development of dementia (Curran, 2008). This change is also influenced by lifestyle, genetics, and socioeconomic status. In the United States, Alzheimer disease (AD) is the most commonly occurring form of dementia, estimated to affect 5.2 million Americans. Projections indicate that by the year 2030, 7.7 million Americans over the age of 65 will have AD. The prevalence of AD in individuals over the age of 80 is at least 40%.

The cause of Alzheimer disease is unknown although there is belief that risk factors other than advancing age may play a role. These risk factors include specific genotypes, obesity, insulin resistance, elevated cholesterol, hypertension, and inflammation. Genetic forms of Alzheimer disease account for less than 7% of all cases (Anderson, 2009).

Numerous treatments for AD have been explored, including ginkgo biloba, estrogen therapy, cholesterol-reducing medications, nonsteroidal anti-inflammatory drugs, and antioxidants. None of these treatments have proven effective. At present there are no therapies that slow the progression of the disease; only symptomatic therapies are available. Cholinesterase inhibitors and N-methyl-D-aspartate antagonists are the only medications approved by the Food and Drug Administration (FDA) to treat cognitive dysfunction. Antidepressants have been used to treat secondary symptoms of depression or mood disorders, which occur in more than 30% of all patients with AD. No special dietary considerations are important in the management of Alzheimer disease (Anderson, 2009).

Premature Menopause

Premature ovarian insufficiency (POI) is a devastating event and is not well understood. It occurs in about 0.1% of women by the age of 30, 0.25% of women by the age of 35, and 1% of women by the age of 40 (Popat & Nelson, 2007). It is defined as 4 to 6 months of no menses in women under the age of 40 years who have elevated FSH and low estradiol levels. Women who receive this diagnosis may not necessarily experience total loss of ovarian function because the rate of progression is variable (Welt, 2008). POI is different from menopause in that women with POI retain intermittent ovarian function, and although difficult, pregnancy may occur. Women with POI who desire pregnancy may experience emotional trauma and require extra sensitivity from caregivers. Concern for the patient's long-term health should be a consideration. Women should be encouraged to engage in weight-bearing exercises for 30 minutes at least 3 days per week to strengthen muscle and maintain bone mass. Adequate intakes of calcium and vitamin D are also important. Premature ovarian insufficiency is treated with estrogen and progesterone therapy and should be monitored annually until discontinuation of treatment at the usual age of menopause (Popat & Nelson, 2007). Other forms of premature menopause occur with anorexia, chemotherapy or radiation treatments, and oophorectomy (surgical removal of the ovaries).

Medical Therapy

Menopausal Hormone Therapy (HT)

Hormone therapy (HT), formerly called *hormone replacement therapy (HRT)*, refers to the administration of specific hormones to alleviate symptoms associated with the changes of menopause. Estrogen therapy (ET) and combined estrogen-progestogen therapy (EPT) are the individual types currently in use. Hormone therapy containing estrogen only is given to women who have undergone a hysterectomy (surgical removal of the uterus), whereas hormone therapy containing estrogen and progestogen (encompasses both progesterone and progestin) is used for women with an intact uterus. Estrogen alone, in a woman with a uterus (unopposed estrogen), increases the risk of endometrial (the lining of the uterus) cancer by eightfold and, therefore, is never given without progesterone in these women.

In 2002 the advisability of HT, specifically EPT, was called into question because of the results of the Women's Health Initiative (WHI) study, which suggested that the risks of HT outweigh its benefits, especially for long-term use, because of the slightly increased risk of breast cancer, thromboembolic disease, and stroke (Writing Group for the Women's Health Initiative Investigators, 2002). Previously HT was thought to provide protection against cardiovascular disease, the number one cause of death for women over age 50. Currently there are studies underway to further define the risks and benefits of HT.

The North American Menopause Society (NAMS), a nonprofit scientific organization, currently recommends that hormone therapy should be considered only when there is an indication for therapy and contraindications for its use have been ruled out. Adequate discussion about the risks and benefits should take place to ensure an informed decision to use HT. HT is a proven therapy for the relief of moderate to severe vasomotor symptoms, vulvar and vaginal atrophy, and dyspareunia (pain with intercourse). Proven risks of HT use include increased risk of venous thrombosis and breast cancer. HT is not currently recommended solely to prevent coronary heart disease. Extended use of HT may be an option for women with a demonstrated reduction in bone mass, whether or not menopausal symptoms exist, to prevent further bone loss or prevent the development of osteoporotic fractures in women when usual therapies are not appropriate or when they cause side effects; and when the benefits of extended use of HT are believed to outweigh the risks (North American Menopause Society [NAMS], 2010).

HT can be prescribed in a number of ways, including orally; transdermally (patch); topically as a gel, lotion, mist, or creams; and through a vaginal ring. It is given in a continuous manner, daily administration of both estrogen and progestogen, or as a cyclic or sequential therapy, with estrogen use daily and a progestogen added on a set sequence (NAMS, 2010). Combination estrogen-progestogen preparations are also available.

Research, though still preliminary, does seem to indicate that postmenopausal women experiencing decreased libido experience improved sexual desire, responsiveness, and frequency when testosterone is added to their HT. Options for providing testosterone in doses low enough for women are still limited and are not approved by the FDA. Estratest, a combined estrogen-androgen pill, is used by some women. Custom-compounded testosterone preparations are available by prescription. Proctor & Gamble has developed a low-dose testosterone transdermal patch for women called Intrinsa that is available by prescription in Europe. Another testosterone product, a gel called LiBiGel, is currently undergoing testing.

A great deal of attention has been given to "bioidentical" hormones lately because of current views, which are not supported by medical literature, that these "more natural" hormones are safer and more effective. A bioidentical hormone refers to a hormone that is structurally identical to those found in the body, more specifically, those produced by the ovaries. These hormones are compounded by a specialty pharmacy and are not approved by the FDA, nor have they been proven to have a better safety profile (Altman, Moore, Speroff, et al., 2009).

In light of the findings from more recent clinical trials and a secondary analysis of the WHI, NAMS convened an advisory panel to develop recommendations about the clinical management of postmenopausal hormone therapy. Among their recommendations they suggested the following (NAMS, 2010):

- The treatment of moderate to severe menopausal vasomotor symptoms (hot flashes and night sweats) is the primary indica-

RESEARCH EVIDENCE IN PRACTICE The Safety of Estrogen/Progesterone Therapy When Initiated Soon After Menopause

CLINICAL QUESTION

Can the timing of the initiation of estrogen/progesterone replacement therapy reduce the known risks associated with postmenopausal hormone therapy?

RESEARCH EVIDENCE

Current guidelines suggest that estrogen therapy for treatment of the symptoms of menopause (e.g., vasomotor symptoms such as hot flashes and night sweats) is associated with an increased risk of breast cancer, thromboembolism, and stroke. If hormone therapy is necessary for the relief of severe symptoms, care standards dictate that therapy be prescribed at the lowest effective dose for the shortest period. Some providers hypothesized that initiating estrogen/progesterone therapy immediately after the onset of postmenopausal symptoms may not carry the same risk of adverse outcomes as delaying treatment. Three large-scale multisite studies involving thousands of postmenopausal women studied the association of disease conditions and the timing of hormone therapy.

Breast cancer and total cancer were both increased in women who took estrogen/progesterone therapy, regardless of the timing of the treatment. Among these women, use of estrogens appeared to produce elevations in venous thromboembolism and stroke. There was a reduction in hip fracture among women undergoing hormone therapy, but it was unrelated to timing.

There has also been a question as to whether estrogen combined with progesterone avoided these outcomes. These studies demonstrated that adding progesterone did not protect the woman from morbidity. In fact, combination therapy increased the long-term risk of breast cancer. Regardless of the timing of initiation of hormone therapy, the longer durations of treatment were associated with a greater increase in breast cancer risk. In some of these women, though, even short durations of hormone therapy were associated with an increase in the breast cancer rate.

WHAT QUESTIONS REMAIN UNANSWERED?

The delivery method of estrogen/progesterone may influence negative outcomes. One European study demonstrated that transdermal estrogen may have the potential for fewer health risks than oral estrogen therapy, but it had a relatively small sample. Replication of this study on a larger sample is needed before any delivery method of estrogen can be recommended.

WHAT IS BEST PRACTICE?

Nonhormonal treatments for the relief of postmenopausal vasomotor symptoms are the standard for safe care. Timing of treatment does not reduce the risk of breast cancer, thromboembolism, and stroke and, in some cases, may increase the long-term risk. Even short periods of treatment increase risk, but longer courses of treatment are clearly associated with increased risk of adverse conditions.

CRITICAL THINKING

What are some nonhormonal interventions that the nurse can offer to the postmenopausal woman to deal with the vasomotor symptoms of menopause?

References

Carroll, N. (2010). A review of transdermal nonpatch estrogen therapy for the management of menopausal symptoms. *Journal of Women's Health, 19*(1), 47–55.

Fournier, A., Mesrine, S., Boutron-Ruault, M., & Clavel-Chapelon, F. (2009). Estrogen-Progestagen menopausal hormone therapy and breast cancer: Does delay from menopause onset to treatment initiation influence risks? *Journal of Clinical Oncology, 27*(31), 5138–5143.

Prentice, R., Manson, J., Langer, R., Anderson, G., Pettinger, M., Jackson, R., . . . Rossouw, J. (2009). Benefits and risks of postmenopausal hormone therapy when it is initiated soon after menopause. *American Journal of Epidemiology, 170*(1), 12–23.

tion for HT. Local vaginal estrogen is generally recommended when HT is considered solely to treat urogenital atrophy.

- Progestogen is prescribed only to protect the endometrium from unopposed estrogen. Thus women with a uterus who are taking estrogen should also have a prescription for adequate progestogen coverage (HT). Women without a uterus who are taking estrogen (ET) should *not* have a progestogen prescribed.
- No estrogen therapy regimen (ET or EPT) should be used solely to prevent coronary heart disease. Alternative prevention regimens should be used instead (weight control, regular exercise, no smoking, healthy diet, etc.).
- HT has been used for the prevention of osteoporosis. However, because of the associated risks, alternative approaches to preventing and treating osteoporosis should be considered first. In certain situations HT may play a role in the treatment of osteoporosis.
- HT use should be limited to the shortest duration feasible in light of treatment goals, benefits, and risks for an individual woman.
- The therapeutic goal should be to prescribe the lowest effective dose of estrogen that is consistent with treatment goals and an analysis of benefits and risks.
- Alternate routes of administration of HT may provide advantages, but at present the long-term risk benefit ratio has not been shown.
- HT may be recommended for women who experience premature menopause and premature ovarian insufficiency at least until they reach the median age of natural menopause.
- Therapy decisions should be made individually based on each woman's symptoms and identified risks.
- Women should be informed of the known risks.

At present, HT is still recognized as the most effective therapy for women who experience moderate to severe menopausal symptoms. For women taking short-term (1 to 4 years) HT therapy to relieve symptoms, the benefits are likely to outweigh the risks.

Before starting HT the woman should undergo a thorough history; physical examination including Pap smear; measurement of cholesterol, lipids, and liver enzyme levels; and baseline mammogram. An initial endometrial biopsy is no longer routinely recommended for all women beginning HT; however, biopsy is indicated for women with an increased risk of endometrial cancer and if excessive, unexpected, or prolonged

Care Plan Activity: Bone Injuries in a Postmenopausal Woman

vaginal bleeding occurs. Caregivers who prescribe HT should teach their patients to report immediately any signs of complications such as headaches, visual changes, signs of thrombophlebitis, or signs of myocardial infarction that are common in women (see later discussion).

Prevention and Treatment of Osteoporosis

Osteoporosis is rapidly becoming a significant health risk for older adults (see Table 4-2). According to the American College of Obstetricians and Gynecologists (ACOG, 2007b) more than 1.5 million fractures occur in the United States each year. Most of these fractures occur in women. Fifty percent of all women over the age of 50 will experience an osteoporosis-related fracture in their lifetime. These numbers are especially worrisome because osteoporosis is a largely preventable disease and a source of significant risk for fracture and subsequent health decline.

Bone mineral density (BMD) testing is useful in identifying individuals who are at risk for osteoporosis. A variety of guidelines are available for BMD testing. ACOG (2008) recommends BMD testing for the following:

- All postmenopausal women aged 65 or older regardless of risk factors
- All postmenopausal women with fractures
- Postmenopausal women under age 65 with one or more risk factors

BMD testing may also be indicated for premenopausal or postmenopausal women with certain medical conditions such as eating disorders, thyroid disorders, leukemia, rheumatoid arthritis, and multiple sclerosis and for those women on certain medications such as corticosteroids or anticonvulsants.

This quick, painless test assesses whether a woman has normal bone mass or has decreased bone density (osteoporosis) or increased bone porosity or softening (osteomalacia). Optimum screening is done using a central dual-energy x-ray absorptiometry (DEXA) scan to measure bone density at the hip and lumbar spine. Figure 4-3 ■ shows a sample bone density testing result.

The woman's height should be measured at each visit, because a loss of height is often an early sign that vertebrae are being compressed because of reduced bone mass. A variety of conditions, including malabsorption syndrome, cancer, cirrhosis of the liver, chronic use of cortisone, and rheumatoid arthritis, can cause secondary arthritis, which resembles osteoporosis. If these secondary causes are ruled out, treatment for osteoporosis is instituted.

Prevention of osteoporosis is the primary goal. It should include encouraging women to adopt lifestyle practices that reduce the risk of bone loss such as regular weight-bearing and muscle-strengthening exercise, smoking cessation, moderation of alcohol intake, and fall prevention strategies (ACOG, 2007b). Women are also advised to maintain an adequate calcium intake. The National Institutes of Health recommends that postmenopausal women have a daily intake of 1200 mg of calcium, increasing to 1500 mg if they are not on hormone therapy. Most women require supplements to achieve this level. Calcium supplementation is most effective when single doses do not exceed 500 mg and when taken with a meal.

Vitamin D is a fat-soluble vitamin that has its greatest effect on maintaining adequate levels of serum calcium. It is primarily metabolized by the body through sunlight or dietary intake. The use of sunscreen can result in decreased production of vitamin D in the skin. Low bone density and certain autoimmune diseases are associated with vitamin D deficiency. It is recommended that adults take a vitamin D supplement of 1000 to 2000 international units per day to reduce the incidence of low bone density (Malone & Kessenich, 2008).

The effectiveness of estrogen in preventing osteoporosis is well documented. Women with no contraindications to estrogen who are showing evidence of bone loss are good candidates for HT. For women who are unable or unwilling to take estrogen, other medications available to treat or help prevent osteoporosis include the following:

1. *Bisphosphonates* have potent antiresorptive effects and are the gold standard in alleviating postmenopausal osteoporosis (Waxman, 2007). These medications are taken upon arising in the morning on an empty stomach with a large glass of water. The woman should sit upright or stand for about 30 minutes after taking the medication and before eating. These medications are dosed daily, once weekly, or once monthly depending on the formulation. New bisphosphonates may offer women alternatives that eliminate the undesirable gastrointestinal side effects. For example, in 2002, an intravenous bisphosphonate, zoledronic acid (Zometa), was approved by the FDA for use in the treatment of metastatic bone cancer. It is the most recent medication approved for the treatment of osteoporosis. The drug, administered intravenously (IV) once a year, seems to achieve the same results in treating osteoporosis as other bisphosphonates taken daily or weekly without the troublesome gastrointestinal side effects. Although many patients may prefer the yearly dosing option, there has been reported increased risk of deterioration of the jaw bone with the use of this medication over extended periods (Waxman, 2007).
2. *Selective estrogen receptor modulators (SERMs)* have estrogen-like properties. The SERM approved for osteoporosis treatment, raloxifene (Evista), acts like estrogen by protecting against osteoporosis but does not stimulate uterine or breast tissue. Raloxifene does not relieve other menopausal symptoms and may increase hot flashes, so it is indicated in asymptomatic women who want preventive therapy for osteoporosis.
3. *Salmon calcitonin* is a calcium regulator that may inhibit bone loss and is approved for use to treat osteoporosis in women who are 5 years postmenopause. Administered as a nasal spray, its value is less clear than that of the other medications listed.
4. *Parathyroid hormone,* a daily subcutaneous injection, activates bone formation, which results in substantial increases in bone density.

The National Osteoporosis Foundation (NOF) provides a wealth of information about osteoporosis diagnosis and management.

Name:	**Doe, Jane**	Sex:	Female	Height:	66.5 in.
Patient ID:	Case A004	Ethnicity:	White	Weight:	165.0 lb
Age:	66	Date of Birth:	09/02/1933	Menopause Age:	53

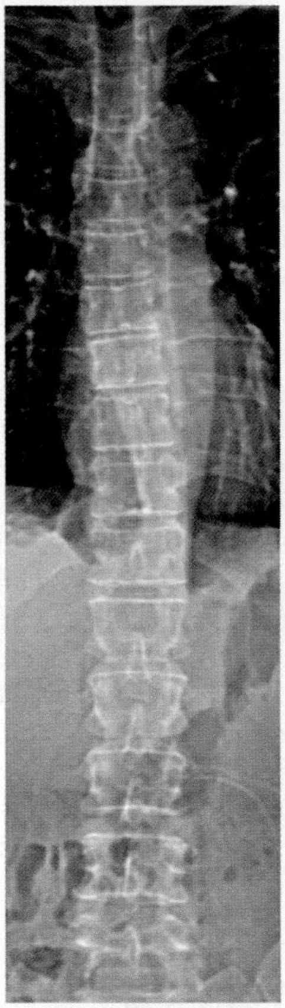

Scan Date: May 01, 2000
Scan ID: A0501000Q
Scan Type: f SE R/L Lateral Image

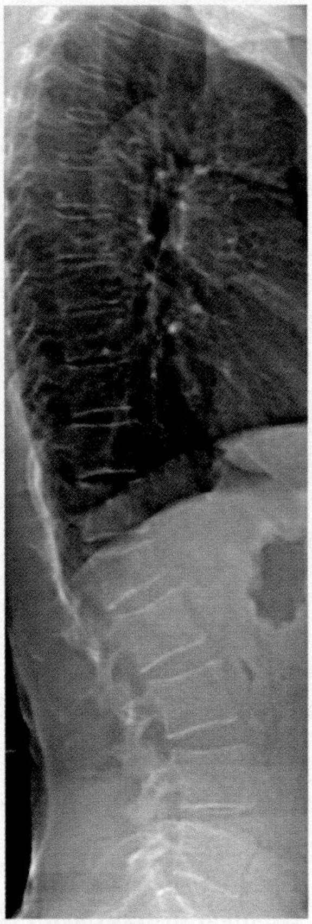

Scan Date: May 01, 2000
Scan ID: A0501000O
Scan Type: f SE AP Image

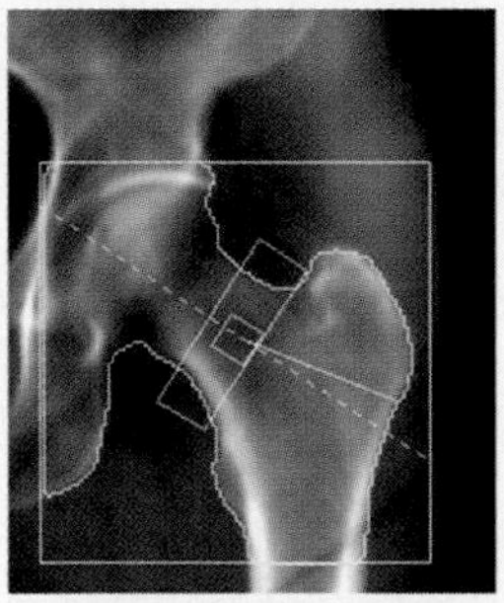

Scan Date: May 01, 2000
Scan ID: A0501000M

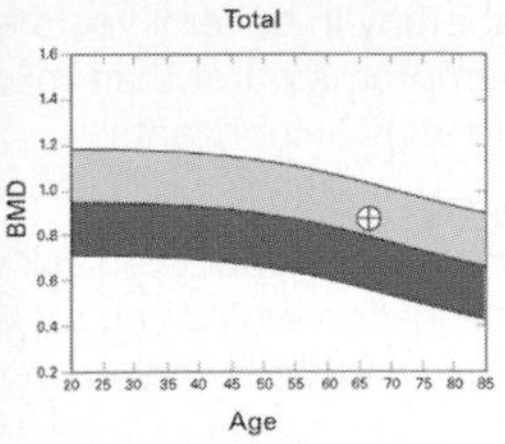

Scan Type: f Left Hip

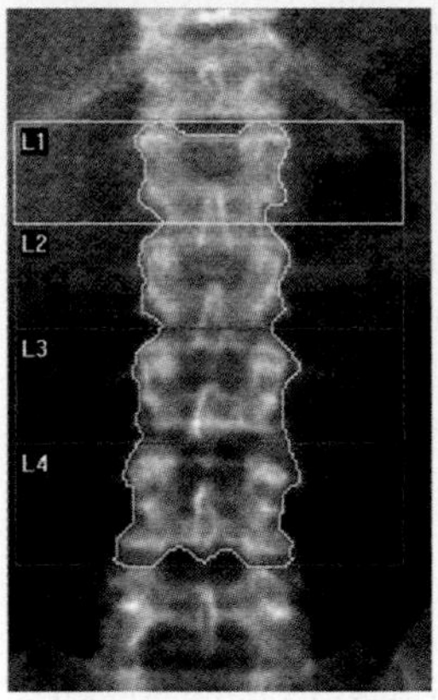

Scan Date: May 01, 2000
Scan ID: A0501000K

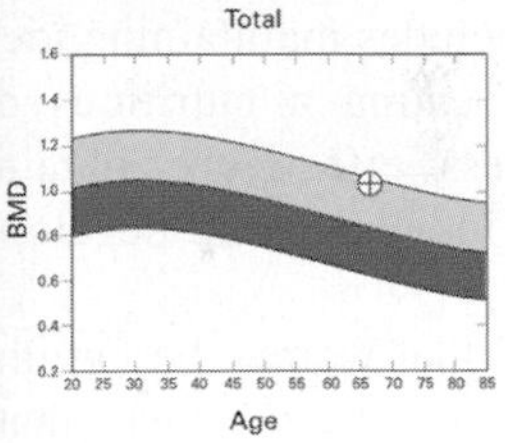

Scan Type: f Lumbar Spine

Results:

	BMD (g/cm^2)	T-Score	PR (%)	Z-Score	AM (%)
Left Hip (Neck)	0.773	-0.7	91	0.9	115
Left Hip (Total)	0.870	-0.6	92	0.7	111
Spine (Total)	1.027	-0.2	98	1.7	122

Total BMD CV 1.0%

Summary:

	Classification
Left Hip BMD (Neck)	Normal
Left Hip BMD (Total)	Normal
Spine BMD (Total)	Normal
Vertebral Evaluation:	Severe Wedge Deformity at L2

A spine fracture indicates 5X risk for subsequent spine fracture and 2X risk for subsequent hip fracture.

World Health Organization criteria for BMD interpretation classify patients as Normal (T-score above -1), Osteopenic (T-score between -1 and -2.5), or Osteoporotic (T-score at or below -2.5).

HOLOGIC®
OSTEOPOROSIS ASSESSMENT

Figure 4-3 ■ For osteoporosis assessment, published studies demonstrate that up to 30% of patients needing treatment are missed using BMD results of the spine and hip alone. The standard of care for assessing osteoporotic fracture risk is combining BMD results with imaging of the thoracic-lumbar spine. The osteoporotic assessment examination presented here shows a 66-year-old postmenopausal woman who has not received hormone replacement therapy because of a personal history of breast cancer. Although her bone mineral density (BMD) results are within normal limits, she does have an identifiable vertebral fracture at L2. This fracture places her at increased risk for future vertebral fractures and, therefore, in need of treatment for osteoporosis.

Source: Scan provided courtesy of Hologic, Inc., Osteoporosis Assessment Division, Bedford, MA. Mary Ann Barrick, Product Specialist, Hologic, Inc., mbarrick@hologic.com

CLINICAL JUDGMENT

Case Study: Janet Turner

Mrs. Turner, a 68-year-old woman, presents for her annual well-woman examination. She is 5 foot 4 inches tall and weighs 120 pounds. In taking her history she states that she has recently gotten out of a cast for a broken wrist. She states that she fell while gardening. She has not used hormone replacement therapy in several years and has no complaints of menopause symptoms other than mild vaginal dryness, which is relieved with vaginal lubricants.

Critical Thinking

What further questions would you ask in your history taking? What recommendation would you make for Mrs. Turner?

See www.nursing.pearsonhighered.com for possible responses.

Prevention of Coronary Heart Disease

Prevention is the key to dealing with CHD. Prevention begins with lifestyle choices and with lifestyle modifications as necessary. This includes maintaining ideal body weight, exercising regularly, eating a nutritious diet, avoiding smoking, managing stress effectively, obtaining regular healthcare screenings as indicated, and developing a strong social support system.

It is critical that women be familiar with the signs of myocardial infarction (heart attack) that are commonly seen in women. These include pain in the neck, back, or epigastric region; loss of appetite; shortness of breath; nausea or vomiting; and weakness in the shoulder, arms, and chest. Research indicates that women are more likely than men to delay seeking treatment. They are also more likely to die from the attack (Rowe, 2007). Thus it is important for nurses to stress the need to seek immediate treatment if symptoms develop.

Complementary and Alternative Therapies

As women evaluate their feelings about the use of HT in light of the recent findings in clinical trials, they may wish to explore alternative therapies for control of their symptoms. A variety of therapeutic modalities have been proposed as alternative or complementary treatment or prevention measures for the discomforts and ailments of the perimenopausal and postmenopausal years. These include nutrition supplements, such as a diet rich in calcium and vitamins E, D, and B complex.

Very little scientific research has been done on complementary alternative therapy for the treatment of menopause. Black cohosh has received the most scientific attention. Mixed results, however, have been found for the use of black cohosh for the relief of hot flashes and night sweats. Experts agree that safety is an issue for women using black cohosh if they have a liver disorder or develop symptoms of liver trouble.

Dong quai has had one randomized clinical study done on it and was not found to have any effect on hot flashes. Dong quai is known to interact with blood thinning medication (warfarin) and can lead to bleeding complications in women taking this medication.

Ginseng, although not helpful for hot flashes, may help with other menopausal symptoms such as moodiness and sleep disturbances. Kava may decrease anxiety, although the FDA has issued a warning about kava for potential liver damage.

Phytoestrogens are plant products that have estrogen-like properties. Examples of foods and botanicals containing phytoestrogens are carrots, yams, soy, and red clover. After five controlled studies, red clover was not found to reduce hot flashes. Soy has had inconsistent results in studies in reducing hot flashes. There is some question that daily intake of soy may reduce slightly the levels of LDL or bad cholesterol. Ongoing studies are underway to examine the effects of soy on women's arteries and bones after menopause (National Center for Complementary and Alternative Medicine [NCCAM], 2008). Women who have endometriosis or uterine fibroids should be cautioned on the use of these products as should women who have had or are at risk for diseases that are affected by hormones, such as breast, uterine, or ovarian cancer (NCCAM, 2008).

DHEA is a dietary supplement that is changed in the body to the hormones estrogen and testosterone. A few small studies have suggested that DHEA might have some benefit for hot flashes and decreased sexual arousal, although randomized controlled trials do not support this. Scientists are not certain whether the use of DHEA increases the risk for breast and prostate cancer (NCCAM, 2008).

A randomized, controlled study of acupuncture treatment for hot flashes was conducted and suggests that this may be an effective therapy to reduce the frequency of hot flashes in some women (Avis et al., 2008).

DEVELOPING CULTURAL COMPETENCE

Filipina Women and Aging

In the Philippines, menopause is viewed as a positive and liberating event. As women age, they are more respected and admired for their years of gained experiences. Older women gain status and importance as they age and are widely embraced by the younger generations within their family. (Comments from a Filipino nursing student.)

Weight-bearing exercise, including such activities as walking, jogging, tennis, and running, is a means of increasing bone mass and potentiating the effect of estrogen on bone mass. Exercise also improves cholesterol profiles and contributes to overall health (Figure 4-4 ■). Pelvic floor, or Kegel, exercises can help maintain vaginal muscle tone and increase blood circulation to the perineal area. Vaginal lubricants and adequate foreplay can be helpful in maintaining a satisfactory sexual experience.

Relaxation techniques, including yoga, meditation, deep breathing, visualization, massage, or acupuncture, may provide a sense of well-being. Menopausal women should avoid foods that may trigger symptoms, including caffeine, alcohol, and spicy foods. Overall, healthy lifestyle, proper nutrition, and adequate exercise will maximize health and decrease health risks and symptoms.

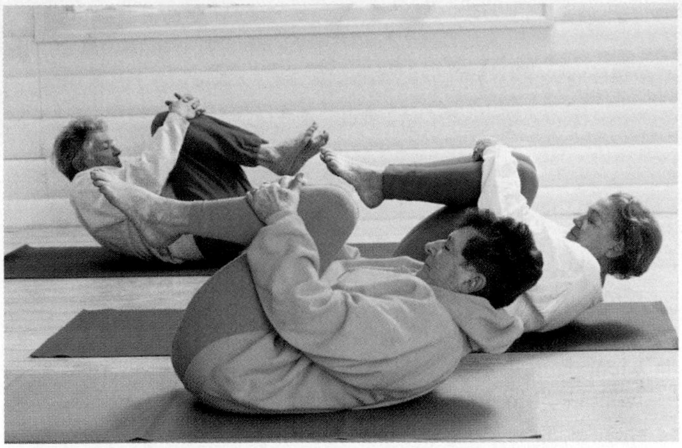

Figure 4-4 ■ Regular exercise is important, especially for postmenopausal women.

Source: Ariel Skelley-CORBIS.

NURSING CARE MANAGEMENT

Some menopausal women may need counseling to adjust successfully to this developmental phase of life. Others have no difficulty with this life transition. Reaction to menopause is determined to a large extent by the kind of life the woman has lived, by the security she has in her feminine identity, by her feelings of self-worth and self-esteem, and by her relationships with others.

Nurses and other healthcare professionals may be able to help the menopausal woman achieve high-level functioning at this time in her life. Of paramount importance is the nurse's ability to understand and provide support for the woman's views and feelings. Whether the woman expresses relief and delight or tearfulness and fear, the nurse needs to use an empathetic approach in counseling, health teaching, or providing physical care.

Women may discuss areas of deep concern, including a history of sexual abuse, current distress, or life problems. Nurses should have appropriate referrals to domestic violence hotlines and to professional therapists who work with women. Women may also be dealing simultaneously with chronically ill parents, divorce or the death of a spouse, troubled or handicapped children, children leaving home, job stressors, and/or generalized fear and anxiety. Nurses can be of assistance with referrals to support groups and counselors who are specific to each woman's need. Although this is a challenge, it is the responsibility of the nurse caring for women to be prepared to meet their needs.

Nurses should explore the question of the woman's comfort during sexual intercourse. In counseling, the nurse may say, "After menopause many women notice that their vaginas seem drier, and sex of any kind can be uncomfortable. Have you noticed any changes?" This gives the woman information and may open discussion. The nurse can then go on to explain that the woman can address dryness and shrinking of the vagina by using a water-soluble lubricant to help provide relief. Use of estrogen, orally or in vaginal creams, may also be indicated. Increased frequency of sexual activity will maintain some elasticity in the vagina. When assessing the menopausal woman, the nurse needs to address the question of sexual activity openly but tactfully, because the woman may have been socialized to be reticent in discussing sex. Heterosexual women who do not wish to become pregnant should be counseled to use a method of contraception for 1 year after their last menstrual period. They should also be advised to report any bleeding after 1 year of amenorrhea because this may indicate a problem and requires evaluation.

The crucial need of women in the perimenopausal period of life is for adequate information about the changes taking place in their bodies and their lives and support in adjusting to the changes that occur. Supplying that information and providing support as needed present both a challenge and an opportunity for nurses.

Additional information about the most current approaches to the management of menopause and the postmenopausal period can be found at the Web site of the North American Menopause Society.

PROFESSIONALISM IN PRACTICE

Personalizing Care During Menopause

Women respond differently to the experience of menopause, so it is important to avoid generalizations. During menopause women are in varying stages of life. In working with menopausal women, being sensitive to their place in life, such as caring for aging parents, empty nest, or change in marital status will personalize their care and offer appropriate measures to help them through this process.

FOCUS YOUR STUDY

- Nurses should provide girls and women with clear information about menstrual issues, such as the use of pads and tampons (including warnings regarding deodorant and absorbency); vaginal spray and douching practices; and self-care comfort measures during menstruation, such as maintaining good nutrition, exercising, and applying heat and massage.
- Dysmenorrhea usually begins at, or a day before, the onset of menses and disappears by the end. Hormone therapy (e.g., combined oral contraceptives), nonsteroidal anti-inflammatory drugs, or prostaglandin inhibitors can alleviate dysmenorrhea. Self-care measures include improving nutrition, exercising, applying heat, and getting extra rest.
- Premenstrual syndrome occurs most often in women over 30. The most pronounced symptoms occur 2 to 3 days before onset of menstruation and subside as menstruation starts, with or without treatment. Medical management usually includes prostaglandin inhibitors and calcium supplementation. Self-care measures include improving nutrition (taking vitamin B complex and E supplements and avoiding methylxanthines, which are found, for example, in chocolate and caffeine), undertaking a program of aerobic exercise, and participating in self-care support groups. In some cases, pharmacologic agents such as selective serotonin reuptake inhibitors may be indicated.
- During her adult years, a healthy woman should make healthful lifestyle choices such as avoiding smoking and exercising regularly. She should also participate in regular health screenings, following a recommended schedule.
- Menopause is a physiologic, maturational change in a woman's life. Physiologic changes include the cessation of menses and a decrease in circulating hormones. Hormonal changes sometimes bring unsettling emotional responses. The more common physiologic symptoms are "hot flashes," palpitations, dizziness, and increased perspiration at night. The woman's anatomy also undergoes changes, such as atrophy of the vagina, reduction in size and pigmentation of the labia, and myometrial atrophy. Osteoporosis becomes an increasing concern.
- Osteoporosis is becoming a significant health problem in the United States. Prevention is the preferred approach to addressing the issue. This includes adequate calcium intake, regular weight-bearing exercise, and HT. For women who have already developed osteoporosis, medications are available as a treatment option.
- Coronary heart disease is the number one killer of women in the United States. Prevention is the goal of therapy.
- Current management of menopause centers on hormone replacement therapy, complementary therapies, and patient healthcare education. Decisions regarding the use of HT should be made individually, based on each woman's symptoms and risks, and women should be advised of the known risks.

CRITICAL THINKING IN ACTION

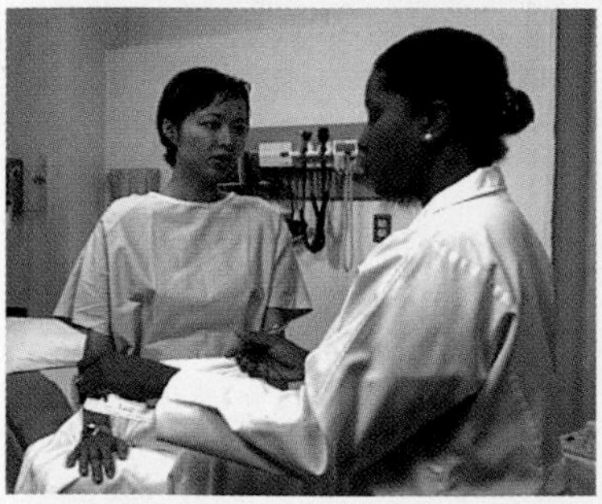

You are working at a local clinic when Joy Lang, age 20, presents for her first pelvic exam. You obtain the following GYN history; menarche age 12 menstrual cycle 28–30 days lasting 4–5 days, heavy one day, then lighter. She tells you that she needs to use superabsorbent tampons on the first day of her period and then she switches to a regular absorbency tampon for the remaining days. She confirms that she changes the tampon every 6 to 8 hours, never leaving it in overnight. She denies premenstrual syndrome, dysmenorrhea, or medical problems and says that she is not taking any medication on a regular schedule. She tells you that she recently got married, but would like to wait before getting pregnant. She'd like to discuss birth control methods. Joy tells you that doctors make her nervous and she admits to being anxious about her first pelvic exam.

1. What steps would you take to reduce Joy's anxiety relating to the pelvic exam?
2. What position is best to relax Joy's abdominal muscles for the pelvic exam?
3. What precaution should be taken when obtaining a Pap smear?
4. Explain the purpose of the Pap smear.
5. What factors do you include in a discussion of the type of birth control that Joy could practice?

See www.nursing.pearsonhighered.com for possible responses.

REFERENCES

Altman, A., Moore, A., Speroff, L., & Wysocki, S. (2009). Tackling the tricky issue of bioidentical hormones. *Women's Health Care: A Practical Journal for Nurse Practitioners, 8*(7), 7–15.

American College of Obstetricians and Gynecologists (ACOG). (2006). *Later childbearing* (ACOG Patient Education Pamphlet No. AP060). Washington, DC: Author.

American College of Obstetricians and Gynecologists (ACOG). (2007a). *Menstruation* (ACOG Patient Education Pamphlet No. AP049). Washington, DC: Author.

American College of Obstetricians and Gynecologists (ACOG). (2007b). *Osteoporosis* (ACOG Patient Education Pamphlet No. AP048). Washington, DC: Author.

American College of Obstetricians and Gynecologists (ACOG). (2008). *Low bone mass (osteopenia) and fracture risk* (ACOG Committee Opinion No. 407). Washington, DC: Author.

Anderson, H. (2009). Alzheimer disease. *eMedicine Neurology.* Retrieved from http://emedicine.medscape .com/article/1134817

Avis, N., Brockwell, S., Randolph, J., Shen, S., Cain, V., Ory, M., & Greendale, G. (2009). *Londitudinal changes in sexual functioning as women transition through menopause: Results from the study of women's health across the nation.* Retrieved from http://www .medscape.com/viewarticle/703258

Avis, N., Legault, C., Coeytaux, R., Pian-Smith, M., Shifren, J., Chen, W., & Valaskatgis, P. (2008). *A randomized, controlled pilot study of acupuncture treatment for menopausal hot flashes.* Retrieved from http://www .medscape.com/viewarticle/583598

Baron, E., Kirkland, E., & Santo Domingo, D. (2008). Advances in photoprotection. *Dermatology nursing.* Retrieved from http://www.medscape.com/viewarticle/ 580643

Blumenthal, P. (2007). Cultural competency in the provision of contraceptive service delivery: Overcoming barriers. *Contraception Online.* Retrieved from http://www.contraceptiononline.org

Camann, W. (2006). Obstetric and anesthetic implications of "body art" (piercing and tattooing). *Medscape OB/GYN & Women's Health, 11,* 1–3. Retrieved from http://www.medscape.com/viewarticle/527920_print

Conway, L., & Green, J. (2009). Metabolic syndrome in Native Americans: Guidelines offer protocols for care. *Advance for Nurse Practitioners, 17*(4), 45–48.

Curran, D. (2008). Menopause. *eMedicine Obstetrics and Gynecology.* Retrieved from http://emedicine .medscape.com/article/264088

Donohoe, M. (2006). Beauty and body modification. *Medscape OB/GYN & Women's Health, 11,* 1–6. Retrieved from http://www.medscape.com/viewarticle/ 529442_print

Endicott, J. (2007). PMDD spotlight: Redefined expectations: Improving quality of life in women with PMDD. *Medscape Ob/Gyn & Women's Health.* Retrieved from http://www.medscape.com/viewarticle.567290_print

Freeman, E. (2007). Epidemiology and etiology of premenstrual syndrome. *Medscape Ob/Gyn & Women's Health.* Retrieved from http://cme.medscape.com/ viewarticle/553603

Freeman, S. (2008). Stuck in between: A closer look at perimenopause. *Advance for Nurse Practitioners, 16*(10), 43–48.

Grubbs, L. (2009). Winning the battle of the bulge: Practical approaches to weight loss. *Advance for Nurse Practitioners, 17*(6), 33–38.

Kohrt, W. (2009). Exercise, weight gain, and menopause. *The North American Menopause Society (NAMS) NAMS Menopause e-consult.* Retrieved from http://www.medscape.com/viewarticle/704909

Malone, R. W., & Kessenich, C. (2008). *Vitamin D deficiency: Implications across the lifespan: Vitamin D: An overview.* Retrieved from http://www.medscape .com/viewarticle/578508_2

Mayo Clinic Staff. (2007). *Premenstrual syndrome.* Retrieved from http://www.mayoclinic.com/health/ premenstrual-syndrome/DS00134

National Center for Complementary and Alternative Medicine (NCCAM). (2008). *Menopausal symptoms and CAM.* Retrieved from http://nccam.nih.gov/health/ menopause/menopausesymptoms.html

National Women's Health Information Center. (2009). *Recommended screenings and immunizations for women at average risk for most diseases.* Washington, DC: Office of Women's Health, U.S. Department of Health and Human Services.

North American Menopause Society (NAMS). (2010). Estrogen and progestogen use in postmenopausal women: 2010 position statement of the North American Menopause Society. *Menopause, 17*(2), 242–255.

Popat, V., & Nelson, L. (2007). Spontaneous primary ovarian insufficiency and premature ovarian failure. *eMedicine Reproductive Endocrinology and Infertility.* Retrieved from http://emedicine.medscape.com/article/255974

Rapkin, A. J. (2008). YAZ® in the treatment of premenstrual dysphoric disorder. *Journal of Reproductive Medicine, 53,* 729–741.

Reiter, S. (2008). *Clinical challenges in women's health in the 21st century: A practice handbook for nurse practitioners.* Cranbury, NJ: NP Communications, LLC.

Rowe, M. (2007). Stop, look, listen: Acute coronary syndrome in women. *Advance for Nurse Practitioners, 15*(10), 81–87.

Speroff, L., & Wysocki, S. (2009). Issues concerning hormonal contraceptive use in perimenopausal women. *Dialogues in Contraception, 11*(4), 5–6.

Sufrin, C., & Korn, A. (2009). Tubal sterilization: A closer look at risk of pregnancy. *Contemporary OB/GYN, 54*(5), 50–55.

Waxman, J. (2007). Making the best use of osteoporosis agents. *The Clinical Advisor,* 23–31.

Welt, C. (2008). Primary ovarian insufficiency: A more accurate term for premature ovarian failure. *Clinical Endocrinology.* Retrieved from http://www.medscape .com/viewarticle/573813

Writing Group for the Women's Health Initiative Investigators. (2002). Risks and benefits of estrogen plus progestin in healthy postmenopausal women: Principal results from the women's health initiative randomized controlled trial. *Journal of the American Medical Association, 288,* 321–333.

CHAPTER 5

Women's Health: Family Planning

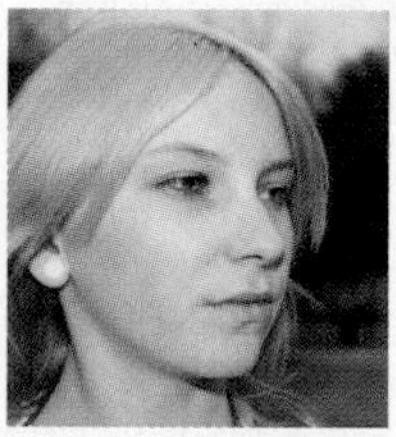

I was 15 when I fell in love with Joe, a handsome, 17-year-old senior on our high school basketball team. My friends were so envious. We didn't plan on becoming sexually involved. It just happened. I knew I should have used some method of birth control, but I didn't know where to go. I couldn't talk to my mother. She wouldn't understand. Joe tried condoms, but he didn't like the way they felt. Several months went by and nothing happened. Then one month my period was late. I was SCARED. It really hit me that a pregnancy would be so hard to handle. I was only a sophomore. My best friend took me to see her nurse practitioner. My pregnancy test was negative. The nurse practitioner encouraged me to talk. She taught me about my body and how to protect myself against an unwanted pregnancy and sexually transmitted infections. She helped me build my self-esteem. I realize now that I'm not ready to be in a sexual relationship yet.

LEARNING OUTCOMES

1. Describe the reasons why women and couples choose to use contraception.
2. Discuss types of fertility awareness-based methods such as natural family planning.
3. List the spermicide preparations currently available in the United States.
4. Compare the barrier methods of contraception with regard to correct use and advantages and disadvantages.
5. Summarize the key points that women who use combined oral contraceptives should know, including the correct procedure for taking pills, common side effects, warning signs, and noncontraceptive benefits.
6. Compare other hormonal methods of birth control, including Depo-Provera, NuvaRing, Ortho Evra, Implanon, and the progestin-only minipill.
7. Identify the appropriate time frame for initiating postcoital emergency contraception (EC).
8. Delineate the advantages and disadvantages of an IUD as a method of contraception.
9. Contrast the forms of sterilization—tubal ligation, Essure, and vasectomy—with regard to risk, effectiveness, advantages, and disadvantages.
10. Compare medical and surgical approaches to pregnancy termination.

KEY TERMS

Coitus interruptus *84*
Combined oral contraceptives (COCs) *90*
Condoms *85*
Depo-Provera *92*
Diaphragm *87*
Fertility awareness-based (FAB) methods *82*
Implanon *92*
Intrauterine devices (IUDs) *88*
Postcoital emergency contraception (EC) *92*
Spermicides *84*
Sterilization *93*
Tubal ligation *93*
Vasectomy *93*

Family planning refers to actions an individual or a couple takes to avoid a pregnancy, to space future pregnancies for a specific reason, or to gain control over the number of children conceived. Thus at a given time a woman may choose one method of contraception and at a later time may elect to use a different method. For example, birth control pills are an excellent method of contraception for women who are healthy and have no medical contraindications. A woman in a stable sexual relationship may choose to use an intrauterine device (IUD), whereas a woman who has no desire for further children may elect permanent sterilization for herself or her male partner may choose such for himself. Although women have several contraceptive methods available, currently, contraceptive methods for men are limited to condoms and vasectomy. This chapter focuses on contraceptive methods currently available, including the advantages and disadvantages of each.

Overview of Family Planning

Demographics

In 2006 there were 66.4 million women in the United States of childbearing age (13 to 46 years) (Guttmacher Institute, 2009). Of these women of childbearing age 62% practiced contraception, whereas 31% did not because they were not sexually active, were infertile, were pregnant or trying to become pregnant, were postpartum, or had never had intercourse. The remaining 7% of these women were not using any contraception (Guttmacher Institute, 2008a.)

Nevertheless in the United States nearly half of all pregnancies are unintended, and of these, 4 in 10 are terminated by abortion. Among women who obtain abortions, 50% are younger than 25—33% are aged 20 to 24 and 17% are teenagers; 30% percent are black, 36% are non-Hispanic white, 25% are Hispanic, and 9% are of other races. About 61% of all abortions are for women who have one or more children (Guttmacher Institute, 2008b).

In 2006, 36.2 million women in the United States were in need of contraceptive services (Guttmacher Institute, 2009). Contraceptive services may be paid for out of pocket, by insurance companies, or by federal employers; contraceptive coverage by insurance companies is mandated in 26 states (Guttmacher Institute, 2008a). Yet, more than 17.5 million women remained in need of publicly funded contraceptive care, with Medicaid continuing to be the largest payer followed by state appropriations. Publicly funded contraceptive services helped prevent 1.94 million pregnancies that could have resulted in 860,000 unintended births and 810,000 abortions (based on statistical projections). For every $1 spent on publicly funded contraceptive care, an average of $4.02 is saved in Medicaid expenditures related to unintended pregnancies, proving the cost-effectiveness of contraceptive care (Guttmacher Institute, 2009).

In the developing world, 137 million women have an unmet need for contraception, and an additional 64 million women have an unmet need for a modern contraceptive method. Although there has been a decline in the unmet needs for contraception across the developing world, it remains high in sub-Saharan Africa, where maternal mortality rates continue to constitute half of all maternal deaths (Sonfield, 2006; World Health Organization [WHO], 2007).

Maternal morbidity and mortality remain a major health challenge in the developing world. Daily 1500 women die or suffer from pregnancy-related problems. In 2005, an estimated 536,000 women died in childbirth or from pregnancy-related problems worldwide; 99% of these deaths occurred in the developing world and many were preventable (WHO, 2007).

HEALTH PROMOTION EDUCATION: CONTRACEPTION

Family planning using a contraceptive method is an important component of women's health. Worldwide, women who are able to use contraception and plan the number of pregnancies they have, as well as the interval between those pregnancies, benefit in several ways (Guttmacher Institute, 2002):

- They enjoy improved health and a lower incidence of sexually transmitted infections, including HIV.
- They have lower rates of induced, sometimes unsafe, abortions.
- They have fewer unwanted pregnancies and births.
- They have the opportunity to get more education and to find jobs, which enhances their economic and social status and improves the well-being of their families.

Most of the causes of maternal mortality are treatable or preventable with adequate health care, including contraceptive services. Thus, it is essential that maternal healthcare services improve if maternal mortality and morbidity are to be reduced. Up to 150,000 maternal deaths per year could be avoided if contraception was available and used by women who did not desire children (United Nations Population Fund [UNPFA], 2008).

Choosing a Method of Contraception

The decision to use a method of contraception may be made individually by a woman (or, in the case of condoms or vasectomy, by a man) or jointly by a couple. Attitudes about contraceptive methods vary considerably. The two leading contraceptive methods in the United States are the combined oral contraceptive pill for women younger than 35 years of age and sterilization for women over the age of 35 (National Center for Health Statistics [NCHS], 2010). Use of the condom and other barrier methods has increased because of the prevalence of sexually transmitted infections (Martinez, Chandra, Abma, et al., 2006).

Decisions about contraception should be made voluntarily with full knowledge of advantages, disadvantages, effectiveness, side effects, contraindications, and long-term effects. Many outside factors influence this choice, including cultural practices, religious beliefs, personality, cost, effectiveness, availability, misinformation, practicality of method, and self-esteem. Different methods of contraception may be appropriate at different times in a person's life (Table 5-1). In choosing a specific method, consistency of use outweighs the absolute reliability of the given method.

TABLE 5-1 Factors to Consider in Choosing a Method of Contraception

- Effectiveness of method in preventing pregnancy
- Safety of the method:
  Are there inherent risks?
  Does it offer protection against sexually transmitted infections (STIs) or other conditions?
- Patient's age and future childbearing plans
- Any contraindications in patient's health history
- Religious or moral factors influencing choice
- Personal preferences, biases
- Lifestyle:
  How frequently does patient have intercourse?
  Does she have multiple partners?
  Does she have ready access to medical care in the event of complications?
- Is cost a factor?
- Partner's support and willingness to cooperate
- Personal motivation to use method

Care Plan Activity: Fertility Awareness

Fertility Awareness-Based Methods

Fertility awareness-based (FAB) methods are based on an understanding of the changes that occur throughout a woman's menstrual cycle and require recording of certain events to identify fertile days. FAB methods take into account the lifespan of sperm (2–7 days) and the ovum (1–3 days) in the female reproductive tract. Maximum fertility for the woman occurs approximately 5 days before ovulation and decreases rapidly the day after. Therefore, the couple must abstain from intercourse, or use a barrier method, during the fertile days (Hatcher et al., 2007).

If the couple using a FAB method also uses a barrier method during fertile days, it is known as fertility awareness-combined methods. If the couple abstains completely from intercourse during fertile days, it is known as natural family planning (NFP) (Hatcher et al., 2007). Other FAB methods include the basal body temperature method, ovulation method, calendar rhythm method, and symptothermal method.

NFP is free, safe, and acceptable to many whose religious beliefs prohibit other methods. It provides an increased awareness of the menstrual cycle, involves no artificial substances or devices, encourages a couple to communicate about sexual activity and family planning, and is useful in helping a couple plan a pregnancy.

To be used effectively, all FAB methods require extensive initial counseling and are best suited for women with regular menstrual cycles. FAB methods may interfere with sexual spontaneity, require the couple to maintain records for several cycles before beginning use, may be difficult or impossible for certain groups of women to use, and may not be as reliable in preventing pregnancy as other methods. Women for whom a FAB method might not be an ideal choice of contraception include those with irregular menstrual cycles, those who are breastfeeding, or those in the perimenopause.

In conjunction with a FAB method or NFP, women may choose to augment identification of their fertile days by use of an over-the-counter ovulation prediction kit (e.g., OvuKit). They may also use a temperature computer (e.g., Bioself 2000) or a hormone computer (e.g., Persona) to help predict fertile days (Hatcher et al., 2007).

Basal Body Temperature Method

The *basal body temperature (BBT)* method is incorporated into the symptothermal method and provides an objective record of fertile days. The BBT method is used to detect ovulation by temperature changes during the menstrual cycle. It requires that the woman take her temperature every morning upon awakening (before any activity) and record the findings on a temperature graph. After 3 to 4 months of recording her temperatures, if she has regular cycles, she should be able to predict when ovulation will occur by a retrospective review of her temperature charts. This method is based on the fact that the temperature almost always rises and remains elevated after ovulation because of the production of progesterone, a thermogenic (heat-producing) hormone, produced by the corpus luteum cyst. Figure 5-1 ■ shows a sample BBT chart.

To avoid conception, the woman and her partner abstain from intercourse, or use a barrier method, on the day of the temperature rise and for 3 days following. Because the temperature rise does not occur until after ovulation, if the woman had intercourse just before the rise she may be at risk of pregnancy.

Ovulation Method

The *ovulation method,* sometimes called the *cervical mucus method* or the *Billings method,* involves the assessment of cervical mucus changes that occur during the menstrual cycle. The amount and character of cervical mucus change because of the influences of estrogen and progesterone. During the follicular phase of the cycle (from the end of menses until just before ovulation) cervical mucus is thick, white, and sticky. This progesterone-dominant mucus is not friendly to sperm and is known as "hostile" mucus. At the time of ovulation, estrogen-dominant mucus is more clear, watery, and stretchable (a quality called *spinnbarkheit*). It has an "egg-white" appearance and is known as "fertile mucus"; it is friendly to sperm, because it assists passage through the cervix and uterus up into the fallopian tubes. It also shows a characteristic fern pattern when placed on a glass slide and allowed to dry. During the luteal phase, cervical mucus is again thick, white, and sticky (progesterone-dominant mucus) and forms a network that traps sperm, making their passage difficult.

Before using the cervical mucus method, the woman abstains from intercourse for one entire menstrual cycle, during which time she assesses her cervical mucus daily for amount, feeling of slipperiness or wetness, color, clearness, and spinnbarkheit. Abstinence is essential during this time, not only so that the woman avoids pregnancy, but also because the presence of ejaculate in the vagina in the hours following intercourse could interfere with the woman's assessment of her cervical mucus.

When using this method, the woman assumes that the peak day of wetness and clear, stretchable mucus is the day of ovulation. However, she abstains from intercourse from the time she *first* notices that the mucus is becoming clearer, more elastic, and slippery until 4 days *after* the peak wet mucus (ovulation) day. Because this method evaluates the effects of hormonal changes, women with irregular cycles can use it.

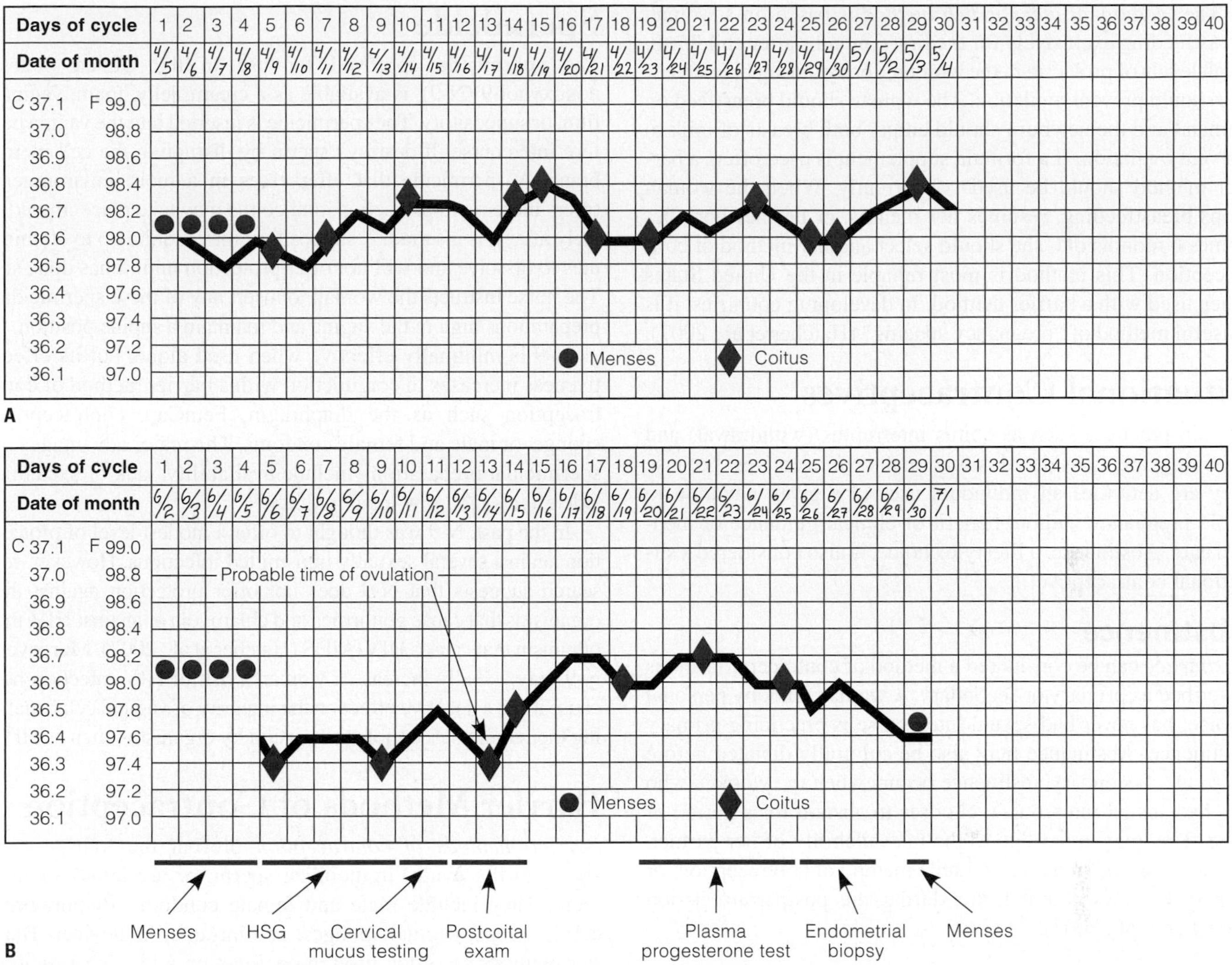

Figure 5-1 ■ A. Monophasic, anovulatory basal body temperature (BBT) chart. B. Biphasic BBT chart illustrating probable time of ovulation, the different types of testing, and the time in the cycle that each would be performed.

Women who feel uncomfortable testing their mucus should be encouraged to use another method.

Calendar Rhythm Method

The *calendar rhythm method (CRM)* is based on the assumption that ovulation tends to occur 14 days (plus or minus 2 days) before the start of the next menstrual period. To use this method, the woman must record her menstrual cycle for 6 months to identify the shortest and longest cycles. The first day of menstruation is the first day of the cycle. The fertile phase is calculated from 18 days before the end of the shortest recorded cycle through 11 days from the end of the longest recorded cycle. For example, if a woman's cycle lasts from 24 to 28 days, the fertile phase would be calculated as day 6 through day 17. Once this information is obtained, the woman can identify the fertile and infertile phases of her cycle. For effective use of this method, she must abstain from intercourse during the fertile phase or use a barrier method. CRM is the *least reliable* of the FAB methods and has largely been replaced by approaches based on objective data.

Symptothermal Method

The *symptothermal method* consists of recording various indicators of fertility by the couple for a number of months. These include: cycle length; frequency and timing of coitus; cervical mucus changes; secondary signs of ovulation such as increased libido, abdominal bloating, mittelschmerz (midcycle abdominal pain); and changes in BBT. In retrospect, using the indicators, the couple learns to recognize signs that indicate ovulation. This combined approach tends to improve the effectiveness of FAB as a method of contraception and is best taught by an expert in the method. For couples interested in the symptothermal method, especially for use as a natural family planning (NFP) method, training courses are available through the Couple to Couple League.

Other Options

The *standard days method* is good for women with regular cycles between 26 and 32 days. Intercourse is avoided, or a barrier method used, between cycle days 8 through 19 (Hatcher et al., 2007).

The *lactational amenorrhea method* is based on a woman breastfeeding exclusively for the first 6 months after childbirth. High levels of prolactin in the woman's body during breastfeeding should prevent ovulation. The woman should breastfeed on demand and the newborn should empty both breasts of milk to prevent ovulation. If a formula supplement is used often, a barrier method should be used concurrently. When the woman stops breastfeeding, resumes her menses, or her newborn becomes 6 months old, she should select another method of contraception. This method is most reliable in the United States when used with a barrier method. In developing countries, it is a useful method of "pregnancy spacing" (Hatcher et al., 2007).

Application: Abstinence Support Resources

Contraception Online

Situational Contraceptives

Certain practices such as coitus interruptus (withdrawal) and douching are considered situational contraceptives because they are activities an individual uses in a given situation to avoid pregnancy without benefit of clinical guidance or medical care. Abstinence, a lifestyle choice, is also considered a situational contraceptive.

Abstinence

Abstinence can be considered a method of contraception and is described as primary or secondary. A woman who, by personal choice, has never had sexual intercourse is practicing primary abstinence. Abstinence may also be culturally dictated before marriage. Secondary abstinence occurs when the woman, who has had sexual intercourse, chooses to abstain for a period of time. This may occur due to the unavailability of her partner, while she waits for a more reliable method of contraception, or it may be the cultural norm during the postpartum period (Hatcher et al., 2007).

Coitus Interruptus

Coitus interruptus, or withdrawal, is one of the oldest methods of contraception. This method requires that the male withdraw from the female's vagina when he feels that ejaculation is impending. He then ejaculates away from the external genitalia of the woman. Failure tends to occur for two reasons:

- This method demands great self-control on the part of the man, who must withdraw just as he feels the urge for deeper penetration with impending orgasm.
- After a recent ejaculation, sperm remain in the urethra. For couples who engage in repeated episodes of orgasm within a short period, this preejaculatory fluid may contain sperm that escape from the penis during the excitement phase before ejaculation. Although the number of sperm is low, this scenario poses the risk of an unintended pregnancy.

Couples who use this method should be aware of postcoital emergency contraceptive options should the man fail to withdraw in time. Such options are discussed later in the chapter.

Douching

Douching after intercourse is an ineffective method of contraception and is *not* recommended. Moreover, it may actually facilitate conception by pushing sperm farther up the birth canal.

Spermicide

The **spermicide** approved for use in the United States, nonoxynol-9 (N-9), is available as a cream, jelly, foam, vaginal film, or suppository. The spermicide is inserted into the vagina before intercourse. It destroys sperm by disrupting the cell membrane. A spermicide that effervesces in a moist environment offers more rapid protection, and coitus may take place immediately after it is inserted. A suppository may require up to 30 minutes to dissolve and will not offer protection until it has done so. The nurse instructs the woman to insert any of these spermicidal preparations high in the vagina and maintain a supine position.

N-9 is minimally effective when used alone, but its effectiveness increases in conjunction with a barrier method of contraception such as the diaphragm, FemCap, contraceptive sponge, or male and female condoms. The major advantages of spermicidal preparations include availability, lack of systemic side effects, and low local toxicity.

In the past, N-9 was thought to offer a modest level of protection against several sexually transmitted infections. However, research suggests that N-9 does not offer protection against the organisms that cause gonorrhea and chlamydia or against HIV, the organism that causes HIV/AIDS (Hatcher et al., 2007). Moreover, N-9 may actually increase a woman's risk of HIV infection because it has a negative effect on the integrity of vaginal cells, making them more susceptible to invasion by organisms such as HIV.

Barrier Methods of Contraception

Barrier methods of contraception prevent the transport of sperm to the ovum, immobilize sperm, or are lethal against them. They include male and female condoms, diaphragms, cervical caps, vaginal sponges, and intrauterine devices. Barrier methods are often used in conjunction with a spermicide, which some authorities consider a form of chemical barrier.

Barrier methods are clearly related to an individual's sexual behavior. Each act of intercourse demands that one or both partners consciously decide whether to use a barrier contraceptive and then take action. Thus these methods require motivation on the part of the user and cooperation from the partner. They may be used less consistently than non–coitus-related methods of contraception, for example, use of the diaphragm only during a woman's fertile days versus taking a pill every day. Because they have few side effects, they are very safe methods and do offer a level of protection against some bacterial sexually transmitted infections.

Barrier methods of contraception are a good choice for women who:

- Have a contraindication to using a specific method such as combined oral contraceptives (COCs), intrauterine devices (IUDs), the subdermal implant (Implanon), and the like.
- Are opposed to taking systemic medications or chemicals such as COCs, injections (Depo-Provera), and so forth.
- Are in the early postpartum period or are lactating.
- Need a backup method of contraception for a period of time such as when beginning COCs, after an IUD has been inserted, or when a male partner has just had a vasectomy.

- Have intercourse rarely or sporadically.
- Are perimenopausal but smoke and thus are not good candidates for COCs.

Before inserting any female barrier contraceptive, a woman should wash her hands with soap and water to prevent the introduction of organisms. Women who use vaginal barrier methods should avoid using oil-based products such as mineral oil or baby oil and vaginal medications such as Monistat cream (for yeast infection) and estrogen creams because they can have a negative effect on latex.

Many barrier methods are made of latex, so women who are allergic should avoid products made of this material and tell their healthcare provider. Nonlatex barrier methods made of silicone, polyurethane, and lambskin are available.

Barrier methods such as the diaphragm, FemCap, and Lea's Shield can be worn for 24 to 48 hours, should be cleaned with soap and water after use, and should not be shared with other women. After the last act of intercourse, these devices should remain in place for a minimum of 6 to 8 hours to prevent pregnancy.

In general, female barrier methods are more effective when used with a male condom. However, a male condom should not be used with a female condom. Women who use barrier methods should be alert for signs of toxic shock syndrome (TSS) such as high fever, sore throat, vomiting and/or diarrhea, faintness, weakness, muscle aches, and a rash (see chapter 7 ∞).

Male Condom

The male **condom** offers a viable means of contraception when used consistently and properly (Figure 5-2 ■). Acceptance has been increasing for two reasons: a growing number of men are assuming responsibility for regulation of fertility, and condoms provide protection from sexually transmitted infections (STIs) for both men and women. For women, regardless of age, an STI increases the risk of pelvic inflammatory disease (PID) and resultant infertility. Many women insist that their sexual partners use condoms, and many women carry condoms with them.

The condom is applied to the erect penis, rolled from the tip to the end of the shaft, before vulvar or vaginal contact. Most condoms have a reservoir tip to allow for collection of ejaculate. When using a condom without a reservoir end, a small space must be left at the end to collect the ejaculate, so that the condom does not break at the time of ejaculation. If the condom or vagina is dry, water-soluble lubricants, such as K-Y jelly or Astroglide, should be used to prevent irritation and possible condom breakage. Care must be taken in removing the condom after intercourse. For optimal effectiveness, the man should withdraw his penis from the vagina while it is still erect and hold the condom rim to prevent spillage. If after ejaculation the penis becomes flaccid while still in the vagina, the man should hold onto the edge of the condom while withdrawing to avoid spilling the semen and to prevent the condom from slipping off.

The effectiveness of male condoms is largely determined by their use. The condom is small, lightweight, disposable, and inexpensive. It has no side effects (if not allergic to latex), requires no medical examination or supervision, and offers visual evidence of effectiveness. Most condoms are made of latex. Thus, their use is contraindicated if the male or his partner has a latex allergy. Polyurethane and silicone rubber condoms are also manufactured and recommended for individuals allergic to latex. Condoms are available with ribbed or smooth sides, tapered or straight-sided, lubricated or unlubricated, with or without spermicide. They come in a variety of colors, sizes, and flavors. "Natural skins" (lambs' intestines) are available; they are used primarily by individuals with latex allergies. All condoms except natural skin condoms offer protection against sexually transmitted infections (STIs). Moreover, a systematic research review indicates that

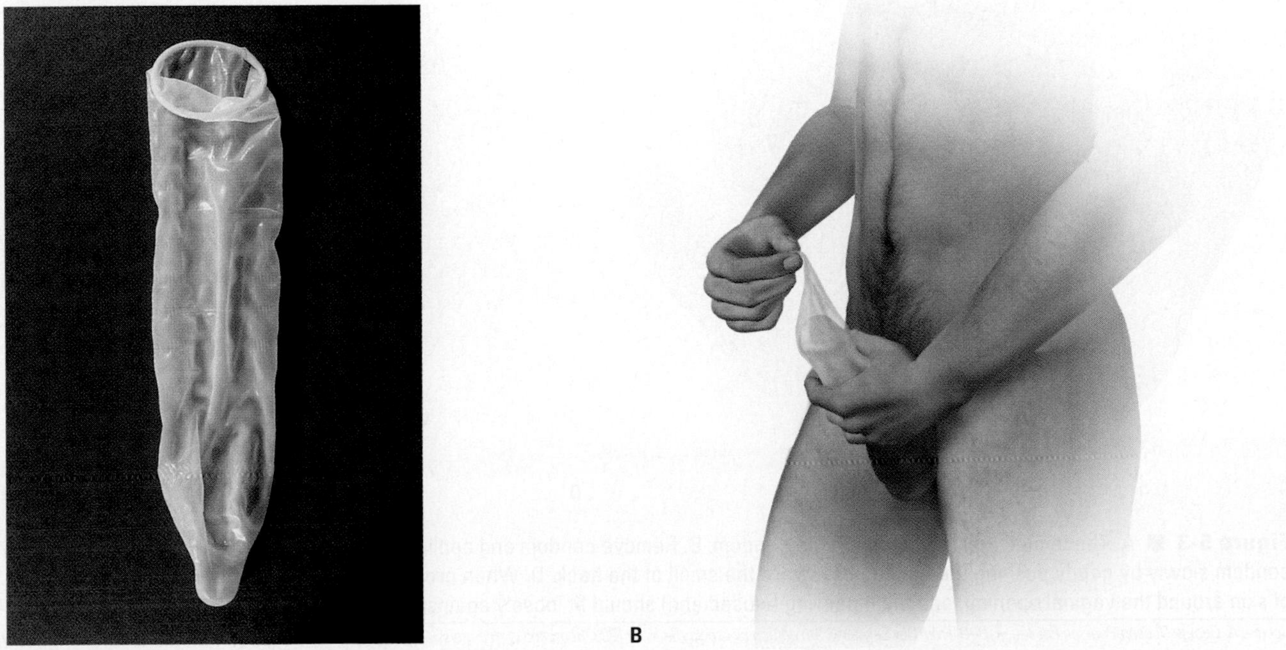

A

B

Figure 5-2 ■ A. An unrolled condom with reservoir tip. B. Correct use.

consistent use of condoms results in an 80% reduction of the incidence of HIV (Weller & Davis-Beatty, 2009). Concurrent use of a vaginal spermicide with the male condom increases the overall effectiveness in the prevention of pregnancy.

Misplacement, risk of breakage, perineal or vaginal irritation, and dulled sensation are possible disadvantages of male condoms. Condoms should not be stored in hot conditions because heat accelerates their deterioration, making them more susceptible to breaking. Thus, men should avoid placing them in their car glove box or in their wallets in a rear pants pocket.

Female Condom

The *Reality female condom* (Figure 5-3 ■) is a thin polyurethane sheath with a flexible ring at each end. The inner ring, at the closed end of the condom, serves as the means of insertion and fits over the cervix like a diaphragm. The second ring remains outside the vagina and covers a portion of the woman's perineum. It also covers the base of the man's penis during intercourse. A woman needs to be careful not to twist the sheath when she inserts the condom because twisting makes male penetration impossible.

Available over the counter and designed for one-time use, the condom may be inserted up to 8 hours before intercourse. The inner sheath is prelubricated but does not contain spermi-

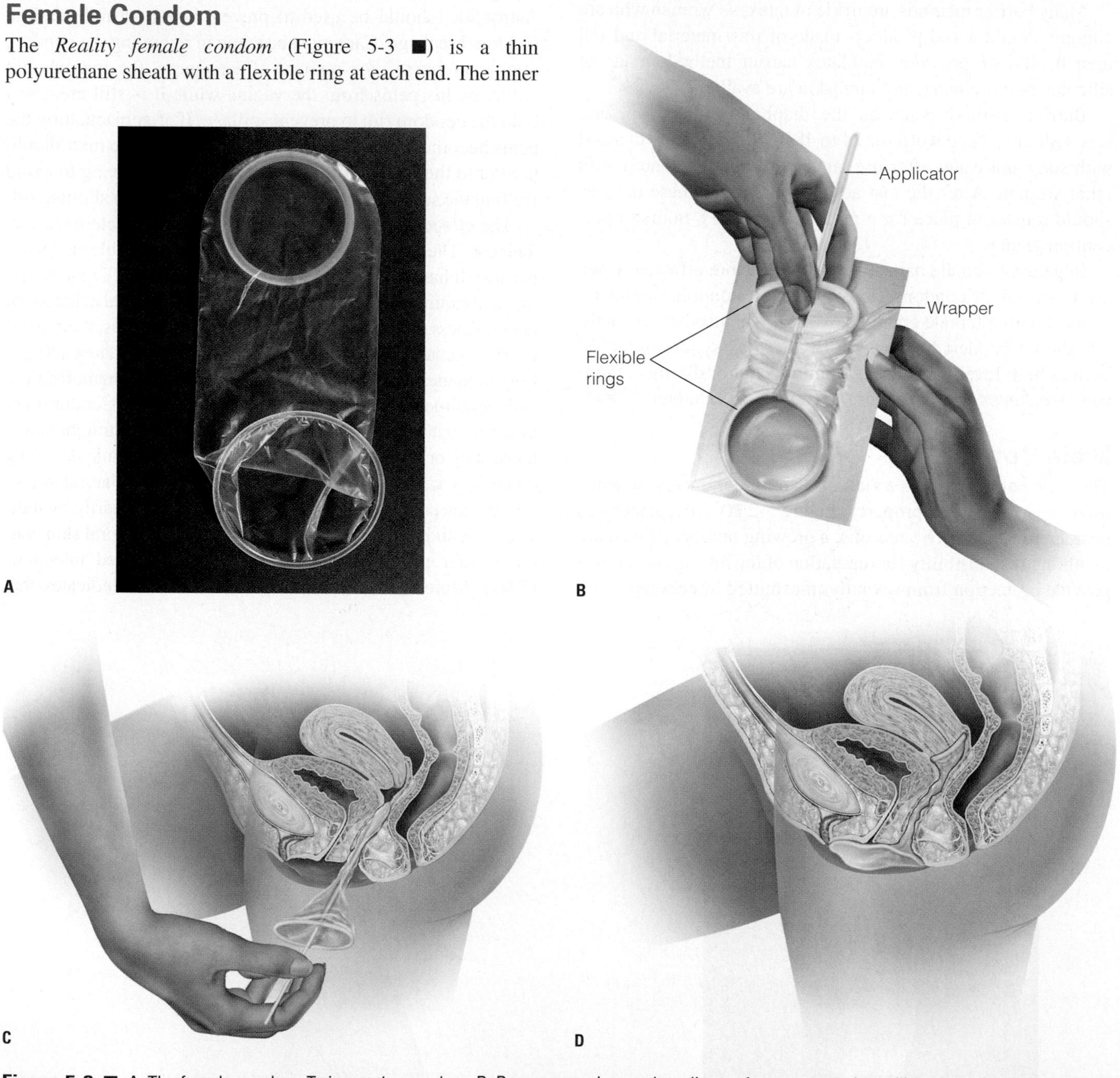

Figure 5-3 ■ A. The female condom. To insert the condom: B. Remove condom and applicator from wrapper by pulling up on the ring. C. Insert condom slowly by gently pushing the applicator toward the small of the back. D. When properly inserted, the outer ring should rest on the folds of skin around the vaginal opening, and the inner ring (closed end) should fit loosely against the cervix.

Source: A. George Dodson/Pearson Education. B–D. From Our Sexuality, 5th edition by Crooks/Baur. © 1993. Reprinted with permission of Wadsworth, a division of Thomson Learning: www.thomsonrights.com

cide and is not designed to be used with a male condom. Because it also covers a portion of the vulva it probably provides better protection than other methods against some of the pathogens that cause STIs. High cost, noisiness during intercourse, and the cumbersome feel of the device make acceptability a problem for some couples.

Diaphragm

The **diaphragm** is a barrier method that consists of a steel band that forms a ring and is covered with latex or silicone so that when the diaphragm is inserted, the ring lodges high in the vagina with the latex or silicone covering the cervix. It is used with spermicidal cream or jelly and offers a good level of protection from conception. Currently it is used by 0.3% of U.S. women (Guttmacher Institute, 2008a).

Three types of diaphragms are available—the flat spring, the coil spring, and the arcing spring. Each type has its own advantages, and the type of coil makes the different diaphragms better suited to some women than to others. A woman must be fitted with a diaphragm and given instructions by trained personnel. The diaphragm should be rechecked for correct size after each childbirth and whenever a woman has gained or lost 10 to 15 pounds or more. Most diaphragms are made of latex; for allergic women, Milex® produces the WIDE-SEAL Silicone Diaphragm.

The diaphragm must be inserted before intercourse, with approximately one teaspoonful (or 1.5 inches from the tube) of spermicidal jelly placed around its rim and in the cup (Figure 5-4 ■). This chemical barrier supplements the mechanical barrier of the diaphragm. The diaphragm is inserted through the vagina and covers the cervix. The last step in insertion is to push the edge of the diaphragm under the pubic symphysis, which may result in a "popping" sensation. When fitted properly and correctly in place, the diaphragm should not cause discomfort to the woman or her partner. Correct placement of the diaphragm can be checked by touching the cervix with a fingertip through the cup. The cervix feels like a small rounded structure and has a consistency similar to that of the tip of the nose. The center of the diaphragm should be located over the cervix.

If more than 6 hours elapse between insertion of the diaphragm and intercourse, additional spermicidal jelly should be inserted into the vagina, although no evidence supports this (Hatcher et al., 2007). It is necessary to leave the diaphragm in place for at least 6 hours after the act of coitus. If intercourse is desired again within the 6 hours, another type of contraception must be used or additional spermicidal jelly placed in the vagina with an applicator, taking care not to disturb the placement of the diaphragm. The diaphragm should not remain in the vagina for more than 24 hours because of the risk of toxic shock syndrome.

Periodically the diaphragm should be held up to the light or filled with water and inspected for tears or holes. If properly maintained, it can last for several years, so it is a cost-effective method of contraception. The diaphragm should be washed and dried well after each use and then stored in a clean, dry container. Talcum powder should not be used with a latex diaphragm because it contributes to the deterioration of the rubber.

Some couples feel that the use of a diaphragm interferes with the spontaneity of intercourse. The nurse can suggest that the partner insert the diaphragm as part of foreplay or the woman may choose to insert it herself before intercourse. Diaphragm use potentially reduces the incidence of cervical gonorrhea and chlamydia. Its use does protect against human papilloma virus (HPV) infection, which can cause cervical neoplasia (Hatcher et al., 2007).

Women who object to touching their genitals to insert the diaphragm, check its placement, and remove it may find this method unsatisfactory. Women who are very obese or who have short fingers may find the diaphragm difficult to insert. It is not recommended for women with a history of urinary tract infection (UTI), because pressure from the diaphragm on the urethra may interfere with complete bladder emptying and lead to recurrent UTIs. These women should be given information about other methods of contraception. As mentioned previously, women with a history of toxic shock syndrome should not use diaphragms or any of the barrier methods left in place for prolonged periods. For the same reason, the diaphragm should not be used during a menstrual period or if a woman has abnormal vaginal discharge.

Cervical Caps

The Prentif Cavity Rim cervical cap or *FemCap* looks like a small sailor's cap and is made of soft silicone. The "dome" of the cap fits over the cervix, while the soft "brim" flares out slightly and conforms to the shape of the vagina. A strap placed over the dome permits easier removal. The cap, which is no longer available in the United States, is available in three sizes and should be used with a spermicide. Advantages, disadvantages, and contraindications are similar to those associated with the diaphragm.

A systematic research review indicates that the FemCap is not as effective as a diaphragm in preventing pregnancy; however, both forms are medically safe to use (Gallo, Grimes, Schulz, et al., 2010).

Lea's Shield is a reusable, silicone, one-size-fits-all vaginal barrier method that completely covers the cervix. It contains a centrally located valve that permits the passage of cervical secretions and air. It is held in place by the vaginal walls. It is available by prescription in the United States. A spermicide should be used with it and it should not be worn for more than 48 hours.

Vaginal Sponge

The Today *vaginal sponge,* available without a prescription, is a pillow-shaped, soft, absorbent synthetic sponge containing a spermicide. It is made with a concave or cupped area on one side, which is designed to fit over the cervix. It has a loop to permit easy removal. The sponge acts as a contraceptive by releasing the spermicide N-9 gradually over a 24-hour period.

The sponge is moistened thoroughly with water before use to activate the spermicide and is then inserted into the vagina

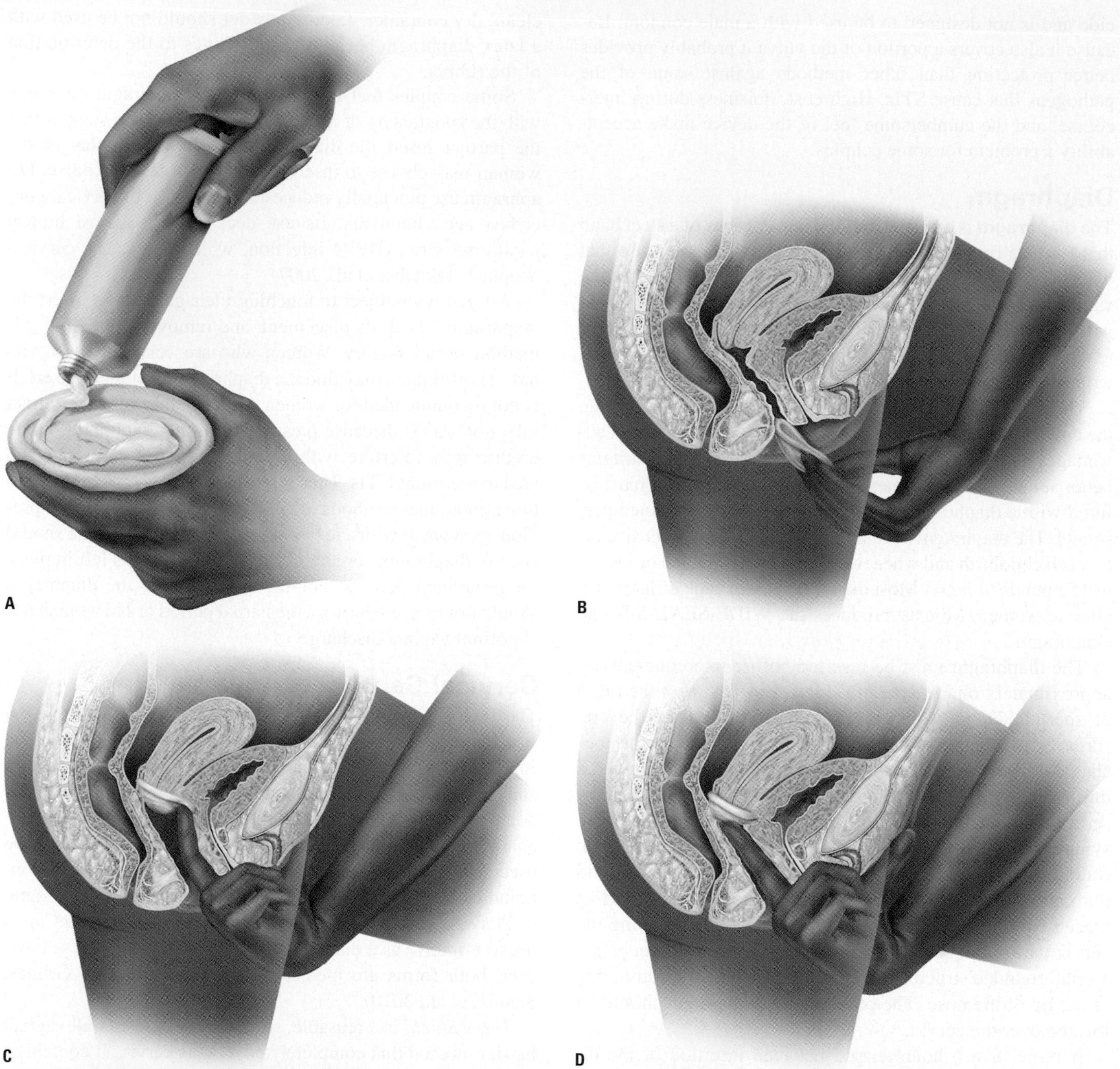

A B C D

Figure 5-4 ■ Inserting the diaphragm. A. Apply jelly to the rim and center of the diaphragm. B. Insert the diaphragm. C. Push the rim of the diaphragm under the pubic symphysis. D. Check placement of the diaphragm. The cervix should be felt through the diaphragm.

so that the cupped side fits snugly against the cervical os (Figure 5-5 ■). This decreases the chance of the sponge being dislodged during intercourse. The sponge may be worn for up to 24 hours. It should be left in place for at least 6 hours after intercourse and then removed and discarded.

Advantages of the sponge include the following: professional fitting is not required; it may be used for multiple acts of coitus for up to 24 hours; one size fits all; and it acts as both a barrier method and a spermicide agent. Problems associated with the sponge include difficulty removing it and irritation or allergic reactions. Some women also report a problem because the sponge absorbs vaginal secretions, contributing to vaginal dryness. For women without children the failure rate is comparable to that of the diaphragm. The failure rate is higher for women who have borne children, possibly because of changes in the shape of the cervix.

Intrauterine Devices

Both of the **intrauterine devices (IUDs)** available in the United States are designed to be inserted into the uterus by a qualified healthcare provider and left in place for an extended period, providing continuous contraceptive protection. The Copper IUD (ParaGard T380A) provides effective contraception for 10 years, whereas the Mirena levonorgestrel intrauter-

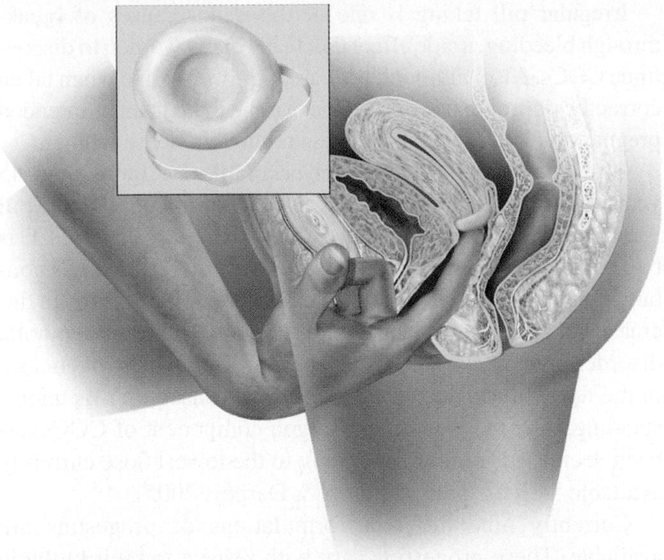

Figure 5-5 ■ The contraceptive sponge is moistened well with water and inserted into the vagina with the concave portion positioned over the cervix.

ine system (LNG-IUS) provides 5 years of protection. The exact mechanism of either IUD is not clearly understood. Traditionally, it was believed to act by preventing the implantation of a fertilized ovum. Thus, it was considered an abortifacient or abortion-causing method. This belief is not accurate; both IUDs are truly contraceptive. The Copper IUD is known to have local inflammatory effects on the endometrium and to impair sperm from functioning properly. The Mirena IUD causes the lining of the uterus (endometrium) to become atrophic. It also produces thick cervical mucus that is "hostile" or unfriendly to sperm. Both IUDs produce a spermicidal intrauterine environment (Speroff & Darney, 2005).

Both IUDs available today, contrary to common myth, do not increase the risk of ectopic pregnancy or cause pelvic inflammatory disease (PID). In reality, infections in IUD users are probably related more to the woman's lifestyle than to the presence of the IUD. Advantages of both IUDs include a high rate of effectiveness, continuous contraceptive protection, non–coitus-related contraception, and relative inexpensiveness over time. Possible adverse reactions to both IUDs include discomfort to the wearer (possible cramping), increased bleeding during menses, increased risk of pelvic infection for about 3 weeks following insertion, perforation of the uterus during insertion, unscheduled bleeding, dysmenorrhea, and expulsion of the device.

The Copper IUD (ParaGard T380A) is a small T-shaped device that has copper covering parts of its stem and arms. This IUD is not an option for women allergic to copper but is an excellent choice for women who have medical conditions that preclude use of other contraceptives, hormonal or barrier. The Mirena (LNG-IUS) (Figure 5-6 ■) is a small, T-shaped frame with a reservoir that releases levonorgestrel on a daily basis. After 3 months of Mirena use, bleeding and length of menstrual cycles are reduced. In fact, 14% to 20% of women have amenorrhea, which they often welcome once they are advised that the absence of menses is safe and not an indication of pregnancy. The

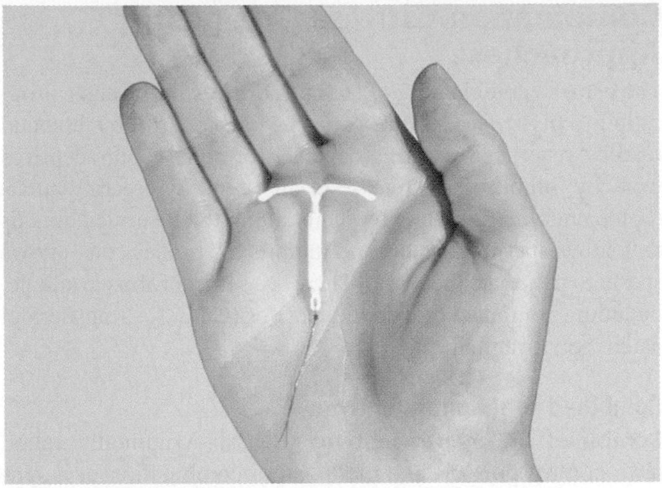

Figure 5-6 ■ The Mirena Intrauterine System, which releases levonorgestrel gradually, may be left in place for up to 5 years.

Source: Courtesy of Berlex Laboratories, Wayne, NJ.

LNG-IUS is an excellent choice for women who are allergic to copper or who have heavy menses and desire amenorrhea.

There are few women for whom either IUD is contraindicated. A current pregnancy or current STI or pelvic infection would be contraindications. Women who have had children have a deeper uterine cavity that accepts placement of either IUD more readily. However, women who have not had children can be candidates for insertion of the IUD if the cavity of their uteri are deep enough (6–9 cm). If the woman has multiple sexual partners, she should be cautioned to use a condom in addition to her IUD. However, because the Mirena causes thick cervical mucus, it may have a protective effect against STIs (Hatcher et al., 2007).

The IUD is inserted into the uterus with its strings protruding through the cervix into the vagina. It may be inserted at any time during the woman's cycle, providing she is not pregnant, or during the 6-week postpartum check. After insertion, the clinician instructs the woman to check for the presence of the strings once a week for the first month and then after each menses. She does this by inserting her index finger or middle finger into her vagina to feel the strings; this ensures the IUD is still in the uterus. She is told that she may have some cramping or bleeding intermittently for 2 to 6 weeks and that her first few menses may be irregular. Follow-up examination is suggested 4 to 8 weeks after insertion.

Women with IUDs should contact their healthcare providers if they are exposed to an STI or if they develop the following warning signs: late period, abnormal spotting or bleeding, dyspareunia (pain with intercourse), abdominal pain, abnormal discharge, signs of infection (fever, chills, malaise), missing strings, or lengthening of the strings. If a woman becomes pregnant with an IUD in place, the device should be removed as soon as possible to prevent infection (Schorge et al., 2008).

Hormonal Contraceptives

Hormonal contraceptives are available in a variety of forms. They may be progestin-only hormones, most often using a synthetic form of progesterone, or a combination of estrogen and a progestin.

Combination Estrogen-Progestin Approaches

The use of a combination of the hormones estrogen and a progestin is a highly successful, very safe birth control method and readily reversible when stopped. Hormonal contraceptives work by inhibiting the release of an ovum, by creating an atrophic endometrium, and by maintaining thick cervical mucus that slows sperm transport and inhibits the process that allows sperm to penetrate the ovum. There are several forms available, including combined oral contraceptives (COCs), a transdermal patch, and a vaginal ring.

Combined Oral Contraceptives

Oral Contraceptive

Combined oral contraceptives (COCs)—commonly called birth control pills or "the pill"—are a combination of a synthetic estrogen and a progestin. COCs are one of the most popular contraceptive options available to women in the United States because they are safe, highly effective, and rapidly reversible. Most COCs are taken daily for 21 or 28 days, following one of these methods:

1. ***Day 1 start.*** The woman begins taking the pill on the first day of her menstrual cycle. This method prevents ovulation in the first cycle, so no backup method of contraception is needed.
2. ***Sunday start.*** The woman begins taking the pill on the Sunday after the first day of the menstrual cycle and ends the packet on a Saturday. In most cases a hormonally mediated menses (known as a "withdrawal" bleed) will occur 1 to 4 days after the last pill is taken. The Sunday start is common because it tends to prevent periods on weekends. However, a backup method of contraception is necessary during the first 7 days of use.
3. ***Quick start.*** The woman begins taking the pill in the practitioner's office if she is reasonably certain she is not pregnant. A backup method is necessary for 7 days. New COC users are more likely to still be using this method 3 months later with this start (Hatcher et al., 2007).

COCs are packaged with 21 or 28 pills. Seven days after taking her last pill, the woman using the 21-day pack of pills restarts the next cycle of pills. The 28-day pack includes seven "blank" pills so that the woman never stops taking a pill and thus never forgets to start a new pack a week later. Women who use either the 21- or 28-day COC pack will always begin a new pack on the same day. The pill should be taken at approximately the same time each day—usually on arising or before retiring in the evening.

Seasonale® and Seasonique® are the two COCs marketed for extended use. Women who choose Seasonale take 84 active pills containing estrogen and a progestin followed by 7 "blank" pills, and those who take Seasonique take 84 active pills and 7 pills with a reduced dosing of estrogen intended to promote less bleeding. Women taking either extended use COC have 4 withdrawal bleeds per year rather than 12. Extended use reduces the side effects of COCs such as bloating, headache, breast tenderness, cramping, and swelling (Hatcher et al., 2007).

Irregular pill taking is one of the major causes of breakthrough bleeding, a side effect that leads many women to discontinue COCs. Also, although they are highly effective when taken correctly, improper use of COCs can contribute to an unintended pregnancy. COCs may also be less reliable in obese women.

Birth control pills have been available for more than 45 years. In the United States, the estrogen component of the pill is either ethinyl estradiol (EE) or mestranol. Of the two, EE is by far the more commonly used estrogen. Initially, COCs contained high levels of estrogen and were linked with an increased risk for myocardial infarction (MI), thromboembolic disorders (blood clots), and stroke. Lowering the estrogen dose in the formulation decreased these risks. Based on this understanding, over the years the estrogen component of COCs has been decreased from 150 mcg/day to the lowest dose currently available—20 mcg/day (Speroff & Darney, 2005).

Currently nine different formulations of progestins are available. These progestins vary with respect to their biologic activity including inhibition of ovulation. Synthetic progestins can have androgenic, antiandrogenic, estrogenic, and antiestrogenic effects. These effects are responsible for the varying progestin-related side effects.

COCs are among the most studied medications available. The current generation of low-dose pills is very safe and would be even safer if smokers over age 35 did not take them. In an effort to reduce complications such as myocardial infarction, stroke, blood clots, and hypertension, regimens have been developed that use very low doses of estrogen (20 or 25 mcg) and progestins that are less androgenic in effect. These very-low-dose pills may result in weaker cycle control, which leads to more irregular or "breakthrough" bleeding. These low-dose pills do provide the same noncontraceptive benefits as the pills that contain 30 to 35 mcg of EE, and it is recommended that smokers of all ages who wish to take the pill be prescribed 20 mcg COCs to reduce serious complications.

Side effects are generally identifiable as estrogen related or progestin related. Thus it is possible to modify some side effects by choosing a different oral contraceptive preparation. The side effects associated with COCs are identified in Table 5-2.

Absolute contraindications to the use of oral contraceptives include pregnancy, previous history of thrombophlebitis or thromboembolic disease, acute or chronic liver disease of cholestatic type with abnormal liver function tests, presence of estrogen-dependent carcinomas, undiagnosed uterine bleeding, heavy smoking, gallbladder disease, hypertension, diabetes, migraine with visual disturbances, hypercoagulable disorders, and hyperlipidemia. Women with relative contraindications may initiate COC use; however, they require close and frequent monitoring. These include women with migraine headaches without visual disturbances, epilepsy, depression, oligomenorrhea, and amenorrhea. Women who choose this method of contraception should be fully advised of the potential side effects and complications. Generic preparations of COCs are as effective as brand-name COCs (Hatcher et al., 2007).

Oral contraceptives have several important noncontraceptive benefits. Many women who use COCs experience relief of uncomfortable menstrual symptoms and premenstrual syndrome;

TABLE 5-2 Side Effects Associated with Oral Contraceptives

ESTROGEN EFFECTS	PROGESTIN EFFECTS
Alterations in lipid metabolism	Acne, oily skin
Breast tenderness, engorgement or increased breast size	Breast tenderness; increased breast size
Cerebrovascular accident	Decreased libido
Changes in carbohydrate metabolism	Decreased high-density lipoprotein (HDL) cholesterol levels
Chloasma	Depression
Fluid retention; cyclic weight gain	Fatigue
Headache	Hirsutism
Hepatic adenomas	Increased appetite; weight gain
Hypertension	Increased low-density lipoprotein (LDL) cholesterol levels
Leukorrhea, cervical erosion, ectropion	Oligomenorrhea, amenorrhea
Nausea	Pruritus
Nervousness, irritability	Sebaceous cysts
Telangiectasia	
Thromboembolic complications—thrombophlebitis, pulmonary embolism	

cramps diminish, flow decreases, and the cycle becomes more regular. Mittelschmerz is eliminated. More important, there is a reduction in the incidence of ovarian cancer, endometrial cancer, colorectal cancer, menstrual migraines, and iron deficiency anemia. In addition, hormonal contraceptives can be effective in improving bone mineral density and in treating acne or hirsutism, pelvic pain due to endometriosis, and bleeding due to leiomyomas (American College of Obstetricians and Gynecologists [ACOG], 2010). Currently, oral contraceptives assist with some of the physiologic changes experienced by women during the perimenopause (such as hot flashes) as well as provide contraception. COCs can be used by nonsmoking women until they transition into menopause, at which time hormone therapy may be necessary to control vasomotor symptoms, such as hot flashes (Hatcher et al., 2007). Because of an increased risk of MI (heart attack), women over age 35 who smoke should not take oral contraceptives.

The woman using oral contraceptives should contact her healthcare provider if she becomes depressed, develops a breast lump, becomes jaundiced, or experiences any of the following warning signs: severe abdominal pain, severe chest pain or shortness of breath, severe headaches, dizziness, changes in vision (vision loss or blurring), speech problems, or severe leg pain.

Transdermal Hormonal Contraception

Combined hormonal contraception can now be provided transdermally using a weekly *contraceptive skin patch* called Ortho Evra, manufactured by Ortho-McNeil-Janssen Pharmaceuticals. Roughly the size of a silver dollar, but square, this patch is applied weekly for 3 weeks on one of four sites: the woman's abdomen, buttocks, upper outer arm, or trunk (excluding the breasts). During the fourth week, no patch is applied and menses typically occurs. The patch is highly effective in women who weigh less than 198 pounds (Hatcher et al., 2007). Patch users apply their first patch on the first day of their menses or on the Sunday following; if the latter is chosen a backup method for 7 days is necessary.

The patch is as safe and effective as COCs and has a better rate of user compliance. Generally, women who are candidates for COCs are candidates for the patch unless they weigh greater than 198 pounds or have skin disorders that may result in reactions at the site of application. Product labeling was changed in 2008 to include a greater risk of venous thromboembolism (VTE) for women using the patch versus those taking COCs. The United States Food and Drug Administration (FDA) considers the patch a safe method of contraception for women not at risk of a VTE (U.S. FDA, 2008).

Vaginal Contraceptive Ring

NuvaRing vaginal contraceptive ring (manufactured by Organon), another form of low-dose, sustained-release combined hormonal contraceptive, is a flexible, soft vaginal ring that is inserted for 3 weeks (Figure 5-7 ■). The ring is left in place for 21 days and then removed for 7 days (Hatcher et al., 2007). This one-size ring fits virtually all women. Women with marked vaginal prolapse should be cautioned to check for expulsion of the ring during early use. Women who use the NuvaRing should begin its use in the same way as described for the patch. Replacement rings should be kept in the refrigerator to maintain integrity.

Progestin Contraceptives

Progestin-Only Pills

Another oral contraceptive is the progestin-only pill, also called the *minipill*. It is used primarily by nursing mothers, because it

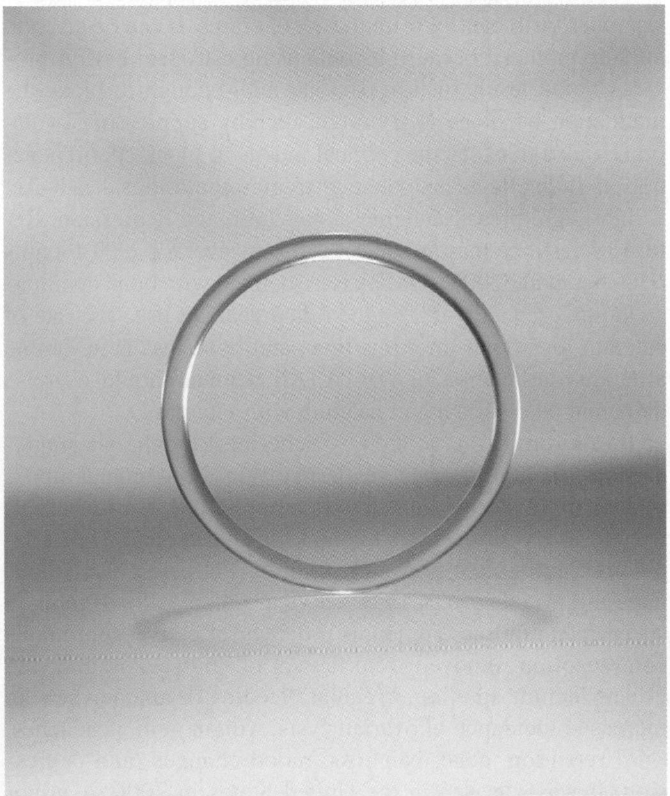

Figure 5-7 ■ The NuvaRing vaginal contraceptive ring.

Source: Merck & Co., Inc. Organon Pharmaceuticals.

does not interfere with breast milk production. It is also used by women who have a contraindication to the estrogen component of the combination preparation, such as history of thrombophlebitis or hypertension or estrogen-related side effects, but are strongly motivated to use this form of contraception. The major problems with progesterone-only pills are amenorrhea or irregular bleeding patterns. They are slightly less effective than a COC. They must be taken consistently at the same time every day (Hatcher et al., 2007).

Long-Acting Progestin Contraceptives

Long-acting progestin-only contraceptives include Depo-Provera and Implanon. Progestin-only contraceptive methods are recommended for lactating women, women who cannot use estrogen or the intrauterine device (IUD), women who forget to take COCs daily, and women who are not bothered by unscheduled bleeding (irregular spotting or bleeding). These are safe, reversible forms of contraception.

Depo-Provera or depot-medroxyprogesterone acetate (DMPA), manufactured by Pfizer, is a long-acting, injectable, progestin-only contraceptive. DMPA is manufactured in 2 dosings: DMPA-IM 150 mg for intramuscular use or DMPA-SC 104 mg for subcutaneous use. Both provide highly effective birth control for 3 months after administration with subsequent injections scheduled every 10 to 14 weeks. DMPA-SC may cause less pain than an intramuscular (IM) injection and could be self-administered, increasing compliance by not having to return every 3 months to the clinic.

DMPA, which acts primarily by suppressing ovulation, is safe, convenient, private, and relatively inexpensive. It also separates birth control from the act of coitus. It can be given to nursing mothers, because it contains no estrogen. DMPA provides blood levels of progesterone high enough to block the luteinizing hormone (LH) surge, thereby suppressing ovulation. It also thickens the cervical mucus to block sperm penetration. Side effects include menstrual irregularities, headache, weight gain, breast tenderness, hair loss, and depression. Return of fertility may be delayed for an average of 9 months (Hatcher et al., 2007). DMPA is associated with bone demineralization, especially during the first 2 years of use. The rate of calcium loss slows after this time, and bone loss is reversible after discontinuation of DMPA. All women should exercise daily and take 1200 mg of calcium with vitamin D.

Implanon, manufactured by Schering-Plough, is a single-capsule implant inserted subdermally in the woman's upper underarm. It is impregnated with etonogestrel, a progestin. It is good as a contraceptive method for 3 years, and its mechanism of action is to prevent ovulation. Implanon also stimulates the production of thick cervical mucus, which inhibits sperm penetration. Implanon provides effective continuous contraception removed from the act of coitus. Possible side effects include spotting, irregular bleeding or amenorrhea, an increased incidence of ovarian cysts, weight gain, headaches, fluid retention, acne, hair loss, mood changes, and depression. It was released in the United States in 2006. A minor surgical procedure is required to insert and remove the implant (Hatcher et al., 2007).

Postcoital Emergency Contraception

Postcoital emergency contraception (EC) is indicated when a woman is worried about pregnancy because of unprotected intercourse, sexual assault, or possible contraceptive failure (e.g., broken condom, slipped diaphragm, missed oral contraceptives, or too long a time between depot-medroxyprogesterone acetate [DMPA] injections). Research indicates that oral hormonal EC taken as soon as possible within 72 hours can reduce the risk of pregnancy after a single act of unprotected intercourse by 75% to 89%.

Two hormonal regimens for EC include a combined hormonal approach (levonorgestrel and ethinyl estradiol), and Plan B, a progestin-only approach (levonorgestrel). Though sometimes called the "morning-after pill," the phrase is misleading because the woman actually takes her first dose as soon after intercourse as possible and a second dose 12 hours later. The combined hormonal approach uses high-dose combined oral contraceptives. The progestin-only approach uses a high dose of one progestin, levonorgestrel. Both methods should inhibit ovulation, although other mechanisms are thought to play a part (Hatcher et al., 2007).

Plan B, manufactured by Duramed as One-Step, is an EC method that is more effective than the combined hormonal EC; it also has a much lower incidence of associated nausea and vomiting. If it is available, it should be used instead of the combined regimen (ACOG, 2007a). Plan B comes as 2 tablets of 0.75 mg levonorgestrel to be taken at once, or as Plan B One-Step, 1 tablet that contains 1.5 mg of levonorgestrel. Both dosings should be taken as soon after coitus as possible. It is available over the counter, without prescription, to any woman 17 years or older.

The combined regimen remains an option because many women knowledgeable about EC can use their unused combined oral contraceptives (COCs) after consulting with their healthcare provider about the appropriate dosing. COCs are prescriptions that must be obtained from a healthcare provider. The high dose of estrogen may lead to nausea and vomiting. A prophylactic antiemetic may be useful.

Both regimens must be initiated within 72 hours after unprotected intercourse, although most research indicates they could be effective up to 5 days after coitus. Emergency contraceptive pills are safe for almost all women. The only contraindication is a diagnosed pregnancy because the pills are ineffective (Hatcher et al., 2007). The woman should have her normal menses 2 weeks after taking EC. If she does not, she should follow up with a pregnancy test. If the pregnancy test is negative, she should be counseled about reliable methods of birth control.

The medical abortion-inducing drug, mifepristone, is very effective in providing emergency contraception. However, its use is highly restricted and it is not currently approved for emergency contraception (Benagiano & vonHertzen, 2010).

Placement of the Copper IUD within 5 days after unprotected intercourse may reduce pregnancy risk by as much as 99% (ACOG, 2007a; ACOG, 2007b; Hatcher et al., 2007).

RESEARCH EVIDENCE IN PRACTICE Emergency Contraception

CLINICAL QUESTION

What are the predictors and outcomes of emergency contraception use after unprotected intercourse?

RESEARCH EVIDENCE

A variety of factors influence the use of emergency contraception to prevent an unintended pregnancy after unprotected intercourse. In one large, multisite study of emergency contraception use, receiving counseling about emergency contraception from a healthcare provider was the strongest predictor of its appropriate use. Yet only 3% of women in this study reported that a clinician had discussed emergency contraception with them in the past year. A woman's likelihood of receiving counseling was further reduced if she was over the age of 30, Hispanic, black, or married.

In a large study of provider attitudes about emergency contraception and subsequent patient counseling, barriers to provision of emergency contraception included staff prejudgment that the woman did not need it, time constraints of office visits, and staff beliefs that the patient did not have the ability to use the method. However, in a study of provider behaviors that enhanced contraception use, the only intervention that was successful in improving use of contraception was providing the woman with contraception during the provider visit.

WHAT QUESTIONS REMAIN UNANSWERED?

Little research has been conducted on the effects of repeated use of emergency contraception as a method of preventing unintended pregnancy. What are the long-term outcomes of emergency contraception for the woman? What is the effect of repetitive emergency contraception on later childbearing?

WHAT IS BEST PRACTICE?

Women are more likely to use emergency contraception if they are counseled about its use by their healthcare provider and if a dose is provided during the clinic visit.

CRITICAL THINKING

How can counseling about emergency contraception be introduced during the routine gynecologic examination? What patient education about emergency contraception will enhance its appropriate use?

References

Cheng, L., Gulmezoglu, A., Piaggio, G., Ezcurra, E., & Van Look, P. (2008). Interventions for emergency contraception. *Cochrane Database of Systematic Reviews*, Issue 2.

Kavanaugh, M., & Schwarz, E. (2008). Counseling about and use of emergency contraception in the United States. *Perspectives on Sexual and Reproductive Health, 40*(2), 81–86.

Kirby, D. (2008). The impact of programs to increase contraceptive use among adult women: A review of experimental and quasi-experimental studies. *Perspectives on Sexual and Reproductive Health. 40*(1), 34–41.

Whittaker, P., Armstrong, K., & Adams, J. (2008). Implementing an advance emergency contraception policy: What happens in the real world? *Perspectives on Sexual and Reproductive Health. 40*(3), 162–170.

Currently there is considerable debate about the best ways to improve access to EC. It is essential that healthcare providers counsel women about the availability of EC during routine screenings and appointments. This approach ensures that women are familiar with the method before an emergency occurs. It is also helpful to have printed literature on EC available in the waiting area. Information about postcoital emergency contraception is available through the Emergency Contraception Hotline (1-888-NOT-2-LATE), and on the World Wide Web.

Operative Sterilization

Operative **sterilization** is an inclusive term that refers to surgical procedures that permanently prevent pregnancy. In the man, sterilization is achieved through a procedure called *vasectomy.* In the woman, sterilization is done by *tubal ligation.*

Before sterilization is performed on either partner, the clinician provides a thorough explanation of the procedure. Each person needs to understand that sterilization is not a decision to be taken lightly or entered into at times of psychologic stress, such as separation or divorce. Even though both male and female procedures are theoretically reversible, the permanency of the procedure should be stressed and understood.

Vasectomy

Male sterilization is achieved through a relatively minor procedure called a **vasectomy**. This involves surgically severing the vas deferens in both sides of the scrotum. It takes about 4 to 6 weeks and 6 to 36 ejaculations to clear the remaining sperm from the vas deferens. During that period, the couple is advised to use another contraceptive method and to bring in two or three semen samples for a sperm count. When the sperm count is negative the couple can safely have unprotected sex. The man is rechecked at 6 and 12 months to ensure that fertility has not been restored by recanalization. Side effects of a vasectomy include pain, infection, hematoma, sperm granulomas, and spontaneous reanastomosis (reconnecting).

Vasectomies can sometimes be reversed by using microsurgery techniques. Restored fertility, as measured by a subsequent pregnancy, ranges from 38% to 82% (Hatcher et al., 2007; Schorge et al., 2008).

Tubal Ligation

Voluntary female sterilization is accomplished by **tubal ligation**. Three procedures are common in the United States:

- Laparotomy following a cesarean birth or other abdominal surgery
- Minilaparotomy in the postpartum period soon after a vaginal birth
- Laparoscopy done postabortion or during an "interval period," when the woman is not pregnant or postpartum

Tubal ligation can be done at any time. However, the postpartal period is an ideal time to perform a tubal ligation because the uterus is enlarged and the tubes are easy to locate. During these procedures the tubes are ligated, clipped, electrocoagulated, banded, or plugged. This interrupts the patency of the fallopian tube, thus preventing the ovum and the sperm from meeting.

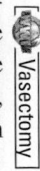

Vasectomy

Case Study: Family Planning | Application: Contraceptive Services for Minors

Complications of female sterilization procedures include coagulation burns on the bowel, bowel perforation, pain, infection, hemorrhage, and adverse anesthesia effects. Reversal of a tubal ligation depends on the type of procedure performed. Achievement of a pregnancy after successful tubal sterilization reversal may vary from 45% to 90%; 10% of women will have an ectopic pregnancy (Schorge et al., 2008).

Nonoperative Sterilization

The *Essure* method of permanent sterilization by Conceptus requires no surgical incision. Under hysteroscopy, a stainless steel microinsert is placed into the proximal section of each fallopian tube. Within 3 months, these microinserts create a benign tissue response that occludes the fallopian tubes. Three months after placement, tubal occlusion is confirmed by hysterosalpingogram. One of the materials used in the production of the implants is a nickel-titanium alloy; therefore, *women allergic to nickel should consult their healthcare provider before placement.* It is the only sterilization method approved in the United States that will yield no surgical scar (Schorge et al., 2008).

Male Contraception

The vasectomy and the condom, discussed previously, are currently the only forms of male contraception available in the United States. Developing reversible methods of contraception for men is a challenge because healthy men produce sperm continuously, whereas women produce eggs cyclically. It is easier to devise a reversible method that interrupts a cyclic process than it is to find ways to interrupt continuous fertility.

Hormonal contraception for men has yet to be developed, although studies are under way using weekly injections of testosterone, a synthetic hormone that significantly inhibits sperm production in most men. Too much testosterone has significant side effects on the man such as feminization, an unfavorable lipid profile, loss of libido, and more, which makes it largely unacceptable. A combination injection of testosterone and DMPA, the progestin found in Depo-Provera, is also under way. If it is successful, injections may only be needed monthly. Investigational approaches include gonadotropin-releasing hormone analogues and sex steroids (Hatcher et al., 2007).

> “I think I'm like a lot of women. During my life I've used a variety of contraceptive methods. I took the pill until I was married and ready to have children, used spermicidal foam without a diaphragm and subsequently had a baby, and later used spermicidal cream and condoms more successfully. I never wanted a tubal, but my husband refuses to consider a vasectomy, so the IUD was a perfect alternative for us. I am 37 and I like using something I don't have to think about every time we want to make love. Maybe someday there will be more contraceptives for men—it seems only fair—but I'm glad that at least I've had some choices.”

NURSING CARE MANAGEMENT

In most cases, the nurse who provides information and guidance about contraceptive methods works with the woman, because most contraceptive methods are female oriented. Because a man can purchase condoms without seeing a healthcare provider, only in the case of vasectomy does a man require counseling and interaction with a nurse. However, men should be encouraged to participate in contraceptive services. The nurse can play an important role in helping a woman and her partner choose a method of contraception that is acceptable to both.

In addition to completing a history and assessing for any medical contraindications to specific methods, the nurse can spend time with a woman learning about her lifestyle, personal attitudes about particular contraceptive methods, religious and cultural beliefs, personal biases, and plans for future childbearing to help the woman select a particular contraceptive method. (See Developing Cultural Competence.)

Once the woman chooses a method, the nurse can help her learn to use it effectively. "Patient Teaching: Using a Method of Contraception" provides guidelines for helping women use a method of contraception effectively.

The nurse also reviews any possible side effects and warning signs related to the method chosen and counsels the woman about what action to take if she suspects she is pregnant. In many cases, the nurse is involved in telephone counseling of women who call with questions and concerns about contraception. Thus it is vital that the nurse be knowledgeable about this topic and have resources available to find answers to less common questions.

Clinical Interruption of Pregnancy

Abortion, the termination of a pregnancy, was legalized in the United States in 1973. However, the associated controversy over moral and legal issues continues. This controversy is as readily apparent in the medical and nursing professions as in other groups.

Many women are strongly opposed to abortion for religious, ethical, cultural, or personal reasons. Other women feel that abortion provides a legally available alternative to a pregnancy. A number of physical and psychosocial factors influence a woman's decision to seek an abortion. The presence of a disease or health state that jeopardizes the mother's life and serious, life-threatening fetal problems are frequently suggested as indications for abortion. In other instances, the timing or cir-

PROFESSIONALISM IN PRACTICE

Using Contraception Resources During Patient Teaching

In your role as teacher, it is important to have resources on hand for women seeking a method of contraception. Have informational handouts available for the various methods of contraception. Describe correct use, side effects, warning signs, and important tips for effective use. Women can then refer to the sheets at home. Be sure to include the office or clinic phone number.

DEVELOPING CULTURAL COMPETENCE
Birth Control Attitudes

Attitudes about birth control may be influenced by cultural factors. Although it is impossible to attribute one attitude to an entire group of people, the following general information may be helpful as a starting point in working with women from a particular ethnic group (Blumenthal, 2007):

- *Deference to authority figures* is not uncommon in traditional Chinese, Arab, Latina, and East Indian women, especially if the nurse is male. The nurse should use active listening when counseling.
- *Gender inequities* may prohibit some Arab, Latina, and Eastern Indian women from seeking out or using a contraceptive method unless their husbands do not object. After being given appropriate information, the nurse may suggest the couple discuss contraceptive options in private.
- *Acquiescence* to the nurse's decision for the woman may occur, especially if the woman is Asian. The nurse should engage the woman in a conversation and use active listening to ascertain *her* attitude toward different contraceptive methods.
- *Attitudes toward bleeding* affect a woman's duties to her family and partner. Vaginal bleeding may be seen as "unclean" by Muslim and Orthodox Jewish women. Any contraceptive method that involves irregular bleeding might not be acceptable. On the other hand, among women who feel a monthly period is necessary, any method that ultimately causes amenorrhea would not be acceptable.
- The Roman Catholic Church considers all artificial methods of contraception unacceptable. Natural family planning might be an acceptable method for women who closely follow the Church's teaching. Among American Catholics, however, attitudes about the proscription regarding birth control may vary, and it is important to determine the woman's beliefs on the subject.
- Large families are valued in many cultures, and contraception may not be desired. Unplanned pregnancies may be welcomed in the Hispanic culture, and unplanned adolescent pregnancies do not necessarily carry a negative stigma for African Americans.

cumstance of the pregnancy creates an inordinate stress on the woman, prompting her to choose an abortion. Some of these situations may involve contraceptive failure, sexual assault, or incest. Usually the decision is best made by the woman or couple involved. A woman whose life is threatened by the pregnancy may choose to continue the pregnancy, whereas one with no obvious threat may choose to have an abortion.

Globally, the legal status of abortion varies greatly, although 1 in 5 pregnancies ends in abortion worldwide. Countries with restrictions on abortion may still have a high rate of abortion. The rate of abortion in Africa, where abortion is illegal, is about the same as it is in parts of Europe, where abortion is permitted. Western and Northern Europe, where abortion is readily available to women, have some of the lowest rates of abortion in the world. Worldwide, between 1995 and 2003, the number of induced abortions declined from nearly 46 million to 42 million, mostly due to the availability of contraceptive methods (Guttmacher Institute, 2008c). The contraceptive needs of women worldwide are a priority.

Medical Interruption of Pregnancy

Medical abortion is now available in the United States and provides an effective alternative to surgical abortion for many women with unintended pregnancies. Three regimens are available: mifepristone combined with misoprostol, methotrexate combined with misoprostol, and misoprostol by itself (Association of Reproductive Health Professionals [ARHP], 2008). The regimen of mifepristone and misoprostol is Food and Drug Administration (FDA) approved for use up to 49 days after the last menstrual period. Mifepristone (Mifeprex or RU 486), an anti-progesterone, and misoprostol, a prostaglandin analogue that causes smooth muscle to contract, lead to complete abortion in approximately 92% of women. Abortion success rates differ when these medications are taken at different gestational ages: 96% to 98% in pregnancies up to 42 days; 91% to 95% in pregnancies from 43 to 49 days' gestation; and less than 85% in pregnancies past 49 days (American College of Obstetricians and Gynecologists [ACOG], 2009). Some clinicians support the use of a slightly modified dosage regimen through 63 days' gestation (ACOG, 2009).

Mifepristone blocks the action of progesterone, thereby altering the endometrium. After the length of the woman's gestation is confirmed, she takes a dose of oral mifepristone in her caregiver's office. One to 3 days (depending on gestation) later she returns to her caregiver and takes an oral or vaginal dose of the prostaglandin misoprostol, which induces contractions that expel the embryo/fetus. About 14 days after taking the misoprostol, the woman is seen a third time to confirm that the abortion was successful.

Endometritis is a risk with any abortion. Since 2001, five deaths may possibly have been related to the oral mifepristone-vaginal misoprostol regimen. Three of these deaths were related to an infection caused by a rare organism, *Clostridium sordelli* (U.S. FDA, 2009). Therefore, *any* woman who has taken the oral mifepristone-vaginal misoprostol regimen and within 24 hours develops stomach pain, weakness, nausea, vomiting, or diarrhea (with or without fever) should contact her healthcare provider *immediately* (U.S. FDA, 2009). Currently, mifepristone is still considered safe, and use of routine prophylactic antibiotics is not recommended.

Although methotrexate is not labeled for medical abortion, 20 years of experience with it has led to its use in the first 7 weeks of pregnancy. Methotrexate stops cell division, and when used with misoprostol, it can be up to 96% effective in terminating a pregnancy (ACOG, 2009). However, ACOG (2009) states that mifepristone-misoprostol regimens are preferable to those using methotrexate-misoprostol or misoprostol alone for medical abortion.

Surgical Interruption of Pregnancy

Surgical abortion in the first trimester (less than 13 weeks' gestation) is technically easier and safer than abortion in the second trimester. The cervix is anesthetized with local anesthesia using a paracervical block. It then must be dilated either mechanically

PATIENT TEACHING Using a Method of Contraception

PATIENT GOALS At the completion of the teaching, the woman will be able to:

1. Confirm for herself that the chosen method of contraception is appropriate for her.
2. List the advantages, disadvantages, and risks of the chosen method.
3. Describe (or demonstrate) the correct procedure for using the chosen method.
4. Cite warning signs that should be reported to the caregiver.

TEACHING PLAN

Content	Teaching Method
Discuss the factors that a woman should consider in choosing a method of contraception (see Table 5-1). Stress that the different methods may be appropriate at different times in the woman's life. Review the woman's reasons for selecting a particular method and confirm any contraindications to specific methods.	Contraception is a personal decision, so the discussion should take place in a private area free of interruptions. Create a supportive, warm, and comfortable atmosphere by attitude and communication style—both verbal and nonverbal. Provide accurate information in an open, nonjudgmental way.
Discuss the advantages, disadvantages, and risks of the chosen method.	Focus on open discussion. It may help to have written information about the method chosen. If a signed permit is required (as with sterilization, an IUD insertion, or Implanon), the provider should also discuss the advantages, disadvantages, and risks.
Describe the correct procedure for using a method. Go through step by step. Periodically stop and have the woman review the information. If a technique is to be learned (as with inserting a diaphragm or charting basal body temperature), demonstrate and then have the woman do a return demonstration as appropriate. (*Note:* If certain aspects are beyond the nurse's level of expertise, the nurse can review the content and confirm that the woman has the opportunity to do a return demonstration. For example, an office nurse who does not do FemCap fittings may cover information on its use, have the woman try inserting the cap herself, and then have the placement checked by the nurse practioner, nurse-midwife, or physician.)	Learning is best accomplished when material is broken down into smaller steps. Have a model or chart available to enable the woman to visualize what is being described. Have a sample of the chosen method available: a package of oral contraceptives, an open IUD, or a symptothermal chart.
Provide information on what the woman should do if unusual circumstances arise (she forgets a pill or misses a morning temperature).	Provide a written handout identifying the warning signs of her chosen method and listing the actions a woman should take. The handout should also cover actions the woman should take if an unusual situation develops. For example, what should she do if she vomits or has diarrhea while taking oral contraceptives?
Stress warning signs that require immediate action on the part of the woman and explain why these signs indicate a risk. Carefully delineate the actions the woman should take.	Arrange to talk with the woman again soon, either on the phone or at a return visit, to determine if she has any questions about the method and to ensure that no problems have arisen.

Evaluation

Evaluate the woman's learning by asking her to describe the method she has chosen, its contraindications and warning signs, and the procedure for using it correctly. In some cases, a return demonstration is useful.

with metal dilators or laminaria or medicinally with misoprostol or mifepristone. A cannula is placed through the cervix and suction is applied to recover all the products of conception. Mechanical scraping of the uterine contents with a sharp curette can be an alternative to suction, or these two procedures can be done together. The major risks include perforation of the uterus, laceration of the cervix, systemic reaction to the anesthetic agent, hemorrhage, retained products of conception, and infection (Schorge et al., 2008).

Second trimester abortion (greater than 13 weeks' gestation) may be done medically or surgically. Medical termination includes the use of a mifepristone-misoprostol regimen, and the woman will need to labor and pass the fetus in the hospital. Surgical termination is done using dilation and evacuation (D&E). This procedure combines vacuum aspiration with the use of appropriate instrumentation to remove the contents of the uterus.

NURSING CARE MANAGEMENT

The woman deciding to terminate a pregnancy may choose to do so based on an unwanted/unintended pregnancy, sexual assault, lack of finances, her health, or the health of the fetus. The nurse should assess the woman's need for support and/or counseling. If the decision was difficult for the woman, the nurse should assist her in finding postprocedure support.

Patient selection is an important factor in medical abortion. Pregnancy needs to be verified early, by 5 weeks' gestation if possible. The woman needs to understand clearly that medical abortion takes time and follow-up is important. Moreover, women need accurate information about the cramping, bleeding, and pain that occur so that they are prepared to deal with both the discomfort and the sight of the blood and possible uterine contents.

In general, important aspects of nursing care for a woman who chooses to have an abortion include providing information about the methods of abortion and associated risks as well as counseling regarding available alternatives to abortion and their implications. Nursing care also includes encouraging the woman to verbalize her feelings; providing support before, during, and after the procedure; monitoring vital signs, intake, and output; providing for physical comfort and privacy throughout the procedure; and teaching the patient self-care, the importance of the postabortion checkup, and use of a reliable contraceptive (including methods that can be started immediately after the procedure).

FOCUS YOUR STUDY

- The fertility awareness-based (FAB) method, natural family planning (NFP), is a "natural," noninvasive method of contraception often used by people whose religious beliefs prevent them from using artificial methods.
- Other FAB methods can be used in conjunction with a barrier method during the woman's fertile days.
- Situational contraceptives such as coitus interruptus (withdrawal) and douching are activities an individual uses in a given situation to avoid pregnancy without benefit of clinical guidance or medical care. Abstinence is also considered a situational contraceptive.
- Barrier contraceptives such as the contraceptive sponge, diaphragm, FemCap, Lea's Shield, and condom act by blocking the transport of sperm. These methods are often used in conjunction with a spermicide.
- N-9, the spermicide available in the United States, is far less effective in preventing pregnancy when it is not used with a barrier method.
- The Copper IUD (intrauterine device) is a mechanical contraceptive. Although its exact method of action is not clearly understood, research suggests it acts by immobilizing sperm or by impeding the progress of sperm from the cervix to the fallopian tubes. In addition, the IUD does have a local inflammatory effect.
- The Mirena levonorgestrel-releasing IUS (LNG-IUS) is both a hormonal and mechanical contraceptive. Its action is similar to that of the Copper IUD; it also secretes a progestin, levonorgestrel, that helps the endometrium to become atrophic, the cervical secretions to become thick, and the menstrual flow to be decreased.
- Combined oral contraceptives (the "pill") are combinations of estrogen and a progestin. When taken correctly, they are one of the most effective and reversible methods of fertility control.
- The progestin-only subdermal implant, Implanon, is an excellent choice for women desiring long-term contraception who cannot take estrogen.
- Other combined hormonal options (estrogen and progestin) such as the patch (Ortho Evra) and the vaginal ring (NuvaRing) have broadened the range of contraceptive options available.
- The "patch" is under investigation for its potential role in increased venous thromboembolism, associated with greater systemic absorption of estrogen, but is still a safe method for women not at risk.
- The long-acting progestin-only injection, Depo-Provera IM 150 mg or Depo-Provera SC 104 mg, is available for lactating women, or those who cannot take estrogen.
- Permanent sterilization is accomplished by tubal ligation for women and vasectomy for men. Although theoretically reversible, patients are advised that the method should be considered irreversible. Essure offers a nonoperative approach to permanent blockage of the fallopian tubes.
- The termination of pregnancy through abortion may now be achieved by either medical or surgical means.

CRITICAL THINKING IN ACTION

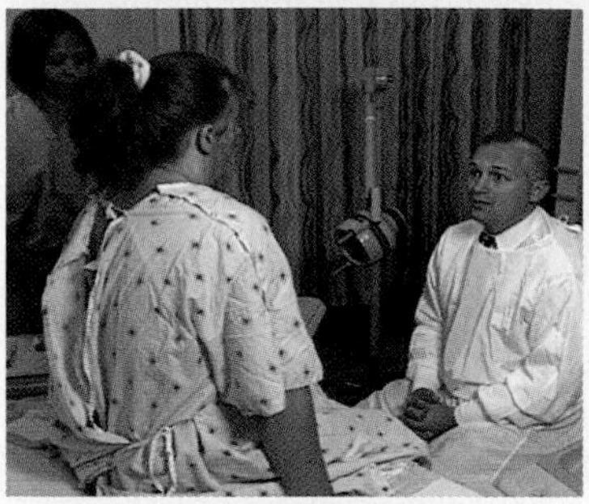

Linda Knoll, 35 years old, presents to you at the GYN clinic for her annual physical and pelvic exam. You obtain the following menstrual history: LMP 8 days ago. Periods occur every 29 days and last 5 days. She tells you that she uses superabsorbent tampons during the first 2 days of her period and then changes to regular absorbency tampons for the duration, and that she currently has an IUD in place for contraception. She tells you that her husband has been complaining for the last few months that she seems irritable, tense, and moody near "that time of the month." Linda admits that she doesn't feel well before her period and describes having low pelvic discomfort, breast tenderness, "bloating," and some constipation. She seems to cry easily 2 to 3 days before her period. She has noticed this pattern over the last 4 or 5 months. You recognize these symptoms as related to premenstrual syndrome (PMS). Linda asks you if these changes are due to female hormones.

1. How would you answer Linda's question concerning female hormones?
2. After reviewing Linda's diet with her, what would you recommend to help?
3. Linda has an IUD in place. What other type of contraceptive might help reduce the symptoms of PMS?
4. What other activities can you suggest to help Linda reduce PMS symptoms?
5. What should you tell Linda about using tampons during heavy menstrual flow?

See www.nursing.pearsonhighered.com for possible responses.

Pearson Nursing Student Resources

Find additional review materials at
www.nursing.pearsonhighered.com

Prepare for success with additional NCLEX®-style practice questions, interactive assignments and activities, Web links, animations and videos, and more!

REFERENCES

American College of Obstetricians and Gynecologists (ACOG). (2007a). *Emergency contraception* (ACOG Practice Bulletin No. 69). Washington, DC: Author.

American College of Obstetricians and Gynecologists (ACOG). (2007b). *Intrauterine device and adolescents* (ACOG Committee Opinion No. 392). Washington, DC: Author.

American College of Obstetricians and Gynecologists (ACOG). (2009). *Medical management of abortion* (ACOG Practice Bulletin No. 67). Washington, DC: Author.

American College of Obstetricians and Gynecologists (ACOG). (2010). *Noncontraceptive uses of hormonal contraceptives* (ACOG Practice Bulletin No. 110). Washington, DC: Author.

Association of Reproductive Health Professionals (ARHP). (2008, April). *What you need to know: The difference between medical abortion and emergency contraceptive pills.* Retrieved from http://www.arhp.org/uploadDocs/mifepristone_ecfactsheet.pdf#search="medical abortion"

Benagiano, G., & von Hertzen, H. (2010). Toward more effective emergency contraception. *The Lancet, 375*(9714), 555–562.

Blumenthal, P. D. (2007). Overcoming cultural barriers to contraceptive care. *Contraception Online* (www.contraceptiononline.org). Houston, TX: Baylor College of Medicine. Retrieved from http://www.baylorcme.org/cme/contraception/monographs/cultural-competency/cultural_competency.pdf

Gallo, M. F., Grimes, D. A., Schulz, K. F., & Lopez, L. M. (2010). Cervical cap versus diaphragm for contraception. *Cochrane Database of Systematic Reviews 2002,* Issue 4. Art. No.: CD003551. doi: 10.1002/14651858.CD003551

Guttmacher Institute. (2002, August). Women and societies benefit when childbearing is planned. *Issues in Brief.* Retrieved from http://www.guttmacher.org/pubs/ib_3-02.html

Guttmacher Institute. (2008a, January). Facts on contraceptive use. *Facts in Brief.* Retrieved from http://www.guttmacher.org/pubs/fb_contr_use.html

Guttmacher Institute. (2008b, July). Facts on induced abortion in the United States. *In Brief.* Retrieved from http://www.guttmacher.org/pubs/fb_induced_abortion.html

Guttmacher Institute. (2008c, October). *Facts on induced abortion worldwide.* Retrieved from http://www.guttmacher.org/pubs/fb_IAW.html

Guttmacher Institute. (2009, February). *Facts on publicly funded contraceptive services in the United States.* Retrieved from http://www.guttmacher.org/pubs/fb_contraceptive_serv.html

Hatcher, R. A., Trussell, J., Nelson, A., Cates, W., Stewart, F., & Kowal, D. (2007). *Contraceptive technology* (19th ed.). New York, NY: Ardent Media, Inc.

Martinez, G. M., Chandra, A., Abma, J. C., Jones, J., & Mosher, W. D. (2006). *Fertility, contraception, and fatherhood: Data on men and women from cycle 6 (2002) of the national survey of family growth.*

National Center for Health Statistics. (2010). Vital Health Stat 23(26). Hyattsville, MD: U.S. Department of Health and Human Services. Retrieved from http:/ /www.cdc.gov/nchs/data/series/sr_23/sr23_026.pdf

National Center for Health Statistics (NCHS). (2010). *Health United States, 2009. With special feature on medical technology.* Hyattsville, MD: Author.

Schorge, J. O., Schaffer, J. I., Halvorson, L. M., Hoffman, B. L., Bradshaw, K. D., & Cunningham, F. G. (2008). *Williams gynecology.* New York, NY: McGraw-Hill Medical.

Sonfield, A. (2006). Working to eliminate the world's unmet need for contraception. *Guttmacher Policy Review, 9*(1), 10–13. Retrieved from http://www.guttmacher.org/pubs/gpr/09/1/gpr090110.html

Speroff, L., & Darney, P. (2005). *A clinical guide for contraception* (4th ed.). Philadelphia, PA: Lippincott Williams & Wilkins.

United Nations Population Fund (UNPFA). (2008). No woman should die giving life. Contraceptives save lives: Meeting the needs for family planning. *Facts and Figures 2.* Washington, DC: Author. Retrieved from http://www.unfpa.org/safemotherhood/mediakit/documents/fs/factsheet2_eng.pdf

United States Food and Drug Administration (U.S. FDA). (2008, January 19). Ortho evra contraceptive transdermal patch. *Safety.* Retrieved from http://www.fda.gov/Safety/MedWatch/SafetyInformation/SafetyAlertsforHumanMedicalProducts/ucm094909.htm

United States Food and Drug Administation (U.S. FDA). (2009, June 26). *Mifeprex (mifepristone) information.* Retrieved from http://www.fda.gov/Drugs/DrugSafety/PostmarketDrugSafetyInformationforPatientsandProviders/ucm111323.htm

Weller, S. C., & Davis-Beatty, K. (2009). Condom effectiveness in reducing heterosexual HIV transmission. *Cochrane Database of Systematic Reviews 2002,* Issue 1. Art. No.: CD003255. doi: 10.1002/14651858.CD003255.

World Health Organization (WHO). (2007). *Maternal mortality.* Geneva, Switzerland: Author. Retrieved from http://www.who.int/making_pregnancy_safer/topics/maternal_mortality/en/index.html

CHAPTER

6

Women's Health: Commonly Occurring Infections

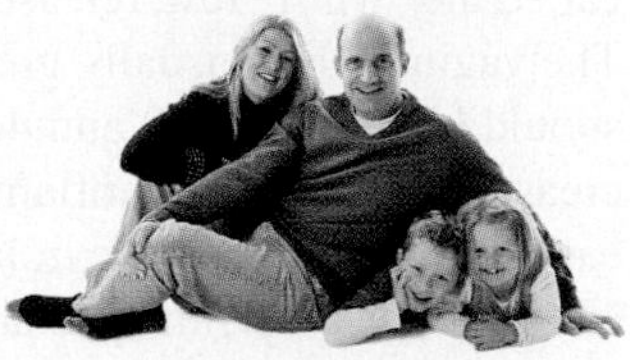

I just wanted to have a good time when I was young. I only had sex with people I "knew" but eventually I got herpes. Now I am 32, with two children, and married to a great man who loves me. He has never had herpes but we are very careful because I don't want him infected because of me. How much simpler life would be if I didn't carry that virus. Too bad that we can't change the past.

LEARNING OUTCOMES

1. Compare vulvovaginal candidiasis and bacterial vaginosis.
2. Summarize modes of transmission, treatments, and descriptions of the most commonly occurring sexually transmitted infections (STIs).
3. Describe the health teaching that a nurse needs to provide to a woman with an STI.
4. Relate the implications of pelvic inflammatory disease (PID) for future fertility to its pathologic origin, signs and symptoms, and treatment.
5. Contrast cystitis and pyelonephritis.
6. Compare the different types of viral hepatitis.

KEY TERMS

Bacterial vaginosis (BV) *100*
Chlamydial infection *104*
Condylomata acuminata *106*
Gonorrhea *105*
Herpes genitalis *105*
Pelvic inflammatory disease (PID) *110*
Sexually transmitted infection (STI) *103*
Syphilis *106*
Trichomoniasis *103*
Urinary tract infection (UTI) *111*
Vulvovaginal candidiasis (VVC) *101*

Many women seek health care because of infections of one sort or another, including those that are sexually transmitted. The nurse caring for a woman with an infection can be most helpful by providing accurate, sensitive, and supportive health care and health information. Additionally, the nurse is uniquely able to provide nonjudgmental health promotion, education, and counseling to influence the woman's future health behaviors positively. To meet the woman's needs, the nurse needs to have up-to-date information about a variety of infections, including how they are spread, diagnosed, and treated, and their long-term implications.

This chapter focuses on several types of infections with an emphasis on sexually transmitted infections. It is designed to provide current information to help nurses provide more effective health care for women and their families.

Care of the Woman with a Lower Genital Tract Infection (Vaginitis)

Centers for Disease Control

Vaginitis is the most common reason women seek gynecologic care. Symptoms of vaginitis, or vulvovaginitis, may include increased vaginal discharge, vulvar irritation and pruritus, external dysuria, dyspareunia (painful sexual intercourse), bleeding with intercourse, or a foul odor. Women with vaginitis may have either infectious abnormal organisms or an abundance or overgrowth of vaginal microorganisms such as *Gardnerella vaginalis, Mycoplasma hominis, Ureasplasma urealyticum, Mobiluncus, Bacteroides,* and *Peptostreptococcus* species (Akhter, Beckmann, & Gorelick, 2009; Centers for Disease Control and Prevention [CDC], 2006b).

Bacterial Vaginosis

Bacterial vaginosis (BV) is the most prevalent form of vaginal infection in the United States and worldwide. BV is more prevalent in sexually active women; however, the debate continues as to whether BV is a sexually transmitted infection, because it has also been detected in virginal women. The etiology of BV is related to a change in the normal vaginal flora. Normal hydrogen peroxide-producing lactobacilli are reduced with an overgrowth of vaginal anaerobes and subsequent rise in vaginal pH.

This process is poorly understood and the causes leading to overgrowth are not clear. Frequent sexual intercourse without condom use (sperm and seminal fluid has pH greater than 7), trauma from douching, cigarette smoking, having a new sexual partner or multiple partners, and an upset in normal vaginal flora are all predisposing or contributing factors. BV can also occur in women who have never had sexual intercourse. Research also suggests that increased psychosocial stress is associated with an increased incidence and greater prevalence of BV (Nansel et al., 2006). In pregnancy, maternal vitamin D deficiency (Bodner, Kohn, & Simhan, 2009) and increased dietary fat intake have been positively associated with BV, while an increased dietary intake of folate, vitamin A, and calcium (Neggers et al., 2007) are inversely related to BV risk. The *Gardnerella vaginalis* and *Mycoplasma hominis* organisms have been found in the vast majority of cases, along with an increased concentration of anaerobic bacteria.

The infected woman often notices an excessive amount of thin, watery, white or gray vaginal discharge with a foul odor sometimes described as "fishy." However, nearly 50% to 75% of women with BV are asymptomatic. (The characteristic "clue cells" are seen on a wet-mount preparation, and leukocytes are conspicuously absent [Figure 6-1 ■]). The addition of a 10% potassium hydroxide (KOH) solution to the vaginal secretions, called the "whiff" test, releases a strong, fishy, amine-like odor. The vaginal pH is usually greater than 4.5 (normal vaginal pH should be between 3.8 and 4.2). Women with BV have an increased risk of pelvic inflammatory disease (PID), HIV disease, abnormal cervical cytology, postoperative cuff infections after hysterectomy, and postabortion PID. BV infections are associated with negative pregnancy outcomes as preterm birth, preterm rupture of the membranes, amniotic infections, and postcesarean endometritis (CDC, 2006b).

The nonpregnant woman who is symptomatic is generally treated with metronidazole (Flagyl) 500 mg orally twice a day for 7 days (see Drug Guide: Metronidazole [Flagyl]) or one full applicator of metronidazole gel, 0.75% intravaginally, once daily for 5 days. Both these routes are equally effective. Alternatively the woman can be treated with 2% clindamycin (Cleocin) vaginal cream, one full applicator at bedtime for 7 days although clindamycin is slightly less effective (CDC, 2006b). It is not recommended that clindamycin be used with latex condoms and diaphragms for 5 days because the cream is oil based and may weaken the barrier method. Follow-up visits are not necessary unless symptoms recur, which occurs in approximately 30% of patients (Chan & Johnson, 2008). Routine treatment of sex partners is not recommended.

For many years, metronidazole was regarded as a potential teratogen, particularly in the first trimester, and its use was generally avoided, especially in early pregnancy. However, the CDC (2006b) now reports that multiple studies have not demonstrated

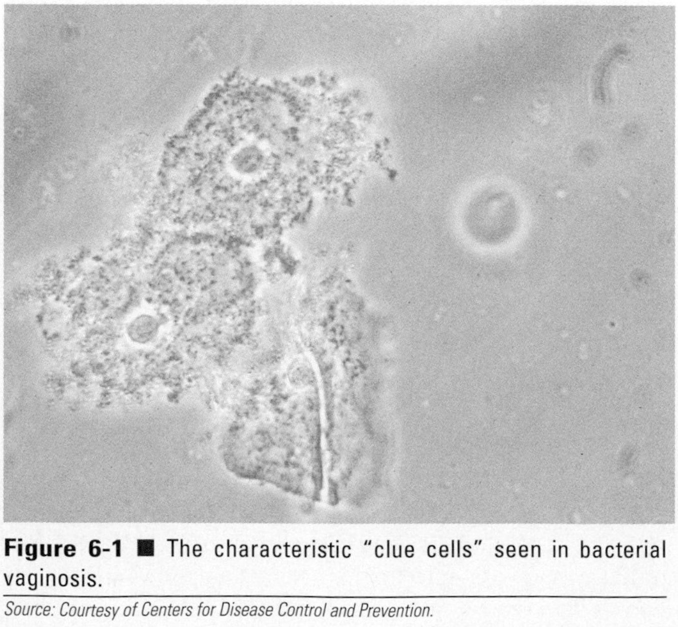

Figure 6-1 ■ The characteristic "clue cells" seen in bacterial vaginosis.

Source: Courtesy of Centers for Disease Control and Prevention.

DRUG GUIDE Metronidazole (Flagyl)

OVERVIEW OF ACTION

Metronidazole is an antiprotozoal and antibacterial agent. It possesses direct trichomonacidal and amebicidal activity against *T vaginalis and E histolytica*. Metronidazole is active in vitro against most obligate anaerobes but does not appear to possess any clinically relevant activity against facultative anaerobes or obligate aerobes. It is used in the treatment of various infections caused by organisms that are sensitive to this drug. It is used predominantly to treat the following infections in women: *T vaginalis,* bacterial vaginosis, endometritis, endomyometritis, tubo-ovarian abscess, and postsurgical vaginal cuff infection (Facts & Comparisons, 2010).

ROUTE, DOSAGE, FREQUENCY

Trichomoniasis—nonpregnant woman: 1 day treatment 2 g orally in a single dose; 7-day treatment: 500 mg orally twice a day for 7 consecutive days (CDC, 2006b).

Amebiasis—Adults: 750 mg orally 3 times a day for 5–10 days; children: 35–50 mg/kg/24 hours orally divided into 3 doses for 10 days.

Bacterial vaginosis—nonpregnant woman: 500 mg orally twice a day for 7 consecutive days or one full applicator of metronidazole gel 0.75% intravaginally once daily for 5 days (CDC, 2006b).

CONTRAINDICATIONS

Blood dyscrasias
Breastfeeding women (drug secreted in breast milk)
Impaired kidney or liver function
Active central nervous system (CNS) disease

SIDE EFFECTS

Convulsive seizures
Peripheral neuropathy
Weakness
Insomnia
Nausea/Vomiting
Headache
Anorexia
Diarrhea
Epigastric distress
Abdominal cramping
Constipation
Metallic taste in mouth
Dizziness
Vertigo
Uncoordination
Ataxia
Confusion
Irritability
Depression
Cystitis
Dysuria
Reversible neutropenia and thrombocytopenia
Flattening of the T wave on electrocardiogram (ECG)
Polyuria
Incontinence
Pelvic pressure
Proliferation of *Candida* in the vagina and mouth
Joint pains
Decreased libido
Dryness in the mouth, vulva, and vagina
Dyspareunia

NURSING CONSIDERATIONS

- Inform the woman about potential side effects.
- Stress the importance of contraceptive compliance during course of treatment.
- Obtain baseline renal and liver function tests as ordered.
- Teach the woman about the signs, symptoms, and treatment of vulvovaginal candidiasis.
- Counsel the woman to avoid alcoholic beverages while taking the medication.
- If the woman is taking oral contraceptives, a backup nonhormonal contraceptive method is recommended during treatment.
- Take a thorough history to rule out the woman's exposure to this medication within the last 6 weeks.
- Teach the woman to monitor the signs and symptoms of her infection.
- Encourage cooperation with the entire course of treatment.

a consistent relationship between metronidazole use during pregnancy and teratogenic effects on the newborn. Nevertheless, some providers still do not treat patients with metronidazole in the first trimester due to the potential for fetal anomalies (Briggs, Freeman, & Yaffe, 2008). Thus, currently the recommended treatment during pregnancy is metronidazole 500 mg orally twice a day or metronidazole 250 mg orally 3 times a day or clindamycin 300 mg orally twice daily. All these regimens should be taken for 7 days (CDC, 2006b). Most providers recommend screening of all pregnant women for BV because it has been associated with preterm labor and birth; others recommend screening only those pregnant women at increased risk for preterm birth. An optimal treatment regimen has not been established. In either case, if a pregnant woman is found to be positive for BV she should be treated.

Vulvovaginal Candidiasis

Vulvovaginal candidiasis (VVC), also known as a candidiasis, or fungal and yeast infection, is a very common vaginal infection. It is estimated that in their lifetime, 75% of women will have at least one episode of VVC, whereas 40% to 45% of women will have two or more episodes (CDC, 2006b; Chan & Johnson, 2008). *Candida albicans* is responsible for the vast majority of vaginal yeast infections. Non-*albicans* species of *Candida,* such as *C glabrata, C tropicalis,* and *C krusei,* can also cause vulvovaginal symptoms and they are becoming more prevalent. There is evidence that some of these strains are developing resistance to therapies such as fluconazole. Predisposing factors to yeast infections include glycosuria, use of oral contraceptives, use of antibiotics, pregnancy, diabetes mellitus, and the use of immunosuppressant drugs.

The woman with VVC often complains of nonmalodorous, thick, white (cottage cheese-like) vaginal discharge, severe itching, dysuria (external versus urethral), and dyspareunia. A male sexual partner may experience a rash or excoriation of the skin of the penis and possibly pruritus. The male can be symptomatic and the female asymptomatic.

On physical examination, the woman's labia may be swollen and excoriated if pruritus has been severe. A speculum examination usually reveals thick, white, tenacious, curd-like patches

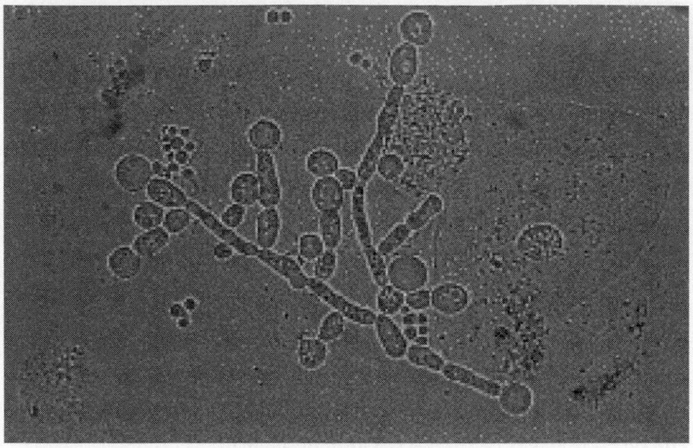

Figure 6-2 ■ Hyphae and spores of *Candida albicans.*

Source: Courtesy of Centers for Disease Control and Prevention.

adhering to the vaginal mucosa. The diagnosis is made by observing mycelia or pseudohyphae upon direct microscopy in a 10% KOH preparation (Figure 6-2 ■). A Gram stain or culture positive for the fungus is a more accurate way of diagnosing the causative organism. The pH of the vagina remains 4 to 4.5 or less (the normal pH of the vagina is about 3.8 to 4.2). This vaginal pH level is in contrast to the pH noted with BV or Trichomonas.

Local vaginal treatment with intravaginal butoconazole, clotrimazole, miconazole, nystatin, terconazole, or tioconazole in the appropriate cream, tablet, or suppository form is recommended. Single-dose and short-course approaches (3 days) are effective for 80% to 90% of women with uncomplicated VVC. One-day regimens include oral fluconazole 150 mg in a single dose, itraconazole capsules (200 mg) twice a day, clotrimazole vaginal tablets 500 mg at bedtime, and tioconazole 6.5% vaginal ointment (5 g) at bedtime (CDC, 2006b). All of these treatments are effective for mild VVC (CDC, 2006b; Chan & Johnson, 2008). There are also 3-day, 5-day, and 7-day treatment regimens. Women with severe symptoms may require a longer course of treatment up to 14 days with vaginal or oral azole agents (Chan & Johnson, 2008). If the vulva is also infected, the cream is applied topically. Women with recurrent infections may be advised to use long-term clotrimazole or fluconazole therapy. The use of vaginal application of lactobacilli products remains unproven and controversial. Some of these medications are available over the counter. They are indicated for women with a history of yeast infections who are able to correctly recognize true VVC symptoms.

Treatment of the male partner is generally not indicated although it may be recommended for partners of women who have recurrent infection. For men who have candidal balanitis (inflammation of the glans penis) treatment with a topical antifungal medication is indicated (CDC, 2006a).

Recurrent VVC, defined as four or more episodes of symptomatic VVC in 1 year, affects less than 5% of women (CDC, 2006b). If a woman experiences frequent recurrences of monilial vaginitis, she should be tested for an elevated blood glucose level to determine whether a diabetic or prediabetic condition is present and evaluated for immunosuppression. Women at high risk for sexually transmitted infections should also be tested for HIV infection. In the absence of other risk factors, recurrent VVC treatment should include confirmation of the organism by culture, followed by an intensive regimen of topical agents for 7 to 14 days or oral doses of fluconazole every third day for 3 doses (days 1, 4, and 7), followed by maintenance antifungal therapy using oral ketoconazole 100 mg every day for 6 months (Chan & Johnson, 2008) or oral fluconazole weekly for 6 months or clotrimazole suppository once weekly for 6 months (CDC, 2006b). Treatment of the sexual partner is not recommended.

Pregnant women with VVC should be treated only with topical azole preparations applied for 7 days (CDC, 2006b). Infection at the time of birth may cause thrush (a *candidal* infection of the mouth) in the newborn.

NURSING CARE MANAGEMENT

Nursing Assessment and Diagnosis

The nurse caring for the woman should suspect VVC if the woman complains of intense vulvar itching and a thick, nonodorous white discharge. Women who are HIV-positive, immunosuppressed, pregnant, or have diabetes mellitus are especially susceptible to this infection; the nurse should be alert for symptoms in these women. In some areas nurses are trained to do speculum examinations and wet-mount preparations and can confirm the diagnosis themselves. In most cases, however, the nurse who suspects a vaginal infection reports it to the woman's healthcare provider.

Nursing diagnoses that might apply to the woman with VVC include the following:

- ***Risk for impaired skin integrity*** related to scratching secondary to discomfort of the infection
- ***Readiness for enhanced knowledge:*** Information about yeast infection related to an expressed desire to know about ways of preventing the development of VVC

Nursing Plan and Implementation

The nurse discusses with the woman the factors that contribute to the development of VVC and suggests ways to prevent recurrences, such as wearing cotton underwear and cotton-crotch pantyhose, avoiding tight-fitting clothing, and avoiding douching and vaginal powders or sprays that can irritate the vulva. Women taking antibiotics should be advised about the possibility of developing VVC and encouraged to seek treatment early if symptoms develop. Some providers encourage women to ingest 8 ounces of yogurt with *Lactobacillus acidophilus* culture daily to reestablish normal vaginal flora (Chan & Johnson, 2008).

Evaluation

Expected outcomes of nursing care include the following:

- The woman's symptoms are relieved, and the infection is cured.
- The woman is able to identify self-care measures to prevent further episodes of VVC.

Care of the Woman with a Sexually Transmitted Infection

The occurrence of **sexually transmitted infection (STI)**, or sexually transmitted disease (STD), has increased over the past few decades. In fact, vaginitis and STIs are the most common reasons for outpatient, community-based treatment of women. More than one STI can occur at the same time. All symptomatic women should be tested for other infections. Table 6-1 provides a summary of vulvovaginal candidiasis (VVC) and bacterial vaginosis (BV) as well as the common STIs.

Prevention of Sexually Transmitted Infections

Effective prevention and control of STIs is based on the following concepts (CDC, 2006b):

1. Education and counseling for people at risk on ways to practice safer sexual behavior.
2. Identification of infected, asymptomatic individuals and of people with symptoms of STI who are not likely to seek diagnostic and treatment services.
3. Effective diagnosis and treatment of people with an STI.
4. Evaluation, treatment, counseling, and education for individuals who are the sex partners of people with an STI.
5. Preexposure vaccination of individuals at risk for vaccine-preventable STIs.
6. Expedited partner therapy (EPT), whereby partners are treated, is recommended by the CDC (2006a). Infected individuals deliver medications or prescriptions to their partners to manage and decrease the reinfection rates of STIs. The legal status of EPT has not been determined in all states.

Individuals are at lowest risk for an STI if they abstain from sexual intercourse (whether vaginal, anal, or oral sex) and if they are in a long-term, monogamous relationship with a partner who is free of infection. Ideally, before entering a new sexual relationship, both partners should be tested for STIs, including HIV infection. If a person decides to have sex without knowing the partner's infection status, a new condom should be used before each act of intercourse (CDC, 2006b).

Nurses can play an important role in educating and counseling individuals who have an STI, who are at risk for one, or who are the partners of an infected individual. Information should be tailored to individual needs and specific risk factors. It can include details about actions a person can take to avoid exposure to an STI or to avoid transmitting one. Nurses need to be nonjudgmental and respectful and draw on their counseling skills in sharing information. In addition, nurses may find teaching opportunities by listening attentively to patients to clarify misconceptions about sexual and reproductive health (Wynn, Foster, & Trussell, 2009).

Trichomoniasis

Trichomoniasis is a commonly occurring STI caused by *Trichomonas vaginalis,* a microscopic motile protozoan that

TABLE 6-1 Summary of Sexually Transmitted Infections*

			TREATMENT	
DISEASE	**ORGANISM**	**DIAGNOSIS**	**NONPREGNANT**	**PREGNANT**
Vulvovaginal candidiasis (VVC)	*Candida albicans*	Wet-mount hyphae	Topically applied azole drugs	Topically applied azole drugs
Bacterial vaginosis (BV)	*Gardnerella vaginalis* and *Mycoplasma hominis*	Wet-mount clue cells	Metronidazole	Metronidazole or clindamycin
Trichomoniasis	*Trichomonas vaginalis*	Wet-mount trichomonads	Metronidazole	Metronidazole
Syphilis	*Treponema pallidum*	Dark-field examination Venereal Disease Research Laboratories (VDRL), Rapid Plasma Reagin (RPR), or microhemagglutination assay-Treponema pallidum (MHA-TP)	Benzathine Penicillin G	Benzathine Penicillin G
Herpes genitalis	Herpes simplex virus	Herpes culture or titer	Acyclovir	Acyclovir
Chlamydia	*Chlamydia trachomatis*	Chlamydia culture	Doxycycline or azithromycin*	Azithromycin or amoxicillin
Gonorrhea	*Neisseria gonorrhoeae*	Gonorrhea culture	Ceftriaxone, cefixime, cefotaxime, ceftizoxime	Ceftriaxone, cefixime, cefotaxime, ceftizoxime
AIDS	HIV	Enzyme-linked immunosorbent assay (ELISA) test and Western blot	Varies	Varies
Condylomata acuminata	Human papilloma virus	Virapap, biopsy, Pap smear, colposcopy	Cryotherapy, trichloroacetic acid (TCA), bichloroacetic acid (BCA), podophyllin, podofilox, excision	Cryotherapy Trichloroacetic acid
Pediculosis pubis	*Phthirus*	Microscopic identification of lice or nits	Permethrin 1% liquid or malathion 0.5% lotion	Permethrin 1% liquid
Scabies	*Sarcoptes scabiei*	Confirmation of symptoms or scraping of furrows	Permethrin 5% cream or crotamiton 10% cream or lotion	Permethrin 5% cream

**Note:* VVC and BV are included for comparison even though they are not spread primarily by sexual contact.

thrives in an alkaline environment. In young, sexually active women, trichomonas is the most common curable sexually transmitted infection with estimates ranging from 3.1% to 13% (Allsworth, Ratner, & Peipert, 2009). The single-celled parasite, called a trichomonad, is an anaerobe that has the ability to generate hydrogen, which combines with oxygen to create an anaerobic environment. Most infections are acquired through sexual intimacy. Fomite transmission by shared bath facilities, wet towels, or wet swimsuits may also be possible. Coinfection with other sexually transmitted infections is common and HIV has been shown to be transmitted more easily with trichomoniasis present (Allsworth et al., 2009).

Often women with trichomoniasis are asymptomatic or have only mild symptoms. More pronounced symptoms of trichomoniasis can include a yellow-green, frothy, odorous discharge and vulvar itching. The woman may also complain of dysuria and dyspareunia. Occasionally, subepithelial hemorrhages on the cervix (strawberry-like red spots) can be seen with the naked eye; smaller areas of hemorrhage are generally visible with a colposcope. Microscopic visualization of mobile trichomonads and increased leukocytes, a vaginal pH of 0.5 or higher, and a positive whiff test are diagnostic of *T vaginalis* (Figure 6-3 ■). Pregnant women with trichomoniasis may be at increased risk for premature rupture of membranes, preterm birth, and low birth weight. Pregnant women who are symptomatic should be treated with a single 2-g dose of metronidazole orally to relieve their symptoms (CDC, 2006b). Some providers prefer to order metronidazole 500 mg twice daily to decrease the risk of gastrointestinal side effects (Chan & Johnson, 2008).

Recommended treatment for trichomoniasis is metronidazole (Flagyl) administered in a single 2-g dose or tinidazole in a single 2-g dose or, alternatively, metronidazole 500 mg twice daily for 7 days for both male and female sexual partners (CDC, 2006b). Tinidazole is equivalent to or superior to metronidazole with less gastrointestinal symptoms but is more costly (CDC, 2006b; Huppert, 2009). Partners should avoid intercourse until both are cured (therapy is completed and both are symptom free). The woman and her partner should be cautioned to avoid alcohol for 24 hours after taking metronidazole and 72 hours after taking tinidazole; the combination has an effect similar to that of alcohol and disulfiram (Antabuse)—abdominal pain, nausea, flushing, or tremors (CDC, 2006b).

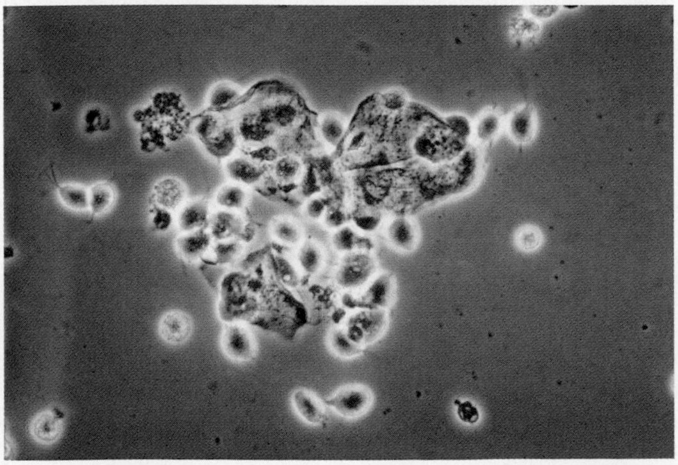

Figure 6-3 ■ Microscopic appearance of *Trichomonas vaginalis.*

Source: Courtesy of Centers for Disease Control and Prevention.

Chlamydial Infection

Chlamydial infection, caused by *Chlamydia trachomatis,* is the most common bacterial STI in the United States (CDC, 2009b). It is found most frequently in sexually active adolescents and young adults. Transmission commonly occurs through vaginal sex. The organism is an intracellular bacterium with different immunotypes. Immunotypes of chlamydia are responsible for lymphogranuloma venereum and trachoma, which is the world's leading cause of preventable blindness.

Chlamydia is a major cause of nongonococcal urethritis (NGU) in men. In women it can cause infections similar to those that occur with gonorrhea. However, asymptomatic infection is common in both men and women. In women, chlamydia can infect the fallopian tubes, cervix, urethra, and Bartholin's glands. Severe sequelae can result from untreated chlamydial infection, including pelvic inflammatory disease (PID), infertility, and ectopic pregnancy. In men, chlamydial infection can result in epididymitis and infertility. In addition, chlamydia infection is associated with an increased risk of acquiring and transmitting HIV infection (CDC, 2009b). In the United States, newborn exposure to chlamydia in the birth canal of the mother is the most common cause of ophthalmia neonatorum (CDC, 2006b). Chlamydial conjunctivitis responds to erythromycin ophthalmic ointment. The newborn may also develop chlamydial pneumonia.

Symptoms of chlamydia include a thin or mucopurulent discharge, cervical ectropia, friable cervix (bleeds easily), burning and frequency of urination, and lower abdominal pain. However, up to 50% of women are asymptomatic (Chan & Johnson, 2008). Of the laboratory tests currently available to diagnose chlamydia, nucleic acid amplification testing (NAAT) is the most sensitive. Other tests used for diagnosis include culture, direct immunofluorescence, enzyme immunoassay (EIA), and nucleic acid hybridization tests (CDC, 2006b). Diagnosis is frequently made after treatment of a male partner for NGU or in a symptomatic woman with a negative gonorrhea culture. Routine screening is recommended in all sexually active women less than 25 years of age (Chan & Johnson, 2008).

The recommended treatment is a single dose of azithromycin 1 g orally or doxycycline 100 mg by mouth twice a day for 7 days. Doxycycline costs less than azithromycin and has been used for a longer period. However, azithromycin administered at the clinic or office visit is an excellent choice for people who do not adhere well with treatment or who are erratic about completing a course of medication. Sexual partners should also be treated and the couple should abstain from intercourse for 7 days after taking the single-dose treatment or for the entire 7 days of the doxycycline therapy (CDC, 2006b). Doxycycline is contraindicated during pregnancy, but azithromycin 1 g orally or amoxicillin 500 mg orally 3 times daily for 7 days may be ordered (CDC, 2006b; Chan & Johnson, 2008). For pregnant women, patients with persisting symptoms, or those with medication nonadherence concerns, repeat testing is recommended 3 weeks after completion of the prescribed medication as a test of cure. Patient education includes information about the need for abstinence for 7 days following treatment (Akhter et al., 2009). Because so many males and females who have chlamydia are asymptomatic, the CDC and medical specialty organizations such as the American College of Obstetricians and Gynecologists (ACOG) recommend screening as the primary method of decreasing the incidence of chlamydia. Specifically, annual screening is recommended for these groups (CDC, 2006b):

- All sexually active adolescent females and women ages 20 to 25 even if they are asymptomatic.
- Women over age 25 who are at risk for chlamydia (history of STIs, multiple sexual partners, new sexual partner, inconsistent use of barrier contraceptives).
- ACOG also recommends screening for high-risk pregnant women at their first prenatal visit or during the third trimester of pregnancy, or both. Practitioners routinely screen all pregnant women.

Screening using a nucleic amplification test can be done on endocervical, urethral, or urine specimens. The urine tests are an attractive alternative for women who are not comfortable with pelvic exams or in clinics where access to gynecologic examination facilities is limited or lacking (Chan & Johnson, 2008).

Gonorrhea

Gonorrhea, an infection caused by the bacterium *Neisseria gonorrhoeae,* is the second most commonly reported STI in the United States with an estimated 336,742 people infected in 2008, with the highest rates in females aged 15 to 24 years of age (CDC, 2009b). Most men seek treatment for gonorrhea early because of symptoms but many women with the infection are asymptomatic until complications such as PID occur. Transmission can occur through vaginal, anal, or oral sex.

If a pregnant woman becomes infected after the third month of gestation, the mucous plug in the cervix generally prevents the infection from ascending, and it remains localized in the urethra, cervix, and Bartholin's glands until the membranes rupture. Then it can spread upward. A newborn exposed to a gonococcal-infected birth canal is at risk of developing ophthalmia neonatorum. Eye prophylaxis for all newborns is provided to prevent this complication.

About 80% of women with gonorrhea are asymptomatic (Little, 2006). Thus it is accepted practice to screen for this infection by doing a cervical culture during the initial prenatal examination. For women at high risk, the culture may be repeated during the last month of pregnancy. Cultures of the urethra, throat, and rectum may also be required for diagnosis, depending on the body orifices used for intercourse.

The most common symptoms of gonorrheal infection, when they occur, include a purulent, greenish-yellow vaginal discharge, dysuria, and urinary frequency. Some women also develop inflammation and swelling of the vulva. The cervix may appear swollen and eroded and may secrete a foul-smelling discharge in which gonococci are present. Bilateral lower abdominal or pelvic pain may also occur.

Treatment for nonpregnant women consists of antibiotic therapy with ceftriaxone 125 mg intramuscularly or cefixime 400 mg orally in a single dose for uncomplicated gonococcal infections of the cervix, urethra, and rectum (CDC, 2007b). For patients with disseminated gonococcal infection the recommended regimen is ceftriaxone 1 g intramuscularly or intravenously every 24 hours (CDC, 2007b). Gonococcal and chlamydial infections often coexist. Treatment recommendations include testing for chlamydia or treatment for chlamydia as previously discussed if chlamydia is not ruled out (CDC, 2007b). Additional treatment may be required if the cultures remain positive 7 to 14 days after completion of treatment. All sexual partners must be treated, or the woman can become reinfected. Pregnant women should be treated with a recommended cephalosporin, usually ceftriaxone intramuscularly or cefixime orally. This is combined with azithromycin or amoxicillin to address the risk of coinfection with chlamydia (CDC, 2006b). As with chlamydia, nurses should recommend abstinence for 7 days following treatment (Akhter et al., 2009).

For uncomplicated gonococcal infections test of cure is not recommended. Retesting is recommended 3 months following treatment secondary to increasing prevalence and the potential for PID (CDC, 2009b). Women should be informed of the need for reculture to verify cure and the need for abstinence or condom use until cure is confirmed. Both sexual partners should be treated if either has a positive test for gonorrhea. Women should also be informed of signs that the infection is worsening (sharp abdominal pain, fever, or chills) and encouraged to seek further care if any of these develop.

Herpes Genitalis

The herpes simplex virus (HSV) causes herpes infections, which are recurrent, lifelong infections. Two serotypes of HSV cause human infections: HSV-1 and HSV-2. HSV-2 causes most cases of recurrent genital herpes and is spread through vaginal, anal, or oral sex. It can also be spread through skin-to-skin contact with an infected site such as a finger (herpetic whitlow). The clinical symptoms and treatment of both types are the same. At least 50 million people in the United States have been diagnosed with genital HSV-2 infection—**herpes genitalis** (Akhter et al., 2009). Even so, most people infected with genital herpes have not been diagnosed because they have mild or unrecognized infections but shed the virus intermittently (CDC, 2006b). HSV-1 infections are often orally acquired as children, while HSV-2 infections are primarily acquired sexually (Akhter et al., 2009); however, genital HSV-1 infections are increasing (Kriebs, 2008).

The primary episode (first outbreak) of herpes genitalis is characterized by the development of single or multiple blister-like vesicles, which usually occur in the genital area and sometimes affect the vaginal walls, cervix, urethra, and anus. The vesicles may appear within a few hours to 20 days after exposure and rupture spontaneously to form very painful, open, ulcerated lesions. Inflammation and pain secondary to the presence of herpes lesions can cause difficult urination and urinary retention. Enlargement of the inguinal lymph nodes may be present. Flulike symptoms and genital pruritus or tingling also may be noticed. Primary episodes usually last the longest and are the most severe. Lesions heal spontaneously in 2 to 4 weeks.

After the lesions heal, the virus enters a dormant phase, residing in the nerve ganglia of the affected area. Some individuals never have a recurrence, whereas others have regular recurrences. Recurrences are usually less severe than the initial episode and seem to be triggered by emotional stress, menstruation, ovulation, pregnancy, and frequent or vigorous intercourse; patients with poor health status, a generally run-down physical condition, or who are immunocompromised can experience more frequent recurrences. Diagnosis is made on the basis of the clinical appearance of the lesions, culture of the lesions, polymerase chain reaction (PCR) identification, and glycoprotein G-based type-specific assays (Herpe Select™, Biokit HSV-2, & Sure Vue HSV-2) (CDC, 2006b).

No known cure for herpes exists; however, medications are available to partially control the symptoms of herpes and prevent complications from secondary infection (Akhter et al., 2009). The recommended treatment of the first clinical episode of genital herpes is oral acyclovir, valacyclovir, or famciclovir. These same medications, in somewhat different dosages, are also recommended for recurrent herpes infection and for daily suppressive therapy for people who have frequent recurrences. Therapy should be started during the prodromal period (time before the onset of lesions) for the greatest benefit (Akhter et al., 2009).

The safety of acyclovir, valacyclovir, and famciclovir in pregnancy has not been established. However, because there is more documented information on acyclovir during pregnancy, it can be administered orally to pregnant women with first episode genital herpes or severe recurrent herpes. Its use in the third trimester may reduce the frequency of cesarean births by decreasing the incidence of recurrences at term (CDC, 2006b). Sometimes 2% lidocaine (Xylocaine) is used to decrease intense pain at the site of the lesions. Keeping the genital area clean and dry, wearing loose clothing, taking sitz baths, and wearing cotton underwear or none at all will promote healing. Primary or recurrent lesions will heal without treatment.

New onset of maternal HSV infections has a 30% to 50% probability of neonatal HSV infection with transmission occurring during labor (85%) (Kriebs, 2008). The majority of providers recommend that women with herpetic lesions intrapartally give birth by cesarean section to prevent neonatal herpes. Note that cesarean birth does not completely prevent the risk of neonatal transmission. See chapter 20 for more detail.

Syphilis

Syphilis is a chronic infection caused by the spirochete *Treponema pallidum.* The rate of primary and secondary syphilis in women is 1.5 cases per 100,000 population; the rate in men is 7.6 cases (CDC, 2009b). Syphilis is commonly acquired through vaginal, oral, or anal sex. Less commonly, it can result from nonsexual exposure to exudates from an infected individual. Congenital transmission through transplacental inoculation may also occur. The incubation period varies from 10 to 90 days, and even though no symptoms or lesions are noted during this time, the blood contains spirochetes and is infectious.

Syphilis is divided into early and late stages. During the early stage (primary), a chancre (painless ulcer) appears at the site where the *T pallidum* organism entered the body. Symptoms include slight fever, loss of weight, and malaise. The chancre persists for about 4 weeks and then disappears. In 6 weeks to 6 months, secondary symptoms appear. Skin eruptions called condylomata lata, which resemble wartlike plaques and are highly infectious, may appear on the vulva. Other secondary symptoms are acute arthritis, enlargement of the liver and spleen, nontender enlarged lymph nodes, iritis, and a chronic sore throat with hoarseness. Transplacentally transmitted syphilis is as high as 95% in the primary and secondary stages but decreases to 10% in the late latent phase. Congenital syphilis can cause intrauterine growth restriction, preterm birth, and stillbirth.

As a result of the disease's impact on the fetus, serologic testing of every pregnant woman is recommended; most state laws require it. Testing is done at the initial prenatal screening and may be repeated in the third trimester. Blood studies may be negative if blood is drawn too early in the pregnancy.

During the early primary stage, the diagnosis is made by dark-field microscopic examination of the chancre for spirochetes and direct fluorescence antibody testing. Blood tests such as Venereal Disease Research Laboratories (VDRL), Rapid Plasma Reagin (RPR), or the more specific fluorescent treponemal antibody absorption test (FTA-ABS) are commonly done. Nontreponemal test antibody titers correlate with disease activity and are used to guide treatment while treponemal tests remain positive for life (CDC, 2006b).

For pregnant and nonpregnant women with syphilis of less than a year's duration (early latent syphilis), the CDC (2006b) recommends 2.4 million units of benzathine penicillin G intramuscularly in a single dose. If syphilis is of long duration (more than 1 year) or of unknown duration, 2.4 million units of benzathine penicillin G are given intramuscularly once a week for 3 weeks. If a woman is allergic to penicillin and nonpregnant, doxycycline or tetracycline can be given. Patients who are allergic to penicillin whose cooperation with treatment and follow-up are questionable should be desensitized to penicillin and then treated with it. Similarly, the pregnant woman with syphilis who is allergic to penicillin should be desensitized and then treated (CDC, 2006b). Maternal serologic testing can remain positive for 8 months, and the newborn can have a positive test for 3 months.

Patients receiving initial treatment for primary or secondary syphilis should be advised that they might experience a Jarisch-Herxheimer reaction within 6 to 12 hours of initial treatment. This reaction is characterized by fever, malaise, sweating, headache, anxiety, and a temporary increase in symptoms, which may be misdiagnosed as an allergic reaction. It generally subsides within 24 hours.

Human Papilloma Virus/Condylomata Acuminata

Condylomata acuminata, also called genital warts, is a common STI caused by the human papilloma virus (HPV) with approximately 60 genotypes that are related to genital warts (McCutcheon, 2009). Transmission can occur through vaginal, oral, or anal sex.

Annually 1 million new cases of condylomata acuminata are diagnosed. Of these, two thirds are in women. Estimates suggest that 1% of sexually active adults have genital warts (Dinh, Sternberg, Dunne, & Markowitz, 2008). Because of the increased evidence of a link between HPV and cervical and anorectal cancers, the condition is receiving increasing attention. Over 120 HPV subtypes have been identified; of these, about 30 types can infect the genital tract (Kennedy & Boardman, 2008). Most HPV infections are unrecognized, asymptomatic, or subclinical. HPV types 6 and 11 most commonly cause 90% of genital warts, but they have a low cancer-causing potential (Dinh et al., 2008). Approximately 15 specific types of HPV are considered high risk for high-grade cervical dysplasia and anogenital cancer (Kennedy & Boardman, 2008). Patients with visible genital warts can be infected concurrently with different HPV types.

Often a woman seeks medical care after noticing single or multiple soft, grayish pink, cauliflower-like lesions in her genital area (D'Ambrogio et al., 2009) (Figure 6-4 ■). These warts are often asymptomatic; however, depending on their location and size, they may cause itching (pruritus), be friable (bleed easily), or be painful. The moist, warm environment of the genital area is conducive to the growth of the warts, which may be present on the vulva, perineum, vagina, cervix, urethra, and anus. The incubation period following exposure is 3 weeks to 3 years, with the average being about 3 months.

Because condylomata sometimes resemble other lesions and can become cancerous, all atypical, pigmented, and persistent warts should be biopsied and treatment instituted promptly. Diagnosis is usually made by visual appearance.

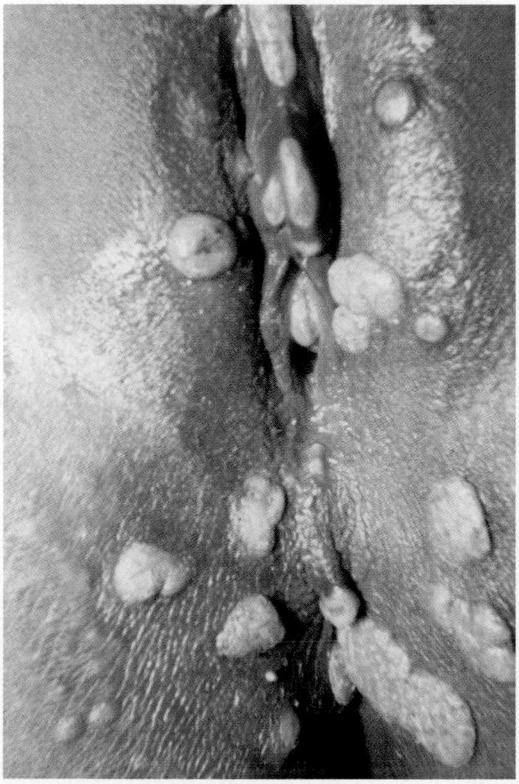

Figure 6-4 ■ Condylomata acuminata on the vulva.

Source: Courtesy of Centers for Disease Control and Prevention.

However, vaginal and cervical warts are more common than warts of the external genitalia. Most of these are flat lesions visible only by colposcopy. Subclinical diagnosis can be made if characteristic changes are present on a Pap smear.

The CDC (2006b) does not specify a treatment of choice for genital warts but recommends that treatment be determined based on patient preference, available resources, and experience of the healthcare provider. No single treatment is best for all types of warts or for all patients. Patient-applied therapies include 0.5% podofilox solution or gel or imiquimod 5% cream. For these methods to be effective, the patient must be able to reach and identify the warts being treated. Provider-administered therapies include cryotherapy with liquid nitrogen or cryoprobe; topical podophyllin (10% to 25%); trichloroacetic acid (TCA); bichloroacetic acid (BCA); and surgical removal by tangential scissors excision, shave excision, curettage, or electrosurgery. Alternative therapies include intralesional interferon or laser surgery (CDC, 2006b). Imiquimod, podophyllin, and podofilox are not used during pregnancy because they are thought to be teratogenic. TCA, BCA, and surgical removal are safe during pregnancy and may be used secondary to the size of the warts and patient discomfort. Genital and vulvar warts do not warrant cesarean birth. More recently, topical sinecatechin ointments, botanicals made from green tea extracts, have demonstrated wart clearance rates of approximately 50% (Tatti et al., 2008). Sinecatechins exert antiviral and antioxidant properties.

Women with HPV infections should have frequent Pap smears to monitor cervical cellular changes. Sex partners are probably infected and do not require treatment unless large exophytic lesions are present. Moreover, no research to date indicates that reinfection plays a role in recurrence (CDC, 2006b). The use of condoms can reduce the risk of transmitting the virus to an uninfected partner. In 2006 the United States Food and Drug Administration approved the first vaccine designed to protect against four HPV types, which, when considered together, are responsible for 90% of genital warts and 70% of cervical cancers. The vaccine—Gardasil®—given in 3 doses over 6 months is approved by the Food and Drug Administration (FDA) for females 9 to 26 years of age (Bornstein, 2009). Gardasil is a quadrivalent vaccine against HPV types 6, 11, 16, and 18. It is injected intramuscularly in the deltoid muscle or the anterolateral thigh. A second vaccine, a bivalent vaccine (Cervarix®) effective against HPV types 16 and 18, received FDA approval in late 2009. At present, both vaccines have demonstrated high antibody levels for greater than 5 years (Bornstein, 2009).

> “I've finally come to terms with the fact that I carry HPV. I know I will always run the risk of recurrence, but it's just a virus. It doesn't define me as a person.”

Case Study: Pediculosis Pubis

Pediculosis Pubis (Pubic or Crab Lice)

Pediculosis pubis is caused by *Phthirus,* a grayish, parasitic “crab” louse that lays eggs that attach to the hair shaft. Transmission is primarily by sexual contact, although shared towels and bed linens are also possible sources.

Symptoms include itching, usually in the pubic area. It is treated by applying 1% permethrin liquid or malathion (0.5%) lotion. Permethrin is applied to clean hair, saturating the hair, removing it after 10 minutes with warm water. Some providers recommend combing the pubic hair with a fine-toothed comb before rinsing off the permethrin. Malathion can be applied to dry hair, massaged in, and allowed to air dry. Because the lotion is flammable due to the high alcohol content, drying with high heat as with a hair dryer is contraindicated (Lehne, 2010). After 20 minutes, the lotion is removed. Over-the-counter medications such as Rid, Nix, and malathione lotion can also be used. Retreatment may be necessary. Both partners must be treated and tested for other STIs. Bed linens, towels, clothing, and other objects should be machine washed and dried in a hot dryer for 20 minutes or dry-cleaned or sealed in an airtight bag for 2 weeks. Sexual contact should be avoided until the woman and her partner(s) have been treated and cured.

Scabies

Sarcoptes scabiei is a parasitic itch mite. The female mite burrows under the skin to deposit her eggs. Transmission by intimate sexual contact is common in adults but scabies in children is not generally sexually acquired (CDC, 2006b).

Symptoms include itching that worsens at night or when the individual is warm. Noticeable erythematous, papular lesions or furrows may be present. The recommended treatment for scabies is permethrin cream 5% applied to all body areas from the neck down and washed off after 8 to 14 hours. Treatment is repeated in 14 days if live mites still exist. Alternate therapy includes crotamiton cream or lotion, which has scabicidal and antipruritic actions. Crotamiton is applied in a thin layer to all areas of the body from the neck down, with attention to body creases, and reapplied 24 hours after the first application. Lindane is no longer recommended as a first line treatment for lice or scabies due to an increased risk of seizures. Permethrin 5% is used in pregnant women. Clothing and bed linens should be washed and dried in a hot dryer or dry-cleaned. Sexual contacts and close household contacts need to be examined and treated for scabies as appropriate.

Viral Hepatitis

Hepatitis is an inflammatory process of the liver caused by infection by one of the five distinct viruses: A, B, C, D, and E. Currently, immunizations are only available for hepatitis A and B. Table 6-2 compares the five forms of viral hepatitis.

Hepatitis A is characterized by symptoms of jaundice, anorexia, nausea, vomiting, malaise, and fever. It is self-limiting and is not a chronic condition. A vaccine is available to prevent hepatitis A.

Hepatitis B, C, and D have symptoms similar to those of hepatitis A and can also include arthralgias, arthritis, and skin eruptions or rash. Unlike hepatitis A infection, those of B, C, and D infections are chronic. See Table 19-5 on page 445 for information about hepatitis B and pregnancy.

Hepatitis E occurs primarily in South Central Asia and the Middle East, and its symptoms are like those of hepatitis A. It is also a self-limiting disease and not a chronic condition.

COMPLEMENTARY AND ALTERNATIVE THERAPIES

Hepatitis C is a common bloodborne infection that is transmitted primarily by contact with infected blood. People at high risk for the infection include intravenous (IV) drug users, healthcare workers who receive a needle stick, and people with multiple sexual partners. To date, no complementary or alternative medical (CAM) therapy has proven effective in treating hepatitis C or its complications, and conventional medical therapy should *not* be replaced with an unproven CAM therapy (National Center for Complementary and Alternative Medicine [NCCAM], 2009).

Milk thistle (*Silybum marianum*), a plant of the aster family, has been used in Europe to treat liver disease since the 16th century. It may offer some protection for the liver by promoting the growth of liver cells. Currently NCCAM is supporting research on the effectiveness of Silymarin for preventing and reversing the complications of chronic hepatitis C (NCCAM, 2009).

Acquired Immunodeficiency Syndrome (AIDS)

Acquired immunodeficiency syndrome (AIDS) is a fatal disorder caused by HIV, which can be transmitted sexually. A medical-surgical text more fully describes this condition. HIV alters the presentation of STIs and can complicate the treatment of an STI. This is a bidirectional relationship because STIs can facilitate the transmission of HIV (Naresh, Beigi, Woc-Colburn, et al., 2009). However, because the diagnosis of HIV/AIDS or the presence of the HIV antibody has implications for a fetus if the woman is pregnant, HIV/AIDS is discussed in greater detail in chapter 19.

TABLE 6-2 Types of Viral Hepatitis

FORM	PRIMARY ROUTE OF TRANSMISSION	INCUBATION PERIOD	CHRONIC INFECTION	IMMUNIZATION AVAILABLE?
Hepatitis A	Fecal-oral, contaminated food/water	15–50 days	No	Yes
Hepatitis B	Blood/body fluids	45–160 days	Yes	Yes
Hepatitis C	Blood/blood products	14–180 days	Yes	No
Hepatitis D	Blood/body fluids	45–160 days	Yes	No
Hepatitis E	Fecal-oral	15–60 days	No	No

NURSING CARE MANAGEMENT

Nursing Assessment and Diagnosis

The nurse working with women must become adept at taking a thorough history and identifying women at risk for STIs. Risk factors include multiple sexual partners; a partner's involvement with other partners; high-risk sexual behaviors, such as intercourse without barrier contraception or anal intercourse; partners with high-risk behaviors; and young age at onset of sexual activity. The nurse should be alert for signs and symptoms of STI and be familiar with diagnostic procedures if it is suspected.

Although each STI has certain distinctive characteristics, the following complaints suggest the possibility of infection and warrant further investigation:

- Presence of a "sore" or lesion on the vulva
- Increased vaginal discharge or malodorous vaginal discharge
- Burning with urination
- Dyspareunia
- Bleeding after intercourse
- Pelvic pain

In many instances the woman is asymptomatic but may report symptoms in her partner, especially painful urination or urethral discharge. It is often helpful to ask the woman whether her partner is experiencing any symptoms.

Nursing diagnoses that may apply to a woman with an STI include the following:

- ***Interrupted family processes*** related to the effects of a diagnosis of sexually transmitted infection on the couple's relationship
- ***Readiness for enhanced knowledge:*** Information on preventing STIs related to an expressed desire to avoid infection

While it is important that nurses learn to effectively communicate with all young adults about STIs, it is especially critical with those of minority groups. Efforts to provide effective screening and treatment of STIs need to be expanded, and teaching and prevention strategies that are culturally sensitive need to be developed. These endeavors will contribute to decreasing the long-term consequences of STIs, such as ectopic pregnancy and infertility, and will also help decrease healthcare costs.

DEVELOPING CULTURAL COMPETENCE

STI Rates in the United States

Racial minorities continue to have the highest rates of STIs in the United States with African Americans most significantly impacted. Gonorrhea rates in blacks are 20 times greater than in whites; rates for chlamydia are similar and reflect the same trends. While blacks represent approximately 12% of the population of the United States, in 2008 they accounted for 71% of reported cases of gonorrhea, 48% of chlamydia, and 49% of syphilis cases (CDC, 2009a & 2009b). American Indian/Native American populations followed by Hispanic populations report significantly greater rates of gonorrhea and chlamydia than whites (CDC, 2009a & 2009b).

Nursing Plan and Implementation

In a supportive, nonjudgmental way, the nurse provides the woman who has an STI with information about the infection, methods of transmission, implications for pregnancy or future fertility, and importance of thorough treatment. If treatment of her partner is indicated, the woman must understand that it is necessary to prevent a cycle of reinfection. She should also understand the need to abstain from sexual activity, if necessary, during treatment.

Some STIs, such as trichomoniasis or chlamydia, may cause a woman concern but once diagnosed are rather simply treated. Other STIs can also be fairly simple to treat medically but may carry a stigma and be emotionally devastating for the woman. Thus the nurse should stress prevention with all women and encourage them to require partners, especially new partners, to use condoms.

The sensitive nurse can be especially helpful in encouraging the woman to explore her feelings about the diagnosis. She may experience anger or feel "betrayed" by a partner; she may feel guilt or see her diagnosis as a form of "punishment"; or she may feel concern about the long-term implications for future childbearing or ongoing intimate relationships. She may experience a myriad of emotions that she never expected. Opportunities to discuss her feelings in a nonjudgmental environment can be especially helpful. The nurse can offer suggestions about support groups, if indicated, and assist the woman in planning for her future with regard to sexual activity.

Care Plan Activity: Gynecologic Infection

PROFESSIONALISM IN PRACTICE

Attitudes About STIs

Many women deal matter-of-factly with an STI diagnosis; other women find it embarrassing and possibly even shameful. The nurse's attitude of straightforward acceptance conveys to the woman that she is still an acceptable person who happens to have an infection and can help the woman deal effectively with her diagnosis and its implications.

Health Promotion Education

Table 6-3 provides a summary of basic information the nurse should share with women who have an STI. STIs that can have an impact on pregnancy or the fetus/newborn are discussed in chapter 20.

Evaluation

Expected outcomes of nursing care include the following:

- The infection is identified and cured, if possible. If not, supportive therapy is provided.
- The woman and her partner can describe the infection, its method of transmission, its implications, and the therapy.
- The woman copes successfully with the impact of the diagnosis on her self-concept.

TABLE 6-3 Health Promotion Education: Preventing STIs and Their Consequences

The risk of contracting an STI increases with the number of sexual partners. Because of the extended time between infection with HIV and evidence of infection, intercourse with an individual exposes a female or male to all the other sexual partners of that individual for the past 5 or more years. Because of this risk, it is important to take the following actions:

- Plan ahead, review decision-making skills, and develop strategies to refuse sex (especially important for adolescents who may be less confident about saying "no" to casual sexual encounters), because abstinence is the best method of preventing STIs.
- Limit the number of sexual contacts and practice mutual monogamy.
- The condom is the best contraceptive method currently available (other than abstinence) for protection from STIs. Use one for every act of vaginal and anal intercourse. Other contraceptives such as the diaphragm, cervical cap, and spermicides also offer some protection against STIs.
- Plan strategies for negotiating condom use with a partner.
- Reduce high-risk behaviors. Use of recreational drugs and alcohol can increase sexual risk taking.
- Refrain from oral sex if your partner has active sores in the mouth, vagina, or anus or on the penis.
- Seek care as soon as you notice symptoms and make sure your partner gets treatment if indicated. Absence of symptoms or disappearance of symptoms does not mean that treatment is unnecessary if you suspect an STI. Take all prescribed medications completely.
- The presence of a genital infection can lead to an abnormal Pap smear. Women with certain infections should have more frequent Pap tests according to a schedule recommended by their caregiver. Ask your health-care provider if you need more frequent Paps.

Care of the Woman with an Upper Genital Tract Infection (Pelvic Inflammatory Disease)

Pelvic inflammatory disease (PID) occurs in approximately 1% of women between ages 15 and 39, although sexually active young women between 15 and 24 have the highest infection rate. In the United States, an estimated 1 million cases of PID are diagnosed annually, and more than 100,000 women become infertile as a result of it (CDC, 2007a).The disease is more common in women who have had multiple sexual partners, a history of PID, early onset of sexual activity, or recent insertion of an intrauterine device (IUD) and in women who douche regularly (CDC, 2007a). In the past, PID infections were primarily caused by gonorrhea and chlamydia trachomata. Newer pathogens that must be considered in the treatment regimen include *Mycoplasma genitalium* and bacterial vaginosis (BV) (Judlin, 2010). PID usually produces a tubal infection (salpingitis) that may or may not be accompanied by a pelvic abscess. However, perhaps the greatest problem of PID is postinfection tubal damage, which is closely associated with infertility.

PID is defined as a clinical syndrome of inflammatory disorders of the upper female genital tract that includes any combination of endometritis, salpingitis, tubo-ovarian abscess, pelvic abscess, and pelvic peritonitis (CDC, 2006b). The organisms most frequently identified with PID include *C trachomatis* and *N gonorrhoeae* with a coinfection rate (both organisms are present) of 60%. Other pathogens associated with PID include *M genitalium*, BV, and multiresistant gonococci (Judlin, 2010). Symptoms of PID include bilateral sharp, cramping pain in the lower quadrants, fever greater than 101°F, chills, mucopurulent cervical or vaginal discharge, irregular bleeding, cervical motion tenderness during intercourse, malaise, nausea, and vomiting. However, it is also possible to be asymptomatic and have normal laboratory values.

Diagnosis consists of a clinical examination to define symptoms. Laboratory tests include vaginal, cervical, and possibly rectal cultures for *N gonorrhoeae*, *C trachomatis*, and other pathogens as well as blood tests, including a complete blood count (CBC) with differential and Rapid Plasma Reagin (RPR) or Venereal Disease Research Laboratories (VDRL) to test for syphilis. A woman with PID often has an elevated C-reactive protein and elevated sedimentation rate. Microscopic examination of the vaginal secretions may reveal white blood cells. Physical examination usually reveals direct abdominal tenderness with palpation and, on bimanual examination, adnexal tenderness, and cervical and uterine tenderness with movement (Chandelier sign). A palpable mass is evaluated with ultrasonography. In confounding cases, laparoscopy can be used to confirm the diagnosis and to enable the examiner to obtain cultures from the fimbriated ends of the fallopian tubes.

Currently, there is no evidence comparing parenteral versus oral treatment, and outpatient treatment is an option. The decision to hospitalize a woman is based on clinical judgment. The woman should be hospitalized if the diagnosis is uncertain, ectopic pregnancy or appendicitis is suspected, the woman is severely ill (nausea, vomiting, high fever, dehydration), there has been little response to oral therapy after 48 to 72 hours, there are complications from pelvic abscesses or pelviperitonitis, the patient is a young adolescent, or the woman is unable to return for follow-up care. Treatment includes intravenous (IV) fluids, pain medication, and administration of IV antibiotics. Intravenous cefotetan (2 g IV every 12 hours) or cefoxitin (2 g IV every 6 hours), plus doxycycline (100 mg IV or by mouth every 12 hours), is one treatment regimen. Intravenous therapy can be discontinued once acute symptoms resolve but oral doxycycline 100 mg twice daily to complete the 14-day therapy must be taken (CDC, 2006b). Ambulatory or outpatient treatment includes ceftriaxone 250 mg intramuscularly once followed by doxycycline 100 mg twice a day for 14 days (CDC, 2006b). Other supportive measures that may be helpful include increased oral fluids (up to 2 liters per day), continued bed rest or pelvic rest, acetaminophen for fever, and pain relievers for abdominal pain. Follow-up visits are important within 48 to 72 hours, sooner if symptoms worsen. The sexual partner should also be treated. If the woman has an IUD, it is generally removed 24 to 48 hours after antibiotic therapy is started.

NURSING CARE MANAGEMENT

Nursing Assessment and Diagnosis

The nurse is alert to factors in a woman's history that put her at risk for PID. Even though fewer types of IUDs are available, there is an upsurge in their use by many women. The nurse should question the woman about possible symptoms, such as aching pain in the lower abdomen, foul-smelling discharge, malaise, and dyspareunia. The woman who is acutely ill has obvious symptoms, but a low-grade infection is more difficult to detect.

Nursing diagnoses that may apply to a woman with PID include the following:

- ***Acute pain*** related to peritoneal irritation
- ***Deficient knowledge*** related to a lack of information about the possible effects of PID on fertility

Nursing Plan and Implementation

The nurse plays a vital role in helping to prevent or detect PID. Accordingly, the nurse spends time discussing risk factors related to this infection. The woman who uses an IUD for contraception and has multiple sexual partners needs to understand clearly the risk she faces.

The nurse should strongly recommend that the IUD be removed and another method of contraception used. The nurse discusses signs and symptoms of PID with women at high risk and stresses the importance of early detection.

The woman who develops PID needs to understand the importance of completing her antibiotic treatment and of returning for follow-up evaluation. She should also understand that one outcome of the infection may be decreased fertility or infertility.

Evaluation

Expected outcomes of nursing care include the following:

- The woman describes her condition, her therapy, and the possible long-term implications of PID on her fertility.
- The woman completes her course of therapy and the PID is cured.

Care of the Woman with a Urinary Tract Infection

Urinary tract infection (UTI) is defined as significant bacteriuria in the presence of symptoms. Approximately 60% of women will experience a UTI in their lifetime (ACOG, 2008). A UTI can be life threatening or a mere inconvenience. Bacteria usually enter the sterile environment of the urinary tract by way of the urethra. The organisms are capable of migrating against the downward flow of urine. The shortness of the female urethra facilitates the passage of bacteria into the bladder. Other conditions that are associated with bacterial entry are relative incompetence of the urinary sphincter, frequent enuresis (bed-wetting) before adolescence, pregnancy, and urinary catheterization. Wiping from back to front after urination may transfer bacteria from the anorectal area to the urethra.

Voluntarily suppressing the desire to urinate is also a predisposing factor. Retention overdistends the bladder and can lead to an infection. There also seems to be a relationship between recurring UTI and new onset of sexual activity. General poor health or lowered resistance to infection can increase a woman's susceptibility to UTI. The rate of urinary tract infections increases as women age. For postmenopausal women, a lifetime history of urinary tract infection is a risk factor for urinary tract infection. Factors that may inhibit bacterial growth include a low pH (5.5 or less) resulting in more acidic urine, high urea concentration, and the presence of organic acids from food such as fruits and proteins. Urinary tract infections can be classified by location or as complicated or uncomplicated.

Application: Preventing Urinary Tract Infections

Asymptomatic bacteriuria (ASB) refers to bacteria in the urine actively multiplying without accompanying clinical symptoms. This becomes especially significant if the woman is pregnant because it is found in up to 11% of pregnancies, and as many as 40% of pregnant women with untreated ASB will develop pyelonephritis (Chan & Johnson, 2008). ASB is almost always caused by one organism. If more than one type of bacteria is cultured, the possibility of urine-culture contamination must be considered. The most common cause of ASB is *Escherichia coli.* Less commonly causative organisms include *Klebsiella* and *Proteus,* and *Pseudomonas* and *Staphylococcus* species.

CLINICAL JUDGMENT

Case Study: Tamara Williams

Tamara Williams, a 16-year-old G2P0, is approximately 14 gestational weeks (GW) when she is first seen by the nurse provider in a community health department prenatal clinic. Tamara's only complaints are occasional nausea, which she indicates has become much better in the last 3 weeks. Her prenatal laboratory results, including blood work and urine testing, reveal a urine sample with greater than 100,000 bacteria. When questioned, she denies urgency, frequency, and dysuria. Her healthcare provider tells her that she has asymptomatic bacteriuria and writes a prescription for nitrofurantoin (Macrodantin) 50 mg by mouth 4 times a day for 7 days.

The nurse overhears Tamara tell another woman in the clinic, "I'm not getting this medication. There's nothing wrong with me."

Critical Thinking

What should the nurse discuss with Tamara about obtaining the medication and taking it?

See www.nursing.pearsonhighered.com for possible responses.

A woman who has had a UTI is susceptible to recurrent infection. Although the role of ASB in pregnancy complications remains controversial, the majority of evidence supports the view that bacteriuria does not, as an isolated factor, lead to low birth weight or prematurity. However, an untreated ASB can progress to a UTI in approximately 30% to 40% of pregnant women (Blackburn, 2007). A number of structural and functional changes occur during pregnancy that predispose pregnant women to urinary tract infections. Ureters elongate and are laterally displaced by the gravid uterus. In addition, progesterone, which relaxes smooth muscles, can facilitate hypertrophy of the distal ureters with resulting ureteral stenosis and dilation, especially in the second half of pregnancy. Though the bladder has an increased capacity in pregnancy, it also has a decreased tone because progesterone relaxes the smooth muscle. Estrogen causes the bladder mucosa to become hyperemic and more susceptible to trauma and infection. Lastly, the intravesical pressure may be

Urinary Tract Infections

RESEARCH EVIDENCE IN PRACTICE **Treatment for Symptomatic Urinary Tract Infections During Pregnancy**

CLINICAL QUESTION

What is the most effective treatment for symptomatic urinary tract infections during pregnancy?

RESEARCH EVIDENCE

Urinary tract infections (UTIs) are among the most common health problems during pregnancy with an incidence between 17% and 20% of pregnancies. Yet they are not innocuous infections. UTI has been associated with premature rupture of the membranes, preterm labor, chorioamnionitis, postpartum fever, and neonatal infections. UTI can lead to serious maternal complications such as aseptic shock, respiratory insufficiency, fluid imbalance, chronic renal insufficiency, and even death.

There are many available drugs for the treatment of UTI. The ideal drug will be of proven effectiveness, active against a broad range of pathogens, inexpensive, well-tolerated, and safe for the fetus. Two large multisite randomized trials and a Cochrane Review focused on the relative effectiveness of five classes of antibiotics used to treat UTI. The cure rates for these treatments have been reported as between 70% and 100%. Drugs in these studies were delivered by IV or oral routes and in single-dose or multi-day regimens.

Only one class of drugs—the cephalosporins—had better cure rates and fewer recurrences than the other drugs. However, the size of difference was small and unlikely to have a broad clinical impact. Among all drugs, a single dose was less effective than a 3-, 5-, or 7-day regimen.

WHAT QUESTIONS REMAIN UNANSWERED?

Do any of these drugs produce effects for the child over the course of time? What is the effect of multiple courses of treatment during pregnancy if the infection is recurrent?

WHAT IS BEST PRACTICE?

Since all treatments had effective cure rates with very rare complications, it is reasonable to give the simplest and least costly available treatment. A single dose in the clinic will be the least effective, so women should be counseled to complete the entire course of treatment.

CRITICAL THINKING

What clinical evaluations can help the provider detect asymptomatic urinary tract infection? What education can help assure the mother will complete the entire medication regimen?

References

Kromery, S., Hromex, J., & Demesova, D. (2001). Treatment of lower urinary tract infection in pregnancy. *International Journal of Antimicrobial Agents, 17,* 279–282.

Stamatiou, K., Alevizos, A., Petrakos, G., Lentzas, I., Papathanasiou, M., & Mariolis, S. (2007). Study of the efficacy of cefaclor for the treatment of asymptomatic bacteriuria and lower urinary tract infections in pregnant women with a history of hypersensitivity to penicillin. *Clinical and Experimental Obstetrics and Gynecology, 34*(2), 85–87.

Vazquez, J., & Villar, J. (2010). Treatments for symptomatic urinary tract infections during pregnancy. *Cochrane Database of Systematic Reviews.* Issue 4. Art. No: CD002256. doi:10.1002/14651858.CD002256

decreased due to the displacement of the bladder and ureters. With micturation, the pressure may increase with urine regurgitating into the ureters. Therefore, changes in the bladder and ureters and hormonal influences both contribute to the propensity of pregnant women to develop urinary tract infections (Blackburn, 2007).

Treatment in pregnant women includes amoxicillin-clavulanate, nitrofurantoin, cefixime, or fosfomycin (Chan & Johnson, 2008).

Lower Urinary Tract Infection (Cystitis and Urethritis)

Because UTIs ascend, it is important to recognize and diagnose a lower UTI early to avoid the sequelae associated with upper UTI. One common lower UTI is cystitis, or infection of the urinary bladder. Several factors place a woman at increased risk for cystitis, including sexual intercourse, the use of a diaphragm and a spermicide, pregnancy, and a history of a recent UTI.

E coli is present in 80% of women with UTIs. *Staphylococcus saprophyticus, Klebsiella, Proteus, Enterobacter,* and *Pseudomonas* are also causative pathogens. Infections without bacteriuria may indicate urethritis and are usually caused by *C trachomatis, N gonorrhoeae,* and herpes simplex.

When cystitis develops, the classic initial symptoms are often acute and include dysuria, specifically at the end of urination, as well as urgency and frequency. Suprapubic or low back pain may also occur. Cystitis is usually accompanied by a low-grade fever (38.3°C, or 101°F, or lower), and hematuria is occasionally seen. Urine specimens often contain an abnormal number of leukocytes and bacteria and may contain protein.

The diagnosis can be made with a urine culture. Bacteriuria dipstick screening tests are quick office screening tests; however, they have high false-positive and false-negative rates. Before treatment, the diagnosis should be confirmed by clinical evaluation and urine culture and sensitivity results. The treatment depends on the causative pathogen. Oral trimethoprim-sulfamethoxazole, trimethoprim, ciprofloxacin, norfloxacin, and levofloxacin are frequently used in twice daily dosing 3-day regimens. Second line drugs may include nitrofurantoin and fosfomycin for 7-day and 1-day regimens, respectively (Lehne, 2010).

Cystitis occurs in 0.3% to 1.3% of pregnant women (Chan & Johnson, 2008). A positive association exists between women with urinary tract infections and preterm birth. Pregnant women complaining of dysuria, urgency, and frequency with a urine culture greater than 10^2/ml from a midstream urine specimen would be diagnosed with cystitis. The most common treatment regimens include (Lehne, 2010):

- Nitrofurantoin (Macrodantin) 100 mg twice a day
- Cefpodoxime (Vantin) 500 mg twice a day to 4 times a day
- Amoxicillin-clavulanate (Augmentin) 500 mg twice a day or 250 mg 3 times a day, all for 3 to 7 days
- Fosfomycin 3 g by mouth as a single dose

For any of these medications, it is important to emphasize completion of the course of treatment.

Upper Urinary Tract Infection (Pyelonephritis)

Pyelonephritis (inflammatory disease of the kidneys) is less common but more serious than cystitis and is often preceded by lower UTI. It is more common during the second and third trimesters (80% to 90%) of pregnancy or early postpartum and poses a serious threat to maternal and fetal well-being (Archabald, Friedman, Raker, & Anderson, 2009). Women with pyelonephritis during pregnancy are at significantly increased risk of preterm labor, preterm birth, development of adult respiratory distress syndrome, and septicemia (Archabald et al., 2009). Acute pyelonephritis has a sudden onset with chills, high temperature of 39.6 to 40.6°C (103 to 105°F), and costovertebral angle tenderness or flank pain, which can be unilateral or bilateral. Nausea, vomiting, and general malaise may ensue. With accompanying cystitis, the woman may experience frequency, urgency, and burning with urination.

Edema of the renal parenchyma or ureteritis with blockage and swelling of the ureter may lead to temporary suppression of urinary output. This is accompanied by severe colicky (spastic, intense) pain, vomiting, dehydration, and ileus of the large bowel. The woman with acute pyelonephritis generally will have significant bacteria in her urine culture, pyuria, and the presence of white blood cell casts.

The woman may be hospitalized depending on the severity of her symptoms and started on intravenous (IV) antibiotics. Therapy also includes IV hydration, urinary analgesics such as Pyridium, pain management, and medication to manage fever. In the case of obstructive pyelonephritis, a blood culture is necessary. The woman is kept on bed rest. If signs of urinary obstruction occur or continue, the ureter may be catheterized to establish adequate drainage.

Initial IV treatment options include ceftriaxone (1 g IV every day), followed with oral ciprofloxacin, ofloxacin, levofloxacin, or gatifloxacin for 10 to 14 days. IV therapy should continue until the woman is afebrile for 48 hours. Oral antibiotics are given to complete the 10 to 14 days of therapy (Chan & Johnson, 2008). With appropriate drug therapy, the woman's temperature should return to normal, the pain subside, and the urine show no bacteria within 2 to 3 days. Follow-up urinary cultures are needed to determine that the infection has been eliminated completely.

NURSING CARE MANAGEMENT

Nursing Assessment and Diagnosis

During the woman's visit, the nurse obtains a medical history, including a sexual history, to determine whether she is at risk for UTI. Additionally, the nurse notes any complaints from the woman of painful urination or other urinary difficulties and systemic complaints such as fever, chills, nausea, vomiting, flank or back pain. A clean-catch urine sample is obtained to evaluate for the presence of bacteriuria.

Nursing diagnoses that may apply to the woman with a UTI include the following:

- ***Acute pain*** related to dysuria, systemic discomforts, flank or back pain secondary to lower or upper urinary tract infection
- ***Deficient knowledge*** related to lack of understanding about ways of preventing UTIs related to an expressed desire to avoid recurrence
- ***Fear*** related to the possible long-term effects of the disease

Nursing Plan and Implementation

Most bacteria enter through the urethra after having spread from the anal area. Therefore, the nurse should make sure that the woman is aware of good hygiene practices and provide information on other ways to avoid UTI (Figure 6-5 ■ and Table 6-4). Additionally, the nurse provides the woman with information to help her recognize the signs and symptoms of a UTI to facilitate early identification and treatment of future infections. The nurse should also reinforce instructions and answer any additional questions the woman may have regarding the prescribed antibiotic and the reasons for

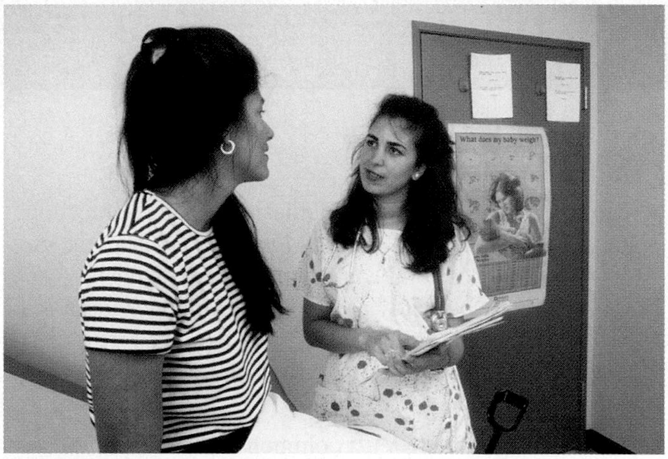

Figure 6-5 ■ The nurse counsels the woman about measures for preventing urinary tract infection.

Source: © Michael Newman/Photo Edit—All rights reserved.

TABLE 6-4 Health Promotion Education: Measures for Preventing Cystitis

- If you use a diaphragm for contraception, try changing methods or using another size diaphragm.
- Avoid bladder irritants, such as alcohol, caffeine products, and carbonated beverages.
- Make regular urination a habit; avoid long waits.
- Practice good genital hygiene, including wiping from front to back after urination and bowel movements.
- Be aware that initial, vigorous, or frequent sexual activity may contribute to urinary tract infection.
- Complete medication regimens even if symptoms decrease.
- Do not use medication left over from previous infections.
- Drink cranberry juice or take cranberry tablets to acidify the urine. This has been found to relieve symptoms in some cases.

these treatments. UTIs usually respond quickly to treatment, but follow-up clinical evaluation and urine cultures are important. Recurrent urinary tract infection can result from reinfection (80%) or relapse (Lehne, 2010). With frequent reinfections, defined as three or more infections yearly, long-term prophylaxis may be needed and can decrease the risk of recurrence by 95% (ACOG, 2008).

Evaluation

Expected outcomes of nursing care include the following:

- The woman implements self-care measures to help prevent recurrent UTI as part of her personal routine.
- The woman completes her prescribed course of antibiotic therapy.
- The woman can identify signs of recurrent UTI or signs and symptoms of worsening urinary symptoms that would require follow-up care.
- The woman's infection is cured.

CLINICAL TIP

Evidence supports the value of drinking cranberry juice or taking cranberry tablets to decrease urinary tract infections (ACOG, 2008).

FOCUS YOUR STUDY

- Vulvovaginal candidiasis (moniliasis), a vaginal infection most often caused by *Candida albicans,* is most common in women who use oral contraceptives, are taking antibiotics, are currently pregnant, are immunosuppressed, or have diabetes mellitus. It is generally treated with intravaginal miconazole or clotrimazole suppositories or fluconazole orally.
- Bacterial vaginosis (BV), a common vaginal infection, is diagnosed by its characteristic fishy odor and by the presence of "clue" cells on a vaginal smear. It is treated with metronidazole.
- Chlamydial infection is difficult to detect in a woman but can result in pelvic inflammatory disease (PID) and infertility. It is treated with antibiotic therapy. It often coexists with gonorrhea.
- Gonorrhea, a common sexually transmitted infection, can be asymptomatic in women initially but can cause PID if not diagnosed early. The treatment of choice is ceftriaxone intramuscularly or cefixime orally. This is combined with azithromycin or amoxicillin to address the risk of coinfection with chlamydia.
- Herpes genitalis, caused by the herpes simplex virus, is a recurrent infection with no known cure. Acyclovir (Zovirax) may reduce the symptoms.
- Syphilis, caused by *Treponema pallidum,* is a sexually transmitted infection that is treatable if diagnosed. The characteristic lesion is the chancre. Syphilis can also be transmitted in utero to the fetus of an infected woman. The treatment of choice is penicillin.
- Condylomata acuminata (genital warts) are transmitted by the human papilloma virus (HPV). Treatment is indicated, because research has identified approximately 15 HPV genotypes linked with cervical cancer. The treatment chosen depends on the size and location of the warts and the woman's reproductive status. A vaccine is now available to prevent several types of HPV.
- Pelvic inflammatory disease can be life threatening and can lead to infertility. The organisms that cause PID most frequently include *C trachomatis* and *N gonorrhoeae. Mycoplasma genitalium* and bacterial vaginosis (BV) are increasingly being noted as pathogens causing PID.
- Women with an abnormal finding on a pelvic examination will need careful explanation of the finding and techniques of diagnosis and emotional support during the diagnostic period.
- The classic symptoms of a lower urinary tract infection (UTI) are dysuria, urgency, frequency, and sometimes hematuria. Oral sulfonamides are the treatment of choice except in middle to late pregnancy.
- An upper UTI is a serious infection that can permanently damage the kidneys if untreated. Generally the woman is acutely ill and may require supportive therapy as well as antibiotics.

CRITICAL THINKING IN ACTION

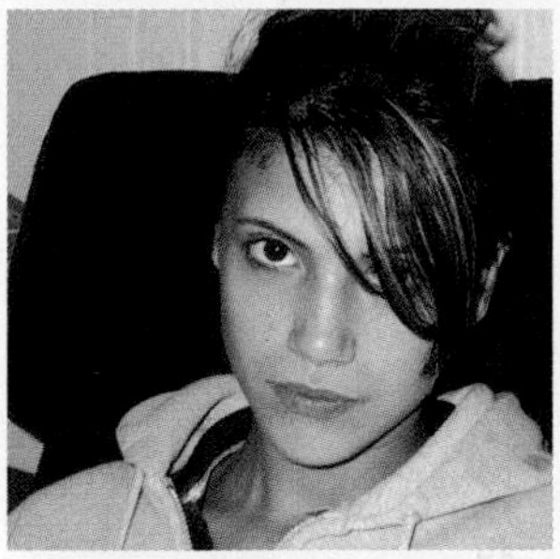

Cherelle Latkowski, age 18, was just diagnosed with gonorrhea by the nurse practitioner at the clinic where you work. Although she had been asymptomatic, she had come in for evaluation after her boyfriend was diagnosed with gonorrhea and started on antibiotics. Cherelle is treated with ceftriaxone administered intramuscularly plus doxycycline by mouth.

1. Cherelle asks you why she received two medications. How would you reply?
2. Cherelle asks you whether she is now immune to gonorrhea. Is she?
3. Cherelle asks whether she can now have sex with her boyfriend. Can she do so?

See www.nursing.pearsonhighered.com for possible responses.

Pearson Nursing Student Resources

Find additional review materials at
www.nursing.pearsonhighered.com

Prepare for success with additional NCLEX®-style practice questions, interactive assignments and activities, Web links, animations and videos, and more!

REFERENCES

Adams, M., & Koch, R. (2010). *Pharmacology: Connections to nursing practice.* Upper Saddle River, NJ: Pearson Education.

Akhter, S., Beckmann, K., & Gorelick, M. (2009). Update on sexually transmitted infections, 2008. *Pediatric Emergency Care, 25*(9), 608–618.

Allsworth, J. E., Ratner, J. A., & Peipert, J. F. (2009). Trichomoniasis and other sexually transmitted infections: Results from the 2001–2004 National Health and Nutrition Examination Surveys. *Sexually Transmitted Diseases, 36*(12), 738–744.

American College of Obstetricians and Gynecologists (ACOG). (2008). Treatment of urinary tract infections in nonpregnant women (ACOG Practice Bulletin No. 91). *Obstetrics & Gynecology, 111,* 758–794.

Archabald, K., Friedman, A., Raker, C., & Anderson, B. (2009). Impact of trimester on morbidity of acute pyelonephritis in pregnancy. *American Journal of Obstetrics & Gynecology, 201*(406e), 1–4.

Blackburn, S. (2007). *Maternal, fetal, & neonatal physiology: A clinical perspective* (3rd ed.). New York, NY: Saunders Elsevier.

Bodner, L. M., Kohn, M. A., & Simhan, H. N. (2009). Maternal vitamin D deficiency is associated with bacterial vaginosis in the first trimester of pregnancy. *The Journal of Nutrition, 139*(6), 1541–1600.

Bornstein, J. (2009). The HPV vaccines—which to prefer? *Obstetrical & Gynecological Survey, 64*(5), 345–350.

Briggs, G., Freeman, R., & Yaffe, S. (2008). *Drugs in pregnancy and lactation* (8th ed.). Philadelphia, PA: Lippincott Williams & Wilkins.

Centers for Disease Control and Prevention (CDC). (2006a). *Expedited partner therapy in the management of sexually transmitted diseases.* Atlanta, GA: Author.

Centers for Disease Control and Prevention (CDC). (2006b). Sexually transmitted diseases treatment guidelines 2006. *Morbidity and Mortality Weekly Report, 55*(RR-11), 1–94.

Centers for Disease Control and Prevention (CDC). (2007a). *CDC fact sheet PID (pelvic inflammatory disease).* Atlanta, GA: Author.

Centers for Disease Control and Prevention (CDC). (2007b). Updated recommended treatment regimens for gonococcal infections and associated conditions—United States, April 2007. *Morbidity and Mortality Weekly Report, 56*(14), 332–336.

Centers for Disease Control and Prevention (CDC). (2009a). *CDC press release. CDC report finds adolescent girls continue to bear a major burden of common sexually transmitted diseases.* Atlanta, GA: Author.

Centers for Disease Control and Prevention (CDC). (2009b). *Sexually transmitted diseases surveillance, 2008.* Atlanta, GA: Author.

Chan, P., & Johnson, S. (2008). *Gynecology and obstetrics.* Blue Jay, CA: Current Clinical Strategies.

D'Ambrogio, A., Yerly, S., Sahli, R., Bouzourene, H., Demartines, N., Cotton, M., & Givel, J. C. (2009). Human papilloma virus type and recurrence rate after surgical clearance of anal condylomata acuminata. *Sexually Transmitted Diseases, 36*(9), 536–540.

Dinh, T., Sternberg, M., Dunne, E., & Markowitz, L. (2008). Genital warts among 18–59 year olds in the United States, National Health and Nutrition Examination Survey, 1999–2004. *Sexually Transmitted Diseases, 35*(4), 357–360.

Facts & Comparisons. (2010). *Drug facts & comparisons 2010.* St. Louis, MO: Wolters Kluwer Health.

Huppert, J. (2009). Trichomoniasis in teens: An update. *Current Opinion in Obstetrics and Gynecology, 21,* 371–378.

Judlin, P. (2010). Current concepts in managing pelvic inflammatory disease. *Current Opinion in Infectious Diseases, 23,* 83–87.

Kennedy, C., & Boardman, L. (2008). New approaches to external genital warts and vulvar intraepithelial neoplasia. *Clinical Obstetrics and Gynecology, 51*(3), 518–526.

Kriebs, J. (2008). Understanding herpes simplex virus: Transmission, diagnosis and considerations in pregnancy management. *Journal of Midwifery & Women's Health, 53*(3), 202–208.

Lehne, R. A. (2010). *Pharmacology for Nurses* (7th ed.). Philadelphia, PA: W. B. Saunders.

Little, J. W. (2006). Gonorrhea: Update. *Oral Surgery, Oral Medicine, Oral Pathology, Oral Radiology, and Endodontology, 101*(2), 137–143.

McCuthcheon, T. (2009). Anal condyloma acuminatum. *Gastroenterology Nursing, 32*(5), 342–349.

Nansel, T. R., Riggs, M. A., Yu, K. F., Andrews, W. W., Schwebke, J. R., & Klebanoff, M. A. (2006). The association of psychosocial stress and bacterial vaginosis in a longitudinal cohort. *American Journal of Obstetrics & Gynecology, 194*(2), 381–386.

Naresh, A., Beigi, R., Woc-Colburn, L., & Salata, R. (2009). The bidirectional interactions of human immunodeficiency virus-1 and sexually transmitted infections. *Infectious Diseases in Clinical Practice, 17*(6), 362–373.

National Center for Complementary and Alternative Medicine (NCCAM). (2009). *CAM and hepatitis: A focus on herbal supplements.* Retrieved from http://nccam.gov/health/hepatitisc/

Neggers, Y., Nansel, T., Andrews, W., Schwebke, J., Yu, K., Goldenberg, R., & Klebanoff, M. (2007). Dietary intake of selected nutrients affects bacterial vaginosis in women. *Journal of Nutrition, 137,* 2128–2133.

Tatti, S., Swinehart, J., Thielert, C., Tawfik, H., Meschder, A., & Beutner, K. (2008). Sinecatechins, a defined green tea extract, in the treatment of external anogenital warts: A randomized controlled trial. *Obstetrics & Gynecology, 111*(6), 1371–1379.

Wynn, L., Foster, A., & Trussell, J. (2009). Misconceptions and ignorance about sexual and reproductive health. *The Female Patient, 34*(11), 29–31.

CHAPTER 7

Women's Health Problems

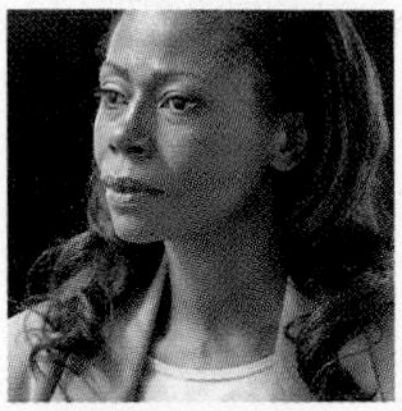

A friend was turning 42 years old a few months ago and knew that it was time for her annual gynecology exam. She had been putting off having her first mammogram because she had heard stories about how much it hurt. Finally, knowing that her nurse practitioner would ask her if she had gotten a mammogram, she scheduled the test the week before her annual gynecology exam. The mammogram detected a suspicious mass and she had a biopsy that confirmed intraductal carcinoma. She never had a palpable lump; she was not considered high risk for breast cancer; and she was an active, health-conscious woman. It never occurred to her that she could get breast cancer.

LEARNING OUTCOMES

1. Contrast the common benign and malignant breast disorders.
2. Describe the emotional reactions a woman may experience in regard to a diagnosis of breast cancer.
3. Summarize behaviors that help to minimize recurrence of some of the common lesions of the vulva.
4. Identify the implications of an abnormal finding during a pelvic examination.
5. Discuss abnormal uterine bleeding and abdominal masses.
6. Describe the role that human papilloma virus plays in abnormal Pap smears.
7. Discuss the importance of an annual Pap smear and appropriate follow-up for an abnormal finding.
8. Identify the risk factors, treatment options, and nursing interventions for a woman with toxic shock syndrome.
9. Discuss the signs and symptoms, medical therapy, and implications for fertility of endometriosis.
10. Discuss the signs and symptoms, diagnosis criteria, treatment options, and health implications of polycystic ovarian syndrome.
11. Compare the signs and symptoms and treatment options of the three forms of pelvic relaxation—cystocele, rectocele, and uterine relaxation.
12. Contrast laparoscope-assisted vaginal hysterectomy and abdominal hysterectomy with regard to indications for use and the advantages and disadvantages of each procedure.
13. Delineate the psychosocial responses a woman may experience when facing any of the common gynecologic procedures.

KEY TERMS

Breast self-examination (BSE) *117*
Colposcopy *132*
Cystocele *139*
Dysfunctional uterine bleeding (DUB) *133*
Dyspareunia *129*
Endometriosis *136*
Fibrocystic breast change *121*
Galactorrhea *121*
Hysterectomy *140*
Mammogram *117*
Pap smear *129*
Polycystic ovarian syndrome (PCOS) *137*
Toxic shock syndrome (TSS) *135*

From early childhood through adolescence, the active reproductive years, into menopause and the years beyond, a woman will likely face a variety of gynecologic or urinary problems. Some may be minor, whereas others have the potential to be quite serious, provoking a wide array of physical and psychologic responses. This chapter provides information about selected gynecologic problems that a woman may encounter during her lifetime with an emphasis on problems commonly addressed in community-based settings. Some of the issues are addressed in detail, and other topics are discussed more briefly. The chapter concludes with a brief description of common gynecologic surgical procedures. For a detailed discussion of gynecologic cancers, for more detailed information on any of the subjects covered in this chapter, or for more in-depth discussion of gynecologic procedures, please consult a specialized text.

Care of the Woman with a Disorder of the Breast

Throughout her lifetime a woman may experience a variety of breast disorders. Some, like mastitis, which is discussed in chapter 38 ∞, are acute disorders, whereas others, such as fibrocystic breast changes, also known as benign breast disease (BBD), are chronic. This section begins with breast screening techniques and then deals with some of the common breast disorders a woman may experience.

Screening Techniques for the Breasts

Despite their limitations, breast examination and mammography remain the most effective screening techniques available for disorders of the breast. However, the American Cancer Society (ACS) now recommends magnetic resonance imaging (MRI) in younger women who are at a higher risk for breast cancer due to gene mutations and/or a strong family history of breast cancer because they often develop breast cancer at a younger age (American Cancer Society [ACS], 2009a).

Breast Examination

Like the uterus, the breast undergoes regular cyclic changes in response to hormonal stimulation. Each month, in rhythm with the cycle of ovulation, the breasts become engorged with fluid in anticipation of pregnancy, and the woman may experience sensations of tenderness, lumpiness, or pain. If conception does not occur, the accumulated fluid drains away via the lymphatic network. *Mastodynia* or *mastalgia* (premenstrual swelling and tenderness of the breasts) is common and usually lasts for 3 to 4 days before the onset of menses. Some women may also experience mastalgia at the time of ovulation, about 14 days into her cycle; for other women the symptoms may persist throughout the month.

After menopause, connective breast tissue atrophies and is replaced by adipose tissue. The breasts lose elasticity and may droop and become pendulous. The recurring breast engorgement associated with ovulation ceases. If hormone therapy (HT) is used to counteract other symptoms of menopause, breast engorgement may resume.

Monthly **breast self-examination (BSE)** has been advocated for years as a good method for detecting breast masses early, and, in truth, a large percentage of women discover their breast cancer accidentally or during a BSE. Women at high risk for breast cancer are specifically encouraged to be attentive to the importance of early detection through routine BSE. BSE may also be of real value for younger women (under age 40) who do not yet get regular mammograms. The value of BSE, however, has been under continual scrutiny. The U.S. Preventive Services Task Force made a recommendation in November 2009 against teaching women breast self-examination. This was based on studies they reviewed that led the task force to believe that BSE did not reduce breast cancer mortality but resulted in additional imaging procedures and biopsies (U.S. Preventive Services Task Force, 2009). The American College of Obstetricians and Gynecologists (ACOG) continues to recommend that women begin performing monthly BSE at age 20 (ACOG, 2009b). The ACS recommends BSE be presented to the patient as an option with close attention to the patient's technique as reviewed at her annual examination (ACS, 2009a). Therefore, even in light of the conflicting recommendations, in the course of a routine physical examination, or during an initial visit to the caregiver, women are generally taught BSE technique. The effectiveness of BSE is determined by the woman's ability to perform the procedure correctly, by her knowledge of her own breast tissue, and by the density of her breast tissue. (See Patient Teaching: Breast Self-Examination.)

Advocates of BSE advise that it be performed on a regular monthly basis about 1 week after the onset of each menstrual period, when the breasts are typically not tender or swollen. BSE is most effective when it uses a dual approach incorporating both inspection and palpation. After menopause, BSE should be performed on the same day each month (chosen by the woman for ease of remembrance). The continuation of BSE during pregnancy and lactation is advised due to the increase in hormonal influence on the breast. Pregnancy-associated breast cancer (PABC) occurs in about 1 in 1000 pregnancies and about 3500 cases of PABC are diagnosed every year in the United States. PABC is classified as such if the diagnosis is made during pregnancy or within one year of giving birth (Logue, 2009).

Clinical breast examination (CBE) by a trained healthcare provider, such as a physician, nurse practitioner, or nurse-midwife, is an essential element of a routine gynecologic examination. Experience in differentiating among benign, suspicious, and worrisome breast changes enables the caregiver to reassure the woman if the findings are normal or move forward with additional diagnostic procedures or referral if the findings are suspicious or worrisome. The ACS (2009a) recommends CBE every 3 years for women age 20 to 39 with no abnormal findings or history of breast-related problems and CBE annually for women age 40 and older. In clinical practice, however, many caregivers advocate annual CBE for all women over age 20, which continues to be the recommendation of ACOG (ACOG, 2009b).

Mammography

A **mammogram** is a soft-tissue x-ray image of the breast taken without the injection of a contrast medium. It can detect lesions in the breast before they can be felt and has gained wide acceptance

Breast Self-Examination

PATIENT TEACHING Breast Self-Examination

PATIENT GOALS At the completion of the teaching, the woman will be able to:

1. Discuss her risk of breast cancer.
2. Describe the use of BSE in breast cancer detection.
3. Demonstrate the correct procedure for BSE.
4. List warning signs of breast cancer to be reported to the caregiver.
5. Incorporate monthly BSE into her personal routine.

TEACHING PLAN

Content	Teaching Method
Discuss the risk factors associated with breast cancer.	Breast cancer should be discussed in a private area free of interruptions. The room needs to have a mirror; a bed, a couch, or an examining table; pillows; a patient gown; and a private area for the woman to disrobe.
Stress the unique risk factors associated with the woman's personal history and lifestyle.	Create a supportive, warm, and comfortable atmosphere by attitude and communication style—both verbal and nonverbal. A discussion of breast cancer may bring forth many emotions in the woman, including grief for previous breast cancer–related losses.
Discuss the use of BSE in breast cancer detection.	Focus on open discussion. A brochure with statistics and illustrations may be useful. Stress the positive outcomes of early detection to counterbalance fears.

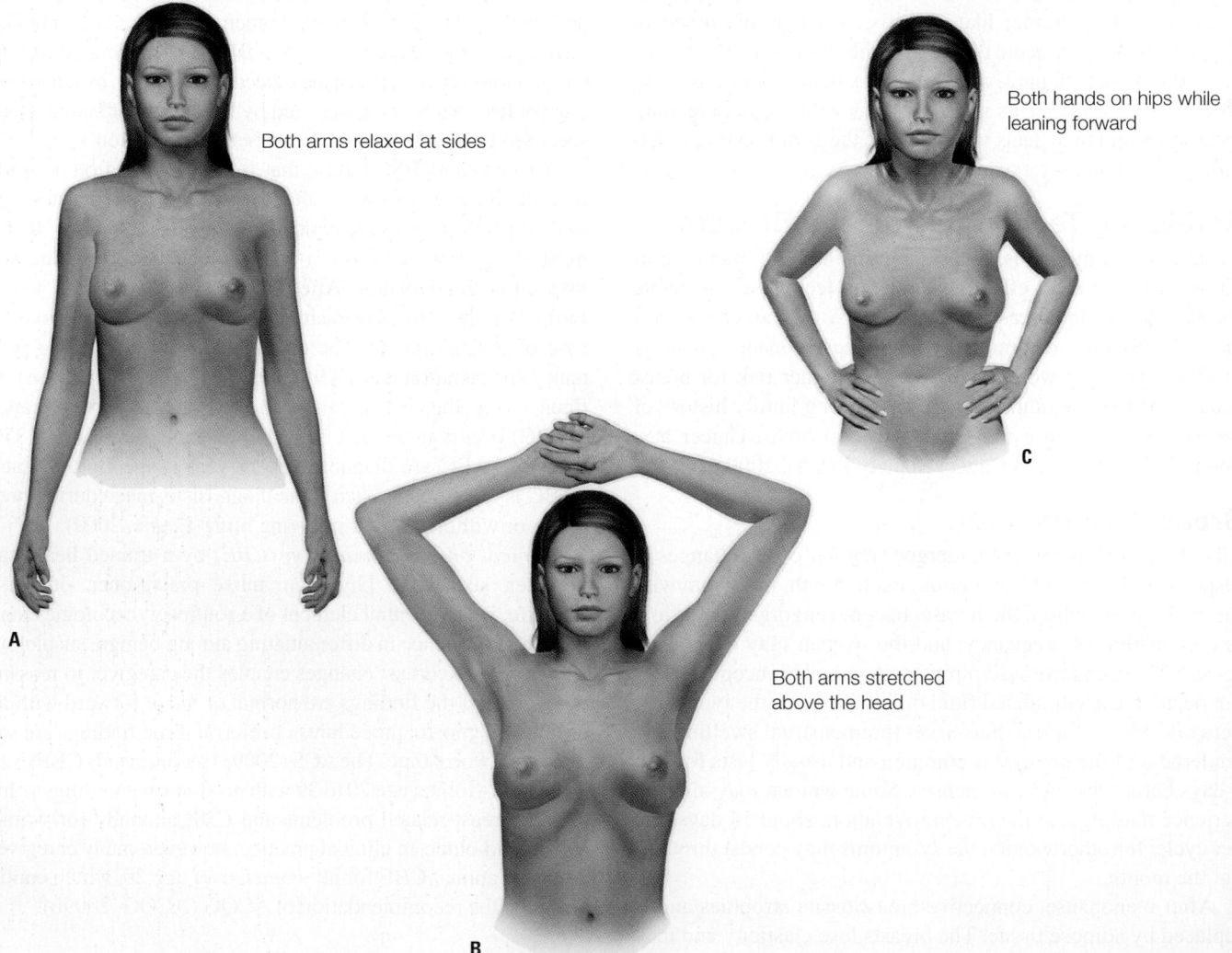

Figure 7-1 ■ Positions for inspection of the breasts. A. Both arms relaxed at sides. B. Both arms stretched above the head. C. Both hands on hips while leaning forward.

PATIENT TEACHING Breast Self-Examination continued

Describe and demonstrate the correct procedure for BSE.

A. Instruct the woman to inspect her breasts by standing or sitting in front of a mirror. She needs to inspect her breasts in three positions: with both arms relaxed down at her sides, both arms stretched straight over her head, and both hands placed on her hips while leaning forward (Figure 7-1 ■).

B. Advise the woman to look at her breasts individually and in comparison with one another. Note and record the following characteristics for each position:

Size and Symmetry of the Breasts

1. Breasts may vary, but the variations should remain constant during rest or movement—note abnormal contours.
2. Some size difference between the breasts is normal.

Shape and Direction of the Breasts

1. The shape of the breasts can be rounded or pendulous with some variation between breasts.
2. The breasts should be pointing slightly laterally.

Color, Thickening, Edema, and Venous Patterns

1. Check for redness or inflammation.
2. A blue hue with a marked venous pattern that is focal or unilateral may indicate an area of increased blood supply due to tumor. Symmetric venous patterns are normal.
3. Skin edema observed as thickened skin with enlarged pores ("orange peel") may indicate blocked lymphatic drainage due to tumor.

Surface of the Breasts

1. Skin dimpling, puckering, or retraction (pulling) when the woman presses her hands together or against her hips suggests malignancy.
2. Striae (stretch marks) red at onset and whitish with age are normal.

Nipple Size and Shape, Direction, Rashes, Ulcerations, and Discharge

1. Long-standing nipple inversion is normal, but an inverted nipple previously capable of erection is suspicious. Note any deviation, flattening, or broadening of the nipples.
2. Check for rashes, ulcerations, or discharge.

C. Instruct the woman to palpate (feel) her breasts as follows:

1. Lie down. Put one hand behind your head. With the other hand, using the three middle fingers with fingers flattened, gently feel your breast (Figure 7-2A ■).
2. Figure 7-2B ■ shows you how to check each breast. Begin as you see in B and follow the arrows, moving in an up and down pattern starting from the underarm and progressing toward the sternum. Be sure to cover all the tissue, going up to the collarbone and down until you feel the ribs. Feel gently for a lump or thickening.
3. Now repeat the same procedure sitting up, with the hand still behind your head (Figure 7-2C ■).
4. Squeeze the nipple between your thumb and forefinger. Look for any discharge—clear or bloody (Figure 7-2D ■).

D. Take the woman's hand and help her to identify her "normal lumps" (e.g., mammary ridge, ribs, and nodularity in the upper outer quadrants).

E. After she examines her breasts and identifies her normal lumps, instruct her to palpate her breasts once more to identify any areas that she may have questions about. If questions arise, the nurse should palpate the area and attempt to identify whether it is normal.

Learning is best accomplished when material is broken down into smaller steps and presented with multiple approaches. Prior to asking the woman to perform BSE, use a model or a chart to demonstrate the procedure. Then have the woman perform BSE. Be very supportive and give a lot of positive feedback because some women may be embarrassed. Demonstrate a nonjudgmental, accepting attitude.

Demonstrate "normal lumps" on the woman herself while guiding her hand and identifying the area. This will increase confidence that she will recognize an abnormal finding. Checking her immediately afterward will positively reinforce her and diminish the fear associated with BSE.

A

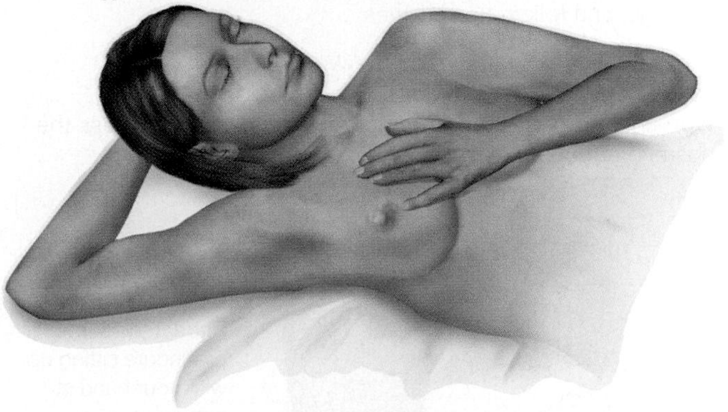

With one hand behind your head, flatten your fingers and press lightly on your breast, feeling gently for a lump or thickening.

B

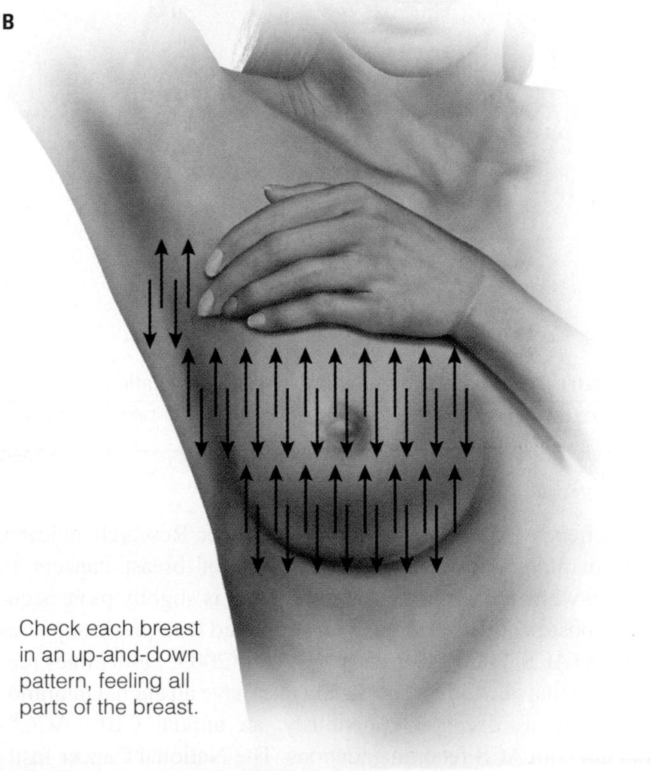

Check each breast in an up-and-down pattern, feeling all parts of the breast.

Figure 7-2 ■ Procedure for breast self-examination.

F. If a breast model is available, instruct the woman to palpate it and identify the lumps.

G. Provide information on the warning signs of breast cancer and what she should do if she identifies any of these signs during BSE.

(continued)

PATIENT TEACHING Breast Self-Examination continued

Timing

Instruct the woman to perform BSE on a monthly basis. Be specific based on whether she is premenopausal, pregnant, postmenopausal, or postmenopausal receiving hormone replacement therapy.

Evaluation

Evaluate the woman's learning through discussion and return demonstration. Learning has occurred if the woman performs BSE correctly and can identify timing, normal and abnormal findings, and follow-up activities.

Provide a written handout on the warning signs of breast cancer. The handout should also cover actions that the woman should take if a warning sign is discovered. Stress the positive effects of early detection.

Provide the woman with a reminder symbol for monthly BSE. The American Cancer Society provides such items to hang in the shower, place on a refrigerator, and so forth. Praise her commitment to do monthly BSE. Give the woman a follow-up telephone number (e.g., American Cancer Society) to use if she needs additional information or has questions.

Documentation

Documentation of patient teaching should include the teaching information discussed, the patient's verbalization of understanding, and specific interventions or warning signs that were given, along with the patient's understanding of follow-up if needed in the future.

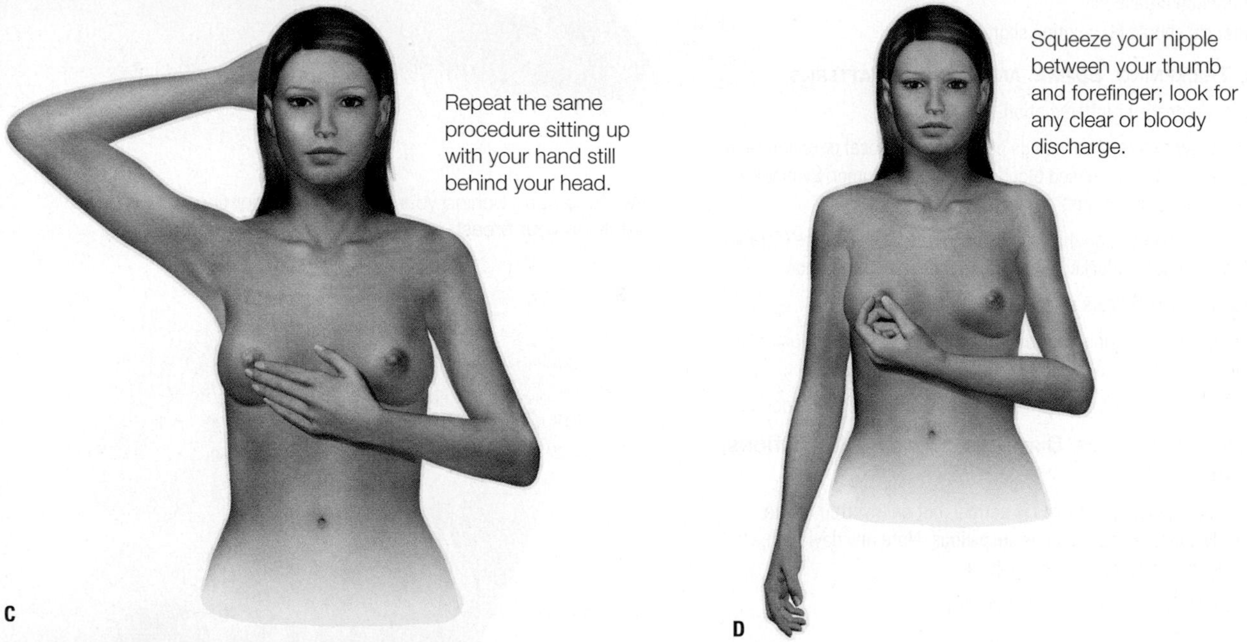
Repeat the same procedure sitting up with your hand still behind your head.
C
Squeeze your nipple between your thumb and forefinger; look for any clear or bloody discharge.
D

Figure 7-2 ■ Procedure for breast self-examination.

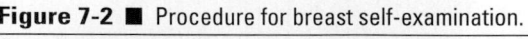

Source: Data from American Cancer Society. (1973). Breast self-examination and the nurse *(No. 3408 PB).*

as an effective screening tool for breast cancer. Research indicates that mammography detects about 90% of breast cancers in women who are symptom free, although it is slightly more accurate in postmenopausal women, as compared with premenopausal women (ACS, 2006). Currently the ACS (2009c) guidelines recommend that all women age 40 and over have an annual mammogram and, as discussed previously, an annual CBE. ACOG concurs with ACS recommendations. The National Cancer Institute (NCI) (2009a) recommends mammograms every 1 to 2 years for women age 40 and older. The NCI also recommends that women who are at higher than average risk of breast cancer should talk with their healthcare providers about whether to have mammograms before age 40 and how often to have them. If a woman has a history of breast cancer in a close relative (i.e., mother, sister) and the cancer was diagnosed before the relative was age 40, many clinicians advocate that the patient begin mammograms 10 years before the age of her close relative's diagnosis.

The sensitivity of mammography in accurately diagnosing a breast cancer increases with age (83% to 92%) and presence of a palpable mass (90%). It decreases in accuracy in women with increased breast density (35%). Overall it carries a 63% to 95% accuracy in women over 40 (Singhal, 2008). This is why clinicians favor the triple assessment protocol in women that starts with clinical breast examination to assess for lumps and lymph nodes. If a lump is found, the examination is then followed by a mammogram or ultrasound for further information on the consistency of the palpable lump. Fine-needle aspiration will follow if the lump in question appears suspicious on imaging (Singhal, 2008).

Breast sensitivity seems to vary from woman to woman and may be a factor in a woman's reluctance to have a mammogram.

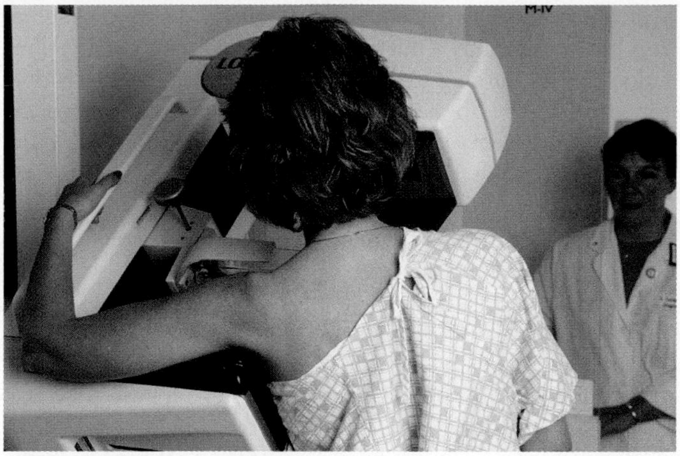

Figure 7-3 ■ Recommended position for mammogram.

Source: Philip Bailey/CORBIS.

To help prevent any discomfort, the nurse can suggest that this x-ray study be scheduled when the woman's breasts are least sensitive, which is about 2 weeks after the onset of menses. In some cases, the woman can obtain relief by reducing caffeine intake from 5 to 7 days before the test. In most cases, a mammogram causes feelings of compression but not pain (Figure 7-3 ■). All women should be instructed to refrain from applying lotions, powders, deodorant, or other cosmetic substances to the torso on the day of the exam because the substances may appear as questionable areas on the mammogram and can interfere with accurate interpretation. The risk of radiation exposure with mammograms is low because strict guidelines are in place to ensure that the equipment is safe and uses the lowest dose of radiation possible. The level of radiation used does not significantly increase the risk for breast cancer (ACS, 2009c).

Benign Breast Conditions

Fibrocystic breast change, also known as benign breast disease (BBD), occurs in 50% to 60% of all women (Lee, 2009). Fibrocystic changes are the most common type of BBD and are most prevalent in women 20 to 50 years of age. Generally fibrocystic changes are not a risk factor for breast cancer. In some rare cases, if the change is proliferative and results in hyperplasia or buildup of the cells of the breast ducts, atypia may occur (Lee, 2009). There is a four- to five-fold increase in the risk of breast cancer in these women (Gordon et al., 2007). Fibrocystic changes may produce an asymptomatic mass but more often are accompanied by pain or tenderness and sometimes nipple discharge. Fluctuations in size and rapid appearance or disappearance of breast masses are common. Bilateral, cyclic breast pain is the most common symptom, and the nodularities may be unilateral or bilateral, often in the upper outer quadrants of the breasts.

The woman often reports pain, tenderness, and swelling that is cyclic, worsening in the late luteal phase of the menstrual cycle (just before menses) and improving about 1 to 2 days into the menstrual cycle. Physical examination may reveal only mild signs of irregularity, or the breasts may feel dense, with areas of irregularity and nodularity. Women often refer to this as "lumpiness." Some women may also experience spontaneous nipple discharge, which should be evaluated separately.

If the woman has a large, fluid-filled cyst, she may experience a localized painful area as the capsule containing the accumulated fluid distends coincident with her cycle. However, if small cysts form, the woman may experience not a solitary tender lump but a diffuse tenderness. Several characteristics help differentiate a cyst from a cancerous lesion. Cysts tend to be mobile and tender and do not cause skin retraction (pulling) in the surrounding tissue, whereas cancerous lesions tend to be fixed and painless and may cause skin retraction.

Mammography, sonography, magnetic resonance imaging (MRI), palpation, and fine-needle aspiration can be used to confirm fibrocystic breast changes. Often, fine-needle aspiration provides treatment as well as relief from the tenderness or pain. Palpable cysts are often treated conservatively with medical management; however, all discrete masses should have a tissue sample sent for biopsy. Women with mild symptoms may benefit from restricting sodium intake and taking a mild diuretic during the week before the onset of menses. This counteracts fluid retention, relieves pressure in the breast, and helps decrease the pain. In other cases, a mild analgesic is necessary. Oral contraceptives help alleviate symptoms for the majority of women, but, unfortunately, symptoms tend to recur when the oral contraceptives are discontinued. Oil of evening primrose is often recommended and may reduce the symptoms of premenstrual breast tenderness (Gordon et al., 2007).

In severe cases, the hormone inhibitor danazol is often helpful although it can cause several undesirable side effects such as nausea, depression, menstrual irregularities, headaches, and masculinization (Gordon et al., 2007). Women who do not respond to other treatment approaches may be given a trial of bromocriptine, a prolactin inhibitor. Some researchers suggest that methylxanthines (found in caffeine products such as coffee, tea, colas, chocolate, and some medications) and the use of tobacco may contribute to the development of fibrocystic breast changes and that limiting use of these substances will help decrease fibrocystic changes.

Fibroadenoma is the second most common benign breast lesion, occurring in 25% of women with the peak incidence at 15 to 35 years. It is an asymptomatic, mobile, well-defined, painless palpable mass with a rubbery texture. Women with no family history and a simple fibroadenoma are at no greater risk for breast cancer than the general population.

Ultrasound is the best method for imaging women under 35 with a palpable mass because of the density of their breast tissue. Most women can be observed and followed every 6 months with ultrasound for 2 years then once yearly thereafter. Some clinicians may prefer surgical excision to prove that it is benign (Lee, 2009).

The term for nipple discharge not associated with lactation (production of milk for breastfeeding) is **galactorrhea**. It is a common breast problem and has been reported in 10% to 15% of women. Nipple discharge can occur in patients of all ages and races and generally is a nonsignificant finding. Nonclinically significant nipple discharge occurs in women who have fibrocystic changes in the breast, who are using contraceptives, or who are on hormone therapy (Azavedo, 2009). Certain medications that are used to treat psychiatric disorders have a side effect of galactorrhea.

The most common types of nipple discharge occur in both breasts, are secreted from several ducts, and vary in color from white to brown. The likelihood of malignancy increases with the presence of a spontaneous discharge arising from a single duct in one breast that is watery or bloody in nature and warrants further investigation. Cytologic evaluation of the fluid can be performed; however, false-positive and false-negative rates have been reported as high as 17.8%. Mammogram is used initially for evaluation. Ultrasound may be used if the nipple discharge is accompanied by a palpable mass or if positive findings are seen on the mammogram (Azavedo, 2009).

Intraductal papillomas are tumors growing in the terminal portion of a duct or, sometimes, throughout the duct system within a section of the breast. Symptoms may include a unilateral mass or a spontaneous, and often bloody, nipple discharge.

The majority of papillomas present as solitary nodules. These small ball-like lesions may be detected on mammography but often are nonpalpable. The presence of a papilloma is often frightening to the woman, because her primary symptom is a discharge from the nipple that may be serosanguineous or brownish green because of old blood. The location of the papilloma within the duct system and its pattern of growth determine whether nipple discharge will be present. They are typically benign but they are generally excised to rule out the possibility of cancer. A solitary papilloma carries a slightly increased risk of developing into a cancer (Lee, 2009).

Duct ectasia (comedomastitis), an inflammation of the ducts behind the nipple, commonly occurs during or near the onset of menopause and is not associated with malignancy. The condition typically occurs in women who have borne and nursed children. It is characterized by a thick, sticky nipple discharge of various colors and by burning pain, pruritus, and inflammation. Nipple retraction may also be noted, especially in postmenopausal women. Treatment is conservative with drug therapy aimed at symptomatic relief. The major central ducts of the breast occasionally have to be excised.

Table 7-1 provides a comparison of the most frequently seen benign breast disorders.

Malignant Breast Disease

Breast cancer constitutes 25% of all cancers in women, making it the most prevalent cancer in females. The lifetime risk of women developing breast cancer in the United States is 1 in 8. Breast cancer accounts for nearly 15% of all cancer deaths in women and is the leading cause of death in women between the ages of 44 and 50 years. Of women who receive a breast cancer diagnosis, 70% to 80% of them will have no family history (ACS, 2009a). The highest incidence of breast cancer occurs in North America and Western Europe with the lowest incidence in South America, Africa, and parts of Asia; immigrants to the United States take on the higher U.S. risk. In the United States it is most common in Caucasian women; African American and Hispanic women have lower occurrence rates (Singhal, 2008).

Predisposing Factors

Factors that predispose a woman to breast cancer include the following:

- Age. Incidence increases steadily with age.
- Female gender.
- History of previous breast cancer.

TABLE 7-1 Summary of Benign Breast Disorders

CONDITION	AGE	PAIN	CANCER RISK	NIPPLE DISCHARGE	LOCATION	CONSISTENCY AND MOBILITY	DIAGNOSIS AND TREATMENT
Fibrocystic breast changes	30–50	Yes	Yes: with proliferative disease and a typical hyperplasia	Varies: none at all or may be clear, milky, straw colored, or green	Upper outer quadrant	Multiple lumps occurring bilaterally, influenced by menstrual cycle, nodular	Needle aspiration, Pap smear of nipple discharge, observation, biopsy if unresolved mass exists or mammographic changes, sonography
Fibroadenoma	15–25, median age 20	No	No	No: but milky discharge in pregnancy	Nipple or upper outer quadrant along the lateral side	Solid, well defined, sharply delineated, rounded rubbery mobile	Mammography, observation, surgical excision
Intraductal papilloma	Menopausal 50–60	Yes: on palpation	Yes: with multiple papillomas	Yes: serous bloody, or brownish green	No specific location	Nonpalpable or small, ball-like, poorly delineated	Pap smear of nipple discharge, mammography ductogram; surgical, excision
Duct ectasia	45–55	Yes: burning and itching around the nipple	No	Yes: in perimenopausal women: thick, sticky, green, greenish brown or bloodstained	Mass behind or around the nipple	Poorly circumscribed inflammation, nipple retraction, axillary lymphadenopathy	Pap smear of breast discharge, mammography, drug therapy for symptoms, surgical excision, observation.

- Have a known BRCA1 or BRCA2 gene mutation, or have a first-degree relative with this gene mutation.
- Family history of mother, sister, or daughter with breast cancer. The lifetime risk is up to 4 times higher if mother or sister is affected (Singhal, 2008).
- Long-term (more than 5 years) postmenopausal combined estrogen and progestin HT (ACS, 2009a).
- Being overweight or obese after menopause.
- Alcohol consumption. This risk increases with the amount of alcohol consumed (ACS, 2009a).
- No history of pregnancy or first pregnancy after age 30.
- Never breastfeeding a child.
- Longer reproductive phase (early menarche [before age 12] and late menopause [after age 50]).
- History of high-dose radiation to the chest between the ages of 10 and 30 (ACS, 2009a).
- Physical inactivity.
- Ashkenazi Jewish descent.

DEVELOPING CULTURAL COMPETENCE

Breast Cancer Survival Rates

While death rates due to breast cancer continue to drop among African American women, the group continues to be diagnosed at advanced stages and have decreased survival rates at each stage of diagnosis compared to their white counterparts (ACS, 2009a).

Prevention

Women should be encouraged to take action to reduce modifiable risks for breast cancer. These include, for example, avoiding obesity, exercising regularly, reducing dietary fat, and limiting alcoholic intake. Women at high risk of breast cancer may choose to begin chemoprevention using the drug tamoxifen. Women at very high genetic risk may consider bilateral prophylactic mastectomy (ACS, 2009b).

Diagnosis

A malignant neoplasm may originate either in a duct or in the epithelium of the breast lobes. About 50% of breast cancers originate in the upper outer quadrant and spread or metastasize to the axillary lymph nodes. Common sites of distant metastasis are the lymph nodes, lungs, liver, brain, and bone.

As previously discussed, a cancerous lump may be discovered by the woman herself, by the clinician who palpates or observes an abnormality, or by mammogram. A painless mass or lump is the most important physical symptom of breast cancer, although up to 10% of women have breast pain but no palpable mass (ACS, 2009a). Early detection greatly improves the treatment options available and increases women's long-term survival rates.

Worrisome findings that point to a higher risk of breast cancer include dimpling of the breast tissue, recent or acute nipple inversion, change in breast size or shape, increase of size in breast mass, skin erosion or ulceration, or presence of an axillary lump. Routine mammography screening detects masses 2 to 3 years before clinical appearance. Other diagnostic modalities include fine-needle biopsy, ultrasonography, and MRI. Biopsy is essential for a diagnosis. Once the diagnosis is made and lymph node involvement is evaluated, clinical staging of the disease is determined and a treatment plan that coincides with the stage is initiated.

Clinical Therapy

Once breast cancer is diagnosed, the woman and her physician make treatment decisions together. The decision is based on a consideration of the following factors:

- Stage of cancer
- Optimal treatment for that stage
- Woman's age
- Personal preferences
- Risks and benefits of each treatment protocol

Most women diagnosed with breast cancer have some form of surgery. The primary goal of the surgery is to remove the cancer from the breast and the lymph nodes, if they are involved. Surgical treatment may consist of *simple* or *total mastectomy,* which involves removal of the entire breast. A *modified radical mastectomy* involves the removal of the breast and the axillary lymph nodes but does not include removal of any of the pectoral muscles of the chest wall. Women who undergo mastectomy are generally given the option of having breast reconstruction surgery. This surgery may be done at the time of the mastectomy or delayed until the prescribed chemotherapy and/or radiation is completed. *Lumpectomy,* or the removal of the cancerous tissue plus a rim of normal tissue, is a breast-sparing approach that is often used for women with stages I or II breast cancer. It is almost always followed by several weeks of radiation therapy to destroy any remaining cancerous cells.

Adjunctive therapy for breast cancer includes chemotherapy, radiation, and hormone therapy. Chemotherapy typically involves a combination of drugs known to combat breast cancer. As indicated previously, radiation is often used to destroy remaining cells following surgery, but it may also be used to reduce the size of a cancerous tumor before surgery. This is termed neoadjuvant therapy. Hormone therapy is based on the knowledge that the hormone estrogen, which is produced by the ovaries, stimulates certain types of breast cancer. Women who have a form of breast cancer that tests positive for estrogen receptors can be given the antiestrogen drug tamoxifen. Tamoxifen counters the effects of circulating estrogen in the body to reduce the risk that the cancer returns or spreads to another area of the body. It is also used for cancer prevention by women who are at high risk for developing breast cancer. This drug has side effects and women taking it need to be monitored closely. Women using tamoxifen are at a higher risk for uterine cancer and should be counseled to follow up with their healthcare provider if they experience any unusual vaginal bleeding or resume menstrual cycles if they are postmenopausal. Blood clots are another risk, and the patient should be counseled about signs and symptoms of this (ACS, 2009b).

Raloxifene, a selective estrogen receptor modulator (SERM), is used to prevent osteoporosis. However, it was shown to be even more effective than tamoxifen in decreasing the risk of breast cancer in postmenopausal women who were taking it for osteoporosis.

Aromatase inhibitors are drugs that stop the body from making estrogen. These are given to postmenopausal women only and to those whose cancers were estrogen receptor positive (ACS, 2009b). These have been shown to prevent the return of breast cancer and are often given in place of tamoxifen or after the 5-year course of tamoxifen for further prevention. The studies show that when given after the completion of tamoxifen therapy, survival clearly improves (Kaunitz, 2008). The side effects of blood clots are much less than with tamoxifen and there is no risk for developing uterine cancer with this medication.

Herceptin, a newer drug, is a man-made version of an immune system protein. A growth-promoting protein called HER2/neu is found in small amounts on the surface of normal breast cells and in large amounts in some breast cancer cells. Herceptin is given to women whose breast cancers have too much HER2/neu to stop this protein from causing breast cancer cell growth. It is also thought to help the immune system better fight the breast cancer (ACS, 2009b).

Some women prefer a combined approach to treatment that draws on both allopathic and complementary medicine. These women elect to use complementary therapies, such as herbal remedies, Therapeutic Touch, acupuncture, aromatherapy, and massage, in combination with medical treatments.

When a woman is confronted with a breast cancer diagnosis, she must decide which therapy is worth what personal risk for her. Although prompt treatment is indicated, a second opinion is encouraged. Care of the woman with breast cancer involves a multidisciplinary approach, including a primary care provider, radiotherapist, surgeon, medical oncologist, and nursing specialists.

Psychologic Adjustment

The emotional feelings a woman experiences can range from fear of the loss of a body part, to fear of the ill effects of treatments, to fear of death and leaving children and family behind. The nurse should encourage the woman to discuss her feelings and concerns, informing her of all procedures, their pros and cons, and alternative options.

The course of adjustment confronting the woman with cancer has been described in four phases: shock, reaction, recovery, and reorientation. In the *shock* phase, women make statements such as "Everything is unreal" or "I can't understand why this is happening to me." Shock generally extends from the discovery of the lump through the process of diagnosis.

Reaction occurs in conjunction with the initiation of treatment. As treatment begins, the woman is compelled to face what has occurred and begins to take in what has happened. Coping mechanisms become evident during this phase. Reaction coincides with the length of treatment. For many women, radiation treatment or chemotherapy prolongs this period to months. Treatment reinforces the diagnosis of cancer and the immediate consequences of the disease. Denial of breast loss, if a mastectomy is done, and denial of the reality of the illness are common responses by the woman during the periods of diagnosis and treatment. Denial protects the woman, making therapy tolerable.

Recovery begins during convalescence following the completion of medical treatment. Anxiety about her illness diminishes and the woman looks to the future once more. She turns outward and gradually resumes her former activities. Conversely, depression and social isolation occur if the woman is unable to negotiate the recovery phase successfully.

A woman's family and friends significantly influence her recovery. Women often perceive their partners as their primary source of support. Both members of a couple must adjust to the woman's condition and its implications as well as to the effect of therapy on their sexual intimacy. Difficulties with psychosocial adjustment to breast cancer tend to be similar for women and their partners except in the area of role adjustments, where women have more difficulties. Many hospitals and community agencies sponsor support groups for women with breast cancer. Online support groups are also available and are of particular value to women in rural areas and in areas that lack adequate community support. In addition, the ACS sponsors support groups for cancer survivors and their families. They also have a highly successful program, "Reach to Recovery," for women following surgery.

Reorientation follows recovery and can be challenging. It is accomplished when the woman can acknowledge that breast cancer is part of her life; yet living, for her, has returned to or perhaps exceeded its former fullness and meaning.

For additional information on breast cancer, refer to a medical-surgical text.

> "The physician also felt the lump and thickening, and now I'm waiting to have my mammogram. My thoughts and feelings since I first felt the lump have been like a roller coaster. I'm 46 and I'm wondering if this is it. Am I dying? Now? I am afraid as I have not been afraid since one of our children was very ill."

NURSING CARE MANAGEMENT

Nursing care of the woman with breast cancer is multidimensional. It involves meeting the educational, psychosexual, and physical needs of the woman and, to a certain extent, those of her family. In meeting these needs, the nurse functions as a caregiver, counselor, educator, liaison, and advocate. Nurses need to support women in their efforts to provide self-care. This increases their self-esteem and sense of control. Nursing care changes as the woman progresses from the period of diagnosis to the period of recovery.

Nursing Assessment and Diagnosis

During the period of diagnosis of any breast disease, the woman may be extremely anxious. The nurse can use therapeutic communication to assess the significance the woman places on her breasts; her current emotional status, coping mechanisms used during periods of stress, and knowledge and beliefs about cancer; and other variables that may influence her coping and adjustment.

Assessment is an ongoing process. Sufficient data must be obtained to provide the nurse and other members of the health-care team with increasing insight into the woman's physical, mental, emotional, and social situation.

Nursing diagnoses that may apply to a woman with a disorder of the breast include the following:

- ***Readiness for Enhanced Knowledge:*** Information about diagnostic procedures for suspected breast cancer related to an expressed wish for information
- ***Anxiety*** related to threat to body image or her life

Nursing Plan and Implementation

During the prediagnosis period, the nurse should provide emotional support, clarify misconceptions, encourage the woman to express her anxiety, and urge her to ask many questions. Once a diagnosis has been made, the nurse should ensure that the woman clearly understands her condition, its association to breast malignancy, and treatment options. The nurse can also locate appropriate resources in the community and encourage the woman to make use of them as she deals with this difficult time. The woman and her partner or support person should discuss the treatment alternatives with her healthcare provider. Nursing advocacy involves supporting the woman's right to make the best treatment decision for her. With the assistance of the nurse, the woman can explore her fears, clarify her values, and identify the treatment options that would be personally acceptable. The nurse can provide psychologic support for the woman with a troublesome diagnosis, supply her with patient education materials, and refer her to professional support groups.

For women who must undergo surgery, nursing care focuses on necessary perioperative interventions. Refer to a medical-surgical nursing textbook for detailed information on these aspects of nursing care.

Evaluation

Expected outcomes of nursing care include the following:

- The woman is able to discuss her fears, concerns, and questions during the period of diagnosis.
- The diagnosis is made quickly and accurately, and treatment is initiated, if indicated.

Care of the Woman During a Pelvic Examination

Women have a pelvic examination performed for a variety of reasons, ranging from health maintenance to disease diagnosis. Many women perceive the pelvic exam as an uncomfortable and embarrassing procedure. These negative feelings may cause women to delay having yearly gynecologic examinations, and this avoidance may pose a threat to life and health.

A woman's first pelvic examination is especially important because a positive experience can help allay anxiety and make subsequent pelvic exams less threatening. Because the initial pelvic examination is typically done when a young woman is a teenager, nurses should be sensitive to a teen's attitudes and concerns. Teens are often shy about revealing their bodies and may feel very embarrassed by the procedure. Nurses can also help by being alert for atypical responses that might indicate a history of sexual abuse.

To make the pelvic exam less threatening, and hopefully improve the woman's health-seeking behavior, it is important to create a trusting atmosphere and incorporate practices that help the woman maintain a sense of control. Additionally, it is important for the nurse to assist in facilitating a nonjudgmental and safe environment in which the woman can be honest in response to the medical providers' inquiries. Some healthcare providers are offering to perform what is called an educational pelvic exam. During this type of exam the woman becomes an active participant and has an opportunity to learn about her body, voice her concerns, and share decisions about her care.

The educational exam includes offering the woman a mirror to watch the procedure, pointing out anatomic parts to her, and positioning and draping her to allow eye-to-eye contact with the practitioner. The woman is encouraged to participate by asking questions and giving feedback. The nurse can assist the woman by encouraging her to relax with specific advice such as "Keep your bottom flat against the table" and "Wiggle your toes if you find yourself beginning to tense your muscles."

Nurse practitioners, certified nurse-midwives, and physicians all perform pelvic examinations. Nurses assist the practitioner and the woman during the examination. Procedure 7-1 provides information on assisting with a pelvic examination.

The pelvic examination consists of three segments: inspection of the vulva; inspection of the vagina and the cervix via a speculum examination; and palpation of the cervix, uterus, and ovaries via a bimanual examination. Often a Papanicolaou (Pap) smear is obtained during the speculum examination. The Pap smear is discussed in the section on abnormal Pap smear results, which begins on page 129.

Vulvar Self-Examination

During the pelvic examination many caregivers also provide education about self-examination of the vulva. This procedure, like breast self-examination (BSE) (discussed previously), permits early detection of abnormalities, thereby maximizing the possibility of early diagnosis and treatment.

Self-examination of the vulva is simple to perform. The woman is advised to assume a sitting position on a bed or a chair. In good light she holds a mirror in one hand and uses the other hand to expose the tissues of her perineum while she carefully inspects and palpates the area. Pregnant or obese women may find it easier to inspect this area in a standing position with one foot elevated on a low stool. Figure 7-4 ■ shows the correct procedure for vulvar self-examination.

Initially, the woman inspects the entire perineum for symmetry, discharge, and lesions. She then gently pushes back the hood of the clitoris to inspect this area. Next she separates the labia to examine the inner tissues. The woman gently palpates the vulva using the flat part of one or two fingers. Then, using her thumb and index finger, the woman palpates the lateral aspects of the genitalia along the length of the vulva, noting any tenderness, masses, or lesions. Lastly, the woman examines the vaginal opening, compressing the tissues between the index

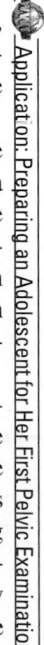

Application: Preparing an Adolescent for Her First Pelvic Examination

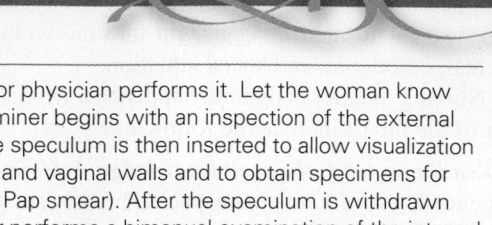

PROCEDURE 7-1 Assisting with a Pelvic Examination

NURSING ACTION

Preparation

- Ensure that the room is sufficiently warm by checking room temperature and adjusting the thermostat if necessary. If overhead heat lamps are available, turn them on.
- Explain the procedure to the woman. If she has never had a pelvic examination, show her the equipment to be used as part of the explanation.

  Rationale: *Explaining the procedure helps reduce anxiety and increase cooperation.*
- Ask the woman to empty her bladder and to remove clothing below the waist.

  Rationale: *An empty bladder promotes comfort during the internal examination.*
- Have padding on the stirrups. If stirrups are not padded, the woman may prefer to leave her shoes on during the procedure.

  Rationale: *Stirrups are padded to ease the pressure of the feet against the metal and to decrease the discomfort associated with cold stirrups. If they are not padded, wearing shoes accomplishes the same purpose.*
- Give the woman a disposable drape or sheet to use during the exam. Ask her to sit at the end of the examining table with the drape opened across her lap.
- Position the woman in the lithotomy position with her thighs flexed and abducted. Place her feet in the stirrups. Her buttocks should extend slightly beyond the edge of the examining table.

  Rationale: *This position provides the exposure necessary to conduct the examination effectively.*
- Drape the woman with the sheet, leaving a flap so that the perineum can be exposed.

  Rationale: *The drape helps preserve the woman's sense of dignity and privacy.*

Equipment and Supplies

- Vaginal specula of various sizes, warmed with water or on a heating pad prior to insertion
- Sterile gloves
- Water-soluble lubricant
- Materials for Pap smear or ThinPrep® Pap test and cultures
- Good light source

Note: *Lubricant may alter the results of tests and cultures and is not used during the speculum examination. Its use is reserved for the bimanual examination.*

Procedure: Sterile Gloves

1. The examiner dons gloves for the procedure. Explain each part of the procedure as the certified nurse-midwife, nurse practitioner, or physician performs it. Let the woman know that the examiner begins with an inspection of the external genitalia. The speculum is then inserted to allow visualization of the cervix and vaginal walls and to obtain specimens for testing (e.g., Pap smear). After the speculum is withdrawn the examiner performs a bimanual examination of the internal organs using the fingers of one hand inserted in the woman's vagina while the other hand presses over the woman's uterus and ovaries. The final step of the procedure is generally a rectal examination.
2. Ask the woman to breathe slowly and regularly and to use any method she finds effective in helping her to remain relaxed.

   Rationale: *Relaxation helps decrease muscle tension. Bearing down helps open the vaginal orifice and relaxes the perineal muscles.*
3. Let her know when the examiner is ready to insert the speculum and ask her to bear down.
4. After the speculum is withdrawn, lubricate the examiner's fingers prior to the bimanual examination.

   Rationale: *Lubrication decreases friction and eases insertion of the examiner's fingers.*
5. After the examiner has completed the examination and moved away from the woman, move to the end of the examination table and face the woman. Cover her with the drape. Apply gentle pressure to her knees and encourage her to move toward the head of the table. Assist her to remove her feet from the stirrups, then offer your hand to her and assist her to sit up.

   Rationale: *Assistance is important because the lithotomy position is an awkward one and many women, especially those women who are pregnant, obese, or older, may find it difficult to get out of the stirrups.*
6. Provide her with tissues to wipe the lubricant from her perineum.

   Rationale: *Vaginal secretions and lubricant may be discharged from the vagina when the woman sits upright.*
7. Provide the woman with privacy while she dresses. Be sure that she is not dizzy and that she is standing or sitting safely before leaving the room.

   Rationale: *Lying supine may cause postural hypotension.*

CLINICAL TIP

With the examiner's consent (obtained beforehand), offer the woman a hand mirror so that she can watch all or part of the examination. This practice removes the "mystery" from the procedure and enables the woman to become familiar with the appearance of her body.

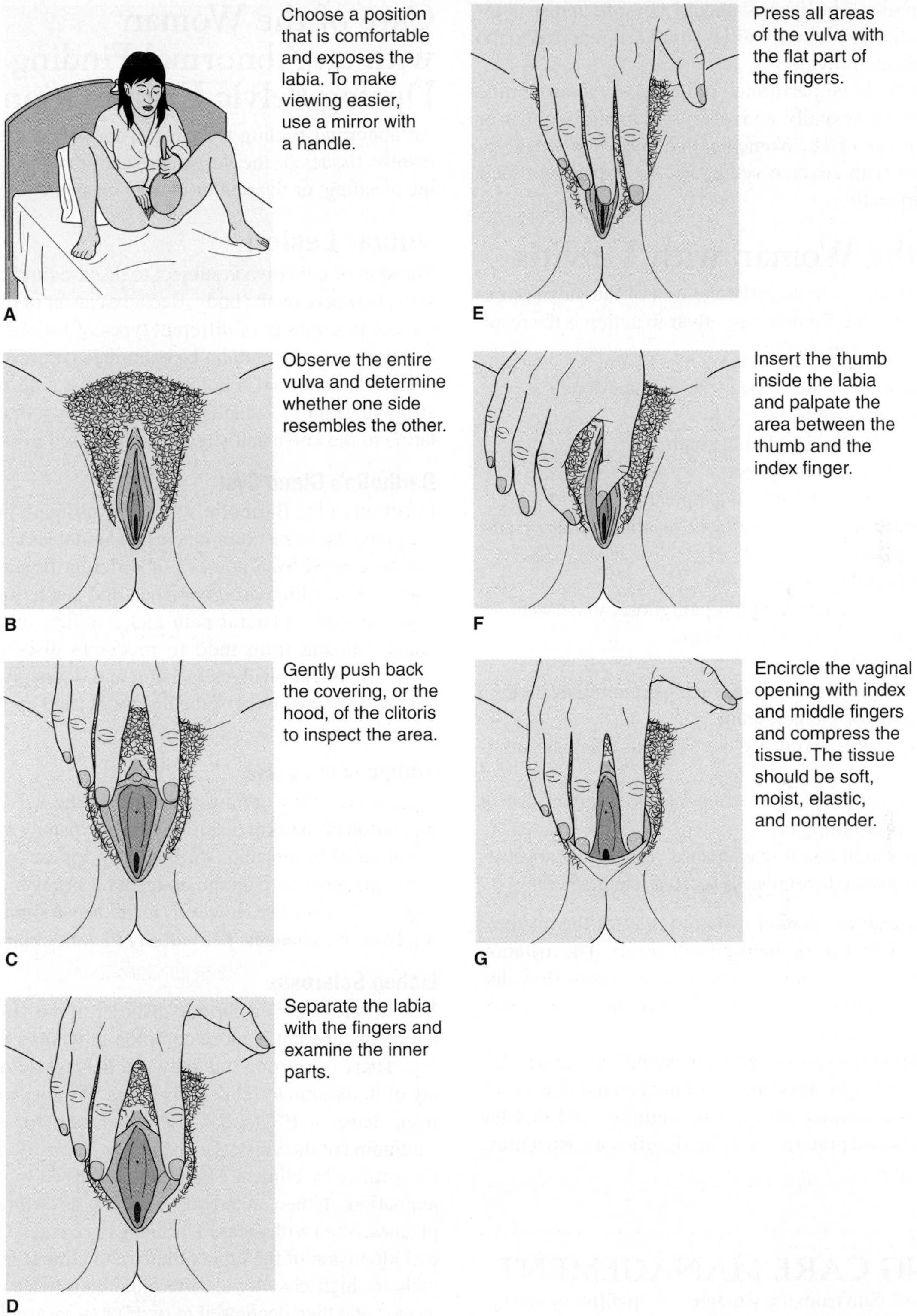
Choose a position that is comfortable and exposes the labia. To make viewing easier, use a mirror with a handle.
A
Observe the entire vulva and determine whether one side resembles the other.
B
Gently push back the covering, or the hood, of the clitoris to inspect the area.
C
Separate the labia with the fingers and examine the inner parts.
D
Press all areas of the vulva with the flat part of the fingers.
E
Insert the thumb inside the labia and palpate the area between the thumb and the index finger.
F
Encircle the vaginal opening with index and middle fingers and compress the tissue. The tissue should be soft, moist, elastic, and nontender.
G

Figure 7-4 ■ Steps to follow to perform vulvar self-examination.

and middle fingers. The tissues should be soft, moist, nontender, and elastic. Any abnormalities should be reported to the woman's healthcare provider.

This exam should be performed monthly, at the same time as the BSE, in all sexually active asymptomatic women or women over the age of 18. Women with a history of vulvar lesions or women with adverse symptoms should inspect their vulva more frequently.

Care of the Woman with Vulvitis

The term *vulvitis* refers to an inflammation of the vulva or external female genitalia. Sometimes vulvar irritation is the result of nonpathologic factors such as:

- Frequent douching or use of over-the-counter douches
- Feminine deodorant spray
- Detergents, harsh soaps, or bubble bath
- Colored or perfumed toilet paper
- Contraceptive creams, foams, or suppositories
- Condoms, possibly related to a latex or nonoxynol-9 (spermicide) sensitivity
- Dye, such as found in new clothing
- Synthetic clothing, such as nylon pantyhose, underwear, or synthetic slacks that may trap moisture
- Tight clothing, such as jeans
- Some repetitive motion exercise, such as running or biking
- Frequent shaving of the perineum
- Frequent intercourse or intercourse without adequate lubrication
- Deodorant menstrual pads or tampons, or frequent use of menstrual pads or tampons
- Estrogen deprivation due to menopause, surgical menopause, or medication-induced menopause (such as chemotherapy)

Other times, external genital irritation may be the result of inflammation or infection of the vagina or cervix. The irritation results when increased vaginal or cervical secretions flow distally and create inflammation of the vulvar tissues. This condition is called *vulvovaginitis*.

Often it is difficult to differentiate, by symptoms alone, vulvitis from vaginitis. The nurse needs to understand that vulvitis can occur as a distinct entity from vaginitis, and that the previously mentioned practices may be significant contributing factors to both.

NURSING CARE MANAGEMENT

The nurse gathers data from the woman to help differentiate behaviors that may cause isolated vulvitis from those that may cause vaginal and cervical inflammation. Once the assessment of vulvitis has been made, the nurse plays a crucial role in providing education about contributing factors that may have led to the development of vulvitis. In addition, educating the woman about behaviors to avoid, strategies or therapies to improve symptoms, and signs of a worsening condition that require further evaluation are all part of the nurse's responsibilities.

Care of the Woman with an Abnormal Finding During Pelvic Examination

An abnormal finding resulting from pelvic examination may involve tissues of the vulva, vagina, or cervix; abnormal uterine bleeding; or ovarian or uterine masses.

Vulvar Lesion

The skin of the vulva is subject to diseases and changes, just as skin elsewhere on the body. Because cancer of the vulva may be present in a variety of different types of lesions, it is important that the external genitalia be examined carefully at the time of pelvic examination. A common benign condition of the vulva, atrophic vaginitis, which is caused by a lack of estrogen stimulation to the vulva and vagina, is discussed in chapter 4 ∞.

Bartholin's Gland Cyst

Infection of the Bartholin's gland resulting in inflammation of the gland itself is a common vulvovaginal lesion. The infection can be caused by a number of different organisms, the most common of which are gonorrhea and staphylococcus. Symptoms include unilateral pain and swelling of the Bartholin's gland, ranging from mild to moderate discomfort to severe pain. Treatment involves incision and drainage of the abscess, culture and sensitivity of the discharge, and appropriate antibiotic therapy.

Vitiligo of the Vulva

Vitiligo is a fairly common finding on the vulva. It is a depigmentation of the skin resulting in white patchy areas because of the absence of melanin. Vitiligo may appear anytime after puberty and anywhere on the body, but it is never associated with a systemic disorder. However, it can cause significant disfiguring cosmetic changes, particularly in dark-skinned individuals.

Lichen Sclerosus

Lichen sclerosus is a chronic disorder of the vulva that can occur at any age but is more common in women in their 40s and 50s. There is a strong link between lichen sclerosus and a variety of autoimmune-related disorders. Women with lichen sclerosus have a 4% to 5% increased risk for squamous cell carcinoma of the vulva (Boardman & Kennedy, 2009). Diagnosis is made by clinical exam and confirmed by biopsy. On examination, lichen sclerosus appears as white papules and plaques, often with areas of bruising or redness. Other finds may include fusion of the labia minora and clitoral hood. Treatment includes high-dose topical steroid cream twice daily for 2 to 3 weeks, and then decreased to once or twice weekly thereafter.

Vulvar Vestibulitis

Women with *vestibulitis* experience local irritation and inflammation of the vulvar vestibule, severe pain with vaginal penetration (tampons or intercourse), burning and itching, and sometimes urinary frequency or dysuria. Proposed precipitating factors are numerous and include history of recurrent vaginal infections; use of oral contraceptives, especially at an early age; and exposure to destructive treatments such as trichloroacetic acid. There is some question if past sexual or physical abuse is a contributing factor. No definitive treatment exists so therapies are directed at comfort measures to relieve symptoms. Therapies include vaginal and introital lubricants; topical anesthetics; local interferon injections; oral antifungal medications; oral tricyclic antidepressants; biofeedback techniques; and in severe cases, surgical intervention (Boardman & Kennedy, 2009).

Malignant Tumors of the Vulva

Cancer of the vulva makes up 3% to 5% of all female genital cancers. It has been identified as 1 of 12 types of cancer that has shown an increase in occurrence with the most pronounced increase in younger women. Two types of vulvar cancer exist. Older women who have vulvar carcinoma have a keratinizing type in which human papilloma virus (HPV) is present in 2% to 23% of all cases. Younger women who develop vulvar carcinoma, however, show a 75% to 100% rate of HPV-related disease (Boardman & Kennedy, 2009). The woman may present with pruritus; a lump; a flat lesion; or, in the case of most HPV-related lesions, may be relatively asymptomatic. Risk factors include chronic vulvar inflammation, immunosuppression from chronic steroid use, smoking, diabetes, HPV infection or HIV, and history of lower genital tract cancer.

Clinical appearance can vary greatly and depends somewhat on the age of the patient. In younger women lesions may occur anywhere on the vulva, including around the anus and urethra. They may appear as flat or raised and may have a rough surface. They can vary in color from brown to white, gray or red. A colposcope, a microscope designed to look at the vulva and cervix (see p. 132), may be used to evaluate the tissue; a biopsy will need to be done. Lesions in older women generally are symptomatic and may include itching, burning, and pain; the woman may complain of chronic ulcerations or bleeding. As the disease becomes more invasive, a distinct tumor may present. Treatment usually involves surgery to remove the lesions and often the tissue surrounding the lesion; however, depending on the extent and degree of the lesion, the rate of reoccurrence is high (Boardman & Kennedy, 2009).

Cervicitis

Acute inflammation of the cervix is usually the result of infection from *Neisseria gonorrhoeae* or *Chlamydia trachomatis*. It may be caused by other organisms such as *Candida, Gardnerella vaginalis, Trichomonas,* herpes, staphylococci, or enterococci. Other causes may include use of intravaginal feminine hygiene products, frequent tampon use, frequent intercourse, or presence of a foreign body (such as an intrauterine device [IUD], contraceptive sponge, diaphragm, or tampon).

Symptoms often include a yellowish white vaginal discharge or copious purulent discharge that is sometimes malodorous, depending on the etiology. **Dyspareunia** (painful intercourse) is a common complaint with postcoital bleeding and occasional irregular vaginal bleeding. Sometimes there is a sense of pelvic heaviness and urinary symptoms such as urgency, frequency, and burning. Diagnosis and evaluation consist of a clinical pelvic examination, wet-mount smear, cultures, and a Pap smear. Treatment depends on the identified problem. It may include antibiotics to treat positive cultures (see chapter 6 ∞), removal of foreign bodies, and in some instances treatment of nonspecific inflammation with local medication (metronidazole gel or clindamycin cream).

Abnormal Pap Smear Results

Women tend to expect a normal Pap smear report but various abnormal findings are common. Notification of an abnormal result may cause significant anxiety in the woman. Therefore, results should be provided in a caring manner with an accurate explanation of the findings; reassurance that early detection of a problem allows early intervention; and information about expected further evaluation, treatment, and follow-up. The woman should be encouraged to ask questions and to voice her concerns.

Pap Smear

The purpose of the Papanicolaou smear (**Pap smear**) is to screen for the presence of cellular abnormalities by obtaining a sample containing cells from the cervix and the endocervical canal. Precancerous and cancerous conditions, as well as atypical findings and inflammatory changes, can be identified by a colposcopy.

Traditionally the test has been performed by preparing a Pap smear slide. However, the smear was often difficult to read because of obscuring factors such as blood, mucus, overlapping cells, and so forth. More recently, another test—the liquid-based medium Pap smear—was approved by the Food and Drug Administration (FDA). In this test, no slide is prepared; instead, the Pap smear is obtained using a speculum to reveal the cervix. The cervix is visualized and a smear is obtained using a plastic spatula on the surface of the cervix and a cytobrush, which is inserted into the cervical os or opening to obtain cells in the cervical canal. The brush and spatula are transferred directly to a vial of preservative fluid, thereby preserving the entire specimen. The specimen is sent to a laboratory where a special processor prepares a slide.

Liquid-based Pap smear preparations have become the method of choice for cervical cancer screening. These types of preparations allow for removal of debris from the sample, such as blood and mucus, thereby increasing the accuracy of the test. Additionally, these preparations allow for HPV screening and for some sexually transmitted infection (STI) screening. The Pap smear is a screening tool. A definitive diagnosis of cervical cancer is made by studying tissue samples obtained by biopsies.

> **PROFESSIONALISM IN PRACTICE**
>
> ***Pap Smear Preparation***
>
> Whenever you teach about pelvic examination and Pap smear, be certain that the woman understands that she should avoid having anything in her vagina for 24 hours before the examination—no intercourse, no tampons, no female hygiene products, and no douching—because this might interfere with the accuracy of the test.

Currently, both the American Cancer Society (ACS) and American College of Obstetricians and Gynecologists (ACOG) recommend that all women begin having Pap smears when they reach the age of 21. Additionally, it is now recommended that screening before the age of 21 be avoided because it may lead to unnecessary evaluation and treatment in women at a very low risk for cervical cancer. ACOG further recommends repeat Pap smears for women between the ages of 21 and 29 years every 2 years. Women aged 30 years and older who have had three consecutive normal Pap smears, who do not have a history of abnormal Pap smears in the past with a precancerous biopsy, who do not have HIV, or were never exposed to diethylstilbestrol (DES) in utero (a hormone given to women to prevent miscarriage in the 1950s and 1960s) may extend the interval to every 3 years (ACOG, 2009a). Some caregivers are reluctant to extend the time between Pap smears, however, because they worry that women may delay the test beyond the recommended time frames.

The Bethesda System

The *Bethesda System* (Table 7-2) is a standardized method of reporting cytologic Pap smear findings. The most widely used method system in the United States for reporting Pap smear results, it provides a uniform format and classification of terminology based on current understanding of cervical disease.

Cervical Abnormalities

Cervical cancer is the second most common cancer in women worldwide with an estimated 400,000 to 500,000 new cases every year (Wysocki, Reiter, & Berman, 2007). However, 50 years ago cervical cancer was the leading type of cancer in women. Since the use of Pap smear screening in the United

TABLE 7-2 The Bethesda System for Classifying Pap Smears

Specimen Type

Indicate conventional smear (Pap smear) vs. liquid based vs. other

Specimen Adequacy

Satisfactory for evaluation *(describe presence or absence of endocervical/transformation zone component and any other quality indicators; e.g., partially obscuring blood inflammation, etc.)*

Unsatisfactory for evaluation *(specify reason)*

Specimen rejected/not processed *(specify reason)*

Specimen processed and examined, but unsatisfactory for evaluation of epithelial abnormality because of *(specify reason)*

General Categorization (optional)

Negative for intraepithelial lesion or malignancy.

Epithelial cell abnormality. See interpretation/result *(specify 'squamous' or 'glandular' as appropriate).*

Other: See interpretation result *(e.g., endometrial cells in a woman* greater than or equal to *40 years of age).*

Automated Review

If case examined by automated device, specify device and result.

Ancillary Testing

Provide a brief description of the test methods and report the result so that it is easily understood by the clinician.

Interpretation/Result

Negative for intraepithelial lesion or malignancy (when there is no cellular evidence of neoplasia, state this in the General Categorization above and/or in the Interpretation/Result section of the report, whether or not there are organisms or other nonneoplastic findings)

ORGANISMS:

Trichomonas vaginalis.

Fungal organisms morphologically consistent with *Candida* spp.

Shift in flora suggestive of bacterial vaginosis.

Bacteria morphologically consistent with *Actinomyces* spp.

Cellular changes associated with herpes simplex virus.

OTHER NONNEOPLASTIC FINDINGS *(Optional to report list not inclusive).*

Reactive cellular changes associated with

—inflammation (includes typical repair)

—radiation

—intrauterine contraceptive device (IUD)

Glandular cells status posthysterectomy

Atrophy

Other

Endometrial cells (in a woman greater than or equal to 40 years of age) *(specify if negative for squamous intraepithelial lesion)*

Epithelial Cell Abnormalities

SQUAMOUS CELL

Atypical squamous cells

—of undetermined significance (ASC-US)

—cannot exclude HSIL (ASC-H)

Low-grade squamous intraepithelial lesion (LSIL)

—encompassing HPV/mild dysplasia/CIN-1

High-grade squamous intraepithelial lesion (HSIL)

—encompassing: moderate and severe dysplasia CIS/CIN-2 and CIN-3

—with features suspicious for invasion (*if invasion is suspected*)

Squamous cell carcinoma

GLANDULAR CELL

Atypical

—endocervical cells *(NOS or specify in comments)*

—endometrial cells *(NOS or specify in comments)*

—glandular cells *(NOS or specify in comments)*

Atypical

—endocervical cells, favor neoplastic

—glandular cells, favor neoplastic

Endocervical adenocarcinoma in situ

Adenocarcinoma

—endocervical

—endometrial

—extrauterine

—not otherwise specified (NOS)

Other Malignant Neoplasms (specify)

Educational Notes and Suggestions (optional)

Suggestions should be concise and consistent with clinical follow-up guidelines published by professional organizations (references to relevant publications may be included).

Source: Courtesy of National Cancer Institute.

States and other countries that have a system of Pap smear screening, the incidence of and mortality due to cervical cancer have decreased dramatically. In 2009, 11,270 new cases of cervical cancer were diagnosed in the United States. Sadly, 4070 cases of cervical cancer related deaths occurred despite the performance of the Pap smear (NCI, 2009b).

Cervical cancer is considered a preventable disease because it is slow-growing, has a lengthy preinvasive state, has inexpensive and available screening programs, and has effective treatment approaches for preinvasive lesions. Unfortunately, several subgroups of women in the United States have never been screened or are not screened at regular intervals. One half of women with newly diagnosed cervical cancer have never had a Pap smear, and 10% have not had a Pap smear in the last 5 years (ACOG, 2009a).

Factors that place a woman at high risk for cervical cancer include:

- Coitus at an early age (first intercourse before 16 years of age increases the risk of cervical cancer twofold)
- History of multiple sexual partners
- Sex partner with a history of numerous sexual partners
- Exposure to STIs
- History of HPV infection
- History of immunosuppressive therapy (chemotherapy) or immunocompromised state (HIV)
- Long-term oral contraceptive use (greater than 5 years)
- Smoking
- Antenatal exposure to diethylstilbestrol (DES)
- History of dysplasia

Virtually all cases of cervical cancer are associated with cervical infection with high-risk HPV and are preceded by high-grade cervical dysplasia (Wysocki et al., 2007). As discussed in chapter 6 ∞, over 120 different types of HPV have been identified; 30 types are known to infect the genital tract.

> **“ Several years ago I was treated for HPV—I got the infection from my husband—and seemed to be doing well. But now I've had some abnormal Pap smears and my doctor is talking about doing a LEEP procedure. I was a virgin when I got married but my husband wasn't. I've done a lot of reading, and I know how common HPV is, so I guess I can't be too hard on the guy. Still I have to admit that I feel a little nudge of resentment—I'm the one with problems. He is symptom free. ”**

The 2001 Bethesda System (ACOG, 2009a) identifies three categories for premalignant squamous cell lesions: atypical squamous cells (ASC), low-grade squamous intraepithelial lesion (LSIL), and high-grade squamous intraepithelial lesion (HSIL), which includes CIN 2 (moderate dysplasia) and CIN 3 (severe dysplasia and carcinoma in situ). The focus of the Pap smear is on the detection of high-grade cervical disease, especially *cervical intraepithelial neoplasia* (CIN). CIN refers to a lesion that may progress to invasive carcinoma (cancer). It is synonymous with the term *dysplasia.* To further support this objective, the ASC category is subdivided into two qualifiers that recognize the importance of detecting HSIL:

- Atypical squamous cells of undetermined significance (ASC-US)
- Atypical squamous cells—cannot exclude HSIL (ASC-H)

The category ASC-H includes those changes that are suggestive of a high-grade lesion but are lacking sufficient criteria for a definitive evaluation and interpretation. An immediate colposcopy is advised because women with this finding have a 20% to 50% risk of having a moderate to severe lesion (ACOG, 2008).

Another cervical cytology result is atypical glandular cells (AGUS), which represents cells that are glandular rather than squamous in origin. These are further subdivided into:

- Atypical endocervical cells
- Atypical endometrial cells
- Atypical glandular cells not otherwise specified

The workup for this type of finding is more aggressive because it may represent a more invasive form of disease (ACOG, 2009a).

The American Society for Colposcopy and Cervical Pathology has further defined the use of HPV genotyping to manage women 30 years and older and has developed an algorithm for clinicians to use. In women with HPV high-risk (HR) positive and negative cytology (normal cells on Pap smear), they can repeat the Pap and HR HPV test in 12 months. When the repeat Pap smear and HPV testing are negative on subsequent Pap smears, they can resume routine screening at 3 years. If the cytology is positive (abnormal cells on Pap smear) with high-risk HPV findings, a colposcopy is performed (ACOG, 2009a).

Evaluation of Abnormal Cytology

The following points summarize the primary guidelines for managing women with abnormal cancer screening results (Wright et al., 2007):

- Women with ASC-US can be treated in one of three ways: (a) referral for colposcopy; (b) repeat the Pap at 6-month intervals until two negative results are obtained with referral for colposcopy if the repeat Pap shows ASC or higher; or (c) deoxyribonucleic acid (DNA) testing for high-risk types of HPV infection with referral for colposcopy if the testing reveals a high-risk strain. If the HPV high-risk testing is negative, the woman should have a repeat Pap in 12 months.
- Women with ASC-H are at greater risk for CIN than women with ASC-US and should be referred directly for colposcopy.
- Women with either LSIL or HSIL are referred directly for loop electrosurgical excision (LEEP) or colposcopy with endocervical assessment. If CIN 2 or 3 is not identified histologically, follow-up may be done by either a diagnostic excisional procedure such as LEEP or conization or observation with colposcopy and Pap at 6-month intervals for a year. A diagnostic excisional procedure is recommended if the colposcopy is unsatisfactory or if the woman is pregnant.

Based on the results of the colposcopy, of endocervical curettage of the tissue, and of biopsy if performed, further treatment may be indicated or follow-up with repeat Pap smears may be recommended. These tests are discussed next.

Colposcopy, the direct, detailed visualization and examination of the cervix, is done in most gynecologic offices. A speculum is placed in the vagina and the cervix is isolated. A 3% acetic acid solution applied on the cervix causes the abnormal epithelial cells to take on a characteristic white appearance. The colposcope, with its bright light and various color filters, provides a 6 to 40 times magnification of the cervical tissues. Lesions or other abnormalities are identified and documented, and directed biopsies can be obtained at this time, if indicated. Sometimes, the biopsy itself can be therapeutic as well as diagnostic if the entire lesion can be removed.

Endocervical curettage (ECC) may also be done at this time to evaluate for extension into the cervical canal. This involves a scraping of the endocervix from the internal os to the external os to obtain endocervical cells for cytology. Histologic evaluation of tissue biopsies and ECC samples is necessary for a definitive diagnosis.

The woman may experience moderate to severe cramplike pains during and after the biopsy and/or ECC. To help alleviate this discomfort, nurses can advise women to premedicate with 600 mg ibuprofen about 30 minutes before the procedure. A small amount of bleeding, initially bright red and then becoming darker, is normal for up to 2 weeks. Bleeding as heavy as a menstrual period is not normal and should be reported to the woman's care provider.

Surgical Treatment for Abnormal Cytology

Premalignant (precancerous) and malignant (cancerous) lesions are often treated with surgical procedures, varying from simple biopsy of the cervix to radical surgery of the pelvic organs, depending on the diagnosis and extent of the disease. A diagnosis of cancer can only be made after a pathologic evaluation of tissue obtained via biopsy. The goals of management are to exclude the presence of invasive cancer, to determine the extent and distribution of noninvasive cancer, and to provide appropriate treatment.

The treatment of cervical cancer depends on the stage of the disease, which is determined by the extent of its spread to other tissues or structures. Surgical treatment of cervical cancer may include a total abdominal hysterectomy (TAH), bilateral salpingo-oophorectomy (BSO), and bilateral lymphadenectomy (discussed further in the section Care of the Woman Requiring Gynecologic Surgery on page 139). It may also include radiation therapy and chemotherapy.

Loop Electrosurgical Excision Procedure

Loop electrosurgical excision procedure (LEEP) can be used to treat cervical, vaginal, and vulvar intraepithelial neoplasia. When an abnormal Pap smear and a colposcopic evaluation indicate a premalignant lesion, a small electrically hot wire loop can be used to excise the entire lesion, squamocolumnar junction, and transformation zone. The cutting effect is created by a steam envelope that develops between the wire loop and the water-laden tissue. This procedure can be performed on an outpatient basis, often in the gynecologic office, under local anesthesia. Complications following LEEP are usually minimal, and it is virtually painless and bloodless. The woman can expect some slight bleeding, and possibly a malodorous dark brown discharge for 1 to 2 weeks after the procedure. The woman needs to know that moderate to heavy bleeding would be abnormal and should be reported to her care provider.

Cryosurgery

Cryosurgery is used to treat women with a small ectocervical lesion who have a negative ECC and no endocervical gland involvement. A double freezing method is advocated, using nitrous oxide or carbon dioxide to freeze the tissue below −20°C (−4°F), resulting in tissue destruction and necrosis. Cryosurgery is less widely used since the development of LEEP because it scars the cervix, making the transformation zone, or squamocolumnar junction, more difficult to evaluate with future colposcopies. It can easily be done in a gynecologic office or clinic without anesthesia. The woman may experience some mild cramping and should be told to expect a thin, watery, persistent, and sometimes heavy vaginal discharge for up to several weeks as the frozen tissue is sloughed. She should avoid tampon use and sexual intercourse while the discharge is present to minimize further damage to the cervix.

Laser Therapy

The carbon dioxide (CO_2) laser is used to treat cervical, vaginal, and vulvar intraepithelial lesions. The laser is used when all boundaries of the lesion are visible on colposcopy and when the ECC is negative. The invisible, highly concentrated beam is absorbed by water in the tissues, elevating the temperature in the tissues to above 100°C (212°F). The targeted tissue "boils" and the exploded cells are vaporized, leaving the normal tissue intact. Laser treatment can be done in outpatient or office settings without anesthesia. The woman may experience mild cramping and a slight discharge for 5 to 7 days; however, bleeding is minimal. She should avoid tampon use, intercourse, and douching for 2 weeks; complete healing may take up to 12 weeks. In many clinical settings, laser therapy has become less common with the advent and effective use of LEEP.

Conization

A cold knife *conization* of the cervix (also known as a "cone") is most commonly performed when the entire lesion cannot be visualized by colposcopic examination or when there is a positive ECC sampling. In this procedure, a cone-shaped section of cervical tissue is excised. The width and depth of the tissue removed varies depending on the extent of the lesion. A large amount of normal tissue is removed, as well as the abnormal tissue, and this procedure can often be diagnostic as well as therapeutic if the entire lesion is excised. Conization is usually done under general anesthesia with the woman in a lithotomy position. Immediate postoperative risks include infection and hemorrhage; long-term risks include spontaneous abortion, incompetent cervix, or preterm labor with future pregnancies. A prolonged or profuse menstrual period may occur in two or three cycles following the procedure. Conization is used less frequently today because of the availability of LEEP.

Abnormal Uterine Bleeding

During the many years of a woman's reproductive period, she is likely to experience some form of abnormal uterine bleeding. It may occur as spotting between periods, missing several cycles followed by a heavy bleed, or menses that occur every 2 to 3 months. Heavy, unpredictable menstrual periods can cause a woman to experience fatigue, anemia, and embarrassment. Abnormal bleeding may be a symptom that accompanies infertility.

Abnormal uterine bleeding (AUB) is a common gynecologic problem. It makes up 5% to 10% of cases in the outpatient setting. It is a reflection of a disruption in the normal cyclic hormonal pattern of ovulation to the endometrium, or lining of the uterus. Many women who experience AUB are exposed to unnecessary surgical treatments before an adequate workup and medical therapy trial is complete. Women who experience repetitive episodes are predisposed to iron deficiency anemia. Endometrial cancer results in 1% to 2% of women with improperly managed anovulatory bleeding (Behera & Price, 2009).

Systemic diseases that cause AUB include coagulation disorders such as von Willebrand's disease, thrombocytopenia, acute leukemia, and advanced liver disease. Endocrine disorders include thyroid, hyperprolactinemia, polycystic ovarian syndrome, and Cushing's syndrome (Gordon et al., 2007).

Medications that may account for AUB include contraception, anticoagulants, antipsychotics, and chemotherapy. Trauma during intercourse or as a result of sexual abuse and foreign bodies may also result in abnormal bleeding (Gordon et al., 2007). Mechanical causes may include leiomyomata (fibroids), endometrial polyps, or adenomyosis.

Infection in the cervix (cervicitis), uterus (endometritis), vagina, or vulva (STI) may be a cause of abnormal bleeding. Endometrial cancer, or cancer of the lining of the uterus, or other genital tract cancers need to be ruled out with the presence of AUB (Gordon et al., 2007).

Evaluation of AUB begins with a thorough history and physical examination including a careful pelvic exam and Pap smear. The diagnosis is made by excluding organic causes, specifically pregnancy, uterine or ovarian pathology, medications, or systemic disease. Based on the information gained, specific laboratory tests such as pregnancy test, liver and renal function tests, thyroid tests, coagulation studies, or prolactin levels may be indicated. Based on the woman's age and findings, other tests that may be indicated include transvaginal ultrasound, saline infusion sonography (SIS), hysteroscopy, magnetic resonance imaging (MRI), and endometrial biopsy. Endometrial biopsy to rule out endometrial cancer is indicated for all women over age 35 (Dodds & Sinert, 2009).

The goals of treatment are to control bleeding, prevent or treat anemia, prevent endometrial hyperplasia or cancer, and restore quality of life. Pharmacologic treatment for AUB varies depending on the woman's desire for pregnancy and whether she is premenopausal, perimenopausal, or postmenopausal. Combined oral contraceptives (COCs) are the most common treatment for women who are not actively trying to conceive. COCs help regulate cycles while also providing contraception. Other options include short-term, high-dose estrogen therapy, cyclic progesterone to regulate cycles in women with contraindications to estrogen therapy, danazol, gonadotropin-releasing hormone (GnRH) therapy, and the levonorgestrel intrauterine system (LNG-IUS) (see chapter 5 ∞). If conservative measures are not effective, the woman and her provider may consider surgical interventions, such as hysteroscope-assisted dilation and curettage (D&C), for the resection of fibroids or endometrial polyps, endometrial ablation, or hysterectomy (Dodds & Sinert, 2009).

Care Plan Activity: Irregular Bleeding in a Perimenopausal Woman

Dysfunctional uterine bleeding (DUB) is characterized by anovulatory cycles with AUB that does not have a demonstrable organic cause. Oligomenorrhea, polymenorrhea, menorrhagia, metrorrhagia, menometrorrhagia, and intermenstrual bleeding are all forms of DUB (see chapter 4 ∞). DUB can occur at any age but is most common at either end of the reproductive age span. Adolescents account for 20% of DUB cases due to hypothalamic immaturity after menarche. Perimenopausal women account for 50% of cases due to waning ovarian function. The remaining cases occur among women of reproductive age, generally as a result of polycystic ovary syndrome, hyperprolactinemia, or hypothalamic dysfunction. It is typically treated medically. Surgical intervention is generally limited to cases in which medical therapy is contraindicated or has failed.

Ovarian (Adnexal) Masses

An *adnexal mass* most commonly refers to an ovarian abnormality but it can also refer to masses found in the fallopian tubes, broad ligament, or bowel, or even a lateral mass of the uterus. Between 70% and 80% of ovarian masses are benign. More than 50% are functional cysts (cysts that develop from ovarian follicles, from the corpus luteum, or from the theca luteum) occurring most commonly in women 20 to 40 years of age. Functional cysts are rare in women who take oral contraceptives.

Ovarian cysts usually represent physiologic variations in the menstrual cycle. Nearly all perimenopausal women have ovarian cysts, and about 15% of postmenopausal women have them. Dermoid cysts (cystic teratomas) comprise 10% of all benign ovarian masses. Cartilage, bone, teeth, skin, or hair can be observed in these cysts. Endometriomas, or "chocolate cysts," are another common type of ovarian mass.

No relationship exists between benign ovarian masses and ovarian cancer. Unfortunately, at present, no adequate techniques exist for ovarian cancer screening. Over 15,000 deaths in the United States occur each year as a result of ovarian cancer. Over 70% of all cases diagnosed are in advanced states. Five-year survival rates for women with advanced disease are 15% to 30%; however, if the disease is diagnosed early, those rates increase to 70% to 90% (Goff & Muntz, 2008). Risk factors for ovarian cancer are:

- Increased age (mean age is 56)
- Nulliparity (never having children)
- History of breast cancer
- Early menarche or late menopause

The risk of ovarian cancer is 5% to 10% for women with family members diagnosed with the disease (Helm & Edwards, 2009).

Family transmission and increased lifetime risk of ovarian cancer account for 5% to 10% of all cases of ovarian cancer. Some cases of ovarian cancer are associated with a mutation in specific genes (BRCA1 and BRCA2 genes). It is now possible to identify many of these mutations. If a mutation of BRCA1 is found, for example, estimates suggest that a woman's lifetime risk of ovarian cancer is between 15% and 45%. If the BRCA2 mutation is present, the lifetime risk of developing ovarian cancer is 10% to 20%. These two mutations are inherited in an autosomal dominant pattern, meaning the gene can come from either parent. Hereditary ovarian cancer tends to occur at a younger age, but the prognosis is generally better. The National Cancer Institute currently recommends that women who are considered high risk should have annual ultrasound examination and a CA 125 blood test (Helm & Edwards, 2009).

In reality, ovarian cancer is the most fatal of all cancers in women because it is difficult to diagnose and often has spread throughout the pelvis before it is detected. Symptoms are often vague and nonspecific and may include:

- Bloating
- Increased abdominal size
- Difficulty eating
- Abdominal or pelvic pain
- Urinary symptoms (urgency and frequency)

Women who have these symptoms daily for several weeks should see a gynecologist for prompt medical evaluation (Goff & Muntz, 2008). The risk of ovarian cancer is decreased significantly by bearing children, taking combined oral contraceptive pills for more than 5 years, or having a tubal ligation (Helm & Edwards, 2009).

A woman with an ovarian mass may be asymptomatic; the mass may be noted on a routine pelvic examination. She may experience a sensation of fullness or cramping in the lower abdomen (often unilateral), dyspareunia, irregular bleeding, or delayed menstruation.

Diagnosis is made on the basis of a palpable mass, with or without tenderness, and other related symptoms. Radiography or ultrasonography may be used to assist or confirm the diagnosis.

The woman is frequently kept under observation for a month or two because most cysts will resolve on their own and are harmless. Oral contraceptives may be prescribed for 1 to 2 months to suppress ovarian function. If this regimen is effective, a repeat pelvic examination should yield normal findings. If the mass is still present after 60 days of observation and oral contraceptive therapy, a diagnostic laparoscopy or laparotomy may be considered. Tubal or ovarian lesions, ectopic pregnancy, cancer, infection, or appendicitis also must be ruled out before a diagnosis can be confirmed.

Surgery is not always necessary but will be considered if the mass is larger than 6 to 7 cm in circumference; if the woman is over 40 years of age with an adnexal mass, a persistent mass, or continuous pain; or if the woman is taking oral contraceptives. Surgical exploration is also indicated when a palpable mass is found in an infant, a young girl, or a postmenopausal woman.

Women may need clear explanations about why the initial therapy is observation. A discussion of the origin and resolution of ovarian cysts may clarify this treatment plan. If a surgical treatment removes or impairs the function of one ovary, the woman needs to be assured that the remaining ovary can be expected to take over ovarian functioning and that pregnancy is still possible.

Uterine Masses

Endometrial polyps are pedunculated (growing on a stalk) overgrowths of the endometrium. They can occur as single or multiple growths. Polyps are common and are often accompanied by symptoms of midcycle bleeding or spotting, bleeding or spotting after intercourse, or prolonged bleeding or spotting with menstrual cycles. Polyps are generally benign, but they can coexist with carcinoma of the endometrium in about 10% of postmenopausal women. Treatment is dilation and curettage (D&C) using the hysteroscope for visualization.

Fibroid tumors, or *leiomyomas,* are among the most common benign disease entities in women. By the age of 50, 70% of Caucasian women and 80% of African American women have fibroids (Parker, 2008b). Fortunately, these tumors progress to a malignancy in fewer than 0.5% of all patients (Flowers, 2008).

Most uterine fibroids are asymptomatic and require no treatment. Treatment is indicated when the fibroids cause symptoms such as lower abdominal pain, fullness or pressure, menorrhagia, metrorrhagia, or increased dysmenorrhea, compelling the woman to seek medical advice. The majority of fibroids will shrink after menopause. In an older woman who experiences uterine growth, pain, or postmenopausal bleeding, a malignancy may be suspected (Parker, 2008b).

On pelvic examination the patient may have an irregular shaped, enlarged uterus. Tentative diagnosis is initially made through pelvic ultrasound for number, size, and location of the fibroid. Occasionally MRI or hysterosonography is used for further evaluation and planning for surgical interventions (Flowers, 2008).

Treatment for uterine fibroids varies from the use of oral contraceptives to control heavy menstrual bleeding to hysterectomy. Myomectomy is a surgical procedure to remove the fibroid without removing the uterus. This is a safe and effective alternative to hysterectomy, which carries more overall risk (Parker, 2008a). GnRH analogs such as Lupron are used off-label to reduce the size and subsequent bleeding due to these tumors. These medications carry with them symptoms of menopause such as hot flashes and reduced bone mineral density. Once discontinued, however, growth of the fibroid can reoccur. Treatment with GnRH analogs may be used before surgery to reduce the size of the fibroid and decrease complications (Flowers, 2008). Uterine artery embolization (UAE) is a relatively new procedure that allows women with symptomatic, moderate-sized (less than 10 cm) fibroids to avoid hysterectomy. It is a radiologic procedure in which a catheter is inserted into the femoral artery and advanced to the uterine arteries. The uterine arteries are then blocked by injecting polyvinyl alcohol particles. This results in diminished blood flow to the uterus and the necrosis of the fibroids (Bradley, 2009). Hysterectomy may be indicated for the treatment of uterine fibroids. This can be performed laparoscopically or abdominally depending on the size of the uterus. A laparoscopic-assisted hysterectomy is less invasive and has a lower risk of surgical and postoperative complication (Parker, 2008a). Myomectomy can be performed to preserve fertility or improve fertility if the location of the fibroid distorts the uterine cavity and would prevent implantation (Parker, 2008a).

Endometrial cancer is the most common female genital tract cancer with over 40,000 new cases annually. It has a high rate of cure if detected early. Although the overall incidence is lower in black women than in white women, black women have a poorer survival rate. This disparity is multifactorial and may be due to barriers to receiving care in the early stages of disease. It may also be related to comorbid conditions such as obesity and diabetes as well as basic genetic differences found in tumors in black women (Allard & Maxwell, 2009).

Risk factors for endometrial cancer include (Gordon et al., 2007):

- White race
- Increased age (mean age is 60)
- Obesity
- Nulliparity
- History of infertility or menstrual irregularities
- History of diabetes
- Hypertension
- Thyroid or gallbladder disease
- Long-term use of unopposed estrogen
- Early menarche or late menopause
- Use of tamoxifen

The majority of endometrial cancer occurs in postmenopausal women. The hallmark sign is vaginal bleeding in postmenopausal women not treated with hormone therapy (HT). Women may present with this complaint or have an incidental finding on a Pap smear of atypical endometrial cells. Generally a pelvic ultrasound is done to evaluate the thickness of the endometrium, and subsequent endometrial biopsy is taken if the thickness is greater than 4 mm. The endometrial biopsy will confirm the suspicion of cancer and the grade of lesion will be reported with pathology. Hysterectomy with bilateral salpingo-oophorectomy (removal of both fallopian tubes and ovaries) is performed and staging of the cancer is done. Although controversy exists in the role of lymph node dissection for staging purposes, in the United States this is generally done in all women with endometrial growths (Fiorelli, Gerzog, & Wright, 2008).

Once staging of the cancer is completed, a plan of treatment is proposed. Hysterectomy may be adequate treatment for stage I disease without lymph node involvement. For more advanced disease, however, adjuvant therapy may be prescribed. Intermediate risk endometrial cancer is generally treated with whole pelvis radiation. Chemotherapy is used in conjunction with radiation for advanced endometrial cancer (Fiorelli et al., 2008).

NURSING CARE MANAGEMENT

Only nurses with special training perform pelvic examinations and Pap smears. In most cases, nursing assessment is directed toward evaluating the woman's understanding of the findings and their implications and her psychosocial response.

The woman needs accurate information on the etiology of the disorder, its symptoms, and treatment options. She should be encouraged to report symptoms and keep appointments for follow-up examination and evaluation. The woman needs realistic reassurance if her condition is benign; she may require counseling and effective emotional support if a malignancy is likely. If the management plan includes surgery, she may need the nurse's support in obtaining a second opinion and making her decision. The nurse can also provide information on available community resources, including support groups.

Care of the Woman with Toxic Shock Syndrome

Case Study: Toxic Shock Syndrome

Although **toxic shock syndrome (TSS)** has been reported in children, postmenopausal women, and men, it is primarily a disease of women in their reproductive years, especially women at or near menses or during the postpartum period. In most cases, the causative organism is a strain of *Staphylococcus aureus*. The use of superabsorbent tampons has been widely related to an increased incidence of TSS. However, occluding the cervical os with a contraceptive device such as a diaphragm or cervical cap, especially if it is left in place for more than 48 hours, may also increase the risk of TSS. The rates of staphylococcal TSS have declined since 1980 because of the decrease in the use of superabsorbent tampons (Totten, 2009).

Early diagnosis and treatment are important in preventing a fatal outcome. For a diagnosis of TSS to be made, certain criteria must be met. The woman must have fever (38.9°C), shock, rash, and multisystem involvement (Totten, 2009). The fever and rash on the trunk present initially, followed by desquamation of the skin, especially the palms and soles, which usually occurs 1 to 2 weeks after the onset of symptoms; hypotension; and dizziness. Systemic symptoms often include vomiting, watery diarrhea, severe myalgia, and inflamed mucous membranes (oropharyngeal, conjunctival, or vaginal). Disorders of the central nervous system, including alterations in consciousness, disorientation, and coma, may also occur. Evidence of renal, hepatic, and hematologic involvement can be seen in abnormal laboratory findings, which reveal elevated blood urea nitrogen (BUN), creatinine, aspartate aminotransferase (AST), alanine aminotransferase (ALT), and total bilirubin, while platelets are often less than $100{,}000/mm^3$.

Women with TSS are generally hospitalized and given supportive therapy, including oxygen, intravenous (IV) fluids to maintain blood pressure, and antibiotics. Severe cases may require administration of vasopressors and intubation. Close follow-up care is necessary because some patients may require dialysis and are also at a higher risk for further episodes. Recurrence rates can be as high as 40% to 50% (Totten, 2009).

> “Two years ago a friend died of toxic shock syndrome. It happened so quickly. Within days she was on life support until the family had it turned off. Until that happened, I was oblivious to the risk factors, especially leaving tampons in too long, one of my big offenses. I have changed that for myself, and I am making it a point to tell other women about toxic shock and ways to prevent it. Such a senseless death!”

NURSING CARE MANAGEMENT

Nurses play a major role in helping to educate women about ways to prevent the development of TSS. Women should understand the importance of avoiding prolonged use of tampons. They should change tampons every 3 to 6 hours, avoid using superabsorbent tampons, and never use more than one tampon at a time. Some women may choose to use other products, such as sanitary pads or minipads. The woman who chooses to continue using tampons may reduce her risk by alternating them with pads and avoiding overnight use of tampons.

Women who are postpartum should avoid the use of tampons for 6 to 8 weeks after childbirth. Women with a history of TSS should be advised of the risk of recurrence and should never use tampons. Women who use diaphragms or cervical caps should not leave them in place for prolonged periods and should not use them during the postpartum period or when they are menstruating. Nurses can also help make women aware of the signs and symptoms of TSS so that they can seek treatment promptly if symptoms occur.

Care of the Woman with Endometriosis

Endometriosis is a condition characterized by the presence of endometrial tissue outside the uterine cavity. The exact prevalence of endometriosis is unknown but it is found in 5% to 15% of reproductive-age women who undergo laparoscopy (Gordon et al., 2007). Endometriosis has been found almost everywhere in the body, including the vagina, lungs, cervix, central nervous system, and gastrointestinal tract. The most common location, however, is the pelvis. This tissue responds to the hormonal changes of the menstrual cycle and bleeds in a cyclic fashion. The bleeding results in inflammation, scarring of the peritoneum, and formation of adhesions.

Endometriosis may occur at any age after puberty, although it is most commonly diagnosed in women between ages 20 and 45 and is rare in postmenopausal women. There is a 20% to 50% prevalence rate of endometriosis in infertile women. A hereditary component also exists with a 10 times greater risk in women with a first-degree relative with endometriosis (Kapoor & Davila, 2008).

The exact cause of endometriosis is unknown. Proposed causative factors include retrograde menstrual flow of the endometrium through the fallopian tubes into the pelvis, lymphatic-vascular (through lymph or blood vessels spreading to lungs, brain, and pericardium), and decrease in cellular immunity (Gordon et al., 2007). Although endometriosis can be asymptomatic, its most common symptom is pelvic pain, which is often dull or cramping although it can be debilitating. It is generally related to the menstrual cycle; however, some women may experience chronic pelvic pain. Dyspareunia may be present due to scarring of the pelvic tissues and organs from the endometrial implants. The condition is often diagnosed when the woman seeks evaluation for infertility. Bimanual examination may reveal a fixed, tender, retroverted uterus and palpable nodules in the cul-de-sac. Diagnosis is confirmed by laparoscopy.

Treatment may be medical or surgical, or a combination of the two. In women with minimal disease and symptoms, treatment includes observation, analgesics, and nonsteroidal anti-inflammatory drugs (NSAIDs). Medical treatment of mild endometriosis does not seem to improve fertility; however, in cases of moderate to severe disease, surgical intervention is indicated (Kapoor & Davila, 2008). Medical therapies include the following:

- ***Combined oral contraceptives (COCs):*** COCs, which suppress menstruation, can be used in women who do not desire fertility.
- ***Progestins:*** Progestins such as medroxyprogesterone acetate (MPA) exert an antiendometriotic effect and ultimate atrophy. The medication is administered intramuscularly every 3 months, and the effectiveness of the treatment is evaluated every 3 to 6 months. Side effects may include nausea, weight gain, fluid retention, and breakthrough bleeding.
- ***Danazol:*** The antiprogestin danazol is sometimes used to treat endometriosis. It suppresses gonadotropin-releasing hormone (GnRH) and has high androgen and low estrogen effects that do not support the growth of the endometrium. It suppresses ovulation and causes amenorrhea. In effect, danazol and the other GnRH analogs (discussed next) induce a “pseudomenopausal” state. Danazol does have some significant side effects, including hirsutism, vaginal bleeding, acne, oily skin, weight gain, reduced libido, voice changes and hoarseness, clitoral enlargement, and decreased breast size.
- ***GnRH analogs:*** GnRH analogs such as nafarelin acetate (given as a metered nasal spray twice daily) and leuprolide acetate (Lupron, given once a month as an intramuscular injection), are gaining popularity because many women tolerate them better than danazol and their results in treating endometriosis are comparable. GnRH analogs suppress the menstrual cycle through estrogen antagonism. This may result in the hypoestrogen side effects of hot flashes, vaginal dryness, headache, breast reduction, and loss of bone density.

Surgical treatment may be conservative (laparoscopy) or definitive (hysterectomy). It is conservative when the uterus and as much of the ovaries as possible are preserved. During the laparoscopic examination, the physician may surgically resect any visible implants of endometrial tissue, taking care to avoid damaging any organs. Laser vaporization can be used for all but the deepest implants. This allows for more exact removal of tissue, less damage of adjacent tissue, and decreased bleeding. There is a 19% recurrence rate for all techniques (Kapoor & Davila, 2008). If the woman is experiencing severe dyspareunia or dysmenorrhea, the surgeon may perform a presacral neurectomy. In advanced cases in which childbearing is not an issue, treatment may be a hysterectomy with bilateral salpingo-oophorectomy (removal of the uterus, fallopian tubes, and ovaries).

Complementary therapies may also play a role in the treatment of endometriosis. These include acupuncture to help with pain control; yoga for relaxation and stress reduction; massage; traditional Chinese herbal medicine for symptomatic relief; and "soul therapies" such as prayer, religious rituals, meditation, and support groups (Kaatz, Solari-Twadell, Cameron et al., 2010).

NURSING CARE MANAGEMENT

Nursing Assessment and Diagnosis

The nurse should be aware of the common symptoms of endometriosis and elicit an accurate history if a woman mentions these symptoms. If a woman is being treated for endometriosis, the nurse should assess the woman's understanding of the condition, its implications, and the treatment alternatives.

Nursing diagnoses that may apply to a woman with endometriosis include the following:

- ***Acute pain*** related to peritoneal irritation secondary to endometriosis
- ***Compromised family coping*** related to depression secondary to infertility

Nursing Plan and Implementation

The nurse can be available to explain the condition, its symptoms, treatment alternatives, and prognosis. The nurse can help the woman evaluate treatment options and make appropriate choices. If the woman begins taking medication, the nurse can review the dosage, schedule, possible side effects, and any warning signs. Women are often advised to avoid delaying pregnancy because of the risk of infertility. The woman may wish to discuss the implications of this decision on her life choices, relationship with her partner, and personal preferences. The nurse can be a nonjudgmental listener and help the woman consider her options. In addition, the nurse can refer the woman to the Endometriosis Association. This group, founded in 1980, offers women support and education.

Evaluation

Expected outcomes of nursing care include the following:

- The woman is able to discuss her condition, its implications for fertility, and her treatment options.
- After considering the alternatives, the woman chooses appropriate treatment options.

Care of the Woman with Polycystic Ovarian Syndrome

Many women struggle with the short-term and long-term effects of a condition known as **polycystic ovarian syndrome**, or **PCOS**. This complex syndrome, with no clear etiology, is the most common endocrine disorder affecting women of reproductive age, with a suggested incidence of 6.5% of women (Guzick & Hoeger, 2009).

As early as 1921, Achard and Thiers cited the link between insulin and elevated androgens in the medical literature in their description of a "bearded woman with diabetes." In 1935, Stein and Leventhal described a triad of symptoms in some women—obesity, hirsutism, and amenorrhea—and additionally, pathologic ovarian findings. As ultrasound techniques became more refined in the 1970s and 1980s, the ability to see polycystic ovaries more clearly further complicated the diagnostic process. Over time, it became evident that not all women with PCOS had polycystic ovaries, and it became recognized that many "normal" women did have polycystic ovaries noted by ultrasound. For these reasons, the term "polycystic ovarian syndrome" is a bit misleading because PCOS is a complex disorder with many confounding variables and multisystem effects.

Signs and Symptoms of PCOS

The most common clinical signs and symptoms of PCOS include menstrual dysfunction since the onset of menstruation, signs of androgen excess (hirsutism or acne), or infertility (Guzick & Hoeger, 2009). Insulin resistance also occurs in women with PCOS.

Menstrual Dysfunction

Irregular menses, including total absence of periods (amenorrhea) or intermittent or infrequent periods (oligomenorrhea), is the hallmark of PCOS (Guzick & Hoeger, 2009). In women of reproductive age, 85% to 90% of oligomenorrhea and 30% to 40% of amenorrhea are attributed to PCOS. Anovulation is usually a chronic problem with PCOS, but it often presents as a long history of menstrual irregularities. However, some women with PCOS can have regular periods and still be chronically anovulatory.

Hyperandrogenism

PCOS is the most common cause of androgen excess in women. Most often it is manifested as *hirsutism*, or an excess of hair growth, and acne. The hair is coarse and appears in a pattern typically seen in adult males. This pattern occurs on the face, chest, between the breasts and on the abdomen. Acne is less prevalent in PCOS than hirsutism; however, most women with severe acne have PCOS (Mason et al., 2008).

Obesity

About 50% of women with PCOS are clinically obese (Guzick & Hoeger, 2009). In women with PCOS who struggle with obesity, it is generally of the android type, with an increased hip-to-waist ratio. PCOS-related obesity is consistent with increased androgen levels, glucose intolerance, insulin resistance, and abnormal lipoprotein profiles. Unfortunately, women with PCOS obesity have difficulty losing weight, which is probably related to hyperinsulinemia and carbohydrate cravings.

Infertility

The majority of women who have been diagnosed with PCOS struggle with some degree of infertility related to anovulation. (See chapter 12 ∞, Special Reproductive Concerns: Infertility and Genetics.)

Insulin Resistance and Diabetes Mellitus

Women with PCOS may be insulin resistant. This is an important long-term clinical manifestation of PCOS. Obese women with PCOS have a higher rate of type 2 diabetes mellitus (7.5%–10%) and glucose intolerance (31%–35%). The rates of glucose intolerance and type 2 diabetes are not as high in women with PCOS who are lean (Guzick & Hoeger, 2009). An estimated 20% of patients with PCOS are lean (ACOG, 2009c).

Diagnosis of PCOS

The National Institutes of Health Androgen Excess Society, the European Society of Human Reproduction and Embryology, and the American Society for Reproductive Medicine (ESHRE/ASRM) agreed in Rotterdam that the diagnosis of PCOS should be based on the presence of two out of three of the following criteria: oligo- or anovulation, clinical and/or biochemical hyperandrogenism, and the appearance of polycystic ovaries on ultrasound. This is known as the Rotterdam Criteria (Barth, Yasmin, & Balen, 2008). If a woman presents with complaints of hirsutism, menstrual irregularities, acne, difficulty conceiving, and unexplained weight gain, several other disorders must be ruled out. Important disorders to consider include hyperthyroidism or hypothyroidism, congenital adrenal hyperplasia, Cushing's syndrome, hyperprolactinemia, and androgen-producing tumors. The diagnostic process is fourfold: history, physical examination, laboratory studies, and imaging. See Table 7-3.

TABLE 7-3 Diagnostic Process for PCOS

History

- Medical history—onset, timing, duration of symptoms (acne, hirsutism, menstrual problems)
- Surgical history
- Menstrual history—frequency, duration, regularity of periods; perception of pain and amount of bleeding
- Medications history (some medications may cause hirsutism, acne, menstrual irregularities)
- Family history—close attention to diabetes, menstrual problems, hirsutism, infertility

Physical

- Blood pressure
- Body mass index (BMI) (weight in kg divided by height in m^2): 25–30 = overweight; over 30 = obese
- Waist circumference: over 35 is abnormal, indicating central fat distribution
- Presence of acne, hirsutism, acanthosis nigricans, androgenic alopecia

Laboratory

- Total testosterone and sex-hormone binding globulin or bioavailable and free testosterone
- Thyroid-stimulating hormone (rules out thyroid disorders)
- Prolactin (rules out hyperprolactinemia)
- 17-hydroxyprogesteron (congenital adrenal hyperplasia)
- 2-hour oral glucose tolerance test using 75 g oral glucose
  fasting glucose less than 110 mg = normal
  110 mg–125 mg = impaired
  greater than 126 mg = type 2 diabetes
  2-hour glucose less than 140 mg = normal
  140 mg–199 mg = impaired
  greater than 200 mg = type 2 diabetes

Ultrasound Examination

- Determination of polycystic ovaries in one or both ovaries
- Identification of endometrial abnormalities

Source: Adapted from American College of Obstetricians and Gynecologists (ACOG). (2009). Polycystic ovary syndrome *(ACOG Practice Bulletin No. 108). Washington, DC: Author.*

Clinical Therapy

Once the diagnosis of PCOS is made, several options are available to the clinician for management. First, the goals for treatment should be established. These include decreasing the effects of hyperandrogenism (hirsutism, acne, etc.); restoring reproductive functioning for women desiring pregnancy; protecting the endometrium (increased risk for uterine cancer); and reducing long-term risks, specifically type 2 diabetes and cardiovascular disease.

If pregnancy is not an immediate goal, menstrual irregularities can be treated with a combined oral contraceptive (COC) or cyclic progesterone. COCs help to regulate menstrual cycles; provide a balance between estrogen and progesterone, thereby protecting the endometrium and decreasing the risk of uterine cancer; and may improve acne by inhibiting ovarian androgen production (Guzick & Hoeger, 2009).

If pregnancy is the immediate goal for the woman and she is overweight or obese, the initiation of a weight loss diet and regular exercise should be the first approach to achieving ovulation. If weight loss does not occur or is not successful in inducing ovulation, the use of clomiphene citrate is the initial therapy of choice for ovulation induction. The starting dose is 50 mg per day usually given on days 5–9 of the menstrual cycle. Approximately 50% of women with PCOS will ovulate on this dose. Ultrasound is done on day 13 to confirm follicle development. If an adequate follicle is present, timed intercourse is then recommended for conception (Guzick & Hoeger, 2009). Although metformin has been used in the past in conjunction with clomiphene citrate, more recent studies show that the combination does not improve ovulatory outcomes and is reserved for women who do not ovulate on clomiphene citrate alone (Guzick & Hoeger, 2009).

Long-Term Implications

PCOS may increase a woman's risk for developing overt type 2 diabetes, dyslipidemia, hypertension, cardiovascular disease, endometrial cancer, breast cancer, and ovarian cancer. Additionally, and very importantly, the woman with PCOS may struggle with significant emotional responses to this chronic disorder. She will likely face, throughout her lifetime, issues related to body image, infertility, problematic menses, and depression.

NURSING CARE MANAGEMENT

The nurse plays a vital role in the identification, evaluation, management, and follow-up when caring for a woman with PCOS. Sometimes it is the nurse who puts the bigger picture together, especially in a community health setting where knowledge of PCOS may be lacking. Women with PCOS may present with complaints such as weight gain, excess hairiness, difficult periods, inability to get pregnant, depression, or expressing feelings like, "What is wrong with me? Why am I not normal like other women?"

Research suggests that the signs of PCOS, especially hirsutism, negatively impact women's feelings of femininity and lead them to invest considerable time and effort in hair removal treatments. Women with PCOS also feel a strong desire to "be normal," with regular menstrual cycles and a more feminine appearance, and struggle with a sense of guilt over their difficulty losing weight (Snyder, 2006). Nurses can help women recognize these feelings and find ways to develop a more positive body image. The nurse also has an important role in providing accurate information, education, and counseling for a woman diagnosed with PCOS. Finally, because the woman with PCOS is at great risk for developing long-term complications, the nurse can play a key role in follow-up and continuity of care throughout the life of a woman facing this challenging disorder.

Care of the Woman with Pelvic Relaxation

The muscles of the pelvic floor form a supportive layer that prevents the abdominal and pelvic organs from prolapsing or sagging downward into the genital tract. If these muscles are weakened or damaged, a variety of conditions may develop, including cystocele, rectocele, and uterine prolapse. Factors that may contribute to diminished pelvic floor muscle tone include damage to these structures related to childbirth; deterioration with age due to estrogen deficiency; metabolic diseases that affect muscle functioning; prolonged lifting; or even chronic coughing due to chronic pulmonary disease, chronic constipation, and obesity (Smith, 2007).

Cystocele

A **cystocele** is the downward displacement of the bladder, which appears as a bulge in the anterior vaginal wall. Arbitrary classifications of mild to severe are frequently given. Genetic predisposition, childbearing, obesity, and increased age are factors that may contribute to cystocele.

Women with a cystocele commonly show symptoms of stress incontinence including loss of urine with coughing, sneezing, laughing, or sudden exertion. The woman may present with complaints of the perception of something "falling out" of her vagina. She may also have urinary retention, problems with sexual dysfunction, or pelvic pressure. If pelvic relaxation is mild, Kegel exercises are helpful in restoring tone (see chapter 16 ∞). The exercises involve contracting and relaxing the pubococcygeal muscle. Women have found these exercises helpful before and after childbirth in maintaining vaginal muscle tone. Estrogen may improve the condition of vaginal mucous membranes—especially in menopausal women. The healthcare provider may refer the woman to a physical therapist who specializes in pelvic floor dysfunction to assist her in learning how to isolate and strengthen the pelvic floor muscles. The use of biofeedback, vaginal weights, electric stimulation, and bladder training may be implemented by the therapist (Rackley, Sandip, Ingber, & Firoozi, 2009). Vaginal pessaries or rings may be used if surgery is undesirable or impossible, or until surgery can be scheduled. Surgery may be considered for cystoceles considered moderate to severe.

The nurse can instruct the woman in the use of Kegel exercises. Providing information on causes and contributing factors and discussing possible alternative therapies greatly assists the woman.

Rectocele

A rectocele may develop if the posterior vaginal wall is weakened. The anterior wall of the rectum protrudes forward, ballooning into the vagina, pushing the weakened posterior wall of the vagina into the vaginal lumen. When the woman strains to have a bowel movement, a pocket of rectum develops that traps stool, and constipation results. The harder a woman with rectocele strains, the larger the pocket becomes. To defecate, women with a rectocele may find it necessary to press the tissue between the vagina and rectum, which elevates the rectocele.

Diagnosis is based on history and physical examination. Decisions about treatment are based on the size of the prolapse, the presence and severity of symptoms, and the woman's individual situation including her overall health status. Surgery is often indicated.

Uterine Prolapse

Because the vagina and the uterus are attached to one another, prolapse of the uterine cervix is associated with prolapse of the upper vagina. The extent of the prolapse is determined by the location of the cervix in the vagina. In severe cases the cervix may prolapse below the vaginal introitus. The woman may report a "dragging" sensation in her groin and a backache over the sacrum, which is caused by pulling on the uterosacral ligaments. Typically these sensations are relieved when the woman lies down. Furthermore, with pronounced prolapse, exposure of the moist vaginal walls may cause a sensation of perineal wetness that the woman might mistake for incontinence. As with cystocele, conservative treatment includes the use of topical or systemic estrogen and vaginal pessaries. Surgery for uterine prolapse often involves hysterectomy and repair of the prolapsed vaginal walls.

Application: Cystocele

Care of the Woman Requiring Gynecologic Surgery

Gynecologic surgeries—particularly hysterectomies—are some of the most common surgical procedures being done in the United States. Many new techniques have been developed for treating a variety of gynecologic and reproductive disorders, and controversy remains as to the high number of procedures being done annually. For these reasons, it is important for the woman considering medical or surgical management of a given gynecologic problem to be well informed.

There are many components to an informed decision to undergo reproductive tract surgery. Questions that should be addressed include, for example: What are the indications for having the surgery? What are the risks? What is the success rate? Are there other alternative therapies to try before proceeding to surgery? An explanation of the surgical procedure and the reasons it is recommended over other possible therapies should be given to the woman. Effects on childbearing ability and potential impact on sexual performance should be addressed as well as the effects on the general functioning of the body. A discussion of the risks and benefits should be presented, and the risks should include the common risks, the nonserious risks, the rare or unusual complications, and the risk of death.

The question of whether to seek a second opinion about the recommended treatment is somewhat controversial. In the case of elective surgery, different physicians may have very different opinions. A woman should be encouraged to consult other physicians when there is controversy about a treatment (as in the treatment of early cervical cancer) or when the surgeon is unknown to the woman. A specialist in gynecology is the preferred source for a second opinion. Some third-party payment plans require second opinions. The woman can analyze the information and discuss her concerns with the nurse or physician before signing a written consent acknowledging that the information has been given and authorizing the surgery.

Other concerns that may influence the decision to have reproductive surgery may be categorized as general concerns about surgery and specific concerns related to gynecologic surgery. General concerns may include:

- Fear of general anesthesia because of loss of control or fear of "not waking up"; fear of regional anesthesia because of possible postoperative problems and concern about being awake during surgery
- Fear of death or disability
- Concerns about limitation of normal functioning and dependency during recovery
- Financial coverage for hospitalization, and potential financial loss if it is necessary to take extensive time off from work
- Concerns about welfare of family members while undergoing surgery (such as child care, loss of wages, help with household work)

Specific concerns related to gynecologic surgery are related to the significance of the reproductive organs for the woman. Surgery to alter or remove reproductive organs may be perceived as a threat to self-concept.

Body image is affected whenever a body part is lost. The degree of mourning for that loss is related to the significance attached to it. Even though there is no outwardly apparent change with a hysterectomy and most other gynecologic procedures, the loss may be felt very strongly. Many women fear postoperative changes such as masculinization, weight gain, loss of sexuality, and permanent loss of the ability to have a child. Reproductive surgery may also be seen as a threat to femininity in any social or cultural group that emphasizes childbearing and motherhood.

Hysterectomy

Hysterectomy is the removal of the uterus. In the United States, approximately 600,000 hysterectomies are performed each year, making it the most common non–pregnancy-related surgical procedure that women in the United States undergo (Gor, 2008).

Removal of the uterus through an abdominal incision is called a *total abdominal hysterectomy (TAH)* and removal of both fallopian tubes and ovaries is called a *bilateral salpingo-oophorectomy (BSO);* when both procedures are done at the same time it is termed a TAH-BSO. When the uterus is removed through the vagina it is termed a *total vaginal hysterectomy (TVH).*

A common technique to perform this surgery is a laparoscopic-assisted vaginal hysterectomy (LAVH). In this technique, the surgeon inserts the laparoscope through an incision near the umbilicus and uses it to assist with visualization and dissection to facilitate vaginal removal of the uterus. The benefit is that the surgeon can achieve results similar to those of a TAH without a large abdominal incision. LAVH shortens the hospital stay, allows for shorter recovery time, and is associated with less postoperative pain. The disadvantage of LAVH is a higher risk of injury to adjacent organs (Domingo & Pellicer, 2009).

Hysterectomy is the usual treatment for several conditions, although there is no medical consensus about absolute indications. Abdominal hysterectomy is generally recommended for cancer of the cervix, endometrium, or ovary; large fibroids; severe endometriosis; chronic pelvic inflammatory disease (PID); and adenomyosis. TAH is preferred when malignancy is suspected or confirmed because the procedure allows exploration of the abdomen and pelvis to determine the degree and extent of involvement. This approach is also helpful when large uterine masses are present, requiring a larger incision. Disadvantages include more scarring, more postoperative pain, slower recovery, and more problems with bowel function.

Vaginal hysterectomy is generally done for pelvic relaxation, abnormal uterine bleeding, or small fibroids. An anterior and posterior repair of the vaginal walls may also be performed during TVH. Sometimes this repair is done when weakened pelvic supports have displaced one or more of the pelvic organs (such as the urethra, bladder, or rectum), sometimes causing urinary incontinence, constipation, or defecation problems. Advantages include earlier ambulation, less postoperative pain, less anesthesia and operative time, less blood loss, no visible scar, and a shorter hospital stay. This approach is preferred for the elderly, obese, or debilitated woman who is a poor risk for abdominal surgery. The major disadvantage is increased risk of trauma to the bladder.

Removal of the ovaries at the time of hysterectomy remains controversial. In premenopausal women, without evidence of ovarian pathology, the ovaries are generally left to avoid forced surgical menopause. Because of the risk of ovarian cancer, some physicians recommend removal of ovaries in all women over 40 years old who undergo hysterectomy. Still others recommend removal of the ovaries in any woman with a family history of ovarian cancer. In any case, removal of the ovaries is not considered routine, and when a BSO is performed in a premenopausal woman, supplemental estrogen replacement therapy is recommended.

Dilation and Curettage

In the United States, dilation and curettage (D&C) is the most frequently performed minor gynecologic procedure. Indications for a D&C may be diagnostic or therapeutic. Diagnostic indications include evaluation for uterine malignancy, infertility evaluation, and investigation of dysfunctional uterine bleeding (DUB). Therapeutic indications include elective abortion, treatment of heavy bleeding, incomplete abortion, dysmenorrhea, and removal of polyps. Sometimes D&C is done after hysteroscopy, which is a procedure that allows visualization of the endometrial cavity and minor surgical procedures. Another procedure that can be done at the time of hysteroscopy is an endometrial ablation, which cauterizes endometrial tissue, preventing regeneration and further bleeding. This procedure is not recommended for women who desire pregnancy, and so a simple D&C may be more appropriate. All of these procedures can be done under general anesthesia, intravenous sedation, and/or regional anesthesia, and most are done as an outpatient procedure.

Uterine Ablation

Several newer techniques and instruments have been developed to treat DUB. One form of therapy gaining wider acceptance is *uterine ablation,* which is a procedure using a variety of specialized instruments to destroy the innermost layer of the endometrium. The instruments often involve some type of heat source, such as cautery or a balloon filled with hot water. In most cases, this procedure is done in a day-surgery setting, and it will often immediately follow a hysteroscopy/D&C, if these procedures confirm the diagnosis of simple endometrial hyperplasia. The success rate varies, depending on the device used and the experience of the operator of the device, but some manufacturers quote as high as a 75% success rate with uterine ablation.

Salpingectomy

The unilateral or bilateral removal of the fallopian tube is called a *salpingectomy*. Indications include diseases of the tubes, sepsis, malignancy, and ectopic pregnancy of the fallopian tube. Salpingectomy for an ectopic pregnancy is generally an emergency procedure. The developing placental tissue erodes the fallopian tube and can cause rupture and hemorrhage once the tube is completely eroded. This procedure can be done via laparoscopy or via an open abdominal approach.

Oophorectomy

Oophorectomy is the unilateral or bilateral removal of the ovary. Indications include severe PID, malignancy, ectopic pregnancy, and symptomatic ovarian cysts. When both ovaries are removed in a premenopausal woman, abrupt surgical menopause occurs. In this case the woman will experience the same symptoms she might in natural menopause: decreased libido, decreased vaginal lubrication, hot flashes and/or night sweats, and decreased sensation in the lower vaginal tract. These symptoms can be treated with estrogen replacement.

Vulvectomy

A *simple vulvectomy* is the removal of the labia majora, labia minora, and clitoris. *Radical vulvectomy* is the removal of the entire vulva, including the skin and the fat of the femoral triangle, and the pelvic lymph nodes. Skin grafts may be necessary. A simple vulvectomy is performed for leukoplakia and intractable pruritus, whereas a radical procedure is done for malignant disease.

This disfiguring procedure is associated with marked psychosexual disturbances. Most women report decreased sexual arousal levels and low self-image. Sexual activity can be resumed within 3 months; however, significant adjustments will be necessary owing to the loss of sensory perception for foreplay. Stimulation of breasts, thighs, buttocks, or anterior abdominal wall can be suggested.

Pelvic Exenteration

A pelvic exenteration is performed for recurrence of cervical cancer. Only about 5% of women with recurrence are candidates for this procedure, which is not performed if there is any evidence of tumor outside the pelvis, if the cancer has metastasized to the lymph nodes, or if all of the tumor cannot be removed.

Exenteration can be of the anterior or posterior pelvis, or of the total pelvis. Anterior exenteration is the removal of the uterus, ovaries, fallopian tubes, vagina, bladder, urethra, and pelvic lymph nodes. Urine is diverted through an ileal conduit. Posterior exenteration is the removal of the uterus, fallopian tubes, ovaries, descending colon, rectum, and anal canal. A colostomy is created. A total exenteration is a combination of the anterior and posterior procedures. A vagina can be reconstructed from split-thickness skin grafts or a segment of small bowel.

Complications associated with exenteration include intestinal and urinary obstruction, thrombophlebitis, pulmonary embolism, pyelonephritis, hypovolemia, peritonitis, pneumonia, and wound infection.

NURSING CARE MANAGEMENT

Nursing Assessment and Diagnosis

Nursing assessment for all of these surgical procedures includes identifying the woman's physiologic, psychosocial, and sexual needs as she approaches her surgery. Additionally, it is important to understand her learning needs about the procedure and its effects. Some factors to consider are the age of the woman, her cultural background and educational level, the attitude of her partner and family, her preoperative status (physically and emotionally), and whether or not this involves a cancer diagnosis. The significance of her reproductive health to her self-image will be reflected in her attitudes about menstruation, childbearing, body image, and sexuality. Many of these procedures have the potential to involve loss, so grieving, anger, sadness, and loss of control are just a few of the feelings the woman may experience.

Nursing diagnoses that may apply to a woman facing gynecologic surgery include the following:

- ***Deficient knowledge*** related to lack of information about preoperative routines, postoperative activities, and expected postoperative changes
- ***Fear*** related to the unknown outcome and long-term implications of the surgery

Nursing Plan and Implementation

Preoperative teaching may be brief in the instance of a simple D&C, or quite extensive in the instances of hysterectomy or pelvic exenteration. In any case, preoperative teaching should include information about the procedure, expected preparation, type of anesthesia to be used, possible risks and complications, postoperative care routines, and expected recovery time. See Figure 7-5 ■.

Routine postoperative care includes monitoring of physiologic responses, emotional responses, and nursing interventions to facilitate physical and emotional well-being specific to the procedure performed. The woman should be aware of potential postoperative complications and when to follow up with her surgeon. Additionally, it is important to discuss those psychosocial issues identified preoperatively, such as support at home, potential for sadness or depression related to the loss she has experienced, and expected sexual and self-image fears. In some instances, it may be necessary to refer the woman to a professional therapist who can help her adjust to these dramatic changes.

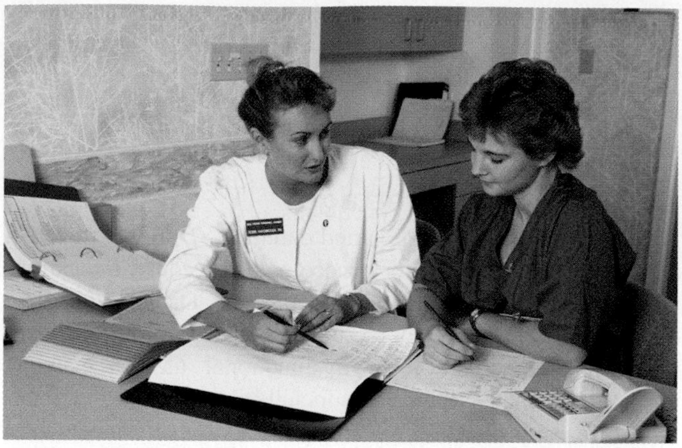

Figure 7-5 ■ The nurse provides information for the woman during preoperative teaching.

Source: Michal Heron/Pearson Education.

Evaluation

Expected outcomes of nursing care include:

- The woman can discuss the reasons for her surgery, the alternatives, and the aspects of self-care after surgery.
- The woman has an uneventful recovery without complications.
- The woman feels she is able to ask questions and obtain support.
- The woman participates in decision making about her care.
- The woman is aware of available resources if she has physical or emotional concerns in the postoperative period.

FOCUS YOUR STUDY

- With fibrocystic breast changes, the cysts tend to be round, mobile, and well delineated. The woman generally experiences increased discomfort premenstrually.
- Because of the increased risk of breast cancer, women with fibrocystic changes should understand the importance of monthly breast self-examination (BSE).
- Galactorrhea (nipple discharge not associated with lactation) should be evaluated with cytologic testing.
- Breast cancer affects one in eight women in the United States. Biopsy is essential for a diagnosis, and prompt treatment is critical.
- Vulvitis is an inflammation of the vulva often caused by external irritants such as tight clothing, feminine hygiene products, and some harsh soaps.
- Vulvar lesions range from slight irritation to vulvar cancer. A common vulvar lesion found in postmenopausal women is atrophic vaginitis. All vulvar lesions should be closely evaluated because cancer of the vulva can have various presentations.
- Pap smear screening is recommended for all women 21 years of age and older. Several factors put a woman at high risk for an abnormal Pap: intercourse at a young age,

multiple partners, history of immunotherapy, long-term combined oral contraceptive (COC) use, smoking, and previous history of dysplasia. Human papilloma virus (HPV) is highly associated with abnormal Pap smears.

- Abnormal uterine bleeding can occur with or without organic pathology. Treatment is geared toward controlling bleeding, preventing anemia, and detecting pathology.
- Toxic shock syndrome, a rare but potentially fatal disease, is usually caused by a toxin of *Staphylococcus aureus* and is most common in women of childbearing age. There is an increased incidence in women who use superabsorbent tampons or barrier methods of contraception, such as the diaphragm and cervical cap, especially if the woman leaves them in place for extended periods of time.
- Endometriosis is a condition in which endometrial tissue occurs outside the endometrial cavity. This tissue bleeds in a cyclic fashion in response to the menstrual cycle. The bleeding leads to inflammation, scarring, and adhesions. The prime symptoms include dysmenorrhea, dyspareunia, and infertility.
- Treatment of endometriosis may be medical or surgical, or a combination of both. For the woman not desiring pregnancy at present, oral contraceptives are used. Women desiring pregnancy are treated with danazol or the gonadotropin-releasing hormone (GnRH) analogs.
- Polycystic ovary syndrome (PCOS) is a disorder of unknown etiology characterized by ovulatory dysfunction, hyperandrogenism, and polycystic ovaries. Women with PCOS often experience infertility, hirsutism, and difficulty controlling their weight. They are at increased risk for type 2 diabetes and cardiovascular disease.
- There are three common forms of pelvic relaxation: A cystocele is a downward displacement of the bladder into the vagina. Often it is accompanied by stress incontinence. Kegel exercises may help restore tone in mild cases. A rectocele is displacement of the rectum into the vagina. Prolapse of the uterus is displacement of the uterine cervix into the vagina.
- Gynecologic surgeries are some of the most common surgical procedures performed in the United States. It is important for the nurse to understand the purpose of the procedure, to know the alternatives to surgery, and to assess the woman's emotional response.

CRITICAL THINKING IN ACTION

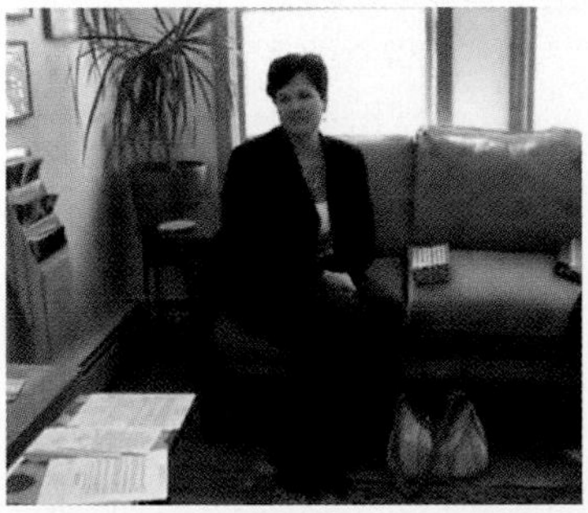

Mercedes de Martini is a 32-year-old gravida 2, para 2 who has a well-documented history of fibrocystic breast changes. Mercedes's breast symptoms typically increase premenstrually, when her breasts become markedly nodular and dense. She is being seen today because she has a palpable "lump" in her left breast that she describes as painful and easily movable. Mercedes reports that her menses is due in 5 days. Based on history and physical examination, the physician suspects that Mercedes has developed a cyst and decides to complete a fine-needle aspiration.

1. Identify findings on examination that might help distinguish a cyst from breast cancer.
2. Why is a fine-needle aspiration done?
3. What steps can Mercedes take to help decrease the discomfort associated with her fibrocystic breast changes?

See www.nursing.pearsonhighered.com for possible responses.

Pearson Nursing Student Resources

Find additional review materials at
www.nursing.pearsonhighered.com

Prepare for success with additional NCLEX®-style practice questions, interactive assignments and activities, Web links, animations and videos, and more!

REFERENCES

Allard, J., & Maxwell, L. (2009). *Race disparities between black and white women in the incidence, treatment, and prognosis of endometrial cancer.* Retrieved from http://www.medscape.com/viewarticle/586336

American Cancer Society (ACS). (2006). *Breast cancer facts and figures 2005–2006.* Atlanta, GA: Author.

American Cancer Society (ACS). (2009a). *Can breast cancer be found early?* Retrieved from http://www.cancer.org/docroot/CRI/content/CRI_2_4_3X_Can_breast_cancer_be_found_early_5.asp?sitearea=

American Cancer Society (ACS). (2009b). *How is breast cancer treated?* Retrieved from http://www.cancer.org/docroot/CRI/content/CRI_2_2_4X_How_Is_Breast_Cancer-Treated_5.asp?mav=cri

American Cancer Society (ACS). (2009c). *Mammograms matter.* Retrieved from http://www.cancer.org/docroot/PED/ped_20_aetna_mammogram.asp

American College of Obstetricians and Gynecologists (ACOG). (2008). *Management of abnormal cervical cytology and histology* (ACOG Practice Bulletin No. 99). Washington, DC: Author.

American College of Obstetricians and Gynecologists (ACOG). (2009a). *Cervical cytology screening* (ACOG Practice Bulletin No. 109). Washington, DC: Author.

American College of Obstetricians and Gynecologists (ACOG). (2009b). *Interpreting the U.S. preventive services task force breast cancer screening recommendations for the general population.* Retrieved from http://www.acog.org

American College of Obstetricians and Gynecologists (ACOG). (2009c). *Polycystic ovary syndrome* (ACOG Practice Bulletin No. 108). Washington, DC: Author.

Azavedo, E. (2009). Breast, nipple discharge evaluation. *E-Medicine Radiology.* Retrieved from http://www.emedicine.medscape.com/article/347305

Barth, J., Yasmin, E., & Balen, A. (2008). *The diagnosis of polycystic ovary syndrome: The criteria are insufficiently robust for clinical research.* Retrieved from http://www.medscape.com/viewarticle/568395

Behera, M., & Price, T. (2009). *Dysfunctional uterine bleeding.* Retrieved from http://www.emedicine.medscape.com/article/257006-overview

Boardman, L., & Kennedy, C. (2009). *Clinical updates in women's health care: Vulvar disorders* (Vol. VIII, No. 2). Washington, DC: The American College of Obstetricians and Gynecologists.

Bradley, L. D. (2009). Uterine fibroid embolization: A viable alternative to hysterectomy. *American Journal of Obstetrics and Gynecology, 201*(2), 127–135.

Dodds, N., & Sinert, R. (2009). *Dysfunctional uterine bleeding: Differential diagnoses & workup.* Retrieved from http://www.emedicine.medscape.com/article/795587-overview

Domingo, S., & Pellicer, A. (2009). *Overview of current trends in hysterectomy: Technique characteristics.* Retrieved from http://www.medscape.com/viewarticle/712569

Fiorelli, J., Gerzog, T., & Wright, J. (2008). *Current treatment strategies for endometrial cancer.* Retrieved from http://www.medscape.com/viewarticle/577643

Flowers, J. (2008). Uterine fibroids: Brief overview of presentation, diagnosis and treatment. *Advance for Nurse Practitioners, 16*(10), 36–40.

Goff, B., & Muntz, H. (2008). Ovarian cancer: Recognizing early symptoms can make a difference. *Contemporary OB/GYN, 53*(3), 26–39.

Gor, H. (2008). *Hysterectomy.* Retrieved from http://www.emedicine.medscape.com/article/267273

Gordon, J., Chan, J., Rydfors, J., Lebovic, D., Druzin, M., Langen, E., . . . el-Sayed, Y. (2007). *Obstetrics, gynecology, & infertility: Handbook for clinicians* (6th ed., pp. 252–259, 280–289, 368–369, 436). Arlington, VA: Scrub Hill Press.

Guzick, D., & Hoeger, K. (2009). *Clinical updates in women's health care. Polycystic ovary syndrome* (Vol. VIII, No. 1). Washington, DC: American College of Obstetricians and Gynecologists.

Helm, W., & Edwards, R. (2009). *Ovarian cancer.* Retrieved from http://emedicine.medscape.com/article/265651-overview

Kaatz, J., Solari-Twadell, P. A., Cameron, J., & Schultz, R. (2010). Coping with endometriosis. *Journal of Obstetric, Gynecologic, and Neonatal Nursing, 39*, 220–226.

Kapoor, D., & Davila, W. (2008). *Endometriosis.* Retrieved from http://www.emedicine.medscape.com/article/271899

Kaunitz, A. (2008). Do aromatase inhibitors extend disease-free survival after tamoxifen therapy in breast cancer survivors? *OBG Management, 20*(7), 20–23.

Lee, E. (2009). Evidence-based management of benign breast diseases. *The American Journal for Nurse Practitioners, 13*(7/8), 22–31.

Logue, K. (2009). *Pregnancy—associated breast cancer.* Retrieved from http://www.medscape.com/viewarticle/588930

Mason, H., Colao, A., Blume-Peytavi, U., Rice, S., Qureshi, A., Pellatt, L., et al. (2008). *Polycystic ovary syndrome (PCOS) trilogy: A translational and clinical review.* Retrieved from http://www.medscape.com/viewarticle/584561

National Cancer Institute (NCI). (2009a). *Mammograms—fact sheet.* Retrieved from http://www.cancer.gov/cancertopics/factsheet/Detection/mammograms

National Cancer Institute (NCI). (2009b). *Cervical cancer.* Retrieved from http://www.cancer.gov/cancertopics/factsheet/types/cervical

Parker, W. (2008a). When necessity calls for treating uterine fibroids. *OBG Management, 20*(6), 49–61.

Parker, W. (2008b). Uterine fibroids: Childbearing, cancer, and hormone effects. *OBG Management, 20*(5), 42–52.

Rackley, R., Sandip, V., Ingber, M., & Firoozi, F. (2009). *Urinary incontinence, nonsurgical therapies.* Retrieved from http://www.emedicine.medscape.com/article/452289

Singhal, H. (2008). *Breast cancer evaluation.* Retrieved from http://www.emedicine.medscape.com/article/263733-overview

Smith, D. (2007). Pelvic organ prolapse. *Advance for Nurse Practitioners, 15*(8), 39–42.

Snyder, B. S. (2006). The lived experience of women diagnosed with polycystic ovary syndrome. *Journal of Obstetric, Gynecologic, & Neonatal Nursing, 35*(3), 385–392.

Totten, B. (2009). *Toxic shock syndrome.* Retrieved from http://emedicine.medscape.com

United States Preventive Services Task Force. (2009). *Screening for breast cancer.* Retrieved from http://www.ahrq.gov/clinic/uspstf/uspsbrca.htm

Wright, T. C., Massad, L. S., Dunton, C. J., Spitzer, M., Wilkinson, E. J., & Solomon, D. (2007). 2006 consensus guidelines for the management of women with abnormal cervical cancer screening tests. *American Journal of Obstetrics and Gynecology, 197*(4), 346–355.

Wysocki, S., Reiter, S., & Berman, N. (2007). Strategies for preventing cervical cancer and HPV-related disease: The role of vaccination. *Women's Health Care: A Practical Journal for Nurse Practitioners, 6*(1), 6–22.

CHAPTER

8

Women's Care: Social Issues

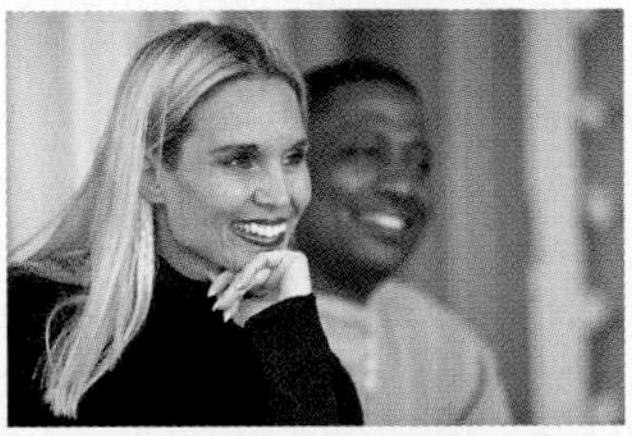

There has never been a more exciting time for women. Although we face many challenges—work, wage, and role issues; safety in pregnancy and childbearing; and conflict over women's rights—we have never been more active and involved in issues that affect us. Moreover, the men who care about us, and recognize the importance of fairness for all, are beginning to join us in speaking out. Together, men and women of integrity and vision are making a difference in women's lives.

LEARNING OUTCOMES

1. Define the phrase *feminization of poverty.*
2. Identify factors that contribute to the wage gap between women and men.
3. Discuss poverty's effect on women's health care.
4. Describe the impact of the Family and Medical Leave Act (FMLA) of 1993 on maternity and paternity leave.
5. Identify environmental hazards that may be present in the workplace or home of a woman of childbearing age.
6. Specify the factors that contribute to older women's economic vulnerability.
7. Identify four different categories of elder abuse.
8. Discuss the implications of aging on women's health and health care.
9. Summarize the five main types of disability.
10. Discuss ways in which a woman's disability may affect her health care.
11. Explain the implications of homophobia for lesbian and bisexual women's health care.
12. Identify types of discrimination commonly faced by lesbian and bisexual women.
13. Discuss the cultural implications of female genital mutilation.

KEY TERMS

Civil unions *160*
Comparable worth *150*
Disability *158*
Domestic partnership *160*
Elder abuse *156*
Environmental toxins *153*
Female genital mutilation (FGM) *161*
Feminization of later life *155*
Feminization of poverty *146*
Polypharmacy *157*

In the 21st century, many women in developed nations are creating and experiencing new opportunities for personal and professional growth. Despite these unparalleled opportunities, other women still struggle daily to overcome poverty, age discrimination, abuse, the economic and interpersonal effects of disability, and unequal treatment because of sexual orientation. Even the most successful and satisfied working women face wage discrimination, lack of safe and nurturing day care for their children, and failure of their governments to support paid maternity and paternity leave.

Every day in their clinical practices, nurses working with women are confronted with these issues and their impact on women's health and well-being. To help nurses better understand their patients' concerns and problems, this chapter addresses some of the serious social issues facing women today.

Case Study: Social Issues Affecting Women

Social Issues Affecting Women Living in Poverty

For impoverished women, life is a day-by-day struggle fraught with anxiety and hardship.

> "I never thought this would happen to me. Two months after I became pregnant with our second child, it was over. My husband left us. Suddenly, I am the sole support of myself and my children. Since he left I haven't been able to get a job, so I don't have medical insurance or any benefits to help with this pregnancy. Applying for Medicaid has to be one of the most humiliating experiences I have ever had. I'm an intelligent woman with a college degree, and yet I couldn't figure out the forms. I felt so dumb. The lines and the impersonal treatment that you hear about are real. I felt like a number, shuttled from one place to the next. I know they don't do it on purpose; they've heard so many awful stories. Still, it hurt. It will take 6 weeks to qualify for assistance, and by then I will be more than halfway through my pregnancy. What's more, only two doctors here accept Medicaid, and they are clear across town—that means three bus transfers with a 2-year-old in tow. I'm thankful that I can get some help, but it is so hard. I never dreamed I'd be in this position. I just never dreamed."

The Feminization of Poverty

The fact that many more women than men live below the poverty level is reflected in the phrase **feminization of poverty**, which was coined by Diana Pearce in 1993. Increasing numbers of U.S. women and their children are attempting to live on $22,050 or less, which is the current income that defines the poverty level for a family of four. In 2008, the number of women living in poverty totaled 14.1 million, or more than 12% of all women 18 years of age or older (Department of Health and Human Services [DHHS], 2009).

Women raising children alone are especially likely to be impoverished. In 2007, only 8.5% of families headed by a married couple lived in poverty, but among households headed by single mothers the percentage was 28.3% (DHHS, 2009). With a divorce rate of approximately 40%, an out-of-wedlock birth rate of about 38.5%, and the median age at first marriage rising for men and women, the reality is that many children will spend at least a portion of their lives in a single-parent family (Centers for Disease Control and Prevention [CDC], 2009b).

The number of children in the United States living in poverty is disturbing. Eighteen percent live below the poverty level. No other age group, not even the elderly, has a higher poverty rate. The two demographic factors most strongly associated with children's poverty are female-headed family and race. Parental gender is important because men earn more money overall than women; women working full time year round earn 78% of what men earn. In 2007, men earned an average of $45,113 per year, whereas women earned $35,102 (U.S. Census Bureau, 2008). More than 43% of impoverished children live in female-headed homes (U.S Census Bureau, 2008). Parental race is related to poverty in children because ethnic minority parents tend to have less education and lower incomes, on average, than Caucasian parents. Twenty-four percent of black children and 21% of Hispanic children live in poverty, but only 12% of Caucasian children do. Currently, two thirds of all poor people in the United States are women and children; in other words, women and children account for most of the people living in poverty (Figure 8-1 ■).

The feminization of poverty is also evident in the rising trend for women to declare bankruptcy. In 2005, new bankruptcy laws were passed that reduced consumer protection and gave lenders more leverage to push for repayment. These new laws have hurt women who are divorced, separated, or widowed, particularly single mothers. Single mothers often work in low-wage jobs and have been shown to be more likely to file for bankruptcy than married parents and 3 times more likely than childless couples. Estimates indicate that 30% of those filing for bankruptcy are single women. In 2008, bankruptcy filings increased 43% in response to an economic recession and heightened unemployment rates (Bankruptcy Action Coalition, 2009).

The feminization of poverty extends beyond the United States. Although there are many scales used to measure global poverty, the Purchasing Power Parity (PPP) scale uses calculations based on money available for purchasing. It is estimated that 1.4 billion people in the world live on less than $1 per day, an additional 2.5 billion live on less than $2 per day, and 80% of the world's population lives on less than $10 per day (UNICEF, 2009; World Bank, 2009). Globally, women must cope with some unique challenges. They typically work more hours than men but are paid less for the same work; they are often expected to bear and raise many children, sometimes in addition to performing a job outside the home; they are frequently abused and beaten in their own homes; and often they have few legal rights.

Both globally and in the United States, poverty has been directly linked to a lack of literacy and educational attainment. In many countries, the literacy rate for females is lower than that for males, and education—when available—is more frequently

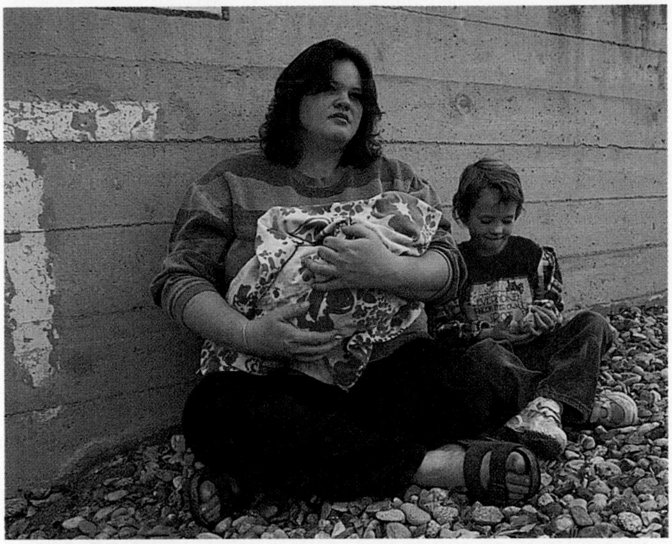

Figure 8-1 ■ Two thirds of Americans living in poverty are women and children.

Source: Photographer, Elena Dorfman.

provided for men even though economic returns on investment in women's education are found to exceed those for men. Also, women who use their skills to increase their income typically invest more in their children's health and education.

Economic Effects of Divorce

The increase in the number of female-headed families is closely associated with divorce. Almost one out of every two marriages ends in divorce. As a result of divorce, a woman's standard of living generally decreases significantly, whereas a man's increases. This dramatic change in the standard of living is usually associated with the lower earning capacity of women, the fact that women receive custody of the children in 75% of cases, and that women often accept lower support payments in exchange for a guarantee of custody (McIntosh & Chisholm, 2008). Although only about one half of divorced women receive the full amount of promised child support payments, tightened enforcement policies at the national level have increased the percentage of men who meet their obligations, either partially or in full, through improved rates of paternity establishment, support order initiation, and support collection. The United States Department of Justice actively investigates and prosecutes individuals who cross state lines to avoid paying child support, and the federal government now intercepts delinquent parents' income tax refunds. To make it easier to track delinquent parents across state lines, employers are required to report all newly hired employees to state agencies, which then transmit the information to the national directory. Moreover, states are required to establish central registries of child support orders and centralized collection and disbursement units. States are permitted to implement tough collection techniques, including garnishing wages, seizing assets, revoking driver's and professional licenses, and, in some cases, requiring mandatory community service of individuals who are delinquent in making child support payment. Information about the enforcement program may be found on the DHHS Office of Child Support Enforcement's Internet home page.

Factors Contributing to Poverty in Working Women

Women have steadily increased their participation in the labor force. In the United States, the number of working women has risen from 5.1 million in 1900, to 18.4 million in 1950, to nearly 68 million in 2008 (U.S. Department of Labor, 2009).

Along with their participation in the labor market, women have steadily increased their earnings; however, a significant wage discrepancy still exists. In 2008, women employed full time earned only about 80% of men's median weekly wages, and for women of color, the gap was wider: African American women earned 63.3%, and Latina women 51.7%, of men's weekly earnings. Although Asian Pacific American women do better, they still earn only 83.5% as much as men (United States Committee on Pay Equality, 2008). The disparity between men's and women's wages may be attributed to several factors:

- About one third of women work in a cluster of "pink collar" occupations, which tend to be poorly paid when compared with male-dominated positions requiring comparable levels of responsibility, skill, and education. When men are employed in these occupations, however, they tend to make more than their female counterparts (Dey & Hill, 2008).
- Women are paid less than men for comparable work in virtually all occupations: In 2008, professional and technical women earned almost 27% less than their male counterparts, whereas women in office and administrative support occupations earned over 12% less. Even women in female-dominated fields (teaching, office work, clerical work) are outearned by male peers (Dey & Hill, 2008).
- Because women are paid less when they work, they receive smaller pensions and social security benefits when they retire. More older women rely on social security payments as their primary source of income than do men. More retired men receive private pensions than do women because, until recent times, fewer women worked in their younger years and thus did not accrue the years of service necessary to participate in a pension program (Employee Benefit Research Institute, 2010). Only 16.4% of older women derive their earnings from employment-based finances compared to 30.5% of older men (Employee Benefit Research Institute, 2007). Part-time workers, who make up 20% of the U.S. workforce, many of whom are women, often have no benefits such as sick leave and health insurance (Shulman, 2009).

For working divorced or single women with children, the issue of child care is especially difficult. Child care is expensive and places a tremendous burden on the single parent's household budget. Moreover, with no partner to bear the burden, divorced or single mothers without social support must miss work when their children become ill, causing employers to view them as unreliable or uncommitted. Currently, more enlightened employers are beginning to recognize and accommodate the needs of mothers in the workforce. Like other areas of reform, however, this trend tends to benefit women in better paying, more secure positions far more than it benefits women who are poor and in low-paying positions.

Public Assistance

The U.S. welfare system was originally designed to provide assistance to those in need, frequently single female heads of households and their children. Unfortunately, the system often failed to provide adequate assistance to raise families above poverty levels and, in many cases, actually provided disincentives for women to work.

In 1996, growing national concern over the failure of the system led to welfare reform via the passage of the Personal Responsibility and Work Opportunity Reconciliation Act. As part of the act, a block grant known as the Temporary Assistance for Needy Families (TANF) was created. The TANF grant replaced the Aid to Families with Dependent Children (AFDC) program, which had provided cash welfare to poor families with children since 1935. The TANF program became the TANF Bureau within the Office of Family Assistance in 2006 and administers all its programs.

TANF is implemented through block grants to the states. States use these funds to operate their own programs in whatever fashion they choose, provided they are congruent with the four TANF purposes set out in federal law:

- Provide assistance to needy families so that children may be cared for in their own homes or in the homes of relatives.
- End the dependence of needy parents on government benefits by promoting job preparation, work, and marriage.
- Prevent and reduce the incidence of out-of-wedlock pregnancies and establish annual numerical goals for preventing and reducing the incidence of these pregnancies.
- Encourage the formation and maintenance of two-parent families.

Under TANF, states are granted unprecedented flexibility in designing welfare programs to meet the needs of their recipients, but they must demonstrate measurable results in moving families toward self-sufficiency and work. With few exceptions, recipients are required to find employment after they have received assistance for 2 years. Work requirements may be met through participation in subsidized or unsubsidized employment, community service, on-the-job training, or 12 months of vocational education. Recipients can also meet the requirement by providing child care services to others who are involved in community service. After 5 cumulative years of assistance, families become ineligible for cash aid, although states can exempt up to 20% of their cases from the time limit provision. States can also choose to use state funds or social security block grant dollars to provide additional noncash assistance and vouchers for families who have reached the time limit. TANF provides $17 billion, which includes child care funding, to enable mothers to provide for adequate child care as they move into jobs. Women on welfare are guaranteed continued healthcare coverage for their families, including at least 1 year of transitional Medicaid as they leave the welfare rolls for work.

The law also mandates that unmarried teenage parents live at home (or in an adult-supervised setting) and stay in school in order to receive assistance (The Urban Institute, 2010). As discussed previously, the act also contains several provisions designed to crack down on noncustodial parents who fail to pay child support.

Several trends have emerged as a result of the welfare reform efforts. A comparison of welfare recipients' pre-TANF status in 1996 to their post-TANF status in 2008 reveals the following: more single women on welfare are living with partners, a decrease in the poverty rate, a decrease in the poverty gap (the amount of income necessary to lift poor families out of poverty), and an increase in the number of families that include at least one working parent (Falk, 2006). Although results appear favorable, it is too early to judge more long-term effects of welfare reform; many parents who have entered the workforce have not yet escaped poverty.

Homelessness

For many people the thought of a homeless person conjures up a vision of an older man curled in a doorway or making a home under a bridge. However, this vision is less accurate today than in the past; today's homeless people have very different characteristics. It is estimated that 3.5 million people, including 1.35 million children, are likely to experience homelessness within a given year. That equates to 6.3% of the population of those living in poverty (National Law Center on Homelessness & Poverty, 2010). Homeless families with children represent the fastest growing group of homeless, having increased to 33% of the homeless population. Children account for 39% of the homeless population and 42% of these children were under the age of 5. Many of these families are composed of single mothers and their children. In addition, single childless women make up 17% of the homeless population (National Coalition for the Homeless, 2008).

Factors Contributing to Homelessness

Because of the nature of homelessness, it is very difficult to come up with a number that reliably reflects the number of people who experience homelessness. Data collected by various local jurisdictions indicates that the homeless population is continuing to increase each year. Approximately 90% of homeless families are headed by a single mother. A major factor contributing to the incidence of homelessness is a lack of housing that low-income people can afford. During the past 20 years, housing costs have increased far more than wages or other income sources, especially for women. In many communities, low-income housing has waiting lists of several hundred families. In addition, federal support for low-income housing has fallen by 49% since 1980 (National Coalition for the Homeless, 2008).

Another factor contributing to homelessness is domestic violence. Research suggests that as many as 22% of homeless women and their children are fleeing from an abusive situation (National Coalition for the Homeless, 2008). Domestic violence and lack of affordable housing are interrelated factors contributing to women's homelessness. Women often return to abusive living situations following unsuccessful attempts to find adequate affordable housing. Many women who have been victims of domestic violence lack rental and employment histories or have poor credit; all are barriers to finding adequate housing and can lead to homelessness.

Other factors that contribute to homelessness include job loss, eroding work opportunities, mortgage foreclosure, low-paying jobs, substance abuse, untreated mental illnesses, domestic violence, poverty, prison release, and changes and cuts in public assistance programs (National Coalition for the Homeless, 2008). Race, education, and the number of children a woman has borne also influence the likelihood that she will experience homelessness. The homeless population consists of 49% African American, 35% Caucasian, 13% Hispanic, 2% Native American, and 1% Asian (National Coalition for Homelessness, 2008). Years of education varied inversely with episodes of homelessness, and women who had given birth to more children experienced homelessness more often than women who had fewer children. The incidence of homelessness is also related to the extent of a woman's social support system. Because middle-class women typically have relatives and friends with more living space and resources, they are able to avoid becoming homeless to a greater extent than poorer women.

A rising concern exists that the nation's weakening economy, bankruptcies of large and small commercial companies, and associated job losses are also having a negative impact on the incidence of homelessness. In 2008, a record number of 3.1 million home foreclosures occurred. In 2009, it was estimated that more than 350,000 foreclosures were occurring monthly (Christy, 2009). These foreclosures dramatically increased the number of homeless families living in the United States. Many of the foreclosures were the result of adjustable rate low-interest or interest-only loans that had adjusted to higher interest rates and thus higher monthly mortgage payments that the borrowers could no longer afford to pay. In addition, the unemployment rate rose during the same period to 8.9%, the highest rate since 1983 (U.S. Bureau of Labor Statistics, 2009). Job losses combined with losses of homes led to a significant increase in homelessness. The demand for shelters and subsidized housing increased rapidly.

Health Risks of Homeless Women and Children

Homeless women and children experience greater health risks and problems than do people in the general population. Malnutrition predisposes homeless people to a variety of respiratory and nutritional disorders. Moreover, a disproportionately high number of homeless women and children have not received preventive healthcare services, such as screening tests and immunizations.

Homeless women who are pregnant are a special challenge for healthcare providers. Inadequate prenatal care, limited access to general health care, poor nutrition, and inadequate housing lead to poor birth outcomes, including an increased incidence of low-birth-weight newborns and a higher rate of infant mortality. In addition, as a group they are at risk for many illnesses that could negatively affect their pregnancies, including substance abuse; sexually transmitted infections; and hepatitis A, B, and C (Bloom et al., 2006).

Even when prenatal care services are available in the community, 75% of homeless pregnant women feel there are barriers to services, including costs, fears, inconvenience, site-related factors, and issues with the provider-patient relationship (Bloom et al., 2006).

Effects of Poverty on Women's Health Care

The effects of poverty on women's health care are extensive. Since 1981, many funding cuts have reduced or eliminated programs that used to help families in poverty access health care. Funding has not been restored, even though adequate nutrition and prenatal care have been proven to yield significant healthcare benefits.

Medicaid is the major U.S. program providing health care to low-income people in four categories: children, adults in families, the elderly, and blind and disabled people. Traditionally Medicaid has played an important role in financing maternity care, covering the costs of about 40% of births in the United States. Because welfare reform measures eliminate the automatic connection between TANF and Medicaid and mandate that women apply for Medicaid separately, the number of women that Medicaid serves may be shown to have decreased over the years since the inception of TANF. Although such an outcome would certainly be undesirable, the overall effect of welfare reform on women's health is not yet clear. Some research suggests that because women on Medicaid are served in managed care programs that typically stress preventive care, poor women's health will improve. TANF recipients are eligible for programs including WIC (Women, Infants and Children nutrition program), nonmedical home visiting for families, and youth development programs aimed at reducing out-of-wedlock births (State Health Department of Minnesota, 2008). A study showed that women enrolled in the Florida Medicaid program had a 2.5% less chance of delivering a small-for-gestational-age infant compared to those not enrolled in Medicaid (Morse, Zheng, Tang, et al., 2009). Investigators in another study found that women enrolled in Medicaid for family-planning services saved over $5.7 billion in pregnancy-related expenditures by not becoming pregnant and attending family planning clinics instead (Frost, Finer, & Tapales, 2008).

Lack of health insurance is also a major problem for the poor. In 2007, 45.7 million people were without health insurance coverage of any kind. The number of people covered by government programs such as Medicaid and The State Children's Health Insurance Program increased from 80.3 million in 2006 to 83 million in 2007. Lack of employment and eligibility for publicly funded programs are responsible for these trends: The percentage of people covered by private health insurance decreased from 67.9% in 2006 to 67.5% in 2007 (Reinberg, 2008). Decreases in health insurance coverage have led to declines in preventive health care that are costing dollars and even lives. Women who do not receive prenatal care are 3 times more likely to have low-birth-weight babies, and the incidence of low-birth-weight babies is increasing. Women who receive adequate prenatal care are less likely to develop severe complications, such as preterm labor. Moreover, lack of prenatal care is a risk factor for infant morbidity and mortality.

The issue of women and poverty is critical, and the implications for childbearing care are very real. A pregnant woman who is suffering economically may also suffer physically and psychologically. In the end, it is often the children who suffer the most, bearing the physical and psychologic scars of their mothers' struggles. As healthcare professionals, nurses should be concerned about the issue of women and poverty. The limited resources available to impoverished women often frustrate nurses' efforts to provide quality care. Nurses need to explore their own beliefs about poverty and public assistance programs and inform others about the barriers poor women face.

Assessing women's financial status is a nursing responsibility, because some women may not have the economic resources to buy infant supplies or other medical supplies that may be needed in the home setting. The nurse asks questions in a sensitive manner and refers women with insufficient resources to social workers or appropriate agencies. A nurse who is knowledgeable about community resources and who can provide the woman with follow-up contacts and phone numbers provides an immeasurable service to impoverished patients.

PROFESSIONALISM IN PRACTICE

Assisting Impoverished Women

Nurses can assist impoverished women by working with community groups and organizations and becoming actively involved in the political process. Nurses can use their work experience to present their views to legislators, support various childbearing programs, and alert legislators to legislation that would benefit mothers and families. Nurse researchers can explore medical and social issues related to the impact of poverty on families.

Social Issues Affecting Women in the Workplace

In 2008, women workers totaled more than 68 million within the U.S. workforce (U.S. Department of Labor, Bureau of Labor Statistics, 2008). Seventy-five percent worked full time, whereas 25% worked part time (U.S. Department of Labor, 2009). As a result of political and social changes that began in the early 1970s, women's career options have expanded dramatically. Although many women still choose careers traditionally entered into by women (office work, nursing, etc.), or choose to stay home full time to raise children, others are entering occupations that until recently were reserved for men. More women than ever have joined the ranks of lawyers and judges, authors and artists, managers and corporate heads, scientists, engineers, legislators, construction workers, plumbers, and electricians, and thus are sharing in the benefits that come with these positions.

Progress has its costs, however. For example, the woman with both a career and a family may experience tremendous day-to-day stress in attempting to fulfill both her professional and mothering roles. The woman who would like nothing more than to be a stay-at-home mother may be forced by financial pressures to work outside the home and entrust the care of her children to others. Women who do stay at home to raise their children sacrifice earnings, retirement savings, and social security benefits, and have decreased opportunities for social contact and intellectual stimulation. In contrast, the woman who has devoted her prime childbearing years to establishing a career rather than a family may feel a deep sense of loss as she ages.

Several social issues affect women in the workplace. Key among these are wage discrepancy, maternity/paternity leave issues, child care, and environmental hazards.

Wage Discrepancy

In 2008, the male-to-female earnings ratio was approximately 79.9%. This means that in that year, women, on average, earned about 79.9 cents for every dollar earned by men (Institute for Women's Policy Research, 2009). To keep this percentage in perspective, however, bear in mind that 40 years ago the wage discrepancy between men and women was much greater. Over the past four decades, women have entered the labor market in great numbers and have also substantially increased their level of educational attainment. For example, in 1970, only 8% of workers classified as professionals (physicians, executives, lawyers, etc.) were women, but by 2008, the percentage had soared to 39%. At the same time, the wage gap between professional workers and blue-collar workers (laborers, service workers, etc.) widened considerably. Consequently, the overall wage discrepancy between men and women declined as women's educational attainment grew and their workforce participation increased. Nevertheless, a wage gap remains, and, ironically, it is widest between well-educated women and men.

Wage disparities begin early in professional women's careers. A study by the American Association of University Women (2009) found that these wage gaps kick in as early as 1 year after college graduation, when female counterparts are making 80% of their male peers' earnings. Within 10 years after college graduation, the percentage drops to 69%. The decreasing, but tenacious, discrepancy between men's and women's wages is thought to be related to a number of factors: deliberate wage discrimination against women, undervaluing of women's work, and women's socialization.

In the past, deliberate and blatant wage discrimination against women was ubiquitous and generally accepted. Women's wages were purposely set lower than men's because it was assumed that men needed substantial funds to support families whereas women did not. In the 1960s and 1970s, women's groups and unions pushed for legislation that would end wage discrimination by mandating that compensation for various types of work be based on **comparable worth**, which means equal pay for work that is of comparable value and requires comparable skills, responsibility, education, and experience. Comparable worth legislation was opposed by business leaders, who argued that wage disparities were rooted not in discrimination against women, but in differences in educational level and seniority, and that basing wages on comparable worth would decrease U.S. manufacturers' ability to compete with foreign manufacturers and reallocate limited salary resources away from lower-class, minority men to middle-class, Caucasian women. Such arguments prevailed, and comparable worth legislation proposed during the Carter administration (1977–1981) was never implemented. Comparable worth has not been raised as a serious issue in recent years, even though research has demonstrated that neither worker nor job characteristics fully account for the wage differences between men and women and that the gender of individuals performing a given job is the best single predictor of the salary associated with that job. Surveys of wage trends show that when the proportion of women in a given occupational field increases, the average weekly salary level decreases. Women commonly are clustered in low-wage jobs such as child care, in which 87% of the workers are women (American Association of University Women, 2009).

Labor classified as "women's work" has been historically undervalued, and that pattern continues and contributes to the wage gap. In 2008 the mean hourly wage for occupations classified under construction and extraction (e.g., brick masons, construction laborers, paving equipment operators), in which male workers predominate, was $20.91. In contrast, the mean hourly wage for the largely female workers in healthcare support occupations (e.g., home health aides, medical assistants, and nursing aides) was $11.68 (U.S. Department of Labor, Bureau of Labor Statistics, 2009). Whether wage discrimination favoring males exists in the nursing profession is not clear. Although it is known that overall, male nurses outearn female nurses, some attribute that phenomenon to the fact that male nurses are overrepresented in high-paying nursing specialties such as anesthesiology. The small numbers of men in the profession make it difficult to determine whether men working in the less well-compensated areas of nursing practice are also better compensated, overall, than women.

Women can combat wage discrimination in several ways. First, they can refuse to contribute to the secrecy about wages that allows some employers to get away with paying women less than men for doing the same job. Women can also actively push for wage equity by making community leaders and legislators aware of wage discrepancies and by urging legislators to support legislation that enhances equal employment and wages for women.

Women's socialization has long been thought to contribute to the wage gap. Although most boys are encouraged to develop a competitive spirit, first in sports and then in other areas of their lives, girls may lack this early introduction to healthy competition, because the willingness and ability to compete has not been seen as an important or desirable trait for a girl to have. Also, some girls learn from their parents, the media, their peers, and others that physical attractiveness, rather than intelligence and hard work, is the key to popularity and success. And, until relatively recently, another significant factor was women's tendency to settle for lower levels of education than men and then choose to work in poorly compensated "women's fields." Since 1982, however, more American women than men have earned bachelor's degrees, and parents, educators, and other concerned citizens have lobbied successfully for programs that encourage girls to explore a wide range of academic pursuits and career options, especially in fields not traditionally seen as welcoming to women. For example, the Department of Labor has developed a mentoring program that encourages schoolgirls to seek nontraditional, higher paying careers.

PROFESSIONALISM IN PRACTICE

Speaking in Public

Speaking out about issues that affect women, children, and families is an integral part of maternal-child nursing. It is difficult for many nurses to do this, so you should practice with friends and family frequently. Be prepared with accurate information, and try various techniques for presenting the information. A friendly, supportive audience helps you get started.

Maternal and Paternal Leave Issues

Combining full-time employment with motherhood has always been challenging. In the past, women who took official or unofficial maternity leave to bear a child often lost benefits, missed out on promotions, or lost their jobs completely. Paternity leave for fathers was unheard of, and remains rare, even in developed countries.

Parenthood and employment became a bit more compatible in 1993 when President Clinton signed the Family and Medical Leave Act (FMLA) into law. FMLA permits employees to take up to 12 weeks of unpaid leave from work following the birth or adoption of a child or the placement of a foster child. Employees may also take leave if faced with serious illness or the illness of a spouse, child, or parent. Health insurance benefits must be continued during the leave, and employees are entitled to return to their former position or one considered comparable. Because the FMLA applies only to companies with 50 or more employees, however, the vast majority of companies are not subject to the law. Moreover, coverage is not mandated for employees who work fewer than 25 hours per week or who have been employed less than 1 year. Thus about 25 million employees are not covered by FMLA and must rely on whatever policies their employers have established. Even though FMLA applies to men as well as women, U.S. fathers often fail to take advantage of it. Studies have shown that American men often forgo paternity leave because they fear that taking it will hinder their careers and that men who do take it feel stigmatized. Companies often send out subtle messages to men that paternity leave exists only on paper; men who do take paternity leave are often seen as pioneers even though the law has been in effect since 1993.

Despite the advances made in this country by the FMLA, parental leave benefits in the United States are meager in comparison with benefits provided in other countries. In other parts of the world, paid parental leave is the rule rather than the exception, and the funding source is often public rather than the private employer. Paid maternity leave, and often paternity leave as well, are standard in most European countries and Canada. The United States remains one of the few countries that have no legislation requiring a national *paid* maternity leave program.

Discrimination Against Pregnant Women

Discrimination against pregnant women by employers who cling to false stereotypes about them (that they cannot do their jobs, that they take more sick leave than other employees, that they fail to return to work after having given birth) remains an issue in some areas. Each year, the Equal Employment Opportunity Commission receives complaints from pregnant women who were turned down for jobs, denied transfers to positions for which they were qualified, or fired unjustly (U.S. Equal Employment Opportunity Commission, 2006). Thus it is important that pregnant women be aware of their legal rights. The Pregnancy Discrimination Act of 1978 guarantees the following:

- A pregnant woman cannot be denied a job if she is able to perform major job functions.
- The same procedure for using sick leave pay or disability benefits must be used for the pregnant woman as for other employees.
- Employee medical coverage must include pregnancy benefits.
- The mother can use all her maternity benefits without penalty.

When a woman is planning a pregnancy, she should acquire information about pregnancy benefits in her work setting. The state in which she lives also has guidelines or regulations about pregnancy.

> “I was thrilled when I found out I was pregnant! Although I had a high-stress job and worked long hours, I rejoiced in the thought of being a mother. As my pregnancy became apparent, my boss started “worrying about me.” He feared I could not keep up with my demanding schedule and that the “emotional strain” would be hard on the baby. By the time I reached 28 weeks, I learned that a coworker would be taking over some of my responsibilities and 2 weeks later I was laid off. My boss felt that my current workload would be too difficult for a “very pregnant woman or a new mother.” I immediately started fighting for my right to keep my position. I was the perfect employee previously with flawless evaluations. Sure there may be legal protection in place, but right now I have no income, am paying high insurance premiums to maintain my health insurance, and am rapidly depleting my savings. I am angry and cry all of the time. I have been diagnosed with depression and am now taking antidepressants. I never missed a minute of work, my performance remained flawless . . . their only complaint, I was pregnant! This should be the happiest time of my life but instead I'm in counseling and taking Prozac; it's so unfair!”

Child Care

Application: How to Find Good Day Care

In 1947, only 12% of mothers with small children were employed. By 2008 that percentage had jumped to 81.5%. The number of families with stay-at-home dads rose to 6.9% in 2008 (U.S. Bureau of Labor Statistics, 2009). Although some fathers are actively involved in meshing work and family responsibilities, child care remains predominantly a woman's issue, both because of the traditional belief that child care is “women's work,” and because of the high percentage of single-parent households headed by a woman (Figure 8-2 ■). In 1970, there were approximately 3 million single mothers heading families. In 2009, there are over 10 million single mothers heading households. Finding high-quality, affordable child care is a critical issue for many American women (National Association of Child Care Resource & Referral [NACCRRA], 2009).

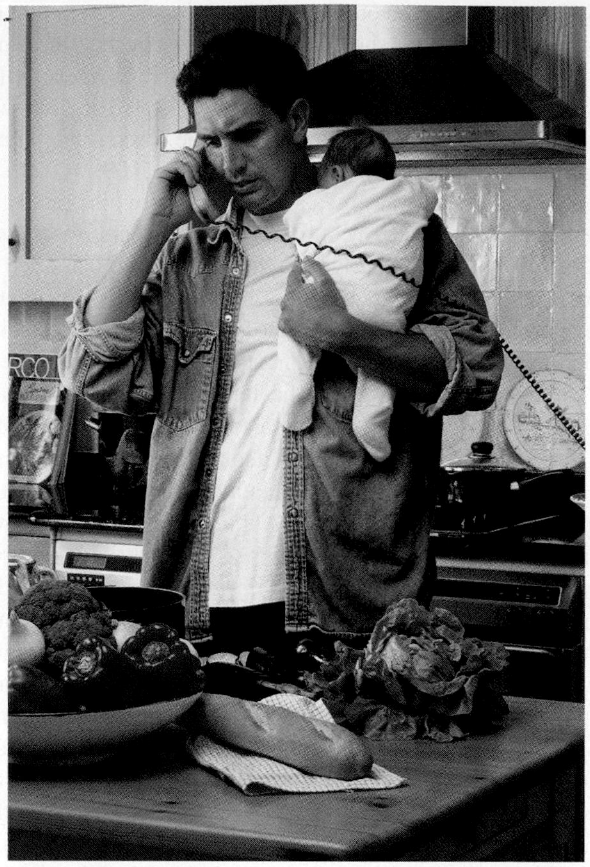

Figure 8-2 ■ Some women rely on the father to provide full-time child care at home while they pursue their career. Stay-at-home fathers provide only 1.5% of care to children under the age of 5 in the United States.

Source: Corbis RF.

> “In contemplating starting a family, I never dreamed that child care would top my list of primary stressors. The decision to work is hard enough, but then you are faced with the inability to find safe, nurturing child care. The turnover is constant, the settings never ideal. I used to think the trick was to pay more. I was wrong there. It doesn't seem to matter how much you pay or how much you investigate, it is an unending struggle. It leaves you wishing away your children's preschool years, just so you can get past the point in their lives when you are constantly dealing with child care!”

Child care costs in the United States range from $4388 to $14,647 per child per year, with an average of $8150 per year per child (BabyCenter.com, 2009). Families with multiple children can quickly consume a large amount of their income on child care costs. These costs hit low-income families especially hard because they are spending a high percentage of their earnings on providing child care.

Numerous studies have demonstrated the benefits of early, high-quality child care that features frequent, positive staff-child

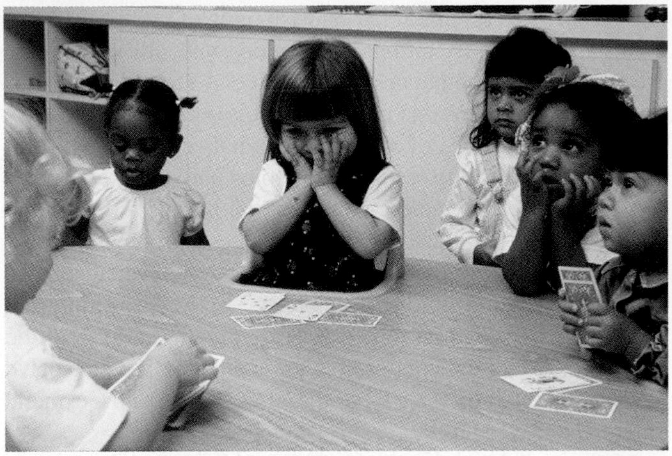

Figure 8-3 ■ Childhood education centers provide preschoolers with advanced skills for early education and provide care while parents work outside of the home.

Source: Tom and Dee Ann McCarthy/CORBIS-NY.

interactions and a strong educational component (Figure 8-3 ■). Children who receive such care tend to do better in school and are more likely to graduate, and they have lower rates of juvenile crime and adolescent pregnancy when they are older. In contrast, low-quality child care is associated with strained maternal-child relationships; higher incidence of insecurity; more problem behaviors; and lower scores on cognitive, language, and school readiness scales (National Institute for Early Education Research, 2009).

Mothers who have a college education and work outside of the home are more likely to enroll their children in education-based child care programs. Currently some employers provide support for employees' child care needs through such mechanisms as referral programs, on-site or near-site centers, or financial assistance programs. Other creative approaches to handling child care are also gaining in popularity: flex-time scheduling, part-time work, job sharing, and telecommuting (working at home via e-mail, phone, and fax) (Figure 8-4 ■). Some parents choose to work alternate shifts to eliminate the need for day care or other forms of nonparental care. Although this option has its advantages, it can be stressful for the family because the parent who is at home may not get enough sleep.

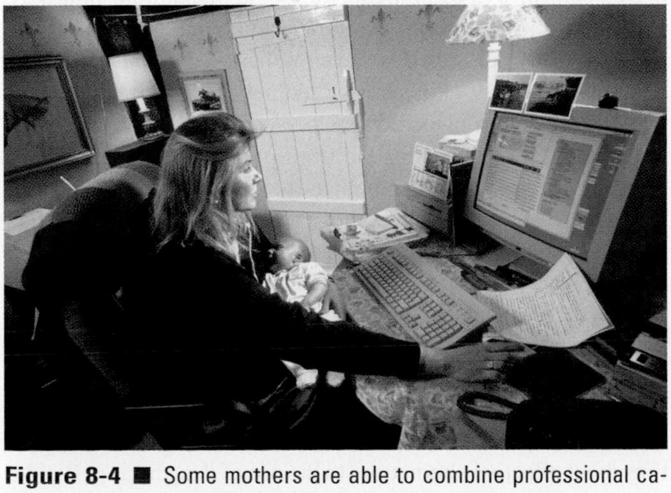

Figure 8-4 ■ Some mothers are able to combine professional careers with motherhood by telecommuting from a home office.

Source: Andrew Errington/Getty Images Inc.—Stone Allstock.

Grandparents can be an invaluable source of child care assistance to working families. In the United States about 8% of grandparents, usually grandmothers, provide extensive care (more than 30 hours per week, or more than 90 nights per year) to their grandchildren. Approximately 4.6 million children live with grandparents who function in the parenting role full time. Grandmothers who take on such daunting responsibility are at risk for neglecting their own health and feeling greater stress than grandmothers who do not act as primary care providers for their grandchildren (Stitof & Stitof, 2009).

Until recently, grandparents and other relatives who assume responsibility for one or more children whose parents are unable to care for them have not been eligible for the financial aid routinely provided to nonrelated foster parents. As of 2004, however, 35 states and the District of Columbia had instituted *Subsidized Guardianship,* a mechanism by which custodial relatives may receive funds through a variety of local, state, and federal programs (National Resource Center for Family-Centered Practice & Permanency Planning, 2009).

Advocacy for Working Women

All women, including nurses, who must balance work and family responsibilities should inquire about maternity and paternity leave; child care benefits; the possibility of working flexible hours; and whether on-site, discounted day care is provided before accepting employment. Women should also inquire about the flexibility of break periods to express their milk for nursing infants. Many employers now have special areas specifically designed for women who need to express milk throughout the workday. Nurses, and women in general, must support other women who are fighting for their rights in the workplace and must demand that legislators pass family- and woman-friendly employment laws. Solidarity and the willingness to actively oppose unfair or discriminatory practices are twin keys to equal rights and treatment for working women.

PROFESSIONALISM IN PRACTICE

Advocating for Working Women

Nurses can act as advocates for working women by serving as role models, providing positive reinforcement and support, and working actively to establish woman-friendly workplace policies.

Environmental Hazards in the Workplace and at Home

Women in developed countries such as the United States are increasingly exposed to **environmental toxins**, chemical compounds found in air, food, and water, whose bioaccumulation can lead to adverse health effects. These substances can affect their reproductive and general health and the health of their children. Toxins of greatest concern include gases that may contaminate indoor air; toxic chemicals to which women may be exposed at work and at home; and various poisonous or otherwise harmful substances that contaminate produce, fish, and meats. Women who are nurses are also exposed to potentially harmful chemical and biologic agents associated with the healthcare industry.

Air pollution is an environmental hazard caused by the release of toxins into the air. Both indoor and outdoor air pollution can cause minor problems such as eye, nose, and throat irritation and headaches as well as serious problems such as lung and heart disease. Indoor air pollution, however, poses the more serious threat to women's health, because most Americans spend 90% of their time indoors. Most indoor air pollution is caused by gases (fumes) released from lit cigarettes, burning candles (especially those scented with synthetic chemicals), wood-burning stoves, kerosene lamps, oil-burning furnaces, cleaning products, paint, varnish, and carpets made from synthetic materials. Pressed-wood products, such as fiberboard, used in flooring, shelving, and paneling, may release a colorless, odorless gas known as *formaldehyde gas,* which is known to cause cancer in animals and may eventually be shown to cause it in humans. *Radon,* a naturally occurring radioactive gas, may seep into homes from certain types of bedrock beneath the foundation and is the second leading cause of lung cancer (smoking is the first), which kills more women than any other type of cancer, including breast cancer. Special kits for detecting radon gas are available, as are devices for removing it from homes. Other common sources of indoor air pollution are cat dander, molds and mildew, dust mites, and cockroaches. Asthma, an increasingly common and serious problem in children, is worsened by most forms of indoor air pollution (MedlinePlus, 2009).

Women may be exposed to potentially harmful chemicals and other toxic substances at work and at home. Of the approximately 80,000 chemicals used today in industry and found in various consumer products, only about 1500 have been tested to find out whether they are likely to cause cancer or have toxic effects on the immune and/or reproductive systems or on children's pre- and postnatal growth and development. Even when testing is done, chemicals are tested individually, not in combination. The interactive and cumulative effects of the thousands of chemicals to which adults and children may be exposed are unknown.

Some types of employment expose women to chemical toxins that may harm them or their unborn children. Women who work around paints, varnishes, sealants, dry cleaning chemicals, synthetic perfumes, hair or clothing dyes, and organic solvents (such as benzene and acetone) are at increased risk.

Women may be exposed to toxic chemicals in their homes as well. Some plastics, such as polyvinyl chloride (PVC), release harmful chemicals (e.g., dioxin and phthalates) when heated. *Dioxin* is a highly toxic compound that occurs as impurities in petroleum-containing pesticides and has been linked to cancer, birth defects, and neurologic disorders. *Phthalates*, salt compounds with known toxic qualities, have been linked to a number of adverse effects on health; they are known carcinogens and sufficient levels of exposure can cause male fetuses to be born with undescended testicles and other abnormalities of the sex organs. They can also lower estrogen and testosterone levels in men (Eco Child's Play, 2009).

Beauty products may also contain harmful chemicals. Studies funded by the nonprofit organization Environmental Working Group have revealed that many brands of nail polish, fragrances, deodorants, lotions, hair spray, and other hair care products contain phthalates. The Food and Drug Administration (FDA) maintains that phthalate levels in cosmetic products are too low to be of concern and does not regulate them, nor does it mandate safety testing of personal care products before they are marketed. Some companies voluntarily submit some or all of their products to the Cosmetic Ingredient Review (CIR) panel for testing. CIR is an industry-established and policed body that has no direct ties to the FDA. According to a study done by the Environmental Working Group, 89% of the nearly 42,000 ingredients used in personal care products have never been tested by the CIR or the FDA (Skin Deep Cosmetic Safety Database, 2009).

Many *pesticides,* chemicals used to kill unwanted pests, are commonly used on public and private lawns and gardens and are potentially dangerous to women and their children. Currently, there are over 1200 such chemicals registered for use in the United States. These chemicals, in various combinations, make up the hundreds of products used by the public to control insects. Of the 30 most frequently used pesticide chemicals, 26 have been found to cause liver or kidney damage; 21 have been linked to various reproductive problems in men or women, or both; 19 have been found to be carcinogenic; 15 are known to be toxic to the nervous system; 13 have been linked with birth defects; and 11 disrupt the hormone systems of human beings (National Coalition for Pesticide-Free Lawns, 2009). Few of us escape exposure to these dangerous chemicals. We may breathe them in if we are downwind when insecticide sprays are being applied to crops or golf courses or along highways, or we may inadvertently consume them when we eat nonorganic fruits and vegetables. We may track them from our lawns into our homes, where they degrade more slowly in the absence of rain and sunlight, and where children who play on the floor will come into contact with them. Pesticide exposure can result in a variety of physical symptoms including headache, elevated body temperature, dizziness, irritability, nausea, vomiting, epigastric pain, myalgia, pain in the limbs and joints, skin irritation, and sweating (Titlic, Josipovic-Jelic, & Punda, 2008). One pesticide chemical subtype, the *organochlorines* (a combination of dioxin, malathion, chlorpyrifos, and lindane) degrade very slowly and remain in the environment for many decades. Thus even if these dangerous pesticides were banned today, exposures would not cease entirely.

The fact that organochlorines persist in the environment has implications for women of childbearing age, because organochlorines can be passed from mothers to babies in the womb and through breast milk. It is imperative that women not increase their own and their children's exposure to pesticides by applying them to their own lawns and gardens. Infants' and children's rapid rates of growth from conception through adolescence make them particularly susceptible to the effects of toxic chemicals. Moreover, children's organ systems are not fully developed and are, therefore, more susceptible to damage from exposures to toxins. The National Coalition for Pesticide-Free Lawns provides information about effective alternatives to the use of dangerous pesticides and herbicides. The plethora of dangerous pesticides sold and used in this country is a problem women should take very seriously. Pesticides and polychlorinated biphenyls are associated with decreased fetal growth and shorter gestations. Exposure to certain pesticides can also increase the risk of developmental delays in children and chronic illness and reduced reproductive capabilities in adults (Stillerman, Mattison, Giudice, et al., 2008).

Produce, fish, and meats can also be contaminated with substances that are not good for women and their children. Nonorganic fruits and vegetables carry *pesticide residue* (trace amounts of pesticides left on produce after washing) on their surfaces. Some fruits and vegetables typically carry more residue than others. Bananas, canned peaches, grape juice, and broccoli tend to have low levels. Organic produce has been shown to have much lower levels of pesticide residue than nonorganic produce; however, it is important to wash all produce before ingesting it.

Nearly all fish and shellfish contain some amount of *mercury*, a silvery white metallic element that can cause birth defects when consumed in large quantities. Most fish do not contain enough mercury to be of concern. Because larger amounts of mercury can harm the nervous systems of fetuses and small children, however, pregnant women and toddlers should not eat the flesh of large, predator fish that can have a large buildup of mercury in their fat; for example, shark, tilefish (white or golden snapper), swordfish, and king mackerel. Because tuna are also large, predator fish, pregnant women should not eat more than 6 ounces of white, albacore tuna per week or more than 12 ounces per week of "light" tuna. Salmon is typically low in mercury, but it may be contaminated with industrial chemicals known as *polychlorinated biphenyls (PCBs)*. PCBs are different types of compounds that are used to replace hydrogen atoms in biphenyls with chlorine. These industrial chemicals were banned 30 years ago, but they still linger in the environment. PCBs are known carcinogens, at least in animals. Farmed salmon contains much higher PCB levels than wild salmon, but wild salmon is available only at certain times of the year and is expensive. The farmed fish industry is being pressured by environmental and consumer groups to lower the PCB levels in its products. Meanwhile, there are still quite a few varieties of tasty, uncontaminated fish; for example, cod, mahi-mahi, ocean perch, whitefish, pollock, halibut, haddock, flounder, sole, tilapia, and striped bass (Gabbe et al., 2008).

Meat animals, such as cattle, hogs, and chicken, are dosed with antibiotics to prevent diseases from spreading because of the generally overcrowded conditions in which these animals are kept. The antibiotics given to farm animals are the same ones used to control disease in human beings—sulfa drugs, penicillin, and others. Because the flesh of commercially raised meat animals contains antibiotic residues, humans who eat meat may develop antibiotic-resistant bacterial strains in their bodies. Organic meats are free of antibiotic residues.

The exposure to various biologic and chemical toxins inherent in providing care for sick people constitutes an occupational hazard for nurses. Exposure to toxoplasmosis, rubella, cytomegalovirus, herpes simplex, and hepatitis B may adversely affect pregnancy and fetal outcome. The risk of exposure to HIV infection via needle sticks and contact with blood and other body fluids also exists. Latex allergy is rapidly becoming a significant problem among healthcare workers, with 5% to 15% demonstrating hypersensitivity symptoms ranging from mild contact dermatitis to severe systemic reactions and anaphylactic shock (American Academy of Allergy, Asthma and Immunology, 2009).

Two governmental agencies have primary responsibility for addressing workplace safety. The Occupational Safety and Health Administration (OSHA), part of the Department of Labor, is responsible for creating and enforcing workplace health and safety regulations. The National Institute for Occupational Safety and Health (NIOSH), which is part of the Department of Health and Human Services, is primarily a research agency. However, it also disseminates information on preventing workplace injury and illness, provides training to occupational safety and health professionals, and investigates potentially hazardous working situations when requested by employers or employees.

PROFESSIONALISM IN PRACTICE

Environmental Risks

Nurses need to educate women and childbearing families about the risks that they face in their environment. Nurses can encourage women to investigate potential hazards in their environment. The Internet can provide information and resources on specific hazards and preventive strategies to decrease risk of exposure. Nurses can also lobby community leaders and legislators to support positions that protect childbearing women from environmental toxins. Nurse researchers can investigate workforce and environmental hazards, recording, analyzing, and publishing findings.

Social Issues Affecting Older Women

In the United States and other developed nations, women tend to outlive men. Thus women are overrepresented in the ranks of older people. This phenomenon is referred to as the **feminization of later life**. As of 2007, there were over 37 million people aged 65 or older living in the United States, 58% of whom are women. Among people aged 80 or older, 65% are female (U.S. Census Bureau, 2007).

Economic Vulnerability of Older Women

The feminization of later life means that older women are more likely than their male counterparts to be widowed, to live alone, to be disabled, and to be poor. However, of all the elderly in the United States, women of color have the highest poverty rates. Factors that contribute to the increased economic vulnerability of women include the following:

- Women must stretch their financial resources further than men because of their longer life expectancy.
- Older women tend to have less educational preparation than older men.
- Historically women have been economically dependent on men and may have intermittent or nonexistent employment histories.
- Women typically earn less than men and often work in jobs without pension benefits or have only limited benefits.

- Intermittent employment is more common in women, which decreases their social security and retirement benefits.
- Women generally have more family caregiving responsibilities than men.
- Historically, public pension systems have been designed with an expectation that men would be the primary economic providers. Older women who worked outside their homes may have only meager pensions.

Middle-class women too face the risk of "cycling into poverty" should they become widows. The current economic difficulties and reductions in stock market holdings have threatened many retirees' incomes that have been saved for their later years. A drastic decline in financial circumstances is particularly likely if a woman's husband had a long, costly illness or if his pension is decreased or discontinued following his death. To help keep elderly women from spending their final years in poverty, it is necessary for governments to develop solutions to the economic concerns caused by a fixed income, to deal with problems of pension inequity, and to address the potentially disastrous effects of staggering health-care costs for the uninsured or underinsured. Because women are living longer than men and the average age has continued to climb, the need for additional income sources is imperative (Table 8-1).

Elder Abuse

Elder abuse includes any deliberate action, or lack of action, that causes harm to an elderly person. It is difficult to determine how many elderly women in the United States are victims of abuse, because perpetrators are usually careful to conceal their behavior, but elderly women are believed to be more at risk than elderly men. Currently in the United States, it is estimated that 3% to 5% of the total elderly population, or approximately 500,000 individuals, are abused annually. Experts anticipate that the problem will continue to grow as the population ages and as illness and financial burdens strain family relationships (National Center on Elder Abuse [NCEA], 2009).

Five different categories of elder abuse have been recognized: psychologic abuse, physical abuse (including sexual abuse), neglect (by self or caregiver), financial abuse, and abandonment (Table 8-2). Multiple forms of abuse may occur simultaneously and tend to intensify with time unless intervention occurs.

The prototypic victim of elder abuse is a white woman over 80 years old who lives in her own home or the home of a family member. The abuser is most often a spouse, followed by family members and then primary caregivers. Elder abuse by staff in nursing homes and long-term care facilities is also well documented. On average, elderly black Americans are more at risk for abandonment than older white Americans. Abandonment statistics are much lower for Asians and Hispanics. Factors that increase the risk of elder abuse include shared living arrangements, family history of violence, lack of financial resources, dependence, isolation, poor health, and cognitive impairment. Substance abuse and stressful events in the life of the abuser may also contribute to the risk (NCEA, 2009).

A full discussion of this growing problem, its identification, and treatment is beyond the scope of this textbook. It is imperative, however, that nurses who care for the elderly be alert for signs of abuse and take steps to address the problem when it is identified.

National Center for Prevention of Elder Abuse

Application: Elder Abuse

TABLE 8-1 Years of Life Expectancy at Birth for Selected Countries, 2008 (Rounded to Nearest Year)

COUNTRY	MALE LIFE EXPECTANCY	FEMALE LIFE EXPECTANCY
Afghanistan	43	43
Argentina	71	79
Australia	78	83
Canada	78	83
China	71	74
Egypt	69	73
Ethiopia	51	54
France	77	84
India	63	66
Japan	79	86
Mexico	73	78
Russia	59	72
Tanzania	51	53
United Kingdom	77	81
United States	75	80

Source: Central Intelligence Agency (CIA). (2008). Adult life expectancy rates: 2008. *Retrieved from http://www.cia.gov/library/publications/the-world-factbook/fields/2102.html*

TABLE 8-2 Definitions of Elder Abuse

Physical abuse: Any physical pain or injury that is intentionally inflicted upon an elderly person by a caregiver or individual who has custody of, or stands in a position of trust with, that elder. Sexual assault, physical attacks, unreasonable physical restraint, and prolonged deprivation of food and water all constitute physical abuse.

Financial abuse: Any theft or misuse of an elderly person's money or property by a caregiver or person in a position of trust.

Neglect: Failure on the part of a caregiver, or any person having custody of an elder, to provide reasonable care, which is the degree of care that a reasonable person would provide. Reasonable care includes, but is not limited to, assistance with personal hygiene; protection from health and safety hazards; and provision of shelter, food, clothing, health needs, and medical care except in instances when the elder refuses treatment.

Self-neglect: Failure to provide adequate self-care because of inability or inattention.

Psychologic abuse: The intentional infliction of mental suffering on an elder by a caregiver or person in a position of trust. Psychologic abuse includes, but is not limited to, verbal assaults, threats, humiliation, intimidation, or isolation of the elder.

Abandonment: The desertion of an elder by any person responsible for the care and custody of that elder, under circumstances in which a reasonable person would continue to provide care.

Source: Adapted from Definitions of Elder Abuse, *2009, with permission from the National Center on Elder Abuse.*

PROFESSIONALISM IN PRACTICE

Elder Abuse

If you suspect elder abuse is occurring, you should immediately report the case to the county social services office of adult protective services.

Implications of Aging for Women's Health and Health Care

Older women often face health problems that become more common as people age: hypertension, coronary artery disease, arthritis, diabetes, osteoporosis, dementia, and depression. Heart disease, cancer, and stroke are the leading causes of death for all women age 65 or older. Among white women, lung disease is the fourth leading cause of death, but for minority women it is diabetes. By age 65, half of all women have developed two or more chronic diseases. Minority and low-income women are more likely than white, higher income women, to have serious health problems.

Unfortunately, older women, particularly those who are poor, face multiple barriers in obtaining adequate healthcare services. For some, lack of transportation to healthcare facilities is an issue. Many older women are no longer able to drive because of failing eyesight or diminished reflexes. Although public transportation may be available in larger cities, many rural areas have no bus, train, or cab service, and even if public transportation is available, poorer women may not be able to afford the costs involved.

Lack of private health insurance coverage or excessive medical costs not covered by Medicare are major problems for many older women. Too often, women on limited incomes must choose between paying rent and purchasing food and paying for needed medicines or other forms of health care. Thus nurses must remain aware of the possibility that a patient's noncompliance may be economically driven.

Another problem common in older women with multiple health problems is a phenomenon known as **polypharmacy**, which means "multiple medicines." A woman who sees two or more specialists for the treatment of multiple medical conditions may well be taking a half-dozen or more powerful drugs, each with its own array of side effects and with the potential for dangerous interactions with one or more of the others, and perhaps several over-the-counter drugs as well. Sometimes polypharmacy is justified by the woman's medical needs, but often it is inadvertent; nurse practitioners and physicians are sometimes unaware that a woman is taking medications prescribed by one or more different providers. Elderly people may not remember what medications they are taking or may not think to keep caregivers informed about them. Also, many people assume that herbs and various other products classified as *nutritional supplements* are safe because they are sold without a prescription. Although such products are generally much less potent than prescription drugs, many can and do interact with drugs elderly people commonly take. For example, the herbal supplement St. John's wort, often taken to relieve mild depression, can increase or decrease the effects of oral contraceptives,

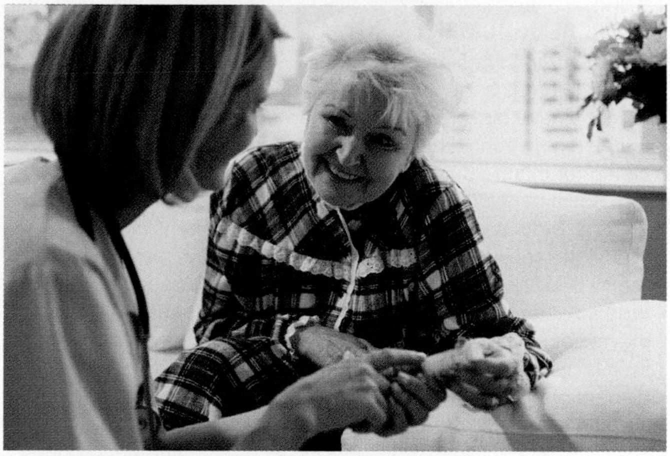

Figure 8-5 ■ Older women are more likely to have multiple medical conditions that require medication. Careful instructions should be given to prevent medication interactions.

Source: Dann Tardif/CORBIS-NY.

blood thinners, and some prescription antidepressants (Barnes, Bloom, & Nahin, 2008).

Sometimes, symptoms in an elderly person are related to drug effects or interactions rather than to disease or illness. Nurses must advise elderly patients to keep a list of the medications they take and provide each of their providers with a copy and to fill all their prescriptions at the same pharmacy. Pharmacists are increasingly alert, aided by computerized systems, to the potential risks posed by multiple drug prescriptions and will warn patients and providers of likely negative effects and interactions (Figure 8-5 ■).

Some drugs have known potential for causing cognitive impairment in elderly persons who have diminished kidney and liver function. Drugs that alter the central nervous system (anticholinergics, antihistamines, antidepressants, anxiolytics, antipsychotics, and antiepileptics) may cause such symptoms as forgetfulness, confusion, disorientation, and inability to concentrate (Waldman, 2008). Nurses can play a key role in identifying older women's concerns as well as the onset of new symptoms. In collaboration with other providers, they can improve an older woman's chances of receiving optimal health care.

Care Plan Activity: Pregnancy in a Patient Who Is Disabled

Social Issues Affecting Women with Disabilities

Approximately 19.1 million U.S. women and girls have some type of mental or physical disability, and of these, 15.4% are unable to perform basic self-care activities. It is estimated that 11.4% to 25.8% of all Americans have some type of disability (CDC, 2009a). Women are more likely than men to be disabled because of longer life expectancy rates, and disabilities are most prevalent in women over the age of 85. The majority of women with disabilities (56%) are in this age group, whereas another 44% are over the age of 65 (National Center on Birth Defects and Developmental Disabilities [NCBDDD], 2009). It is estimated that there are 19.9 to 28.6 million women living in the United States who have some type of a disability (CDC, 2010).

CLINICAL JUDGMENT

Case Study: Tanesia Ford

Tanesia Ford is a 24-year-old with an intellectual disability who recently gave birth to a baby girl named Ruby Rose. Tanesia finished high school and has experience in the church nursery caring for infants during church services. Her husband, Ben, also has a mild intellectual disability but has several younger siblings and has some experience with newborns and toddlers. Tanesia's parents live 1.5 miles away from the young family and are willing to provide assistance as needed. Ben works full time for a large grocery store and Tanesia will be staying at home with Ruby to care for her. Tanesia states "I love taking care of Ruby, I don't even mind changing her diapers or breastfeeding her."

Critical Thinking

Discuss what resources you would recommend for this young family based on the parents' intellectual disability and family circumstances.

See www.nursing.pearsonhighered.com for possible responses.

Definitions of Disability

A **disability** is a chronic physical or mental health problem or impairment that restricts an individual's ability to perform one or more major activities. Whether a given activity is considered major depends on the circumstances and responsibilities of the woman in question. For example, if a middle-aged woman cannot care for her home and children because of a disability, that disability would be considered major. If an elderly woman's disability makes independent self-care impossible, that disability would be considered major. Disabilities may also be categorized as "work" and "severe." *Work disabilities* restrict individuals from employment; a nurse who sustains a back injury that becomes chronic and prevents her from returning to her position as a staff nurse has a work disability. *Severe disabilities* prohibit individuals from performing basic activities of daily living without assistance.

Types of Disabilities

Disabilities are categorized as physical, developmental, learning, neurologic, psychiatric, and sensory. *Developmental disabilities* such as autism, cerebral palsy, epilepsy, and spina bifida are ongoing and manifest before the age of 22. They create severe limitations in three or more of the following areas: self-care, receptive and expressive language, learning, mobility, self-direction, ability to live alone, and financial independence. More than 4 million individuals are affected with some type of developmental disability, and *intellectual disability* (formerly referred to as mental retardation) is the most common (Figure 8-6 ■) (NCBDDD, 2009).

In the early- to mid-20th century, women with intellectual disabilities were often faced with mandatory sterilization at the request of family members or caregivers as a means to prevent pregnancy and thus contamination of the gene pool. This mentality led to the involuntary sterilization of many individuals without their consent. In recent years, the need for sexual health choices have become a norm as the human rights movement has evolved (Eastgate, 2008). While some women with intellectual disability may find themselves with an unplanned pregnancy, others are now choosing pregnancy and parenting as a basic human right.

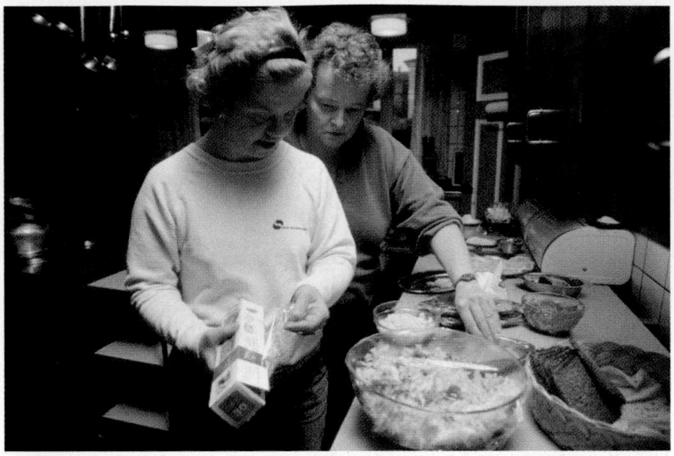

Figure 8-6 ■ Intellectual disability is the most common developmental disability.

Source: Stephanie Maze/CORBIS-NY.

Women with intellectual disability may pursue prenatal care services later than other women. It is also common for women with intellectual disability to request termination services after the gestational age limit due to significant barriers with reproductive choices (Burgen, 2010). Among women with intellectual disability who do give birth, one quarter of those will become involved with Child Protective Services (Burgen, 2010). Those who choose to parent need additional social support and parenting education offerings. Peer support often provides an effective means of learning and educating these mothers (Australian Family & Disability Studies Research Collaboration, 2007). Caregivers should give concise easy to understand directions at multiple times to ensure information is understood clearly and accurately.

Learning disabilities, such as dyslexia and attention-deficit hyperactivity disorder, can inhibit educational attainment and employment. *Common neurologic disabilities* include spina bifida, cerebral palsy, multiple sclerosis, and Alzheimer's disease. Spina bifida, or congenital malformation of the spinal cord, can cause partial paralysis. Multiple sclerosis, which affects a disproportionately high number of women in comparison with men, can cause severe mental and physical disability through degeneration of nerve fibers in the brain and spinal cord. Alzheimer's disease causes ongoing, incurable dementia that culminates in death. *Psychiatric disabilities* can cause significant impairment and significantly alter an individual's quality of life. Women's rates of depression, anxiety, panic disorders, and phobic disorders are 50% higher than men's. *Sensory disabilities* such as hearing loss and visual impairments can dramatically impair a woman's ability to interact socially and to live independently (CDC, 2009c).

Economic Vulnerability of Women with Disabilities

Only about 31% of women with disabilities are employed, in contrast with 62% of men with disabilities. Many women with disabilities can only manage part-time employment, which severely restricts their income potential. An additional problem is that people with disabilities face formidable barriers to employment: Some cannot drive or easily access public transportation. Many buildings are still without ramps and wide door openings that facilitate wheelchair access, and employers are sometimes reluctant to hire persons with disabilities. The Americans with Disabilities Act (ADA) of 1990 was intended to reduce such barriers by mandating modest improvements in building accessibility and forbidding unjustified hiring discrimination against persons with disabilities (Waldman, 2008). Although the ADA has brought about some improvements, many barriers to employment still exist.

Even when women with disabilities are able to work and find work, they typically do not earn as much as women who are not disabled. A greater number of women who are disabled live in poverty than men who are disabled or women without a disability. Many women who are disabled live in less expensive rural areas where unemployment rates are also higher (Waldman, 2008). When women with disabilities cannot work, or cannot find a job, they often lose the ability to care for themselves and their families financially. Although many people assume that social security benefits keep individuals with disabilities out of poverty, this is simply not the case. More than a fourth of all women with disabilities live in poverty (Waldman, 2008).

Violence Against People with Disabilities

Both men and women with developmental disabilities are 4 to 10 times more likely to be victims of crime than people without disabilities. Women who have intellectual disabilities are 50% more likely to be sexually assaulted in their lifetime than women of normal intelligence. Women with intellectual disabilities are sexually assaulted by caregivers, family members, residential care staff, or transportation personnel in 97% to 99% of all cases of sexual abuse (Association of Retarded Citizens [ARC], 2010). Women who are disabled may have difficulties escaping from or fighting off an attacker, may be unable to communicate well enough to report crimes, and/or may be unable to positively identify an attacker because of sensory or cognitive limitations (National Women's Health Information Center, 2009a).

Effects of Disability on Women's Health Care

Women with disabilities need routine gynecologic care and preventive health education, as do all women, but healthcare services for women who are disabled are often suboptimal. Many women with disabilities report that various barriers prevent them from obtaining routine healthcare services. Overall, women who are disabled receive less preventive care than women without disabilities but have 2.5 times the yearly health expenditures of women without disabilities (Waldman, 2008).

An additional problem is that many healthcare providers assume incorrectly that women with severe disabilities are not sexually active. Because of these false assumptions, many women who are disabled are not offered screening for sexually transmitted infections (STIs), education regarding STI prevention, contraceptive counseling, or preconception counseling. Women with intellectual disabilities are more likely to develop osteoporosis and need appropriate screening (Wilkinson & Cerrato, 2008).

Social Issues Affecting Lesbian and Bisexual Women

Various social issues can detract from lesbian and bisexual women's quality of life. These include employment and housing discrimination, discrimination involving domestic life and parenting issues, and general social discrimination based on the stigma associated with homosexuality. In addition, lesbian and bisexual women face perceived and actual discrimination on the part of healthcare providers that negatively affects both access to and quality of health care.

Employment Discrimination

Employment discrimination is the most frequent complaint the American Civil Liberties Union (ACLU) receives from gay and lesbian individuals. An act that would have prohibited termination of employment on the basis of sexual orientation, the 1997 Employment Non-Discrimination Act, was defeated by one vote. An updated version of the bill was introduced in 2007 but has yet to be passed. Table 8-3 lists those states that do provide legal protection for homosexual employees. In addition, Indiana, Kansas, Michigan, Ohio and Arizona, Delaware, Montana, Virginia, and Pennsylvania have executive orders prohibiting public employers from discrimination based on sexual orientation (Lambda Legal Defense Fund, 2009).

Discrimination exists not only in the private sector, but also in the military. The battle over homosexuals in the military has raged on since President Clinton enacted the "don't ask, don't tell" policy in 1994. Although this legislation removed sexual orientation as a contraindication to military service, it has been far from successful in protecting gay and lesbian service members from expulsion; homosexual conduct is still grounds for terminating their service. Homosexual conduct includes not only homosexual acts, but also statements that demonstrate a

TABLE 8-3 States with Legislation Protecting Homosexual Workers Against Discrimination by Public and Private Employers

California	Nevada
Connecticut	New Hampshire
Colorado	New Jersey
District of Columbia	New Mexico
Hawaii	New York
Iowa	Oregon
Illinois	Rhode Island
Maine	Vermont
Maryland	Washington
Massachusetts	Wisconsin
Minnesota	

propensity or intent to engage in homosexual acts. In short, lesbian women can serve in the military, but if their sexual orientation becomes known, they can be asked to resign. In 2006, the number of military discharges based on sexual orientation was lower (612) than at any time since 1996, comprising a small fraction of total unplanned discharges (Tyson, 2007).

Spousal Benefits

Lesbians face additional discrimination in the area of spousal benefits. Under federal statutory laws, civil marriage grants 1138 federal provisions designed to support and protect family life, therefore excluding most lesbian couples (American College of Obstetricians and Gynecologists [ACOG], 2009). Although individuals who are legally married can receive health insurance coverage, life insurance benefits, retirement pensions, and disability coverage for their partners, lesbian partners who are not legally married (the vast majority) cannot. Currently, only six states—Massachusetts, Vermont, Maine, New Hampshire, Iowa, and Connecticut, plus the District of Columbia—recognize marriage between same-sex individuals. In May 2008, California passed a law allowing same-sex marriage that was later repealed in the November 2008 elections. In August 2010, however, a federal district court struck down the ban on California same-sex marriage, and the issue is currently being debated anew.

New Jersey permits **civil unions**, which are legally recognized partnerships that involve rights and responsibilities comparable with those enjoyed by married couples. Other states offer limited recognition to same-sex couples, including Hawaii, Maryland, and Washington state. Couples who enter into civil unions are generally subject to the same laws and processes regarding inheritance, property rights, child custody, and medical decision making as married couples. Same-sex couples who wish to enter into a civil union must obtain a special license and have a solemnization ceremony. Civil union dissolution proceedings are handled in much the same manner as divorces (Lambda Legal Defense Fund, 2009).

Domestic partnership recognition is another mechanism by which public and private employers can provide insurance coverage and pension rights benefits to the partners of gay and lesbian employees. Both California and Oregon provide such benefits to employees, as do increasing numbers of city and county governments and private employers (Lambda Legal Defense Fund, 2009).

Housing Discrimination

Lesbians also face housing discrimination. Although *Fair Housing laws* protect members of various groups (minorities, pregnant women, and families with children) from being denied housing, they do not generally apply to homosexuals. Except in the few states and municipalities in which antidiscrimination-in-housing laws cover sexual orientation, landlords can refuse to rent, and homeowners can refuse to sell, to gay and lesbian people. The mechanisms by which housing discrimination on the basis of sexual orientation work are often subtle; leases may forbid "immoral" (code for homosexual) activities and/or restrict occupancy to those "related by blood or marriage." Some homeowner association boards reserve the right to refuse prospective purchasers on the basis of "inappropriate lifestyle." In one study of gay and lesbian couples, 34% had been turned away from either renting or purchasing a home due to their sexual orientation (Lamda Legal Defense Fund, 2009). Another housing-related problem gay and lesbian couples face is that, unlike married couples, they may not be able to use their combined income to determine their eligibility for a mortgage and may have to settle for cheaper housing than they can actually afford. Ironically, gay and lesbian couples who are not well off often wind up at the bottom of eligibility lists for public housing because they are not considered to constitute a "family."

Parenting Issues

Many lesbian women wish to become adoptive parents. Both single women and couples often desire the presence of children in their lives, and women who are coparenting their partner's child may want to formally adopt that child. Gay and lesbian people who wish to adopt, however, often face formidable barriers. Some child placement agencies have policies restricting adoption to married couples and in a few states (Florida, Virginia, Mississippi, Nebraska, Oklahoma, and Utah), legislation specifically bars homosexuals from adopting. Even in the absence of such policies or statutes, however, prejudice on the part of judges, social workers, and others who make decisions about child placement often makes it almost impossible for gay and lesbian people to adopt children or even become foster parents. Foreign adoptions may be no easier, because some agencies that facilitate them refuse gay and lesbian applicants; other countries ban single women from adopting. A small number of states, however, have laws prohibiting child custody or adoption discrimination against homosexuals, and some states make what is known as *second parent adoption* available to lesbian women who are coparenting the biologic children of their partners. This option allows coparents to adopt children legally, thus ensuring stability for them, should the biologic parent become incapacitated or die (ACOG, 2009).

Although there are societal concerns about children who are being raised by same-sex parents, there is no objective evidence supporting such concern. The American Academy of Pediatrics (AAP) reviewed decades of research data on children raised by heterosexual parents and children raised by lesbian or gay parents, and in 2002 it issued a policy statement stating that no differences were observed (AAP, 2009) (Figure 8-7 ■).

Although sexual orientation per se has no effect on the quality of parenting, discriminatory tax laws can adversely affect lesbian couples' ability to provide for their children. If one of the partners is employed and the other remains at home to care for the children, the working partner may not be able to claim either her partner or their children as dependents because the partners are not legally married. Lesbian couples are typically not eligible to access the family Medical Leave Act to care for their partner or their partner's children (ACOG, 2009).

Social Barriers

Lesbian and gay individuals and couples often face discrimination—and even danger. They may be treated rudely in stores; motels; restaurants; and other public facilities and ostracized by business networks, churches, neighbors, and even families. There

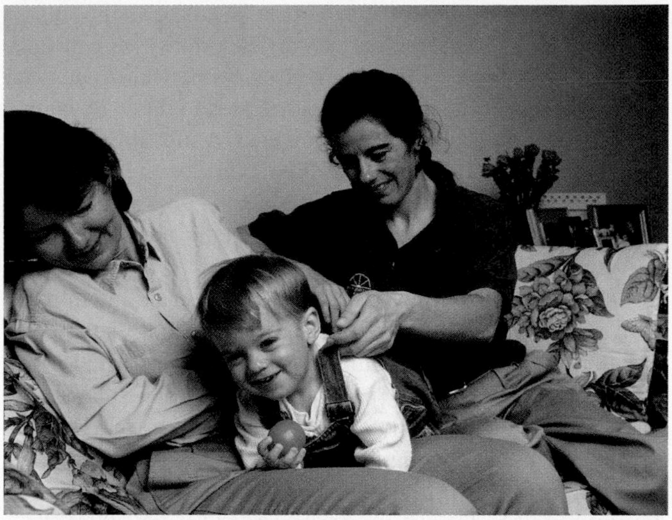

Figure 8-7 ■ Lesbian families face discrimination that more traditional families do not commonly encounter.

Source: Vanessa Vick/Photo Researchers, Inc.

are reports of newspapers having refused to accept advertisements from gay people or gay organizations. When homosexual people are made to feel uncomfortable in establishments that cater to the general public, they are forced to congregate in gay bars or other venues, where they may become inviting targets for violently homophobic individuals. In 2006, 1415 hate crimes based solely on sexual orientation (16.4% of total hate crimes) were reported to the Federal Bureau of Investigation (Johnson, 2008). Although those numbers may seem relatively small, it must be kept in mind that hate crime reporting by law enforcement officials is voluntary, and hate crimes motivated by homophobia are considered to be significantly underreported. Many lesbian women are reluctant to be open about their lifestyle because of social discrimination and the possibility of violence.

Although the goal of equality for all women is still unmet and the burden of discrimination is even greater for lesbian than heterosexual women, there is reason for optimism. Acceptance of gay men and lesbian women is on the rise with sympathetic portrayals in the media. Ongoing research by CNN Politics indicates that 44% of Americans now believe homosexual people should be allowed to marry (CNN Politics, 2009).

Effects of Discrimination on Lesbian and Bisexual Women's Health Care

In its *Healthy People 2010* action plan, the U.S. Department of Health and Human Services acknowledged sexual orientation as a risk factor for inferior health care, citing reasons such as lack of insurance, fear of discrimination on the part of providers, and provider ignorance of gay and lesbian people's healthcare needs. The first two factors limit access to health care, and the third has a negative effect on healthcare quality.

Lesbian and bisexual women are less likely than heterosexual women to have health insurance because, unlike heterosexual women, they are usually not eligible for insurance benefits based on a partner's employment. Lack of coverage can cause women to forgo health screening procedures such as Pap smears and mammography, and delay treatment until illnesses have become serious. The fear that providers may harbor anti-gay sentiments, or be uncomfortable around gay people, is common, despite position statements from multiple healthcare organizations advocating for lesbian rights. The assumption of heterosexuality, revealed daily in questions such as *What kind of birth control do you use?* and intake forms that list only *single, married, widowed, or divorced* as lifestyle options, can alienate lesbian women and may cause them to conceal their sexual orientation. Lesbian women's reluctance to disclose their sexual orientation can lower the quality of health care they receive. For example, women who do not admit that they live with a partner will not be screened for domestic violence, which is a routine screening for women in heterosexual relationships.

An additional problem that lesbian women face is that providers tend to not be knowledgeable about lesbian women's healthcare needs. Providers may not realize, for example, that lesbians are thought (but not yet proven) to be at increased risk for breast cancer because they are more likely than heterosexual women to have never given birth, to be overweight, to be stressed, and to smoke and drink alcohol. Many providers also believe that lesbian women are not at risk for sexually transmitted infections (STIs) and cervical cancer, both of which are untrue. Lesbian sexual contact can transmit a number of STIs and the virus that causes cervical cancer, because it involves exposure to vaginal secretions.

Female Genital Mutilation (FGM)

Female genital mutilation (FGM), also known as *female genital cutting, female circumcision,* and *genital circumcision,* refers to the practice of removing all or parts of a girl's or woman's genitalia for cultural reasons. It is a phenomenon with which nurses who provide health care to women, especially immigrant women from certain parts of the world, must be familiar. The damage done to a woman's anatomy in the more severe versions of the practice can cause a variety of health problems, including bleeding, infection, infertility, painful intercourse, and difficulties related to childbearing.

Origin and Demographics of FGM

FGM is a very old practice; evidence of it is present in the female mummies of Egyptian royalty. It survives in at least 28 countries in Northern Africa, parts of the Middle East (Oman, Yemen, United Arab Emirates), and Asia (Indonesia, Malaysia, Sri Lanka, India). In 18 African countries, more than 50% of women undergo the procedure (Turner, 2007). In other countries, a high percentage of women undergo the procedure, and in others only a minority does. FGM is not associated with any particular religion and is found among Christians, Muslims, Animists, and one Jewish sect. FGM is practiced in male-dominated societies in which patriarchal authority and control of women's bodies and fertility are taken for granted. In such societies, girls receive little education and are valued primarily as sources of labor and for their future role as producers of children. Fathers in many such societies sell their daughters into marriage, the payment being known as the *brideprice.*

The original reason for FGM is thought to have been the prevention of sexual intercourse before or outside of marriage, thus ensuring men that the children their wives bear are theirs. In societies in which genital mutilation has become the norm, the procedure has become heavily enculturated and is supported by both men and women. It is women, in fact, who actively promote and carry out FGM. Myths about the clitoris (that it will grow very long if not amputated; that if it touches a baby during childbirth, the baby will die) are widely believed, and uncircumcised women are seen as impure, unclean, and ugly. They are generally cut off from marriage, motherhood, and full female identity and may be ostracized. Because FGM is so closely associated with female identity, even the educated women in a given society may support it. The age at which FGM procedures are performed varies from culture to culture, with the most common range being from 5 to 12 years. A few societies carry out the procedure on infants or on teenagers just before marriage (Turner, 2007).

Nature of the Procedure(s)

In the most extreme form of FGM, known as *infibulation,* the clitoris, the labia minora, and most of the labia majora are removed and the raw surfaces of the remaining stumps of the labia majora are sewn together over the vaginal opening, leaving only a small hole for the passage of urine and menstrual blood. The opening is widened (deinfibulated) somewhat at the time of marriage, either rapidly, with a knife, or gradually, to permit sexual intercourse. Infibulation accounts for 15% of women with FGM (Shah, Susan, & Furcroy, 2009). Further deinfibulation is done to permit childbirth, and women are sewn up again afterward. Of all circumcised women in Djibouti, the Sudan, and Somalia, 80% to 90% are infibulated. The least extreme form of FGM is *partial clitoridectomy,* in which the tip of the clitoris is removed. The most common procedure (80% to 85% of all procedures) involves complete removal of the clitoris with partial or complete removal of the labia minora (Shah et al., 2009).

FGM procedures are generally carried out in villages, by a female birth attendant or elder, as part of an elaborate ritual. Very primitive instruments may be used and no anesthesia is provided. The procedure lasts approximately 20 to 30 minutes, depending on its nature and the skill of the person carrying it out. Girls are restrained by female relatives, usually including their mothers. Young girls generally do not realize what is about to happen to them; older girls may undergo the procedure willingly to conform to societal expectations.

Health Implications

Data on the number of deaths from shock and infection that occur following FGM are hard to come by, because mortality is often attributed to some other cause. Hemorrhage is the most common immediate complication of all procedures, followed by pain, infection, and urinary retention related to swelling. In developing countries, HIV transmission can occur from the use of unsterilized instruments (O'Connor, 2008). Infibulation causes the most severe long-term complications, most of which are related to the urinary tract and childbirth. Chronic urinary infections caused by inadequate emptying of the bladder are common; although a woman with intact genitalia can usually empty her bladder in 5 to 10 seconds, it may take an infibulated woman as long as 5 minutes to do so. Many women have meatal obstruction or urinary strictures. Some women develop chronic reproductive tract infections related to retained vaginal fluid and blood. Such infections can lead to infertility, which is thought to affect 25% to 30% of infibulated women. Urinary incontinence in the form of dribbling is another common problem, as is genital pain. Many infibulated women experience pain during sexual intercourse (dyspareunia), some because they have developed a neuroma in their scar tissue and introital and vaginal stenosis (Turner, 2007). Infibulation-related complications associated with childbirth include obstructed labor, nonreassuring fetal status, postpartum hemorrhage, and postpartum sepsis. The psychologic trauma caused by FGM may persist throughout a woman's life. It is related not only to personal suffering, but also to knowing that daughters and granddaughters will undergo the procedure too (Turner, 2007).

Efforts to Eradicate FGM

FGM has been denounced as a form of child abuse by the World Health Organization and by many other international and national organizations. Healthcare-related organizations, including the American Medical Association and the American Nurses Association, have denounced it as well. FGM has been outlawed in 14 African countries and some Arab countries in which it has traditionally been practiced. It is illegal in many North American and European countries that have sizable immigrant populations. The United States and Great Britain have laws forbidding parents from taking girls to another country for the purpose of having an FGM procedure performed. Grassroots organizations in many countries combat FGM by providing education about its dangers to parents and village elders. Nevertheless, FGM persists, even in countries in which it is illegal. Entrenched cultural values and practices are exceedingly difficult to change and can only be changed from within a given society. In time, FGM will no doubt go the way of foot-binding in China, but until it does, nurses must respond appropriately and professionally to women who have been subjected to it (Turner, 2007).

Responding Appropriately to Circumcised Women

It is estimated that as many as 140,000 women worldwide have had an FGM procedure (Shah et al., 2009). Given the increasingly multicultural nature of American society, it is likely that nurses who provide physical care to female patients will encounter women and/or girls whose genitalia have been surgically altered. Nurses must be prepared for this eventuality and refrain from behavior that may insult or alienate the patient. Exhibiting shock, revulsion, or pity at the sight of altered genitalia, for example, is inappropriate. Nurses must also understand that women brought up in cultures in which FGM is a fact of life may not consider themselves to have been mutilated or victimized. In fact, such a woman may be offended if her nurse uses the term *mutilation* or expresses disapproval of genital alteration. If a woman shares her indecision regarding some aspect of FGM, for example, whether to be sewn up again after delivery, the nurse should listen nonjudgmentally.

FOCUS YOUR STUDY

- The number of women living in poverty is increasing. Childbearing women seem to be at particular risk because of current trends in the divorce rate, the frequency with which the mother gains custody of children, and factors in the work environment that make it difficult for women to earn an adequate wage.
- The number of homeless families is increasing.
- Women's wages have always been lower than men's because of demand, education, skills, discrimination, and underlying philosophies that deem women's work less valuable. Many people are working to change the wage system by pushing for comparable worth legislation.
- Employee benefits that affect women include maternity leave, paternity leave, and child care. The Family and Medical Leave Act mandates parental leave for childbirth or adoption but applies only to companies with 50 or more employees. Insurance coverage for childbirth varies by company.
- Elder abuse includes physical abuse, financial abuse, neglect, self-neglect, psychologic abuse, and abandonment.
- Older women may face multiple barriers when obtaining health care, including transportation difficulties; lack of health coverage; lack of research regarding chronic conditions affecting women; and symptom-specific, rather than holistic, care.
- There are multiple types of disabilities. All have the potential for limiting a woman's quality of life, her ability to care for herself, and the quality of her health care.
- Lesbian and bisexual women face various forms of discrimination, some of which can negatively affect their health and health care.
- Nurses must provide culturally sensitive care to women who have undergone procedures involving genital mutilation.

CRITICAL THINKING IN ACTION

DOMESTIC VIOLENCE IN THE ELDERLY

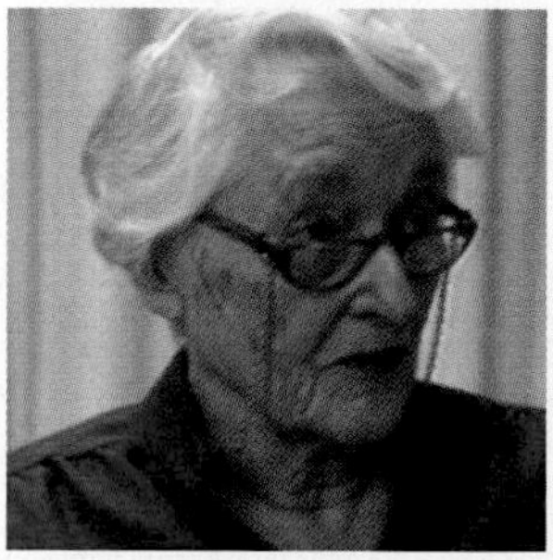

Grace Abbey, an 83-year-old woman, presents for irregular bleeding to the gynecologist. Mrs. Abbey, a widow, has been living with her son, a 54-year-old unemployed retail manager, for the last 2 years since her husband died. Her son accompanies her to the visit and is reluctant to leave his mother's side. You ask the son to wait in the waiting room and begin your assessment of Mrs. Abbey. When you roll up her sleeve to take her blood pressure, you note bruises on her wrist and forearm. When you question her about the etiology of the bruises, she looks down at the floor and avoids making eye contact. She then states she cannot remember how the bruises occurred. After obtaining her vital signs, you escort her into the exam room and note additional bruises on her back as you assist her with her gown. When you question her about those bruises, she breaks down sobbing, saying. "Don't say anything. Don't tell my son you saw them."

1. Discuss how you would assess Mrs. Abbey for other forms of elder abuse.
2. Mrs. Abbey describes physical violence that started occurring after her son lost his job and his wife left him. She admits. "I have been more trouble with my health problems lately." What factors can increase the risk of elder abuse?
3. Mrs. Abbey begins crying and says, "I know this has never happened to anyone else. I don't understand why this is happening." What is your reply?

See www.nursing.pearsonhighered.com for possible responses.

Pearson Nursing Student Resources

Find additional review materials at

www.nursing.pearsonhighered.com

Prepare for success with additional NCLEX®-style practice questions, interactive assignments and activities, Web links, animations and videos, and more!

REFERENCES

American Academy of Allergy, Asthma and Immunology. (2009). *Allergy statistics.* Retrieved from http://www.aaaai.org/media/statistics/allergy-statistics.asp#latex_allergy

American Academy of Pediatrics (AAP). (2009). Technical report: Coparent or second-parent adoption by same-sex parents. *AAP Policy Statement, 109*(2), 341–344.

American Association of University Women (AAUW). (2009). *The paycheck fairness act.* Retrieved from http://www.aauw.org/advocacy/issue_advocacy/actionpages/paycheckfairness.cfm

American College of Obstetricians and Gynecologists (ACOG). (2008). *Legal status: Health impact for lesbian couples.* ACOG Committee Opinion No. 428. Washington, DC: Author.

American College of Obstetricians and Gynecologists (ACOG). (2009). *Same-sex couples and their families should have same legal protections and benefits as married heterosexuals.* Retrieved from http://www.acog.org/from_home/publications/press_releases/nr01-23-09.cfm

Association of Retarded Citizens (ARC). (2010). *People with intellectual disabilities and sexual violence.* Retrieved from http://www.thearc.org/NetCommunity/Document.Doc?&id=155

Australian Family & Disability Studies Research Collaboration. (2007). *Understanding and planning support: A collaborative approach to assessing parents' support needs.* Retrieved from http://www.afdsrc.org/parents/completed/support.php#ss19

BabyCenter.com. (2009). *How much you'll spend on childcare.* Retrieved from http://www.babycenter.com/0_how-much-youll-spend-on-childcare_1199776.bc

Bankruptcy Action Coalition. (2009). *Bankruptcy statistics.* Retrieved from http://www.bankruptcyaction.com/USbankstats.htm

Barnes, P., Bloom, B., & Nahin, R. (2008). Complementary and alternative medicine use among adults and children: United States, 2007. *National Health Statistics Reports, 12*(10), 1–18.

Bloom, K. C., Bednarzk, M. S., Devitt, D. L., Renault, R. A., Teaman, V., Loock, D. M., et al. (2006). Barriers to prenatal care of homeless pregnant women. *Journal of Obstetric, Gynecologic, and Neonatal Nursing, 33*(4), 428–435.

Burgen, C. (2010). *Policy research brief.* Retrieved from http://ici.umn.edu/products/prb/172/default.html

Centers for Disease Control and Prevention (CDC). (2009a). *Disability and health.* Retrieved from http://www.cdc.gov/ncbddd/dh/disabilityprevalence.htm

Centers for Disease Control and Prevention (CDC). (2009b). *Faststats: Unmarried childbearing.* Retrieved from http://www.cdc.gov/nchs/FASTATS/unmarry.htm

Centers for Disease Control and Prevention (CDC). (2009c). *Faststats: Disabilities or limitations.* Retrieved from http://www.cdc.gov/omhd/Populations/Disability/Disability.htm

Centers for Disease Control and Prevention (CDC). (2010). *Women and disabilities.* Retrieved from http://www.cdc.gov/ncbddd/women/default.htm

Christy, L. (2009, January 23). *Flood of foreclosures: It's worse than you think.* Retrieved from http://money.cnn.com/2009/01/21/real_estate/ghost_inventory/

CNN Politics. (2009). *Same-sex marriage rights a step closer in District of Columbia.* Retrieved from http://cnn.site.printthis.clickability.com/pt/cpt?action=cpt&title=Same-sex-marriage+rights/a/step+

Department of Health and Human Services (DHHS). (2009). *Women's health, USA 2008.* Retrieved from http://mchb.hrsa.gov/whusa08/popchar/pages/104wp.html

Dey, J. G., & Hill, C. (2008). *Behind the pay gap.* Washington, DC: American Association of University Women Educational Foundation.

Eastgate, G. (2008). Sexual health for people with intellectual disability. *Salud Publica de Mexico, 50*(2), s255–s259.

Eco Child's Play. (2009). *Rubber duckies cause lower sperm count.* Retrieved from http://ecochildsplay.com/2009/01/30/rubber-duckies-cause-lower-sperm-count/

Employee Benefit Research Institute. (2007). Retirement trends in the United States over the past quarter century. Retrieved from http://www.ebri.org/pdf/publications/facts/0607fact.pdf

Employee Benefit Research Institute, (2010). Income And benefits: Health insurance coverage. Retrieved from http://www.ebri.org/pdf/FFE152.27Jan10.Final.pdf

Falk, G. (2006). *Temporary assistance for needy families (TANF) block grant: FY 2007 budget proposals. Congressional Research Service Report for Congress.* Washington, DC: Library of Congress.

Frost, J. J., Finer, L. B., & Tapales, A. (2008). The impact of publicly funded family planning clinic services on unintended pregnancies and government cost savings. *Journal of Health Care for the Poor and Underserved, 19*(3), 778–796.

Gabbe, S. G., Simpson, J. L., Niebyl, J. R., Galan, H., Goetzl, L. Jauniaux, E. R. M., et al. (2008). *Obstetrics: Normal and problem pregnancies* (5th ed.). Philadelphia, PA: Churchhill Livingstone.

Institute for Women's Policy Research. (2009). *Women's economic status of the states: Wide disparities by race, ethnicity, and region.* Retrieved from http://www.iwpr.org/states2004/index.htm

Johnson, R. (2008). *Hate crimes and sexual orientation.* Retrieved from http://gaylife.about.com/od/hatecrimes/a/statistics.htm

Lambda Legal Defense Fund. (2009). *Partial summary of domestic partner benefit legislation.* Retrieved from http://www.lambdalegal.org/our-work/issues/marriage-relationships-family/same-sex-relationships/details-about-domestic.html

McIntosh, J., & Chisholm, R. (2008). Cautionary notes on the shared care of children in conflicted parental separation. *Journal of Family Studies, 14*(1), 37–52.

MedlinePlus. (2009). *Asthma in children.* Retrieved from http://www.nlm.nih.gov/medlineplus/asthmainchildren.html

Morse, S. B., Zheng, H., Tang, Y., & Roth, J. (2009) Early school age outcomes of late preterm infants. *Pediatrics, 123(4)*, e622–e629.

National Association of Child Care Resource & Referral (NACCRRA). (2009). *Child care in America.* Retrieved from www.naccrra.org/news/facts-and-figures

National Center on Birth Defects and Developmental Disabilities (NCBDDD). (2009). *Women with disabilities.* Retrieved from http://www.cdc.gov/ncbddd/women/links/ctrresearch.htm

National Center on Elder Abuse (NCEA). (2009). *What is abuse?* Retrieved from http://www.ncea.aoa.gov/ncearoot/Main_Site/pdf/publication/NCEA_WhatIsAbuse.doc

National Coalition for Pesticide-Free Lawns. (2009). *Pesticide alert.* Retrieved from http://www.beyondpesticides.org/lawn/factsheets/30health.pdf

National Coalition for the Homeless. (2008). *How many people experience homelessness?* Retrieved from http://www.nationalhomeless.org/factsheets/How-Many.html

National Institute for Early Education Research. (2009). *Economics of early education: Benefits & costs of quality early childhood education.* Retrieved from http://nieer.org/docs/index.php?DocID=151

National Law Center on Homelessness & Poverty, 2010). Federal plan to end homelessness released. Retrieved from http://www.nlchp.org/news.cfm?id=1

National Resource Center for Family-Centered Practice & Permanency Planning. (2009). *All children deserve a permanent home: Subsidized guardianship as a common sense solution for children in long-term foster care.* Retrieved from http://www.hunter.cuny.edu/socwork/nrcfcpp/info_services/guardianship.html

National Women's Health Information Center. (2009a). *Illness and disabilities.* Retrieved from http://www.4women.gov/WWD

O'Connor, M. (2008). Restructuring the hymen: Mutilation or restoration? *Journal of Law and Medicine, 16*(1), 161–175.

Reinberg, S. (2008, August 26). Number of uninsured Americans drops. *US News & World Report.* Retrieved from http://health.usnews.com/articles/health/healthday/2008/08/26/number-of-uninsured-americans-drops.html

Shah, G., Susan, L., & Furcroy, J. (2009). Female circumcision: History, medical and psychological complications, and initiatives to eradicate the practice. *The Canadian Journal of Urology, 16*(2), 4576–4579.

Shulman, B. (2009, February 9). Respect low for part-time workers. *News Services.* Retrieved from http://www.ajc.com/hotjobs/content/printedition/2009/02/09/shulmaned0209.html

Skin Deep Cosmetic Safety Database. (2009). *Safety guide to cosmetics and personal care products.* Retrieved from http://www.cosmeticsdatabase.com/research/

State Health Department of Minnesota. (2008). *TANF grant guidelines.* Retrieved from http://www.health.state.mn.us/divs/fh/mch/fhv/admin/tanfgrantguide.pdf

Stillerman, K. P., Mattison, D. R., Giudice, L. C., & Woodruff, T. J. (2008). Environmental exposures and adverse pregnancy outcomes: A review of the literature. *Reproductive Sciences, 15*(7), 631–650.

Stitof, S., & Stitof, B. (2009). *Raising grandkids: A growing trend.* Retrieved from http://marriage.about.com/cs/grandparenting/a/raisinggrandkids.htm

Titlic, M., Josipovic-Jelic, Z., & Punda, A. (2008). Headache caused from pesticides: A review of the literature. *Acta Medica Coatica, 62*(2), 233–236.

Turner, D. (2007, August/September). Female genital cutting: Implications for nurses. *Nursing for Women's Health,* 367–372.

Tyson, A. S. (2007). *Sharp drop in gays discharged from military tied to war need.* Retrieved from http://www.washingtonpost.com/wp-dyn/content/article/2007/03/13/AR2007031301174.html

UNICEF. (2009). *Poverty facts and statistics.* Retrieved from http://www.globalissues.org/article/26/poverty-facts-and-stats

Urban Institute. (2010). *Children and youth.* Retrieved from http://www.urban.org/adolescents/index.cfm

U.S. Bureau of Census Bureau. (2008). USDL news release, Average Annual Pay by State and Industry, annual through 2000 data; 2002 Annual Wages for All Covered Workers by State; thereafter Employment and Wages, Annual Averages, 2007, Bulletin 2718. Source: Author: Washington, D.C.

United States Committee on Pay Equality. (2008). *U.S. current population survey.* Retrieved from http://www.pay-equity.org/PDFs/PayEquityFactSheet_May2008.pdf

U.S. Bureau of Labor Statistics. (2009). *Employment characteristics of families summary.* Retrieved from http://www.bls.gov/news.release/famee.nr0.htm

U.S. Bureau of Labor Statistics. (2009). *Occupational earnings tables: United States, December 2007—January 2009.* Retrieved from http://www.bls.gov/ncs/ncswage2008.htm#Wage_Tables

U.S. Census Bureau. (2007). *United States: Population 65 and over in the United States.* Retrieved from http://quickfacts.census.gov/qfd/states/00000.html

U.S. Department of Labor, Bureau of Labor Statistics. (2008). *Employment and earnings, 2008 annual averages and the monthly labor review, November 2007.* Retrieved from http://www.dol.gov/wb/stats/main.htm

U.S. Department of Labor, Bureau of Labor Statistics. (2009). *Quick stats on women workers.* Retrieved from http://www.dol.gov/wb/stats/main.htm

U.S. Equal Employment Opportunity Commission. (2006). *Pregnancy discrimination charges.* Retrieved from http://www.eeoc.gov/stats/pregnanc.html

Waldman, S. (2008, November 1). Women dentists and women with disabilities. *The Exceptional Parent,* 54–62.

Wilkinson, J. E., & Cerreto, M. C. (2008). Primary care for women with intellectual disabilities. *Journal of the American Board of Family Medicine, 21*(3), 215–222. doi:10.3122/jabfm.2008.03.070197

World Bank. (2009). *World Bank's poverty estimates.* Retrieved from http://www.globalissues.org/article/4/poverty-around-the-world#WorldBanksPovertyEstimatesRevised

CHAPTER 9

Violence Against Women

My friends believe I'm living the American dream. My husband has a great job in his company and our life looks ideal. Even if I told them about the occasional slap, the shove, the forced sex, and the angry words, they would probably think it was worth it. Sometimes I think about leaving, but it would mean admitting I failed. I know it doesn't make sense—he does the hitting, but I feel ashamed. I'm not a battered wife; I can't be. My husband just has a quick temper.

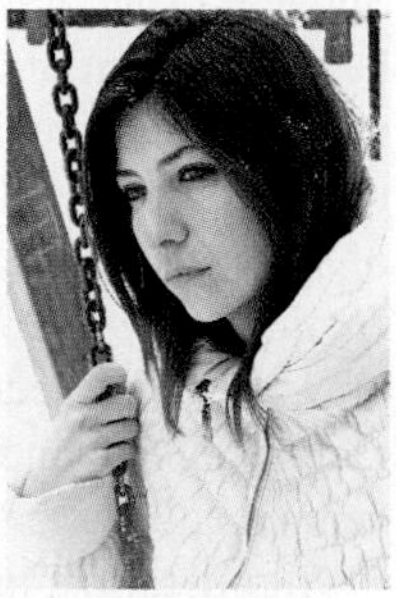

LEARNING OUTCOMES

1. Describe the social, psychologic, political, and cultural factors that contribute to the occurrence of domestic violence and sexual assault.
2. Identify factors that contribute to domestic violence.
3. Identify the phases of the cycle of violence.
4. Summarize the characteristics of batterers and perpetrators of sexual assault.
5. Delineate the role of the nurse in caring for women who have experienced partner abuse.
6. Specify physical and psychologic signs that may indicate a woman is in an abusive relationship.
7. Describe the needs that women with abusive partners and their children may have beyond the healthcare setting.
8. Identify the phases of the rape trauma syndrome.
9. Discuss the nurse's role as patient advocate with domestic violence and sexual assault survivors.
10. Summarize the procedures for collecting and preserving physical evidence of sexual assault.
11. Discuss the legal responsibilities of the community to prevent and address violence against women.

KEY TERMS

Acquaintance rape *178*
Cycle of violence *169*
Date rape *178*
Domestic violence *166*
Post-traumatic stress disorder (PTSD) *179*
Rape *176*
Rape trauma syndrome *178*
Sexual assault *176*

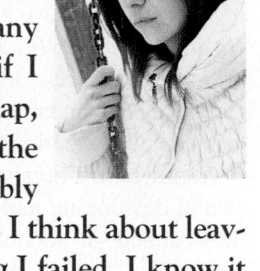

Violence against women has become endemic in society today. Experts suggest that as many as one in three women will be abused at some time in their lives. Violence affects women of all ages, races, ethnic backgrounds, and religions, from all socioeconomic levels, all educational levels, and all walks of life. Two of the most common forms of societal violence are domestic violence (also called *intimate partner violence (IPV)* or *relationship violence*) and sexual assault, the topics of this chapter. Perhaps surprisingly, these two types of violence are primarily perpetrated by intimate partners or persons known to the victim. Further, evidence indicates that a significant proportion of all female homicide victims are killed by their intimate partners. For example, national statistics indicate that in 2007 24% of female homicide victims were murdered by a spouse or ex-spouse and an additional 21% were killed by a boyfriend or girlfriend. Specifically, 1640 females were killed by an intimate partner. It is somewhat encouraging to note that between 1993 and 2007 the total number of female homicide victims killed by an intimate partner decreased by 26% (Figure 9-1 ■) (Catalano, Smith, Snyder, et al., 2009).

Between 1993 and 2008 nonfatal violence against a female by an intimate partner declined 53% from a rate of 9.4 per 1000 females age 12 or older to 4.3 per 1000. Specifically, in 2008 nonfatal violence against women by an intimate partner resulted in 552,000 victimizations. Nevertheless, estimates suggest that fewer than half (49%) of acts of intimate partner violence against females are reported to police (Catalano et al., 2009). In addition to injuries sustained during violent episodes, physical, sexual, and psychologic violence are linked to a number of adverse physical and mental health outcomes. The estimated health-related costs of violence against women exceed $8.3 billion *annually* in the United States. This cost includes medical care, mental health services, and lost productivity (e.g., time away from work) (Centers for Disease Control and Prevention [CDC], 2006).

Individuals who are controlling of their partners are much more likely to be physically assaultive, sending partners for

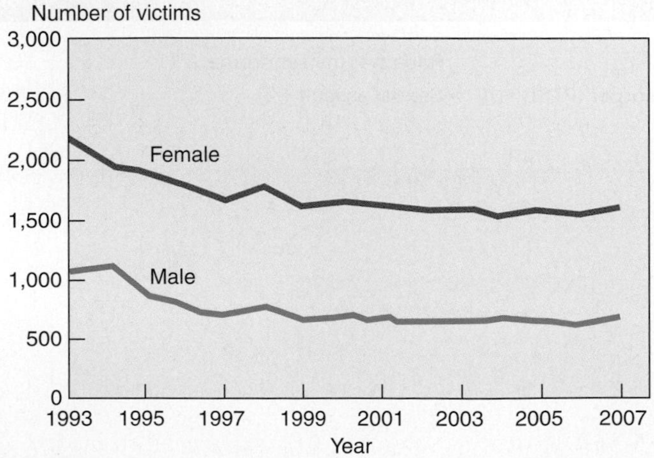

Figure 9-1 ■ Homicides of intimate partners by gender of victim, 1993–2007.

Source: Catalano, S., Smith, E., Snyder, H., & Rand, M. (2009). Female victims of violence. Bureau of Justice statistics: Selected findings. *Retrieved from http://bjs.ojp.usdoj.gov/content/pub/pdf/fw.pdf*

visits to emergency departments and often leading to future homicides (Felson & Outlaw, 2007). Healthcare providers can play a critical role in identifying and reducing violence, even in homicide prevention efforts.

Since the early 1980s healthcare providers and organizations have recognized the importance of their role and have worked to address this issue. Over the past three decades there have been a number of notable changes in healthcare policy and practices aimed at responding to violence against women. In 1985 the U.S. Surgeon General identified intimate partner violence as a public health problem of epidemic proportions. In 1990 the Joint Commission on Accreditation of Healthcare Organizations mandated the development of protocols for the identification and treatment of women who have been abused by their intimate partners. *Healthy People 2010*, a national health promotion and disease prevention project, identifies IPV as a problem crossing racial/ethnic boundaries and socioeconomic strata and cites intervention and prevention for violent behavior as a national priority.

Significantly, nursing has played and continues to play a key role in developing and evaluating innovative healthcare practices aimed at identifying and reducing violence against women. In 1991 the American Nurses Association (ANA) authored a position statement, which was revised in 2000, advocating education for all nurses in identifying and preventing violence against women, assessment of women for evidence of violence in community settings and healthcare institutions, and research on violence against women (ANA, 2002).

Historic Factors Contributing to Violence Against Women

Violence against women is not new. Throughout history, for thousands of years in patriarchal societies, women have been victims of violence. Within the institution of marriage, wives were considered the property of husbands, subject to their wishes and demands. A husband had the right—even the duty—to "keep her in line," to have sex on demand, even to kill her. Outsiders were expected to "keep out of it"; battering and sexual assault were family matters. The legal status of women has improved over the years in many cultures. However, many people still hold to the traditional views of male dominance in marriage or any intimate relationship, which can contribute to the occurrence of domestic violence and sexual assault.

Traditionally, rape outside of marriage was not viewed as an act of a man against a woman, but as an act of aggression against another man—the woman's husband, father, or brother, whoever was considered her "owner."

Worldwide, women today are at great risk. Violence against women and girls is increasingly being used as a weapon of war, stigmatizing, humiliating, and terrifying women and their families. And yet, according to the United Nations, it has been the least condemned war crime (Plan UK, 2007).

Domestic Violence

Domestic violence is defined as a pattern of coercive behaviors and methods used to gain and maintain power and control by one individual over another in an adult intimate relationship. This chapter focuses on domestic violence experienced by women in heterosexual relationships, although gay and lesbian individuals do experience domestic violence in their relationships as well. Among heterosexual couples, estimates indicate that in at least 95% of all domestic violence cases the perpetrators are men. Domestic violence occurs in relationships in which the partners are dating, living together, married, separated, or divorced.

Domestic violence is staggeringly common in the United States. In the United States, one in four women will experience domestic violence (CDC, 2008a). Forms of abuse vary but are typically described as falling into the following categories, which the batterer uses to maintain control over his partner's behavior and the relationship: psychologic abuse, physical abuse, sexual abuse, and threats of physical or sexual violence. In addition, stalking, a course of conduct directed at a specific person that would cause a reasonable person to feel fear, is another way that women with abusive partners are threatened.

Psychologic abuse includes a range of behaviors such as:

- ***Emotional abuse:*** putting her down, making her feel bad about herself, calling her names, negatively comparing her to other women, making unreasonable demands, using things that matter to her against her.
- ***Isolation:*** controlling who she sees and where she goes, using jealousy to justify restricting her actions, interfering with her job, forbidding her to see family and friends, limiting her outside involvement.
- ***Obfuscation:*** denying responsibility for his actions, blaming her, minimizing her concerns, distorting the truth, lying to her.
- ***Using others:*** using the children against her, using visitation to harass her, threatening to take the children away from her, using religion to control her.
- ***Male privilege:*** treating her like a servant, defining rigid men's and women's roles, making all of the decisions or rules in the household.
- ***Economic abuse:*** preventing her from getting or keeping a job, making her ask for money, controlling her money, destroying her property, making all the financial decisions.
- ***Coercion threats:*** making and/or carrying out threats to harm her or her family and friends, threatening to commit suicide, pressuring her to drop charges, threatening negative consequences if she does not cooperate with his wishes, pressuring her with gifts/promises/apologies.
- ***Intimidation:*** making her afraid through looks and gestures, smashing things, harming pets, displaying weapons, yelling, stalking her, driving recklessly.

Often, in addition to psychologic abuse, the batterer will use physical and sexual abuse to maintain power and control within the relationship. Physical abuse can include acts such as pushing, shoving, slapping, hitting the woman with a fist or object, kicking, choking, threatening with a gun or knife, or using a gun or knife against her. Sexual abuse occurs any time the batterer forces or tries to force sex (including vaginal, oral, or anal

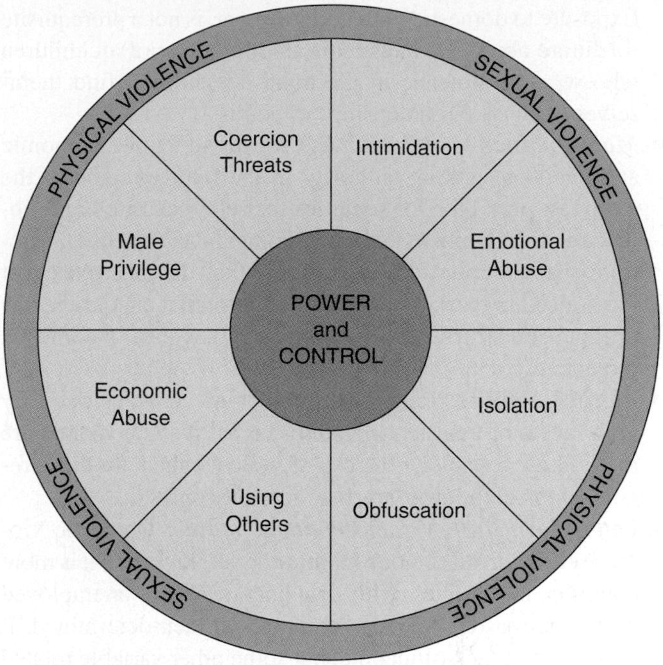

Figure 9-2 ■ The power and control wheel.

Source: Adapted from the Domestic Abuse Intervention Project, Duluth, Minnesota.

intercourse). It also includes the forced use of objects, or forcing a woman to have sex with someone else against her will. Figure 9-2 ■, the power and control wheel, illustrates how batterers use these tactics in relationships.

Typically these forms of abuse begin slowly and subtly after some form of commitment, such as engagement, onset of a sexual relationship, marriage, pregnancy, first childbirth, or first statement of commitment. Sometimes the woman will not recognize that she is in an abusive relationship.

The consequences of the abuse can be profound. In addition to the physical consequences, which are outlined later in this chapter, a woman may experience adverse psychologic consequences, such as symptoms of post-traumatic stress disorder, depression, antisocial behavior, anxiety, suicidal behavior, low self-esteem, and fear of intimacy. Women sometimes face social consequences as well, including restricted access to services, isolation from social networks, and strained relationships with health providers and employers (CDC, 2008a). Clearly it is important to understand the factors that contribute to domestic violence and the role of the nurse in caring for women who have experienced battering.

Contributing Factors

Domestic violence is a result of the complex and dynamic interaction of social, cultural, political, and psychologic factors. Although none of these factors alone is sufficient to explain why domestic violence occurs, there is substantial research to suggest that the following factors are significantly related to experiences of domestic violence.

- ***Childhood experiences:*** Children who witness or experience abuse and battering are more likely to become batterers (men) or to be abused (women) in their own relationships.

Exposure to domestic violence, however, is not a prerequisite for future abuse. Perhaps more importantly, not all children who witness violence in the home as children find themselves in abusive relationships as adults.

- *Male dominance in the family:* Worldwide, male economic and decision-making authority in the family is one of the strongest predictors of societies that demonstrate high violence against women, including domestic violence. This notion is also supported by research that demonstrates that men raised in patriarchal families (those that encourage traditional gender roles) are more likely to engage in domestic violence.
- *Marital conflict:* Relationships that are characterized by high levels of conflict, including verbal disagreements, are more likely to include the use of violence than are those relationships with lower levels of marital conflict.
- *Unemployment/low socioeconomic status:* Domestic violence occurs in all socioeconomic classes; however, it is more common in families with low incomes and unemployed men. The reasons for this have not yet been determined. It may not be a lack of income, but some other variable related to living in poverty—stress, frustration, feelings of inadequacy in filling the male role of provider, overcrowding, or a lack of community institutions and norms that would create quality community social interactions—that explains this relationship.
- *Traditional definitions of masculinity/hypermasculinity:* Cultures that link definitions of manhood to dominance, toughness, or male honor are more likely to demonstrate violence against women. This may result because socialization into traditional male norms includes telling young boys to be tough, not to shy away from violence, and to hide their feelings, particularly those that are associated with traditional notions of femininity.

Often healthcare providers view domestic violence as primarily a problem of younger women and believe that the violence decreases with age. Research indicates, however, that domestic violence does exist in older couples and that it will become an ever-increasing health problem as the population of baby boomers ages (Straka, 2006).

Common Myths About Battering and Women with Abusive Partners

Both professionals and the public believe numerous myths about battering and about women with abusive partners. These myths often reinforce misunderstanding of battering, furthering a woman's sense of victimization. Nurses need to recognize and counteract these myths. Some commonly accepted myths are discussed here.

Application: Domestic Violence

- *Battering occurs in a small percentage of the population:* The statistics on reported cases underrepresent the true incidence. As many as 1 in 3 women may be the victim of assault by her partner in her lifetime; however, it is estimated that only 1 in 10 women will report battering assaults.
- *Women who are abused provoke men to beat them; women push men beyond the breaking point and incite physical violence:* It is important to recognize that people are individually responsible for their own behavior. Batterers become violent because of their own internal inadequacies, not because of what their partners did or did not do.
- *Alcohol and drug abuse cause battering:* Studies do show a relationship between battering incidents and alcohol or drug use by batterers, and many batterers have a history of alcoholism or drug addiction. However, claims that substance abuse *causes* domestic violence are false and only serve to shift the responsibility away from the batterer. Some researchers suggest that batterers use alcohol as an excuse to carry out a violent act and shift the blame from themselves to the alcohol. Others suggest that alcohol or drugs reduce the batterer's inhibitions, increasing the likelihood of violent acts. Battered women sometimes think that the abuse will stop if their partners stop drinking or using drugs. Unfortunately, this usually does not happen.
- *Battered women can easily leave the situation:* Leaving is easier said than done. Society encourages women to take greater responsibility for their marriages and children. In addition, battered women may still love their partners or husbands and believe the promises of change, rely on them for financial support, and feel their children need a father. Women with physically abusive partners nearly always experience psychologic abuse as well and have been told repeatedly by their batterers that the family's problems are their fault. They often are isolated by their abuser from family, friends, and agencies that could assist them. Women may also experience a lack of support from family members, friends, and their religious community. Others may not believe the woman's accounts or blame her for the violence she experiences. Many women with children have no place to go, and shelters sometimes have long waiting lists. Moreover, battered women are at greatest risk for injury or domestic homicide when they leave the abuser. A woman may fear for her safety, her children's safety, and the safety of those who help her.
- *Domestic violence is a low-income or minority issue:* Domestic violence occurs among all sectors of society. It happens to women of all socioeconomic statuses, races, ethnicities, and religious faiths. It is true that lower income women are more likely to seek assistance from public agencies, such as hospitals and emergency departments, because they have fewer private resources than women with greater incomes do. Therefore, they are more likely to be counted in various reporting statistics.
- *Battered women will be safer when they are pregnant:* Battering may occur for the first time during pregnancy or may escalate in intensity if the woman is already being abused. The injury is frequently aimed at the breasts, abdomen, or vagina. Many researchers and advocates believe that batterers are threatened by a pregnancy because the fetus interferes with the abuser's ability to maintain power and control within the relationship. Pregnancy is often a time during which a woman receives extra attention from family, friends, and healthcare providers. The intensified violence that some women experience merits serious attention.

> "Miles hit me for the first time when I was 5 months pregnant. I was stunned. My father never laid a hand on my mother or any of us. Women who stayed in abusive situations had always appalled me but suddenly I found myself making excuses for him and rationalizing that he hadn't meant it, that he would never do it again. Three months later he shoved me so hard I fell against an end table. I was pretty bruised, but I didn't go into labor. Somehow I found the courage to call my dad. He came and got me that night. My baby is 3 months old now and Miles keeps calling, telling me how sorry he is and that he loves me. Oh, how I want to believe him when he says he is changed, but I just can't take the chance."

Cycle of Violence

Walker (1984), in an effort to better explain the experience of battered women, developed the theory of the **cycle of violence**, which postulates that battering takes place in a cyclic fashion through three phases.

1. In the *tension-building phase,* the batterer demonstrates power and control. This phase is characterized by anger, arguing, blaming the woman for external problems, and possibly minor battering incidents. As the stress builds and communications break down, the woman often senses growing danger. She may also blame herself for the battering and believe she can prevent the escalation of the batterer's anger by her own actions, hoping that the relationship will somehow change for the better. The length of this phase varies considerably across individual cases, ranging from weeks to years.
2. The *acute battering incident* is typically triggered by some external event or internal state of the batterer. It is an episode of acute violence distinguished by lack of predictability and major destructiveness. The batterer blames the woman for the abuse, and the woman may accommodate him in order to survive, believe that escape is futile, or escape and return when the crisis is over. This is generally the briefest of the three phases, lasting from a few hours to a few days.
3. The *tranquil phase* is also sometimes called the *honeymoon period.* This phase may be characterized by extremely loving, kind, and contrite behaviors by the batterer as he tries to make up with the woman, or it may simply be manifested by an absence of tension and violence. The couple or family is often relieved that the crisis is past, and the woman may accept the batterer's promises and gifts because she is worn down and wants to believe that the violence will not happen again. Without intervention this phase will end at some point, and the cycle of violence will repeat. Over time, the cycle of violence often increases in severity and frequency.

Characteristics of Batterers

Batterers come from all racial, ethnic, and religious groups and all professions, occupations, and socioeconomic strata. They may have only a sixth-grade education or hold a doctorate. What they have in common are feelings of insecurity, inferiority, powerlessness, and helplessness that conflict with their assumptions of male supremacy. Because they tend to be emotionally immature and aggressive, they have a tendency to express their overwhelming feelings of inadequacy through violence.

Many batterers feel undeserving of their partners, yet they blame and punish the very person they value. Extreme jealousy and possessiveness are the hallmarks of abusers. They characteristically express their ambivalence by alternating episodes of unmerciful beatings with periods of remorse and loving attention. Extremes in behavior and overreacting are typical patterns.

Batterers may be very calculating and select a partner they feel may be vulnerable. Over time they slowly and purposefully isolate the woman, creating a situation of increased dependence.

Women often describe their abusive husbands or partners as lacking respect toward women in general, having come from homes where they have witnessed abuse of their mothers or were themselves abused as children, and having a hidden rage that erupts occasionally. Batterers accept conventional "macho" values, yet when they are not angry or aggressive, they may appear childlike, dependent, seductive, manipulative, and in need of nurturing. They may be well respected in the community. This is important because it is one of the reasons why women are sometimes not believed or taken seriously when they seek support and assistance from friends, family members, and other resources. This dual personality of batterers reflects the conflict between their belief that they must live up to their macho image and their feelings of inadequacy and insecurity in the role of husband or provider. Combined with low tolerance for frustration and poor impulse control, the batterers' pervasive sense of powerlessness leads them to strike out at life's inequities by abusing women.

Care Plan Activity: Suspicious Injury and Bruises

NURSING CARE MANAGEMENT

Increased publicity, public sensitivity, and heightened awareness of domestic violence are encouraging women with abusive partners to seek resources and community assistance. In the past decade, many communities have developed domestic violence programs, shelters, and resources for women with abusive partners. However, the needs of women who have been abused and their children are still insufficiently met.

Women in abusive relationships enter the healthcare system in many different settings. Nurses may see them in the physician's office with minor trauma or in the emergency department with multiple severe injuries. They are frequently seen in obstetric services because battering often begins or escalates during pregnancy. Nurses in psychiatric-mental health services frequently counsel women who have been battered, and community health nurses may find women reporting abuse during home visits. Universal screening is advocated as an effective approach to identify women in such situations, and nurses must recognize that being so identified requires both caring concern and follow-up practices.

Nurses in many different healthcare settings often come in contact with women who have experienced abuse but fail to recognize them, especially if they have no visible injuries.

Nurses who wish to help battered women need advanced knowledge of the dynamics of battering; assessment skills for recognizing and documenting abuse; and appropriate intervention skills in counseling, safety planning, and referral.

Working with women who have been abused is sometimes frustrating, and many healthcare providers feel puzzled when women return to their abusive situations. Nurses must realize that they cannot rescue women with abusive partners; women must decide on their own how to handle the situation, which is often incredibly complex and dangerous. Research has shown that women's risk for homicide and additional violence are greatest during separation or attempts at separation. The effective nurse provides women who have been abused with information that empowers them in decision making and provides critical assistance in safety planning for women and their children.

Nursing Assessment and Diagnosis

Domestic violence is very prevalent and yet frequently remains unidentified by healthcare providers. Though experts and caregivers now advocate universal screening of all female patients at every healthcare encounter, impediments to universal screening range from a lack of institutional or organizational support to the attitudes of individual nurses.

A majority of the reasons cited by nurses indicate a lack of education about domestic violence in general and a lack of confidence in their own skills specific to domestic violence intervention. This fact underscores the importance of and need for comprehensive domestic violence education and training for healthcare providers, a policy recommendation that was affirmed by the 2000 National Violence Against Women (NVAW) Survey and the ANA Position Statement on Physical Violence Against Women (ANA, 2000). In addition to factual information about domestic violence and its impact on women's physical, psychologic, and sexual health, comprehensive education and training should include opportunities to practice skill development (e.g., in screening, assessment, empathic listening, diagnosis, planning, and communication across diverse age and ethnic/cultural groups) as well as opportunities to explore one's personal responses, attitudes, and values related to abuse.

Nurses may also be hesitant to ask because they presume the woman may be offended by the questions. However, women are rarely offended by questions about abuse, particularly if prefaced by a statement such as, "Because violence is so common in many people's lives, I've begun routinely asking all the women I care for about it." Showing knowledge about and familiarity with the issue of domestic violence not only increases a nurse's effectiveness in identifying women who have experienced abuse, but also fulfills an important health education function for women who have not experienced abuse.

Four basic screening questions, identified in Figure 9-3 ■, are useful in identifying women who are experiencing abuse. If a woman responds affirmatively to the questions, she is asked to mark the area(s) of injury on the body map. Screening for women experiencing domestic violence must be done privately, with only the nurse and patient present, in a safe and quiet place (Figure 9-4 ■). The nurse needs to reassure the woman that her responses will be kept confidential. The nurse should also strive for a calm and reassuring tone. Although tone, body language, and other nonverbal signs are important in establishing trusting relationships with all women, nurses should be especially aware of these issues in interventions with women from cultural and linguistic minority groups. Women from cultural and linguistic minority groups are often sensitized to these cues because they have used them as a survival strategy against discrimination and prejudice.

A number of signs that may not be related to a woman's presenting injuries can indicate the possibility that a woman is in a violent relationship. Although no single one of these signs necessarily indicates abuse, the occurrence of several of these signs certainly merits an at-risk diagnosis. Nurses must exercise their professional judgment and communicate their conclusions to their patients. Signs that may indicate a woman is in an abusive relationship include the following:

- ***Neurologic signs:*** Headaches, including headache following trauma or concussion, tension headache, and migraines; dizziness; paresthesias; unexplained stroke from strangulation; hearing loss; detached retina
- ***Gynecologic signs:*** Dyspareunia (painful intercourse), sexually transmitted infections (STIs), frequent vaginal infections, sexual dysfunction, menstrual disorders, pelvic pain
- ***Obstetric signs:*** Late onset of prenatal care, premature labor, low-birth-weight infant, excessive concern over fetal well-being, recurrent therapeutic abortion, recurrent spontaneous abortion
- ***Gastrointestinal signs:*** Dyspepsia, irritable bowel syndrome, globus (sensation of a lump in the throat)
- ***Musculoskeletal signs:*** Arthralgias (painful joints), chronic pain, osteoarthritis, fibromyalgia
- ***Psychiatric signs:*** Anxiety, panic, post-traumatic stress disorder, mood disorders, depression, suicide attempts, somatization, eating disorders, substance abuse, child abuse and neglect
- ***Constitutional signs:*** Fatigue, weight loss, weight gain, multiple somatic complaints, contusions, abrasions, sleep and appetite disturbances, decreased concentration, frequent use of pain medication or tranquilizers
- ***Trauma:*** Any injury to the female organs, extensive accident history, old fractures, sexual trauma
- ***Other signs:*** History of missed appointments or frequently changed appointments; low self-esteem, as seen in the woman's dress, her appearance, and the way she relates to healthcare providers

When a woman seeks care for an injury, the nurse should be alert to the following cues of abuse:

- Hesitation in providing detailed information about the injury and how it occurred
- Inappropriate affect for the situation
- Defensive injuries
- Delayed reporting of symptoms or of seeking care for injuries
- Pattern of injury consistent with abuse, including multiple injury sites involving bruises, abrasions, or contusions to the head (eyes and back of neck), throat, chest, breast, abdomen, or genitals (Nonbattered women's injuries are usually lo-

Abuse Assessment Screen

Universal Screening is recommended for all women during ED visits, Hospital admission, Prenatal visits, Routine PE and GYN screening, and Well Child visits of children to their pediatricians.

Note: Some agencies have nurses and/or physicians verbally ask questions, others include them in a written health questionnaire given to all patients, and others do both.

INTRODUCTION AND QUESTIONS:

Because violence is so common in many people's lives, I've begun to ask all my patients about it routinely:

1. **WITHIN THE LAST YEAR**, have you been hit, slapped, kicked, or otherwise physically hurt by someone? YES NO

   If YES, by whom? ________

   Total number of times ______

2. **SINCE YOU'VE BEEN PREGNANT**, have you been hit, slapped, kicked, or otherwise physically hurt by someone? YES NO

   If YES, by whom? ________

   Total number of times ______

MARK THE AREA OF INJURY ON THE BODY MAP
SCORE EACH INCIDENT ACCORDING TO THE FOLLOWING SCALE

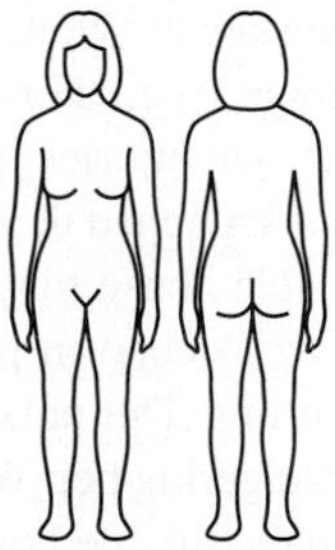

	SCORE
1 = Threats of abuse including use of a weapon	______
2 = Slapping, pushing; no injuries and/or lasting pain	______
3 = Punching, kicking, bruises, cuts, and/or continuing pain	______
4 = Beating up, severe contusions, burns, broken bones	______
5 = Head injury, internal injury, permanent injury	______
6 = Use of weapon; wound from weapon	______

If any of the descriptions for the higher number apply, use the higher number.

3. **WITHIN THE LAST YEAR**, has anyone forced you to have sexual activities? YES NO

   If YES, by whom? ________

   Total number of times ______

4. Are you afraid of anyone at home or an ex-partner? YES NO

Developed by the Nursing Research Consortium on Violence and Abuse.
Readers are encouraged to reproduce and use this assessment tool.

Figure 9-3 ■ Abuse assessment screen.

Source: Developed by the Nursing Research Consortium on Violence and Abuse. Reprinted from the Web site of the Nursing Network on Violence Against Women International (http://www.nnvawi.org).

cated at one or two sites and on the extremities, such as sprains and strains. Women in abusive relationships may have scars and evidence of old injuries that have healed.)

- Inappropriate explanation for the injuries, such as being "accident prone"
- Vague complaints without accompanying pathology
- Lack of eye contact
- Signs of increased anxiety in the presence of the possible batterer, who frequently does most of the talking or hovers around the woman

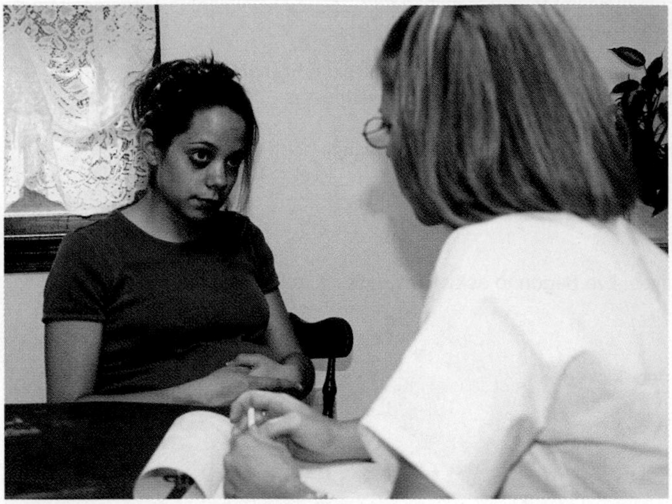

Figure 9-4 ■ Screening for domestic violence should be done privately.

Source: Al Dodge, Photographer.

As with the universal screening, if the nurse observes these potential cues, then the nurse should arrange for a private place in which the woman can feel safe. If a man is with the woman, the nurse should tell him to remain in the waiting room while the woman is examined. It is good practice to ask the same of family members or friends because it can be difficult for women in abusive relationships to talk candidly about their situation with others present. The nurse can encourage the woman to talk about her injuries and home situation by asking, "How did this happen to you?" or by saying, "We often see injuries like yours when a woman has been beaten. Has this happened to you?" Directly confronting the injuries and possible abuse may provide an opening for the woman who is trying to cope in private. A woman may continue to deny her battering. The nurse should encourage her to talk but should avoid badgering her. When culturally appropriate, it is important to maintain eye contact and avoid excessive note taking. The nurse should assure the woman that her privacy will be respected. It is essential that the nurse remains nonjudgmental; creates a warm, caring climate conducive to sharing; and demonstrates a willingness to talk about violence. A woman will often interpret the nurse's willingness to discuss violence as permission for her to discuss it as well.

> “No one had ever asked me about my "injuries" until I was in the ER one night and the nurse asked me right out if I had been beaten. It gave me real hope to think that people might see what was happening to me.”

Assessment is a complex process. It is important for the nurse to gather information about the woman's history of abuse. Getting a sense of the pattern of abuse is key to determining the degree of danger she might face. The nurse can help the woman assess whether or not the cycle of violence is becoming more frequent or severe. Determining whether or not there are weapons in the home, and whether or not her batterer has used or threatened to use weapons might also be warranted. In cases of severe abuse, it is important for the nurse to address the connection between homicide and domestic violence. Finally, the nurse should ask about the presence of sexual abuse within the relationship, another factor that indicates severe abuse.

Equally important, however, the assessment of the woman who may be experiencing abuse should include information about her strengths and her support system. Strengths may include education, employment history, activities in the home, community involvement, and her ability to cope with past problems. The woman's support system may include her family, friends, neighbors, and community agencies or organizations. It is helpful to consider assessing a woman's strengths in a cultural context. If the nurse is aware of strong values that a particular cultural group holds, then he or she should look for opportunities to recognize and affirm those strengths as valuable.

> **CLINICAL TIP**
>
> In seeking ways to help a woman feel less helpless, consider actually recording a woman's strengths in her medical record and showing her that they are an official part of the record. This action lets her know that you believe that her strengths are as significant as any problems that were noted.

During the assessment phase, the nurse begins building a relationship with the woman based on trust, understanding, and advocacy. A woman may feel ashamed and embarrassed about her injuries and her situation. It is important to tell her the purpose of the assessment and to communicate what level of confidentiality she can expect. Clearly, nurses need to be informed about the confidentiality policies of the organization where they work and aware of any mandatory reporting policies that exist. Trust begins as the nurse conveys an attitude of unconditional acceptance, empathy, and positive regard for the woman's worth and dignity. Nurses should show that they recognize the woman's feelings and accept her right to feel as she does.

In cases in which the woman states she has been beaten, kicked, punched, or attacked but does not identify the assailant, the nurse should record the extent of injuries (e.g., size, shape, color, where they are located on her body), note the woman's exact words, and describe the incident with a diagnosis of probable battering. Full documentation of specific information is critical, because the nurse might be called to testify in court or the medical records might be subpoenaed as evidence in legal proceedings such as custody disputes, stay-away/restraining orders, or other civil or criminal proceedings. Moreover, documenting the abuse works to ensure a woman's continuity of care. Those cases in which the woman states she was beaten by a husband or partner may be diagnosed as battering with all evidence recorded, including the woman's statements. In both cases, taking photographs of the injuries can be of great value. However, to further protect the woman's confidentiality and safety, it is critical that the nurse or other medical personnel do not refer to domestic violence or abuse on any discharge papers.

When abuse or battering is suspected or determined, the nurse should formulate nursing diagnoses based on the assessment findings. Nursing diagnoses related to nonphysical components of abuse or battering may include the following:

- ***Risk for powerlessness*** related to feelings of worthlessness secondary to ongoing psychologic partner abuse.
- ***Readiness for enhanced knowledge:*** Information about community resources to assist battered women related to an expressed desire to learn about alternatives to remaining in an abusive situation.

Nursing Plan and Implementation

A woman who is experiencing abuse needs to reestablish a feeling of control over her world. She needs to regain a sense of predictability by knowing what to expect from her disclosure. The nurse should provide sufficient information about what to expect in terms the woman can understand. Simple explanations about how long she will stay, whom she will see, and what will be done are important. Giving the woman control can be accomplished by asking her permission before any activities or procedures and by providing her with choices whenever possible.

Supportive counseling and reassurance are professional skills nurses use throughout each phase of the nursing process with a battered woman. The nurse should do the following:

- Acknowledge and support the woman for discussing her situation. Reporting abuse is a risk.
- Let the woman work through her story, problems, and situation at her own pace.
- Let the woman know that she is believed and that her feelings are reasonable and normal.
- Anticipate her ambivalence in the love-hate relationship with the batterer. She knows he may be loving and contrite after the incident if she has been through the cycle of violence before.
- Respect the woman's capacity to change and grow when she is ready.
- Assist her in identifying specific problems, and support realistic ideas for reducing or eliminating those problems.
- Help clarify the woman's beliefs and myths; provide information to change her false beliefs.
- Stress that no one should be abused and that the abuse is not her fault.

The appropriate intervention is not to tell an abused woman what to do but to explore options and resources with her, allowing her to make her own decisions. Even advising or encouraging a woman to leave an abusive situation is not always in the woman's best interest; leaving the home is a major decision with long-lasting consequences. The woman may be economically unable to leave the situation, especially if she has young children. If the woman leaves and then later returns home, both husband and wife may become more frustrated, increasing the possibility of further beatings and even homicide. The most acceptable course of action is one that the woman freely chooses. It often takes many interventions before a woman gains enough courage and skill to leave an abusive situation.

DEVELOPING CULTURAL COMPETENCE

Cultural Factors Influencing Survivors of Violence

Providing nursing care to women who are from a different cultural community, who speak a different language, or who are immigrants can be challenging. This is especially true when providing care to women who are in abusive relationships. When assisting survivors from different cultural or linguistic backgrounds, consider the following:

- It is often difficult for women in certain cultural communities to seek help outside their families for a variety of reasons, ranging from cultural notions about the role of women, to fear of being ostracized within or isolated from her community, to a loss of social respect that includes her entire family (Tahirih Justice Center, 2009).
- Language can be a powerful barrier to effective communication. Patients with comparable needs require comparable service. Thus it is important to have bilingual nurses and personnel available and to translate assessment tools, such as those found in Figure 9-2 (The Joint Commission, 2008).
- Have information available about language-specific and culturally appropriate community resources, including legal services that specialize in family and immigration law, individual and family counseling services, and shelters with bilingual and bicultural staff.
- Immigrant women may have inaccurate perceptions of law enforcement and the legal system, either because of negative experiences with law enforcement in their country of origin or because of misinformation about the U.S. legal system from their abusers (Tahirih Justice Center, 2009).
- Abusers may threaten women with deportation if they seek help for the abuse. Women may be fearful of jeopardizing their financial or immigration status and that of their children, their family, or their abuser. For a more complete list of tactics used to control immigrant women experiencing domestic violence, see Table 9-1.
- Women in some cultures may have deeply held religious beliefs that conflict with standard legal remedies. It is vital to find creative remedies that do not ask a woman to choose between religious and spiritual convictions and much needed legal remedies (Tahirih Justice Center, 2009).
- Avoid cultural stereotyping—there are many subcultures and traditions within any cultural community. Create a safe space for the woman to share her needs, fears, and any cultural barriers that she must overcome.
- Educate yourself. Become aware of your own biases and stereotypes and make a commitment to learn about the practices of others from various minority communities.

Health Promotion Education

If the woman returns to an abusive situation, the nurse should encourage her to develop an exit, or safety, plan for herself and her children, if she has any. As part of the plan, she should pack a change of clothes for herself and the children, including toilet articles and an extra set of car and house keys. She should store these away from the house with a friend or neighbor and ask a neighbor to call the police if violence begins. If possible,

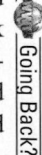

Going Back?

TABLE 9-1 Tactics Used to Control Immigrant Women in Abusive Relationships

Isolation	Keeping her isolated from family, friends, community and religious leaders, or people who speak her native language; not allowing her to learn English.
Threats	Threatening to report the victim to the U.S. Immigration and Naturalization Service (INS) or threatening to withdraw a petition to legalize immigration status. The abuser often threatens to seek sole custody of the children if the woman reports the abuse or attempts to leave.
Intimidation	Hiding or destroying important papers such as passports and green cards, documentation for the children; destroying her only property from the country of origin such as mementos or photographs.
Citizenship or Residency Privilege	Failing to file papers to legalize immigration status and/or withdrawing such papers altogether; lying to the woman that her immigration is legal.
Economic Abuse	Not letting her obtain job training, work, or schooling; threatening to report the victim for working "under the table"; taking money she wants to send abroad to family; forcing the woman to work illegally.
Emotional Abuse	Lying about immigration status; threatening to harm the children or other family members; calling her racist or abusive names.
Spiritual Abuse	Misusing religious teachings and/or personal beliefs and values.

Source: From Immigrant Victims of Domestic Violence, *National Coalition Against Domestic Violence (NCADV). Reprinted with permission.*

she should have money, identification papers (driver's license, social security cards), checkbook, bank account information, other financial records (such as mortgage papers, rent and utility receipts, automobile title, insurance policies and numbers), and information about the children to help her enroll them in school. She should also plan where she will go, regardless of the day or time. It is also helpful to identify friends and family who know about the situation and will help her. Ask that she establish a code word for danger with those family and friends. The nurse should ensure that the woman has a planned escape route and emergency telephone numbers she can call, including personal numbers, the local police, a phone hotline, and a women's shelter if one is available in the community.

National Coalition Against Domestic Violence

Community-Based Nursing Care

Besides offering emotional support, medical treatment, and counseling, the nurse should inform any woman who may be in an abusive situation of the services available in the hospital, through agencies, and in the community. The nurse can also provide the woman with the phone number of any local resources, as well as the number for the National Domestic Violence Hotline (1-800-799-SAFE).

Specifically, a woman who has been abused may need:

- Medical treatment for injuries
- Temporary shelter to provide a safe environment for herself and her children
- Legal assistance for protection or prosecution of the batterer
- Financial assistance to provide shelter, food, and clothing
- Job training or employment counseling
- Counseling to raise her self-esteem and help her understand the dynamics of domestic violence, or an ongoing support group for herself and her children

A network of community agencies can meet the numerous, varied needs of women, children, and batterers. It is important that employees in these agencies understand the complex dynamics of domestic violence as well as how their services and those of other agencies can assist women and their children. An overview of resources available to women with abusive partners and their children is presented in the following sections.

Emergency Department Services

Many women who are experiencing abuse are first seen and diagnosed in the emergency departments (EDs) of their neighborhood hospitals. ED nurses and personnel need to be alert to symptoms of battering, recognize these cues, and encourage women to seek assistance from community agencies. The most innovative and effective domestic violence programs in hospitals and urgent care facilities work collaboratively with domestic violence service agencies, develop a comprehensive community referral network, and work with multidisciplinary intervention teams. Some states require that suspected cases of abuse and battering be reported to the legal authorities or social service agencies. Domestic violence forensic examinations are now available at many large community hospitals, allowing for needed forensic gathering of evidence for possible future legal use by the survivor.

Shelter

Because domestic violence has been recognized as a major social problem, many community agencies have sought federal and state funds to provide shelters. These shelters differ in the services they provide, depending on the governing body, financial resources and funding agencies, organizational structure, staff qualifications, and range of available community services. Typical shelters provide women in abusive relationships and their children with a room, beds, food, clothing, and other basic necessities. If professional staff is available, the shelter may offer crisis counseling; individual and group counseling; and information about community agencies such as legal aid, welfare, job training, financial and employment agencies, and women's counseling or support groups.

For safety reasons, the location of most shelters is undisclosed, but they can be contacted through a community crisis line. Admission requirements vary from shelter to shelter, so it is wise for nurses to become familiar with all local shelters and other resources available in case one or more shelters are full and the woman and her children are in need of a safe place to stay.

Legal Services and Options

During incidents of domestic violence, the woman or her neighbors may summon the police. Domestic violence often occurs on the weekend or in late evening, when most social service agencies are closed; therefore, the police department is one of the first major agencies involved, in addition to those that provide medical services.

RESEARCH EVIDENCE IN PRACTICE Advocacy Interventions to Reduce Intimate Partner Violence Against Women

CLINICAL QUESTION

Are either brief or intensive advocacy interventions effective in reducing or stopping intimate partner abuse or its associated morbidity?

RESEARCH EVIDENCE

The World Health Organization estimates that between 10% and 50% of women worldwide report having been assaulted physically or sexually by an intimate partner at some time in their lives. This number escalates when emotional and financial abuse are included. Domestic violence affects the physical and mental well-being of its victims and often continues throughout pregnancy. Intimate partner abuse is one of the most common causes of non–fatal injury in women and makes up between a third and a half of all murders of women in the United States and Canada.

A variety of interventions have been proposed to prevent or alleviate intimate partner abuse. Advocacy interventions are considered secondary interventions, in that these efforts seek to prevent further abuse once it has begun. Advocacy interventions vary, but in general they aim to empower women and link them to community resources that might assist them in avoiding abuse. The core activities of advocacy are provision of legal, housing, and financial advice; facilitation of access to community resources such as refuges or shelters; and the provision of safety planning advice. Advocacy may be brief, such as that delivered in an emergency department, or more intensive, involving group and/or individual therapies over time. Advocacy interventions are based on the concept of empowerment and seek to help women make decisions and find solutions rather than directing or prescribing certain actions.

Trials involving more than 1500 women demonstrated evidence that intensive advocacy for women recruited into domestic violence shelters has a beneficial effect on the women's physical and psychosocial well-being. However, it does not appear that even intensive advocacy services are effective for women who continue to live with abusive partners. Brief advocacy may have a positive effect on reducing minor physical abuse in women in emergency settings or who present for antenatal care, but there is no evidence to suggest that brief interventions result in a reduction of more severe abuse. Neither appears to affect the long-term rate of depression or post-traumatic stress disorder, two common conditions that accompany intimate partner abuse.

WHAT QUESTIONS REMAIN UNANSWERED?

What interventions can be offered to the abusive partner that might alleviate the pattern of abuse? What advocacy interventions will help a woman take the step of leaving an abusive relationship?

WHAT IS BEST PRACTICE?

Intensive interventions to empower women to take advantage of community services such as refuges and shelters hold the most promise for ending a pattern of domestic violence. In the absence of intensive interventions, brief interventions in emergency settings can help reduce the effects of minor injuries.

CRITICAL THINKING

How are the effects of intimate partner violence detected in the clinic or emergency setting? How can intensive interventions be initiated in these settings?

References

Constantino, R., Kim Y., & Crane, P. (2005). Effects of a social support intervention on health outcomes in residents of a domestic violence shelter. *Issues in Mental Health Nursing, 26*, 575–590.

McFarlane, J., Groff, J., O'Brien, J., & Satson, K. (2006). Secondary prevention of intimate partner violence: A randomized controlled trial. *Nursing Research, 55*, 52–61.

Ramsay, J., Carter, Y., Davidson, L., Dunne, D., Eldridge, S., Hegarty, K., . . . Feder, G. (2009). Advocacy interventions to reduce or eliminate violence and promote the physical and psychosocial well-being of women who experience intimate partner abuse. *Cochrane Database of Systematic Reviews*. Issue 3. Art. No.: CD005043. doi: 10.1002/14651858.CD005043.pub2

PROFESSIONALISM IN PRACTICE

Legislative Advocacy

Patient advocacy is a nursing responsibility that extends beyond individual nurse-patient relationships. Nurses can follow and become involved in legislative advocacy for issues related to domestic violence and other issues related to women's health through participation in their local and state chapters of the American Nurses Association, by being aware of current issues, by following the progress of specific bills online, by writing to their legislators, and by exercising their right to vote.

Legal options for women with abusive partners vary according to state laws and services. In some states a woman may seek a restraining (or protective) order from the family court or a domestic relations court to protect herself from the batterer. This restraining/protective order specifies the type of contact, if any, allowed between the batterer and the victim. Unfortunately, many abusive men violate the restraining/protective order and continue to stalk, harass, intimidate, and abuse their female partners. The case then becomes a criminal matter. If the woman decides to prosecute, and if her case meets the legal requirements for an indictment, the case is usually heard in criminal court, which handles crimes of assault, harassment, and battery. Criminal court hearings may result in a fine, probation, or a jail sentence if the batterer is convicted, giving the man a criminal record. The prosecution process is often lengthy and may last more than a year. Some state judicial systems are introducing other options, such as mandatory counseling in a Batterer Intervention Program (BIP) in lieu of prosecution. Unfortunately, this counseling does not show great promise for permanent change. Divorce is another legal recourse a woman may choose, but divorce takes time and may cause added financial burdens for the woman.

Many women who are abused are unaware of their legal options. They fear further beatings if they prosecute the batterer. Limited financial resources may also keep them from seeking legal assistance. Some women report lack of sensitivity or awareness about domestic violence on the part of some members of the legal and criminal justice systems, further limiting their ability or willingness to seek help. Currently, some communities provide legal advocacy services to help women understand the judicial process, their options within that system, and the possible consequences for the woman, her children, and the batterer.

Financial Services
Once women who have been in battering relationships leave their homes or seek legal assistance, they usually receive no financial support from their batterers. Without funds, women and their children are at the mercy of community social service agencies, and it usually takes weeks for papers to be processed before any money is forthcoming. Agencies that may provide financial assistance include their county welfare department; federal programs (e.g., Temporary Assistance for Needy Families); the United Way; women's support groups; religious organizations; and, possibly, the Salvation Army. There may be other local groups who assist abused women in other ways, such as by providing food or clothing.

Employment Training or Placement
Some women who experience abuse are full-time mothers who may lack advanced education, training, and job experience. Minimal or out-of-date skills and inadequate transportation often make it difficult for these women to obtain employment with an adequate salary. Women who have children must consider where to place them during working hours as well as the added cost of child care. Often, the woman's choice is restricted to accepting welfare or taking a low-paying job. Either choice usually means lowering the standard of living to mere subsistence.

Some women do seek job training if the opportunities are available, but training provides no guarantee of future job placement. A woman may still have to arrange for financial support and child care while obtaining advanced employment skills or an education.

Counseling or Advocacy
Women who have experienced domestic violence may be offered a variety of counseling and advocacy services, such as crisis intervention, short-term individual therapy, group therapy, or peer support groups, over an extended period. Specially trained nurses, social workers, psychologists, mental health specialists, or clergy may provide counseling and therapy.

Evaluation

Expected outcomes of nursing care include the following:

- The woman receives compassionate, respectful, and individualized medical attention.
- The woman recovers from the physical effects of physical and sexual abuse.
- The woman has the information she needs to make a decision about her future based on thoughtful consideration of alternatives.
- The woman is able to identify culturally appropriate community resources available to her and develops strategies for keeping herself, her children, and her family as safe as possible.
- If the woman chooses to apply for a restraining order or to prosecute her assailant, all necessary documentation is recorded in her medical records, leading to a more successful prosecution.

Sexual Assault

Sexual assault is a broad term that refers to a variety of types of unwanted sexual touching or penetration without consent, from unwanted sexual contact or touching of an intimate part of another person to forced anal, oral, or genital penetration. Rape is, therefore, one type of sexual assault. Although the specific definition of rape varies from state to state, the Bureau of Justice Statistics (2009) defines it as follows: **Rape** is "forced sexual intercourse including both psychologic coercion as well as physical force. Forced sexual intercourse means vaginal, anal or oral penetration by the offender(s). This category also includes incidents where the penetration is from a foreign object such as a bottle" (p. 2). The rapist may be a stranger, acquaintance, spouse or other relative, or an employer. Rape is an act of violence expressed sexually—most commonly, a man's need for power and control acted out against a woman (Tjaden & Thoennes, 2006).

Sexual assault remains one of the most underreported violent crimes in the United States. The Rape, Abuse, and Incest National Network (RAINN) (2009) estimates that someone is sexually assaulted in the United States every 2 minutes. Research indicates that one in six American women over age 12 will be the victim of an attempted or completed sexual assault or rape in her lifetime (Tjaden & Thoennes, 2006). In 2008, 551,590 women were the victims of a reported rape or sexual assault; however, only an estimated 47% of incidents were reported to the police, making the actual number significantly higher (Catalano et al., 2009).

Reporting varies by the type of rape or sexual assault. Rapes and sexual assaults committed by strangers are more likely to be reported to the police than rapes and sexual assaults committed by "nonstrangers," including intimate partners, other relatives, and friends or acquaintances. Women injured during a rape incident are also much more likely to report it to the police. Much research suggests that only 2% to 20% of sexually victimized women report the incidents to the police (Thompson, Sitterle, Clay, et al., 2007; RAINN, 2009).

Although both men and women can be sexually assaulted, the National Crime Victimization Survey reported that 9 out of every 10 rape victims were female (RAINN, 2009). Sexual violence often occurs early in life. Over half (60.4%) of all female victims were first raped before age 18; of these, 25.5% occur before age 12 (CDC, 2008a). No woman of any age, cultural or ethnic background, or socioeconomic status is immune, but statistics indicate that young, unmarried women; women who are unemployed or have low family income; and students have the highest incidence of sexual assault or attempted assault.

Common Myths About Rape

As with domestic violence, many myths about rape exist. These myths can have a negative impact on women who are assaulted and can hinder their ability to receive optimum health care following their attack. Some of the most commonly cited myths include the following:

- ***Only certain types of women are raped:*** No woman is safe from a rape attempt. Women of all ages, races, ethnicities, classes, religious backgrounds, occupations, ability levels, sexual and gender identities, or appearances are raped; rape is a very "democratic" form of violence.

- ***Men rape women because that is men's nature and biologic role:*** Rape is not universal to all societies and not all men rape women. This suggests that rape is an act that can be encouraged or discouraged. Generally, violent societies that encourage aggression in boys and men tend to have more reports of sexual violence.
- ***Women who party hard, drink, and do drugs are setting themselves up to be sexually assaulted:*** No one asks for or deliberately "sets herself up" to be sexually violated. The misunderstanding that rape is about sex perpetrates this myth. Rape is sexual violence and a crime of power. Blaming the victim for the crime is not only inappropriate, it serves to excuse the behavior of the perpetrator. Because alcohol and drugs may affect judgment, feelings, and perceptions, as well as lower inhibitions, a woman may be in a more vulnerable position when she engages in these activities. However, it is not a crime to wear particular clothes, show naivete, use poor judgment, or even engage in reckless behavior. The victim's behavior before the crime is irrelevant.
- ***If a woman just relaxes, it will all be over with soon. She might even find it isn't so bad after all:*** Rape is an act of violence in which the perpetrator uses sex as a weapon to control, intimidate, and violate the victim. Rape involves persistent pressure, taking advantage of a person's inability to say "no"; calculated drugging with alcohol or other substances; and/or threats, sometimes against the woman's life, her livelihood, her academic career, even her family members and friends. Many survivors recall being in fear for their lives, even if a weapon was not present.
- ***Most rapes are interracial:*** The overwhelming majority of rapes and other sexual assaults involve people of the same racial background. Unfortunately, media reports and the entertainment industry tend to emphasize incidents that are interracial, which may encourage racist misconceptions in our society.
- ***A rapist is easy to spot in a crowd:*** There is no way to distinguish men who commit sexual assault from men who do not on the basis of race, ethnicity, socioeconomic status, educational level, or religious background. They can be large or small, able-bodied or disabled, married or single.
- ***Women lie about rape as an act of revenge or guilt:*** False rape charges are infrequent. According to the Federal Bureau of Investigation (FBI), false charges are reported at the same rate for rape as for other felonies; that is, about 2% to 6% of all rape reports. Furthermore, it is important to remember that simply because there is not enough evidence to prosecute, it *does not* mean the woman was lying.
- ***Fighting back incites a rapist to violence:*** Most assailants pick out potential victims they believe may be good targets without a fight. They may even test women nonverbally or verbally before determining whether or not to assault. Both verbal and physical resistance may actually lessen the severity of injury in some instances. Women who recognize that they have options for responding to their assailant are less likely to be paralyzed by fear and more likely to resist. Each incident is unique. Only the targeted person knows her abilities and can assess the assailant's behavior. Evaluating her options realistically may help the survivor understand that submission is also a viable form of self-protection.

Characteristics of Perpetrators

Like their victims, rapists come from all ethnic, racial, and religious backgrounds; socioeconomic statuses; educational levels; and professions. Clinicians and researchers who work with rapists, both convicted and not convicted, report that many rapists are married and engage in regular sexual relationships, both inside and outside of marriage. A substantial number of perpetrators are quite young. Most research studies indicate that sex offenders are often under the age of 18, while the largest number is between 18 and 25 years of age. Unfortunately, so few perpetrators are arrested and convicted that clear characterizations of assailants are not available.

Attitudes toward women do seem to influence who is likely to be a rapist and who is not, especially when it comes to believing that men have a right to sexual access of women. Perpetrators tend to be impulsive and have antisocial tendencies. They may prefer impersonal sex and feel hostility toward women. Additional individual risk factors for perpetration include being male, alcohol and drug use, having friends who are sexually aggressive, an emotionally unsupportive family environment, childhood history of witnessing or experiencing violence, and a belief in societal norms or shared beliefs that support male entitlement and sexual violence (CDC, 2009).

Parental Sexual Abuse

Types of Rape

Rape has been categorized in different ways, which are not mutually exclusive. Specifically, rape may be categorized according to the rapist's possible motives or purposes for the assault, according to the relationship between the victim and perpetrator, or according to the number of assailants.

- In *power rape,* the purpose of the assault is control or mastery. The assailant uses sexual intercourse to place a woman in a powerless position so that he can feel dominant, potent, and strong. He often believes that his victim enjoys the assault, and he exerts only the amount of force necessary to subdue his victim. Often power rape is a planned stranger attack, but most acquaintance rapes are also power rapes. The vast majority of all rapes are motivated by this need for power and control.
- In *anger rape,* the sexual assault is used to express feelings of rage and to retaliate for what the attacker perceives as wrongs against him. These perceived wrongs most often have nothing to do with the rape victim. Considerable brutality and degradation can characterize this type of rape. Attacks on older women often are a form of anger rape.
- In *sadistic rape,* the assailant has an antisocial personality and delights in torture and mutilation. In this type of rape, the victim and assailant are generally strangers, and the assault is planned. Sadistic rapes cause the most injuries, including homicide.

- In *stranger rape,* the assailant and victim are strangers, and the rape is often a blitz-style attack—sudden and unexpected. The rapist is more likely to use a weapon and threaten violence or murder.
- In **acquaintance rape** *or nonstranger rape,* the assailant is someone with whom the victim has had previous nonviolent interaction. The attacker uses deception and trust to gain access to the victim and then betrays that trust. Marital rape and date rape are included in this category. In **date rape**, the male has usually planned to have sex and will do what he feels is necessary if denied. Between 70% and 80% of rapes are committed by someone the victim knows—an acquaintance, a friend, a relative, a coworker, or an intimate partner (Victim Rights Law Center, 2009).
- In *gang rape,* the rape is used as a reinforcing mechanism for membership in a particular group of men (such as a street gang, fraternity, athletic team, or other known group). Often responding to peer pressure from the group leader, participation in the rape provides a means for individuals to demonstrate their power by forcing sex on a woman, thus proving their status in the group. Often gang rape can escalate to severe violence as the young men resort to mob mentality.

> “I always knew that rape was a terrifying experience physically but I never really thought about the horror that comes from being helpless and in someone else's control.”

Role of Substances in Sexual Assault

Application: Rohypnol

In some cases, a perpetrator uses alcohol or other drugs to sedate his intended victim—*alcohol or drug-facilitated sexual assault.* While alcohol is the most common and most easily obtained drug, flunitrazepam (Rohypnol), a potent sedative-hypnotic that is legal in 80 countries worldwide but illegal in the United States, has received considerable attention as the "date rape drug of choice" since the late 1990s. Typically Rohypnol, which dissolves easily and is odorless, is slipped into the drink of an unsuspecting woman. Gamma hydroxybutyrate (GHB), ketamine, MDMA (Ecstasy), clonazepam, and scopolamine have also been identified as date rape drugs that are used to incapacitate a woman. More recently, prescription drugs have been used in combination with alcohol to facilitate many sexual assaults. Because these drugs frequently produce amnesia, the woman may be unable to remember details of her assault, thereby making prosecution more difficult. She may be left uncertain about the perpetrator's identity, the events of the assault, the presence of birth control or a condom, and possible injury or risk for contracting sexually transmitted infections (STIs). See Table 9-2 for indicators of possible drug-facilitated sexual assault.

TABLE 9-2 Indicators of Possible Drug-Facilitated Sexual Assault

- Becoming intoxicated very rapidly, especially after accepting a drink from someone else or drinking a drink she left unattended.
- Having just one or two drinks, and then suddenly feeling "very drunk"; feeling more intoxicated than usual after drinking an amount of alcohol she is used to consuming.
- Feeling drowsy, dizzy, agitated, weak, confused, or nauseous; experiencing an increased heart rate or blood pressure, slurred speech, or a lack of motor coordination.
- Waking up suspecting she may have been raped because of vaginal soreness, finding herself in an unfamiliar place, or other indicators.
- Being told that she suddenly appeared drunk; drowsy; dizzy; or confused with impaired motor skills, judgment, and amnesia or partial amnesia.

Rape Trauma Syndrome

Rape is viewed as a situational crisis; that is, an unanticipated traumatic event that the victim generally is unprepared to handle because it is unforeseen. Following rape, the survivor may experience a cluster of symptoms originally described by Burgess and Holmstrom (1979) as the **rape trauma syndrome**. Burgess and Holmstrom described this syndrome as having two phases: the acute phase and the adjustment, or reorganization, phase. Other authors added a third phase: an intermediate, outward adjustment phase. A fourth phase—integration and recovery—has also been suggested, which serves to complete the syndrome (Holmes, 1998). Although the phases of response are discussed individually in the following sections, they often overlap, as do individual responses and their duration.

Acute Phase (Disorganization)

The acute phase of rape trauma syndrome begins during the rape and may last for a few days or up to 3 weeks. The woman may experience fear; shock; disbelief; and, sometimes, denial. The woman may feel humiliated, guilty, and unclean; her wish to cleanse herself by bathing or douching may be overpowering, even if she knows that by doing so she is destroying evidence. She may feel angry or anxious, powerless or helpless.

The rape survivor may suppress her emotions or may reveal them by crying, sobbing, or acting tense and restless. Survivors who control or mask their emotions may appear calm, composed, or subdued. Many rape survivors also experience alterations in sleep patterns, such as insomnia, nightmares, or crying out at night.

Outward Adjustment Phase (Denial)

Once the acute stage has passed, the survivor may appear adjusted. She returns to work or school and resumes her usual roles. But although she appears composed, she is actually coping by denial and suppression. The survivor needs the outward adjustment phase to cope with the experience of rape; it is a means of regaining control of her life. During this time, she may move to a different residence or may institute security measures, such as installing extra locks or requesting an unlisted telephone number. She may buy a weapon or take a course in self-defense. These activities do not resolve her emotional trauma; they simply push it further into her subconscious. In addition she may get less support from others who perceive her as being "over it."

Reorganization

Denial and suppression cannot sustain the survivor for long. As these coping mechanisms deteriorate, she becomes depressed and anxious and feels a strong urge to talk about the rape. At this point, the woman enters the reorganization phase of the rape trauma syndrome. She must alter her self-concept and resolve her feelings about the rape.

During this phase, the rape survivor may develop phobias. Fears of being indoors or outdoors or of being attacked from behind—depending on how the attack took place—are common. Because of these fears, the woman may alter her lifestyle. If she is afraid of crowds, of being out after dark, or of returning to an empty house, she may become a virtual recluse.

Rape survivors frequently report menstrual or other gynecologic disorders as well as sexual dysfunction. Some women become totally averse to sexual activity. Those who do try to engage in sex often report a decrease in vaginal lubrication, an inability to be aroused, unusual sensations in the genital area, and an inability to achieve orgasm.

There are a number of long-term physical and psychologic health consequences of sexual assault. Long-term physical consequences include pregnancy, chronic pain, gastrointestinal disorders, headaches, and sexually transmitted infections. Chronic psychologic consequences include depression, fear and anxiety, difficulty trusting others, eating disorders, attempted or completed suicide, post-traumatic stress disorder, and/or unhealthy behaviors (e.g., smoking, alcohol abuse, use of drugs, and risky sexual behavior) (National Center for Injury Prevention and Control [NCIPC], 2007). Sleep disorders persist. Survivors report repeated nightmares in which they either relive the rape or thwart the rapist's attempt. In either case the dream contains disturbing violence. The woman repeatedly replays the role of victim until she comes to terms with the experience.

Integration and Recovery

This final phase brings resolution for the woman. She is able to recognize that the blame for her assault lies with her assailant. She begins to trust others again and begins to feel safe in her life and day-to-day activities. She may be filled with a sense of righteous anger and become an advocate for other women (Holmes, 1998).

Silent Reaction

Women who do not report the rape go through the phases of the rape trauma syndrome without using available support systems. Their reasons for keeping silent vary. A woman may be embarrassed, she may accept society's "temptress view" and blame herself, or she may fear retaliation. Her experience may be discovered much later, perhaps when she seeks professional help in resolving a different crisis.

Some women seek medical help for their physical injuries without disclosing that a rape was the cause. The nurse who suspects that a woman has been raped should seek validation through sympathetic questioning.

Sexual Assault as a Cause of Post-Traumatic Stress Disorder

Sexual assault survivors may exhibit high levels of **post-traumatic stress disorder (PTSD)**, the same disorder that developed in many of the veterans of the Vietnam War. To be diagnosed as having PTSD, a person must:

- Have been exposed to a traumatic event that triggered feelings of intense fear, horror, or helplessness.
- Reexperience the event in recurrent, intrusive thoughts, images, perceptions, and flashbacks.
- Persistently avoid stimuli associated with the trauma and demonstrate a generalized "numbing" of responsiveness.
- Demonstrate persistent signs of increased arousal, such as exaggerated startle response, difficulty falling asleep, hypervigilance or outbursts of anger, emotional detachment, and sleep disturbances that were not present before the trauma occurred.

PTSD is marked by varying degrees of intensity depending on prior mental health issues and the woman's own resiliency. Sexual assault victims with PTSD are 13 times more likely than nonvictims to have alcohol-related problems and 26 times more likely to have two or more serious drug abuse problems. Compared to victims of other types of traumatic events, sexual assault victims are the largest single group of PTSD sufferers (Victim Rights Law Center, 2009).

PTSD is difficult to treat. Because the symptoms keep an individual from addressing the problem, she cannot integrate the event into her life and healing is blocked. Recovery depends on empowering the woman to seek to regain control of her life within the context of healing relationships and professional counseling.

Physical Care of the Sexual Assault Survivor

Following a sexual assault, a primary purpose of care is to meet the needs of the survivor. This is accomplished by evaluating and treating injuries; conducting prompt examinations; providing support, crisis intervention, and advocacy; providing prophylaxis against STIs; assessing for pregnancy risk and discussing treatment options; and providing follow-up care for medical and emotional needs. As many as 31.5% of women who are sexually assaulted sustain injuries although often the injuries are minor; more severe physical consequences may also occur (CDC, 2008b; Tjaden & Thoennes, 2006).

Hope for Healing

Sexual assault victims tend to have more medical complaints and to access healthcare services more than those who have not been victimized. Both emotional and physical symptoms manifest themselves in the aftermath of an assault, sometimes immediately and sometimes for a lengthy period postassault. Research indicates that between 45% and 77% of women who were actual victims of rape did not define their experience as rape. Even without such an acknowledgment, these women experience physical health concerns, including headaches, stomachaches, distress, menstrual difficulties, and sexual functioning difficulties (Conoscenti & McNally, 2006). All healthcare settings must be alert to this phenomenon and assess patients carefully.

Because sexual assault is a crime as well as a traumatic emergency, however, the other purpose of health care is to collect and preserve legal evidence for use in prosecuting the assailant. It is important to note that even though evidence is collected, it does not necessarily mean that the survivor has to prosecute; the survivor always has the right to reconsider her decisions. In collecting legal evidence, healthcare providers must respect the rights of the survivor. Sexual assault survivors have the right to immediate, compassionate, and comprehensive medical-legal examination and treatment by a trained professional who has the experience to anticipate their needs during this time of crisis.

As a result of the reauthorization and new provisions of the Violence Against Women Act of 2005, additional services have been available to all victims of sexual assault. Beginning in January 2009 all victims of rape, sodomy, and other penetrating types of sexual assault have been able to receive a forensic examination at specially equipped medical settings without the requirement to first participate in the criminal justice system or cooperate with law enforcement. This new law has given greater freedom to victims to access forensic care whether or not they choose to report to police. Specific procedures have been created in all jurisdictions to accomplish this new right and provide expert, timely medical services to victims who otherwise may not have chosen to access services. With the passage of this law, there is a hope that more victims will eventually report their crimes to the police since they no longer must do so within those first few hours following the incident, while at the same time obtaining needed services for future prosecutorial efforts.

Unfortunately, in many communities the treatment of a woman immediately following a sexual assault has been almost as traumatic as the assault itself. Often referred to as "the second rape" or as "secondary victimization," it is reflected in victim blaming and insensitive and prying care. To address this concern, many emergency departments use multidisciplinary teams to provide effective care to sexual assault survivors and their families. Sexual assault nurse examiner (SANE) programs and sexual assault response teams (SART) (composed of law enforcement and prosecution professionals, forensic examiners and/or healthcare providers, and victim advocates) are two examples of successful multidisciplinary community programs that coordinate teams of medical, legal, and social service professionals with effective advocacy on behalf of sexual assault survivors.

Other communities provide rape victim advocates, who help survivors in hospital emergency departments (EDs) and in dealing with the police. Research suggests that rape survivors who have the assistance of an advocate in the ED report less emotional distress from the experience, have fewer negative interactions with hospital staff, and receive more medical services such as prophylaxis against STIs and emergency contraception (Campbell, 2006).

Detailed History

Obtaining a detailed history is an essential first step in acquiring necessary medical and forensic data, but it can also be a therapeutic tool if done in a sensitive, caring way. Because a sexual assault survivor may appear relaxed and normal when first seen, caregivers may underestimate her needs, but it is essential that she receive immediate attention. Immediately after the woman has received any necessary emergency care, the nurse takes an explicit history of the event in the woman's own words to aid in evidence collection and examination of injuries. Many agencies use a standardized forensic chart containing a history flow sheet to record information obtained. The caregiver should use a nonjudgmental approach and must avoid leading or coaching the woman.

Collection of Evidence

The collection of evidence may, in itself, be traumatic for the woman. It is valuable to have someone available to provide support and act as an advocate. This person may be a family member or close friend, but often it is a nurse. An interpreter should also be provided as necessary.

The woman should receive a thorough explanation of the procedures to be carried out and should sign an informed consent form. An important legal concept when dealing with rape survivors is the need to preserve the *chain of evidence,* meaning that all physical evidence and specimens must remain in the hands of a professional until they are turned over to a police officer. The evidence that the nurse or forensic examiner collects has four primary uses (Ledray, 1999): (1) to confirm recent sexual contact; (2) to show that force or coercion was used; (3) to identify the assailant; and (4) to corroborate the survivor's story. Most agencies have special sexual assault kits that contain all necessary supplies for collecting and labeling evidence.

A careful examination of the entire body is necessary. Vaginal and rectal examinations are performed, along with a complete physical examination for trauma. Any lacerations of the vaginal wall are repaired and noted. A colposcope with photographic capability can be used to document injuries to the genitalia.

CLOTHING Each piece of clothing and foreign material dislodged from clothing is marked, placed in an individual paper bag, sealed, and labeled.

SWABS OF STAINS AND SECRETIONS Swabs of body stains and secretions are analyzed for semen or sperm. The absence of sperm, however, does not signify that no sexual assault has occurred. Many assailants do not ejaculate because of sexual dysfunction, or they may use a condom. Because victims are often forced to commit fellatio, oral swabs are also examined for semen. Gonorrhea and chlamydia cultures also are taken from vaginal, rectal, and oral cavities.

HAIR AND SCRAPINGS Clippings or scrapings of the woman's fingernails are examined for blood or tissue from the assailant. Approximately 20 to 25 hairs are pulled from her head and pubic area to analyze the root structure and identify foreign hairs. Her pubic hair is also combed to check for loose hairs that may have been transferred from the rapist.

BLOOD SAMPLES Blood is drawn to test for syphilis and to determine the woman's blood type. Additional blood may be drawn for a pregnancy test if the woman indicates that she wants to take emergency contraception (see discussion in chapter 5) to prevent pregnancy. She has to have a negative pregnancy test to receive the medication.

URINE SAMPLES Urine should be collected in cases in which a drug-facilitated sexual assault is suspected and the drug was ingested within 96 hours of the evidentiary exam. It is important to document in the record the time the survivor believes that the drug was ingested and the number of urinations between the ingestion and the exam. A forensic laboratory with the capability of conducting toxicology tests should be identified because not all crime laboratories have the specialized equipment needed to test for rape drugs. Moreover, because of the increased sensitivity of deoxyribonucleic acid (DNA) tests, many jurisdictions are extending the standard cutoff time for evidence collection in their jurisdictions (U.S. Department of Justice, 2004).

PHOTOGRAPHS Photographs should be taken of injured areas if possible. Before taking any photos, the healthcare provider should ask the woman to sign an informed consent form.

Prevention of Sexually Transmitted Infections

Among women who have been sexually assaulted, trichomoniasis, bacterial vaginosis, gonorrhea, and chlamydia are the most frequently diagnosed infections. Thus, during the initial examination, cultures for *Neisseria gonorrhoeae* and *Chlamydia trachomatis* should be obtained from any body sites of penetration or attempted penetration. However, because these infections are fairly prevalent among sexually active women, the diagnosis of one or more of these infections following an assault does not necessarily indicate that it was acquired during the assault. If any STI is diagnosed, it is treated (CDC, 2007). Most clinicians recommend routine preventive therapy after a sexual assault with follow-up referral to a clinic specializing in the treatment of STIs to evaluate the effectiveness of the therapy. The CDC (2007) recommends a prophylaxis regimen that includes a single dose of ceftriaxone intramuscularly plus a single oral dose of metronidazole and a single oral dose of azithromycin. If the survivor chooses not to receive prophylactic antibiotic treatment, the nurse should instruct her to be seen by her caregiver in 2 weeks for assessment for any STIs. In addition, because hepatitis B is a risk, the woman who has never been immunized should be given hepatitis B immune globulin; she should also begin the hepatitis B 3-dose immunization series immediately (CDC, 2007).

If the assailant's HIV status is not known, consideration should be given to offer postexposure prophylaxis with HIV antiviral medications. If postexposure HIV prophylaxis is considered, consultation with an HIV specialist is advised (CDC, 2007).

Prevention of Pregnancy

The woman is questioned about her menstrual cycle and contraceptive practices. If she is at risk for pregnancy and a pregnancy test is negative, she should receive information about her treatment options. Women of different ages, social, cultural, and religious/spiritual backgrounds will have diverse feelings about acceptable treatment options. The nurse needs to be sensitive and nonjudgmental when discussing various reproductive health services. If the woman wishes, emergency postcoital contraception is provided. (See chapter 5 for further discussion.)

NURSING CARE MANAGEMENT

Sexual assault survivors frequently enter the healthcare system by way of the ED; thus nurses are often the first to provide services to them. Because the caregiver's values, attitudes, and beliefs will necessarily affect the competence and focus of the care, nurses who work with survivors must understand their own attitudes and beliefs about sexual assault and sexual assault survivors and resolve any conflicts that may exist, ensuring nonjudgmental patient support.

In addition to examining their own attitudes and beliefs, nurses must be mindful of the potential for increased complexity of treatment with sexual assault survivors who are members of different ethnic or cultural backgrounds. For example, a woman's membership in a particular ethnic or cultural group could affect her willingness to disclose all the details of an assault, her willingness to follow up with community resources or to seek counseling, and her willingness to prosecute. Being aware of potential cultural differences is important when discussing future courses of action available.

Nursing Assessment and Diagnosis

Policies for admitting and examining sexual assault survivors vary among institutions, but clinical guidelines and protocols for the health care of sexual assault victims have been issued by many national medical agencies to create consistency in treatment in healthcare facilities across the United States. A woman who has been assaulted is under great stress and needs the sensitive care of professionals who are aware of her special needs. The first priority is creating a safe, secure environment. Professionals should gather admission information from the victim in a quiet, private room and reassure the woman that she is not alone, will not be abandoned, and is safe from a second attack.

A full mental status examination should be performed, both for the purpose of planning care and as possible courtroom evidence. Scrupulous documentation is essential because the victim's medical record is often used in the courtroom to verify her testimony if the rapist is prosecuted.

Examples of nursing diagnoses that may apply to the sexual assault victim include the following:

- ***Fear*** related to invasion of personal space secondary to assault
- ***Powerlessness*** related to inability to regain sense of control secondary to assault

Nursing Plan and Implementation

Table 9-3 outlines the general nursing actions that are appropriate during each of the phases of recovery. It is imperative that control be returned to the woman as quickly as possible. When feasible, the woman should decide on the sequence of forensic events, such as pulling her own hair (head and pubic), having blood drawn after clothes are collected rather than before, and so forth. In this way the nurse helps her deal with her crisis in small, manageable increments. The nurse should encourage the woman to express her feelings and reassure her that anger and fear are normal, appropriate responses. The nurse can also address expressed or unexpressed guilt by assuring the woman that the sexual assault was not her fault.

By explaining the general health or forensic examination and the sequence of events in the ED, the nurse can alleviate the patient's anxiety related to fear of the unknown. The woman should know what is going to happen and why and how she can assist in each phase of the examination. Throughout the experience, the

Case Study: Teenage Rape Victim

TABLE 9-3 Nursing Actions Appropriate to Phases of Recovery Following Rape

Acute Phase	Create a safe environment.
	Explain the sequence of events in the healthcare facility.
	Allow the woman to grieve and express her feelings.
	Provide care for significant others.
Outward Adjustment Phase	Provide advocacy and support at the level requested by the woman.
	Provide assistance to significant others.
Reorganizational Phase	Establish a trusting relationship.
	Assist the woman to understand her role in the assault.
	Clarify and enhance the woman's feelings.
	Assist the woman in planning for her future.
Integration and Recovery	Acknowledge the victim's success in overcoming trauma; support advocacy efforts.

nurse acts as the survivor's advocate, providing support without usurping decision making. The nurse need not agree with all the survivor's decisions but should respect and defend her right to make them. A victim also has the right to have a victim advocate, family member, or friend with her throughout the examination process.

The family members or friends on whom the survivor calls also need nursing care. Like those of the victim, the reactions of the family will depend on the values to which they ascribe. Some family members or partners may blame the survivor for the sexual assault and feel angry with her for not having been more careful. They may also incorrectly view the assault as a sexual act rather than as an act of violence. They may feel personally wronged or attacked and see the survivor as being devalued or unclean. Their reactions may compound the victim's crisis. By spending some time with family members before their first interaction with the survivor, the nurse can reduce their anxiety and help them examine and reconcile their feelings, sparing the woman further trauma. In most cases, the nurse should contact and/or refer them to a sexual assault advocate who can help them address their needs. Hospital-based advocates, if available, should be called to the ED to provide support services. Community victim advocates are on call in most areas of the United States to respond 24 hours a day and be of assistance throughout the medical and/or forensic examinations as well as providing crisis intervention and advocacy in future criminal justice process involvement.

PROFESSIONALISM IN PRACTICE

Remaining Nonjudgmental

Strive to listen and respond nonjudgmentally. Allowing your own beliefs to interfere with care can make the difference in a victim's readiness to disclose the full details of her assault and to begin the recovery process. Hindering that ability is detrimental to the mental health of the woman and can decrease the possibility of identifying a sex offender.

Community-Based Nursing Care

As the woman enters the reorganization phase, she usually feels a strong urge to discuss and resolve her feelings about herself and her assailant. During this phase, the victim may benefit from talking with a specially trained sexual assault advocate or counselor. The nurse offers the services of the responding sexual assault advocate to the patient and introduces the advocate as soon as is possible, preferably prior to any physical examination. If she is not certain that she wants added support, or denies any need for counseling or advocacy, it is appropriate to respect her current wishes and to provide her with referral information for possible future use.

Information and support, provided by qualified nurses or other service providers, is a valuable tool in helping the sexual assault victim come to terms with her attack and its impact on her life. The woman should be encouraged to explore and identify her feelings and determine appropriate actions to resolve her problems and concerns. It is important for the provider to assist the woman to realize that the sexual assault was not her fault. The fault always lies with the perpetrator. With the provider/advocate, the woman explores her thoughts and feelings about self-care and celebrates her victories. It is important to emphasize that the loss of control that occurred during the assault was temporary and that she *does* have control over other aspects of her life.

Health Promotion Education

Local high schools, colleges, or rape awareness groups may offer courses in preventive strategies. Some classes focus on increasing women's awareness of situations in which they are at risk, whereas others are concerned with changing societal and men's attitudes about sexual assault and sexual assault survivors. Because sexual assault is a considerable risk for any woman, courses in what to do during and after an attack and how family members and friends can support a survivor are also helpful. Table 9-4 provides general guidelines for helping victims of sexual assault. Nurses who have completed addi-

TABLE 9-4 General Guidelines for Helping Victims of Sexual Assault

- Believe the victim—one of the greatest fears of sexual assault survivors is that they will not be believed.
- Listen and be patient—let the person talk and tell the story at her/his own pace.
- Reinforce the fact that the sexual assault was not the victim's fault.
- For recent assaults, encourage the victim to report the assault and preserve evidence.
- Encourage the person to seek medical attention.
- Suggest seeking counseling and other support services.
- Help the victim to organize her/his thoughts, but let the survivor make her/his own decision on how to proceed.
- Take care of yourself—assisting a friend or family member can be stressful. Set aside time for yourself so that you don't feel overwhelmed by the survivor's problems.
- Acknowledge your limits and realistically identify your abilities to assist the survivor.

Source: From General Guidelines for Helping Victims of Sexual Assault. *George Mason University Office of Sexual Assault Services. Reprinted with permission.*

tional education and are thoroughly prepared are well qualified to initiate or participate in preventive instruction.

Sexual Assault Advocacy and Information
Most sexual assault crisis centers operate 24 hours a day, 7 days a week. Their services are invaluable. Properly trained advocates and counselors can help the victim regain control early in the crisis. Many sexual assault crisis centers offer free services to victims or can refer them to qualified counselors within the community. Information on STIs and pregnancy alternatives may also be obtained from these centers. In addition, there are many Internet resources that provide information for survivors and their family members and friends as well as for professionals seeking information about how to better assist victims of sexual assault. See www.nursing.pearsonhighered.com for a list of hotline information and Internet-based resources about sexual assault.

Evaluation

Expected outcomes of quality nursing care include the following:

- The woman receives prompt, compassionate, respectful, and individualized medical attention.
- The woman recovers from the physical effects of the sexual assault.
- The woman is able to verbalize her recognition that sexual assault is a crime of violence expressed sexually.
- The woman is able to identify culturally appropriate community resources available to her as she works to adjust psychologically to the assault.
- The woman makes a decision about whether to prosecute her assailant.

CLINICAL JUDGMENT

Case Study: Sally Smith

Sally is a 19-year-old college student who has just transferred to her university. In order to make some new friends, Sally decided to go to an off-campus party that was advertised on a poster hanging in her residence hall lobby. She accepted a ride to the party with one of her new schoolmates. Once there, she became separated from her new friend and became isolated in the basement by a few males she had just met. She began drinking some of the punch the party-givers had made and soon felt very disoriented. Someone escorted her to a bedroom on the third floor to "sleep it off." The next thing Sally remembers is awaking to an unknown male on top of her having sex with her. Her slacks and panties were around her ankles. She tried to push him away but before she could get him off her body, he ejaculated inside of her. He then left the room, and she went downstairs to wait for her ride back to the residence hall. When she got back to her room, she told her roommate what happened, and the roommate drove her to the nearest hospital to get an exam.

Critical Thinking

As the nurse responding to this young woman, what are the presenting issues that must be addressed before an examination should begin?

What will be important for you to include in the history of this patient?

See www.nursing.pearsonhighered.com for possible responses.

- If a victim decides to prosecute her assailant, all necessary forensic evidence will have been collected, leading to a more successful investigation and prosecution.

Prosecution of the Assailant

Legally, sexual assault, like any criminal action, is considered a crime against the state rather than against the victim. Therefore, prosecution of the assailant is a community responsibility in which the prosecuting attorney will act on the victim's behalf. The victim, however, must initiate the process by reporting the crime and pressing charges against her assailant. Once authorities have apprehended the alleged attacker, the judicial system is set into motion.

Procedures vary from state to state. A judge or magistrate generally conducts a hearing to determine whether there is sufficient evidence to hold the defendant over for a trial. If indicted, a defendant must stand trial unless he waives this right. Either a judge or a jury will find the defendant guilty or not guilty, and he will be retained or set free accordingly.

Many sexual assault survivors who have gone through the judicial process refer to it as a second rape—and sometimes a more damaging one. The victim must identify the assailant and repeat the details of the assault. Delays can further frustrate the victim and increase her fear. Publicity may intensify her feelings of humiliation, and if the perpetrator is released on bail pending trial, she may fear retaliation.

During the trial itself, cross-examination by the defendant's attorney can be a severely degrading and intimidating experience for the victim. The defense attorney may try to discredit her testimony, causing a second victimization. Fortunately, rape shield laws are quite common, and nearly every state prohibits the publicizing of a victim's sexual history. Moreover, despite the difficulties of prosecution, many victims feel a sense of justice in taking their case to court.

The nurse involved with any sexual assault victim needs to be aware of the judicial sequence to anticipate rising tension and frustration in the victim and her support system. They will need consistent, effective support at this crucial time.

Responding to Violence Against Women: Vicarious Trauma

Vicarious trauma, or secondary trauma effect, can occur as a result of working with people who are trauma victims. It refers to a gradual internal transformation that can negatively affect commitment to one's work, reduce any sense of accomplishment, and lead to a questioning of personal belief systems. Nurses who treat and assist domestic violence and sexual assault survivors should be aware of this phenomenon so that they are able to periodically assess the effect of their work on their lives. When the lives of nurses—and indeed of all healthcare professionals—are balanced and there is equal time for self, family, friends, work, play, and rest, then they are better able to provide compassionate and sensitive health care.

FOCUS YOUR STUDY

- Domestic violence is very common. One in three to one in four women will experience violence at the hands of an intimate partner during their lifetime.
- Batterers use psychologic, physical, and sexual abuse to maintain power and control in abusive relationships.
- Battering occurs in a cyclic pattern called the cycle of violence, which increases in frequency and severity over time.
- Women in abusive relationships who belong to cultural and linguistic minority communities and immigrant women face additional barriers when attempting to access services. The nurse must work to provide culturally aware and competent care.
- Nurses are in an excellent position to intervene and assist women with abusive partners by recognizing their cues, diagnosing their problems appropriately, and understanding the complex dynamics of the battering family. The nurse provides information about available culturally appropriate community resources, medical attention, and emotional support.
- Estimates suggest that the majority of sexual assaults are not reported to the police. Rapes and sexual assaults committed by strangers are more likely to be reported to the police than rapes or sexual assaults committed by nonstrangers, including intimate partners, other relatives, and friends or acquaintances.
- Rape is an act of violence acted out sexually. Most sexual assaults are expressions of a need for power and control.
- Following sexual assault, the victim will usually experience an assortment of symptoms known as rape trauma syndrome. Recent research also links the effects of rape to post-traumatic stress disorder. Nursing actions to assist rape victims are encompassed in the roles of healthcare provider, advocate, and educator.
- Nurses inform the woman of the sequence of events involved in providing her care and developing the chain of evidence, and support the victim's decisions.
- Widespread education is needed to abolish societal myths surrounding domestic violence and sexual assault.

CRITICAL THINKING IN ACTION

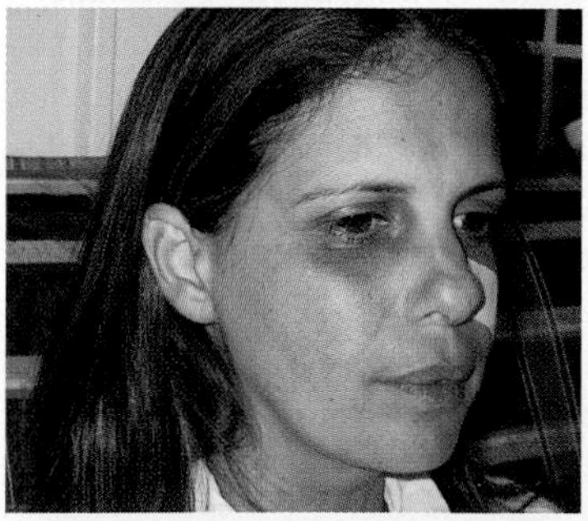

Marishka Devonowski, a 28-year-old G2P2, has a 9-year-old daughter and a 3-month-old daughter at home. Mrs. Devonowski has been seen at the emergency department several times for a variety of problems including a broken arm, sprained ankle, and multiple contusions from reportedly "walking into a door" when she got up during the night but did not turn on a light. She describes herself as clumsy and accident-prone. At each visit her husband, a computer analyst, who appears thoughtful and protective of his wife, accompanies her.

Today she is being seen for a severe laceration of her cheek and a mild concussion. You observe that she also has a black eye and bruising of her upper arm and chest. At each previous visit the nurse had managed to spend time alone with Mrs. Devonowski and had asked specifically about domestic violence. However, Marishka denied it vehemently each time. Today, when you are alone with her you ask about abuse. This time she admits that her husband caused her injuries. She states, "His job is so stressful and sometimes he just loses his temper. But he seems to get more angry no matter what I do. I hate it but I can't leave him. I don't know how I would manage alone."

1. In talking with Marishka, what information would you focus on initially?
2. What specific information should you share about preparing an exit or safety plan?

See www.nursing.pearsonhighered.com for possible responses.

Pearson Nursing Student Resources

Find additional review materials at **www.nursing.pearsonhighered.com**

Prepare for success with additional NCLEX®-style practice questions, interactive assignments and activities, Web links, animations and videos, and more!

REFERENCES

American Nurses Association (ANA). (2000). *Position statement: Violence against women.* Retrieved from http://www.nursingworld.org/SocialCausesHealthCare

American Nurses Association (ANA). (2002). *Intimate partner violence: Implications for nursing.* Retrieved from http://nursingworld.org/ANAMarketplace/ANAPeriodicals/OJINhtm

Bureau of Justice Statistics. (2009). *Terms and definitions: Victims.* Retrieved from http://bjs.ojp.usdoj.gov/index.cfm?ty=tdtp&tid=9

Burgess, A. W., & Holmstrom, L. L. (1979). *Rape: Crisis and recovery.* Englewood Cliffs, NJ: Prentice Hall.

Campbell, R. (2006). Rape survivors' experiences with the legal and medical systems: Do rape victim advocates make a difference? *Violence Against Women, 12*(1), 30–45.

Catalano, S., Smith, E., Snyder, H., & Rand, M. (2009). *Female victims of violence. Bureau of Justice statistics: Selected findings.* Retrieved from http://bjs.ojp.usdoj.gov/content/pub/pdf/fw.pdf

Centers for Disease Control and Prevention (CDC). (2006). *Understanding intimate partner violence fact sheet.* Retrieved from http://www.cdc.gov/ViolencePrevention/pdf/IPV-FactSheet.pdf

Centers for Disease Control and Prevention (CDC). (2007). Sexually transmitted diseases treatment guidelines. *Morbidity and Mortality Weekly Report, 2006, 55*(RR–11).

Centers for Disease Control and Prevention (CDC). (2008a). Adverse health conditions and health risk behaviors associated with intimate partner violence, *Morbidity and Mortality Weekly Report.* Retrieved from http://www.cdc.gov/mmwr/preview/mmwrhtml/mm5705a1.htm

Centers for Disease Control and Prevention (CDC). (2008b). *Sexual violence: Facts at a glance.* Retrieved from http://cdc.gov/violenceprevention/pdf/SV-DataSheet-a.pdf

Centers for Disease Control and Prevention (CDC). (2009). *Understanding sexual violence.* Retrieved from http://cdc.gov/violenceprevention/pdf/SV_factsheet-a.pdf

Conoscenti, L., & McNally, R. (2006). Health complaints in acknowledged and unacknowledged rape victims, *Journal of Anxiety Disorders, 20,* 372–379.

Felson, R., & Outlaw, M. (2007). The control motive and marital violence. *Violence and Victims, 22*(4), 387–407.

Holmes, M. M. (1998). The clinical management of rape in adolescents. *Contemporary OB/GYN, 43*(5), 62–78.

Ledray, L. E. (1999). *Sexual assault nurse examiner (SANE) development and operations guide.* Washington, DC: US Department of Justice, Office for Victims of Crime; and Minneapolis, MN: Sexual Assault Resource Service.

National Center for Injury Prevention and Control (NCIPC). (2007). *Sexual violence: Fact sheet.* Retrieved from http://www.cdc.gov/ncipc/pub-res/images/SV%20Factsheet.pdf

Plan UK. (2007). *Because I am a girl: The state of the world's girls 2007.* Retrieved from http://www.planusa.org/becauseiamagirl/docs/becauseiamagirl.pdf

Rape, Abuse, and Incest National Network (RAINN). (2009). *Statistics.* Retrieved from http://www.rainn.org/statistics

Straka, S. M. (2006). Responding to the needs of older women experiencing domestic violence. *Violence Against Women, 12*(3), 251–267.

Tahirih Justice Center. (2009). *Know the facts brochure.* Retrieved from http://www.tahirih.org

The Joint Commission and the Crosswalk of the Office of Minority Health National Standards for Culturally and Linguistically Appropriate Services (CLAS). (2008). Retrieved from http://www.jointcommission.org/NR/rdonlyres/02E99D6E-E4EA-4F6A-A31F-4A10CAE691DC/0/2009OMHJCCLASXwalkHAP.pdf

Thompson, M., Sitterle, D., Clay, G., & Kingree, J. (2007). Reasons for not reporting victimizations to the police: Do they vary for physical and sexual incidents? *Journal of American College Health, 55*(5).

Tjaden, P., & Thoennes, N. (2006). *Extent, nature, and consequences of rape victimization: Findings from the national violence against women survey* (NCJ 210346). Retrieved from http://www.ncjrs.gov/pdffiles1/nij/210346.pdf

U.S. Department of Justice, Office on Violence Against Women. (2004). *National protocol for sexual assault medical forensic examinations: Adults/adolescents* (NCJ-206554). Washington, DC: Author.

Victim Rights Law Center. (2009). *How focusing on the perpetrators' actions prior to assault benefit prevention.* Paper presented at the Men Can Stop Rape's National Conference: Men and Women as Allies, Washington, DC.

Walker, L. (1984). *The battered woman syndrome.* New York, NY: Springer.

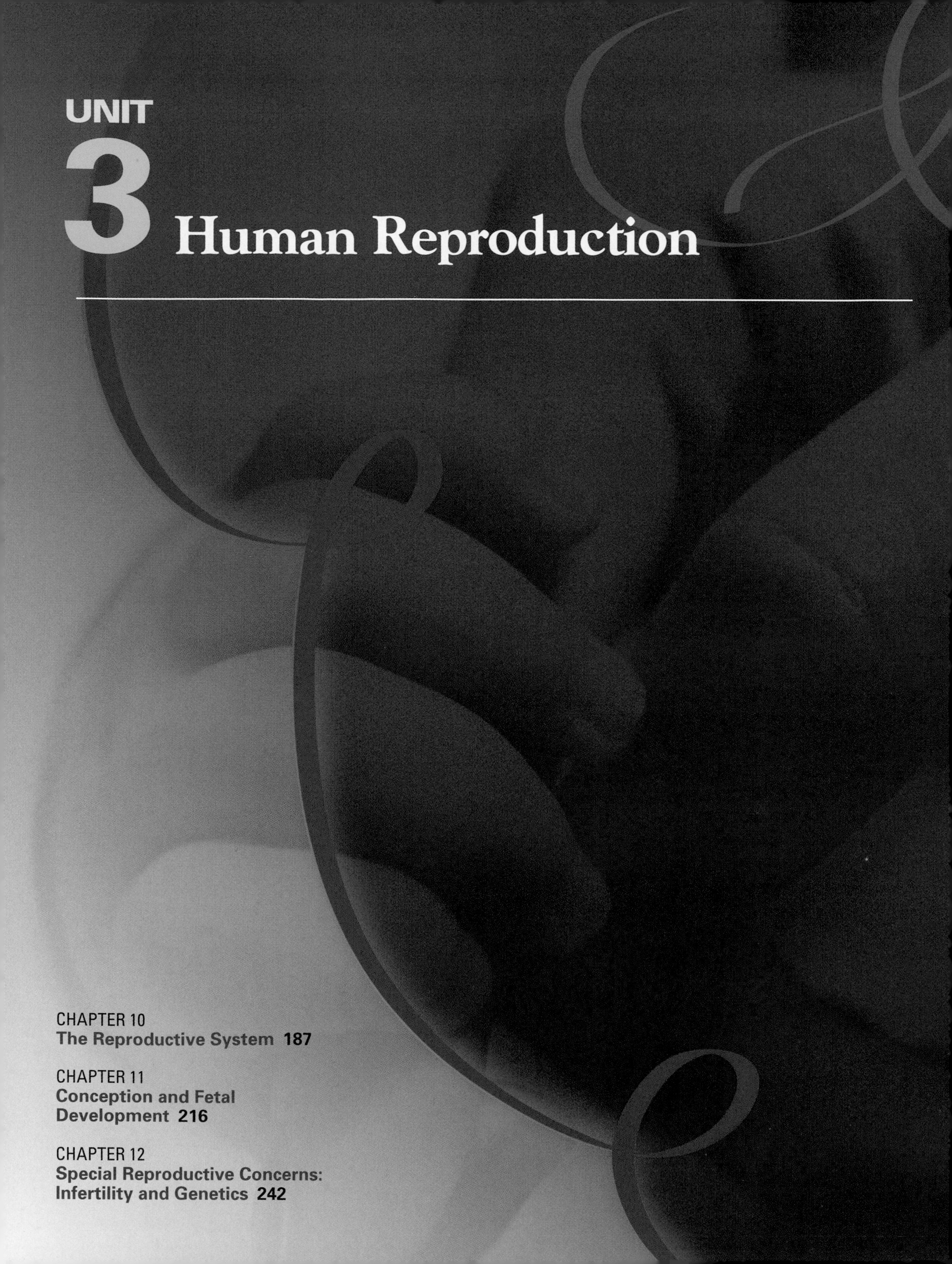

UNIT 3 Human Reproduction

The Reproductive System

10 CHAPTER

I always thought it was so boring to study anatomy and physiology. Who cares how many bones there are in the pelvis or the muscles involved. But now I'm with mothers having babies, and now it all makes sense.

—A Nursing Student

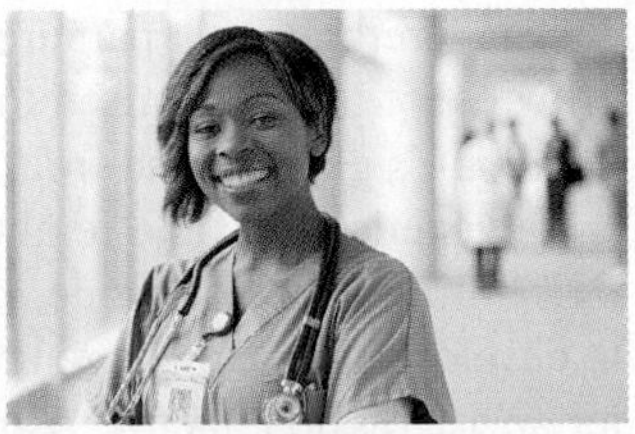

LEARNING OUTCOMES

1. Describe the differentiation of the male and female reproductive organs during embryonic development.
2. Summarize the major changes in the reproductive system that occur during puberty.
3. Identify the structures and functions of the female reproductive system.
4. Identify the structures and functions of the male reproductive system.
5. Discuss the significance of specific female reproductive structures during pregnancy and childbirth.
6. Summarize the actions of the hormones that affect reproductive functioning.
7. Identify the two phases of the ovarian cycle and the changes that occur in each phase.
8. Describe the phases of the menstrual cycle, their dominant hormones, and the changes that occur in each phase.

KEY TERMS

Ampulla *197*
Areola *204*
Breasts *203*
Broad ligament *196*
Cardinal ligaments *196*
Cervix *195*
Conjugate vera *201*
Cornua *194*
Corpus *194*
Corpus luteum *207*
Diagonal conjugate *201*
Endometrium *195*
Estrogens *206*
Fallopian tubes *197*
False pelvis *200*
Female reproductive cycle (FRC) *205*
Fimbria *197*
Follicle-stimulating hormone (FSH) *190*
Fundus *194*
Gonadotropin-releasing hormone (GnRH) *190*
Graafian follicle *207*
Human chorionic gonadotropin (hCG) *207*
Infundibulopelvic ligament *197*
Ischial spines *198*
Isthmus *197*
Luteinizing hormone (LH) *190*
Myometrium *195*
Nidation *195*
Nipple *204*
Obstetric conjugate *201*
Oogenesis *188*
Ovarian ligaments *196*
Ovaries *197*
Ovulation *207*
Pelvic cavity *199*
Pelvic diaphragm *198*
Pelvic inlet *201*
Pelvic outlet *201*
Perimetrium *195*
Perineal body *192*
Progesterone *206*
Prostaglandins (PGs) *206*
Puberty *188*
Pubis *198*
Round ligaments *196*
Sacral promontory *198*
Spermatogenesis *188*
Symphysis pubis *198*
Testosterone *211*
Transverse diameter *201*
True pelvis *200*
Uterosacral ligaments *197*
Uterus *193*
Vagina *192*
Vulva *190*

Understanding childbearing requires more than understanding sexual intercourse or the process by which the female and male sex cells unite. The nurse must also become familiar with the structures and functions that make childbearing possible and the phenomena that initiate it. This chapter considers the anatomic, physiologic, and sexual aspects of the female and male reproductive systems. It also provides information regarding basic embryonic development of the reproductive structures.

The female and male reproductive organs are *homologous;* that is, they are fundamentally similar in function and structure. The primary functions of both the female and male reproductive systems are to produce sex cells and transport them to locations where their union can occur. The sex cells, called *gametes,* are produced by specialized organs called *gonads.* A series of ducts and glands within both the male and female reproductive systems contributes to the production and transport of the gametes.

Embryonic Development of Reproductive Structures and Processes

Although the genetic sex of an embryo is determined at fertilization, the male and female reproductive systems are undifferentiated for about the first 8 weeks of gestation. This undifferentiated period is followed by a period of rapid, dramatic changes as the reproductive organs differentiate into recognizable structures.

Ovaries and Testes

During the 5th week of gestation, a primitive gonad arises from the intermediate mesoderm tissue known as gonadal ridges (Figure 10-1 ■ top image). The gonad develops a medulla (inner part of the organ) and cortex (outer part of the organ), which appear in the underlying mesenchyme (embryonic tissue from which connective and muscle tissue arises; see Table 11-2 on page 224). In genetic males during the 7th and 8th weeks, the medulla develops into a testis, and the cortex regresses. In genetic females by about the 10th week, the cortex develops into an ovary, and the medulla regresses.

Every egg available for maturation in a woman's reproductive life is present at her birth. During fetal life the ovary produces oogonia, cells that become primitive eggs called *oocytes,* by the process of **oogenesis** (see chapter 11 ∞). No oocytes are formed after fetal development. About 150,000 oocytes are contained in the ovaries at birth.

Each testis produces the male gametes, called *spermatozoa* or *sperm,* by a process called **spermatogenesis**. This process is described in chapter 11 ∞. Spermatogenesis of mature sperm does not occur until the onset of puberty. Figure 10-1 illustrates the embryologic development of the gonads and other internal reproductive organs.

Other Internal Structures

During the undifferentiated period—the first 7 weeks—two pairs of genital ducts develop: the mesonephric and paramesonephric ducts (Cunningham et al., 2010).

In genetic females the fallopian tubes are formed from the unfused portions of the paramesonephric ducts, and the fused portions give rise to the epithelium and uterine glands. The endometrial stroma and the myometrium (thick layer of smooth muscle in the wall of the uterus) develop from the adjacent mesenchyme.

The vagina is derived from more than one embryologic structure. The vaginal epithelium develops from the endoderm of the urogenital sinus, and the musculature develops from the uterovaginal primordium.

The urethral and paraurethral glands develop from outgrowths of the urethra into the surrounding mesenchyme. Bartholin's glands arise from similar structures.

In genetic males the fetal testes secrete two hormones. The first hormone, testosterone, stimulates the mesonephric ducts to develop into the male genital tract. The other hormone, Müllerian regression factor, suppresses the development of the paramesonephric ducts, which would otherwise develop into the female genital tract.

From the mesonephric ducts comes development of the efferent ductule, vas deferens, epididymis, seminal vesicle, and ejaculatory duct. Both the prostate and the bulbourethral glands develop from endodermal outgrowths of the urethra.

External Structures

Genetic males and females possess the same external genitals until the end of the 9th week. By the 12th week, differentiation of the external genitals is complete.

If fetal testosterone is not present, the undifferentiated external genitals are feminized. The phallus becomes the clitoris, and the urogenital folds remain open, forming the labia minora. The labioscrotal folds form the labia majora.

If fetal testosterone is present, the undifferentiated external genitals become masculine. The phallus elongates, forming the penis. The fusion of the urogenital folds on the ventral surface of the penis forms the penile urethra with the urethral meatus moving forward toward the glans penis.

Puberty

The term **puberty** refers to the developmental period between childhood and attainment of adult sexual characteristics and functioning. Generally, boys mature physically about 2 years later than girls. Puberty lasts from 1.5 to 5 years and involves profound physical, psychologic, and emotional changes. These changes include an altered body image, changing roles, and changing societal expectations and responses as the child matures into an adult.

Major Physical Changes

In both girls and boys, puberty is preceded by an accelerated growth rate called adolescent spurt. Widespread body system changes occur, including maturation of the reproductive organs.

Girls experience a broadening of the hips, then budding of the breasts, the appearance of pubic and axillary hair, and the onset of menstruation, called menarche. The average time between breast development and menarche is 2.3 years.

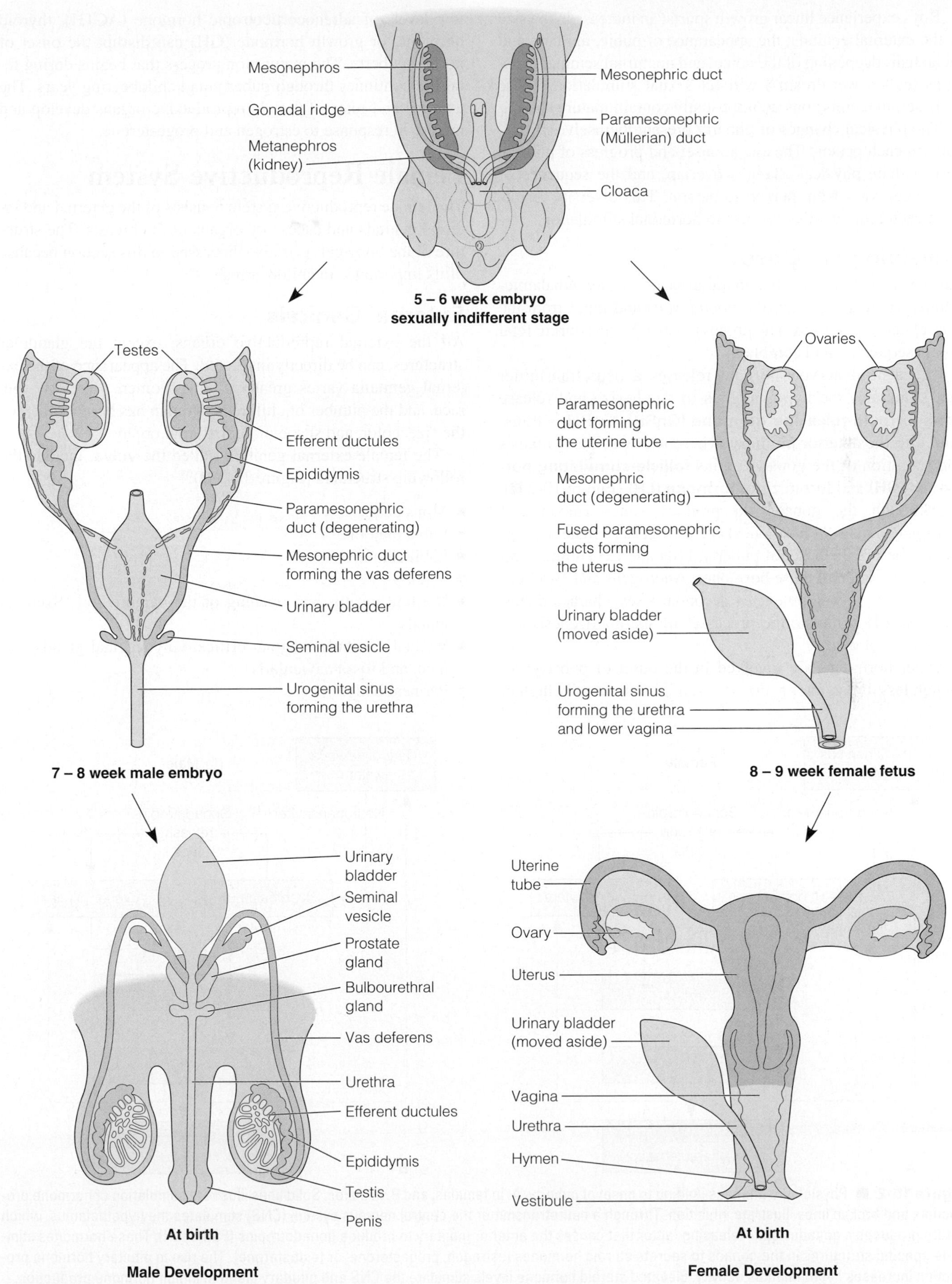

Figure 10-1 ■ Embryonic differentiation of male and female internal reproductive organs.

Boys experience linear growth spurts; an increase in the size of the external genitals; the appearance of pubic, axillary, and facial hair; deepening of the voice; and nocturnal seminal emissions (called wet dreams) without sexual stimulation. These early seminal emissions do not usually contain mature sperm.

The physical changes of puberty present themselves differently in each person. The age at onset and progress of puberty vary widely, physical changes overlap, and the sequence of events can vary from person to person. This diversity results from each individual's response to hormonal stimulation.

Physiology of Onset

Puberty is initiated by the maturation of the hypothalamic-pituitary-gonad complex (the *gonadostat*) and input from the central nervous system. The process, which begins during fetal life, is sequential and complex.

The central nervous system releases a neurotransmitter that stimulates the hypothalamus to synthesize and release **gonadotropin-releasing hormone (GnRH)**. GnRH is transmitted to the anterior pituitary, where it causes the synthesis and secretion of the gonadotropins **follicle-stimulating hormone (FSH)** and **luteinizing hormone (LH)** (Figure 10-2 ■).

Although the gonads do produce small amounts of *androgens* (male sex hormones) and *estrogens* (female sex hormones) before the onset of puberty, FSH and LH stimulate increased secretion of these hormones. Androgens and estrogens influence the development of secondary sex characteristics. FSH and LH stimulate the processes of spermatogenesis and maturation of ova.

Other hormones are involved in the onset of puberty; although less direct, their action is essential. Abnormally high or low levels of adrenocorticotropic hormone (ACTH), thyroid hormone, or growth hormone (GH) can disrupt the onset of normal puberty. The maturation process that begins during fetal life continues through puberty and childbearing years. The external and internal female reproductive organs develop and mature in response to estrogen and progesterone.

Female Reproductive System

The female reproductive system consists of the external and internal genitals and accessory organs of the breasts. The structure of the bony pelvis is also discussed in this section because of its importance in childbearing.

External Genitals

All the external reproductive organs, except the glandular structures, can be directly inspected. The appearance of the external genitalia varies greatly among women. Heredity, age, race, and the number of children a woman has borne influence the size, color, and shape of her external organs.

The female external genitals, called the **vulva**, include the following structures (Figure 10-3 ■):

- Mons pubis
- Labia majora
- Labia minora
- Clitoris
- Urethral meatus and opening of the paraurethral (Skene's) glands
- Vaginal vestibule (vaginal orifice, vulvovaginal glands, hymen, and fossa navicularis)
- Perineal body

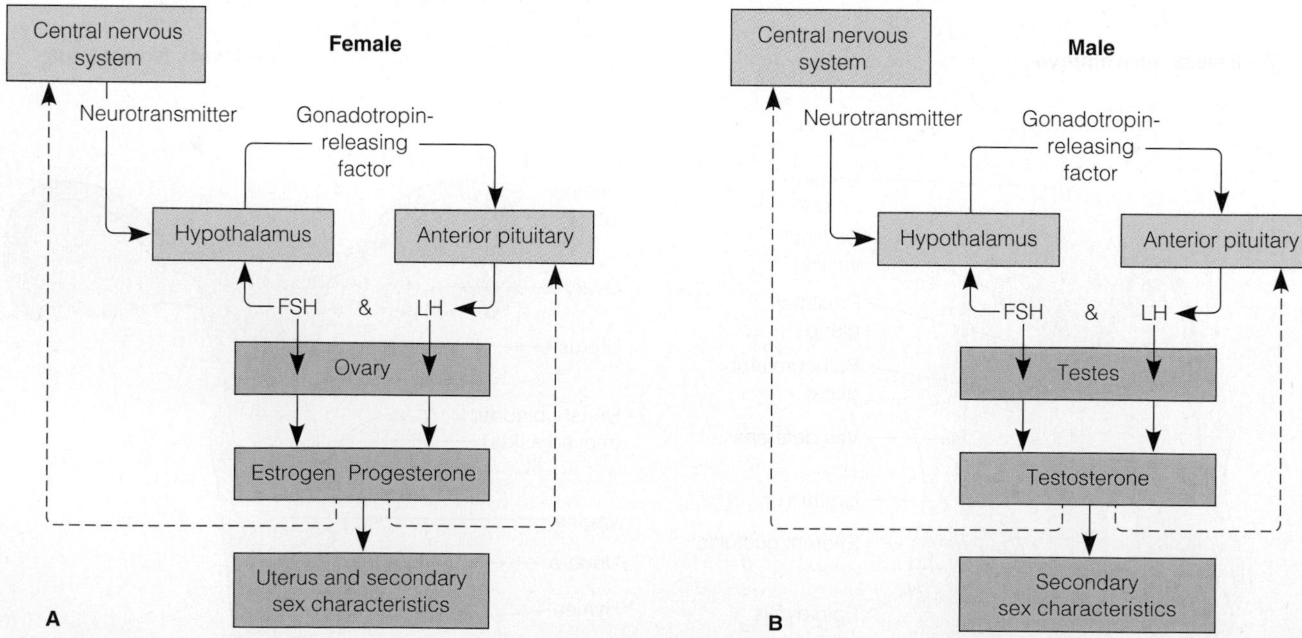

Figure 10-2 ■ Physiologic changes leading to onset of puberty. A. In females; and B. in males. Solid lines illustrate stimulation of hormone production, and broken lines illustrate inhibition. Through a neurotransmitter the central nervous system (CNS) stimulates the hypothalamus, which in turn produces a gonadotropin-releasing factor that causes the anterior pituitary to produce gonadotropins (FSH or LH). These hormones stimulate specific structures in the gonads to secrete steroid hormones (estrogen, progesterone, or testosterone). The rise in pituitary hormone production increases hypothalamus activity. Elevated steroid hormone levels stimulate the CNS and pituitary gland to inhibit hormone production.

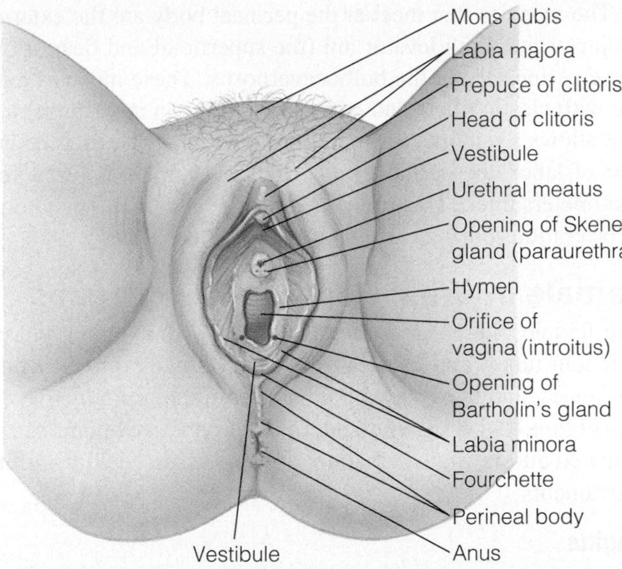

Figure 10-3 ■ Female external genitals, longitudinal view.

Although they are not true parts of the female reproductive system, the urethral meatus and perineal body are considered here because of their proximity and relationship to the vulva. The vulva has a generous supply of blood and nerves. As a woman ages, estrogen secretions decrease, causing the vulvar organs to atrophy.

Mons Pubis

The *mons pubis* is a softly rounded mound of subcutaneous fatty tissue beginning at the lowest portion of the anterior abdominal wall (see Figure 10-3). Also known as the mons veneris, this structure covers the anterior portion of the symphysis pubis. The mons pubis is covered with pubic hair, typically with the hairline forming a transverse line across the lower abdomen. The hair is short in all women. It can vary from sparse and fine in Asian women to heavy, coarse, and curly in women of African descent. The mons pubis protects the pelvic bones, especially during coitus.

Labia Majora

The *labia majora* are longitudinal, raised folds of pigmented skin, one on either side of the vulvar cleft (see Figure 10-3). As the pair descends, they narrow, enclosing the vulvar cleft, and merge to form the posterior junction of the perineal skin. Their chief function is to protect the structures lying between them. The labia majora are covered by stratified squamous epithelium containing hair follicles and sebaceous glands with underlying adipose and muscle tissue. The dartos muscle sheath is responsible for the wrinkled appearance of the labia majora as well as for their sensitivity to heat and cold. The inner surface of the labia majora in women who have not had children is moist and looks like mucous membrane, whereas after many births it is more skinlike. With each pregnancy the labia majora become less prominent.

Because of the extensive venous network in the labia majora, varicosities may occur during pregnancy, and birth trauma or sexual trauma may cause hematomas. The labia majora share an extensive lymphatic supply with the other structures of the vulva, which can facilitate the spread of cancer in the female reproductive organs. Because nerves from the first lumbar and third sacral segment of the spinal cord supply the labia majora, certain regional anesthesia blocks will affect them and cause numbness.

Labia Minora

The *labia minora* are soft folds of skin within the labia majora that converge near the anus, forming the *fourchette* (see Figure 10-3). Each labium minus has the appearance of a shiny mucous membrane, moist and devoid of hair follicles. The labia minora are rich in sebaceous glands, which lubricate and waterproof the vulvar skin and provide bactericidal secretions. Because sebaceous glands do not open into hair follicles but directly onto the surface of the skin, sebaceous cysts commonly occur in this area. The labia minora are composed of erectile tissue and involuntary muscle tissue. Vulvovaginitis in this area is very irritating because the labia minora have many tactile nerve endings. The labia minora increase in size at puberty and decrease after menopause because of changes in estrogen levels.

Clitoris

The *clitoris,* located between the labia minora, is about 5 to 6 mm long and 6 to 8 mm across. Its tissue is essentially erectile (see Figure 10-3). The glans of the clitoris is partly covered by a fold of skin called the *prepuce,* or clitoral hood (an extension of the labia minora). This area resembles an opening to an orifice and may be confused with the urethral meatus. Accidental attempts to insert a catheter in this area produce extreme discomfort. The clitoris has very rich blood and nerve supplies and is the primary erogenous organ of women. It secretes *smegma,* which, along with other vulval secretions, has a unique odor that may be sexually stimulating to the male. In some cultures, the clitoris is removed (see discussion in chapter 8 ∞).

Urethral Meatus and Paraurethral Glands

The *urethral meatus* is located 1 to 2.5 cm beneath the clitoris in the midline of the vestibule; it often appears as a puckered, slitlike opening (see Figure 10-3). At times the meatus is difficult to visualize because of the presence of blind dimples, small mucosal folds, or wide variations in location.

The paraurethral glands, or *Skene's glands,* open into the posterior wall of the urethra close to its opening (see Figure 10-3). Their secretions help lubricate the vaginal vestibule, facilitating sexual intercourse.

Vaginal Vestibule

The vaginal vestibule is a boat-shaped depression enclosed by the labia majora and visible when they are separated (see Figure 10-3). The vestibule contains the vaginal opening, or *introitus,* which is the border between the external and internal genitals.

The *hymen* is a thin, elastic collar or semicollar of tissue that surrounds the vaginal opening. The appearance of the hymen changes during the woman's lifetime. The hymen is essentially avascular. For thousands of years, some societies have perpetuated the belief that the hymen covers the vaginal opening and thus that an intact hymen is a sign of virginity. However, modern studies of female genital anatomy have revealed that the hymen surrounds rather than entirely covers the vaginal opening, and can be torn not only through sexual intercourse, but also through strenuous physical activity, masturbation, menstruation, or the use of tampons, thus dispelling old beliefs. For discussion of the nurse's role in discussing these topics see chapter 4 ∞.

External to the hymen at the base of the vestibule are two small papular elevations containing the openings of the ducts of the *vulvovaginal (Bartholin's) glands.* They lie under the constrictor muscle of the vagina. These glands secrete a clear, thick, alkaline mucus that enhances the viability and motility of sperm deposited in the vaginal vestibule. These gland ducts can harbor *Neisseria gonorrhoeae* and other bacteria, which can cause suppuration and abscesses in the Bartholin's glands.

The vestibular area is innervated mainly by the perineal nerve from the sacral plexus. The area is not sensitive to touch generally; however, the hymen contains numerous free nerve endings as receptors to pain.

Perineal Body

The **perineal body** is a wedge-shaped mass of fibromuscular tissue measuring about 4 × 4 × 4 cm, found between the lower part of the vagina and the anus (see Figure 10-3). The superficial area between the anus and the vagina is referred to as the *perineum.*

The muscles that meet at the perineal body are the external sphincter ani, both levator ani (the superficial and deep transverse perineal), and the bulbocavernosus. These muscles mingle with elastic fibers and connective tissue in an arrangement that allows a remarkable amount of stretching. During the last part of labor, the perineal body thins out until it is just a few centimeters thick. This tissue is often the site of an episiotomy or lacerations during childbirth (see chapter 28 ∞).

Female Internal Reproductive Organs

The female internal reproductive organs—the vagina, uterus, fallopian tubes, and ovaries—are target organs for estrogenic hormones, and they play a unique part in the reproductive cycle (Figure 10-4 ■). Certain internal reproductive organs can be palpated during vaginal examination and assessed with various instruments.

Vagina

The **vagina** is a muscular and membranous tube that connects the external genitals with the uterus (see Figure 10-4). It extends from the vulva to the uterus in a position nearly parallel to the plane of the pelvic brim. The vagina is often referred to as the *birth canal* because it forms the lower part of the axis through which the fetus must pass during birth.

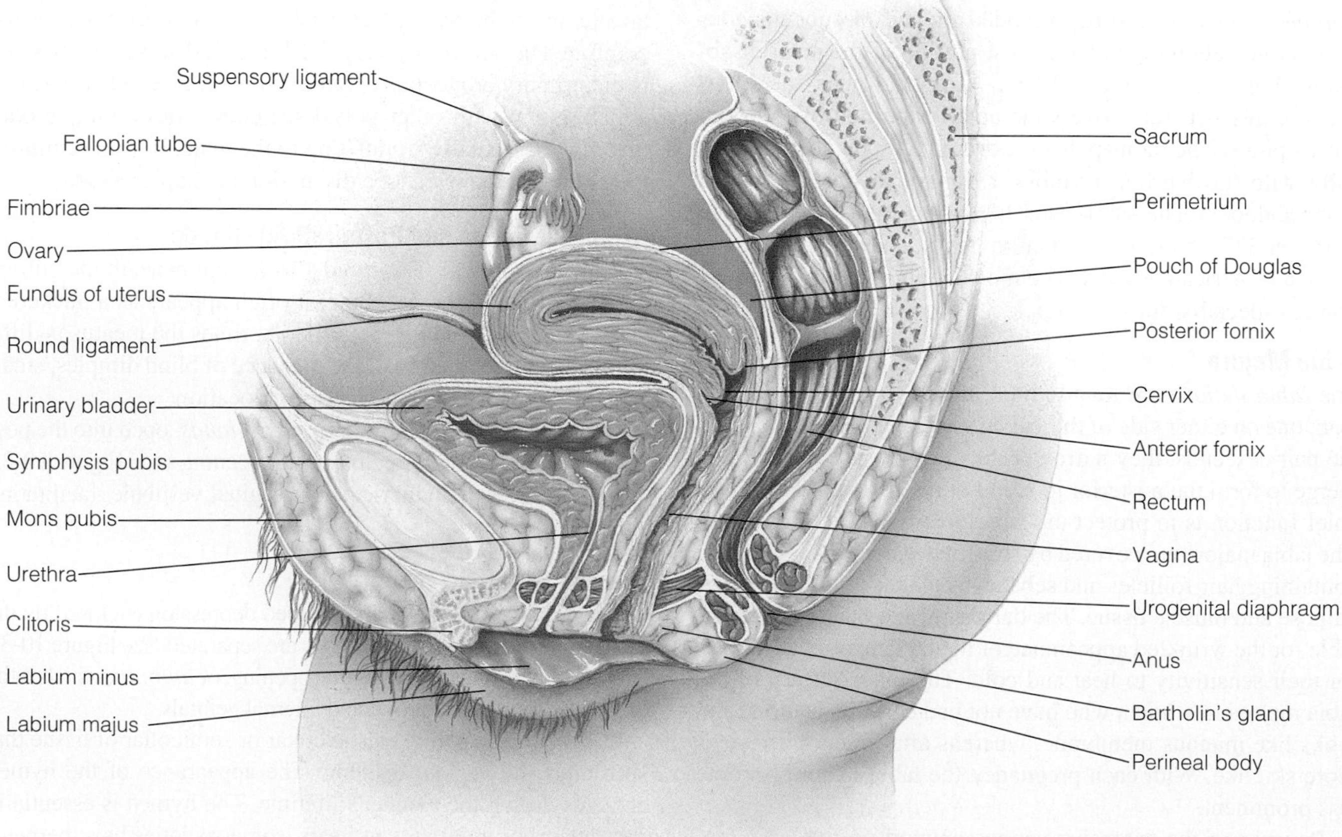

Figure 10-4 ■ Female internal reproductive organs.

Because the cervix of the uterus projects into the upper part of the anterior wall of the vagina, the anterior wall is approximately 2.5 cm shorter than the posterior wall. Measurements range from 6 to 8 cm for the anterior wall and 7 to 10 cm for the posterior wall.

In the upper part of the vagina, which is called the *vaginal vault*, there is a recess or hollow around the cervix. This area is called the vaginal fornix. Because the walls of the vaginal vault are very thin, various structures can be palpated through them, including the uterus, a distended bladder, the ovaries, appendix, cecum, colon, and the ureters. The upper fourth of the vagina is separated from the rectum by the pouch of Douglas (sometimes referred to as the cul-de-sac of Douglas). This deep pouch or recess is posterior to the cervix.

When a woman lies on her back after intercourse, the space in the fornix permits the pooling of semen. The collection of a large number of sperm near the cervix at or near the time of ovulation in the woman increases the chances of pregnancy.

The walls of the vagina are covered with ridges, or *rugae*, crisscrossing each other. These rugae allow the vaginal tissues to stretch enough for the fetus to pass through during childbirth as well as stretch for accommodation during coitus. A rich blood supply is needed to maintain a high glycogen content in the epithelial cells as well as to nourish the underlying musculofascial layer, through which the vaginal vault has strong attachments to the cervix. These muscle layers are continuous with the superficial muscle fibers of the uterus. A thin band of striated muscle, the sphincter vaginae, is found at the lowest extremity of the vagina. However, the levator ani is the principal muscle that closes the vagina.

During a woman's reproductive life, the vaginal environment is normally acidic (pH 4 to 5). Secretion from the vaginal epithelium provides a moist environment. The acidic environment is maintained by a symbiotic relationship between lactic acid-producing bacilli (Döderlein's bacillus or lactobacillus) and the vaginal epithelial cells. These cells contain glycogen, which is broken down by the bacilli into lactic acid. The amount of glycogen is regulated by the ovarian hormones. Any interruption of this process can destroy the normal self-cleansing action of the vagina. Such interruption may be caused by antibiotic therapy, douching, or use of vaginal sprays or deodorants. For further discussion, see chapter 4 ∞. The acidic vaginal environment is normal only during the mature reproductive years and in the first days of life, when maternal hormones are operating in the infant. A relatively neutral pH of 7.5 is normal from infancy until puberty and after menopause.

Each third of the vagina is supplied by a distinct vascular and lymphatic pattern. Although one would expect venous drainage to go directly to the heart and then the lungs, anastomoses of veins are present and make it possible for a pelvic embolism or carcinoma to bypass the heart and lungs and lodge in the brain, spine, or other remote part of the body.

Vaginal lymphatics drain into the external and internal iliac nodes, the hypogastric nodes, and the inguinal glands. The posterior wall drains into nodes lying in the rectovaginal septum. Any vaginal infection follows these routes.

The pudendal nerve supplies what relatively little somatic innervation there is to the lower third of the vagina. Thus vaginal sensation during sexual excitement and coitus is minimal, as is vaginal pain during the second stage of labor.

The vagina has the following functions:

- To serve as the passageway for sperm during coitus and for the fetus during birth
- To provide passage for the menstrual blood flow from the uterine endometrium to the outside of the body
- To protect against trauma from sexual intercourse and infection of the uterus, ovaries, and pelvis from pathogenic organisms

Uterus

As the core of reproduction and hence continuation of the human race, the uterus, or womb, has been endowed with a mystical aura. Numerous customs, taboos, mores, and values have evolved about women and their reproductive function. Although scientific knowledge has replaced much of this folklore, remnants of old ideas and superstitions persist. To provide effective care, nurses must be cognizant of their own attitudes and beliefs as well as those of their patients.

The **uterus** is a hollow, muscular, thick-walled organ shaped like an upside-down pear (Figure 10-5 ■). It lies in the center of the pelvic cavity between the base of the bladder and the rectum and above the vagina (see Figure 10-4). It is level with or slightly below the brim of the pelvis with the external opening of the cervix (the external os) about the level of the ischial spines. The uterus of the mature women weighs about 40 to 70 g and is 6 to 8 cm long (Cunningham et al., 2010).

Many uterine anomalies are thought to be congenital. A normal uterus requires two symmetric, parallel, equal-sized paramesonephric ducts to meet in the midline. Their ultimate midline fusion gives rise to the fallopian tubes, uterine fundus, cervix, and upper vagina. Anomalies represent the absence of either one

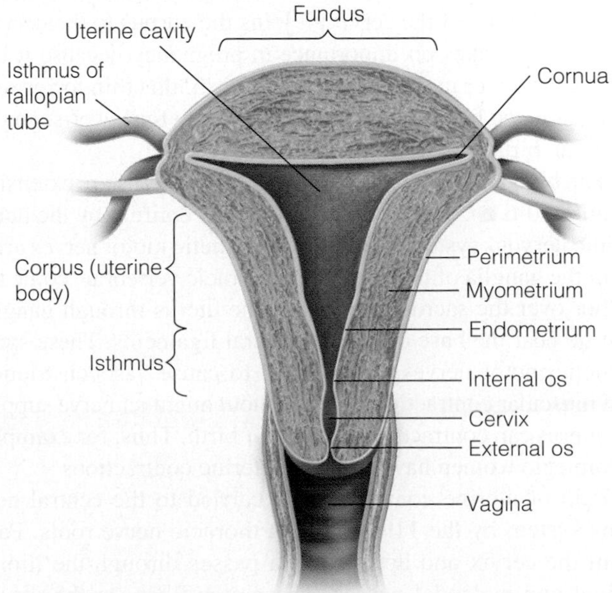

Figure 10-5 ■ Structures of the uterus.

or both of the ducts, degrees of failure to fuse, or canalization defects. Uterine malformations such as the uterus bicornuate ("two-horned") and uterus didelphys ("double uterus") are associated with habitual abortion. Because both the urinary and reproductive systems develop from the common urogenital fold in the embryo, anomalies in one system are frequently accompanied by anomalies in the other. Problems of infertility and premature labor and birth are common.

About a fourth of women exposed to diethylstilbestrol (DES) in utero have structural variations of the cervix, uterus, and vagina (Cunningham et al., 2010). These women have increased incidence of miscarriage, ectopic pregnancy, cervical incompetency, and preterm births.

The body of the uterus can move freely forward or backward. Only the cervix is anchored laterally. Thus the position of the uterus can vary, depending on a woman's posture, number of children borne, bladder and rectal fullness, and even normal respiratory patterns. Generally, the uterus bends forward, forming a sharp angle with the vagina. If there is a bend in the area of the isthmus of the uterus, and from there the cervix points downward, the uterus is said to be anteverted or anteflexed. Four pairs of ligaments (i.e., cardinal, uterosacral, round, and broad) support the uterus. Single anterior and posterior ligaments also support the uterus.

The uterus is divided into two major parts: an upper triangular portion called the **corpus**, or uterine body, and a lower cylindric portion called the cervix (see Figure 10-5). The corpus comprises the upper two thirds of the uterus and is composed mainly of a smooth muscle layer (myometrium). The lower third is the cervix, or neck. The rounded uppermost portion of the corpus that extends above the points of attachment of the fallopian tubes is called the **fundus**. The elongated portion of the uterus where the fallopian tubes enter is called the **cornua**.

The *isthmus* is that portion of the uterus between the internal cervical os and the endometrial cavity. The isthmus is about 6 mm above the uterine opening of the cervix (the internal os), and it is in this area that the uterine lining changes into the mucous membrane of the cervix; it joins the corpus to the cervix. The isthmus takes on importance in pregnancy because it becomes the lower uterine segment. At birth, this thin lower segment, situated behind the bladder, is the site for lower-segment cesarean births (see chapter 28 ∞).

The blood and lymphatic supplies to the uterus are extensive (Figure 10-6 ■). The uterus is innervated entirely by the autonomic nervous system. Efferent sympathetic motor nerves arise from the ganglia of the 5th to 10th thoracic vertebrae, come together over the sacrum, and reach the uterus through ganglia that lie near the base of the uterosacral ligaments. These sympathetic motor nerves are believed to cause vasoconstriction and muscular contraction. Even without an intact nerve supply, the uterus can contract adequately for birth. Thus, for example, hemiplegic women have adequate uterine contractions.

Pain of uterine contractions is carried to the central nervous system by the 11th and 12th thoracic nerve roots. Pain from the cervix and upper vagina passes through the ilioinguinal and pudendal nerves. The motor fibers to the uterus arise from the 7th and 8th thoracic vertebrae. Because the sen-

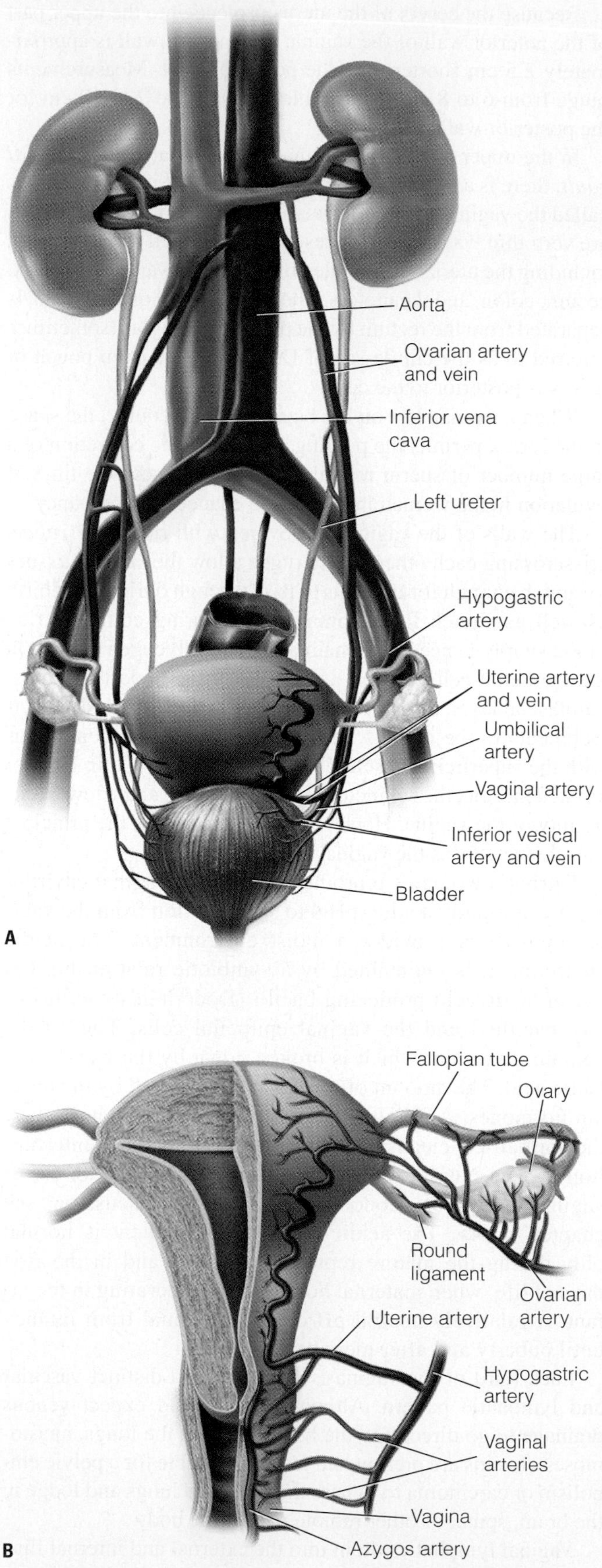

Figure 10-6 ■ Blood supply to internal reproductive organs: A. Pelvic blood supply. B. Blood supply to the vagina, ovary, uterus, and fallopian tube.

sory and motor levels are separate, epidural anesthesia can be used during labor and birth.

The function of the uterus is to provide a safe environment for fetal development. The uterine lining is cyclically prepared by steroid hormones for implantation of the embryo, a process known as **nidation**. Once the embryo is implanted, the developing fetus is protected until it is expelled.

Both the body of the uterus and the cervix are changed permanently by pregnancy. The body never returns to its prepregnant size, and the external os changes from a circular opening of about 3 mm to a transverse slit with irregular edges.

UTERINE CORPUS The uterine corpus is made up of three layers. The outermost layer is the *serosal layer,* or **perimetrium**, which is composed of peritoneum. The middle layer is the *muscular uterine layer,* or **myometrium**. This muscular uterine layer is continuous with the muscle layer of the fallopian tubes and with that of the vagina. This characteristic helps the organs present a unified reaction to various stimuli—ovulation, orgasm, or the deposit of sperm in the vagina. These muscle fibers also extend into the ovarian, round, and cardinal ligaments and minimally into the uterosacral ligaments, which helps explain the vague but disturbing pelvic "aches and pains" reported by many pregnant women.

The myometrium has three distinct layers of uterine (smooth) involuntary muscles (Figure 10-7 ■). The outer layer, found mainly over the fundus, is made up of longitudinal muscles that cause the descent of the fetus, which places pressure on the cervical fibers leading to cervical effacement and delivery of the fetus. The thick middle layer is made up of interlacing muscle fibers in figure-eight patterns that assist the longitudinal fibers in expelling the fetus. These muscle fibers surround large blood vessels, and their contraction produces a hemostatic action (a tourniquet-like action on blood vessels to stop bleeding after birth). The inner muscle layer consists of circular fibers that form sphincters at the fallopian tube attachment sites and at the internal os. The internal os sphincter inhibits the expulsion of the uterine contents during pregnancy but relaxes in labor as cervical dilatation occurs. An incompetent cervical os can be caused by a torn, weak, or absent sphincter at the internal os. The sphincters at the fallopian tubes prevent menstrual blood from flowing backward into the fallopian tubes from the uterus.

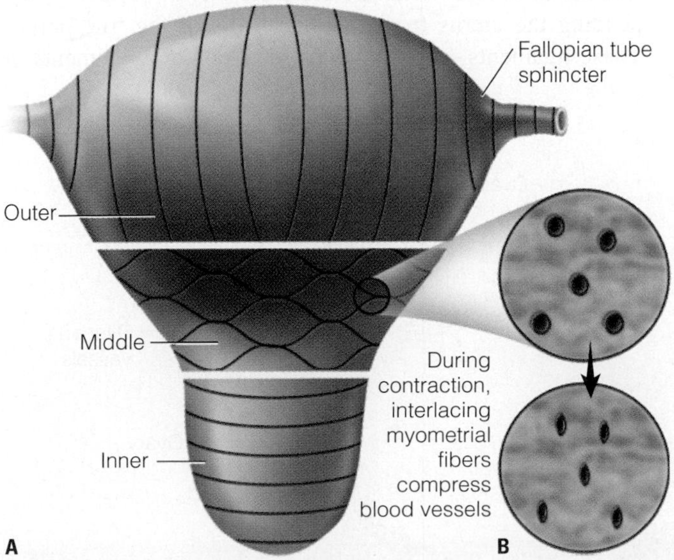

Figure 10-7 ■ Myometrium uterine muscle layers placement and function. A. Outer layer (longitudinal muscles) suited to expel fetus. B. Middle layer (interlacing muscle fibers in figure-eight pattern) surround and constrict blood vessels to stop bleeding, C. Inner layer (circular muscle fibers form sphincters at fallopian tubes and internal os) to prevent backflow menstrual blood into fallopian tubes and cervical dilatation during labor/delivery.

Although each layer of muscle has been discussed as having a unique function, it must be remembered that the uterine musculature works as a whole. The uterine contractions of labor are responsible for the dilatation of the cervix and provide the major force for the passage of the fetus through the pelvic and vaginal canal at birth.

The innermost layer of the uterine corpus is the *mucosal layer,* or **endometrium**, which is composed of a single layer of columnar epithelium, glands, and stroma. From menarche to menopause, the endometrium undergoes monthly renewal and degeneration in the absence of pregnancy. As it responds to a governing hormonal cycle and prostaglandin influence as well, the endometrium varies in thickness from 0.5 to 5 mm.

The glands of the endometrium produce a thin, watery, alkaline secretion that keeps the uterine cavity moist. This endometrial milk not only helps sperm travel to the fallopian tubes but also nourishes the developing embryo before it implants in the endometrium (see chapter 11 ∞).

The blood supply to the endometrium is unique. In the myometrium, the radial arteries branch off from the arcuate arteries at right angles. Once inside the endometrium, they become the basal arteries supplying the zona basalis (a layer of the endometrium) and ultimately become the coiled arteries supplying the zona functionalis (also part of the endometrium). The basal arteries are not sensitive to cyclic hormonal control; hence, the zona basalis portion remains intact and is the site of new endometrial tissue generation. The coiled arteries are extremely sensitive to cyclic hormonal control. Their response is alternate relaxation and constriction during the ischemic, or terminal, phase of the menstrual cycle. These differing responses allow for part of the endometrial tissue to remain intact while other endometrial tissue is shed during menstruation.

When pregnancy occurs and the endometrium is not shed, the reticular stromal cells surrounding the endometrial glands become the decidual cells of pregnancy. The stromal cells are highly vascular, channeling a rich blood supply to the endometrial surface.

CERVIX The distal end of the uterus is the **cervix**. It meets the body of the uterus at the internal os and descends about 2.5 cm to connect with the vagina at the external os (see Figure 10-5). Thus it provides a protective portal for the body of the uterus. The cervix is divided by its line of attachment into the vaginal and supravaginal areas. The vaginal cervix projects into the vagina at an angle from 45 to 90 degrees. The *supravaginal* cervix is surrounded by the attachments that give the uterus its main support: the uterosacral ligaments, the transverse ligaments of the cervix (Mackenrodt's ligaments), and the pubocervical ligaments.

The vaginal cervix appears pink and ends at the external os. The cervical canal appears rosy red and is lined with columnar ciliated epithelium, which contains mucus-secreting glands. Most cervical cancer begins at this *squamocolumnar junction.* The specific location of the junction varies with age and number of pregnancies. Figure 10-8 ■ shows this junction at various stages of a woman's life.

Elasticity is the chief characteristic of the cervix. Its ability to stretch is due to the high fibrous and collagenous content of the supportive tissues and also to the vast number of folds in the cervical lining.

The cervical mucosa has three functions:

- To provide lubrication for the vaginal canal
- To act as a bacteriostatic agent
- To provide an alkaline environment to shelter deposited sperm from the acidic vaginal secretions

At ovulation, cervical mucus is clearer, thinner, and more alkaline than at other times.

Uterine Ligaments

The uterine ligaments support and stabilize the various reproductive organs. The ligaments shown in Figure 10-9 ■ are described in this section.

- The **broad ligament** keeps the uterus centrally placed and provides stability within the pelvic cavity. It is a double layer that is continuous with the abdominal peritoneum. The broad ligament covers the uterus anteriorly and posteriorly and extends outward from the uterus to enfold and stabilize the fallopian tubes. The round and ovarian ligaments are at the upper border of the broad ligament. At its lower border, the broad ligament forms the cardinal ligaments. Between the folds of the broad ligament are connective tissue, involuntary muscle, blood and lymph vessels, and nerves.
- The **round ligaments** keep the uterus in place. The round ligaments arise from the sides of the uterus near the fallopian tube insertions. They extend outward between the folds of the broad ligament, passing through the inguinal ring and canals and eventually fusing with the connective tissue of the labia majora. The round ligaments are made up of longitudinal muscle and enlarge during pregnancy. During labor the round ligaments steady the uterus, pulling downward and forward, so that the presenting part of the fetus is forced into the cervix.
- The **ovarian ligaments** anchor the lower pole of the ovary to the cornua of the uterus. They are composed of muscle fibers, which allow the ligaments to contract. This contractile ability influences the position of the ovary to some extent, thus helping the fimbriae of the fallopian tubes to "catch" the ovum as it is released each month.
- The **cardinal ligaments** are the chief uterine supports, suspending the uterus from the side walls of the true pelvis. These ligaments, also known as Mackenrodt's ligaments or

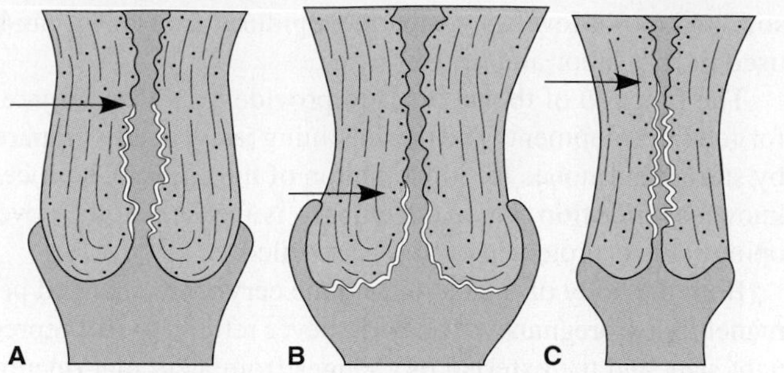

Figure 10-8 ■ Changes in squamocolumnar junction (arrows) at various stages of life: A. Childhood. B. Reproductive years. C. Postmenopausal years.

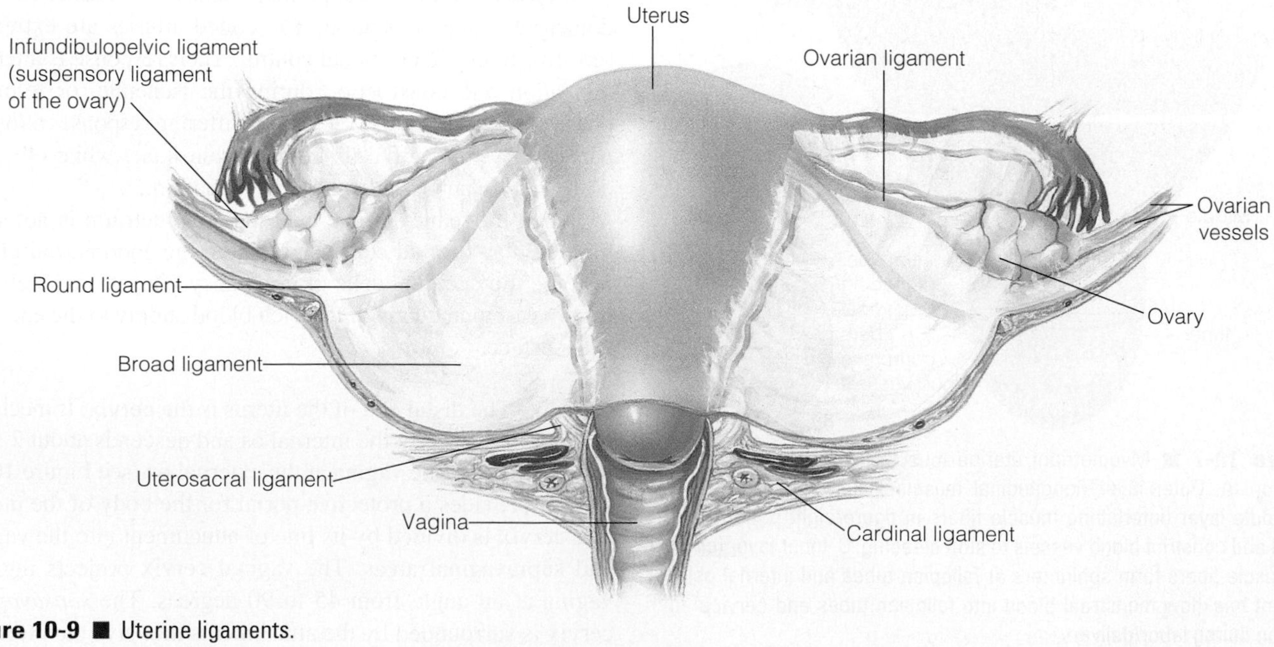

Figure 10-9 ■ Uterine ligaments.

transverse cervical ligaments, arise from the sides of the pelvic walls and attach to the cervix in the upper vagina. These ligaments prevent uterine prolapse and also support the upper vagina.

- The **infundibulopelvic ligament** suspends and supports the ovaries. Arising from the outer third of the broad ligament, the infundibulopelvic ligament contains the ovarian vessels and nerves.
- The **uterosacral ligaments** provide support for the uterus and cervix at the level of the ischial spines. Arising on each side of the pelvis from the posterior wall of the uterus, the uterosacral ligaments sweep back around the rectum and insert on the sides of the first and second sacral vertebrae. The uterosacral ligaments contain smooth muscle fibers, connective tissue, blood and lymph vessels, and nerves. They also contain sensory nerve fibers that contribute to dysmenorrhea (painful menstruation; see chapter 4 ∞).

Fallopian Tubes

The two **fallopian tubes**, also known as *oviducts* or *uterine tubes,* arise from each side of the uterus and reach almost to the side of the pelvis, where they turn toward the ovaries (Figure 10-10 ■). Each tube is approximately 8 to 13.5 cm long. A short section of each fallopian tube is inside the uterus; its opening into the uterus is 1 mm in diameter. The fallopian tubes link the peritoneal cavity with the uterus and vagina. This linkage increases a woman's vulnerability to disease processes.

Each fallopian tube may be divided into three parts: the isthmus, the ampulla, and the infundibulum or fimbria. The fallopian tube **isthmus** is straight and narrow, with a thick muscular wall and an opening (lumen) 2 to 3 mm in diameter. It is the site of tubal ligation (a surgical procedure to prevent pregnancy; see chapter 5 ∞).

Next to the isthmus is the curved **ampulla**, which comprises the outer two thirds of the tube. Fertilization of the secondary oocyte by a spermatozoon usually occurs here. The ampulla ends at the **fimbria**, which is a funnel-like enlargement with many moving fingerlike projections (fimbriae) reaching out to the ovary. The longest of these, the *fimbria ovarica,* is attached to the ovary to increase the chances of intercepting the ovum as it is released.

The wall of the fallopian tube is made up of four layers: peritoneal (serous), subserous (adventitial), muscular, and mucous tissues. The peritoneum covers the tubes. The subserous layer contains the blood and nerve supply, and the muscular layer is responsible for the peristaltic movement of the tube. The mucosal layer, immediately next to the muscular layer, is composed of ciliated and nonciliated cells with the number of ciliated cells more abundant at the fimbria. Nonciliated cells secrete a protein-rich, serous fluid that nourishes the ovum. The constantly moving tubal cilia propel the ovum toward the uterus. Because the ovum is a large cell, this ciliary action is needed to assist the tube's muscular layer peristalsis. Any malformation or malfunction of the tubes could result in infertility, ectopic pregnancy, or even sterility.

A well-functioning tubal transport system involves active fimbriae close to the ovary, peristalsis of the tube created by the muscular layer, ciliated currents beating toward the uterus, and the proximal contraction and distal relaxation of the tube caused by different types of prostaglandins.

A rich blood and lymph supply serves each fallopian tube. Thus the fallopian tubes have an unusual ability to recover from any inflammatory process.

The fallopian tubes have three functions:

- To provide transport for the ovum from the ovary to the uterus (transport through the fallopian tubes varies from 3 to 4 days)
- To provide a site for fertilization
- To serve as a warm, moist, nourishing environment for the ovum or zygote (a fertilized egg; see also chapter 11 ∞)

Ovaries

The **ovaries** are two almond-shaped glandular structures just below the pelvic brim. One ovary is located on each side of the pelvic cavity. Their size varies among women and according to the stage of the menstrual cycle. Each ovary weighs 6 to 10 g and is 1.5 to 3 cm wide, 2 to 5 cm long, and 1 to 1.5 cm thick.

Activities: Female Reproductive System

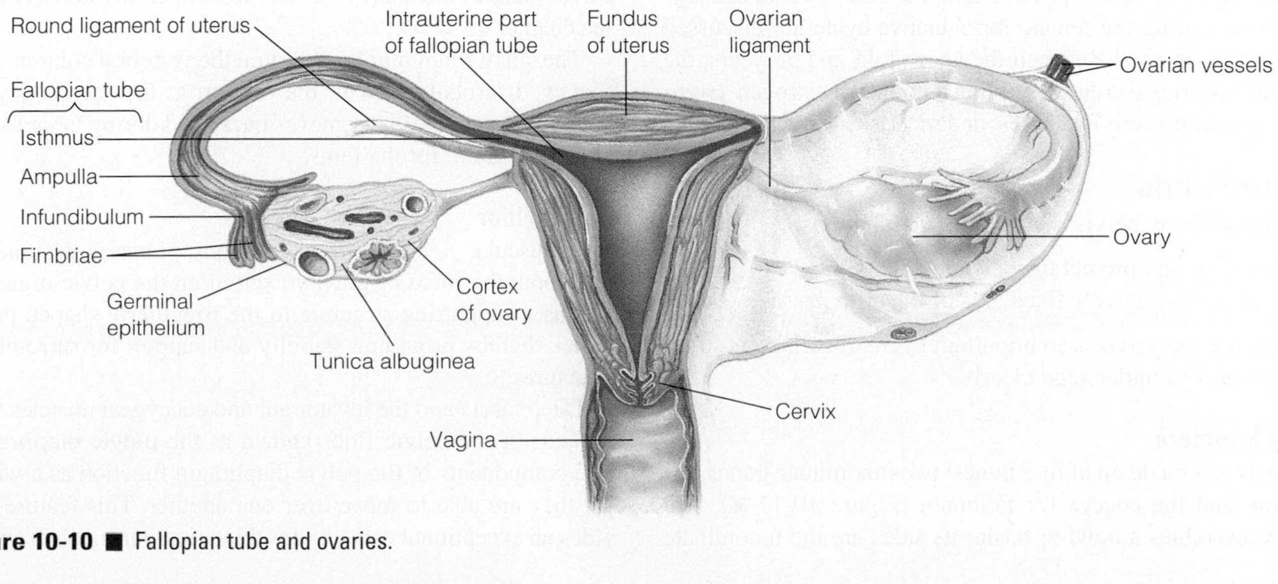

Figure 10-10 ■ Fallopian tube and ovaries.

The ovaries of girls are small, but they become larger after puberty and then decrease in size following menopause. They also change in appearance from smooth-surfaced, dull white organs to pitted gray organs as the woman ages. The pitting appearance on their surface is the result of scarring after ovulation. It is rare for both ovaries to be at the same level in the pelvic cavity. The ovary is held in place by the ovarian, broad, and infundibulopelvic ligaments (see Figure 10-9), discussed earlier in the chapter.

There is no peritoneal covering for the ovaries. Although this lack of covering assists the mature ovum to erupt, it also allows easier spread of malignant cells from cancer of the ovaries. A single layer of cuboidal epithelial cells, called the germinal epithelium, covers the ovaries. The ovaries are composed of three layers: the tunica albuginea, the cortex, and the medulla. The *tunica albuginea* is dense and dull white and serves as a protective layer. The *cortex* is the main functional part, containing ova, graafian follicles, corpora lutea, degenerated corpora lutea (corpora albicantia), and degenerated follicles. The *medulla* is completely surrounded by the cortex and contains the nerves and the blood and lymphatic vessels.

The ovaries are the primary source of two important hormones: the estrogens and progesterone. *Estrogens* are associated with characteristics contributing to femaleness, including breast alveolar lobule growth and duct development. The ovaries secrete large amounts of estrogens; the adrenal cortex (extraglandular sites) produces minute amounts of estrogens in nonpregnant women and the fat cells produce a secondary estrogen.

Progesterone is often called the *hormone of pregnancy* because it inhibits uterine contractions and relaxes smooth muscle to cause vasodilation, allowing pregnancy to be maintained. The placenta is the primary source of progesterone during pregnancy. This hormone also inhibits the action of prolactin in α-lactalbumin synthesis, thereby preventing lactation during pregnancy (Lawrence & Lawrence, 2009).

The interplay between the ovarian hormones and other hormones such as follicle-stimulating hormone (FSH) and luteinizing hormone (LH) is responsible for the cyclic changes that allow pregnancy to occur. The hormonal and physical changes that occur during the female reproductive cycle are discussed later in this chapter. Between the ages of 45 and 55 years, the woman's ovaries secrete decreasing amounts of estrogen. Eventually ovulatory activity ceases, and menopause occurs.

Bony Pelvis

Application: Pelvic Structures

The female bony pelvis has two unique functions:

- To support and protect the pelvic contents
- To form the relatively fixed axis of the birth passage

Because the pelvis is so important to childbearing, its structures should be understood clearly.

Bony Structure

The pelvis is made up of four bones: two innominate bones, the sacrum, and the coccyx (or tailbone) (Figure 10-11 ■). The pelvis resembles a bowl or basin; its sides are the innominate bones, and its back is composed of the sacrum and coccyx. Lined with fibrocartilage and held tightly together by ligaments, the four bones join at the symphysis pubis, the two sacroiliac joints, and the sacrococcygeal joints.

The *innominate* bones, also known as the hip bones or os coxae, are made up of three separate bones: the ilium, the ischium, and the pubis. These bones fuse to form a circular cavity, the *acetabulum,* which articulates with the femur.

The *ilium* is the broad, upper prominence of the hip. The *iliac crest* is the margin of the ilium. The ischial spines, the foremost projections nearest the groin, are the site of attachment for ligaments and muscles.

The *ischium,* the strongest bone, lies under the ilium and below the acetabulum. The L-shaped ischium ends in a marked protuberance, the *ischial tuberosity,* on which the weight of a seated body rests. The **ischial spines** arise near the junction of the ilium and ischium and jut into the pelvic cavity. The shortest diameter of the pelvic cavity is located between the ischial spines. The ischial spines can serve as a reference point during labor to evaluate the descent of the fetal head into the birth canal. (See chapter 22 ∞ and Figure 22-7 on page 535).

The **pubis** forms the slightly bowed front portion of the innominate bone. Extending medially from the acetabulum to the midpoint of the bony pelvis, the two pubic bones meet to form a joint, the **symphysis pubis**. The triangular space below this junction is known as the pubic arch. The fetal head passes under this arch during birth. The symphysis pubis is formed by heavy fibrocartilage and the superior and inferior pubic ligaments. The mobility of the inferior ligament increases during the first pregnancy and to a greater extent in subsequent pregnancies.

The sacroiliac joints also have a degree of mobility that increases near the end of pregnancy and results in an upward gliding movement. The pelvic outlet may be increased by 1.5 to 2 cm in the squatting and sitting positions. Relaxation of the pelvic joints is induced by relaxin, one of the hormones of pregnancy.

The *sacrum* is a wedge-shaped bone formed by the fusion of five vertebrae. On the anterior upper portion of the sacrum is a projection into the pelvic cavity known as the **sacral promontory**. This projection is another obstetric guide in determining pelvic measurements. (For discussion of pelvic measurements, see chapter 15 ∞).

The small triangular bone last on the vertebral column is the coccyx. It articulates with the sacrum at the sacrococcygeal joint. The coccyx usually moves backward during labor to provide more room for the fetus.

Pelvic Floor

The muscular *pelvic floor* of the bony pelvis is designed to overcome the force of gravity exerted on the pelvic organs. It acts as a supporting structure to the irregularly shaped pelvic outlet, thereby providing stability and support for surrounding structures.

Deep fascia and the levator ani and coccygeal muscles form the part of the pelvic floor known as the **pelvic diaphragm**. The components of the pelvic diaphragm function as a whole, yet they are able to move over one another. This feature provides an exceptional capacity for dilatation during birth and re-

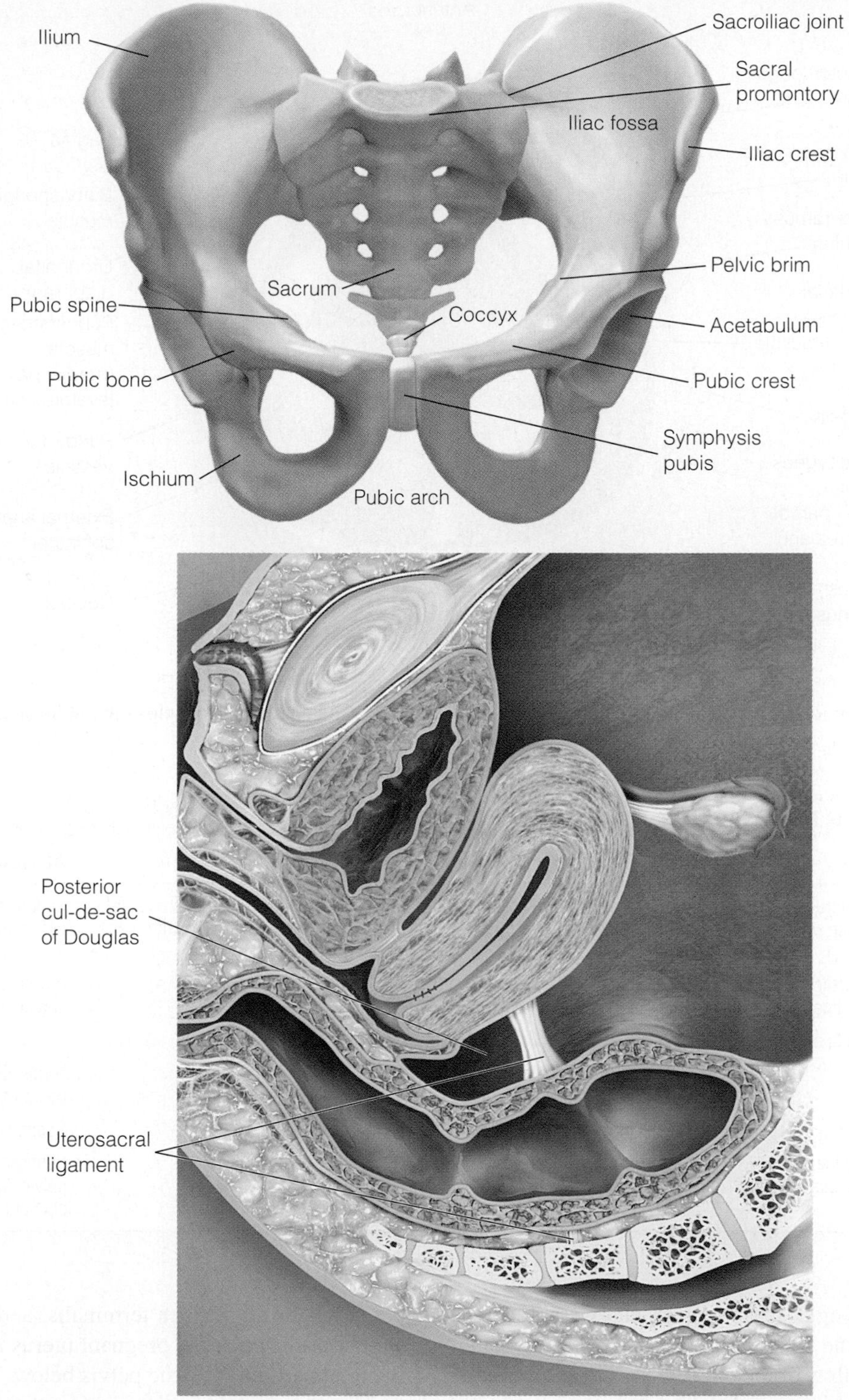

Figure 10-11 ■ Pelvis: A. Pelvic bones. B. Midsagittal view in supine position with uterosacral ligament attachment.

turn to prepregnancy condition following birth. Above the pelvic diaphragm is the **pelvic cavity**; below and behind it is the perineum. The sacrum is located posteriorly.

The levator ani muscle makes up the major portion of the pelvic diaphragm. It consists of four muscles: the iliococcygeus, pubococcygeus, puborectalis, and pubovaginalis muscles. The iliococcygeal muscle, a thin muscular sheet underlying the sacrospinous ligament, helps the levator ani support the pelvic organs. Muscles of the pelvic floor are shown in Figure 10-12 ■ and discussed in Table 10-1.

Endopelvic fascia covers the pelvic diaphragm and allows the pelvic diaphragm components to function as a whole, yet allows them to move over one another. This feature provides the pelvic diaphragm with the exceptional capacity for dilatation during birth and facilitates the return to prepregnant condition following birth.

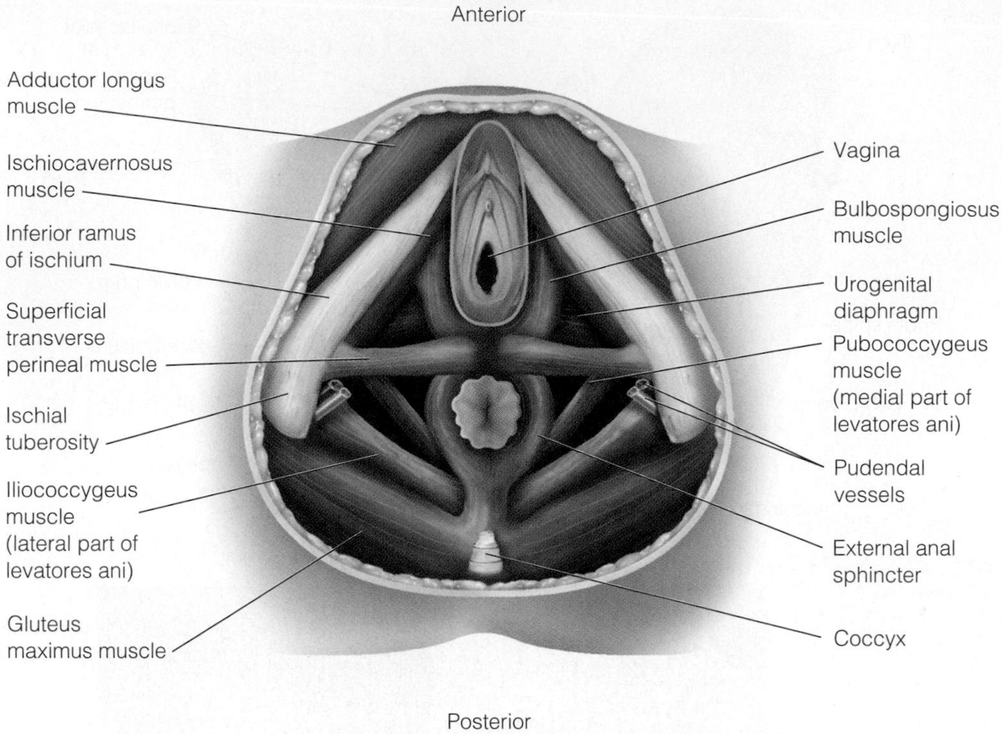

Figure 10-12 ■ Muscles of the pelvic floor. (The puborectalis, pubovaginalis, and coccygeal muscles cannot be seen from this view.)

TABLE 10-1 Muscles of the Pelvic Floor

MUSCLE	ORIGIN	INSERTION	INNERVATION	ACTION
Levator ani	Pubis, lateral pelvic wall, and ischial spine	Blends with organs in pelvic cavity	Inferior rectal, second and third sacral nerves, plus anterior rami of third and fourth sacral nerves	Supports pelvic viscera; helps form pelvic diaphragm
Iliococcygeus	Pelvic surface of ischial spine and pelvic fascia	Central point of perineum, coccygeal raphe, and coccyx		Assists in supporting abdominal and pelvic viscera
Pubococcygeus	Pubis and pelvic fascia	Coccyx		
Puborectalis	Pubis	Blends with rectum; meets similar fibers from opposite side		Forms sling for rectum, just posterior to it; raises anus
Pubovaginalis	Pubis	Blends into vagina		Supports vagina
Coccygeus	Ischial spine and sacrospinous ligament	Lateral border of lower sacrum and upper coccyx	Third and fourth sacral nerves	Supports pelvic viscera; helps form pelvic diaphragm; flexes and abducts coccyx

The urogenital triangle (diaphragm) is external to the pelvic diaphragm, in the triangular area between the ischial tuberosities and the hollow of the pubic arch. The most important muscles in this region are the deep transverse perineal muscles, which are flat bands of muscle arising from the ischiopubic rami and intertwining in the midline to form a seam, or raphe. These muscles are modified to encircle both the urinary meatus and the vaginal orifice, forming the urethral and vaginal sphincters.

Pelvic Division

The pelvic cavity is divided into the false pelvis and the true pelvis (Figure 10-13 ■). The **false pelvis** is the portion above the pelvic brim, or linea terminalis, and serves to support the weight of the enlarged pregnant uterus and direct the presenting fetal part into the true pelvis below.

The **true pelvis** is the portion that lies below the pelvic brim. The bony circumference of the true pelvis is made up of the sacrum, coccyx, and innominate bones and represents the bony limits of the birth canal. It measures about 5 cm at its anterior wall at the symphysis pubis and about 10 cm at its posterior wall. When a woman is standing upright, the upper portion of the pelvic cavity or canal is directed downward and backward; its lower portion, downward and forward. This forms a curved canal through which the presenting part of the baby must pass during birth (see Figure 10-13). The inclina-

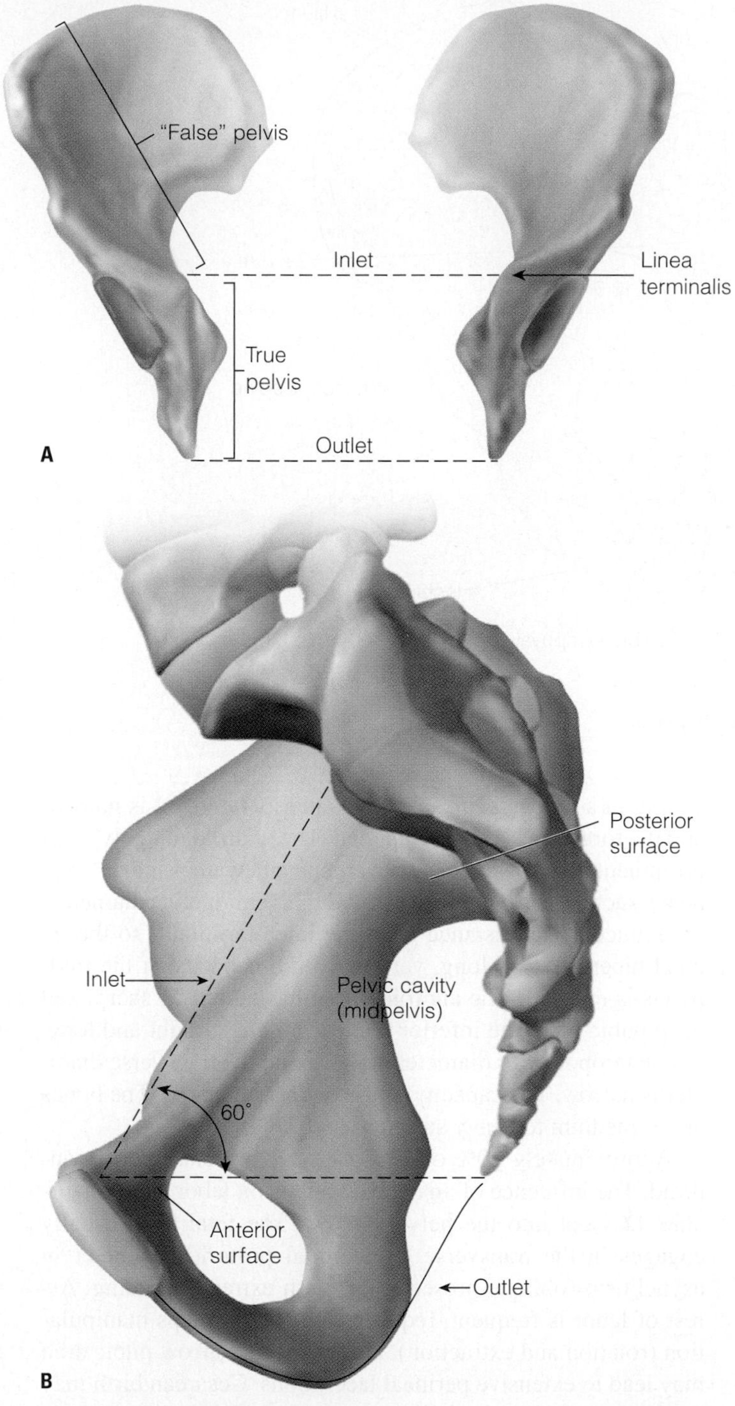

Figure 10-13 ■ Female pelvis: A. The false pelvis is the shallow cavity above the inlet; the true pelvis is the deeper portion of the cavity below the inlet. B. The true pelvis consists of the inlet, cavity (midpelvis), outlet, and pelvic angle of inclination when the woman is standing.

tion of the pelvis is the angle formed by two planes: a horizontal plane passing through the tip of the coccyx and the superior border of the symphysis pubis, and an inclined plane passing through the sacral promontory and the superior border of the symphysis pubis. This pelvic angle of inclination usually measures 50 to 60 degrees.

The relationship of the fetal head to the true pelvic cavity is of paramount importance. The size and shape of the true pelvis must be adequate for normal fetal passage during labor and at birth. The true pelvis consists of three parts: the inlet, the pelvic cavity, and the outlet. Each part has distinct measurements that aid in evaluating the adequacy of the pelvis for childbirth. Measurement techniques are discussed in chapter 15 ∞. The effects of inadequate or abnormal pelvic diameters on labor and birth are considered in chapter 27 ∞.

The **pelvic inlet** is the upper border of the true pelvis and typically is round in the female. The size and shape of the pelvic inlet are determined by assessing three anteroposterior diameters: the diagonal conjugate, obstetric conjugate, and conjugate vera (Figure 10-14 ■). (For an in-depth discussion, see chapter 15 ∞). The **diagonal conjugate** extends from the subpubic angle to the middle of the sacral promontory and is typically 12.5 cm. The diagonal conjugate can be measured manually during a pelvic examination. The **obstetric conjugate** extends from the middle of the sacral promontory to an area approximately 1 cm below the pubic crest. Its length is estimated by subtracting 1.5 cm from the diagonal conjugate. The fetus passes through the obstetric conjugate, and the size of this diameter determines whether the fetus can move down into the birth canal in order for engagement to occur. The true (anatomic) conjugate, or **conjugate vera**, extends from the middle of the sacral promontory to the middle of the pubic crest (superior surface of the symphysis). One additional measurement, the transverse diameter, helps determine the shape of the inlet. The **transverse diameter** is the largest diameter of the inlet and is measured by using the linea terminalis as the point of reference.

The *pelvic cavity* (canal) is a curved canal with a longer posterior than anterior wall. A change in the lumbar curve can increase or decrease the pelvic inclination and can influence the progress of labor, because the fetus has to adjust itself to this curved path as well as to the different diameters of the true pelvis.

The **pelvic outlet** is at the lower border of the true pelvis. The size of the pelvic outlet can be determined by assessing the *transverse diameter.* The anteroposterior diameter of the pelvic outlet increases during birth as the presenting part pushes the coccyx posteriorly at the mobile sacrococcygeal joint. Decreased mobility, a large fetal head, and/or a forceful birth can cause the coccyx to break. As the infant's head emerges, the long diameter of the head (occipital frontal) parallels the long diameter of the outlet (anteroposterior).

The transverse diameter *(bi-ischial or intertuberous)* extends from the inner surface of one ischial tuberosity to the other. It is the shortest diameter of the pelvic outlet and becomes even shorter if the woman has a narrowed pubic arch. The pubic arch has great importance because the baby must pass under it during birth. If it is narrow, the baby's head may be pushed backward toward the coccyx, making the extension of the head difficult. This situation, known as *outlet dystocia,* may require the use of forceps or a cesarean birth. The shoulders of a large baby may also get stuck under the pubic arch, making birth more difficult. The clinical assessment of each of these obstetric diameters is discussed further in chapter 15 ∞.

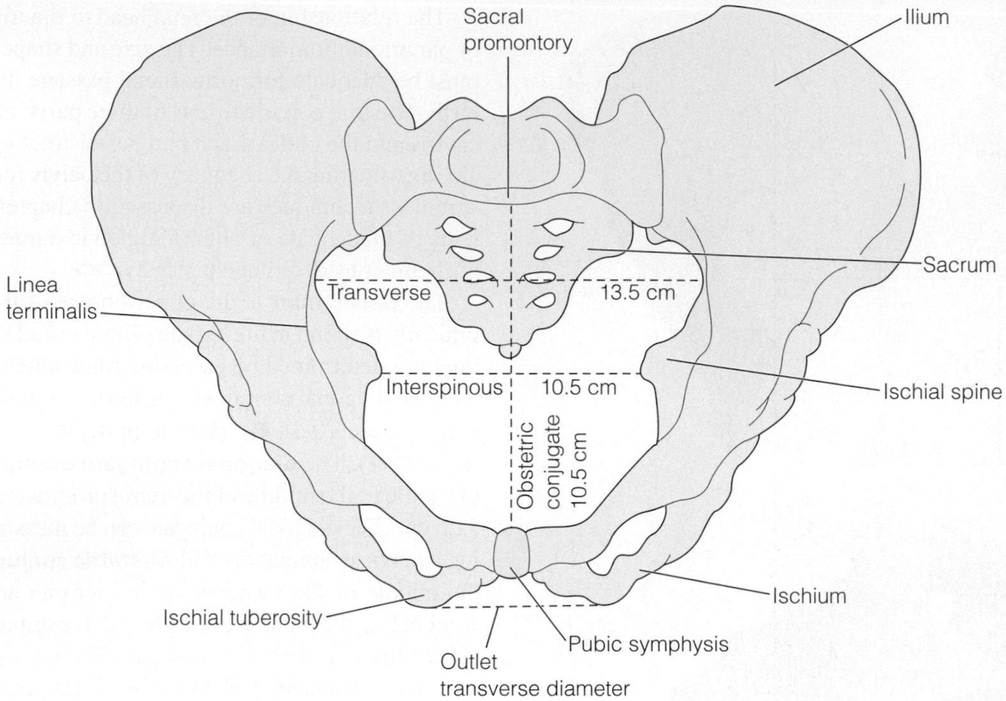

Figure 10-14 ■ Pelvic planes: coronal section and diameters of the bony pelvis.

Pelvic Types

The Caldwell-Moloy classification of pelves (Figure 10-15 ■) is widely used to differentiate types of bony pelves (Caldwell & Moloy, 1933). *Gynecoid, android, anthropoid,* and *platypelloid* are the four basic types. However, variations in the female pelvis are so great that classic types are not usual. Each type of pelvis has a characteristic shape, and each shape has implications for labor and birth. The types are described briefly here, and their implications for labor and birth are discussed in detail in chapter 22 ∞.

GYNECOID PELVIS The most common female pelvis is the gynecoid type. The inlet is rounded with the anteroposterior diameter a little shorter than the transverse diameter. All of the inlet diameters are at least adequate. The posterior segment is broad, deep, and roomy, and the anterior segment is well rounded. The gynecoid midpelvis has nonprominent ischial spines; straight and parallel side walls; and a wide, deep sacral curve. The sacrum is short and slopes backward. All of the midpelvic diameters are at least adequate. The gynecoid pelvic outlet has a wide and round pubic arch; the inferior pubic rami are short and concave. The anteroposterior diameter is long; the transverse diameter, adequate. The capacity of the outlet is adequate. The bones are of medium structure and weight. Approximately 50% of female pelves are classified as gynecoid.

ANDROID PELVIS The normal male pelvis is the android type; however, it occasionally is seen in females. The inlet is heart shaped. The anteroposterior and transverse diameters are adequate for birth, but the posterior sagittal diameter is too short, and the anterior sagittal diameter is long. The posterior segment is shallow because the sacral promontory is indented, resulting in a reduced capacity. The anterior segment is narrow, and the forepelvis is sharply angled. The android midpelvis has prominent ischial spines; convergent sidewalls; and a long, heavy sacrum inclining forward. All of the midpelvic diameters are reduced. The distance from the linea terminalis to the ischial tuberosities is long, yet the overall capacity of the midpelvis is reduced. The android outlet has a narrow, sharp, and deep pubic arch; the inferior pubic rami are straight and long. The anteroposterior diameter is short, and the transverse diameter is narrow. The capacity of the outlet is reduced. The bones are of medium to heavy structure and weight.

Approximately 20% of female pelves are classified as android. The influence of an android pelvis on labor is not favorable. Descent into the pelvis is slow. The fetal head usually engages in the transverse or occipital posterior diameter in asynclitism (oblique presentation) with extreme molding. Arrest of labor is frequent, requiring difficult forceps manipulation (rotation and extraction), and the deep, narrow pubic arch may lead to extensive perineal lacerations. Cesarean birth may be required.

ANTHROPOID PELVIS The inlet of an anthropoid pelvis is oval, with a long anteroposterior diameter and an adequate but rather short transverse diameter. Both the posterior and anterior segments are deep; the posterior sagittal diameter is extremely long, as is the anterior sagittal diameter. The anthropoid midpelvis has variable ischial spines, straight side walls, and a narrow and long sacrum that inclines backward. The midpelvic diameters are at least adequate, making its capacity adequate. The anthropoid outlet has a normal or moderately narrow pubic arch; the interior pubic rami are long and narrow. The outlet capacity is adequate, and the bones are of medium weight

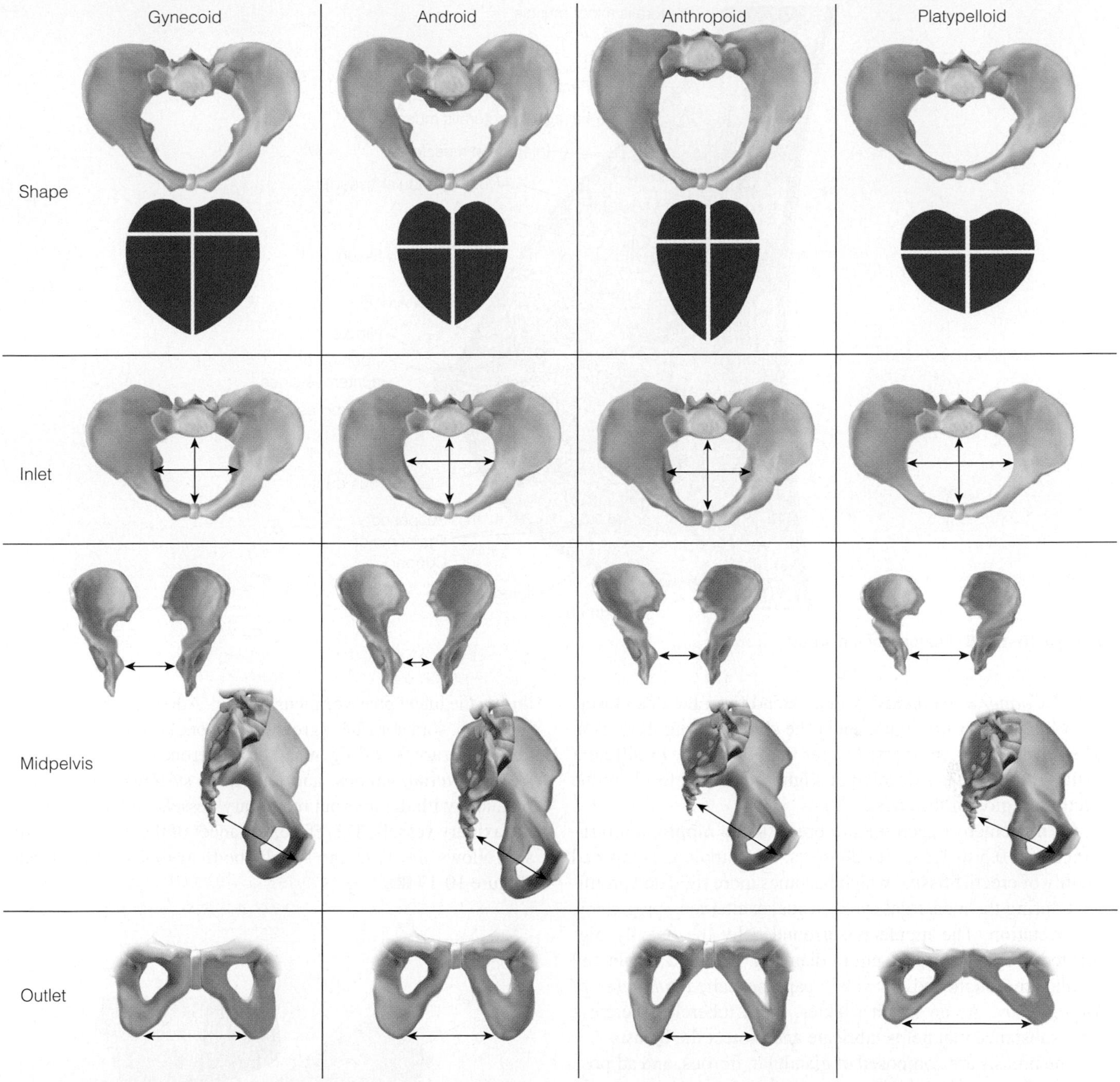

Figure 10-15 ■ Comparison of Caldwell-Moloy pelvic types.

and structure. Approximately 25% of female pelves are classified as anthropoid.

PLATYPELLOID PELVIS The platypelloid type refers to the flat female pelvis. The inlet is a distinctly transverse oval with a short anteroposterior and extremely short transverse diameter. The posterior sagittal and anterior sagittal diameters are short. Both the anterior and posterior segments are shallow. The platypelloid midpelvis has variable ischial spines, parallel side walls, and a wide sacrum with a deep curve inward. Only the transverse diameter is adequate; thus the midpelvic capacity is reduced. The platypelloid outlet has an extremely wide pubic arch; the inferior pubic rami are straight and short. The transverse diameter is wide, but the anteroposterior diameter is short. The outlet capacity may be inadequate. The platypelloid bones are similar to the gynecoid type. Only 5% of female pelves are classified as platypelloid.

Breasts

The **breasts**, or *mammary glands,* considered accessories of the reproductive system, are specialized sebaceous glands. They are conical and symmetrically placed on the sides of the chest. The greater pectoral and anterior serratus muscles underlie each breast. Suspending the breasts are fibrous tissues,

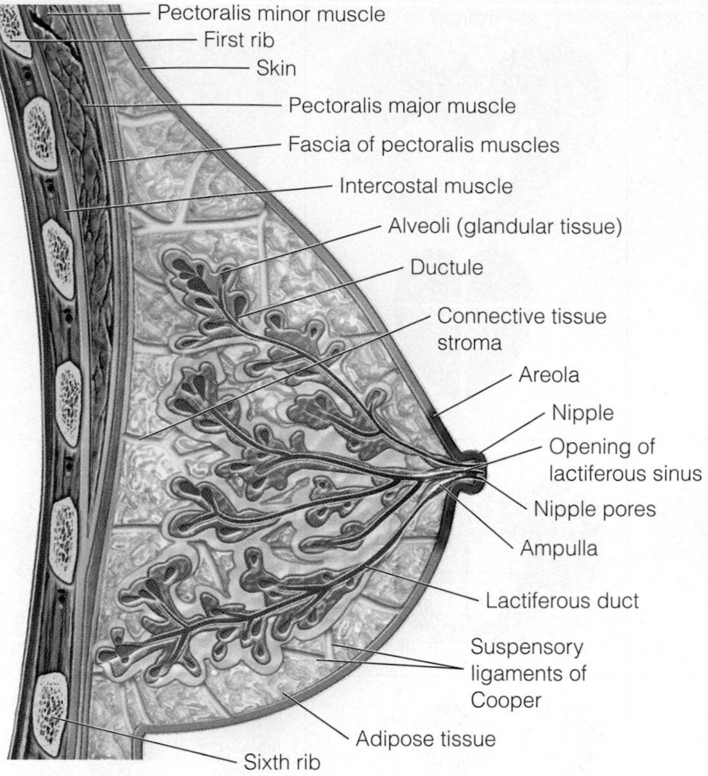

Figure 10-16 ■ Anatomy of the breast.

called *Cooper's ligaments,* which extend from the deep fascia in the chest outward to just under the skin covering the breast. The left breast is frequently larger than the right. In different racial groups breasts develop at slightly different levels in the pectoral region of the chest.

In the center of each mature breast is the **nipple**, a protrusion about 0.5 to 1.3 cm in diameter. The nipple is composed mainly of erectile tissue, which becomes more rigid and prominent during the menstrual cycle, sexual excitement, pregnancy, and lactation. The nipple is surrounded by the heavily pigmented **areola**, 2.5 to 10 cm in diameter. Both the nipple and areola are roughened by small papillae called *tubercles of Montgomery.* As an infant suckles, these tubercles secrete a fatty substance that helps lubricate and protect the breasts.

The breasts are composed of glandular, fibrous, and adipose tissue. The glandular tissue consists of acini, or alveoli (Figure 10-16 ■), which are arranged in a series of 15 to 24 lobes separated from each other by adipose and fibrous tissue.

Each lobe is made up of several lobules, which are made up of many grapelike clusters of alveoli around tiny ducts. They are lined with a single layer of cuboidal epithelium, which secretes the various components of milk. The ducts from several lobules combine to form larger lactiferous ducts and then join to form the lactiferous sinuses, which serve as reservoirs for milk collection and open on the surface of the nipple. The smooth muscle of the nipple causes erection of the nipple on contraction.

Cyclic hormonal control of the mature breast is complex. Essentially, estrogenic hormones stimulate the growth and development of the ductal epithelium. Progesterone, in association with estrogen, is responsible for the acinar and lobular development during the luteal phase of menstruation. Adrenal corticosteroids, prolactin, somatotropin (growth hormone), and thyroxine are also necessary for estrogen and progesterone to act.

The arterial, venous, and lymphatic systems communicate medially with the internal mammary vessels and laterally with the axillary vessels. Therefore, in cancer of the breast, metastasis follows the vascular supply both medially and laterally (Figure 10-17 ■).

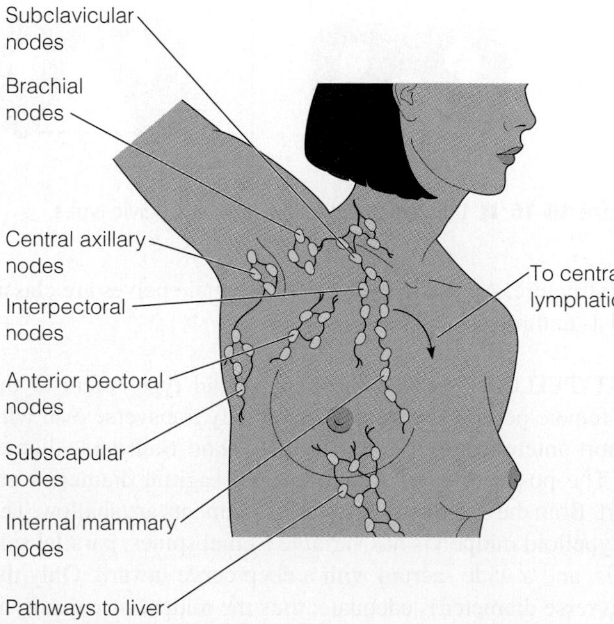

Figure 10-17 ■ Lymphatic vessels draining the breast.

The biologic function of the breasts is to provide nourishment and protective maternal antibodies to infants through the lactation process. They are also a source of pleasurable sexual sensation.

Female Reproductive Cycle

The **female reproductive cycle (FRC)** is composed of the ovarian cycle, during which ovulation occurs, and the menstrual cycle, during which menstruation occurs. These two cycles take place simultaneously (Figure 10-18 ■).

Effects of Female Hormones

After menarche, a woman undergoes a cyclic pattern of ovulation and menstruation for a period of 30 to 40 years. An orderly process under neurohormonal control, this cyclic pattern

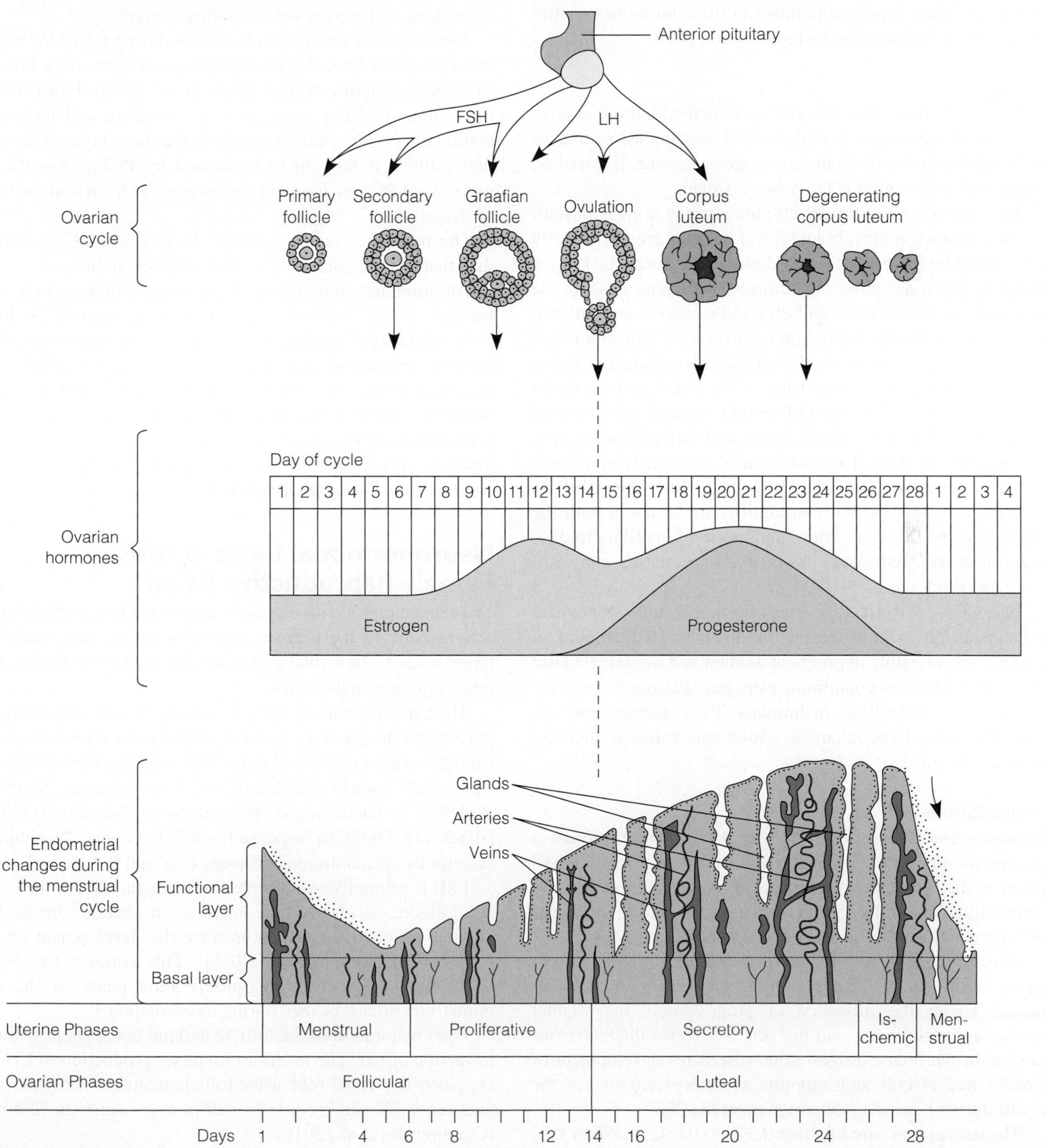

Figure 10-18 ■ Female reproductive cycle: interrelationships of hormones, the four phases of the uterine cycle, and the two phases of the ovarian cycle.

is disrupted only by pregnancy. Each month, multiple oocytes mature, with one rupturing from the ovary and entering the fallopian tube. The ovary, vagina, uterus, and fallopian tubes are major target organs for female hormones.

The ovaries produce mature gametes (see discussion in chapter 11) and secrete hormones. Ovarian hormones include the estrogens, progesterone, and testosterone. The ovary is sensitive to follicle-stimulating hormone (FSH) and luteinizing hormone (LH). The uterus is sensitive to estrogen and progesterone. The relative proportions of these hormones control the events of both ovarian and menstrual cycles.

Estrogens

Estrogens are hormones that are associated with those characteristics contributing to "femaleness." The major estrogenic effects are due primarily to three estrogens: estrone, β-estradiol, and estriol. β-Estradiol is the major estrogen.

Estrogens control the development of the female secondary sex characteristics: breast development, growth of body hair, widening of the hips, and deposits of tissue (fat) in the buttocks and mons pubis. In addition, estrogens assist in the maturation of the ovarian follicles and cause the endometrial mucosa to proliferate following menstruation. The amount of estrogens is greatest during the proliferative (follicular or estrogenic) phase of the menstrual cycle. Estrogens cause the uterus to increase in size and weight because of increased glycogen, amino acids, electrolytes, and water. Blood supply is expanded as well. The endometrial mucosa is in a ready state as a result of estrogenic influence. Under the influence of estrogens, myometrial contractility increases in both the uterus and the fallopian tubes, and uterine sensitivity to oxytocin increases. Estrogens inhibit FSH production and stimulate LH production.

Activity: Ovulation

Estrogens have effects on many hormones and other carrier proteins, such as contributing to the increased amount of protein-bound iodine in pregnant women and women who use oral contraceptives containing estrogen. Estrogens may increase libidinal feelings in humans. They decrease the excitability of the hypothalamus, which may cause an increase in sexual desire.

Progesterone

Progesterone is secreted by the corpus luteum and is found in greatest amounts during the secretory (luteal or progestational) phase of the menstrual cycle. It decreases uterine motility and contractility caused by estrogens, thereby preparing the uterus for implantation after the ovum is fertilized.

This hormone is often called the *hormone of pregnancy* because its effects on the uterus allow pregnancy to be maintained. Under the influence of progesterone, the vaginal epithelium proliferates, and the cervix secretes thick, viscous mucus. In the breast progesterone stimulates development of lobules and alveoli and supports secretory function of the breast during lactation (Cunningham et al., 2010).

The temperature rise of about 0.3°C to 0.6°C (0.5°F to 1°F) that accompanies ovulation and persists throughout the secretory phase of the menstrual cycle is due to progesterone.

Prostaglandins

Prostaglandins (PGs) are oxygenated fatty acids that are produced by the cells of the endometrium and are also classified as hormones. Prostaglandins have varied actions in the body. The two primary types of prostaglandins are groups E and F. Generally, PGE relaxes smooth muscles and is a potent vasodilator; PGF is a potent vasoconstrictor and increases the contractility of muscles and arteries. Although their primary actions seem antagonistic, their basic regulatory functions in cells are achieved through an intricate pattern of reciprocal events.

Prostaglandin production increases during follicular maturation, is dependent on gonadotropins, and seems to be critical to follicular rupture (Cunningham et al., 2010). Extrusion of the ovum, resulting from follicular swelling and increased contractility of the smooth muscle in the theca layer of the mature follicle, is thought to be caused by $PGF_{2\alpha}$. Significant amounts of PGs are found in and around the follicle at the time of ovulation.

During the late secretory phase, the level of $PGF_{2\alpha}$ is higher than that of PGE (Blackburn, 2007). This event increases vasoconstriction and contractility of the myometrium, which contributes to the ischemia preceding menstruation. A high concentration of PGs may also account for the vasoconstriction of the endometrium venous lacunae, allowing for platelet aggregation at vascular rupture points, thereby preventing a rapid blood loss during menstruation. The menstrual flow's high concentration of PGs may also facilitate the process of tissue digestion, which allows for an orderly shedding of the endometrium during menstruation.

Neurohormonal Basis of the Female Reproductive Cycle

The female reproductive cycle is controlled by complex interactions between the nervous and endocrine systems and their target tissues. These interactions involve the hypothalamus, anterior pituitary, and ovaries.

The hypothalamus secretes *gonadotropin-releasing hormone (GnRH)* to the pituitary gland in response to signals received from the central nervous system. This releasing hormone is often called follicle-stimulating hormone-releasing hormone (FSHRH) or luteinizing hormone-releasing hormone (LHRH) (Blackburn, 2007). In response to GnRH, the anterior pituitary secretes the gonadotropic hormones *FSH* and *LH*.

FSH is primarily responsible for the maturation of the ovarian follicle. As the follicle matures, it secretes increasing amounts of estrogen, which enhance the development of the follicle (Cunningham et al., 2010). (This estrogen also is responsible for the rebuilding/proliferation phase of the endometrium after it is shed during menstruation.)

Final maturation of the follicle will not come about without the action of LH. The anterior pituitary's production of LH increases 6-fold to 10-fold as the follicle matures. The peak production of LH can precede ovulation by as much as 12 hours (Cunningham et al., 2010).

LH is also responsible for "luteinizing" the increase in production of progesterone by the granulosa cells of the follicle.

As a result, estrogen production declines and progesterone secretion continues. Thus, estrogen levels fall a day before ovulation; tiny amounts of progesterone are in evidence. **Ovulation** takes place following the very rapid growth of the follicle—as the sustained high level of estrogen diminishes and progesterone secretion begins.

The ruptured follicle undergoes rapid change, complete luteinization is accomplished, and the mass of cells becomes the **corpus luteum**. The lutein cells secrete large amounts of progesterone with smaller amounts of estrogen. (Concurrently, the excessive amounts of progesterone are responsible for the secretory phase of the uterine cycle.) On day 7 or 8 following ovulation, the corpus luteum begins to involute, losing its secretory function. The production of both progesterone and estrogen is severely diminished. The anterior pituitary responds with increasingly large amounts of FSH; a few days later, LH production begins. New follicles become responsive to another ovarian cycle and begin maturing.

Ovarian Cycle

The ovarian cycle has two phases: the *follicular phase* (days 1 to 14) and the *luteal phase* (days 15 to 28 in a 28-day cycle). Figure 10-19 ■ depicts the changes that the follicle undergoes during the ovarian cycle. In women whose menstrual cycles vary, usually it is only the length of the follicular phase that varies, because the luteal phase is of fixed length. During the follicular phase, the immature follicle matures as a result of FSH. Within the follicle, the oocyte grows.

A mature **graafian follicle** appears about the 14th day under dual control of FSH and LH. It is a large structure, measuring about 5 to 10 mm, and produces increasing amounts of estrogen. In the mature graafian follicle, the cells surrounding the fluid-filled antral cavity are called granulosa cells. The mass of granulosa cells surrounding the oocyte and follicular fluid is called the *cumulus oophorus*. In the fully mature graafian follicle, the zona pellucida, a thick elastic capsule, develops around the oocyte. Just before ovulation, the mature oocyte completes its first meiotic division (see chapter 11 for a description of meiosis). As a result of this division, two cells are formed: a small cell called a *polar body,* and a larger cell called the *secondary oocyte.* The secondary oocyte matures into the ovum.

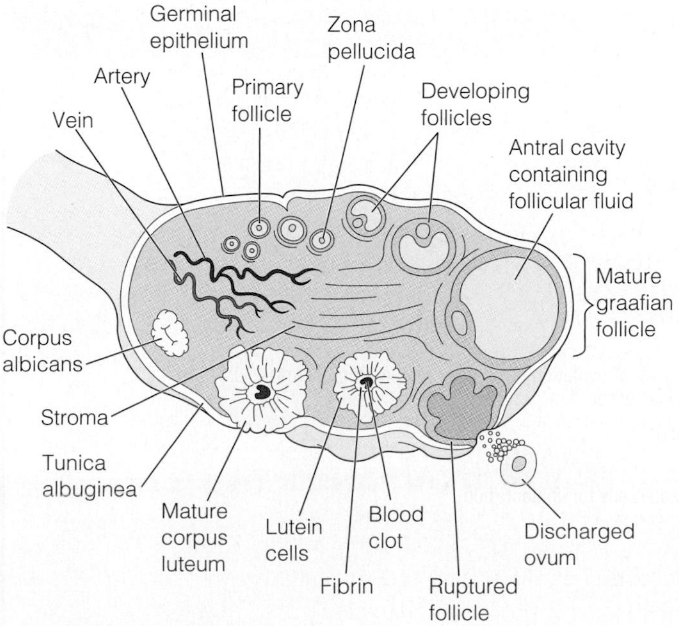

Figure 10-19 ■ Various stages of development of the ovarian follicles.

As the graafian follicle matures and enlarges, its walls thin and it travels outward to the surface of the ovary. This surface has a blisterlike protrusion 10 to 15 mm in diameter, where the secondary oocyte, polar body, and follicular fluid are pushed out. The ovum is discharged near the fimbria of the fallopian tube and is pulled into the tube to begin its journey toward the uterus. (See Figure 11-5 on page 223.)

In some women, ovulation is accompanied by midcycle pain, known as *mittelschmerz.* This pain may be caused by a thick tunica albuginea or by a local peritoneal reaction to the expelling of the follicular contents. Vaginal discharge may increase during ovulation, and a small amount of blood (midcycle spotting) may be discharged as well.

Application: Ovarian Cycle

The body temperature increases about 0.3°C to 0.6°C (0.5°F to 1°F) 24 to 48 hours after the time of ovulation. It remains elevated until the day before menstruation begins. There may be an accompanying sharp basal body temperature drop just before the increase. These temperature changes are useful clinically to determine the approximate time ovulation occurs (Blackburn 2007).

Generally the ovum takes several minutes to travel through the ruptured follicle to the fallopian tube opening. The contractions of the tube's smooth muscle and its ciliary action propel the ovum through the tube. The ovum remains in the ampulla, where, if it is fertilized, cleavage can begin. The ovum is thought to be fertile for only 6 to 24 hours. It reaches the uterus 72 to 96 hours after its release from the ovary.

The luteal phase begins when the ovum leaves its follicle. Under the influence of LH, the corpus luteum develops from the ruptured follicle. Within 2 or 3 days the corpus luteum becomes yellowish and spherical and increases in vascularity. If the ovum is fertilized and implants in the endometrium, the fertilized egg begins to secrete **human chorionic gonadotropin (hCG)**, which is needed to maintain the corpus luteum. If fertilization does not occur, within about a week after ovulation, the corpus luteum begins to degenerate, eventually becoming a connective tissue scar called the *corpus albicans.* With degeneration comes a decrease in estrogen and progesterone. This allows for an increase in LH and FSH, which triggers the hypothalamus.

Uterine (Menstrual) Cycle

Menstrual Cycle Central

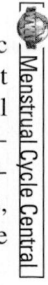

Menstruation is cyclic uterine bleeding in response to cyclic hormonal changes. Menstruation occurs when the ovum is not fertilized and begins about 14 days after ovulation (in an ideal 28-day cycle), in the absence of pregnancy. The menstrual discharge, also referred to as the *menses* or *menstrual flow,* is composed of blood mixed with cervical and vaginal secretions, bacteria, mucus, leukocytes, and other cellular debris. The menstrual discharge is dark red and has a distinctive odor.

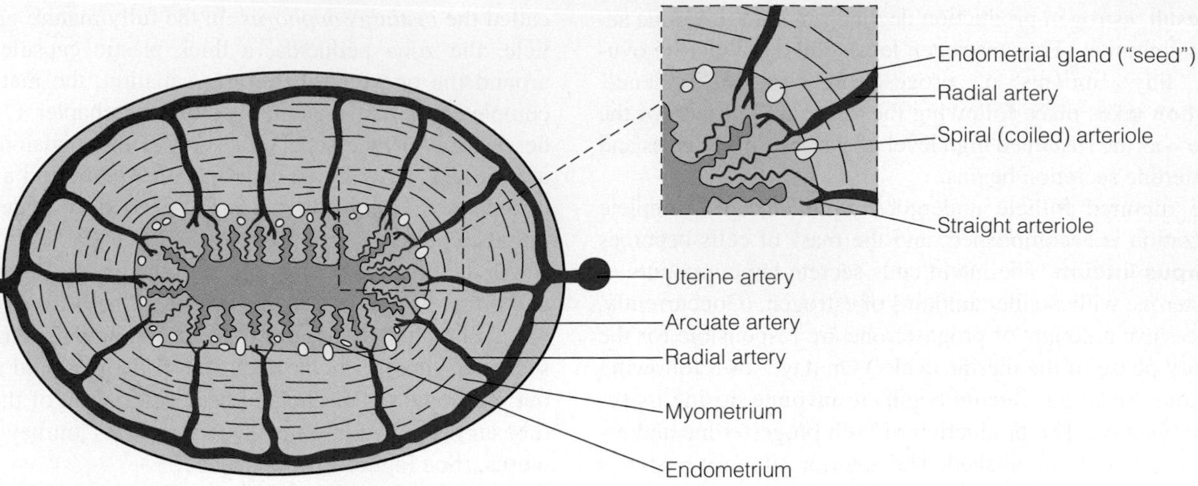

Figure 10-20 ■ Blood supply to the endometrium (cross-sectional view of the uterus).

Frequently, ovulation does not occur in early menstrual cycles; these are called anovulatory cycles. Early cycles also are often irregular in frequency, amount of flow, and duration. Within several months to 2 to 3 years, a regular cycle becomes established.

Menstrual parameters vary greatly among individuals. Generally, menstruation occurs every 29 days but varies from 21 to 35 days. Some women normally have longer cycles, which can skew standard calculations of the estimated date of birth (EDB) when they become pregnant. Emotional and physical factors such as illness, excessive fatigue, stress or anxiety, and rigorous exercise programs can alter the cycle interval. Certain environmental factors such as temperature and altitude may also affect the cycle. The duration of menses is from 2 to 8 days, with the blood loss averaging 25 to 60 ml and the loss of iron averaging 0.5 to 1 mg daily.

Care Plan Activity: Irregular Menses in a Patient with Anxiety

A review of the endometrium and its arterial blood supply will provide further understanding of the menstrual process (Figure 10-20 ■). Blood flow from the spiral arterioles in the superficial endometrium is reduced, leading to a lack of blood and oxygen, which in turn produces tissue death (necrosis) and discharge of the superficial endometrium (menses). At the same time, the straight arterioles provide the basal endometrium with sufficient blood flow to maintain this layer of the endometrium and the endometrial glands (or seeds) that are responsible for the generation of the endometrium in the next female reproductive or menstrual cycle (see Figure 10-18). Bleeding is controlled by vasospasm of the straight basal arterioles, resulting in coagulative necrosis at the vessel tips.

The uterine (menstrual) cycle has four phases: the menstrual phase, proliferative phase, secretory phase, and ischemic phase (Table 10-2). Menstruation occurs during the *menstrual phase.*

TABLE 10-2 Characteristics of Menstrual Cycle and Ovulation

Menstrual phase (days 1–6)	Estrogen levels are low.
	Cervical mucus is scanty, viscous, and opaque.
	Endometrium is shed.
Proliferative phase (days 7–14)	Endometrium and myometrium thickness increases.
	Estrogen peaks just before ovulation.
	Cervical mucus at ovulation: Is clear, thin, watery, and alkaline Is more favorable to sperm Has elasticity (spinnbarkheit) greater than 5 cm Shows ferning pattern on microscopic exam
	Just prior to ovulation body temperature drops; then at ovulation basal body temperature increases 0.3°C to 0.6°C, and mittelschmerz and/or midcycle spotting may occur.
Secretory phase (days 15–26)	Estrogen drops sharply, and progesterone dominates.
	Vascularity of entire uterus increases.
	Tissue glycogen increases, and the uterus is made ready for implantation.
Ischemic phase (days 27–28)	Both estrogen and progesterone levels fall.
	Spiral arteries undergo vasoconstriction.
	Endometrium becomes pale.
	Blood vessels rupture.
	Blood escapes into uterine stromal cells.

Some endometrial areas are shed, whereas others remain. Some of the remaining tips of the endometrial glands begin to regenerate. The endometrium is in a resting state following menstruation. Estrogen levels are low, and the endometrium is 1 to 2 mm deep. During this part of the cycle the cervical mucus is scanty, viscous, and opaque.

The *proliferative phase* begins when the endometrial glands enlarge, becoming twisted and longer, in response to increasing amounts of estrogen. The blood vessels become prominent and dilated, and the endometrium increases in thickness sixfold to eightfold. This gradual process reaches its peak just before ovulation. The cervical mucus becomes thin, clear, watery, and more alkaline, making the mucus more favorable to spermatozoa. As ovulation nears, the cervical mucus shows increased elasticity, called *spinnbarkheit.* At ovulation, the mucus will stretch more than 5 cm. The cervical mucosa pH increases from below 7 to 7.5 at the time of ovulation. On microscopic examination, the mucus shows a characteristic ferning pattern (see Figure 12-4B on page 249). This ferning pattern is a useful aid in assessment of ovulation time (Table 10-2). For an in-depth discussion, see chapter 12 ∞.

The *secretory phase* follows ovulation. The endometrium, under estrogenic influence, undergoes slight cellular growth. Progesterone, however, causes such marked swelling and growth that the epithelium is warped into folds (Figure 10-21 ■). The amount of tissue glycogen increases. The glandular epithelial cells begin to fill with cellular debris, and the glands become tortuous and dilate. The glands secrete small quantities of endometrial fluid in preparation for a fertilized ovum. The vascularity of the entire uterus increases greatly, providing a nourishing bed for implantation. If implantation occurs, the endometrium, under the influence of progesterone, continues to develop and becomes even thicker (Figure 10-22 ■). See chapter 11 ∞ for an in-depth discussion of implantation.

If fertilization does not occur, the *ischemic phase* begins. The corpus luteum begins to degenerate, and as a result both estrogen and progesterone levels fall. Areas of necrosis appear under the epithelial lining. Extensive vascular changes also occur. Small blood vessels rupture, and the spiral arteries constrict and retract, causing a deficiency of blood in the endometrium, which becomes pale. This ischemic phase is characterized by the escape of blood into the stromal cells of the uterus. The menstrual flow begins, thus beginning the menstrual cycle again. After menstruation, the basal layer remains so that the tips of the glands can regenerate the new functional endometrial layer. See Table 10-3 for a summary of the female reproductive cycle.

Male Reproductive System

The primary reproductive functions of the male genitals are to produce and transport the male sex cells (sperm) through and eventually out of the genital tract into the female genital tract. The male reproductive system consists of the external and internal genitals (Figure 10-23 ■).

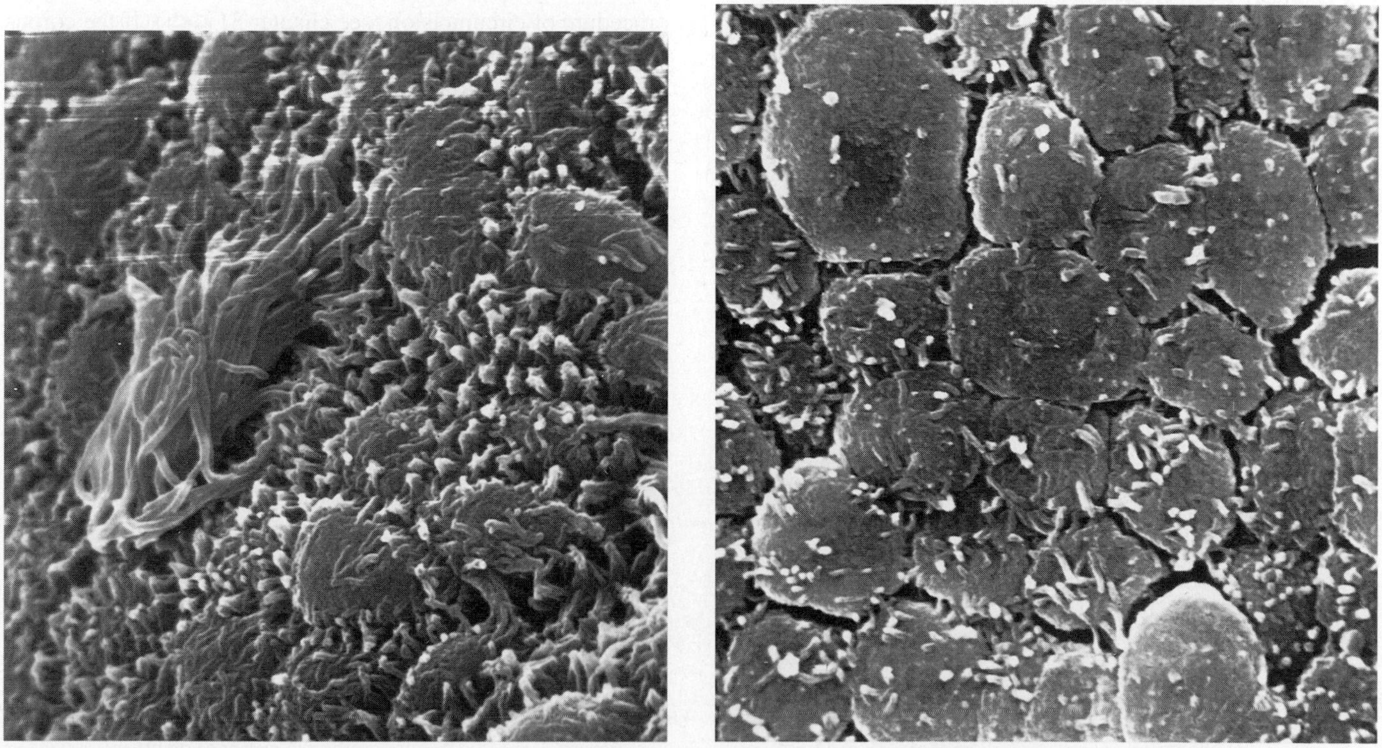

A B

Figure 10-21 ■ Scanning electron micrographs of the uterine lining during different phases of the uterine cycle. A. During the luteal phase, some of the cells have cilia, and some are secreting droplets. The secreting cells are covered with microvilli. B. In the secretory phase, microvilli are still present on the surface of the secreting cells, but the general surface of the lining has a lumpier appearance than during the proliferative phase, and the cilia appear shorter and less numerous. The named phases refer to the uterine condition at the time the photographs were taken.

Source: Courtesy of Dr. E.S.E. Hafez, Wayne State University, Detroit, Michigan.

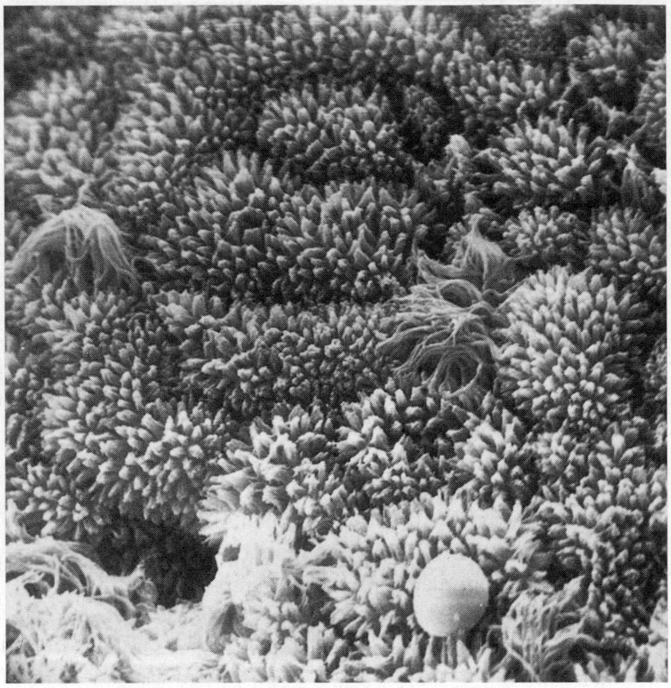

Figure 10-22 ■ Scanning electron micrograph of the inner lining of the uterus at the time of blastocyst implantation. The blastocyst is an embryo at an early stage of development.

Source: Courtesy of Dr. E.S.E. Hafez, Wayne State University, Detroit, Michigan.

TABLE 10-3 Summary of Female Reproductive Cycle

Ovarian Cycle

Follicular phase (days 1–14): Primordial follicle matures under influence of FSH and LH up to the time of ovulation.

Luteal phase (days 15–28): Ovum leaves follicle, corpus luteum develops under LH influence and produces high levels of progesterone and low levels of estrogen.

Menstrual Cycle

Menstrual phase (days 1–6): Estrogen levels are low, cervical mucus is scant, viscous, and opaque.

Proliferative phase (days 7–14): Estrogen peaks just prior to ovulation. Cervical mucus at ovulation is clear, thin, watery, alkaline, and more favorable to sperm; shows ferning pattern; and has spinnbarkheit greater than 5 cm. At ovulation body temperature drops, then rises sharply and remains elevated under influence of progesterone.

Secretory phase (days 15–26): Estrogen drops sharply, and progesterone dominates.

Ischemic phase (days 27–28): Both estrogen and progesterone levels drop.

External Genitals

The two external reproductive organs are the penis and the scrotum.

Penis

The *penis* is an elongated, cylindrical structure consisting of a body, termed the *shaft,* and a cone-shaped end called the *glans.* The penis lies in front of the scrotum. The shaft of the penis is made up of three longitudinal columns of erectile tissue: the paired *corpora cavernosa* and a third, the *corpus spongiosum.* These columns are covered by a dense, fibrous connective tissue and then enclosed by an elastic tissue. The penis is covered by a thin outer layer of skin.

The corpus spongiosum contains the urethra and becomes the glans at the distal end of the penis. The urethra widens within the glans and ends in a slitlike orifice, located in the tip of the glans, called the *urethral meatus.* A circular fold of skin arises just behind the glans and covers it. Known as the *prepuce,* or *foreskin,* it is frequently removed by the surgical procedure of circumcision (see chapter 31 ∞). If the corpus spongiosum does not surround the urethra completely, the urethral meatus may occur on the ventral aspect of the penile shaft (hypospadias) or on the dorsal aspect (epispadias).

The penis is innervated by the pudendal nerve. Sexual stimulation causes the penis to elongate, thicken, and stiffen, a process called *erection.* The penis becomes erect when its blood vessels become engorged, a consequence of parasympathetic nerve stimulation. If sexual stimulation is intense enough, the forceful and sudden expulsion of semen occurs

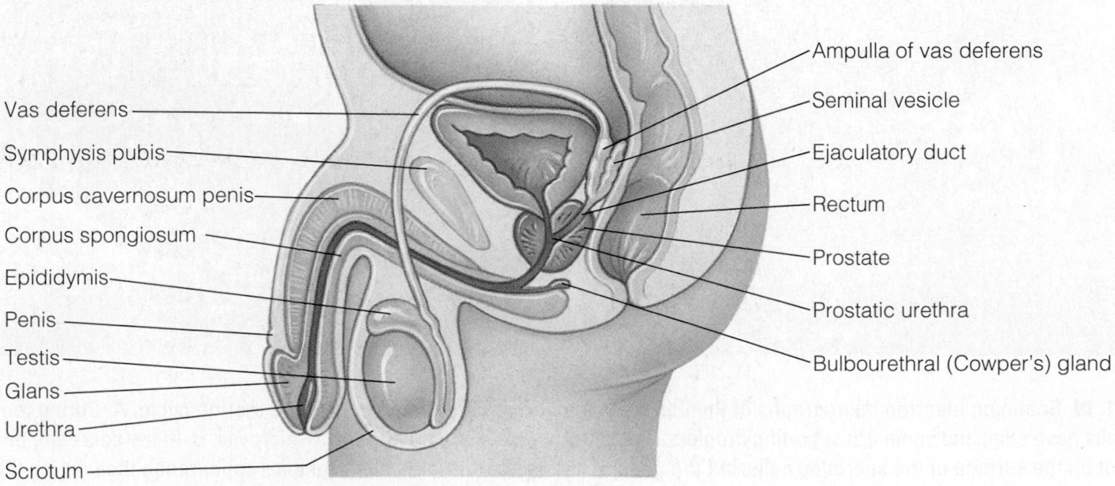

Figure 10-23 ■ Male reproductive system, sagittal view.

through the rhythmic contractions of the penile muscles. This phenomenon is called *ejaculation.*

The penis serves both the urinary and reproductive systems. Urine is expelled through the urethral meatus. The primary reproductive function of the penis is to deposit sperm in the female vagina during sexual intercourse so that fertilization of the ovum can occur.

Scrotum

The *scrotum* is a pouchlike structure that hangs in front of the anus and behind the penis. Composed of skin and the *dartos muscle,* the scrotum shows increased pigmentation and scattered hairs. The sebaceous glands open directly onto the scrotal surface; their secretion has a distinctive odor. Contraction of the dartos and cremasteric muscles shortens the scrotum and draws it closer to the body, thus wrinkling its outer surface. The degree of wrinkling is greatest in young men and at cold temperatures and is least in older men and at warm temperatures.

Inside the scrotum are two lateral compartments. Each compartment contains a testis with its related structures. Because the left spermatic cord grows longer, the left testis and its scrotal sac hang lower than the right. A ridge (raphe) on the external scrotal surface marks the position of the medial septum and continues anteriorly on the urethral surface of the penis but disappears in the perineal area.

The function of the scrotum is to protect the testes and the sperm by maintaining a temperature lower than that of the body. Spermatogenesis will not occur if the testes fail to descend and thus remain at body temperature. Because it is sensitive to touch, pressure, temperature, and pain, the scrotum defends against potential harm to the testes.

Male Internal Reproductive Organs

The male internal reproductive organs include the gonads (testes or testicles), a system of ducts (epididymis, vas deferens, ejaculatory duct, and urethra), and accessory glands (seminal vesicles, prostate gland, bulbourethral glands, and urethral glands). See Table 10-4 for a summary of male reproductive organ functions.

Testes

The *testes* are a pair of oval compound glandular organs contained in the scrotum (Figure 10-24 ■). In the sexually mature male, they are the site of spermatozoa (male gamete) production and the secretion of several male sex hormones.

Each testis is 4 to 6 cm long, 2 to 3 cm wide, and 3 to 4 cm deep and weighs 10 to 15 g. Each testis is covered by a serous membrane and an inner capsule that is tough, white, and fibrous. The connective tissue sends projections inward to form septa, dividing the testis into 250 to 400 lobules. Each lobule contains one to three tightly packed, convoluted *seminiferous tubules* containing sperm cells in all stages of development.

The seminiferous tubules are surrounded by loose connective tissue, which houses abundant blood and lymph vessels and the *interstitial (Leydig's) cells.* The interstitial cells produce testosterone, the primary male sex hormone. The tubules also contain Sertoli's cells, which nourish and protect

TABLE 10-4 Summary of Male Reproductive Organ Functions

- The testes house seminiferous tubules and the gonads.
- Seminiferous tubules contain sperm cells in various stages of development and undergoing meiosis.
- Sertoli's cells nourish and protect spermatocytes (phase between spermatids and spermatozoa).
- Leydig's cells are the main source of testosterone.
- Epididymides provide an area for maturation of sperm and a reservoir for mature spermatozoa.
- The vas deferens connects the epididymis with the prostate gland and then connects with ducts from the seminal vesicle to become an ejaculatory duct.
- Ejaculatory ducts provide a passageway for semen and seminal fluid into the urethra.
- Seminal vesicles secrete yellowish fluid rich in fructose, prostaglandins, and fibrinogen. This provides nutrition that increases motility and fertilizing ability of sperm. Prostaglandins also aid fertilization by making the cervical mucus more receptive to sperm.
- The prostate gland secretes thin, alkaline fluid containing calcium, citric acid, and other substances. Alkalinity counteracts acidity of ductus and seminal vesicle secretions.
- Bulbourethral (Cowper's) glands secrete alkaline, viscous fluid into semen, aiding in neutralization of acidic vaginal secretions.

the spermatocytes. The seminiferous tubules come together to form the 20 or 30 straight tubules, which in turn form an anastomosing network of thin-walled spaces, the rete testis. The rete testis forms 10 to 15 efferent ducts that empty into the duct of the epididymis.

WebMD Anatomy

Most of the cells lining the seminiferous tubules undergo *spermatogenesis,* a process of maturation in which spermatocytes become spermatozoa. (See chapter 11 for further discussion of spermatogenesis.) Sperm production varies among and within the tubules, with cells in different areas of the same tubule undergoing different stages of spermatogenesis. The sperm are eventually released from the tubules into the epididymis, where they mature further.

Like the female reproductive cycle, the process of spermatogenesis and other functions of the testes are the result of complex neural and hormonal controls. The hypothalamus secretes releasing factors, which stimulate the anterior pituitary to release the gonadotropins—follicle-stimulating hormone (FSH) and luteinizing hormone (LH). These hormones cause the testes to produce testosterone, which maintains spermatogenesis, increases sperm production by the seminiferous tubules, and stimulates production of seminal fluid.

Testosterone is the most prevalent and potent of the testicular hormones. It is also responsible for the development of secondary male characteristics and certain behavioral patterns. The effects of testosterone include structural and functional development of the male genital tract, emission and ejaculation of seminal fluid, distribution of body hair, promotion of growth and strength of long bones, increased muscle mass, and enlargement of the vocal cords. The action of testosterone on the central nervous system is thought to produce aggressiveness and sexual drive. The action of testosterone is constant, not cyclic like that of the female hormones.

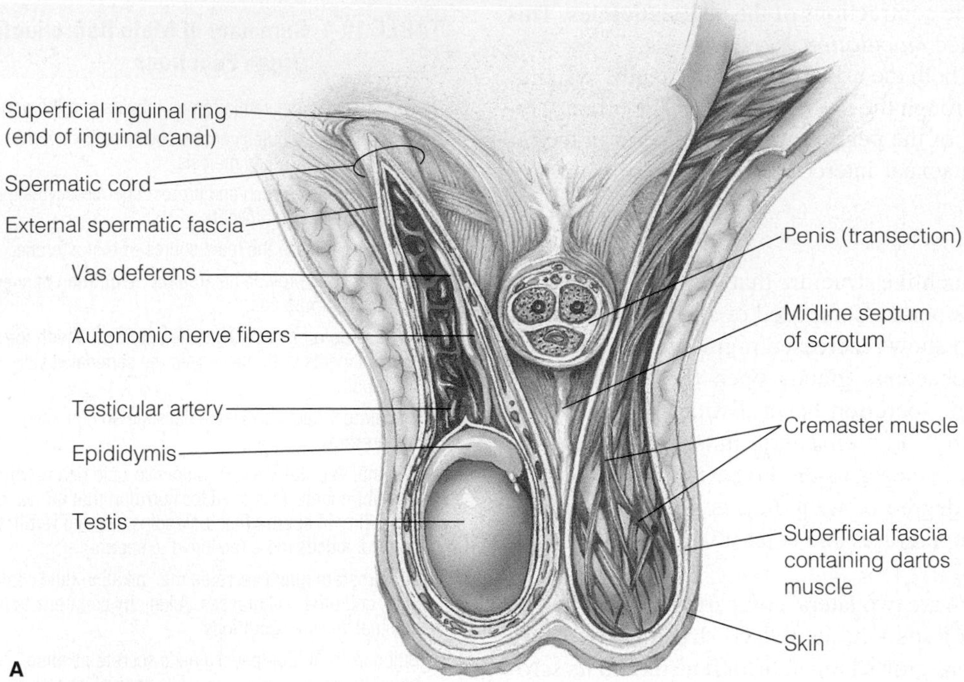

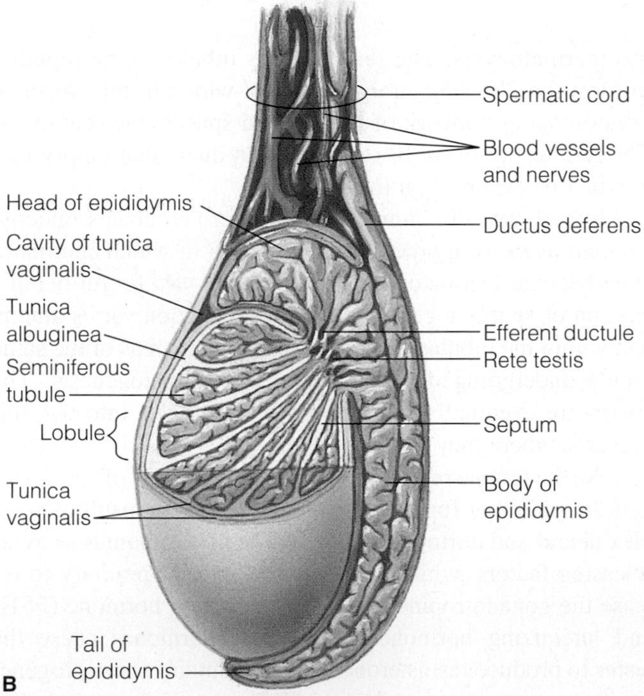

Figure 10-24 ■ The testes: A. External view. B. Sagittal view showing interior anatomy.

Activities: Male Reproductive System

Its production is not limited to a certain number of years but is thought to decrease with age.

The testes have two primary functions:

- To serve as the site of spermatogenesis
- To produce testosterone

Epididymis

The *epididymis* (plural, *epididymides*) is a duct about 5.6 m long although it is convoluted into a compact structure about 3.75 cm long. An epididymis lies behind each testis. It arises from the top of the testis, extends downward, and then passes upward, where it becomes the vas deferens.

The epididymis provides a reservoir where spermatozoa can survive for a long period. When discharged from the seminiferous tubules into the epididymis, the sperm are immobile and incapable of fertilizing an ovum. The spermatozoa usually remain in the epididymis for 2 to 10 days but can be stored in the body for up to 42 days. As the sperm are transported along the tortuous course of the epididymis, they become both motile and fertile.

Vas Deferens and Ejaculatory Ducts

The *vas deferens,* also known as the *ductus deferens,* is about 40 cm long and connects the epididymis with the prostate (see Figure 10-23). One vas deferens arises from the posterior border of each testis. It joins the spermatic cord and weaves over and between several pelvic structures until it meets the vas deferens from the opposite side. Each vas deferens terminus expands to form the *terminal ampulla.* It then unites with the seminal vesicle duct (a gland) to form the ejaculatory duct, which enters the prostate gland and ends in the prostatic urethra. The ejaculatory ducts serve as a passageway for semen and fluid secreted by the seminal vesicles. The main function of the vas deferens is to rapidly squeeze the sperm from their storage sites (the epididymis and distal part of the vas deferens) into the urethra.

Men who choose to take total responsibility for birth control may elect to have a vasectomy. In this procedure, the scrotal portion of the vas deferens is surgically incised or cauterized. Although sperm continue to be produced for the next several years, they can no longer reach the outside of the body. Eventually, the sperm deteriorate and are reabsorbed.

Urethra

The *male urethra* is a passageway for urine and semen. The urethra begins in the bladder and passes through the prostate gland, where it is called the *prostatic urethra.* The urethra emerges from the prostate gland to become the *membranous urethra.* It terminates in the penis, where it is called the *penile urethra.* In the penile urethra, goblet secretory cells are present, and smooth muscle is replaced by erectile tissue.

Accessory Glands

The male accessory glands secrete a unique and essential component of the total seminal fluid in an ordered sequence.

The *seminal vesicles* are two glands composed of many lobes. Each vesicle is about 7.5 cm long. They are situated between the bladder and rectum and immediately above the base of the prostate. The epithelium lining the seminal vesicles secretes an alkaline, viscous, clear fluid rich in high-energy fructose, prostaglandins, fibrinogen, and amino acids. During ejaculation this fluid mixes with sperm in the ejaculatory ducts. This fluid helps provide an environment favorable to sperm motility and metabolism.

The prostate gland encircles the upper part of the urethra and lies below the neck of the bladder. Made up of several lobes, it measures about 4 cm in diameter and weighs 20 to 30 g. The prostate is made up of both glandular and muscular tissue. It secretes a thin, milky, alkaline fluid containing high levels of zinc, calcium, citric acid, and acid phosphatase. This fluid protects the sperm from the acidic environment of the vagina and the male urethra, which could be spermicidal.

The *bulbourethral glands (Cowper's glands)* are a pair of small round structures on either side of the membranous urethra. The glands secrete a clear, thick, alkaline fluid rich in mucoproteins that becomes part of the semen. This secretion also lubricates the penile urethra during sexual excitement and neutralizes the acid in the male urethra and the vagina, thereby enhancing sperm motility.

The *urethral glands (Littre's glands)* are tiny mucus-secreting glands found throughout the membranous lining of the penile urethra. Their secretions add to those of the bulbourethral glands.

Semen

The male ejaculate, *semen* or *seminal fluid,* is made up of spermatozoa and the secretions of all the accessory glands. The seminal fluid transports viable and motile sperm to the female reproductive tract. Effective transportation of sperm requires adequate nutrients, an adequate pH (about 7.5), a specific concentration of sperm to fluid, and an optimal osmolarity.

A spermatozoon is made up of a head and a tail (Figure 10-25 ■). The head's main components are the acrosome and the nucleus. The head carries the male's haploid number of chromosomes (23), and it is the part that enters the ovum at fertilization (see chapter 11 ∞). The tail, or *flagellum,* is specialized for motility. The tail is divided into the middle and end piece.

Sperm may be stored in the male genital system up to 42 days, depending primarily on the frequency of ejaculations. The average volume of ejaculate following abstinence for several days is 2 to 5 ml but may vary from 1 to 10 ml. Repeated ejaculation results in decreased volume. Once ejaculated, sperm can live only 2 or 3 days in the female genital tract.

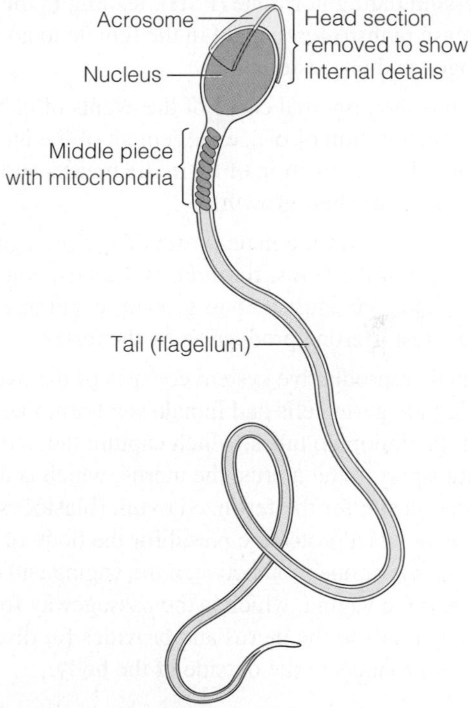

Figure 10-25 ■ Schematic illustration of a mature spermatozoon.

Case Study: Sex Education for Teens

FOCUS YOUR STUDY

- The genetic sex of an embryo is determined at fertilization. The male and female reproductive systems are undifferentiated initially. By the 12th week the external genitals are fully differentiated.
- Reproductive activities require complex interactions between the reproductive structures; the central nervous system; and such endocrine glands as the pituitary, hypothalamus, testes, and ovaries.
- At puberty, an alteration in brain sensitivity leads to an increased release of gonadotropin-releasing hormone (GnRH), which stimulates luteinizing hormone (LH) and follicle-stimulating hormone (FSH), leading in the male to an increase in testosterone and in the female to an increase in estrogen and progesterone.
- Estrogen is the principal cause of the events of puberty in females (maturation of ova, enlargement of the uterus and fallopian tubes, deposition of fat in the breasts and hips, and characteristic hair growth).
- Puberty changes for the male (onset of spermatogenesis; enlargement of the penis, scrotum, and testes; voice changes; and characteristic hair growth) occur as a result of increased testosterone production by the testes.
- The female reproductive system consists of the ovaries, where female germ cells and female sex hormones are formed; the fallopian tubes, which capture the ovum and allow transport to the uterus; the uterus, which is the implantation site for the fertilized ovum (blastocyst); the cervix, which is a protective portal for the body of the uterus and the connection between the vagina and the uterus; and the vagina, which is the passageway from the external genitals to the uterus and provides for discharge of menstrual products to the outside of the body.
- The female reproductive cycle may be described in terms of the ovarian cycle, during which ovulation occurs, and the menstrual cycle, during which menstruation occurs. These two cycles take place simultaneously and are under neurohormonal control.
- The ovarian cycle has two phases: the follicular phase and the luteal phase. During the follicular phase, the primordial follicle matures under the influence of FSH and LH until ovulation occurs. The luteal phase begins when the ovum leaves the follicle and the corpus luteum develops under the influence of LH. The corpus luteum produces high levels of progesterone and low levels of estrogen.
- The menstrual cycle has four phases: menstrual, proliferative, secretory, and ischemic. Menstruation is the actual shedding of the endometrial lining, when estrogen levels are low. The proliferative phase begins when the endometrial glands begin to enlarge under the influence of estrogen and cervical mucosal changes occur; the changes peak at ovulation. The secretory phase follows ovulation, and, influenced primarily by progesterone, the uterus increases its vascularity to make ready for possible implantation. The ischemic phase is characterized by degeneration of the corpus luteum, decreases in both estrogen and progesterone levels, constriction of the spiral arteries, and escape of blood into the stromal cells of the endometrium.
- The male reproductive system consists of the testes, where male germ cells and male sex hormones are formed; a series of continuous ducts through which spermatozoa are transported outside the body; accessory glands that produce secretions important to sperm nutrition, survival, and transport; and the penis, which serves as the reproductive organ of intercourse.

CRITICAL THINKING IN ACTION

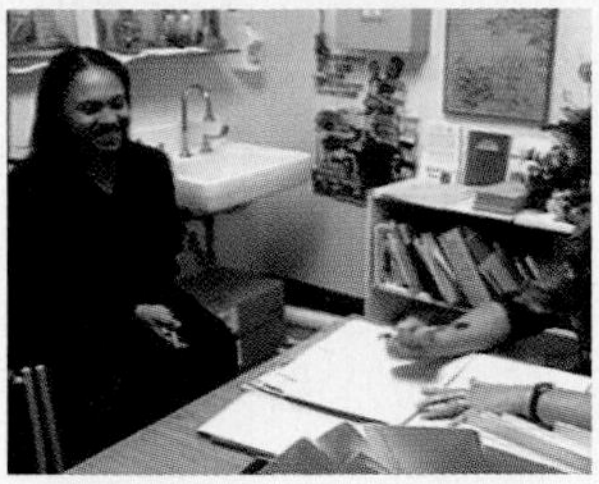

You are working in the OB/GYN clinic when Sally Smith, a 17-year-old teenager, comes in complaining of irregular menses. She believes her periods are really "messed up" and interfering with her active schedule. She wants them to be more regular and asks you for birth control. She tells you that she is a member of the swimming team and is a senior in high school. She says she is planning to start community college next year to obtain an associate degree in computer technology. You assess Sally's history as follows: menarche began at age 12; periods occur every 28 to 32 days. She usually experiences cramping in the first 2 days and the flow lasts 4 to 5 days. She uses an average of 4 to 5 tampons a day during her period. She has never been hospitalized, has no prior medical problems, and is up-to-date on her immunizations except for meningitis.

1. Based on your knowledge of menstruation, how would you describe Sally's menstrual cycle?
2. What is your primary goal in discussing Sally's menstrual cycle with her?
3. What information would you give Sally relating to her menstrual cycle?
4. What important request does Sally have?
5. Sally expresses problems dealing with the cramping she experiences with the first 2 days of her menses. What would you suggest to Sally to cope with the discomfort?

See www.nursing.pearsonhighered.com for possible responses.

REFERENCES

Blackburn, S. T. (2007). *Maternal, fetal, & neonatal physiology: A clinical perspective* (3rd ed.). St. Louis, MO: Saunders.

Caldwell, W. E., & Moloy, H. C. (1933). Anatomical variations in the female pelvis and their effect on labor with a suggested classification [Historical article]. *American Journal of Obstetrics & Gynecology, 26*, 479–505.

Cunningham, F. G., Leveno, K. J., Bloom, S. L., Hauth, J. C., Rouse, D. J., & Spong, C. Y. (2010). *Williams obstetrics* (23rd ed.). New York, NY: McGraw-Hill.

Lawrence, R. M., & Lawrence, R. A. (2009). The breast and the physiology of lactation. In R. K. Creasy, R. Resnik, J. D. Iams, C. J. Lockwood, & T. R. Moore (Eds.), *Creasy & Resnik's maternal-fetal medicine: Principles and practice* (6th ed.). St. Louis, MO: Saunders.

CHAPTER 11

Conception and Fetal Development

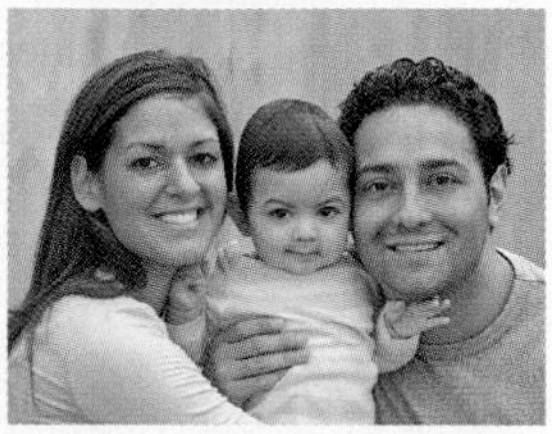

My friends tease me when I say this, but I know the moment my daughter was conceived. My husband and I had both been so busy at work, but we finally went away for a long weekend together. It was wonderful—we got back some of the magic as we took long walks and talked and talked. Until that weekend, whenever we discussed having children it was always "maybe someday." On the second night we decided to skip the birth control for the first time ever. Our lovemaking seemed so special that evening, a true reflection of the emotional closeness we had recaptured. I never went back to using birth control after that weekend, but I am convinced that Jennifer is the result of that night together!

LEARNING OUTCOMES

1. Differentiate between mitotic cellular division and meiotic cellular division.
2. Compare the processes by which ova and sperm are produced.
3. Analyze the components of the process of fertilization as to how each may impact fertilization.
4. Analyze the processes that occur during the cellular multiplication and differentiation stages of intrauterine development and their effects on the structures that form.
5. Compare the factors and processes by which fraternal (dizygotic) and identical (monozygotic) twins are formed.
6. Describe the development, structure, and functions of the placenta and umbilical cord during intrauterine life (embryonic and fetal development).
7. Summarize the significant changes in growth and development of the fetus at 4, 6, 12, 16, 20, 24, 28, 32, 36, and 40 weeks' gestation.
8. Identify the factors that influence congenital malformations of the organ systems and the resulting congenital malformations.

KEY TERMS

Acrosomal reaction *221*
Amnion *223*
Amniotic fluid *223*
Bag of waters (BOW) *223*
Blastocyst *222*
Capacitation *221*
Chorion *223*
Chromosomes *217*
Cleavage *221*
Cotyledon *228*
Decidua basalis *223*
Decidua capsularis *223*
Decidua vera (parietalis) *223*
Diploid number of chromosomes *217*
Ductus arteriosus *231*
Ductus venosus *231*
Ectoderm *223*
Embryo *234*
Embryonic membranes *223*
Endoderm *223*
Fertilization *220*
Fetus *236*
Foramen ovale *231*
Gametes *219*
Gametogenesis *219*
Haploid number of chromosomes *219*
Lanugo *224*
Meiosis *219*
Mesoderm *223*
Mitosis *217*
Morula *221*
Placenta *227*
Postconception age periods *233*
Teratogen *239*
Trophoblast *222*
Umbilical cord *225*
Vernix caseosa *238*
Wharton's jelly *225*
Zygote *219*

The human genome contains *genes*, which are units of genetic information. Genes are encoded in the deoxyribonucleic acid (DNA) that makes up the chromosomes in the nucleus of each cell. These chromosomes, which determine the structure and function of organ systems and traits, are of the same biochemical substances. How then does each person become unique? The answer lies in the physiologic mechanisms of heredity, the processes of cellular division, and the environmental factors that influence our development from the moment we are conceived. This chapter explores the processes involved in conception and fetal development—the basis of human uniqueness.

Chromosomes

Human (body) cells contain within their nuclei threadlike bodies known as **chromosomes**, which are composed of strands of deoxyribonucleic acid (DNA) and protein. Each chromosome contains two longitudinal halves called *chromatids,* which are joined together at a point called the *centromere* (Figure 11-1A ■). Chromosomes are classified according to their length and to the position of their centromere. When the centromere is centrally located, the longitudinal halves are divided into one short arm region and one long arm region, and the chromosome resembles an X. This is the shape of most human chromosomes.

Every body (somatic) cell in the human body contains 46 chromosomes, referred to as the **diploid number of chromosomes**. These are divided into 23 pairs. There are 22 pairs of similar cells in both males and females, called *autosomes,* and one pair of sex chromosomes (XX in females, XY in males). One chromosome of each pair is contributed by the individual's mother, and the other is contributed by the father. The two chromosomes carrying matching genetic information that make up each pair are called *homologous chromosomes* or *homologs.*

Genes are regions in the DNA strands that contain coded information used to determine the unique characteristics—or *traits*—of an individual. Genes in the autosomes determine such traits as hair color or blood type, whereas genes in the sex chromosomes determine the individual's gender. Genes are arranged in linear order on the chromosomes and can be numbered and studied accordingly.

Each homologous chromosome pair carries genes coding for similar traits in identical locations on the chromosomes. Genes that are similar are called *homozygous* genes, whereas dissimilar genes are referred to as *heterozygous* genes (Figure 11-1B ■). When an individual is homozygous for a particular trait, he or she has inherited similar genes for that trait from each parent. Genetics is discussed in greater detail in chapter 12 ∞.

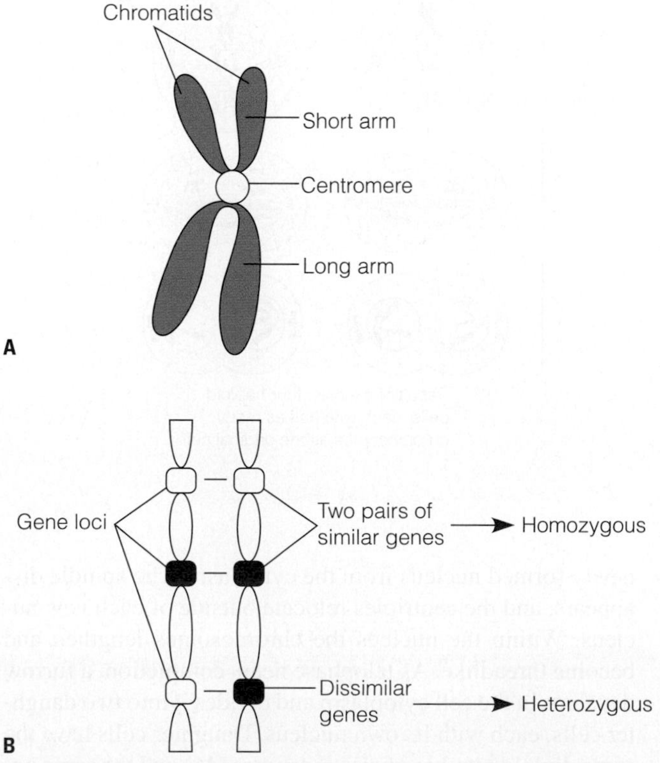

Figure 11-1 ■ A. Chromosomes contain two longitudinal halves called *chromatids,* which are joined together at a point called the *centromere.* B. One pair of homologous chromosomes with similar (homozygous) genes and dissimilar (heterozygous) genes.

Cellular Division

Each human begins life as a single cell called a fertilized ovum or zygote. This single cell reproduces itself, and in turn each new cell also reproduces itself in a continuing process. The new cells are similar to the cells from which they came. Cells are reproduced either by mitosis or meiosis, two different but related processes.

Mitosis

Mitosis is a process of cell division that results in daughter cells that are exact copies of the original cell. During mitosis, the cell undergoes several changes, ending in cell division. As the last phase of cell division nears completion, a furrow develops in the cell cytoplasm, which divides it into two daughter cells, each with its own nucleus. They are identical to the parent cell and to each other. These cells contain a full set of chromosomes or genetic material and are called diploid because of this. Mitosis makes growth and development possible, and in mature individuals it is the process by which the (somatic) body cells continue to divide and replace themselves.

Although mitosis is a continuous process, it is generally divided into five stages: interphase, prophase, metaphase, anaphase, and telophase (Figure 11-2A ■).

Interphase: Before cell division takes place during interphase, the deoxyribonucleic acid (DNA) within the chromosomes replicates so that the genes will be doubled. Mitosis begins when the cell enters prophase.

Prophase: During prophase, the chromosomes condense and form the shape we usually recognize as a chromosome. Next comes the appearance of a mitotic apparatus known as a spindle, in which fine threads extend from the top and bottom poles of the nucleus. At each pole of the spindle, a body known as the *centrosome* is formed, so the threads of the spindle extend from one centrosome to the other. Next the nuclear membrane, which separates the nucleus from the cytoplasm,

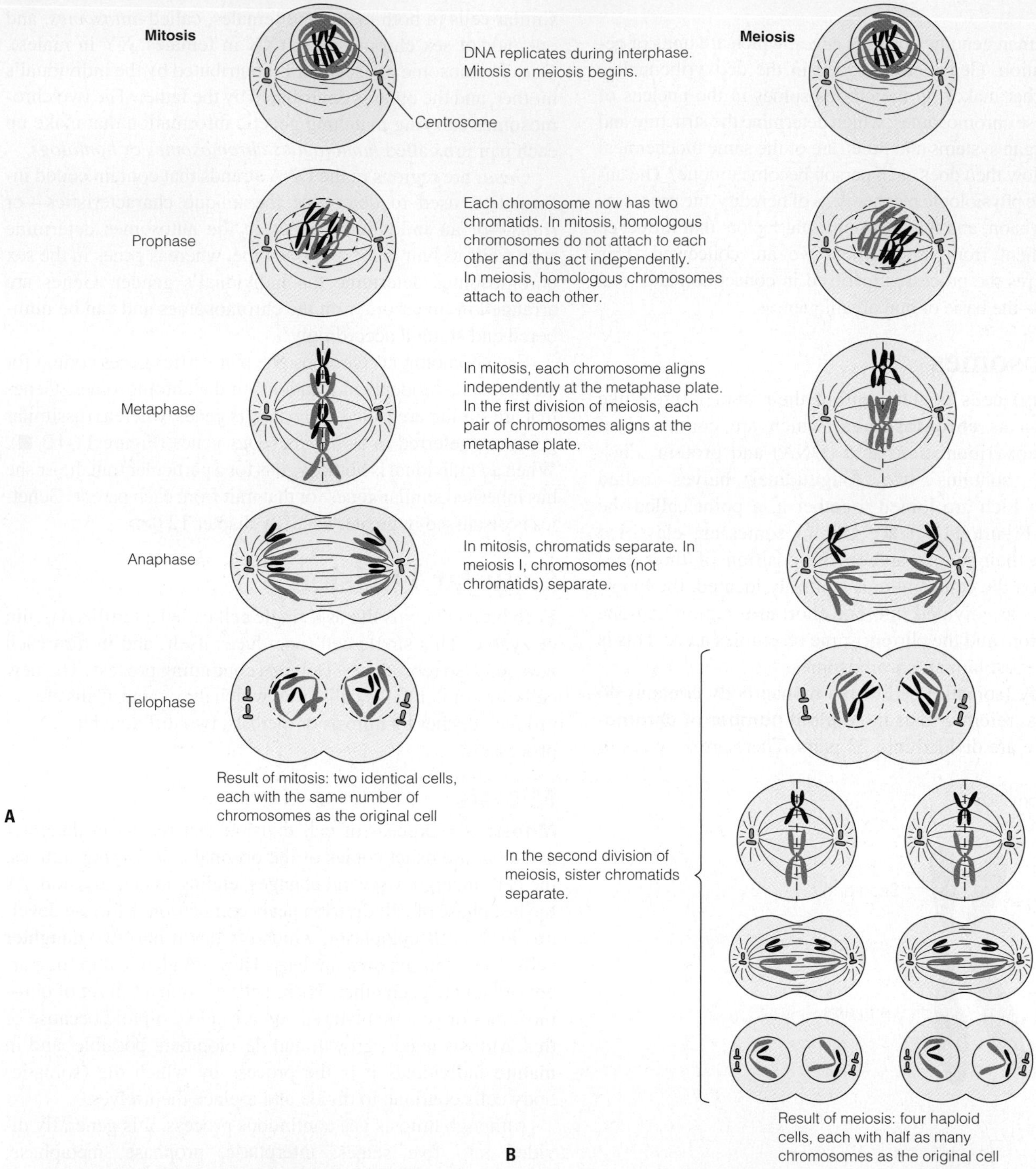

Mitosis
Meiosis
DNA replicates during interphase. Mitosis or meiosis begins.
Centrosome
Prophase
Each chromosome now has two chromatids. In mitosis, homologous chromosomes do not attach to each other and thus act independently. In meiosis, homologous chromosomes attach to each other.
Metaphase
In mitosis, each chromosome aligns independently at the metaphase plate. In the first division of meiosis, each pair of chromosomes aligns at the metaphase plate.
Anaphase
In mitosis, chromatids separate. In meiosis I, chromosomes (not chromatids) separate.
Telophase
Result of mitosis: two identical cells, each with the same number of chromosomes as the original cell
A
In the second division of meiosis, sister chromatids separate.
Result of meiosis: four haploid cells, each with half as many chromosomes as the original cell
B

Figure 11-2 ■ Comparison of: A. Mitosis. B. Meiosis.

disappears, the nucleus as a separate entity disappears, and the cell enters metaphase.

Metaphase: During metaphase, the chromosomes line up at the equator (midway between the poles) of the spindle. Metaphase is followed by anaphase.

Anaphase: During anaphase the two chromatids of each chromosome separate and move to opposite ends of the spindle, where they cluster in masses near the two poles of the cell.

Telophase: Essentially the opposite of prophase, during telophase a new nuclear membrane forms, separating each newly formed nucleus from the cytoplasm. The spindle disappears, and the centrioles relocate outside of each new nucleus. Within the nucleus the chromosomes lengthen and become threadlike. As telophase nears completion, a furrow develops in the cell cytoplasm and divides it into two daughter cells, each with its own nucleus. Daughter cells have the same diploid number of chromosomes (46) and the same genetic makeup as the cell from which they came. At the end of mitosis, a cell with 46 chromosomes results in two identical cells, each with 46 chromosomes.

Meiosis

Meiosis is a special type of cell division by which diploid cells give rise to **gametes** (sperm and ova). These cells are different from other somatic (body) cells because they contain half the genetic material of the parent cell—only 23 chromosomes—the **haploid number of chromosomes**.

Meiosis consists of two successive cell divisions (see Figure 11-2B ■). In the first division, the chromosomes replicate. Next a pairing takes place between homologous chromosomes (Sadler, 2010). Instead of separating immediately, as in mitosis, the similar chromosomes become closely intertwined. At each point of contact, there is a physical exchange of genetic material between the chromatids (arms of the chromosomes). New combinations are provided by the newly formed chromosomes; these combinations account for the wide variation of traits, such as hair or eye color. The chromosome pairs then separate, each member of a pair moving to opposite sides of the cell. (In contrast, during mitosis the chromatids of each chromosome separate and move to opposite poles.) The cell divides, forming two daughter cells, each with 23 double-structured chromosomes—the same amount of DNA as a normal somatic cell. In the second division, the chromatids of each chromosome separate and move to opposite poles of each of the daughter cells. Cell division occurs, resulting in the formation of four cells, each containing 23 single chromosomes, the haploid number of chromosomes. These daughter cells contain only half the DNA of a normal somatic cell (Sadler, 2010).

The process of meiosis is important for the following reasons:

- It maintains the *constancy of the chromosome number* from one generation to the next by reducing the chromosome number from diploid to haploid, thereby producing haploid gametes.
- It allows random assortment of *maternal and paternal chromosomes* between the gametes.
- It relocates segments of maternal and paternal chromosomes by *crossing over of chromosome segments,* which "shuffles" the genes and produces a recombination of genetic material.

Mutations may occur during the second meiotic division if two of the chromatids do not move apart rapidly enough when the cell divides. The still-paired chromatids are carried into one of the daughter cells and eventually form an extra chromosome. This condition is referred to as an *autosomal nondisjunction* (chromosomal mutation) and is harmful to the offspring that may result should fertilization occur. Another type of chromosomal mutation can occur if chromosomes break during meiosis. If the broken segment is lost, the result is a shorter chromosome; this is known as a *deletion.* If the broken segment becomes attached to another chromosome, a harmful mutation called a *translocation* is the result. The effects of nondisjunction and translocation are described in chapter 12 ∞. See Table 11-1 for a comparison of meiosis and mitosis.

Gametogenesis

Meiosis occurs during **gametogenesis**, the process by which germ cells, or gametes (ovum and sperm), are produced. These cells contain only half the genetic material of a typical body cell. The gametes must have a haploid number (23) of chromosomes so that when the female gamete (egg or ovum) and the male gamete (sperm or spermatozoon) unite to form the **zygote** (fertilized ovum), the normal human diploid of chromosomes (46 chromosomes)—half of it from the mother and half from the father, is reestablished.

TABLE 11-1 Comparison of Meiosis and Mitosis

Meiosis	
Purpose	Produce reproductive cells (gametes). Reduction of chromosome number by half (from diploid [46] to haploid [23]), so that when fertilization occurs the normal diploid number is restored. Introduces genetic variability.
Cell Division	Two-stage reduction.
Number of Daughter Cells	Four daughter cells, each containing one half the number of chromosomes as the mother cell, or 23 chromosomes. Nonidentical to original cell.
Mitosis	
Purpose	Produce cells for growth and tissue repair. Cell division characteristic of all somatic cells.
Cell Division	One-stage cell division.
Number of Daughter Cells	Two daughter cells identical to the mother cell, each with the diploid number (46 chromosomes).

Oogenesis

Oogenesis is the process that produces the female gamete, called an ovum (egg). As discussed in chapter 10 ∞, the ovaries begin to develop early in the fetal life of the female. All the ova that the female will produce in her lifetime are present at birth. The ovary gives rise to oogonial cells, which develop into oocytes. Meiosis (cell replication by division) begins in all oocytes before the female infant is born but stops before the first division is complete and remains in this arrested phase until puberty. During puberty the mature primary oocyte continues through the first meiotic division in the graafian follicle of the ovary.

The first meiotic division produces two cells of unequal size with different amounts of cytoplasm but with the same number of chromosomes. One of these cells is the *secondary oocyte* and the other is a minute *polar body.* Both the secondary oocyte and the first polar body contain 22 double-structured autosomal chromosomes and one double-structured sex chromosome (X).

At the time of ovulation, the second meiotic division begins immediately and proceeds as the oocyte moves down the fallopian tube. Division is again not equal, and the secondary oocyte moves into the metaphase stage of cell division, where its meiotic division is arrested until and unless the oocyte is fertilized.

When the secondary oocyte completes the second meiotic division after fertilization, the result is a mature ovum with

Oogenesis
Spermatogenesis
Oogenesis and Spermatogenesis Compared

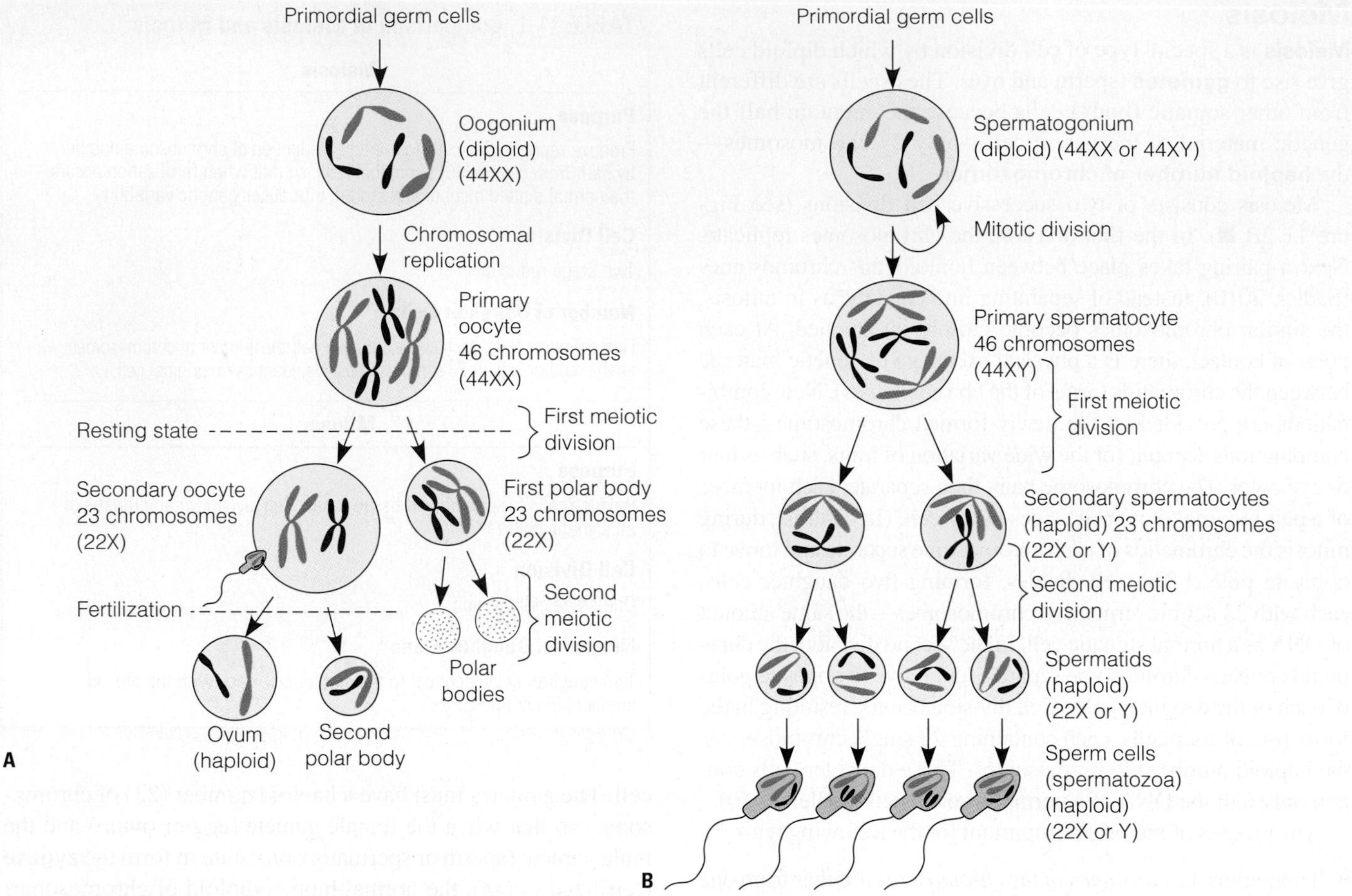

Figure 11-3 ■ Gametogenesis involves meiosis within the ovary and testis. A. During meiosis, each oogonium produces a single haploid ovum once some cytoplasm moves into the polar bodies. B. Each spermatogonium, in contrast, produces four haploid spermatozoa.

Activity: Matching Oogenesis and Spermatogenesis

the haploid number of chromosomes and virtually all the cytoplasm. In addition, the second polar body (also haploid) forms at this time (Figure 11-3A ■). The first polar body has now also divided, producing two additional polar bodies. Thus when meiosis is completed, four haploid cells have been produced: three small polar bodies, which eventually disintegrate, and one ovum (Sadler, 2010).

Spermatogenesis

During puberty, the germinal epithelium in the seminiferous tubules of the testes begins the process of spermatogenesis, which produces the male gametes (sperm). The diploid spermatogonium replicates before it enters the first meiotic division, during which it is called the *primary spermatocyte.* During this first meiotic division, the spermatogonium replicates and forms two haploid cells termed *secondary spermatocytes,* each of which contains 22 double-structured autosomal chromosomes and either a double-structured X sex chromosome or a double-structured Y sex chromosome. During the second meiotic division, they divide to form four spermatids, each with the haploid number of chromosomes (see Figure 11-3B ■). The spermatids undergo a series of changes during which they lose most of their cytoplasm and become sperm (spermatozoa). The nucleus becomes compacted into the head of the sperm, which is covered by a cap called an acrosome that is, in turn, covered by a plasma membrane. A long tail is produced from one of the centrioles.

The Process of Fertilization

Fertilization is the process by which a sperm fuses with an ovum to form a new diploid cell, or zygote. The zygote begins life as a single cell with a complete set of genetic material, 23 chromosomes from the mother's ovum and 23 chromosomes from the father's sperm for a total of 46 chromosomes. The following events lead to fertilization.

Preparation for Fertilization

The mature ovum and spermatozoa have only a brief time to unite. Ova are considered fertile for about 12 to 24 hours after ovulation. Sperm can survive in the female reproductive tract for 48 to 72 hours but are believed to be healthy and highly fertile for only about the first 24 hours.

The ovum's cell membrane is surrounded by two layers of tissue. The layer closest to the cell membrane is called the *zona pellucida.* It is a clear, noncellular layer whose thickness influences the fertilization rate. Surrounding the zona pellucida is a ring of elongated cells, called the *corona radiata,* because they radiate from the ovum like the gaseous corona around the sun. These cells are held together by hyaluronic acid. The ovum has no power of movement of its own. During ovulation, high estrogen levels increase peristalsis within the fallopian tubes, which helps move the ovum through the tube toward the uterus. The high estrogen levels also cause a thinning of the cervical mucus, easing passage of the sperm through the cervix, into the uterus, and up the fallopian tube.

The process of fertilization usually takes place in the ampulla (outer third) of the fallopian tube. In a single ejaculation, the male deposits approximately 200 to 500 million spermatozoa in the vagina, of which only hundreds of sperm actually reach the ampulla (Sadler, 2010). Fructose in the semen, secreted by the seminal vesicles, is the energy source for the sperm. The spermatozoa propel themselves up the female tract by the flagellar movement of their tails. Transit time from the cervix into the fallopian tube can be as short as 5 minutes but usually takes an average of 2 to 7 hours after ejaculation (Sadler, 2010). Prostaglandins in the semen may increase uterine smooth muscle contractions, which help transport the sperm. The fallopian tubes have a dual ciliary action that facilitates movement of the ovum toward the uterus and movement of the sperm from the uterus toward the ovary.

The sperm must undergo two processes before fertilization can occur: capacitation and the acrosomal reaction. **Capacitation** is the removal of the plasma membrane and glycoprotein coat overlying the spermatozoa's acrosomal area and the loss of seminal plasma proteins. If the glycoprotein coat is not removed, the sperm will not be able to fertilize the ovum (Sadler, 2010). Capacitation occurs in the female reproductive tract (aided by uterine enzymes) and is thought to take about 7 hours. Sperm that undergo capacitation take on three characteristics: (1) the ability to undergo the acrosomal reaction, (2) the ability to bind to the zona pellucida, and (3) the acquisition of hypermotility.

The **acrosomal reaction** follows capacitation. The acrosome caps of the sperm surrounding the ovum release their enzymes (hyaluronidase, a protease called acrosin, and trypsin-like substances). These enzymes break down the hyaluronic acid that holds the elongated cells of corona radiata, the outer layer of the ovum, together (Sadler, 2010). Hundreds of acrosomes must rupture to clear enough hyaluronic acid for even a single sperm to penetrate the ovum successfully.

At the moment of penetration by a fertilizing sperm, the zona pellucida undergoes a reaction that prevents additional sperm from entering a single ovum. This is known as the *block to polyspermy.* This cellular change is mediated by release of materials from the cortical granules, organelles found just below the ovum's surface, and is called the *cortical reaction* (Figure 11-4 ■).

The Moment of Fertilization

After the sperm enters the ovum, a chemical signal prompts the secondary oocyte to complete the second meiotic division, forming the nucleus of the ovum and ejecting the second polar body. Then the nuclei of the ovum and sperm swell and approach each other. The true moment of fertilization occurs as the nuclei unite. Their individual nuclear membranes disappear, and their chromosomes pair up to produce the diploid zygote. Because each nucleus contains a haploid number of chromosomes (23), this union restores the diploid number (46). The zygote contains a new combination of genetic material that results in an individual different from either parent and from anyone else.

It is also at the moment of fertilization that the sex of the zygote is determined. The two chromosomes (the sex chromosomes) of the 23rd pair—either XX or XY—determine the sex of an individual. X chromosomes are larger and bear more genes than Y chromosomes. Females have two X chromosomes, and males have an X and a Y chromosome. The mature ovum produced by oogenesis can have only one type of sex chromosome—an X—while spermatogenesis produces two sperm with an X chromosome and two sperm with a Y chromosome. When each gamete contributes an X chromosome, the resulting zygote is female. When the ovum contributes an X chromosome and the sperm contributes a Y, the resulting zygote is male. As discussed in chapter 12 ∞, certain traits are termed *sex-linked* because they are controlled by the genes on the X sex chromosome. Two examples of sex-linked traits are color blindness and hemophilia.

DEVELOPING CULTURAL COMPETENCE

Iraqi Childbirth Customs

"My sister, she did not have baby for very, very long time, you see. This is very sad where I am from [Iraq]. Her husband's family wanted him to leave her and we so feared he would. Then my sister became pregnant and it was very nice, we all so happy you see. Then I learned my sister birthed a baby girl and I cried and cried for a week. My mother cried too, so sad all this time no baby come and then finally to have a girl. I still feel sad for her."

Source: Excerpt from author's interview with an Iraqi woman on childbirth customs in Iraq.

Preembryonic Stage

The first 14 days of human development, starting on the day the ovum is fertilized (conception), are referred to as *the preembryonic stage,* or *the stage of the ovum.* Development after fertilization can be divided into two phases: cellular multiplication and cellular differentiation. These phases are characterized by rapid cellular multiplication and differentiation and the establishment of the primary germ layers and embryonic membranes. Synchronized development of both the endometrium and embryo is a prerequisite for implantation to succeed (Moore & Persaud, 2008). These phases and the process of implantation (nidation), which occurs between them, are discussed next.

Cellular Multiplication

Cellular multiplication begins as the zygote moves through the fallopian tube toward the cavity of the uterus. This transportation takes 3 days or more and is accomplished mainly by a very weak fluid current in the fallopian tube resulting from the beating action of the ciliated epithelium that lines the tube.

The zygote now enters a period of rapid mitotic divisions called **cleavage**, during which it divides into two cells, four cells, eight cells, and so on. These cells, called *blastomeres,* are so small that the developing cell mass is only slightly larger than the original zygote. The blastomeres are held together by the zona pellucida, which is under the corona radiata. The blastomeres will eventually form a solid ball of 12 to 16 cells called the **morula**.

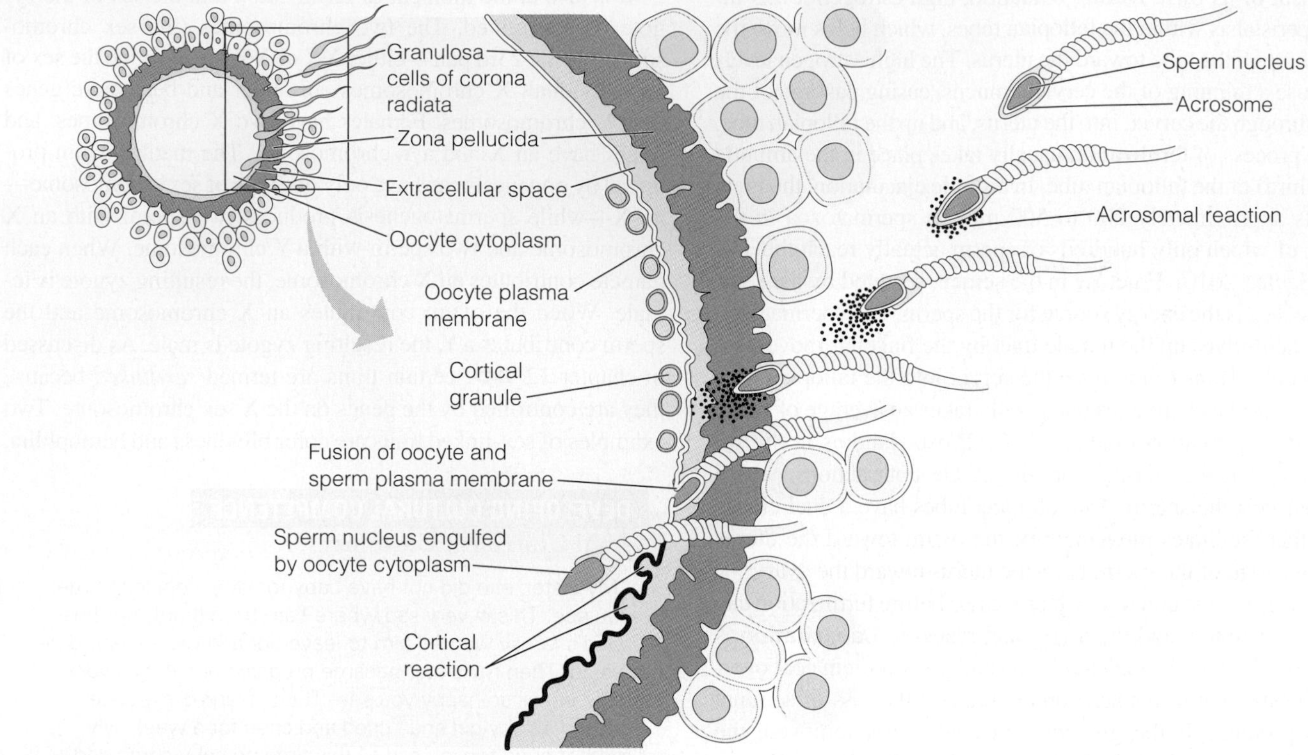

A

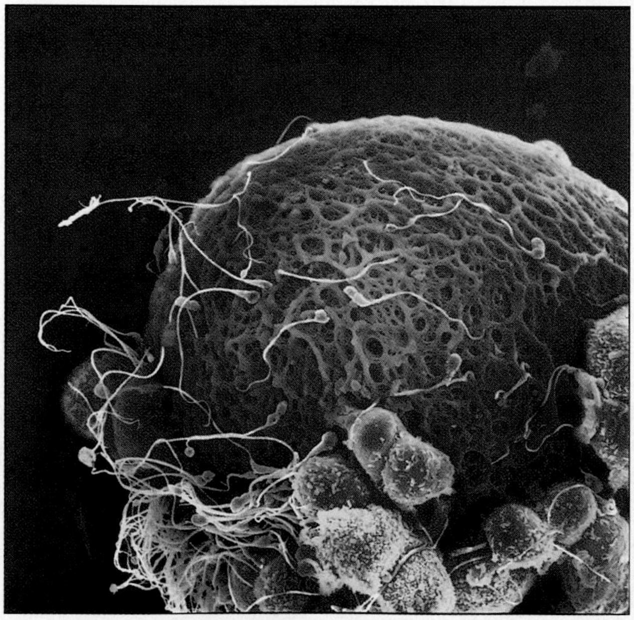

B

Figure 11-4 ■ Sperm penetration of an ovum. A. The sequential steps of oocyte penetration by a sperm are depicted moving from top to bottom. B. Scanning electron micrograph of human sperm surrounding a human oocyte (750×). The smaller spherical cells are granulosa cells of the corona radiata.

Source: B. Used with permission from Nilsson, L. (1990). A child is born. *New York, NY: Dell Publishing.*

As the morula enters the uterus, two things happen: the intracellular fluid in the morula increases, and a central cavity forms within the cell mass. Inside this cavity is an inner solid mass of cells called the **blastocyst**. The outer layer of cells that surround the cavity and have replaced the zona pellucida is the **trophoblast**. Eventually, the trophoblast develops into one of the embryonic membranes, called the chorion. The blastocyst develops into a double layer of cells called the *embryonic disc,* from which the embryo and the amnion (embryonic membrane) will develop. The journey of the fertilized ovum to its destination in the uterus is illustrated in Figure 11-5 ■.

Early pregnancy factor (EPF), an immunosuppressant, is secreted by the trophoblastic cells. EPF appears in the maternal serum within 24 to 48 hours after fertilization and forms the basis of a pregnancy test during the first 10 days of development (Moore & Persaud, 2008).

Implantation (Nidation)

While floating in the uterine cavity, the blastocyst is nourished by the uterine glands, which secrete a mixture of lipids, mucopolysaccharides, and glycogen. The trophoblast attaches itself to the surface of the endometrium for further nourishment. The most frequent site of attachment is the upper part of the posterior uterine wall (Figure 11-5). Between days 7 and 10 after fertilization, the zona pellucida disappears, and the blastocyst implants itself by burrowing into the uterine lining and penetrating down toward the maternal capillaries until it is completely covered (Moore & Persaud, 2008). The lining of the uterus thickens below the implanted blastocyst, and the cells of the trophoblast grow down into the thickened lining, forming processes called chorionic villi.

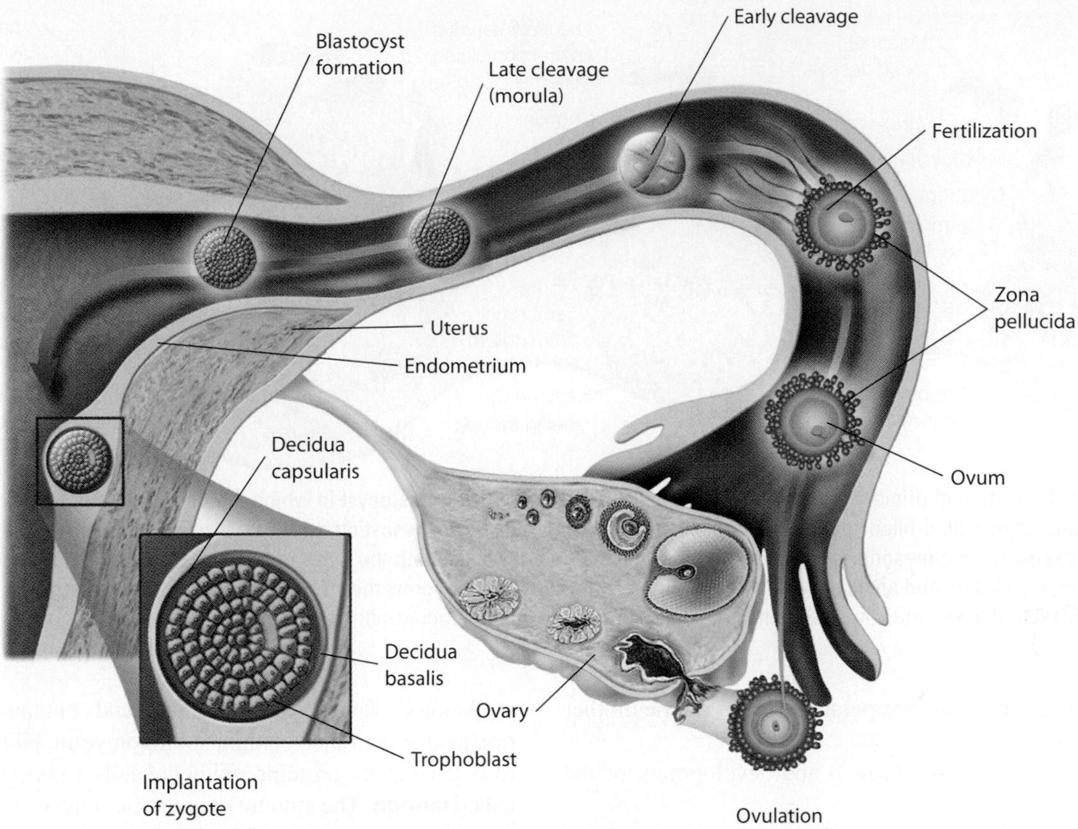

Figure 11-5 ■ During ovulation, the ovum leaves the ovary and enters the fallopian tube. Fertilization generally occurs in the outer third of the fallopian tube. Subsequent changes in the fertilized ovum from conception to implantation are depicted.

Under the influence of progesterone, the endometrium increases in thickness and vascularity in preparation for implantation and nourishment of the ovum. After implantation, the endometrium is called the decidua. The portion of the decidua that covers the blastocyst is called the **decidua capsularis**; the portion directly under the implanted blastocyst is the **decidua basalis**; and the portion that lines the rest of the uterine cavity is the **decidua vera (parietalis)** (see Figure 11-5, inset) (Benirschke, 2009a). The maternal part of the placenta develops from the decidua basalis, which contains large numbers of blood vessels. The chorionic villi (discussed shortly) in contact with the decidua basalis will form the fetal portion of the placenta.

Cellular Differentiation

Primary Germ Layers

About 10 to 14 days after conception, the homogenous mass of blastocyst cells differentiates into the primary germ layers. These layers—the **ectoderm**, **mesoderm**, and **endoderm** (see Figure 11-6 ■)—are formed at the same time as the embryonic membranes. All tissues, organs, and organ systems will develop from these primary germ cell layers (Table 11-2). For example, differentiation of the endoderm results in the formation of the epithelium lining the respiratory and digestive tracts (Figure 11-7 ■).

Embryonic Membranes

The **embryonic membranes** begin to form at the time of implantation (Figure 11-8 ■). These membranes protect and support the embryo as it grows and develops inside the uterus. The first and outermost membrane to form is the **chorion**. This thick membrane develops from the trophoblast and has many fingerlike projections, called *chorionic villi,* on its surface. These chorionic villi can be used for early genetic testing of the embryo at 8 to 11 weeks' gestation by chorionic villi sampling (see chapter 21 ∞). As the pregnancy progresses, the villi begin to degenerate, except for those just under the embryo, which grow and branch into depressions in the uterine wall, forming the fetal portion of the placenta. By the fourth month of pregnancy, the surface of the chorion is smooth except at the place of attachment to the uterine wall.

The second membrane, the amnion, originates from the ectoderm, a primary germ layer, during the early stages of embryonic development. The **amnion** is a thin protective membrane that contains amniotic fluid. The space between the amniotic membrane and the embryo is the *amniotic cavity.* This cavity surrounds the embryo and yolk sac, except where the developing embryo (germ layer disc) attaches to the trophoblast via the umbilical cord. As the embryo grows, the amnion expands until it comes in contact with the chorion. These two slightly adherent membranes form the fluid-filled amniotic sac, also called **bag of waters (BOW)**, which protects the floating embryo.

Amniotic Fluid

The primary functions of **amniotic fluid** are to:

- Act as a cushion to protect the embryo against mechanical injury.

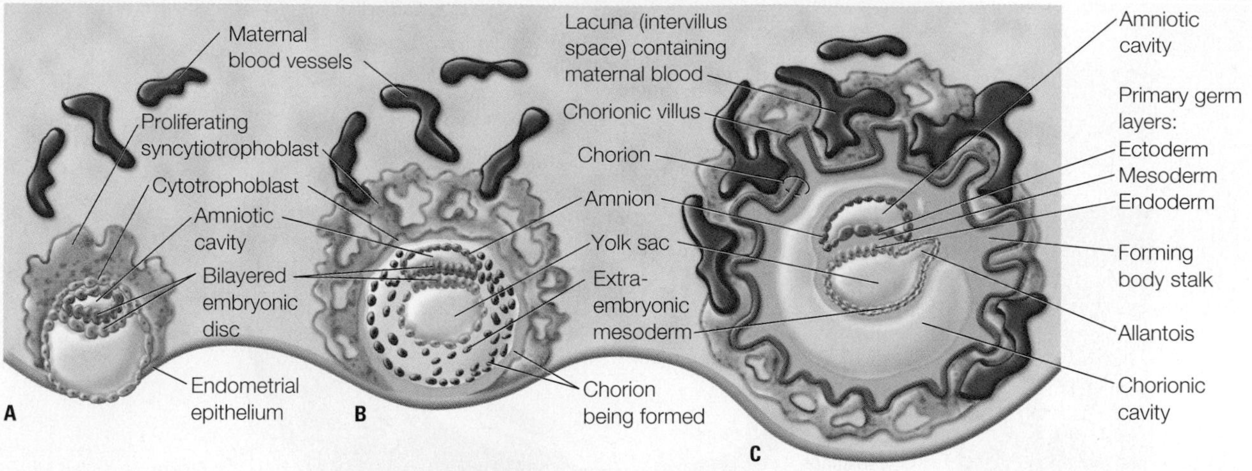

Figure 11-6 ■ Formation of primary germ layers. A. Implantation of a 7 1/2-day blastocyst in which the cells of the embryonic disc are separated from the amnion by a fluid-filled space. The erosion of the endometrium by the syncytiotrophoblast is ongoing. B. Implantation is completed by day 9, and extraembryonic mesoderm is beginning to form a discrete layer beneath the cytotrophoblast. C. By day 16, the embryo shows all three germ layers, a yolk sac, and an allantois (an outpouching of the yolk sac that forms the structural basis of the body stalk, or umbilical cord). The cytotrophoblast and associated mesoderm has become the chorion, and chorionic villi are developing.

- Help control the embryo's temperature (relies on the mother to release heat).
- Permit symmetric external growth and development of the embryo.
- Act as an extension of fetal extracellular space (hydropic infants have increased amniotic fluid).
- Prevent adherence of the embryo-fetus to the amnion (decreases chance of amniotic band syndrome) to allow freedom of movement so that the embryo-fetus can change position (flexion and extension), thus aiding in musculoskeletal development.
- Allow the umbilical cord to be relatively free of compression.
- Act as a wedge during labor.
- Provide fluid for analysis to determine fetal health and maturity.

Amniotic fluid is slightly alkaline and contains albumin, urea, uric acid, creatinine, lecithin, sphingomyelin, bilirubin, fat, fructose, leukocytes, proteins, epithelial cells, enzymes, and fine hair called **lanugo**. The amount of amniotic fluid at 10 weeks is about 30 ml and increases to 350 ml at 20 weeks. After 20 weeks the volume ranges from 700 to 1000 ml. The amniotic fluid volume is constantly changing as the fluid moves back and forth across the placental membrane. Water and solutes must pass between the amniotic fluid and fetus. As the pregnancy continues, the fetus contributes to the volume of amniotic fluid by excreting urine. The fetus also swallows up to 262 ml/kg/day. Approximately 400 ml of amniotic fluid flows out of the fetal lungs each day (Gilbert, 2007). Abnormal variations in amniotic fluid volume are *oligohydramnios* (less than 400 ml of amniotic fluid) and *hydramnios* (more than 2000 ml or amniotic fluid index greater

TABLE 11-2 Derivation of Body Structures from Primary Cell Layers

ECTODERM	MESODERM	ENDODERM
Epidermis	Dermis	Respiratory tract epithelium
Sweat glands	Wall of digestive tract	Epithelium (except nasal), including pharynx, tongue, tonsils, thyroid, parathyroid, thymus tympanic cavity
Sebaceous glands	Kidneys and ureter (suprarenal cortex)	Lining of digestive tract
Nails	Reproductive organs (gonads, genital ducts)	Primary tissue of liver and pancreas
Hair follicles	Connective tissue (cartilage, bone, joint cavities)	Urethra and associated glands
Lens of eye	Skeleton	Urinary bladder (except trigone)
Sensory epithelium of internal and external ear, nasal cavity, sinuses, mouth, anal canal	Muscles (all types)	Vagina (parts)
Central and peripheral nervous systems	Cardiovascular system (heart, arteries, veins, blood, bone marrow)	
Nasal cavity	Pleura	
Oral glands and tooth enamel	Lymphatic tissue and cells	
Pituitary gland	Spleen	
Mammary glands		

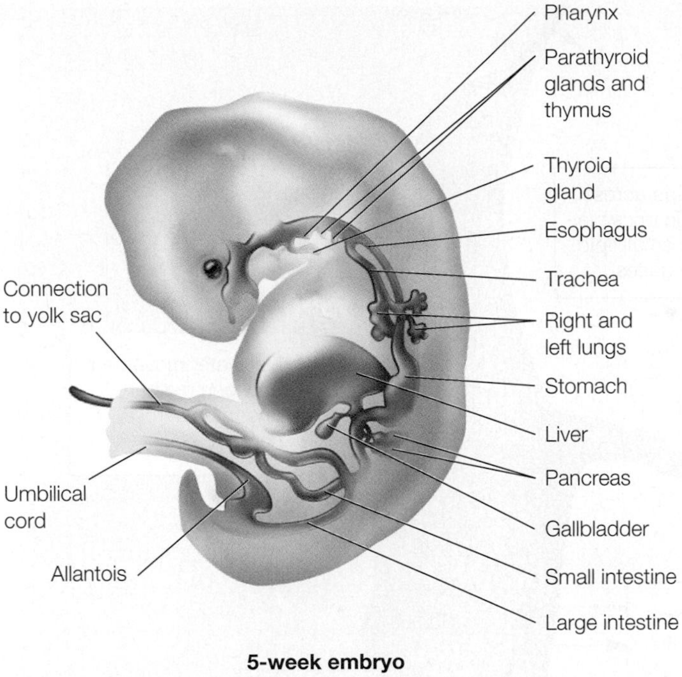

Figure 11-7 ■ Endoderm differentiates to form the epithelial lining of the digestive and respiratory tracts and associated glands.

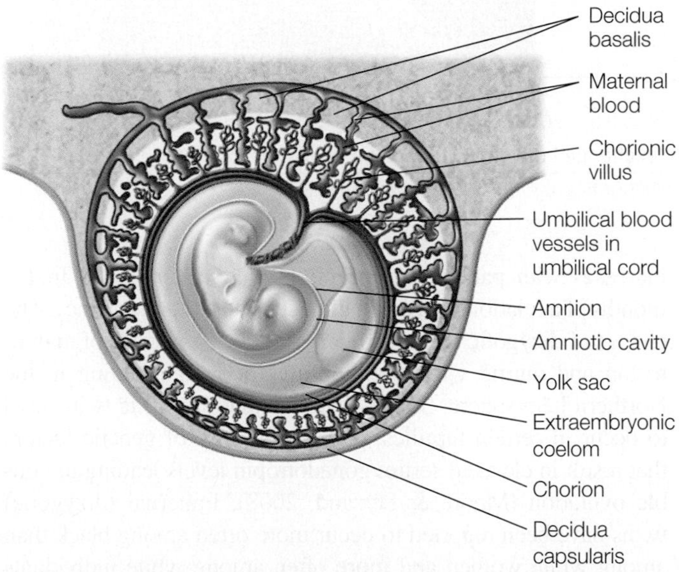

Figure 11-8 ■ Early development of primary embryonic membranes. At 4 1/2 weeks, the decidua capsularis (placental portion enclosing the embryo on the uterine surface) and decidua basalis (placental portion encompassing the elaborate chorionic villi and maternal endometrium) are well formed. The chorionic villi lie in blood-filled intervillous spaces within the endometrium. The amnion and yolk sac are well developed.

than 97.5 percentile for the corresponding gestational age). Hydramnios is also called *polyhydramnios.* Chapter 27 ∞ discusses alterations in amniotic fluid volume. Figure 11-9 ■ summarizes the major pathways of exchange.

Early in the first trimester of pregnancy, amniotic fluid is isoosmolar with fetal and maternal plasma and is secreted from the developing trophoblast or embryo. Water and solutes move freely across the fetal skin before the time of skin keratinization. After 23 to 25 weeks, thickening of the fetal skin inhibits this diffusion. During the rest of the pregnancy, the fetal kidneys are the major source of fluid that enters the amniotic sac. Abnormalities of fetal urine production can result in changes in amniotic fluid volume. For example, with obstruction of urine outflow, as in Potter's syndrome, oligohydramnios develops. Conversely, Bartter's syndrome results in a fetal diuresis and hydramnios. The fetal lungs are also significant contributors to amniotic fluid. Fetal breathing movements are associated with the bidirectional flow of fluid through the trachea. Net outflow from the fetal lungs averages 4.3 ml/kg/hr or 10% of body weight per day. This outflow of lung and tracheal fluid is used as the basis for amniotic fluid tests of fetal lung maturity.

The major mechanism by which amniotic fluid is removed in the last half of the pregnancy is fetal swallowing, which occurs mostly during periods of fetal breathing movements. In pregnancy, when the fetus does not swallow normal amounts of amniotic fluid (as in esophageal atresia and anencephalus), hydramnios will result. A potential route of amniotic fluid removal is by the transmembranous pathway; that is, the movement of fluid across the amniochorion and into the maternal circulation within the uterine wall. Another major regulator of amniotic fluid volume and composition is the intramembranous pathway. This pathway causes amniotic water and/or solutes to be absorbed by the fetal blood that perfuses the fetal surface of the placenta.

Yolk Sac

In humans the yolk sac is small and functions only in early embryonic life. It develops as a second cavity in the blastocyst, about day 8 or 9 after conception, and forms primitive red blood cells during the first 6 weeks of development until the embryo's liver takes over the process. As the embryo develops, the yolk sac is incorporated in the umbilical cord, where it can be identified as a degenerate structure after birth.

Umbilical Cord

As the placenta is developing, the **umbilical cord** is also being formed from the amnion. The *body stalk,* which attaches the embryo to the yolk sac, contains blood vessels that extend into the chorionic villi. The body stalk fuses with the embryonic portion of the placenta to provide a circulatory pathway from the chorionic villi to the embryo (see Figure 11-9). As the body stalk elongates to become the umbilical cord, the vessels in the cord decrease to one large vein and two smaller arteries. About 1% of umbilical cords have only two vessels, an artery and a vein; this condition may be associated with congenital malformations, primarily of the renal, cardiovascular, and gastrointestinal systems. A specialized connective tissue known as **Wharton's jelly** surrounds the blood vessels in the umbilical cord. This tissue, plus the high blood volume pulsating through the vessels, prevents compression of the umbilical cord in utero. The umbilical cord has no sensory or motor innervation, so cutting the cord after birth is not painful. At term (38 to 42 weeks' gestation), the average cord is 2 cm (0.8 in.) across and about 55 cm (22 in.) long. The cord can attach

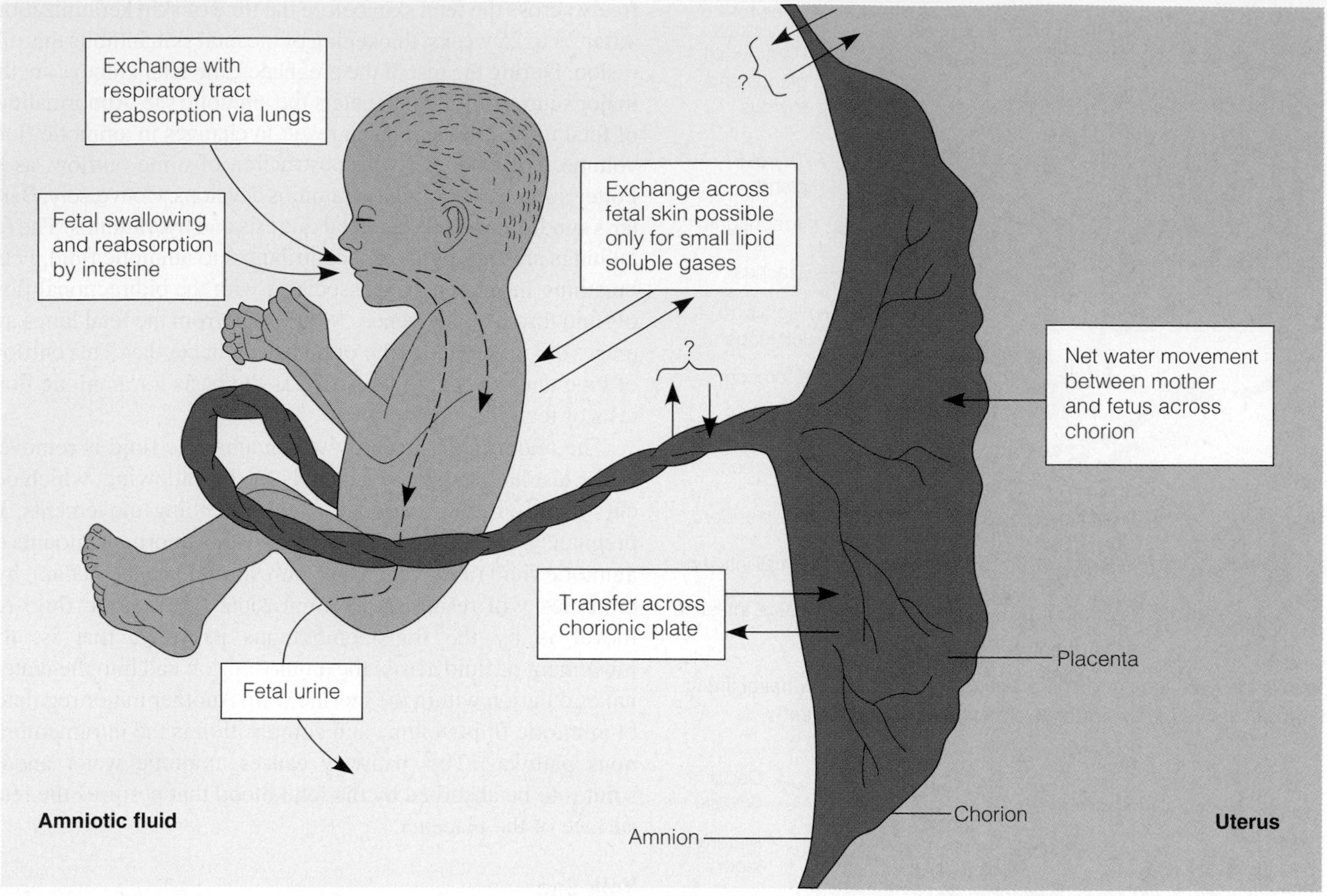

Figure 11-9 ■ Summary of the significant pathways of water and solute exchange between the amniotic fluid and fetus.

Source: Used with permission from Seeds, A. E. (1980, November). Current concepts of amniotic fluid dynamics. American Journal of Obstetrics and Gynecology, 138, *575.*

itself to the placenta at various sites. Central insertion into the placenta is considered normal. (Chapter 26 ∞ discusses the various attachment sites.)

Umbilical cords appear twisted or spiraled. This is most likely caused by fetal movement. A true knot in the umbilical cord rarely occurs; if it does, the cord is usually long. More common are so-called false knots caused by the folding of cord vessels. A nuchal cord exists when the umbilical cord encircles the fetal neck.

Care Plan Activity: Client Fearful of Multiple Gestations

Application: Fraternal or Identical Twins

Twins

Twinning occurs in approximately 1 in 43 pregnancies, and triplets in 1 in 1341 pregnancies (Benirschke, 2009b). Among all groups, as parity (having given birth to a viable infant) increases, so does the chance for multiple births.

Twins may be either fraternal or identical (Figure 11-10 ■). If they are fraternal, they are dizygotic, which means they arise from two separate ova fertilized by two separate spermatozoa. There are two placentas, two chorions, and two amnions; however, the placentas sometimes fuse and look as if they are one. Despite their birth relationship, fraternal twins are no more similar to each other than they would be to siblings born singly. They may be the same or different sex.

Dizygotic twinning increases with maternal age up to about 35 years and then decreases abruptly. The chance of dizygotic twins increases with parity, in conceptions that occur in the first 3 months of a relationship, and with increased coital frequency. The chance of dizygotic twinning decreases during periods of malnutrition and during winter and spring for women living in the Northern hemisphere. Studies indicate that dizygotic twins tend to occur in certain families, perhaps because of genetic factors that result in elevated serum gonadotropin levels leading to double ovulation (Moore & Persaud, 2008). Fraternal (dizygotic) twins have been reported to occur more often among black than among white women and more often among white individuals than among women of Asian origin (Moore & Persaud, 2008).

Identical, or monozygotic, twins develop from a single fertilized ovum. They are of the same sex and have the same phenotype (appearance). Identical twins usually have a common placenta (see Figure 11-10). Monozygosity is not affected by environment, race, physical characteristics, or fertility.

Monozygotic twins originate from division of the fertilized ovum at different stages of early development, after the zygote consists of thousands of cells. Complete separation of the cellular mass into two parts is necessary for twin formation. The number of amnions and chorions present depends on the timing of the division.

- If division occurs within 3 days of fertilization (before the inner cell mass and chorion are formed), two embryos, two amnions,

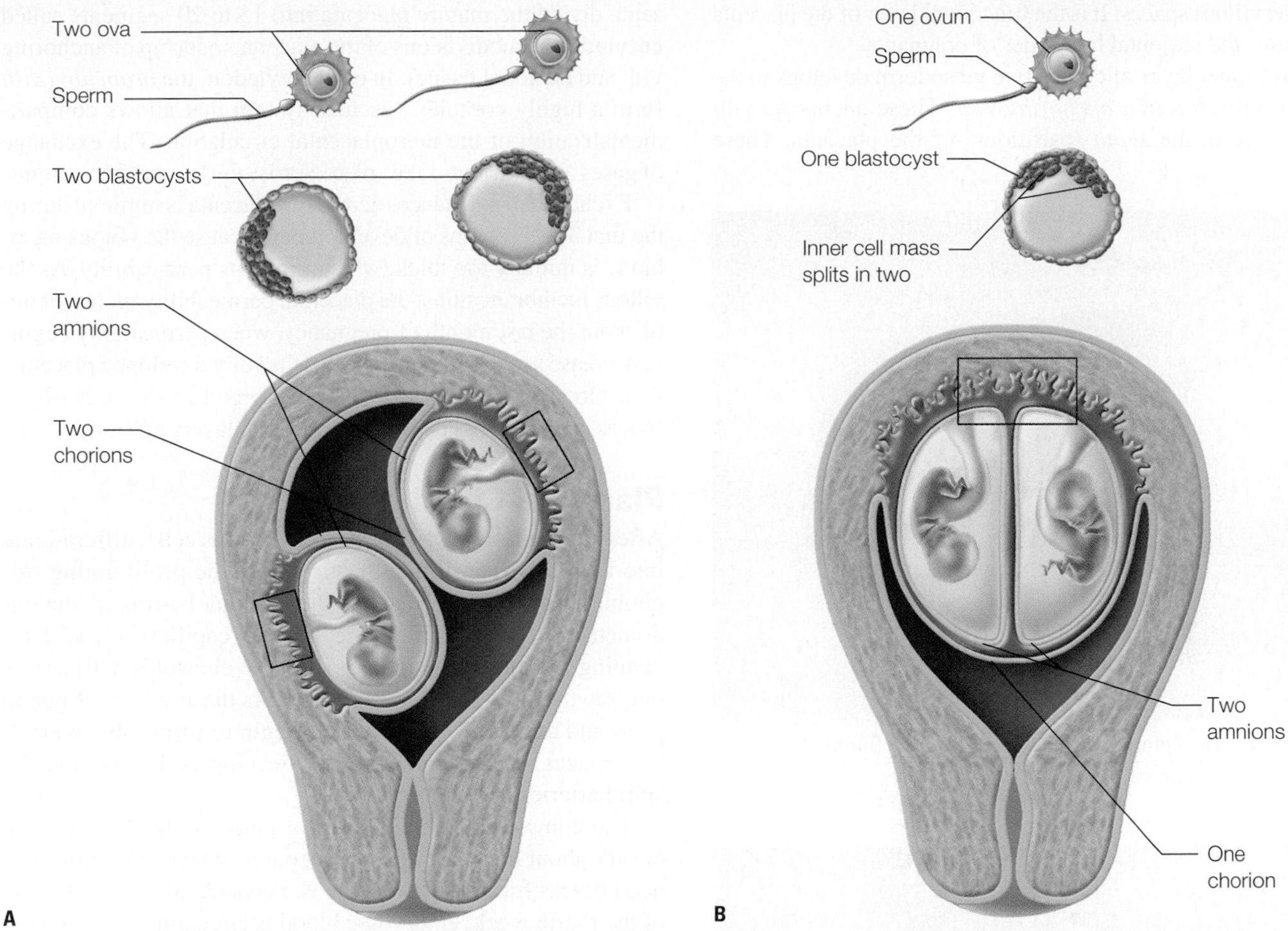

Figure 11-10 ■ A. Formation of fraternal twins. (Note separate placentas.) B. Formation of identical twins.

and two chorions will develop. This dichorionic-diamniotic situation occurs about 20% to 30% of the time, and there may be two distinct placentas or a single fused placenta.

- If division occurs about 5 days after fertilization (when the inner cell mass is formed and the chorion cells have differentiated but those of the amnion have not), two embryos develop with separate amnion sacs. These sacs will eventually be covered by a common chorion; thus there will be a monochorionic-diamniotic placenta.
- If the amnion has already developed approximately 7 to 13 days after fertilization, division results in two embryos with a common amnion sac and a common chorion. This type occurs rarely.

Monozygotic twinning is considered a random event and occurs in approximately 3.5 per 1000 live births (Benirschke, 2009b). The survival rate of monozygotic twins as a group is 10% lower than that of dizygotic twins, and congenital anomalies are more prevalent. Both twins may have the same malformation.

Development and Functions of the Placenta

The **placenta** is the means of metabolic and nutrient exchange between the embryonic and maternal circulations. Placental development and circulation does not begin until the third week of embryonic development. The placenta develops at the site where the developing embryo attaches to the uterine wall. Expansion of the placenta continues until about 20 weeks, when it covers about half the inside of the uterus. After 20 weeks' gestation, the placenta becomes thicker but not wider. At 40 weeks' gestation, the placenta is about 15 to 20 cm (5.9 to 7.9 in.) in diameter and 2.5 to 3 cm (1 to 1.2 in.) in thickness. It weighs approximately 400 to 600 g (14 to 21 oz).

The placenta has two parts: the maternal portion and the fetal portion. The maternal portion consists of the decidua basalis and its circulation. Its surface is red and fleshlike (often called *Dirty Duncan*). The fetal portion consists of the chorionic villi and their circulation. The fetal surface of the placenta is covered by the amnion, which gives it a shiny, gray appearance (often called *Shiny Schultz*) (Figures 11-11 ■ and 11-12 ■).

The placenta begins to form at implantation when the trophoblastic cells of the chorionic villi form spaces in the tissue of the decidua basalis. These spaces fill with maternal blood, and the chorionic villi grow into these spaces. As the chorionic villi differentiate, two trophoblastic layers appear: an outer layer called the *syncytium* (consisting of syncytiotrophoblasts), and an inner layer known as the *cytotrophoblast* (Figure 11-13 ■). The cytotrophoblast thins out and disappears about the fifth month, leaving only a single layer of syncytium covering the chorionic villi. The syncytium is in direct contact with the maternal blood

Formation of Placenta

in the intervillous spaces. It is the functional layer of the placenta and secretes the placental hormones of pregnancy.

A third, inner layer of connective mesoderm develops in the chorionic villi, forming *anchoring villi.* These anchoring villi eventually form the *septa* (partitions) of the placenta. These septa divide the mature placenta into 15 to 20 segments called **cotyledons** (subdivisions of the placenta made up of anchoring villi and decidual tissue). In each cotyledon, the *branching villi* form a highly complex vascular system that allows compartmentalization of the uteroplacental circulation. The exchange of gases and nutrients takes place across these vascular systems.

Exchange of substances across the placenta is minimal during the first 3 to 5 months of development because the villous membrane is initially too thick, which limits its permeability. As the villous membrane thins, the placental permeability increases until about the last month of pregnancy, when permeability begins to decrease as the placenta ages. In the fully developed placenta, fetal blood in the villi and maternal blood in the intervillous spaces are separated by three to four thin layers of tissue.

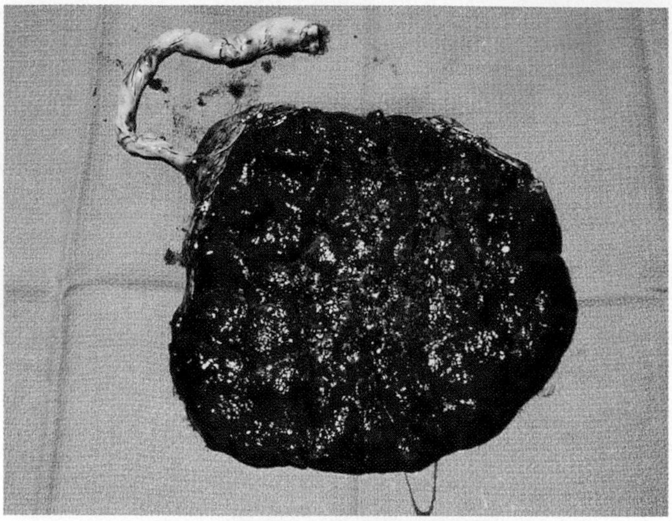

Figure 11-11 ■ Maternal side of placenta (Dirty Duncan).

Source: Photo courtesy of M. London.

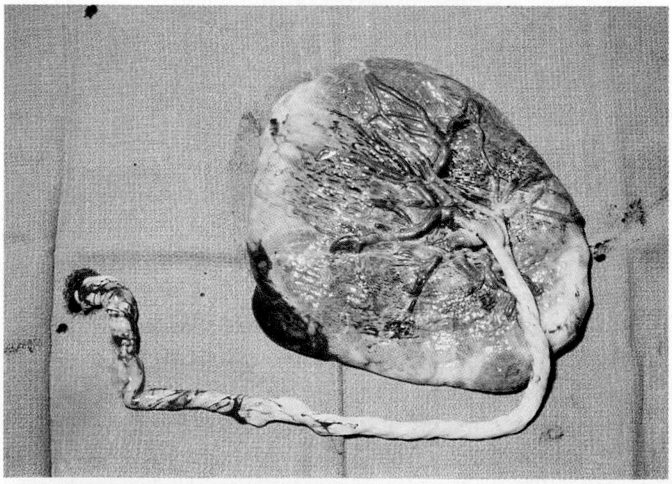

Figure 11-12 ■ Fetal side of placenta (Shiny Schultz).

Source: Photo courtesy of M. London.

Placental Circulation

After implantation of the blastocyst, the cells differentiate into fetal cells and trophoblastic cells. The proliferating trophoblast successfully invades the decidua basalis of the endometrium, first opening the uterine capillaries and later opening the larger uterine vessels. The chorionic villi are an outgrowth of the blastocystic tissue. As these villi continue to grow and divide, the fetal vessels begin to form. The intervillous spaces in the decidua basalis develop as the endometrial spiral arteries are opened.

The completion of the maternal-placental-fetal circulation occurs about 17 days after conception, when the embryonic heart begins functioning (Moore & Persaud, 2008). By the end of the fourth week, embryonic blood is circulating between the embryo and the chorionic villi. In the intervillous spaces, maternal blood supplies oxygen and nutrients to the embryonic capillaries in the villi. The placenta has begun to function as a means of metabolic exchange between embryo and mother. Waste products and carbonic dioxide diffuse into the maternal blood. By 14 weeks the placenta is a discrete organ. It has grown in thickness as a result of growth in the length and size of the chorionic villi and accompanying expansion of the intervillous space.

The *cotyledons* of the maternal surface contain branches of a single placental mainstream villus, allowing for some compartmentalization of the uteroplacental circulation. Each cotyledon is a vascular unit containing branching vessels that are distributed throughout a particular lobule and partially separated from other lobules by the cotyledon's thin septal partitions.

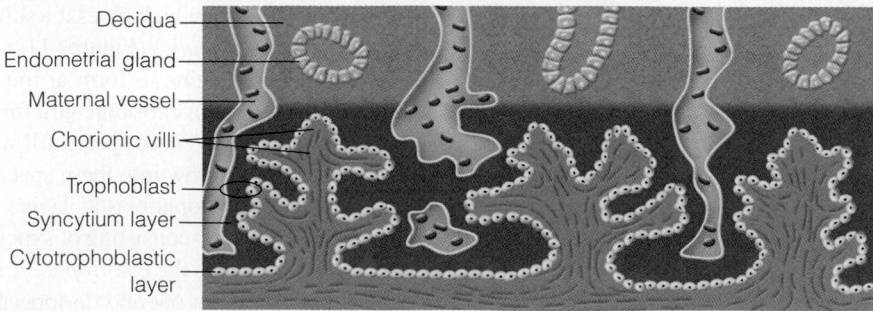

Figure 11-13 ■ Longitudinal section of placental villus. Spaces formed in the maternal decidua are filled with maternal blood; chorionic villi proliferate into these maternal blood-filled spaces and differentiate into a syncytium layer and a cytotrophoblast layer.

The capillaries of the villi are lined with an extremely thin endothelium and are surrounded by a layer of mesenchymal (connective) tissue. This connective tissue is covered by chorionic epithelium consisting of cytotrophoblast and syncytiotrophoblast (see Figure 11-13). As previously discussed, the cytotrophoblast thins out and disappears after the fifth month.

In the fully developed placenta's umbilical cord, fetal blood flows through the two umbilical arteries to the capillaries of the villi, and oxygen-enriched blood flows back through the umbilical vein to the fetus (Figure 11-14 ■). Late in pregnancy, a soft blowing sound (*funic souffle*) can be heard over the area of the umbilical cord of the fetus. The sound is synchronous with the fetal heartbeat and the flow of fetal blood through the umbilical arteries.

Maternal blood, rich in oxygen and nutrients, moves from the arcuate artery to the radial artery to the uterine spiral arteries and then spurts into the intervillous spaces. These spurts are produced by the maternal blood pressure. The spurt of blood is directed toward the chorionic plate, and as the blood flow loses pressure, it becomes lateral (spreads out). Fresh blood continually enters and exerts pressure on the contents of the intervillous spaces, pushing blood toward the exits in the basal plate. Blood is then drained through the uterine and other pelvic veins. A *uterine souffle* is also heard in the latter months of pregnancy. This uterine souffle, which is timed precisely with the mother's pulse and heard just above the mother's symphysis pubis, is caused by the augmented blood flow entering the dilated uterine arteries.

Circulation within the intervillous spaces depends on maternal blood pressure producing a gradient between arterial and venous channels. The lumen of the spiral uterine artery is narrow when it pierces the chorionic plate and enters the intervillous space, resulting in an increased blood pressure. The pressure in the arteries forces the blood into the intervillous spaces and bathes the numerous small villi in oxygenated blood. As the pressure decreases, the blood flows back from the chorionic plate toward the decidua, where it enters the endometrial veins.

Braxton Hicks contractions (see chapter 14 ∞) are believed to facilitate placental circulation by enhancing the movement of blood from the center of the cotyledon through the intervillous space. Placental blood flow is thought to be enhanced when the woman is lying on her left side, because the venous return from the lower extremities is not compromised (Blackburn, 2007).

Placental Functions

Placental exchange functions occur only in those fetal vessels that are in intimate contact with the covering syncytial membrane. The syncytium villi have brush borders containing many microvilli, which greatly increase the exchange rate between maternal and fetal circulation (Sadler, 2010).

The placental functions, many of which begin soon after implantation, include fetal respiration, nutrition, and excretion. To carry out these functions, the placenta is involved in metabolic and transfer activities. In addition, it has endocrine functions and special immunologic properties (see discussion later in this section).

Metabolic Activities

The placenta produces glycogen, cholesterol, and fatty acids continuously for fetal use and hormone production. The placenta also produces numerous enzymes required for fetoplacental transfer

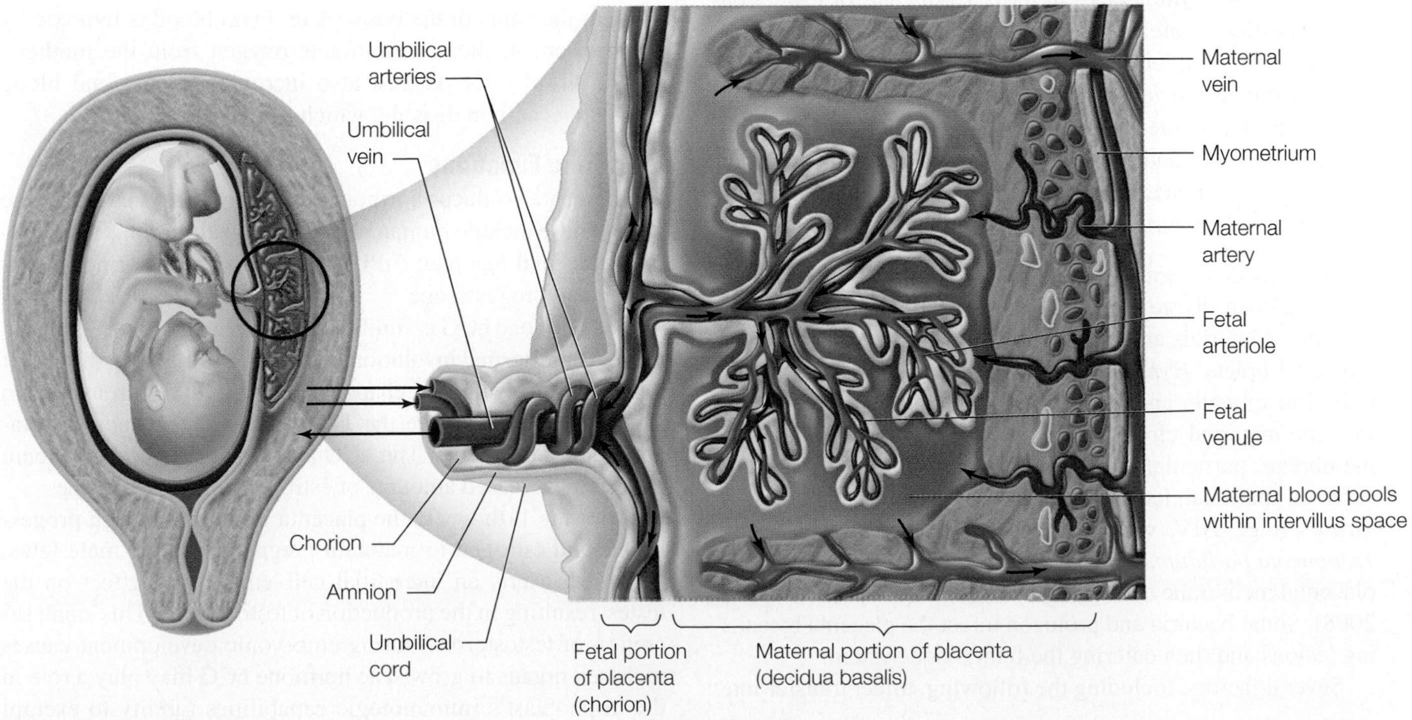

Figure 11-14 ■ Vascular arrangement of the placenta. Arrows indicate the direction of blood flow. Maternal blood flows through the uterine arteries to the intervillous spaces of the placenta and returns through the uterine veins to maternal circulation. Fetal blood flows through the umbilical arteries into the villous capillaries of the placenta and returns through the umbilical vein to the fetal circulation.

such as sulfatase, which enhances excretion of fetal estrogen precursors, and insulinase, which increases the barrier to insulin. It breaks down certain substances, such as epinephrine and histamine (Blackburn, 2007). In addition it stores glycogen and iron.

Transport Functions

The placental membranes actively control the transfer of a wide range of substances by a variety of transport mechanisms.

1. *Simple diffusion* moves substances from an area of higher concentration to an area of lower concentration. Substances that move across the placenta by simple diffusion include water, oxygen, carbon dioxide, electrolytes (sodium and chloride), anesthetic gases, and drugs. Insulin and steroid hormones originating from the adrenal glands and thyroid hormones also cross the placenta but at a very slow rate. The rate of oxygen transfer across the placental membrane is greater than that allowed by simple diffusion, indicating that oxygen is also transferred by some type of facilitated diffusion. Unfortunately many substances of abuse, such as cocaine and heroin, cross the placenta via simple diffusion.
2. *Facilitated transport* involves a carrier system to move molecules from an area of greater concentration to an area of lower concentration. Molecules such as glucose, galactose, and some oxygen are transported by this method. The glucose level in the fetal blood is ordinarily 20% to 30% lower than the glucose level in the maternal blood, because glucose is being metabolized rapidly. This in turn causes rapid transport of additional glucose from the maternal blood into the fetal blood.
3. *Active transport* can work against a concentration gradient, allowing molecules to move from areas of lower concentration to areas of higher concentration. Amino acids, calcium, iron, iodine, water-soluble vitamins, and glucose are transferred across the placenta this way. The measured amino acid content of fetal blood is greater than that of maternal blood, and calcium and inorganic phosphate occur in greater concentration in fetal blood than in maternal blood (Blackburn, 2007).

Other modes of transport also exist. *Pinocytosis* is important for transferring large molecules, such as albumin and gamma globulin. Materials are engulfed by amoeba-like cells forming plasma droplets. *Hydrostatic and osmotic pressures* allow the bulk flow of water and some solutes. Fetal red blood cells pass into the maternal circulation through breaks in the placental membrane, particularly during labor and birth. Certain cells, such as maternal leukocytes, and microorganisms, such as viruses (e.g., HIV, which causes AIDS) and the bacterium *Treponema pallidum,* which causes syphilis, can also cross the placental membrane under their own power (Moore & Persaud, 2008). Some bacteria and protozoa infect the placenta by causing lesions and then entering the fetal blood system.

Several factors, including the following, affect transfer rate:

- Molecular size
- Electrical charge
- Lipid solubility
- Placental surface area
- Diffusion distance
- Maternal-placental-fetal blood flow
- Blood saturation with gases and nutrients
- pK_a of the substance
- Maternal-placental-fetal metabolism of the substance

Substances that have a molecular weight of 1000 daltons or more have difficulty crossing the placenta by simple diffusion. Therefore, heparin, with a molecular weight above 6000, does not cross the placenta, but warfarin sodium (Coumadin), which has a molecular weight in the 300 to 400 range, crosses easily. Electrically charged molecules cross the placenta more slowly. An example is the muscle relaxant succinylcholine. A lipid-soluble substance moves quickly across the placenta into the fetal circulation.

Reduction of the placental surface area, as with abruptio placentae (partial or complete premature separation of a normally implanted placenta), will lessen the area that is functional for exchange. Placental diffusion distance also affects exchange. In conditions such as diabetes and placental infection, edema of the villi increases the diffusion distance, thus increasing the distance the substance has to be transferred.

Blood flow alteration changes the transfer rate of substances, the ratio of blood on each side of the placenta, and the binding and dissociation abilities of carrier molecules in the blood. Decreased intervillous space blood flow is seen during labor and with certain maternal disease conditions such as hypertension. Mild fetal hypoxia increases the umbilical blood flow, but severe hypoxia results in decreased blood flow.

As the maternal blood picks up fetal waste products and carbon dioxide, it drains back into the maternal circulation through the veins in the basal plate. Fetal blood is hypoxic by comparison; it, therefore, attracts oxygen from the mother's blood. Affinity for oxygen also increases as the fetal blood gives up its carbon dioxide, which decreases its acidity.

Endocrine Functions

The placenta produces hormones that are vital to survival of the fetus. These include human chorionic gonadotropin (hCG); human placental lactogen (hPL); and two steroid hormones, estrogen and progesterone.

The hormone hCG is similar to luteinizing hormone (LH) and prevents the normal involution of the corpus luteum at the end of the menstrual cycle (see chapter 10). If the corpus luteum stops functioning before the 11th week of pregnancy, spontaneous abortion occurs. The hCG also causes the corpus luteum to secrete increased amounts of estrogen and progesterone.

After the 11th week, the placenta produces enough progesterone and estrogen to maintain pregnancy. In the male fetus, hCG also exerts an interstitial cell–stimulating effect on the testes, resulting in the production of testosterone. This small secretion of testosterone during embryonic development causes male sex organs to grow. The hormone hCG may play a role in the trophoblast's immunologic capabilities (ability to exempt the placenta and embryo from rejection by the mother's system). This hormone is used as a basis for pregnancy tests (for discussion of pregnancy tests, see chapter 14).

The hormone hCG is present in maternal blood serum 8 to 10 days after fertilization, just as soon as implantation has occurred, and is detectable in maternal urine at the time of the missed menses. Chorionic gonadotropin reaches its maximum level at 50 to 70 days' gestation and then begins to decrease as placental hormone production increases.

Progesterone is a hormone essential for pregnancy. It increases the secretions of the fallopian tubes and uterus to provide appropriate nutritive matter for the developing morula and blastocyst. It also appears to aid in ovum transport through the fallopian tube. Progesterone causes decidual cells to develop in the uterine endometrium, and it must be present in high levels for implantation to occur. Progesterone also decreases the contractility of the uterus, thus preventing uterine contractions from causing spontaneous abortion.

Before hCG stimulation, the production of progesterone by the corpus luteum reaches a peak about 7 to 10 days after ovulation. Implantation occurs at about the same time as this peak. At 16 days after ovulation, the production of progesterone reaches a level between 25 and 50 mg per day and continues to rise slowly in subsequent weeks. After 11 weeks, the placenta (specifically, the syncytiotrophoblast) takes over the production of progesterone and secretes it in tremendous quantities, reaching levels of more than 250 mg per day late in pregnancy.

By 7 weeks, the placenta produces more than 50% of the estrogens in the maternal circulation. *Estrogens* serve mainly a proliferative function, causing enlargement of the uterus, breasts, and breast glandular tissue. Estrogens also have a significant role in increasing vascularity and vasodilation, particularly in the villous capillaries, near the end of pregnancy. Placental estrogens increase markedly toward the end of pregnancy to as much as 30 times the daily production in the middle of a normal monthly menstrual cycle. The primary estrogen secreted by the placenta is different from that secreted by the ovaries. The placenta secretes mainly *estriol,* whereas the ovaries secrete primarily estradiol. The placenta cannot synthesize estriol by itself. Essential precursors such as dehydroepiandrosterone sulfate (DHEA-S) is provided by the fetal adrenal glands, processed by the fetal liver, and transported to the placenta for the final conversion to estrone, estradiol, and estriol (Blackburn, 2007).

The hormone hPL (human placental lactogen; sometimes referred to as human chorionic somatomammotropin, or hCS) is similar to human pituitary growth hormone; hPL stimulates certain changes in the mother's metabolic processes. These changes ensure that more protein, glucose, and minerals are available for the fetus. Secretion of hPL can be detected by about 4 weeks.

Immunologic Properties

The placenta and embryo are transplants of living tissue within the same species and are, therefore, considered *homografts.* Unlike other homografts, the placenta and embryo appear exempt from immunologic reaction by the host. Most recent data suggest that the placental hormones (progesterone and hCG) suppress cellular immunity during pregnancy. One theory posits that chorionic villi syncytiotrophoblastic tissue is immunologically inert. The chorionic villi may lack major histocompatibility (HC) antigens and thus do not evoke rejection responses. It does, however, protect against antibody formation. Extravillous trophoblast (EVT) cells, which invade the uterine decidas, have human leukocyte antigen G (HLA-G), which is not readily recognized by sensitized T lymphocytes and natural killer cells (Cunningham et al., 2010).

Development of the Fetal Circulatory System

The circulatory system of the fetus has several unique features that, by maintaining the blood flow to the placenta, provide the fetus with oxygen and nutrients while removing carbon dioxide and other waste products.

Most of the blood supply bypasses the fetal lungs because they do not carry out respiratory gas exchange. The placenta assumes the function of the fetal lungs by supplying oxygen and allowing the fetus to excrete carbon dioxide into the maternal bloodstream. Figure 11-15 ■ shows the fetal circulatory system. The blood from the placenta flows through the umbilical vein, which enters the abdominal wall of the fetus at the site that, after birth, is the umbilicus (belly button). As umbilical venous blood approaches the liver, a small portion of the blood enters the liver sinusoids, mixes with blood from the portal circulation, and then enters the inferior vena cava via hepatic veins. Most of the umbilical vein's blood flows through the **ductus venosus** directly into the inferior vena cava, bypassing the liver. This blood then enters the right atrium, passes through the **foramen ovale** into the left atrium, and pours into the left ventricle, which pumps it into the aorta. Some blood returning from the head and upper extremities by way of the superior vena cava is emptied into the right atrium and passes through the tricuspid valve into the right ventricle. This blood is pumped into the pulmonary artery, and a small amount passes to the lungs and provides nourishment only. The larger portion of blood passes from the pulmonary artery through the **ductus arteriosus** into the descending aorta, bypassing the lungs. Finally, blood returns to the placenta through the two umbilical arteries, and the process is repeated.

Fetal Circulation

The fetus receives oxygen via diffusion from the maternal circulation because of the gradient difference of Po_2 of 50 mmHg in maternal blood in the placenta to a 30 mmHg Po_2 in the fetus. At term the fetus receives oxygen from the mother's circulation at a rate of 20 to 30 ml/min (Sadler, 2010). Fetal hemoglobin facilitates obtaining oxygen from the maternal circulation because it carries as much as 20% to 30% more oxygen than adult hemoglobin. For further discussion, see chapter 29 ∞.

Fetal circulation delivers the highest available oxygen concentration to the head, neck, brain, and heart (coronary circulation) and a lesser amount of oxygenated blood to the abdominal organs and the lower body. This circulatory pattern leads to cephalocaudal (head-to-tail) development in the fetus.

Fetal Heart

The heart of the fetus, as in the adult, is under the control of its own pacemaker. The sinoatrial (SA) node sets the rate and is supplied by the vagus nerve. Bridging the atrium and the ventricle is

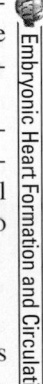

Embryonic Heart Formation and Circulation

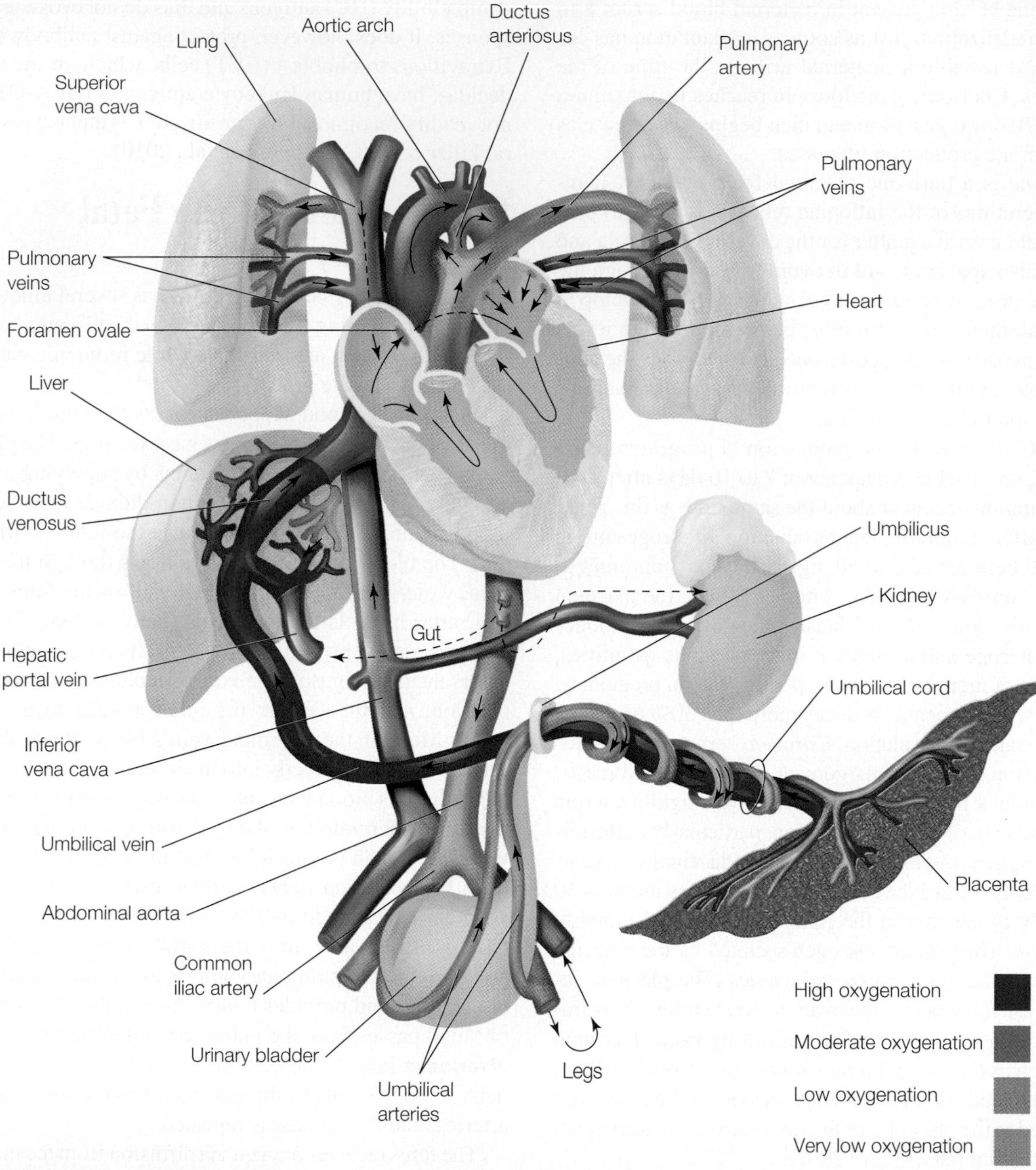

Figure 11-15 ■ Fetal circulation. Blood leaves the placenta and enters the fetus through the umbilical vein. After circulating through the fetus, the blood returns to the placenta through the umbilical arteries. The ductus venosus, the foramen ovale, and the ductus arteriosus allow the blood to bypass the fetal liver and lungs.

the atrioventricular (AV) node, also supplied by the vagus nerve. Baseline changes in the fetal heartbeat have been shown to be under the influence of this nerve. Atropine will block this effect.

When the fetus is stressed, the sympathetic nervous system causes the release of norepinephrine, which increases the fetal heart rate. To counteract the increase in blood pressure, baroreceptors, which respond to the increase pressure, are present in the vessel walls at the junction of the internal and external carotid arteries. When stimulated, these receptors, under the influence of the vagus and glossopharyngeal nerves, cause the heart rate to slow.

Chemoreceptors in the fetal peripheral and central nervous systems respond to decreased oxygen tensions and to increased carbon dioxide tensions, leading to fetal tachycardia and an increase in blood pressure. The central nervous system (CNS) also has control over heart rate. Increased activity of the fetus in a wakeful period is exhibited in an *increase in the beat-to-beat variability* of the fetal heart baseline. Sleep patterns demonstrate a *decrease in the beat-to-beat baseline variability.* In cases of severe hypoxia, increased levels of epinephrine and norepinephrine act on the fetal heart to produce a faster and stronger rate.

Embryonic and Fetal Development

Pregnancy is calculated to last an *average* of 10 lunar months: 40 weeks, or 280 days. This period of 280 days is calculated from the beginning of the last normal menstrual period to the time of birth. Estimated date of birth (EDB), sometimes referred to as the *estimated date of delivery (EDD),* is usually calculated by this method. Most fetuses are born within 10 to 14 days of the calculated date of birth. The fertilization age (or postconception age) of the fetus is calculated to be *about* 2 weeks less, 266 days (38 weeks) or 9 1/2 calendar months. The latter measurement is more accurate because it measures time from the fertilization of the ovum, or conception.

The basic events of organ development in the embryo and fetus are outlined in Table 11-3. The time periods used in Table 11-3 are **postconception age periods**. During the period from fertilization to the end of the embryonic period (8 weeks), age is often expressed in days but can be given in weeks. During the fetal period (9th week until birth), age is given in weeks (Moore & Persaud, 2008). For a detailed discussion of each body system's development, see chapter 28 ∞; the foldout poster in the middle of the book summarizes fetal development.

In review, human development follows three stages. The preembryonic stage just discussed consists of the first 14 days

TABLE 11-3 Summary of Organ System Development

Age: 2–3 Weeks

Length: 2 mm C–R (Crown to rump).
Nervous system: Groove forms along middle back as cells thicken; neural tube forms from closure of neural groove.
Cardiovascular system: Beginning of blood circulation; tubular heart begins to form during third week.
Gastrointestinal system: Liver begins to function.
Genitourinary system: Formation of kidneys beginning.
Respiratory system: Nasal pits forming.
Endocrine system: Thyroid tissue appears.
Eyes: Optic cup and lens pit have formed; pigment in eyes.
Ears: Auditory pit is now enclosed structure.

Age: 4 Weeks

Length: 4–6 mm C–R.
Weight: 0.4 g.
Nervous system: Anterior portion of neural tube closes to form brain; closure of posterior end forms spinal cord.
Musculoskeletal system: Noticeable limb buds.
Cardiovascular system: Tubular heart beats at 28 days, and primitive red blood cells circulate through fetus and chorionic villi.
Gastrointestinal system: Mouth: formation of oral cavity; primitive jaws present; esophagotracheal septum begins division of esophagus and trachea. Digestive tract: stomach forms; esophagus and intestine become tubular; ducts of pancreas and liver forming.

Age: 5 Weeks

Length: 8 mm C–R.
Weight: Only 0.5% of total body weight is fat (to 20 weeks).
Nervous system: Brain has differentiated and cranial nerves are present.
Musculoskeletal system: Developing muscles have innervation.
Cardiovascular system: Atrial division has occurred.

Age: 6 Weeks

Length: 12 mm C–R.
Musculoskeletal system: Bone rudiments present; primitive skeletal shape forming; muscle mass begins to develop; ossification of skull and jaws begins.
Cardiovascular system: Chambers present in heart; groups of blood cells can be identified.
Gastrointestinal system: Oral and nasal cavities and upper lip formed; liver begins to form red blood cells.
Respiratory system: Trachea, bronchi, and lung buds present.
Ears: Formation of external, middle, and inner ear continues.
Sexual development: Embryonic sex glands appear.

Age: 7 Weeks

Length: 18 mm C–R.
Cardiovascular system: Fetal heartbeats can be detected.
Gastrointestinal system: Mouth: tongue separates; palate folds. Digestive tract: stomach attains final form.
Genitourinary system: Separation of bladder and urethra from rectum.
Respiratory system: Diaphragm separates abdominal and thoracic cavities.
Eyes: Optic nerve formed; eyelids appear, thickening of lens.
Sexual development: Differentiation of sex glands into ovaries and testes begins.

Age: 8 Weeks

Length: 2.5–3 cm C–R.
Weight: 2 g.
Musculoskeletal system: Digits formed; further differentiation of cells in primitive skeleton; cartilaginous bones show first signs of ossification; development of muscles in trunk, limbs, and head; some movement of fetus now possible.
Cardiovascular system: Development of heart essentially complete; fetal circulation follows two circuits—four extraembryonic and two intraembryonic. Heartbeat can be heard with Doppler at 8–12 weeks.
Gastrointestinal system: Mouth: completion of lip fusion. Digestive tract: rotation in midgut; anal membrane has perforated.
Ears: External, middle, and inner ear assuming final forms.
Sexual development: Male and female external genitals appear similar until end of ninth week.

Age: 10 Weeks

Length: 5–6 cm C–R.
Weight: 14 g.
Nervous system: Neurons appear at caudal end of spinal cord; basic divisions of brain present.
Musculoskeletal system: Fingers and toes begin nail growth.
Gastrointestinal system: Mouth: separation of lips from jaw; fusion of palate folds. Digestive tract: developing intestines enclosed in abdomen.
Genitourinary system: Bladder sac formed.
Endocrine system: Islets of Langerhans differentiated.
Eyes: Eyelids fused closed; development of lacrimal duct.
Sexual development: Males: production of testosterone and physical characteristics between 8 and 12 weeks.

Age: 12 Weeks

Length: 8 cm C–R; 11.5 cm C–H (crown to heel).
Weight: 45 g.
Musculoskeletal system: Clear outlining of miniature bones (12–20 weeks); process of ossification is established throughout fetal body; appearance of involuntary muscles in viscera.
Gastrointestinal system: Mouth: completion of palate. Digestive tract: appearance of muscles in gut; bile secretion begins; liver is major producer of red blood cells.
Respiratory system: Lungs acquire definitive shape.
Skin: Pink and delicate.
Endocrine system: Hormonal secretion from thyroid; insulin present in pancreas.
Immunologic system: Appearance of lymphoid tissue in fetal thymus gland.

Age: 16 Weeks

Length: 13.5 cm C–R; 15 cm C–H.
Weight: 200 g.
Musculoskeletal system: Teeth beginning to form hard tissue that will become central incisors.
Gastrointestinal system: Mouth: differentiation of hard and soft palate. Digestive tract: development of gastric and intestinal glands; intestines begin to collect meconium.
Genitourinary system: Kidneys assume typical shape and organization.
Skin: Appearance of scalp hair; lanugo present on body; transparent skin with visible blood vessels; sweat glands developing.
Eyes, ears, and nose: Formed.
Sexual development: Sex determination possible.

(continued)

TABLE 11-3 Summary of Organ System Development continued

Age: 18 Weeks

Musculoskeletal system: Teeth beginning to form hard tissue (enamel and dentine) that will become lateral incisors.
Cardiovascular system: Fetal heart tones audible with fetoscope at 16–20 weeks.

Age: 20 Weeks

Length: 19 cm C–R; 25 cm C–H.
Weight: 435 g (6% of total body weight is fat).
Nervous system: Myelination of spinal cord begins.
Musculoskeletal system: Teeth beginning to form hard tissue that will become canine and first molar. Lower limbs are of final relative proportions.
Gastrointestinal system: Fetus actively sucks and swallows amniotic fluid; peristaltic movements begin.
Skin: Lanugo covers entire body; brown fat begins to form; vernix caseosa begins to form.
Immunologic system: Detectable levels of fetal antibodies (immunoglobin G [IgG] type).
Blood formation: Iron is stored and bone marrow is increasingly important.

Age: 24 Weeks

Length: 23 cm C–R; 28 cm C–H.
Weight: 780 g.
Nervous system: Brain looks like mature brain.
Musculoskeletal system: Teeth are beginning to form hard tissue that will become the second molars.
Respiratory system: Respiratory movements may occur (24–40 weeks). Nostrils reopen. Alveoli appear in lungs and begin production of surfactant; gas exchange possible.
Skin: Reddish and wrinkled, vernix caseosa present.
Immunologic system: IgG levels reach maternal levels.

Age: 28 Weeks

Length: 27 cm C–R; 35 C–H.
Weight: 1200–1250 g.
Nervous system: Begins regulation of some body functions.
Skin: Adipose tissue accumulates rapidly; nails appear; eyebrows and eyelashes present.
Eyes: Eyelids open (26–29 weeks).
Sexual development: Males: testes descend into inguinal canal and upper scrotum.

Age: 32 Weeks

Length: 31 cm C–R; 38–43 cm C–H.
Weight: 2000 g.
Nervous system: More reflexes present.

Age: 36 Weeks

Length: 35 cm C–R; 42–48 cm C–H.
Weight: 2500–2750 g.
Musculoskeletal system: Distal femoral ossification centers present.
Skin: Pale; body rounded, lanugo disappearing, hair fuzzy or woolly; few sole creases; sebaceous glands active and helping to produce vernix caseosa (36–40 weeks).
Ears: Earlobes soft with little cartilage.
Sexual development: Males: scrotum small and few rugae present; descent of testes into upper scrotum to stay (36–40 weeks). Females: labia majora and minora equally prominent.

Age: 38–40 Weeks

Length: 40 cm C–R; 48–52 C–H.
Weight: 3200+ g (16% of total body weight is fat).
Respiratory system: At 38 weeks, lecithin-sphingomyelin (L/S) ratio approaches 2:1 (indicates decreased risk of respiratory distress from inadequate surfactant production if born now).
Skin: Smooth and pink; vernix present in skin folds; moderate to profuse silky hair; lanugo on shoulders and upper back; nails extend over tips or digits; creases cover sole.
Ears: Earlobes firmer due to increased cartilage.
Sexual development: Males: rugous scrotum. Females: labia majora well developed and minora small or completely covered.

Note: Age refers to postfertilization or postconception age.
Source: Data from Sadler, T. W. (2010). Langman's medical embryology *(11th ed). Philadelphia, PA: Lippincott, Williams & Wilkins.*

of development after the ovum is fertilized; the embryonic stage covers the period from day 15 until approximately the end of the eighth week postconception; and the fetal stage extends from the end of the eighth week until birth. (See the detailed discussion of the embryonic and fetal stages next.)

Embryonic Stage

The stage of the **embryo** starts on day 15 (beginning of the third week after conception) and continues until approximately 8 weeks or until the embryo reaches a crown-to-rump (C–R) length of 3 cm (1.2 in.). This length is usually reached about 56 days after fertilization (the end of the eighth gestational week). During the embryonic stage, tissue differentiates into essential organs, and the main external features develop (Figure 11-16 ■). The embryo is most vulnerable to teratogens during this period. These are discussed in more depth later in the chapter.

Three Weeks

In the third week, the embryonic disc becomes elongated and pear-shaped, with a broad cephalic end and a narrow caudal end. The ectoderm has formed a long cylindrical tube called the notochord for brain and spinal cord development. The gastrointestinal tract, created from the endoderm, appears as another tubelike structure communicating with the yolk sac. The most advanced organ is the heart. At 3 weeks, a single tubular heart forms just outside the body cavity of the embryo.

Four to Five Weeks

During days 21 to 32, *somites,* a series of mesodermal blocks, form on either side of the embryo's midline. The vertebrae that form the spinal column will develop from these somites. Before 28 days, arm and leg buds are not visible, but the tail bud is present. The pharyngeal arches—which will form the lower jaw (mandibular arch), hyoid bone, and cartilage of the larynx—develop at this time. The pharyngeal pouches appear now; these pouches will form the eustachian tube and cavity of the middle ear, the tonsils, and the parathyroid and thymus glands. The primordia of the ear and eye are also present (Figure 11-17 ■). By the end of 28 days, the tubular heart is beating at a regular rhythm and pushing its own primitive blood cells through the main blood vessels.

During the fifth week, the optic cups and lens vesicles of the eye form and the nasal pits develop. Partitioning in the heart occurs with the dividing of the atrium. The embryo has a marked C-shaped body, accentuated by the rudimentary tail and the large head folded over a protuberant trunk (Figure 11-18 ■). By

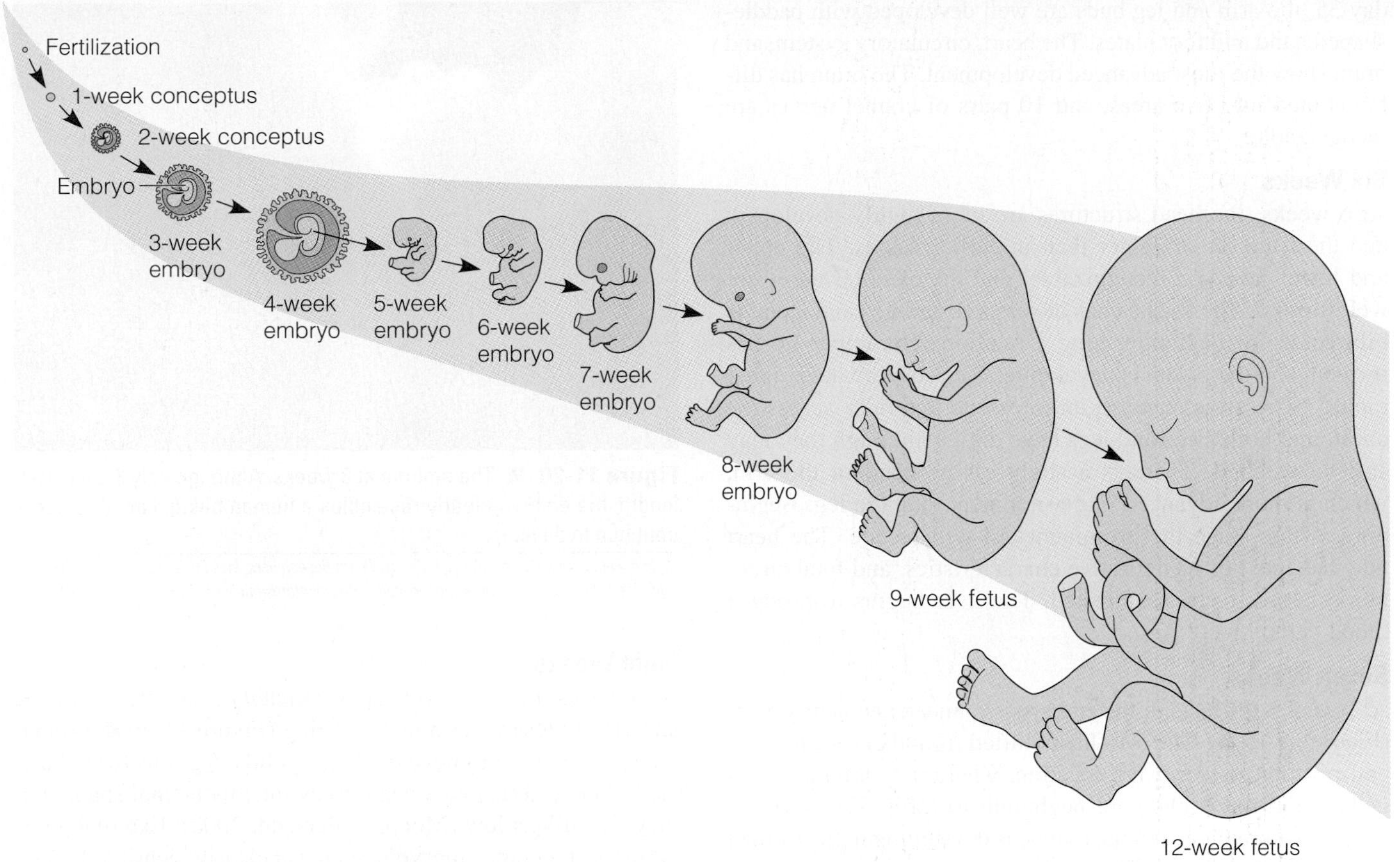

Figure 11-16 ■ The human conceptus from fertilization to the early fetal stage. The embryonic stage begins in the third week after fertilization; the fetal stage begins in the ninth week.

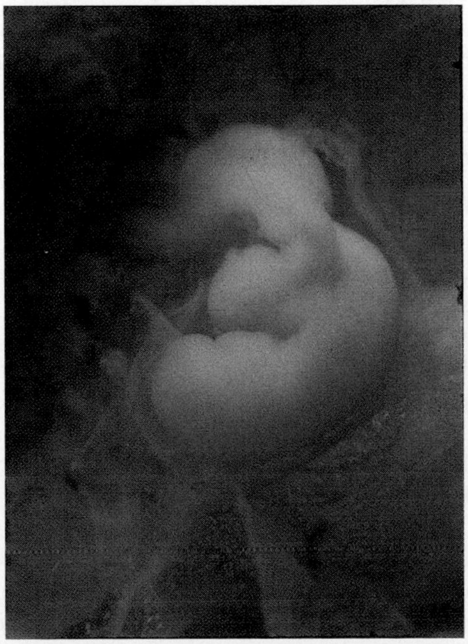

Figure 11-17 ■ The embryo at 4 weeks. Pharyngeal arches, pharyngeal pouches, and primordia of the ear and eye are present.

Source: Petit Format/Nestle/Science Source/Photo Researchers, Inc., 60 East 56th Street, New York, NY 10022, www.photoresearchers.com, info@photoresearchers.com

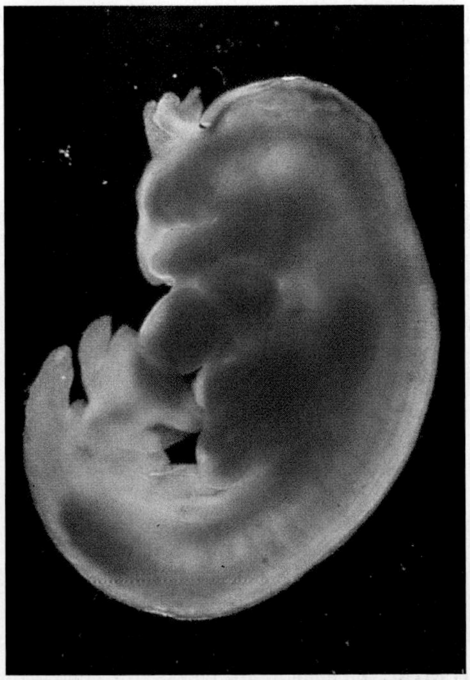

Figure 11-18 ■ The embryo at 5 weeks. The embryo has a marked C-shaped body and a rudimentary tail.

Source: Petit Format/Nestle/Science Source/Photo Researchers, Inc., 60 East 56th Street, New York, NY 10022, www.photoresearchers.com, info@photoresearchers.com day 35, the arm and leg buds are well developed with paddle-shaped hand and foot plates. The heart, circulatory system, and brain show the most advanced development. The brain has differentiated into five areas, and 10 pairs of cranial nerves are recognizable.

Six Weeks

At 6 weeks, the head structures are more highly developed, and the trunk is straighter than in earlier stages. The upper and lower jaws are recognizable, and the external nares are well formed. The trachea has developed, and its caudal end is bifurcated for beginning lung formation. The upper lip has formed, and the palate is developing. The ears are developing rapidly. The arms have begun to extend ventrally across the chest, and both arms and legs have digits, although they may still be webbed. There is a slight elbow bend in the arm, which is more advanced in development than the leg. Beginning at this stage the prominent tail will recede. The heart now has most of its definitive characteristics, and fetal circulation begins to be established. The liver begins to produce blood cells.

Seven Weeks

At 7 weeks, the head of the embryo is rounded and nearly erect (Figure 11-19 ■). The eyes have shifted from their original lateral position to a forward location, where they are closer together, and the eyelids are beginning to form. The palate is nearing completion, and the tongue is developing in the formed mouth. The gastrointestinal and genitourinary tracts undergo significant changes during the seventh week. Before this time the rectal and urogenital passages formed one tube that ended in a blind pouch; they now separate into two tubular structures. The intestines enter the extraembryonic coelom in the area of the umbilical cord (called umbilical herniation) (Moore & Persaud, 2008). The beginnings of all essential external and internal structures are present.

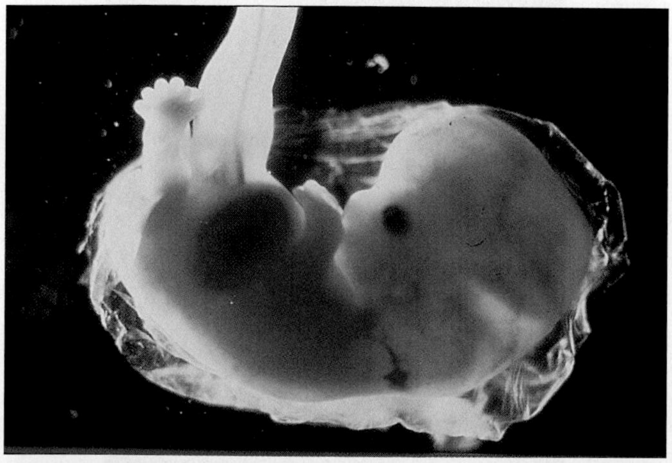

Figure 11-19 ■ The embryo at 7 weeks. The head is rounded and nearly erect. The eyes have shifted forward and are closer together, and the eyelids begin to form.

Source: Petit Format/Nestle/Science Source/Photo Researchers, Inc., 60 East 56th Street, New York, NY 10022, www.photoresearchers.com, info@photoresearchers.com

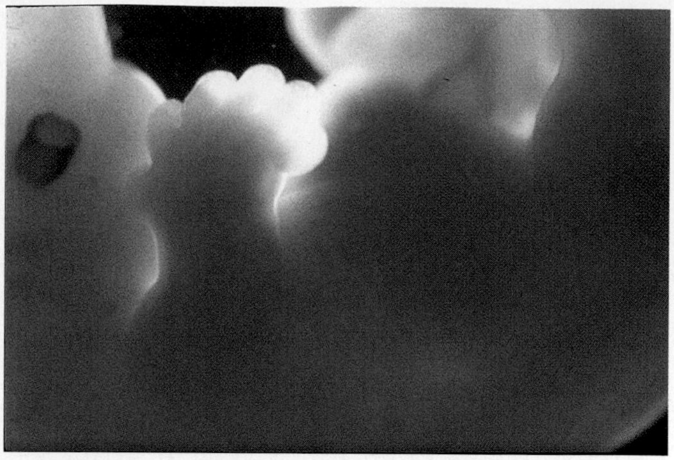

Figure 11-20 ■ The embryo at 8 weeks. Although only 3 cm in C–R length, the embryo clearly resembles a human being. Facial features continue to develop.

Source: Petit Format/Nestle/Science Source/Photo Researchers, Inc., 60 East 56th Street, New York, NY 10022, www.photoresearchers.com, info@photoresearchers.com

Eight Weeks

At 8 weeks, the embryo is approximately 3 cm (1.2 in.) C–R and clearly resembles a human being (Figure 11-20 ■). Facial features continue to develop. The eyelids begin to fuse. Auricles of the external ears begin to assume their final shape, but they are still set low (Moore & Persaud, 2008). External genitals appear, but the embryo's sex is not clearly identifiable. The rectal passage opens with the perforation of the anal membrane. The circulatory system through the umbilical cord is well established. Long bones are beginning to form, and the large muscles are now capable of contracting.

Fetal Stage

By the end of the eighth week, the embryo is sufficiently developed to be called a **fetus**. Every organ system and external structure that will be found in the full-term newborn is present. The remainder of gestation is devoted to refining structures and perfecting function.

Nine to Twelve Weeks

By the end of the ninth week, the fetus reaches a C–R length of 5 cm (2 in.) and weighs about 14 g (0.5 oz). The head is large and comprises almost half of the fetus's entire size (Figure 11-21 ■).

At 12 weeks, the fetus reaches an 8 cm (3.2 in.) C–R length and weighs about 45 g (1.6 oz). The face is well formed, with the nose protruding, the chin small and receding, and the ears acquiring a more adult shape. The eyelids close at about the 10th week and will not begin to reopen until about the 26th to 29th week. Some movements of the lips suggestive of the sucking reflex have been observed at 3 months. Tooth buds now appear for all 20 of the child's first teeth (baby teeth). The limbs are long and slender with well-formed digits. The fetus can curl the fingers toward the palm and make a tiny fist. The legs are still shorter and less developed than the arms. The urogenital tract completes its development, well-differentiated genitals appear, and the kidneys begin to produce urine. Red blood cells are produced primarily by the liver. Spontaneous movements of

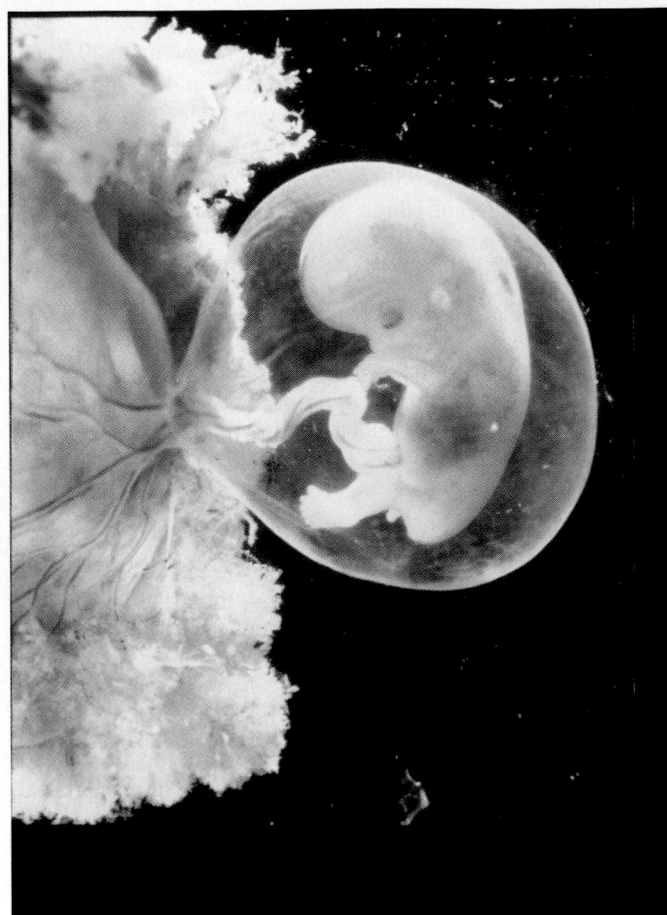

Figure 11-21 ■ The fetus at 9 weeks. Every organ system and external structure is present.

Source: Used with permission from Nilsson, L. (1990). A child is born. *New York, NY: Dell Publishing.*

the fetus occur. Fetal heart tones (the sound of the heartbeat) can be ascertained by electronic devices between 8 and 12 weeks. The heart rate is 120 to 160 beats per minute.

Thirteen to Sixteen Weeks

This is a period of rapid growth. At 13 weeks, the fetus weighs 55 to 60 g (1.9 to 2.1 oz) and is about 9 cm (3.6 in.) in C–R length. Lanugo, or fine hair, begins to develop, especially on the head. Blood vessels are clearly visible beneath transparent skin. More muscle tissue and body skeleton have developed, which holds the fetus more erect (Figure 11-22 ■). Active movements are present—the fetus stretches and exercises its arms and legs. It makes sucking motions, swallows amniotic fluid, and produces meconium in the intestinal tract. Bronchial tubes are branching out in the primitive lungs, and sweat glands are developing. The liver and pancreas now begin production of their appropriate secretions. By the beginning of week 16, skeletal ossification is clearly identifiable.

Twenty Weeks

The fetus doubles its C–R length and now measures about 19 cm (8 in.). Fetal weight is between 435 and 465 g (15.2 and 16.3 oz). Lanugo covers the entire body and is especially prominent on the shoulders. Subcutaneous deposits of brown fat, which has a rich

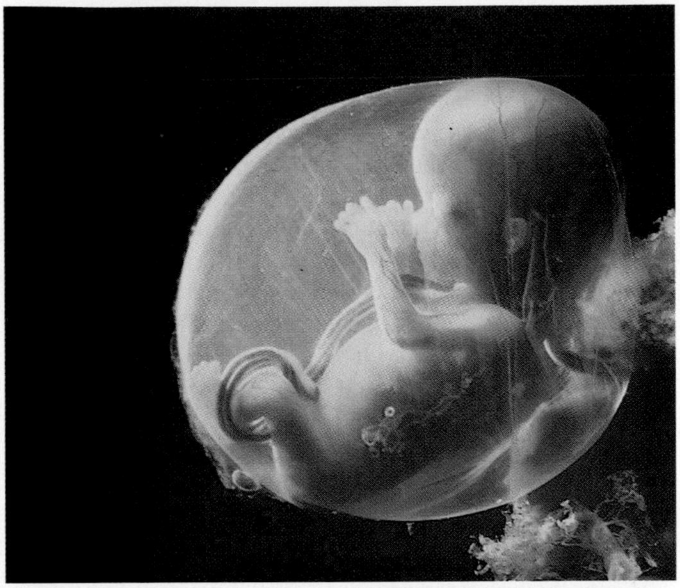

Figure 11-22 ■ The fetus at 14 weeks. During this period of rapid growth, the skin is so transparent that blood vessels are visible beneath it. More muscle tissue and body skeleton have developed, which holds the fetus more erect.

Source: Used with permission from Nilsson, L. (1990). A child is born. *New York, NY: Dell Publishing.*

blood supply, make the skin a little less transparent. Nipples now appear over the mammary glands. The head is covered with fine, "woolly" hair, and the eyebrows and eyelashes are beginning to form (Figure 11-23 ■). Nails are present on both fingers and toes. Muscles are well developed, and the fetus is active. Fetal movement, known as quickening, is felt by the mother. The fetal

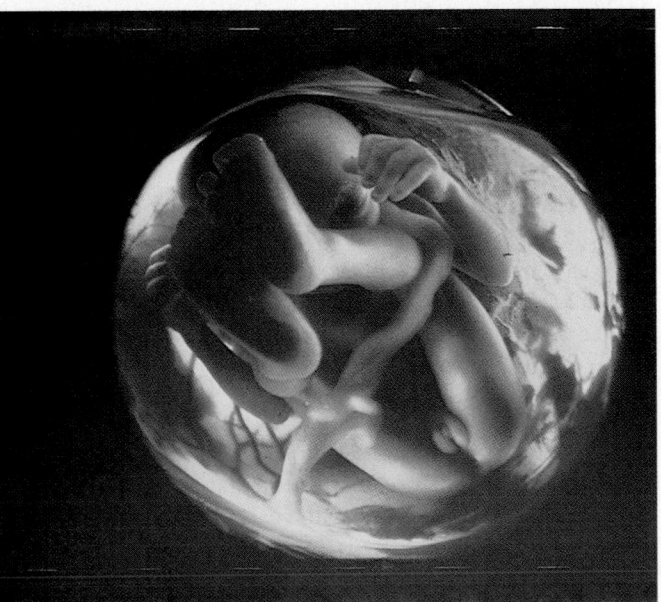

Figure 11-23 ■ The fetus at 20 weeks. The fetus weighs approximately 435 to 465 g and measures about 19 cm. Subcutaneous deposits of brown fat make the skin less transparent. "Woolly" hair covers the head, and nails have developed on the fingers and toes.

Source: Used with permission from Nilsson, L. (1990). A child is born. *New York, NY: Dell Publishing.*

heartbeat is audible through the fetoscope. Quickening and fetal heartbeat can help in validating the EDB.

Twenty-Four Weeks

The fetus at 24 weeks reaches a crown-to-heel (C–H) length of 28 cm (11.2 in.). It weighs about 780 g (1 lb 10 oz). The hair on the head is growing long, and eyebrows and eyelashes have formed. The eyes are structurally complete and will soon open. The fetus has a reflex hand grip (grasp reflex) and, by the end of 6 months, a startle reflex. Skin covering the body is reddish and wrinkled, with little subcutaneous fat. Skin on the hands and feet has thickened, with skin ridges on palms and soles forming distinct footprints and fingerprints. The skin over the entire body is covered with a protective cheeselike fatty substance, called **vernix caseosa**, secreted by the sebaceous glands. The alveoli in the lungs are just beginning to form.

Twenty-Five to Twenty-Eight Weeks

At about 25 weeks, the fetal skin is still red, wrinkled, and covered with vernix caseosa. The brain is developing rapidly, and the nervous system is complete enough to provide some degree of regulation of body functions. The eyelids open and close under neural control. The fetus has nails on both fingers and toes. If the fetus is a male, the testes begin to descend into the scrotal sac. Even though the lungs are still physiologically immature, they are sufficiently developed to provide gas exchange. A fetus born at this time will require immediate and prolonged intensive care to survive and then to decrease the risk of major handicap. The fetus at 28 weeks is about 27 cm (10.8 in.) C–R or 35 to 38 cm (14 to 15 in.) long C–H and weighs 1200 to 1250 g (2 lb 10.5 oz to 2 lb 12 oz).

Twenty-Nine to Thirty-Two Weeks

At 30 weeks, the pupillary light reflex is present (Moore & Persaud, 2008). The fetus is gaining weight from an increase in body muscle and fat and weighs about 2000 g (4 lb 6.5 oz) with a C–R of 31 cm (12.4 in.) or C–H length of about 38 to 43 cm (15 to 17 in.) by 32 weeks of age. The central nervous system (CNS) has matured enough to direct rhythmic breathing movements and partially control body temperature. However, the lungs are not yet fully mature. Bones are now fully developed but are soft and flexible. The fetus begins storing iron, calcium, and phosphorus. In males, the testicles may be located in the scrotal sac but are often still high in the inguinal canals.

Application: Fetal Development

Thirty-Five to Thirty-Six Weeks

The fetus is beginning to get plump with less-wrinkled skin covering the deposits of subcutaneous fat. Lanugo hair is beginning to disappear, and the nails reach the edge of the fingertips. By 35 weeks, the fetus has a firm grasp and exhibits spontaneous orientation to light. By 36 weeks of age, the weight is usually 2500 to 2750 g (5 lb 12 oz to 6 lb 11.5 oz), and the C–H length of the fetus is about 42 to 48 cm (17 to 19 in.) or C–R 35 cm (14 in.). An infant born at this time has a good chance of surviving but may require some special care, especially if there is intrauterine growth restriction.

Fetal Development Overview

Thirty-Eight to Forty Weeks

The fetus is considered full term at 38 weeks and up to 40 weeks after conception. The C–H length varies from 48 to 52 cm (19 to 21 in.) or C–R of 40 cm (16 in.), with males usually longer than females. Males also usually weigh more than females. The weight at term is about 3000 to 3600 g (6 lb 10 oz to 7 lb 15 oz) and varies in different ethnic groups. The skin has a smooth, polished look. The only lanugo left is on the upper arms and shoulders. The hair on the head is no longer woolly but coarse and about an inch long. Vernix caseosa is present, with heavier deposits remaining in creases and folds of the skin. The body and extremities are plump, with good skin turgor, and the fingernails extend beyond the fingertips. The chest is prominent but still a little smaller than the head, and mammary glands protrude in both sexes. The testes are in the scrotum or are palpable in the inguinal canals.

As the fetus enlarges, amniotic fluid diminishes to about an average of 500 ml, and the fetal body mass fills the uterine cavity (Beall & Ross, 2009). The fetus assumes what is called its *position of comfort,* or lie. The head is generally pointed downward, following the shape of the uterus (and also possibly because the head is heavier than the feet). The extremities and often the head are well flexed. After 5 months, feeding patterns, sleeping patterns, as well as activity patterns become established, so the fetus at term has its own body rhythms and individual style of response. See Table 11-4 for important developmental milestones. For a detailed discussion of each body system's transition to and their functioning in the newborn see chapter 29.

TABLE 11-4 Embryonic and Fetal Development: What Parents Want to Know

4 weeks	The fetal heart begins to beat.
8 weeks	All body organs are formed.
8–12 weeks	Fetal heart tones can be heard by Doppler device.
16 weeks	Baby's sex can be seen. Although thin, the fetus looks like a baby.
20 weeks	Heartbeat can be heard with fetoscope. Mother feels movement (quickening). Baby develops a regular schedule of sleeping, sucking, and kicking. Hands can grasp. Baby assumes a favorite position in utero. Vernix (lanolin-like covering) protects the body, and lanugo (fine hair) keeps oil on skin. Head hair, eyebrows, and eyelashes present.
24 weeks	Weighs 780 g (1 lb 10 oz). Activity is increasing. Fetal respiratory movements begin.
28 weeks	Eyes begin to open and close. Baby can breathe at this time. Surfactant needed for breathing at birth is formed. Baby is two thirds its final size.
32 weeks	Baby has fingernails and toenails. Subcutaneous fat is being laid down. Baby appears less red and wrinkled.
38+ weeks	Baby fills total uterus. Baby gets antibodies from mother.

Factors Influencing Embryonic and Fetal Development

Factors that may affect embryonic development include the quality of the sperm or ovum from which the zygote was formed, the genetic code established at fertilization, and the adequacy of the intrauterine environment. If the environment is unsuitable before cellular differentiation occurs, all the cells of the zygote are affected. The cells may die, which causes spontaneous abortion, or growth may be slowed, depending on the severity of the situation. When differentiation is complete and the fetal membranes have formed, an injurious agent has the greatest effect on those cells undergoing the most rapid growth. Thus the time of injury is critical in the development of anomalies.

Because organs are formed primarily during embryonic development, the growing organism is considered most vulnerable to hazardous agents during the first months of pregnancy. Table 11-5 lists potential malformations related to the time of insult. Any agent (e.g., drug, virus, or radiation) that can cause development of abnormal structures in an embryo is referred to as a **teratogen**. It is important to remember that the effects of teratogens depend on the (1) maternal and fetal genotype, (2) stage of development when exposure occurs, and (3) dose and duration of exposure of the agent (Chambers & Weiner, 2009). Chapter 14 discusses the effects of specific teratogenic agents on the developing fetus.

Adequacy of the maternal environment is also important during the periods of rapid embryonic and fetal development. Maternal nutrition can affect brain and neural tube development. The period of maximum brain growth and myelination begins with the fifth lunar month before birth and continues during the first 6 months after birth, when there is a twofold increase in myelination (Volpe, 2008). Amino acids, glucose, and fatty acids are considered to be the primary dietary factors in brain growth. A subtle type of damage that affects the associative capacity of the brain, possibly leading to learning disabilities, may be caused by nutritional deficiency at this stage. Vitamins and folic acid supplements taken before conception can reduce the incidence of neural tube defects (Volpe, 2008). Maternal nutrition may also predispose to the development of adult coronary heart disease, hypertension, and diabetes in babies who were small or disproportionate at birth. Maternal nutrition is discussed in depth in chapter 18. Cigarette smoking during pregnancy negatively impacts neurodevelopment of the fetus (Shea & Steiner, 2008).

TABLE 11-5 Developmental Vulnerability Timetable

WEEKS SINCE CONCEPTION	POTENTIAL TERATOGEN-INDUCED MALFORMATION
3	Ectromelia (congenital absence of one or more limbs)
	Ectopia cordis (heart lies outside thoracic cavity)
4	Omphalocele (herniation of abdominal viscera into the umbilical cord)
	Tracheoesophageal fistula (abnormal connection between trachea and esophagus) (4–5 weeks)
	Hemivertebra (4–5* weeks)
5	Nuclear cataract
	Microphthalmia (abnormally small eyeballs) (5–6* weeks)
	Facial clefts
	Carpal or pedal ablation (5–6* weeks)
6	Gross septal or aortic abnormalities
	Cleft lip, agnathia (absence of the lower jaw)
7	Interventricular septal defects
	Pulmonary stenosis
	Cleft palate, micrognathia (smallness of the jaw)
	Epicanthus
	Brachycephalism (shortness of the head) (7–8* weeks)
	Mixed sexual characteristics
8	Persistent ostium primum (persistent opening in atrial septum)
	Digital stunting (shortening of fingers and toes)

*May occur in several periods after conception.

Source: Modified with permission from Danforth, D. N., & Scott. J. R. (1986). Obstetrics and gynecology *(5th ed., p. 319). Copyright © 1986 Lippincott Williams & Wilkens.*

CLINICAL JUDGMENT

Case Study: Melodie Chong

Melodie Chong, in her third week of pregnancy, develops a fever of 104°F (40°C) and flulike symptoms but refuses to take any medication because she is afraid that drugs will harm her baby. Many factors—maternal, fetal, and environmental—may affect prenatal growth.

Critical Thinking

What would you advise Melodie about use of medication in this situation and to do during her pregnancy to decrease her chances of problems?

Melodie asks when her baby is most vulnerable for abnormal growth or structure. How would you answer?

See www.nursing.pearsonhighered.com for possible responses.

Another prenatal influence on the intrauterine environment is maternal hyperthermia associated with sauna baths or hot tub use. Studies of the effects of maternal hyperthermia during the first trimester have raised concern about possible spontaneous abortion, central nervous system (CNS) defects, and failure of neural tube closure (see Table 11-5). Maternal substance abuse also affects the intrauterine environment and is discussed in chapter 19 and chapter 32.

[redacted]

FOCUS YOUR STUDY

- Humans have 46 chromosomes, which are divided into 23 pairs—22 pairs of autosomes and 1 pair of sex chromosomes.
- Mitosis is the process by which additional somatic (body) cells are formed. It provides growth and development of the organs and replacement of body cells.
- Meiosis produces cells called gametes (ova and sperm) that are necessary for reproduction of the species. It occurs during gametogenesis (oogenesis and spermatogenesis) and consists of two successive cell divisions (reduction division), which produce a gamete with 23 chromosomes (22 chromosomes and 1 sex chromosome)—the haploid number of chromosomes.
- Gametes must have a haploid number (23) of chromosomes so that when the female gamete (ovum) and the male gamete (spermatozoon) unite to form the zygote, the normal human diploid number of chromosomes (46) is reestablished.
- An ovum is considered fertile for about 12 to 24 hours after ovulation, and the sperm is believed to be capable of fertilizing the ovum for about 24 hours after it is deposited in the female reproductive tract.
- Fertilization usually takes place in the ampulla (outer third) of the fallopian tube. Both capacitation and the acrosomal reaction must occur for the sperm to fertilize the ovum. Capacitation is the removal of the plasma membrane, which exposes the acrosomal covering of the sperm head. The acrosomal reaction is the deposit of hyaluronidase in the corona radiata, which allows the sperm head to penetrate the ovum.
- Sex chromosomes are referred to as X and Y. Females have two X chromosomes, and males have an X and a Y chromosome. Y chromosomes are carried only by the sperm. To produce a female child, both the mother and the father contribute an X chromosome. To produce a male child, the mother contributes an X chromosome and the father contributes a Y chromosome.
- Intrauterine development first proceeds via cellular multiplication in which the zygote undergoes rapid mitotic division called cleavage. As a result of cleavage, the zygote divides and multiplies into cell groupings called blastomeres, which are held together by the zona pellucida. The blastomeres will eventually become a solid ball of cells called the morula. When a cavity forms in the morula cell mass, the inner solid cell mass is called the blastocyst.
- Implantation usually occurs in the upper part of the posterior uterine wall when the blastocyst burrows into the uterine lining.
- After implantation, the endometrium is called the decidua. Decidua capsularis is the portion that covers the blastocyst. Decidua basalis is the portion that is directly under the blastocyst. Decidua vera is the portion that lines the rest of the uterine cavity.
- Embryonic membranes are called the amnion and the chorion. The amnion is formed from the ectoderm and is a thin protective membrane that contains the amniotic fluid and the embryo. The chorion is a thick membrane that develops from the trophoblast and encloses the amnion, embryo, and yolk sac.
- Amniotic fluid cushions the fetus against mechanical injury, controls the embryo's temperature, allows symmetric external growth, prevents adherence to the amnion, and permits freedom of movement.
- Primary germ layers will give rise to all tissues, organs, and organ systems. The three primary germ cell layers are the ectoderm, endoderm, and mesoderm.
- The umbilical cord contains two umbilical arteries, which carry deoxygenated blood from the fetus to the placenta, and one umbilical vein, which carries oxygenated blood from the placenta to the fetus. The umbilical cord has a central insertion into the placenta. Wharton's jelly, a specialized connective tissue, prevents compression of the umbilical cord in utero.
- Twins are either dizygotic (fraternal) or monozygotic (identical). Dizygotic twins arise from two separate ova fertilized by two separate spermatozoa. Monozygotic twins develop from a single ovum fertilized by a single spermatozoon.
- The placenta, which develops from the chorionic villi and the decidua basalis, has two parts. The maternal portion, consisting of the decidua basalis, is red and flesh-looking; the fetal portion, consisting of chorionic villi, is covered by the amnion and appears shiny and gray. The placenta is made up of 15 to 20 segments called cotyledons.
- The placenta serves metabolic functions, endocrine functions (production of human placental lactogen (hPL), human chorionic gonadotropin (hCG), estrogen, and progesterone), and immunologic functions. It acts as the fetus's respiratory organ, is an organ of excretion, and aids in the exchange of nutrients.
- Fetal circulation is a specially designed circulatory system that provides for oxygenation of the fetus while bypassing the fetal lungs.
- Stages of fetal development include the preembryonic stage (the first 14 days of human development starting at

fertilization), the embryonic stage (from day 15 after fertilization, or the beginning of the third week, until approximately 8 weeks after conception), and the fetal stage (from 8 weeks until birth at approximately 38 weeks postconception).

- Significant events that occur during the embryonic stage are that at 4 weeks the fetal heart begins to beat and at 6 weeks fetal circulation is established.
- The fetal stage is devoted to refining structures and perfecting function. The following are some significant developments during the fetal stage:

  At 8 to 12 weeks, all organ systems are formed and now require maturation.

  At 16 weeks, the sex of the fetus can be determined visually.

  At 20 weeks, fetal heartbeat can be auscultated by a fetoscope, and the mother can feel movement (quickening).

  At 24 weeks, vernix caseosa covers the entire body.

  At 26 to 28 weeks, the eyes reopen.

  At 32 weeks, skin appears less wrinkled and red because subcutaneous fat has been laid down.

  At 35 weeks, fingernails reach the ends of fingers.

  At 38 weeks, vernix caseosa is apparent only in creases and folds of skin, and lanugo remains on upper arms and shoulders only.
- The embryo is particularly vulnerable to teratogenesis during the first 8 weeks of cell differentiation and organ system development.

CRITICAL THINKING IN ACTION

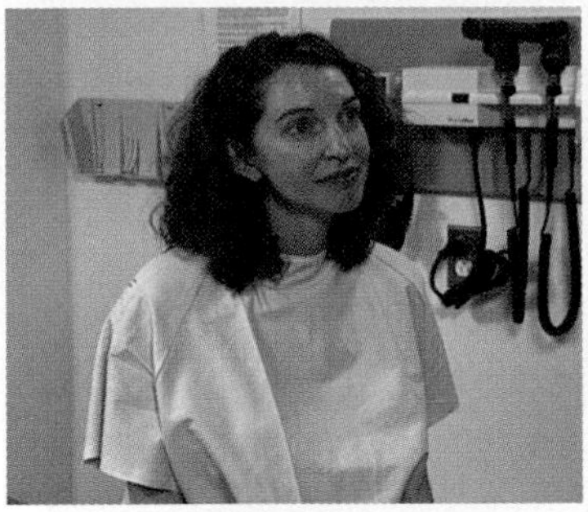

You are working at the local clinic when Frances, a 28-year-old G2 P1001 at 11 weeks' gestation, comes into the office. Frances tells you that early in the first trimester, her husband experienced a flulike syndrome and that he was later diagnosed with cytomegalovirus (CMV) pneumonia. She tells you that his physician found an enlarged supraclavicular lymph node and an ulcer on one tonsil. Laboratory testing revealed elevated liver enzymes. Further testing led to the discovery of positive cytomegalovirus (CMV) lgM levels. She has come today with symptoms including night sweats, persistent sore throat, joint pain, headache, vomiting, and fatigue. You obtain vital signs of temperature 90°F, pulse 90, respirations 14, BP 110/70. Her physical exam is normal; no lymphadenopathy are present. Her weight gain is 2 lb even with nausea and some vomiting. She is worried that her husband's illness could be related to her current symptoms.

1. How would you respond to Frances's concern?
2. Frances asks you if her baby is formed. How would you discuss the three stages of development?
3. Frances asks when her baby is most vulnerable for abnormal growth or structure. How would you answer?
4. Frances asks what stage her baby is in. What would you tell her?

See www.nursing.pearsonhighered.com for possible responses.

Pearson Nursing Student Resources

Find additional review materials at
www.nursing.pearsonhighered.com

Prepare for success with additional NCLEX®-style practice questions, interactive assignments and activities, Web links, animations and videos, and more!

REFERENCES

Beall, M. H., & Ross, M. G. (2009). Amniotic fluid dynamics. In R. K. Creasy, R. Resnik, J. D. Iams, C. J. Lockwood, & T. R. Moore (Eds.), *Creasy & Resnik's maternal-fetal medicine: Principles and practice* (6th ed., pp. 47–54). Philadelphia, PA: Saunders Elsevier.

Benirschke, K. (2009a). Normal early development. In R. K. Creasy, R. Resnik, J. D. Iams, C. J. Lockwood, & T. R. Moore (Eds.), *Creasy & Resnik's maternal-fetal medicine: Principles and practice.* (6th ed., pp. 37–45). Philadelphia, PA: Saunders Elsevier.

Benirschke, K. (2009b). Multiple gestation: The biology of twinning. In R. K. Creasy, R. Resnik, J. D. Iams, C. J. Lockwood, & T. R. Moore (Eds.), *Creasy & Resnik's maternal-fetal medicine: Principles and practice.* (6th ed., pp. 55–68). Philadelphia, PA: Saunders Elsevier.

Blackburn, S. T. (2007). *Maternal, fetal, & neonatal physiology: A clinical perspective* (3rd ed.). St. Louis, MO: Saunders.

Chambers, C., & Weiner, C. P. (2009). Teratogenesis and environmental exposure. In R. K. Creasy, R. Resnik, J. D. Iams, C. J. Lockwood, & T. R. Moore (Eds.), *Creasy & Resnik's maternal-fetal medicine: Principles and practice.* (6th ed., pp. 347–359). Philadelphia, PA: Saunders Elsevier.

Cunningham, F. G., Leveno, K. J., Bloom, S. L., Hauth, J. C., Rouse, D. J., & Spong, C. Y. (2010). *Williams obstetrics* (23rd ed.). New York, NY: McGraw-Hill.

Gilbert, W. M. (2007). Amniotic fluid disorders. In S. G. Gabbe, J. R. Niebyl, & J. L. Simpson (Eds.), *Obstetrics: Normal and problems pregnancies* (5th ed., pp. 834–845). Philadelphia, PA: Churchill Livingstone Elsevier.

Moore, K. L., & Persaud, T. V. N. (2008). *The developing human: Clinical oriented embryology* (8th ed.). Philadelphia, PA: Saunders.

Sadler, T. W. (2010). *Langman's medical embryology* (11th ed.). Philadelphia, PA: Lippincott Williams & Wilkins.

Shea, A. K., & Steiner, M. (2008). Cigarette smoking during pregnancy. *Nicotine & Tobacco Research, 10*(2), 267–278. doi:10.1080/14622200701825908

Volpe, J. J. (2008). *Neurology of the newborn* (5th ed.). Philadelphia, PA: Saunders.

CHAPTER 12

Special Reproductive Concerns: Infertility and Genetics

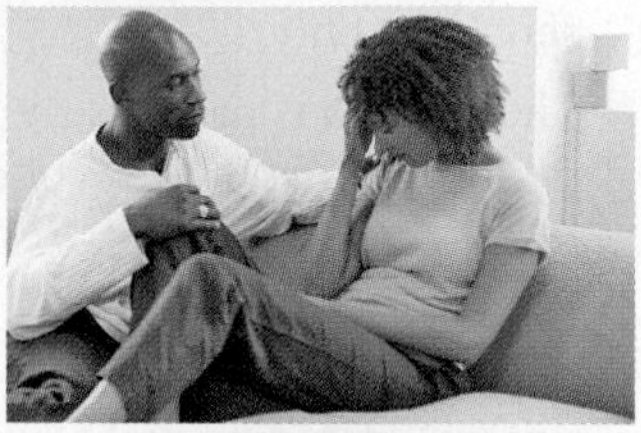

As we sat in the waiting room at the in vitro clinic, I felt great apprehension. For 4 years we had been unable to conceive. I'd been through two surgeries, dozens of blood tests, and hormone drugs that made me irrational and emotional. It was difficult at times—I blamed myself, felt out of control, and had surprisingly painful reactions to seeing mothers with babies. After many long talks we decided that if in vitro didn't work for us, we would adopt. Still, we felt that we wanted to experience childbirth together.

LEARNING OUTCOMES

1. Identify the components of fertility.
2. Describe the elements of the preliminary investigation of infertility and the nurse's role in supporting/teaching patients during this phase.
3. Summarize the indications for the tests and associated treatments, including assisted reproductive technologies, that are done in an infertility workup.
4. Relate the physiologic and psychologic effects of infertility on a couple to the nursing care management of the couple.
5. Describe the nurse's roles as counselor, educator, and advocate during infertility evaluation and treatment.
6. Identify couples who may benefit from preconceptual chromosomal analysis and prenatal testing.
7. Identify the characteristics of autosomal dominant, autosomal recessive, and X-linked (sex-linked) recessive disorders.
8. Compare prenatal and postnatal diagnostic procedures used to determine the presence of genetic disorders.
9. Explain the nurse's role in supporting the family undergoing genetic counseling.
10. Discuss the emotional impact on a couple coping with the birth of a baby with a genetic disorder and the nurse's role in supporting the family.

KEY TERMS

Autosomes *263*
Basal body temperature (BBT) *245*
Chromosomes *262*
Endometrial biopsy (EMB) *247*
Ferning capacity *248*
Gamete intrafallopian transfer (GIFT) *258*
Genotype *266*
Hysterosalpingography (HSG) *251*
Infertility *243*
In vitro fertilization (IVF) *257*
Karyotype *263*
Laparoscopy *251*
Mendelian (single-gene) inheritance *266*
Monosomies *264*
Mosaicism *264*
Nonmendelian (multifactorial) inheritance *266*
Pedigree *267*
Phenotype *266*
Recurrent pregnancy loss (RPL) *261*
Secondary infertility *243*
Spinnbarkheit *248*
Subfertility *243*
Therapeutic insemination *256*
Transvaginal ultrasound *247*
Trisomies *263*
Tubal embryo transfer (TET) *259*
Zygote intrafallopian transfer (ZIFT) *259*

Most couples who want children conceive with little difficulty. Pregnancy and childbirth usually take their normal course, and a healthy baby is born. But some less fortunate couples are unable to fulfill their dream of having a healthy baby because of infertility or genetic problems.

This chapter explores two particularly troubling reproductive problems facing some couples: the inability to conceive and the risk of bearing babies with genetic problems.

Infertility

Infertility is defined by the failure to achieve a successful pregnancy after 12 months or more of regular unprotected intercourse (American Society for Reproductive Medicine [ASRM], 2008b). It has a profound emotional, psychologic, and economic impact on both the affected couple and society. *Sterility* is a term applied when there is an absolute factor preventing reproduction. **Subfertility** is used to describe a couple having difficulty conceiving because both partners have reduced fertility. The term **secondary infertility** is applied to couples who have been unable to conceive after one or more successful pregnancies. The medical causes are similar to those of infertility in general.

Approximately 10% to 15% of couples in their reproductive years are infertile in the United States (Wright & Johnson, 2008). Public perception is that the incidence of infertility is increasing, but in fact there has been no significant change in the proportion of infertile couples in the United States. What has changed is the composition of the infertile population; the infertility diagnosis has increased in the age group 25 to 44 years because of delayed childbearing and the entry of the baby-boom cohort into this age range in Western society. The mean age for a first birth is now 4.5 years older than that of women 2 decades ago (Balen & Rutherford, 2007).

Many factors affect male and female fertility, including environmental factors such as weight, sexually transmitted infections, stress, and smoking. Cigarette smoking in females can delay time to conception and increase the risk for spontaneous abortion, preterm labor, and low birth weight. The quantity and quality of male sperm is also affected by cigarette smoking (ASRM, 2008k). The ASRM promotes maintenance of a healthy weight and body mass index (BMI) to protect fertility in women. Women weighing >120% or <95% of their predicted ideal body weight can alter the production and storage of sex steroid hormones, which in turn affect a woman's reproductive cycle. It is estimated that 12% or more of infertile couples have an abnormal body weight as the cause of their infertility and 70% of women will conceive spontaneously if their weight disorder is corrected (ASRM, 2008f). Male obesity is associated with increased incidence of low sperm concentration and poor sperm motility (ASRM, 2008e). Sexually transmitted infections, such as *Chlamydia trachomatis*, can cause salpingitis and subsequent tubal obstruction, leading to infertility or ectopic pregnancy (ASRM, 2008h).

Endocrine disrupting chemicals (EDC) are common environmental pollutants and exposures to natural and synthetic chemicals that can affect reproductive health. Some of the common EDCs include bisphenol A (BPA), phthalates, and certain pesticides. Maternal and paternal exposure to these compounds can affect fertility and the ability to reproduce. Heavy metals, such as lead, are known to cause decreased fertility and increased pregnancy loss. Preconceptual exposure to pesticides in agricultural and horticultural settings has also been associated with infertility (Woodruff, Carlson, Schwartz et al., 2008).

The perception that infertility is on the rise may be related to the following factors:

- The deferring of marriage and then the desire to have a family shortly after marriage
- The increase in assisted reproduction techniques
- The increase in availability and use of infertility services
- The increase in insurance coverage of some socioeconomic groups for diagnosis of and treatment for infertility
- The increased number of childless women over 35 seeking medical attention for infertility

Essential Components of Fertility

Understanding the elements essential for normal fertility can help the nurse identify the many factors that may cause infertility. The components necessary for normal fertility are correlated with possible causes of deviation in Table 12-1. In addition, adequate reproductive hormones must be present.

With the intricacies of timing and environment playing such a crucial role, it is an impressive natural phenomenon that the majority of couples in the United States are able to conceive. The remaining couples experience infertility due to a male factor (20%), a female factor (40%), or either an unknown cause (unexplained infertility) or a problem with both partners (30% to 40%) (ASRM, 2008g). Professional intervention can help approximately 65% of infertile couples achieve pregnancy.

Young couples with no history that is suggestive of reproductive disorders should be referred for infertility evaluation if they have been unable to conceive after at least 1 year of attempting to achieve pregnancy. An earlier workup is indicated in couples with positive history for fertility-lowering disease or advancing maternal age (Wright & Johnson, 2008). In women over 35 years of age, it is appropriate to refer the couple after only 6 months of unprotected intercourse without conception or earlier if clinically indicated (ASRM, 2008b). The most important determinant of a couple's fertility is the age of the woman. The cumulative conception rate for women up to age 25 is 60% at 6 months and 85% at 1 year (Balen & Rutherford, 2007).

Initial Investigation: Physical and Psychosocial Issues

The easiest and least intrusive infertility testing approach is used first. Extensive testing is avoided until data confirm that the timing of intercourse and the length of coital exposure have been adequate. The nurse informs the couple of the most fertile times to have intercourse during the menstrual cycle. Teaching the couple factors that influence fertility, the signs and timing of ovulation, and the most effective timing

TABLE 12-1 Possible Causes of Infertility

NECESSARY NORMS	DEVIATIONS FROM NORMAL
Female	
Favorable cervical mucus	Cervicitis, cervical stenosis, use of coital lubricants, antisperm antibodies (immunologic response)
Clear passage between cervix and tubes	Myomata, adhesions, adenomyosis, polyps, endometritis, cervical stenosis, endometriosis, congenital anomalies (e.g., septate uterus, diethylstilbestrol [DES] exposure)
Patent tubes with normal motility	Pelvic inflammatory disease, peritubal adhesions, endometriosis, intrauterine device [IUD], salpingitis (e.g., chlamydia, recurrent sexually transmitted infections [STIs]), neoplasm, ectopic pregnancy, tubal ligation
Ovulation and release of ova	Primary ovarian failure, polycystic ovarian disease, hypothyroidism, pituitary tumor, lactation, periovarian adhesions, endometriosis, premature ovarian failure, hyperprolactinemia, Turner syndrome
No obstruction between ovary and tubes	Adhesions, endometriosis, pelvic inflammatory disease
Endometrial preparation	Anovulation, luteal phase defect, malformation, uterine infection, Asherman syndrome
Male	
Normal semen analysis	Abnormalities of sperm or semen, polyspermia, congenital defect in testicular development, mumps after adolescence, cryptorchidism, infections, gonadal exposure to x-rays, chemotherapy, smoking, alcohol abuse, malnutrition, chronic or acute metabolic disease, medications (e.g., morphine, aspirin [ASA], ibuprofen), cocaine use, marijuana use, constrictive underclothing, heat
Unobstructed genital tract	Infections, tumors, congenital anomalies, vasectomy, strictures, trauma, varicocele
Normal genital tract secretions	Infections, autoimmunity to semen, tumors
Ejaculate deposited at the cervix	Premature ejaculation, impotence, hypospadias, retrograde ejaculation (e.g., diabetic), neurologic cord lesions, obesity (inhibiting adequate penetration)

TABLE 12-2 Suggestions for Improving Fertility

- Avoid douching and artificial lubricants (gels, oils, saliva) that can alter sperm mobility. Prevent alteration of pH of vagina and introduction of spermicidal agents.
- Promote retention of sperm. The male superior position with the female remaining recumbent for at least 20–30 minutes after intercourse maximizes the number of sperm reaching the cervix.
- Avoid leakage of sperm. Elevate the woman's hips with a pillow after intercourse for 20–30 minutes to allow liquefaction of seminal fluid and motility of the sperm toward the egg. Avoid getting up to urinate, shower, or douche for 1 hour after intercourse.
- Maximize the potential for fertilization. Instruct the couple that it is optimal if sexual intercourse occurs every other day during the fertile period. Because each woman's menstrual cycle varies in length, the fertile period can extend from cycle day (CD) 7 through CD 17. Note: CD 1 is considered the first day of actual menstrual flow.
- Avoid emphasizing conception during sexual encounters to decrease anxiety and potential sexual dysfunction.
- Maintain adequate nutrition and reduce stress. Stress reduction techniques and good nutritional habits increase sperm production.
- Explore other methods to increase fertility awareness, such as home assessment of cervical mucus and basal body temperature (BBT) recordings.
- Seek counsel and advice from a valued friend or family member.
- Consider incorporating culturally appropriate methods to enhance fertility.

for intercourse within the cycle may solve the problem (Table 12-2). Primary assessment, including a comprehensive history (with a discussion of genetic conditions) and physical examination for any obvious causes of infertility, is done before a costly, time-consuming, and emotionally trying investigation is initiated.

The initial infertility evaluation offers nurses a unique opportunity to initiate preconception counseling, thereby helping infertile couples maximize their chances of delivering a healthy baby. Prenatal vitamins are often one of the earliest recommendations for women planning to conceive. Studies show that folic acid supplementation of at least 400 micrograms (0.4 mg/day) taken 1 to 3 months preconceptually and continued through the first trimester greatly reduces the incidence of neural tube defects such as anencephaly and spina bifida. Preconception is the optimal time to review the importance of rubella and varicella immunity and the risk of congenital anomalies associated with exposure. It also provides the opportunity to address risks associated with alcohol, tobacco, and medications. Women may warrant a change in medications or stricter management of chronic illnesses.

The mutual desire to have children is a cornerstone of many marriages. A fertility problem is a deeply personal, emotion-laden area in a couple's life. The self-esteem of one or both partners may be threatened if the inability to conceive is seen as a lack of virility or femininity (Paterno, 2008). It is never easy to discuss one's sexual activity, especially when potentially irreversible problems with fertility may exist. The nurse can provide comfort to couples by offering a sympathetic ear, a nonjudgmental approach, and appropriate information and instructions throughout the diagnostic and therapeutic process (McGrath, Samra, Zukowsky, et al., 2010). Because counseling includes discussion of very personal matters, nurses who are comfortable with their own sexuality are more capable of establishing rapport and eliciting relevant information from couples with fertility problems.

The first interview should involve both partners and include a comprehensive history and a physical examination. Table 12-3 lists the items in a complete infertility physical workup and laboratory evaluation for both partners. Because

TABLE 12-3 Initial Infertility Physical Workup and Laboratory Evaluations

FEMALE	MALE
Physical Examination Assessment of height, weight, blood pressure, temperature, and general health status Endocrine evalution of thyroid for exophthalmos, lid lag, tremor, or palpable gland Optic fundi evaluation for presence of increased intracranial pressure, especially in oligomenorrheal or amenorrheal women (possible pituitary tumor) Reproductive features (including breast and external genital area) Physical ability to tolerate pregnancy **Pelvic Examination** Papanicolaou (PAP) smear Culture for gonorrhea if indicated and possibly chlamydia or mycoplasma culture (opinions vary) Signs of vaginal infections (see chapter 6) Shape of escutcheon (e.g., does pubic hair distribution resemble that of a male's?) Size of clitoris (enlargement caused by endocrine disorders) Evaluation of cervix: old lacerations, tears, erosion, polyps, condition and shape of os, signs of infections, cervical mucus (evaluate for estrogen effect of spinnbarkheit and cervical ferning) **Bimanual Examination** Size, shape, position, and motility of uterus Presence of congenital anomalies Presence of endometriosis Evaluation of adnexa: ovarian size, cysts, fixations, or tumors **Rectovaginal Examination** Presence of retroflexed or retroverted uterus Presence of rectouterine pouch masses Presence of possible endometriosis **Laboratory Examination** Complete blood count Sedimentation rate if indicated Serology Urinalysis Rh factor and blood grouping Rubella immunoglobulin (IgG) Follicle-stimulating hormone (FSH) level regardless of age and regularity of menstrual cycles If indicated depending on age and regularity of menstrual cycles: thyroid-stimulating hormone (TSH), prolactin levels (PRL), glucose tolerance test, hormonal assays including estradiol (E_2), luteinizing hormone (LH), midluteal progesterone (MLP), dehydroepiandrosterone sulfate (DHEAS), androstenedione, testosterone, 17 α-hydroxyprogesterone (17-OHP).	**Physical Examination** General health (assessment of height, weight, blood pressure) Endocrine evaluation (e.g., presence of gynecomastia) Visual fields evaluation for bitemporal hemianopia (blindness in one-half of the visual field) Abnormal hair patterns **Urologic Examination** Presence or absence of phimosis Location of urethral meatus Size and consistency of each testis, vas deferens, and epididymis Presence of varicocele **Rectal Examination** Size and consistency of the prostate with microscopic evaluation of prostate fluid for signs of infection Size and consistency of seminal vesicles **Laboratory Examination** Complete blood count Sedimentation rate if indicated Serology Urinalysis Rh factor and blood grouping Semen analysis If indicated, testicular biopsy, buccal smear Hormonal assays, FSH, LH, prolactin

at least 20% of infertility is due to a male factor, a semen analysis should be one of the first diagnostic tests performed before moving on to the more invasive diagnostic procedures involving the woman. Figure 12-1 ■ outlines the historic database, diagnostic tests usually performed, and healthcare interventions in cases of infertility.

Assessment of the Woman's Fertility

After a thorough history and physical examination, both partners may undergo tests to identify causes of infertility. A thorough evaluation of the woman's fertility includes assessment of the hypothalamic-pituitary axis in terms of ovulatory function as well as structure and function of the cervix, uterus, fallopian tubes, and ovaries.

Evaluation of Ovulatory Factors

Ovulation problems account for approximately 25% of couples' infertility. For review of the characteristics of the female reproductive cycle, see Table 12-4 and Figure 12-2 ■. For an in-depth discussion on female reproductive cycle characteristics, see chapter 10.

BASAL BODY TEMPERATURE RECORDING One basic test of ovulatory function is the **basal body temperature (BBT)** recording, which aids in identifying follicular and luteal phase abnormalities. At the initial visit, the nurse instructs the woman in the technique of recording BBT on a special form. The woman is instructed to begin a new chart on the first day of every monthly cycle. The temperature can be taken with a standard oral or rectal thermometer calibrated by tenths of a degree, making slight temperature changes readily apparent. A special kind of thermometer (BBT) may be used to measure temperature only between 35°C and 37.8°C (96°F and 100°F). In addition to traditional or digital thermometers, tympanic thermometry, which provides a reading in only a few seconds, may also be a valid method.

Activity: Ovulation

The woman records daily variations on a temperature graph. The temperature graph typically shows a biphasic pattern

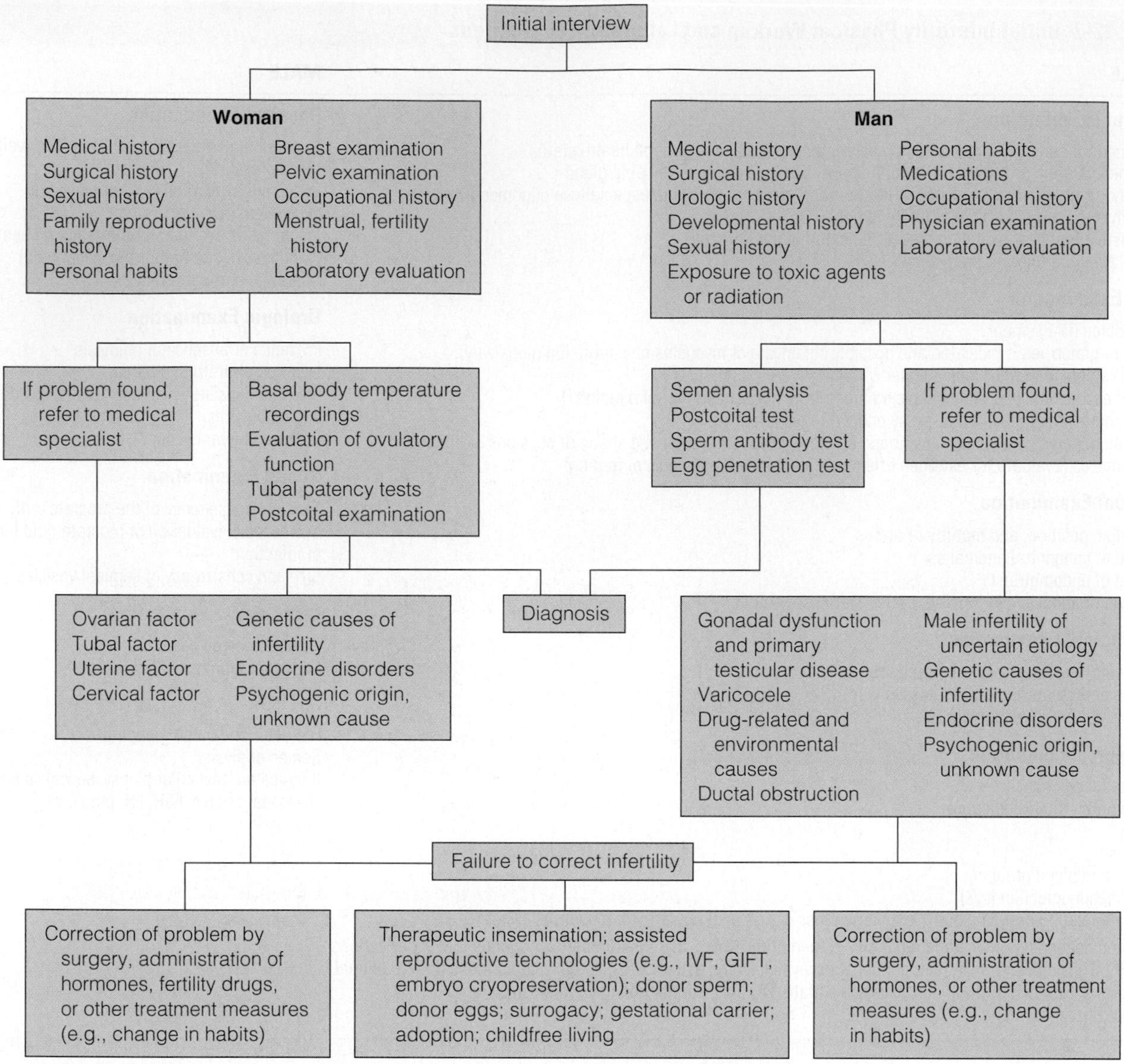

Figure 12-1 ■ Flow chart for management of the infertile couple.

TABLE 12-4 Female Reproductive Cycle

OVARIAN CYCLE	MENSTRUAL CYCLE
Follicular phase (days 1–14): Primordial follicle matures under influence of FSH and LH up to the time of ovulation. *Luteal phase* (days 15–28): Ovum leaves follicle, corpus luteum develops under LH influence and produces high levels of progesterone and low levels of estrogen.	*Menstrual phase* (days 1–6): Estrogen levels are low; cervical mucus is scant, viscous, and opaque. *Proliferative phase* (days 7–14): Estrogen peaks just before ovulation. Cervical mucus at ovulation is clear, thin, watery, alkaline, and more favorable to sperm; shows ferning pattern; and has spinnbarkheit greater than 8 cm. At ovulation body temperature drops then rises sharply and remains elevated under influence of progesterone. *Secretory phase* (days 15–26): Estrogen drops sharply and progesterone dominates. *Ischemic phase* (days 27–28): Both estrogen and progesterone levels drop.

during ovulatory cycles, whereas in anovulatory cycles it remains monophasic. The woman uses the readings on the temperature graph to detect ovulation and direct the timing of intercourse (Figure 12-3A ■).

Basal temperature for females in the preovulatory (follicular) phase is usually below 36.7°C (98°F). As ovulation approaches, production of estrogen increases and at its peak may cause a slight drop, then rise, in the basal temperature. The slight drop in temperature before ovulation is often difficult to capture on the BBT chart. After ovulation there is a surge of luteinizing hormone (LH), which stimulates production of progesterone. Because progesterone is thermogenic (produces heat), it causes a 0.3°C to 0.6°C (0.5°F to 1°F) sustained rise in basal temperature during the second half of the menstrual cycle (luteal phase). Immediately before or coincident with the onset of menses, the temperature falls below 36.7°C (98°F). These changes in the basal temperature create the typical biphasic pattern. Figure 12-3B ■ shows a biphasic ovulatory BBT chart. Temperature elevation does not predict the day of

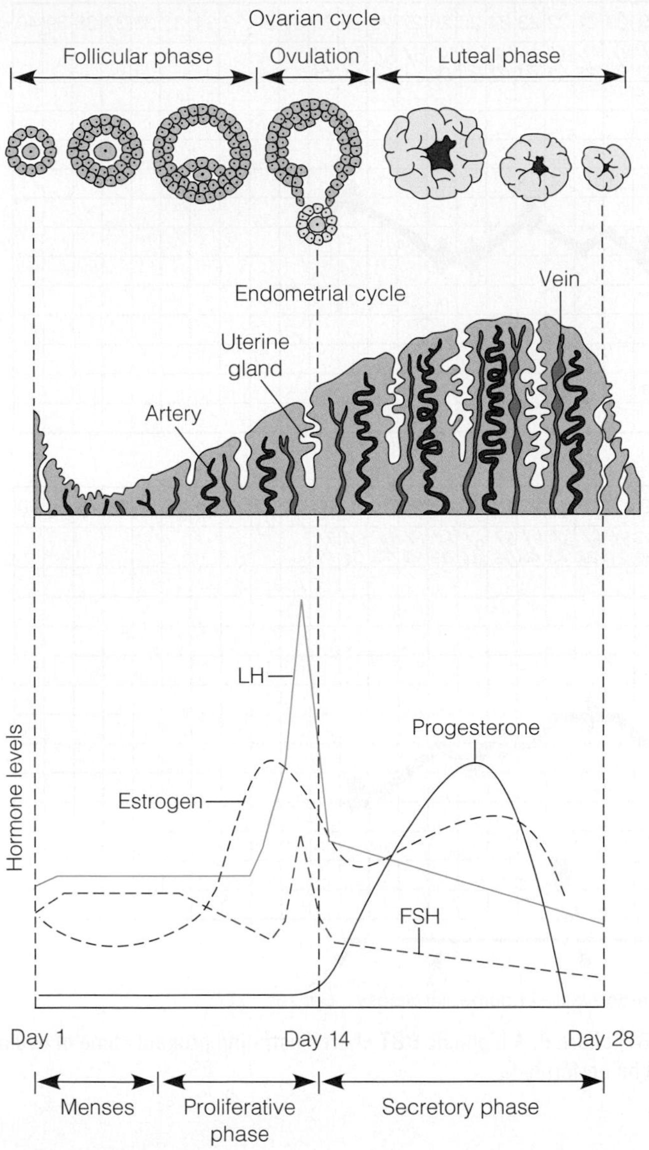

Figure 12-2 ■ Sequence of events in a normal reproductive cycle showing the relationship of hormone levels to events in the ovarian and endometrial cycles.

ovulation but provides supportive evidence of ovulation about a day after it has occurred.

Although there are other, more reliable methods to detect ovulatory function, BBT offers couples a low-tech, noninvasive, and inexpensive option. Based on serial BBT charts, the clinician might recommend sexual intercourse *every other day* beginning 3 to 4 days before and continuing for 2 to 3 days after the expected time of ovulation. See Patient Teaching: Methods of Determining Ovulation on pages 250–251.

HORMONAL ASSESSMENTS OF OVULATORY FUNCTION Hormonal assessments of ovulatory function fall into the following categories:

1. *Gonadotropin levels (FSH, LH):* Baseline hormonal assessment of follicle-stimulating hormone (FSH) and luteinizing hormone (LH) provides valuable information about normal ovulatory function. Measured on cycle day (CD) 3, FSH is the single most valuable test in assessing ovarian reserve (number of remaining oocytes or follicles in the ovary) and function. FSH should always be measured, particularly in women over 30, to predict the potential for successful treatment with ovulation induction treatment cycles (Wright & Johnson, 2008). LH levels may be measured early in the cycle to rule out disorders associated with androgen excess, causing a disruption in normal follicular development and oocyte maturation. Daily sampling of serum LH at midcycle can detect the LH surge. The day of the LH surge is believed to be the time of maximum fertility. Ovulation occurs 24 to 26 hours after the onset of the LH surge and 10 to 12 hours after the peak of the LH surge. Urine LH ovulation prediction and serum LH assay (predictor) kits (such as First Response Ovulation Test ©) are available for home use to better time postcoital testing, insemination, and intercourse (Kumar, Ghadir, Eskandari et al., 2007).
2. *Progesterone assays:* Progesterone levels furnish the best evidence of ovulation and corpus luteum function. Serum levels begin to rise with the LH surge and peak about 8 days later. A level of 3 ng/ml 3 days after the LH surge generally confirms ovulation (Wright & Johnson, 2008). On day 21 (7 days postovulation) a level of 10 ng/ml or higher generally indicates an adequate luteal phase.
3. *Prolactin:* Elevated levels of the anterior pituitary hormone prolactin are a frequent cause of ovulatory dysfunction, which may range from a luteal phase defect to anovulation to amenorrhea.
4. *Thyroid-stimulating hormone (TSH):* Thyroid hormone is necessary for most body functions, not only metabolism but also specific tissue activities. TSH stimulates prolactin secretion by the pituitary gland. Hypothyroidism may have a dramatic effect on ovulatory function and cause menstrual irregularities and bleeding irregularities.
5. *Androgen levels (testosterone, DHEAS, androstenedione):* Androgen excess can originate from the adrenal glands, ovaries, or peripheral tissue. Despite the origin, it usually results in specific clinical symptoms such as acne, hirsutism, virilization, and ovulatory dysfunction—which can range from oligomenorrhea to anovulation to amenorrhea.

ENDOMETRIAL BIOPSY **Endometrial biopsy (EMB)** provides information about the effects of progesterone produced by the corpus luteum after ovulation and endometrial receptivity. EMB is reliable for determining the presence of ovulation. Histologic evidence of a secretory endometrium detected by endometrial biopsy shows ovulation and corpus luteum formation. However, it is not effective for diagnosing luteal phase deficiency (Wright & Johnson, 2008).

TRANSVAGINAL ULTRASOUND **Transvaginal ultrasound** is the method of choice for follicular monitoring of women undergoing ovulation induction cycles, for timing ovulation for insemination and intercourse, for retrieving oocytes for in vitro fertilization (IVF), and for monitoring early pregnancy. The use of transvaginal color flow Doppler to investigate uterine

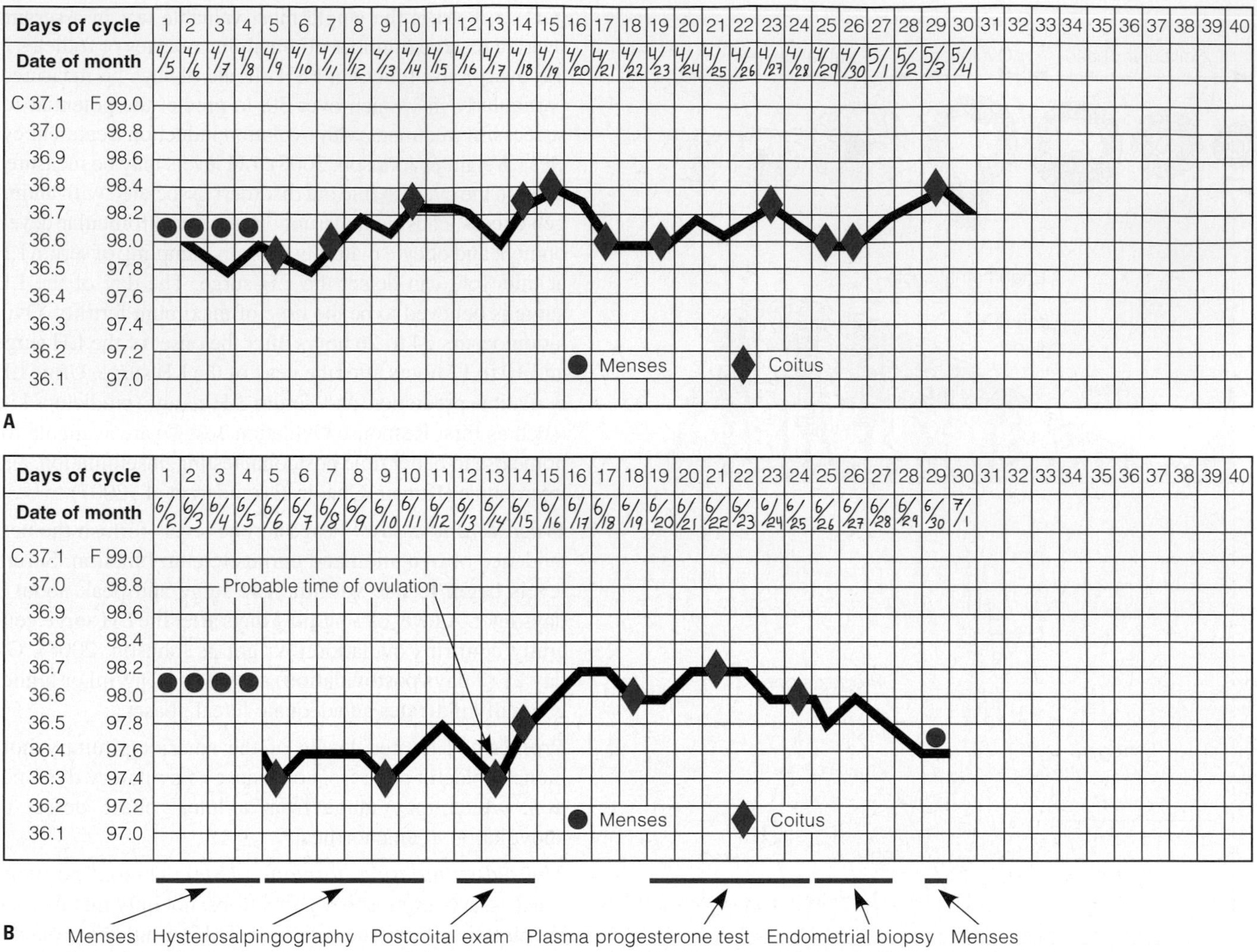

Figure 12-3 ■ A. A monophasic, anovulatory basal body temperature (BBT) chart. B. A biphasic BBT chart illustrating probable time of ovulation, the different types of testing, and the time in the cycle that each would be performed.

blood flow may in the future help the endocrinologist evaluate the adequacy of the developing follicle, further assessing oocyte maturity and endometrial development and patterns, and improve the diagnosis of luteal phase defects. For the procedure, the woman does not need to have a full bladder. In addition, if the woman finds it more comfortable to do so, she can insert the lubricated transvaginal probe herself (Thomas & Van Voorhis, 2008).

Evaluation of Cervical Factors

The mucus cells of the endocervix consist predominantly of water. As ovulation approaches, the ovary increases its secretion of estrogen and produces changes in the cervical mucus. The amount of mucus increases 10-fold, and the water content rises significantly. At ovulation, mucus elasticity, called **spinnbarkheit**, increases to at least 5 cm in length and the viscosity decreases. Excellent spinnbarkheit exists when the mucus can be stretched 8 to 10 cm or longer. Mucus elasticity is determined by using two glass slides (Figure 12-4A ■) or by grasping some mucus at the external os. (See Patient Teaching: Methods of Determining Ovulation.)

The **ferning capacity** (crystallization) (Figure 12-4B ■ and C ■) of the cervical mucus also increases as ovulation approaches. Ferning is caused by decreased levels of salt and water interacting with the glycoproteins in the mucus during the ovulatory period and is thus an indirect indication of estrogen production. To test for ferning, mucus from the cervical os is spread on a glass slide, allowed to air dry, and then examined under the microscope. Within 24 to 48 hours postovulation, rising levels of progesterone cause a marked decrease in the quantity of cervical mucus and an increase in viscosity and cellularity. The resulting absence of spinnbarkheit and ferning capacity decreases sperm survival.

To be receptive to sperm, cervical mucus must be thin, clear, watery, profuse, alkaline, and acellular. As shown in Figure 12-5 ■, the mazelike microscopic mucoid strands align in a parallel manner to allow for easy sperm passage. The mucus is termed *inhospitable* if these changes do not occur.

Cervical mucus inhospitable to sperm survival can have several causes, some of which are treatable. For example, estrogen secretion may be inadequate for the development of receptive mucus. Cone biopsy, electrocautery, or cryosurgery of the cervix may remove large numbers of mucus-producing glands, creating

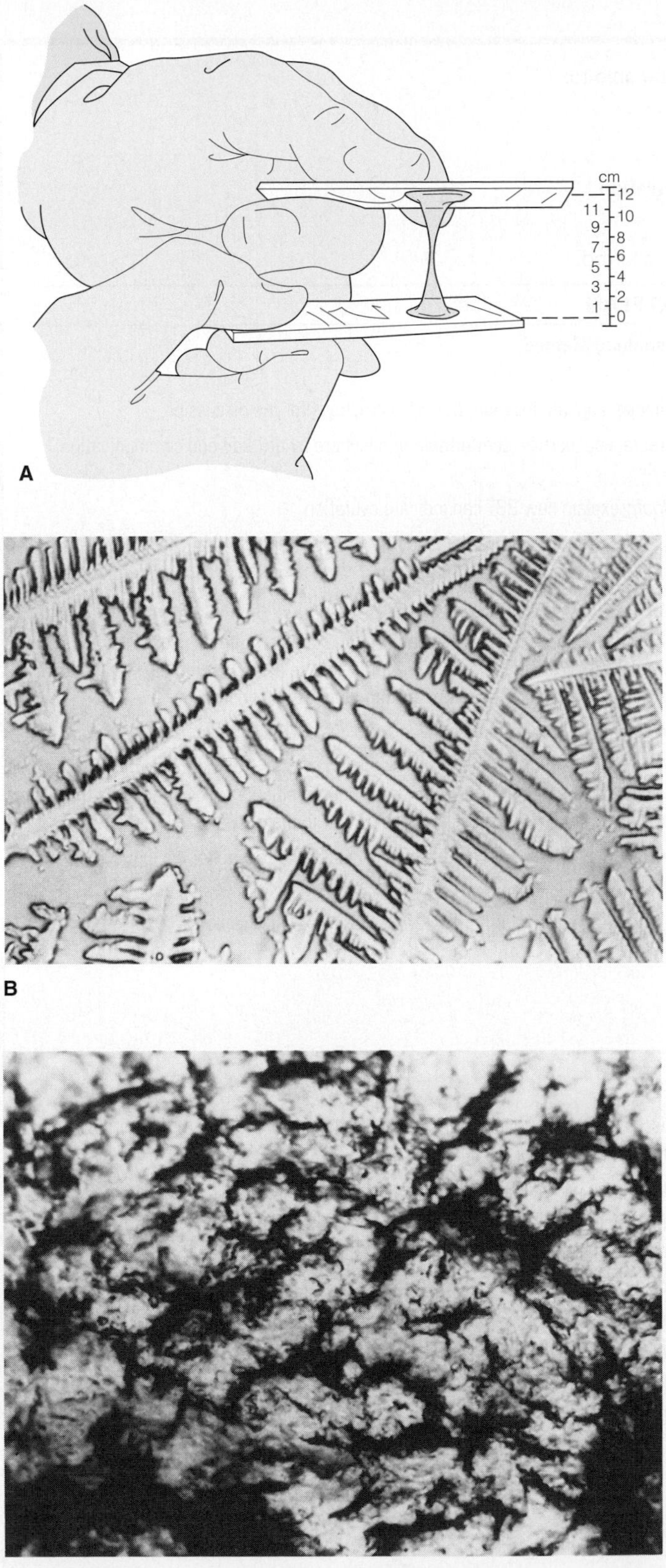

Figure 12-4 ■ A. Spinnbarkheit (elasticity). B. Ferning pattern. C. Lack of ferning pattern.

Source: B. Courtesy of Lavena Porter OB/GYN NP. C. From Clinical gynecologic endocrinology and infertility, *5e, by L. Speroff, et al., p. 818. Copyright 1994 Lippincott, Williams & Wilkins. Reprinted with permission.*

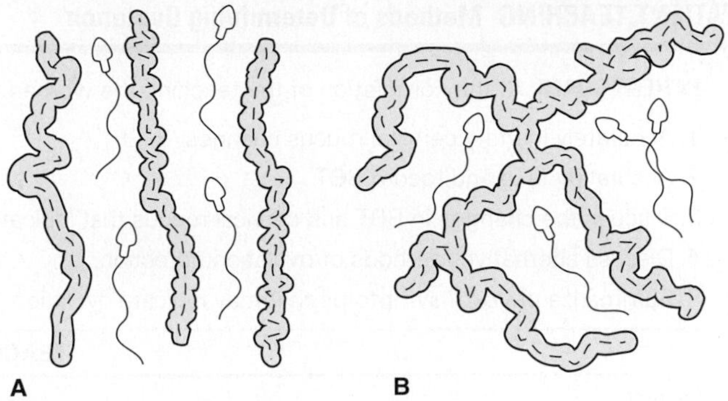

Figure 12-5 ■ Sperm passage through cervical mucus. A. Appearance at the time of ovulation with channels favoring efficient sperm penetration and migration upward. B. Unfavorable mazelike configuration found at other times of the menstrual cycle.

Source: Corson, S. (1990). Conquering infertility *(p. 16). A guide for couples (4th ed.). Vancouver, BC: EMIS-Canada.*

a "dry cervix" that decreases sperm survival. Treatment with clomiphene citrate may have deleterious effects on cervical mucus because of its antiestrogenic properties. Therapy with supplemental estrogen for approximately 6 days before expected ovulation is sometimes employed to encourage formation of suitable spinnbarkheit. However, intrauterine insemination (IUI) is more often the most appropriate therapy to overcome these obstacles. When mucosal hostility to sperm is due to cervical infection, antimicrobial therapy may be effective.

The cervix can also be the site of secretory immunologic reactions in which antisperm antibodies are produced, causing agglutination or immobilization of sperm. The most widely used serum sperm bioassay to detect specific classes of antibodies in serum and seminal fluid is direct immunobead binding testing (IBT) (Lu, Huang, & Lu, 2008). The IBT is considered clinically significant when 50% of the sperm are coated with immunobeads. The treatment for antisperm antibodies may include IUI of the male's washed sperm to bypass the cervical factor.

The *postcoital test (PCT),* also called the Huhner test, is performed 1 or 2 days before the expected date of ovulation as determined by previous BBT charts, the length of prior cycles, or urinary LH kit. This examination evaluates the cervical mucus, the number of active sperm in the cervical mucus, and the length of sperm survival (in hours) after intercourse. Its use is controversial and has limited use in infertility workups because its value in assessing cervical hostility to sperm has never been proven (Wright & Johnson, 2008). Tests that can potentially predict the fertilizing ability of sperm include the zona-free hamster egg penetration assay and the hemizona test.

Evaluation of Uterine Structures and Tubal Patency

Uterine abnormalities are a relatively uncommon cause of infertility but should always be considered. A few tests offer the ability to evaluate the uterine cavity and tubal patency simultaneously. These tests are usually done after BBT evaluation, semen analysis, and the other less invasive tests. Tubal patency and uterine assessment are usually evaluated by hysterosalpingography or laparoscopy. Other invasive tests used to evaluate only the uterine cavity are hysteroscopy and sonohysterography.

PATIENT TEACHING Methods of Determining Ovulation

PATIENT GOALS At the completion of the teaching the woman will be able to:

1. Accurately identify cervical mucus changes.
2. Accurately take and record BBT.
3. Discuss the changes in BBT and cervical mucus that indicate ovulation.
4. Discuss alternative methods of ovulation detection.
5. Summarize physical symptoms that may indicate ovulation has occurred.

TEACHING PLAN

Basal Body Temperature (BBT) Method

Content

The basal body temperature (BBT) method relies on assessing the woman's temperature pattern.

Describe the expected findings with an ovulatory (biphasic) cycle and stress the need to monitor BBT for 3 to 4 months to establish a pattern. BBT can be used to time intercourse if pregnancy is desired or as a method of natural family planning. Describe the timing of intercourse to achieve or avoid pregnancy.

Procedure for Measuring BBT:

- Using a BBT thermometer, the woman chooses one site (oral, vaginal, or rectal), which she uses consistently.
- The woman takes her temperature every day before arising and before starting any activity, including smoking. Any activity can produce an increase in body temperature.

Note: Read and follow manufacturers' instructions for each type of BBT thermometer in regard to amount of time needed for accurate reading.

- The result is then recorded immediately on a special BBT chart, and the temperature dots for each day are connected to form a graph.
- The woman then shakes the thermometer down in preparation for use the next day.

Explain that certain situations can disturb body temperature such as large alcohol intake, sleeplessness, fever, warm climate, jet lag, shift work, the use of an electric blanket, or use of a heated waterbed.

Teaching Method

Choose a private location, free of distractions for the discussion.

Create a supportive, comfortable atmosphere by attitude and communication style.

Briefly explain how BBT can indicate ovulation.

Use pictures or graphs to demonstrate the BBT changes that indicate ovulatory and ovulatory cycles.

Break content down into smaller steps to facilitate learning.

Show the woman the BBT thermometer and demonstrate its use. *Note:* A tympanic (ear) electric thermometer may also be used. Remind the woman to use the same type of thermometer throughout the menstrual cycle.

Provide a blank chart. Ask the woman to chart 3 days' findings using temperature results you identify.

Remind the woman that BBT charts are not a prediction of ovulation and that the temperature rise is a response to ovulation that has already occurred.

Provide the woman with an example of LH testing results for comparison.

Provide a handout summarizing the procedure.

Provide frequent opportunities for questions and discussion.

Cervical Mucus Method

Content

Explain that cervical mucus characteristics change throughout a woman's menstrual cycle, and that the quality of the mucus can be used to predict ovulation.

Procedure for Assessing Cervical Mucus Changes:

- Every day when she uses the bathroom the woman checks her vagina, either by dabbing the vaginal opening with toilet paper or by putting a finger in the opening.
- She notes the wetness (presence of mucus), collects some mucus, determines its color and consistency, and records her findings on a chart. For discussion of mucus characteristics, see page 248.
- She washes her hands before and after the procedure.

Teaching Method

Discuss the various characteristics of the mucus throughout the menstrual cycle and the rationale for the changes.

Explore the woman's feelings about using the procedure.

Show pictures of the mucus changes, including spinnbarkheit of different degrees of elasticity.

Encourage the woman to ask questions.

Stress that it may take several cycles for the woman to become familiar with the pattern.

Explain that the presence and consistency of the mucus are altered by vaginal infection, vaginal medications, spermicides, lubricants, douching, sexual arousal and semen.

LH Predictor Kit Method

Content

Explain that LH kits are a good predictor of ovulation for a woman with a history of regular menstrual cycles.

Describe the procedures for using an LH predictor kit:

- Determine the length of the woman's menstrual cycle. Use a calendar to determine the cycle day the woman will initiate testing.
- The testing must occur the same time daily. The morning is recommended, because the LH concentration is highest upon wakening.
- Begin testing with the first morning urine void and examine the test strips for color changes that indicate if ovulation has occurred or is close to occurring.

PATIENT TEACHING Methods of Determining Ovulation continued

TEACHING PLAN

Content	Teaching Method
Mittelschmerz	
Explain that mittelschmerz (midcycle pain) located in the lower pelvis is a common symptom of ovulation.	
Encourage the woman to document this occurrence (or absence) on her BBT chart.	

Evaluation	Documentation
Evaluate the learning by providing time for discussion, questions, and practice using the charts and thermometer. Ask the woman to describe the selected procedure in her own words. Provide a written handout describing the process and findings so that the woman has information readily available. Review at a follow-up visit the BBT and cervical mucus assessment from the previous cycle(s).	The nurse should document the information that was given, the type of teaching method used, indicate if the patient performed BBT thermometer assessment, if it was demonstrated, or if verbal or written directions were given. Verbalization of understanding and clarification of any information should be documented. Safety issues and instruction were reviewed.

Hysteroscopy may be performed earlier in the evaluation if the woman's history suggests the potential for adhesive disease or uterine abnormalities.

HYSTEROSALPINGOGRAPHY Hysterosalpingography (HSG), or hysterogram, involves an instillation of a radiopaque substance into the uterine cavity. In addition, the oil-based dye and injection pressure used in HSG may have a therapeutic effect. This effect may be caused by the flushing of debris, breaking of adhesions, or induction of peristalsis produced by the instillation.

The HSG should be performed in the follicular phase of the cycle to avoid interrupting an early pregnancy. This timing also avoids the lush secretory changes in the endometrium that occur after ovulation, which may prevent the passage of the dye through the tubes and present a false picture of obstruction of the entry point of the fallopian tube into the uterus. HSG causes moderate discomfort. The pain is referred from the peritoneum (which is irritated by the subdiaphragmatic collection of gas) to the shoulder. The cramping may be decreased if the radiopaque dye is warmed to body temperature before instillation. Women can take an over-the-counter (OTC) prostaglandin synthesis inhibitor (such as ibuprofen) 30 minutes before the procedure to decrease the pain, cramping, and discomfort. HSG can also cause serious recurrence of pelvic inflammatory disease, so prophylactic antibiotics are recommended to prevent infection that could be triggered by the procedure (Wright & Johnson, 2008).

HYSTEROSCOPY *Hysteroscopy* is the definitive method for both diagnosis and treatment of intrauterine pathology (Speroff & Fritz, 2005). Hysteroscopy allows the physician to further evaluate any areas of suspicion within the uterine cavity revealed by HSG. It can be done in conjunction with a laparoscopy or independently in the office and does not require general anesthesia. A fiberoptic instrument called a hysteroscope is placed into the uterus and allows direct visualization of the size; shape; and location of any intrauterine pathology, such as polyps, myomata (fibroids), or structural variations (Goldstein, 2008). The newest generation hysteroscope allows for minor operative procedures to be performed in the office setting.

LAPAROSCOPY Laparoscopy enables direct visualization of the pelvic organs; it is not routinely advised after a normal HSG unless symptoms suggest the need for earlier evaluation (Wright & Johnson, 2008). Diagnostic laparoscopy is an outpatient procedure requiring the use of general anesthesia. Generally a three-puncture approach is used; entry is made through the umbilical area, and supporting instruments are inserted in two suprapubic incisions. The peritoneal cavity is distended with carbon dioxide gas, and the pelvic organs can be directly visualized with a fiberoptic instrument. Tube patency can be assessed by instilling dye into the uterine cavity through the cervix. The pelvis is evaluated for endometriosis, adhesions, organ fixations, pelvic inflammatory disease, tumors, and cysts. The intraperitoneal gas is usually manually expressed at the end of the procedure. In routine preanesthesia instructions, the woman is told that she may have some discomfort from organ displacement and shoulder to chest pain caused by gas in the abdomen. She should be informed that she can resume normal activities as tolerated after 24 hours. Using postoperative pain medication and assuming a supine position may help relieve residual shoulder and chest discomfort caused by any remaining gas.

Activity: Infertility Testing

Assessment of the Man's Fertility

Male infertility can be caused by numerous factors, some of which can be identified and are reversible, such as ductal obstruction and varicocele. Varicocele, which is an abnormal dilation of scrotal veins, is present in 15% of the normal population and accounts for approximately 40% of male infertility (ASRM, 2008j). Other identifiable conditions are not reversible, such as bilateral testicular atrophy secondary to viral orchitis and congenital bilateral absence of the *vas deferens* (CBAVD). Idiopathic male factor infertility occurs when the etiology of an abnormal semen analysis is not identifiable.

If a male infertility factor is present, it is usually defined by the findings of an abnormal semen analysis (ASRM, 2008c). A semen analysis of sperm quality, quantity, and motility is the single most important diagnostic study of the man. It should be done early in the couple's evaluation, before invasive testing of the woman.

To obtain accurate results, the specimen is collected after 2 to 3 days of abstinence and usually by masturbation to avoid contamination or loss of any ejaculate. If the man has difficulty producing sperm by masturbation, special medical grade condoms are available to collect the sperm during intercourse. Regular latex and nonlatex condoms should not be used because they contain agents that impair the mobility of sperm and because sperm can be lost in the condom. Most lubricants also are spermicidal and should not be used unless approved by the andrology laboratory. If the specimen is obtained at home, it needs to be brought to the laboratory within 1 hour and kept at body temperature so as not to impair motility.

Both seasonal and incidental variability may be seen in count and motility in successive semen samples from the same person. Thus a repeat semen analysis may be required to assess the man's fertility potential adequately; a minimum of two separate analyses is recommended for confirmation. In a case in which a known testicular insult has occurred, such as infection, high fevers, or surgery, a repeat analysis may not be done for at least 2.5 months to allow for new sperm maturation.

Semen analysis provides information about sperm motility and morphology as well as a determination of the absolute number of spermatozoa present (Table 12-5). Although it is known that low numbers and motility may indicate compromised fertility, other parameters such as morphology, volume, motion patterns, viscosity, pH, and progression are important prognostic indicators. Values previously thought to indicate subfertility may in fact be compatible with normal fertility when these factors are considered. The quality of sperm decreases with increasing paternal age and may result in chromosomal damage. For example, fathers older than 40 years may be at an increased risk for offspring with chromosome abnormalities or new gene mutations (Toriello & Meck, 2008).

TABLE 12-5 Normal Semen Analysis

FACTOR	VALUE
Volume	Greater than 2 ml
pH	7 to 8
Total sperm count	Greater than 20 million/ml
Liquefaction	Complete in 1 hour
Motility	50% or greater forward progression
Normal forms	30% or greater
Round cells	Less than 5 million/ml
White cells	Less than 1 million/ml

Source: Courtesy of the World Health Organization. (1999). WHO Laboratory Manual for the Examination of Human Semen and Sperm-Cervical Mucus Interaction *(4th ed., pp. 9–106). Cambridge, UK: Cambridge University Press.*

Genetic factors may affect male fertility. Men with oligospermia (semen with a low concentration of sperm) and nonobstructive azoospermia (impaired or nonexistent sperm production) have an increased risk for chromosome abnormalities and Y chromosome deletions. The chance of detecting one of these abnormalities is approximately 10% in oligospermic men and 30% in azoospermic men (ASRM, 2008c). Men with obstructive azoospermia, such as congenital bilateral absence of the vas deferens (CBAVD) have an up to 80% risk for cystic fibrosis genetic mutations (ASRM, 2008c).

Spermatozoa have been shown to possess intrinsic antigens that can provoke male immunologic infertility. Any disruption in the blood-testes barrier, such as vasectomy reversals, or genital trauma, such as testicular torsion, can lead to the production of antisperm antibodies (ASA) (Lee et al., 2009). Treatment for antisperm antibodies is directed toward preventing the formation of antibodies or arresting the underlying mechanism that compromises sperm function. Therapies such as immunosuppression with corticosteroids and IUI have not proved effective. The treatment of choice for clinically significant antisperm antibodies is intracytoplasmic sperm injection (ICSI) in conjunction with IVF.

Tests such as the hamster sperm penetration assay (SPA), hemizona (HZA), acrosome reaction assay, and sperm density evaluation may be performed, but their usefulness is controversial. If the man's history indicates, he may be referred to a urologist for further testing.

Methods of Managing Infertility

Methods of managing infertility include pharmacologic agents, therapeutic insemination, IVF, and other assisted reproductive techniques. In addition, many couples choose adoption as their preferred response to infertility.

Pharmacologic Agents

This section provides a brief overview of the drugs commonly used for ovarian stimulation in the follicular phase, control of midcycle release, and luteal phase support. The pharmacologic treatment chosen depends on the specific cause of the infertility. Table 12-6 lists some of the drugs commonly used and indications for use.

CLOMIPHENE CITRATE If a woman has normal ovaries, a normal prolactin level, and an intact pituitary gland, *clomiphene citrate* (Clomid, Serophene) is often used as first-line therapy to induce ovulation. See Drug Guide: Clomiphene Citrate. This medication induces ovulation in 70% of women by action at both the hypothalamic and ovarian levels; 30% to 40% of these women will become pregnant. Approximately 10% of women develop multiple gestation pregnancies, almost exclusively twins (Storment, 2006). Clomiphene citrate works by stimulating the hypothalamus to secrete more gonadotropin-releasing hormone (GnRH), which increases the secretion of FSH and LH. These stimulate follicular growth and facilitate the release of ova (Speroff & Fritz, 2005).

For the first course the woman usually takes 50 mg/day orally for 5 days from cycle day (CD) 3 to day 7 or CD 5 to day 9. In nonresponders, the dose may be increased to 100 mg/day

TABLE 12-6 Drugs Commonly Used to Treat Infertility

	INDICATIONS	
DRUGS	**WOMEN**	**MEN**
Clomiphene citrate (Clomid, Serophene)	• Polycystic ovarian syndrome (PCOS) • Hyperandrogenemia • Premature follicle rupture	• Low levels of gonadotropins • Hypothalamic hypogonadism
Human menopausal gonadotropin (hMG) (Repronex, Bravelle)	• Hypothalamic ovulatory dysfunction (after failure of clomiphene) • Hypopituitarism • PCOS (rarely) • Luteinized unruptured follicle syndrome (after failure of hCG alone) • Inadequate cervical mucus • In vitro fertilization, gamete intrafallopian transfer (GIFT), zygote intrafallopian transfer (ZIFT) • Controlled superovulation	• Hypothalamic pituitary failure due to Kallmann syndrome or delayed puberty • Hypogonadotrophic hypogonadism (deficiency of FSH and LH)
Recombinant follicle-stimulating hormone (rFSH) (Follistim, Gonal-F)	• PCOS • Too long cycles • In vitro fertilization, GIFT, ZIFT	
Human chorionic gonadotropin (hCG) (Pregnyl, Novarel, A.P.L.)	• Induces dominant follicle to release egg • Luteinized unruptured follicle syndrome	
Bromocriptine (Parlodel) Cabergoline (Dostinex)	• Pituitary adenoma • Hyperpituitarism	• Hyperprolactinemia (functional or pituitary adenoma)
Gonadotropin releasing hormone (GnRh) (Factrel, Lutre-pulse)	• Hypothalamic ovulatory dysfunction—to ensure a pulsatile release of GnRH by a small pump	• Hypothalamic pituitary failure due to Kallmann syndrome or delayed puberty (pulsed infusion)
GnRh Analogs • Leuprolide acetate (Lupron) • Nafarelin acetate (Synarel) • Goserelin acetate (Zoladex)	• Premature follicular rupture • In vitro fertilization, GIFT, ZIFT • Endometriosis	• Hypogonadotrophic hypogonadism
GnRH Antagonists • Ganirelix acetate (Antagon)	• Same as GnRH analogs	
Progesterone (Crinone, Prometrium, progesterone in oil)	• Luteal phase dysfunction • Luteal phase support	

Source: Adapted from American Society for Reproductive Medicine Booklet. (2006). Medications for inducing ovulation—A guide for patients. *Retrieved from http://www.asrm.org/Patientbooklets/ovulation_drugs.pdf; Shane, J. (1993). Evaluation and treatment of infertility.* Clinical Symposia, 45, 2; *Wilson, B. A., Shannon, M. T., & Shields, K. M. (2010).* Prentice Hall nurse's drug guide 2010. *Upper Saddle River, NJ: Pearson Education.*

to a maximum of 250 mg/day, although doses in excess of 100 mg/day are not approved by the Food and Drug Administration (FDA) (Wilson, Shannon, & Shields, 2010). The woman may need to take estrogen simultaneously if a decrease in cervical mucus occurs.

The woman is informed that if ovulation occurs, it is expected to occur 5 to 9 days after the last dose. The nurse determines if the couple has been advised to have sexual intercourse every other day for 1 week, beginning 5 days after the last day of medications. Upon a negative pregnancy test, another trial of clomiphene can be initiated. After the first treatment cycle, a pelvic ultrasound should be done to rule out ovarian enlargement, ovarian cysts, or hyperstimulation. Ovarian enlargement and abdominal discomfort (bloating) may result from follicular growth and the formation of multiple corpus lutea. Persistence of ovarian cysts is a contraindication for subsequent treatment cycles. Other side effects include hot flashes, abdominal distention, bloating, breast discomfort, nausea and vomiting, vision problems (such as visual spots), headache, and dryness or loss of hair (Wright & Johnson, 2008). Supplemental low-dose estrogen may be given to ensure appropriate quality and quantity of cervical mucus, or IUI may be employed to overcome this obstacle. Women can assess the presence of ovulation and possible response to clomiphene therapy by doing BBT and urinary LH tests. The woman should be knowledgeable about side effects and call her healthcare provider if they occur. When visual disturbances (flashes, blurring, spots) occur, the woman should avoid bright lighting. This side effect disappears within a few days or weeks after discontinuation of therapy. Hot flashes may be due to the antiestrogenic properties of clomiphene citrate. The woman can obtain some relief through increasing intake of fluids and using fans. Fecundability (the ability to become pregnant) declines with advancing age as described earlier; therefore, prolonged treatment with clomiphene is unjustified in women in their later reproductive years. Clomiphene treatment should generally be limited to the minimum effective dose and to no more than six ovulatory cycles. Failure to conceive after clomiphene induction is an indication to expand the diagnostic evaluation or to change the overall treatment plan if evaluation is complete.

DRUG GUIDE Clomiphene Citrate (Clomid, Milophene, Serophene)
Pregnancy Category: X

OVERVIEW OF ACTION

Clomiphene citrate stimulates follicular growth by stimulating the release of FSH and LH. Ovulation is expected to occur 5 to 9 days after the last dose. Used when anovulation is caused by hypothalamic dysfunction, luteal phase dysfunction, or oligo-ovulation, as seen in polycystic ovary syndrome (PCOS).

ROUTE, DOSAGE, FREQUENCY

Administered orally. Treatment should begin with a low dose, 50 mg/day (one tablet) for 5 days from cycle day 3 to day 7 or cycle day 5 to day 9. In nonresponders, the dose may be increased to 100 mg/day to a maximum of 250 mg/day, although doses in excess of 100 mg/day are not approved by the FDA (Wilson et al., 2010). May need to give estrogen simultaneously if decrease in cervical mucus occurs.

CONTRAINDICATIONS

Presence of ovarian enlargement, ovarian cysts, hyperstimulation syndrome, liver disease, visual problems, pregnancy. *Interaction:* Herbal: Black cohosh may antagonize infertility treatments (Wilson et al., 2010).

SIDE EFFECTS

Antiestrogenic effects may cause decrease in cervical mucus production and endometrial lining development. Other side effects include vasomotor flushes; abdominal distention and ovarian enlargement secondary to follicular growth (bloating) and multiple corpus luteum formation; pain, soreness, breast discomfort; nausea and vomiting; visual symptoms (spots, flashes); headaches, dryness or loss of hair; multiple pregnancies.

NURSING CONSIDERATIONS

- Determine if the couple has been advised to have sexual intercourse every other day for 1 week, beginning 5 days after the last day of medications. If insemination is the preferred treatment strategy ascertain that this is appropriately timed within the ovulatory window (24 to 36 hours of an LH surge).
- Instruct the couple on use of the BBT chart to assess whether ovulation has occurred, or instruct on the use of urinary LH kits to predict the onset of LH surge. Also inform the couple that plasma progesterone, cervical mucus, and postcoital tests may be done. Remind couples of the need to confirm the outcome with a pregnancy test with either a home pregnancy test or a serum blood test. Clomiphene cycle may be cancelled for ovarian hyperstimulation and subsequent risk of a high-order multiple pregnancy.

INSULIN SENSITIZING AGENTS Insulin resistance and hyperinsulinemia are now recognized as a common feature of polycystic ovary syndrome (PCOS) and a contributing cause of chronic anovulation. Anovulatory women with PCOS are hyperinsulinemic and subsequently are more resistant to clomiphene treatment. Recently, studies have shown that oral hypoglycemia agents (e.g., metformin and rosiglitazone) can induce ovulation in women with PCOS. Clinical trials are under way to determine the appropriateness of oral hypoglycemic agents with and without clomiphene in the infertility setting.

GONADOTROPINS Therapy using *human menopausal gonadotropins (hMG)*, which include menotropins (Repronex and Menopur) and urofollitropin (Bravelle), is indicated as a first line of therapy for the anovulatory infertile woman with low to normal levels of gonadotropins (FSH and LH) and as a second line of therapy in women who fail to ovulate or conceive with clomiphene citrate therapy and in women undergoing controlled ovarian stimulation with assisted reproduction. Menotropin is a mixture of FSH and LH, and urofollitropin is a further purified form and contains mainly FSH with trace amounts of LH. Immediately before injection, the powder is reconstituted with a diluent and injected subcutaneously.

More recently, however, recombinant gonadotropins (rFSH and rLH) have been produced through genetic engineering, giving rise to more consistent preparations. Recombinant FSH is homogenous and free of contaminants by proteins. It is marketed under the names Gonal-F (follitropin alpha) and Follistim (follitropin beta). Luveris, a recombinant form of LH, is used concomitantly with recombinant FSH in women with profound LH deficiency such as hypogonadotropic hypogonadism. It is thought that the use of recombinant gonadotropins will eventually become the preferred preparation and that the use of urinary preparations will be phased out (Figure 12-6 ■).

Gonadotropin therapy requires close observation with serum estradiol levels and ultrasound. Follicle development must be monitored to minimize the risk of multiple pregnancy and to avoid ovarian hyperstimulation syndrome. The daily dose of medication given is titrated based on serum estradiol and ultrasound findings. Then once optimal follicle growth has occurred, human chorionic gonadotropin (hCG) may be administered by either intramuscular or subcutaneous injection to induce final follicular maturation and stimulate ovulation. The couple is advised to have intercourse 24 to 36 hours after hCG administration and for the next 2 days. Women who elect to undergo ovarian stimulation with gonadotropins have usually passed through all other forms of management without conceiving. Strong emotional support and thorough education are needed because of the numerous office visits and injections. Often the partner is instructed, with return demonstration, to administer the daily injections.

BROMOCRIPTINE High prolactin levels may impair production of FSH and LH or block their action on the ovaries. When hyperprolactinemia accompanies anovulation, the infertility may be treated with bromocriptine (Parlodel). This medication acts directly on the prolactin-secreting cells in the anterior pituitary. It inhibits the pituitary's secretion of prolactin—thus

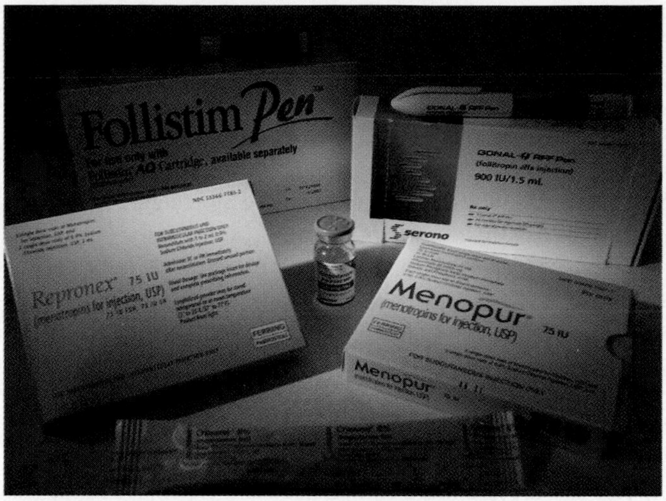

A

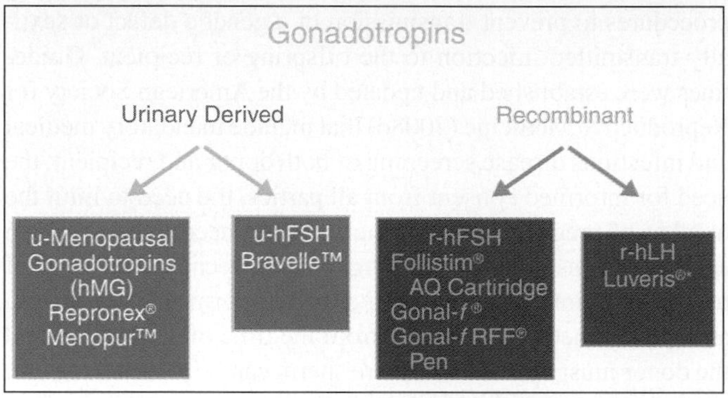

B

Figure 12-6 ■ A. A selection of commonly prescribed medications for ovulation induction. B. Derivation of gonadotropin medications.

Source: A. Courtesy of PENN Fertility Care, Philadelphia, PA. B. Courtesy of Serono, Inc., Rockland, MA.

preventing suppression of the pulsatile secretion of FSH and LH. This restores normal menstrual cycles and induces ovulation by allowing FSH and LH production. If treatment is successful, the tests of ovulatory function will indicate that ovulation is occurring with a normal luteal phase. Bromocriptine should be discontinued if pregnancy is suspected or at the anticipated time of ovulation because of its possible teratogenic effects. Other side effects, which include nausea, diarrhea, dizziness, headache, and fatigue, can be attributed to the dopaminergic action of bromocriptine. To mimimize side effects for women who are extremely sensitive, treatment may be initiated with a dose of 1.25 mg, slowly building tolerance toward the usual dose of 2.5 mg bid. Intravaginal administration also has been shown to decrease the occurrence of side effects (Wright & Johnson, 2008).

DANAZOL When endometriosis is determined to be the cause of the infertility, *danazol* (Danocrine) may be given to suppress ovulation and menstruation and to affect atrophy of the ectopic endometrial tissue. Temporary suppression has been shown to result in healing of the endometriosis. The treatment regimen may last for 6 to 12 months or longer, depending on the severity of the disease. Other pharmacologic treatments involve use of the oral contraceptives or oral medroxyprogesterone acetate, and GnRH agonists. For in-depth discussion of the management and care needed for endometriosis, see chapter 7 ∞.

GONADOTROPIN-RELEASING HORMONE (GNRH) *GnRH* is a therapeutic tool for inducing ovulation, but its use is limited to women who have insufficient endogenous release of GnRH. Administration is usually by continuous intravenous infusion accomplished by a portable infusion pump with a pulsatile mechanism worn on a belt around the waist. The length of treatment varies from 2 to 4 weeks, and hCG is also given to stimulate ovulation. The risk of multiple gestation and hyperstimulation of the ovaries is less than with gonadotropin therapy, and the treatment is also less expensive. Significant patient education and support are necessary for effective use of the pump. Some women find the pump cumbersome.

GnRH agonists (Lupron) and antagonists (Cetrotide and Ganirelix) are often used adjunctively with gonadotropin therapy to suppress the pituitary secretion of endogenous LH and FSH. This is often referred to as down-regulation.

PROGESTERONE Treatment of luteal phase defects may include the use of progesterone to augment luteal phase progesterone levels or the use of ovulation induction agents, such as clomiphene citrate or gonadotropins (discussed previously), which will augment proliferative phase FSH production of the developing follicle. Women with luteal phase defects have been found to have decreased FSH production in the proliferative phase. This is associated with a decline in luteal phase progesterone and estrogen production and is manifested by an out-of-phase endometrial biopsy. It is also common to use progesterone supplementation in conjunction with these ovulation induction agents for luteal phase support, thereby increasing endometrial receptivity for embryonic implantation. The initiation of progesterone (vaginal or rectal suppositories, intramuscular injections, or orally) occurs after the hCG injection in ovulation induction cycles or IVF cycles with gonadotropins; the treatment continues until pregnancy testing and may continue further if pregnancy testing is positive. Occasionally, hCG therapy may be used in the luteal phase to stimulate corpus luteum production of progesterone.

COMPLEMENTARY AND ALTERNATIVE THERAPIES FOR INFERTILITY Couples experiencing infertility may seek out alternative treatments. Some common treatments include acupuncture and herbs.

Acupuncture: Acupuncture is a therapy used in traditional Chinese medicine (TCM), and has become a popular complementary treatment. Acupuncture involves inserting sterile needles into specific points on the body to control the flow of chi, or life energy. Acupuncture treatment would focus on balancing the flow of chi in the kidneys and adrenal glands. Several clinical studies have shown acupuncture to be effective in treating infertility in both men and women (Cheong, Hung Yu Ng, & Ledger, 2008).

Herbal treatments: Herbs frequently recommended to treat infertility include ginseng and astragalus. Herbalists cite the healing and hormone-balancing effects of these herbs.

Ginseng has historically been used in TCM to enhance male virility and fertility. Several studies also cite ginseng, as well as astragalus, in enhancing in vitro sperm motility (Skidmore-Roth, 2010).

The nurse should be alert for signs that the couple is pursuing complementary therapies out of desperation. A sensitive, nonjudgmental approach will go a long way toward comforting a couple and assuring them that many complementary therapies used are helpful and not harmful.

Therapeutic Insemination

Therapeutic insemination has replaced the previously used term *artificial insemination* and involves depositing sperm at the cervical os or in the uterus by mechanical means. *Therapeutic donor insemination* (*TDI*) is the current term for use of donor semen, and *therapeutic husband insemination* (*THI*) is the current term for use of the husband's semen.

THI is generally indicated for such seminal deficiencies as oligospermia (low sperm count), asthenospermia (decreased motility), and teratospermia (low percentage, abnormal morphology); for anatomic defects that are accompanied by inadequate deposition of sperm, such as hypospadias (a congenital abnormal male urethral opening on the underside of the penis); and for ejaculatory dysfunction, such as retrograde ejaculation. THI is also indicated in unexplained infertility and some cases of female factor infertility, specifically infertility due to cervical factors, such as scant or inhospitable mucus, persistent cervicitis, or cervical stenosis. In such cases, IUI would be indicated to bypass the cervical factor. Because the seminal fluid contains high levels of prostaglandins, IUI prevents the violent reaction of nausea, severe cramps, abdominal pain, and diarrhea that can result from the absorption of prostaglandins by the uterine lining. Sperm preparation for IUI involves washing sperm from the seminal plasma. IUI, with or without ovulation induction therapy, is an option for many couples before more aggressive treatments such as IVF are employed.

TDI is considered in cases of azoospermia (absence of sperm), severe oligospermia or asthenospermia, inherited male sex-linked disorders, and autosomal dominant disorders. In the past several years, indications for donor insemination have expanded to include single women or lesbians desirous of pregnancy. Some states have specified the parental rights of the single woman and the donor, but most are silent on this issue.

TDI has become more complicated and expensive in the last decade because of the need for strict screening and processing procedures to prevent transmission of a genetic defect or sexually transmitted infection to the offspring or recipient. Guidelines were established and updated by the American Society for Reproductive Medicine (2008d) that include mandatory medical and infectious disease screening of both donor and recipient, the need for informed consent from all parties, the need to limit the number of pregnancies per donor, and the need to establish an accurate means of record keeping. Finally, because of the risk of transmitting infectious disease, donated sperm must be frozen and quarantined for 6 months from the time of acquisition and the donor must be retested before sperm can be released for use.

RESEARCH EVIDENCE IN PRACTICE: Cervical Insemination Versus Intrauterine Insemination of Donor Sperm

CLINICAL QUESTION

Which method of insemination of sperm results in the best pregnancy rate with the lowest costs and risks?

RESEARCH EVIDENCE

One out of ten couples is considered subfertile, in that they cannot conceive spontaneously within a year. Subfertility may be due to severe male factor infertility, and for these couples, insemination with donor sperm is a viable option. Insemination may be the only option for single women or same-sex female couples. There are two techniques for insemination—cervical and intrauterine. In cervical insemination, sperm is deposited near the cervix. In intrauterine insemination, the sperm is deposited in the uterine cavity. It has been assumed that intrauterine insemination is superior because the sperm is deposited more closely to the fallopian tubes and, therefore, has a better chance of fertilizing the ovum, resulting in a successful pregnancy. However, intrauterine insemination requires an invasive procedure of dilating the cervix and inserting instrumentation into the uterus. This procedure is more costly than cervical insemination, can be painful, and carries the risk of uterine perforation and infection.

In a systematic review published in the Cochrane Collaborative (a strong source of high-quality research evidence) and a meta-analysis of studies, intrauterine insemination was found to be superior to cervical insemination in terms of achievement of pregnancy. There were no differences in the two approaches in adverse outcomes or complications.

WHAT QUESTIONS REMAIN UNANSWERED?

Intrauterine insemination requires laboratory preparation of cryosperm and administration of follicle-stimulating drugs in the mother. Cervical insemination often uses live sperm with no stimulating drugs. Would the less invasive method be as effective if follicle-stimulating drugs were administered?

WHAT IS BEST PRACTICE?

Intrauterine insemination with cryopreserved sperm, preceded by follicle-stimulating drugs for the mother, has the most successful pregnancy rate without increased adverse complications.

CRITICAL THINKING

Are there couples for whom the less invasive cervical procedure may be as effective? How can the woman be counseled about the risks and benefits of each procedure?

References

Besselink, D., Farquhar, C., Kremer, J., Marjoribanks, J., & O'Brien, P. (2008). Cervical insemination versus intra-uterine insemination of donor sperm for subfertility. *Cochrane Database of Systematic Reviews,* Issue 2. Art. No.: CD000317. doi:10.1002/14651858.CD001838.pub3

Ferrara, I., Balet, R., & Grudzinskas, J. (2002). Intrauterine insemination with frozen donor sperm: Pregnancy outcome in relation to ovarian stimulation regime. *Human Reproduction, 17*(9), 2320–2324.

VanWeert, J., Repping, S., VanVoorhis, B., VanderVeen, F., Bossuyt, P., & Mol, B. (2004). Performance of postwash total motile sperm count as a predictor of pregnancy: A meta-analysis. *Fertility and Sterility, 2*(3), 612–620.

Numerous factors must be evaluated before TDI is performed. Has every possible effort been made to diagnose and treat the cause of the male infertility? Do tests indicate normal ovulation and sperm/ovum transport in the woman? Has the couple had an opportunity to discuss this option with an infertility counselor to explore the issues of secrecy, disclosure, and potential feelings of loss that the couple (particularly the male partner) may feel because of their inability to have a genetic child? After making the decision, the couple should allow themselves time to assess their concerns further and explore their feelings individually and together to ensure that this option is acceptable to both.

In Vitro Fertilization

In vitro fertilization (IVF) is selectively used in cases in which infertility has resulted from tubal factors, mucus abnormalities, male infertility, unexplained infertility, male and female immunologic infertility, and cervical factors. In IVF, a woman's eggs are collected from her ovaries, fertilized in the laboratory, and placed into her uterus after normal embryo development has begun. If the procedure is successful, the embryo continues to develop in the uterus, and pregnancy proceeds naturally.

DEVELOPING CULTURAL COMPETENCE
Infertility Treatments

The acceptance of infertility treatments varies widely around the world. Some belief systems do not allow various treatments, because using a treatment is considered interfering with God's design or because the treatment itself is seen as tainted or sinful. For example, fertility practices in Arab cultures are influenced by traditional Arab Bedouin values that support tribal dominance and beliefs that "God decides family sizes." In Arab cultures, procreation is the purpose of marriage.

If a couple is infertile, the approved methods for treating infertility are limited to use of therapeutic insemination using the husband's sperm and IVF involving the fertilization of the wife's ovum by the husband's sperm because of lineage concerns (Purnell & Paulanka, 2008).

Sterility in a woman can lead to rejection and divorce. Also with the advent of ICSI (intracytoplasmic sperm injection), male-initiated divorce is becoming more common for aging wives of infertile husbands (Inhorn, 2006). Contemporary Islamic religious opinion forbids any kind of egg, embryo, or semen donation, as well as surrogacy (Inhorn, 2006).

In Jewish cultures, infertile couples are to try all possible means to have children, including egg and sperm donation. However, Orthodox Jewish opinion is virtually unanimous in prohibiting artificial insemination when the semen donor is a Jewish man other than the woman's husband, because it may constitute adultery (Purnell & Paulanka, 2008). If the infertility is because of a male factor, artificial insemination with sperm from a non-Jewish sperm donor is acceptable because "Jewishness" is conferred through the matriline. IVF and embryo transfer (ET) are also acceptable artificial insemination methods because they do not involve putting sperm into another's wife (Schenker, 2010).

The potential for a successful pregnancy with IVF is maximized by replacing three to four embryos (rather than one). For this reason, fertility drugs are used to induce ovulation before the process. Follicular growth is monitored frequently with ultrasound and hormonal assays. Monitoring usually begins around cycle day 5, and medications are titrated according to individual response. When the follicles have grown to an appropriate size, hCG is given to induce final egg maturation and control the induction of ovulation. Egg retrieval is performed approximately 35 hours later, before ovulation occurs.

In the majority of cases, egg retrieval is performed by a transvaginal approach under ultrasound guidance (Figure 12-7A ■). It is an outpatient procedure performed with intravenous sedation and a cervical block for anesthesia. A needle guide that helps direct the aspirating needle through the posterior vaginal wall into the follicle is attached to the vaginal ultrasound probe (Figure 12-7B ■). Many follicles can be aspirated with only one puncture, and the procedure generally lasts no more than 30 minutes. Once the eggs are fertilized and progress to the embryo stage, the

Application: In Vitro Fertilization

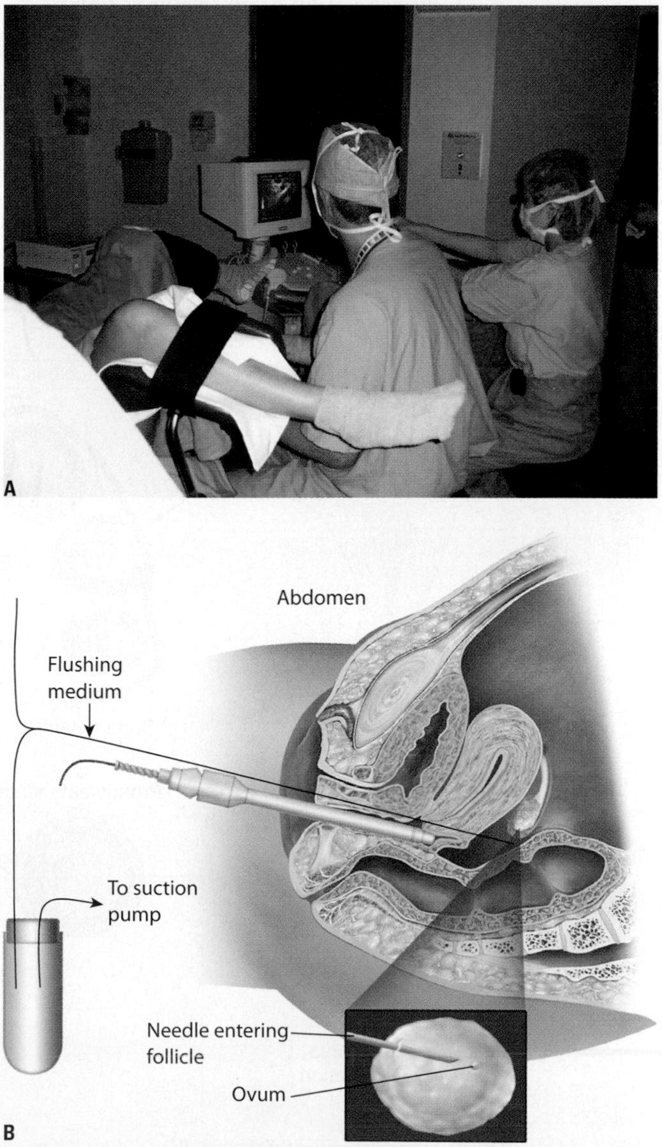

Figure 12-7 ■ A. Operating room setup for ultrasound-guided oocyte retrieval. B. Transvaginal ultrasound-guided oocyte retrieval.

Source: A. Courtesy of PENN Fertility Care, Philadelphia, PA. B. Courtesy of Serono, Inc., Rockland, MA.

embryos are placed in the uterus. This occurs 1 to 2 days after conception. After the procedure, the woman is advised to engage in only minimal activity for 12 to 24 hours. Progesterone supplementation is prescribed to promote implantation and support the early pregnancy; therefore, the woman will not have a period even if she is not pregnant (the pregnancy is usually determined by transvaginal ultrasound).

Sperm used to fertilize the eggs in vitro can be obtained naturally or surgically via microsurgical epididymal sperm aspiration (MESA) and testicular sperm aspiration (TESA). These are procedures that address severe male factor infertility. MESA and TESA involve the retrieval of sperm from the gonadal tissue of men who have azoospermia or an ejaculatory disorder. Percutaneous epididymal sperm aspiration (PESA) and TESA are replacing MESA as the preferred techniques for retrieval of sperm because they are not surgical procedures. ICSI is a microscopic procedure to inject a single sperm into the outer layer of an ovum so that fertilization will occur (Devine, 2008).

Success with IVF depends on many factors, the two most important of which are the woman's age and the indication. Women with an average of three cycles of IVF have a good chance of achieving pregnancy. Many couples find the emotional, physical, and financial costs of going beyond three cycles too great. Costs vary by treatment and by region of the country (ASRM, 2010). Clinical birth rates in the United States reported by the Society of Assisted Technology (SART) were 50% per egg donation for women regardless of age or indication (ASRM, 2008d). The increase in maternal and neonatal morbidity associated with IVF because of the multiple gestation rates remains an issue.

Other Assisted Reproductive Techniques

Other assisted reproductive techniques include procedures for transferring gametes, zygotes, or embryos; cryopreservation of embryos; IVF using donor oocytes; micromanipulation techniques; and use of a gestational carrier (Figure 12-8 ■).

GAMETE INTRAFALLOPIAN TRANSFER **Gamete intrafallopian transfer (GIFT)** involves the retrieval of oocytes by laparoscopy; immediate placement of the oocytes in a catheter with washed, motile sperm; and placement of the gametes into the fimbriated end of the fallopian tube. Fertilization occurs in the fallopian tube as with normal conception (in vivo), rather than in the laboratory (in vitro). The fertilized egg then travels through the fallopian tube to the uterus for implantation as in normal reproduction. GIFT may be more acceptable than other procedures such as ZIFT to adherents of some religions (Roman Catholic), because fertilization does not occur outside the woman's body.

GIFT has proven to be a very effective therapy for couples whose infertility results from various seminal deficiencies, unexplained factors, cervical factors, immunologic factors, and endometriosis when less aggressive means of therapy have failed. In cases of male factor infertility, GIFT offers an opportunity for

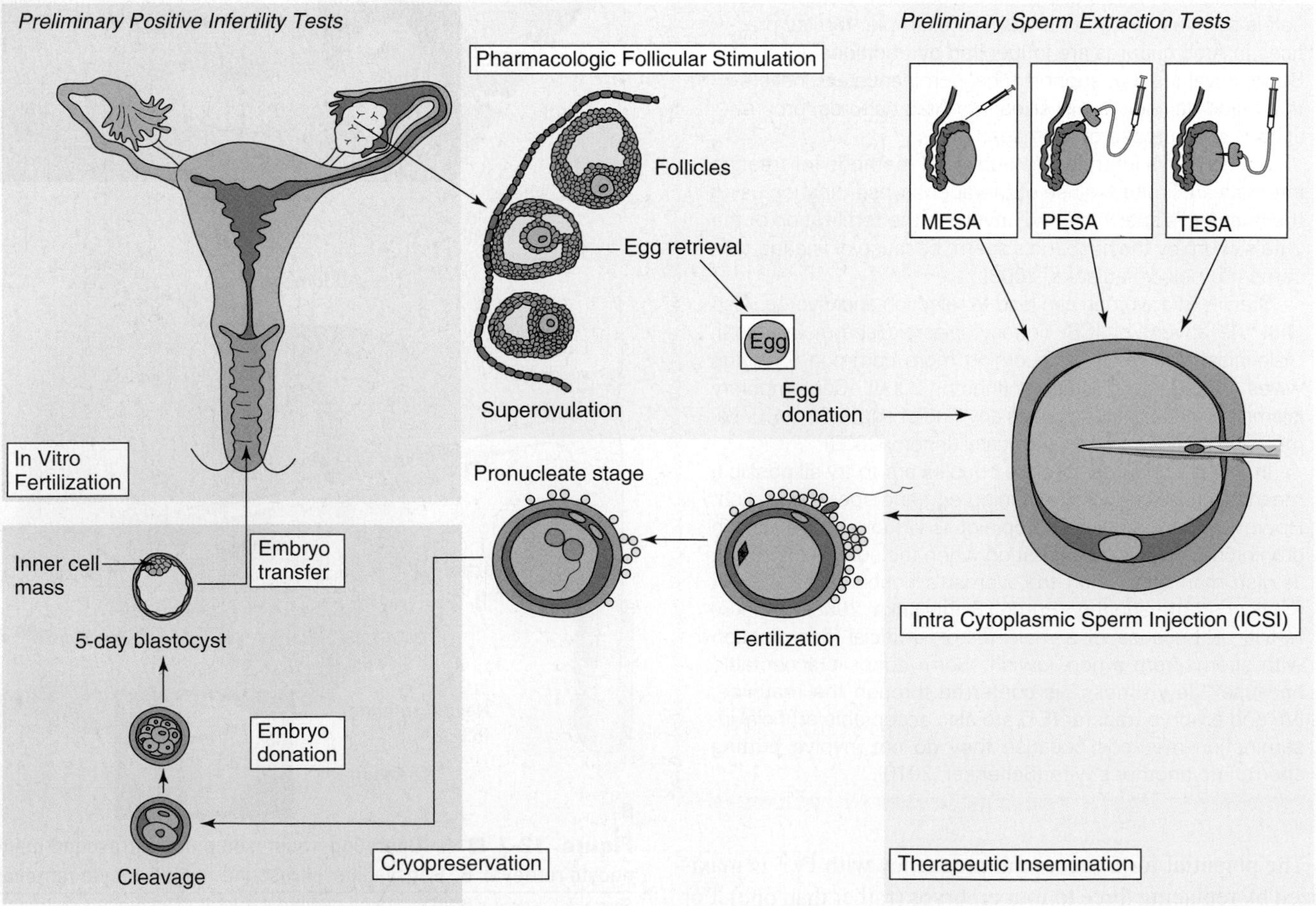

Figure 12-8 ■ Assisted reproductive techniques.

the egg and an adequate concentration of sperm to meet in the fallopian tube; with coitus, in contrast, sperm with low count or motility may never reach the tube. The major prerequisite for GIFT is the presence of at least one normal fallopian tube. It is not an appropriate therapy for any woman with a history of pelvic inflammatory disease, tubal disease, or ectopic gestation because the passage of the fertilized ova to the uterus is slowed, thereby increasing the chance of sustaining an ectopic tubal pregnancy.

From the GIFT technology evolved several other transfer procedures such as **zygote intrafallopian transfer (ZIFT)** and **tubal embryo transfer (TET)**. In these procedures eggs are retrieved and incubated with the man's sperm. However, the eggs are transferred back to the woman's body at a much earlier stage of cell division than in IVF and, as in GIFT, are placed in the fallopian tube or tubes and not in the uterus. In TET, the placement is done at the embryo stage. These procedures allow fertilization to be documented, which is not possible with GIFT, and the pregnancy rate is theoretically increased when the fertilized ovum is placed in the fallopian tube.

When considering IVF and the transfer procedures, several factors must be weighed. IVF success rates approximate those that have been achieved with the transfer procedures, and IVF is a much less invasive and costly procedure. For these reasons, the transfer procedures have lost some acceptance and IVF techniques are more often used.

EMBRYO CRYOPRESERVATION Research has shown that replacing three to four embryos in a treatment cycle offers the best chances for pregnancy. Replacing more than four only increases the chance for a multiple pregnancy. To minimize this risk, excess embryos may be stored using freezing, or cryopreservation. Should a pregnancy not ensue, frozen embryos can be thawed. After they are maintained in culture for a short time to confirm resumption of growth, they are replaced in the woman's uterus at the appropriate time in her menstrual cycle. Thus freezing affords the couple another attempt at pregnancy without having to undergo stimulation and egg retrieval again.

Ethical issues to consider in this situation include the following: Who has legal custody of the embryos? How long can they be frozen? What options does the couple have in the event of divorce, if one or both partners die, or if they do not wish to use the embryos at a later date? These issues must be addressed with all couples so that they can make informed decisions when executing their consent forms and legal statements. Reproductive endocrine nurses need to be involved in establishing standards and guidelines for assisted reproduction technologies. Clinically, the reproductive endocrine nurse is instrumental in providing support, education, and counseling to couples considering assisted reproductive methods. The nurse assesses the couple for personal, marital, and parenting difficulties and initiates interventions that help establish family roles and bonds. Follow-up care mechanisms can be set, thereby aiding in individual growth, marital stability, and family development.

IN VITRO FERTILIZATION USING DONOR OOCYTES The use of donor eggs, a natural extension of IVF, is reserved for women who do not produce viable eggs because of premature ovarian failure, surgical removal of the ovaries, advanced maternal age, chemotherapy or radiation exposure, or inherent oocyte defects but who do have a functional uterus. Women with normal ovarian function may also benefit from egg donation if they have an autosomal dominant or sex-linked genetic disorder such as hemophilia or Duchenne muscular dystrophy.

Oocyte donors may be either known or anonymous. In either case, both donors and recipients undergo psychologic evaluation and counseling to ensure that all parties have explored and discussed potential issues and are comfortable with the process. The donors are subject to extensive medical and genetic testing. The FDA has instituted screening and testing requirements for all tissue donors, which includes donors of oocytes, sperm, and embryos (ASRM, 2008d). The nurse functions as a case manager by coordinating the many tests, procedures, and educational and counseling sessions that are involved for the donor and recipient couple.

Once donor eggs are available, they are inseminated with the sperm of the recipient's partner. After fertilization has occurred and embryo development has begun, the embryos are placed in the recipient's uterus. Pregnancies can be achieved and maintained in these women with an estrogen/progesterone replacement protocol. When pregnancy occurs, hormonal support is continued until the placenta is capable of supporting the pregnancy, usually at 10 to 12 weeks.

EMBRYO DONATION Much like egg donation, embryo donation offers couples another option in creating a family. Couples who have gone through assisted reproductive technology (ART) and have completed their family may choose to donate their cryopreserved embryos to another couple. There are two types of donation, known or directed donation and anonymous donation. Couples interested in being the recipients of these donations include those with severe or untreatable male and female factor infertility, those who have experienced repeated treatment failures or multiple pregnancy losses not due to implantation problems, and those at risk for transmitting genetic diseases to their offspring. Screening and assessment guidelines have been established by the American Society of Reproductive Medicine (2008d).

MICROMANIPULATION AND BLASTOMERE ANALYSIS Micromanipulation allows individual eggs and sperm to be handled through the use of very fine, specialized instruments. Using the micromanipulators allows the clinician to handle cells under the microscope with magnification of 200 to 400 times and to inject a sperm cell directly into an egg. This procedure, known as *ICSI,* has revolutionized the treatment of severe male factor infertility. The procedure has achieved fertilization in cases of extremely low sperm concentrations, in cases of absence of motility, and in cases where previous IVF therapy failed.

Assisted embryo hatching is another micromanipulation procedure that has proved to be an effective adjunct therapy in IVF. It is indicated for women in whom the normal "hatching" process may be impeded because of a hardening or thickening of the zona pellucida, most commonly seen in women of advanced maternal age. Assisted hatching involves creating a small opening in the zona pellucida of the embryo using micromanipulators (Figure 12-9 ■).

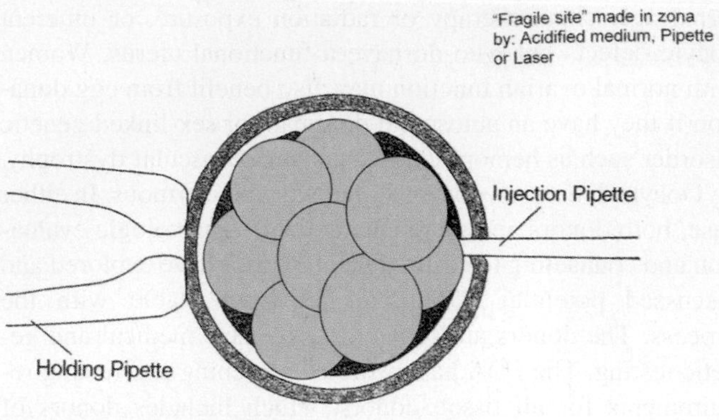

Figure 12-9 ■ Assisted hatching of embryo.

Source: Courtesy of Serono, Inc., Rockland, MA.

The small opening may facilitate the natural hatching process, allowing the embryo to escape from the zona pellucida and interact with the endometrium for implantation.

PREIMPLANTATION GENETIC DIAGNOSIS (PGD) Other recent advances in micromanipulation allow a single cell to be removed from the oocyte (polar body) or embryo (blastomere or trophoectoderm cells) for genetic study. Couples at risk for having a detectable single gene or chromosomal anomaly may wish to undergo such preimplantation genetic testing. *Preimplantation genetic diagnosis* (PGD) is a term used when one or both genetic parents carry a gene mutation or balanced chromosome rearrangement and testing is performed to determine whether that mutation or unbalanced chromosomal compliment has been passed to the oocyte or embryo (ASRM, 2008i). Preimplantation genetic screening (PGS) is a term used when the genetic parents are known or presumed to have normal chromosomes, and their embryos are screened for aneuploidy with the purpose of increasing the likelihood of a viable pregnancy with normal chromosomes (ASRM, 2008i). Specific genetic disorders or chromosome abnormalities can be tested for using the polymerase chain reaction (PCR) technique or fluorescence in situ hybridization (FISH). The cell's deoxyribonucleic acid (DNA) is amplified 1,000,000 times and examined so that embryos affected with a particular genetic disease or chromosome abnormality are not placed in the mother. Results of genetic testing on the preimplantation embryos are available in 4 to 24 hours, so unaffected embryos may still be transferred during the required biologic window of time without the need for cryopreservation. Both PGD and PGS can produce false positive and false negative results. Prenatal diagnostic testing to confirm the results is strongly encouraged (ASRM, 2008i).

The diagnosis of genetic disorders before implantation provides couples with the option of forgoing the attempt to establish a pregnancy and thereby avoiding a difficult decision about terminating an affected pregnancy (Kuliev & Verlinsky, 2010). This technology also raises several ethical issues, including the following:

- Identification of couples at risk. There is a need for criteria that identify couples at risk for diseases that constitute significant hardship and suffering so that "wrongful birth" cases can be avoided.
- Availability of and access to centers providing PGD. Should society provide access for those at risk for genetic transfer of disease but without the financial resources to pay for the services?
- Analysis of blastomeres for sex chromosome testing when a genetic disorder carried on the sex chromosomes is suspected. In X-linked diseases, this may mean selecting against the blastomere with the Y chromosome.
- Identification of late-onset diseases. The Human Genome Project has aided in the identification of genetic markers for late-onset disease. Couples may wish to choose to implant blastomeres that do not carry these markers.
- Effect on the offspring as a result of removing cells from the embryo.
- Selection for nonmedical reasons and potential concern of eugenics "designer babies."

SPERM SORTING Sperm sorting is a technology designed to separate sperm that primarily produce females or those that primarily produce males. Sorted sperm enriched with male- or female-producing sperm is then used for IUI or IVF. The accuracy depends on the laboratory that performs the sorting and the technology it uses. Study data indicate that 9 out of 10 patients sorting for a girl will conceive a female. Approximately 3 out of 4 patients that sort for a boy will conceive a male. This technology is used to increase the likelihood of having a child of a particular gender in couples at risk for an X-linked genetic disorder or for couples interested in family balancing (gender selection when a couple has two or more children of the same gender) (Gleicher & Nakajima, 2009).

IN VITRO FERTILIZATION USING A GESTATIONAL CARRIER A *gestational carrier* is a woman who has contracted with the infertile woman or couple to carry an embryo/fetus that is not genetically her own offspring. This must be distinguished from surrogate motherhood, wherein the surrogate is both gestational carrier and gamete donor. IVF using a gestational carrier is appropriate for the infertile woman who is able to produce her own eggs but unable to carry a pregnancy because of (1) congenital absence or surgical removal of her uterus; (2) a reproductively impaired uterus, myomas, uterine synechiae (adhesion of uterus), or any other congenital abnormalities; or (3) a medical condition that might be life threatening during pregnancy such as diabetes; immunologic problems; or a severe heart, kidney, or liver disease. Use of a gestational carrier allows a couple with any of these conditions to have a child who is a genetic relation (American College of Obstetricians and Gynecologists [ACOG], 2008). All participants are required to have medical and psychologic screening as well as legal counsel before acceptance into the program.

Adoption

Infertile couples consider various alternatives for resolving their infertility; adoption is one option that will be considered at several points during the treatment process. As couples begin to consider adoption, an important aspect of this exploration is the reading of books, magazines, and informational Web sites such as the National Adoption Information Clearinghouse; attending adoption support groups and conferences; and meeting with adoptive parents to discuss their experiences with adoption.

The adoption of an infant in the United States can be difficult and frustrating, often involving long waiting periods, continual setbacks, and high costs. Thus many couples seek international adoptions or consider adopting older children, children with disabilities, or children of mixed racial parentage, because the adoption process in such cases is quicker and more children are available. Nurses in the community can assist couples considering adoption by providing information on community resources for adoption as well as by providing support throughout the adoption process. Informational books, Web sites, and support groups such as San Francisco RESOLVE's "Living Without Children" are available for couples who remain childless by choice or circumstances.

Pregnancy After Infertility

The feeling of being infertile does not necessarily disappear with pregnancy. Although there may be initial ecstasy, the couple may also face a whole new arena of fear and anxieties, and the parents-to-be often do not know where they "fit in." They may feel a great sense of loss and isolation because those who have had no trouble conceiving cannot relate to the physical and emotional pain they endured to achieve the pregnancy. Contact with their past "infertile" support system may vanish when peers learn that the couple has resolved their infertility. Although the desperation to become pregnant may have superseded the couple's ability to acknowledge their concerns about undergoing various treatments or procedures, questions about the repeated cycle of fertility drugs or the achievement of pregnancy through IVF technology or cryopreservation may now arise. The expectant couple may be very concerned about the potential of these treatments for adverse effects on the fetus (McGrath et al., 2010; Wright & Johnson, 2008). Couples may need much reassurance throughout the pregnancy to allay these anxieties. The nurse can assist couples who conceive after infertility by acknowledging their past experience of infertility treatment; validating their fears and anxieties as they face childbirth classes, birth, and parenting issues; and providing education and support regarding what to anticipate physically and emotionally throughout the pregnancy. The nurse can also counsel couples that infertility due to nonstructural causes may correct itself following a successful pregnancy and delivery; therefore, postdelivery contraception counseling may be warranted. These interventions will go a long way toward normalizing the experience for the couple.

Recurrent Pregnancy Loss

Recurrent pregnancy loss (RPL) is a disease distinct from infertility, defined by two or more failed pregnancies (ASRM, 2008b). Estimates suggest that RPL occurs in 0.5% to 1% of fertile couples attempting pregnancy (Warren & Silver, 2008). There are several etiologies, including maternal medical complications, chromosome abnormalities and other genetic conditions, autoimmune disorders, and thrombotic causes. However, in up to 50% of couples with RPL, an etiology will not be identified.

Maternal medical complications associated with RPL include luteal phase defects or progesterone deficiency and congenital uterine abnormalities. Autoimmune disorders such as antiphospholipid antibody syndrome, alloimmune factors, and blood group isoimmunization have been associated with RPL. Chromosome abnormalities such as recurrent aneuploidy and parental chromosome abnormalities are associated with RPL. One partner will have a balanced chromosome rearrangement in 3% to 5% of couples with RPL (Warren & Silver, 2008). Single gene disorders such as alpha-thalassemia major, some metabolic diseases, and some X-linked dominant disorders that are lethal *in utero* in males can account for RPL. Hereditary thrombophilias, such as factor V Leiden, prothrombin gene, protein C or S deficiency, and antithrombin III deficiency are known to predispose individuals to pregnancy complications including RPL.

Internet Resources

NURSING CARE MANAGEMENT

Care Plan Activity: Infertile Couple

Infertility therapy taxes a couple's financial, physical, and emotional resources. Treatment can be costly, and often insurance coverage is limited. Years of effort and numerous evaluations and examinations may take place before a conception occurs, if one occurs at all. In a society that values children and considers them to be the natural result of marriage, infertile couples may face a myriad of tensions and discrimination.

The clinic nurse needs to be constantly aware of the emotional needs of the couple confronting infertility evaluation and treatment. Often an intact marriage will become stressed with the intrusive but necessary infertility procedures and treatments. Constant attention to temperature charts and instructions about their sex life from a person outside the relationship naturally affect the spontaneity of a couple's interactions.

Tests and treatments may heighten feelings of frustration or anger between partners. The need to share this intimate area of a relationship, especially when one or the other is identified as "the cause" of infertility, may precipitate feelings of guilt or shame. Infertility often becomes a central focus for role identity, especially for women (Devine, 2008).

The couple may experience feelings of loss of control, feelings of reduced competency and defectiveness, loss of status and ambiguity as a couple, a sense of social stigma, stress on the marital and sexual relationship, and a strained relationship with healthcare providers. The nurse's roles can be summarized as those of counselor, educator, and advocate.

Tasks of the infertile couple and appropriate nursing interventions are summarized in Table 12-7. Throughout the evaluation process, nurses can play a key role in lessening the stress these couples must endure by providing them with appropriate resources and accurate information about what treatment entails and what physical, emotional, and financial demands they can anticipate throughout the process (Paterno, 2008).

The nurse's ability to assess and respond to emotional and educational needs is essential to give infertile couples control and help them negotiate the treatment process. An assessment tool such as an infertility questionnaire (Table 12-8) can be helpful. Extensive and repeated explanations and written instruction may be necessary because the couple's anxiety often overwhelms

TABLE 12-7 Tasks of the Infertile Couple

TASKS	NURSING INTERVENTIONS
Recognize how infertility affects their lives and express feelings (may be negative toward self or mate)	Supportive: help to understand and facilitate free expression of feelings
Grieve the loss of potential offspring	Help to recognize feelings
Evaluate reasons for wanting a child	Help to understand motives
Decide about management	Identify alternatives; facilitate partner communication

Source: Reprinted with permission from Sawatzky, M. (1981). Tasks of the infertile couple. Journal of Obstetric, Gynecologic, and Neonatal Nursing, 10, *132. Copyright by the Association of Women's Health, Obstetric and Neonatal Nurses. All rights reserved.*

their ability to retain all the information given. It is important to use a nursing framework that recognizes the multidimensional needs of the infertile individual or couple within physical, social, psychologic, spiritual, and environmental contexts.

Infertility may be perceived as a loss by one or both partners. Affected individuals have described this as loss of their relationship with spouse, family, or friends; their health; their status or prestige; their self-esteem and self-confidence; their security; and the potential child. Any one of these types of losses may lead to depression and, in many cases, the crisis of infertility evokes feelings similar to ones associated with all these losses (Paterno, 2008). Each couple passes through several stages, not unlike those identified by Kübler-Ross: surprise, denial, anger, isolation, guilt, grief, and resolution. The impact of these feelings on the couple and how fast they move into resolution, if ever, may depend on the cause and duration of treatment. Each partner may progress through the stages at different rates (McGrath et al., 2010). Nonjudgmental acceptance and a professional, caring attitude on the nurse's part can go far to dissipate the negative emotions the couple may experience while going through these stages.

This is also a time when the nurse may assess the quality of the couple's relationship: Are they able and willing to communicate verbally and share feelings? Are they mutually supportive? The answers to these questions may help the nurse identify areas of strength and weakness and construct an appropriate plan of care.

Referral to mental health professionals is helpful when the emotional issues become too disruptive in the couple's relationship or life. Couples should be made aware of infertility support and education organizations such as RESOLVE (National Infertility Association), which may help meet some of these needs and validate their feelings. Finally, individual or group counseling with other infertile couples may help the couple resolve feelings brought about by their own difficult situation.

TABLE 12-8 Infertility Questionnaire

Self-Image

1. I feel bad about my body because of our inability to have a child.
2. Since our infertility, I feel I can do anything as well as I used to.
3. I feel as attractive as before our infertility.
4. I feel less masculine/feminine because of our inability to have a child.
5. Compared with others, I feel I am a worthwhile person.
6. Lately, I feel I am sexually attractive to my wife/husband.
7. I feel I will be incomplete as a man/woman if we cannot have a child.
8. Having an infertility problem makes me feel physically incompetent.

Guilt/Blame

1. I feel guilty about somehow causing our infertility.
2. I wonder if our infertility problem is due to something I did in the past.
3. My spouse makes me feel guilty about our problem.
4. There are times when I blame my spouse for our infertility.
5. I feel I am being punished because of our infertility.

Sexuality

1. Lately I feel I am able to respond to my spouse sexually.
2. I feel sex is a duty, not a pleasure.
3. Since our infertility problem, I enjoy sexual relations with my spouse.
4. We have sexual relations for the purpose of trying to conceive.
5. Sometimes I feel like a "sex machine," programmed to have sex during the fertile period.
6. Impaired fertility has helped our sexual relationship.
7. Our inability to have a child has increased my desire for sexual relations.
8. Our inability to have a child has decreased my desire for sexual relations.

Note: The questionnaire is scored on a Likert scale, with responses ranging from "strongly agree" to "strongly disagree." Each question is scored separately, and the mean score is determined for each section (Self-Image, Guilt/Blame, and Sexuality). The total mean score is then divided by 3. A final mean score of greater than 3 indicates distress.

Source: Reproduced with permission from AWHONN. (1985). Bernstein, J., Potts, N., and Mattox, J. H., Assessment of psychological dysfunction association with infertility. Journal of Obstetric, Gynecologic, and Neonatal Nursing. 14*(Suppl.), 64S, Table 1. Washington, DC: Author. © 1985 by the Association of Women's Health, Obstetric and Neonatal Nurses. All rights reserved.*

Genetic Disorders

Even when conception has been achieved, families can have special reproductive concerns. The desired and expected outcome of any pregnancy is the birth of a healthy, "perfect" baby. Parents experience grief, fear, and anger when they discover that their baby has been born with a defect or a genetic disease. Such an abnormality may be evident at birth or may not appear for some time. The baby may have inherited a disorder from one parent or both, creating guilt and strife within the family.

Regardless of the type or scope of the problem, parents will have many questions: "What did I do?" "What caused it?" "How do I cope with it?" "Will it happen again?" The nurse must anticipate the parents' questions and concerns, direct the family to the appropriate resources, and support the family. To do so, the nurse must have a basic knowledge of genetics and genetic counseling. Professional nurses can help expedite this questioning process if they understand the principles involved and can direct the family to the appropriate resources.

Chromosomes and Chromosomal Analysis

All hereditary material is carried on tightly coiled strands of deoxyribonucleic acid (DNA) known as **chromosomes**. The

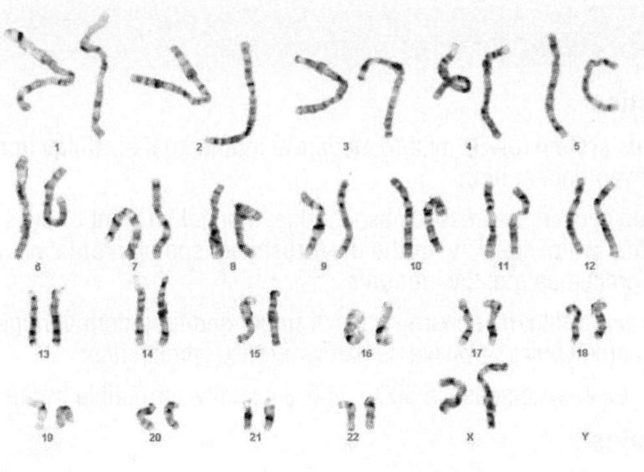

Figure 12-10 ■ Normal female karyotype.

Source: Courtesy of Susan Olson, PhD., The Oregon Health & Science University Cytogenics Laboratory.

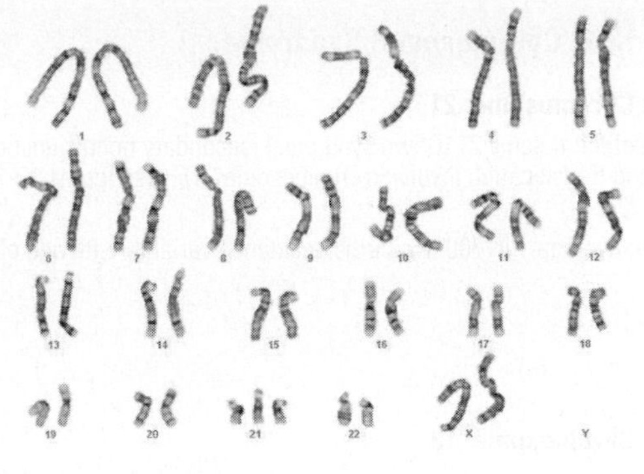

Figure 12-12 ■ Karyotype of a female who has trisomy 21, Down syndrome. Note the extra chromosome 21.

Source: Courtesy of Susan Olson, PhD., The Oregon Health & Science University Cytogenics Laboratory.

chromosomes carry the *genes,* the smallest unit of inheritance, as discussed in greater detail in chapter 11 ∞. The Human Genome Project has made remarkable advances toward determining the exact DNA sequence of human genes and the precise genes that are associated with certain abnormalities, such as fragile X syndrome and cystic fibrosis, as discussed later in this chapter (Ward, 2008).

All *somatic* (*body*) *cells* contain 46 chromosomes, which is the *diploid* number; the sperm and egg contain half as many (23) chromosomes, or the *haploid* number (see chapter 11 ∞). There are 23 pairs of homologous chromosomes (a matched pair of chromosomes, one inherited from each parent). Twenty-two of the pairs are known as **autosomes** (nonsex chromosomes), and one pair is the sex chromosome, X and Y. A normal female has a 46, XX chromosome constitution, the normal male, 46, XY (Figures 12-10 ■ and 12-11 ■).

The **karyotype**, or pictorial analysis of an individual's chromosomes, is usually obtained from specially treated and stained peripheral blood lymphocytes. Placental tissue or amniotic fluid can be obtained prenatally and sent for karyotyping of the fetus.

Chromosome abnormalities can occur in either the autosomes or the sex chromosomes and can be divided into two categories: abnormalities of number and abnormalities of structure. Even small alterations in chromosomes can cause problems, especially those associated with delayed growth and

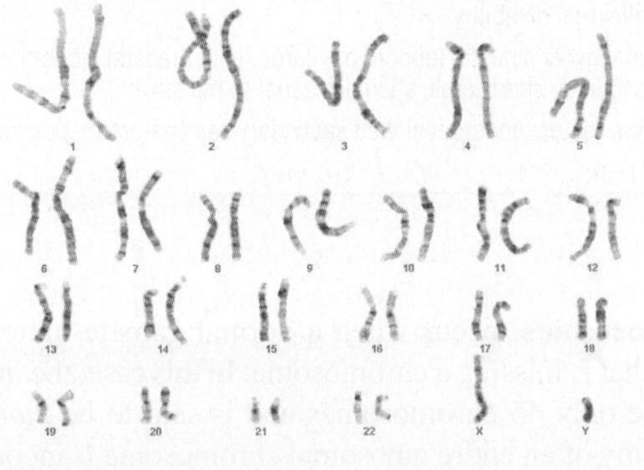

Figure 12-11 ■ Normal male karyotype.

Source: Courtesy of Susan Olson, PhD., The Oregon Health & Science University Cytogenics Laboratory.

development. Some of these abnormalities can also be passed on to other offspring. Thus, in some cases, chromosomal analysis is appropriate even if clinical manifestations are mild.

Abnormalities of Chromosome Number

Abnormalities of chromosome number are most commonly seen as trisomies, monosomies, and as mosaicism. In all three cases, the abnormality is most often caused by nondisjunction, a failure of paired chromosomes to separate during cell division. If nondisjunction occurs in either the sperm or the egg before fertilization, the resulting zygote (fertilized egg) will have an abnormal chromosome makeup in all of the cells (trisomy or monosomy). If nondisjunction occurs after fertilization, the developing zygote will have cells with two or more different chromosome makeups, evolving into two or more different cell lines (mosaicism).

Trisomies are the product of the union of a normal gamete (egg or sperm) with a gamete that contains an extra chromosome. The individual will have 47 chromosomes and be trisomic (have three copies of the same chromosome) for whichever chromosome is extra (Table 12-9). Down syndrome is the most common trisomy abnormality seen in children (Figure 12-12 ■). The presence of the extra chromosome 21 produces distinctive clinical features (Figure 12-13 ■). Although children born with Down syndrome can have a variety of physical ailments, advances in medical science and early intervention services have improved their quality of life and extended their life expectancy.

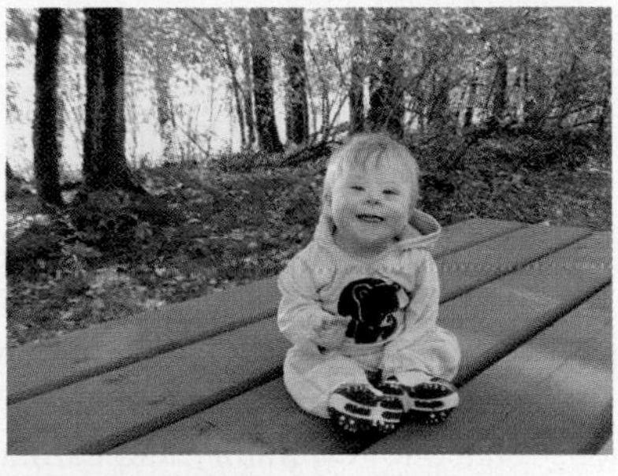

Figure 12-13 ■ A boy with Down syndrome.

Source: Mariah Buhman, photographer.

TABLE 12-9 Chromosomal Syndromes

Altered Chromosome: 21	**Characteristics**
Genetic defect: trisomy 21 (Down syndrome) (secondary nondisjunction or unbalanced translocation involving chromosome 21) (see Figures 12-12 and 12-13) Incidence: average 1 in 700 live births, incidence variable with age of woman	Central nervous system (CNS): mild to moderate intellectual disability (mental retardation); hypotonia at birth Head: flattened occiput; depressed nasal bridge; mongoloid slant of eyes; epicanthal folds; white specking of the iris (Brushfield spots); protrusion of the tongue; high, arched palate; low-set ears Hands: broad, short fingers; abnormalities of finger and foot; dermal ridge patterns (dermatoglyphics); transverse palmar crease (simian line) Other: congenital heart disease in 30% to 60%, usually correctible by surgery.
Altered Chromosome: 18	**Characteristics**
Genetic defect: trisomy 18 Incidence: 1 in 3000 live births	CNS: intellectual disability; severe hypotonia Head: prominent occiput; low-set ears; corneal opacities; ptosis (drooping of eyelids) Hands: third and fourth fingers overlapped by second and fifth fingers; abnormal dermatoglyphics; syndactyly (webbing of fingers) Other: congenital heart defects (>90%); renal abnormalities; single umbilical artery; gastrointestinal tract abnormalities; rocker-bottom feet; cryptorchidism; various malformations of other organs
Altered Chromosome: 13	**Characteristics**
Genetic defect: trisomy 13 Incidence: 1 in 5000 live births	CNS: intellectual disability; severe hypotonia; seizures; anatomic defects of the brain (holoprosencephaly) in 60% Head: microcephaly; microphthalmia and/or coloboma (keyhole-shaped pupil); malformed ears; aplasia of external auditory canal; micrognathia (abnormally small lower jaw); cleft lip and palate Hands: polydactyly (extra digits); abnormal posturing of fingers; abnormal dermatoglyphics Other: omphalocele; congenital heart defects; hemangiomas; gastrointestinal tract defects; kidney defects; various malformations of other organs
Altered Chromosome: 5p	**Characteristics**
Genetic defect: deletion of short arm of chromosome 5 (cri du chat, or cat cry, syndrome) (see Figure 12-17) Incidence: 1 in 20,000 live births	CNS: severe intellectual disability; a catlike cry in infancy Head: microcephaly; hypertelorism (widely spaced eyes); epicanthal folds; low-set ears Other: failure to thrive; various organ malformations
Altered Chromosome: X (sex chromosome)	**Characteristics**
Genetic defect: only one X chromosome in female (Turner syndrome) Incidence: 1 in 5000 live female births (see Figure 12-18)	CNS: no intellectual impairment; some perceptual difficulties Head: low hairline; webbed neck Increased risk for intrauterine fetal death (IUFD) (>95% of all conceptions) Trunk: short stature; cubitus valgus (increased carrying angle of arm); excessive nevi (congenital discoloration of skin due to pigmentation); broad shieldlike chest with widely spaced nipples; puffy feet; no toenails Other: fibrous streaks in ovaries; underdeveloped secondary sex characteristics; primary amenorrhea; usually infertile; renal anomalies; coarctation of the aorta
Altered Chromosome: XXY (sex chromosome)	**Characteristics**
Genetic defect extra X chromosome in male (Klinefelter syndrome) Incidence: 1 in 1000 live male births	CNS: mild intellectual disability Trunk: occasional gynecomastia (abnormally large male breasts); abnormal body proportions (long legs, short trunk, shoulder equal to hip size) Other: small firm testes; underdeveloped secondary sex characteristics; reduced fertility

The other two common trisomies are trisomy 18 and trisomy 13 (see Table 12-9 and Figures 12-14 ■ and 12-15 ■). The prognosis for both trisomy 18 or 13 is extremely poor. Most children (70%) die within the first 3 months of life as a result of complications related to respiratory and cardiac abnormalities. However, 10% survive the first year of life; therefore, the family needs to plan for the possibility of long-term care of a severely affected infant and for family support.

Monosomies, occur when a normal gamete unites with a gamete that is missing a chromosome. In this case, the individual will have only 45 chromosomes and is said to be *monosomic*. Monosomy of an entire autosomal chromosome is incompatible with life. The only monosomy of an entire chromosome that is compatible with life is 45, X (Turner syndrome).

Mosaicism occurs after fertilization and results in an individual with two different cell lines, each having a different

A

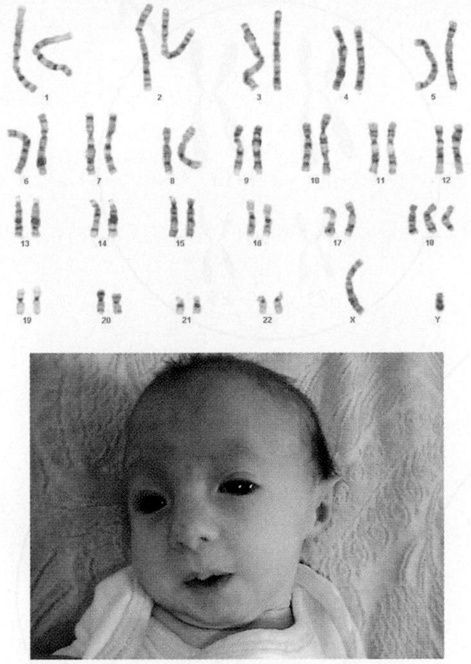

B

Figure 12-14 ■ A. Karyotype of a male who has trisomy 18. B. Infant girl with trisomy 18.

Source: Courtesy of Susan Olson, PhD., The Oregon Health & Science University Cytogenics Laboratory.

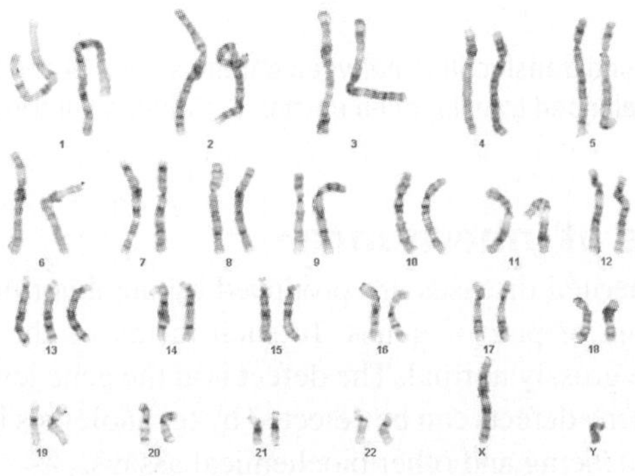

Figure 12-15 ■ Karyotype of a male with trisomy 13.

Source: Courtesy of Susan Olson, PhD., The Oregon Health & Science University Cytogenics Laboratory.

chromosomal number. Mosaicism tends to be more common in the sex chromosomes; when it does occur in the autosomes, it is most common in Down syndrome.

Abnormalities of Chromosome Structure

Abnormalities of chromosome structure involve only parts of the chromosome and generally occur in the form of translocation, deletions, or duplications. Most (>95%) children born with Down syndrome have trisomy 21, whereas some (<5%) have an abnormal rearrangement of chromosomal material known as *translocation.* Clinically, the two types of Down syndrome are indistinguishable; the only way to distinguish them is to do a chromosome analysis.

A translocation is the transfer of a segment of one chromosome to another chromosome. If the two chromosomes are nonhomologous the translocation is *reciprocal.* Reciprocal translocations are relatively common and are found in 1 in 600 newborns. If there is no deletion or duplication of chromosome material, the translocation is considered to be *balanced.* Individuals with a balanced translocation generally do not have any health concerns related to the rearrangement. However, they can have offspring with an *unbalanced* translocation. If there is chromosome material deleted or duplicated, the translocation is considered *unbalanced* and can lead to pregnancy loss, congenital anomalies, intellectual disability (mental retardation)/developmental disabilities, or other health concerns. Translocations that involve two acrocentric chromosomes (chromosomes 13, 14, 15, 21, and 22) that fuse near the centromere regions with loss of the short (p) arms are called *Robertsonian translocations*. An individual with a balanced Robertsonian translocation will have 45 chromosomes, including the translocation chromosome, which is made up of the long arms of two chromosomes (Figure 12-16 ■). For example, the two most common Robertsonian translocations are 13q14q (the long arm of one chromosome 13 is fused to the long arm of one chromosome 14) and 14q21q. The translocation involving 13q and 14q is found in about 1 person out of 1300 and is the most common chromosome rearrangement in humans. Individuals with Robertsonian translocations are at risk to have offspring with unbalanced translocations. This may lead to pregnancy loss or offspring with trisomy 13 or trisomy 21.

Structural abnormality is also caused by *duplications* or *deletions* of chromosomal material. Any portion of a chromosome may be lost or added, generally leading to some adverse effect. Depending on how much chromosomal material is involved, the clinical effects may be mild or severe. Many types of duplications and deletions have been described, such as a deletion of the short arm of chromosome 5 (cri du chat, or cat cry, syndrome [Figure 12-17 ■]). Table 12-9 lists other chromosomal syndromes.

Abnormalities of the Sex Chromosome

To better understand abnormalities of the sex chromosomes, the nurse should know that in females, at an early embryonic stage, one of the two normal X chromosomes becomes inactive. This phenomenon is called *X-inactivation* or *Lyonization.* The inactive X chromosome forms a dark-staining area known as the *Barr body,* or sex chromatin body. The typical female has one Barr body because one of her two X chromosomes has been inactivated. The typical male has no Barr bodies because he has only one X chromosome.

The most common sex chromosome abnormalities are Turner syndrome in females (45, X with no Barr bodies present) and Klinefelter syndrome in males (47, XXY with one Barr body present). See Figure 12-18 ■ and Table 12-9 for clinical descriptions of these abnormalities.

There is a concern that children born as a result of intracytoplasmic sperm injection (ICSI) might be at increased risk for chromosomal and other major congenital anomalies, cancer, or infertility, because ICSI may override natural safeguards that serve to prevent fertilization. Therefore it is strongly recommended that karyotyping and Y chromosome deletion analysis be offered to all men with severe male factor infertility who are candidates for in vitro fertilization (IVF) with ICSI (ASRM, 2008a).

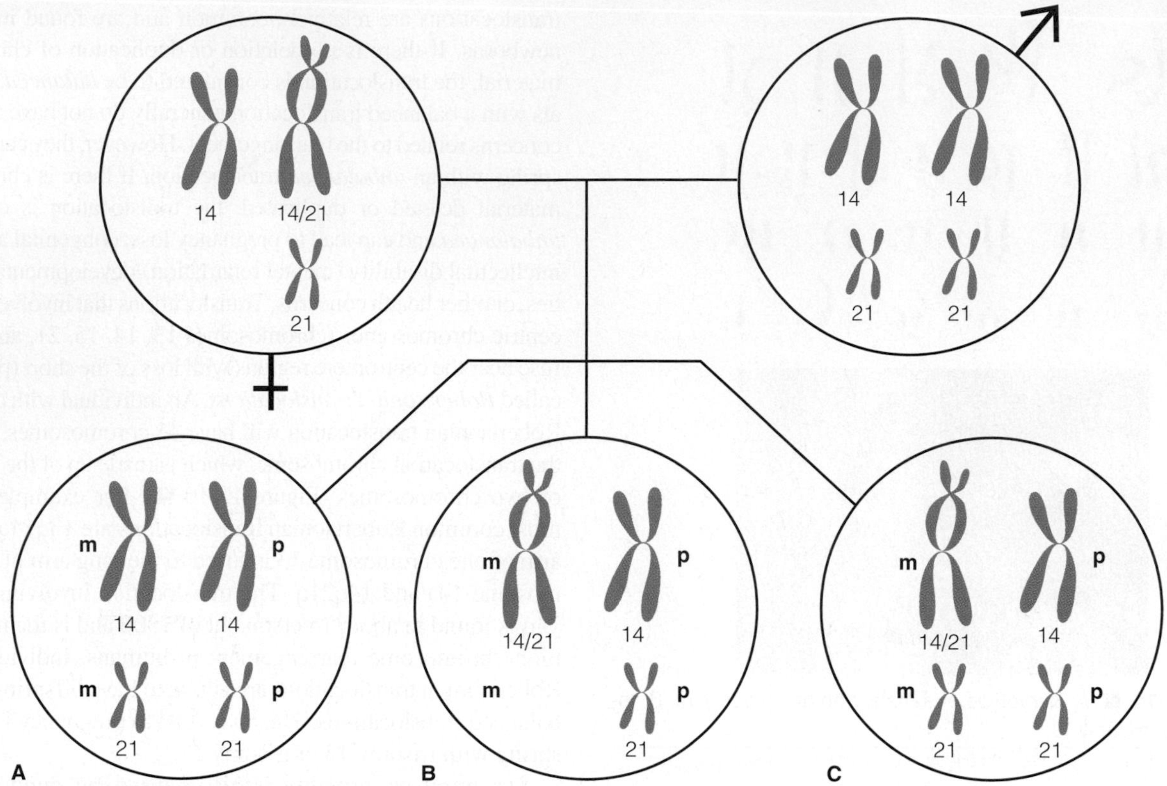

m = maternal origin
p = paternal origin

Figure 12-16 ■ Diagram of various types of offspring when the mother has a balanced translocation between chromosomes 14 and 21 and the father has a normal arrangement of chromosomal material. A. Normal offspring. B. Balanced translocation carrier. C. Unbalanced translocation. Child has Down syndrome.

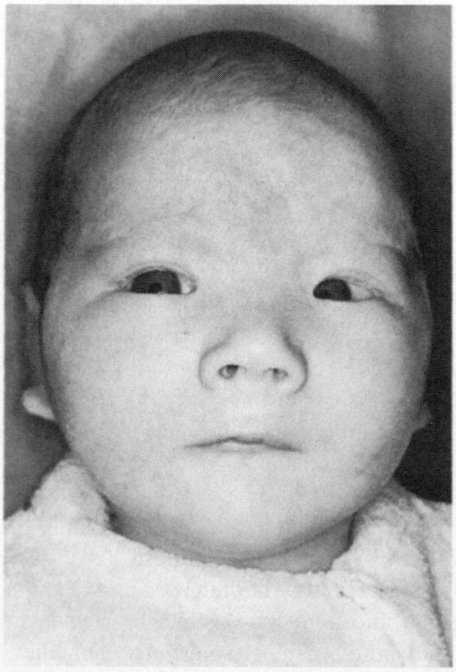

Figure 12-17 ■ Infant with cri du chat syndrome resulting from deletion of part of the short arm of chromosome 5. Note characteristic facies with hypertelorism, epicanthus, and retrognathia.

Source: Reprinted from Genetics in Medicine, 5e, *by J. S. Thompson & M. W. Thompson, Copyright 1991, with permission from Elsevier.*

Modes of Inheritance

Many inherited diseases are produced by an abnormality in a single gene or pair of genes. In such instances the chromosomes are grossly normal. The defect is at the gene level. Some of these gene defects can be detected by technologies including DNA sequencing and other biochemical assays.

There are two major categories of inheritance: **mendelian (single-gene) inheritance** and **nonmendelian (multifactorial) inheritance**. Each single-gene trait is determined by a pair of genes working together. These genes are responsible for the observable expression of the traits (e.g., brown eyes, dark skin), referred to as the **phenotype**. The total genetic makeup of an individual is referred to as the **genotype** (pattern of the genes on the chromosomes).

One of the genes for a trait is inherited from the mother; the other, from the father. Individuals who have two identical genes at a given locus are considered to be *homozygous* for that trait. Individuals are considered to be *heterozygous* for a particular trait when they have two different alleles (alternate forms of the same gene) at a given locus on a pair of homologous chromosomes.

The best known modes of single-gene inheritance are autosomal dominant, autosomal recessive, and X-linked (sex-linked).

Autosomal Dominant Inheritance

A person is said to have an autosomal dominantly inherited disorder if the disease trait is heterozygous; that is, the abnormal

A

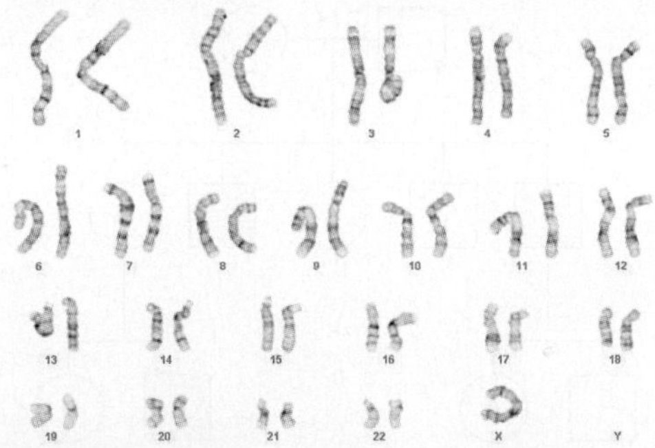

B

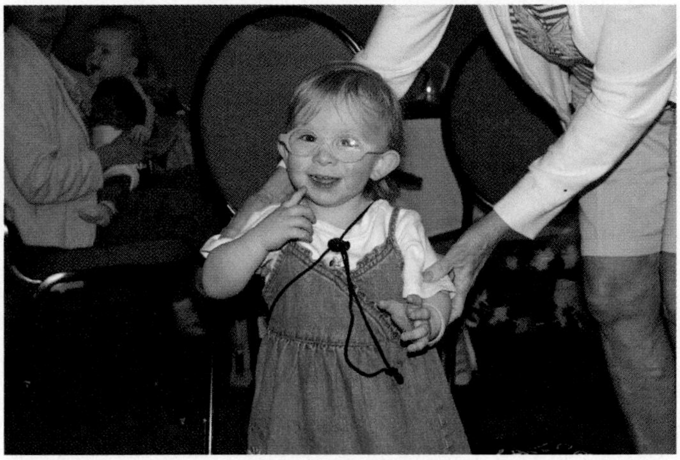

Figure 12-18 ■ A. Karyotype of a female with Turner syndrome. B. Toddler girl with Turner syndrome.

Source: Courtesy of Susan Olson, PhD., The Oregon Health & Science University Cytogenics Laboratory. B. Courtesy of the Turner Syndrome Society, U.S.A.

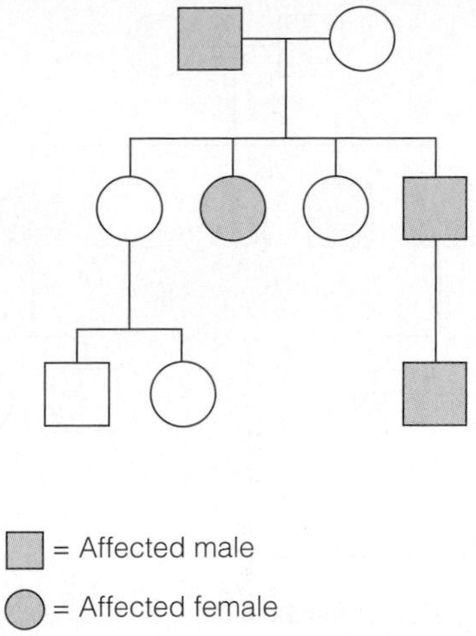

Figure 12-19 ■ Autosomal dominant pedigree. One parent is affected. Statistically, 50% of offspring will be affected, regardless of sex.

gene overshadows the normal gene of the pair to produce the trait. The genetic condition may be familial, meaning it was passed to an individual from one of his or her parents; or it may be the result of a *de novo* (new) mutation that occurred during meiosis of the egg or sperm that created the individual, and he or she is the first and only affected person in the family. In autosomal dominant inheritance, the following occurs:

- An affected individual may have an affected parent. The family **pedigree** (graphic representation of a family tree) usually shows multiple generations having the disorder.
- Affected individuals have a 50% chance of passing on the abnormal gene to each of their children (Figure 12-19 ■).
- Males and females are equally affected, and a father can pass the abnormal gene on to his son. This is an important principle when distinguishing autosomal dominant disorders from X-linked disorders.
- Autosomal dominant inherited disorders have varying degrees of presentation. This is an important factor when counseling families concerning autosomal dominant disorders. Although a parent may have a mild form of the disease, the child may have a more severe form.

Some autosomal dominant conditions have differences in their expression and can lead to difficulties in diagnosis. These differences in expression are known as reduced penetrance, variable expressivity, and pleiotropy. *Penetrance* is the possibility that a gene will have any phenotypic expression at all. When an individual with the genetic trait for a condition fails to express features of the disorder, the gene is said to show reduced penetrance. *Expressivity* is the severity of expression of the phenotype. When the severity of the condition differs in people who have the same genotype, the phenotype is said to have variable expressivity. When a single abnormal gene produces diverse phenotypic effects, such as which organ systems are affected and which symptoms occur, the expression is said to be *pleiotropic*.

Some autosomal dominant disorders are caused by a phenomenon known as *anticipation*. Anticipation occurs when a trinucleotide repeat expands during meiosis, resulting in a gene passed from generation to generation with a larger and larger number of triplet repeats. A larger number of repeats is associated with phenotypic expression of the condition and, typically, the larger the number of repeats the more severe the condition. More than a dozen diseases are known to result from triplet repeat expansion, including autosomal dominant disorders such as Huntington disease and myotonic dystrophy, fragile X syndrome (an X-linked disorder), and Friedreich ataxia (an autosomal recessive disorder).

Autosomal Recessive Inheritance

In an autosomal recessively inherited disorder, the individual must have two abnormal genes to be affected. A *carrier* is an individual who is heterozygous for the abnormal gene and clinically normal. It is not until two carriers mate and pass on the same abnormal gene that affected children may appear. In autosomal recessive inheritance, the following occurs:

- An affected individual can have clinically normal parents, but both parents are generally carriers of the abnormal gene (Figure 12-20 ■).
- In the case where both parents are carriers, there is a 25% chance that the abnormal gene will be passed on to any of their offspring. Each pregnancy has a 25% chance of resulting in an affected child.
- If the child of two carrier parents is clinically normal, there is a two-thirds chance that the child is a carrier of the gene.

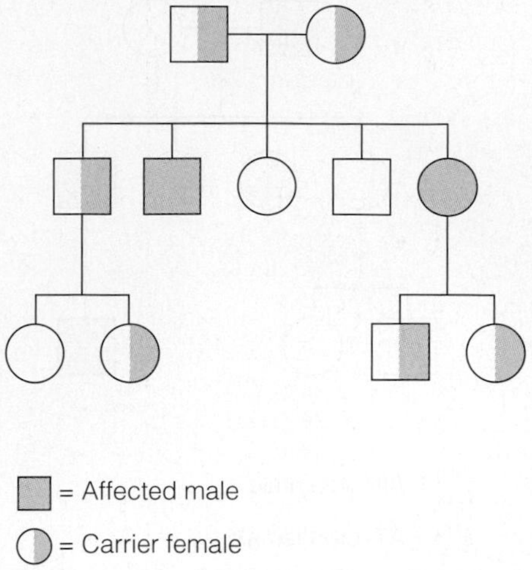

Figure 12-20 ■ Autosomal recessive pedigree. Both parents are carriers. Statistically, 25% of offspring will be affected, regardless of sex.

- Both males and females are equally affected.
- There is an increased history of consanguineous matings (mating of blood relatives).

Some common autosomal recessive inherited disorders are cystic fibrosis, phenylketonuria (PKU), galactosemia, sickle cell anemia, Tay-Sachs disease, and many metabolic disorders.

X-Linked Recessive Inheritance

X-linked, or sex-linked, disorders are those for which the abnormal gene is carried on the X chromosome. Thus an X-linked disorder is manifested in a male who carries the abnormal gene on his only X chromosome and is considered *hemizygous* for the condition. Approximately two thirds of the time, the mother of a male with an X-linked disorder will be a carrier. Most carrier females (known as *heterozygous females*) do not have symptoms of the condition. However, in some X-linked conditions heterozygous females can manifest symptoms of the disorder due to skewed Lyonization, but the symptoms tend to be milder and have later onset. In X-linked recessive inheritance, the following occurs:

- There is no male-to-male transmission. Affected males are related through the female line (Figure 12-21 ■).
- There is a 50% chance that a carrier mother will pass the abnormal gene to each of her sons, who will thus be affected.
- There is a 50% chance that a carrier mother will pass the normal gene to each of her sons, who will thus be unaffected.
- There is a 50% chance that a carrier mother will pass the abnormal gene to each of her daughters, who become carriers.
- Fathers affected with an X-linked disorder cannot pass the disorder to their sons, but all their daughters become carriers of the disorder.

Common X-linked recessive disorders are hemophilia, Duchenne muscular dystrophy, and some forms of color blindness. Fragile X syndrome is an X-linked recessive disorder that exhibits anticipation. This condition is the most common form of inherited intellectual disability (mental retardation) second only to Down syndrome. It is caused by an increased number of CGG trinucleotide repeats in the *FMR1* gene, located at a "fragile site"

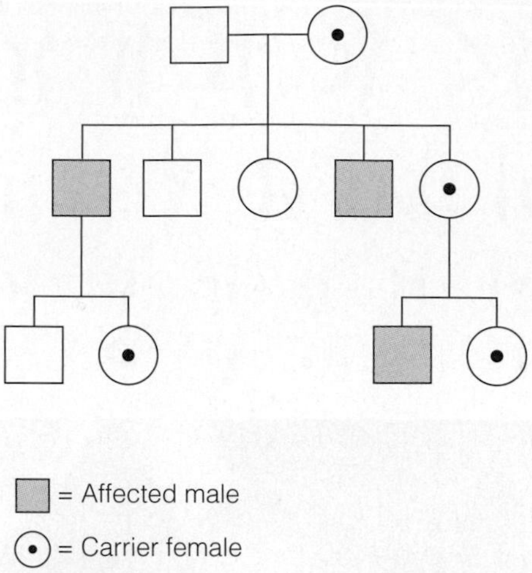

Figure 12-21 ■ X-linked recessive pedigree. The mother is the carrier. Statistically, 50% of male offspring will be affected, and 50% of female offspring will be carriers.

on the long arm of the X chromosome. The normal number of CGG repeats is up to 60. Individuals with a repeat number ranging between 60 and 200 have a *premutation* allele, meaning the copy number can increase during maternal (but not paternal) meiosis. If the CGG repeat number increases over 200, the individual (particularly hemizygous males) can have fragile X syndrome. Approximately one third of females with over 200 CGG repeats will be affected with fragile X syndrome, one third will have mild developmental or learning disabilities, and one third will have no symptoms at all.

X-Linked Dominant Inheritance

X-linked dominant disorders are rare, the most common being vitamin D–resistant rickets. When X-linked dominance does occur, the pattern is similar to X-linked recessive inheritance except that heterozygous females can also be affected. In X-linked dominant inheritance, there is no male-to-male transmission. Affected fathers will have affected daughters but no affected sons. Some types of X-linked dominant disorders are so severe that they can be lethal in utero or in the newborn period in hemizygous males (e.g., Rett syndrome or severe forms of otopalataldigital [OPD] syndrome).

Multifactorial Inheritance

Many common congenital malformations, such as cleft palate, heart defect, spina bifida, dislocated hips, clubfoot, and pyloric stenosis do not follow a clear pattern of mendelian inheritance. They are generally caused by an interaction of many genes and environmental factors and are considered to have "multifactorial" inheritance. In multifactorial inheritance, the following occurs:

- The malformations may vary from mild to severe. For example, spina bifida may range in severity from mild, as spina bifida occulta, to more severe, as a myelomeningocele. The risk may be greater when the disorder is severe.
- There is often a sex bias, and the risk is higher for relatives of a patient of the sex in which the condition is less common. Pyloric stenosis is more common in males, whereas cleft palate is more common among females. When a member of the less

commonly affected sex shows the condition, a greater number of genes must usually be present to cause the defect.

- Not only is increased risk greatest among closest relatives and decreases with distance of relationship, but the risk is increased when multiple family members are affected.

Although most congenital malformations are multifactorial, a careful family history should always be taken because, occasionally, cleft lip and palate, certain congenital heart defects, and other malformations can also be inherited as autosomal dominant or recessive traits. Other disorders thought to be within the multifactorial inheritance group are diabetes, hypertension, some heart diseases, and mental illness.

Prenatal Diagnostic Tests

Parent-child and family-planning counseling have become a major responsibility of professional nurses. To be effective counselors, nurses need to have the most current knowledge available concerning prenatal testing options. Appropriate counseling should occur before prenatal screening or diagnostic testing is done. It is essential that the couple be completely informed as to the known and potential risks of each of the genetic diagnostic procedures. The prescreening counseling should include the conditions detectable by the screen, diagnostic test available if the screen is positive, risk to mother and pregnancy if the test is performed, accuracy of the test, and limitations of the test (Lashley, 2007). The nurse needs to recognize the emotional impact on the family of a decision to undergo or not to undergo a genetic diagnostic procedure. The ability to diagnose certain genetic diseases by various diagnostic tools has enormous implications for the practice of preventive health care. Several methods are available for prenatal diagnosis, although some are still experimental.

Genetic Ultrasound

Ultrasound may be used to assess the fetus for genetic or congenital problems. With ultrasound, one can visualize the fetal head for abnormalities in size, shape, and structure. (For a detailed discussion of ultrasound technology, see chapter 21 ∞.) Craniospinal defects (anencephaly, microcephaly, hydrocephalus), gastrointestinal malformations (omphalocele, gastroschisis), renal malformations (dysplasia or obstruction), and skeletal malformations (caudal regression, conjoined twins) are only some of the disorders that can be diagnosed in utero by ultrasound. Screening by ultrasound for congenital anomalies is best done at 18 to 20 weeks, when fetal structures have completed development. With the addition of fetal nuchal translucency measurement at 10 to 13 weeks, there is high correlation with fetal chromosome abnormalities (ACOG, 2007). The nuchal translucency is a fluid-filled space at the back of the fetal neck. An increased amount of fluid is associated with an increased risk for chromosome abnormalities, birth defects, genetic syndromes, and poor pregnancy outcome—the larger the nuchal translucency, the higher the risk for abnormalities. The nuchal translucency should only be measured by a specifically trained sonographer or physician. There is no information documenting harm to the fetus or long-term effects with exposure to ultrasound. However, there is no guarantee of complete safety; therefore, the practitioner and the parents must evaluate the risks against the benefits on an individual basis.

Screening and invasive diagnostic testing for chromosome abnormalities should be available to all women who present for prenatal care before 20 weeks of pregnancy regardless of maternal age (ACOG, 2007). Women should be counseled regarding the differences between screening and invasive diagnostic testing. Screening tests, such as the nuchal translucency ultrasound and maternal serum screening, are designed to gather information about the risk that the pregnancy could have chromosome abnormalities or open spina bifida. If the risk is increased above a specific cutoff, the woman is offered invasive prenatal diagnosis. Prenatal diagnostic techniques, such as amniocentesis and chorionic villus sampling (CVS), obtain cells from the pregnancy to rule out or diagnose a chromosome abnormality or certain genetic disorders. They are associated with a small risk of pregnancy complications, including miscarriage.

Maternal Serum Screening

Measuring specific hormones and proteins in the maternal serum during the first and/or second trimester can determine the risk for Down syndrome, trisomy 18, or open spina bifida. In the first trimester, the nuchal translucency measurement is often added to improve the detection rate for Down syndrome and trisomy 18. Detection and false-positive rates differ depending on the type of screening test that is performed and may also differ depending on the laboratory that performs the screening.

Genetic Amniocentesis

A major method of prenatal diagnosis is genetic amniocentesis (Figure 12-22 ■). The procedure is described in chapter 21 ∞. The risk for pregnancy complications, including infection and miscarriage, are thought to be less than 0.5%.The indications for genetic amniocentesis include the following:

- *Maternal age 35 or older:* Women 35 or older are at greater risk for having children with chromosome abnormalities. Chromosomal abnormalities due to maternal age are trisomy 21, 13, 18, XXX, or XXY. The risk of having a live-born infant with a chromosome problem is 1 in 200 for a 35-year-old woman; the risk for trisomy 21 is 1 in 365. At age 45 the risks are 1 in 20 and 1 in 40, respectively (Ward, 2008).
- *Previous child born with a chromosomal abnormality:* Couples who have had a child with trisomy 21, 18, or 13 have approximately a 1% risk or their age-related risk, whichever is higher, of a future child having a chromosome abnormality.
- *Parent carrying a chromosomal abnormality (balanced translocation):* These couples are at an increased risk to have conceptions with an unbalanced translocation. Depending on the chromosomes involved in the translocation, there may be an increased risk for pregnancy loss or a viable offspring with congenital anomalies and/or intellectual disability. For example, a woman who carries a balanced 14/21 translocation has a risk of approximately 10% to 15% that her children will be affected with the unbalanced translocation of Down syndrome; if the father is a carrier, there is a 2% to 5% risk.
- *Mother carrying an X-linked disease:* Prenatal diagnosis may be available for families in which the woman is a known

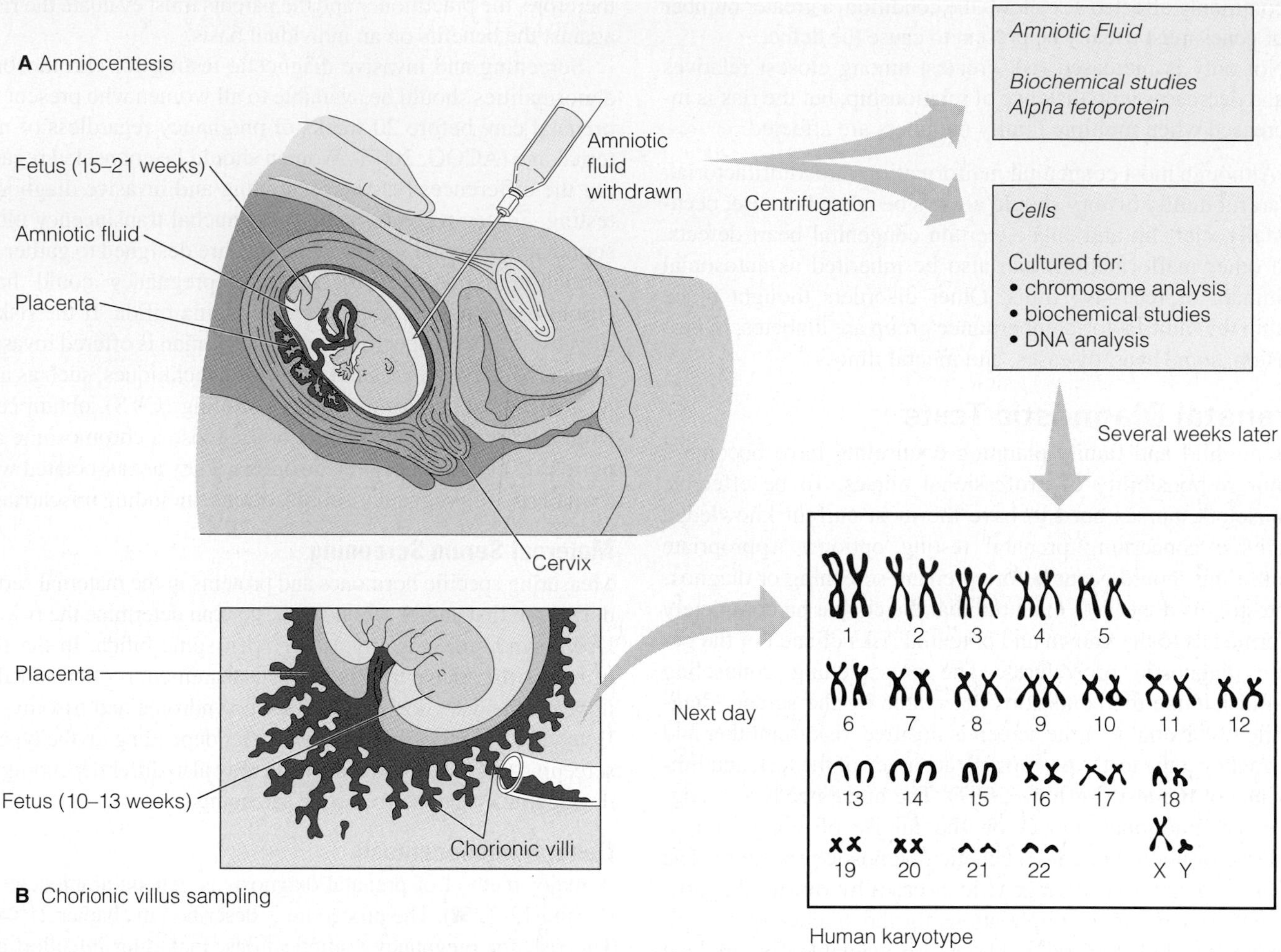

Figure 12-22 ■ A. Genetic amniocentesis for prenatal diagnosis is done at 15–21 weeks' gestation. B. Chorionic villus sampling is done at 10–13 weeks, and the cells are cultured and karyotyped. Results generally take 7–14 days.

or possible carrier of an X-linked disorder, such as Duchenne muscular dystrophy or hemophilia A or B. For a known female carrier, the risk of having an affected male fetus is 25%. DNA testing may make it possible to distinguish affected males from nonaffected males in some disorders.

- ***Parents carrying an inborn error of metabolism that can be diagnosed in utero:*** Many metabolic disorders are detectable *in utero* by DNA analysis or biochemical testing. Examples include argininosuccinicaciduria, cystinosis, Fabry disease, galactosemia, Gaucher disease, homocystinuria, Hunter syndrome, Hurler disease, Krabbe disease, Lesch-Nyhan syndrome, maple syrup urine disease, Niemann-Pick disease, Pompe disease, Sanfilippo syndrome, and Tay-Sachs disease.
- ***Both parents carrying an autosomal recessive disease:*** When both parents are carriers of an autosomal recessive disease, there is a 25% risk for *each pregnancy* that the fetus will be affected. Autosomal recessive diseases identified by amniocentesis include hemoglobinopathies such as sickle cell anemia or thalassemia and cystic fibrosis.
- ***Family history of neural tube defects:*** Genetic amniocentesis is available to those couples who have had a child with neural tube defects or who have a family history of these conditions, which include anencephaly, spina bifida, and myelomeningocele. The diagnosis is made by measuring amniotic fluid alpha-feto protein (AFP) and a neurotransmitter called acetylcholinesterase. Neural tube defects are usually multifactorial traits.

Chorionic Villus Sampling

Chorionic villus sampling (CVS) is a technique that obtains chorionic villi tissue from the placenta either transabdominally or transcervially. Its diagnostic capability is similar to that of amniocentesis. Its advantages are that diagnostic information is available at 10 to 13 weeks' gestation. The risk for pregnancy complications, including infection and pregnancy loss, is estimated to be around 1%. (For further discussion, see chapter 21 ∞.)

Percutaneous Umbilical Blood Sampling

Percutaneous umbilical blood sampling (PUBS) is a technique that obtains blood from the umbilical cord during pregnancy. Obtaining fetal blood cells allows for more rapid chromosome diagnosis, or for transfusion for Rh isoimmunization or hydrops fetalis. (For more in-depth discussion, see chapter 21 ∞.)

Noninvasive Prenatal Diagnosis (NIPD)

In the near future, noninvasive methods of prenatal diagnosis for chromosome abnormalities or genetic disorders will be available by obtaining maternal blood as early as 8 weeks of pregnancy. Fetal ribonucleic acid (RNA) and/or DNA can be isolated in the maternal serum to test for specific disorders. This technology is currently used for fetal Rh determination in women who are Rh negative. Commercial biotechnology companies plan to introduce this testing, particularly for the diagnosis of chromosomal trisomies such as Down syndrome. Preliminary data estimate that the accuracy of the test is >99%.

Implications of Prenatal Diagnostic Testing

It is imperative that counseling precede any procedure for prenatal diagnosis. Many questions and points must be considered if the family is to reach a satisfactory decision.

With the advent of diagnostic techniques such as amniocentesis and CVS, at-risk couples who would not otherwise have a first child or additional children can decide to conceive. Following prenatal diagnosis a couple can decide not to have a child with a genetic disease. For many couples, prenatal diagnosis is not selected because abortion is not an option for them. The decision whether to use prenatal diagnosis can be made only by the family. Even when termination is not an option, prenatal diagnosis can give parents an opportunity to prepare for the birth of a child with special needs, to contact other families with children with similar problems, or to contact support services before the birth.

It is important to remember that prenatal screening and diagnosis are optional and not required as part of routine prenatal care. Nurses should present these options to patients using a nondirective manner. *Nondirective counseling* is a technique designed to allow patients or clients to talk about their problems or emotional difficulties and reach a decision best for themselves or their families with a minimum of direction from the person serving as their counselor. While it is imperative that nurses give their patients accurate, up-to-date information about the various prenatal screening and diagnostic testing options, they must remain impartial and not recommend any specific course of action. It is also important for nurses to remember that the language they use when discussing these options with patients matters (see Table 12-10 Health Promotion Education: Couples Who May Benefit From Prenatal Diagnosis). For example, when discussing prenatal screening for Down syndrome, terms such as *handicapped* or *retarded* should be replaced with *disabled* and/or *developmentally/cognitively/intellectually disabled*. Instead of using the word *risk*, consider using the terms *chance* or *possibility*.

Every pregnancy has a 3% to 5% risk of resulting in an infant with a birth defect, chromosome abnormality, genetic disease, or developmental disability. When an abnormality is detected or suspected, an attempt is made to determine the diagnosis by assessing the family health history (via the pedigree) and the pregnancy history and by evaluating the fetal anomaly or anomalies via ultrasound. Experts on a specific disorder are consulted, and health-care professionals can then present the parents with information and options. Treatment of prenatally diagnosed disorders may begin during the pregnancy, thus possibly preventing irreversible damage. In light of the philosophy of preventive health care, information on what data can be obtained prenatally should be made available to all couples who are expecting a baby or who are contemplating pregnancy.

TABLE 12-10 Health Promotion Education: Couples Who May Benefit from Prenatal Diagnosis

- Women age 35 or over at time of birth
- Couples with a balanced translocation (chromosomal abnormality)
- Family history of known or suspected mendelian genetic disorder (e.g., cystic fibrosis, hemophilia A & B; Duchenne muscular dystrophy)
- Couples with a previous child with chromosomal abnormality
- Couples in which either partner or a previous child is affected with, or in which both partners are carriers for, a diagnosable metabolic disorder
- Family history of birth defects and/or intellectual disability (mental retardation) (e.g., neural tube defects, congenital heart disease, cleft lip and/or palate).
- Ethnic groups at increased risk for specific disorders (see Developing Cultural Competence: Genetic Screening Recommendations for Various Ethnic and Age Groups)
- Couples with a history of two or more first trimester spontaneous abortions
- Women with an abnormal maternal serum screening test
- Women with a teratogenic risk secondary to an exposure or maternal health condition (e.g., diabetes)

Postnatal Diagnosis

Human Genome Project

Questions concerning genetic disorders (cause, treatment, and prognosis) are most often first discussed in the newborn nursery or during the infant's first few months of life. When a child is born with anomalies, has a stormy neonatal period, or does not progress as expected, a genetic evaluation may well be warranted. Accurate diagnosis and an optimal treatment plan incorporate the following:

- Complete and detailed histories to determine whether the problem is prenatal (congenital), postnatal, or familial in origin.
- Thorough physical and dysmorphology examination by a trained clinical geneticist.
- Laboratory analysis, which includes chromosome analysis; enzyme assay for inborn errors of metabolism (see chapter 33 for further discussion on these specific tests); DNA studies (both direct and by linkage); and antibody titers for infectious teratogens, such as toxoplasmosis, rubella, cytomegalovirus, and herpes virus (TORCH syndrome) (see chapter 19).

To make an accurate diagnosis, the geneticist consults with other specialists and reviews the current literature. This lets the geneticist evaluate all the available information before arriving at a diagnosis and plan of action.

PROFESSIONALISM IN PRACTICE

2008 Prenatally and Postnatally Diagnosed Conditions Act

The Prenatally and Postnatally Diagnosed Conditions Act was signed into law in 2008. This law requires that medical providers give parents accurate, updated, and scientific information regarding their child's diagnosis, prognosis, treatment, and life expectancy. Nurses are often an important source of information and support when a prenatal or postnatal diagnosis of a genetic condition or birth defect is made.

The Human Genome Project will have significant implications for the identification and management of inherited disorders. Once genes have been identified, it will be possible to detect their presence in carriers and lead to better genetic counseling. However, concerns have been voiced about ethical considerations with genetic research. What guidelines are needed to protect children and families so that genetic testing does not lead to discrimination in future employment or health insurance? Who should be tested for genetic diseases, and who should have access to the results? Because children cannot yet give informed consent for genetic testing (see chapter 1 ∞ for discussion of informed consent), it is recommended that children and adolescents should have genetic testing *only* when medical treatment could help if the disease is identified, or when another family member might benefit from the knowledge for his or her own health and the child will not be harmed by the testing (American Academy of Pediatrics, Committee on Genetics, 2000, reaffirmed 2009). Whenever genetic testing is performed, counseling about the results must be available.

Genetic Counseling

Genetic counseling is a communication process in which the genetic counselor, physician, or specially trained and certified nurse helps a family or individuals understand and adapt to the medical, psychologic, and familial implications of genetic contributions to disease (National Society of Genetic Counselors [NSGC], 2005).

Referral

Genetic counseling referral is advised for any of the following categories:

- ***Congenital abnormalities, including intellectual disability:*** Any couple who has a child or a relative with a congenital malformation may be at an increased risk and should be so informed. If intellectual disability of unidentified cause has occurred in a family, there may be an increased risk of recurrence. In some cases, the genetic counselor will identify the cause of a malformation as a teratogen (see chapter 16 ∞). The family should be aware of teratogenic substances so they can avoid exposure during any subsequent pregnancy.
- ***Familial disorders:*** Families should be told that certain diseases may have a genetic component and that the risk of their occurrence in a particular family may be higher than that for the general population. Such disorders as diabetes, heart disease, cancer, and mental illness fall into this category.
- ***Known inherited diseases:*** Families may know that diseases are inherited but not know the mechanism or the specific risk for them. An important point to remember is that family members who are not at risk for passing on a disorder should be as well informed as family members who are at risk.
- ***Metabolic disorders:*** Any families at risk for having a child with a metabolic disorder or biochemical defect should be referred for genetic counseling. Because most inborn errors of metabolism are autosomal recessively inherited ones, a family may not be identified as at risk until the birth of an affected child. Carriers of the sickle cell trait can be identified before pregnancy is begun, and the risk of having an affected child can be determined.
- ***Chromosomal abnormalities:*** As discussed previously, any couple who has had a child with a chromosomal abnormality may be at an increased risk of having another child similarly affected. This group includes families in which there is concern for a possible translocation.

After the couple has been referred to the genetic clinic, they are sent a form requesting information on the health status of various family members. This information assists the genetic counselor in creating the family's pedigree. The pedigree and health history facilitate identification of other family members who might also be at risk for the same disorder (Figure 12-23 ■). The couple being counseled may wish to notify those relatives at risk so that they, too, can be given genetic counseling. When done correctly, the family history and pedigree are two of the most powerful and useful tools for determining a family risk.

Initial Session

During the initial session, the counselor gathers additional information about the pregnancy, the affected child's growth and development, and the family's understanding of the problem. The counselor also elicits information concerning ethnic background and family origin. Many genetic disorders are more common among certain ethnic groups or in particular geographic areas.

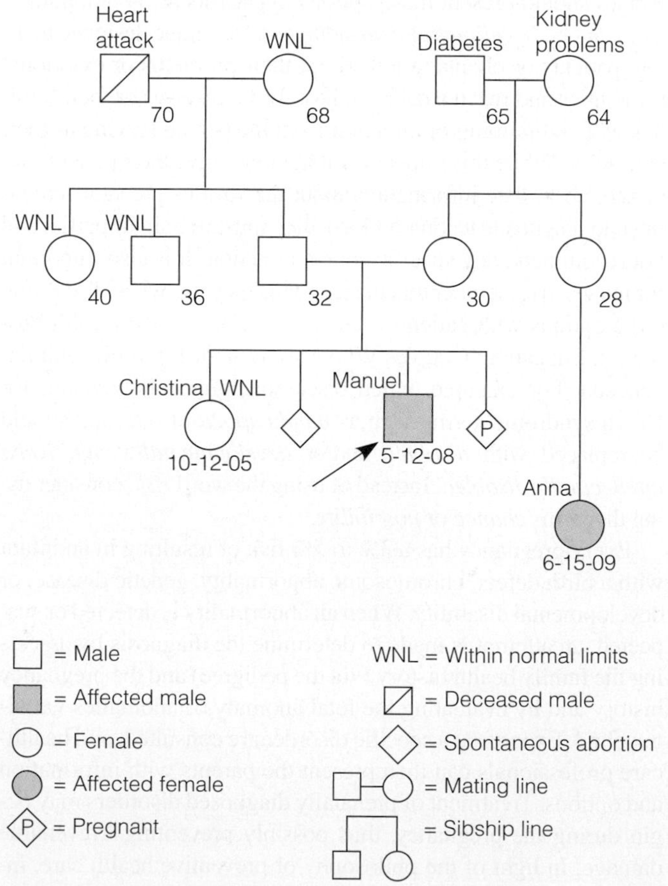

Figure 12-23 ■ Screening pedigree. Arrow indicates the nearest family member affected with the disorder being investigated. Numbers refer to the ages or birth dates of family members.

DEVELOPING CULTURAL COMPETENCE
Consanguineous Marriages

In the United States, marriage between related individuals is generally taboo. In Western medicine, there is a concern that a child conceived by people who are related by blood may have an increased risk for birth defects. This has not, however, been supported by recent research unless the relationship is closer than first cousins. In many other cultures, marriage of first cousins and others who are related by blood is acceptable and even common. Egypt has a high rate of consanguineous (blood relationship) marriages. Reasons for consanguineous marriage include: "increase family links," "they knew each other and everything would be clear before marriage," "customs and traditions," and "less cost." The most common type of consanguineous marriage in Egypt is between first cousins.

For example, families from the British Isles are at higher risk of having children with neural tube defects; Ashkenazi Jews (from eastern Europe) and French Canadians are at higher risk for Tay-Sachs disease; people of African descent for sickle cell anemia; Mennonites for maple syrup urine disease; and people of Mediterranean heritage for thalassemias. (See Developing Cultural Competence: Genetic Screening Recommendations for Various Ethnic and Age Groups.)

Generally the child is given a physical examination. Other family members may also be examined. If any laboratory tests, such as chromosomal analysis, genetic testing, metabolic studies, or viral titers, are indicated, they are performed at this time. The genetic counselor may then give the family some preliminary information based on the data at hand.

Follow-Up Counseling

When all the data have been carefully examined and analyzed the family returns for a follow-up visit. At this time the parents are given all the information available, including the medical facts, diagnosis, probable course of the disorder, and any available management; the inheritance pattern for this particular family and their risk of recurrence; and the options or alternatives for dealing with the risk of recurrence. The remainder of the counseling session is spent discussing the course of action that seems appropriate to the family in view of their risk and family goals. For couples who desire to become parents or who want a subsequent child, options include prenatal diagnosis; early detection and treatment; and, in some cases, adoption, preimplantation genetic diagnosis or other assisted reproduction techniques, or delayed childbearing.

The couple may consider assisted reproduction techniques, such as therapeutic donor insemination (TDI), discussed earlier in this chapter. This alternative is appropriate in several instances; for example, if the man has an autosomal dominant disease, TDI would decrease to zero the risk of having an affected child (if the sperm donor is not at risk) because the child would not inherit any genes from the affected parent. If the man is affected with an X-linked disorder and does not wish to continue the gene in the family (all his daughters will be carriers), TDI would be an alternative to terminating all pregnancies with a female fetus. If the man is a carrier for a balanced translocation and if termination of pregnancy is against family ethics, TDI is an appropriate alternative. If both parents are carriers of an autosomal recessive disorder, TDI lowers the risk to a very low level or to zero if a carrier test is available. Finally, TDI may be appropriate if the family is at high risk for a multifactorial disorder.

DEVELOPING CULTURAL COMPETENCE
Genetic Screening Recommendations for Various Ethnic and Age Groups

Background of Population at Risk	Disorder	Screening Test	Definitive Test
Ashkenazi Jewish, French-Canadian, Cajun	Tay-Sachs disease	Decreased serum hexosaminidase-A or DNA mutation analysis	CVS* or amniocentesis for hexosaminidase-A assay or DNA mutation analysis
Ashkenazi Jewish	Cystic fibrosis, Canavan disease, familial dysautonomia, several other disorders	DNA mutation analysis	CVS or amniocentesis for DNA mutation analysis
African; Hispanic from Caribbean, Central America, or South America; Arab, Egyptian; Asian Indian	Sickle cell anemia	Presence of sickle cell hemoglobin; confirmatory hemoglobin electrophoresis	CVS or amniocentesis for DNA mutation analysis
Greek, Italian	Beta-thalassemia	Mean corpuscular volume less than 80% confirmatory hemoglobin electrophoresis	CVS or amniocentesis for DNA mutation analysis
Southeast Asian (Vietnamese, Laotian, Cambodian), Filipino	Alpha-thalassemia	Mean corpuscular volume less than 80%; confirmatory hemoglobin electrophoresis	CVS or amniocentesis for DNA mutation analysis or gene deletion studies
Women over age 35 (all ethnic groups)	Chromosomal trisomies	Prenatal serum and/or ultrasound screening	CVS or amniocentesis for cytogenetic analysis
Women of any age (all ethnic groups; particularly suggested for women from British Isles, Ireland)	Neural tube defects and selected other anomalies	Maternal serum alpha-fetoprotein (MSAFP)	Amniocentesis for amniotic fluid alpha-fetoprotein (AFP) and acetylcholinesterase assays
Caucasian (northern European, Celtic population), Ashkenazi Jewish	Cystic fibrosis	DNA mutation analysis of the cystic fibrosis transmembrane regulation (CFTR) gene	CVS or amniocentesis for DNA mutation analysis

*Chorionic villus sampling.

TABLE 12-11 Nursing Responsibilities in Genetic Counseling

- Identify families at risk for genetic problems.
- Determine how the genetic problem is perceived and what information is desired before proceeding.
- Assist families in acquiring accurate information about the specific problem.
- Act as liaison between family and genetic counselor.
- Assist the family in understanding and dealing with information received.
- Provide information on support groups.
- Aid families in coping with this crisis.
- Provide information about known genetic factors.
- Ensure continuity of nursing care to the family.

Couples who are young and at risk may decide to delay childbearing for a few years. These couples may find in a few years that prenatal diagnosis will be available or that a disease can be detected and treated early to prevent irreversible damage.

When the parents have completed the counseling sessions, the counselor sends them and their physician a letter, detailing the contents of the sessions. The family keeps this document for reference. See Table 12-11 for a list of nursing responsibilities in genetic counseling.

NURSING CARE MANAGEMENT

In both prospective and retrospective genetic counseling, timely nursing intervention is a crucial factor. During annual examinations and other clinical appointments, the nurse should interview all women of childbearing age to determine any family history or other risk factors for genetic disorders. If the woman is planning to conceive, genetic counseling should be encouraged before discontinuation of contraception.

The nurse has a key role in preventing recurrence. One cannot expect a couple who has just learned that their child has a birth defect or Down syndrome to take in any information concerning future risks. However, the couple should never be "put off" from genetic counseling for so long that they conceive another affected child because of lack of information. The perinatal nursing team frequently has the first contact with the family who has a newborn with a congenital abnormality. At the birth of an affected child, the nurse can inform the parents that before they attempt having another child, genetic counseling is available. After genetic counseling, the nurse with the appropriate knowledge of genetics is in an ideal position to help families review what has been discussed during the sessions and to answer any additional questions they might have. As the family returns to the daily aspects of living, the nurse can provide helpful information on the day-to-day aspects of caring for the child, answer questions as they arise, support parents in their decisions, and refer the family to other health and community agencies.

The family may return to the genetic counselor a number of times to air their questions and concerns, especially if the couple is considering having more children, or if siblings want information about their affected brother or sister. It is most desirable for the nurse working with the family to attend many or all of these counseling sessions. Because the nurse has already established a rapport with the couple, the nurse can act as a liaison between the family and the genetic counselor. Hearing directly what the genetic counselor says helps the nurse clarify issues for the family, which in turn helps them formulate questions. Many genetic centers have found the public health nurse to be the ideal health professional to provide such follow-up care.

Nurses must be careful not to assume a diagnosis, determine carrier status or recurrence risks, or provide genetic counseling without adequate information and training. Inadequate, inappropriate, or inaccurate information may be misleading or harmful. Healthcare professionals need to learn the appropriate referral systems and options for care in their region.

FOCUS YOUR STUDY

- A couple is considered infertile when they do not conceive after 1 year of unprotected coitus.
- At least 8% of couples in the United States are infertile.
- A thorough history and physical of both partners is essential as a basis for infertility investigation.
- General fertility investigations include evaluation of ovarian function, cervical mucus adequacy and receptivity to sperm, sperm number and function, tubal patency, general condition of the pelvic organs, and certain laboratory tests.

- Among cases of infertility, 20% involve male factors, 40% involve female factors, and 30% to 40% involve either an unknown cause (unexplained infertility) or a problem with both partners.
- Medications may be prescribed to induce ovulation, facilitate cervical mucus formation, reduce antibody concentration, increase sperm count and motility, and suppress endometriosis.
- The emotional aspect of infertility may be more difficult for the couple than the testing and therapy.
- The nurse needs to be prepared to provide accurate information about infertility and dispel myths.
- The nurse assesses coping responses and initiates counseling referrals as indicated.
- In autosomal dominant disorders, an affected parent has a 50% chance of having an affected child. Such disorders equally affect both males and females. The characteristic presentation will vary in each individual with the gene. Some of the common autosomal dominant inherited disorders are Huntington disease, polycystic kidney disease, and neurofibromatosis (von Recklinghausen disease).
- Autosomal recessive disorders are characterized by both parents being carriers; each offspring has a 25% chance of having the disease, a 25% chance of not being affected, and a 50% chance of being a carrier. Males and females are equally affected. Some common autosomal recessive inheritance disorders are cystic fibrosis, phenylketonuria (PKU), galactosemia, sickle cell anemia, Tay-Sachs disease, and most metabolic disorders.
- X-linked recessive disorders are characterized by no male-to-male transmission; effects limited to males; a 50% chance that a carrier mother will pass the abnormal gene to her sons; a 50% chance that her daughters will be carriers; and a 100% chance that daughters of affected fathers will be carriers. Common X-linked recessive disorders are hemophilia, some forms of color blindness, and Duchenne muscular dystrophy.
- Multifactorial inheritance disorders include cleft lip and palate, spina bifida, dislocated hips, clubfoot, and pyloric stenosis.
- Some genetic conditions that can currently be diagnosed prenatally are neural tube and cranial defects, renal malformations, hemophilia, fragile X syndrome, thalassemia, cystic fibrosis, and many inborn errors of metabolism such as Tay-Sachs disease. This list expands daily as new technology allows more conditions to be detected.
- The chief tools of prenatal diagnosis are ultrasound, maternal serum alpha-fetoprotein testing, amniocentesis, chorionic villus sampling, and percutaneous umbilical blood sampling.
- Based on sound knowledge about common genetic problems, the nurse should prepare the family for counseling and act as a resource person during and after the counseling sessions. Many nurses with advanced training are entering the field of genetic counseling.

CRITICAL THINKING IN ACTION

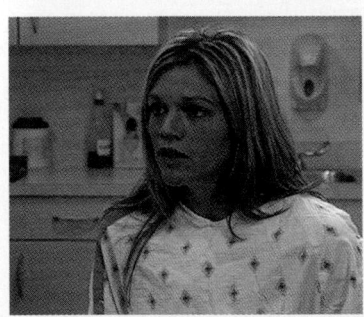

Source: George Dodson/Pearson Education.

Marie Neives, age 19, presents while you are working at a Planned Parenthood Clinic. She is there for a GYN exam and tells you that she is sexually active with her boyfriend but doesn't want to become pregnant. Since she lives at home with her parents, she does not want to use "the pill" because her mother might find out. Marie tells you she has a family history of cystic fibrosis and is concerned that she will pass the disease on. Marie asks you for information concerning fertility awareness. You obtain a menstrual history as follows: menarche age 12, cycle every 28 days for 5 days, dysmenorrhea the first 2 days with moderate flow. She has had one sexual partner. She states her boyfriend doesn't like to use condoms and that she has been lucky so far in not getting pregnant. You assist the nurse practitioner with a physical and pelvic exam. The results show that Marie is essentially healthy. The nurse practitioner asks you to review with Marie the basal body temperature (BBT) method of fertility awareness.

1. Explore with Marie "natural family planning." How would you explain this to her?
2. Briefly explain why the basal body temperature (BBT) method can predict ovulation.
3. How would you describe to Marie the procedure for obtaining BBT?
4. After figuring out her menstruation cycle, to avoid conception when would you tell Marie to abstain from unprotected intercourse?

See www.nursing.pearsonhighered.com for possible responses.

REFERENCES

American Academy of Pediatrics, Committee on Genetics. (2000). Molecular genetic testing in pediatric practice: A subject review. *Pediatrics, 106*, 1494–1497. Statement of Reaffirmation, May 2009. doi:10.1542/peds106.6.1494

American College of Obstetricians and Gynecologists (ACOG). (2007). ACOG practice bulletin #77: Screening for fetal chromosomal abnormalities. *Obstetrics & Gynecology, 109*(1), 217–227.

American College of Obstetricians and Gynecologists (ACOG). (2008). ACOG committee opinion #397: Surrogate motherhood. *Obstetrics & Gynecology, 111*(2, Pt. 1), 465–470.

American Society for Reproductive Medicine (ASRM). (2008a). *Assisted reproductive technologies: A guide for parents*. Retrieved from http://www.asrm.org/patientbooklets/

American Society for Reproductive Medicine. (2008b). Definitions of infertility and recurrent pregnancy loss. *Fertility & Sterility, 90*(3), S60. doi:10.1016/j.fertnstert.2008.08.065

American Society for Reproductive Medicine. (2008c). Evaluation of the azoospermic male. Practice committee of the ASRM in collaboration with the Society for Male Reproduction and Urology. *Fertility & Sterility, 90*(Suppl. 3), S74–S77. doi:10.1016/j.fertnstert.2008.08.092

American Society for Reproductive Medicine. (2008d). Guidelines for gamete and embryo donation: A practice committee report. *Fertility & Sterility, 90*(3), S30–S44. doi:10.1016/j.fertnstert.2008.08.090

American Society for Reproductive Medicine. (2008e). Male obesity and alteration in sperm parameters. *Fertility & Sterility, 90*(6), 2222–2225. doi:10.1016/j.fernstert.2007.10.011

American Society for Reproductive Medicine. (2008f). Obesity and reproduction: An educational bulletin. *Fertility & Sterility, 90*(3), S21–S29. doi:10.1016/j.fertnstert.2008.08.005

American Society for Reproductive Medicine. (2008g). Optimizing natural fertility. *Fertility & Sterility, 90*(3), S1–S6. doi:10.1016/j.fertnstert.2008.08.122

American Society for Reproductive Medicine. (2008h). *Patient fact sheet: Ectopic pregnancy*. Retrieved from http://www.asrm.org/Patients/FactSheets/EctopicPregnancy.pdf

American Society for Reproductive Medicine. (2008i). Preimplantation genetic testing: A practice committee opinion. *Fertility & Sterility, 90*(3) s136–143. doi:10.1016/j.fertnstert.2008.08.062

American Society for Reproductive Medicine. (2008j). Report on varicocele and infertility. *Fertility & Sterility, 90*(3), S247–S249. doi:10.1016/j.fertnstert.2008.08.050

American Society for Reproductive Medicine. (2008k). Smoking and infertility. *Fertility & Sterility, 90*(3), S254–S259. doi:10.1016/j.fertnstert.2008.08.035

American Society of Reproductive Medicine (ASRM). (2010). *Frequently asked questions about infertility*. Retrieved from http://www.asrm.org/patients/faqs.htm

Balen, A. H., & Rutherford, A. J. (2007). Management of infertility. *British Medical Journal, 335*, 608–611. doi:10.1136/bmj.39324.662049.80

Cheong, Y. C., Hung Yu Ng, E., & Ledger, W. L. (2008). Acupuncture and assisted conception. *Cochrane Database of Systematic Reviews* (4). Art. No. CD006920.

Devine, K. S. (2008). *Challenges and management of infertility, including assisted reproductive technologies*. White Plains, NY: March of Dimes Foundation.

Gleicher, N., & Nakajima, S. T. (2009). Should a woman undergoing IVF be allowed to select the baby's gender. *Contemporary OB/Gyn, 54*(8), 46–53.

Goldstein, S. R. (2008). Abnormal bleeding. In R. S. Gibbs, B. Y. Karlan, A. F. Haney, & I. Nygaard (Eds.), *Danforth's obstetrics and gynecology* (10th ed., chap. 37, pp. 664–671). Philadelphia, PA: Lippincott, Williams & Wilkins.

Inhorn, M. C. (2006). "Making Muslim babies: Ivf and gamete donation in sunni versus shi'a islam. *Cultural Medical Psychiatry, 30*(4), 427–450. doi: 10.1007/s11013-006-9027-x

Kuliev, A., & Verlinsky, Y. (2010). Preimplantation diagnosis for genetic disorders. *Sexuality, Reproductive & Menopause, 8*(1), 9–13.

Kumar, A., Ghadir, S., Eskandari, N., & DeCherney, A. H. (2007). Infertility. In A. H. DeCherney, L. Nathan, T. M. Goodwin, & N. Laufer (Eds.), *Current diagnosis and treatment: Obstetrics & gynecology* (10th ed.). Boston, MA: McGraw-Hill.

Lashley, F. R. (2007). *Essentials of clinical genetics in nursing practice*. New York, NY: Springer.

Lee, R., Goldstein, M., Ullery, B. W., Ehrlich, J., Soares, M., Razzano, R. A., . . . Witkin, S. S. (2009). Value of serum antisperm antibodies in diagnosing obstructive azoospermia. *The Journal of Urology, 181*, 264–269.

Lu, J.-C., Huang, Y.-F., & Lu, N.-Q. (2008). Antisperm immunity and infertility. *Expert Review Clinical Immunology, 4*(1), 113–126.

McGrath, J. M., Samra, H. A., Zukowsky, K., & Baker, B. (2010). Parenting after infertility: Issues for families and infants. *American Journal of Maternal/Child Nursing, 35*(3), 156–165.

National Society of Genetic Counselors. (2005). *Genetic counseling as a profession*. Retrieved from http://www.nsgc.org/about/definition/cfm

Paterno, M. T. (2008). Families of two: Meeting the needs of couples experiencing male infertility. *Nursing for Women's Health, 12*(4). doi: 300-306. 10.1111/j.1751-486X.2008.00344x

Purnell, L. D., & Paulanka, B. J. (2008). *Guide to culturally competent health care*. Philadelphia, PA: F. A. Davis.

Schenker, J. G. (2010). *Infertility evaluation and treatment according to Jewish law*. Retrieved from http://www.obgyn.net/women/women.asp?page=/eago/art13

Skidmore-Roth, L. (2010). *Mosby's handbook of herbs & natural supplements* (4th ed.). St. Louis, MO: Elsevier Mosby.

Speroff, L., & Fritz, M. (2005). *Clinical gynecologic endocrinology and infertility*. Philadelphia, PA: Lippincott, Williams & Wilkins.

Storment, J. M. (2006). Infertility and recurrent pregnancy loss. In M. G. Curtis, S. Overholt, & M. P. Hopkins (Eds.), *Glass' office gynecology* (6th ed.). Philadelphia. PA: Lippincott, Williams & Wilkins.

Thomas, M., & Van Voorhis, B. J. (2008). Gynecologic ultrasound. In R. S. Gibbs, B. Y. Karlan, A. F. Haney, & I. E. Nygaard (Eds.), *Danforth's obstetrics and gynecology* (10th ed., pp. 540–554). Philadelphia, PA: Lippincott, Williams & Wilkins.

Toriello, H. V., & Meck, J. M. (2008). ACMG practice guidelines: Statement on guidance for genetic counseling in advanced paternal age. *Genetics in Medicine, 10*(6), 457–460. doi: 10.1097/GIM.0b013e318176fabb

Ward, K. (2008). Genetics in obstetrics and gynecology. In R. S. Gibbs, B. Y. Karlan, A. F. Haney, & I. E. Nygaard (Eds.), *Danforth's obstetrics and gynecology* (10th ed., pp. 88–110). Philadelphia, PA: Lippincott, Williams & Wilkins.

Warren, J. E., & Silver, R. M. (2008). Genetics of pregnancy loss. *Clinical Obstetrics & Gynecology, 51*(1), 84–95. doi: 10.1097/GRF.0b013e318161719c

Wilson, B. A., Shannon, M. T., & Shields, K. M. (2010). *Prentice Hall nurse's drug guide—2010*. Upper Saddle River, NJ: Pearson Education.

Woodruff, T. J., Carlson, A., Schwartz, J. M., & Guidice, L. C. (2008). Proceedings of the Summit on Environmental Challenges to Reproductive Health and Fertility: Executive summary. *Fertility & Sterility, 89*(2), 281–300.

Wright, K. P., & Johnson, J. (2008). Infertility. In R. S. Gibbs, B. Y. Karlan, A. F. Haney, & I. E. Nygaard (Eds.), *Danforth's obstetrics and gynecology* (10th ed., pp. 705–715). Philadelphia, PA: Lippincott, Williams & Wilkins.

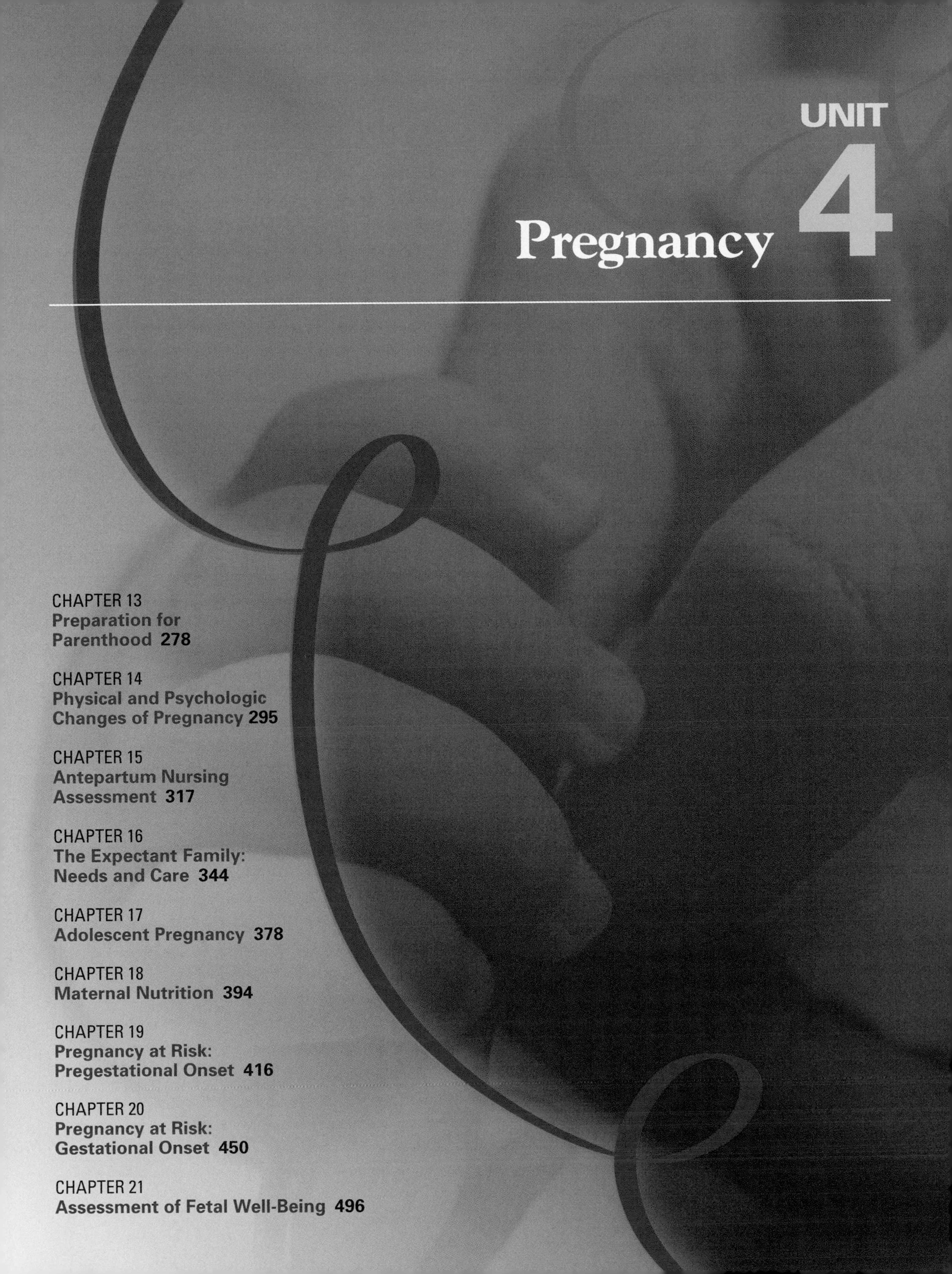

UNIT 4

Pregnancy

CHAPTER 13

Preparation for Parenthood

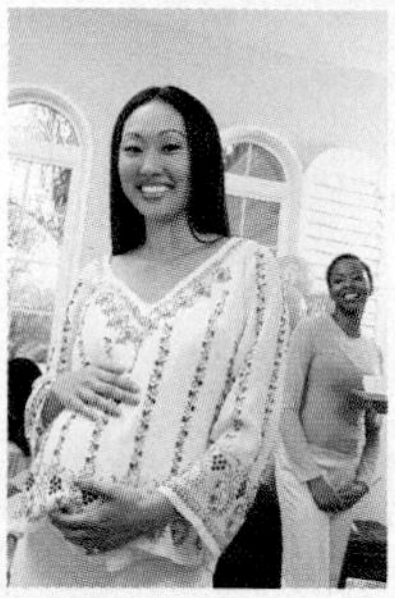

I couldn't wait to begin our childbirth classes. Attending the classes with the other expectant parents made the pregnancy and upcoming labor seem so much more real. Our childbirth educator helped ease our anxiety and gave us guidance on how to make the most of the birth. I still keep in contact with a few of my classmates and send an annual holiday greeting card with my son's photograph to our instructor.

LEARNING OUTCOMES

1. Apply the nursing process to help couples prepare for childbirth.
2. Identify the various issues related to preconception counseling, pregnancy, labor, and birth that require decision making by parents.
3. Discuss the basic goals of childbirth education.
4. Summarize the role of the doula/labor companion during labor and birth.
5. Describe the types of prenatal education programs available to expectant couples and their families.
6. Delineate the childbirth educator's role in promoting relaxation for pregnant women.
7. Compare methods of childbirth preparation.

KEY TERMS

Birth plan *281*
Centering *283*
Childbearing decisions *281*
Disassociation relaxation *291*
Doula *284*
Effleurage *292*
Labor support *284*
Prenatal education *284*
Progressive relaxation *290*
Touch relaxation *291*

Preparation for parenthood begins with one's own birth into a family. Attitudes, feelings, and fears about pregnancy, birth, and parenthood are molded by numerous factors, including relationships within and outside one's own family, cultural conditioning, personal history, and discussions with healthcare providers, friends, and other women.

A person's experiences with parenting or children may have been pleasant or uncomfortable. A person's information about parenthood and related areas may or may not be accurate. Because people bring their beliefs and fears with them to the childbearing period, the nurse can do much to correct misconceptions and calm fears about pregnancy, childbirth, and early parenting. Although some women may approach labor and birth with great excitement and anticipation, others may view it as a fearful, unpleasant experience. One way that people can cope with feelings about impending parenthood is to assume an active, participatory role during the preconception, prenatal, intrapartum, and postpartum periods. This involvement offers them a degree of control over what could otherwise be an overwhelming experience.

Some of the decisions that the childbearing family must consider are presented in this chapter. These include the decision to have a baby; choice of care provider; type of childbirth preparation; type of prenatal care including group or individual care, place of birth, activities during the birth, method of infant feeding, and choices surrounding the care of the newborn. The chapter also considers the role of the nurse, who provides information that enables the family to make informed decisions.

Throughout this chapter the term "childbearing family" is used to include all family types. In today's society, the childbearing family may be composed of a man and a woman joined by marriage or simply by mutual personal commitment, a single woman living alone or with a friend or family member, or a lesbian couple. No matter what the family structure and configuration, the expectant woman and her support person have similar concerns and educational needs during this time.

Today's professional nurse has many opportunities to help the childbearing family make the decisions that are part of pregnancy and birth. The nurse can help families seek preconceptual counseling, select a healthcare provider, find prenatal classes that meet their needs, and make informed choices. Even more important, as the family members work through these decisions, the nurse is able to affirm their decision-making abilities and their ability to take on parenting roles. For first-time parents in particular, the decisions may seem numerous, complicated, and sometimes overwhelming. The nurse has a unique opportunity to help these families establish a pattern of decision making that will serve them well in their years as parents (Figure 13-1 ■).

Preconception Counseling

Care Plan Activity: Preconception Counseling

One of the first questions a couple should ask before conception is whether they wish to have children. This involves consideration of each person's goals, expectations of their relationship, and desire to be a parent. At times one individual wishes to have a child, whereas the other does not. In such situations, an open discussion is essential to reach a mutually acceptable decision. In some cases, professional counseling for the couple may be necessary.

Couples who wish to have children face a decision about the timing of pregnancy. At what point in their lives do they believe it would be best to become parents? Pregnancy comes as a surprise even when the decision about timing is made, but at least the couple has some control over it.

For couples who have religious beliefs that do not support contraception or who feel that family planning is unnatural and wrong, planning the timing of pregnancy is unacceptable and

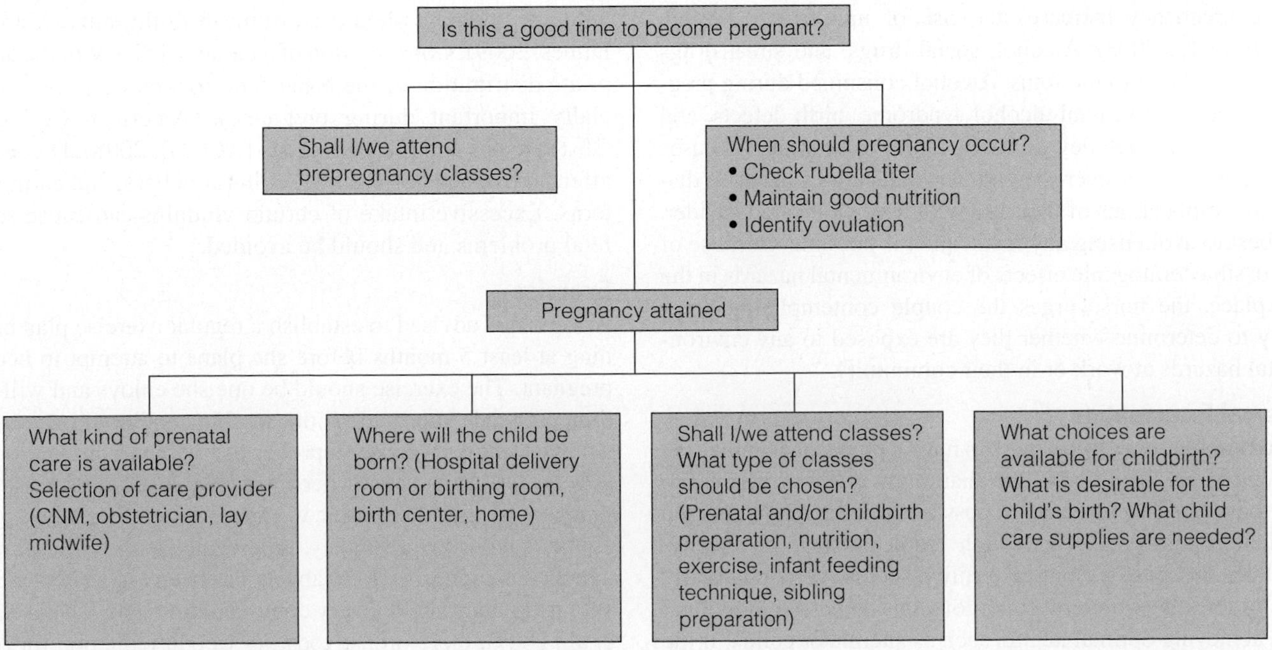

Figure 13-1 ■ Pregnancy decision tree.

irrelevant. These couples can still take steps to ensure that they are in the best possible physical and mental health when pregnancy occurs.

Ideally, the decision to become pregnant and have a child should be a conscious one; however, this is not always the case. Nearly half of the pregnancies in the United States are unintended or unplanned (Jones, Zolna, Henshaw, et al., 2008). Couples with unplanned pregnancies may need additional support from the nurse, such as information about community resources available for the couple and their infant. Encouragement and reassurance are especially needed for these families.

Case Study: Preparing for Pregnancy

Preconception Health Measures

The professional role of the nurse working with women or couples during the preconception period includes conveying information about known or suspected health risks. After a thorough assessment, the nurse advises the woman to cease smoking if possible, or to at least limit her cigarette intake. Placenta previa, abruptio placentae, preterm rupture of membranes, and pregnancy loss are risk factors that are increased in mothers who smoke. According to the Centers for Disease Control and Prevention (CDC), 13% of women reported smoking during the last 3 months of pregnancy. Furthermore, pregnant women exposed to secondhand smoke have 20% higher odds of giving birth to a low-birth-weight baby (CDC, 2009). Secondhand smoke has been found to increase the risk of small-for-gestational-age infants; therefore, partners of pregnant women should refrain from smoking in the woman's presence. Research has found that smoking during pregnancy is a significant risk factor in the incidence of sudden infant death syndrome (SIDS) (Einarson & Riordan, 2009). (See chapter 37 ∞ for a detailed discussion on SIDS prevention.)

The effects of caffeine are less clearly understood; however, as a precaution the woman is advised to avoid caffeine or limit her intake. Research shows that high doses of caffeine ingested during pregnancy increases the risk of miscarriage (Weng, Odouli, & Li, 2008). Alcohol, social drugs, and street drugs pose a real threat to the fetus. Alcohol consumed during pregnancy can result in fetal alcohol syndrome, birth defects, and low birth weight (Bailey & Sokol, 2008). A woman who uses any prescription or over-the-counter medications needs to discuss the implications of their use with her healthcare provider. It is best to avoid using any medication if possible. Because of the possible teratogenic effects of environmental hazards in the workplace, the nurse urges the couple contemplating pregnancy to determine whether they are exposed to any environmental hazards at work or in their community.

Physical Examination

It is advisable for both partners to have a physical examination to identify any health problems that might affect pregnancy so that they can be corrected if possible. These might include medical conditions, such as high blood pressure or obesity; problems that pose a threat to fertility, such as certain sexually transmitted infections; or conditions that keep the individual from achieving optimal health, such as anemia or colitis. If the family history indicates previous genetic disorders, or if the couple is planning pregnancy when the woman is over age 35, the healthcare provider may suggest that the couple consider genetic counseling.

In addition to the history and physical exam, the woman may have the following laboratory tests: urinalysis, complete blood count, blood type and Rh factor, venereal disease research laboratory (VDRL) test, Pap smear, gonorrhea culture, chlamydia screen, and rubella and hepatitis screens. Women who are nonimmune to rubella should be counseled about the possible effects on the fetus should infection occur during the first trimester of pregnancy. If a woman decides to receive the rubella vaccine, the nurse must inform her to wait 3 months before conceiving to eliminate the risk of prenatal infection. These women should be counseled to use contraception during the 3-month period to prevent pregnancy. Before conception, the woman is also advised to have a dental examination and any necessary dental work completed to avoid exposure to x-rays and the risk of infection.

Women should also be asked questions regarding their psychologic history and assessed for mental illness. Certain classes of medications may be contraindicated during pregnancy and drug changes may be needed prior to conception to prevent adverse maternal or fetal effects.

Nutrition

Before conception, it is advisable for the woman to be at an average weight for her body build and height. The nurse can discuss nutrition and recommend that the woman follow a nutritious diet that contains ample quantities of all the essential nutrients. Some nutritionists advocate emphasizing the following nutrients: calcium, protein, iron, B complex vitamins, vitamin C, magnesium, and folic acid. Folic acid supplementation should be initiated before conception because it decreases the incidence of neural tube defects in infants. (See the discussion in chapter 18 ∞.) The Institute of Medicine recommends that women of childbearing age consume 4 milligrams of folic acid per day before conception, and women who are pregnant should consume 6 milligrams (March of Dimes, 2009). Consumption of a balanced diet with the appropriate distribution of the basic food pyramid groups is especially important during pregnancy (American College of Obstetricians and Gynecologists [ACOG], 2008). Diet can be affected by food preferences, cultural beliefs, and eating patterns. Excessive intake of certain vitamins can cause severe fetal problems and should be avoided.

Exercise

A woman is advised to establish a regular exercise plan beginning at least 3 months before she plans to attempt to become pregnant. The exercise should be one she enjoys and will continue. It needs to provide some aerobic conditioning and some general toning. Exercise improves the woman's circulation and general health and tones her muscles. Once an exercise program is well established, the woman is generally encouraged to continue it during pregnancy. Prepregnancy obesity, defined as a body mass index of 30 or above, has been associated with severe pregnancy and delivery complications (Jain, Denk, Kruse, et al., 2007); therefore, advocating weight reduction for obese women who want to become pregnant is advisable.

Contraception

A woman who takes birth control pills is advised to stop the pill and have two or three normal menses before attempting to conceive. This allows the natural hormonal cycle to return and facilitates dating the subsequent pregnancy. A woman using an intrauterine device is advised to have it removed and wait 1 month before attempting to conceive. This allows the endometrium to be resterilized. Other methods of contraception that women can use during the waiting period include a variety of barrier methods of contraception (condoms, diaphragm, or cervical cap with a spermicide).

Conception

Most preconception recommendations focus on helping the couple attain their best possible health state so that they do not enter pregnancy with unnecessary risks. Conception is a personal and emotional experience and, even if a couple is prepared, the individuals may feel some ambivalence. This is a normal response, but they may require reassurance that the ambivalence will pass. The prospective parents may get so caught up in preparation and in their efforts to "do things right" that they lose sight of the pleasure they derive from each other and their lives together and cease to value the joy of spontaneity in their relationship. It is often helpful for the healthcare provider to remind an overly zealous couple that moderation is always appropriate and that there is value in "taking time to smell the roses."

Childbearing Decisions

Childbearing decisions are decisions parents face about their childbirth preferences and experiences. A method that has assisted many couples in making these choices is called a birth plan. In the **birth plan**, prospective parents identify aspects of the childbearing experience that are most important to them. (A sample birth plan is presented in Figure 13-2 ■.) The birth plan helps identify available options and becomes a tool for communication among the expectant parents, the healthcare providers, and the healthcare professionals at the birth setting.

The birth plan also helps pregnant women and couples set priorities. Using the plan, they identify areas that they want to incorporate in their own birth experience. Then they can take the birth plan to a visit with their certified nurse-midwife (CNM) or other care provider and use it in discussing and comparing their wishes with the philosophy and beliefs of the provider. It is imperative that the couple discuss their preferences at a prenatal visit before labor. Sometimes couples may include requests that need clarification. For example, if the couple states they do not want any external monitoring, the provider needs to explain that intermittent monitoring could be provided but that eliminating all monitoring during labor could jeopardize both the mother and the fetus. Possible obstetric interventions that may be needed should also be part of the birth plan. They can also take the birth plan to the birth setting and use it as a basis for communicating their wishes during the childbirth experience.

Today, there are many more choices that pregnant women and couples make. Some of these are explored in Table 13-1. Although most birth experiences are close to the desired experience, at times expectations cannot be met. This may be because of the unavailability of some choices in the community or unexpected problems during pregnancy or birth. It is important for nurses to help expectant parents keep sight of what is realistic for their situation. Maternal satisfaction is obviously important when outcomes of childbirth are considered. However, it must not be seen as separate from, or a greater priority than, the physical safety of both mother and child (Bailey, Crane, & Nugent, 2008).

Sample Birth Plan

Choice	*Choice*
Care provider:	Position during birth:
Certified nurse-midwife	On side
Obstetrician	Hands and knees
Family physician	Kneeling
Lay midwife	Squatting
Birth setting:	Birthing chair
Hospital:	Birthing bed
Birthing room	Other:
Delivery room	Family present (sibs)
Birth center	Filming of birth (videotaping)
Home	Photography of birth
Support during labor and birth:	Leboyer
Partner present	Episiotomy
Doula present	No sterile drapes
During labor:	Partner to cut umbilical cord
Ambulate as desired	Hold baby immediately after birth
Shower if desired	Breastfeed immediately after birth
Wear own clothes	No separation after birth
Use hot tub	Save the placenta
Use own rocking chair	Collect cord blood for banking
Have perineal prep	Newborn care:
Have enema	Eye treatment for the baby
Water birth	Vitamin K injection
Electronic fetal monitor	Heptovac injection
Membranes:	Breastfeeding
Rupture naturally	Formula feeding
Amniotomy if needed	Pacifier use
Labor stimulation if needed	Glucose water
Medication:	Circumcision
Identify type desired	Postpartum care:
Fluids or ice as desired	Short stay
Music during labor and birth	48-hour stay after vaginal birth
Massage	Home visits after discharge
Therapeutic touch	Home doula
Healing touch	Other:

Figure 13-2 ■ Birth plan for childbirth choices. The columns list various choices that the couple may consider during their childbirth experience. Once the couple has considered each of the choices, they may circle the items they desire.

Healthcare Provider

One of the first decisions facing expectant parents is the selection of a healthcare provider. The nurse assists them by explaining the various options and outlining what can be expected from each. A thorough understanding of the differences of educational preparation, skill level, practice style, and general philosophy and characteristics of practice of certified nurse-midwives, obstetricians, family practice physicians, and lay midwives is essential. The nurse can encourage expectant parents to investigate the care provider's credentials, basic and special education and training, fee schedule, and availability to new patients; this is often accomplished by telephoning the provider's office.

Childbirth Solutions

TABLE 13-1 Benefits and Risks of Some Consumer and Medical Decisions During Pregnancy, Labor, and Birth

ISSUE	BENEFITS	RISKS
Breastfeeding	• No additional expense • Contains maternal antibodies • Decreases incidence of infant otitis media, vomiting, and diarrhea, hospitalizations during the first year of life, and allergies • Easier to digest than formula • Immediately after birth, promotes uterine contractions and decreases incidence of postpartum hemorrhage • Promotes maternal-infant bonding	• Transmission of maternal infections to newborn, such as HIV • Irregular ovulation and menses can cause false sense of security and nonuse of hormonal contraceptives • Increased nutritional requirement in mother

Ambulation during labor	• Comfort for laboring woman
	• May assist in labor progression by
	  • Stimulating contractions
	  • Allowing gravity to help descent of fetus
	  • Giving sense of independence and control
		• Cord prolapse with rupture of membranes unless engagement has occurred
		• Birth of infant in undesirable locations (hallways, outdoors, waiting area)
		• Inability to monitor fetal heart rate (FHR) unless telemetry unit available

Electronic fetal monitoring	• Helps evaluate fetal well-being • Helps identify fetal stress • Useful in diagnostic testing • Helps evaluate labor progress	• Supine postural hypotension • Intrauterine perforation (with internal uterine pressure device) • Infection (with internal monitoring) • Decreases personal interaction with mother because of attention paid to the machine • Mother is unable to ambulate or change her position freely
Whirlpool (jet hydrotherapy)	• Increased relaxation • Decreased anxiety • Stimulation of labor • Provides pain relief • Slight decrease in blood pressure (BP) • Increased diuresis • Decreased incidence of vacuum and forceps deliveries • Increased pain threshold • Higher satisfaction with birth • Decreased use of pain medication (Stark, Rudell, & Haus, 2008)	• May slow contractions if used before active labor is established • Possible risk of infection if membranes are ruptured • Slight increase in maternal temperature and pulse in tub • Hypothermia • Increases fetal heart rate (FHR) by 10–20 beats/min
Analgesia	• Maternal relaxation facilitates labor	• All drugs reach the fetus in varying degrees and with varying effects
Episiotomy	• Decreases irregular tearing of perineum • Easier to repair for practitioner	• Increased pain after birth and for 1–3 months following birth • Dyspareunia • Infection • Increased frequency of third- and fourth-degree lacerations (Frankman, Wang, Bunker, et al., 2009)

The nurse can also help the woman/couple develop a list of interview questions for their first visit to a care provider. These could include the following:

- Who is in practice with you, or who covers for you when you are unavailable?
- At what point after admission do you come to the hospital or birth setting to provide support?
- How do your partners' philosophies compare to yours?
- How do you feel about my partner, other support person, or other children coming to the prenatal visits?
- Do you offer centering (group care) or individual prenatal care visits?
- What weight gain do you recommend and why?
- What are your feelings about (fill in special desires for the birth event, such as different positions assumed during labor, avoidance of an episiotomy, induction of labor, other people present during the birth, pain control measures, breastfeeding immediately after the birth, no separation of infant and parents following birth, and so on)?
- If a cesarean is necessary, can my partner be present?
- What are your feelings regarding complementary treatments during labor (herbs to augment labor, use of acupressure/massage/hypnosis, use of oils for perineal massage, and so on)?

Expectant parents also need to discuss the qualities they want in a care provider for the newborn. They may want to visit several pediatric healthcare providers before the birth to select someone who will meet their needs and those of their child.

PROFESSIONALISM IN PRACTICE

Referrals

The nurse provides referrals to appropriate providers, hospitals, and clinics as needed to ensure that the woman receives competent, professional medical care.

Prenatal Care Services

The nurse can assist expectant parents in obtaining the type of prenatal care services that are most appropriate for their personal needs. Most practitioners offer individual prenatal care services in which the woman or the woman and her family attend a clinic or office visit on a regular basis depending on her stage of pregnancy. Recently, the concept of **centering**, or group prenatal care, has begun to evolve.

In the centering model, expectant women and their families or support persons attend a group session with other women in the same stage of pregnancy. During each session, women voice their questions and gather support from their pregnant peers. The practitioner meets with each woman individually before the group to perform basic assessments and examinations as appropriate; however, women benefit greatly from the group support and learning that occurs in the centering groups. Women who opt for the centering model of prenatal care typically experience more satisfaction with their prenatal care experience (Robertson, Aycock, & Darnell, 2009). Women express a sense of empowerment and benefit from the group interaction. In addition, centering has shown to be an effective model for both adolescents and immigrant women (Robertson et al., 2009). Outcomes are the same as traditional prenatal care, making it both cost effective and safe for participants.

Birth Setting

The nurse can help expectant parents choose a birth setting by suggesting they tour facilities and talk with nurses there as well as talk with friends or acquaintances who are recent parents. Questions that may be asked of new parents include the following:

- What kind of support did you receive during labor? Was it what you wanted?
- If the setting has both labor and delivery rooms and birthing rooms, was a birthing room available when you wanted it?
- Were you encouraged to be mobile during labor or to do what you wanted to do (walking, sitting in a rocking chair, remaining in bed, sitting in a hot tub, standing in a shower, and so on)?
- How was your labor partner or coach treated?
- Were you allowed to take an active role in decision making throughout the birth process?
- If you had a doula, was her role respected? Was she welcome in the birth setting?
- Was your birth plan respected? Did you share it with the facility before the birth? If something did not work, why do you think there were problems?
- Did the nurse offer suggestions regarding comfort measures?
- Did the healthcare team provide emotional support?
- How were medications handled during labor? Were you comfortable with this?
- Were siblings welcomed in the birth setting? At the birth? After the birth?
- Did you feel you were given ample time to spend with your baby immediately after childbirth?
- Was the nursing staff helpful after the baby was born? Did you receive self-care and infant care information? Was it in a usable form? Did you have a choice about what information you got? Did they let you decide what information you needed?
- Did you feel your choice of feeding method was supported?

The nurse helps expectant parents understand the array of choices available to them. The nurse can encourage them to consider options early in the pregnancy to allow time for talking with other parents and touring facilities.

> “What I've seen time and again is that the technology of the hospital overwhelms patients' natural instincts; they are intimidated, afraid of appearing stupid or clumsy or sentimental in a surrounding that seems too efficient and immaculate and intelligent.”
>
> — *A Midwife's Story*

Nurses involved in childbirth education need to include the concept of individuality when providing information to expectant parents about the process of childbirth and their own pattern of coping. The wave of the future in childbirth education is to encourage women to incorporate their natural responses into coping with the pain of labor and birth. Alternative self-care activities should be explored with the expectant couple to identify preferences.

Nurses should encourage expectant women and couples to personalize the birth setting. The woman might plan, for example, to bring items from home to enhance relaxation and comfort, such as warm socks, slippers, bath powder, lotion, or a favorite blanket. She may wish to bring photographs of children, parents, or friends who cannot be there to share the birth experience. Many expectant parents enjoy listening to tapes of favorite music or watching home videotapes or favorite films. Such personalization of the birth setting may give expectant parents feelings of increased serenity and empowerment.

> **CLINICAL TIP**
>
> Call the birthing facilities in your community and inquire about what choices are available in each facility so that you can answer expectant parents' questions.

Labor Support Person

Some of the first formal childbirth preparation classes were patterned after a book entitled *Husband Coached Childbirth* by Dr. Robert Bradley, published in 1965. Since that time, husbands and other partners of expectant women have been very involved in acting as "coaches" or support persons during childbirth classes, labor, and birth. Although some men or support persons welcome the role and look forward to providing emotional and physical support, others do not. Some men may become anxious and fearful. These feelings can be related to past experiences and/or cultural factors. In these situations, the nurse provides encouragement and support to both the woman and her support person. Women who had continuous intrapartum support were less likely to have intrapartum analgesia, operative birth, or to report dissatisfaction with their childbirth experiences (Hodnett, Gates, Hofmeyr, et al., 2007). A woman's satisfaction with childbirth is directly affected by the relationship with the caregiver, the support she received from caregivers, personal expectations, and her involvement with decision making. Clearly, the role of the nurse cannot be overestimated.

Doulas of North America

Application: Benefits of Having a Doula

For centuries, women have been serving and assisting other women in childbirth. Out of this need for companionship and special support in the birthing journey, the role of the **doula** has evolved. *Doula* is a Greek word that means "woman's servant." In the birthing environment, a doula is a companion who provides support but does not perform any clinical tasks. The doula provides **labor support**, which includes emotional, physical, and informational support and acts as an advocate for the woman and her family by verbalizing their wishes to the nurses and physicians or certified nurse-midwives. Continuous labor support facilitates birth; enhances the mother's memory of the experience; strengthens mother-infant bonding; increases breastfeeding success; and significantly reduces many forms of medical intervention, including cesarean delivery and the use of analgesia, anesthesia, vacuum extraction, and forceps (McGrath & Kennell, 2008). A doula may also be trained to provide support and care during the postpartum period. Later postpartum benefits include increased bonding/interaction with the infant and decreased symptoms of depression. The doula may accompany the childbearing couple on a volunteer basis or may be paid a fee by the family. Another support person who has been involved in labor and birthing is a monitrice. *Monitrice* is a French word that refers to a specially trained nurse who provides assessment, nursing care, and support. The role of monitrice is not common in the United States.

Siblings at Birth

Some couples decide to have their other children present at the birth. Children who will attend a birth can be prepared through books, audiovisual materials, models, discussion, and sibling classes. Nurses can assist parents with sibling preparation by helping them understand the stresses a child may experience. For example, the child may feel left out when there is a new child to love or disappointed if a brother is born when a sister is expected.

It is imperative that the child has his or her own support person or coach whose sole responsibility is tending to the needs of that child during the labor and birth experience. The support person should be familiar to the child, warm, sensitive, flexible, knowledgeable about the birth process, and comfortable with sexuality and birth. This person must be prepared to interpret to the child what is happening and to intervene when necessary. The support person should not be one who would hesitate to leave the birthing room (such as a maternal grandmother) but should be amenable to the child's desire to leave. The support person for the child should assume responsibility for providing distractions when needed. Trips to the cafeteria, visits to the nursery window, outdoor walks, and other age-appropriate activities should be available for the child.

Children should be given the option of relating to the birth in whatever manner they choose as long as it is not disruptive. Children should understand that it is their own choice to be there and that they may stay or leave the room as they choose. To help children recognize their needs and desires, the nurse may wish to elicit exactly what they expect from the experience. Children need to feel free to ask questions and express feelings.

In general, the presence of siblings at birth engenders feelings of interest (Kuramoto, 2008) and the desire to nurture "our" baby, as opposed to jealousy and rivalry directed at "Mom's" baby. The mother does not disappear mysteriously into the hospital and return with a demanding outsider. Instead, the family attending the birth together finds a new opportunity for closeness and growth by sharing in the birth of a new member.

DEVELOPING CULTURAL COMPETENCE

Female Relatives as Caregivers

In most Middle Eastern countries, childbirth is exclusively attended to by women. A woman in labor is most commonly surrounded by female relatives and friends. It is customary for the husband to be excluded from the delivery room. In Iran, full segregation is mandated by law. Women can only be cared for by female healthcare providers.

Classes for Family Members During Pregnancy

Childbirth classes are routinely taught by certified childbirth educators (CBEs or CCEs). These are individuals who have received specific educational preparation related to pregnancy, labor, birth, and postpartum/newborn care and issues. Many CBEs are also registered nurses; however, nursing training is not required. The majority of the certification programs do, however, require witnessing a minimum number of births.

The CBE should consider elements developed by authoritative organizations such as the Coalition for Improving Maternity Services (CIMS) when developing their own Philosophy of Childbirth for their classes. The "Mother-Friendly Childbirth Initiative" was created in 1996 by the CIMS, a national alliance of more than 50 childbirth organizations and many prominent individuals. The coalition's mission is to promote a wellness model of maternity care that will improve birth outcomes and substantially reduce costs. The philosophic cornerstones of mother-friendly care are: (1) normalcy of the birthing process, (2) empowerment, (3) autonomy, (4) do no harm, and (5) responsibility (Coalition for Improving Maternity Services [CIMS], 2009).

Prenatal education programs provide important opportunities to share information about pregnancy, childbirth, coping mechanisms, and choices available for the woman and her support person. Studies have shown that prepared childbirth education programs can have a beneficial effect on performance in labor and delivery. The prenatal period should be used to expose the prospective parents to information about labor and delivery, pain relief, obstetric complications and procedures, breastfeeding, normal newborn care, and postpartum adjustment. Along with this information, women need up-to-date, evidence-based information to help them make decisions regarding their choices during pregnancy and childbirth (Lothian, 2008). The content of each class is generally directed by the overall goals of the program. For example, in classes that aim to provide preconception information, preparations for becoming pregnant would be the major topics. Other classes may be directed toward childbirth choices available today, preparation of the mother for pregnancy and birth, preparation for cesarean birth, preparation for vaginal birth after cesarean, preparation for couples who desire an unmedicated birth, and preparation of specific people such as grandparents or siblings for the birth. The nurse who knows the types of prenatal programs available in the community can direct expectant parents to programs that meet their special needs and learning goals. Childbirth preparation classes usually contain information about changes in the woman and the developing baby (Table 13-2).

From the expectant parents' point of view, class content is best presented in chronology with the pregnancy (Figure 13-3 ■). It is important that the classes begin by identifying the parents' needs, goals, and learning styles. Although both parents expect to learn breathing and relaxation techniques and infant care, fathers usually expect facts and mothers expect coping strategies. Women's goals commonly include gaining information, reducing anxiety/increasing confidence, having their partner present and involved, and having a positive emotional experience in childbirth. Classes that provide an environment supportive of practicing newly learned techniques and the freedom to ask questions and receive explanations are beneficial in helping class participants obtain these goals. By the end of the class, parents should feel that they will be able to make appropriate and informed decisions by participating in a class where information is given in a nonjudgmental, nonthreatening environment. Classes may be divided into early and late classes so specific needs can be addressed.

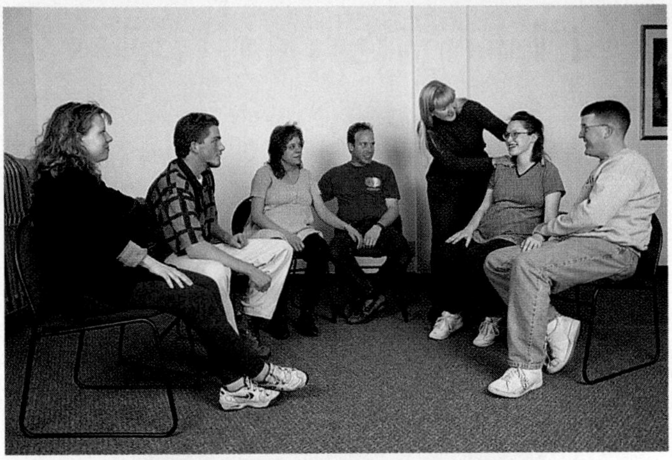

Figure 13-3 ■ In a group setting with a nurse-instructor, expectant parents share information about pregnancy and childbirth.

TABLE 13-2 Possible Content of Classes for Childbirth Preparation

Early Classes (First Trimester)
Early gestational changes
Self-care during pregnancy including diet and exercise
Fetal development, environmental dangers for the fetus
Sexuality in pregnancy
Birth settings and types of care providers
Nutrition, rest, and exercise suggestions
Relief measures for common discomforts of pregnancy
Psychologic changes in pregnancy
Information for getting pregnancy off to a good start
Danger signs that warrant immediate medical attention
Choosing a pediatrician
Feeding choices/benefits of breastfeeding
Depression and other psychologic disorders that can occur with pregnancy
Later Classes (Second and Third Trimesters)
Preparation for birth process
Postpartum self-care
Common birthing procedures (episiotomy, medications, fetal monitoring, perineal prep, enema, etc.)
Relaxation techniques
Breathing techniques
Alternative therapies in pregnancy and labor
Newborn care (feeding, bathing, dressing)
How to recognize when the baby is ill
Infant stimulation
Newborn safety issues, such as car seats and sleeping positions
Adolescent Preparation Classes
Stresses specific to adolescents
Newborn care
Health dangers for the baby
Weight gain issues and nutrition
How to recognize when the baby is ill
Baby care: physical and emotional
Sexuality
Peer relationships
Breastfeeding Programs
Advantages and disadvantages
Medical benefits of breastfeeding
Maternal nutrition
Techniques of breastfeeding (positions, latching on, engorgement, etc.)
Involvement of fathers in the feeding process
Cultural considerations

Early Classes: First Trimester

Early prenatal classes may include prepregnant women and couples as well as those in early pregnancy. As shown in Table 13-2, the classes cover early gestational changes; self-care during pregnancy; fetal development and environmental dangers for the fetus; sexuality in pregnancy; birth settings and types of care providers; nutrition, rest, and exercise suggestions; common discomforts of pregnancy and relief measures; psychologic changes in pregnancy for the woman and man; and getting the pregnancy off to a good start by following a healthful lifestyle, learning methods of coping with stress, and avoiding alcohol and smoking. Early classes should provide information about factors that place the woman at risk for preterm labor and about how to recognize symptoms of preterm labor. Early classes should also present the advantages and disadvantages of formula feeding or breastfeeding. The majority of women (50% to 80%) have made their infant feeding decision before the sixth month of pregnancy.

Later Classes: Second and Third Trimesters

The later classes focus on preparation for the birth, infant care and feeding, postpartum self-care, common birthing procedures (episiotomy, medications, fetal monitoring, perineal prep, enema, and so forth), and newborn safety issues. Many childbirth education programs now provide labor preparation classes that focus on preparation for the birth, birth options, and postpartum self-care with expectant parents attending separate classes that focus singly on breastfeeding or newborn care. Subjects such as emergency situations or labor and birth complications should be reviewed during the class. This includes information regarding assisting with an unattended birth when the couple fails to reach the hospital in a timely manner.

Through the Eyes of a Nurse
Childbirth Education

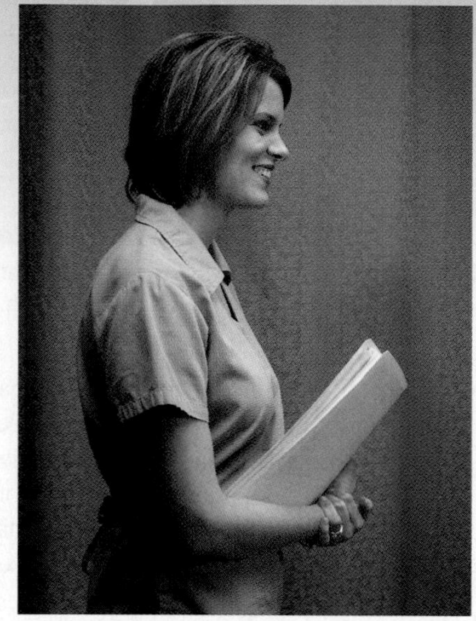

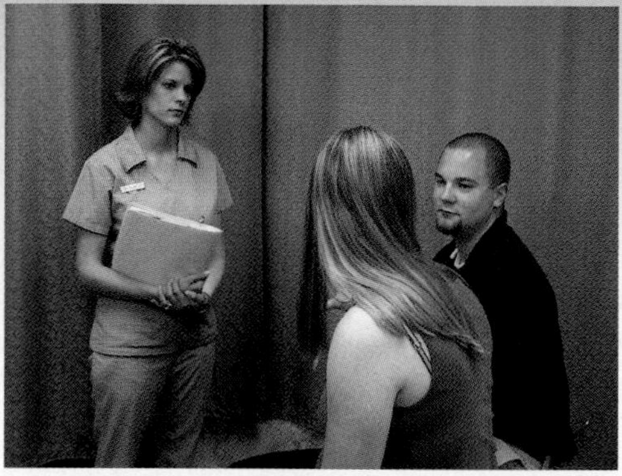

Family Experience

"I can't help but be nervous about labor and the pain I will feel. All my friends are asking me what childbirth preparation method I am going to use. I did some research on the Internet; there are a ton of different opinions. It is almost overwhelming!"

Nurse's Response

"Many women are anxious about the labor and birth process. These are normal feelings and your concerns are very common. It is helpful to use a method of childbirth preparation because it will give you some sense of control.

"Many couples, especially first-time parents, enroll in childbirth education courses. I can give you information about the classes offered at the birthing center, the hospital, and the community center. These classes tell you about pregnancy and teach relaxation and breathing techniques that can help you in labor. If you take classes, I encourage you to practice these techniques at home. Some families choose to gain information from instructional videos, books, or the Internet. There are even Web-based specialty programs that address specific needs, such as vaginal birth after cesarean (VBAC), or breastfeeding interventions for women who are having problems with nursing."

Nurse's Actions and Rationale

The nurse provides information about educational opportunities such as classes, videos, books, and the Internet. Some couples may not be able to attend classes due to financial restraints, child care issues, or work conflicts. Providing alternatives to traditional classroom instruction enables the family to pursue other educational sources. Recent studies have examined alternative resources like Web-based childbirth classes and found that they are effective in teaching couples childbirth education information and relaxation practice techniques (Wang, Chung, Sung, et al., 2006). The nurse bases advice to the family on evidence-based practice and current research.

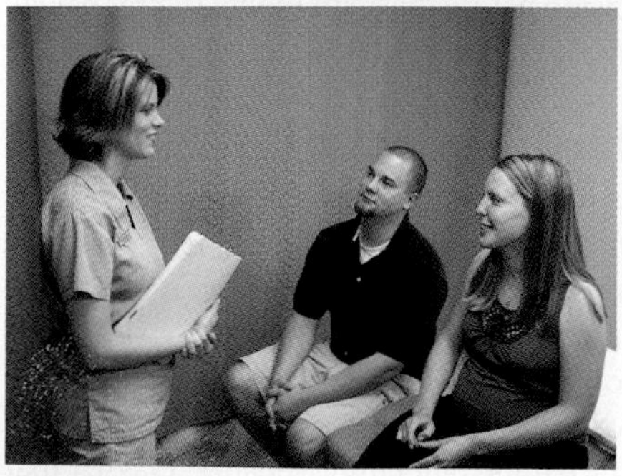

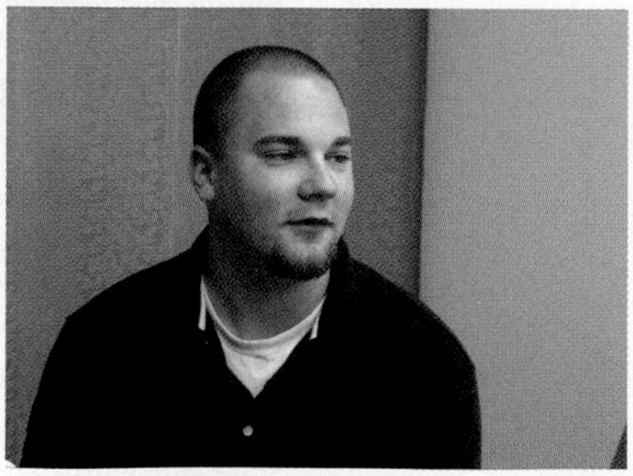

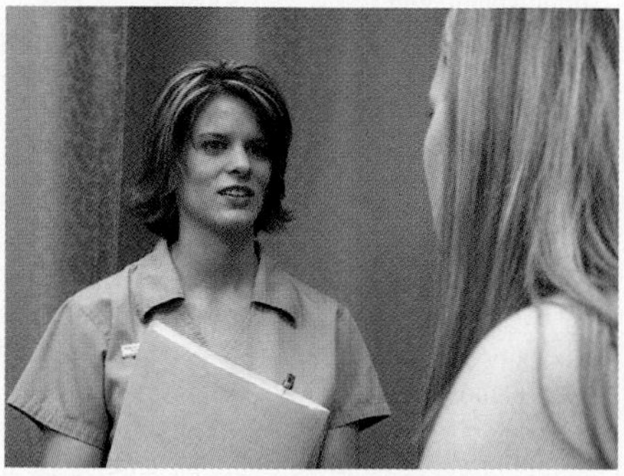

> **"** As a childbirth educator, I find one of the least favorite topics to discuss in class is unexpected outcomes, a topic that introduces the topic of grief that may be related to various situations. This can apply to patients who feel that they did not experience their envisioned perfect birth, or on a much more serious note, those who have a baby who is ill, has a disability, or those who have experienced a fetal loss. I have found it helpful to share a short story written by Emily Pearl Kingsley, a mother who explains her journey raising a child with special needs. She says it is rather like leaving on a trip to Italy that you have planned in detail for a long time, but instead of landing in Italy, you find yourself in Holland. . . . It is not bad, it is just different. She explains that if you spend the rest of your life mourning the fact you didn't get to Italy, you may never be free to enjoy the very special, the very lovely things about Holland. **"**
>
> — *(Amis & Green, 2002)*

Infant stimulation concepts can easily be incorporated into infant care class content. This will aid in the development of parenting skills and enhance prenatal and neonatal bonding. Stimulation methods that can be used include tactile, vestibular, auditory, and visual stimulation. Parents who use these methods may have better parenting skills and higher self-esteem. Infant massage classes are becoming very popular as an instructional series that parents attend after pregnancy with their infants to learn and practice different massage strokes to use on their infant as she or he grows. Vimala McClure, the founder of the International Association of Infant Massage, states that infant massage has physiologic and psychologic benefits for babies and their caregivers, providing colic relief, parent-infant bonding, as well as other benefits. Numerous studies support its use in infants. Infants who receive infant massage have exhibited decreased stress levels, increased weight gain, and improved motor function when compared with nonmassaged controls (Gonzalez et al., 2009).

Tactile stimulation can be discussed when maternal physiology is being presented. As the uterine wall thins during the pregnancy, the mother and father are better able to feel the baby, and the fetus can sense the parents' stroking and patting through the abdominal wall. *Effleurage* (a light, stroking movement made with the fingertips) can also be used over the abdominal wall to provide tactile stimulation to the fetus. Vestibular stimulation through movement of the fetus is provided while the expectant woman does the pelvic-tilt exercise. Rocking in a rocking chair is also a comfortable way to provide relaxation for the expectant woman and vestibular stimulation for the fetus. Auditory stimulation can be provided by playing music. Classical music (such as Vivaldi, Mozart, Beethoven, and Bach) is found to be pleasing to the fetus. In the prenatal period, actual visual stimulation for the fetus is not possible.

Adolescent Parenting Classes

Adolescents have special learning needs during pregnancy. Adolescents often need more support and more extensive teaching during pregnancy (Devito, 2007). Pregnant teens face a myriad of both psychologic and physical risks throughout pregnancy. Prenatal education and mentoring are essential. The childbirth educator should consider the teenager's need for privacy, acceptance, and respect. For this reason, classes designed specifically for the teenage population are highly desirable because many teenagers may feel that they may not receive this in a standard adult-centered childbirth class. Often teenage mothers face pregnancy and childbirth without adequate support from a partner or parents. Prenatal education classes specifically designed for teens can provide a forum for verbalization of fears and concerns. The nurse can also identify community resources for young mothers and their infants.

Breastfeeding Programs

Programs offering information on breastfeeding are increasing. For decades, a primary source of information has been La Leche League. Information can also be obtained from lactation consultants, peer counselors, labor and postpartum nurses, birthing centers, hospitals, and health clinics. Rates of breastfeeding in the United States are well below the *Healthy People 2010* objective of 75% (Cramton, Zain-Ul-Abideen, & Whalen, 2009). Breastfeeding education and support is positively correlated to successful breastfeeding. A goal of the surgeon general's national breastfeeding conference is to have 25% of women breastfeeding their infants a minimum of 1 full year by 2010 compared with the current data showing most mothers wean before the recommended 6 months (Forste & Hoffmann, 2008). Dennis's (2002) data stated that this was because of perceived difficulties with breastfeeding rather than because of maternal choice. Lack of education and knowledge, both on the part of caregivers and mothers, is the biggest barrier to breastfeeding; therefore, outpatient pediatric healthcare providers can be instrumental in preventing early weaning (Geraghty, Riddle, & Shaikh, 2008).

The father's support and encouragement of the mother is vital, so it is important to include him in the educational program and involve him in the decision making. Some fathers may feel negative and resentful about breastfeeding and need opportunities in the prenatal period for discussion and sharing of information. The decision to breastfeed is strongly related to the father's feeding preference.

Sibling Preparation: Adjustment to a Newborn

The birth of a new sibling is a significant event in a child's life. Positive adjustment can be enhanced by attendance at formal sibling preparation classes (Figure 13-4 ■). Typically, the classes are attended by children ages 3 to 12 years. Children younger than 3 tend to have shorter attention spans and may have difficulty participating in the class; however, many facilities will allow younger children to attend, especially if an older sibling is enrolled in the class. These classes can assist with decreasing sibling rivalry and reducing children's anxiety. They help children

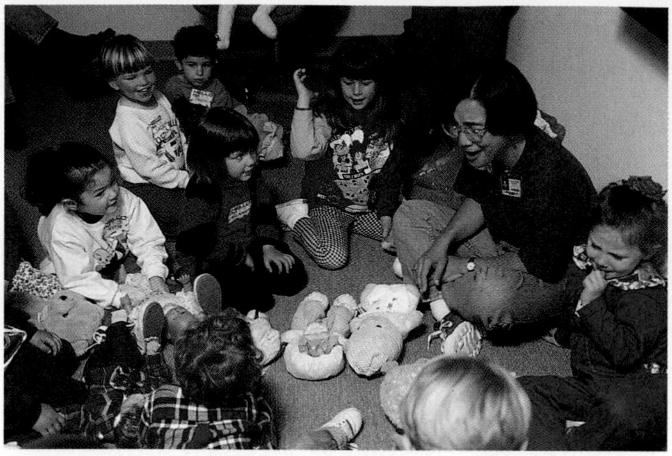

Figure 13-4 ■ It is especially important that siblings be well prepared when they are going to be present at the birth. However, even siblings who will not be present at the birth can benefit from information about birth and the new baby ahead of time.

feel that they are part of the birthing process. The classes also enable parents to identify children's concerns related to the new baby. They provide a means to facilitate communication and explore children's feelings. They also provide basic information about pregnancy, childbirth, and the characteristics and behavior of newborns.

Typically, parents and their children attend the class together. Many activities are devised to help each child feel special. Time is usually allotted at the end of the class for talking with parents about coping skills and providing hints about dealing with sibling jealousy. Class content typically includes care and behavior of new babies, a practice session holding anatomically correct dolls, changing diapers, and a tour of the "bedroom" and the nursery where Mom and baby will stay. Many times, a newborn is held up at the nursery window so the children can see a "real baby." Some facilities give the children a special gift for attendance or a trip to the cafeteria for a special treat.

Sibling preparation can be addressed through a formal class like the one just described, or in a less formal way by preparing a booklet for parents that addresses issues affecting both parents and children. Also, several excellent books and videos are available to help children prepare for a new sibling.

Classes for Grandparents

Grandparents are an important source of support and information for prospective and new parents. They are now being included in the birthing process more frequently. Prenatal programs for grandparents can address current roles, transitioning to a new role, beliefs regarding childbirth, and ways to support the new family unit. Grandparents can also benefit from educational information, such as the benefits of breastfeeding, and updates on infant care, such as proper infant sleep positions and when to introduce foods. If they plan to be integral members of the labor and birth team, they will need information about being coaches.

Education of the Family Having Cesarean Birth

Cesarean birth is an alternative method of birth via an abdominal and uterine incision.

Preparation for Cesarean Birth

Because one out of every three or four births is a cesarean, preparation for this possibility should be an integral part of every childbirth education curriculum. The national cesarean rate has rebounded to 31.1% (Lothian, 2008). The instructor should treat cesarean birth as a normal event and present factual information that allows expectant parents to make choices and be full participants in their birth experience. The instructor can emphasize the similarities between cesarean and vaginal births to minimize undertones of "normal" versus "abnormal" birth. This helps diminish the feelings of anger, loss, and grief that often accompany cesarean births.

Cesarean birth classes should cover what the parents can expect to happen during a cesarean birth, what they will feel, and what they can do. All pregnant women and couples should be encouraged to discuss with their certified nurse-midwife or physician what the approach would be in the event of a cesarean. They can also discuss their needs and preferences regarding the following:

- Participating in the choice of anesthetic.
- Father (or significant other) being present during the birth.
- Planning initial contact with their newborn.

> "As a nurse midwife, I felt extremely disappointed when I learned I would have to have a cesarean birth with my second child. I had great expectations about how much easier my second birth would be, and how I would "do everything different this time." I was amazed at how satisfied and happy I was immediately after the cesarean birth. During the birth, I asked the physician if the baby was almost out and how things were progressing. In the end, I had a beautiful, healthy baby and it turned out to be even a better experience than my first birth. I always try to comfort women who have medically indicated cesarean births by telling them it is still an amazing experience and a wonderful birthday!"

Preparation for Repeat Cesarean Birth

When expectant parents are anticipating a repeat cesarean birth, they have time to plan and prepare. Many hospitals or local groups (such as C-Sec, Inc.) provide preparation classes for cesarean birth. Parents who have had previous negative experiences need an opportunity to describe what contributed to their feelings. They should be encouraged to identify what they would like to change and to list interventions that would make the experience more positive. Those who have had positive experiences need reassurance that their needs and desires will be met in the same manner. In addition, all parents are encouraged to air any fears or anxieties.

A specific concern of the woman facing a repeat cesarean is anticipation of pain. She needs reassurance that subsequent cesareans are often less painful than the first. If her first cesarean was preceded by a long or strenuous labor, she will not experience the same fatigue. Giving this information will help her cope more effectively with all stressful stimuli, including pain. The nurse can remind the woman that she has already had experience with how to prevent, cope with, and alleviate painful stimuli.

Preparation for Parents Desiring Vaginal Birth After Cesarean Birth

Parents who are anticipating a vaginal birth after cesarean birth (VBAC) have unique needs. Because they may have unresolved questions and concerns about the last birth, it is helpful to begin the series of classes with an informational session. During this session, they can ask questions, share experiences, and begin to form bonds with one another. The nurse can supply information regarding the criteria necessary to attempt a trial of labor and identify decisions regarding the birth experience. Concerns regarding the complications associated with VBAC can also be discussed. Some women may wish to undergo a repeat cesarean birth to avoid the risk of uterine rupture associated with a trial of labor. Some certified childbirth educators (CBEs) find it helpful to have the parents prepare two birth plans: one for vaginal birth and one for cesarean birth. The preparation of the two plans seems to help parents take more control of the birth experience and tends to increase the positive aspects of the experience.

After an informational session, the classes may be divided according to the needs of the expectant parents. Those with recent coached childbirth experiences may need only refresher classes, whereas others may need complete training. Some parents may choose to attend regular classes after participating in the informational session.

Methods of Childbirth Preparation

Application: Lamaze

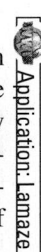

Various methods of childbirth preparation are taught in North America. The most common methods of this type are Lamaze (psychoprophylactic), Kitzinger (sensory memory), Bradley (partner-coached childbirth), and HypnoBirthing. Many hospital-based classes use a combination of these methods and are education focused. See Table 13-3 for differentiating characteristics of each method.

TABLE 13-3 Summary of Selected Childbirth Preparation Methods

METHOD	PURPOSE OR PHILOSOPHY	GOALS	TECHNIQUES	CLASS CONTENT
Bradley	To have the best, safest, and most rewarding birth experience possible.	• Natural childbirth. • Active participation of the husband as coach. • Excellent nutrition. • Breastfeeding, beginning at birth.	• Working in harmony with your body using controlled breathing and deep abdominopelvic breathing (Bradley, 1974) • Promoting general body relaxation (Bradley, 1974)	• Nutrition • Coach's role • Introduction to stages of labor • Birth planning • Variations and complications of labor • Postpartum preparation • Advanced first- and second-stage techniques • Preparation for your new family
Lamaze	Childbirth education empowers women to make informed choices in health care, to assume responsibility for their health, and to trust their inner wisdom.	• Birth is normal, natural, and healthy. • The experience of birth profoundly affects women and their families. • Women's inner wisdom guides them through birth. • Women have the right to give birth free from routine medical interventions.	• Disassociation relaxation • Controlled muscular relaxation • Breathing patterns	• Nutrition • Gestational changes • Labor and birth techniques for easing pain • Breathing techniques • Positioning during labor
Kitzinger	Sheila Kitzinger campaigns for women to have the information they need to make choices about childbirth. She is a strong believer in the benefits of home birth for women who are not high risk.	• Uses sensory memory to help the woman understand and work with her body in preparation for birth.	• Uses chest breathing in conjunction with abdominal relaxation • Incorporates elements of the Stanislavesky method of acting in a way to teach relaxation	• Antenatal care • Birth plans • Therapeutic touch during labor • Post-traumatic stress following childbirth • Breastfeeding
HypnoBirthing	HypnoBirthing is about eliminating fear and experiencing birth in a stress-free, calm, and gentle environment that most resembles nature's own design.	• With both mind and body relaxed, the muscles of the uterus work in complete neuromuscular harmony. • When in a relaxed state, the body releases endorphins, the body's natural anesthesia.	• Relaxation techniques • Deep breathing • Slow breathing • Breathing your baby down • Maintaining comfort and eliminating pain	• HynoBirthing philosophy • Rapid, progressive relaxation/ deepening techniques for transition • Visualizations for labor • Composing a birth plan • Early signs of labor • Birthing companion's integral role in labor • Pushing techniques • Postnatal bonding of parents with baby

The programs in prepared childbirth share some similarities. All have an educational component to help eliminate fear and teach coping mechanisms. The classes vary in coverage of subjects related to the maternity cycle, but all teach relaxation techniques and all prepare the participants for what to expect during labor and birth. Most methods also feature exercises to condition muscles and use breathing patterns needed in labor. The greatest differences among the methods lie in the theories of why they work and in the relaxation techniques and breathing patterns they teach.

There are several advantages to these methods of childbirth preparation. The most important is that the baby may be healthier because of the reduced need for analgesics and anesthetics. Another is the satisfaction of the parents for whom childbirth becomes a shared and profound emotional experience over which they feel a sense of control. In addition, each method has been shown to shorten labor. All nurses must know how these methods differ, so that they can support each birth experience effectively.

The International Childbirth Education Association (ICEA) is a well-known organization that provides antepartum education. Although this is not a method of preparation, it offers education and resources to the certified childbirth educator (CBE) with a philosophy grounded in providing support to the individual couple's choices and decisions. Many couples find ICEA classes appealing because they discuss all alternatives and choices that are available. Many hospital-based childbirth education programs now use this approach.

Body-Conditioning Exercises

Some body-conditioning exercises, such as the pelvic tilt, pelvic rock, and Kegel exercises, are taught in childbirth preparation classes. Other exercises strengthen the abdominal muscles for the expulsive phase of labor. (See chapter 16 ∞ for a description of recommended exercises.)

Relaxation Exercises

Relaxation during labor allows the woman to conserve energy and allows the uterine muscles to work more efficiently. Without practice it is very difficult to relax the whole body in the midst of intense uterine contractions. However, many people can quickly master one or more of the following exercises.

Progressive Relaxation

In **progressive relaxation** exercises, the woman learns how to tense and then relax one muscle group at a time. An example follows:

- Lie down on your back or side. (The left side position is best for pregnant women.)

TABLE 13-4 Touch Relaxation

Practice is vital to the following exercises, which require that the pregnant woman and her partner work very closely together. Tell the woman, "With practice you will train yourself to release not only in response to your partner's touch, but also to the touch of doctors or nurses as they examine you. This technique will also help you to be more comfortable with your own body."

Goals

(For her) To recognize and release tension in response to partner's touch; to be able to do this automatically and spontaneously.

(For partner) To recognize her tension in its very early stages; to learn how to touch in a firm yet sensitive way; to concentrate on her problem areas.

Tools

(For her) Conscious relaxation, comfortable positioning, and trust.

(For partner) Sensitivity, patience, and warm hands!

Procedure

She tenses.

Partner touches.

She immediately releases toward touch.

Partner strokes "drawing" tension from her.

She releases all residual tension.

Sequence

- Contract muscles of the scalp and raise eyebrows. Partner cups hands on either side of the scalp. Immediately release tension in response to the pressure of your partner's touch. Then release any residual tension as your partner strokes your head.
- Frown, wrinkle nose, and squeeze eyes shut. Partner rests hands on brow and then strokes down over temples. Release.
- Grit teeth and clench jaw. Partner rests hands on either side of jaw. Release.
- Press shoulder blades back. Partner rests hands on front of shoulders. Release.
- Pull abdominal wall toward spine. Partner rests hands on sides of abdomen and then strokes down over her hips. Partner might also stroke the lower curve of abdomen across pubic symphysis. Release.
- Press thighs together. Partner touches outside of each leg. Relax and let legs move apart. Partner strokes firmly down outside of leg with light strokes up on inner thigh.
- Press legs outward, still flexed but forcing thighs apart. Partner rests hands with fingers pointing downward, on inner thighs. Firmly strokes down to knees, then lightly strokes upward on outside of leg. Release.
- Tense arm muscles. Partner places hands on the upper arm and shoulder area, one on the inside and one on the outside of the arm. Strokes down to the elbow and then down forearm to wrist, and over fingertips. Release. Repeat with other arm.
- Tighten leg muscles, being careful not to cramp them. Partner touches foot around the instep, firmly without tickling. Release whole leg. Partner moves hands up, placing one on either side of the thigh, stroking down to the knee then down the calf to the foot and over the toes. Release. Repeat with other leg.
- Change to the Sims, lateral, or side-lying position. Raise chin, contracting the muscles at the back of the neck. Partner rests hand on nape of neck and massages. Release.
- Curl into fetal position, drawing shoulders forward. Partner applies pressure to back of shoulders. Strokes upper back. Release.
- Hollow the small of back by arching back. Partner rests hands against either side of spine and follows with stroking down over buttocks. Release.
- Press buttocks together. Partner rests one hand on each buttock. After initial release, strokes down toward thighs.

Source: O'Halloran, S. (1984). Pregnant and prepared: A guide to preparing for childbirth *(p. 45). Wayne, NJ: Avery Publishing Group.*

- Tighten your muscles in both feet. Hold the tightness for a few seconds, and then relax the muscles completely, letting all the tension drain out.
- Tighten your lower legs, hold for a few seconds, and then relax the muscles, letting all the tension drain out.
- Continue tensing and relaxing parts of your body, moving up the body as you do so.

Touch Relaxation

Another type of relaxation exercise, called **touch relaxation**, requires cooperation between the woman and her coach. It is particularly useful in working together during labor. An example is provided in Table 13-4.

Disassociation Relaxation

An additional exercise, **disassociation relaxation**, is used in both Lamaze and Bradley methods. The woman is taught to become familiar with the sensation of contracting and relaxing the voluntary muscle groups throughout her body. She then learns to contract a specific muscle group and relax the rest of her body. This process of isolating the action of one group of voluntary muscles from the rest of the body is called *neuromuscular disassociation.* The exercise conditions the woman to relax uninvolved muscles while the uterus contracts, creating an active relaxation pattern (Table 13-5).

Although it is not possible to simulate the pain of uterine contractions, the coach may use one of two methods to induce some discomfort so the woman can practice the relaxation exercises:

1. The coach places both hands in a grasping position firmly on the upper arm and turns them in opposite directions to create a burning sensation. This is begun slowly and gently and increased at the direction of the woman as she continues to practice relaxation breathing techniques (Figure 13-5 ■).
2. The coach places a hand on the woman's inner thigh just above the knee and pinches the area.

While practicing, the coach checks the woman's neck, shoulders, arms, and legs for relaxation. As tense areas are found, the coach encourages the woman to relax those particular body parts. The woman learns to respond to her own perceptions of tense muscles and also to the suggestion from others.

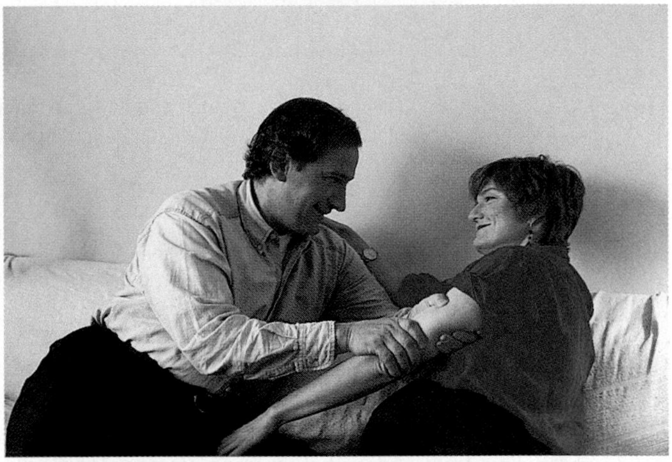

Figure 13-5 ■ To help the woman practice relaxing in the presence of discomfort, the coach can induce discomfort by "twisting" the skin of her upper arm or by pinching her inner thigh.

TABLE 13-5 Disassociation Relaxation

The uterus, an involuntary muscle over which you have no control, will work most efficiently and effectively when the rest of your body is free from tension. The following exercises will give you further practice in conscious release. They will also give you and your partner a way to evaluate your progress.

Goals

During pregnancy, disassociation relaxation will teach you consciously to release certain sets of muscles, while contracting others, and to disassociate yourself from voluntary tension. During labor, this technique will release all voluntary muscles of your body at will, while the uterus contracts. This conserves energy and fights fatigue.

Tools

Body awareness, touch release, and concentration.

Procedure

Partner gives consistent suggestions.
Partner checks relaxation using touching.

Example

Partner: "Contraction begins."
Mother: Relaxation breath (following with a comfortable rate of breathing).
Partner: [See suggested sequence.]
Mother: Relaxation breath.

Sequence

"Contract right arm. Hold. Release."
"Contract left arm. Hold. Release."
"Contract right leg. Hold. Release."
"Contract left leg. Hold. Release."
"Contract both arms. Hold. Release."
"Contract both legs. Hold. Release."
"Contract right side (arm and leg). Hold. Release."
"Contract left side (arm and leg). Hold. Release."
"Contract right arm and right leg. Hold. Release."
"Contract left arm and left leg. Hold. Release."

For Variety

"Contract right arm and left leg."
"Release left leg. Contract right leg. Release right arm. Contract left arm."
"Release."

Source: O'Halloran, S. (1984). Pregnant and prepared: A guide to preparing for childbirth *(pp. 45–46). Wayne, NJ: Avery Publishing Group.*

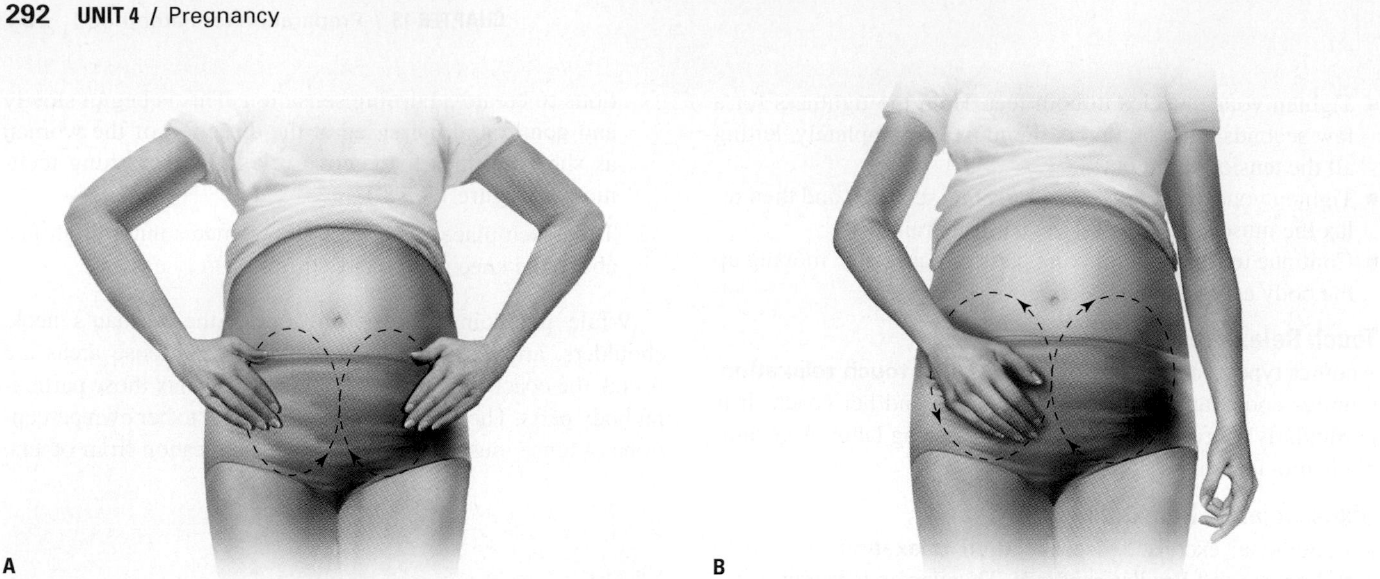

Figure 13-6 ■ Effleurage is light stroking of the abdomen with the fingertips. A. Starting at the symphysis, the woman lightly moves her fingertips up and around in a circular pattern. B. An alternative approach involves using one hand in a figure-eight pattern. This light stroking can also be done by the support person.

The suggestion can come verbally or from touch. The exercises are usually practiced each day so that they become comfortable and easy to do.

Other Relaxation Techniques

A specific type of cutaneous stimulation called abdominal **effleurage** is used before the transitional phase of labor (Figure 13-6 ■). This light abdominal stroking effectively relaxes the woman experiencing mild to moderate pain. Deep pressure over the sacrum is more effective for relieving back pain.

Additional modalities that may be used to promote relaxation in labor include guided imagery, hypnosis, meditation, music, massage, aromatherapy, therapeutic touch, biofeedback, transcutaneous electrical nerve stimulation (TENS) unit, acupressure, and acupuncture. In addition to these measures, the nurse can promote relaxation by encouraging and supporting the patient's controlled breathing.

Individualization is essential when choosing appropriate relaxation techniques. The nurse should encourage techniques that are comfortable for the woman. Some techniques that may be beneficial are as follows:

- Vocalization or "sounding" to relieve tension in pregnancy and labor.
- Massage (light touch) to facilitate relaxation.
- Breathing in any manner that seems to bring relief. No specific pattern is followed.
- Use of warm water for showers or bathing during labor.
- Visualization (imagery).
- Relaxing music and subdued lighting.

Breathing Techniques

Breathing techniques are a key element of most childbirth preparation programs. They help keep the mother and her unborn baby adequately oxygenated and help the mother relax and focus her attention appropriately (Table 13-6). Breathing techniques are best taught during the final trimester of pregnancy when the expectant mother's attention is focused on the birth experience. The nurse then supports the mother's use of breathing techniques during labor. Breathing techniques are described in detail in chapter 24 ∞.

TABLE 13-6 Goals of Breathing Techniques

- Provide adequate oxygenation of mother and baby, open maternal airways, and avoid inefficient use of muscles.
- Increase physical and mental relaxation.
- Decrease pain and anxiety.
- Provide a means of focusing attention.
- Control inadequate ventilation patterns that are related to pain and stress.
- Provide a sense of control for the mother.

CLINICAL TIP

Practice the techniques for relaxation yourself. This practice will prepare you to help expectant parents and laboring women.

Vocalization Techniques

With the increased use of analgesics and epidural anesthesia, many nurses have become unfamiliar with and may be uncomfortable about natural sounds made by laboring women. Vocalization or *sounding* during uterine contractions can be encouraged to promote relaxation and relieve tension. The nurse should encourage the woman to relax, drop her jaw to her chest, and make low-pitched sounds. Suggesting that the woman try to sound like a man or a mother bear can help her to produce the appropriate pitch. These low, moaning sounds open the glottis, helping the woman to relax, breathe freely, and feel confident and strong. In contrast, high-pitched sounds can promote tension, closure of the glottis, and a feeling of fear.

FOCUS YOUR STUDY

- Preconception counseling can be used to identify risk factors and unhealthy behaviors before a pregnancy occurs. Healthful lifestyle changes can be employed.
- Childbearing decisions include the healthcare provider, birth setting, support persons, and whether to include siblings in the birth experience.
- Prenatal education programs vary in their goals, content, leadership techniques, and method of teaching. The major childbirth preparation methods are Lamaze, Kitzinger, Bradley, and HypnoBirthing.
- Prenatal classes may be offered early or late in the pregnancy. The class content varies depending on the type of class and the individual offering it. Expectant parents tend to want information in chronologic sequence with the pregnancy.
- Breastfeeding programs in the prenatal period offer encouragement, practical instruction, and resources for the breastfeeding family.
- Siblings are now included in the whole birthing process, and classes for them are available from many sources.
- Grandparents have unique information needs that are addressed in grandparents' classes.
- Information regarding cesarean birth is included in antepartum classes to help prepare all parents for this alternative method of birth.
- Most childbirth classes include information on body-toning exercises, relaxation techniques, breathing method, and vocalization techniques.

CRITICAL THINKING IN ACTION

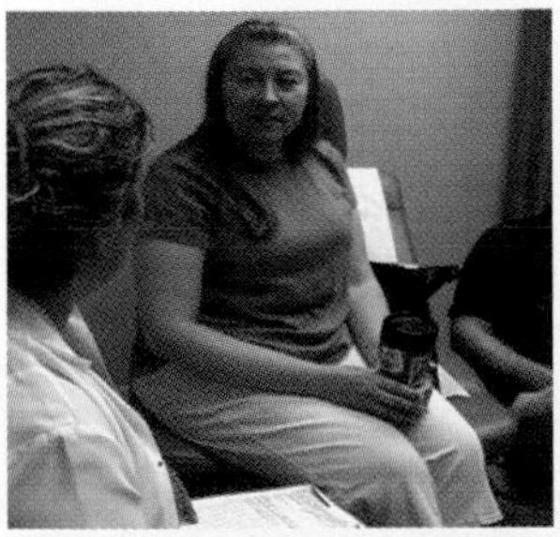
Source: George Dodson/Pearson Education.

Terry Dole, a 38-year-old G1 P0000, at 6 weeks' gestation, presents to you at the OB clinic for her first prenatal visit with the certified nurse-midwife (CNM). One of the first decisions facing Terry is the selection of a healthcare provider. The midwife explains the various options available to Terry at the clinic related to the differences in educational preparation, skill level, practice characteristics, and general philosophy of CNMs and obstetricians. Terry tells you that she has been married for 6 years and works as a massage therapist. You obtain the following data: BP 110/70, temperature 97.0° F, pulse 76, respirations 12, weight 140 lb, height 5'7". The physical and pelvic exams are essentially normal. The CNM asks you to teach Terry about birth plans.

1. Discuss the advantages of a birth plan.
2. Discuss the disadvantages of a birth plan.
3. Explain the role of a doula.
4. What gender differences are there in moving toward parenthood?

See www.nursing.pearsonhighered.com for possible responses.

Pearson Nursing Student Resources

Find additional review materials at
www.nursing.pearsonhighered.com

Prepare for success with additional NCLEX®-style practice questions, interactive assignments and activities, Web links, animations and videos, and more!

REFERENCES

American College of Obstetricians and Gynecologists (ACOG). (2008). *Nutrition during pregnancy.* Retrieved from http://www.acog.org/publications/patient_education/bp001.cfm

Amis, D., & Green, J. (2002). *Prepared childbirth: The educator's guide.* Plano, TX: The Family Way Publications.

Bailey, B. A., & Sokol, R. J. (2008). Pregnancy and alcohol use: Evidence and recommendations for prenatal care. *Clinical Obstetrics and Gynecology, 51*(2), 436–444.

Bailey, J. M., Crane, P., & Nugent, C. E. (2008). Childbirth education and birth plans. *Obstetrics & Gynecology Clinics of North America, 35*(3), 497–509.

Bradley, R. A. (1965). *Husband-coached childbirth.* New York, NY: Harper Row.

Bradley, R. A. (1974). *Husband-coached childbirth* (3rd ed.). New York, NY: Harper Row.

Centers for Disease Control and Prevention (CDC). (2009). *Tobacco use and pregnancy.* Retrieved from http://www.cdc.gov/reproductivehealth/tobaccousepregnancy/index.htm

Coalition for Improving Maternity Services (CIMS). (2009). *Principles.* Retrieved from http://www.motherfriendlyorg/mfci.php

Cramton, R., Zain-Ul-Abideen, M., & Whalen, B. (2009). Optimizing successful breastfeeding in the newborn. *Current Opinion in Pediatrics, 21*(3), 386–396.

Dennis, C. L. (2002). Breastfeeding initiation and duration: A 1990–2000 literature review. *Journal of Obstetric, Gynecologic, & Neonatal Nursing, 31,* 12–32.

Devito, J. (2007). Self-perceptions of parenting among adolescent mothers. *The Journal of Perinatal Education, 16*(1), 16–23.

Einarson, A., & Riordan, S. (2009). Smoking in pregnancy and lactation: A review of risks and cessation strategies. *European Journal of Clinical Pharmacology, 65*(4), 325–330.

Forste, R., & Hoffmann, J. P. (2008). Are U.S. mothers meeting the *Healthy People 2010* breastfeeding targets for initiation, duration, and exclusivity? The 2003 and 2004 National Immunization Survey. *Journal of Human Lactation, 24*(3), 278–288.

Frankman, E. A., Wang, L., Bunker, C. H., & Lowder, J. L. (2009). Episiotomy in the United States: Has anything changed? *American Journal of Obstetrics & Gynecology, 200*(5), e1–7.

Geraghty, S. R., Riddle, S. W., & Shaikh, U. (2008). The breastfeeding mother and the pediatrician. *Journal of Human Lactation, 24*(3), 335–339.

Gonzalez, A. P., Vasquez-Mendoza, G., Garcia-Vela, A., Guzman-Ramirez, A., Salazar-Torres, M., & Romero-Gutierrez, G. (2009). Weight gain in preterm infants following parent-administered Vimala massage: A randomized controlled trial. *American Journal of Perinatology, 26*(4), 247–252.

Hodnett, E. D., Gates, S., Hofmeyr, G. J., & Sakala, C. (2007). Continuous support for women during childbirth. *The Cochrane Database of Systemic Reviews, 3.* (Article No. CD003766).

Jain, N. J., Denk, C. E., Kruse, L. K., & Dandolu, V. (2007). Maternal obesity: Can pregnancy weight gain modify risk of selected adverse pregnancy outcomes? *American Journal of Perinatology, 24*(5), 291–298.

Jones, R. K., Zolna, M. R., Henshaw, S. K., & Finer, L. B. (2008). Abortion in the United States: Incidence and access to services, 2005. *Perspectives on Sexual and Reproductive Health, 40*(1), 6–16.

Kuramoto, N. (2008). Children present at the birth of a younger sibling, and the meaning of this experience. *Journal of Japan Academy of Midwifery, 22*(2), 124–135.

Lothian, J. A. (2008). Childbirth education at the crossroads. *The Journal of Perinatal Education, 17*(2), 45–49.

March of Dimes. (2009). *Folic acid: How much folic acid does a woman need? And do women need folic acid throughout pregnancy?* Retrieved from http://www.marchofdimes.com/professionals/14332_1151.asp

McGrath, S. K., & Kennell, J. H. (2008). A randomized controlled trial of continuous labor support for middle-class couples: Effect on cesarean delivery rates. *Birth: Issues in Perinatal Care, 35*(2), 92–97.

Robertson, B., Aycock, D. M., & Darnell, L. A. (2009). Comparison of centering pregnancy to traditional care in Hispanic mothers. *Maternal & Child Health Journal, 13*(3), 407–414.

Stark, M. A., Rudell, B., & Haus, G. (2008). Observing position and movements in hydrotherapy: A pilot study. *Journal of Obstetric, Gynecologic, & Neonatal Nursing (JOGNN), 37*(1), 116–122.

Wang, H. H., Chung, U. L., Sung, M. S., & Wu, S. M. (2006). Development of a web-based childbirth education program for vaginal birth after cesarean (VBAC) mothers. *Journal of Nursing Research, 14*(1), 1–8.

Weng, X., Odouli, R., & Li, D. K. (2008). Maternal caffeine consumption during pregnancy and the risk of miscarriage: a prospective cohort study. *American Journal of Obstetrics & Gynecology, 198*(3), 279.e1–8.

CHAPTER 14

Physical and Psychologic Changes of Pregnancy

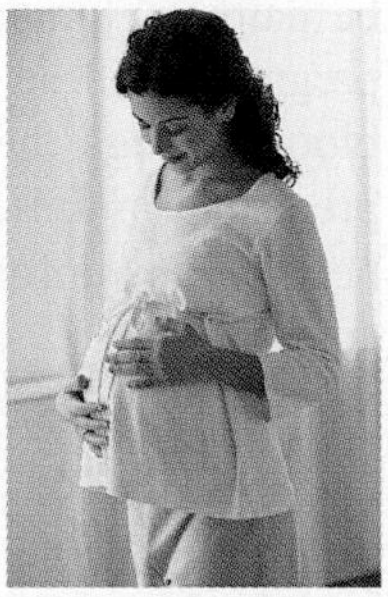

The atmosphere of approval in which I was bathed—even by strangers on the street, it seemed—was like an aura I carried with me . . . This is what women have always done.

—Adrienne Rich, *Of Woman Born*

LEARNING OUTCOMES

1. Identify the anatomic and physiologic changes that occur during pregnancy.
2. Relate the physiologic and anatomic changes that occur in the body systems during pregnancy to the signs and symptoms that develop in the woman.
3. Compare subjective (presumptive), objective (probable), and diagnostic (positive) changes of pregnancy.
4. Contrast the various types of pregnancy tests.
5. Discuss the emotional and psychologic changes that commonly occur in a woman, her partner, and her family during pregnancy.
6. Summarize cultural factors that may influence a family's response to pregnancy.

KEY TERMS

Ballottement *304*
Braxton Hicks contractions *296*
Chadwick's sign *296*
Chloasma (melasma gravidarum) *299*
Colostrum *297*
Couvade *312*
Goodell's sign *296*
Hegar's sign *303*
Linea nigra *299*
McDonald's sign *303*
Morning sickness *303*
Mucous plug *296*
Physiologic anemia of pregnancy *298*
Quickening *303*
Striae *297*
Supine hypotensive syndrome (vena caval syndrome, aortocaval compression) *298*

Through modern technology and highly evolved research methods, we know a great deal about how pregnancy occurs and what happens to the fetus and the woman's body during gestation. Yet no matter how much we learn about this event, it never ceases to amaze us. First, it is nothing short of a miracle that the union of two microscopic entities—an ovum and a sperm—can produce a living being. Second, the woman's body must undergo extraordinary physical changes to sustain a pregnancy. A pregnant woman's body changes in size and shape, and all her organ systems modify their functions to create an environment that protects and nurtures the growing fetus.

Pregnancy is divided into three trimesters, each a 3-month period. Each trimester has its own predictable developments in both the fetus and the mother. This chapter describes both obvious and subtle physical and psychologic changes caused by pregnancy. It also discusses the various cultural factors that can affect a woman's well-being during pregnancy.

Anatomy and Physiology of Pregnancy

The changes that occur in the pregnant woman's body are caused by several factors. Many changes are the result of hormonal influences, some are caused by the growth of the fetus inside the uterus, and some are a result of the mother's physical adaptation to the changes that are occurring.

Reproductive System

Uterus

The changes in the uterus during pregnancy are phenomenal. Before pregnancy the uterus is a small, almost solid, pear-shaped organ measuring approximately 7.5 × 5 × 2.5 cm and weighing about 60 g (2 oz). At the end of pregnancy the dimensions are approximately 28 × 24 × 21 cm with an organ weight of approximately 1100 g (2.5 lb). Its capacity increases from 10 to 5000 ml (5 L) or more (Cunningham et al., 2010).

The enlargement of the uterus is primarily a result of an increase in size (hypertrophy) of the preexisting myometrial cells. Only a limited increase in cell number (hyperplasia) occurs. The amount of fibrous tissue between the muscle bands increases markedly, which adds to the strength and elasticity of the muscle wall.

The uterine walls become considerably thicker during the first few months of pregnancy than during the nonpregnant state. The initial changes are stimulated by increased estrogen and progesterone levels and not by mechanical distention (enlargement) by the fetus, placenta, and amniotic fluid. In general, the uterus enlarges more around the placental insertion site and in the upper portion of the uterus, the *fundus* (Cunningham et al., 2010). After approximately the third month, the uterine contents begin to exert intrauterine pressure. The myometrial hypertrophy continues during the first few months of pregnancy. Then the musculature begins to distend, resulting in a thinning of the muscle wall to a thickness of about 1.5 cm or less at term (38 through 41 weeks of gestation). The ease of palpating the fetus through the abdominal wall attests to this thinning.

The circulatory requirements of the uterus increase as the uterus enlarges and the fetus and placenta develop. The size and number of the blood and lymphatic vessels within the uterine layers increase greatly. By the end of pregnancy, one sixth of the total maternal blood volume is contained within the vascular system of the uterus.

Braxton Hicks contractions—irregular contractions of the uterus—occur intermittently throughout pregnancy. They may be palpated bimanually beginning about the fourth month of pregnancy. These contractions help stimulate the movement of blood through the intervillous spaces of the placenta. In late pregnancy as these contractions increase in frequency, they can become uncomfortable and may be confused with true labor contractions.

CLINICAL TIP

Beginning early in pregnancy, have the woman feel her uterus periodically so that she becomes familiar with the size and the way it feels. As her pregnancy progresses she then will be more likely to identify Braxton Hicks contractions and preterm labor should it occur.

Cervix

The major component of cervical tissue is connective tissue, which is rearranged as pregnancy progresses. At term its strength is 1/12 of its prepregnant strength, facilitating cervical changes during labor (Cunningham et al., 2010).

Estrogen stimulates the glandular tissue of the cervix, which increases in cell number and becomes hyperactive. The endocervical glands occupy about half the mass of the cervix at term, as compared with a small fraction in the nonpregnant state. They secrete a thick, tenacious mucus, which accumulates and thickens to form the **mucous plug** that seals the endocervical canal and prevents the ascent of bacteria or other substances into the uterus. This plug is expelled when cervical dilatation begins. The hyperactive glandular tissue also causes an increase in the normal physiologic mucorrhea, at times resulting in a profuse discharge. Increased vascularization causes both the softening of the cervix (**Goodell's sign**) and a blue-purple discoloration of the cervix (**Chadwick's sign**). Increased vascularization is a result of hypertrophy and engorgement of the vessels below the growing uterus.

Ovaries

The ovaries cease ovum production during pregnancy. Many follicles develop temporarily but never to the point of maturity. The cells lining these follicles, the thecal cells, become active in hormone production and have been called the interstitial glands of pregnancy.

During early pregnancy human chorionic gonadotropin (hCG) maintains the corpus luteum, which persists and produces hormones until about weeks 6 to 8 of pregnancy. The corpus luteum engulfs approximately a third of the ovary at its peak of hypertrophy. By the middle of pregnancy it has regressed to almost complete obliteration. The corpus luteum secretes progesterone to maintain the endometrium until the placenta produces enough progesterone to maintain the pregnancy; then the corpus luteum disintegrates slowly.

Vagina

The vaginal epithelium undergoes hypertrophy, increased vascularization, and hyperplasia during pregnancy. As with the cervical changes, these changes are estrogen induced and result in a thickening of mucosa, a loosening of connective tissue, and an increase in vaginal secretions. The secretions are thick, white, and acidic (pH 3.5 to 6). The acid pH plays a significant role in preventing infections. However, it also favors the growth of yeast organisms, resulting in moniliasis, a common vaginal infection during pregnancy.

As in the uterus, the smooth muscle cells of the vagina hypertrophy, with an accompanying loosening of the supportive connective tissue. By the end of pregnancy, the vaginal wall and perineal body have become sufficiently relaxed to permit distention of the tissues and passage of the infant.

Because the blood flow to the vagina increases, it may show the same blue-purple color (Chadwick's sign) seen in the cervix.

Breasts

Soon after the woman first misses her menstrual period, estrogen- and progesterone-induced changes occur in the mammary glands. Increases in breast size and nodularity are the result of glandular hyperplasia and hypertrophy in preparation for lactation. By the end of the second month, superficial veins are prominent, nipples are more erectile, and pigmentation of the areola is obvious. Pigmentation tends to be more pronounced in women with dark complexions. Hypertrophy of Montgomery's follicles is noted within the primary areola. **Striae** (purplish stretch marks that slowly turn silver after childbirth) may develop as the pregnancy progresses. Breast changes are often most noticeable in the woman who is pregnant for the first time.

Colostrum, an antibody-rich, yellow secretion, may be expressed manually by the 12th week and may leak from the breasts during the last trimester of pregnancy. Colostrum gradually converts to mature milk during the first few days following childbirth.

Respiratory System

Pulmonary function is modified throughout pregnancy. Pregnancy induces a small degree of hyperventilation as the tidal volume (amount of air breathed with ordinary respiration) increases steadily throughout pregnancy. There is a 30% to 40% rise from nonpregnant values in the volume of air breathed each minute. Between weeks 16 and 40, oxygen consumption increases approximately 15% to 20% to meet the increased needs of the mother as well as those of the fetus and placenta. The vital capacity (maximum amount of air that can be moved in and out of the lungs with forced respiration) increases slightly, while lung compliance (elasticity) and pulmonary diffusion remain constant. Measurements of airway resistance show a marked decrease in pregnancy in response to elevated progesterone levels. The diaphragm is elevated and the subcostal angle is increased as a result of pressure from the enlarging uterus. This change causes the rib cage to flare with a decrease in the vertical diameter and increases in the anteroposterior and transverse diameters. The circumference of the chest may increase by as much as 6 cm. The increase compensates for the elevated diaphragm, and there is no significant loss of intrathoracic volume. Breathing changes from abdominal to thoracic as pregnancy progresses. Overall, pulmonary function is not impaired by pregnancy. Many women experience an increased awareness of the need to breathe, however, starting early in pregnancy. This may be perceived as dyspnea and is thought to be due to the increased tidal volume, which causes a slight decrease in blood PCO_2. Actual lung disease may be aggravated by pregnancy because of the increased need for oxygen by the woman and her fetus (Cunningham et al., 2010).

Nasal stuffiness and congestion, referred to as rhinitis of pregnancy, are not uncommon. Epistaxis (nosebleeds) may also occur. They are primarily the result of estrogen-induced edema and vascular congestion of the nasal mucosa.

Cardiovascular System

The growing uterus exerts pressure on the diaphragm, pushing the heart upward and to the left and rotating it forward. This lateral displacement makes the heart appear somewhat enlarged on x-ray examination. A systolic murmur can be heard in 90% of pregnant women, and the first and third heart sounds are louder.

Blood volume progressively increases throughout pregnancy, beginning in the first trimester, and increases rapidly until about 30 to 34 weeks, then plateaus until birth at about 40% to 50% above nonpregnant levels. This increase is due to increases in both plasma and erythrocytes (Gordon, 2007). No increase occurs in pulmonary capillary wedge pressure or in central venous pressure despite the increase in blood volume. This is due to decreases in both systemic vascular resistance and pulmonary vascular resistance, which enable the circulation to adapt to higher blood volume while maintaining normal vessel pressures. Cardiac output begins to increase early in pregnancy and peaks at 25 to 30 weeks' gestation at 30% to 50% above prepregnant levels. It generally remains elevated in the third trimester.

During pregnancy, organ systems receive additional blood flow according to their increased workload. Thus blood flow to the uterus, placenta, and breasts increases, whereas hepatic and cerebral flow remains unchanged.

The pulse rate frequently increases during pregnancy, although the amount varies from almost no increase to an increase of 10 to 15 beats per minute. The blood pressure decreases slightly during pregnancy, reaching its lowest point during the second trimester. The blood pressure then gradually increases during the third trimester and is near prepregnant levels at term (when the baby is due).

The femoral venous pressure slowly rises as the uterus exerts increasing pressure on return blood flow. There is an increased tendency toward stagnation of blood in the lower extremities, with a resulting dependent edema and tendency toward varicose vein formation in the legs, vulva, and rectum late

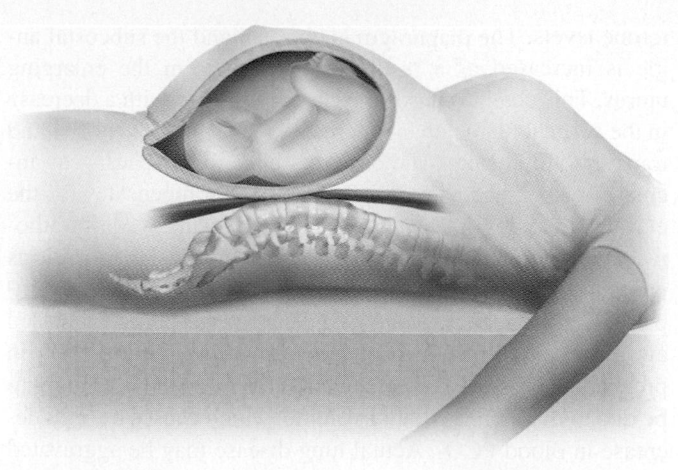

Figure 14-1 ■ Vena caval syndrome. The gravid uterus compresses the vena cava when the woman is supine. This reduces the blood flow returning to the heart and may cause maternal hypotension.

in pregnancy. In addition to the effects of increased femoral venous pressure, a reduction of plasma colloid osmotic pressure resulting from a reduction in plasma albumin further maintains the presence of fluid in the extravascular space. The pregnant woman becomes more prone to develop postural hypotension because of the increased blood volume in the lower extremities.

During pregnancy the enlarging uterus may put pressure on the vena cava when the woman is supine, resulting in **supine hypotensive syndrome**, also called **vena caval syndrome** or **aortocaval compression**. This pressure interferes with returning blood flow and produces a marked decrease in blood pressure with accompanying dizziness, pallor, and clamminess, which can be corrected by having the woman lie on her left side. Research indicates that the enlarging uterus may press on the aorta and its collateral circulation as well (Cunningham et al., 2010) (Figure 14-1 ■).

The total erythrocyte volume increases by about 30% in women who receive iron supplementation but increases only about 18% without iron supplements. This increase is necessary to transport the additional oxygen required during pregnancy. The increase in plasma volume averages about 50%. Because the plasma volume increase (50%) is greater than the erythrocyte increase (30%), however, the hematocrit, which measures the portion of whole blood that is composed of erythrocytes, decreases slightly (Gordon, 2007). This decrease is sometimes referred to as the **physiologic anemia of pregnancy** (pseudoanemia).

Iron is necessary for hemoglobin formation, and hemoglobin is the oxygen-carrying component of erythrocytes. Thus the increase in erythrocyte levels results in an increased need for iron by the pregnant woman. Even though the gastrointestinal absorption of iron is moderately increased during pregnancy, it is usually necessary to add supplemental iron to the diet to meet the expanded red blood cell and fetal needs.

Leukocyte production equals or is slightly greater than the increase in blood volume. The average cell count is 5600 to 12,200/mm^3, with an occasional woman developing a physiologic leukocytosis of 15,000/mm^3. During labor and the early postpartum period, these levels may reach 20,000 to 30,000/mm^3 or higher (Gordon, 2007). The reason for this dramatic increase remains unknown, but similar leukocyte changes occur with physiologic stress such as vigorous exercise. It probably represents the return to the circulation of mature leukocytes that had been shunted out of the circulatory system (Cunningham et al., 2010).

The platelet count does not change much in pregnancy, but the plasma fibrinogen has been known to increase by as much as 50%. The increased fibrinogen accounts for the nonpathologic rise of the sedimentation rate. Although the clotting time of the pregnant woman does not differ significantly from that of the nonpregnant woman, blood factors VII, VIII, IX, and X are increased so that pregnancy becomes a somewhat hypercoagulable state. These changes, coupled with venous stasis in late pregnancy, place the pregnant woman at increased risk of developing venous thrombosis.

Gastrointestinal System

Many of the discomforts of pregnancy are attributed to changes in the gastrointestinal system. Nausea and vomiting during the first trimester are sometimes associated with the hCG secreted by the implanted blastocyst and with a change in carbohydrate metabolism that occurs in early pregnancy. Peculiarities of taste and smell are common and can further aggravate gastrointestinal discomfort. Gum tissue may become hyperemic and softened and may bleed when only mildly traumatized. The secretion of saliva may increase or become excessive (ptyalism).

During the second half of pregnancy, numerous gastrointestinal symptoms are attributable to the pressure of the growing uterus and smooth muscle relaxation due to elevated progesterone levels. The intestines are moved laterally and posteriorly and the stomach superiorly. Heartburn (pyrosis) is caused by the reflux of acidic secretions from the stomach into the lower esophagus as a result of relaxation of the cardiac sphincter. Gastric emptying time and intestinal motility are delayed, leading to frequent complaints of bloating and constipation, which can be aggravated by the smooth muscle relaxation and increased electrolyte and water reabsorption in the large intestine. Hemorrhoids frequently develop if constipation is a problem or, in the second half of pregnancy, from pressure on vessels below the level of the uterus.

Only minor liver changes occur with pregnancy. Plasma albumin concentrations and serum cholinesterase activity decrease with normal pregnancy as with certain liver diseases.

The emptying time of the gallbladder is prolonged during pregnancy as a result of smooth muscle relaxation from progesterone. Hypercholesterolemia may follow, and it can predispose the woman to gallstone formation. Pruritus (itching) caused by retained bile salts may also occur (Cunningham et al., 2010).

Urinary Tract

During the first trimester, the growing uterus puts pressure on the bladder, producing urinary frequency until the second trimester, when the uterus becomes an abdominal organ. Near term, when the presenting part engages in the pelvis, pressure is again exerted on the bladder. This pressure can impair the drainage of blood and lymph from the hyperemic bladder, rendering it more susceptible to infection and trauma. The bladder, normally a convex organ, becomes concave from the external pressure, and its capacity is greatly reduced.

Dilation of the kidneys and ureter may occur, most frequently on the right side above the pelvic brim, because of the lie of the uterus. This dilation is accompanied by elongation and curvature of the ureter. There appears to be no single factor accounting for this anatomic variation; instead a combination of ureteral atonia and hypoperistalsis, probably caused by pressure from the enlarging fetus with some progesterone effects, seems to be involved. The presence of amino acids and glucose in the urine in conjunction with the tendency toward ureteral atonia and stasis of urine in the ureters may increase the risk of urinary tract infection.

The glomerular filtration rate (GFR) and renal plasma flow (RPF) increase early in pregnancy. The GFR rises by as much as 50% by the beginning of the second trimester and remains elevated until birth. The increase in RPF is slightly less and decreases somewhat during the third trimester (Cunningham et al., 2010). The mechanism for these rises remains unclear.

An increased renal tubular reabsorption rate compensates for the increased glomerular activity. Amino acids and water-soluble vitamins are excreted in greater amounts than in the nonpregnant woman. Glycosuria is not uncommon or necessarily pathogenic during pregnancy but is merely a reflection of the kidneys' inability to reabsorb all of the glucose filtered by the glomeruli. However, pregnancy can be diabetogenic, so the possibility of diabetes mellitus cannot be disregarded.

The increased renal function during pregnancy results in an increased clearance of urea and creatinine and in a lowering of the blood urea and nonprotein nitrogen values. Because of this, measurement of creatinine clearance provides an accurate test of renal functioning during pregnancy.

Skin and Hair

Changes in skin pigmentation commonly occur during pregnancy. These changes are thought to be stimulated by increased estrogen, progesterone, and α-melanocyte-stimulating hormone levels.

Pigmentation of the skin increases primarily in areas that are already hyperpigmented: the areolae, the nipples, the vulva, the perianal area, and the linea alba. The linea alba refers to the midline of the abdomen from the pubic area to the umbilicus and above. During pregnancy increased pigmentation may cause this area to darken. It is then referred to as the **linea nigra** (Figure 14-2 ■). Some women also develop facial **chloasma** (or **melasma gravidarum**), the "mask of pregnancy." This is an irregular pigmentation of the cheeks, forehead, and nose that occurs in many women during pregnancy and is accentuated by sun exposure. Similar changes may occur in women who are taking oral contraceptives. Facial melasma is more prominent in dark-haired women and is occasionally disfiguring. Fortunately, it fades or at least regresses soon after birth when the hormonal influence of pregnancy has stopped.

Striae, or stretch marks, are reddish, wavy, depressed streaks that may occur over the abdomen, breasts, and thighs as pregnancy progresses. They are caused by reduced connective tissue strength due to elevated adrenal steroid levels.

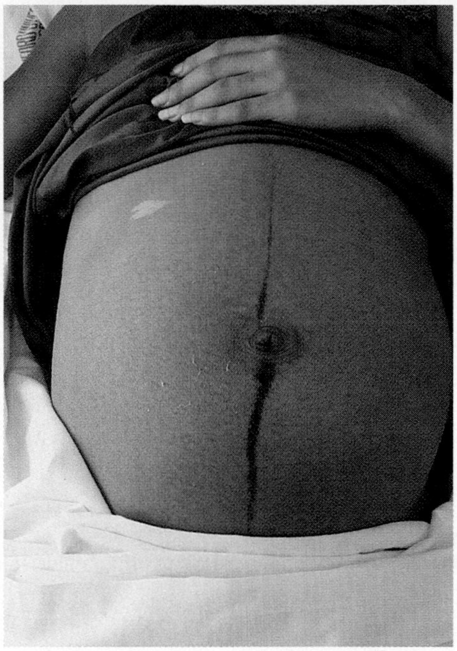

Figure 14-2 ■ Linea nigra.
Source: George Dodson/Pearson Education.

Vascular spider nevi may develop on the chest, neck, face, arms, and legs. They are small, bright-red elevations of the skin radiating from a central body. They may be caused by increased subcutaneous blood flow in response to increased estrogen levels. This condition is of no clinical significance and disappears after pregnancy ends.

The rate of hair growth may decrease during pregnancy, and the number of hair follicles in the resting or dormant phase also decreases. After birth the number of hair follicles in the resting phase increases sharply, and the woman may notice increased shedding of hair for 1 to 4 months. Practically all hair is replaced within 6 to 12 months, however (Cunningham et al., 2010).

Finally, the sweat and sebaceous glands are frequently hyperactive during pregnancy. Some women may notice heavy perspiration, night sweats, and/or the development of acne even if they have never experienced these symptoms before.

Musculoskeletal System

No demonstrable changes occur in the teeth of the pregnant woman. No demineralization takes place. The fairly common occurrence of dental caries during pregnancy has led to the myth "a tooth for every pregnancy." The dental caries that may accompany pregnancy is likely to be caused by inadequate oral hygiene and dental care.

The sacroiliac, sacrococcygeal, and pubic joints of the pelvis relax in the later part of the pregnancy, presumably as a result of hormonal changes. This often causes a waddling gait. A slight separation of the symphysis pubis can often be demonstrated on radiologic examination.

As the pregnant woman's center of gravity gradually changes, the lumbodorsal spinal curve is accentuated, and the woman's

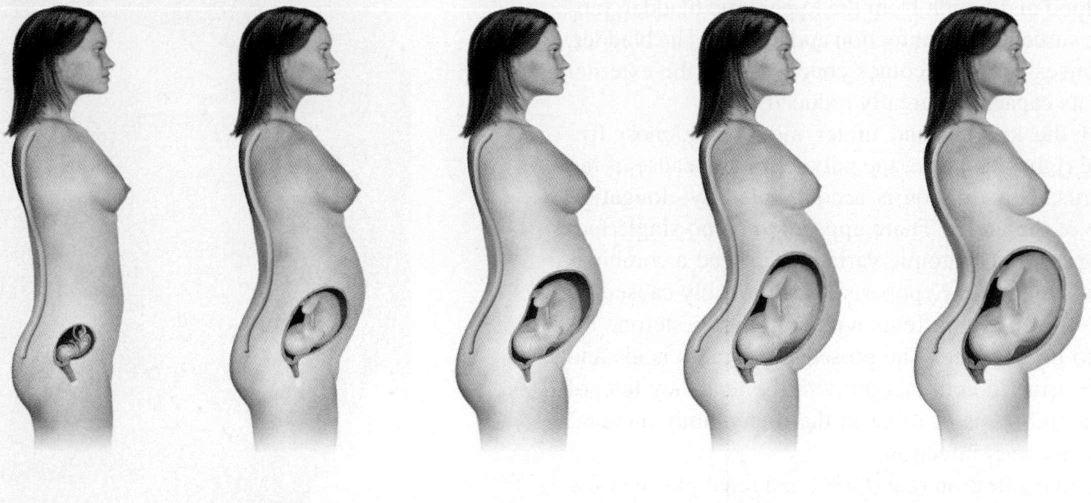

Figure 14-3 ■ Postural changes during pregnancy. Note the increasing lordosis of the lumbosacral spine and the increasing curvature of the thoracic area.

posture changes (Figure 14-3 ■). This posture change compensates for the increased weight of the uterus anteriorly and frequently results in low backache. Late in pregnancy, aches in the neck, shoulders, and upper extremities may occur because of shoulder slumping and anterior flexion of the neck accompanying the lumbodorsal lordosis. Paresthesias of the extremities may occur late in pregnancy as a result of pressure on peripheral nerves.

Often pressure of the enlarging uterus on the abdominal muscles causes the rectus abdominis muscle to separate, producing *diastasis recti.* If the separation is severe and muscle tone is not regained postpartally, subsequent pregnancies will not have adequate support, and the woman's abdomen may appear pendulous.

Eyes

Two changes generally occur in the eyes during pregnancy. First, intraocular pressure decreases, probably as a result of increased vitreous outflow. Second, a slight thickening of the cornea occurs, which is generally attributed to fluid retention. Although these changes are not readily perceived, some pregnant women experience difficulty wearing previously comfortable contact lenses (Cunningham et al., 2010). The change in the corneas generally disappears by 6 weeks postpartum.

Central Nervous System

Pregnant women frequently describe decreased attention, concentration, and memory during and shortly after pregnancy, but few studies have explored this phenomenon. One study did compare a group of pregnant women against a control group, finding a decline in memory that could not be attributed to depression, anxiety, sleep deprivation, or other physical changes of pregnancy. This memory loss disappeared soon after childbirth. Another study found that sleep problems are common in pregnancy. These include difficulty going to sleep, frequent awakenings, fewer hours of night sleep, and reduced sleep efficiency (Cunningham et al., 2010).

Metabolism

Most metabolic functions accelerate during pregnancy to support the additional demands of the growing fetus and its support system. The expectant mother must meet her own tissue replacement needs, those of the fetus, and those preparatory for labor and lactation. No other event in life induces such profound metabolic changes.

Weight Gain

Growth of the uterus and its contents, growth of the breasts, and increases in intravascular fluids account for most of the weight gain in pregnancy. In addition, extra water, fat, and protein are stored; these are usually called *maternal reserves.*

The recommended total weight gain during pregnancy for a woman of normal weight before pregnancy is 11.5 to 16 kg (25 to 35 lb); for women who were overweight before becoming pregnant, the recommended gain is 6.8 to 11.5 kg (15 to 25 lb). Obese women are advised to limit weight gain to 5 to 9 kg (11 to 20 lb). Underweight women are advised to gain 12.7 to 18.1 kg (28 to 40 lb) (Institute of Medicine [IOM], 2009). Weight may decrease slightly during the first trimester because of nausea, vomiting, and food intolerances of early pregnancy. The lost weight is soon regained, and the IOM (2009) recommends that a normal weight woman gain 0.5 to 2 kg (1.1 to 4.4 lb) during the first trimester, followed by an average gain of about 0.45 kg (1 lb) per week during the last two trimesters.

Adequate nutrition and weight gain are important during pregnancy. Maternal nutrition is discussed in detail in chapter 18 ∞.

Water Metabolism

Increased water retention is a basic chemical alteration of pregnancy. Several interrelated factors cause this phenomenon. The increased level of steroid sex hormones affects sodium and fluid retention. The lowered serum protein also influences the fluid balance, as do the increased intracapillary pressure and permeability.

The extra water is needed for the products of conception—the fetus, placenta, and amniotic fluid—and the mother's increased blood volume, interstitial fluids, and enlarged organs.

Nutrient Metabolism

The fetus makes its greatest protein and fat demands during the second half of gestation, doubling in weight in the last 6 to 8 weeks. The increased protein retention that begins in early pregnancy is initially used for hyperplasia and hypertrophy of maternal tissues, such as the uterus and breasts. Protein must also be stored during pregnancy to maintain a constant level within the breast milk and to avoid depletion of maternal tissues.

Fats are more completely absorbed during pregnancy, resulting in a marked increase in the serum lipids, lipoproteins, and cholesterol and decreased elimination through the bowel. Fat deposits in the fetus increase from about 2% at midpregnancy to almost 12% at term. The excess nitrogen and lipidemia are considered to be a preparation for lactation. In addition, the woman's body switches from glucose metabolism to lipid metabolism once glucose from food intake has been used up. This leads to an increased tendency to develop ketosis between meals and overnight. The demand for carbohydrate increases, especially during the last two trimesters. Intermittent glycosuria is not uncommon during pregnancy. When it is not accompanied by a rise in blood sugar levels, glycosuria is a physiologic entity secondary to the increased glomerular filtration rate. Fasting blood sugar levels tend to fall slightly, returning to more normal levels by the sixth postpartal month. The oral glucose tolerance test shows no change with pregnancy.

The possibility of diabetes must not be overlooked during pregnancy. Plasma levels of insulin increase during pregnancy (probably because of hormonal changes that cause increased tissue resistance) and rapid destruction of insulin takes place within the placenta. Insulin production must be increased by the mother during the second trimester, and any marginal pancreatic function quickly becomes apparent. The woman with diabetes often experiences increased exogenous insulin demands during pregnancy.

The demand for iron during pregnancy is accelerated, and the pregnant woman needs to guard against anemia. Iron is necessary for the increase in erythrocytes, hemoglobin, and blood volume, as well as for the increased tissue demands of both woman and fetus.

Iron transfer takes place at the placenta in only one direction—toward the fetus. It has been demonstrated that approximately five sixths of the iron stored in the fetal liver is assimilated during the last trimester of pregnancy. This stored iron in the fetal liver compensates in the first 4 months of neonatal life for the normal inadequate amounts of iron available in breast milk and non–iron-fortified formulas.

The progressive absorption and retention of calcium during pregnancy has been noted. The maternal plasma concentration of bound calcium decreases as the levels of bindable plasma proteins fall. Approximately 30 g of calcium is retained in maternal bone for fetal deposition late in pregnancy.

Pregnancy produces little change in the metabolism of most other minerals, other than retention of amounts needed for fetal growth.

Endocrine System

Thyroid

Pregnancy influences the thyroid gland's size and activity. Often a palpable change is noted, which represents an increase in vascularity and hyperplasia of glandular tissue. Total serum thyroxine (T_4) increases in early pregnancy, and thyroid-stimulating hormone (TSH) decreases. The elevated levels of total T_4 continue until several weeks postpartum, although the level of free serum T_4 returns to normal after the first trimester (Cunningham et al., 2010). Increased thyroxine-binding capacity is evidenced by an increase in serum protein-bound iodine (PBI), probably due to the increased levels of circulating estrogens.

The basal metabolic rate (BMR) increases by as much as 20% to 25% during pregnancy. The increased oxygen consumption is due primarily to fetal metabolic activity.

Application: Endocrine Hormones

Parathyroid

The concentration of the parathyroid hormone and the size of the parathyroid glands increase, paralleling the fetal calcium requirements. Parathyroid hormone concentration reaches its highest level of approximately twofold between 15 and 35 weeks of gestation, returning to a normal or even subnormal level before childbirth.

Pituitary

During pregnancy, the pituitary gland enlarges somewhat, but it returns to normal size after birth. There is no significant change in the posterior lobe of the gland, although the anterior lobe increases in weight with each successive pregnancy.

Pregnancy is made possible by the hypothalamic stimulation of the anterior pituitary hormones: follicle-stimulating hormone (FSH), which stimulates follicle growth within the ovary, and luteinizing hormone (LH), which effects ovulation. Pituitary stimulation prolongs the corpus luteal phase of the ovary, which maintains the secretory endometrium for development of the pregnancy.

Two additional pituitary hormones, thyrotropin and adrenotropin, alter maternal metabolism to support the pregnancy. Prolactin, also an anterior pituitary secretion, is responsible for initial lactation. Its levels increase 10-fold during pregnancy and then, somewhat surprisingly, decrease after childbirth, even in breastfeeding women. (Continued lactation depends on the suckling of the infant.)

The posterior pituitary contains the mechanism for the release of oxytocin and vasopressin, which exert oxytocic, vasopressor, and antidiuretic effects. The main effects of oxytocin are the promotion of uterine contractility and the stimulation of milk ejection from the breasts. Vasopressin causes vasoconstriction, which results in increased blood pressure; it also has an antidiuretic effect and plays an important role in the regulation of water balance. Vasopressin secretion is controlled by changes in plasma osmolarity and blood volume.

Adrenals

Little structural change occurs in the adrenal glands during a normal pregnancy. Estrogen-induced increases in the levels of circulating cortisol result primarily from lowered renal excretion.

The circulating cortisol levels regulate carbohydrate and protein metabolism. A normal level resumes 1 to 6 weeks postpartum.

The adrenals secrete increased levels of aldosterone by the early part of the second trimester. The levels of secretion are even more elevated in the woman on a sodium-restricted diet. This increase in aldosterone in a normal pregnancy may be the body's protective response to the increased sodium excretion associated with progesterone (Cunningham et al., 2010).

Pancreas

The pregnant woman has increased insulin needs. The islets of Langerhans are stressed to meet this increased demand, and a latent deficiency may become apparent during pregnancy, producing symptoms of gestational diabetes (see chapter 19 ∞).

Hormones in Pregnancy

Several hormones are required to maintain pregnancy. Most of these are produced initially by the corpus luteum; production is then assumed by the placenta. (For an in-depth discussion of placental hormones, see chapter 11 ∞.)

HUMAN CHORIONIC GONADOTROPIN The trophoblast secretes hCG in early pregnancy. This hormone stimulates progesterone and estrogen production by the corpus luteum to maintain the pregnancy until the placenta is developed sufficiently to assume that function.

HUMAN PLACENTAL LACTOGEN Also called human chorionic somatomammotropin (hCS), human placental lactogen (hPL) is produced by the syncytiotrophoblast. This hormone is an antagonist of insulin; it increases the amount of circulating free fatty acids for maternal metabolic needs and decreases maternal metabolism of glucose to favor fetal growth.

ESTROGEN Secreted originally by the corpus luteum, estrogen is produced primarily by the placenta as early as the seventh week of pregnancy. Estrogen stimulates uterine development to provide a suitable environment for the fetus. It also helps to develop the ductal system of the breasts in preparation for lactation.

PROGESTERONE Progesterone, also produced initially by the corpus luteum and then by the placenta, plays the greatest role in maintaining pregnancy. It maintains the endometrium and also inhibits spontaneous uterine contractility, thus preventing early spontaneous abortion due to uterine activity. In addition, progesterone helps develop the acini and lobules of the breasts in preparation for lactation.

RELAXIN Relaxin is detectable in the serum of a pregnant woman by the time of the first missed menstrual period. Relaxin inhibits uterine activity, diminishes the strength of uterine contractions, aids in the softening of the cervix, and has the long-term effect of remodeling collagen. Its primary source is the corpus luteum, but small amounts are believed to be produced by the placenta and uterine decidua throughout pregnancy.

Prostaglandins in Pregnancy

Prostaglandins (PGs) are lipid substances that can arise from most body tissues but occur in high concentrations in the female reproductive tract and are present in the decidua during pregnancy. The exact functions of PGs during pregnancy are still unknown, although it has been proposed that they are responsible for maintaining reduced placental vascular resistance. Decreased PG levels may contribute to hypertension and preeclampsia. Prostaglandins are also believed to play a role in the complex biochemistry that initiates labor, although their specific functions are still being defined.

Signs of Pregnancy

Many of the changes women experience during pregnancy are used to diagnose the pregnancy itself. They are called the subjective (or presumptive) changes, the objective (or probable) changes, and the diagnostic (or positive) changes of pregnancy.

Subjective (Presumptive) Changes

The subjective changes of pregnancy are the symptoms the woman experiences and reports. They can be caused by other conditions (Table 14-1) and, therefore, cannot be considered proof of pregnancy. The following can be diagnostic clues when other signs and symptoms of pregnancy are also present.

Amenorrhea is the earliest symptom of pregnancy. In a healthy woman whose menstrual cycles are regular, missing one or more menstrual periods leads to the consideration of pregnancy.

Nausea and vomiting of pregnancy (NVP) are experienced by almost half of all pregnant women during the first 3 months of pregnancy and may be the result of elevated human chorionic gonadotropin (hCG) levels and changed carbohydrate me-

TABLE 14-1 Differential Diagnosis of Pregnancy—Subjective Changes

SUBJECTIVE CHANGES	POSSIBLE ALTERNATIVE CAUSES
Amenorrhea	Endocrine factors: early menopause; lactation; thyroid, pituitary, adrenal, ovarian dysfunction Metabolic factors: malnutrition, anemia, climatic changes, diabetes mellitus, degenerative disorders, long-distance running Psychologic factors: emotional shock, fear of pregnancy or sexually transmitted infection, intense desire for pregnancy (pseudocyesis), stress Obliteration of endometrial cavity by infection or curettage Systemic disease (acute or chronic), such as tuberculosis or malignancy
Nausea and vomiting	Gastrointestinal disorders Acute infections such as encephalitis Emotional disorders such as pseudocyesis or anorexia nervosa
Urinary frequency	Urinary tract infection Cystocele Pelvic tumors Urethral diverticula Emotional tension
Breast tenderness	Premenstrual tension Chronic cystic mastitis Pseudocyesis Hyperestrogenism
Quickening	Increased peristalsis Flatus ("gas") Abdominal muscle contractions Shifting of abdominal contents

tabolism. Further research is being conducted to determine other causes for nausea and vomiting. The woman may feel merely a distaste for food or may suffer extreme vomiting, which may be accompanied by dehydration and ketosis. Because these symptoms frequently occur in the early part of the day and disappear within a few hours, they are commonly called **morning sickness**. In reality, symptoms may occur at any time. This gastrointestinal disturbance usually appears about 6 weeks after the first day of the last menstrual period (LMP) and usually disappears spontaneously 6 to 12 weeks later, although it may be prolonged in some instances. Research suggests that women who experience NVP often have a more favorable pregnancy outcome than those who do not.

> “I believed that the nausea and vomiting would only occur in the morning because everyone called it morning sickness. I soon realized that it could occur at any time of the day or night. I was exhausted all the time and nauseated. Everyone told me the nausea was a sign of a healthy baby, which was reassuring I guess but I was so relieved when I started my second trimester and the nausea ended. The rest of my pregnancy was a breeze.”

Excessive fatigue may be noted within a few weeks after the first missed menstrual period and may persist throughout the first trimester.

Urinary frequency is experienced during the first trimester as the enlarging uterus exerts pressure on the bladder. The increased vascularization and pelvic congestion that occur in each pregnancy can also cause frequent voiding. This symptom decreases during the second trimester, when the uterus is an abdominal organ, but reappears during the third trimester, when the presenting part descends into the pelvis.

Changes in the breasts are frequently noted in early pregnancy. Some women report significant breast changes even before missing their first menses. Engorgement of the breasts due to the hormone-induced growth of the secretory ductal system results in the subjective symptoms of tenderness and tingling, especially of the nipple area. The veins also become more visible and form a bluish pattern beneath the skin in fair-skinned women.

Quickening, or the mother's perception of fetal movement, occurs about 18 to 20 weeks after the LMP in a primigravida (a woman who is pregnant for the first time) but may occur as early as 16 weeks in a multigravida (a woman who has been pregnant more than once). Quickening is a fluttering sensation in the abdomen that gradually increases in intensity and frequency.

CLINICAL TIP

Some women suggest that it is easiest to imagine the fluttering associated with quickening by letting the outer tips of the eyelashes brush a finger and then imagining that same sensation deep inside the abdomen.

TABLE 14-2 Differential Diagnosis of Pregnancy—Objective Changes

OBJECTIVE CHANGES	POSSIBLE ALTERNATIVE CAUSES
Changes in pelvic organs	Increased vascular congestion
Goodell's sign	Estrogen-progestin oral contraceptives
Chadwick's sign	Vulvar, vaginal, cervical hyperemia
Hegar's sign	Excessively soft walls of nonpregnant uterus
Uterine enlargement	Uterine tumors
Braun von Fernwald's sign	Uterine tumors
Piskacek's sign	Uterine tumors
Enlargement of abdomen	Obesity, ascites, pelvic tumors
Braxton Hicks contractions	Hematometra, pedunculated, submucous, and soft myomas
Uterine souffle	Large uterine myomas, large ovarian tumors, or any condition with greatly increased uterine blood flow
Pigmentation of skin	Estrogen-progestin oral contraceptives
Chloasma (melasma)	Melanocyte hormonal stimulation
Linea nigra	
Nipples/areola	
Abdominal striae	Obesity, pelvic tumor
Ballottement	Uterine tumors/polyps, ascites
Pregnancy tests	Increased pituitary gonadotropins at menopause, choriocarcinoma, hydatidiform mole
Palpation for fetal outline	Uterine myomas

Objective (Probable) Changes

An examiner can perceive the objective changes that occur in pregnancy. They are more diagnostic than the subjective symptoms. However, their presence does not offer a definite diagnosis of pregnancy (Table 14-2).

Changes in the pelvic organs caused by increased vascular congestion are the only physical signs detectable within the first 3 months of pregnancy. These changes are noted on pelvic examination. There is a softening of the cervix, called Goodell's sign. Chadwick's sign is the deep red to purple or bluish coloration of the mucous membranes of the cervix, vagina, and vulva due to increased vasocongestion of the pelvic vessels. **Hegar's sign** is a softening of the isthmus of the uterus, the area between the cervix and the body of the uterus, which occurs at 6 to 8 weeks of pregnancy. This area may become so soft that on a bimanual exam there seems to be nothing between the cervix and the body of the uterus (Figure 14-4 ■).

Ladin's sign is a soft spot anteriorly in the middle of the uterus near the junction of the body of the uterus and cervix (Figure 14-5A ■). **McDonald's sign** is an ease in flexing the body of the uterus against the cervix.

The uterus assumes an irregular globular shape during the early months of pregnancy. Irregular softening and enlargement at the site of implantation, known as *Braun von Fernwald's sign,* occurs about the fifth week (Figure 14-5B ■). Occasionally an almost tumorlike, asymmetric enlargement

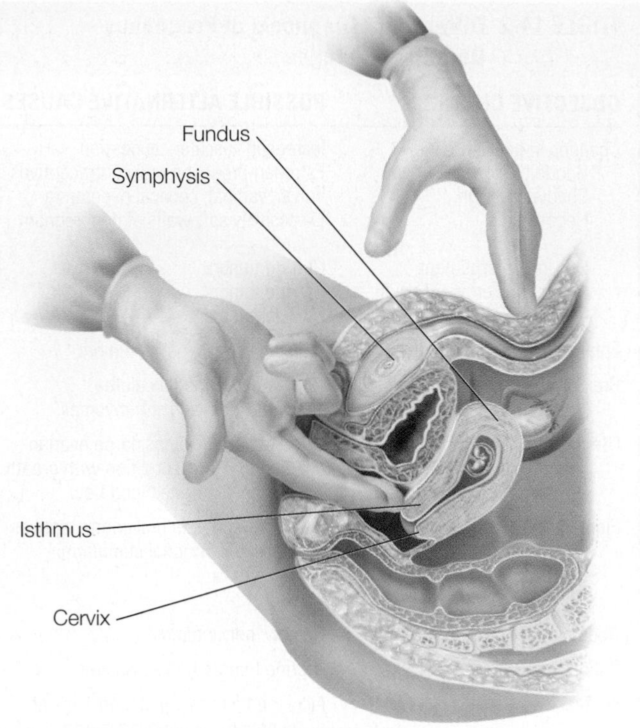

Figure 14-4 ■ Hegar's sign, a softening of the isthmus of the uterus, can be determined by the examiner during a vaginal examination.

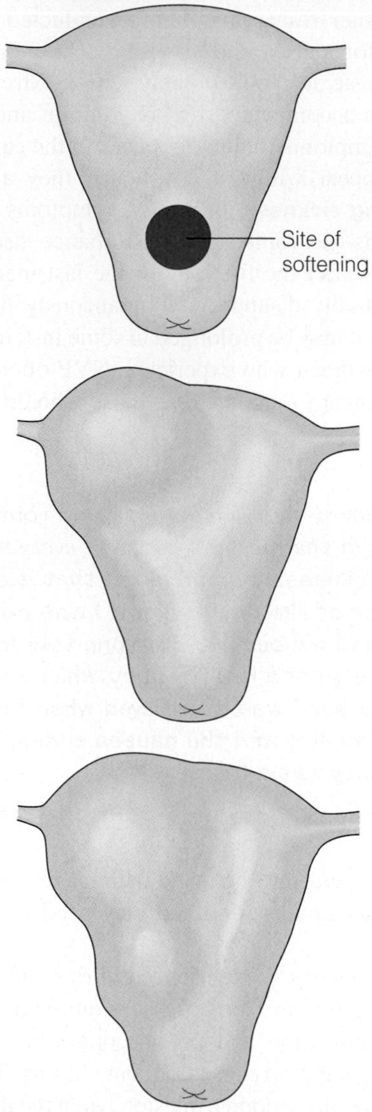

Figure 14-5 ■ Early uterine changes of pregnancy. A. Ladin's sign: a soft spot anteriorly in the middle of the uterus near the junction of the body of the uterus and the cervix. B. Braun von Fernwald's sign: irregular softening and enlargement at the site of implantation. C. Piskacek's sign: a tumorlike asymmetric enlargement.

occurs, called *Piskacek's sign* (Figure 14-5C ■). Generalized enlargement and softening of the body of the uterus are present after the eighth week of pregnancy. The fundus of the uterus is palpable just above the symphysis pubis at approximately 10 to 12 weeks' gestation and at the level of the umbilicus at 20 to 22 weeks' gestation (Figure 14-6 ■).

Enlargement of the abdomen during the childbearing years is usually regarded as evidence of pregnancy, especially if the enlargement is progressive and is accompanied by a continuing amenorrhea. It is generally more pronounced in a woman whose abdominal musculature has lost some of its tone because of previous childbirth.

As mentioned earlier, *Braxton Hicks* contractions are irregular, ordinarily painless contractions that occur at irregular intervals throughout pregnancy but are felt with abdominal palpation after week 28. As the woman approaches the end of the pregnancy, these contractions often become more uncomfortable and are then called *false labor.*

Uterine souffle may be heard when auscultating the abdomen over the uterus. It is a soft blowing sound at the same rate as the maternal pulse and is due to the increased uterine vascularization and the blood pulsating through the placenta. It is sometimes confused with the *funic souffle,* which is a soft blowing sound of blood pulsating through the umbilical arteries. The funic souffle is at the same rate as the fetal heart rate.

Changes in pigmentation of the skin and the *appearance of abdominal striae* are common manifestations in pregnancy. Facial melasma (chloasma) occurs in varying degrees after week 16. The pigmentation of the nipple and areola may darken, especially in primigravidas and dark-haired women. The Montgomery glands of the areola may become enlarged. The skin in the midline of the abdomen may develop a pigmented line, the linea nigra (Figure 14-2). As pregnancy progresses, striae appear on the abdomen and buttocks.

The *fetal outline* may be identified by palpation in many pregnant women after 24 weeks of gestation, becoming easier to distinguish as term approaches. **Ballottement** is the passive fetal movement elicited by pushing up against the cervix with two fingers. This pushes the fetal body up and, as it falls back, the examiner feels a rebound.

Pregnancy tests are based on analysis of maternal blood or urine for the detection of hCG, the hormone secreted by the trophoblast. These tests are not considered positive signs of pregnancy because the similarity of hCG and the pituitary-secreted luteinizing hormone (LH) occasionally results in cross-reactions.

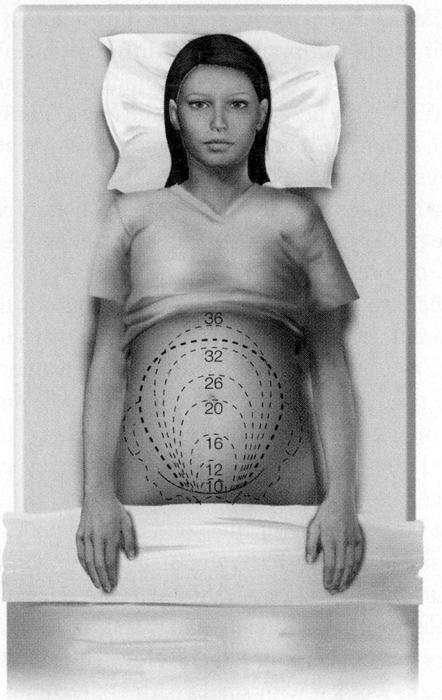

Figure 14-6 ■ Approximate height of the fundus at various weeks of pregnancy.

In addition, certain conditions other than pregnancy can cause elevated levels of hCG.

Clinical Pregnancy Tests

A variety of assay techniques are available to detect hCG in either blood or urine during early pregnancy. Companies that manufacture pregnancy tests provide instructions for performance and interpretation of the test as well as test accuracy. It is important to remember that the presence of hCG in the serum or urine is not always the result of an intrauterine pregnancy. Historically, the following two tests were commonly used urine pregnancy tests.

- *Hemagglutination-inhibition test,* an immunoassay, is based on the fact that no clumping of cells occurs when the urine of a pregnant woman is added to the hCG-sensitized red blood cells of sheep.
- *Latex agglutination test,* also an immunoassay, is based on the fact that latex particle agglutination is inhibited in the presence of urine containing hCG.

The hemagglutination-inhibition test and the latex agglutination test are approximately 95% accurate in diagnosing pregnancy and 98% accurate in determining the absence of pregnancy. The tests become positive approximately 10 to 14 days after the first missed menstrual period. The specimen used for the tests is the first early morning midstream urine because it is adequately concentrated for accuracy. The presence of protein substances (such as blood) in the specimen should be avoided because false-positive results may occur.

Several newer types of pregnancy tests are available, including the following (Buster & Carson, 2002):

- *β-Subunit radioimmunoassay* (RIA) uses an antiserum with specificity for the β-subunit of hCG in blood plasma. This is a very accurate pregnancy test that becomes positive a few days after presumed implantation, thereby permitting earlier diagnosis of pregnancy. This test is also used in the diagnosis of ectopic pregnancy or trophoblastic disease. However, because it requires several hours to perform and has only limited sensitivity, it is being replaced by other, simpler tests such as the immunoradiometric assay.
- *Immunoradiometric assay* (IRMA) uses a radioactive antibody to identify the presence of hCG in the serum. This test can identify very low concentrations of hCG and requires only about 30 minutes to perform. Because this test requires a gamma counter, many laboratories are switching to the enzyme-linked immunosorbent assays.
- *Enzyme-linked immunosorbent assay* (ELISA) does not use radioisotopes but a substance that results in a color change after binding. A blue color develops, the intensity of which is related to the amount of hCG present. This assay, which may be done on urine or blood, is sensitive and quick. It can detect hCG levels as early as 7 to 9 days after ovulation and conception, which is 5 days before the first missed period.
- *Fluoroimmunoassay* (FIA) uses an antibody tagged with a fluorescent label to detect serum hCG. The test, which takes about 2 to 3 hours to perform, is extremely sensitive and is used primarily to identify and follow hCG concentrations.

Over-the-Counter Pregnancy Tests

Home pregnancy tests (HPTs) are available over the counter at a reasonable cost. These enzyme immunoassay tests are quite sensitive and detect even low levels of hCG in urine. Home pregnancy tests are convenient, provide privacy, and allow women to diagnose pregnancy prior to visiting a provider.

Pregnancy Resource Center

Multiple brands and types of HPTs are available, which differ in use and instructions. The newer HPTs claim to be 99% accurate at the time of the missed menses and to have the ability to detect pregnancy 4 days prior to the expected period. This accuracy has been questioned by researchers. Nevertheless, an HPT with a sensitivity of 1.2–5 international units/L hCG will detect 98% of pregnancies close to the time of missed menses (Cole & Ladner, 2009).

There are many variables that may affect the accuracy of home pregnancy test results. Most HPT instructions do not meet recommended compliance with plain language guidelines, including use of wording and language at a reading level above the 6th grade level (Wallace, Zite, Homewood, 2009). Women may not comprehend the HPT instructions, which can affect the accuracy results. It is important that nurses, providers, and patients remember that the tests are not always accurate.

The false-positive rate of these tests is quite low but can also occur in certain situations such as early pregnancy loss, protein in the urine, or the presence of background hCG production. False-negative results are more common and more concerning and should be followed up in the presence of pregnancy symptoms. False-negative results typically occur when the test is completed too early or too late. If the results are negative, the woman should repeat the test in 1 week if she has not started her menstrual period; at that time the test may become positive. Unfortunately, a false-negative result may lead to delays in beginning prenatal care and obtaining guidance, which could negatively impact the pregnancy and fetus. It is important that women using home pregnancy tests understand that a positive result merely indicates growing trophoblastic tissue and not necessarily a uterine pregnancy. If the woman delays seeking prenatal care after pregnancy is confirmed, an early ectopic pregnancy may be missed.

Diagnostic (Positive) Changes

The positive signs of pregnancy are completely objective, cannot be confused with pathologic states, and offer conclusive proof of pregnancy.

The *fetal heartbeat* can be detected with a fetoscope by approximately weeks 17 to 20 of pregnancy. With the electronic Doppler device it is possible to detect the fetal heartbeat as early as weeks 10 to 12. The fetal heart rate is between 120 and 160 beats per minute and must be counted and compared with the maternal pulse for differentiation. Auscultation of the abdomen may reveal sounds other than that of the fetal heart. The maternal pulse, emanating from the abdominal aorta, may be unusually loud, or a uterine souffle may be heard.

Fetal movement is actively palpable by a trained examiner after about 20 weeks' gestation. The movements vary from a faint flutter in the early months to more vigorous movements late in pregnancy.

Visualization of the fetus by ultrasound confirms a pregnancy. The gestational sac can be observed by 4 to 5 weeks' gestation (2 to 3 weeks after conception). Fetal parts and fetal heart movement can be seen as early as 8 weeks. Recently, ultrasound using a vaginal probe has been used to detect a gestational sac as early as 10 days after implantation (Cunningham et al., 2010).

Psychologic Response of the Expectant Family to Pregnancy

Application: Internet Pregnancy Information

Pregnancy is a developmental challenge, a turning point in a family's life accompanied by stress and anxiety whether the pregnancy is desired or not. Pregnancy confirms one's biologic capabilities to reproduce. It is evidence of one's participation in sexual activity and as such is an affirmation of one's sexuality. For beginning families, pregnancy is the transition period from childlessness to parenthood. If the pregnancy terminates in the birth of a child, the couple enters a new stage of their life together, one that is irreversible and characterized by awesome responsibilities.

The expectant couple may be unaware of the physical, emotional, and cognitive states peculiar to pregnancy. The couple may anticipate no problem from such a normal event as pregnancy and, therefore, may be confused and distressed by new feelings and behaviors that are generally considered normal.

If the expectant woman is married or has a stable partner, she no longer is only a mate but also must assume the role of mother. Her partner will also assume a parenting role. Career goals and mobility may be altered or thwarted for one or both partners. Each partner begins to see the other in a different light. Their relationship takes on a different meaning to them and within the larger family and community. Their lifestyle changes. With each pregnancy, routines and family dynamics are altered, requiring readjustment and realignment.

If a pregnant woman is without a stable partner, she will still experience changes in role identity and psychobiologic maturation. She must deal alone with the role changes, fears, and adjustments of pregnancy or seek support from family and friends. She also faces the reality of planning for the future as a single parent. Even if the pregnant woman plans to relinquish her infant, she must still deal with the adjustments of pregnancy. She is no longer a separate individual; she must consider the needs of another being who depends on her totally, at least during the pregnancy. This adjustment can be especially difficult without a good support system.

In most pregnancies, whether of a mother with a supportive partner, a single mother, or a relinquishing mother, finances are an important consideration. Traditional lore relegates to the father the role of primary breadwinner, and, indeed, finances are often a very real concern for fathers. However, in today's society even pregnant women with stable partners recognize the financial impact of a child and may feel concern about financial issues. For the single mother, finances may be a major source of concern.

Decisions about financial matters need to be made at this time. Will the woman work during the pregnancy and return to work after the baby is born? Who will provide child care if she works? Decisions may also need to be made about the division of tasks within the home. Any differences of opinion must be discussed openly and resolved so that the family can meet its members' needs.

The couple must face the realities of labor and birth. Many nonparents have little idea what labor entails. Their information is frequently based on contacts with visual or print media and on experiences related to them by family members or friends, and these tales are often fraught with myths and exaggerations. Classes in prepared childbirth can help them address this lack of information or misinformation.

Labor is threatening in many respects. Pain, disfigurement, disruption of bodily function, and even death are potential threats for the woman. The partner faces the threat of the woman's disfigurement, impairment of her health, or her death. Both fear that the baby may be ill or disfigured. The expectant couple is subject to anxiety during this period because no one can provide total reassurance about the outcome.

Pregnancy can be viewed as a developmental stage with its own distinct developmental tasks. It can be a time of support or conflict for a couple, depending on the amount of adjustment each is willing to make to maintain the family's equilibrium. Family dynamics are an important factor in adjusting to pregnancy. Family strengths include the ability of the couple to talk about issues that are important to them, to resolve conflicts and make compromises, and to seek and receive assistance and support from loved ones.

During pregnancy, the woman and her partner plan together for the first child's arrival, collecting information on how to be parents. At the same time, each continues to participate in some

Case Study: Prenatal Education

separate activities with friends or family members. The availability of social support is an important factor in psychosocial well-being during pregnancy. Most pregnant women turn to their partners as their primary source of social support. In addition, the broader social network often is a major source of advice for the pregnant woman. However, evidence indicates that both sound and unsound information is given.

The expectant mother and her partner both face significant changes during pregnancy and must deal with major psychosocial adjustments (Table 14-3). Other family members, especially other children of the woman or couple, and the grandparents-to-be, must also adjust to the pregnancy.

In late pregnancy, the concerns of expectant fathers tend to focus most on the health of the unborn child and the safety of the mother. The concerns of expectant mothers center on the health of the baby and their ability to handle labor and birth. Couples typically agree on the primary concern, the health of the unborn child. Nurses can use this focus as a springboard for discussing other concerns. Couples can then come to understand the differences between their second most important concerns. A woman worries about how she will handle labor and birth but has little concern for her own safety; the father's expression of his fear for her safety can be seen as evidence that he cares enough to worry about her. This response may allow the mother to depend on him more during the vulnerable time of late pregnancy and birthing. Sharing his views gives the father a chance to express his love and concern for mother and child, encouraging the development of stronger marital and paternal relationships.

For some couples, pregnancy is more than a developmental stage; it is a crisis. *Crisis* can be defined as a disturbance or conflict in which the individual cannot maintain a state of equilibrium. Pregnancy can be considered a *maturational crisis* because it is a common event in the normal growth and development of the family. During such a crisis, the individual or family is in disequilibrium. The period of disequilibrium and disorganization is marked by abortive attempts to solve the perceived problems. If the crisis is not resolved, it will result in maladaptive behaviors in one or more family members and possible disintegration of the family. Families who are able to resolve a maturational crisis successfully will return to normal functioning and can even strengthen the bonds in the family relationship.

Mother

Pregnancy is a condition that alters body image and also necessitates a reordering of social relationships and changes in roles of family members. The way a particular woman meets the

TABLE 14-3 Parental Reactions to Pregnancy

FIRST TRIMESTER	SECOND TRIMESTER	THIRD TRIMESTER
Mother's Reactions	**Mother's Reactions**	**Mother's Reactions**
Informs father secretively or openly. Feels ambivalent toward pregnancy, anxious about labor and responsibility of child. Is aware of physical changes; daydreams of possible miscarriage. Develops special feelings for and renewed interest in her own mother, with formation of a personal identity.	Remains regressive and introspective; projects all problems with authority figures onto partner; may become angry if she perceives his lack of interest as a sign of weakness in him. Continues to deal with feelings as a mother; shops for nursery furniture as something concrete to do. May experience anxiety or, alternately, may be extremely lackadaisical and wait until 9th month to look for furniture and clothes for baby. Feels movement and is aware of fetus and incorporates it into herself. Dreams that partner will be killed; telephones him often for reassurance. Experiences more distinct physical changes; sexual desires may increase or decrease.	Experiences more anxiety and tension, with physical awkwardness. Feels much discomfort and insomnia from physical condition. Prepares for birth, assembles layette; picks out names. Dreams often about misplacing baby or not being able to give birth; fears birth of deformed baby. Feels ecstasy and excitement; has spurt of energy during last month.
Father's Reactions	**Father's Reactions**	**Father's Reactions**
Differ according to age, parity, desire for child, economic stability. Acceptance of pregnant woman's attitude or complete rejection and lack of communication. Is aware of his sexual feelings; may develop more or less sexual arousal. Accepts, rejects, or resents mother-in-law. May develop new hobby outside of family as sign of stress.	If he can cope, will give her extra attention she needs; if he cannot cope, will develop a new time-consuming interest outside of home. May develop a creative feeling and a "closeness to nature." Many become involved in pregnancy and buy or make furniture. Feels for movement of baby, listens to heartbeat, or remains aloof, with no physical contact. May have fears and fantasies about himself being pregnant; may become uneasy with this feminine aspect in himself. May react negatively if partner is too demanding; may become jealous of physician and of physician's importance to partner and her pregnancy.	Adapts to alternative methods of sexual contact. Becomes concerned over financial responsibility. May show new sense of tenderness and concern, treats partner like doll. Daydreams about child as if older and not newborn; dreams of losing partner. Renewed sexual attraction to partner. Feels he is ultimately responsible for whatever happens.

stresses of pregnancy is influenced by her emotional makeup, her sociologic and cultural background, and her acceptance or rejection of the pregnancy. However, many women manifest similar psychologic and emotional responses during pregnancy, including ambivalence, acceptance, introversion, mood swings, and changes in body image.

Intendedness

Many pregnancies are unintended, but not all unintended pregnancies are unwanted. For some women, an unintended pregnancy has more psychologic and social advantages than disadvantages. It provides purpose and direction to life and allows a woman to test the devotion and love of her partner and family. However, an unintended pregnancy can be a risk factor for depression. Women with an unintended pregnancy may perceive life events as being more stressful than women with an intended pregnancy—another contributor to depression. Depression, in turn, can negatively impact a pregnant woman's health choices and behaviors (Messer, Dole, Kaufman, et al., 2005).

Ambivalence

Initially, even if the pregnancy is planned, the mother may experience a sense of surprise that conception has actually occurred. This may be coupled with a feeling that pregnancy is desirable "someday" but "not now." Such ambivalence may be related to feelings that the timing is somehow "wrong," worries about the need to modify existing relationships or career plans, fears about assuming a new role, unresolved emotional conflicts with the woman's own mother, and fears about pregnancy, labor, and birth. Indirect evidence of ambivalence includes complaints about prolonged or frequent depression, considerable physical discomfort, significant dissatisfaction with body shape, excessive mood swings, and difficulty accepting the life changes resulting from the pregnancy (Lederman & Weis, 2009).

Such feelings may be even more pronounced if the pregnancy is unintended or unwanted. Women who view their pregnancy as unwanted are more likely to delay prenatal care and to experience complications. The support and opinion of the woman's current partner, even if he is not the father of the child, have a major impact on pregnancy wantedness. Financial and emotional support from the partner are essential to the woman's positive attitude. Involving the partner in the prenatal care may help promote a supportive attitude. During the early months, the pregnant woman may consider the possibility of a therapeutic abortion if the pregnancy is unwanted. In the event of religious conflicts about induced abortion, the woman may experience guilt feelings about her thoughts or may tend to focus on the possibility of spontaneous abortion (miscarriage). Even when the pregnancy is planned, thoughts of abortion and miscarriage arise. Concurrently, the pregnant woman may feel guilty for having such negative thoughts and may worry that in some way these thoughts will harm the baby.

Acceptance

Acceptance of pregnancy is influenced by many factors. Lower acceptance tends to be related to an unplanned pregnancy and greater evidence of fear and conflict. The woman carrying an unplanned pregnancy tends to experience more physical discomfort and depression. When a pregnancy is well accepted, the woman demonstrates feelings of happiness and pleasure in the pregnancy. She experiences less physical discomfort and shows a high degree of tolerance for the discomforts associated with the third trimester (Lederman & Weis, 2009).

Conflicts about adapting to pregnancy are no more pronounced for older pregnant women (age 35 and older) than for younger ones. Moreover, older pregnant women tend to be less concerned about the normal physical changes of pregnancy and are confident about handling issues that arise during pregnancy and parenting. This may be because mature pregnant women have more experience with problem solving. However, mature pregnant women may have fewer pregnant peers and thus may have fewer people with whom to share concerns and expectations.

For some women, an unintended pregnancy has more psychologic and social advantages than disadvantages. It provides purpose and direction to life and allows a woman to test the devotion and love of her partner and family.

> **"I didn't expect to get pregnant, but my baby seems like a gift from God. Suddenly I feel like I have a purpose in life. I know I have to do the right things so the baby will be okay. Being pregnant made me grow up in a hurry, but I don't regret it—not at all."**

During the *first trimester,* evidence of pregnancy is often limited to amenorrhea and to the word of the caregiver that the pregnancy test was positive. Unless the woman has the opportunity to see the gestational sac during an ultrasound, her baby may not seem real. Consequently, she may tend to focus on herself and her pregnancy. In an effort to verify her condition, a woman may become minutely conscious of changes in her body that could validate the pregnancy.

The *second trimester* is relatively tranquil. Morning sickness generally passes, the threat of spontaneous abortion diminishes, and the woman begins to accept the reality of her pregnancy. It is not unusual for an enthusiastic primigravida to don maternity clothes at the beginning of this trimester even when it is not truly necessary. The clothing serves as a verification of her pregnant state.

The highlight of the second trimester is quickening, which generally occurs about week 20—midway through the pregnancy. Actual perception of fetal movement frequently produces dramatic changes in the woman. She now perceives her baby as a real person and generally becomes excited about the pregnancy even if she has not been before this time.

As quickening and her altered physical appearance confirm her pregnant state, the woman adjusts to the idea of change and begins to prepare for her new role and her new set of relationships—with her partner and family, the child-to-be and other children, friends, and loved ones. When the pregnancy is well accepted, the woman takes pleasure in the sensations of pregnancy and attempts to picture her baby in order to know him or her better. She may seek out other women who are pregnant or have recently given birth. She feels well, is excited, and may exhibit the "glow" so often attributed to pregnant women.

The *third trimester* combines a sense of pride with anxiety about what is to come in order for the child to be born. During this time, the special prerogatives of pregnancy may be most marked. As her protruding abdomen proclaims her advanced pregnancy, the woman may find that others become more solicitous, that a chair may be offered in a crowded room, that others may carry her parcels. The woman may actually need this help, she may simply enjoy the attention as a privilege of pregnancy, or she may reject it if she fears that such gestures indicate she is helpless.

During the final trimester, physical discomforts again increase, and adequate rest becomes a necessity. The woman makes final preparation for the baby and may spend long periods considering names for the child. During this time she worries more about the health and safety of her unborn child and may have concerns that she will not behave well during childbirth.

The woman may feel vulnerable to rejection, loss, or insult. She may worry about a variety of things and may withdraw into the security and quiet of her home. Toward the end of this period many women report bursts of energy in which they vigorously clean and organize their homes ("nesting").

Introversion

Introversion, or turning in on oneself, is a common occurrence in pregnancy. An active, outgoing woman may become less interested in previous activities and more concerned with needs for rest and time alone. This concentration of attention permits the woman to plan, adjust, adapt, build, and draw strength in preparation for her child's birth. As she becomes more aware of herself, her partner may feel she is being overly sensitive. Her partner may perceive her introversion and passivity as exclusionary and may in turn become unable to interact with her, either verbally or physically, or to provide the affection, support, and consideration she requires. This change may result in disequilibrium and stress for the entire family. It is essential that the couple work together to establish new, mutually acceptable patterns of response to overcome these blocks to communication.

Fantasies about the unborn child are quite common among pregnant women. However, the themes of the fantasies (baby's appearance, gender, traits, impact on parents, and so forth) vary by trimester and also differ between women pregnant for the first time and women who already have children.

Mood Swings

Throughout pregnancy, the emotions of many women are characterized by mood swings, from great joy to deep despair. Frequently, the woman will become tearful with little apparent cause. When asked why she is crying, she may find it difficult or impossible to give a reason. The situation may be extremely unsettling for the partner, causing him to feel confused and inadequate. Because the man may feel unable to handle the woman's tears, he often reacts by withdrawing and ignoring the problem. Because the pregnant woman needs increased love and affection, she may perceive his reaction as unloving and nonsupportive. Once the couple understands that this behavior is characteristic of pregnancy, it becomes easier for them to deal with it more effectively—although it will be a source of stress to some extent throughout pregnancy.

Changes in Body Image

Pregnancy produces marked changes in a woman's body within a relatively short time. With these changes, women also experience changes in body image. The degree of this change is related to a certain extent to personality factors, social network responses, and attitudes toward pregnancy. Changes in body image are normal but can be very stressful for the pregnant woman. Explanation and discussion of the changes may help both the woman and her partner deal with the stress associated with this aspect of pregnancy.

> **"I'm due in 2 weeks and I can't wait. These last few weeks have been hard on my self-image. I can't see my feet anymore and I feel awkward and lumbering, not graceful at all."**

Psychologic Tasks of the Mother

Rubin (1984) identified four major tasks that the pregnant woman undertakes to maintain her intactness and that of her family and at the same time incorporate her new child into the family system. These tasks form the basis for a mutually gratifying relationship with her baby:

1. ***Ensuring safe passage through pregnancy, labor, and birth:*** The pregnant woman feels concern for both her unborn child and herself. She seeks competent maternity care to provide a sense of control. She may also seek knowledge from literature, observation of other pregnant women and new mothers, and discussion with others. The pregnant woman also seeks to ensure safe passage by engaging in self-care activities related to diet, exercise, alcohol consumption, and so forth. In the third trimester, as her movements slow and her body mass increases, she becomes aware of external threats in the environment—a toy on a stair, the awkwardness of an escalator—that pose a threat to her intactness and represent hazards to be overcome. She may worry if her partner is late or if she is home alone. Sleep becomes difficult, and she begins to long for the baby's birth, even though it, too, is frightening.
2. ***Seeking of acceptance of this child by others:*** The birth of a child alters a woman's primary support group, her family, and her secondary affiliative groups. The family generally makes the transition, and the woman slowly and subtly alters her secondary network to meet the needs of her pregnancy. In this adjustment the woman's partner is the most important figure. The partner's support and acceptance influence her completion of her maternal tasks and the formation of her maternal identity. If there are other children in the home, the mother also works to ensure their acceptance of the coming child. Accepting the coming change in exclusive relationships—woman and

partner or mother and first child—can be stressful, and the woman will often work to maintain some special time with her partner or older child. Achieving social acceptance of the child and of herself as mother may be more difficult for the adolescent mother or single woman. The child to come is not always wanted, and the woman often must direct her energies to changing this situation.

3. ***Seeking of commitment and acceptance of self as mother to the infant (binding-in):*** During the first trimester, the child remains a rather abstract concept. With quickening, however, the child begins to become a real person, and the mother begins to develop bonds of attachment. The mother experiences the movement of the child within her in an intimate, exclusive way, and out of this experience bonds of love form. The mother develops a fantasy image of her ideal child. This binding-in process, characterized by its strong emotional component, motivates the pregnant woman to become competent in her role and provides satisfaction for her in her role of mother (Mercer, 2004). This possessive love increases her maternal commitment to protect her fetus now and her child after she or he is born.
4. ***Learning to give of oneself on behalf of one's child:*** Childbirth involves many acts of giving. The man "gives" a child to a woman; she in turn "gives" a child to the man. Life is given to an infant; a sibling is given to older children of the family. The woman begins to develop a capacity for self-denial and learns to delay immediate personal gratification to meet the needs of another. Baby showers and baby gifts are acts of giving that help the mother's self-esteem while also helping her acknowledge the separateness and needs of the coming baby.

Accomplishment of these tasks helps the expectant woman develop her self-concept as mother. The expectant mother who was well nurtured by her own mother may view her mother as a role model and emulate her; the woman who views her own mother as a "poor mother" may worry that she will make similar mistakes (Lederman & Weis, 2009). A woman's self-concept as mother expands with actual experience and continues to grow through subsequent childbearing and childrearing. Occasionally, a woman never accepts the mother role but plays the role of babysitter or older sister.

Father

Until fairly recently, the expectant father was often viewed as a "bystander" or observer of his partner's pregnancy. He was necessary for conception, for bill paying, and for providing male guidance as his child matured. This view has changed, and the father of today is expected to fulfill the role of nurturing, caring, involved parent as well as provider. In response to societal pressures, the influence of the feminist movement, and the economic pressures that result in more women employed outside the home, shared parenting and breadwinning have become more commonplace. Many men have actively sought to be more involved in the experience of childbirth and parenting.

Expectant fathers experience many of the same feelings and conflicts experienced by expectant mothers when the pregnancy has been confirmed. Initially, expectant fathers may feel pride in their virility, which pregnancy confirms, but also have ambivalent feelings. The extent of ambivalence depends on many factors, including the father's relationship with his partner, his previous experience with pregnancy, his age, his economic stability, and whether the pregnancy was planned. The expectant father must first deal with the reality of the pregnancy and then struggle to gain recognition as a parent from his partner, family, friends, coworkers, society—and from his baby as well. The expectant mother can help her partner be a participant and not merely a helpmate to her if she has a definite sense of the experience as their pregnancy and their infant and not her pregnancy and her infant.

Men whose partners are pregnant following a previous pregnancy loss may experience a variety of emotions attributable to the loss. These emotions might include an increased sense of risk, feelings of increased concern about the outcome of the current pregnancy, the recognition that something could go wrong again, and the sense that increased vigilance is essential. These fathers may call home more often to check on the mother's condition and the baby and may also feel an increased need to be involved more actively in the current pregnancy. They wish to be acknowledged as more than just a support person; they want their important role as family protector recognized (O'Leary & Thorwick, 2006).

In general, the expectant father faces psychologic stress as he makes the transition from nonparent to parent or from parent of one to parent of two or more. Sources of stress include financial issues, unexpected events during pregnancy, concern that the baby will not be healthy and normal, worry about the pain the partner will experience in childbirth, and his role during labor and birth. Other sources of stress for expectant fathers include concern over the changing relationship with their partners, diminished sexual responsiveness in their partners or in themselves, change in relationships with their families or male friends, and their ability to parent. Most men handle the transition to fatherhood well, and generally any anxieties they feel resolve over time. Fathers' feelings of anxieties often stem from inadequate preparation and can be addressed by recognizing paternal needs and including fathers more in antepartal education (Deave, Johnson, & Ingram, 2008).

The expectant father must establish a fatherhood role just as the woman develops a motherhood role. The mother experiences biologic changes of pregnancy that aid in the transition to motherhood. Fathers may feel left out because they are unable to experience what their partner is experiencing. Fathers who are most successful at developing a fatherhood role generally like children, are excited about the prospect of fatherhood, are eager to nurture a child, have confidence in their ability to be a parent, and share the experiences of pregnancy and childbirth with their partners (Lederman & Weis, 2009).

First Trimester

After the initial excitement of the announcement of the pregnancy to friends and relatives and receipt of their congratulations, an expectant father may begin to feel left out of the

Through the Eyes of a Nurse
Psychologic Changes in Pregnancy

Family's Experience

"I am dealing with a lot of shifting emotions right now. One minute I feel happy and elated, and then suddenly I am so blue. I feel like I am on an emotional roller coaster! I find myself tearful for no reason and can't even explain to my husband why I am crying. When he doesn't act supportive, I feel unloved and angry like I am the one dealing with all of these changes while my family stands by, unaffected."

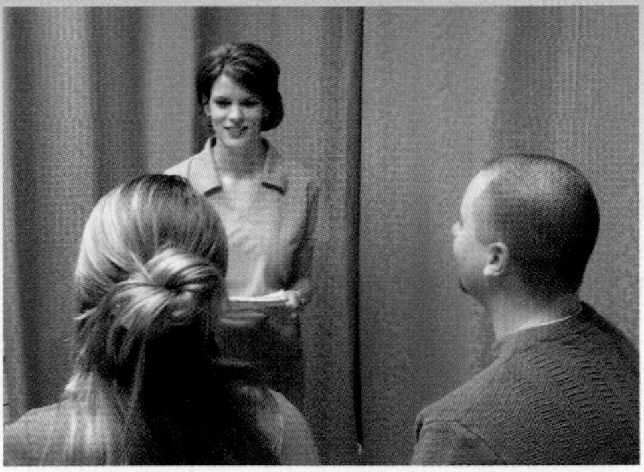

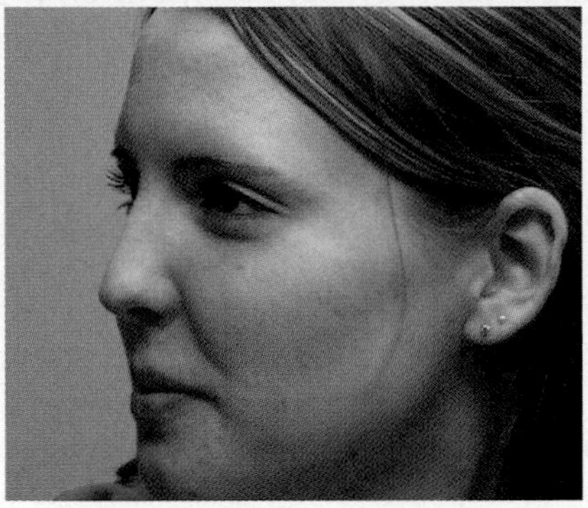

Nurse's Response

"Even though each woman is different in her reactions to pregnancy and every pregnancy is different, mood swings with extremes in emotions are common. So what you are describing is pretty typical but it can be hard to handle, and you may feel overwhelmed at times.

"During pregnancy, women experience a wide variety of responses such as ambivalence, mood swings, and changes in body image. Because your emotional well-being is so important during pregnancy, we will assess your adjustment to pregnancy at each visit, much like we routinely monitor your blood pressure, the baby's movements, and the size of your uterus.

"It might help if you express your feelings to your family and ask them for additional support when you are sad, overwhelmed, or ambivalent about the pregnancy. Also, I would be glad to talk to your husband about these changes and suggest ways for him to be supportive if you feel that would help."

Nurse's Actions and Rationale

The nurse validates the woman's feelings and provides reassurance that the feelings she is experiencing are normal. The nurse also takes the opportunity to provide teaching about the common emotional responses that occur during pregnancy. The father's actions can be a positive influence during a woman's pregnancy and postpartum so it is important to seek opportunities to provide him with interventions to ease the adjustment process for his partner.

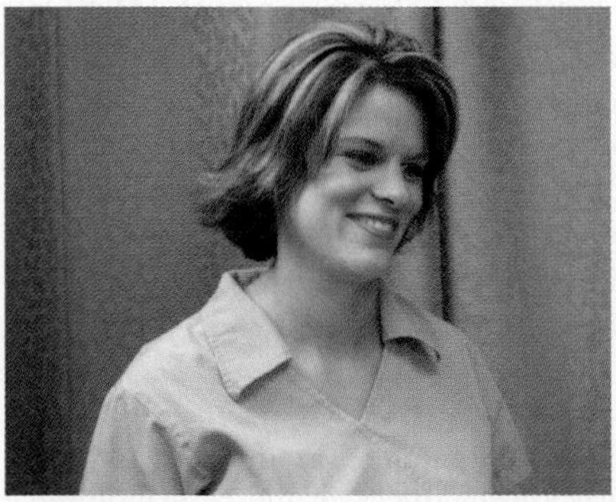

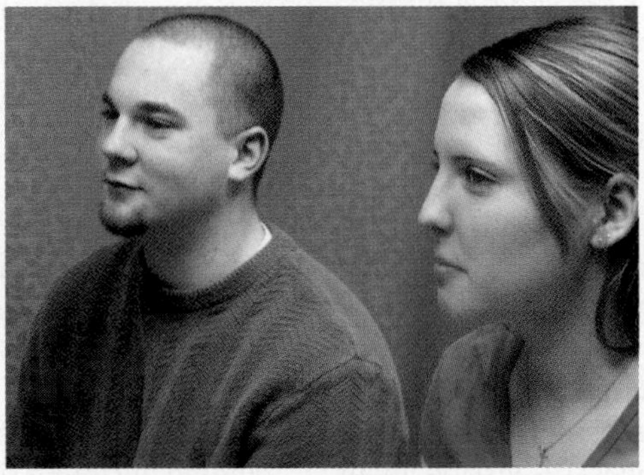

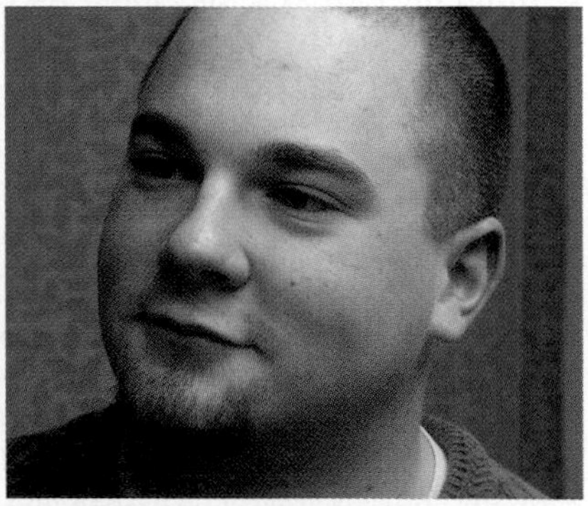

pregnancy. He is also often confused by his partner's mood changes and perhaps bewildered by his responses to her changing body. He may resent the attention given to the woman and the need to change their relationship as she experiences fatigue and a decreased interest in sex.

During this time, his child is a "potential baby." Fathers often picture interacting with a child of 5 or 6 rather than a newborn. Even the pregnancy itself may seem unreal until the woman shows more physical signs.

Second Trimester

The father's role in the pregnancy is still vague in the second trimester, but his involvement can be increased by his watching and feeling fetal movement. It is helpful if the father, as well as the mother, has the opportunity to hear the fetal heartbeat. That requires a visit to the nurse-midwife's or physician's office. Involvement of fathers in antepartal care is increasing and may even be an expectation of their partner. For many men, seeing the infant on ultrasound is an important experience in accepting the reality of the pregnancy.

Like expectant mothers, expectant fathers need to confront and resolve some of their own conflicts about the fathering they received. A father needs to sort out those behaviors in his own fathering that he wants to imitate and those he wishes to avoid. Research indicates that a father's beliefs about the fathering role are a strong predictor of his competence in parenting (Schoppe-Sullivan, Brown, Cannon, et al., 2008).

> "I was excited about the chance to be the kind of father who was involved and available. However, I also wanted to provide adequately for my child, support my wife, and still have time to do the things I loved to do. I was surprised by how excited my father was about becoming a grandfather. He even talked to me about the regrets he had about not being around as I was growing up. I think the experience will help to bring my dad and me closer as he tries to be a great grandfather and I understand more about his struggles as a father."

The father-to-be's anxiety is lessened if both parents agree on the support role the man is to assume during pregnancy and on his projected paternal role. For example, if both see his role as that of breadwinner, the man's stress is low. However, if the man views his role as that of breadwinner and the woman expects him to be actively involved in preparations and child care, his stress increases. An open and honest discussion about the expectations each parent has about their roles will help the father-to-be to determine his transition to fatherhood (Goodman, 2005).

The woman's appearance begins to alter at this time too, and men react differently to the physical change. For some it decreases sexual interest; for others it may have the opposite effect. Both partners experience a multitude of emotions, and it continues to be important for them to communicate and accept each other's feelings and concerns. In situations in which the expectant mother's demands dominate the relationship, the expectant father's resentment may increase to the point that he is spending more time at work, involved in a hobby, or with his friends. The behavior is even more likely if the expectant father did not want the pregnancy and/or if the relationship was not a good one before the pregnancy.

Care Plan Activity: Preparing Siblings for New Baby

Third Trimester

If the couple have communicated their concerns and feelings to one another and grown in their relationship, the third trimester is a special and rewarding time. A more clearly defined role evolves at this time for the expectant father, and it becomes more obvious how the couple can prepare together for the coming event. They may become involved in childbirth education classes and make concrete preparations for the arrival of the baby, such as shopping for a crib, car seat, and other equipment. If the expectant father has developed a detached attitude about the pregnancy before this time, however, it is unlikely that he will become a willing participant even though his role becomes more obvious.

Concerns and fears may recur. Many men are afraid of hurting the unborn baby during intercourse. The father may also begin to have anxiety and fantasies about what could happen to his partner and the unborn baby during labor and birth and feels a great sense of responsibility. The questions asked earlier in pregnancy emerge again. What kind of parents will he and his partner be? Will he really be able to help his partner in labor? Can they afford to have a baby?

Couvade

The term **couvade** traditionally referred to the observance of certain rituals and taboos by the male to signify the transition to fatherhood. This observance affirms his psychosocial and biophysical relationship to the woman and child. These taboos may have taken specific form—for example, the man may have been forbidden to eat certain foods or carry certain weapons before and immediately after the birth. More recently, the term has been used to describe the unintentional development of physical symptoms, such as fatigue, increased appetite, difficulty sleeping, depression, headache, or backache by the partner of the pregnant woman. Men who demonstrate couvade syndrome tend to have a higher degree of paternal role preparation and be involved in more activities related to this preparation.

Siblings

The introduction of a new baby into the family is often the beginning of sibling rivalry. Sibling rivalry results from children's fear of change in the security of their relationships with their parents. Some of the behaviors demonstrating feelings of sibling rivalry may even be directed toward the mother during the pregnancy as she experiences more fatigue and less patience with her toddler, for example. Parents who recognize the situation early in pregnancy and begin constructive actions can help minimize the problems of sibling rivalry.

Preparation of the young child begins several weeks before the anticipated birth and is designed according to the age and experience of the child. Because they do not have a clear concept of time, young children should not be told too early about the pregnancy. From the toddler's point of view "several weeks" is an extremely long time. The mother may let the child feel the baby moving in her uterus, explaining that this is "a special place where babies grow." The child can help the parents put the baby clothes in drawers or prepare the baby's room.

Consistency is important in dealing with young children. They need reassurance that certain people, special things, and familiar places will continue to exist after the new baby arrives. The crib is an important though transient object in a child's life. If it is to be given to the new baby, the parents should thoughtfully help the child adjust to this change. Any move from crib to bed or from one room to another should precede the baby's birth by several weeks or more. If the new baby is to share a room with siblings, the parents must discuss this with the older child or children.

Some parents advocate cosleeping or bed sharing (one or both parents sleeping with their baby or young child), and so the crib is less of an issue. Cosleeping, which is common in many non-Western cultures, is on the increase in the United States. Opinion varies sharply about the advantages and risks of the practice. In 2005 the American Academy of Pediatrics (AAP) issued a policy statement recommending against cosleeping because of the increased risk of sudden infant death syndrome (SIDS). This policy statement was reaffirmed by the AAP in January 2009. The AAP stresses that the infant can be brought to the bed to be comforted or for breastfeeding but should be placed supine in a separate bed ("back to bed") to sleep. (See the discussion in chapter 37 ∞.) Parents who choose to cosleep must make decisions about the sleeping arrangements of other siblings following the birth of the baby.

If the child is ready for toilet training, it is most effectively done several months before or after the baby's arrival. Parents should know that the older, toilet-trained child may regress to wetting or soiling because he or she sees the new baby getting attention for such behavior. The older, weaned child may want to drink from the breast or bottle again after the new baby comes. If the new mother anticipates these behaviors, they will be less frustrating during her early postpartum days.

During the pregnancy, older children should be introduced to a new baby for short periods to get an idea of what a new baby is like. This introduction dispels fantasies that the new arrival will be big enough to be a playmate. Pregnant women may also find it helpful to bring their children to a prenatal visit after they have been told about the expected baby. The children are encouraged to become involved in prenatal care and to ask any questions they may have. They are also given the opportunity to hear the baby's heartbeat, either with a stethoscope or with the Doppler. This helps make the baby more real to them.

If siblings are school-age children, the pregnancy should be viewed as a family affair. Teaching about the pregnancy should be based on the child's level of understanding and interest. Overeager parents may go into lengthier and more in-depth responses than the child is able to understand. Some children are more curious than others. Books at their level of understanding can be made available in the home. Involvement in family discussions, attendance at sibling preparation classes, encouragement to feel fetal movement, and an opportunity to listen to the fetal heart supplement the learning process and help make the school-age child feel part of the pregnancy. Sibling preparation classes assist in the transition process for both parents and children. After attending the classes, children often exhibit less anxiety and increased ability to express their feelings.

Older children or adolescents may appear to have a sophisticated knowledge base, but it may be intermingled with many misconceptions. Thus the parents should make opportunities to discuss their concerns and should involve the children in preparation for the new baby.

Even after the birth, siblings need to feel that they are part of a family affair. Changes in hospital regulations allowing siblings to be present at the birth or to visit their mother and the new baby facilitate this process. Participation in special programs for siblings may help in this process. On arrival at home, siblings can share in "showing off" the new baby.

Sibling preparation for the arrival of a new baby is essential, but other factors are equally important. These include the amount of parental attention focused on the new arrival, the amount of parental attention given the older child after the birth of the new arrival, and parental skill in dealing effectively with regressive and/or aggressive behavior.

Grandparents

The first relatives told about a pregnancy are usually the grandparents. Although relationships with parents can be very complex, the expectant grandparents often become increasingly supportive of the expectant couple, even if conflicts previously existed. But it can be difficult for even sensitive grandparents to know how deeply to become involved in the childrearing process.

Because grandparenting can occur over a wide expanse of years, people's response to this role can vary considerably. Younger grandparents leading active lives may not demonstrate as much interest as the young couple would like. In other cases, expectant grandparents may give advice and gifts unsparingly. For grandparents, conflict may be related to the expectant couple's need to feel in control of their lives, or it may stem from events that signal changing roles in the grandparents' own lives (e.g., retirement, financial concerns, menopause, or death of a friend). Some parents of expectant couples may already be grandparents with a developed style of grandparenting. This influences their response to the pregnancy.

Childbearing and childrearing practices are very different for today's childbearing couple. It helps family cohesiveness for young couples to share with interested grandparents what today's practices are and why they feel they are effective. At the same time, it is important for young couples to listen to any differences expectant grandparents want to explain. When grandparents give advice, it helps to remember that they care. When their recommendations seem effective, it is significant to grandparents that young couples do listen and follow their advice.

Occasionally young couples feel they are receiving more advice than they can tolerate. Too often they perceive parents' suggestions as criticizing their ability to prepare adequately for the childbearing process—and later as criticizing their care of the newborn. It is useful for the young couple to discuss the problem and agree on a plan of action. The role of the helping grandparents when the new baby is brought home needs to be clarified before the event to ensure a comfortable situation for all.

In some areas, classes for grandparents provide information about changes in birthing and parenting practices. These classes help familiarize grandparents with new parents' needs and may offer suggestions for ways in which the grandparents can support the childbearing woman or couple.

Cultural Values and Pregnancy

A universal tendency exists to create ceremonial rituals and rites around important life events. Thus pregnancy, childbirth, marriage, and death are often tied to ritual (Spector, 2009). The rituals, customs, and practices of a group are a reflection of the group's values. In many developed countries such as the United States, Canada, England, Germany, and so forth, populations are becoming more and more ethnically diverse as the number of immigrants continues to grow. It is not realistic or appropriate to assume that people who are new to a country or area will automatically abandon their ways and adopt the practices of the dominant culture (Dean, 2010). Consequently the identification of cultural values is useful in planning and providing culturally sensitive care.

Generalizations about cultural characteristics or cultural values are difficult because not every individual in a culture may display these characteristics. Just as variations are seen among cultures, variations are also seen within cultures. These variations are often related to social and economic factors such as class, income, and education. For example, because of their exposure to the American culture, a third-generation Chinese American family might have very different values and beliefs from those of a traditional Chinese family who has recently immigrated to America. For this reason, the nurse needs to supplement a general knowledge of cultural values and practices with a complete assessment of the individual's values and practices. The Developing Cultural Competence box summarizes the key actions a nurse can take to become more culturally aware.

DEVELOPING CULTURAL COMPETENCE

Providing Culturally Sensitive Care

Nurses who are interacting with expectant families from a different culture or ethnic group can provide more effective, culturally sensitive nursing care by:

- Critically examining their own cultural beliefs.
- Identifying personal biases, attitudes, stereotypes, and prejudices.
- Making a conscious commitment to respect and study the values and beliefs of others.
- Using sensitive, current language when describing others' cultures.
- Learning the rituals, customs, and practices of the major cultural and ethnic groups with whom they have contact.
- Including cultural assessment and assessment of the family's expectations of the healthcare system as a routine part of prenatal nursing care.
- Incorporating the family's cultural and spiritual practices into prenatal care as much as possible.
- Fostering an attitude of respect for and cooperation with alternative healers and caregivers whenever possible.
- Providing for the services of an interpreter if language barriers exist.
- Learning the language (or at least several key phrases) of at least one of the cultural groups with whom they interact.
- Recognizing that ultimately it is the woman's right to make her own healthcare choices.
- Evaluating whether the patient's healthcare beliefs have any potential negative consequences for her health.

Cultural assessment is an important aspect of prenatal care (see Figure 2-8 ∞ on page 38). Healthcare professionals are becoming increasingly aware of the importance of addressing cultural, physiologic, and psychologic needs in the prenatal assessment in order to provide culture-specific health care during pregnancy. The nurse needs to identify the main beliefs, values, and behaviors that relate to pregnancy and childbearing. This includes information about ethnic background, amount of affiliation with the ethnic group, patterns of decision making, religious preferences, language, communication style, and common etiquette practices. The nurse can also explore the woman's (or family's) expectations of the healthcare system. Once this information is gathered, the nurse can then plan and provide care that is appropriate and responsive to the family's needs. These topics are discussed in detail in chapter 2 ∞.

FOCUS YOUR STUDY

- Virtually all systems of a woman's body are altered in some way during pregnancy. Blood pressure decreases slightly during pregnancy. It reaches its lowest point in the second trimester and gradually increases to near normal levels in the third trimester. The enlarging uterus may exert pressure on the vena cava when the woman lies supine, causing a drop in blood pressure. This is called the vena caval syndrome or supine hypotension.
- A physiologic anemia may occur during pregnancy because the total plasma volume increases more than the total number of erythrocytes. This produces a drop in the hematocrit.
- The glomerular filtration rate increases during pregnancy. Glycosuria may be caused by the body's inability to reabsorb all the glucose filtered by the glomeruli.
- Changes in the skin include the development of chloasma; linea nigra; darkened nipples, areolae, and vulva; striae; and spider nevi.
- Insulin needs increase during pregnancy. A woman with a latent deficiency state may respond to the increased stress on the islets of Langerhans by developing gestational diabetes mellitus.
- The subjective (presumptive) signs of pregnancy are those symptoms experienced and reported by the woman, such as amenorrhea, nausea and vomiting, fatigue, urinary frequency, breast changes, and quickening.
- The objective (probable) signs of pregnancy can be perceived by the examiner but may be caused by conditions other than pregnancy.
- The diagnostic (positive) signs of pregnancy can be perceived by the examiner and can be caused only by pregnancy.
- During pregnancy the expectant woman may experience ambivalence, acceptance, introversion, emotional lability, and changes in body image.
- Rubin (1984) identified four developmental tasks for the pregnant woman: (1) ensuring safe passage through pregnancy, labor, and birth; (2) seeking acceptance of this child by others; (3) seeking commitment and acceptance of self as mother to the infant; and (4) learning to give of oneself on behalf of one's child.
- Fathers also face a series of adjustments as they accept their new role.
- Siblings of all ages require assistance in dealing with the birth of a new baby.
- Cultural values, beliefs, and behaviors influence a couple's response to childbearing and the healthcare system.
- A cultural assessment should focus on factors that will influence the practices of the childbearing family with regard to their health needs.

CRITICAL THINKING IN ACTION

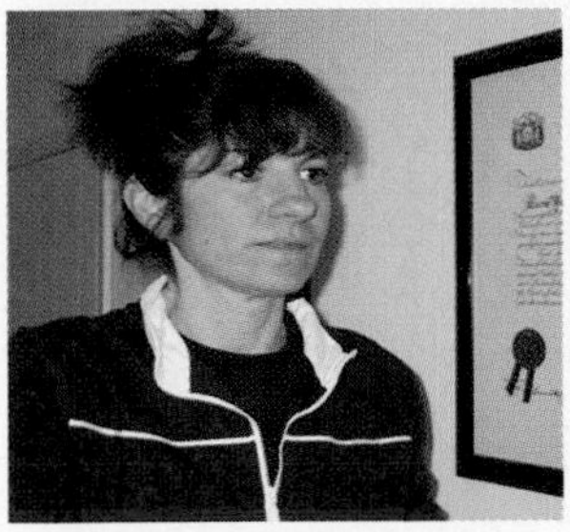
Source: George Dodson/Pearson Education.

Twenty-two-year-old Jean Simmons is an aerobics instructor, G0, P0000 in her first trimester of pregnancy. She presents to you at the local clinic complaining of frequent nausea, urinary frequency, and fatigue. You obtain her vital signs as: BP 108/60, temperature 97° F, pulse 68, respirations 12, weight 125 lb, height 64 inches. Her urine tests negative for ketones, albumin, leukocytes, and sugar. You note that Jean has lost 3 lb since her last visit. You assist the certified nurse-midwife with a physical exam, the findings of which are essentially normal. Jean says that while she knows it could become an issue, she would like to continue working as an aerobic instructor for as long as she possibly can during the pregnancy. You identify Jean's complaints as normal discomforts of pregnancy, and proceed with prenatal education.

1. What advice would you suggest to cope with the nausea of pregnancy?
2. What advice might you suggest to cope with urinary frequency?
3. What teaching would be important relating to exercise in pregnancy?
4. What symptoms related to exercise should Jean report to her physician?

See www.nursing.pearsonhighered.com for possible responses.

REFERENCES

American Academy of Pediatrics (AAP). (2005, Reaffirmed 2009). Policy statement: The changing concept of sudden infant death syndrome: Diagnostic coding shifts, controversies regarding the sleeping environment, and new variables to consider in reducing risk. *Pediatrics, 116*(5), 1245–1255.

Buster, J. E., & Carson, S. A. (2002). Endocrinology and diagnosis of pregnancy. In S. G. Gabbe, J. R. Niebyl, & J. L. Simpson (Eds.), *Obstetrics: Normal and problem pregnancies* (4th ed.). New York, NY: Churchill Livingstone.

Cole, A. C., & Ladner, D. G. (2009). Background hCG in non-pregnant individuals: Need for more sensitive point-of-care and over-the-counter pregnancy tests. *Clinical Biochemistry, 42*, 168–175.

Cunningham, F. G., Leveno, K. J., Bloom, S. L., Hauth, J. C., Rouse, D. J., & Spong, C. Y. (2010). *Williams obstetrics* (23rd ed.). New York, NY: McGraw-Hill.

Dean, R. A. K. (2010). Cultural competence: Nursing in a multicultural society. *Nursing for Women's Health, 14*(1), 51–60.

Deave, T., Johnson, D., & Ingram, J. (2008). Transition to parenthood: The needs of parents in pregnancy and early parenthood. *Pregnancy and Childbirth, 8*, 30–35.

Goodman, J. H. (2005). Becoming an involved father of an infant. *Journal of Obstetric, Gynecologic, & Neonatal Nursing, 34*(2), 190–200.

Gordon, M. C. (2007). Maternal physiology in pregnancy. In S. G. Gabbe, J. R. Niebyl, & J. L. Simpson (Eds.), *Obstetrics: Normal and problem pregnancies* (5th ed.). New York, NY: Churchill Livingstone.

Institute of Medicine (IOM). (2009). *Weight gain during pregnancy: Reexamining the guidelines.* Washington, DC: National Academies Press.

Lederman, R. P., & Weis, K. (2009). *Psychosocial adaptation to pregnancy* (3rd ed.). New York, NY: Springer.

Mercer, R. T. (2004). Becoming a mother versus maternal role attainment. *Journal of Nursing Scholarship, 36*(3), 226–232.

Messer, L. C., Dole, N., Kaufman, J. S., & Savitz, D. A. (2005). Pregnancy intendedness, maternal psychosocial factors and preterm birth. *Maternal and Child Health Journal, 9*(4), 403–412.

O'Leary, J., & Thorwick, C. (2006). Fathers' perspectives during pregnancy, postperinatal loss. *Journal of Obstetric, Gynecologic, & Neonatal Nursing, 35*(1), 78–86.

Rubin, R. (1984). *Maternal identity and the maternal experience.* New York, NY: Springer.

Schoppe-Sullivan, S. J., Brown, G. L., Cannon, E. A., Mangelsdorf, S. C., & Sokolowski, M. S. (2008). Maternal gatekeeping, coparenting quality, and fathering behavior in families with infants. *Journal of Family Psychology, 22*(3), 389–398.

Spector, R. E. (2009). *Cultural diversity in health and illness* (7th ed.). Upper Saddle River, NJ: Pearson/Prentice Hall.

Wallace, L. S., Zite, N. B., & Homewood, V. J. (2009) Making sense of home pregnancy test instructions. *Journal of Women's Health, 13*(3), 363–368.

15 CHAPTER

Antepartum Nursing Assessment

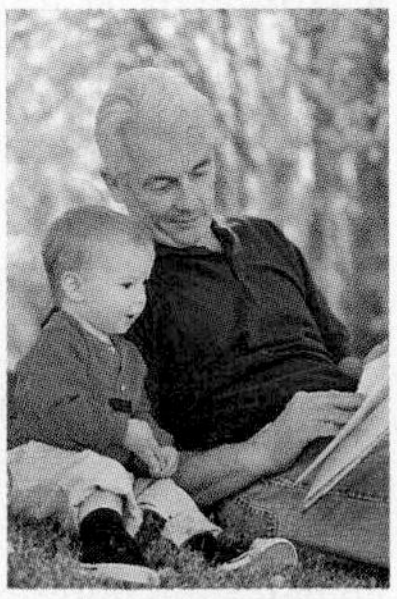

The father of the late 1950s . . . Main objective: Get your wife to the hospital on time. Check her in and find the father's waiting lounge. You won't be needed until the baby is born. Fathers are really useless at this time. Try not to be nervous. Coffee is available. Lots of coffee.

More coffee, pacing, no sleep, waiting for word. What a drain on the father. . . . The baby finally comes. "It's a beautiful, healthy baby girl. Mother and baby are doing fine. You can see them now, but only for 5 minutes." What a relief. The pressure is finally off. Isn't nature wonderful?

Today's father, my grandson. Attends most of the prenatal visits. Schooled in Lamaze. Drives his wife to the hospital. Coaches her through her labor. Helps her push. His digital camera is ready. The baby is born. He cuts the cord. He sends e-mail & pictures of the baby to everyone. Isn't nature wonderful?

—The father of one of the book authors

LEARNING OUTCOMES

1. Summarize the essential components of a prenatal history.
2. Define common obstetric terminology found in the history of maternity patients.
3. Identify factors related to the father's health that should be recorded on the prenatal record.
4. Describe the normal physiologic changes one would expect to find when performing a physical assessment on a pregnant woman.
5. Explain the use of Nägele's rule to determine the estimated date of birth.
6. Develop an outline of the essential measurements that can be determined by clinical pelvimetry.
7. Describe areas that should be evaluated as part of the initial assessment of psychosocial factors related to a woman's pregnancy.
8. Relate the danger signs of pregnancy to their possible causes.

KEY TERMS

Abortion *318*
Antepartum *318*
Diagonal conjugate *332*
Estimated date of birth (EDB) *323*
Gestation *318*
Gravida *318*
Intrapartum *318*
Multigravida *318*
Multipara *318*
Nägele's rule *329*
Nulligravida *318*
Nullipara *318*
Obstetric conjugate *332*
Para *318*
Postpartum *318*
Postterm labor *318*
Preterm or premature labor *318*
Primigravida *318*
Primipara *318*
Risk factors *320*
Stillbirth *318*
Term *318*

Today nurses are assuming a more important role in prenatal care, particularly in the area of assessment. The certified nurse-midwife has the education and skill to perform in-depth prenatal assessments with the opportunity to care for women during labor, birth, and the postpartum period. The nurse practitioner may also share the assessment responsibilities of women during their prenatal care. The primary roles of a nurse in an office or prenatal clinic are to counsel, educate, and meet the psychologic needs of the expectant family and perform other nursing care functions and assessments.

The nurse needs to establish an environment of comfort and open communication at each prenatal visit, conveying concern for the woman as an individual and being available to listen to and discuss the woman's concerns and needs. A supportive atmosphere coupled with the information found in the prenatal assessment guides in this chapter will enable the nurse to identify needed areas of education and counseling for each individual patient.

Initial Patient History

The course of a pregnancy depends on a number of factors, including the past pregnancy history (if this is not a first pregnancy), prepregnancy health of the woman, presence of disease/illness states, emotional status, and past health care. Ideally, antenatal care is a continuation of established care that the woman has been receiving to ensure a status of health outside of pregnancy. For some women, however, this may be the only health care that they have received in many years. One important method of determining the adequacy of a woman's prepregnancy care is by completing a thorough history.

Definition of Terms

The following terms are used in recording the obstetric history of maternity patients:

- **Antepartum:** Time between conception and onset of labor, usually used to describe the period during which a woman is pregnant; used interchangeably with *prenatal.*
- **Intrapartum:** Time from onset of labor until the birth of the infant and placenta.
- **Postpartum:** Time from birth until the woman's body returns to an essentially prepregnant condition.
- **Gestation:** The number of weeks since the first day of the last menstrual period (LMP).
- **Abortion:** Birth that occurs before 20 weeks' gestation or the birth of a fetus-newborn who weighs less than 500 g (Cunningham et al., 2010).
- **Term:** The normal duration of pregnancy (38 to 42 weeks' gestation).
- **Preterm or premature labor:** Labor that occurs after 20 weeks but before the completion of 37 weeks of gestation.
- **Postterm labor:** Labor that occurs after 42 weeks of gestation.
- **Gravida:** Any pregnancy, regardless of duration, including present pregnancy.
- **Nulligravida:** A woman who has never been pregnant.
- **Primigravida:** A woman who is pregnant for the first time.
- **Multigravida:** A woman who is in her second or any subsequent pregnancy.
- **Para:** Birth after 20 weeks' gestation, regardless of whether the infant is born alive or dead.
- **Nullipara:** A woman who has not given birth at more than 20 weeks' gestation.
- **Primipara:** A woman who has had one birth at more than 20 weeks' gestation, regardless of whether the infant is born alive or dead.
- **Multipara:** A woman who has had two or more births at more than 20 weeks' gestation.
- **Stillbirth:** A fetus born dead after 20 weeks' gestation.

The terms *gravida* and *para* refer to pregnancies, not to the fetus. Thus, traditionally, twins, triplets, and other multiple fetuses are counted as one pregnancy and one birth. This approach is confusing because it fails to identify the number of children a woman may actually have. Consequently, to provide more comprehensive data, a detailed approach is now used by many healthcare team members. Using this detailed system, *gravida* keeps the same meaning but the use of *para* changes because the detailed system counts *each infant born* rather than the number of pregnancies carried to viability (Varney, Kriebs, & Gegor, 2004). Thus in the traditional approach, twins would count as *one* pregnancy and *one* birth. In the detailed system, twins count as *one* pregnancy but *two* babies. A useful acronym for remembering the system is TPAL.

T: number of *term* infants born (number of infants born at the completion of 37 weeks' gestation or beyond)

P: number of *preterm* infants born (number of infants born after 20 weeks' but before the completion of 37 weeks' gestation, whether living or stillborn)

A: number of pregnancies ending in either spontaneous or therapeutic *abortion*

L: number of currently *living* children to whom the woman has given birth

The following examples delineate the differences between the two systems.

1. Jean Sanchez has one child born at 38 weeks' gestation and became pregnant for a second time. The second pregnancy ended in a miscarriage at 15 weeks' gestation. Using the *traditional approach* her obstetric history would be recorded as "gravida 2 para 1 ab 1." Using the *detailed approach,* her obstetric history would be recorded as "gravida 2 para 1011."
2. Tracy Hopkins is pregnant for the fourth time. At home she has a child who was born at term. Her second pregnancy ended at 10 weeks' gestation. She then gave birth to twins at 35 weeks. One of the twins died soon after birth. Using the *traditional approach* her obstetric history would be recorded as gravida 4 para 2 ab 1. Using the *detailed approach* her obstetric history would be recorded as "gravida 4 para 1212."

Occasionally a fifth digit is added to indicate the number of pregnancies that ended in multiple births (Varney et al., 2004). Thus, using the five-digit system, Tracy Hopkins would be gravida 4 para 12121. Some practice settings seem to have adopted variations of these two approaches. Consequently, to avoid confusion, it is best for practicing nurses to clarify the recording system used at their facilities (Figure 15-1 ■).

Name	Gravida	Term	Preterm	Abortions	Living Children
Jean Sanchez	2	1	0	1	1
Tracy Hopkins	4	1	2	1	2

Figure 15-1 ■ The TPAL approach provides more detailed information about the woman's pregnancy history.

Patient Profile

The patient's history is a screening tool that identifies factors that can affect the course of a pregnancy. For optimal prenatal care, the nurse should obtain the following information for each maternity patient at the initial prenatal assessment:

1. ***Current pregnancy***
   - First day of last normal menstrual period (LMP). Is this a sure date or uncertain? Within days? Does she know the last month of menses? Do her cycles normally occur every 28 days, or do her cycles tend to be longer or shorter? Does she have monthly menses? Was the LMP normal in duration and bleeding? Was she using any form of contraception?
   - Presence of cramping, bleeding, or spotting since LMP.
   - Woman's opinion about time when conception occurred and when infant is due? Was she charting her cycles?
   - Woman's attitude toward pregnancy. (Is pregnancy planned or unplanned? Wanted?)
   - Date of positive pregnancy test; date of negative pregnancy test.
   - Any pregnancy discomforts since LMP, such as nausea, vomiting, urinary frequency, fatigue, breast tenderness, constipation, fever, headaches.
2. ***Past pregnancies***
   - Number of pregnancies.
   - Number of abortions, spontaneous or therapeutic.
   - Number of living children.
   - History of previous pregnancies: length of pregnancy, length of labor and birth, type of birth (vaginal, forceps or vacuum-assisted birth, cesarean), location of birth, type of anesthesia/medication used (if any), woman's perception of the experience, complications (antepartal, intrapartal, postpartal).
   - Neonatal status of previous children: Apgar scores, birth weights, general development, complications, feeding method (breast, formula, or both). If breastfed, how long?
   - Loss of a child (miscarriage, elective or medically indicated abortion, stillbirth, neonatal death, relinquishment, death after the neonatal period). Cause of loss? What was the experience like for her? What coping skills helped? How did her partner, if involved, respond?
   - Blood type and Rh factor. (If Rh negative, was Rh immune globulin received after birth/miscarriage/abortion?)
   - Prenatal education classes, resources (books, Web sites).
3. ***Gynecologic history***
   - Date of last Pap smear; result? History of abnormal Pap results? Colposcopy? Loop electrosurgical excision procedure (LEEP)? Human papilloma virus (HPV)?
   - Previous infections: vaginal, cervical, pelvic inflammatory disease (PID), sexually transmitted.
   - Previous surgery (uterine, ovarian).
   - Age of menarche.
   - Regularity, frequency, and duration of menstrual flow.
   - History of dysmenorrhea.
   - History of infertility.
   - Sexual history.
   - Contraceptive history. (If hormonal method was used, did pregnancy immediately follow cessation of method? If not, how long after? When was contraception last used?)
4. ***Current medical history***
   - Weight (prepregnancy and current), height, body mass index (BMI) (determine recommended weight gain).
   - Blood type and Rh factor.
   - General health, including nutrition (dietary practices or problems such as vegetarianism, lactose intolerance, food allergies), regular exercise program (type, frequency, duration), monthly breast exams, eye exam, dental exam.
   - Any medication use (nonprescription, homeopathic, or herbal medications); medications taken since LMP?
   - Previous or present use of alcohol, tobacco, or caffeine (if yes, ask about amounts consumed each day); planning cessation?
   - Illicit drug use or abuse (specific drugs such as cocaine, crack, marijuana, methamphetamines); planning cessation?
   - Drug allergies, latex allergy or sensitivities: what type of reaction?
   - Potential teratogenic insults to this pregnancy, such as viral infections, medications, x-ray examinations, surgery, or cats in the home (source of toxoplasmosis).
   - Presence of chronic disease conditions, such as diabetes, hypertension, asthma, cardiovascular disease, renal problems, or thyroid disorders.
   - Infections or illnesses since LMP (flu, measles).
   - Record of immunizations (especially rubella); up to date?
   - Presence of any abnormal signs/symptoms.
5. ***Past medical history***
   - Childhood diseases (varicella).
   - Past treatment for any disease condition. Any hospitalizations? Major accidents?
   - Surgical procedures.
   - Presence of bleeding disorders or tendencies.
   - Blood transfusion history? Will she accept blood transfusion?
6. ***Family medical history***
   - Presence of diabetes, cardiovascular disease, hypertension, hematologic disorders, tuberculosis, thyroid disease.
   - Occurrence of multiple births.
   - History of congenital diseases or deformities.
   - History of mental illness.
   - Occurrence of cesarean births and cause, if known.
   - Cause of death of deceased parents or siblings.

7. *Genetic history (patient, father of child [FOC], and both families)*
   - Birth defects.
   - Recurrent pregnancy loss.
   - Stillbirth.
   - Down syndrome, mental retardation, developmental delay, chromosomal abnormalities.
   - Ethnic background (Mediterranean decent, Jewish, Asian).
   - Genetic disorders (cystic fibrosis, sickle cell disease/trait, muscular dystrophy).
8. *Religious/cultural history*
   - Does the woman wish to specify a religious preference on her chart? Does she have any spiritual beliefs or practices that might influence her health care or that of her child, such as prohibition against receiving blood products, dietary considerations, or other practices?
   - What practices are important to maintain her spiritual well-being?
   - Are there practices in her culture or that of her partner that might influence her care or that of her child?
9. *Occupational history*
   - Occupation.
   - Physical demands. (Does she stand all day, or are there opportunities to sit and elevate her legs? Does she do any heavy lifting?)
   - Exposure to lead, chemicals, or other harmful substances.
   - Opportunity for regular meals and breaks for nutritious snacks.
   - Provision for maternity or family leave.
10. *History of the FOC*
    - Presence of genetic conditions or diseases in him or in his family history.
    - Age.
    - Significant health problems.
    - Previous or present alcohol intake, drug use, or tobacco use.
    - Blood type and Rh factor.
    - Occupation.
    - Educational level; methods by which he learns best.
    - Thoughts/feelings regarding pregnancy.
11. *Personal information about the woman (social history)*
    - Age.
    - Relationship status (married? partner involved?).
    - Educational level; methods by which she learns best.
    - Race or ethnic group (to identify need for prenatal genetic screening or counseling).
    - Housing; stability of living conditions.
    - Economic level.
    - Any history of emotional or physical deprivation or abuse of herself or children. (Does she experience any abuse in her current relationship? Has she been hit, slapped, kicked, or hurt within the past year or since she has been pregnant? Is she afraid of her partner or anyone else? If yes, of whom is she afraid?)
    - History of emotional/mental health disorder (depression in general, postpartum depression, anxiety).
    - Support systems available to her.
    - Overuse or underuse of healthcare system.
    - Personal preferences about the birth (expectations of both the woman and her partner, presence of others, and so on). (See chapter 13 ∞.)
    - Plans for care of child following birth.
    - Feeding method for the baby (breast milk, formula, or both).

Obtaining Data

In many settings, nurses use standardized questionnaires to obtain the necessary data for the initial prenatal visit. The questionnaire developed by the American College of Obstetricians and Gynecologists (ACOG), for example, is commonly used in many clinical settings. The woman should fill out the questionnaire in a quiet place with a minimum of distractions and be provided ample time to complete all questions.

The nurse can review the questionnaire and obtain further information in a direct interview with the patient. This allows the pregnant woman to expand or clarify her responses to questions and allows the nurse to gather additional information or clarify data provided. The initial interview provides the nurse and the woman the opportunity to begin developing a healthy relationship. The expectant partner should be encouraged to attend the initial and subsequent prenatal visits. He or she is often able to contribute information to the history and may use this opportunity to ask questions and express concerns that may be of particular importance to him or her.

> “I didn't know what to expect when I went for my first prenatal visit. I'm clean now and wanted to be honest, but I was afraid they would yell if I told them about some of the really dumb things I did in high school—the drinking, the marijuana, the sex and stuff. I really liked the nurse-midwife who was taking care of me, so I decided to be straight with her—for the baby's sake, you know. She was great about everything and really made me feel okay.”

Prenatal Risk-Factor Screening

A highly significant part of the prenatal assessment is screening for risk factors. **Risk factors** are any findings that have been shown to have a negative effect on pregnancy outcomes either for the woman or her unborn child. Many risk factors can be identified during the initial prenatal assessment, while others may be detected during subsequent visits through subjective and objective data collection. Identification of risk factors allows for education to promote change and to initiate interventions to reduce risk and avoid poor outcomes (Jordan & Murphy, 2009).

All risk factors do not threaten the pregnancy to the same degree. The nurse needs to be aware of potential risk factors and the impact that they might have on the pregnancy. It is possible that a pregnancy may begin as low risk and change to high risk because of current or developed risk factors. Risk is also assessed intrapartally and postpartally. Ideally, the initial risk assessment should occur prior to pregnancy when changes can be made to decrease risks during pregnancy.

Table 15-1 identifies the major prenatal risk factors currently recognized. The table describes potential maternal and fetal/neonatal implications should the risk be present in the pregnancy. In addition to the factors listed, the perinatal health team also needs to evaluate psychosocial factors, including ethnic background; occupation; education; financial status; environment, including living arrangements and location; and the woman's and her family's concept of health, which might influence her attitude toward seeking health care. Women's health status and risk is continually evaluated at every healthcare team encounter.

TABLE 15-1 Prenatal High-Risk Factors

FACTOR	MATERNAL IMPLICATIONS	FETAL/NEONATAL IMPLICATIONS
Social-Personal		
Low income level/or low educational level	Insufficient antenatal care or late antenatal care ↑ risk preterm birth Poor nutrition ↑ risk of preeclampsia	Low birth weight Prematurity Intrauterine growth restriction (IUGR)/small for gestational age (SGA)
Poor diet	↑ Inadequate nutrition/inadequate Poor weight gain ↑ risk preterm labor/birth ↑ risk anemia ↑ risk preeclampsia	Fetal malnutrition Prematurity IUGR/SGA
Living at high altitude	↑ hemoglobin	Prematurity IUGR ↑ hemoglobin (polycythemia)
Multiparity greater than 3	↑ risk antepartum or postpartum hemorrhage	Anemia Fetal death
Weight less than 45.5 kg (100 lb)	Poor nutrition Cephalopelvic disproportion Prolonged labor	IUGR Hypoxia associated with difficult labor and birth
Weight greater than 91 kg (200 lb)	↑ risk hypertension ↑ risk cephalopelvic disproportion ↑ risk diabetes	↓ fetal nutrition/perfusion ↑ risk macrosomia
Age less than 16	Poor nutrition Insufficient/late antenatal care ↑ risk preeclampsia ↑ risk cephalopelvic disproportion	Low birth weight ↑ fetal demise
Age greater than 35	↑ risk preeclampsia ↑ risk cesarean birth Psychosocial issues	↑ risk congenital anomalies ↑ chromosomal abnormalities
Smoking one pack/day or more	↑ risk hypertension ↑ risk cancer	↓ placental perfusion → ↓ O_2 and nutrients available Low birth weight IUGR/SGA Preterm birth
Use of addicting drugs	↑ risk poor nutrition ↑ risk of infection with intravenous (IV) drugs ↑ risk HIV, hepatitis C ↑ risk abruptio placentae	↑ risk congenital anomalies ↑ risk low birth weight Neonatal withdrawal Lower serum bilirubin
Excessive alcohol consumption	↑ risk poor nutrition Possible hepatic effects with long-term consumption	↑ risk fetal alcohol syndrome (FAS)
Preexisting Medical Disorders		
Diabetes mellitus	↑ risk preeclampsia, hypertension Episodes of hypoglycemia and hyperglycemia ↑ risk cesarean birth	Low birth weight Macrosomia Neonatal hypoglycemia ↑ risk congenital anomalies ↑ risk respiratory distress syndrome
Cardiac disease	Cardiac decompensation Further strain on mother's body ↑ maternal death rate	↑ risk fetal demise ↑ perinatal mortality
Anemia: hemoglobin less than 11 g/dl less than 32% hematocrit	Iron deficiency anemia Low energy level Decreased oxygen-carrying capacity	Fetal death Prematurity Low birth weight
Hypertension	↑ vasospasm ↑ risk central nervous system (CNS) irritability ↑ risk convulsions ↑ risk cerebrovascular accident (CVA) ↑ risk renal damage	↓ placental perfusion → low birth weight Preterm birth

(continued)

TABLE 15-1 Prenatal High-Risk Factors continued

FACTOR	MATERNAL IMPLICATIONS	FETAL/NEONATAL IMPLICATIONS
Thyroid disorder Hypothyroidism Hyperthyroidism	↑ infertility ↓ basal metabolic rate (BMR), goiter, myxedema ↑ risk miscarriage ↑ risk preterm labor/birth ↑ risk preeclampsia ↑ risk postpartum hemorrhage ↑ risk preeclampsia Danger of thyroid storm	↑ spontaneous abortion ↑ risk congenital goiter ↑ risk IUGR/SGA ↑ risk anemia ↑ risk stillbirth Mental retardation → cretinism ↑ incidence congenital anomalies ↑ IUGR/SGA ↑ neonatal hyperthyroidism
Renal disease (moderate to severe)	↑ risk renal failure	↑ risk IUGR/SGA ↑ risk preterm birth
Diethylstilbestrol (DES) exposure	↑ Infertility, spontaneous abortion ↑ cervical incompetence ↑ risk breech presentation	↑ risk preterm birth
Obstetric Considerations		
Previous Pregnancy		
Stillborn	↑ emotional/psychologic distress	↑ risk IUGR/SGA ↑ risk preterm birth
Habitual abortion	↑ emotional/psychologic distress	↑ risk abortion
Cesarean birth	↑ possibility repeat cesarean birth Risk of uterine rupture	↑ risk preterm birth ↑ risk respiratory distress
Rh or blood group sensitization		Hydrops fetalis Icterus gravis Neonatal anemia Kernicterus Hypoglycemia
Current Pregnancy		
Large for gestational age (LGA)	↑ risk cesarean birth ↑ risk gestational diabetes ↑ risk operative birth	↑ risk birth injury Hypoglycemia
Gestational diabetes mellitus	↑ risk operative birth ↑ risk preeclampsia ↑ risk extensive lacerations ↑ risk primary pulmonary hypertension (PPH) ↑ risk shoulder dystocia	Macrosomia Hyperbilirubinemia ↑ risk birth injury
Rubella (first trimester)		Congenital heart disease Cataracts Nerve deafness Bone lesions Prolonged virus shedding
Rubella (second trimester)		Hepatitis Thrombocytopenia
Cytomegalovirus		IUGR Encephalopathy
Herpesvirus type 2	Severe discomfort Concern about possibility of cesarean birth, fetal infection	Neonatal herpesvirus type 2 Hepatitis with jaundice Neurologic abnormalities
Syphilis	↑ incidence abortion	↑ fetal demise Congenital syphilis
Urinary tract infection	↑ risk preterm labor Uterine irritability	↑ risk preterm birth
Abruptio placentae and placenta previa	↑ risk hemorrhage Bed rest Extended hospitalization	Fetal/neonatal anemia Intrauterine hemorrhage ↑ fetal demise
Preeclampsia/eclampsia	See hypertension	↓ placental perfusion → low birth weight
Multiple gestation	↑ risk postpartum hemorrhage ↑ risk gestational diabetes ↑ risk preeclampsia ↑ risk placenta previa	↑ risk preterm labor/birth ↑ risk stillbirth ↑ risk fetal demise ↑ risk IUGR/SGA ↑ risk malpresentation
Elevated hematocrit (greater than 41%)	Increased viscosity of blood	Fetal death rate 5 times normal rate
Spontaneous premature rupture of membranes	↑ risk uterine infection	Preterm birth Fetal demise

Initial Prenatal Assessment

The initial prenatal assessment focuses on the woman holistically by considering physical, cultural, and psychosocial factors that influence her health. During this visit she and her primary support person are also evaluating the health team that they have chosen. The establishment of the nurse-patient relationship will help the woman evaluate the health team and also provide the nurse with a basis for developing an atmosphere that is conducive to interviewing, support, and education. Because many women are excited and anxious at the first antepartal visit, the initial psychosocial-cultural assessment is of a general nature.

As part of the initial psychosocial-cultural assessment the nurse discusses with the woman any religious, cultural, or socioeconomic factors that may influence the woman's expectations of the childbearing experience. It is especially helpful if the nurse is familiar with common practices of various religious and cultural groups who reside in the community. Gathering the data in a tactful, caring way can help make the childbearing woman's experience a positive one and provides opportunity for a partnership in care to develop.

After the history is obtained, the nurse prepares the woman for the physical examination. The physical examination begins with assessment of vital signs followed by the head-to-toe examination with the pelvic examination completed last. It is important for the nurse or caregiver to provide anticipatory guidance and reassurance when completing the physical exam because this may be the patient's first gynecologic examination.

Before the examination, the woman should provide a clean urine specimen for screening. When her bladder is empty, the patient will be more comfortable during the pelvic examination, and the examiner can palpate the pelvic organs more easily. After the woman has emptied her bladder, the nurse asks her to disrobe and gives her a gown and sheet or some other protective covering to provide modesty, comfort, and warmth.

CLINICAL TIP

Use of Gloves

Gloves are worn for procedures that involve contact with body fluids such as drawing blood for laboratory work, handling urine specimens, and conducting pelvic examinations. Because of the increased incidence of latex allergies, it is becoming more common for latex-free gloves to be used. It is important to inquire about latex allergies with any patient before beginning the exam.

Thoroughness and a systematic procedure are the most important considerations when performing the physical portion of an antepartal examination (see Assessment Guide: Initial Prenatal Assessment). To promote completeness, the assessment guide is organized into three columns that address the areas to be assessed, the variations or alterations that may be observed, and nursing responses to the data. The nurse should be aware that certain organs and systems are assessed concurrently with other systems during the physical portion of the examination.

PROFESSIONALISM IN PRACTICE

Physical Exams and Scope of Practice

Increasing numbers of nurses, such as certified nurse-midwives and other advanced practice nurses are educationally prepared to perform physical examinations. The nurse who has not yet fully developed these specific assessment skills obtains the woman's vital signs, explains the procedures to allay apprehension, positions her for examination, and assists the examiner as necessary. Each nurse is responsible for operating at expected professional standards within his or her skill level, educational preparation, and knowledge base.

Initial Prenatal Assessment

DEVELOPING CULTURAL COMPETENCE

Using Cultural Information Effectively

During prenatal assessment, it is important for nurses to avoid stereotyping women based on race or ethnicity. However, race and ethnicity may provide valuable information about cultural, behavioral, environmental, and medical factors that might affect a pregnant woman's health (American College of Obstetricians and Gynecologists [ACOG], 2005a).

Nursing interventions based on assessment of the normal physical and psychosocial changes, as well as the cultural influences associated with pregnancy and patient teaching and counseling needs that have been mutually defined, are discussed further in chapter 16 ∞.

Determination of Due Date

Application: Ovulation Calculator

Childbearing families are generally eager to know the "due date," or the date around which childbirth will occur. Determination of the due date should be attempted at the initial visit. Historically, the due date has been called the *estimated date of confinement (EDC)*. The concept of confinement is rather negative, however, and there is a trend among caregivers to avoid it by referring to the birth date as the *estimated date of delivery (EDD)*. Childbirth educators often stress that babies are not "delivered" like a package but rather they are *born* or *birthed by the mother*. In keeping with a view that emphasizes the normality of the process, we have chosen to refer to the due date as the **estimated date of birth (EDB)** throughout this text.

It is crucial to know the first day of the woman's LMP when calculating the EDB. The LMP is sometimes not known because some women have episodes of irregular bleeding or amenorrhea or they may fail to keep track of their menstrual cycles. Thus there are other techniques to help determine how far along a woman is in her pregnancy or how many weeks' gestation she is. Other techniques that can be used include evaluating uterine size, establishing when quickening occurs (or occurred), using early ultrasound (US), and auscultating the fetal heart rate. An early ultrasound should be obtained if a precise LMP is not available to help establish an accurate EDB. See Research Evidence in Practice.

ASSESSMENT GUIDE Initial Prenatal Assessment

Physical Assessment/Normal Findings	Alterations and Possible Causes*	Nursing Responses to Data†
VITAL SIGNS		
Blood Pressure (BP): Less than or equal to 135/85 mmHg	High BP (essential hypertension; renal disease; pregestational hypertension, apprehension or anxiety, preeclampsia if initial assessment not done until after 20 weeks' gestation)	BP greater than 140/90 requires immediate consideration; establish woman's BP; refer to healthcare provider if necessary. Assess woman's knowledge about high BP; counsel on self-care and medical management.
Pulse: 60–90 beats/min; rate may increase10 beats/min during pregnancy	Increased pulse rate (excitement or anxiety, dehydration, infection, cardiac disorders)	Count for 1 full minute; note irregularities. Evaluate temperature, increase fluids.
Respirations: 12–22 breaths/min (or pulse rate divided by 4); pregnancy may induce a degree of hyperventilation; thoracic breathing predominant	Marked tachypnea or abnormal patterns	Assess for respiratory disease.
Temperature: 36.2°–37.6°C (97°–99.6°F)	Elevated temperature (infection)	Assess for infection process or disease state if temperature is elevated; refer to healthcare provider.
HEIGHT AND WEIGHT		
Depends on body build	Weight less than 45 kg (100 lb) or greater than 91 kg (200 lb); rapid, sudden weight gain (preeclampsia)	Evaluate need for nutritional counseling; obtain information on eating habits, cooking practices, food regularly eaten, income limitations, need for food supplements, food allergies, pica and other abnormal food habits. Note initial weight to establish baseline for weight gain throughout pregnancy. Determine body mass index (BMI) and recommended weight gain for pregnancy.
SKIN		
Color: Consistent with racial background; pink nail beds	Pallor (anemia); bronze, yellow (hepatic disease; other causes of jaundice)	Tests to perform: complete blood count (CBC), bilirubin level, urinalysis, and blood urea nitrogen (BUN).
	Bluish, reddish, mottled; dusky appearance or pallor of palms and nail beds in dark-skinned women (anemia)	If abnormal, refer to healthcare provider.
Condition: Absence of edema (slight edema of lower extremities is normal during pregnancy)	Edema (preeclampsia, normal pregnancy changes); rashes, dermatitis (allergic response)	Counsel on relief measures for slight edema. Initiate preeclampsia assessment; refer to healthcare provider.
Lesions: Absence of lesions	Ulceration (varicose veins, decreased circulation)	Further assess circulatory status; refer to healthcare provider if lesion is severe.
Spider nevi common in pregnancy	Petechiae, multiple bruises, ecchymosis (hemorrhagic disorders; abuse)	Evaluate for bleeding or clotting disorder. Provide opportunities to discuss abuse if suspected.
	Change in size or color (carcinoma)	Refer to healthcare provider.
Moles		
Pigmentation: Pigmentation changes of pregnancy include linea nigra, striae gravidarum, melasma		Assure woman that these are normal manifestations of pregnancy and explain the physiologic basis for the changes.
Café-au-lait spots	Six or more (Albright syndrome or neurofibromatosis)	Consult with healthcare provider.
NOSE		
Character of Mucosa: Redder than oral mucosa; in pregnancy nasal mucosa is edematous in response to increased estrogen, resulting in nasal stuffiness (rhinitis of pregnancy) and nosebleeds	Olfactory loss (first cranial nerve deficit)	Counsel woman about possible relief measures for nasal stuffiness and nosebleeds (epistaxis); refer to healthcare provider for olfactory loss.
MOUTH		
May note hypertrophy of gingival tissue because of estrogen	Edema, inflammation (infection); pale in color (anemia)	Assess hematocrit for anemia; counsel regarding dental hygiene habits. Refer to healthcare provider or dentist if necessary. Routine dental care appropriate during pregnancy.
NECK		
Nodes: Small, mobile, nontender nodes	Tender, hard, fixed, or prominent nodes (infection, carcinoma)	Examine for local infection; refer to healthcare provider.
Thyroid: Small, smooth, lateral lobes palpable on either side of trachea; slight hyperplasia by third month of pregnancy	Enlargement or nodule tenderness (hyperthyroidism)	Test to perform: thyroid-stimulating hormone (TSH). Listen over thyroid for bruits, which may indicate hyperthyroidism. Question woman about dietary habits (iodine intake). Ascertain history of thyroid problems; refer to healthcare provider.
	*Possible causes of alterations are identified in parentheses.	†This column provides guidelines for further assessment and initial intervention.

ASSESSMENT GUIDE Initial Prenatal Assessment continued

Physical Assessment/Normal Findings	Alterations and Possible Causes*	Nursing Responses to Data†
CHEST AND LUNGS		
Chest: Symmetric, elliptic, smaller anteroposterior (AP) than transverse diameter	Increased AP diameter, funnel chest, pigeon chest (emphysema, asthma, chronic obstructive pulmonary disease [COPD])	Evaluate for emphysema, asthma, pulmonary disease (COPD).
Ribs: Slope downward from nipple line	More horizontal (COPD)	Evaluate for COPD. Evaluate for fractures.
	Angular bumps	Consult healthcare provider.
	Rachitic rosary (vitamin C deficiency)	Consult nutritionist.
Inspection and Palpation: No retraction or bulging of intercostal spaces (ICS) during inspiration or expiration; symmetric expansion	ICS retractions with inspirations, bulging with expiration; unequal expansion (respiratory disease)	Do thorough initial assessment. Refer to healthcare provider.
Tactile fremitus	Tachypnea, hyperpnea, Cheyne-Stokes respirations (respiratory disease)	Refer to healthcare provider.
Percussion: Bilateral symmetry in tone	Flatness of percussion, which may be affected by chest wall thickness	Evaluate for pleural effusions, consolidations, or tumor.
Low-pitched resonance of moderate intensity	High diaphragm (atelectasis or paralysis), pleural effusion	Refer to healthcare provider.
Auscultation: Upper lobes—bronchovesicular sounds above sternum and scapulas; equal expiratory and inspiratory phases	Abnormal if heard over any other area of chest	Refer to healthcare provider.
Remainder of Chest: Vesicular breath sounds heard; inspiratory phase longer (3:1)	Rales, rhonchi, wheezes; pleural friction rub; absence of breath sounds; bronchophony, egophony, whispered pectoriloquy	Refer to healthcare provider.
BREASTS		
Supple: Symmetric in size and contour; darker pigmentation of nipple and areola; may have supernumerary nipples, usually 5–6 cm below normal nipple line	"Pigskin" or orange-peel appearance, nipple retractions, swelling, hardness (carcinoma); redness, heat, tenderness, cracked or fissured nipple (infection)	Encourage monthly self-examination; instruct woman how to examine her own breasts (see chapter 7 ∞).
Axillary nodes nonpalpable or pellet sized	Tenderness, enlargement, hard node (carcinoma); may be visible bump (infection)	Refer to healthcare provider for evaluation of abnormal breast findings. Plan ultrasound/mammogram/ magnetic resonance imaging (MRI) of breasts.
Pregnancy Changes: 1. Size increase noted primarily in first 20 weeks. 2. Become nodular. 3. Tingling sensation may be felt during first and third trimester; woman may report feeling of heaviness. 4. Pigmentation of nipples and areolae darkens. 5. Superficial veins dilate and become more prominent. 6. Striae seen in multiparas. 7. Tubercles of Montgomery enlarge. 8. Colostrum may be present after 12th week. 9. Secondary areola appears at 20 weeks, characterized by series of washed-out spots surrounding primary areola. 10. Breasts less firm, old striae may be present in multiparas.		Discuss normalcy of changes and their meaning with the woman. Teach and/or institute appropriate relief measures. Encourage use of supportive, well-fitting brassiere.
HEART		
Normal rate, rhythm, and heart sounds	Enlargement, thrills, thrusts, gross irregularity or skipped beats, gallop rhythm or extra sounds (cardiac disease)	Complete an initial assessment. Explain normalcy pregnancy-induced changes. Refer to healthcare provider if indicated.
Pregnancy Changes: 1. Palpitations may occur due to sympathetic nervous system disturbance. 2. Short systolic murmurs that increase in held expiration are normal due to increased volume.		
ABDOMEN		
Normal appearance, skin texture, and hair distribution; liver nonpalpable; abdomen nontender	Muscle guarding (anxiety, acute tenderness); tenderness, mass (ectopic pregnancy, inflammation, carcinoma)	Assure woman of normalcy of diastasis. Provide initial information about appropriate prenatal and postpartum exercises. Evaluate woman's anxiety level. Refer to healthcare provider.
	*Possible causes of alterations are identified in parentheses.	†This column provides guidelines for further assessment and initial intervention.

(continued)

ASSESSMENT GUIDE Initial Prenatal Assessment continued

Physical Assessment/Normal Findings	Alterations and Possible Causes*	Nursing Responses to Data†
Pregnancy Changes:		
1. Purple striae may be present (or silver striae on a multipara) as well as linea nigra.		
2. Diastasis of the rectus muscles late in pregnancy.		
3. Size: Flat or rotund abdomen; progressive enlargement of uterus due to pregnancy. 10–12 weeks: Fundus slightly above symphysis pubis. 16 weeks: Fundus halfway between symphysis and umbilicus. 20–22 weeks: Fundus at umbilicus. 28 weeks: Fundus three finger breadths above umbilicus. 36 weeks: Fundus just below ensiform cartilage.	Size of uterus inconsistent with length of gestation (intrauterine growth restriction [IUGR], multiple pregnancy, fetal demise, incorrect estimated date of birth (EDB), abnormal amniotic fluid, hydatidiform mole)	Reassess menstrual history regarding pregnancy dating. Evaluate increase in size using McDonald's method. Use ultrasound to establish diagnosis.
4. Fetal heart rate: 110–160 beats/min may be heard with Doppler at 10–12 weeks' gestation; may be heard with fetoscope at 17–20 weeks.	Failure to hear fetal heartbeat with Doppler (fetal demise, hydatidiform mole)	Refer to healthcare provider. Administer pregnancy tests. Use ultrasound to establish diagnosis.
5. Fetal movement palpable by a trained examiner after the 18th week.	Failure to feel fetal movements after 20 weeks' gestation (fetal demise, hydatidiform mole)	Refer to healthcare provider.
6. Ballottement: During fourth to fifth month fetus rises and then rebounds to original position when uterus is tapped sharply.	No ballottement (oligohydramnios)	Refer to healthcare provider.
EXTREMITIES		
Skin warm, pulses palpable, full range of motion; may be some edema of hands and ankles in late pregnancy; varicose veins may become more pronounced; palmar erythema may be present	Nonpalpable or diminished pulses (arterial insufficiency); marked edema (preeclampsia)	Evaluate for other symptoms of heart disease; initiate follow-up if woman mentions that her rings feel tight. Discuss prevention and self-treatment measures for varicose veins; refer to healthcare provider if indicated.
SPINE		
Normal Spinal Curves: Concave cervical, convex thoracic, concave lumbar	Abnormal spinal curves; flatness, kyphosis, lordosis	Refer to healthcare provider if indicated.
In pregnancy, lumbar spinal curve may be accentuated	Backache	May have implications for administration of spinal anesthetics; see chapter 25 for relief measures.
Shoulders and iliac crests should be even	Uneven shoulders and iliac crests (scoliosis)	Refer very young women to healthcare provider; discuss back-stretching exercise with older women.
REFLEXES		
Normal and symmetric	Hyperactivity, clonus (preeclampsia)	Evaluate for other symptoms of preeclampsia.
PELVIC AREA		
External Female Genitals: Normally formed with female hair distribution; in multiparas, labia majora loose and pigmented; urinary and vaginal orifices visible and appropriately located	Lesions, hematomas, varicosities, inflammation of Bartholin's glands; clitoral hypertrophy (masculinization)	Explain pelvic examination procedure. Encourage woman to minimize her discomfort by relaxing her hips. Provide privacy.
Vagina: Pink or dark pink, vaginal discharge odorless, nonirritating; in multiparas, vaginal folds smooth and flattened; may have episiotomy scar	Abnormal discharge associated with vaginal infections	Obtain vaginal smear. Provide understandable verbal and written instructions about treatment for woman and partner, if indicated.
Cervix: Pink color; os closed except in multiparas, in whom os admits fingertip	Eversion, reddish erosin, nabothian or retention cysts, cervical polyp; granular area that bleeds (carcinoma of cervix); lesions (herpes, human papilloma virus [HPV]); presence of string or plastic tip from cervix (intrauterine device [IUD] in uterus)	Provide woman with a hand mirror and identify genital structures for her; encourage her to view her cervix if she wishes. Refer to healthcare provider if indicated. Advise woman of potential serious risks of leaving an IUD in place during pregnancy; refer to healthcare provider for removal.
Pregnancy Changes:		
1–4 weeks' gestation: Enlargement in anteroposterior diameter		
4–6 weeks' gestation: Softening of cervix (Goodell's sign); softening of isthmus of uterus (Hegar's sign); cervix takes on bluish coloring (Chadwick's sign)	Absence of Goodell's sign (inflammatory conditions, carcinoma)	Refer to healthcare provider.
8–12 weeks' gestation: Vagina and cervix appear bluish violet in color (Chadwick's sign)		
Uterus: Pear shaped, mobile; smooth surface	Fixed (pelvic inflammatory disease [PID]); nodular surface (fibromas)	Refer to healthcare provider.
Ovaries: Small, walnut shaped, nontender (ovaries and fallopian tubes are located in the adnexal areas)	Pain on movement of cervix (PID); enlarged or nodular ovaries (cyst, tumor, tubal pregnancy, corpus luteum of pregnancy)	Evaluate adnexal areas; refer to healthcare provider. Plan ultrasound to evaluate mass.
	*Possible causes of alterations are identified in parentheses.	†This column provides guidelines for further assessment and initial intervention.

ASSESSMENT GUIDE Initial Prenatal Assessment continued

Physical Assessment/Normal Findings	Alterations and Possible Causes*	Nursing Responses to Data†
PELVIC MEASUREMENTS		
Internal Measurements:	Measurement below normal	Vaginal birth may not be possible if deviations are present.
1. Diagonal conjugate at least 11.5 cm (see Figure 15-6) 2. Obstetric conjugate estimated by subtracting 1.5–2 cm from diagonal conjugate	Disproportion of pubic arch	
3. Inclination of sacrum	Abnormal curvature of sacrum	
4. Motility of coccyx; external intertuberosity diameter greater than 8 cm	Fixed or malposition of coccyx	
ANUS AND RECTUM		
No lumps, rashes, excoriation, tenderness; cervix may be felt through rectal wall	Hemorrhoids, rectal prolapse; nodular lesion (carcinoma)	Counsel about appropriate prevention and relief measures; refer to healthcare provider for further evaluation.
LABORATORY EVALUATION		
Hemoglobin: 12–16 g/dl; women residing in areas of high altitude may have higher levels of hemoglobin	Less than 11 g/dl (anemia)	Hemoglobin less than 12 g/dl requires nutritional counseling; less than 11 g/dl requires iron supplementation.
ABO and Rh Typing: Normal distribution of blood types	Rh negative	If Rh negative, check for presence of anti-Rh antibodies. Check partner's blood type; if partner is Rh positive, discuss with woman the need for Rh immune globulin administration at 28 weeks, management during the intrapartal period, and possible need for Rh immune globulin after childbirth. (See chapter 20 ∞.)
Complete Blood Count (CBC)		
Hematocrit: 38%–47% physiologic anemia (pseudoanemia) may occur	Marked anemia or blood dyscrasias	Perform CBC and Schilling differential cell count.
Red Blood Cells (RBC): 4.2–5.4 million/microliter		
White Blood Cells (WBC): 5000–12,000/microliter	Presence of infection; may be elevated in pregnancy and with labor	Evaluate for other signs of infection.
Differential Neutrophils: 40%–60% Bands: up to 5% Eosinophils: 1%–3% Basophils: up to 1% Lymphocytes: 20%–40% Monocytes: 4%–8%		
Syphilis Tests: Serologic tests for syphilis (STS), complement fixation test, venereal disease research laboratory (VDRL) test—nonreactive	Positive reaction STS—tests may have 25%–45% incidence of biologic false-positive results; false results may occur in individuals who have acute viral or bacterial infections, hypersensitivity reactions, recent vaccinations, collagen disease, malaria, or tuberculosis	Positive results may be confirmed with the fluorescent treponemal antibody-absorption (FTA-ABS) test; all tests for syphilis give positive results in the secondary stage of the disease; antibiotic tests may cause negative test results. Refer to healthcare provider for treatment.
Gonorrhea Culture: Negative	Positive	Refer for treatment.
Urinalysis (u/a): Normal color, specific gravity; pH 4.6–8	Abnormal color (porphyria, hemoglobinuria, bilirubinemia): alkaline urine (metabolic alkalemia, *Proteus* infection, old specimen)	Repeat u/a; refer to healthcare provider.
Negative for protein, red blood cells, white blood cells, casts	Positive findings (contaminated specimen, kidney disease)	Repeat u/a; refer to healthcare provider.
Glucose: Negative (small degree of glycosuria may occur in pregnancy)	Glycosuria (low renal threshold for glucose, diabetes mellitus)	Assess blood glucose level; test urine for ketones.
Rubella Titer: Hemagglutination-inhibition (HAI) test–1:10 or above indicates woman is immune	HAI titer less than 1:10	Immunization will be given postpartum. Instruct woman whose titers are less than 1:10 to avoid children who have rubella. Educate regarding prevention measures and need for immunization after birth.
Hepatitis B Screen for hepatitis B surface antigen (HbsAg): negative	Positive	If positive, refer to physician. Infants born to women who test positive are given hepatitis B immune globulin soon after birth followed by first dose of hepatitis B vaccine.
HIV Screen: Offered to all women; encouraged for those at risk; negative	Positive	Refer to healthcare provider.
	*Possible causes of alterations are identified in parentheses.	†This column provides guidelines for further assessment and initial intervention.

(continued)

ASSESSMENT GUIDE **Initial Prenatal Assessment** continued

Physical Assessment/Normal Findings	Alterations and Possible Causes*	Nursing Responses to Data†
LABORATORY EVALUATION (continued)		
Illicit Drug Screen: Offered to all women; negative	Positive	Refer to healthcare provider.
Sickle-Cell Screen for Patients of African Descent: Negative	Positive; test results would include a description of cells	Refer to healthcare provider.
Pap Smear: Negative	Test results that show abnormal cells with negative or positive high-risk human papilloma virus (HPV).	Refer to healthcare provider. Discuss with the woman the meaning of the findings and the importance of follow-up. Plan colposcopy if indicated by results.
Cultural Assessment	**Variations to Consider***	**Nursing Responses to Data†**
Determine the woman's fluency in written and oral English.	Woman may be fluent in language other than English.	Work with a knowledgeable translator to provide information and answer questions.
How does she prefer to be addressed? Nickname?	Some women prefer informality; others prefer to use titles.	Address the woman according to her preference. Maintain formality in introducing oneself if that seems preferred.
Determine customs and practices regarding prenatal care:	Practices are influenced by individual preference, cultural expectations, or religious beliefs.	Honor a woman's practices and provide for specific preferences unless they are contraindicated because of safety.
• Are there certain practices she expects to follow when she is pregnant?	Some women believe that they should perform certain acts related to sleep, activity, or clothing.	Have information printed in the language of different cultural groups that live in the area.
• Are there any activities she cannot do while she is pregnant?	Some women have restrictions or taboos they follow related to work, activity, sexual, environmental, or emotional factors.	Respect the woman's food preferences, help her plan an adequate prenatal diet within the framework of her preferences, and refer to a dietitian if necessary.
• Are there certain foods she is expected to eat or avoid while she is pregnant? Determine whether she has lactose intolerance or food allergies.	Foods are an important cultural factor. Some women may have certain foods they must eat or avoid; many women have lactose intolerance and have difficulty consuming sufficient calcium.	
• Is the caregiver's gender of concern to her?	Some women are comfortable only with a female caregiver.	Arrange for a female caregiver if it is the woman's preference.
• What amount or type of partner involvement in her pregnancy does she expect or want? This includes her mother, other family members, and friends.	A woman may not want her partner involved in the pregnancy. For some the role falls to the woman's mother or a female relative or friend.	Respect the woman's preferences about her partner or husband's involvement; avoid imposing personal values or expectations.
• What type of support and counseling resources are available to her?	Some women seek advice from family members, *curanderas,* tribal healers, or religious leaders.	Respect and honor the woman's sources of support.
PSYCHOLOGIC STATUS		
Excitement and/or apprehension, ambivalence	Marked anxiety (fear of pregnancy diagnosis, fear of medical facility or providers) Apathy; display of anger with pregnancy diagnosis	Establish lines of communication. Active listening is useful. Establish trusting relationship. Encourage woman to take active part in her care. Establish communication and begin counseling. Use active listening techniques.
EDUCATIONAL NEEDS		
May have questions about pregnancy or may need time to adjust to reality of pregnancy		Establish educational, supporting environment that can be expanded throughout pregnancy.
SUPPORT SYSTEM		
Can identify at least two or three individuals with whom woman is emotionally intimate (partner, parent, sibling, friend)	Isolated (no telephone, unlisted number); cannot name a neighbor or friend whom she can call on in an emergency; does not perceive parents as part of her support system	Institute support system through community groups. Help woman to develop trusting relationship with healthcare professionals.
FAMILY FUNCTIONING		
Emotionally supportive Communications adequate Mutually satisfying Cohesiveness in times of trouble	Long-term problems or specific problems related to the pregnancy, potential stressors within the family, pessimistic attitudes, unilateral decision making, unrealistic expectations of the pregnancy or child	Help identify the problems and stressors, encourage communication, and discuss role changes and adaptations. Refer to counseling as indicated.
ECONOMIC STATUS		
Source of income is stable and sufficient to meet basic needs of daily living and medical needs	Limited prenatal care; poor physical health; limited use of healthcare system; unstable economic status	Discuss available resources for health maintenance and the birth. Institute appropriate referral for meeting expanding family's needs (food stamps, WIC [a federally funded nutrition program for women, infants, and children], and so forth)
STABILITY OF LIVING CONDITIONS		
Adequate, stable housing for expanding family's needs	Crowded living conditions; questionable supportive environment for newborn	Refer to appropriate community agency. Work with family on self-help ways to improve situation.
	*Possible causes of alterations are identified in parentheses.	†This column provides guidelines for further assessment and initial intervention.

RESEARCH EVIDENCE IN PRACTICE — Ultrasound for Pregnancy Viability, Dating, and Location

CLINICAL QUESTIONS

Is routine diagnostic ultrasound in early pregnancy effective in identifying the viability and location of a pregnancy? Is ultrasound an accurate method of determining the baby's due date?

RESEARCH EVIDENCE

Determining whether a pregnancy is viable, and doing so early in the pregnancy, is of intense interest to many potential parents. Additionally, the determination of the location of a pregnancy can help identify mothers who may be at risk for the serious complications of an ectopic pregnancy. While ultrasound is of clear benefit for monitoring fetal well-being, it is unclear how early ultrasound may reveal a viable pregnancy and its location. Its role in determining the due dates of a pregnancy has also been questioned.

A Cochrane Collaborative Systematic Review appraised 11 randomized trials including 37,505 women to study the effectiveness of ultrasound as a diagnostic tool. One of the study questions was the use of ultrasound for accurate dating of a pregnancy. These studies were conducted over a period of 3 decades and so provide evidence of effectiveness as well as longitudinal data about long-term effects of this diagnostic method. A secondary application tested in multiple international studies involved the use of ultrasound early in pregnancy to determine viability. These studies, involving more than 1500 women, focused on the effectiveness and optimal timing of ultrasound scans to assess the location of a pregnancy (uterine vs. ectopic) and the viability of the fetus.

The routine use of diagnostic ultrasound improved gestational dating and, subsequently, reduced the rate of inductions of labor for postterm pregnancy. The earliest that ultrasound appears to be effective in confirming fetal viability is 42 days; prior to that time, ultrasound may reveal an amniotic sac but cannot confirm viability. Diagnosis of the location of the pregnancy, that is, ectopic or uterine, continues to involve a combination of clinical examination and ultrasound. The presence of an adnexal mass combined with the absence of an intrauterine gestational sac are the best indicators of an ectopic pregnancy.

WHAT QUESTIONS REMAIN UNANSWERED?

There continues to be a lack of standardization as to how early and how often ultrasounds should be conducted. What is the optimal time to begin ultrasound assessment? How often should they be conducted during a normal pregnancy?

WHAT IS BEST PRACTICE?

Routine diagnostic ultrasound can be conducted in early pregnancy to determine adequate dating of the pregnancy. Diagnostic ultrasound scans are probably not useful before 40 days of gestation, and clinical examination is still required to adequately diagnose the location of the pregnancy.

CRITICAL THINKING

How can the nurse assure the mother that routine diagnostic ultrasound is a safe and useful prenatal assessment?

References

Bottomley, C., Van Belle, V., Mukri, F., Kirk, E., Van Huffel, S., Timmerman, D., & Bourne, T. (2009). The optimal timing of an ultrasound scan to assess the location and viability of an early pregnancy. *Human Reproduction, 24*(8), 1811–1817.

Perriera, L., & Reeves, M. (2008). Ultrasound criteria for diagnosis of early pregnancy failure and ectopic pregnancy. *Seminars in Reproductive Medicine, 26*(5), 373–382.

Tuladhar, A., Tuladhar, A., Karki, D., Shrestha, A., & Pradhan. S. (2009). Role of ultrasound in early pregnancy in differentiating normal and abnormal pregnancies. *Nepal Medical College Journal, 11*(2), 127–129.

Whitworth, M., Bricker, L., Neilson, J., & Dowswell, R. (2010). Ultrasound for fetal assessment in early pregnancy. *Cochrane Database of Systematic Reviews*, Issue 4. Art. No.: CD007058. doi:10.1002/14651858

Nägele's Rule

The most common method of determining the EDB is by **Nägele's rule**. To use this method, begin with the first day of the LMP, subtract 3 months, and add 7 days. The following is an example of Nagele's rule:

First day of LMP	July 20
Subtract 3 months	− 3 months
	April 20
Add 7 days	+ 7 days
EDB	April 27 (of the next year)

It is simpler to change the months to numeric terms:

July 20 becomes	07 − 20
Subtract 3 months	− 3
	04 − 20
Add 7 days	+ 7
EDB	04 − 27 (of next year)

A gestation calculator or "wheel" permits the caregiver to calculate the EDB even more quickly (Figure 15-2 ■).

Nägele's rule can be a fairly accurate determiner of EDB if a woman has a history of menses every 28 days, has an accurate LMP, and was not utilizing hormonal contraception prior to conception. Some women, however, may have cycles that

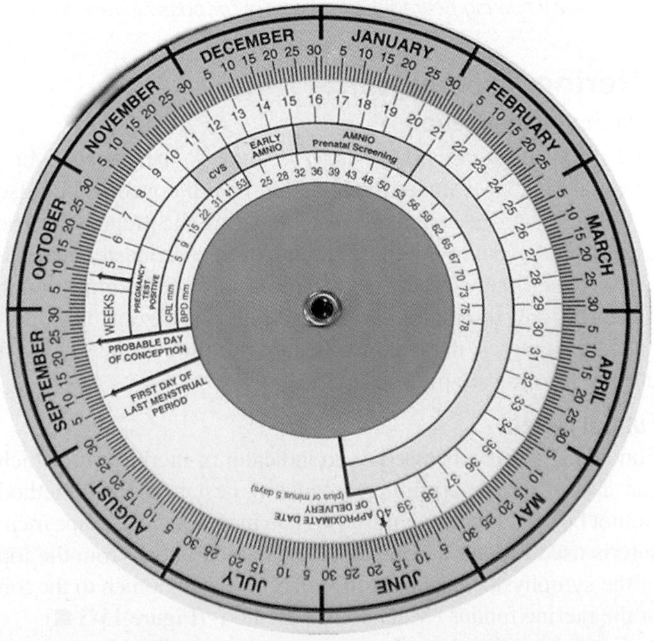

Figure 15-2 ■ The EDB wheel can be used to calculate the due date. To use it, place the arrow labeled "first day of last period" on the date of the woman's LMP. Then read the EDB at the arrow labeled 40. In this case, the LMP is September 8th and the EDB is June 17th.

last from 35 to 40 days in length, which will cause ovulation to be delayed by several days. Ovulation usually occurs 14 days before the onset of the next menses, not 14 days after the previous menses. In cases of unsure LMP, irregular menstrual cycles, breastfeeding women, amenorrhea, or hormonal contraception use, an ultrasound is done to visualize the gestational sac and obtain measurements of the embryo/fetus to determine EDB. (See the discussion of ultrasound in chapter 21 ∞.)

Thus Nägele's rule, although helpful, is not always accurate. It is of no use in calculating EDB for (1) women with markedly irregular periods that include one or more months of amenorrhea, (2) women who have amenorrhea but are ovulating and conceive while breastfeeding, or (3) women who conceive before regular menstruation is established following discontinuation of oral contraceptives or termination of a pregnancy (Varney et al., 2004). An estimation of EDB can be made using other subjective and objective findings such as fundal height, uterine size, auscultation of fetal heart tones, and timing of quickening. Despite these assessments, an ultrasound should be completed as early as possible if Nägele's rule cannot be used.

CLINICAL JUDGMENT

Case Study: Davia Mankovitz

Davia Mankovitz is a 27-year-old G1P0 who presents with her husband for her initial prenatal visit. She is at 13 weeks' gestation based on her LMP. She has a history of irregular menses. She has been trying to get pregnant for 2 years and had a visit scheduled with the infertility clinic next month to be evaluated. She and her husband are very excited about the pregnancy. She reports feeling baby movement for 3 weeks. Her fundal height today is 22 cm.

Critical Thinking

What are your initial impressions about her pregnancy status?
See www.nursing.pearsonhighered.com for possible responses.

Uterine Assessment

Physical Examination

The initial physical examination is done at the patient's first prenatal visit to evaluate for potential health concerns but also to evaluate uterine size to assist with dating the pregnancy. The exam could occur in the first, second, or third trimester depending on when the woman seeks care initially. It becomes much more difficult to accurately evaluate uterine size as the pregnancy progresses, in obese women, in multiple gestations, or if uterine fibroids are present.

Fundal Height

Fundal height may be used as an indicator of uterine size, which can assist with determining pregnancy gestation. This method cannot be used for dating purposes late in pregnancy. A tape measure is used to measure the distance in centimeters from the top of the symphysis pubis over the curve of the abdomen to the top of the uterine fundus (McDonald's method) (Figure 15-3 ■).

Fundal height in centimeters correlates well with weeks of gestation between 22 weeks and 34 weeks. At 26 weeks' gestation, for example, fundal height is probably about 26 cm. Typically, ±2 cm is considered normal. To be most accurate, fundal height should be measured by the same examiner each time. Maternal position (trunk elevation, knee flexion) may influence fundal height measurement. If the woman is very tall or very short, fundal height may also differ. In the third trimester, variations in fetal weight decrease the accuracy of fundal height measurements. Unfortunately, this method of dating a pregnancy can be quite inaccurate in the following situations:

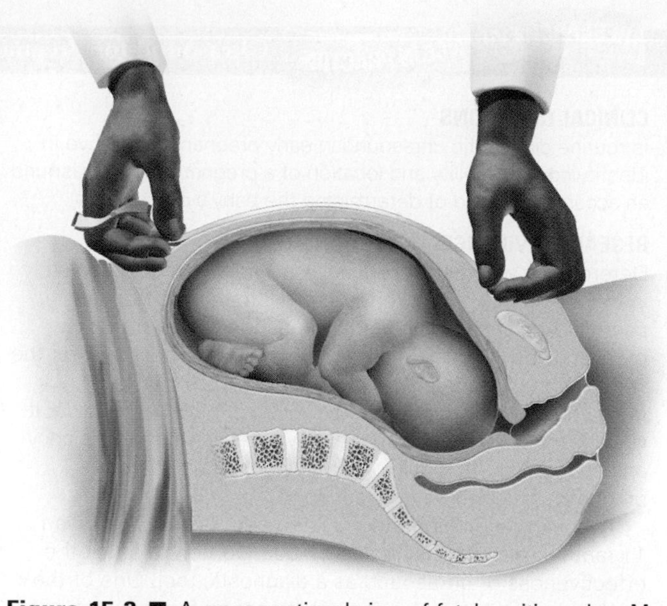

Figure 15-3 ■ A cross-sectional view of fetal position when McDonald's method is used to assess fundal height.

- Obese women (because of difficulty palpating the fundus accurately)
- Women with uterine fibroids (because uterine size may be distorted)
- Women who develop hydramnios (because the excess fluid increases uterine size, leading the examiner to conclude the fetus is larger than it is)

CLINICAL TIP

The woman should empty her bladder before measuring fundal height. A full bladder may impact the accuracy of the measurement.

Measurements of fundal height from month to month and week to week may yield other information as well. For example, a lag in the progression of fundal height may indicate intrauterine growth restriction (IUGR), or oligohydraminos, and a sudden increase in height may indicate the presence of twins, polyhydramnios, or a large for gestational age (LGA) fetus. Abnormal fundal height measurements should be assessed by ultrasound to determine possible cause.

Assessment of Fetal Development

Quickening

Fetal movements felt by the mother or perception of life—*quickening*—may give some indications that the fetus is nearing 20 weeks' gestation. Quickening may be experienced between 16 and 22 weeks' gestation, so this is not a completely accurate method to date a pregnancy. Because multiparous women have experienced quickening before, they often report fetal movement earlier than a primigravida does. It is good to note this milestone, but it should not be used solely for determining an EDB.

CLINICAL TIP

Early fetal movement may be described by the mother as feeling butterfly movements, gas, flicking sensations, or bubbles.

Fetal Heartbeat

The ultrasonic Doppler device (Figure 15-4 ■) is the primary tool for assessing fetal heartbeat. It may detect fetal heartbeat at about 10 to 12 weeks' gestation. The normal range for fetal heart tones (FHT) is 110–160. An ultrasound should be completed if the nurse is unable to auscultate between 10 and 12 weeks, because there may be a discrepancy of EDB, twins, or a missed abortion. In the case of twins or the obese woman, it may be later before the fetal heartbeat can be detected.

> “I went with my daughter to her prenatal visit, which included an ultrasound. I was not only able to hear the heartbeat of my first grandchild, I was also able to see the baby. What a blessing to be part of this experience! It was a special moment for me as a soon-to-be grandfather.”

Ultrasound

In the first trimester, transabdominal ultrasound can detect a gestational sac as early as 4 to 5 weeks after the LMP, fetal heart activity by 6 to 7 weeks, and fetal breathing movements by 10 to 11 weeks of pregnancy. Crown-to-rump measurements can be completed for assessment of fetal age until the fetal head can be defined. Crown-to-rump length can be used for gestational age from 4 days up to 12 weeks. Biparietal diameter (BPD) measurements can be made by approximately 14 weeks and are most accurate between 14 and 26 weeks, when rapid growth in biparietal diameter occurs. The BPD predicts EDB within 7 to 10 days. Both of these measurements can provide a gestational age for EDB determination or to compare with LMP dating. (See chapter 21 ∞ for an in-depth discussion of ultrasound scanning of the fetus.)

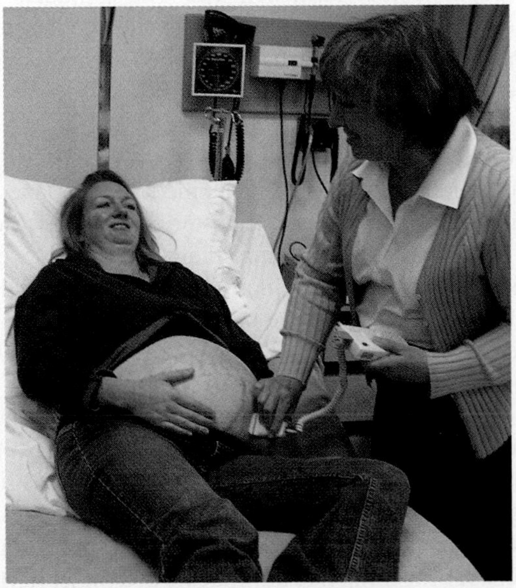

Figure 15-4 ■ Listening to the fetal heartbeat with a Doppler device.

CLINICAL TIP

An ultrasound should be ordered or completed at the initial prenatal visit if the EDB is unknown. The ultrasound is more accurate in dating the pregnancy the earlier it is completed.

Assessment of Pelvic Adequacy

By performing a series of assessments and measurements, the examiner assesses the pelvis vaginally to determine whether the size and shape are adequate for a vaginal birth. This procedure, called *clinical pelvimetry,* is typically performed by physicians and advanced practice nurses during the pelvic exam. Clinical pelvimetry should not be used to determine if a patient is appropriate to attempt a vaginal birth. All women should be allowed a trial of labor despite clinical pelvimetry findings. For a detailed description of clinical pelvimetry, refer to a nurse-midwifery text. This section provides general information about the assessment of the inlet, midpelvis, and outlet. These terms are defined in chapter 10 ∞.

Pelvic Inlet

The important anteroposterior diameters of the inlet for childbearing are the diagonal conjugate, the obstetric conjugate, and the conjugata vera, or true conjugate (Figure 15-5 ■).

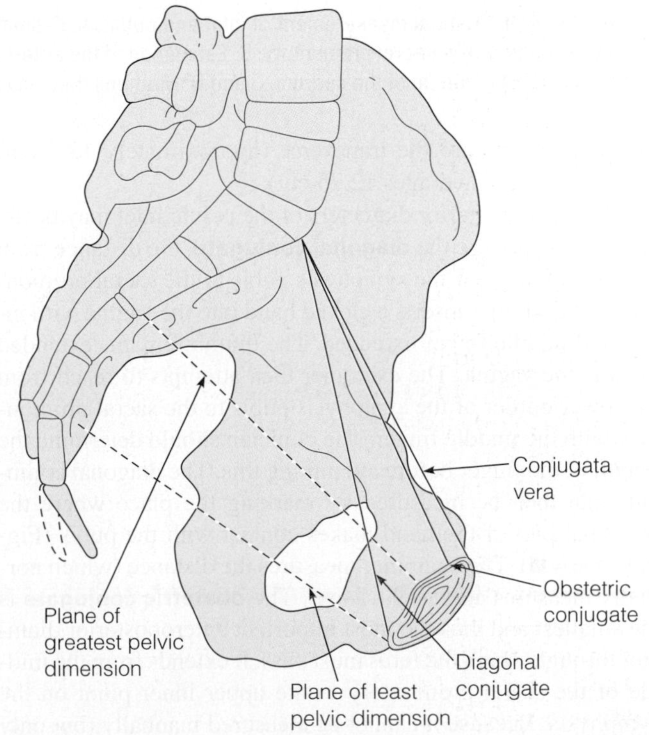

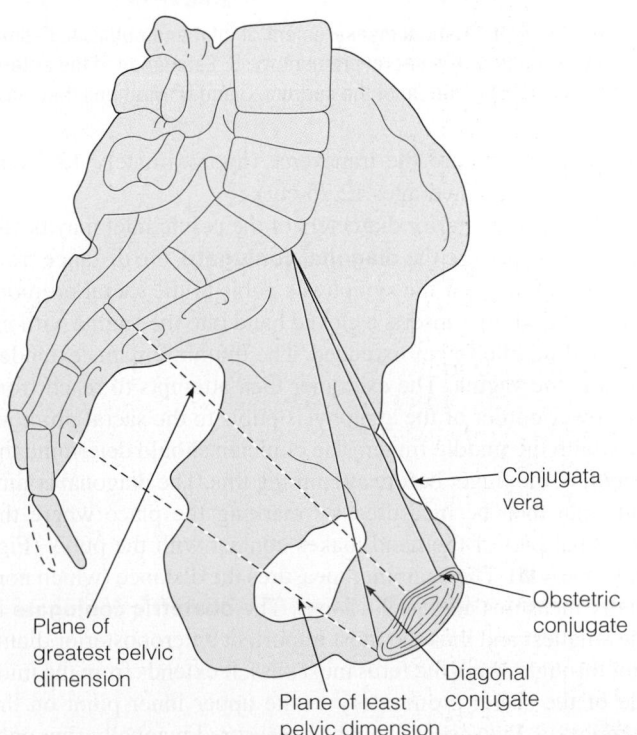

Figure 15-5 ■ Anteroposterior diameters of the pelvic inlet and their relationship to the pelvic planes.

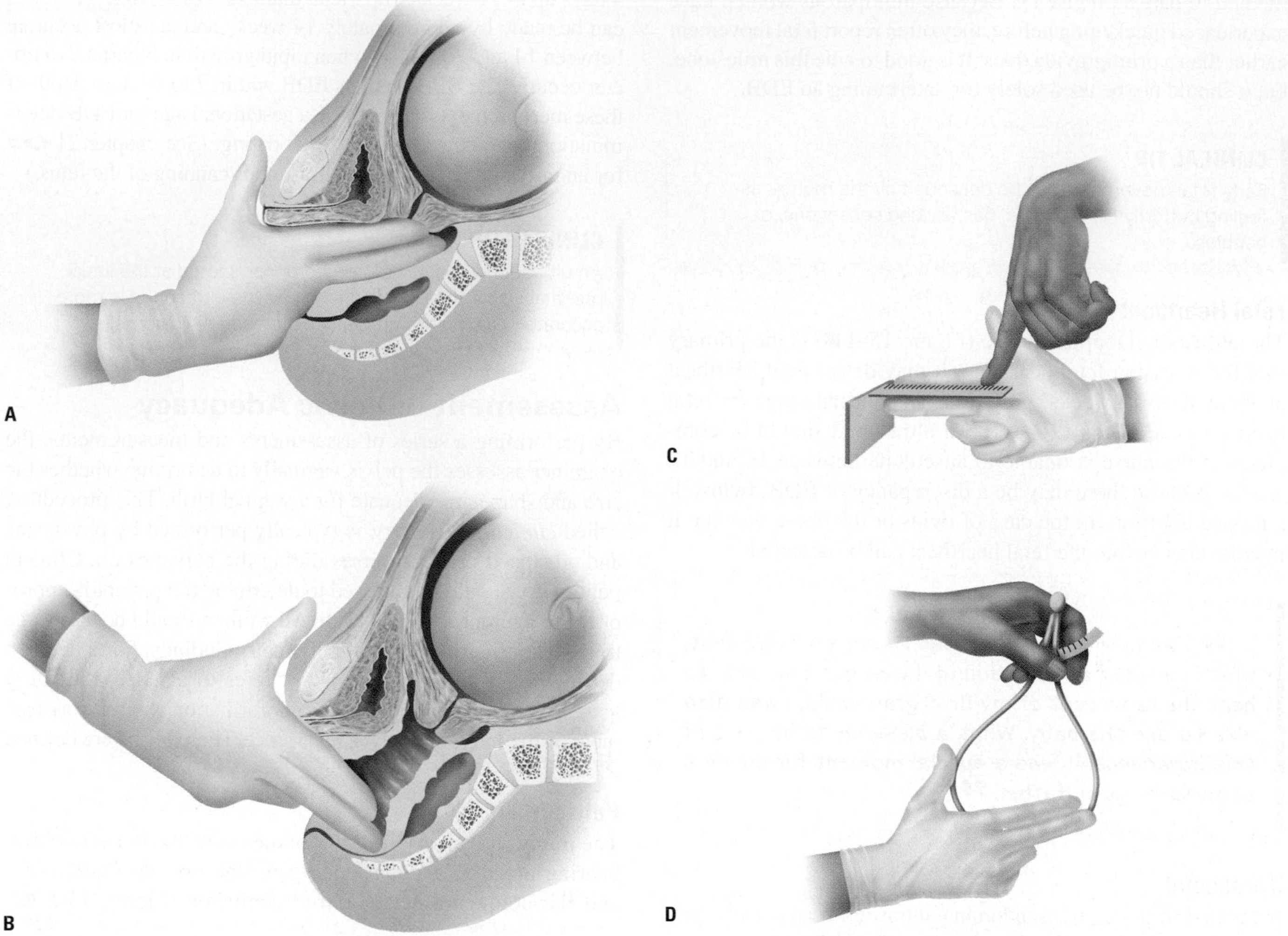

Figure 15-6 ■ Manual measurement of inlet and outlet. A. Estimation of the diagonal conjugate, which extends from the lower border of the symphysis pubis to the sacral promontory. B. Estimation of the anteroposterior diameter of the outlet, which extends from the lower border of the symphysis pubis to the tip of the sacrum. C and D. Methods that may be used to check the manual estimation of anteroposterior measurements.

Other diameters are the transverse (approximately 13.5 cm) and the oblique (averages 12.75 cm).

The anteroposterior diameters of the pelvic inlet may be assessed. To measure the **diagonal conjugate**, the distance from the lower border of the symphysis pubis to the sacral promontory, the examiner inserts a gloved hand into the vagina with index and middle finger extended. The thumb remains extended outside the vagina. The examiner then attempts to reach from the lower border of the symphysis pubis to the sacral promontory with the middle finger. The clinician should determine the length of the finger before attempting this. The diagonal conjugate can then be measured by marking the place where the proximal part of the hand makes contact with the pubis (Figure 15-6A ■). The examiner measures the distance (which normally measures at least 11.5 cm). The **obstetric conjugate** is the smallest and thus the most important anteroposterior diameter through which the fetus must pass. It extends from the middle of the sacral promontory to the upper inner point on the symphysis. Because it cannot be measured manually (but only by x-ray examination), it is estimated by subtracting 1.5 to 2 cm from the length of the diagonal conjugate. It should measure 10 cm or more in order for an average size baby (7.5 to 8 lb) to pass through without difficulty. The true conjugate extends from the upper border of the symphysis pubis to the middle of the sacral promontory. It can be determined by subtracting 1 cm from the diagonal conjugate.

Pelvic Cavity (Midpelvis)

Important midpelvic measurements include the plane of least dimension, or midplane (anteroposterior diameter, normally 11.5 to 12 cm; posterior sagittal diameter, 4.5 to 5 cm; and transverse diameter [interspinous], 10 cm). It is shown in Figure 15-5. The planes of the midpelvis cannot be accurately measured by clinical examination. An evaluation of adequacy is made based on the prominence of the ischial spines and degree of convergence of the side walls.

Location of the sacrospinous ligament, a firm ridge of tissue, makes location of the ischial spines easier. When this ligament is located, the examiner should run the fingers along it laterally toward the anterior portion of the pelvis. The spines may range from a small, firm bump like the knuckle of a finger (termed *not encroaching*) to a very prominent bone (called *encroaching*).

The sacrosciatic notch should admit two fingers. A wide notch means that the sacrum curves posteriorly, giving the anteroposterior diameter of the midpelvis a greater length. A narrow notch indicates a decreased diameter. The width of the sacrosciatic notch is more accurately evaluated through x-ray examination but can be estimated through vaginal exam. The length of the sacrospinous ligament is measured by tracing the ligament from its origin on the ischial spines to its insertion on the sacrum. It is usually 4 cm, or two to three finger breadths long.

The capacity of the cavity can be assessed by sweeping the fingers down the side walls bilaterally to evaluate the shape of the pelvic side walls. They may be termed *convergent* (closer together at the outlet than the inlet, like a funnel), *divergent* (side walls farther apart at the outlet, which typically means the pubic arch will have a wide angle), or *straight* (normal finding). The curvature, inclination, and hollowness of the sacrum help indicate the capacity of the posterior pelvis. It is estimated digitally by palpating the sacrococcygeal junction and by inching up toward the promontory. The examiner then estimates the hollowness of the sacrum. A flat or shallow sacrum has less room; a hollow sacrum is considered normal. The plane of greatest pelvic dimensions represents the largest portion of the pelvic cavity and has no obstetric significance.

Pelvic Outlet

The anteroposterior diameter of the pelvic outlet (9.5 to 11.5 cm), which extends from the lower border of the symphysis pubis to the tip of the sacrum, can be measured digitally (Figure 15-6B ■). The transverse diameter of the outlet is measured by placing the fist between the ischial tuberosities. It usually measures 8 to 10 cm (Figure 15-7 ■). The posterior sagittal diameter, the third important outlet diameter, normally measures at least 7.5 cm.

The mobility of the coccyx is determined by pressing down on it with the forefinger and middle finger during the initial vaginal examination. An immobile coccyx can decrease the diameter of the outlet.

The subpubic angle is estimated by palpating the bony structure externally with two fingers placed side by side at the border of the symphysis (Figure 15-8A ■). It should be 85 to 90 degrees. The angle is probably less if the examiner cannot separate his or her fingers.

The length and shape of the pubic rami affect the transverse diameter of the outlet. The pubic ramus is expected to be short and concave inward, as opposed to straight and long.

The height and inclination of the symphysis pubis are measured, and the contour of the pubic arch is estimated. Excessively long or angulated bone structure shortens the diameter of the obstetric conjugate. Height can be determined by placing the index finger of the gloved hand up to the superior border of the symphysis (Figure 15-8B ■). The examiner should measure the length of the first phalanx of the index finger (normally about 2.5 cm). Inclination can be determined by externally placing one finger on the top of the symphysis while the internal finger palpates the internal margin (Figure 15-8C ■). An imaginary line is drawn between the fingers, and the angle is estimated.

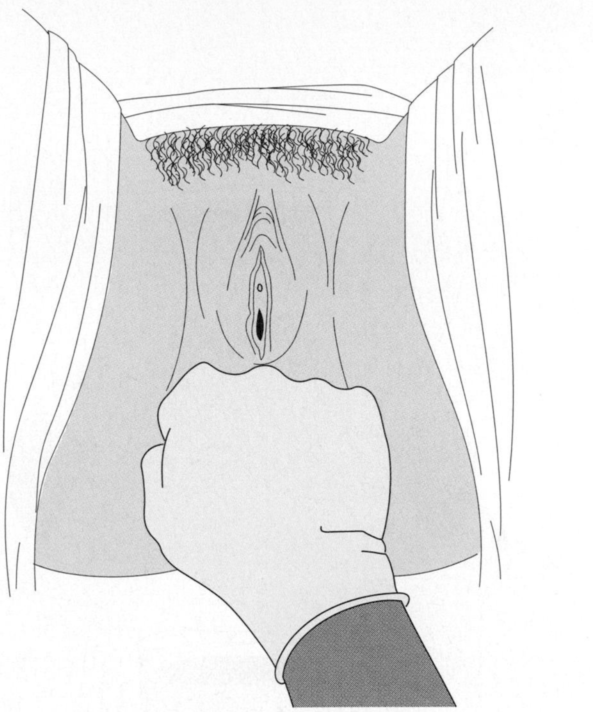

Figure 15-7 ■ Use of a closed fist to measure the outlet. Most examiners know the distance between their first and last proximal knuckles. If they do not, they can use a measuring device.

Care Plan Activity: Initial Assessment of Primigravida

A posterior inclination with the lower border of the pubis slanting inward decreases the anteroposterior diameter. The anteroposterior sagittal diameter is the most significant diameter of the outlet because it is the shortest diameter through which the infant must pass. The examiner uses two fingers to determine the contour of the pubic arch. This provides information on the width of the angle at which these bones come together (Figure 15-8D ■). The pubic arch has obstetric importance; if it is narrow, the infant's head may be pushed backward toward the coccyx, making extension of the fetal head difficult, which may lengthen the second stage of labor.

Screening Tests

Many screening tests are routinely performed during pregnancy, either at the initial prenatal visit or at specified times during pregnancy. Tests completed at the initial visit include a Pap smear, complete blood count, HIV screening, rubella titer, ABO and Rh typing, urine culture, and hepatitis B screen, as well as testing for sexually transmitted infections such as syphilis, HIV, chlamydia, and gonorrhea. Additional tests are completed at certain gestational ages throughout the pregnancy.

Women are routinely screened for gestational diabetes mellitus (GDM). Several methods may be used. Typically, between 24 and 28 weeks' gestation a 50-g 1-hour glucose screen is completed to detect GDM. The cutoff range may vary between 130 mg/dl, 135 mg/dl, or 140 mg/dl depending on the specific laboratory. If the screen is abnormal, a 3-hour glucose tolerance test (gtt) is then completed for diagnosis (see chapter 19 ∞). A hemoglobin or hematocrit is also completed at this time to evaluate for iron deficiency anemia.

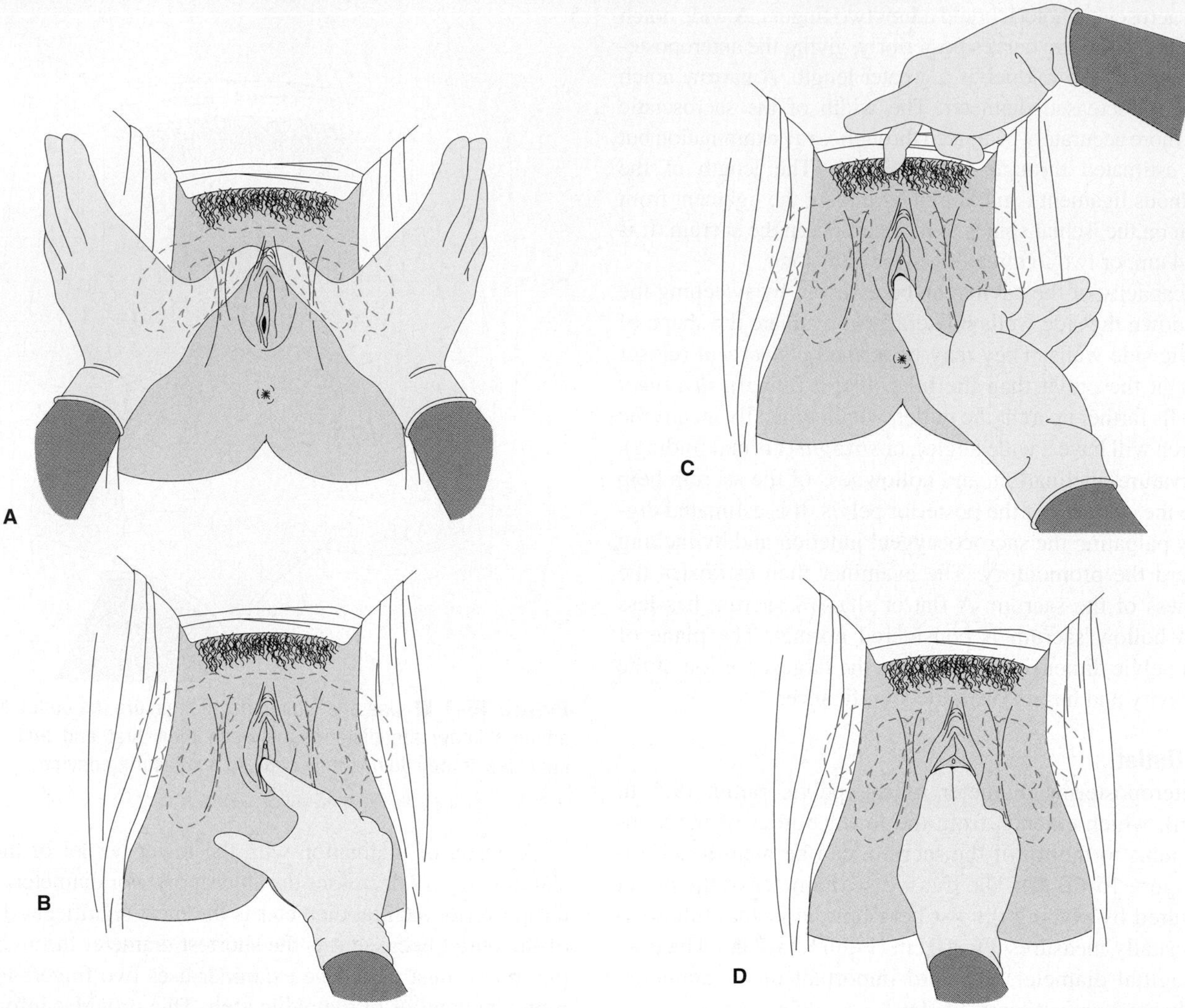

Figure 15-8 ■ Evaluation of the outlet. A. Estimation of the subpubic angle. B. Estimation of the length of the pubic ramus. C. Estimation of the depth and inclination of the pubis. D. Estimation of the contour of the subpubic angle.

Group B streptococcus (GBS) testing is completed between 35 and 37 weeks. GBS is a leading cause of serious neonatal infections. For this reason, a rectal and vaginal swab of the mother is obtained to screen for presence of the bacteria. Women with GBS in the urine at any time during the pregnancy are considered to be positive and do not need a culture completed. Intrapartum prophylaxis with antibiotics is recommended for women with positive GBS status.

Certain screening tests should be offered to women based on risk findings that become apparent from the history and/or physical evaluation. For example, a hemoglobin electrophoresis should be performed in women of African, Southeast Asian, and Mediterranean descent to evaluate for sickle cell disease and thallasemias. Appropriate treatment and counseling can then be arranged based on the laboratory findings. Women who have not received varicella immunization or report a negative disease history should also be evaluated for varicella immunity. If they do not have documented immunity, plans should be made for the woman to be immunized after pregnancy. A tuberculin test (PPD) should also be completed on women who are considered to be high risk. High-risk populations include women who are foreign born, have a known exposure to tuberculosis, and healthcare workers who care for patients with tuberculosis. Lastly, additional tests are completed in the event of pathologic findings or known disease states. For example, a woman with known chronic hypertension should have a 24-hour urine, metabolic panel, and uric acid completed.

Additional genetic screening tests may be offered to pregnant women. Prenatal screening for cystic fibrosis (CF) is available. Originally the screening was offered before conception or in early pregnancy to Caucasian couples (including Ashkenazi Jews) because the condition is most common in these populations. However, ACOG (2005b) now recommends that cystic fibrosis carrier screening be offered to all couples regardless of ethnicity or race during preconception or early in pregnancy. It is important that families are counseled about the limitations of CF screening, including the fact that a risk of positive CF carrier status is still present after negative results because the test does not screen for all possible mutations.

Through the Eyes of a Nurse
Prenatal Testing in Pregnancy

Family's Experience

"I know there are things that can go wrong in pregnancy. Maybe I have just read too much, but I am really scared something is going to go wrong. How will you know if there is a problem?"

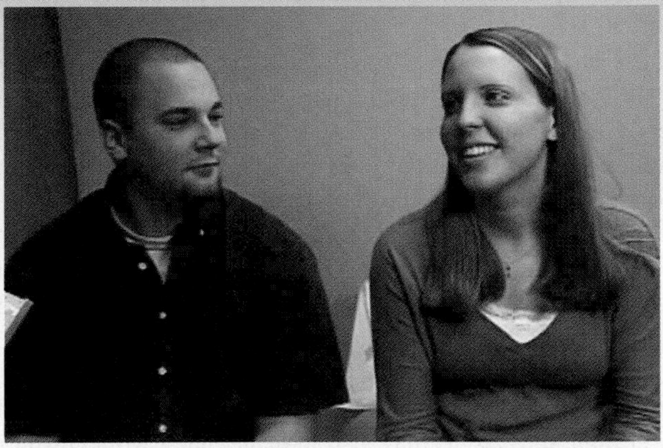

Nurse's Response

"It is not uncommon to be nervous or scared about the baby and yourself. At your first visit, you remember that we asked you a lot of medical information and questions about your medical history, the medical history of the father of the baby, and questions about your social situation and environmental factors in your everyday life. This provides us with information to determine if there are problems that you may be at risk for developing.

"The physical exam and lab tests you have had done also allow us to look for underlying or developing complications. So far, all of your test results have been normal. We will continue monitoring you and the baby throughout the pregnancy to make sure things are progressing normally and that there are no concerns."

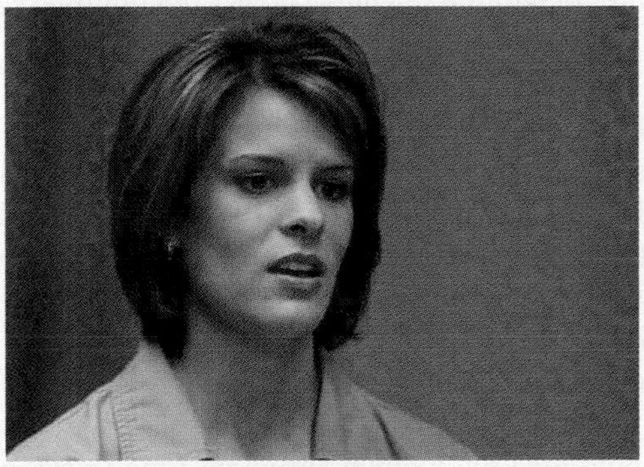

Nurse's Actions and Rationale

The nurse validates the woman's feelings and provides reassurance that feeling concerned and worried about problems that can occur during pregnancy are normal responses. In the beginning of pregnancy, a physical examination is performed to determine a baseline physical assessment. The assessment guide in this chapter reviews the physical examination, along with laboratory tests that are commonly performed. The nurse should also assess for cultural, educational, psychologic, and financial needs or concerns. A family assessment (discussed in chapter 2 ∞) should also be performed during the pregnancy.

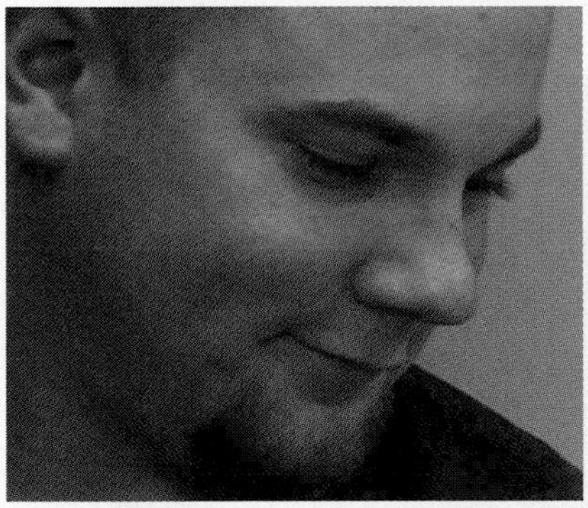

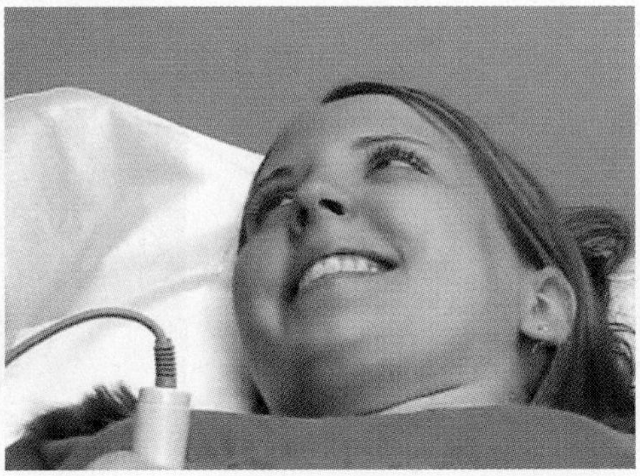

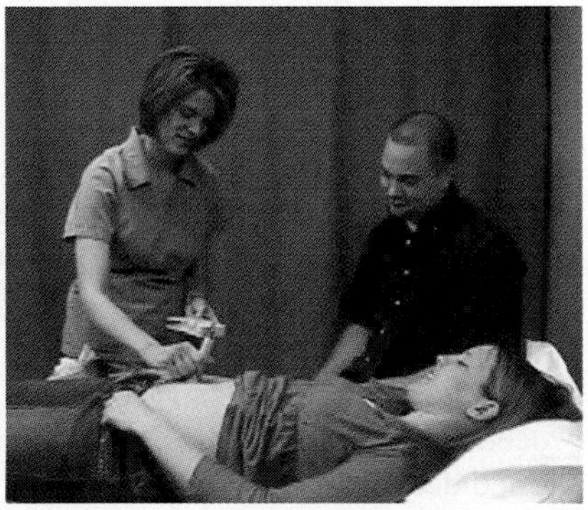

Women and family members should be counseled about the process of screening, interpretation of outcomes, and limitations of testing.

Universal screening for certain birth defects including neural tube defects, Down syndrome, and trisomy 18 is offered to all women during pregnancy. The goal of screening is to identify women who will benefit from diagnostic testing and to decrease the need for invasive procedures (Rappaport, 2008).

The *quadruple screen* (quad screen) is a safe, useful screening test performed on the mother's serum between 15 and 21 weeks of pregnancy. The test is used to detect levels of specific serum markers—alpha-fetoprotein (AFP), human chorionic gonadotropin (hCG), unconjugated estriol (UE), and inhibin-A (a placental hormone). Test results that reveal higher than normal AFP levels indicate an increased risk of a fetal neural tube defect, a multiple gestation, or a pregnancy that is farther along than believed. Lower than normal AFP could indicate that the woman is at risk for having a baby with Down syndrome or trisomy 18. Higher than normal levels of hCG and inhibin-A and lower than normal UE may also indicate that a woman is at increased risk of having a baby with Down syndrome. An accurate gestational age must be determined when using the quad screen. The more accurate the EDB estimation, the better the screening performance (Saller & Canick, 2008).

First trimester ultrasound assessment of the thickness (presence of fluid) in the fetal nuchal fold (called *nuchal translucency [NT]*) is a positive marker for Down syndrome and an early presenting feature of fetal chromosomal, genetic, and structural abnormalities. Ultrasound evaluation of NT combined with a serum screen of pregnancy-associated plasma protein A (PAPP-A) and free B-hCG completed between 11 and 13 weeks has an 85% detection rate for Down syndrome (Saller & Canick, 2008). These tests are generally combined with second trimester serum screening and may be called either a sequential or an integrated test depending on the sequence of evaluation. NT evaluations may not be available in all areas due to lack of NT certified sonographers (Rappaport, 2008). Neural tube defect screening should be offered in the second trimester to women who complete the first trimester screening.

It is important for healthcare professionals to provide parents with factual information about the results of screening tests that detect chromosomal defects or fetal anomalies including detection rates, false-positive results, advantages, disadvantages, limitations, risks, and benefits of diagnostic procedures (ACOG, 2007). This allows patients to make informed decisions when choosing to complete screening or diagnostic testing. The goal of screening is to identify women who might benefit from diagnostic testing based on screening results. Parents need to decide on any course of action based on their own spiritual, cultural, and personal beliefs prior to initiating diagnostic or screening testing. It is important to remember that some patients will decline genetic screening for personal reasons. This decision must be respected and supported by the nurse.

Subsequent Patient History

At subsequent prenatal visits, the nurse continues to gather data about the family's adjustment to the pregnancy and the course of the pregnancy to date. Each subsequent visit includes a chart review, history and physical examination, laboratory studies as indicated, and explanations and teaching appropriate to the woman's needs and gestational age. A chart review should be completed before starting the subsequent visit. This allows the nurse to determine the gestational age of the woman, evaluate laboratory results, and identify any problems or risks that may be present. The nurse can subsequently address important findings and investigate findings as needed. Once the chart review is completed, the nurse should obtain a basic revisit history, which should indicate complications or discomforts that the women may be experiencing. The nurse inquires about physical changes that relate directly to the pregnancy.

At prenatal visits, the nurse should evaluate the psychosocial needs of the woman and the adjustment and expectations of the support person and other children in the family. As the pregnancy progresses, the nurse assesses preparations that the family has made for the new baby and provides anticipatory guidance as needed. Taking time to address psychosocial issues is necessary in helping the nurse assess the family's success in meeting their developmental tasks.

Danger signs and signs of preterm labor that a woman should report immediately are discussed during the initial prenatal visit and reviewed at each subsequent prenatal visit (Figure 15-9 ■). Many caregivers also provide printed information on the subject written in lay terms. Table 15-2 identifies the danger signs of pregnancy and possible causes for each. Table 15-3 lists the signs of preterm labor.

The interchange between the nurse and woman will be facilitated if it takes place in a friendly, trusting environment. The nurse should give the woman sufficient time to ask questions and to voice concerns. If the nurse provides the time and

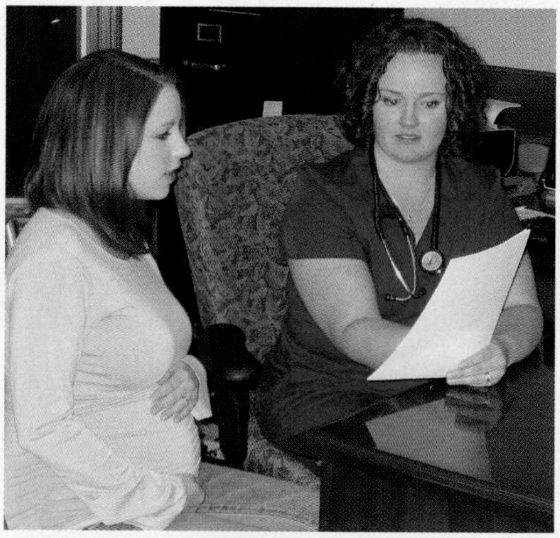

Figure 15-9 ■ The nurse reviews the danger signs in pregnancy at the initial prenatal visit and at each subsequent visit.

TABLE 15-2 Danger Signs in Pregnancy

The woman should report the following danger signs in pregnancy immediately.

DANGER SIGN	POSSIBLE CAUSE
Sudden gush of fluid from vagina	Premature rupture of membranes
Vaginal bleeding	Abruptio placentae, placenta previa Lesions of cervix or vagina "Bloody show" Cervical, vaginal infection Irritation of cervix from intercourse
Abdominal pain	Premature labor, abruptio placentae
Temperature above 38.3°C (101°F) and chills	Infection
Dizziness, blurring of vision, double vision, spots before eyes	Hypertension, preeclampsia
Persistent nausea and vomiting	Hyperemesis gravidarum
Severe headache	Hypertension, preeclampsia
Edema of hands or face	Preeclampsia
Seizures or convulsions	Preeclampsia, eclampsia
Epigastric pain	Preeclampsia, ischemia in major abdominal vessel
Dysuria	Urinary tract infection
Absent or decreased fetal movement	Maternal medication, obesity, fetal death, fetal distress

TABLE 15-3 Signs of Preterm Labor

- Painful menstrual-like cramps
- Dull low backache
- Suprapubic pain or pressure
- Pelvic pressure or heaviness
- Change in character or amount of vaginal discharge (bloody, thinner, thicker)
- Diarrhea
- Uterine contractions felt every 10 minutes for 1 hour
- Leaking of water from vagina

demonstrates genuine interest, the woman will feel more at ease bringing up questions that she may believe are silly or concerns that she has been afraid to verbalize. The nurse who has an accurate understanding of all the changes of pregnancy is most able to answer questions and provide information. See the foldout color chart, "Maternal-Fetal Development," for vivid illustrations of some of this information.

CLINICAL TIP

The woman and her partner should be encouraged to bring a list of questions or concerns to subsequent prenatal visits. This helps ensure that the needs and concerns of the woman and her family are addressed.

The nurse should be sensitive to religious, spiritual, cultural, and socioeconomic factors that may influence a family's response to pregnancy as well as to the woman's expectations of the healthcare system. The nurse can avoid stereotyping simply by asking each woman about her expectations for the antepartal period. Although many women's responses may reflect what are thought to be traditional norms, other women will have decidedly different views or may have expectations that represent a blending of beliefs or cultures.

During the prenatal period, it is essential that the nurse begin assessing the developing readiness of the woman and her partner to take on the responsibilities of parenthood successfully. Table 15-4 identifies areas for assessment and provides some sample questions the nurse might use to obtain necessary information. If the woman's responses are primarily negative, the nurse can plan interventions for the prenatal and postpartal periods.

Depression during and after pregnancy is a common problem, one that is gaining increased attention worldwide. The challenges of pregnancy and motherhood can be overwhelming for women experiencing perinatal depression (Baisch, Carey, Conway, et al., 2010). Infants of depressed women are at increased risk for delayed cognitive, neurologic, psychologic, and motor development (Gjerdingen & Yawn, 2007). Although ACOG reports that there is not sufficient evidence to recommend universal screening for depression at this time, women who have a history of depression or who are currently depressed need to be evaluated and monitored closely (ACOG, 2010).

Subsequent Prenatal Assessment

The Subsequent Prenatal Assessment Guide, which begins on page 340, provides a systematic approach to the regular physical examinations the pregnant woman should undergo for optimal prenatal care and a model for evaluating both the pregnant woman and the expectant partner, if he or she is involved in the pregnancy.

CLINICAL TIP

When assessing blood pressure, have the pregnant woman sit up with her arm resting on a table so that her arm is at the level of her heart. Expect a decrease in her blood pressure from baseline during the second trimester because of normal physiologic changes.

The woman's individual needs and the assessment of her risks should determine the frequency of subsequent visits. Generally, the recommended frequency of prenatal visits is as follows:

- Every 4 weeks for the first 28 weeks of gestation
- Every 2 weeks until 36 weeks' gestation
- After week 36, every week until childbirth

During the subsequent antepartal assessments, most women demonstrate ongoing psychologic adjustment to pregnancy and ever-improving coping skills. However, some women may exhibit signs of psychologic problems. These signs may include one or more of the following:

- Increasing anxiety
- Depression or feelings of sadness
- Inability to establish communication
- Inappropriate responses or actions
- Denial of pregnancy
- Inability to cope with stress
- Intense preoccupation with the sex of the baby
- Failure to acknowledge quickening
- Failure to plan and prepare for the baby (for example, living arrangements, clothing, feeding methods)
- Indications of substance abuse

If the woman's behavior indicates possible psychologic problems, the nurse should provide ongoing support and counseling and also refer the woman to appropriate professionals as indicated.

DEVELOPING CULTURAL COMPETENCE

Pregnant Women Who Decline Blood Products

At the first prenatal visit, it is important to evaluate your patient's willingness to receive blood products in the event of an emergency. Some women and families decline blood products based on religious, cultural, or personal beliefs. Jehovah's Witnesses make up the largest population of individuals who typically refuse blood products. Women who are Jehovah's Witnesses have a 6 times increased risk for maternal death and have 3.1 times increased risk for serious maternal morbidity compared to the general population (Van Wolfswinkel et al., 2009).

A woman's decision to decline blood products should be respected; however, the woman needs to understand the potential consequences of this decision including increased risk of a hysterectomy or death. It is important to determine which blood products the patient will accept, obtain a healthcare proxy, obtain an advance directive, complete a blood refusal consent form, avoid anemia during the pregnancy, and provide the necessary counseling so that the patient can make informed decisions. The obstetrician and anesthesiologist (if needed) should be aware of the woman's decision. A multidisciplinary team approach is indicated to ensure that appropriate care is provided to avoid serious complications.

TABLE 15-4 Guide to Prenatal Assessment of Parenting

AREAS ASSESSED	SAMPLE QUESTIONS
I. Perception of complexities of mothering A. Desires baby for itself Positive: 1. Feels positive about pregnancy Negative: 1. Wants baby to meet own needs such as someone to love her, someone to get her out of unhappy home	1. Did you plan on getting pregnant? 2. How do you feel about being pregnant? 3. Why do you want this baby?
B. Expresses concern about impact of mothering role on other roles (wife, career, school) Positive: 1. Realistic expectations of how baby will affect job, career, school, and personal goals 2. Interested in learning about child care Negative: 1. Feels pregnancy and baby will make no emotional, physical, or social demands on self 2. Has no insight that mothering role will affect other roles or lifestyle	1. What do you think it will be like to take care of a baby? 2. How do you think your life will be different after you have your baby? 3. How do you feel this baby will affect your job, career, school, and personal goals? 4. How will the baby affect your relationship with your partner? 5. Have you done any reading, baby-sitting, or made any things for a baby?
C. Gives up routine habits because "not good for baby" (e.g., quits smoking, adjusts time schedule) Positive: 1. Gives up routines not good for baby (quits smoking, adjusts eating habits)	
II. Attachment A. Strong feelings regarding sex of baby. Why? Positive: 1. Verbalizes positive thoughts about the baby Negative: 1. Baby will be like negative aspects of self and partner	1. Why do you prefer a certain sex? (Is reason inappropriate for a baby?) 2. Note comments patient makes about baby not being normal and why patient feels this way.
B. Interested in data regarding fetus (e.g., growth and development, heart tones) Positive: 1. As above	

TABLE 15-4 Guide to Prenatal Assessment of Parenting continued

AREAS ASSESSED	SAMPLE QUESTIONS
Negative: 1. Shows no interest in fetal growth and development, quickening, and fetal heart tones 2. Expresses negative feelings about fetus by rejecting counseling regarding nutrition, rest, hygiene	
C. Fantasies about baby Positive: 1. Follows cultural norms regarding preparation 2. Time of attachment behaviors appropriate to her history of pregnancy loss Negative: 1. Bonding conditional depending on sex, age of baby, and/or labor and birth experience 2. Woman considers only own needs when making plans for baby 3. Exhibits no attachment behaviors after critical period of previous pregnancy 4. Failure to follow cultural norms regarding preparation	1. What did you think or feel when you first felt the baby move? 2. Have you started preparing for the baby? 3. What do you think your baby will look like—what age do you see your baby at? 4. How would you like your new baby to look?
III. Acceptance of child by significant others	
A. Acknowledges acceptance by significant other of the new responsibility inherent in child Positive: 1. Acknowledges unconditional acceptance of pregnancy and baby by significant others 2. Partner accepts new responsibility inherent with child 3. Timely sharing of experience of pregnancy with significant others Negative: 1. Significant others not supportively involved with pregnancy 2. Conditional acceptance of pregnancy depending on sex, race, age of baby 3. Decision making does not take in needs of fetus (e.g., spends food money on new car) 4. Takes no/little responsibility for needs of pregnancy, woman/fetus	1. How does your partner feel about this pregnancy? 2. How do your parents feel? 3. What do your friends think? 4. Does your partner have a preference regarding the baby's sex? Why? 5. How does your partner feel about being a parent? 6. What do you think he/she will be like as a parent? 7. What do you think he/she will do to help you with child care? 8. Have you and your partner talked about how the baby might change your lives? 9. Who have you told about your pregnancy?
B. Concrete demonstration of acceptance of pregnancy/baby by significant others (e.g., baby shower, significant other involved prenatal education) Positive: 1. Baby shower 2. Significant other attends prenatal class with patient	1. Note if partner attends clinic with patient (degree of interest; e.g., listens to heart tones). 2. Does your partner plan to be with you during labor and birth? 3. Is your partner contributing financially?
IV. Ensures physical well-being	
A. Concerns about having normal pregnancy, labor and birth, and baby 1. Preparing for labor and birth, attends prenatal classes, interested in labor and birth 2. Aware of danger signs of pregnancy 3. Seeks and uses appropriate health care (e.g., time of initial visit, keeps appointments, follows through on recommendations) Negative: 1. Denies signs and symptoms that might suggest complications of pregnancy 2. Verbalizes extreme fear of labor and birth—refuses to talk about labor and birth 3. Misses appointments, fails to follow instructions, refuses to attend prenatal classes	1. What have you heard about labor and birth? 2. Note data about patient's reaction to prenatal class.
B. Family/patient decisions reflect concern for health of mother and baby (e.g., use of finances, time) Positive: 1. As above	

Source: Modified and used with permission of the Minneapolis Health Dept., Minneapolis, MN.

Note: When "Negative" is not listed in a section, the reader may assume that negative is the absence of positive responses.

ASSESSMENT GUIDE Subsequent Prenatal Assessment

Physical Assessment/Normal Findings	Alterations and Possible Causes*	Nursing Responses to Data†
VITAL SIGNS		
Temperature: 36.2°–37.6°C (97°–99.6°F)	Elevated temperature (infection)	Evaluate for signs of infection. Refer to healthcare provider.
Pulse: 60–90/min Rate may increase 10 beats/min during pregnancy	Increased pulse rate (anxiety, cardiac disorders)	Note irregularities. Assess for anxiety and stress.
Respiration: 12–22/min	Marked tachypnea or abnormal patterns (respiratory disease)	Refer to healthcare provider.
Blood Pressure: Less than or equal to 135/85 (falls in second trimester)	Greater than 140/90 or increase of 30 mm systolic and 15 mm diastolic (preeclampsia)	Assess for edema, proteinuria, and hyperreflexia. Refer to healthcare provider. Schedule appointments more frequently.
WEIGHT GAIN		
First Trimester: .05–2 kg (1.1–4.4 lb)	Inadequate weight gain (poor nutrition, nausea, intrauterine growth restriction [IUGR])	Discuss appropriate weight gain.
Second Trimester: 5.5–6.8 kg (12–15 lb)	Excessive weight gain (excessive caloric intake, edema, preeclampsia)	Provide nutritional counseling. Assess for presence of edema or anemia. Refer to dietitian as needed.
Third Trimester: 5.5–6.8 kg (12–15 lb)		
EDEMA		
Small amount of dependent edema, especially in last weeks of pregnancy	Edema in hands, face, legs, and feet (preeclampsia)	Identify any correlation between edema and activities, blood pressure, or proteinuria: Refer to healthcare provider if indicated.
UTERINE SIZE		
See "Assessment Guide: Initial Prenatal Assessment" for normal changes during pregnancy	Unusually rapid growth (multiple gestation, hydatidiform mole, hydramnios, miscalculation of estimated date of birth [EDB])	Evaluate fetal status. Determine height of fundus (page 330). Use diagnostic ultrasound.
FETAL HEARTBEAT		
120–160/min	Absence of fetal heartbeat after 20 weeks' gestation (maternal obesity, fetal demise)	Evaluate fetal status.
Funic soufflé		
LABORATORY EVALUATION		
Hemoglobin: 12–16 g/dl Pseudoanemia of pregnancy	Less than 11 g/dl (anemia)	Provide nutritional counseling. Hemoglobin is repeated at 7 months' gestation. Women of Mediterranean heritage need a close check on hemoglobin because of the possibility of thalassemia.
Quad Marker Screen: Blood test performed at 15–21 weeks' gestation. Evaluates four factors—maternal serum alpha-fetoprotein (MSAFP), unconjugated estriol (UE), human chorionic gonadotropin (hCG), and inhibin-A: normal levels	Elevated MSAFP (neural tube defect, underestimated gestational age, multiple gestation). Lower than normal MSAFP (Down syndrome, trisomy 18). Higher than normal hCG and inhibin-A (Down syndrome). Lower than normal UE (Down syndrome)	Offered to all pregnant women. If quad screen abnormal further testing such as ultrasound or amniocentesis is offered.
Indirect Coombs Test done on Rh negative women: Negative (done at 28 weeks' gestation)	Rh antibodies present (maternal sensitization has occurred)	If Rh negative and unsensitized, Rh immune globulin given (see chapter 20 ∞). If Rh antibodies present, Rh immune globulin not given; fetus monitored closely for isoimmune hemolytic disease. Refer for a diagnostic 100-g oral glucose tolerance test. Discuss implications of gestational diabetes mellitus (GDM) if diagnosis is made. Refer to healthcare provider.
50-g 1-hour glucose screen (done between 24 and 28 weeks' gestation)	Plasma glucose level greater than 130–140 depending on the facility are abnormal. Be aware of your institution's guidelines	
Urinalysis: See "Assessment Guide: Initial Prenatal Assessment" for normal findings	See "Assessment Guide: Initial Prenatal Assessment" for deviations	Urinalysis and culture is completed at initial visit and at subsequent visits as indicated.
Protein: Negative	Proteinuria, albuminuria (contamination by vaginal discharge, urinary tract infection, preeclampsia)	Obtain dipstick urine sample. Refer to healthcare provider if deviations are present.
Glucose: Negative **Note:** Glycosuria may be present due to physiologic alterations in glomerular filtration rate and renal threshold	Persistent glycosuria (diabetes mellitus)	Refer to healthcare provider.
	*Possible causes of alterations are identified in parentheses.	†This column provides guidelines for further nursing assessment and initial intervention.

ASSESSMENT GUIDE Subsequent Prenatal Assessment continued

Physical Assessment/Normal Findings	Alterations and Possible Causes*	Nursing Responses to Data†
Screening for Group B Streptococcus (GBS): Rectal and vaginal swabs obtained at 35–37 weeks' gestation for all pregnant women	Positive culture (maternal infection)	Explain maternal and fetal/neonatal risks (see chapter 20). Refer to healthcare provider for therapy.
Cultural Assessment	**Variations to Consider***	**Nursing Responses to Data†**
Determine the mother's (and family's) attitudes about the sex of the unborn child.	Some women have no preference about the sex of the child; others do. In many cultures, boys are especially valued as firstborn children.	Provide opportunities to discuss preferences and expectations; avoid a judgmental attitude to the response.
Ask about the woman's expectations of childbirth. Will she want someone with her for the birth? Whom does she choose? What is the role of her partner?	Some women want their partner present for labor and birth; others prefer a female relative or friend. Some women expect to be separated from their partner once labor begins.	Provide information on birth options but accept the woman's decision about who will attend.
Ask about preparations for the baby. Determine what is customary for the woman.	Some women may have a fully prepared nursery; others may not have a separate room for the baby.	Explore reasons for not preparing for the baby. Support the mother's preferences and provide information about possible sources of assistance if the decision is related to a lack of resources.
EXPECTANT MOTHER ***Psychologic Status***	Increased stress and anxiety	Encourage woman to take an active part in her care.
First Trimester/Period of Adjustment: Incorporates idea of pregnancy; may feel ambivalent or anxious, especially if she must give up desired role; usually looks for signs of verification of pregnancy, such as increase in abdominal size or fetal movement ***Second Trimester/Period of Radiant Health:*** Baby becomes more real to woman as abdominal size increases and she feels movement; she begins to turn inward, becoming more introspective ***Third Trimester/ Period of Watchful Waiting:*** Begins to think of baby as separate being; may feel restless, uneasy, and may feel that time of labor will never come; remains self-centered and concentrates on preparing place for baby. Fears well-being for herself and baby	Inability to establish communication; inability to accept pregnancy; inappropriate response or actions; denial of pregnancy; inability to cope	Establish lines of communication. Discuss and provide anticipatory guidance regarding normalcy of feelings and actions. Establish a trusting relationship. Counsel as necessary. Refer to appropriate professional as needed.
Educational Needs		
Self-care Measures and Knowledge About the Following: Health promotion Breast care Hygiene Rest Exercise Nutrition Relief measures for common discomforts of pregnancy Danger signs in pregnancy (see Table 15-2) Signs of preterm labor (see Table 15-3)	Inadequate information	Provide information and counseling.
Sexual Activity: Woman knows how pregnancy affects sexual activity	Lack of information about effects of pregnancy and/or alternative positions during sexual intercourse	Provide counseling.
Preparation for Parenting: Appropriate preparation	Lack of preparation (denial, failure to adjust to baby, unwanted child)	Counsel. If lack of preparation is due to inadequacy of information, provide information.
Preparation for Childbirth		If couple chooses particular technique, refer to classes (see chapter 13 for description of childbirth preparation techniques).
Patient Aware of the Following: 1. Prepared childbirth techniques 2. Normal processes and changes during childbirth	Continued abuse of drugs and alcohol; denial of possible effect on self and baby	Encourage prenatal class attendance. Educate woman during visits based on current physical status. Provide reading list for more specific information.
3. Problems that may occur as a result of drug and alcohol use and of smoking		Review danger signs that were presented on initial visit.
	*Possible causes of alterations are identified in parentheses.	†This column provides guidelines for further nursing assessment and initial intervention.

(continued)

ASSESSMENT GUIDE Subsequent Prenatal Assessment continued

Physical Assessment/Normal Findings	Alterations and Possible Causes*	Nursing Responses to Data†
Woman has met other physician or nurse-midwife who may be attending her birth in the absence of primary caregiver	Introduction of new individual at birth may increase stress and anxiety for woman and partner	Introduce woman to all members of group practice.
Impending Labor ***Patient Knows Signs of Impending Labor:*** 1. Uterine contractions that increase in frequency, duration, and intensity 2. Bloody show 3. Expulsion of mucous plug 4. Rupture of membranes	Lack of information	Provide appropriate teaching, stressing importance of seeking appropriate medical assistance.
EXPECTANT PARTNER ***Psychologic Status***		
First Trimester: May express excitement over confirmation of pregnancy and of his virility; concerns move toward providing for financial needs; energetic, may identify with some discomforts of pregnancy and may even exhibit symptoms	Increasing stress and anxiety; inability to establish communication; inability to accept pregnancy diagnosis; withdrawal of support; abandonment of the mother	Encourage expectant partner to come to prenatal visits. Establish line of communication. Establish trusting relationship.
Second Trimester: May feel more confident and be less concerned with financial matters; may have concerns about wife's changing size and shape, her increasing introspection		Counsel. Let expectant partner know that it is normal for him to experience these feelings.
Third Trimester: May have feelings of rivalry with fetus, especially during sexual activity; may make changes in his physical appearance and exhibit more interest in himself; may become more energetic; fantasizes about child but usually imagines older child; fears mutilation and death of woman and child		Include expectant partner in pregnancy activities as he desires. Provide education, information, and support. Increasing numbers of expectant partners are demonstrating desire to be involved in many or all aspects of prenatal care, education, and preparation.
	*Possible causes of alterations are identified in parentheses.	†This column provides guidelines for further nursing assessment and initial intervention.

FOCUS YOUR STUDY

- A complete history forms the basis of prenatal care and is reevaluated and updated as necessary throughout the pregnancy.
- The initial prenatal assessment is a careful and thorough physical examination and cultural and psychosocial assessment designed to identify variations and potential risk factors.
- Laboratory tests completed at the initial visit, such as a complete blood count, ABO and Rh typing, urinalysis/culture, Pap smear, chlamydia culture, gonorrhea culture, rubella titer, and various blood screens (such as rapid plasma reagin [RPR], HIV, and hepatitis B), provide information about the woman's health during early pregnancy and also help detect potential problems.
- The estimated date of birth (EDB) can be calculated using Nägele's rule. Using this approach, one begins with the first day of the last menstrual period, subtracts 3 months, and adds 7 days. A "wheel" may also be used to calculate the EDB.
- Accuracy of the EDB may be evaluated by physical examination to assess uterine size, measurement of fundal height, and ultrasound. Perception of quickening and auscultation of fetal heartbeat are also useful tools in confirming the gestation of a pregnancy.

- The diagonal conjugate is the distance from the lower posterior border of the symphysis pubis to the sacral promontory. The obstetric conjugate is estimated by subtracting 1.5 to 2 cm from the length of the diagonal conjugate.
- As part of the assessment of the pelvic cavity (midpelvis), the prominence of the ischial spines is assessed, the sacrosciatic notch and the length of the sacrospinous ligament are measured, and the shape of the pelvic side walls is evaluated. Finally, the hollowness of the sacrum is determined.
- The anteroposterior diameter of the pelvic outlet is determined, the mobility of the coccyx is assessed, the suprapubic angle is estimated, and the contour of the pubic arch is evaluated to assess the adequacy of the pelvic outlet.
- The nurse begins evaluating the woman psychosocially during the initial prenatal assessment. This assessment continues and is modified throughout the pregnancy.
- Cultural and ethnic beliefs may strongly influence the woman's attitudes and apparent cooperation with care during pregnancy.

CRITICAL THINKING IN ACTION

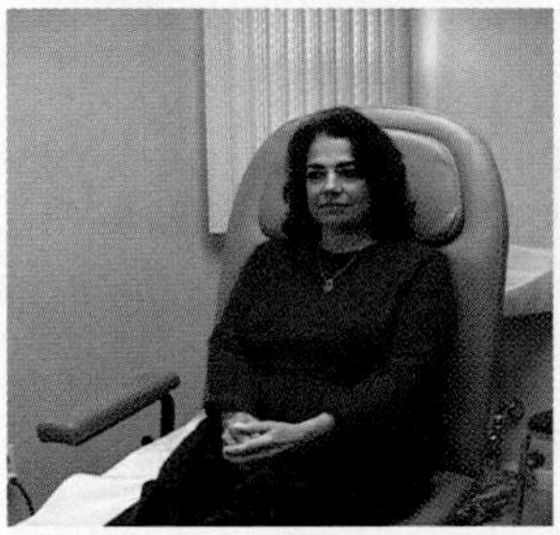

Source: George Dodson/Pearson Education.

Wendy Stodard, age 40, G3, P0020 comes to the obstetrician's office where you are working for a prenatal visit. Wendy has experienced two spontaneous abortions followed by a D & C at 14 and 15 weeks' gestation during the previous year. She has a history of *Chlamydia trachomatis* infection 3 years ago, which was treated with azithromycin. She is at 10 weeks' gestation. Wendy tells you that she is afraid of losing this pregnancy as she did previously. She says that she has been experiencing some mild nausea, breast tenderness, and fatigue, which did not occur with her other pregnancies. You assist the obstetrician with an ultrasound. The gestational sac is clearly seen, fetal heartbeat is observed, and crown-to-rump measurements are consistent with gestational age of 10 weeks. The pelvic exam demonstrates a closed cervix, and positive Goodell's, Hegar's, and Chadwick's signs. You discuss with Wendy the signs of a healthy pregnancy.

1. What signs are reassuring with this pregnancy?
2. What symptoms should be reported to the obstetrician immediately?
3. What is the frequency of antepartal visits?

See www.nursing.pearsonhighered.com for possible responses.

Pearson Nursing Student Resources

Find additional review materials at
www.nursing.pearsonhighered.com

Prepare for success with additional NCLEX®-style practice questions, interactive assignments and activities, Web links, animations and videos, and more!

REFERENCES

American College of Obstetricians and Gynecologists (ACOG). (2005a). *Racial and ethnic disparities in women's health* (ACOG Committee Opinion No. 317). Washington, DC: Author.

American College of Obstetricians and Gynecologists (ACOG). (2005b). *Update on carrier screening for cystic fibrosis* (ACOG Committee Opinion No. 325). Washington, DC: Author.

American College of Obstetricians and Gynecologists (ACOG). (2007). *Screening for fetal chromosomal abnormalities* (ACOG Practice Bulletin No. 77). Washington, DC: Author.

American College of Obstetricians and Gynecologists (ACOG). (2010). *Screening for depression during and after pregnancy* (ACOG Committee Opinion, No. 453). Washington, DC: Author.

Baisch, M. J., Carey, L. K., Conway, A. E., & Mounts, K. O. (2010). Perinatal depression: A health marketing campaign to improve screening. *Nursing for Women's Health, 14*(1), 18–33.

Cunningham, F. G., Leveno, K. J., Bloom, S. L., Hauth, J. C., Gilstrap, L. C., III, & Wenstrom, K. D. (2010). *Williams's obstetrics* (23rd ed.). New York, NY: McGraw-Hill.

Gjerdingen, D. K., & Yawn, B. P. (2007). Postpartum depression screening: Importance, methods, barriers, and recommendations for practice. *Journal of the American Board of Family Medicine, 20,* 280–288.

Jordan, R. G., & Murphy, P. A. (2009). Risk assessment and risk distortion: Finding the balance. *Journal of Midwifery & Women's Health, 54*(3), 191–200.

Rappaport, V. J. (2008). Prenatal diagnosis and genetic screening—integration into prenatal care. *Obstetrics and Gynecology Clinics of North America, 35,* 435–458.

Saller, D. N., & Canick, J. A. (2008). Current methods of prenatal screening for Down syndrome and other fetal abnormalities. *Clinical Obstetrics and Gynecology, 51*(1), 24–36.

Van Wolfswinkel, M. E., Zwart, J. J., Schutte, J. M., Duvekot J. J., Pel, M., & Van Roosmalen, J. (2009). Maternal mortality and serious maternal morbidity in Jehovah's witnesses in the Netherlands. *British Journal of Obstetrics and Gynecology, 116*(8), 1103–1110.

Varney, H., Kriebs, J. M., & Gegor, C. L. (2004). *Varney's midwifery* (4th ed.). Sudbury, MA: Jones & Bartlett.

CHAPTER 16

The Expectant Family: Needs and Care

I don't know how I timed it, but my nursing program OB rotation finishes up right about my due date. Watching all the births during my clinicals has been really exciting. The labor and delivery nurses laugh and say my hormones should be hopping now, but I think this baby is subliminally telling me that we won't "hatch" until I take my final exam!

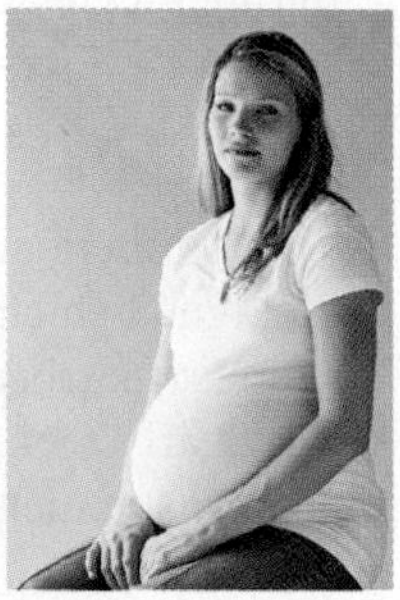

LEARNING OUTCOMES

1. Describe the significance of using the nursing process to promote health in the woman and her family during pregnancy.
2. Describe actions the nurse can take to help maintain the well-being of the expectant father and siblings during a family's pregnancy.
3. Discuss the significance of cultural considerations in managing nursing care during pregnancy.
4. Identify the common discomforts of pregnancy and their causes.
5. Summarize appropriate measures to alleviate the common discomforts of pregnancy.
6. Delineate self-care actions a pregnant woman and her family can take to maintain and promote well-being during each trimester of pregnancy.
7. Identify some of the concerns that an expectant couple may have about sexual activity.
8. Describe factors that have contributed to the increased incidence of pregnancy in women over age 35.
9. Compare similarities and differences in the needs of expectant women in various age groups.

KEY TERMS

Fetal alcohol syndrome (FAS) *371*
Fetal movement record (FMR) *358*
Kegel exercises *365*
Leukorrhea *353*
Lightening *357*
Pelvic tilt *363*
Ptyalism *353*
Teratogens *369*

From the moment a woman finds out that she is pregnant, she faces a future marked by dramatic changes. Her appearance will be altered. Her relationships will change. She will experience a variety of unique physical changes throughout the pregnancy. Even her psychologic state will be affected. In coping with these changes she needs to make adjustments in her daily life.

Her family must also adjust to the pregnancy. Roles and responsibilities of family members will change as the woman's ability to perform certain activities changes. They too must adapt psychologically to the situation.

The expectant woman and her family will probably have many questions about the pregnancy and its impact on her and the other members of the family. In addition, the daily activities and healthcare practices of the woman become of concern when she and her family realize that what she does can affect the well-being of the unborn child.

Nurses caring for pregnant women need a clear understanding of pregnancy and the changes it brings if they are to be effective in managing nursing care. With this in mind, chapter 14 ∞ provides a database for the nurse by presenting material related to the normal physical, psychologic, social, and cultural changes of pregnancy. Chapter 15 ∞ then uses that database to begin a discussion of nursing care management by focusing on patient assessment. This chapter further addresses nursing care management as it relates to the needs of the expectant woman and her loved ones.

Nursing Care During the Prenatal Period

Nursing Diagnosis

The nurse may see a pregnant woman only once every 4 to 6 weeks during the first several months of her pregnancy. To ensure continuity of care, therefore, a written care plan that incorporates assessment data, nursing diagnoses, and patient goals is essential.

The nurse can anticipate that, for many women with a low-risk pregnancy, certain nursing diagnoses will be made more frequently than others. Nursing diagnoses will, of course, vary from woman to woman and according to the time in the pregnancy. Examples of common nursing diagnoses include the following:

- *Constipation* related to the physiologic effects of pregnancy
- *Ineffective Sexuality Patterns* related to discomfort during late pregnancy

After formulating an appropriate diagnosis, the nurse establishes related goals to guide the nursing plan and interventions.

Nursing Plan and Implementation

Once nursing diagnoses have been identified, the next step is to establish priorities of nursing care. Sometimes priorities of care are based on the most immediate needs or concerns perceived by the woman. For example, during the first trimester, a woman is probably not ready to hear about labor and birth because she is likely to have more immediate concerns, such as nausea or concerns about sexual intimacy with her partner.

At other times priorities may develop as a result of findings during a prenatal visit. For example, the nurse may stress the need for frequent rest periods for a woman who is showing signs of preeclampsia (a pregnancy complication discussed in chapter 20 ∞). However, the woman may feel well physically and find it difficult to accept the nurse's emphasis on rest. It is the responsibility of medical and nursing professionals to help the woman and her family understand the significance of a problem and to plan appropriate interventions to deal with it.

The intervention methods most used by nurses in caring for the expectant woman and her family are communication techniques and teaching-learning strategies. These intervention methods are often used in groups, such as early pregnancy classes and childbirth education classes, but the nurse in the prenatal setting also applies these techniques with individuals.

Community-Based Nursing Care

Prenatal care, especially for women with low-risk pregnancies, is community based, typically in a clinic or private office. The healthcare community recognizes the value of providing a primary care nurse in these settings to coordinate care for each childbearing family. The nurse in a clinic or health maintenance organization (HMO) may be the only source of continuity for the woman, who may see a different physician or certified nurse-midwife at each visit. The nurse can be extremely effective in working with the expectant family by answering their questions; providing them with complete information about pregnancy, appropriate prenatal self-care measures, and community resources or referral agencies; and supporting the healthcare activities of the woman and her family. Communities often have a wealth of services and educational opportunities available for pregnant women and their families, and the knowledgeable nurse can help the woman access these services. This allows the family to assume equal responsibility with healthcare providers in working toward their common goal of a positive childbearing experience.

HOME CARE Home care can be of benefit to any pregnant woman, but it is especially effective in removing barriers for women who have difficulty accessing health care. These barriers may include lack of locally available healthcare facilities, problems with transportation to the facility, or schedule conflicts with available appointment times because of employment hours or family responsibilities.

In-home nursing assessments vary according to the scope of practice of the nurse and include current history and those screening procedures typically completed in an office or clinic: vital signs, weight, urine screen, physical activity, and dietary intake. Advanced practice nurses can also assess reflexes, perform tests of fetal well-being, and even do cervical examinations. Once the assessments are completed, the nurse can determine the level of follow-up home care or telephone contact needed.

A prenatal home care visit or phone contact can also be useful for women who anticipate a short inpatient stay after childbirth. At the prenatal contact, the nurse explains the postpartum program and answers any questions the woman or her family has.

Although the use of home care for women with uncomplicated pregnancies is growing, it is most often used for women with prenatal complications that can be managed without hospitalization if effective nursing assessment and care are provided in the home (see chapters 19 and 20).

HEALTH PROMOTION EDUCATION

Throughout the prenatal period the nurse provides informal and formal teaching to the childbearing family designed to help the family carry out self-care when appropriate and to report changes that may indicate a possible health problem. The teaching is most effective if timed to coincide with the woman's (couple's) readiness and needs (Table 16-1). The nurse also provides anticipatory guidance to help the family plan for changes that will occur following childbirth. The expectant couple should discuss issues that could be possible sources of postpartal stress. Issues to be resolved beforehand may include the sharing of infant and household chores, help in the first few days, reapportionment of family finances, options for baby-sitting to allow the mother (and couple) some free time, the mother's return to work after the baby's birth, and sibling rivalry.

TABLE 16-1 Topics for Patient Teaching During Pregnancy

All Three Trimesters
- Discomforts of pregnancy (see Table 16-3)
- Nutrition and weight gain
- Sexual activity
- Sibling preparation

First Trimester
- Attitude toward pregnancy
- Exercise and rest
- Smoking; use of alcohol and other drugs
- Traveling
- Fetal growth and development
- Danger signals associated with spontaneous abortion
- Employment
- Early pregnancy classes

Second Trimester
- Concerns related to changes in body
- Fetal growth and development
- Fetal movement
- Clothing
- Care of skin and breasts
- Beginning preparation for care of the infant (equipment and room)
- Decisions about infant feeding

Third Trimester
- Exercise and rest
- Traveling
- Danger signals
- Preparation for labor and birth
- Completion of preparation in home for new baby
- Decisions about the infant (circumcision, method of feeding, and so forth)
- Decision making for the early postpartum period
- Education about psychologic and physical expectations in the early postpartum period

Care of the Pregnant Woman's Family

Relieving the expectant woman's discomforts, maintaining her physical health, and providing anticipatory guidance are important parts of nursing care management. In addition, the nurse helps meet the needs of the woman's family to better maintain the harmony and integrity of the family unit. The nurse does this by providing support and prenatal education. If the nurse is effective, family members may gain greater problem-solving ability, self-esteem, self-confidence, and ability to participate in health care.

Care of the Father

Although the father of the baby is generally present, his presence cannot be assumed. If he is not a part of the family structure, it is important to assess the woman's support system to determine what significant persons in her life will play a major role during this childbearing experience.

When the father is part of the family or support system, providing anticipatory guidance to him is a necessary part of any plan of care. He may need information about the anatomic, physiologic, and emotional changes that occur during pregnancy and postpartum, the couple's sexuality and sexual response, and the reactions that he may experience. He may wish to express his feelings about breastfeeding versus formula-feeding, the sex of the child, and other topics. If it is culturally acceptable to the couple and personally acceptable to him, the nurse refers the couple to expectant parents' classes. These classes provide valuable information about pregnancy and childbirth using a variety of teaching strategies such as discussion, films, demonstrations with educational models, and written handouts. Some classes even give fathers the opportunity to get a "feel" for pregnancy by wearing a pregnancy simulator (Figure 16-1 ■).

The nurse assesses the father's intended degree of participation during labor and birth and his knowledge of what to ex-

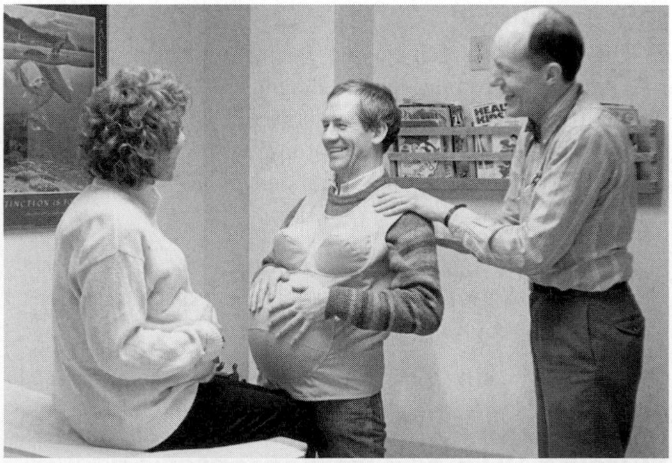

Figure 16-1 ■ The Empathy Belly® is a pregnancy simulator that allows males and females to experience some of the symptoms of pregnancy. The "belly," which weighs 33 lb, produces symptoms such as shortness of breath, bladder pressure, shift in the center of gravity with resulting waddling gait, increased lordosis and backache, and fatigue. It can also simulate fetal kicking movements.

Source: Used with permission from Birthways Childbirth Resource Center.

pect. If the couple prefers that his participation be minimal or restricted, the nurse supports their decision and does not try to impose personal values. Research indicates that increased focus on the father's needs during prenatal care aids his transition to fatherhood and also improves the mother's emotional status in the postpartum period (Condon, 2006). With this type of consideration and collaboration, the father is less apt to develop feelings of alienation, helplessness, and guilt during the pregnancy. Assessing and fostering progress in the father's journey to becoming a parent has significant long-term benefits for the man, his partner, and their child (Condon, 2006).

Care of Siblings and Other Family Members

In the plan for prenatal care, the nurse considers the effect of the pregnancy on any other children the couple may have. For example, the nurse may initiate a discussion about the ambivalence that older children may feel about the pregnancy. Parents who are unprepared for the older child's feelings of anger, jealousy, and rejection may respond inappropriately in their confusion and surprise. The nurse emphasizes that open communication between parents and children (or acting out feelings with a doll if the child is too young to verbalize) helps children master their feelings and may prevent them from hurting the baby when they are unsupervised. Children may feel less neglected and more secure if they know that their parents are willing to listen to their expressions of sadness or to help with their anger and aggressiveness.

Parents may be encouraged to bring their children to antepartal visits. Seeing what is involved and listening to the fetal heartbeat may make the pregnancy more real to siblings. Many agencies also provide sibling classes geared to different ages and levels of understanding. Relationship changes with in-laws should be addressed as well as the woman's or couple's expectations of the grandparents. Although some grandparents are eager to assist with child care by baby-sitting, others are not. The parents should also give some thought to the best ways of dealing with possible conflicts with the grandparents over childrearing approaches. Couples resolve these issues in different ways; however, postpartal adjustment is easier for a couple who agrees on the issues beforehand than for a couple who does not confront and resolve these issues.

Cultural Considerations in Pregnancy

As discussed in chapter 2 ∞, the increasingly diverse population in the United States, Canada, and in other countries around the world, requires a more inclusive approach—culturally competent care—to the delivery of care to people who belong to diverse and multicultural groups. The cultural competence approach allows care providers to include patients' cultural backgrounds in their care; this approach, however, does not examine the role of individual experience in people's health-related values, beliefs, and behaviors. The concept of *cultural humility* has been proposed as a more suitable goal in multicultural education. Cultural humility focuses on the process of intercultural exchange, paying explicit attention to clarifying the care provider's values and beliefs through self-reflection and self-critique—in other words, identifying the caregiver's own biases; additionally, it incorporates the characteristics of both the care provider and the patient into a mutually beneficial and balanced relationship (Community Partnership for Older Adults, 2007). Being open to cultural differences and learning from patients about their beliefs, values, and practices helps caregivers build relationships based on similarities.

By assessing each woman individually, the cultural humility approach removes the need to know the cultural features of every diverse group. Consequently, prenatal care should always include a discussion that clarifies each woman's health-related values and beliefs.

DEVELOPING CULTURAL COMPETENCE

Pregnant Women of African American Heritage

In caring for pregnant women of African American heritage, it is helpful to consider the following general points (Purnell, 2009):

- African American pregnant women may be guided by their extended family into common practices such as geophagia, the ingestion of dirt or clay, which is believed to alleviate mineral deficiencies. This practice has implications for the focus of teaching a nurse offers.
- Many African American families are matriarchal. Women are respected and heeded in decision making and often stress good behavior and firm parenting with their children, especially to keep them safe in dangerous situations.
- Three-generation extended families are common, and the grandmother is often highly respected for her wisdom. She may play a critical role in the care of the children.
- Certain taboos may exist, such as the belief in the necessity to avoid taking pictures during pregnancy to prevent stillbirths. Some women of African American descent may also believe that the purchase of infant clothing or supplies can result in a stillbirth. Thus they may appear to be unprepared for the arrival of the baby.

This conversation allows the nurse to adapt to the specific healthcare needs of each perinatal patient. Using the nursing process, the nurse can then formulate a transcultural nursing diagnosis that is focused on the cultural beliefs of the specific woman. The nursing diagnosis should reflect cultural sensitivity and build on the strengths of the patient, such as "***Anxiety*** related to culturally unusual expectations for behavior and treatment" (Mattson, 2004).

A major goal of transcultural nursing is to understand and assist people of diverse cultural groups with their healthcare needs. Culturally sensitive nurses recognize that each childbearing family, shaped by culture and life experience, has expectations of both its members and the healthcare system during pregnancy and birth.

Pregnancy and childbirth are recognized as special or transitional events in virtually all cultures (Lauderdale, 2008). Additionally, specific actions during pregnancy are often determined by cultural beliefs. According to Mattson (2004), these beliefs can be divided into three types:

- Prescriptive beliefs or requirements that describe expected behaviors

- Restrictive beliefs, which are stated negatively and limit behaviors
- Taboo beliefs, which refer to specific supernatural consequences

These activities are viewed as having the potential to impact the outcome of the pregnancy either positively or negatively. Table 16-2 describes activities that are encouraged (prescriptive) or forbidden (restrictive) or taboo by specific cultures. The table is not meant to be all-inclusive but rather to offer a few examples of cultural activities that may be important to some patients during the prenatal period.

In working with patients of another culture, the healthcare professional should be as open as possible to other beliefs. If certain activities are not harmful, there is no need to impose one's beliefs and practices on a person of another culture. If the activities are proving to be harmful, the nurse can consult or work with someone within the culture or someone aware of the cultural beliefs and values to see whether the patient's behavior can be modified (Figure 16-2 ■). See Nursing Care Plan: Language Barriers at First Prenatal Visit.

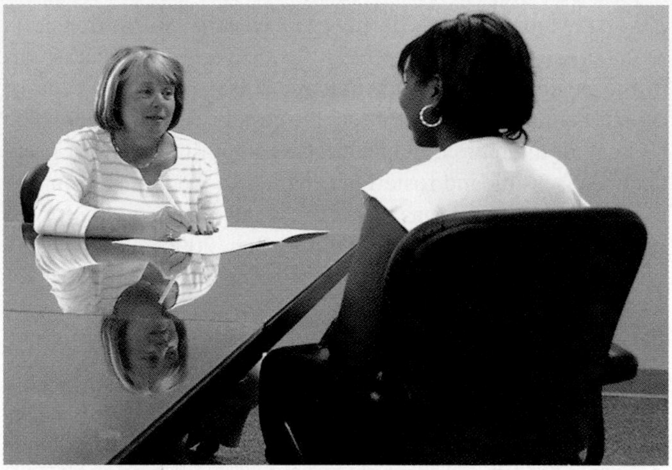

Figure 16-2 ■ The culturally competent nurse respects the culture and values of the pregnant woman.

TABLE 16-2 Cultural Beliefs and Practices During Pregnancy

These are a few examples of cultural beliefs and practices related to pregnancy. It is important not to make assumptions about a patient's beliefs, because cultural norms vary greatly within a culture and from generation to generation. The nurse should observe the patient carefully and take the time to ask questions. Patients will benefit greatly from the nurse's increased awareness of their cultural beliefs and practices.

BELIEF OR PRACTICE	NURSING CONSIDERATION
Home Remedies	
Pregnant women of Native American background may use herbal remedies. An example is the dandelion, which contains a milky juice in its stem believed to increase breast milk flow in mothers who choose to breastfeed (Spector, 2009). Patients of Chinese descent may drink ginseng tea for faintness after childbirth or as a sedative when mixed with bamboo leaves. Some people of African heritage may use self-medication for pregnancy discomforts—for example, laxatives to prevent or treat constipation (Purnell, 2009).	Find out what medications and home remedies your patient is using, and counsel your patient regarding overall effects. It is common for individuals to avoid telling healthcare workers about home remedies; the patient may feel this will be judged unfavorably. Phrase your questions in a sensitive, accepting way. In some cases, you might want to suggest remedies that may be more effective—for example, eating high-fiber foods to reduce constipation. If the home remedy is not harmful, there is no reason to ask a patient to discontinue this practice.
Nutrition	
Some women of Italian background may believe that it is necessary to satisfy desires for certain foods in order to prevent congenital anomalies. Also, they may believe that they must eat food that they smell, or else the fetus will move "inside," which will result in a miscarriage. Pregnant women of Vietnamese descent are considered to be in a weak, cold state and must correct this by eating and drinking hot foods during the first trimester (Purnell, 2009).	Discuss the patient's beliefs and practices in regard to nutrition during pregnancy. Obtain a diet history from the patient. Discuss the importance of a well-balanced diet during pregnancy with consideration of the patient's cultural beliefs and practices.
Alternative Healthcare Providers	
Pregnant women of Mexican background may choose to seek out the care of a *partera* (midwife) for prenatal and intrapartal care. A partera speaks their language, shares a similar culture, and can care for pregnant women at home or in a birthing center instead of a hospital. Some people in Hispanic American communities may use the *curandero,* the folk healer. The curanderos are believed to have received their gift from God and may prescribe over-the-counter medications (Purnell, 2009).	Discuss the variety of choices of healthcare providers available to the pregnant woman. Contrast the benefits and risks of different settings for prenatal care and birth. Provide reassurance that the goal of health care during pregnancy and birth is a healthy outcome for mother and baby with respect for the specific cultural beliefs and practices of the patient.
Exercise	
Pregnant women of Korean descent may work hard toward the end of pregnancy to increase the chances of delivering a small baby (Purnell, 2009). Some people of European, African, and Mexican descent believe that reaching over the head during pregnancy can harm the baby.	Ask your patient whether there are any activities she is afraid to do because of the pregnancy. Assure her that reaching over her head will not harm the baby, and evaluate other activities to their effect on the pregnancy.
Spirituality	
Navajo Indians are aware of the mind-soul connection and may try to follow certain practices to have a healthy pregnancy and birth. Practices could include focus on peace and positive thoughts as well as certain types of prayers and ceremonies. A traditional healer may assist them (Purnell, 2009). Some people of European background may tend to pay more attention to spirituality in their life to alleviate fears and ensure a safe birth.	Encourage the use of support systems and spiritual aids that provide comfort for the mother.

NURSING CARE PLAN Language Barriers at First Prenatal Visit

INTERVENTION	RATIONALE
1. Nursing Diagnosis: Ineffective Health Maintenance related to alteration in verbal and written communication skills **Goal:** Patient will demonstrate understanding of health information received during prenatal visits.	
■ If no interpreter is available, refer to posters with pictures to explain routine care and procedures during the prenatal examination.	■ Posters put words into verbal images and are helpful in communicating information.
■ Provide handouts and brochures about prenatal care in the woman's native language.	■ Translated handouts provide information that the patient can refer to at home. This reinforces information discussed during the visit and helps the family understand what the woman will experience during the pregnancy and at each visit.
■ Use teaching models to demonstrate procedures. Teaching models may include plastic pelvis, knitted uterus, fetal model, breast model, birth control devices, ultrasound equipment, and so forth.	■ Visual aids help to communicate information during the examination.
■ Schedule an interpreter for subsequent prenatal visits.	■ If a family member cannot translate the health information to the patient, an independent translator is essential to ensure that information is accurately provided. When an interpreter is used (especially a family member), the nurse should be sure that the interpreter is translating information received from the woman and not simply answering the questions for her.
■ Refer the woman to prenatal classes taught in her own language, if available.	■ Prenatal classes taught in the woman's language enable her to receive health information that is easily understood, which will prove a better understanding of what she should expect during pregnancy, birth, and postpartum. Prenatal classes may also provide a social outlet for patients.
■ Involve other members of the healthcare team in planning and providing care.	■ Cultures vary in language, nonverbal expression, dietary habits, use of time, spatial expectations, and so forth. Use of medication and blood products may also be influenced by cultural beliefs. Social workers who are familiar with the patient's cultural beliefs, for example, may help the patient adjust to different healthcare practices while providing suggestions to ensure prenatal care that is more in line with the woman's cultural beliefs. Dietitians may help the woman plan meals that are aligned with her cultural practices while meeting the nutritional needs of pregnancy.

EXPECTED OUTCOME: Effective communication occurs. The patient will gain an understanding of basic prenatal information as evidenced by using hand gestures, by pointing to pictures on posters and translated phrases on handouts, and through an interpreter, if one is available.

PROFESSIONALISM IN PRACTICE

In providing effective, culturally sensitive care, nurses can use the following strategies (College of Nurses of Ontario, 2009):

- Take actions that help break down language barriers.
- Explain the reasons for suggestions made to the woman or couple.
- Integrate folk treatments and Western medicine as much as possible.
- Enlist the family caretaker and others as needed.
- Get permission or consent to act from the right person.
- Provide printed materials in the patient's language.

Relief of the Common Discomforts of Pregnancy

Healthcare professionals often refer to the common discomforts of pregnancy as minor discomforts. These discomforts, however, are not minor to the pregnant woman.

Most of the discomforts of pregnancy are a result of physiologic and anatomic changes and are fairly specific to either the first trimester or to the second and third trimesters. Table 16-3 identifies the common discomforts of pregnancy, their possible causes, and the self-care measures that might relieve the discomfort.

TABLE 16-3 Health Promotion Education: Self-Care Measures for Common Discomforts of Pregnancy

DISCOMFORT	INFLUENCING FACTORS	SELF-CARE MEASURES
First Trimester		
Nausea and vomiting	Increased levels of human chorionic gonadotropin Changes in carbohydrate metabolism Emotional factors Fatigue	Avoid odors or causative factors. Eat dry crackers or toast before arising in morning. Have small but frequent meals. Avoid greasy or highly seasoned foods. Take dry meals with fluids between meals. Drink carbonated beverages.
Urinary frequency	Pressure of uterus on bladder in both first and third trimesters	Void when urge is felt. Increase fluid intake during the day. Decrease fluid intake *only* in the evening to decrease nocturia.
Fatigue	Specific causative factors unknown May be aggravated by nocturia due to urinary frequency	Plan time for a nap or rest period daily. Go to bed earlier. Seek family support and assistance with responsibilities so that more time is available to rest.
Breast tenderness	Increased levels of estrogen and progesterone	Wear well-fitting, supportive bra.
Increased vaginal discharge	Hyperplasia of vaginal mucosa and increased production of mucus by the endocervical glands due to the increase in estrogen levels	Promote cleanliness by daily bathing. Avoid douching, nylon underpants, and pantyhose; cotton underpants are more absorbent; powder can be used to maintain dryness if not allowed to cake.
Nasal stuffiness and nosebleed (epistaxis)	Elevated estrogen levels	May be unresponsive, but cool-air vaporizer may help; avoid use of nasal sprays and decongestants.
Ptyalism (excessive, often bitter salivation)	Specific causative factors unknown	Use astringent mouthwashes, chew gum, or suck hard candy.
Second and Third Trimesters		
Heartburn (pyrosis)	Increased production of progesterone, decreasing gastrointestinal motility and increasing relaxation of cardiac sphincter, displacement of stomach by enlarging uterus, thus regurgitation of acidic gastric contents into the esophagus	Eat small and more frequent meals. Use low-sodium antacids. Avoid overeating, fatty and fried foods, lying down after eating, and sodium bicarbonate.
Ankle edema	Prolonged standing or sitting Increased levels of sodium due to hormonal influences Circulatory congestion of lower extremities Increased capillary permeability Varicose veins	Practice frequent dorsiflexion of feet when prolonged sitting or standing is necessary. Elevate legs when sitting or resting. Avoid tight garters or restrictive bands around legs.
Varicose veins	Venous congestion in the lower veins that increases with pregnancy Hereditary factors (weakening of walls of veins, faulty valves) Increased age and weight gain	Elevate legs frequently. Wear supportive hose. Avoid crossing legs at the knees, standing for long periods, garters, and hosiery with constrictive bands.
Hemorrhoids	Constipation (see following discussion) Increased pressure from gravid uterus on hemorrhoidal veins	Avoid constipation. Apply ice packs, topical ointments, anesthetic agents, warm soaks, or sitz baths; gently reinsert into rectum as necessary.
Constipation	Increased levels of progesterone, which cause general bowel sluggishness Pressure of enlarging uterus on intestine Iron supplements Diet, lack of exercise, and decreased fluids	Increase fluid intake, fiber in the diet, and exercise. Develop regular bowel habits. Use stool softeners as recommended by physician.
Backache	Increased curvature of the lumbosacral vertebrae as the uterus enlarges Increased levels of hormones, which cause softening of cartilage in body joints Fatigue Poor body mechanics	Use proper body mechanics. Practice the pelvic-tilt exercise. Avoid uncomfortable working heights, high-heeled shoes, lifting heavy loads, and fatigue.
Leg cramps	Imbalance of calcium/phosphorus ratio Increased pressure of uterus on nerves Fatigue Poor circulation to lower extremities Pointing the toes	Practice dorsiflexion of feet to stretch affected muscle. Evaluate diet. Apply heat to affected muscles. Arise slowly from resting position.

TABLE 16-3 Health Promotion Education: Self-Care Measures for Common Discomforts of Pregnancy continued

DISCOMFORT	INFLUENCING FACTORS	SELF-CARE MEASURES
Second and Third Trimesters		
Faintness	Postural hypotension Sudden change of position causing venous pooling in dependent veins Standing for long periods in warm area Anemia	Avoid prolonged standing in warm or stuffy environments. Evaluate hematocrit and hemoglobin.
Dyspnea	Decreased vital capacity from pressure of enlarging uterus on the diaphragm	Use proper posture when sitting and standing. Sleep propped up with pillows for relief if problem occurs at night.
Flatulence	Decreased gastointestinal motility leading to delayed emptying time Pressure of growing uterus on large intestine Air swallowing	Avoid gas-forming foods. Chew food thoroughly. Get regular daily exercise. Maintain normal bowel habits.
Carpal tunnel syndrome	Compression of median nerve in carpal tunnel of wrist Aggravated by repetitive hand movements	Avoid aggravating hand movements. Use splint as prescribed. Elevate affected arm.

CLINICAL TIP
At each prenatal visit, focus your teaching on changes or possible discomforts the woman might encounter during the coming month and the next trimester. If the pregnancy is progressing normally, spend a few minutes describing her baby at this stage of development.

First Trimester

The dramatic hormonal changes of the first trimester account for many of the discomforts experienced in this period. These discomforts tend to abate by the beginning of the fourth month of pregnancy.

Nausea and Vomiting

Nausea and vomiting of pregnancy (NVP) are early, very common symptoms. These symptoms appear sometime after the first missed menstrual period and usually cease by the fourth missed menstrual period. Research indicates that approximately 70% to 85% of pregnant women experience NVP (American College of Obstetricians and Gynecologists [ACOG], 2004). Some women develop an aversion only to specific foods. Many experience nausea on arising in the morning, and others experience nausea only in the evening.

The exact cause of NVP is unknown but is believed to be multifactorial. Research has identified possible hormonal, metabolic, neurologic, and psychosomatic factors contributing to its development. Relaxation of the smooth muscle of the stomach contributes to this common discomfort (Johnson, Gregory, & Niebyl, 2007). Human chorionic gonadotropin (hCG) is often cited as a major factor because it begins to be present in the body at about the time symptoms of morning sickness usually begin, and hCG levels are subsiding when the discomfort of nausea and vomiting usually ends. Changes in carbohydrate metabolism, fatigue, and emotional factors may also play a role in the development of NVP.

HEALTH PROMOTION EDUCATION Treatment of nausea and vomiting is not always successful, but the symptoms can be reduced. To decrease the potential for development of hyperemesis gravidarum, ACOG (2004) recommends the initiation of prompt treatment for nausea and vomiting. It is beneficial for the healthcare professional to provide empathetic recognition of the pregnant woman's symptoms and distress as well as provide safe and effective treatment suggestions (Locock, Alexander, & Rozmovits, 2008; Wills & Forster, 2008).

The nurse needs to assess the onset, frequency, duration, and severity of symptoms and actual nutritional intake to be helpful in suggesting methods of relief or necessary medical care (Lacasse, Rey, Ferreira, et al., 2009; McParlin, Graham, & Robson, 2008). Physical assessment of the woman should include particular attention to skin color, texture, and turgor as well as vital signs and bowel sounds. For some women, simply avoiding the odor of certain foods or other conditions that precipitate the problem may relieve nausea. If nausea occurs most frequently during early morning, the woman may find it helpful to eat dry crackers or toast before arising and to rise from bed slowly. Rising slowly and avoiding sudden position changes throughout the day may also help prevent nausea due to hypotensive episodes. In addition, the nurse can suggest that the woman avoid brushing her teeth right after eating, because this, too, may trigger vomiting. Evidence suggests that a pregnant woman should start a multivitamin before reaching 6 weeks' gestation to reduce the effects of nausea and vomiting (ACOG, 2004).

Generally, it is helpful to eat small meals every 2 to 3 hours during the day and to avoid greasy or highly seasoned foods. Food may be salted to taste. The salt increases the palatability of the food and replaces any chloride lost when the woman vomits hydrochloric acid from the stomach. Eating dry meals and taking all liquids, including soups, between meals may help some women by avoiding overdistention of the stomach. Sudden changes in blood sugar levels can be avoided if the small meals are high in low-fat protein or complex carbohydrates. Some women find that slowly sipping herbal tea (peppermint, chamomile, or spearmint) or a carbonated beverage helps reduce nausea.

In addition to common self-care measures, certain complementary or alternative therapies may be useful. For example, many women find that acupressure applied to pressure points in the wrists is helpful (Figure 16-3 ■). ACOG (2004) reports that the

Case Study: First Trimester Patient

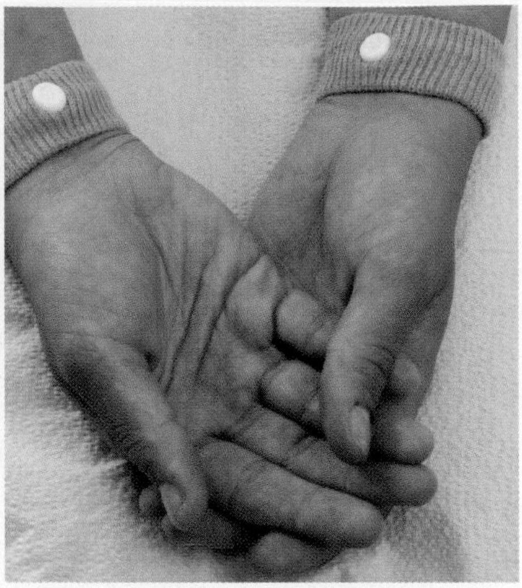

Figure 16-3 ■ Acupressure wristbands are sometimes used to help relieve nausea during early pregnancy.

Source: Patrick Watson/Pearson Education.

evidence supporting or refuting the use of acupressure for nausea and vomiting of pregnancy is unclear. Ginger may also relieve NVP. Ginger, long used in traditional Chinese medicine for a variety of maladies ranging from gastrointestinal problems to headaches, is a popular, effective, and safe treatment for NVP (Ozgoli, Goli, & Simbar, 2009). Pyridoxine (vitamin B_6) alone or in combination with doxylamine (Unisom), an over-the-counter antihistamine, is considered a first-line treatment. See Research Evidence in Practice.

Antihistamine H_1 receptor blockers, benzamines, and phenothiazines are considered safe and effective for treating refractory cases. In very severe cases, methylprednisolone, a steroid, may be used, but as a last resort because it poses a potential risk to the fetus (ACOG, 2004).

Although some nausea is common, the woman who suffers from extreme nausea coupled with vomiting requires further assessment. She should be advised to contact her care provider if she vomits more than once per day or shows signs of dehydration, such as dry mouth, decreased amounts of highly concentrated urine, and the like. In such cases, the physician or certified nurse-midwife (CNM) may order antiemetics. However, antiemetics should be avoided if at all possible during the first trimester because of the danger of teratogenic effects on embryo development.

Nausea and vomiting symptoms generally decrease by the 16th week of pregnancy. If they do not, hyperemesis gravidarum, which occurs in 1% to 3% of pregnancies must be considered (Johnson et al., 2007). Hyperemesis symptoms include weight loss, dehydration, and nutrition imbalance (Katz, 2008).

RESEARCH EVIDENCE IN PRACTICE: Ginger as a Treatment for the Nausea and Vomiting of Pregnancy

CLINICAL QUESTIONS

Is ginger an effective treatment for the nausea and vomiting of early pregnancy? Is the use of ginger free of side effects for mother and baby?

RESEARCH EVIDENCE

The most common unpleasant symptom that presents during early pregnancy is nausea and vomiting, particularly upon arising. This condition can have effects on family and personal life, as well as implications for work life. However, most of the medications used to treat nausea and vomiting are not safe to use in early pregnancy, and so nonpharmacologic treatments are desirable. A large number of women—more than 75% in one large study—use alternative therapies during pregnancy, frequently without informing their physicians or midwives. However, many of these therapies have not been tested for efficacy or safety.

Ginger has demonstrated a positive effect in calming the gastrointestinal system and has been posed as an alternative to traditional medications in the treatment of nausea and vomiting. It is classified as a nutritional supplement by the Food and Drug Administration and is listed as a safe herbal preparation.

Vitamin B_6 has also been proposed as a potential treatment for nausea and vomiting, and it is considered a nutritional supplement that is safe to use during pregnancy. However, neither ginger nor vitamin B_6 has been thoroughly evaluated as to its relative effectiveness, the optimal dosage for symptom control, or the most appropriate form of administration.

In one strong randomized trial, ginger was more effective than vitamin B_6 in treating the nausea and vomiting of early pregnancy, although both were effective in reducing episodes of vomiting. A separate randomized trial focused on the optimal daily dosage. Women who ingested 250 mg of ginger, administered in capsules 4 times a day, had fewer episodes of vomiting and less reported nausea than women who had smaller doses or who were given a placebo. No adverse effects were reported for mothers or babies who used either ginger or vitamin B_6.

WHAT QUESTIONS REMAIN UNANSWERED?

Is it necessary to administer the ginger in separate doses throughout the day, or could a single dose be effective? If a woman chooses to use vitamin B_6 instead of ginger, what is the optimal dosage?

WHAT IS BEST PRACTICE?

Women who are experiencing nausea and vomiting in early pregnancy can be encouraged to take 250 mg ginger capsules 4 times daily to minimize their symptoms. They can be reassured that the treatment will have no ill effects on their babies. Vitamin B_6 may also be recommended to control vomiting but with the caution that it may be less effective in controlling nausea than ginger.

CRITICAL THINKING

What are alternative ways of ingesting ginger if capsules or repetitive dosing is not effective? How can the pregnant woman's diet be modified to ingest both ginger and vitamin B_6 naturally and safely?

References

Ensiyeh, J., & Mohammad-Alizadeh, C. (2009). Comparing ginger and vitamin B_6 for the treatment of nausea and vomiting in early pregnancy: a randomized controlled trial. *Midwifery, 25*, 649–653.

Holst, L., Wright, D., Haavik, S., & Hedvig, N. (2009). The use and the user of herbal remedies during pregnancy. *The Journal of Alternative and Complementary Therapies, 15*(7), 787–792.

Ozgoli, G., Goli, M., & Simbar, M. (2009). Effects of ginger capsules on pregnancy, nausea, and vomiting. *The Journal of Alternative and Complementary Therapies, 15*(3), 243–246.

Urinary Frequency

Urinary frequency, a common discomfort of pregnancy, occurs early in pregnancy and again during the third trimester because of the pressure of the enlarging uterus on the bladder. Approximately 40% to 50% of pregnant women experience urinary incontinence, particularly, in the third trimester (Johnson et al., 2007). Although the glomerular filtration rate increases in pregnancy, it does not cause a significant increase in urine output. Urinary frequency is considered normal during the first and third trimesters; however, the nurse should advise the woman to contact her healthcare provider if she experiences any signs of bladder infection such as painful urination (dysuria), burning with voiding, or blood in the urine (hematuria).

HEALTH PROMOTION EDUCATION There are no methods of decreasing the frequency of urination in pregnancy. Fluid intake should never be decreased to prevent frequency. The woman should be encouraged to maintain an adequate fluid intake: at least 2000 ml per day. She should also be encouraged to empty her bladder frequently (approximately every 2 hours while awake).

Frequent bladder emptying helps decrease the incidence of leakage of urine. Because frequency often results in several trips to the bathroom each night, it is important to remind the woman to consider safety factors in the home, such as a clear path to the bathroom, the use of a night-light, and the like. The woman who leaks urine may choose to wear pantyliners during the day. If she does, she should change them as soon as they become damp to avoid perineal excoriation and to avoid contamination of the perineum from the rectal area if the pads move back and forth as she walks. Tightening of the pubococcygeus muscle, which supports internal organs and controls voiding, can help maintain good perineal tone. This procedure, known as Kegel exercise, is discussed later in this chapter.

Fatigue

Marked fatigue, often out of proportion to the woman's normal pattern, is so common in early pregnancy that it is considered a presumptive sign of pregnancy. The sleep-inducing effects of progesterone may play a role in the development of this sign (Cunningham et al., 2010). It is aggravated if the woman has to arise several times each night because of urinary frequency. Typically, it resolves soon after the end of the first trimester.

HEALTH PROMOTION EDUCATION Scheduling activities to allow for napping is helpful. Women should be encouraged to use every opportunity available to rest, including going to bed earlier in the evening. The woman's partner needs to understand that the fatigue is normal and will subside. The partner can be encouraged to assume more home responsibilities to support the woman and enable her to rest.

Breast Tenderness

Sensitivity of the breasts occurs early and continues throughout the pregnancy. Increased levels of estrogen and progesterone contribute to the soreness and tingling felt in the breasts and to the increased sensitivity of the nipples.

HEALTH PROMOTION EDUCATION A well-fitting, supportive brassiere gives the most relief for this discomfort. The qualities of a properly supportive brassiere are discussed in "Breast Care" later in this chapter.

Increased Vaginal Discharge

Increased whitish vaginal discharge, called **leukorrhea**, is common in pregnancy. It occurs as the result of hyperplasia of vaginal mucosa and increased production of mucus by the endocervical glands. In addition, the increased acidity of the secretions encourages the growth of *Candida albicans,* and the woman is thus more susceptible to monilial vaginitis.

HEALTH PROMOTION EDUCATION Cleanliness is important in preventing excoriation and vaginal infections. Daily bathing is adequate; douching is avoided during pregnancy. The woman should avoid nylon underpants and pantyhose because they retain heat and moisture in the genital area; absorbent cotton underpants should be worn to help prevent problems. The nurse can advise the pregnant woman to report any change in vaginal discharge, any irritation in the perineal area, and intense vaginal itching. These changes frequently indicate vaginal infections.

Nasal Stuffiness and Epistaxis

Once pregnancy is well established, elevated estrogen levels may produce edema of the nasal mucosa, resulting in nasal stuffiness, nasal discharge, and obstruction (rhinitis of pregnancy). *Epistaxis* (nosebleed) may also result.

HEALTH PROMOTION EDUCATION Cool air vaporizers and normal saline nose drops may be helpful. However, the problem is often unresponsive to treatment. Women experiencing these problems find it difficult to sleep and may resort to medicated nasal sprays and decongestants to relieve the problem. Such interventions may provide relief initially but can actually increase the nasal stuffiness over time. The use of any medication in pregnancy should be avoided if possible.

Ptyalism

Ptyalism is a rare discomfort of pregnancy in which excessive, often bitter, saliva is produced. Its cause has not been established, although it may be related to the ingestion of starch (Cunningham et al., 2010). Effective treatments are limited.

HEALTH PROMOTION EDUCATION Using astringent mouthwashes, chewing gum, or sucking on hard candy may minimize the problem of ptyalism. It may also be helpful to reduce or limit starch intake.

Second and Third Trimesters

It is difficult to classify discomforts as specifically occurring in the second or third trimester because their timing varies because of individual variations in women. The symptoms discussed in this section usually do not appear until the third trimester in primigravidas but may occur earlier with each succeeding pregnancy.

Heartburn (Pyrosis)

Heartburn is the regurgitation of acidic gastric contents into the esophagus. It creates a burning or irritating sensation in the esophagus and radiates upward, sometimes leaving a bad taste

Through the Eyes of a Nurse Physical Symptoms in the First Trimester of Pregnancy

Family's Experience

"I know that each pregnancy is different and some women have nausea and some don't but I feel so sick! I have a lot of nausea and feel awful most of the time. I am not really worried because I haven't lost weight, and I only throw up occasionally, but I would like to find better ways of handling this. I eat dry crackers in the morning and during the day but that only helps a little."

Nurse's Response

"Nausea and vomiting frequently occur in the first trimester of pregnancy as a result of changes in the gastrointestinal system as well as changes in carbohydrate metabolism. The nausea and vomiting commonly begin at 6 weeks and can continue another 6 to 12 weeks. Try small, frequent meals, avoiding hot and spicy foods. The use of antiemetic medication has been shown to reduce nausea. You might want to discuss that with your nurse-midwife. Some studies have also shown that vitamin B_6 reduces the severity of vomiting. Other studies have shown that ginger reduces nausea and vomiting, so you may want to consider taking that. We have also found that some women have found relief with acupressure bands. You can purchase these bands at any pharmacy. I would try these things and see if they help.

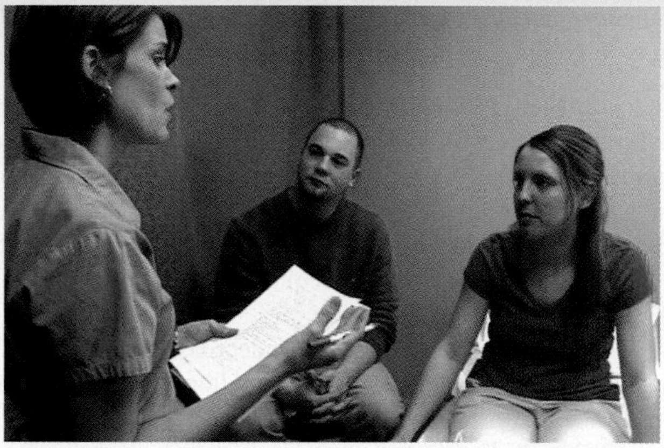

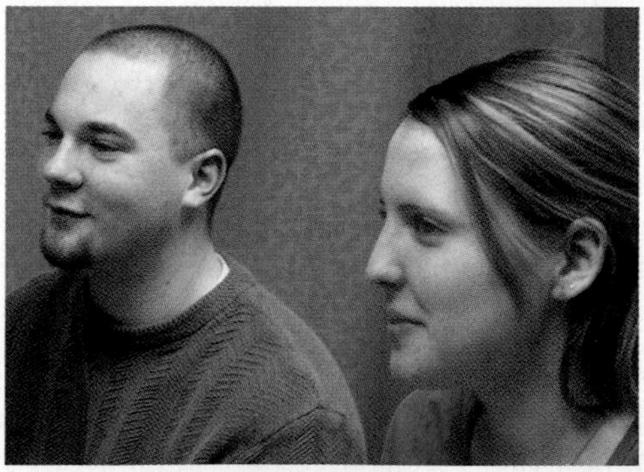

"We are monitoring your weight at each visit and checking your urine for ketones. You actually gained a pound and your urine is negative for ketones, so those are both good signs. Please let us know if the nausea and vomiting become so severe that you are unable to keep anything down within a 24-hour period. If you have questions or concerns, you can call us."

Nurse's Actions and Rationale

The nurse explains the physiologic process that leads to nausea and provides evidence-based information on ways of relieving or reducing nausea and vomiting (ACOG, 2004). As discussed in this chapter, interventions such as ginger, acupressure wrist bands, and vitamin B_6 are often helpful. The nurse also provides reassurance and explains how the woman will be monitored to ease the family's anxiety. Finally the nurse reassures the woman that she can call if questions arise and reviews the parameters for the woman to follow as to when to call the healthcare provider.

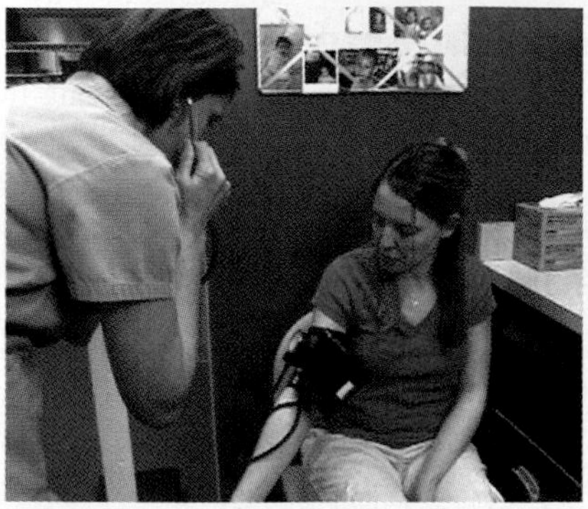

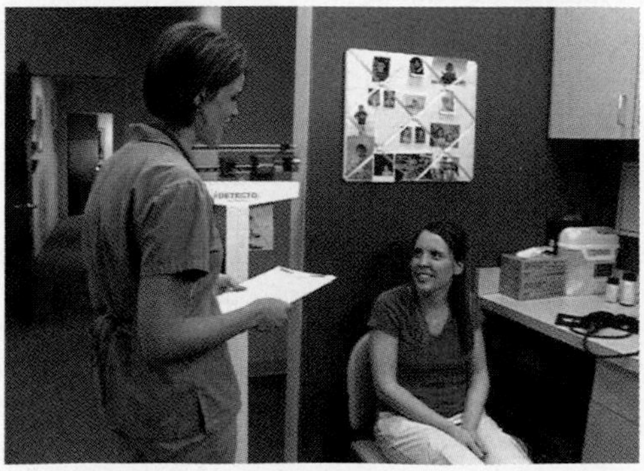

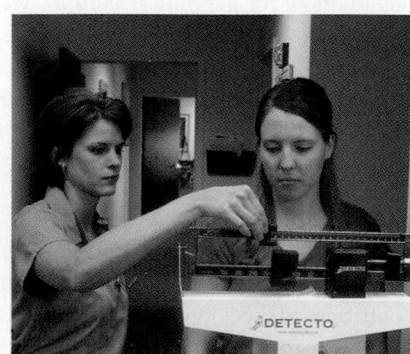

in the mouth. Heartburn appears to be primarily a result of the displacement of the stomach by the enlarging uterus. The increased production of progesterone in pregnancy, decreases in gastrointestinal motility, and relaxation of the cardiac (esophageal) sphincter also contribute to heartburn.

HEALTH PROMOTION EDUCATION Heartburn is aggravated by overeating, ingesting fatty and fried foods, and lying down soon after eating. The woman should, therefore, avoid these situations. The woman should be encouraged to drink an adequate amount of fluid (8 to 10 8-oz glasses) each day and to eat smaller, more frequent meals to accommodate the decreased size of her stomach. Good posture is important because it allows more room for the stomach to function. Some women choose complementary and alternative medicine (CAM) approaches to relieving their heartburn (see chapter 3 for more information about CAM).

The caregiver may recommend the liquid form of a low-sodium antacid, such as aluminum hydroxide (Amphojel) or a combination of aluminum hydroxide and magnesium hydroxide (Maalox). Because aluminum alone tends to cause constipation, and magnesium alone is associated with diarrhea, the combined approach is more desirable (Katz, 2008). Sodium bicarbonate (baking soda) and Alka-Seltzer should be avoided because of the potential for electrolyte imbalance.

If maternal heartburn is severe, not relieved by antacids, and accompanied by gastrointestinal reflux, an antisecretory agent (H_2-blocker) such as ranitidine (Zantac), cimetidine (Tagamet), or omeprazole (Losec) may be necessary. Research to date has not linked these medications with an excessive risk of birth defects, preterm birth, or intrauterine growth restriction.

Ankle Edema

Most women experience ankle edema in the last part of pregnancy because of the increasing difficulty of venous return from the lower extremities. Prolonged standing or sitting and warm weather increase the edema. It is also associated with varicose veins. Ankle edema becomes a concern only when accompanied by hypertension or proteinuria or when the edema is not postural in origin.

HEALTH PROMOTION EDUCATION The aggravating conditions just mentioned should be avoided. If the woman has to sit or stand for long periods, frequent dorsiflexion of her feet will help contract muscles, thereby squeezing the fluid back into circulation. The pregnant woman should not wear tight garters or other restrictive bands around her legs. During rest periods, the woman should elevate her legs and hips as described in the following section on varicose veins.

Varicose Veins

Varicose veins are a result of weakening of the walls of veins or faulty functioning of the valves. Poor circulation in the lower extremities predisposes the woman to varicose veins in the legs and thighs, as does prolonged standing or sitting. The weight of the gravid uterus on the pelvic veins aggravates the development of varicosities in the legs and pelvic area by preventing good venous return. Increased maternal age, excessive weight gain, a large fetus, heredity, and multiple gestation can all contribute to the problem. Symptoms may range from mildly unpleasant cosmetic effects to chronic pain and superficial thrombophlebitis.

Vulvar varicosities may also be a problem in pregnancy, although they are less common. Varicosities in the vulva and perineum cause aching and a sense of heaviness.

Treatment of varicose veins is not generally recommended during pregnancy (Cunningham et al., 2010). The woman should be aware that treatment might be needed after pregnancy because the problem will be aggravated by a succeeding pregnancy.

HEALTH PROMOTION EDUCATION Regular exercise, such as swimming, cycling, or walking, promotes venous return, which helps prevent varicosities. Avoiding factors that contribute to venous stasis is also helpful. The pregnant woman should avoid standing or sitting for prolonged periods. She should also avoid crossing her legs at the knees because of the pressure on her veins. She should not wear garters or hosiery with constricting bands, such as knee-high hose. However, supportive hose or elastic stockings may be extremely helpful. Supportive hose should be put on in the morning and should be washed daily with soap and warm water to help retain elasticity.

The pregnant woman should be encouraged to elevate her legs level with her hips when she sits. She can enhance comfort by supporting the entire leg rather than simply propping her feet up on a stool, which may lead to hyperextension of the knees. The woman who sits or stands for long periods should walk around frequently to promote venous return to the heart. She can also be encouraged to dorsiflex her feet, hold the position for 3 seconds, then release, with 8 to 10 repetitions several times each day. Venous return is most effectively promoted if the woman lies down with her feet elevated several times a day. To avoid difficulty related to pressure of the uterus on the vena cava, the woman can lie with her legs elevated on pillows and a pillow placed under one hip to displace the uterus to one side (Figure 16-4 ■).

Wearing one of the foam rubber commercial products that is placed across the perineum and held in place by a sanitary pad–type belt can provide support for vulvar varicosities (Cunningham et al., 2010). Elevation of only the legs aggravates vulvar varicosities by creating stasis of blood in the pelvic area. Therefore, it is important that the pelvic area also be elevated to promote venous drainage into the trunk of the body. More than one firm pillow under the hips may be needed to accomplish this elevation. Near the end of pregnancy, this position may be extremely awkward; the woman may best relieve uterine pressure on the pelvic veins by resting on her side. Blocks may also be placed under the foot of her bed to elevate it slightly.

Flatulence

Flatulence results from decreased gastrointestinal motility, leading to delayed emptying, and from pressure on the large intestine by the growing uterus. Air swallowing may also contribute to the problem.

HEALTH PROMOTION EDUCATION The woman should be advised to avoid gas-forming foods and to chew her food thoroughly. Regular bowel habits and exercise can also decrease flatulence.

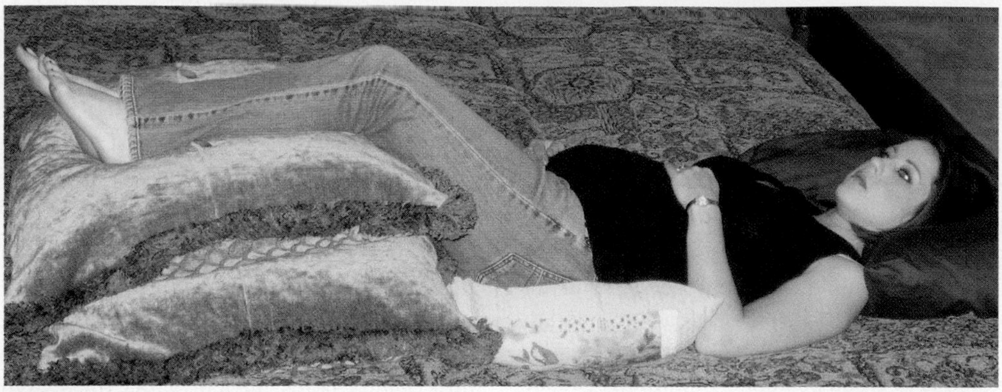

Figure 16-4 ■ Swelling and discomfort from varicosities can be decreased by lying down with the legs and one hip elevated (to avoid compression of the vena cava).

Hemorrhoids

Hemorrhoids are varicosities of the veins in the lower end of the rectum and anus. During pregnancy, the gravid uterus presses on the veins and interferes with venous circulation. As the pregnancy progresses, the straining that accompanies constipation can contribute to the development of hemorrhoids.

Hemorrhoids may not bother some women until the second stage of labor, when the hemorrhoids appear as they push just before birth. Hemorrhoids that occur in pregnancy or at birth usually become asymptomatic after the early postpartum period.

Symptoms of hemorrhoids include itching, swelling, pain, and bleeding. Internal hemorrhoids are located above the anal sphincter and are responsible for bleeding, usually with defecation. They are not usually painful unless they protrude from the anus. External hemorrhoids are located outside the anal sphincter. They are not usually the source of bleeding or pain; however, thrombosis of the hemorrhoids can occur, and in that case they become extremely painful. The thrombosis may resolve itself in 24 hours, or the physician can treat it by incising and evacuating the blood clot. Women who have hemorrhoids before pregnancy frequently experience more difficulties with them during pregnancy.

HEALTH PROMOTION EDUCATION Relief can be achieved by gently and carefully reinserting the hemorrhoids. The woman lies on her side or in the knee to chest position. She places some lubricant on her finger and presses against the hemorrhoids, pushing them inside. She holds them in place for 1 to 2 minutes and then gently withdraws her finger. The anal sphincter should then hold them inside the rectum. The woman will find it especially helpful if she can then maintain a side-lying (Sims') position for a time, so this procedure is best done before bed or before a daily rest period.

Avoiding constipation is important in preventing or relieving the discomfort of hemorrhoids. Relief measures for existing hemorrhoid symptoms include ice packs, use of topical ointments and anesthetic agents, and warm soaks.

The woman should contact her healthcare provider if the hemorrhoids become hardened and noticeably tender to touch. Rectal bleeding that is more than spotting following defecation should also be reported.

Constipation

Conditions in pregnancy that predispose the woman to constipation include general bowel sluggishness caused by increased progesterone and steroid metabolism; displacement of the intestines, which increases with the growth of the fetus; and oral iron supplements, which most pregnant women need.

HEALTH PROMOTION EDUCATION Increased fluid intake (at least 2000 ml/day), adequate roughage or bulk in the diet, regular bowel habits, and adequate daily exercise can often maintain good bowel function in women who have not had previous problems. The addition of dietary fiber, such as Metamucil, or surface active agents, such as Colace, can decrease constipation (Johnson et al., 2007). Some women find it helpful to drink a warm beverage or glass of prune juice in the morning. Women should leave sufficient time following breakfast so that the natural action of the body will produce defecation.

In severe or preexisting cases of constipation, the woman may need a mild laxative, stool softeners, or suppositories as recommended by her caregiver.

Backache

Over 50% of pregnant women experience backache during pregnancy (Johnson et al., 2007). Backache is due primarily to the increased curvature of the lumbosacral vertebrae that occurs as the uterus enlarges and becomes heavier. Circulating steroid hormones cause a softening and relaxation of pelvic joints, contributing to the problem. If the woman does not learn how to correct this curvature, the strain on the muscles and ligaments will cause backache. Low backache can occur at any point during pregnancy.

HEALTH PROMOTION EDUCATION An exercise called the pelvic tilt can help restore proper body alignment. As the anterior pelvis is tilted upward, the curvature of the back is automatically decreased, relieving much of the discomfort. There are many exercises that can be done by the pregnant woman to relieve symptoms of low back pain (Jeffcoat, 2008). See "Exercises to Prepare for Childbirth" later in this chapter.

The use of proper posture and good body mechanics throughout pregnancy is important. The pregnant woman

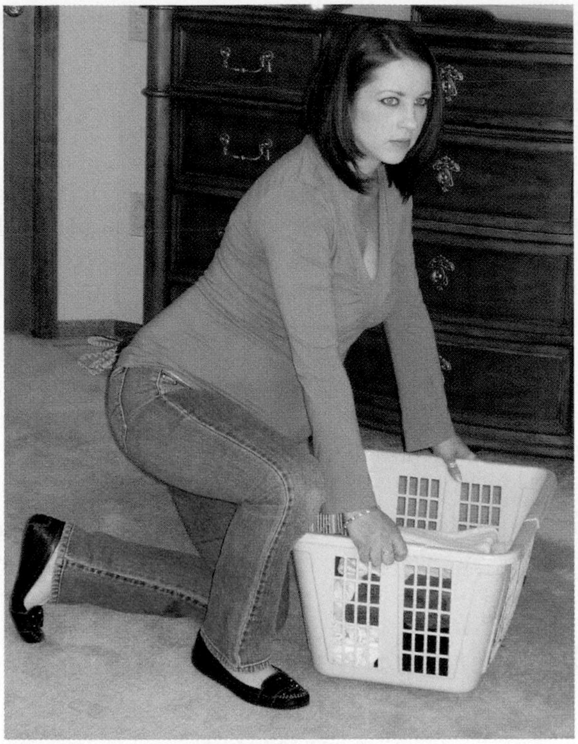

Figure 16-5 ■ When picking up objects from floor level or lifting objects, the pregnant woman must use proper body mechanics.

should avoid bending over to lift or pick up items from the floor. The strain is felt in the muscles of the back. Leg muscles should be used to do the work instead. The woman can keep her back straight by bending her knees to lower her body into the squatting position (Figure 16-5 ■). She should place her feet 12 to 18 inches apart to maintain body balance. When lifting a heavy object, such as a child, she should place one foot flat on the floor, slightly in front of the other foot, and lower herself to the other knee. The object is held close to her body for lifting. This same principle of keeping the back straight and bending the knees applies when the woman sits down or gets out of a chair. Work heights that require constant bending can contribute to backache and should be adjusted as necessary.

A pendulous abdomen contributes to backache by increasing the curvature of the spine. Although maternity support belts have been typically used to decrease low back pain in pregnancy, there is inadequate evidence to conclude that wearing them is effective (Ho, Yu, Lao, et al., 2009). The use of a supportive maternity girdle is discussed later in this chapter, as is the role of high-heeled shoes in increasing the lumbosacral curvature.

Leg Cramps

Nearly half of pregnant women experience recurrent, painful muscle spasms in the lower extremities (Katz, 2008).They occur most frequently at night after the woman has gone to bed but may occur at other times. Extension of the foot can often cause leg cramps. The nurse should warn the pregnant woman not to extend the foot during childbirth preparation exercises or during rest periods.

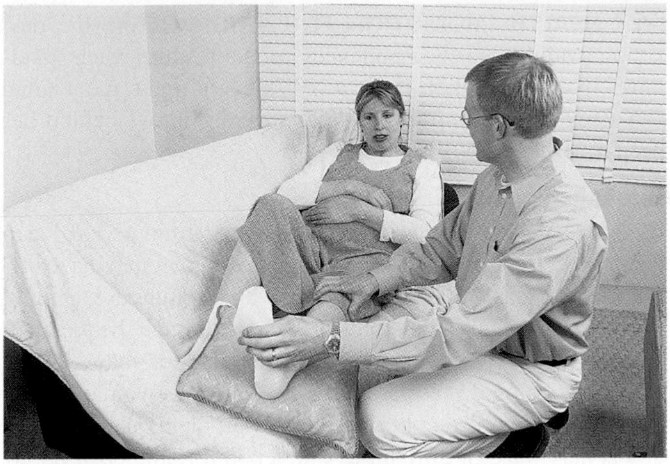

Figure 16-6 ■ The expectant father can help relieve the woman's painful leg cramps by flexing her foot and straightening her leg.

HEALTH PROMOTION EDUCATION The woman can achieve immediate relief of the muscle spasm by stretching the muscle. With the woman lying on her back, another person can press the woman's knee down to straighten her leg while pushing her foot toward her leg (Figure 16-6 ■). The woman may also stand and put her foot flat on the floor. Massage and warm packs can be used to alleviate discomfort from leg cramps. Stretching exercises before bedtime may help prevent leg cramps.

Faintness

Many pregnant women occasionally feel faint, especially in warm, crowded areas. Faintness is caused by a combination of changes in the blood volume and postural hypotension due to venous pooling of blood in the dependent veins. Sudden change of position or standing for prolonged periods can cause this sensation, and fainting can occur.

HEALTH PROMOTION EDUCATION The nurse should first be certain that the pregnant woman understands the symptoms of faintness. These include slight dizziness, a "swirling" or "floating" sensation, and a decreased ability to hear or focus attention. If a woman feels faint from prolonged standing or from being in a warm, crowded room, she should sit down and lower her head between her knees. If this procedure does not help, the woman should be assisted to an area where she can lie down and get fresh air. When arising from a resting position, she should move slowly. Women whose jobs require standing in one place for long periods should march in place regularly to increase venous return from the legs.

Care Plan Activity: Common Discomforts of Pregnancy

Shortness of Breath

Shortness of breath occurs as the uterus rises into the abdomen and causes pressure on the diaphragm. This problem worsens in the last trimester as the enlarged uterus presses directly on the diaphragm, decreasing vital capacity. The primigravida experiences considerable relief from shortness of breath in the last few weeks of pregnancy, when **lightening** occurs, and the fetus and uterus move down in the pelvis. Because the multigravida does not usually experience lightening until labor, shortness of breath will continue throughout her pregnancy.

HEALTH PROMOTION EDUCATION During the day, sitting straight in a chair and using proper posture when standing help provide relief. If distress is great at night, the woman can sleep propped up in bed with several pillows behind her head and shoulders.

Difficulty Sleeping

From 12 weeks of pregnancy into the postpartum period, sleep disturbances are common. The pregnant woman may have difficulty falling asleep or she may wake up throughout the night, resulting in fewer overall hours of sleep. Although the pregnant woman may experience difficulty sleeping for many of the same psychologic reasons as the nonpregnant woman, many physical factors also contribute to this problem. The enlarged uterus may make it difficult to find a comfortable position for sleep, and an active fetus may aggravate the problem. The other discomforts of pregnancy such as urinary frequency, shortness of breath, and leg cramps may also be contributing factors.

HEALTH PROMOTION EDUCATION The nurse should conduct a thorough assessment of the sleep habits of the pregnant woman and offer information about habits and activities that help promote restful sleep. The pregnant woman may find it helpful to drink a warm (caffeine-free) beverage before bed and may benefit from a soothing backrub given by her partner or a family member. Pillows may be used to provide support for her back, between her legs, or for her upper arm when she lies on her side. Relaxation techniques may also help. The woman should avoid caffeine products, stimulating activity, and sleeping medication.

Restless Leg Syndrome

Approximately 25% of pregnant women develop restless leg syndrome (RLS), particularly in the second half of pregnancy. RLS is characterized by the need to move the legs and tingling or other sensations in the calves, usually as the woman falls asleep (Katz, 2008).

HEALTH PROMOTION EDUCATION RLS has been associated with iron deficiency anemia, so iron supplements may decrease leg restlessness. Also, to avoid increasing RLS symptoms, pregnant women should avoid caffeine products later in the day (Katz, 2008).

Round Ligament Pain

As the uterus enlarges during pregnancy, the round ligaments stretch, hypertrophy, and lengthen as the uterus rises up in the abdomen. Round ligament pain is attributed to this stretching.

HEALTH PROMOTION EDUCATION The woman may feel concern when she first experiences round ligament pain because it is often intense and causes a "grabbing" sensation in the lower abdomen and inguinal area. The nurse should warn women of this possible discomfort. Few treatment measures really alleviate this discomfort, but understanding the cause will help decrease anxiety. Once the caregiver has ascertained that the cause of the discomfort is not related to a medical complication such as appendicitis or gallbladder disease, the woman may find that a heating pad applied to the abdomen brings some relief. She may also benefit from bringing her knees up on her abdomen.

Carpal Tunnel Syndrome

Carpal tunnel syndrome (CTS), characterized by numbness and tingling of the hand near the thumb, occurs in about 25% to 50% of pregnant women (Johnson et al., 2007). It is caused by compression of the median nerve in the carpal tunnel of the wrist. The syndrome is commonly bilateral but may be more pronounced in the dominant hand and is characterized by numbness, tingling, or burning in the fleshy part of the palm near the thumb. The syndrome is aggravated by repetitive hand movements, such as typing/keyboarding, and may disappear following birth. Treatment involves splinting, avoiding aggravating movements, and in severe cases injecting steroids into the carpal tunnel. Surgery is indicated in severe cases.

HEALTH PROMOTION EDUCATION Although the condition is not preventable, the woman should be advised to avoid aggravating activities and use her splint as directed.

Health Promotion Education During Pregnancy

The pregnant woman is faced with the important responsibility of maintaining her health not only for her sake but also for the sake of her fetus. Nurses can help promote maternal and fetal well-being by providing expectant couples with accurate and complete information about health behaviors that can affect pregnancy and childbirth. Some women prefer to gather their own information. The nurse can refer these women to a variety of sources, including the National Women's Health Information Center, which is sponsored by the U.S. Public Health Service's Office on Women's Health.

Fetal Activity Monitoring

Many caregivers encourage pregnant women to monitor their unborn child's well-being by regularly assessing fetal activity beginning at 28 weeks' gestation. Research has documented a good positive correlation between maternal perception of fetal movement and fetal movement confirmed by ultrasound monitoring (Cunningham et al., 2010). Vigorous fetal activity generally provides reassurance of fetal well-being, whereas a marked decrease in activity or cessation of movement may indicate possible fetal compromise requiring immediate evaluation. Sound, drugs, cigarette smoking, fetal sleep state, and time of day affect fetal activity. At times, a healthy fetus may be minimally active or inactive.

A variety of methods for assessing fetal activity have been developed. They focus on having the woman keep a **fetal movement record (FMR)**, such as the Cardiff Count-to-Ten Method (Figure 16-7 ■). An FMR is a noninvasive technique that enables the pregnant woman to monitor and record fetal well-being easily and without expense. The woman's perceptions of fetal movements are influenced by her activity level, medications, and the presence of obesity (Johnson et al., 2007). Her commitment to completing a movement record may be increased when the woman understands the purpose of the as-

Sample Cardiff Count–to–Ten scoring card

Month: ________ Week of gestation at beginning of month: ________

	9:00 AM	9:30	10:00	10:30	11:00	11:30	12:00 PM	12:30	1:00	1:30	2:00	2:30	3:00	3:30	4:00	4:30	5:00	5:30	6:00	6:30	7:00	7:30	8:00	8:30	9:00
1																									
2																									
3																									
4																									
5																									
6																									
7																									
8																									
9																									
10																									
11																									
12																									
13																									
14																									
15																									
16																									
17																									
18																									
19																									
20																									
21																									
22																									
23																									
24																									
25																									
26																									
27																									
28																									
29																									
30																									
31																									

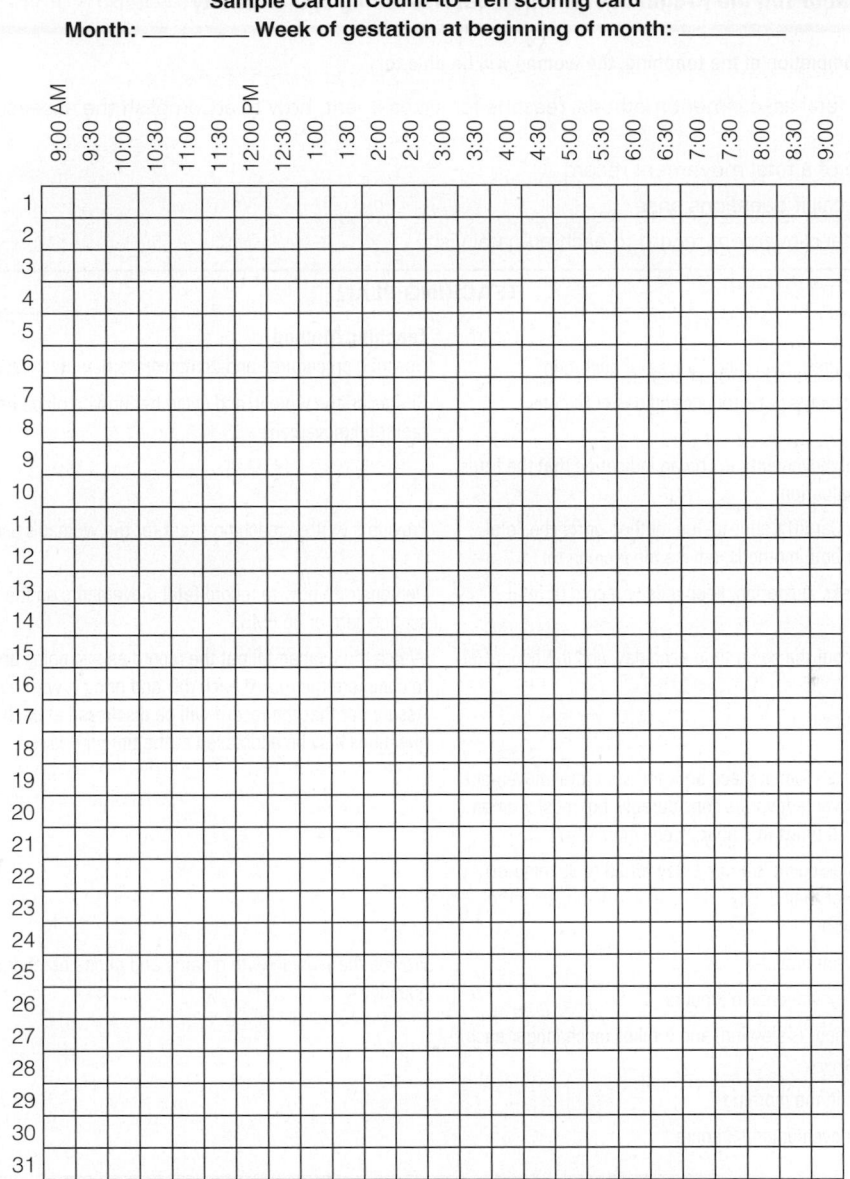

Figure 16-7 ■ An adaptation of the Cardiff Count-to-Ten scoring card for fetal movement assessment.

sessment, how to complete the form, whom to call with questions, and what to report and has the opportunity for follow-up during each visit. See Patient Teaching: What to Tell the Pregnant Woman About Assessing Fetal Activity.

> **“I like doing the fetal movement counts each day. It gives me a “time out,” when I can focus on my baby and really enjoy this special time in my life.”**

Breast Care

Whether the pregnant woman plans to formula-feed or breastfeed her infant, proper support of the breasts is important to promote comfort, retain breast shape, and prevent back strain, particularly if the breasts become large and pendulous. The sensitivity of the breasts in pregnancy is also relieved by good support.

A well-fitting, supportive brassiere has the following qualities:

- The straps are wide and do not stretch (elastic straps soon lose their tautness because of the weight of the breasts and frequent washing).
- The cup holds all breast tissue comfortably.
- The brassiere has tucks or other devices that allow it to expand, thus accommodating the enlarging chest circumference.
- The brassiere supports the nipple line approximately midway between the elbow and shoulder. At the same time, the brassiere is not pulled up in the back by the weight of the breasts.

Cleanliness of the breasts is important, especially as the woman begins producing colostrum. Colostrum that crusts on

PATIENT TEACHING What to Tell the Pregnant Woman About Assessing Fetal Activity

PATIENT GOALS At the completion of the teaching, the woman will be able to:

1. Discuss the types of fetal assessment methods, reasons for assessment, how to accomplish the assessment, and methods of record keeping.
2. Demonstrate the use of a fetal movement record.
3. Identify resources to call if questions arise.
4. Agree to bring the fetal movement record to each prenatal visit.

TEACHING PLAN

Content	Teaching Method
Explain that fetal movements are first around 18 weeks' gestation.	Describe procedures and demonstrate how to assess fetal movement.
From that time the fetal movements get stronger and easier to detect.	Sit beside the woman and show her how to place her hand on the fundus to feel fetal movement.
A slowing or stopping of fetal movement may be an indication that the fetus needs some attention and evaluation.	
Explain the procedure for the Cardiff Count-to-Ten method or for the Fetal Movement Record (FMR). For both methods, advise the woman to:	Provide a written teaching sheet for the woman's use at home.
■ Beginning at about 28 weeks' gestation, keep a daily record of fetal movement.	Demonstrate how to record fetal movements on the Cardiff Count-to-Ten scoring card or on FMR.
■ Try to begin counting at about the same time each day, about 1 hour after a meal if possible. ■ Lie quietly in a side-lying position.	Watch the woman fill out the record as examples are provided. Encourage her to complete the record each day and bring it with her to each prenatal visit. Assure her that the record will be discussed at each prenatal visit, and questions may be addressed at the time if desired.
Using the Cardiff card, have the woman place an X for each fetal movement until she has recorded 10. Movement varies considerably, but most women feel fetal movement at least 10 times in 3 hours (see Figure 16-7).	
Using the FMR have the woman count 3 times a day for 20 to 30 minutes each session. If there are fewer than 3 movements in a session, have the woman count for 1 hour or more.	
Explain when to contact the care provider: ■ If there are fewer than 10 movements in 3 hours ■ If overall the fetus's movement is slowing, and it takes much longer each day to note 10 movements ■ If there are no movements in the morning ■ If there are fewer than 3 movements in 8 hours	Provide the woman with a name and phone number in case she has further questions.

Evaluation	Documentation
Evaluate learning by having the woman explain the method and by asking the woman to fill the card in using a fictitious situation. At each prenatal visit review the expectant woman's record. Review of the record provides opportunities for questions and clarification.	Document the information given to the woman, including specifics on when to contact her healthcare provider (specify if written instructions were provided in addition to verbal ones) and the type of teaching method used. Indicate if the woman practiced counting fetal movements. Document the woman's verbalization of understanding and your clarification of any information.

the nipples should be removed with warm water. The woman planning to breastfeed should not use soap on her nipples because of its drying effect.

Some women have flat or inverted nipples. True nipple inversion, which is rare, is usually diagnosed during the initial antepartal assessment. Occasionally, a nipple appears inverted at all times. In other cases, the nipple appears normal initially, but pressure on the areola with the examiner's thumb and finger causes the nipple to retract. The normal or flat nipple protrudes when this is done (Figure 16-8 ■). Breast shields designed to correct inverted nipples can be effective but some women gain little or no benefit from them (Figure 16-9 ■).

More information on breastfeeding can be found on the Web sites of La Leche League, the American Academy of Pediatrics, the National Organization of Mothers of Twins Club, and other breastfeeding-focused sites.

Clothing

Traditionally, maternity clothes have been constructed with fuller lines to allow for the increase in abdominal size during

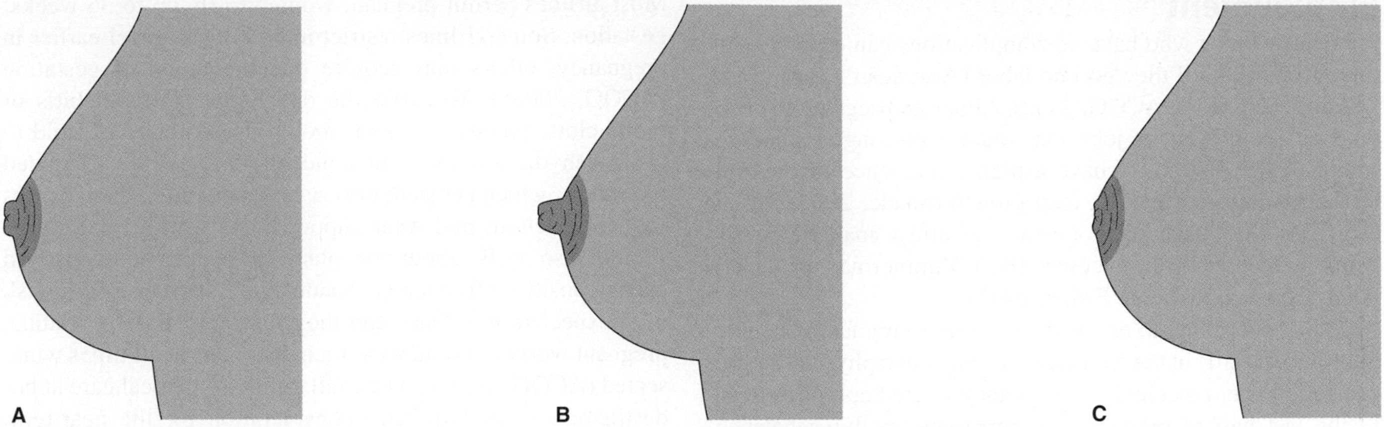

Figure 16-8 ■ A. When not stimulated, normal and inverted nipples often look alike. B. When stimulated, the normal nipple protrudes. C. When stimulated, the inverted nipple retracts. However, great variation exists; in some women, for example, one or both nipples always appear inverted, even when not stimulated.

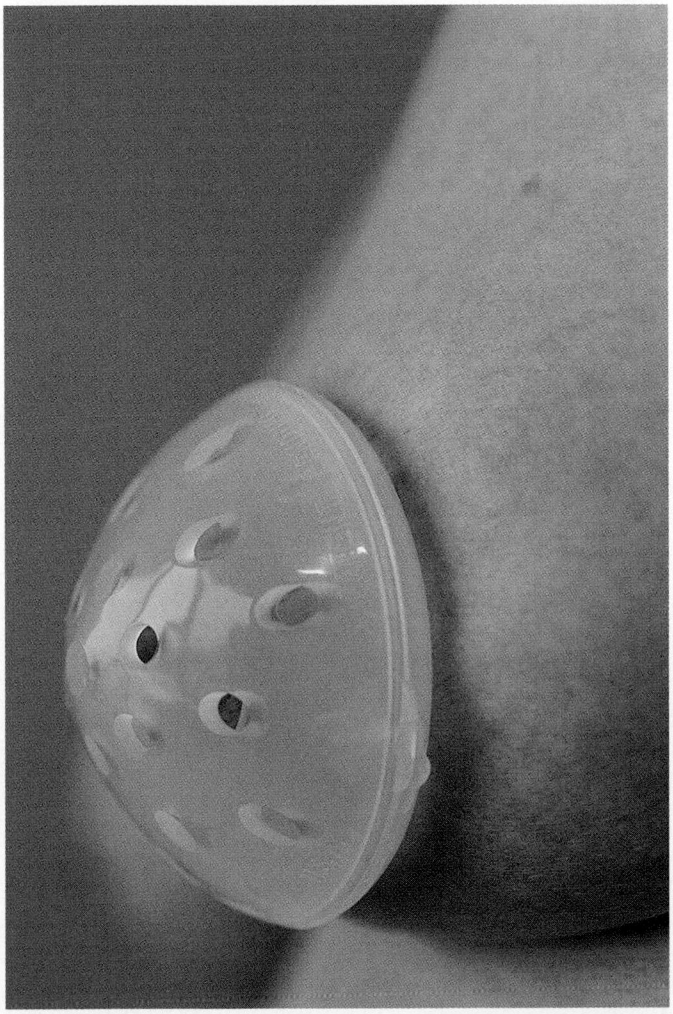

Figure 16-9 ■ This breast shield is designed to increase the protractility of inverted nipples. Worn the last 3 to 4 months of pregnancy, they exert gentle pulling pressure at the edge of the areola, gradually forcing the nipple through the center of the shield. They may be used after birth if necessary.

Source: Photographer, Elena Dorfman.

pregnancy. Skirts and slacks have soft elastic waistbands and a stretchable panel over the abdominal area. However, maternity wear has changed in recent years and now also includes clothes that are more fitted, with little attempt to hide the pregnant abdomen. Maternity clothing is expensive, however, and is worn for a relatively short time. Women can economize by sharing clothes with friends, sewing their own garments, or buying used maternity clothing.

Clothing should be loose and nonconstricting. Women with large, pendulous abdomens may benefit from a well-fitting, supportive girdle. Without this support, the pendulous abdomen increases the curvature of the spine and is a source of backache and general discomfort. Tight leg bands on girdles should be avoided.

High-heeled shoes aggravate back discomfort by increasing the curvature of the spine. They should not be worn if the woman experiences backache or problems with her balance. Shoes should fit properly and feel comfortable.

Bathing

Daily bathing is important because of the increased perspiration and mucoid vaginal discharge that occurs during pregnancy. Practices related to cleansing the body are often influenced by cultural norms; thus a pregnant woman may choose to cleanse only some portions of her body daily or may elect to take a daily shower or tub bath. Caution is needed during tub baths because balance becomes a problem as pregnancy advances. Rubber tub mats and handgrips are valuable safety devices. Moreover, vasodilation due to the warm water may cause the woman to experience some faintness when she attempts to get out of the tub. Thus she may require assistance, especially in the third trimester. To avoid introducing infection, tub baths are contraindicated in the presence of vaginal bleeding or when the membranes are ruptured. During the first trimester, pregnant women should avoid hyperthermia associated with the use of a hot tub or whirlpool bath, such as a Jacuzzi®, because it may increase the risk for neural tube defects (Cunningham et al., 2010).

Employment

Pregnant women who have no complications can usually continue to work until they go into labor (American Academy of Pediatrics [AAP] & ACOG, 2008). Although pregnant women who are employed in jobs that require prolonged standing (more than 5 hours) do have a higher incidence of preterm birth, this has no effect on fetal growth (Saade, 2007). However, the workplace environment can affect maternal well-being as well as birth outcomes (Bell, Zimmerman, & Diehr, 2008; Cooklin, Rowe, & Fisher, 2007).

Major deterrents to employment during pregnancy include fetotoxic hazards in the environment, excessive physical strain, overfatigue, and medical- or pregnancy-related complications. In the last half of pregnancy, occupations involving balance should be adjusted to protect the mother.

Fetotoxic hazards in the environment are always a concern to the expectant couple. If the pregnant woman or the woman contemplating pregnancy is working in industry, she should contact her company physician or nurse about possible hazards in her work environment and should do her own reading and research on environmental hazards as well. Similarly, her partner can seek information about hazards in his workplace that might affect his sperm, if he has not already done this before conception.

Application: Exercise During Pregnancy

Travel

If medical or pregnancy complications are not present, there are no restrictions on travel. Pregnant women should avoid travel if there is a history of bleeding or preeclampsia or if multiple births are anticipated.

Travel by automobile can be especially fatiguing, aggravating many of the discomforts of pregnancy. The pregnant woman needs frequent opportunities to get out of the car and walk. (A good pattern to follow is to stop every 2 hours and walk around for approximately 10 minutes.) A pregnant woman should use a seat belt, specifically a properly positioned three-point restraint. She should wear both lap and shoulder belts. The lap belt should fit snugly and be positioned under the abdomen and across the upper thighs. The shoulder belt should be positioned snugly between the breasts. Seat belts play an important role in preventing fetal and maternal mortality and morbidity with subsequent fetal death (Cunningham et al., 2010). Fetal death in car accidents is also caused by placental separation (abruptio placentae) as a result of uterine distortion. Use of the shoulder belt decreases the risk of traumatic flexion of the woman's body, thereby decreasing the risk of placental separation. Thus it clearly is important for nurses to provide information about car safety early in the prenatal period.

As pregnancy progresses, travel by airplane or train is generally recommended for long distances. Currently, occasional flying is considered safe in the absence of any obstetric or medical complications (ACOG, 2009a). However, those women who have medical or obstetric complications, such as poorly controlled diabetes, sickle cell disease, or preeclampsia, and those women with placental abnormalities or who are at risk for preterm birth are advised to avoid flying during pregnancy. Before flying, the pregnant woman should check with her particular airline to see if it has any travel restrictions. Most airlines permit pregnant women to fly up to 36 weeks' gestation. Some airlines restrict international travel earlier in pregnancy; others may require documentation of gestation (ACOG, 2009a). To avoid the development of phlebitis or blood clots, pregnant women should drink plenty of fluid to avoid dehydration and hemoconcentration; avoid caffeinated beverages, which act as diuretics, and smoking, which causes vasoconstriction; and wear support hose while flying. They should also walk about the plane at regular intervals and change positions frequently (Saade, 2007). Because of the risk of unexpected turbulence and the subsequent risk for trauma, pregnant women should wear their seat belts at all times while seated (ACOG, 2009a). The availability of medical care at her destination is an important consideration for the near-term woman who travels. A copy of the woman's medical records can be helpful to have for extensive travel (Johnson et al., 2007). Prior to international travel, pregnant women should consult with their healthcare providers about specific preventive strategies (McGovern, Boyce, & Fischer, 2007).

Activity and Rest

Exercise during pregnancy helps maintain maternal fitness and muscle tone, leads to improved self-image, increases energy, improves sleep, relieves tension, helps control weight gain, promotes regular bowel function, and is associated with improved postpartum recovery. Regular aerobic exercise maintains or improves a pregnant woman's general physical fitness and body image (Kramer, 2006). Normal participation in regular exercise can continue and, in fact, is encouraged throughout an uncomplicated pregnancy.

Exercise may play a role in the prevention of maternal and fetal complications (Gavard & Artal, 2008). For women who are morbidly obese, exercise may assist in the prevention of gestational diabetes. Exercise is also recommended by the American Diabetes Association to assist in glycemic control for women with gestational diabetes (Katz, 2008). Exercise in pregnancy may also provide long-term healthcare benefits to the woman with weight reduction and overall cardiovascular fitness (Gavard & Artal, 2008).

CLINICAL JUDGMENT

Case Study: Ana Gonzalez

Ana Gonzalez, a 24-year-old G1P0, is 11 weeks pregnant when she presents for her first prenatal exam. She has been a long-distance runner for 6 years. Because of her low body fat, her menses have always been irregular, and it had not occurred to Ana that she might be pregnant. Ana says she has been told that it is fine to continue any physical activity at which one is proficient and says that she would like to continue running long distances while pregnant.

Critical Thinking

What should the nurse advise Ana about running long distances?
See www.nursing.pearsonhighered.com for possible responses.

Before beginning an exercise program, a pregnant woman should be examined by her certified nurse-midwife or physician. A pregnant woman who is already in an exercise program can discuss her degree of participation with her caregiver. If a woman has not been physically active before her pregnancy, she should gradually increase her exercise period. However, maximum benefit of exercise for pregnant women is derived for those who have been physically fit before conception.

Women should seek the opinion of their healthcare provider about taking part in contact sports (Pivarnik & Mudd, 2009). In general, the skilled sportswoman is no longer discouraged from participating in these activities if her pregnancy is uncomplicated. However, pregnant women should not participate in physical activities that have a high risk for blunt trauma (Pivarnik & Mudd, 2009). Certain conditions do contraindicate exercise. Absolute contraindications to exercise include the following (ACOG, 2002):

- Rupture of the membranes
- Preeclampsia-eclampsia
- Incompetent cervix (cerclage)
- Persistent vaginal bleeding in the second or third trimesters
- Multiple gestation at risk for preterm labor
- History of preterm labor in the prior or current pregnancy
- Placenta previa after 26 weeks' gestation
- Chronic medical conditions that might be negatively impacted by vigorous exercise such as significant heart disease or restrictive lung disease

Research related to the effects of maternal exercise on the fetus is reassuring. Moderate exercise has not been demonstrated to increase maternal core temperature; cause fetal hyperthermia; or increase the rate of malformations such as miscarriage, retardation, or growth restriction (Katz, 2008).

The following guidelines are helpful in counseling pregnant women about exercise:

- Even mild to moderate exercise is beneficial during pregnancy. Regular exercise—at least 30 minutes of moderate exercise daily or at least most days of the week—is preferred (Penney, 2008).
- After the first trimester, women should avoid exercising in the supine position. In most pregnant women, the supine position is associated with decreased cardiac output. Because uterine blood flow is reduced during exercise as blood is shunted from the visceral organs to the muscles, the remaining cardiac output is further decreased. Similarly, women should avoid standing motionless for prolonged periods (ACOG, 2002; Penney, 2008).
- Because decreased oxygen is available for aerobic exercise during pregnancy, women should modify the intensity of their exercise based on their symptoms, should stop when they become fatigued, and should avoid exercising to the point of exhaustion. Non–weight-bearing exercises, such as swimming or cycling, are recommended because they decrease the risk of injury and provide fitness with comfort.
- As pregnancy progresses and the woman's center of gravity changes, especially in the third trimester, she should avoid exercises in which the loss of balance could pose a risk to her or her fetus. Similarly, the woman should avoid any type of exercise that has a high potential for physical contact such as basketball, soccer, and ice hockey because it could result in trauma to the woman or her fetus.
- A normal pregnancy requires an additional 300 kcal per day. Women who exercise regularly during pregnancy should be careful to ensure that they consume an adequate diet.
- To augment heat dissipation, especially during the first trimester, pregnant women who exercise should wear appropriate clothing, ensure adequate hydration, and avoid prolonged overheating (Katz, 2008). As a result of the cardiovascular changes of pregnancy, heart rate is not an accurate indicator of the intensity of exercise for pregnant women. If a pregnant woman is unable to talk or feels unable to breathe, then the exercise effort is too high (Saade, 2007).

In addition, the nurse may suggest that the woman wear a supportive bra and appropriate shoes when exercising. She should be advised to warm up and stretch to help prepare the joints for activity and cool down with a period of mild activity to help restore circulation and avoid pooling of blood. A moderate, rhythmic exercise routine involving large muscle groups such as swimming, cycling, or brisk walking is best. Jogging or running is acceptable for women already conditioned to these activities as long as they avoid exercising at maximum effort and overheating.

Warning signs include the following: pain of any kind, vaginal bleeding, uterine contractions, decreased or absent fetal movement, fluid loss from the vagina, dizziness, headache, dyspnea before exertion, and muscle weakness (ACOG, 2002). The woman should stop exercising if any of these symptoms occur and modify her exercise program. If the symptoms persist, the woman should contact her caregiver.

Adequate rest in pregnancy is important for both physical and emotional health. Women need more sleep throughout pregnancy, particularly in the first and last trimesters, when they tire easily. Without adequate rest, pregnant women have less resilience.

Finding time to rest during the day may be difficult for women who work outside the home or have small children. The nurse can help the expectant mother examine her daily schedule to develop a realistic plan for short periods of rest and relaxation.

Sleeping becomes more difficult during the last trimester because of the enlarged abdomen, increased frequency of urination, and greater activity of the fetus. Finding a comfortable position becomes difficult for the pregnant woman. Figure 16-10 ■ shows a position most pregnant women find comfortable. Progressive relaxation techniques similar to those taught in prepared childbirth classes can help prepare the woman for sleep.

Exercises to Prepare for Childbirth

Certain exercises help strengthen muscle tone in preparation for birth and promote more rapid restoration of muscle tone after birth. The woman can reduce some physical changes of pregnancy considerably by faithfully practicing prescribed body-conditioning exercises. Many body-conditioning exercises for pregnancy are taught; a few of the more common ones are discussed here.

The **pelvic tilt**, or pelvic rocking, helps prevent or reduce back strain and strengthens abdominal muscle tone. To do the pelvic tilt, the pregnant woman lies on her back and puts her feet flat on the floor. This bent position of the knees helps prevent strain and discomfort. She decreases the curvature in her back by pressing her spine toward the floor. With her back pressed to

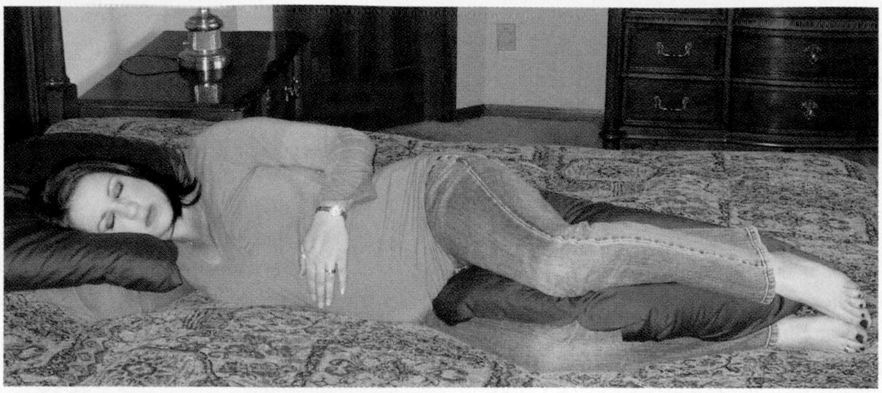

Figure 16-10 ■ Position for relaxation and rest as pregnancy progresses.

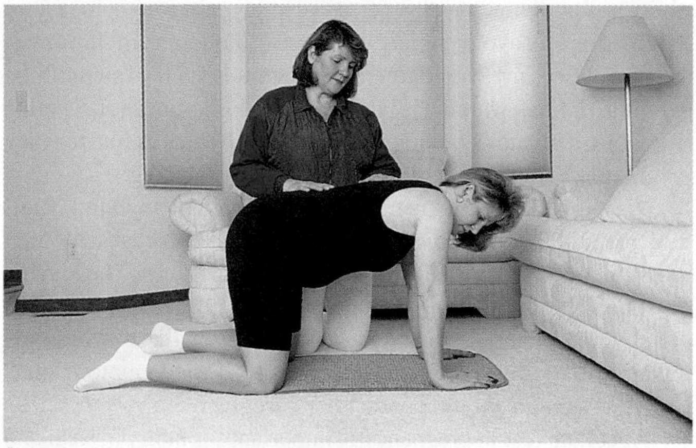

A

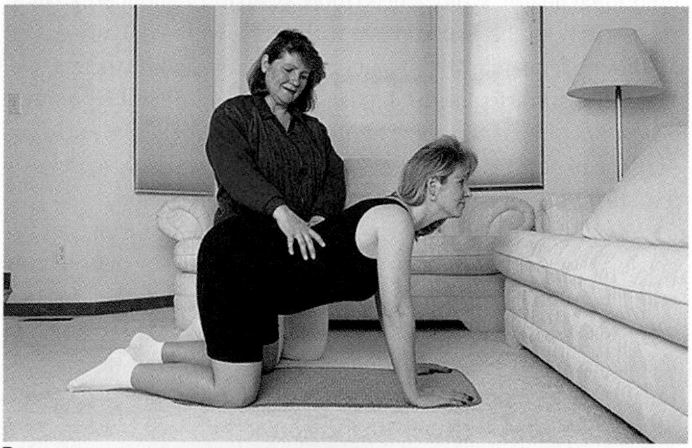

B

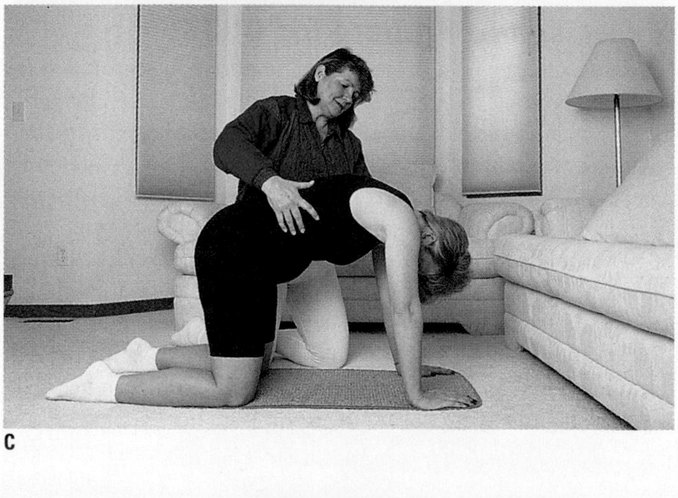

C

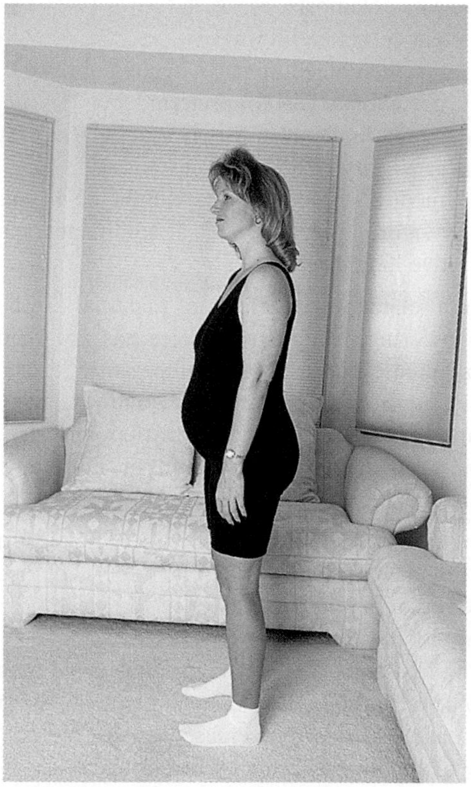

D

Figure 16-11 ■ A. Starting position when the pelvic tilt is done on hands and knees. The back is flat and parallel to the floor, the hands are under the head, and the knees are directly under the buttocks. B. A prenatal yoga instructor offers pointers for proper positioning for the first part of the tilt: head up, neck long and separated from the shoulders, buttocks up, and pelvis thrust back, allowing the back to drop and release on an inhaled breath. C. The instructor helps the woman assume the correct position for the next part of the tilt. It is done on a long exhalation, allowing the pregnant woman to arch her back, drop her head loosely, push away from her hands, and draw in the muscles of her abdomen to strengthen them. Note that in this position the pelvis and buttocks are tucked under, and the buttock muscles are tightened. D. Proper posture. The knees are slightly bent but not locked, the pelvis and buttocks are tucked under, thereby lengthening the spine and helping support the weighty abdomen. With her chin tucked in, this woman's neck, shoulders, hips, knees, and feet are all in a straight line perpendicular to the floor. Her feet are parallel. This is also the starting position for doing the pelvic tilt while standing.

Source: Photographer, Elena Dorfman.

the floor, the woman tightens her buttocks and abdominal muscles as she tucks in her buttocks. The pelvic tilt can also be performed on hands and knees (Figure 16-11 ■), while sitting in a chair, or while standing with the back against a wall. The body alignment achieved when the pelvic tilt is correctly done should be maintained as much as possible throughout the day.

CLINICAL TIP

Doing the pelvic tilt on hands and knees may aggravate back strain. Teach women with a history of minor back problems to do the pelvic tilt only in the standing position.

Abdominal Exercises

A basic exercise to increase abdominal muscle tone is tightening abdominal muscles with each breath. It can be done in any position, but it is best learned while the woman lies supine. With knees flexed and feet flat on the floor, the woman expands her abdomen and slowly takes a deep breath. As she slowly exhales, she gradually pulls in her abdominal muscles until they are fully contracted. She relaxes for a few seconds and then repeats the exercise.

Partial sit-ups strengthen abdominal muscle tone and are done according to individual comfort levels. When doing a partial sit-up, the woman lies on the floor as just described (Figure 16-12 ■). The exercise is done with the knees bent and the feet flat on the floor to avoid undue strain on the lower back. She stretches her arms toward her knees as she slowly pulls her head and shoulders off the floor to a comfortable level. (If she has poor abdominal muscle tone, she may not be able to pull up very far.) She then slowly returns to the starting position, takes a deep breath, and repeats the exercise. To strengthen the oblique abdominal muscles, she repeats the process but stretches the left arm to the side of her right knee, returns to the floor, takes a deep breath, and then reaches with the right arm to the left knee.

These exercises can be done approximately 5 times in a sequence, and the sequence can be repeated several times during the day as desired. It is important that the woman do the exercises slowly to prevent muscle strain and overtiring.

Perineal Exercises

Perineal muscle tightening, also referred to as **Kegel exercises**, strengthens the pubococcygeus muscle and increases its elasticity (Figure 16-13 ■). This muscle helps support the pelvic organs, including the uterus and bladder. A strong pubococcygeus muscle

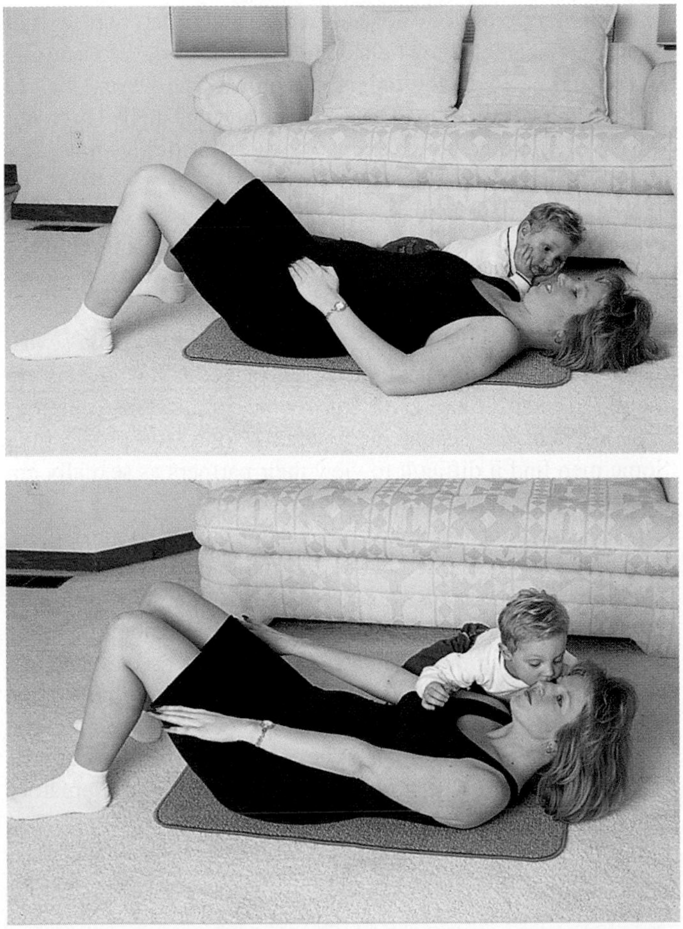

Figure 16-12 ■ The pregnant woman can strengthen her abdominal muscles by doing partial sit-ups.

Source: Photographer, Elena Dorfman.

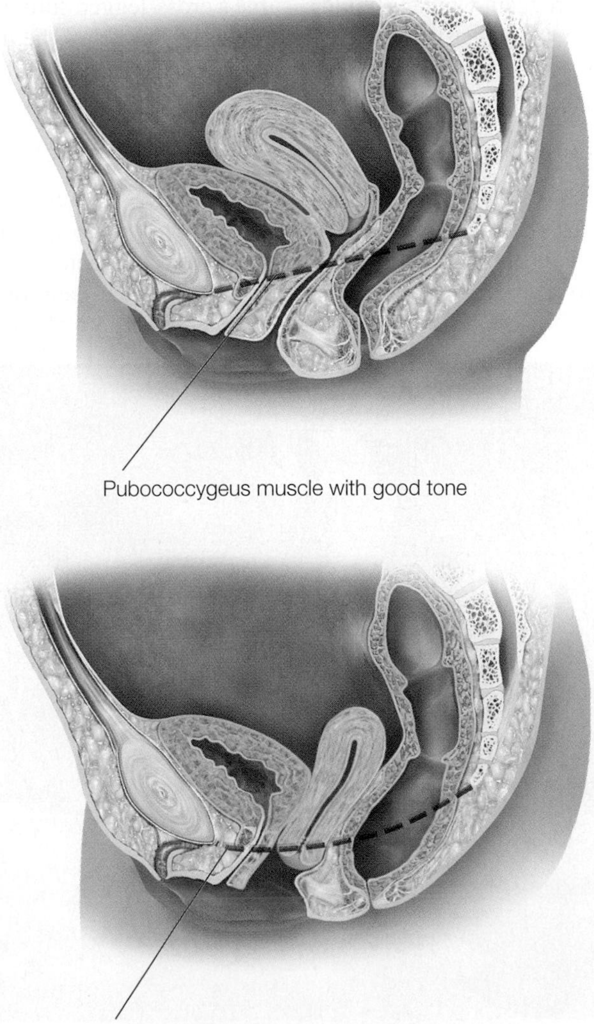

Figure 16-13 ■ Kegel exercises. The woman tightens the pubococcygeus muscle to improve support to the pelvic organs.

helps prevent stress incontinence, cystocele, rectocele, and uterine prolapse in women following childbirth.

The woman can feel the specific muscle group to be exercised by stopping urination midstream. However, doing Kegel exercises while urinating is discouraged because this practice has been associated with urinary stasis and urinary tract infection.

Childbirth educators sometimes use the following technique to teach Kegel exercises. They tell the woman to think of her perineal muscles as an elevator. When she relaxes, the elevator is on the first floor. To do the exercises, she contracts, bringing the elevator to the second, third, and fourth floors. She keeps the elevator on the fourth floor for a few seconds, and then gradually relaxes the area. If the exercise is properly done, the woman does not contract the muscles of the buttocks and thighs.

Kegel exercises can be done at almost any time. Some women use ordinary events—for instance, stopping at a red light—as a cue to remember to do the exercise. Others do Kegel exercises while waiting in a checkout line, talking on the telephone, or watching television.

Inner Thigh Exercises

The pregnant woman should assume a cross-legged sitting position whenever possible. This "tailor sit" stretches the muscles of the inner thighs in preparation for labor and birth (Figure 16-14 ■).

Sexual Activity

As a result of the physiologic, anatomic, and emotional changes of pregnancy, the couple usually has many questions and concerns about sexual activity during pregnancy. Often these questions are about possible injury to the baby or the woman during intercourse and about changes in the desire each partner feels for the other.

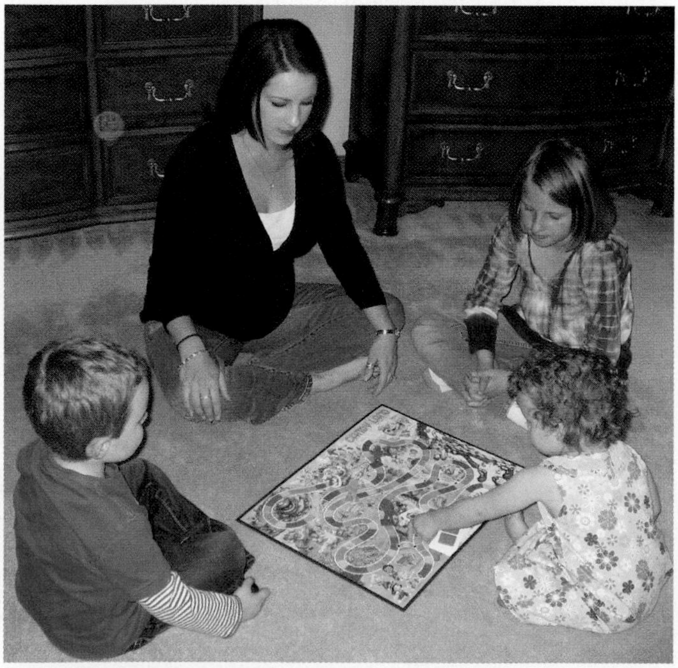

Figure 16-14 ■ To help prepare her inner thigh muscles for labor and birth, the pregnant woman should assume a cross-legged sitting position whenever possible during the day.

In the past, couples were frequently warned to avoid sexual intercourse during the last 6 to 8 weeks of pregnancy to prevent complications such as infection or premature rupture of the membranes. However, these fears seem to be unfounded. In a healthy pregnancy, there is no medical reason to limit sexual activity. Intercourse is contraindicated if the membranes are ruptured or if placenta previa is diagnosed (Katz, 2008).

The expectant mother may experience changes in sexual desire and response. Often these are related to the various discomforts that occur throughout pregnancy. For instance, during the first trimester, fatigue or nausea and vomiting may decrease desire, and breast tenderness may make the woman less responsive to fondling of her breasts. During the second trimester, many of the discomforts have lessened, and with the vascular congestion of the pelvis the woman may experience even greater sexual satisfaction than she experienced before pregnancy.

During the third trimester, interest in coitus may again decrease as the woman becomes more uncomfortable and fatigued. In addition, shortness of breath, painful pelvic ligaments, urinary frequency, and decreased mobility may lessen sexual desire and activity. If they are not already using them, the couple should consider coital positions other than male superior, such as side-by-side, female superior, and vaginal rear entry.

Sexual activity does not have to include intercourse. Cuddling, kissing, and being held can satisfy many of the nurturing and sexual needs of the pregnant woman. The warm, sensual feelings that accompany these activities can be an end in themselves. Her partner, however, may need to masturbate more frequently than before.

The sexual desires of men are also affected by many factors in pregnancy. These include the previous relationship with the partner, acceptance of the pregnancy, attitudes toward the partner's change of appearance, and concern about hurting the expectant mother or baby. Some men may withdraw from sexual contact because of a belief that sex with a pregnant woman is immoral. This may be especially true for the couple whose religious beliefs teach that sexual intercourse is only for procreation. Some men find it difficult to view their partners as sexually appealing while they are adjusting to the concept of her as a mother. Other men feel their partner's pregnancy is arousing and experience feelings of increased happiness, intimacy, and closeness.

The expectant couple should be aware of their changing sexual desires, the normality of these changes, and the importance of communicating these changes to each other so that they can make nurturing adaptations. The nurse has an important role in addressing the sexuality concerns of the expectant couple. The couple must feel free to express concerns about sexual activity, and the nurse must be able to respond and give anticipatory guidance in a comfortable manner. See Patient Teaching: Sexual Activity During Pregnancy.

Dental Care

No evidence suggests that pregnancy causes or accelerates the development of dental caries. Nevertheless, in spite of such discomforts as nausea and vomiting, gum hypertrophy and tenderness,

PATIENT TEACHING Sexual Activity During Pregnancy

PATIENT GOALS At the completion of the teaching, the woman will be able to:

1. Relate the changes in sexuality and sexual response that may occur during pregnancy to changes in technique, frequency, and response that may be indicated.
2. Explore personal attitudes, beliefs, and expectations about sexual activity during pregnancy.
3. Cite maternal factors that would contraindicate sexual intercourse.

TEACHING PLAN

Content	Teaching Method
Begin by explaining that the pregnant woman may experience changes in desire during the course of pregnancy. During the first trimester, discomforts such as nausea, fatigue, and breast tenderness may make intercourse less desirable for many women. In the second trimester, as symptoms decrease, desire may increase. In the third trimester, discomfort and fatigue may lead to decreased desire in the woman.	Universal statements that give permission, such as "Many couples experience changes in sexual desire during pregnancy. What kind of changes have you experienced?" are often effective in starting discussion. Depending on the woman's (or couple's) level of knowledge and sophistication, part or all of this discussion may be necessary.
Explain that men may notice changes in their level of desire, too. Among other things, this change may be related to feelings about his partner's changing appearance, his belief about the acceptability of sexual activity with a pregnant woman, or concern about hurting the woman or fetus. Some men find the changes of pregnancy erotic; others must adjust to the notion of their partners as mothers.	If the partner is present, approach him in the same nonjudgmental way used above. If not, ask the woman if she has noticed any changes in her partner or if he has expressed any concerns.
Explain that the woman may notice that orgasms are much more intense during the last weeks of pregnancy and may be followed by cramping. Because of the pressure of the enlarging uterus on the vena cava, the woman should not lie flat on her back for intercourse after about the fourth month. If the couple prefers that position, a pillow should be placed under her right hip to displace the uterus. Alternate positions such as side-by-side, female superior, or vaginal rear entry may become necessary as her uterus enlarges.	Deal with any specific questions about the physical and psychologic changes that the couple may have.
Stress that sexual activities that both partners enjoy are generally acceptable. It is not advisable for couples who favor anal sex to go from anal penetration to vaginal penetration because of the risk of introducing *Escherichia coli* into the vagina.	Discussion about various sexual activities requires that you be comfortable with your sexuality and that you be tactful.
Suggest that alternative methods of expressing intimacy and affection such as cuddling, holding and stroking each other, and kissing may help maintain the couple's feelings of warmth and closeness. If the man feels desire for further sexual release, his partner may help him masturbate to ejaculation, or he may prefer to masturbate in private. Advise the woman who is interested in masturbation as a form of gratification that the orgasmic contractions may be especially intense in later pregnancy.	The couple may be content with these approaches to meeting their sexual needs, or they may require assurance that such approaches are indeed "normal."
Stress that sexual intercourse in contraindicated once the membranes are ruptured or if bleeding is present. Women with a history of preterm labor may be advised to avoid intercourse because the oxytocin that is released with orgasm stimulates uterine contractions and may trigger preterm labor. Because oxytocin is also released with nipple stimulation, fondling the breasts may also be contraindicated in those cases.	An explanation of the contraindications accompanied by their rationale provides specific guidelines that most couples find helpful.
A discussion of sexuality and sexual activity should stress the importance of open communication so that the couple feels comfortable expressing feelings, preferences, and concerns.	Some couples are skilled at expressing their feelings about sexual activity. Others find it difficult and can benefit from specific suggestions. The nurse should provide opportunities for discussion throughout the talk. Specific handouts on sexual activity are also helpful for couples and may address topics that were not discussed.

Evaluation

Evaluate the learning by assessing the woman's (or couple's) response to information throughout the discussion. Ask the woman to express information such as the contraindications to intercourse in her own words. Follow-up sessions and questions from the woman also provide information about teaching effectiveness.

Documentation

Document the information given to the woman, including specifics on contraindications to sexual activity (specify if written instructions were provided in addition to verbal ones) and the type of teaching method used. Document the woman's verbalization of understanding and your clarification of any information.

possible ptyalism, and heartburn, it is important for pregnant women to maintain regular oral hygiene.

Ensuring a healthy oral environment is essential to overall health. Women should be advised to do the following:

- Have extensive dental work done before becoming pregnant if possible.
- Eat a healthy diet including foods high in protein; calcium; phosphorus; and vitamins C, A, and D.
- Take prenatal vitamins daily.
- Maintain good oral hygiene by brushing at least twice a day and flossing daily.
- Use an antibacterial fluoride mouth rinse.
- If morning sickness occurs, brush teeth following vomiting to prevent tooth erosion caused by stomach acids.
- Have teeth cleaned every 6 months.

Ideally, a woman should have a dental examination as part of preconception planning. If that does not occur, the pregnant woman is encouraged to have a dental checkup early in her pregnancy. She should inform her dentist of her pregnancy so that she is not exposed to teratogenic substances. Dental x-rays are permitted during pregnancy as long as the woman's abdomen is shielded with a lead apron (Guilbeau & Hurst, 2009). The second trimester is considered the most appropriate time for dental treatment because the risk of pregnancy loss tends to be lower and the woman tends to be more comfortable (Russell & Mayberry, 2008). Extensive dental care during pregnancy requires consultation between the dentist and the woman's healthcare professional.

Immunizations

Ideally, women of childbearing age should receive immunizations prior to becoming pregnant to avoid unnecessary fetal exposure (ACOG, 2009b). All women of childbearing age need to be fully aware of the risks of receiving specific immunizations if pregnancy is possible. Expectant women, especially those who intend to travel internationally, should be aware of the immunizations that are contraindicated during pregnancy. Immunizations with attenuated live viruses, such as rubella vaccine, should not be given in pregnancy because of the possible teratogenic effect of the live virus (ACOG, 2009b; Katz, 2008). The most current recommendations on vaccines related to pregnancy may be obtained from the Centers for Disease Control and Prevention Web site. Recommendations for immunizations during pregnancy are summarized in Table 16-4.

COMPLEMENTARY AND ALTERNATIVE THERAPIES

According to the National Center for Complementary & Alternative Medicine (NCCAM) (2008), the use of complementary and alternative medicine (CAM) is more common in women and in those with higher levels of education and higher incomes. Many women are electing to use CAM therapies, such as homeopathy, herbal medicine (phytomedicine), acupressure, acupuncture, biofeedback, Therapeutic Touch, massage, and chiropractic, as part of a holistic approach to their healthcare regimens. Nurses are in a unique position to bridge the gap between conventional therapies and CAM therapies. As patient advocates, nurses are able to provide patients with information needed to make informed decisions about their health and health care. Utilizing a nonjudgmental approach, the nurse should inquire about the use of CAM as part of a routine antepartal assessment. It is important that nurses working with pregnant women and their families develop a general understanding of the more commonly used therapies to be able to answer questions and provide resources as needed. See chapter 3 ∞ for an in-depth discussion of CAM.

Homeopathy

Homeopathy means "like suffering." Homeopathic medicine is based on the theory that a miniscule amount of a substance can cure symptoms in a sick person that are similar to the symptoms the substance causes in healthy people. Thus, for example, ipecac, which induces vomiting, may be used to treat a

TABLE 16-4 Recommendations for Immunization During Pregnancy

LIVE ATTENUATED VIRUS VACCINES	INACTIVATED BACTERIAL VACCINES	HYPERIMMUNE GLOBULINS
Measles—contraindicated	Pneumococcal—if indicated	Hepatitis B—postexposure prophylaxis: give along with hepatitis B vaccine initially, then vaccine alone at 1 and 6 months
Mumps—contraindicated	Meningococcal—if indicated	Rabies—postexposure prophylaxis
Rubella—contraindicated	Typhoid—not recommended	Tetanus—postexposure prophylaxis
Varicella-zoster—contraindicated		Varicella—consider for postexposure within 96 hr
Poliomyelitis—no longer recommended		
Yellow fever—high-risk areas only		
Smallpox—contraindicated		
INACTIVATED VIRUS VACCINES	**TOXOIDS**	**POOLED IMMUNE SERUM GLOBULINS**
Influenza—same as nonpregnant	Tetanus-diptheria—same as nonpregnant	Hepatitis A—postexposure prophylaxis
Rabies—same as nonpregnant		Measles—postexposure prophylaxis
Hepatitis A and B—same as nonpregnant		
Enhanced poliomyelitis (IPV-e)—risk of exposure		
Human papilloma virus (HPV)—contraindicated		

Source: K. J. (2001). Williams Obstetrics, *21st ed. New York: McGraw-Hill. Reproduced with permission of the McGraw-Hill Companies.*

person who is vomiting, such as a pregnant woman with severe nausea and vomiting.

Homeopathic therapies are available for pregnancy-related symptoms such as musculoskeletal disorders, anemia, nausea, ptyalism, pica, threatened miscarriage, and preterm labor. According to homeopathic theory, homeopathic remedies either help an individual or have no effect. However, a healing crisis or aggravation of symptoms can occur if the remedy is given in too high a potency or repeated too frequently.

Herbal Medicine

Herbal medicine uses therapies derived from plants. Many have been used for centuries in different parts of the world and are well recognized.

In the United States, herbs are categorized as dietary supplements rather than drugs. It is important for the pregnant woman to understand that herbs are considered dietary supplements and are not regulated as prescription or over-the-counter drugs through the Food and Drug Administration (FDA). Due to limited scientific evaluation of potential harmful effects on the fetus, herbal supplements should be avoided, particularly in the first trimester (Yankowitz, 2008).

In general, it is best to advise pregnant women not to ingest any herbs, except ginger, during the first trimester of pregnancy (Yankowitz, 2008). Pregnant women need to avoid certain categories of herbs such as abortifacient (abortion-inducing) herbs, herbs that induce menstruation, nervous system stimulants, stimulant laxatives, and so forth. Lists identifying common herbs that women are advised to avoid or use with caution during pregnancy and lactation are available; an example is shown in Table 16-5.

For a reliable source of information about herbs, homeopathic therapies, and other alternative options, consumers or healthcare providers can access the National Center for Complementary and Alternative Medicine Web site and the Office of Dietary Supplements Web site.

Some alternative therapies are safe and effective during pregnancy. In fact, some have been shown to be even more effective than traditional remedies. For nausea in early pregnancy, acupuncture, acupressure, ginger root (250-mg capsules 4 times a day), and vitamin B_6 (pyridoxine, 25 mg 2 or 3 times a day) work well (Cleveland Clinic, 2006). For backache, chiropractic manipulation holds the best track record, but other successful alternative therapies include yoga, massage, and reflexology that utilize light, gentle pressure. For turning a breech baby, exercise, hypnosis, and a traditional Chinese treatment called moxibustion (burning an incense-like substance on the fifth toe) have proven to be beneficial (Cleveland Clinic, 2006).

TABLE 16-5 Common Herbs to Avoid in Pregnancy*

Blue cohosh	Goldenseal
Black cohosh	Ginkgo biloba
Chamomile, Valeria	Ginseng
Comfrey	Horehound
Dong quai	Horseradish (fresh)
Ephedra (ma huang)	
Use with caution:	
Garlic	
Turmeric	

*Avoid excessive consumption relative to usual and customary food use.

Source: Hardy, M. (2000). *Herbs of special interest to women.* Journal of the American Pharmaceutical Association, 40(2), 234–242. Copyright American Pharmacists Association (APhA). Reprinted by permission APhA.

Centering Pregnancy

When empowering women to choose health-promoting behaviors, it may be helpful to consider a relatively new, innovative model for prenatal care called Centering Pregnancy. Centering Pregnancy integrates the three major components of care—health assessment, education, and support—into a unified program providing complete prenatal care to women within a group setting. This model replaces the traditional one-on-one visits in an examination room with a healthcare provider. Instead, group meetings are held where mothers-to-be and their partners receive care and education and form a sense of community with other group members.

Patients begin meeting in small groups at 12 to 16 weeks' gestation and continue to meet monthly for the first 4 months, and biweekly as their due dates approach. Each group session begins with the expectant mothers taking their own blood pressure, monitoring weight gain, checking urine samples, and recording data on medical charts under their provider or nurse's guidance. The provider then reviews each group member's information and completes any further assessments that are indicated. After all assessments are completed, the group members convene in a circle to discuss topics such as nutrition, fetal development, common discomforts of pregnancy and possible remedies, exercise, relaxation, labor and birth procedures, parenting and relationship issues, contraception, and infant care (Reid, 2007). Prenatal assessment, knowledge and skills development, and support occur in an atmosphere that facilitates learning, encourages free exchange, and develops mutual support (Massey, Schindler Rising, & Ickovics, 2006). Both mothers and fathers report an increased investment in the pregnancy and self-care after attending group sessions. Studies conclude that women in group sessions are less likely to have suboptimal prenatal care and are more likely to have significantly better prenatal knowledge, feel better prepared for labor and delivery, and have greater satisfaction with their care (Ickovics et al., 2007).

Teratogenic Substances

Substances that adversely affect the normal growth and development of the fetus are called **teratogens**. Many of these effects are readily apparent at birth, but others may not be identified for years. A well-known example is the development of cervical cancer in adolescent females whose mothers took diethylstilbestrol (DES) during pregnancy.

Developmental defects may result from genetic, environmental, or unknown causes (Niebyl & Simpson, 2007). Environmental exposure to toxins may occur by inhalation, eye contact (e.g., chemical splash), ingestion and absorption through the gastrointestinal tract (e.g., foods containing pesticides or contaminated water), exposure through the skin (e.g., pesticides, chemicals found in cosmetics, etc.), maternal-fetal transfer, and through breastfeeding (Chalupka & Chalupka, 2010).

Medications are perhaps the most likely documented teratogens, but other factors can also harm the fetus, including certain infections such as rubella, syphilis, herpes virus type 2, toxoplasmosis, and cytomegalovirus (CMV). During pregnancy, women need to have adequate information available and a realistic perspective on potential environmental hazards. Factors that are suspected to be hazardous to the general population should be avoided if possible.

Medications

The use of medications during pregnancy, including prescriptions, over-the-counter drugs, and herbal remedies, is of great concern because maternal drug and chemical exposure is thought to account for at least 10% of birth defects (Yankowitz, 2008). Over 60% of American women receive at least one prescription during pregnancy (Katz, 2008). Many pregnant women need medication for therapeutic purposes, such as the treatment of infections, allergies, or other pathologic processes. Known teratogenic agents are not prescribed and usually can be replaced by medications considered safe. Even when a woman is highly motivated to avoid taking any medications, she may have taken potentially teratogenic medications before her pregnancy was diagnosed, especially if she had an irregular menstrual cycle.

The greatest potential for gross abnormalities in the fetus occurs during the first trimester of pregnancy, when fetal organs are first developing. Many factors influence teratogenic effects, including the specific identity and dose of the teratogen, the state of embryo development, and the genetic sensitivity of the mother and fetus. For example, the commonly prescribed acne medication isotretinoin (Accutane) is associated with a high incidence of spontaneous abortion and congenital malformations if taken early in pregnancy. Valproic acid, an anticonvulsant, is associated with an increased risk of neural tube defects (Katz, 2008) and cleft lip (Niebyl & Simpson, 2007).

To provide information for caregivers and patients, the Food and Drug Administration (FDA) has developed the following classification system for medications administered during pregnancy:

Category A. Controlled studies in women have demonstrated no associated fetal risk. Few drugs fall into this category. Vitamin C is cited as a category A drug as long as its use does not exceed the recommended dietary allowance.

Category B. Either animal studies show no risk, but there are no controlled studies in women; or animal studies indicate a risk, but controlled human studies fail to demonstrate a risk. The penicillins fall into this category.

Category C. Either (1) no adequate studies, either in animals or women, are available; or (2) animal studies show teratogenic effects, but no controlled studies in women are available. Many drugs fall into this category, and the lack of information poses a problem for caregivers. Zidovudine, a drug used to decrease perinatal transmission of HIV, falls into this category.

Category D. Evidence of human fetal risk does exist, but the benefits of the drug in certain situations are thought to outweigh the risks. Examples in this category include tetracycline, vincristine, lithium, and hydrochlorothiazide.

Category X. The demonstrated fetal risks clearly outweigh any possible benefit. An example of a drug in this category is isotretinoin (Accutane), the acne medication, which can cause multiple central nervous system (CNS), facial, and cardiovascular anomalies.

If a woman has taken a drug in category D or X, she should be informed of the risks associated with that drug and of her alternatives. Similarly, a woman who has taken a drug in the safer categories can be reassured. For up-to-date information on the risks associated with specific drugs, women can contact drug information centers, either by telephone or by using online databases.

The FDA system, although useful, has been criticized because the letter system suggests a risk grading that is not necessarily accurate. More important, not all drugs in a category have the same risk level. While the FDA is working to develop a new evidence-based system, slow progress has prompted experts to recommend teratogen information databases as an alternative resource (Niebyl & Simpson, 2007; Yankowitz, 2008).

Although the first trimester is the critical period for teratogenesis, some medications are known to have teratogenic effect when taken in the second and third trimesters. For example, tetracycline taken in late pregnancy is commonly associated with staining of teeth in children and has been shown to depress skeletal growth, especially in preterm infants. Warfarin (Coumadin), a commonly prescribed anticoagulant, is associated with CNS defects following fetal exposure during the second and third trimesters (Niebyl & Simpson, 2007). Because heparin does not cross the placenta, it is safer for the fetus than warfarin and other anticoagulants.

Pregnant women should avoid all medication—prescribed, homeopathic, or over the counter—if possible. If a medication is necessary during pregnancy, the benefits must clearly outweigh the risks. If no alternative exists, it is wisest to select a well-known medication rather than a newer drug whose potential teratogenic effects may not be known. When possible, the oral form of the drug should be used, and it should be prescribed in the lowest possible therapeutic dose for the shortest time possible. Finally, the caregiver should carefully consider the multiple components of the medication.

A woman clearly has a right to the most comprehensive information available concerning medications. The nurse can assist her by suggesting appropriate references and helping her research information. Some excellent reference books on drugs and pregnancy are currently available and should be part of the library of every office and clinic that provides prenatal care. In addition, several online databases that provide information on teratogens are available for convenient reference.

The nurse should remind the woman of the need to check with her caregiver about medications she was taking when pregnancy occurred and about any nonprescription drugs she is contemplating using. Any medication with possible teratogenic effects must be avoided.

Tobacco

In the United States, smoking during pregnancy is one of the most significant, modifiable causes of poor pregnancy outcomes. Smoking during pregnancy has a strong association with low-birth-weight infants. In addition, mothers who smoke have an increased risk of infertility, spontaneous abortion, intrauterine growth restriction (IUGR), placentae previa, abruptio placentae, premature rupture of membranes, and preterm birth (ACOG, 2005; Niebyl & Simpson, 2007; Kahn, Hobbins, & Galan, 2008; Hartmann et al., 2007). Pregnant women who smoke as well as participate in other unhealthy behaviors, such as alcohol use, further increase their risk for low-birth-weight infants (Kahn et al., 2008; Martin et al., 2008). Research also links maternal smoking, both during pregnancy and afterward, with more than 3 times the risk of sudden infant death syndrome (SIDS) than that of nonsmokers (Wisner et al., 2007). Children exposed to tobacco smoke prenatally and environmentally have an increased risk of learning disabilities (Anderko, Braun, & Auinger, 2010). Maternal smoking also exposes young children to other risks of secondhand smoke including middle ear infections, acute and chronic respiratory tract illnesses, and behavioral disabilities (Niebyl & Simpson, 2007; Martin et al., 2008).

The ingredients in cigarette smoke, such as carbon monoxide, nicotine, lead, and cotinine, are toxic to the fetus. Carbon monoxide decreases availability of oxygen to maternal and fetal tissue, while nicotine decreases uteroplacental blood flow to the fetus (Niebyl & Simpson, 2007).

In response to public health education campaigns in the United States, smoking during pregnancy has decreased significantly. In fact, approximately 46% of women who smoke quit during pregnancy. Unfortunately, 60% to 80% of women who quit smoking during their pregnancy resume smoking within a year after birth (ACOG, 2005). This finding suggests that although women are aware of the potential impact of smoking on the fetus, they may be less knowledgeable about the effects of passive smoke on the baby.

Smoking cessation programs decrease the number of women who smoke in pregnancy and, therefore, the incidence of low-birth-weight infants and preterm births ((Johnson et al., 2007). Studies demonstrate that any decrease in smoking during pregnancy improves fetal outcome, and researchers continue to explore approaches designed to help women quit smoking. ACOG (2005) suggests a 5- to 15-minute intervention with women who smoke fewer than 20 cigarettes a day to be most effective. This program and other programs encourage healthcare providers to use the five As:

- *Ask* about tobacco use.
- *Advise* to quit smoking.
- *Assess* willingness to quit.
- *Assist* in attempt to quit.
- *Arrange* for follow-up care.

The nurse can play an important role in counseling women about the importance of smoking cessation during pregnancy and can be actively involved in offering smoking cessation programs.

If smoking cessation efforts are not successful in pregnant women who smoke more than 10 cigarettes per day, the healthcare provider might consider prescribing nicotine replacement therapy (NRT), which is available as gum, lozenge, patch, nasal spray, or inhaler. This approach, while still somewhat controversial, delivers less nicotine than cigarettes and avoids exposure to the other substances found in tobacco smoke (Galic & Martino, 2010). Medications such as bupropion and varenicline have been approved for smoking cessation therapy in the general population, but their safety in pregnancy has not been demonstrated (Forest, 2010). ACOG (2005) suggests that NRT or bupropion be considered for pregnant and lactating women if other efforts at cessation fail.

Application: Smoking Cessation Plan

Many educational resources are available for healthcare providers and consumers on smoking cessation programs. Organizations that might be helpful include the following:

- American Lung Association
- March of Dimes
- American Cancer Society
- Healthy Mothers, Healthy Babies

Alcohol

Application: Smoking Cessation Plan

Alcohol is now considered one of the primary teratogens in the Western world. Fetuses of women who are heavy drinkers are at increased risk for developing **fetal alcohol syndrome (FAS)**. Currently FAS, characterized by growth restriction; behavioral disturbances; craniofacial abnormalities; and brain, cardiac, and spinal defects, is the most common preventable cause of intellectual disability (mental retardation) in the United States. The Centers for Disease Control and Prevention (CDC) analysis of the 2002 Behavioral Risk Factor Surveillance System (BRFSS) survey revealed that 10% of pregnant women used alcohol, and approximately 2% engaged in binge drinking (Floyd, Ebrahim, Tsai, et al., 2006). The incidence of fetal alcohol syndrome is approximately 1 in every 100 births (Wisner et al., 2007).

The effects of moderate consumption of alcohol during pregnancy are unclear. Research suggests an increased incidence of lowered birth weight and some neurologic effects, such as attention deficit disorder. Evidence suggests that the risk of teratogenic effects increases proportionately with increased average daily intake of alcohol. Although an occasional drink during pregnancy does not carry any known risk, no safe level of drinking during pregnancy has been identified, and caregivers should recommend that pregnant women abstain from all alcohol during pregnancy (Katz, 2008). In 2005, the U.S. surgeon general issued an advisory on alcohol use in pregnancy to increase public awareness about this serious health concern (CDC, 2005).

Alcohol passes the placental barrier within minutes after consumption, with fetal blood alcohol levels becoming equivalent to maternal blood alcohol levels. The effects of alcohol consumption vary according to the stage of fetal development. During the first trimester, alcohol probably alters embryonic development; throughout pregnancy, alcohol may interfere with cell division and growth; in the third trimester, the time of most rapid brain growth, alcohol may alter CNS development and contribute to growth retardation (Cunningham et al., 2010). The risk of neurologic damage decreases with the cessation of heavy drinking in the third trimester. Decreased consumption of alcohol in midpregnancy is associated with a lower incidence of growth restriction.

Assessment of alcohol intake is a chief part of each woman's medical history with questions asked in a direct, nonjudgmental manner. All women of childbearing age who are sexually active and not using an effective method of birth control should be advised of the tetratogenic effect of alcohol (CDC, 2005). Because the most profound impact of alcohol occurs in the first weeks after conception, however, nurses and other healthcare providers will see the most dramatic decrease in the effects of alcohol during pregnancy by increasing their teaching efforts in the period before conception. In a study of pregnant women with a positive alcohol screening assessment who received educational intervention, nearly two thirds decreased their risk of an alcohol exposed pregnancy (Floyd et al., 2006). If heavy consumption is involved, women should be referred early to an alcoholic treatment program. Because the drug disulfiram (Antabuse), which is often used in the treatment of alcoholism, is a suspected teratogen, a woman in such a program should inform her counselor if she becomes pregnant.

Caffeine

Current research reveals no evidence that moderate levels of caffeine are linked to birth defects. However, high caffeine intake may be linked to an increased rate of spontaneous abortion (Weng, Odouli, & Li, 2008). Furthermore, an increased risk of decreased birth weight has been found in infants of mothers who consume greater than 300 mg of caffeine daily (CARE Study Group, 2008). (The average cup of brewed coffee has 100 mg, a cup of tea has 50 mg, a regular cola drink has up to 40 mg, and a normal-sized chocolate bar has up to 50 mg.) Until more definitive data are available, nurses should advise women of common sources of caffeine, including coffee, tea, colas, and chocolate, and suggest they limit their caffeine intake to about 300 mg/day (Cunningham et al., 2010).

Marijuana

Research reveals that approximately 15% of pregnant women use marijuana. The prevalence of marijuana use in our society raises concerns about its effect on the fetus, but to date no teratogenic effects of marijuana use during pregnancy have been documented (Schempf, 2007; Wisner et al., 2007). Research on marijuana use in pregnancy is difficult, however, because it is an illegal drug. Unreliability of reporting, lack of a representative population, inability to determine strength or composition of the marijuana used (including the presence of herbicides), and use of other drugs at the same time are major factors complicating the research being done.

Cocaine

Research indicates that 2.8% of pregnant women use illicit substances; 1% of those women use cocaine at some point in their pregnancy (Wisner et al., 2007). A woman who uses cocaine is at increased risk for acute myocardial infarction, cardiac arrhythmias, ruptured ascending aorta, seizures, cerebrovascular accidents, hypertension, bowel ischemia, and sudden death (Cunningham et al., 2010). Cocaine use during pregnancy has been related to abruptio placentae, premature rupture of the membranes, preterm birth, low birth weight, neonatal irritability, and neonatal depression (Schempf, 2007) as well as SIDS (March of Dimes [MOD], 2009; Wisner et al., 2007). Studies indicate normal intelligence levels despite exposure in utero. However, subtle learning and behavioral problems may occur as a result of prenatal cocaine exposure (MOD, 2009; Wisner et al., 2007). Several congenital anomalies have been linked to maternal cocaine use, including genitourinary anomalies, congenital heart defects, limb reduction defects, CNS anomalies, prune belly syndrome (congenital absence of abdominal muscles), and segmental intestinal atresia (Cunningham et al., 2010).

As cocaine becomes more widely used by women of childbearing age, healthcare providers need to be alert to early signs of cocaine use. It is often difficult for a healthcare provider to face the fact that a patient may be using cocaine, but ongoing alertness and an open, nonjudgmental approach are important in early detection. Maternal urine screening for cocaine is valuable, but because cocaine is metabolized rapidly, the drug screen is negative within 24 to 48 hours after cocaine use. Thus it is probable that many expectant mothers who use cocaine are not identified. However, the newborn may also be screened to document maternal cocaine use. It is important for the nurse to promote early detection of fetal exposure to cocaine in order to provide appropriate newborn care.

Evaluation

Throughout the antepartum period, evaluation is an essential part of effective nursing care. As nurses ask questions of the pregnant woman and her family or make observations of physical changes, they are evaluating the results of previous interventions. In evaluating the effectiveness of the interventions, the nurse should not be afraid to try creative solutions if they are logical and carefully thought out. This is especially important in dealing with families from other cultures. If a practice is important to a woman and not harmful, the culturally competent nurse will not discourage it.

In completing an evaluation, the nurse must also recognize situations that require referral for further evaluation. For example, a woman who has gained 4 lb in 1 week probably does not require counseling about nutrition; she needs further assessment for preeclampsia. The nurse who has a sound knowledge of theory will recognize this and act immediately.

The ongoing and cyclic nature of the nursing process is especially evident in the prenatal setting. Throughout the course of pregnancy nurses can use certain criteria to determine the quality of care provided. In essence, nursing care has been effective if the following have been met:

- The common discomforts of pregnancy are quickly identified and are relieved or lessened effectively.
- The woman is able to discuss the physiologic and psychologic changes of pregnancy.

- The woman implements appropriate self-care measures, if they are indicated, during pregnancy.
- The woman avoids substances and situations that pose a risk to her well-being or that of her child.
- The woman seeks regular prenatal care.

Care of the Expectant Couple Over 35

Today an increasing number of women are choosing to have their first baby after age 35 (Table 16-6). In fact, in 2006, 1 in 5 women in the United States had her first child after the age of 35 (MOD, 2009). The birth rates for women between the ages of 35 and 39 (47.3 births per 1000 women) and between the ages of 40 and 44 (9.4 per 1000) are the highest in more than three decades (Martin et al., 2009). Many factors contribute to this trend, including the following:

- The availability of effective birth control methods
- The expanded roles and career options available for women
- The increased number of women obtaining advanced education, pursuing careers, and delaying parenthood until they are established professionally
- The increased incidence of later marriage and second marriage
- The high cost of living, which causes some young couples to delay childbearing until they are more secure financially
- The increased number of women in this older reproductive age group because of the baby boom between 1946 and 1964
- The increased availability of specialized fertilization procedures, which offers opportunities for women who had previously been considered infertile

There are advantages to having a first baby after the age of 35. Single women or couples who delay childbearing until they are older tend to be well educated and financially secure.

Usually their decision to have a baby was deliberately and thoughtfully made (Figure 16-15 ■). Because of their greater life experiences, they are also more aware of the realities of having a child than younger women, and they recognize what it means to have a baby at their age. This delay in family allows for women to pursue advanced educational degrees and prepare financially for the impact children will have on their lives. Some women are ready to make a change in their lives, desiring to stay home with a new baby. Those who plan to continue working are typically able to afford good child care.

TABLE 16-6 Pregnancy in Women over Age 35

- Couples who choose pregnancy at a later age are usually financially secure and have made a thoughtful, planned choice.
- If the woman has no existing health problems, her risk during pregnancy is not appreciably higher than that of the general population.
- The decreased fertility of women over age 35 may make conception more difficult.
- The incidence of Down syndrome increases somewhat in women over age 35 and significantly in those over age 40.
- The couple may choose to have amniocentesis or chorionic villus sampling to gain information about the health of their fetus.

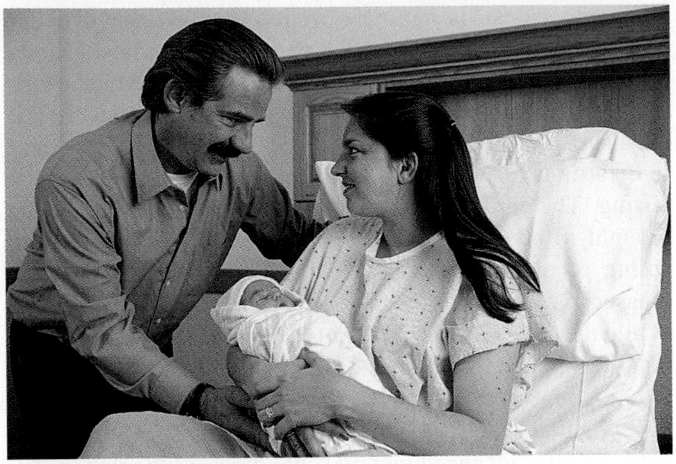

Figure 16-15 ■ For many older couples, the decision to have a child may be a very rewarding one.

Source: Photographer, Elena Dorfman.

Medical Risks

In the United States and Canada over the past 30 years, the risk of death has declined dramatically for women of all ages as a result of advances in maternal health and obstetric practice. However, the risk for maternal death is significantly higher for women over age 35 and even higher for women age 40 and older. These women also are more likely to have chronic medical conditions. Preexisting medical conditions, such as hypertension or diabetes, probably play a more significant role than age in maternal well-being and the outcome of pregnancy. The incidence of low-birth-weight infants and preterm births is higher among women age 35 or older (Delbaere et al., 2007). In addition, the rate of miscarriage is significantly higher in older women. Women over age 35 who become pregnant also have an increased risk for gestational diabetes mellitus, hypertension, placenta previa, difficult labor, and newborn complications (MOD, 2009).

The cesarean birth rate is also increased in pregnant women over 35. This practice may be related to increased concern by the woman and physician about the pregnancy outcome (MOD, 2009).

The risk of conceiving a child with Down syndrome does increase with age, especially over age 35. ACOG (2007) recommends that all pregnant women, regardless of age, be screened for Down syndrome. Research has focused on the use of quadruple screening to detect Down syndrome and trisomy 18 (see chapter 15 ∞). First trimester ultrasound assessment of the thickness of fetal nuchal folds (nuchal translucency, or NT) combined with serum screens of free beta-human chorionic gonadotropin (hCG) and pregnancy-associated plasma protein A (PAPP-A), is increasing the detection of Down syndrome, trisomy 18, and trisomy 13. If the screening results are not in the normal range, follow-up testing using ultrasound and amniocentesis is often indicated (Cleveland Clinic, 2006).

Amniocentesis is routinely offered to all women over age 35 to permit the early detection of several chromosomal abnormalities, including Down syndrome. Routine genetic testing has not been offered to couples in which the only risk is advanced paternal age, because there is no sufficient evidence to determine a specific paternal age at which to start genetic testing. The chromosomal mutations that occur with age are thought to be responsible for the increased risk of the offspring of older fathers having reduced fertility and an increased risk of birth defects (Bray, Gunnel, & Smith, 2006). While the causes of stillbirth in the over-40 age group are not known, a number of studies have found that women over age 40 are about 2 to 3 times as likely as women in their 20s to have a stillborn baby (MOD, 2009; Warren & Silver, 2008). Additionally, advanced paternal age increases the risk for genetic aberrations, especially if the father is 50 or older at the time of conception (Johnson et al., 2007).

Special Concerns of the Expectant Couple over 35

No matter what their age, most expectant couples have concerns regarding the well-being of the fetus and their ability to parent. The older couple has additional concerns related to their age, especially the closer they are to 40. Some couples are concerned about whether they will have enough energy to care for a new baby. Of greater concern is their ability to deal with the needs of the older child as they, themselves, age.

> “I didn't really think I would get married but then I met Antonio and fell hard. I was 35 and he was 43, a widower with no children. We both really wanted a baby, so here I am, 36 and pregnant. How I pray that this baby will be healthy.”

The financial concerns of an older couple are usually different from those of a younger couple. The older couple is generally more financially secure than the younger couple. However, when their “baby” is ready for college, the older couple may be near retirement and might not have the means to provide for their child.

While considering their financial future and future retirement, the older couple may be forced to face their own mortality. Certainly this is not uncommon in midlife, but instead of confronting this issue at 40 to 45 years of age or later, the older expectant couple may confront the issue several years earlier as they consider what will happen as their child grows.

The older couple facing pregnancy following a late or second marriage or after therapy for infertility may find themselves somewhat isolated socially. They may feel “different” because they are often the only couple in their peer group expecting their first baby. In fact, many of their peers are likely to be parents of adolescents or young adults and may be grandparents as well.

The response of older couples who already have children to learning that the woman is pregnant may vary greatly depending on whether the pregnancy was planned or unexpected. Other factors influencing their response include the attitudes of their children, family, and friends to the pregnancy; the impact on their lifestyle; and the financial implications of having another child. Sometimes couples who had previously been married to other mates will choose to have a child together. The concept of blended family applies to situations in which “her” children, “his” children, and “their” children come together as a new family group.

Healthcare professionals may treat the older expectant couple differently than they would a younger couple. Older women may be offered more medical procedures, such as amniocentesis and ultrasound, than younger women. An older woman may be prevented from using a birthing room or birthing center even if she is healthy, because her age is considered to put her at risk.

The woman who has delayed pregnancy may be concerned about the limited amount of time that she has to bear children. When pregnancy does not occur as quickly as she hoped, the older woman may become increasingly anxious as time slips away on her “biological clock.” When an older woman becomes pregnant but experiences a spontaneous abortion, her grief for the loss of her unborn child is exacerbated by her anxiety about her ability to conceive again in the time remaining to her.

NURSING CARE MANAGEMENT

Nursing Assessment and Diagnosis

In working with a woman in her 30s or 40s who is pregnant, the nurse makes the same assessments as are appropriate in caring for any woman who is pregnant. These include assessing physical status, the woman's understanding of pregnancy and the changes that accompany it, any health teaching needs that exist, the degree of support the woman has available to her, and her knowledge of infant care. In addition, the nurse explores the woman's and her partner's attitudes about the pregnancy and their expectations of the impact a baby will have on their lives.

The nursing diagnoses that are applicable to any pregnant woman apply to the pregnant woman who is over the age of 35. Examples of other nursing diagnoses that may apply include the following:

- ***Decisional Conflict*** related to unexpected pregnancy
- ***Impaired Social Interaction*** related to changes associated with pregnancy

Nursing Plan and Implementation

Once an older couple has decided to have a child, it is the nurse's responsibility to respect and support them in this decision. As with any patient, the nurse needs to discuss risks, identify concerns, and promote strengths. The woman's age should not be made an issue. To promote a sense of well-being, the nurse should treat the pregnancy as "normal" unless specific health risks are identified.

As the pregnancy continues, the nurse should identify and discuss concerns that the woman may have related to her age or to specific health problems. The older woman who has made a conscious decision to become pregnant often has carefully thought through potential problems and may actually have fewer concerns than a younger woman or one with an unplanned pregnancy.

Childbirth education classes are important in promoting adaptation to the event of childbirth for expectant couples of any age. However, older expectant couples, who are still in the minority, often feel uncomfortable in classes where the majority of participants are much younger. Because of the differences in age and life experiences, many of the needs of the older couple may not be met in the class. Consequently, classes for expectant parents over age 35 are now available in many communities. Women who are over 35 years of age and having their first baby tend to be better educated than other healthcare consumers. These patients frequently know the kind of care and services they want and are assertive in their interactions with the healthcare system. The nurse should neither be intimidated by these patients nor assume that they do not need anticipatory guidance and support. Instead, the nurse should support the couple's strengths and be sensitive to their individual needs.

A particularly difficult issue that older expectant couples face is the possibility of bearing an unhealthy child. Because of the risk of Down syndrome in these families, amniocentesis is encouraged. Chorionic villus sampling may also be suggested if available in the area. The decision to have amniocentesis can be difficult to make merely on the basis of its possible risks to the fetus. But that becomes almost a minor concern when the couple thinks of the implications of the possible findings of Down syndrome or other chromosomal abnormalities. The finding of abnormalities means that the couple may be faced with an even more difficult decision about continuing the pregnancy.

A couple's decision to have amniocentesis is usually related to their beliefs and attitudes about abortion. Generally, amniocentesis is not even considered by couples who are strongly opposed to abortion for any reason. Health professionals must respect the couple's decision, take a nonjudgmental approach, and provide them with emotional support throughout the pregnancy.

The decision to have an abortion is a painful one even when couples are not opposed to abortion on political or philosophic grounds. Even though the couple may believe that terminating a high-risk pregnancy is an option for their family, they may feel a great deal of ambivalence about amniocentesis. If the results are such that the couple elects to have an abortion, they will usually feel much grief for their loss.

Many health professionals assume that the couple who agrees to amniocentesis will also elect to have an abortion if Down syndrome or another condition is diagnosed. This is not necessarily the case. Some couples choose not to have an abortion after being informed that their unborn child has genetic abnormalities.

For couples who decide to have amniocentesis, the first few months of pregnancy are a difficult time. Amniocentesis cannot be done until 14 weeks of pregnancy, and the chromosomal studies take roughly 2 weeks to complete. Their fear that the fetus is at risk may delay the successful completion of the psychologic tasks of early pregnancy.

The nurse can support couples who decide to have amniocentesis in several ways:

- The nurse should make sure that the couple is aware of the risks of amniocentesis and why it is being performed.
- The nurse who is present during the amniocentesis procedure can offer comfort and emotional support to the expectant woman. The nurse can also provide information about the procedure as it is being performed.
- The nurse can facilitate a support group for women during the difficult waiting period between the procedure and the results.
- If the results indicate that the fetus has Down syndrome or another genetic abnormality, the nurse can ensure that the couple has complete information about the condition, its range of possible manifestations, and its developmental implications.
- The nurse can support the couple in their decision about continuing or terminating the pregnancy. It is essential that the nurse and other health professionals involved with the couple not impose their philosophic or political beliefs about abortion on the couple. The decision is the couple's, and it should be based on their belief system and a nonbiased presentation of risks and choices from caregivers.

Amniocentesis is discussed further in chapter 21 ∞.

Evaluation

Expected outcomes of nursing care include the following:

- The woman and her partner are knowledgeable about the pregnancy and make appropriate healthcare choices.
- The expectant couple is able to cope successfully with the pregnancy and its implications for the future.
- The woman receives effective health care throughout her pregnancy and during birth and the postpartum period.
- The woman and her partner develop skills in child care and parenting as necessary.

FOCUS YOUR STUDY

- Providing anticipatory guidance about childbirth, the postpartum period, and childrearing is a primary responsibility of the nurse caring for women in an antepartal setting.
- The nurse assesses the expectant father's knowledge level and intended degree of participation and then works with the couple to help ensure a satisfying experience.
- Culturally based practices and taboos may have a major impact on the childbearing family.
- The common discomforts of pregnancy occur as a result of physiologic and anatomic changes. The nurse provides the woman with information about self-care activities aimed at reducing or relieving discomfort.
- To make appropriate self-care choices and ensure healthful habits, a pregnant woman requires accurate information about a range of subjects from exercise to sexual activity, from bathing to immunization.
- Maternal assessment of fetal activity keeps the woman "in touch" with her fetus and provides ongoing assessment of fetal status.
- Teratogenic substances are substances that adversely affect the normal growth and development of the fetus.
- A pregnant woman should avoid taking nonessential medications or using over-the-counter preparations during pregnancy.
- Evidence confirms that smoking, consuming alcohol, or using social drugs during pregnancy may be harmful to the fetus.
- Childbirth among women over 35 is becoming increasingly common. It poses fewer health risks than previously believed and offers advantages for the woman or couple who makes the choice.
- A major risk for the older expectant couple relates to the increased incidence of Down syndrome in children born to women over age 35. Amniocentesis can provide information as to whether the fetus has Down syndrome. The couple can then decide whether they wish to continue the pregnancy.

CRITICAL THINKING IN ACTION

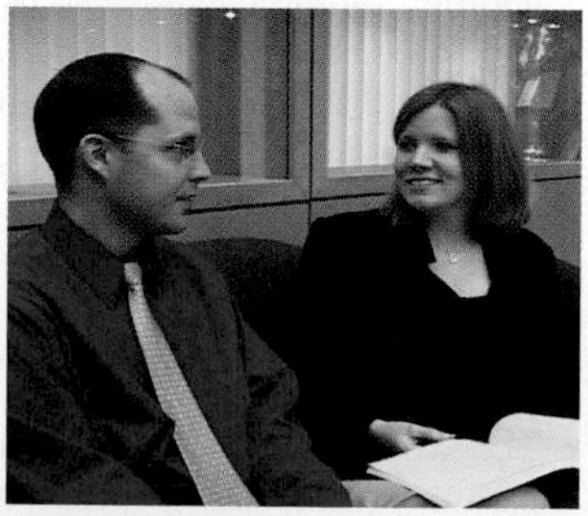

Thirty-seven-year-old Cathy Sommers, G1, P0000, presents to you, with her husband, at the OB physician's office at 32 weeks' gestation. Cathy tells you that she and her husband are practicing lawyers with their own firm. The couple delayed starting a family because it has been important to them to advance their careers and establish their firm. Cathy had an amniocentesis at 18 weeks' gestation because of her advanced maternal age, and the results ruled out chromosomal abnormalities. The couple knows that the baby is a boy, and are anticipating a vaginal birth. Cathy tells you that she is experiencing more fatigue, leg cramps, and shortness of breath when climbing stairs. The physical exam including a negative Homan's sign is within normal limits with the exception of slight ankle edema. Her weight is 150 lb, temperature 98.6°F, pulse 88, respirations 16, BP 126/70. You discuss pregnancy discomforts in the third trimester with Cathy and her husband.

1. What measures can you suggest to cope with fatigue?
2. Discuss measures to decrease leg cramps.
3. Discuss the physiologic changes underlying dyspnea.
4. Review Braxton Hicks contractions.

See www.nursing.pearsonhighered.com for possible responses.

Pearson Nursing Student Resources

Find additional review materials at
www.nursing.pearsonhighered.com

Prepare for success with additional NCLEX®-style practice questions, interactive assignments and activities, Web links, animations and videos, and more!

REFERENCES

American Academy of Pediatrics (AAP) and the American College of Obstetricians and Gynecologists (ACOG). (2008). *Guidelines for perinatal care* (6th ed.). Elk Grove Village, IL: Author.

American College of Obstetricians and Gynecologists (ACOG). (2002). *Exercise during pregnancy and the postpartum period* (ACOG Technical Bulletin No. 267). Washington, DC: Author.

American College of Obstetricians and Gynecologists (ACOG). (2004). *Diagnosis and treatment of nausea and vomiting of pregnancy* (ACOG Practice Bulletin No. 52). Washington, DC: Author.

American College of Obstetricians and Gynecologists (ACOG). (2005). *Smoking cessation during pregnancy* (ACOG Committee Opinion No. 316). Washington, DC: Author.

American College of Obstetricians and Gynecologists (ACOG). (2007). *Screening for fetal chromosomal abnormalities* (ACOG Practice Bulletin No. 77). Washington DC: Author.

American College of Obstetricians and Gynecologists (ACOG). (2009a). *Air travel during pregnancy* (ACOG Committee Opinion No. 443). Washington, DC: Author.

American College of Obstetricians and Gynecologists (ACOG). (2009b). *Update on immunization and pregnancy: Tetanus, diphtheria, and pertussis vaccination* (ACOG Committee Opinion No. 438). Washington, DC: Author.

Anderko L., Braun, J., & Auinger, P. (2010). Contribution of tobacco smoke exposure to learning disabilities. *JOGNN: Journal of Obstetric, Gynecologic, and Neonatal Nursing, 39*(1), 111–117.

Bell, J. F., Zimmerman, F. J., & Diehr, P. K. (2008). Maternal work and birth outcome disparities. *Maternal Child Health Journal, 12*, 415–426.

Bray, I., Gunnel, D., & Smith, G. D. (2006). Advanced paternal age: How old is too old? *Journal of Epidemiology and Community Health, 60*, 851–853.

CARE Study Group. (2008). Maternal caffeine intake during pregnancy and the risk of fetal growth restriction: A large prospective observational study. *British Medical Journal, 337*, a2332.

Centers for Disease Control and Prevention (CDC). (2005). Surgeon general's advisory on alcohol use in pregnancy. *Morbidity and Mortality Weekly Report, 54*, 229.

Chalupka, S., & Chalupka, A. N. (2010). The impact of environmental and occupational exposures on reproductive health. *Journal of Obstetric, Gynecologic, and Neonatal Nursing,39*(1), 84–100.

Cleveland Clinic. (2006). Quad marker screen. Retrieved from http://my.clevelandclinic.org/services/Quad_Marker_Screen/hic_Quad_Marker_Screen.aspx

College of Nurses of Ontario. (2009). *Culturally sensitive care* (Publication No. 41040). Toronto, Ontario, Canada: Author.

Community Partnership for Older Adults. (2007). *Cultural competence vs. cultural humility*. Retrieved from Robert Wood Johnson Foundation Web site: http://www.partnershipsforolderadults.org/resources/levelthree.aspx?sectionGUID=774e17bd-fa1e-4253-8d6d-34d808334fb0

Condon, J. (2006). What about dad? Psychosocial and mental health issues for new fathers. *Australian Family Physician, 35*, 690–692.

Cooklin, A. R., Rowe, H. J, & Fisher, J. (2007). Employee entitlements during pregnancy and maternal psychological well-being. *Australian and New Zealand Journal of Obstetrics and Gynaecology, 47*, 483–490.

Cunningham, F. G., Leveno, K. J., Bloom, S. L., Hauth, J. C., Rouse, D. J., & Spong, C. Y. (2010). *Williams obstetrics* (23rd ed.). New York, NY: McGraw-Hill.

Delbaere, I., Verstraelen, H., Goetgeluk, S., Martens, G., De Backer, G., & Temmerman, M. (2007). Pregnancy outcome in primiparae of advanced maternal age. *European Journal of Obstetrics, Gynecology, and Reproductive Biology, 135*(1), 41–46.

Floyd, R. L., Ebrahim, S., Tsai, J., O'Connor, M., & Sokol, R. (2006). Strategies to reduce alcohol-exposed pregnancies. *Maternal Child Health, 10*, 149–151.

Forest, S. (2010). Controversy and evidence about nicotine replacement therapy in pregnancy. *MCN: The American Journal of Maternal-Child Nursing, 35*(2), 89–95.

Galic, V., & Martino, M. (2010). Smoking cessation in the female patient. *The Female Patient, 35*(3), 28–31.

Gavard, J. A., & Artal, R. (2008). Effect of exercise on pregnancy. *Clinical Obstetrics and Gynecology, 51*(2), 467–480.

Guilbeau, J. R., & Hurst, H. (2009). Brush up: Periodontal disease and pregnancy. *Nursing for Women's Health, 13*(6), 496–499.

Hartmann, K. E., Wechter, M. E., Payne, P., Salisbury, K., Jackson, R. D., & Melvin, C. L. (2007). Best practice smoking cessation and resource needs of prenatal care providers. *Obstetrics and Gynecology, 110*(4), 765–770.

Ho, S. S., Yu, W. W., Lao, T. T., Chow, D. H., Chung, J. W., & Li, Y. (2009). Garment needs of pregnant women based on content analysis of in-depth interviews. *Journal of Clinical Nursing, 18*(17), 2426–2435.

Ickovics, J., Kershaw, T., Westdahl, C., Magriples, U., Massey, Z., Reynolds, H., & Rising, S. (2007). Group prenatal care and perinatal outcomes: A randomized trial. *Obstetrics and Gynecology, 110*(2, Pt. 1), 330–339.

Jeffcoat, H. (2008). Exercises for low back pain in pregnancy. *International Journal of Childbirth Education, 23*(3), 9–12.

Johnson, T. R., Gregory, K. D., & Niebyl, J. R. (2007). Preconception and prenatal care: Part of the continuum. In S. G. Gabbe, J. R. Niebyl, Y. J. L. Simpson (Eds.), *Obstetrics: Normal and problem pregnancies* (5th ed., pp. 111–137). Philadelphia, PA: Churchill Livingstone.

Kahn, B. F., Hobbins, J. C., & Galan, H. L. (2008). Intrauterine growth restriction. In R. Gibbs, B. Karlan, A. Haney, & I. Nygaard (Eds.), *Danforth's obstetrics and gynecology* (10th ed., pp. 198–219). Philadelphia, PA: Lippincott, Williams & Wilkins.

Katz, V. (2008). Prenatal care. In R. Gibbs, B. Karlan, A. Haney, & I. Nygaard (Eds.), *Danforth's obstetrics and gynecology* (10th ed., pp. 1–21). Philadelphia, PA: Lippincott, Williams & Wilkins.

Kramer, M. S. (2006). Aerobic exercise for women during pregnancy. *Cochrane Library* (1). (Article 2006 No. CD 000180).

Lacasse, A., Rey, E., Ferreira, E., Morin, C., & Berard, A. (2009). Determinants of early medical management of nausea and vomiting of pregnancy. *Birth, 36*(1), 70–77.

Lauderdale, J. (2008). Transcultural perspectives in childbearing. In M. Andrews (Ed.), *Transcultural concepts in nursing* (5th ed., pp. 95–131). Philadelphia, PA: Lippincott, Williams & Wilkins.

Locock, L., Alexander, J., & Rozmovits, L. (2008). Women's responses to nausea and vomiting in pregnancy. *Midwifery, 24*, 143–152.

March of Dimes (MOD). (2009). Pregnancy after 35. Retrieved from http://www.marchofdimes.com/printableArticles/14332_1155.asp

Martin, J. A., Hamilton, B. E., Sutton, P. D., Ventura, M. L., Menacker, F., Kirmeyer, S., & Mathews, T. J. (2009). Births: Final data for 2006. *National Vital Statistics Reports, 57*(7), 1–102.

Martin, L. T., McNamara, M., Milot, A., Bloch, M., Hair, E. C., & Halle, T. (2008). Correlates of smoking before, during, and after pregnancy. *American Journal of Health Behavior, 32*(3), 272–282.

Massey, Z., Schindler Rising, S., & Ickovics, J. (2006). Centering pregnancy group prenatal care: Promoting relationship-centered care. *Journal of Obstetric, Gynecologic, and Neonatal Nursing, 35*(2), 286–294.

Mattson, S. (2004). Ethnocultural considerations in the childbearing period. In S. Mattson & J. E. Smith (Eds.), *Core curriculum for maternal-newborn nursing* (3rd ed.). St. Louis, MO: Elsevier Saunders.

McGovern, L. M., Boyce, T. G., & Fischer, P. R. (2007). Congenital infections associated with international travel during pregnancy. *Journal of Travel Medicine, 14*(2), 117–128.

McParlin, C., Graham, R. H., & Robson, S. C. (2008). Caring for women with nausea and vomiting in pregnancy: New approaches. *British Journal of Midwifery, 16*(5), 280–285.

Nation Center for Complementary and Alternative Medicine (NCCAM). (2008, December). The use of complementary and alternative medicine in the United States. Retrieved from http://nccam.nih.gov/news/camstats/2007/camsurvey_fs1.htm

Niebyl, J. R., & Simpson, J. L. (2007). Drugs and environmental agents in pregnancy and lactions: Embryology, teratology, epidemiology. In S. E. Gabbe, J. R. Niebyl, & J. L. Simpson (Eds.), *Obstetrics: Normal and problem pregnancies* (5th ed.). New York, NY: Churchill-Livingstone.

Ozgoli, G., Goli, M., & Simbar, M. (2009). Effects of ginger capsules on pregnancy, nausea, and vomiting. *Journal of Alternative and Complementary Medicine, 15*(3), 243–246.

Penney, D. S. (2008). The effects of vigorous exercise during pregnancy. *Journal of Midwifery and Women's Health, 53*(2), 155–159.

Pivarnik, J. M., & Mudd, L. (2009). Oh baby! Exercise during pregnancy and the postpartum period. *ACSM's Health and Fitness Journal, 13*(3), 8–13.

Purnell, L. D. (2009). *Guide to culturally competent health care*. Philadelphia, PA: F. A. Davis.

Reid, J. (2007). Centering pregnancy: A model for group prenatal care. *Nursing for Women's Health, 11*(4), 383–388.

Russell, S. L., & Mayberry, L. J. (2008). Pregnancy and oral health. *MCN: The American Journal of Maternal/Child Nursing, 33*(1), 59–68.

Saade, G. R. (2007). Occupational hazards. *Contemporary OB/Gyn, 52*(3), 59–68.

Schempf, A. H. (2007). Illicit drug use and neonatal outcomes: A critical review. *Obstetrical & Gynecological Survey, 62*(11), 749–757.

Spector, R. E. (2009). *Cultural diversity in health and illness* (7th ed.). Upper Saddle River, NJ: Prentice-Hall Health.

Warren, J., & Silver, R. (2008). Genetics of pregnancy loss. *Clinical Obstetrics and Gynecology, 51*(1), 84–95.

Weng, X., Odouli, R., & Li, D. K. (2008). Maternal caffeine consumption during pregnancy and the risk of miscarriage. *American Journal of Obstetrics and Gynecology, 198*, 279el–279e8.

Wills, G., & Forster, D. (2008). Nausea and vomiting in pregnancy: What advice do midwives give? *Midwifery, 24*, 390–398.

Wisner, K. L., Sit, D. K. Y., Reynolds, M. A., Altemus, M., Bogen, D. L., Sunder, K. R., Misra, D., & Perel, J. M. (2007). Psychiatric disorders. In S. G. Gabbe, J. R. Niebyl, & J. L. Simpson (Eds.), *Obstetrics: Normal and problem pregnancies* (5th ed., pp. 1249–1288). Philadelphia, PA: Churchill Livingstone.

CHAPTER 17

Adolescent Pregnancy

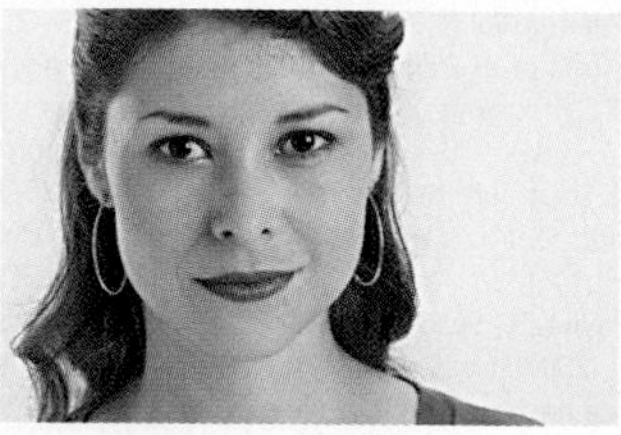

I am a freshman in college, and so is my daughter. I had her when I was 15, and that forced me to grow up in a hurry. For years I've thought about being a nurse, and now is my chance. Please understand, my daughter is very precious to me, but a part of me knows that if I had it to do over, I would change so much of my life—if only I had known!

LEARNING OUTCOMES

1. Discuss the physical and psychosocial changes of adolescence.
2. Compare the three stages of adolescence: early adolescence, middle adolescence, and late adolescence.
3. Summarize the developmental tasks of adolescence and the impact that pregnancy superimposes on these tasks.
4. Describe the major factors that contribute to teenage pregnancy.
5. Identify the impact of cultural factors on the desirability of early pregnancy.
6. Identify the physical, psychologic, and sociologic risks faced by an adolescent who is pregnant.
7. Delineate characteristics of the fathers of children of adolescent mothers.
8. Discuss the reactions of the adolescent's family and social support groups to her pregnancy.
9. Formulate a plan of care to meet the needs of a pregnant adolescent.
10. Describe successful community approaches to adolescent pregnancy prevention.

KEY TERMS

Early adolescence *380*
Emancipated minors *387*
Late adolescence *380*
Middle adolescence *380*

Adolescent pregnancy is a health and social issue with no single cause or cure. For a teen, pregnancy comes at a time when her physical development and the developmental tasks of adolescence are incomplete. She may not be prepared physically, psychologically, or economically for parenthood. Thus both she and her child are at high risk for a number of adverse outcomes. Compared with women of similar socioeconomic status who postpone childbearing, teen mothers are less likely to finish high school, less likely to go to college, more likely to be single, and more likely to end up on welfare. Babies of adolescent mothers are often born prematurely and of low birth weight. In addition, children of teen mothers are at increased risk for intellectual disability (mental retardation), poverty, welfare dependency, and poor school performance. They are also more likely to grow up without a father. In addition, they suffer higher rates of abuse and neglect than would occur if their mothers had delayed childbearing (National Campaign to Prevent Teen and Unplanned Pregnancy [NCPTUP], 2010).

Each year, an estimated 750,000 U.S. adolescents ages 15 to 19 years become pregnant, and approximately 442,000 children are born to teens. Of these pregnancies, about 27% are terminated by therapeutic abortion (Alan Guttmacher Institute [AGI], 2010a). A portion of pregnancies end in miscarriage but more than half the teens who become pregnant give birth and keep their babies.

The teenage pregnancy rate dropped 40% from 1990 to 2005, from 61.8 per 1000 women to an historic low of 40.5 per 1000 women ages 15 to 19 years. Rates fell much more for younger than for older teenagers. However, the birth rate for teenagers ages 15 to 19 years rose 3% in 2006 and 1% more in 2007 to 42.5 per 1000, interrupting the long-term decline that had extended from 1991 through 2005 (NCPTUP, 2010). See Figure 17-1 ■. This increase was halted in 2008, when the birth rate for teens fell 2% to 41.5 per 1000 (Hamilton, Martin, & Ventura, 2010).

The U.S. teenage birth rate remains the highest of any industrialized nation, almost twice as high as those of England, Wales, and Canada and 8 times as high as those of the Netherlands and Japan (AGI, 2006). The incidence of sexual activity among teens in other countries is as high as in the United States. These countries may have lower adolescent pregnancy rates because of family influences, a greater openness about sexuality, better access to contraceptives, and a more comprehensive approach to sex education.

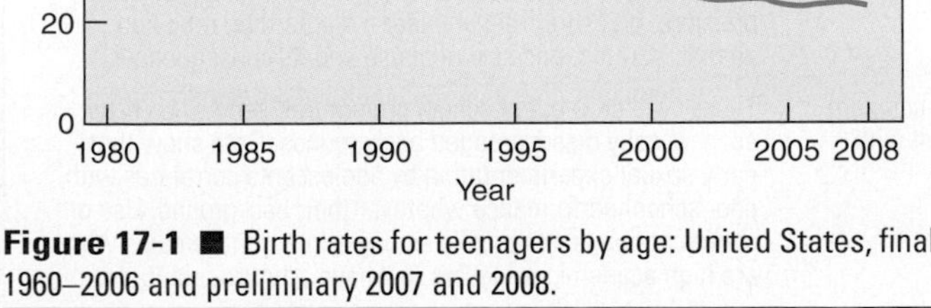

Figure 17-1 ■ Birth rates for teenagers by age: United States, final 1960–2006 and preliminary 2007 and 2008.

Source: U. S. Department of Health and Human Services. (2010). Births: preliminary data for 2008. National Vital Statistics Report, 58(15).

This chapter explores the incidence, risk factors, and consequences of adolescent pregnancy. It then presents the role of the nurse in meeting the special needs and concerns of pregnant adolescents and their families and concludes with a discussion of efforts to prevent adolescent pregnancy.

Overview of Adolescence

Physical Changes

Adolescence is the period of development during which an individual makes the psychologic and physiologic transition from childhood to young adulthood, usually between 13 and 20 years of age. Puberty, the period during which an individual becomes capable of reproduction, is a maturational process that can last from 1.5 to 6 years and generally coincides with adolescence. The major physical changes of puberty include a growth spurt, weight change, and the appearance of secondary sexual characteristics. *Menarche,* or the time of the first menstrual period, usually occurs in the last half of puberty, with the average age between 12 and 13.

The initial menstrual cycles are usually irregular and often anovulatory for the first 12 to 18 months; however, this is not true for all females. Some adolescents do not use contraception during this time because they falsely assume that they cannot get pregnant. Even if their initial menstrual cycles are anovulatory, there is no certainty about when the first ovulatory cycle will occur; thus, contraception is important during this time for all adolescents who are sexually active.

Psychosocial Development

Although it is well documented that the onset of puberty now occurs at a younger age than it did 50 years ago, there are no data to indicate that psychosocial development, particularly cognitive development, occurs at an earlier age. Developmental tasks of adolescence have been described by many writers and are based on a variety of classic theories. These tasks are issues that individuals may struggle with at other times in their lives, but they are especially significant during adolescence to help ensure a successful transition from childhood to adulthood. The following are major developmental tasks of this period (Steinberg, 2010):

- Developing an identity.
- Gaining autonomy and independence.
- Developing intimacy in a relationship.
- Developing comfort with one's own sexuality.
- Developing a sense of achievement.

Resolving these tasks is a developmental process that occurs over time. This developmental process is reflected in the behaviors of youths during early, middle, and late adolescence.

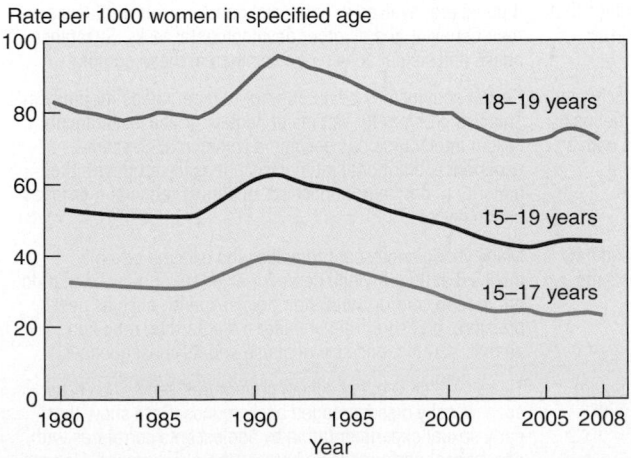

During adolescence, there is a need to "try on" various roles in a process of experimentation and exploration as adolescents grapple with ideas about who they want to be and how they want to live. This developmental process occurs in youths during all stages of adolescence and is affected by many factors, including culture, religion, and socioeconomic status.

Teens work to separate themselves from their parents to establish their own identity and they begin to express themselves with music, clothing, and hairstyles. Some choose peer-identity behaviors such as body modifications (body piercing) and body art (tattoos). Although these forms of peer identity have been around for thousands of years, they are gaining popularity, especially among teens and preteens. See the discussion in chapter 4 ∞.

During **early adolescence** (age 14 and under), psychosocial development is marked by rapid physical changes that engender self-centeredness and initiate the struggle for independence. The teen at this age still sees authority as resting with the parents. She perceives her locus of control as external; that is, her destiny is controlled by others, such as parents and school authorities. However, she begins the process of "leaving the family" by spending more time with friends, especially friends of the same sex. Conformity to peer group standards is reflected in her behavior and her clothing. She may lack impulse control, which can result in risk-taking behaviors. During this phase, the adolescent has a rich fantasy life. She is also struggling to become comfortable with her changing body and body image and to fit this image with her fantasy life. Much time is spent in front of the mirror. The adolescent in this phase is very egocentric and is a concrete thinker. She has only minimal ability to see herself in the future or foresee the consequences of her behavior.

Middle adolescence (15 to 17 years) is the time for challenging authority. Experimentation with drugs, alcohol, and sex is a common method of rebellion. As the middle adolescent seeks independence, she turns increasingly to her peer group, identifying with and conforming to them in her choice of dress, makeup, hairstyle, and music. These years are often a time of great turmoil for the family as the adolescent struggles for independence and challenges the family's values and expectations.

The middle adolescent wants to be treated as an adult. However, fear of adult responsibility may cause fluctuation in behavior. At times she seems like a child; at other times she is surprisingly mature. She is beginning to move from concrete thinking to formal operational thought but is not yet able to anticipate the long-term implications of all her actions. She may even believe that she is invincible and will not suffer negative consequences from risk-taking behaviors.

In **late adolescence** (18 to 19 years), the young woman is more at ease with her individuality and decision-making ability. She can think abstractly and anticipate consequences. During this time, she becomes more confident of her personal identity. The late adolescent is capable of formal operational thought. She is learning to solve problems, to conceptualize, and to make decisions. These abilities help her see herself as having control, which leads to the ability to understand and accept the consequences of her behavior.

Table 17-1 describes successful resolution of each of the developmental tasks of adolescence and identifies high-risk factors for adolescent pregnancy.

TABLE 17-1 Developmental Tasks of Adolescence

TASKS	DESCRIPTION OF SUCCESSFUL RESOLUTION	HIGH-RISK FACTORS FOR TEEN PREGNANCY
Developing an identity	As individuals enter puberty, their physical appearance begins to change, and others begin to respond differently to them. The media present idealized images of the teenage female. Self-esteem may fluctuate, and hormonal changes create awareness of sexual desire. Adolescents experience confusion about their self-image. This is a time of experimentation until they become comfortable with whom they are.	If the young adolescent feels she cannot live up to parents' expectations or is in a dysfunctional family situation, she may adopt a negative identity. She may become rebellious and actively involved in risk-taking behaviors, such as substance abuse and early sexual activity.
Gaining independence	Adolescents gradually move away from parental control and are influenced by peers. Eventually, they develop values that help govern their behavior responsibly without extrinsic control of peers or parents.	Peer pressure is highest during early and middle adolescence. If peers are involved in antisocial behavior, this influences their behavior and all other developmental tasks. Substance abuse and sexual activity are common in these groups.
Developing emotional intimacy in relationships	Adolescents begin to develop a close emotional attachment with another individual. They can share innermost feelings and have empathy for the other. This usually begins with a friend of the same sex and eventually develops into a trusting and loving relationship with someone of the opposite sex.	Sexual activity may be an attempt to meet needs for intimacy. This is a problem for victims of neglect or abuse. Although sexual intercourse has become a common adolescent experience, emotional intimacy is not associated with the majority of dating relationships, and most teenage marriages end in divorce.
Developing comfort with their sexuality	Puberty causes a new awareness of sexual desire and new meaning about physical contact with others. Adolescents learn to express sexual feelings appropriately and comfortably in a relationship.	Many young adolescent females who become sexually involved at an early age do so for a variety of reasons that do not lead to comfort with their own sexuality, such as peer pressure, pressure from an older male partner, rebellion against parents, and sexual abuse and its consequences.
Gaining a sense of achievement	Adolescents begin to look toward the future and compare talents, work skills, and/or academic achievement with reality in preparing for adult working roles.	Those who drop out of school prematurely tend to be from economically disadvantaged backgrounds. Data show that early sexual experimentation by adolescents correlates with poor school performance whatever their background. Use of contraception is more likely among adolescent females who are high academic achievers and have a future orientation.

Source: Adapted from Steinberg, L. (2010). Adolescence *(9th ed.). New York, NY: McGraw-Hill.*

Factors Contributing to Adolescent Pregnancy

Teenagers rarely plan pregnancy. *Pregnancy risk taking* (sexual activity without use of pregnancy prevention measures) is believed to stem from a complex variety of factors, the most important of which are discussed next.

Socioeconomic and Cultural Factors

Nearly all young people experience pressure of some kind to be sexually active and are, therefore, at risk of pregnancy and its consequences. It is not the case that only one group of teens, only one ethnic group, or only low-income teens engage in sex and become pregnant. Sexual activity, pregnancy, and the risk for sexually transmitted infections cut across all of these groups (NCPTUP, 2007).

Poverty is both a cause and a consequence of teen pregnancy and childbearing. For many years it was believed that poverty and its manifestations, such as drop-out rates, were the *consequence* of early childbearing. However, recent research has associated poverty and social disorganization as among the *causes* of teen childbearing as well (NCPTUP, 2007). Adolescents who do not have access to middle-class opportunities tend to maintain their pregnancies, because they see pregnancy as their only option for adult status; 85% of births to unmarried teens occur to those from poor or low-income families (AGI, 2006). Not surprisingly, research indicates that the more time high school students spend without adult supervision, the greater their level of sexual activity.

In the United States, the adolescent birth rate is higher among African American and Hispanic teens than among white teens. To some degree, the higher teenage pregnancy rate in these groups reflects the impact of poverty, because a disproportionately higher number of African American and Hispanic youths live in poverty. Research has shown that minority teens are most vulnerable to early sexual activity with subsequent pregnancy (Talashek, Alba, & Patel, 2006). Pregnancy prevention programs cannot affect race or ethnicity but sometimes in collaboration with other programs they can help reduce minority poverty or minority cultural values that may contribute to sexual risk (NCPTUP, 2007).

Low educational achievement is another major risk factor for adolescent pregnancy. Teenage pregnancy is the leading reason why adolescent women drop out of school. An estimated 30% to 40% of female teenage dropouts are mothers. Teens who grow up in poor neighborhoods with inferior schools are likely to have the view that employment and educational opportunities are limited whether they are pregnant or not. Family obligations, which compete with the time and energy needed to attend school, and a lack of vocational opportunities may influence poor teens' misuse of contraception and, if they do become pregnant, their decision to carry their babies to term. Unlike middle-class teens, whose college and career plans would be inconvenienced by having a child, motherhood may become a rite of passage to adulthood for disadvantaged teens. Although many studies show discouraging results for adolescents who become pregnant, for others, pregnancy may lead the way to more responsible and mature behaviors (SmithBattle, 2007).

The younger the teen when she first gets pregnant, the more likely she is to have another pregnancy in her teens. Moreover, the likelihood of repeat pregnancies increases when the teen is living with her sexual partner and has dropped out of school. Additionally, girls whose sister had a baby in her early teens and girls whose mother and sister both gave birth as teens are significantly more likely to have a teenage pregnancy themselves (East, Reyes, & Horn, 2007).

High-Risk Behaviors

Developmentally, adolescents, especially younger ones, are not yet able to foresee the consequences of their actions. As a result, they may have a sense of invulnerability that leads to the mistaken idea that harm will not befall them. This sense of invulnerability may also result in an overly optimistic view of the outcomes of the risks associated with their actions (King-Jones, 2008).

Among American adolescents there is tremendous peer pressure to become sexually active during the teen years. Premarital sexual activity is commonplace and teenage pregnancy is more socially acceptable today than it was in the past. In fact, nearly half (46%) of all teenagers 15 to 19 have had sex at least once (AGI, 2010a).

Sexual innuendo permeates every aspect of the popular media, including music, music videos, television, and movies. Research shows that adolescents spend an average of 8 hours per day engaged in mass media including approximately 3 to 4 hours per day watching TV. Sexual content dominates many programs most popular with adolescents, and they frequently use television as a source of their sexual information (Pinkleton, Austin, Cohen, et al., 2008).

The Internet provides teens with unlimited access to information about sex as well as a steady supply of people willing to discuss it with them. These experiences and images feed the adolescent's rich fantasy life and may glamorize unprotected intercourse as proof of "true love." At the same time, media aimed at teens largely ignore issues of sexual responsibility and fail to convey the physical, emotional, financial, and social costs of pregnancy risk-taking behaviors. Of particular note is the current blend of "sex and tech" in which teens and young adults use electronic activity to send or post sexually suggestive text and images. Statistics show that 20% of teens have sent or posted nude or semi-nude pictures or videos of themselves; 39% of teens say they are sending or posting sexually suggestive messages via e-mail or phone; and 48% of teens say they have received such messages. Seventy-five percent of teens say they know that sending such messages can have serious consequences and even know that such messages are often shared with people other than the intended receiver. Another alarming outcome in the research shows that sending or posting sexually suggestive text or images has made teens personally more forward and aggressive in cyberspace than they are in their real lives (NCPTUP, 2008).

In addition to vaginal intercourse, many adolescents engage in other sexual behaviors. The incidence of oral sex is increasing. Initiation of oral sex generally occurs soon after first vaginal intercourse and up to 82% of adolescents who had engaged in vaginal intercourse went on to engage in oral sex within 6 months (Lindberg, Jones, & Santelli, 2008). The increase has occurred, especially among young and early-middle adolescents, because of the pressure to have sex coupled with the fear of pregnancy.

The question of whether "oral sex" is really "sex" has led adolescents to perceive that they are still virgins if they have not had vaginal-penile sexual activity. Adolescents believe that they are less likely to get a bad reputation, get into trouble, or feel bad about themselves if they have oral rather than vaginal sex. However, they typically underestimate the risks of contracting chlamydia, HIV, and other sexually transmitted infections (STIs).

High-risk sexual behaviors, including, for example, multiple partners and lack of contraceptive use, are of concern. Research indicates that young people ages 15 to 24 constitute 25% of the sexually experienced population in the United States. However, they account for 48% of the new cases of STIs. This is particularly worrisome because many STIs, including HIV, are asymptomatic. Thus, apparently healthy young people who are infected may not seek health care (Weinstock, Berman, & Cates, 2004).

Statistics have demonstrated an increased use of condoms among the adolescent population, probably because of widespread educational efforts related to HIV. The condom is the most common contraceptive method used at first intercourse with 66% of females and 71% of males reporting its use (AGI, 2006). Nevertheless, adolescents remain inconsistent contraceptive users. Barriers to consistent contraceptive use include denial of their status as being sexually active when they may have had intercourse only once or twice; not considering the consequences of unprotected sexual activity; and embarrassment while talking about the topic with healthcare providers, their parents, and their partners. Teens reported feeling challenged when discussing contraception, unless it was with same age and gender peers, and, therefore, they avoided discussing it with their sexual partners who "seemed so opposed to it" (Lemay, Cashman, Elfenbein, et al., 2007). Many teens lack accurate and adequate knowledge about contraceptive options. This is a common topic of sex education programs; however, debate continues about the appropriateness of such programs in schools. Proponents advocate early sex education to provide teens with the knowledge they need to avoid unwanted pregnancy and the risk of STIs. Opponents feel that sex education is the responsibility of parents and worry that sex education in the schools will promote sexual activity. However, evaluations of comprehensive sex education and HIV/STI prevention programs show that they do not increase rates of sexual initiation, do not lower the age at which youth initiate sex, and do not increase the frequency of sex or the number of sex partners among sexually active youth. Conversely, when only abstinence programs are provided, the limited education can mean that teens are less likely to get STI testing and less likely to use a condom or contraception when they do have sex. Other factors affecting the use of contraception include access or availability, cost of supplies, and concern regarding confidentiality.

Adolescent sexuality is not pathologic but a part of normal development as a human being. Emphasizing sexual health rather than discussing sex exclusively as a behavior that has only bad consequences results in more effective work with adolescents (Kelly, Lesser, & Smoots, 2005).

Psychosocial Factors

Family dysfunction and poor self-esteem are also major risk factors for adolescent pregnancy. Some young teenagers deliberately plan to get pregnant. The adolescent girl may use pregnancy for various subconscious or conscious reasons: to punish her father and/or mother, to escape from an undesirable home situation, to gain attention, or to feel that she has someone to love and to love her. In these cases, pregnancy may in a sense be the young woman's form of delinquency. Like delinquent males, pregnant adolescents often have a history of troubled family relationships, poor school achievement, and drug abuse. For others, however, pregnancy marks an important milestone that leads to positive lifestyle changes and healthier behaviors (Pinkleton et al., 2008).

More teens who become pregnant, compared with teens who have not been pregnant, have been physically, emotionally, or sexually abused. Many teens have been exposed to intimate partner violence or have lived with someone who has substance abuse, has mental illness, or is involved in criminal activity. These experiences often lead the teen herself to engage in risk-taking behaviors such as smoking and alcohol consumption and may lead to mental health problems such as depression. Children born to these mothers have a higher risk of psychologic problems, which can lead to a multigenerational risk of mental health disability (Magill & Wilcox, 2007).

Teenage pregnancy can result from an incestuous relationship. In the very young adolescent, incest or sexual abuse should be suspected as a possible cause of pregnancy. Sex at a young age with an older partner can be associated with poor reproductive health outcomes because of the younger teen's undeveloped decision-making and negotiation skills, power imbalances, and exploitation by an older partner (Manlove, Terry-Humen, & Ikramullah, 2006).Teenage pregnancy could also be caused by other nonvoluntary sexual experiences such as acquaintance rape.

International Perspective

Globally about 16 million girls ages 15 to 19 give birth each year. One in 10 babies worldwide is born to an adolescent mother with almost 95% of adolescent mothers living in developing countries. The highest birth rates are found in sub-Saharan Africa and in some parts of Latin America and south Asia. Age at marriage is an important consideration. The majority of adolescent mothers are married; in developing countries, about 90% of births to adolescent mothers occur in marriage and three out of four pregnancies are planned. Despite this, however, statistics show that 4 million adolescents become pregnant unintentionally (World Health Organization [WHO], 2008a).

Cultural factors often play a significant role in the desirability of early pregnancy. Specifically, adolescent women are more likely to welcome a pregnancy in a country where Islam is the predominant religion, where large families are desired, where social change is slow in coming, and where most childbearing occurs within marriage. Early pregnancy is less desired in countries where the reverse is true.

In the past 2 to 3 decades the rates of adolescent childbirths have dropped significantly in most regions and countries. At the same time, in most countries, educational levels for girls have risen and job opportunities have increased (WHO, 2008b). In addition, in many parts of the world, young women now have goals in their lives beyond marriage and motherhood.

Growing evidence suggests that a significant number of girls in developing countries have experienced coercive (forced) sex.

Although the actual magnitude of the problem and its implications for women's health are not well known, several negative consequences have been identified. These include unintended pregnancy and abortion, increased incidence of STIs including HIV, low self-esteem, depression, and substance abuse (Population Council, 2004).

Risks to the Adolescent Mother

Physiologic Risks

Adolescents over age 15 who receive early, thorough prenatal care are at no greater risk during pregnancy than women over 20 years. Unfortunately, many adolescents fail to seek early prenatal care. Those who do seek care may fail to cooperate with recommendations. In addition, teenage mothers are more likely to smoke than older pregnant women and less likely to gain sufficient weight during their pregnancy. Thus risks for pregnant adolescents include preterm births, low-birth-weight (LBW) infants, preeclampsia-eclampsia and its sequelae, iron deficiency anemia, and cephalopelvic disproportion (CPD). In the adolescent age group, prenatal care is the critical factor that most influences pregnancy outcome.

DEVELOPING CULTURAL COMPETENCE
Educational Level and Childbearing

Throughout the world, the higher a woman's educational level, the more likely she is to delay marriage and childbirth.

Iron deficiency anemia is a problem in all pregnant women. The adolescent who begins her pregnancy already anemic, however, is at increased risk and must be followed closely and counseled carefully regarding nutrition during pregnancy. The increased risk of CPD is a concern in adolescent pregnancy, especially with the early adolescent, because of a lack of pelvic maturity.

Teenagers 15 to 19 years old have a high incidence of STIs including herpes virus, syphilis, and gonorrhea. The incidence of chlamydial infection is also increased in this age group. The presence of such infections during a pregnancy greatly increases the risk to the fetus (see chapter 20). Other problems seen in adolescents are alcohol and drug use. By the time pregnancy is confirmed in young women, the fetus may already be harmed by these substances.

Application: Preeclampsia in an Adolescent Patient

Psychologic Risks

The most profound psychologic risk to the adolescent who maintains her pregnancy is the interruption of progress in her developmental tasks. Although adolescents have become sexually active at an earlier age and the incidence of adolescent pregnancy has decreased, the developmental tasks of this age group remain the same. Add to this the tasks of pregnancy, and the young woman has an overwhelming amount of psychologic work to do, the success of which will affect her own and her newborn's future.

Table 17-2 identifies typical behaviors of the early, middle, and late adolescent when she becomes aware of her pregnancy. In reviewing these behaviors, the nurse should realize that other factors may influence the age at which the behaviors are seen.

TABLE 17-2 Initial Reaction to Awareness of Pregnancy

AGE	ADOLESCENT BEHAVIOR	NURSING IMPLICATIONS
Early adolescent (14 and under)	Fears rejection by family and peers. Enters healthcare system with an adult, most likely mother (parents still seen as locus of control). Value system still closely reflects that of parents, so still turns to parents for decision or approval of decision. Pregnancy probably not result of intimate relationship. Is self-conscious about normal adolescent changes in body. Self-consciousness and low self-esteem likely to increase with rapid breast enlargement and abdominal enlargement of pregnancy.	Be nonjudgmental in approach to care. Focus on needs and concerns of adolescent, but if parent accompanies daughter, include parent in plan of care. Encourage both to express concerns and feelings regarding pregnancy and options: abortion, maintaining pregnancy, adoption. Be realistic and concrete in discussing implications of each option. During physical exam of adolescent, respect increased sense of modesty. Explain in simple and concrete terms physical changes that are produced by pregnancy versus puberty. Explain each step of physical exam in simple and concrete terms.
Middle adolescent (15–17 years)	Fears rejection by peers and parents. Unsure in whom to confide. May seek confirmation of pregnancy on own with increased awareness of options and services, such as over-the-counter pregnancy kits and Planned Parenthood. If in an ongoing, caring relationship with partner (peer), may choose him as confidant. Economic dependence on parents may determine if and when parents are told. Future educational plans and perception of parental support or lack of support are significant factors in decision regarding termination or maintenance of the pregnancy. Possible conflict in parental and own developing value system.	Be nonjudgmental in approach to care. Reassure the adolescent that confidentiality will be maintained. Help adolescent identify significant individuals in whom she can confide to help make a decision about the pregnancy. Be aware of state laws regarding requirement of parental notification if abortion intended. Also be aware of state laws regarding requirements for marriage: usually, minimum age for both parties is 18; 16- and 17-year-olds are, in most states, allowed to marry only with consent of parents. Encourage adolescent to be realistic about parental response to pregnancy.
Late adolescent (18–19 years)	Most likely to confirm pregnancy on own and at an earlier date due to increased acceptance and awareness of consequences of behavior. Likely to use pregnancy kit for confirmation. Relationship with father of baby, future educational plans, and own value system are among significant determinants of decision about pregnancy.	Be nonjudgmental in approach to care. Reassure the adolescent that confidentiality will be maintained. Encourage adolescent to identify significant individuals in whom she can confide. Refer to counseling as appropriate. Encourage adolescent to be realistic about parental response to pregnancy.

TABLE 17-3 The Early Adolescent's Response to the Developmental Tasks of Pregnancy

STAGE	DEVELOPMENTAL TASKS OF PREGNANCY	EARLY ADOLESCENT'S RESPONSE TO PREGNANCY	NURSING IMPLICATIONS
First trimester	Pregnancy confirmation. Seeking early prenatal care as a confirmation tool. Begins to evaluate her diet and general health habits. Initial ambivalence common. Usually supportive partner.	May delay confirmation of pregnancy until late part of first trimester or later. Reasons for delay may include lack of awareness that she is pregnant, fear of confiding in anyone, or denial. Rapid enlargement and sensitivity of breasts are embarrassing and frightening to early adolescent—may be perceived as changes of puberty. If confiding in mother, may be experiencing family turmoil in response to pregnancy.	Explain physiologic changes of pregnancy versus those associated with puberty. Explain that ambivalence is normal with any pregnancy, but recognize it as a much greater concern with adolescent pregnancy. Emphasize need for good nutrition as important for her well-being as much as infant's (prevention of preeclampsia and anemia). Use simple explanations and lots of audiovisuals. Have adolescent listen to fetal heart rate (FHR) with Doppler.
Second trimester	Changes in physical appearance begin, and fetal movement is experienced, causing pregnancy to be experienced as a reality. Begins wearing maternity clothes to accommodate the physical changes. As a result of quickening she perceives her fetus as a real baby and begins preparing for the maternal role and new relationships with her partner and members of her family.	Some teenagers may delay validation of pregnancy until now, with family turmoil occurring at this time. Abdominal enlargement and quickening may be perceived as loss of control over body image. May try to maintain prepregnant weight and wear restrictive clothing to control and conceal changing body. Becomes dependent on her own mother for support. Egocentric; unable to develop a maternal role at this time.	Continue to discuss importance of good nutrition and adequate weight gain as noted above. Discuss ways of utilizing common teenage clothing (large sweatshirts, blouses) to promote comfort but preserve adolescent image to some degree. Discuss plans being made for baby, continued educational plans, and role of teen's parents.
Third trimester	At end of second trimester begins to view fetus as separate from self. Buys baby clothes and supplies. Prepares a place for the baby. Realistic about what baby is like. Prepares to give birth to infant. Anxiety increases as labor and birth approach and has concerns about well-being of fetus.	May focus on "wanting it to be over." May have trouble individuating fetus. May have fantasies, dreams, or nightmares about childbirth. Natural fears of labor and birth greater than with older primigravida. Probably has not been in a hospital, and may associate this with negative experiences.	Assess whether adolescent is preparing for baby by buying supplies and preparing a place in the home. Childbirth education important. Provide hospital tour. Assess for discomforts of pregnancy, such as heartburn and constipation. Adolescent may be uncomfortable mentioning these and other problems.

Table 17-3 identifies the early adolescent's response to the developmental tasks of pregnancy. The early adolescent's response reflects her level of development, with pregnancy as an interruption of the normal process of development. The middle and late adolescent responds differently, reflecting her maturational progress through the developmental tasks. In addition to her maturational level, the amount of nurturing the pregnant adolescent receives is also a critical factor in the way she handles pregnancy and motherhood.

Sociologic Risks

A substantial body of research indicates that the adolescent mother is at higher risk for social and economic disadvantages than her teenage counterpart who is not pregnant and lives in the same social environment. Being forced into adult roles before completing adolescent developmental tasks causes a series of events that may result in a prolonged dependence on parents, lack of stable relationships with the opposite sex, and lack of economic and social stability. Many teenage mothers drop out of school during their pregnancy and then are less likely to complete their schooling. Similarly they are less likely to go to college, more likely to have big families, and more likely to be single. Lack of education in turn reduces the quality of jobs available. Childbearing at an early age is a strong predictor that the children of teenage mothers will live in poverty (Kirby, 2007).

Some pregnant adolescents choose to marry the father of the baby, who may also be a teen. Unfortunately, the majority of adolescent marriages end in divorce. This fact is not surprising because pregnancy and marriage interrupt the partners' "childhood" and basic education. Failure to be self-supporting logically follows lack of education and lost career goals. Lack of maturity in dealing with an intimate relationship also contributes to marital breakdown in this age group.

Dating violence is often an issue for teens, especially for younger girls dating older boys. These younger teens may interpret such actions as hitting, pushing, and making verbal threats as signs of love, caring, and a deep commitment to the relationship that will ultimately produce long-term positive results. Research suggests that up to half of teenage mothers experience domestic violence before, during, or just after their pregnancies (National Coalition Against Domestic Violence [NCADV], 2007).

In the United States, the results of teenage childbearing cost taxpayers $7 billion each year (Pinkleton et al., 2008). Simply delaying these births could result in significant savings because of the improvement in both education and occupational status of these young women.

The increased incidence of maternal complications, premature birth, and LBW babies among adolescent mothers also has an impact on society because many of these mothers are on welfare. The need for increased financial support for good prenatal care and nutritional programs remains critical.

Risks for Her Child

Children of adolescent parents are at a disadvantage in many ways because teens are not developmentally or economically prepared to be parents. In general, children of teenage mothers are at a developmental disadvantage compared with children whose mothers were older at the time of their birth. Many factors contribute to these differences, especially the adverse social and economic conditions many teenage mothers face.

These factors result in high rates of family instability, disadvantaged neighborhoods, and high rates of behavior problems. In addition, often these children do not do as well in school and are less likely to complete high school. Children born to adolescent mothers also have higher rates of abuse and neglect and are more likely to become adolescent parents themselves (Klein & The Committee on Adolescence, 2005).

Partners of Adolescent Mothers

Statistics indicate that approximately two thirds of the male partners of adolescent mothers are not teens themselves but are 20 years of age or older. In particular, teens in poorer, recently immigrant populations have considerably older partners (Males, 2004).

Adolescent males tend to become sexually active at an earlier age than females, and they have more sexual partners in their teenage years. When the father is an adolescent, he, too, generally has not yet completed the developmental tasks of his age group and is no better prepared psychologically to deal with the consequences of pregnancy than the adolescent mother. Research also suggests that, when compared to sons of older fathers, sons of adolescent fathers are at greater risk of becoming adolescent fathers themselves, creating an intergenerational cycle of adolescent fathering (Sipsma, Biello, Cole-Lewis, et al., 2010).

The adolescent who attempts to assume his responsibility as a father faces many of the same psychologic and sociologic risks as the adolescent mother. The mother and father are generally from similar socioeconomic backgrounds and have similar educational levels.

Although not married, many adolescent couples are involved in meaningful relationships. Adolescent fathers may be very involved in the pregnancy and may be present for the birth. Although relationships among fathers, teenage mothers, and their infants appear prone to deterioration over time, research suggests that many young fathers genuinely want to be involved with their children and would have more contact and input if they could. Issues such as conflicts with the teen mother or maternal grandparents and a lack of financial resources may act as additional barriers for the young father.

The lack of responsibility shown by some unwed fathers has caused a shift in cultural and community attitudes. Fathers are being included on birth certificates far more frequently today than in the past. This helps ensure the father's rights and encourages him to meet his responsibilities to his child. In addition, legal paternity gives children access to military and social security benefits and to medical information about their fathers.

In some situations, the pregnant adolescent may not want to identify or contact the father of the baby, and the father may not readily acknowledge paternity. Those situations include rape, exploitative sexual relations, incest, and casual sexual relations. If healthcare providers suspect any of the first three causes, further investigation into the situation is important for the well-being of the pregnant adolescent, and referral to other resources should be made as appropriate.

In situations in which the adolescent father wants to assume some responsibility, healthcare providers should support him in his decision. It is important, however, that the pregnant adolescent have the opportunity to decide whether she wants the father to participate in her health care.

If the adolescents perceive that they have a caring relationship, the adolescent father may want to be supportive and protective but probably does not understand the physical and psychologic changes that his partner is experiencing. The young man will need education regarding pregnancy, childbirth, child care, and parenting. Mentoring programs can be useful tools in helping teen fathers who do not have good role models to understand the role of a father and support their children.

Even if the adolescent father has been included in the health care of the young woman throughout the pregnancy, it is not unusual for her to want her mother as her primary support person during labor and birth. This is especially true with younger adolescents. It is important both to support her wishes and also to acknowledge and support the adolescent father's wishes as appropriate.

As a part of counseling, the nurse should assess the young man's stressors, his support systems, his plans for involvement in the pregnancy and childbearing, and his future plans. He should be referred to social services for an opportunity to be counseled regarding his educational and vocational future. When the father is involved in the pregnancy, the young mother feels less deserted, more confident in her decision making, and better able to discuss her future.

Reactions of Family and Social Supports to Adolescent Pregnancy

The reactions of family members and social supports to adolescent pregnancy are as varied as the motivation and cause of the pregnancy. In families who foster educational and career goals for their children, adolescent pregnancy is often a shock. Anger, shame, and sorrow are common reactions. The majority of pregnant adolescents from these families are most likely to use contraception or choose abortion, with the exception of those teens whose cultural and religious beliefs prevent them from seeking an abortion.

Some adolescent fathers also face negative reactions from people, including their own families and the families of their young partners. They may experience others' anger, shame, and disappointment. Their relationships with their peers may be altered as well.

In populations in which adolescent pregnancy is more prevalent and more socially acceptable, family and friends may be more supportive of the adolescent parents. In many cases, friends as well as the teen's mother are present at the birth. The expectant couple may also have friends who are already teen parents. For some male partners of these adolescent mothers, pregnancy and the birth of a baby are seen as a sign of adult status and increased sexual prowess—a sense of pride.

The mother of the pregnant adolescent is usually among the first to be told about the pregnancy. She typically becomes involved with decision making, especially with the younger adolescent, about issues such as maintaining the pregnancy, abortion, and dealing with the father-to-be and his family. As discussed previously, the pregnant adolescent may not want to identify or contact the father of the baby, especially in situations where rape or other exploitative sex was involved, or with casual sexual relationships. Family input in these matters is important in the adolescent's decision making.

Once the decision about the pregnancy has been made, it is usually the mother who helps the teen access health care and accompanies her to her first visit. If the pregnancy is maintained, the mother may participate in prenatal care classes and can be an excellent support system for her daughter. She should be encouraged to participate if the mother-daughter relationship is positive. If the baby's father is involved in the pregnancy, he and the pregnant teen's mother may be able to work together to support the teenage mother. The nurse can update the pregnant teen's mother on childbearing practices to clarify any misconceptions she might have. During labor and birth, the mother may be a key figure for her daughter, offering reassurance and instilling confidence in the teen.

The younger the adolescent when she gives birth, the more she needs her mother's support. Children of adolescent parents experience more negative outcomes, including more aggressive behavior at a young age, when the adolescent is in constant conflict with her mother and becomes less involved in parenting.

> “Miranda left for college back East in September. She was just 18 and I thought she had the world in front of her. At Thanksgiving she came home to tell us she was 4 months pregnant and planned to keep the baby even though she and Tony had broken up and he wanted no part of fatherhood. She finished the semester, then moved back home and transferred to a state college near us. Tina was born 2 days after her mom finished the spring semester. Now Miranda's life is a juggling act—part-time job, part-time school, full-time mom. We help all we can. I am so sorry that my child has lost out on so much but I am proud of the woman she has become.”

NURSING CARE MANAGEMENT

In working with adolescents, the nurse should remember that oftentimes the nurse is the first contact with the healthcare system that the adolescent has. Adolescents think differently than adults. Adolescents, especially younger adolescents, tend to be more concrete thinkers and may not plan ahead for more than a few days. As a result, nurses need to recognize that missed appointments are not unusual. Missed appointments may also be caused by other factors such as a lack of transportation, especially for those teens not old enough to drive. Teens may avoid health care because they are underinsured, uninsured, or lack the funds to pay for care. Many adolescents have never before accessed health care without a parent. They may fear that using their healthcare insurance for reproductive health visits will be discovered by their parents. If they are unable to share their concerns with a parent, they must be highly motivated to seek health care independently for purposes of contraception, treatment of sexually transmitted infections (STIs), diagnosis of pregnancy, or prenatal care.

Nursing Assessment and Diagnosis

The nurse begins her care of the pregnant adolescent by establishing a database to plan interventions for the adolescent mother and family. Areas of assessment include history of family health and personal physical health, developmental level and impact of pregnancy, and emotional and financial support. The nurse also assesses the family and social support network and the father's degree of involvement in the pregnancy. It is important for the nurse to demonstrate a sincere sense of caring for the young woman and the outcome of her pregnancy during early prenatal visits. Pregnant adolescents are different from other groups of pregnant women in their physical and psychologic response. Professionals need to equip themselves with awareness, knowledge, and skills to meet the needs of the pregnant teen (Tilghman, 2008). Listening more and talking less may be the best tool the nurse can use to develop an effective relationship with the pregnant adolescent.

As with all pregnant women, it is important to have information on the teen's general physical health. This may be the first time many adolescents have ever provided a health history. The nurse may find it helpful to ask very specific questions and give examples if the young woman appears confused about a question. The nurse may find that the teen's mother is best able to answer questions about family history because the adolescent is often unaware of this information.

The following areas should be assessed:

- Family and personal health history
- Medical history
- Menstrual history
- Obstetric and gynecologic history
- Substance abuse history

It is important to assess the maturational level of each individual. The adolescent's development level and the impact of pregnancy are reflected in the degree to which the teen recognizes the realities and responsibilities involved in pregnancy and parenting. The mother's self-concept (including body image), her relationship with the significant adults in her life, her attitude toward her pregnancy, and her coping methods in the situation are just a few of the significant factors that need to be assessed. It is important for the nurse to ask specifically about dating violence. Teens are not likely to reveal dating violence unless they are asked about it.

Adolescent lifestyles and support systems vary greatly. It is imperative that the interdisciplinary health team have information about the expectant adolescents' feelings and perceptions about themselves, their sexuality, and the coming baby; their knowledge of, attitude toward, and anticipated ability to care for and support the infant; their maturational level and needs; and the family, social, and financial support available to them.

The nursing diagnoses that are applicable to any pregnant woman apply to the pregnant adolescent. Other nursing diagnoses are influenced by the adolescent's age, support systems, socioeconomic situation, health, and maturity. Examples of nursing diagnoses more specific to the pregnant adolescent may include the following:

- ***Imbalanced Nutrition: Less than Body Requirements*** related to poor eating habits
- ***Risk for Situational Low Self-Esteem*** related to unanticipated pregnancy

Nursing Plan and Implementation

Early, thorough prenatal care is the strongest and most critical determinant for reducing risk for the adolescent mother and her newborn. When an adolescent presents for health care, her needs must be met and she must be treated as an individual who can make decisions about her own health care. The pregnant adolescent may perceive the nurse who attempts to exert control over her health care as threatening to her independence and will terminate communication. The nurse needs to be vigilant to laying aside personal biases and assumptions when caring for the pregnant teen (King-Jones, 2008).

Community-Based Nursing Care

Many new and innovative community-based agencies have evolved to provide care for high-risk patients throughout the childbearing experience and beyond. Nurses in all community-based agencies can help adolescents access the healthcare system as well as social services and other support services (i.e., food banks and the Special Supplemental Food Program for Women, Infants, and Children [WIC]). Best practice research shows that teaching adolescents in groups according to their ages may be more effective for learning, because younger adolescent mothers may lack parenting skills and have different emotional needs than older adolescent mothers. Soliciting ideas from the teens themselves and identifying their values may also contribute to better education and success of programs for pregnant teens (Broussard & Broussard, 2009). In addition, many teens prefer teaching aids that are visual and that they can handle, such as realistic fetal models. Pregnant teens with low reading levels tend to prefer handouts and posters that have visual interest, short sentences, bulleted lists, and white space (Broussard & Broussard, 2010).

> **PROFESSIONALISM IN PRACTICE**
>
> ***Avoiding Stereotypical Assumptions***
>
> Nurses occasionally make comments regarding the age and immaturity of adolescent mothers, questioning their readiness to become parents. King-Jones (2008) emphasized that nurses need to provide individualized care that is free from "stereotypical assumptions" (p. 117), which stigmatize adolescent mothers. Discussions about patients with other nurses to brainstorm and problem solve in order to improve care are appropriate, but discussions without the patient's best interest in mind are inappropriate in the professional setting. Nurses should serve as role models if they find themselves in this situation. Comments such as "I wonder what we could do to help increase her confidence with her baby?" or "Perhaps she would benefit from talking about her concerns" may help to steer nonproductive conversations in a professional direction.

Nurses working with pregnant adolescents are also involved extensively in counseling and patient teaching. During their interactions, several challenges typically arise, including safeguarding the patient's confidentiality, winning her trust, and helping to build her sense of self-esteem. These and other challenges of adolescent prenatal care are discussed here.

Issues of Confidentiality and Consent to Care

Most states in the United States have passed legislation that confirms the right of some minors to assume the rights of adults. These adolescents are referred to as **emancipated minors**. An adolescent may be considered emancipated if he or she is self-supporting and living away from home, married, pregnant, a parent, or in the military. Even if a minor has not become formally emancipated, all 50 states have passed legislation that enables teens to consent to care without a parent's knowledge for certain "medically emancipated" conditions. These conditions vary from state to state. For example, all 50 states permit minors to consent to STI services but just over half (26) of the states explicitly permit minors (12 and older) to consent to contraception without a parent's knowledge or consent. Currently 32 states allow minors to consent to prenatal care; 4 states specify that "mature" minors can consent; 13 states have no relevant law or policy. All states either explicitly allow minors to give consent for their children's medical care or have no explicit policy about it (AGI, 2010b).

> **PROFESSIONALISM IN PRACTICE**
>
> ***Emancipated Minors***
>
> It is important to remember that if a pregnant minor is considered emancipated, she has the right and responsibility to consent to health care for herself and later for her child. She is entitled to respect and confidentiality in her dealings with healthcare providers. Only with her consent can other adults, including her parents, be included in communication.

Development of a Trusting Relationship with the Pregnant Adolescent

The first visit to the clinic or office may cause anxiety for the young woman. She may be nervous not only because of her situation, but also because this may be her first exposure to the healthcare system since early childhood. Making this experience as positive as possible for the young woman will encourage a favorable attitude toward health care and increase the likelihood that she will return for follow-up visits, whether she chooses to terminate or maintain the pregnancy.

Depending on how young the adolescent is, this may be her first pelvic examination, an anxiety-provoking experience for any woman. The nurse can help provide a thorough explanation of the procedure. A gentle and thoughtful examination technique will help the young woman to relax.

> **CLINICAL TIP**
>
> During the initial pelvic examination, with the consent of the examiner, offer the teen the opportunity to visualize her external genitalia and cervix with a handheld mirror. A mirror is helpful in enabling the young woman to see her cervix, thus educating her about her anatomy. It also gives her an active role in the exam if she so desires.

Developing a trusting relationship with the pregnant adolescent is essential. Honesty and respect for the individual and a caring attitude promote self-esteem. As the nurse develops a trusting relationship with the young woman, the nurse's attitudes about self-care and responsibility affect the adolescent's maturation process. Building a partnership with the adolescent, respecting her unique situation, and appreciating her values will assist the young mother to care for herself and her baby (Broussard & Broussard, 2009).

Promotion of Self-Esteem and Problem-Solving Skills

The nurse assists the adolescent in her decision-making and problem-solving skills so that she can proceed with her developmental tasks and begin to assume responsibility for her own as well as her newborn's life. An overview of what the young woman will experience over the prenatal course, along with thorough explanations and rationale for each procedure as it occurs, will foster the adolescent's understanding and give her some measure of control. Actively involving the young woman in her care gives her a sense of participation and responsibility (Figure 17-2 ■).

Adolescents tend to be egocentric, and even if they realize that their health-related behaviors affect their fetus, they might not feel that this is important. In light of this fact, it is often more helpful to emphasize the effects of these practices on the patient *herself.* Because of their immature cognitive development, they also need help in problem solving, in visualizing themselves in the future, and in imagining what the consequences of their actions might be.

Promotion of Physical Well-Being

Baseline weight and blood pressure measurements will be valuable in assessing weight gain and predisposition to preeclampsia-eclampsia. The adolescent may be encouraged to take part in her care by measuring and recording her weight. The nurse may use this time as an opportunity for assisting the young woman in problem solving: "Have I gained too much or too little weight?" "What influence does my diet have on my weight?" "How can I change my eating habits?"

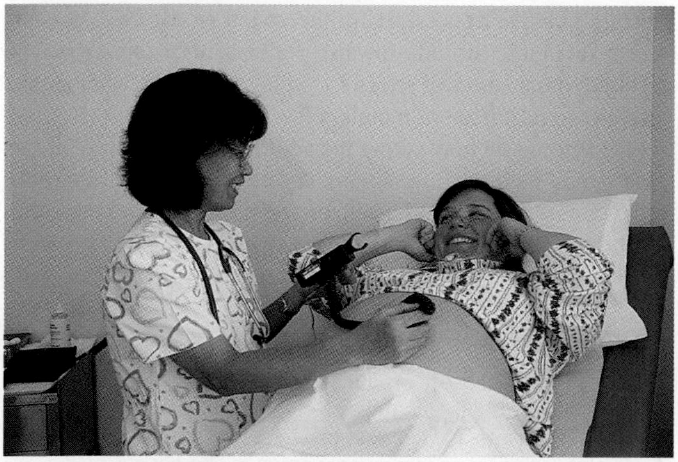

Figure 17-2 ■ The nurse gives a young mother an opportunity to listen to her baby's heartbeat.

Source: Photographer, Elena Dorfman.

The nurse can also introduce the subject of nutrition during measurement of baseline and subsequent hemoglobin and hematocrit values. Because the adolescent is at risk for anemia, she will need education regarding the importance of iron in her diet. Indeed, basic education about nutrition is a critical component of care for pregnant teens.

Preeclampsia-eclampsia is one of the most common, serious complications of pregnancy in general. It also represents the most prevalent medical complication of pregnant adolescents. Preeclampsia-eclampsia is typically characterized by high blood pressure, proteinuria, and edema. In adult women, a blood pressure reading of 140/90 mmHg is often used as evidence of hypertension. However, it is sometimes difficult to recognize hypertension in adolescent females. Women ages 14 to 20 years without evidence of high blood pressure usually have diastolic readings between 50 and 66 mmHg. Gradual increases from the prepregnant diastolic readings, along with excessive weight gain, proteinuria, and sudden edema, must be evaluated as precursors to preeclampsia. Blood pressure readings of 140/90 mmHg are not acceptable as the determinant of preeclampsia in teens. This is one reason why early prenatal care is vital to the effective management of the adolescent.

Adolescents have an increased incidence of STIs. The initial prenatal examination should include gonococcal and chlamydial cultures and wet prep for *Candida, Trichomonas,* and *Gardnerella.* Tests for syphilis should also be done. Education about STIs is important, as is careful observation for herpetic lesions or other symptoms throughout the young woman's pregnancy. Although today's teens are knowledgeable about AIDS, they know much less about other STIs, especially with regard to symptoms and risk reduction. If the adolescent's history indicates that she is at increased risk for HIV, she should be given information about it and offered HIV screening.

The nurse should also discuss substance abuse with adolescents. It is important to review the risks associated with the use of tobacco, caffeine, drugs, and alcohol. The young woman should be aware of the effects of these substances on her development as well as on the development of the fetus.

Ongoing care includes the same assessments that the older woman receives. Special attention should be paid to evaluating fetal growth by determining when quickening occurs and by measuring fundal height, fetal heart tones, and fetal movement. Comparing the dates of auscultating fetal heart tones with the date of the last menstrual period and quickening can be helpful in determining correct estimates of time of birth. If, when measuring fundal height, there is a question of size-date discrepancy by 2 cm either way, an ultrasound is warranted to establish fetal age so that instances of intrauterine growth restriction (IUGR) may be diagnosed and treated early. To ensure the most accurate dating possible, an ultrasound is also warranted early in pregnancy if the date of the last menstrual period is not known.

Promotion of Family Adaptation

The nurse assesses the family situation during the first prenatal visit and ascertains the level of involvement the adolescent desires from each of her family members and the father of the child as well as her perception of their present support. A sensitive approach to daughter-mother relationships helps motivate their communication. If the mother and daughter agree, the mother should be included in the patient's care. Pregnancy may change a teen's relationship with her mother from one of antagonism to one of understanding and empathy. The opportunity to renew or establish a positive relationship with their mothers is welcomed by most teens. It symbolizes approval, acceptance, and support from the individual who would serve as her role model for mothering.

The nurse should also help the mother assess her daughter's needs and assist her in meeting them. Some adolescents become more dependent during pregnancy, and some become more independent. The mother can ease and encourage her daughter's self-growth by understanding how best to respond and support the adolescent.

Finally, the father of the adolescent's infant can be included to promote the family's successful adaptation to the pregnancy. He may be asked to attend prenatal visits, classes, and health teaching and to be present at the birth itself and involved to the extent that he wishes and that is acceptable to the teenage mother. He should also have the opportunity to express his feelings and concerns and to have his questions answered.

Facilitation of Prenatal Education

Some school systems are currently attempting to meet prenatal education needs in a variety of ways. The most effective method appears to be mainstreaming the pregnant adolescent in academic classes with her peers and adding classes appropriate to her needs during pregnancy and initial parenting experiences. Classes about growth and development, beginning with the newborn and early infancy, can help teenage parents have more realistic expectations of their infants and may help decrease child abuse. Mainstreaming pregnant adolescents in school is also an ideal way to help them complete their education while learning the skills they need to cope with childbearing and parenting. Vocational guidance in this setting is also most beneficial to their future. Some schools provide infant and toddler child care facilities on their premises, which may allow the mother to continue her education without the added difficulty of finding appropriate child care.

As stated previously, early adolescents especially tend to be oriented to the present and to be concrete thinkers. As a result, teaching needs to be simple, direct, and responsive to their more immediate needs. Teens also responded positively when there were more hands-on experiences during childbirth preparation classes with less lecture and more one-on-one interaction (Broussard & Broussard, 2009).

For example, teaching about preparation for birth is most effective in the last weeks of pregnancy when this topic is of greater concern and teens are more motivated to practice breathing and relaxation techniques for labor. Although some childbirth educators believe that older couples can be role models for pregnant adolescents, most believe that prenatal classes with other teens are generally preferable even though these classes can be challenging to teach (Figure 17-3 ■). Attendance may be sporadic. The pregnant teen may be accompanied by

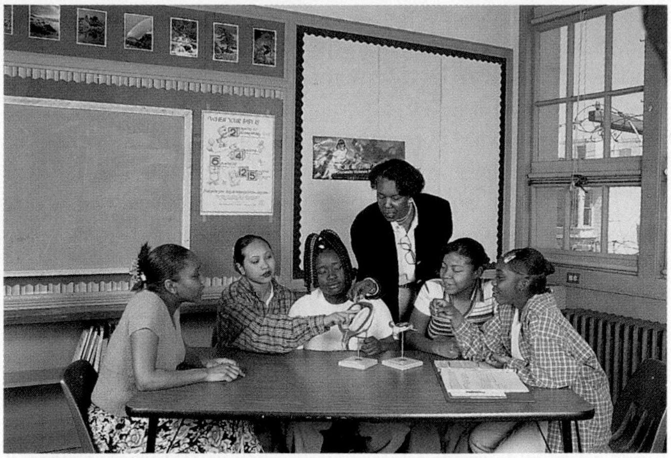

Figure 17-3 ■ Young adolescents may benefit from prenatal classes designed specifically for them.

Source: Jerry Thomas Photography.

her mother, her boyfriend, or her girlfriends. Those who bring girlfriends may bring a different one each time. In such cases, giggling and side conversations may occur. Such activity reflects the short attention span of the teen and is fairly typical. Thus, to keep the attention of the participants, it is important to use a variety of teaching strategies, including age-appropriate audiovisual aids, demonstrations, and games.

Case Study: Late Detection of Adolescent Pregnancy

Goals for prenatal classes may include some or all of the following:

- Providing anticipatory guidance about pregnancy.
- Preparing the participants for labor and birth.
- Helping participants identify the problems and conflicts of teenage pregnancy and parenting.
- Increasing self-esteem.
- Providing information about available community resources.
- Helping participants develop more adaptive coping skills.

During prenatal classes, nurses can also share information on breastfeeding, which has significant health benefits for both the adolescent mother and her infant. Adolescents often do not choose a feeding method until later in pregnancy, so early education can help ensure success for the adolescent who chooses to breastfeed her infant. As many infants of adolescents are born prematurely, it is important for the young mother to know that breast milk is the optimal nutrition for premature infants.

Care Plan Activity: Adolescent's Response to Pregnancy

Topics on parenting, although sometimes included in prenatal classes for adolescents, tend to be less effective, again because adolescents tend to be oriented to the present. Parenting skills are crucial, but adolescents generally are not ready to learn about these skills until birth makes the newborn a reality.

Hospital-Based Nursing Care

The adolescent in labor has the same care needs as any pregnant woman. However, the importance of a sustained presence for her cannot be overemphasized. Adolescents want their care provider to be respectful, caring, and supportive. The nurse must be readily available and should answer questions simply and honestly, using lay terminology. Adolescents need their caregiver to provide education to guide their choices. The nurse can also help the adolescent's support people understand their roles in assisting the teen. If the father is involved, the nurse can encourage him to work within his own level of comfort to play an active role in all phases of the birth process, perhaps by feeding ice chips to the mother, timing her contractions, and coaching her with her breathing. The nurse can also let the couple know that holding hands, backrubs, and supportive touching are acceptable and therapeutic. Chapter 24 ∞ provides further information on care of the adolescent during labor and birth.

During the postpartum period, most teens do not foresee that they will become sexually active in the near future and are often adamant about the fact that they will not become pregnant again for an extended period. However, the statistics demonstrate a different reality. Thus, contraception remains a critical part of the national effort to decrease adolescent pregnancy. Before discharge, it is important for the nurse to provide information about the resumption of ovulation and the importance of contraception. It is especially helpful to do this teaching with the sexual partner present.

Several safe and effective contraceptive options are available for adolescents. Condoms are by far the most common method of contraception among teens and, when used consistently and correctly, they offer the added advantage of protection against STIs. Healthcare providers often recommend a dual approach to prevent pregnancy and STIs—a condom combined with a second method of contraception, typically a hormonal method such as a combined oral contraceptive (Hillard, 2005). The American College of Obstetricians and Gynecologists (ACOG) (2007) supports the use of intrauterine devices (IUDs) as a safe, first-line contraceptive choice for adolescents, stating that the IUD does not increase the adolescent's risk of pelvic inflammatory disease (PID) or affect her fertility. The benefits and convenience of long-acting oral contraceptives also make them an appropriate choice for sexually active adolescents. In general, all methods used for healthy adults are potentially appropriate for adolescents providing they make educated decisions and understand what the use of various contraceptive methods entails.

National Campaign to Prevent Teen Pregnancy

Areas to discuss with the adolescent include the nature of her sexual relationship with her partner, the behaviors in which they are engaged, their ability to comply with the use of certain contraceptive devices, the costs of various methods, the teen's religious beliefs, and her partner's potential cooperation (Bearinger, Sieving, Ferguson, et al., 2007). As part of discharge planning, the nurse should ensure that the teen is aware of community resources available to assist her and her family. Postpartum classes and new-mother support groups, especially with peers, can be extremely beneficial. Such classes address a variety of topics, including postpartum adaptation, infant and child development, and parenting skills.

> **CLINICAL JUDGMENT**
>
> **Case Study: Rachel Kalaras**
>
> Rachel Kalaras is an 18-year-old G1PO who is 16 weeks pregnant when she arrives for her prenatal visit. When discussing her plans for the pregnancy, Rachel indicates that she is considering adoption. She has not discussed this plan with anyone but is seeking information about the process of relinquishment.
>
> **Critical Thinking**
>
> What should you consider in discussing this issue with Rachel?
> *See www.nursing.pearsonhighered.com for possible responses.*

Evaluation

Expected outcomes of nursing care include the following:

- A trusting relationship is established with the pregnant adolescent.
- The adolescent is able to use her problem-solving abilities to make appropriate choices.
- The adolescent follows the recommendations of the healthcare team and receives effective health care throughout her pregnancy, the birth, and the postpartum period.
- The adolescent, her partner (if he is involved), and their families are able to cope successfully with the effects of the pregnancy.
- The adolescent is able to discuss pregnancy, prenatal care, and childbirth.
- The adolescent demonstrates developmental and pregnancy progression within established normal parameters.
- The adolescent develops skill in child care and parenting.

Prevention of Adolescent Pregnancy

At the individual level, balanced, realistic sexuality education, which includes information on both abstinence and contraception, can delay teens' onset of sexual activity, increase the use of contraception by sexually active teens, and reduce the number of their sexual partners. The American Academy of Pediatrics (2007) has issued a policy statement on contraception and adolescents that addresses the role of healthcare providers in working with adolescents. The statement stresses the importance of encouraging abstinence while also providing counseling on risk-reduction approaches including the use of latex condoms for every act of sexual intercourse. It also emphasizes the need to ensure ready access to contraceptive services and appropriate follow-up.

Key strategies for prevention of unintended teen pregnancy and sexual health promotion that have been suggested include the provision of services that ensure accessible and high-quality reproductive health care; sex education programs that provide developmentally appropriate, evidence-based curricula; and youth development strategies to enhance life skills, connection to supportive adults, and educational and economic opportunities (Bearinger et al., 2007).

At the national level, the National Campaign to Prevent Teen and Unplanned Pregnancy (NCPTUP), a private, nonprofit organization made up of a broad spectrum of religious, political, social, human services, health, and academic organizations, is working to reduce teenage pregnancy by one third between 2006 and 2015 (NCPTUP, 2010). The Association of Women's Health, Obstetric and Neonatal Nurses (AWHONN) is one of the many professional organizations that joined this group and made a commitment to focus on adolescent pregnancy prevention. Not surprisingly, the task forces have found that adolescent pregnancy is a multifaceted problem with no easy answers. The best approach is local and is based on strong, community-wide involvement with a variety of programs directed at the multiple causes of the problem.

One of the major problems in local communities continues to be intense conflict among different groups about how to approach adolescent pregnancy prevention. Some parents and communities advocate abstinence-only programs, and, until recently, abstinence-only programs were funded by the government. Critics argue that these curricula are ineffective and insulting and tell teens what to think, not how to think for themselves (Taverner, 2007). Other parents advocate an "abstinence-plus" approach that stresses abstinence as the best approach but includes information on condoms and contraception for those teens who do not abstain.

Most Americans support providing education in junior and senior high schools with information about protection against unplanned pregnancy and sexually transmitted infections (STIs). Youth development programs that focus on meeting the needs of adolescents by building on young people's capacities, assisting them to cultivate their own talent and to increase their feelings of self-worth, ease their transition into adulthood and can reduce sexual risk behaviors and unintended teen pregnancy (Advocates for Youth, 2008).

The National Campaign's task forces have identified characteristics shared by all successful programs, regardless of the type of offering or community. Effective adolescent pregnancy prevention programs are long term and intensive. They also involve adolescents in program planning, include good role models from the same cultural and racial backgrounds, and focus on the adolescent male (Kirby, 2007). See Research Evidence in Practice for additional information on effective programs.

The National Campaign has identified a list of recommendations for parents that are designed to help teens avoid pregnancy. Nurses can use this information in working with parents (NCPTUP, 2008):

1. Parents should be clear about their own sexual attitudes and values in order to communicate clearly with children.
2. Parents need to talk with their children about sex early and often and be specific in the discussions.
3. Parents should supervise and monitor their children and teens with well-established rules, expectations, curfews, and standards of behavior.

RESEARCH EVIDENCE IN PRACTICE: Interventions for Preventing Unintended Adolescent Pregnancy

CLINICAL QUESTION

What interventions are effective in preventing unintended pregnancy during the adolescent years?

RESEARCH EVIDENCE

Early childbearing carries significant health risks for both the teen mother and the baby. In addition, adolescents with unintended pregnancies face a number of challenges such as abandonment by their partners, peer social isolation, and an inability to complete their education, which has lifelong employment and economic consequences.

A review sponsored by the Cochrane Collaborative, one of the most rigorous sources of evidence reviews, appraised the results of more than 40 randomized controlled trials with more than 95,000 adolescent subjects. Some of the studies (11) were pooled into a meta-analysis that used statistical analysis to determine the clinical importance of the effects of treatments.

Interventions that are multifaceted have the strongest evidence for effectiveness. Specifically, a combination of educational and contraceptive interventions appears to reduce unintended pregnancy among adolescents. The education that was most effective did not focus solely on sexual factors, but rather included skills training and personal development as well. The most successful programs engaged stakeholders, including pregnant teens, parents, healthcare providers, schools, and churches, to design and implement programs that are practical, evidence based, and culturally appropriate. Involving teens in program design resulted in education that was more readily accepted by the target population.

Educational interventions were most effective when coupled with the promotion of the effective use of contraception. There was little evidence to show that either of these interventions alone was as effective as the integration of both education and contraception in preventing pregnancy.

WHAT QUESTIONS REMAIN UNANSWERED?

While these interventions have demonstrated effectiveness in reducing pregnancy, effects on other aspects of teen sexuality—timing of initial sexual intercourse, use of birth control, and sexually transmitted infections—was not conclusive. More research is needed to determine if there are successful interventions to prevent these additional adolescent risk behaviors.

WHAT IS BEST PRACTICE?

Multifaceted programs that educate teens about sexuality and personal skills development, coupled with promotion of appropriate contraceptive use, are most effective in preventing unintended pregnancies in adolescents.

CRITICAL THINKING

How can the nurse participate effectively in the design and development of effective pregnancy prevention programs for adolescents? How can the nurse apply these principles to the individual care and counseling of teens in preventing pregnancy?

References

Boyer, C., Shafer, M., Shaffer, R., Brocine, S., Pollack, L., & Betsinger, K. (2005). Evaluation of a cognitive-behavioral group, randomized controlled trials to prevent sexually transmitted infections and unintended pregnancies in young women. *Preventive Medicine, 40*, 420–431.

Henderson, M., Wright, D., Raab, G., Abraham, C., Parkes, S., Scott, S., & Hart, G. (2007). Impact of a theoretically based sex education programme delivered by teachers on NHS registered conceptions and terminations: Final results of cluster randomized trial. *British Medical Journal, 334*, 133–138.

Oringanje, C., Meremikwu, M., Edo, H., Esu, E., Meremikwu, A., & Ehiri, J. (2009). Interventions for preventing unintended pregnancies among adolescents. *Cochrane Database of Systematic Reviews,* Issue 4. Art. No.: CD005215. doi:10.1002/14651858

Piepert, J., Redding, C., Blume, J., Allsworth, J., Matteson, K., Lozowski, F., . . . & Rossi, J. (2008). Tailed intervention to increase contraceptive method use: A randomized trial to reduce unintended pregnancies and sexually transmitted infections. *American Journal of Obstetrics and Gynecology, 198*, 630.e1–630.e8.

4. Parents should know their children's friends and their families.
5. Parents need to clearly discourage early dating as well as frequent and steady dating.
6. Parents should take a strong stand against allowing a daughter to date a much older boy; similarly they should not allow a son to develop an intense relationship with a much younger girl.
7. Parents need to help children set goals for their future and have options that are more attractive than early pregnancy and childrearing.
8. Parents should show their children that they value education and take school performance seriously.
9. Parents need to monitor what their children are reading, listening to, and watching.
10. It is especially important that parents build a strong, loving relationship with their children from an early age by showing affection clearly and regularly, spending time with them doing age-appropriate activities, building children's self-esteem, and have meals together as a family often.

In summary, although it is sometimes difficult for adults, it is important to address topics related to healthy relationships, abstinence, birth control, responsible sexual behavior, and the possible consequences of unsafe practices honestly and in a way that reflects adolescents' knowledge level, perspectives, and personal experience. Discussion about teenage pregnancy needs to reflect an awareness of teens' priorities related to the costs and rewards of having a baby. All such discussions need to be honest, frank, and open and based on recognition of the developmental level of the teen (Herman, 2008).

FOCUS YOUR STUDY

- Birth rates for teens ages 15 to 19 have decreased from 61.8 per 1000 females in 1991 to 41.5 in 2008. Although this is a significant improvement, the U.S. teenage pregnancy rate is the highest of any industrialized nation.
- Many factors contribute to the high teenage pregnancy rate, including earlier age of first sexual intercourse, lack of knowledge about conception, lack of easy access to contraception, lessened stigma associated with adolescent pregnancy in some populations, poverty, early school failure, and early childhood sexual abuse.
- The major psychologic risk the pregnant adolescent faces is the interruption of her own developmental tasks.
- Physical risks of adolescent pregnancies include preterm births, low-birth-weight infants, cephalopelvic disproportion, iron deficiency anemia, and preeclampsia and its sequelae.
- Almost half of the fathers of infants of adolescent mothers are age 20 or older, but they are often similar to adolescent fathers psychosocially and are no more likely to be able to support the mother.
- Factors affecting an adolescent's response to pregnancy include her degree of achievement of the developmental tasks of adolescence (which can be closely associated with age) as well as cultural, religious, and socioeconomic factors.
- Nurses working with pregnant adolescents face many challenges, including safeguarding the patient's confidentiality, winning her trust, and helping to build her sense of self-esteem.
- Often the adolescent has little understanding of pregnancy, childbirth, or parenting. Consequently, education is a primary responsibility of the nurse.
- Adolescent pregnancy prevention programs should be multifaceted, target males as well as females, and involve community-wide approaches.

CRITICAL THINKING IN ACTION

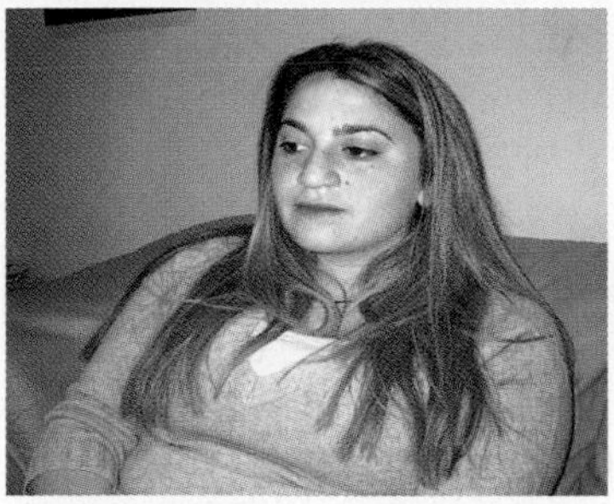

Source: George Dodson/Pearson Education.

Sixteen-year-old Linda Perez and her mother present to you at the OB clinic for Linda's first prenatal visit. You determine that Linda is 20 weeks pregnant. Her weight is 135 lb, height 5′4″, T 98°F, P 80, R 14, BP 100/64. You assess that Linda's mother has type 2 diabetes, and that her siblings are healthy. Linda admits to having one sexual partner and says she has never been hospitalized. Her immunizations are up to date and she's never used tobacco or recreational drugs. To date, the father of the baby is not involved. Mrs. Perez is clearly upset that Linda's pregnancy is so far advanced without her knowledge. Linda is quiet and speaks only when questioned directly. You do your best to try to establish a trusting relationship with Linda and her mother by providing an atmosphere where issues can be discussed.

1. What psychologic factors contribute to teenage pregnancy?
2. Explore reasons why teenagers delay prenatal care.
3. Linda's mother asks you what factors facilitate adolescent pregnancies.
4. You assess that Linda has some anxiety concerning the birth process. She states she is not interested in prenatal classes because she is single and does not want to have natural childbirth. Your best response would be:

See www.nursing.pearsonhighered.com for possible responses.

Pearson Nursing Student Resources

Find additional review materials at
www.nursing.pearsonhighered.com

Prepare for success with additional NCLEX®-style practice questions, interactive assignments and activities, Web links, animations and videos, and more!

REFERENCES

Advocates for Youth. (2008). *Teenage pregnancy, the case for prevention: An updated analysis of recent trends and federal expenditures associated with teenage pregnancy* (2nd ed.). Retrieved from http://www.advocatesforyouth.org/index.php?option=com_content&task=view&id=387&l

Alan Guttmacher Institute (AGI). (2006). *U.S. teenage pregnancy statistics: National and state trends and trends by race and ethnicity.* Retrieved from http://www.guttmacher.org

Alan Guttmacher Institute (AGI). (2010a). *Facts on American teens' sexual and reproductive health.* Retrieved from http://www.guttmacher.org/pubs/FB-ATSRH.pdf

Alan Guttmacher Institute (AGI). (2010b). *State policies in brief: An overview of minors' consent law.* Retrieved from http://www.guttmacher.org/statecenter/spibs/spib-OMCL.pdf

American Academy of Pediatrics. (2007). Policy statement: Contraception and adolescents. *Pediatrics, 120*(5), 1135–1148.

American College of Obstetricians and Gynecologists (ACOG). (2007). *Intrauterine device and adolescents* (ACOG Committee Opinion No. 392). Washington, DC: Author.

Bearinger, L., Sieving, R., Ferguson, J., & Sharma, V. (2007). Global perspectives on the sexual and reproductive health of adolescents: Patterns, prevention, and potential. *The Lancet, 369,* 1220–1231.

Broussard, A. B., & Broussard, B. S. (2009, Spring). Designing and implementing a parenting resource center for pregnant teens. *Journal of Perinatal Education, 18*(2), 40–47.

Broussard, A. B., & Broussard, B. S. (2010). Teaching pregnant teens: Lessons learned. *Nursing for Women's Health, 14*(2), 104–111.

East, P. L., Reyes, B. T., & Horn, E. J. (2007). Association between adolescent pregnancy and a family history of teenage births. *Perspectives on Sexual and Reproductive Health, 39*(2), 108–115.

Hamilton, B. E., Martin, J. A., & Ventura, S. J. (2010). Births: Preliminary data for 2008. *National Vital Statistics Reports, 58*(16), 1–17.

Herman, J. W. (2008). Adolescent perceptions of teen births. *JOGNN: Journal of Obstetric, Gynecologic, and Neonatal Nursing, 37*(1), 42–50.

Hillard, P. J. A. (2005). Contraceptive behaviors in adolescents. *Pediatric Annals, 34*(10), 794–802.

Kelly, P. J., Lesser, J., & Smoots, A. (2005). Tailoring STI & HIV prevention programs for teens. *The American Journal of Maternal-Child Nursing, 30*(4), 237–244.

King-Jones, T. (2008). Pregnant adolescents: Perils and pearls of communication. *Nursing for Women's Health, 12*(2), 114–119.

Kirby, D. (2007). *Emerging answers: Research findings on programs to reduce teen pregnancy and sexually transmitted diseases.* Retrieved from http://www.thenationalcampaign.org/EA2007/EA2007-sum.pdf

Klein, J. D., & The Committee on Adolescence. (2005). Adolescent pregnancy: Current trends and issues. *Pediatrics, 116,* 281–286.

Lemay, C., Cashman, S., Elfenbein, D., & Felice, M. (2007). Adolescent mothers' attitudes toward contraceptive use before and after pregnancy. *Journal of Pediatric Adolescence and Gynecology, 20,* 233–240.

Lindberg, L., Jones, R., & Santelli, J. (2008). Non-coital sexual activities among adolescents. *Journal of Adolescent Health, 43*(3), 231–238.

Magill, M., & Wilcox, R. (2007). Adolescent pregnancy and associated risks: Not just a result of maternal age. *American Family Physician, 75*(9), 1310–1311.

Males, M. (2004). *Teens and older partners. Resource Center for Adolescent Pregnancy Prevention (ReCAPP).* Retrieved from http://www.etr.org/recap/research/AuthoredPapOlderPrtnrs0504.htm

Manlove, J., Terry-Humen, E., & Ikramullah, E. (2006). Young teenagers and older sexual partners: Correlates and consequences for males and females. *Perspectives on Sexual and Reproductive Health, 38*(4), 197–207.

National Campaign to Prevent Teen and Unplanned Pregnancy (NCPTUP). (2008). *Ten tips for parents.* Retrieved from http://www.thenationalcampaign.org/resources/pdf/pubs/10Tips_final.pdf

National Campaign to Prevent Teen and Unplanned Pregnancy (NCPTUP). (2010). *Our mission: Goal.* Retrieved from http://www.thenationalcampaign.org/about-us/our-mission.aspx

National Campaign to Prevent Teen and Unplanned Pregnancy (NCPTUP). (2007). *What's it going to take? Extending the research base to improve teen pregnancy prevention.* Retrieved from http://www.thenationalcampaign.org/resources/pdfexec_summary.pdf

National Coalition Against Domestic Violence (NCADV). (2007). *Reproductive health and pregnancy: Why it matters.* NCADV Public Policy Office. Washington, DC: Author.

Pinkleton, B., Austin, E., Cohen, M., Chen, Y.-C., & Fitzgerald, E. (2008). Effects of a peer-led media literacy curriculum on adolescents' knowledge and attitudes toward sexual behavior and media portrayals of sex. *Health Communication, 23,* 462–472.

Population Council. (2004). The adverse health and social outcomes of sexual coercion: Experiences of young women in developing countries. Retrieved from http://www.popcouncil.org

Sipsma, H., Biello, K. B., Cole-Lewis, H., & Kershaw, T. (2010). Like father, like son: The intergenerational cycle of adolescent fatherhood. *American Journal of Public Health, 100*(3), 517–524.

SmithBattle, L. (2007). "I wanna have a good future": Teen mothers' rise in educational aspirations, competing demands, and limited school support. *Youth Society, 38*(3), 348–371.

Steinberg, L. (2010). *Adolescence* (9th ed.). New York, NY: McGraw-Hill.

Talashek, M., Alba, M., & Patel, A. (2006). Untangling the health disparities of teen pregnancy. *Journal for Specialists in Pediatric Nursing, 11*(1), 14–27.

Taverner, B. (2007). Reclaiming 'abstinence' in comprehensive sex education. *Contemporary Sexuality, 41*(4), 9–14.

Tilghman, J. (2008). Prenatal care: The adolescents' perspective. *Journal of Perinatal Education, 17*(2), 50–53.

Weinstock, H., Berman, S., & Cates, W. (2004). Sexually transmitted diseases among American youth: Incidence and prevalence estimates, 2000. *Perspectives on Sexual and Reproductive Health, 36*(1), 6–10.

World Health Organization (WHO). (2008a, August). Making pregnancy safer. Reducing maternal mortality by improving care for pregnant adolescents. *Hot Topics* (6).

World Health Organization (WHO). (2008b). *Why is giving special attention to adolescents important for achieving Millennium Development Goal 5?* Retrieved from http://www.who.int/making_pregnancy_safer_/events/2009/10_02_2009/en/

CHAPTER

18 Maternal Nutrition

I'm trying to be very careful about what I eat. I've had more salads and fresh fruit than I can remember. Sometimes, though, I get a "cookie attack" and indulge myself. My husband says I should eat oatmeal cookies so I could feel that my cravings were nutritionally sound!

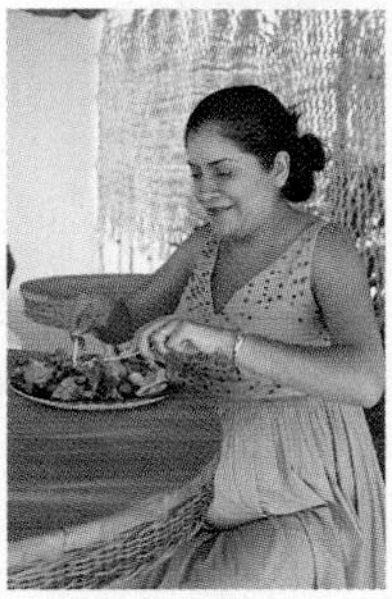

LEARNING OUTCOMES

1. Identify the role of specific nutrients in the diet of the pregnant woman.
2. Compare nutritional needs during pregnancy, postpartum, and lactation with nonpregnant requirements.
3. Discuss effects of maternal nutrition on fetal outcomes.
4. Evaluate adequacy and pattern of weight gain during different stages of pregnancy.
5. Plan adequate prenatal vegetarian diets based on nutritional requirements of pregnancy.
6. Describe ways in which various physical, psychosocial, and cultural factors can affect nutritional intake and status.
7. Compare recommendations for weight gain and nutrient intakes in the pregnant adolescent with those for the mature pregnant adult.
8. Describe basic factors a nurse should consider when offering nutritional counseling to a pregnant adolescent.
9. Compare nutritional counseling issues for breastfeeding and formula-feeding mothers.
10. Formulate a nutritional care plan for pregnant women based on a diagnosis of nutritional problems.

KEY TERMS

Adequate intake (AI) *395*
Calorie (cal) *398*
Dietary reference intakes (DRIs) *395*
Folic acid *403*
Kilocalorie (kcal) *398*
Lactase deficiency (lactose intolerance) *406*
Lacto-ovovegetarians *405*
Lactovegetarians *405*
Pica *408*
Recommended dietary allowance (RDA) *395*
Vegans *405*

A woman's nutritional status before and during pregnancy can significantly influence her own health and that of her unborn child. In most prenatal clinics and offices, nurses provide nutritional counseling directly or work closely with dietitians in providing any necessary nutritional assessment and teaching.

This chapter focuses on the nutritional needs of a normal pregnant woman. Special sections consider the nutritional needs of the pregnant adolescent and the woman after birth.

Many factors influence a woman's ability to achieve good prenatal nutrition, including the following:

- ***General nutritional status before pregnancy.*** Good prenatal nutrition is the result of proper eating throughout life, not just during pregnancy, although pregnancy may motivate a woman to improve poor eating habits. Nutritional deficits at conception and during the early prenatal period may influence the outcome of the pregnancy.
- ***Maternal age.*** An expectant adolescent must meet the nutritional needs for her own growth in addition to the nutritional needs of pregnancy.
- ***Maternal parity.*** A mother's nutritional needs and the outcome of her pregnancy are influenced by the number of pregnancies she has had and by the intervals between them.

A mother's nutritional status does affect her fetus. Factors influencing fetal well-being are interrelated, but nutrient deficiencies alone can produce measurable effects on cell and organ growth of the developing fetus. Fetal growth occurs in three overlapping stages: (1) growth by increase in cell number, (2) growth by increase in cell number and cell size, and (3) growth by increase in cell size alone. The nutritional problems that interfere with cell division may have permanent consequences. If the nutritional insult occurs when cells are mainly enlarging, the changes are usually reversible when normal nutrition resumes.

Growth of fetal and maternal tissues requires increased quantities of nutrients. These are listed in the **dietary reference intakes (DRIs)** as specific allowances for pregnant and lactating women (Table 18-1). The DRIs distinguish between pregnant women and pregnant adolescents because of the greater nutrient needs of the adolescent. The DRIs are subdivided into the **recommended dietary allowance (RDA)** and **adequate intake (AI)**. An RDA is the daily dietary intake that is considered sufficient to meet the nutritional requirements of nearly all individuals in a specific life stage and gender group. An AI is a value cited for a nutrient when the data are not sufficient to calculate an estimated average requirement.

Maternal Weight

Prepregnancy Weight

Prepregnancy weight is an important factor for both mothers and their babies. Women who are underweight before pregnancy, especially younger adolescents, have a higher risk of giving birth to a low-birth-weight infant than women who begin pregnancy at normal weight for height. Obesity during pregnancy is associated with many complications, including gestational diabetes, gestational hypertension, preeclampsia, birth defects, cesarean birth, fetal macrosomia, perinatal deaths, and postpartum anemia (Waller et al., 2007). Babies of obese women may be at a higher risk of becoming obese themselves as they age.

Maternal Weight Gain

Case Study: Maternal Weight Gain

Maternal weight gain is an important factor in fetal growth and in infant birth weight. An adequate weight gain over time indicates an adequate caloric intake. It does not, however, ensure that the woman has a sufficient nutrient intake. The diet may not be of high enough nutritional quality even though its caloric content supports the recommended weight gain. The pregnant woman must maintain the nutritional quality of her diet as her weight gain progresses.

Weight gain, even in women with a healthy pregnancy outcome, tends to be quite variable. Optimal weight gain depends on the woman's weight for height (body mass index [BMI]) and her prepregnant nutritional state. The Institute of Medicine (IOM) (2009) recommends weight gain in terms of optimum ranges based on prepregnant BMI (Table 18-2). Studies continue to show that weight gain within the IOM recommended weight ranges are associated with improved pregnancy outcomes, avoidance of excessive maternal postpartum weight retention, and reduction of risk of chronic disease later in life (American Dietetic Association [ADA], 2008).

The pattern of weight gain during pregnancy is also important. For example, inadequate prenatal weight gain during the second trimester is closely associated with reduced birth weight in the newborn. For women of normal weight, assuming a gain of 0.5 to 2 kg (1.1 to 4.4 lbs) during the first trimester, the recommended gain during the second and third trimesters is .45 kg (1 lb) per week. The rate of weight gain in the second and third trimesters needs to be slightly higher for underweight women and slightly lower for overweight women (IOM, 2009). A maternal weight gain of 1.5 lb per week has been suggested for normal-weight women during the second half of a twin pregnancy. Underweight women should strive for a gain of 1.75 lb per week after 20 weeks' gestation.

The average maternal weight gain is distributed as follows:

5 kg (11 lb)	Fetus, placenta, amniotic fluid
0.9 kg (2 lb)	Uterus
1.8 kg (4 lb)	Increased blood volume
1.4 kg (3 lb)	Breast tissue
2.3 to 4.5 kg (5 to 10 lb)	Maternal stores

Obesity is becoming increasingly prevalent in the United States and in many developed countries. Because pregnant women who are obese are at risk for many pregnancy complications, it is recommended these women receive counseling on strategies to move toward and to remain at a healthful weight prior to conceiving (ADA & the American Society for Nutrition, 2009).

TABLE 18-1 Dietary Reference Intakes (DRIs) for Nonpregnant Females and for Pregnant and Lactating Females

	AGE	VITAMIN A (MCG/D)	VITAMIN D (MCG/D)	VITAMIN E (MG/Dα-TOCOPHEROL)	VITAMIN K (MCG/D)	VITAMIN C (MG/D)	THIAMINE (MG/D)	RIBOFLAVIN (MG/D)
Females	9–13 y	600	5*	11	60*	45	0.9	0.9
	14–18 y	700	5*	15	75*	65	1.0	1.0
	19–30 y	700	5*	15	90*	75	1.1	1.1
	31–50 y	700	5*	15	90*	75	1.1	1.1
	50–70 y	700	10*	15	90*	75	1.1	1.1
	Greater than 70 y	700	15*	15	90*	75	1.1	1.1
Pregnancy	Less than or equal to 18 y	750	5*	15	75*	80	1.4	1.4
	19–30 y	770	5*	15	90*	85	1.4	1.4
	31–50 y	770	5*	15	90*	85	1.4	1.4
Lactation	Less than or equal to 18 y	1200	5*	19	75*	115	1.4	1.6
	19–30 y	1300	5*	19	90*	120	1.4	1.6
	31–50 y	1300	5*	19	90*	120	1.4	1.6

*Values are adequate intakes (AIs) rather than recommended dietary allowances (RDAs). All other values on chart are RDAs.

Source: All data from the Institute of Medicine (1997–2006). Dietary reference intakes, Washington, DC: National Academy Press.

TABLE 18-2 Recommendations for Total Weight Gain During Pregnancy

PRE-PREGNANCY BMI	BMI (KG/M^2)	TOTAL WEIGHT GAIN (LBS)	RATES OF WEIGHT GAIN IN 2ND AND 3RD TRIMESTER (LBS/WEEK)
UNDERWEIGHT	<18.5	28–40	1 (1–1.3)
NORMAL WEIGHT	18.5–24.9	25–35	1 (0.8–1)
OVERWEIGHT	25.0–29.9	15–25	0.6 (0.5–0.7)
OBESE	>30	11–20	0.5 (0.4–0.6)

Source: Institute of Medicine. (2009). Weight Gain During Pregnancy: Reexamining the Guide. *Reprinted with permission from the National Academies Press, Copyright © 2009, National Academy of Sciences.*

Because of the association between maternal weight gain and pregnancy outcome, most caregivers pay close attention to weight gain during pregnancy (Figure 18-1 ■). Weight gain charts can be useful in monitoring the rate of weight gain over time. If a significant deviation from the anticipated pattern occurs, the cause should be determined and appropriate interventions planned with the woman.

As mentioned earlier, weight gain alone does not guarantee adequate nutrition. A diet may be high in energy (calories) but low in vitamins, minerals, or complex carbohydrates and protein. Pregnancy is not a time to diet, and severe caloric restriction during pregnancy can result in maternal ketosis. Counseling the pregnant woman to eat a variety of nutrients from each of the food groups places less emphasis on the amount of her weight gain and more on the quality of her intake. MyPyramid offers users a colorful plan that emphasizes variety, proportions, moderation, and physical activity (Figure 18-2 ■). "MyPyramid for Moms" is also available through the U.S. Department of Agriculture's MyPyramid Web site to provide food plans that meet the energy needs of

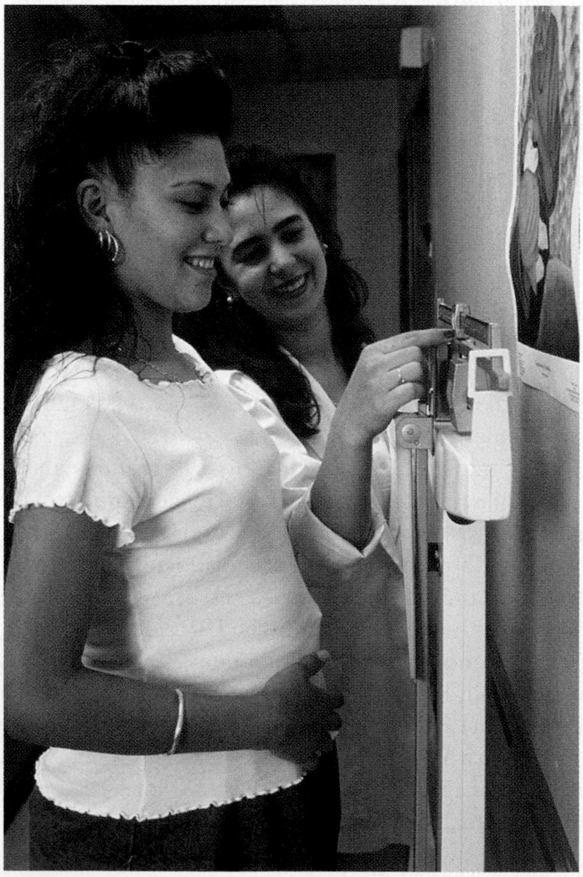

Figure 18-1 ■ It is important to monitor a pregnant woman's weight over time.

Source: Michael Newman/Photo Edit Inc.

NIACIN (MG/D)	VITAMIN B_6 (MG/D)	FOLATE (MCG/D)	VITAMIN B_{12} (MCG/D)	CALCIUM (MG/D)	PHOSPHORUS (MG/D)	MAGNESIUM (MG/D)	IRON (MG/D)	ZINC (MG/D)	IODINE (MCG/D)	SELENIUM (MCG/D)
12	1	300	1.8	1300*	1250	240	8	8	120	40
14	1.2	400	2.4	1300*	1250	360	15	9	150	55
14	1.3	400	2.4	1000*	700	310	18	8	150	55
14	1.3	400	2.4	1000*	700	320	18	8	150	55
14	1.5	400	2.4	1200*	700	320	8	8	150	55
14	1.5	400	2.4	1200*	700	320	8	8	150	55
18	1.9	600	2.6	1300*	1250	400	27	12	220	60
18	1.9	600	2.6	1000*	700	350	27	11	220	60
18	1.9	600	2.6	1000*	700	360	27	11	220	60
17	2	500	2.8	1300*	1250	360	10	13	290	70
17	2	500	2.8	1000*	700	310	9	12	290	70
17	2	500	2.8	1000*	700	320	9	12	290	70

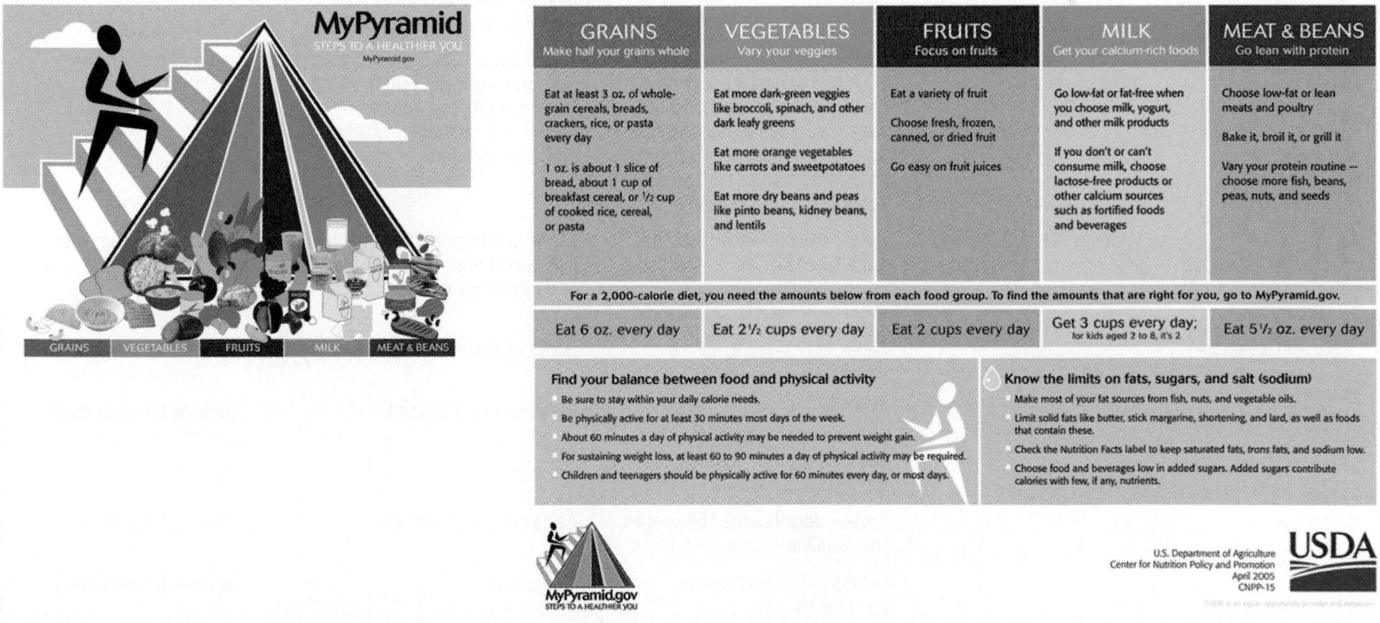

Figure 18-2 ■ MyPyramid: Steps to a Healthier You identifies the basic food groups and provides guidance about healthful eating. Grains, vegetables, fruits, and dairy products are emphasized with slightly less emphasis on protein. The narrow yellow bar is designated for fats, sugar, and salt. People are encouraged to have most of their fat intake come from fish, nuts, and vegetable oils while limiting solid fats like butter, margarine, shortening, and lard. The emphasis is also placed on limiting added sugars, which contribute calories but few, if any, nutrients.

Source: US Department of Agriculture; US Department of Health and Human Services.

pregnant women, as recommended by the dietary reference intakes, and promote healthier food choices (U.S. Department of Agriculture [USDA], 2009). The MyPyramid for Moms is a customized approach. At the Web site the pregnant woman answers a series of questions about her gestation, activity level, age, and so forth. Based on the information she provides, a specific plan is developed for her.

The pregnant woman can obtain most of the recommended nutrients by eating a well-balanced diet each day. The basic food groups and recommended amounts during pregnancy and lactation are presented in Table 18-3.

> **CLINICAL TIP**
>
> Consider factors that may cause variations in weight. Weight varies with time of day, amount of clothing, inaccurate scale adjustment, or weighing error. Consequently, do not overemphasize a single weight but pay attention to the pattern of weight gain.

TABLE 18-3 Daily Food Plan for Pregnancy and Lactation

FOOD GROUP	NUTRIENTS PROVIDED	FOOD SOURCE	RECOMMENDED DAILY AMOUNT DURING PREGNANCY	RECOMMENDED DAILY AMOUNT DURING LACTATION
Dairy products	Protein; riboflavin; vitamins A, D, and others; calcium; phosphorus; zinc; magnesium	Milk—whole, 2%, low-fat, skim, dry, buttermilk Cheeses—hard, semisoft, cottage Yogurt—plain, low-fat Soybean milk—canned, dry	Four (8 oz) cups (five for teenagers) used plain or with flavoring, in shakes, soups, puddings, custards, cocoa Calcium in 1 cup milk equivalent to 1 1/2 cups cottage cheese, 1 1/2 oz hard or semisoft cheese, 1 cup yogurt, 1 1/2 cups ice cream (high in fat and sugar)	Four (8 oz) cups (five for teenagers); equivalent amount of cheese, yogurt, and so forth
Meat and meat alternatives	Protein; iron; thiamine, niacin, and other vitamins; minerals	Beef, pork, veal, lamb, poultry, animal organ meats, fish, tofu; eggs; legumes; nuts, seeds, peanut butter, grains in proper vegetarian combination (vitamin B_{12} supplement needed)	Three servings (one serving = 2 oz), combination in amounts necessary for same nutrient equivalent (varies greatly)	Two servings
Grain products, whole grain or enriched	B vitamins; iron; whole grain also has zinc, magnesium, and other trace elements; provides fiber	Breads and bread products such as cornbread, muffins, waffles, hotcakes, biscuits, dumplings, cereals, pastas, rice	Six to 11 servings daily: one serving = one slice bread, 3/4 cup or 1 oz dry cereal, 1/2 cup rice or pasta	Same as for pregnancy
Fruits and fruit juices	Vitamins A and C; minerals; raw fruits for roughage	Citrus fruits and juices, melons, berries, all other fruits and juices	Two to four servings (one serving for vitamin C): one serving = one medium fruit, 1/2–1 cup fruit, 4 oz orange or grapefruit juice	Same as for pregnancy
Vegetables and vegetable juices	Vitamins A and C; minerals; provides roughage	Leafy green vegetables; deep yellow or orange vegetables such as carrots, sweet potatoes, squash, tomatoes; green vegetables such as peas, green beans, broccoli; other vegetables such as beets, cabbage, potatoes, corn, lima beans	Three to five servings (one serving of dark green or deep yellow vegetable for vitamin A): one serving = 1/2–1 cup vegetable, two tomatoes, one medium potato	Same as for pregnancy
Fats	Vitamins A and D; linoleic acid	Butter, cream cheese, fortified table spreads; cream, whipped cream, whipped toppings; avocado, mayonnaise, oil, nuts	As desired in moderation (high in calories): one serving = 1 tbsp butter or enriched margarine	Same as for pregnancy
Sugar and sweets		Sugar, brown sugar, honey, molasses	Occasionally, if desired	Same as for pregnancy
Desserts		Nutritious desserts such as puddings, custards, fruit whips, and crisps; other rich, sweet desserts and pastries	Occasionally, if desired	Same as for pregnancy
Beverages		Coffee, decaffeinated beverages, tea, bouillon, carbonated drinks	As desired, in moderation	Same as for pregnancy
Miscellaneous		Iodized salt, herbs, spices, condiments	As desired	Same as for pregnancy

Note: The pregnant woman should eat regularly, three meals a day, with nutritious snacks of fruit, cheese, milk, or other foods between meals if desired. (More frequent but smaller meals are also recommended.) Four to 6 (8 oz) glasses of water and a total of 8 to 10 (8 oz) cups total fluid intake should be consumed daily. Water is an essential nutrient.

Nutritional Requirements

The requirements for calories and almost all nutrients increase during pregnancy, although the amount of increase varies with each nutrient. These increases reflect the additional requirements of both the mother and the developing fetus (see Table 18-1).

Calories

The term **calorie (cal)** stands for the amount of heat required to raise the temperature of 1 gram of water 1 degree centigrade. The **kilocalorie (kcal)** is equivalent to 1000 cal and is the unit used to express the energy value of food.

The dietary reference intakes for total energy indicate energy requirements do not change during the first trimester. During the second and third trimesters, pregnant women should consume an extra 300 kcal per day (American College of Obstetricians and Gynecologists [ACOG], 2009). Weight gains should be monitored regularly, and dietary recommendations should be individualized to help the pregnant woman meet her caloric needs. Prepregnant weight, height, maternal age, activity, and health status all affect caloric requirements.

PATIENT TEACHING Helping the Pregnant Woman Add 300 kcal to Her Diet

PATIENT GOALS At the completion of the teaching, the woman will be able to:

1. Identify the MyPyramid for Moms categories and the foods included in each.
2. Cite the increase in kilocalories indicated during pregnancy.
3. Discuss the most nutritionally sound way to use the additional calories.
4. Use the information she has gained to plan a nutritionally sound sample menu.

TEACHING PLAN

Content	Teaching Method
Describe the basic food groups, which include the following: Grains: 6 to 11 servings (one serving = 1 slice bread, 1/2 hamburger roll, 1 oz dry cereal, 1 tortilla, 1/2 cup pasta, rice, grits) Fruits: Two to four servings; one should be a good source of vitamin C (one serving = 1 medium-sized piece of fruit, 1/2 cup juice) Vegetables: Three to five servings (one serving = 1 cup raw vegetable, 1 cup green leafy vegetable, 1/2 cup cooked vegetable) Dairy: Two to three servings (one serving = 1 cup milk or yogurt, 1.5 oz hard cheese, 2 cups cottage cheese, 1 cup pudding made with milk) Meats and alternatives: Two to three servings (one serving = 2 oz cooked lean meat, poultry, or fish; 2 eggs, 1/2 cup cottage cheese; 1 cup cooked legumes [kidney, lima, garbanzo, or soybeans, split peas]; 6 oz tofu; 2 oz nuts or seeds; 4 tbsp peanut butter)	Ask the woman if she has received nutritional information using this approach before. Discuss her understanding of it. Use that information to plan the amount of detail you will use. Use a chart or colorful handout to explain the basic food groups and to give examples of equivalent foods.
Point out that not all foods that are nutritionally equivalent have the same number of calories; it is important to consider that when making food choices.	Use a calorie-counting guide to compare the calories in a variety of foods that are equivalent, such as 2 oz beef and 2 oz fish or 1 cup low-fat milk and 1 cup whole milk.
Explain the design of MyPyramid for Moms.	
MyPyramid for Moms is designed to represent the food groups needed to make a balanced diet throughout pregnancy. The grain, fruit, vegetable, and dairy groups are the widest color bands of the pyramid and should account for the majority of the food selections. Fewer servings of meat or meat alternatives are required in the diet. Fats, oils, sweets, and sodium do not have a high nutritional value and should be used sparingly.	Use a similar approach to evaluate the calories in fats, oils, and sweets, but also evaluate their nutrient content, especially levels of nutrients such as vitamin C, iron, and calcium. Discuss the MyPyramid for Moms recommendations about the importance of regular exercise in controlling weight gain and maintaining good health.
Emphasize that a woman only has to add 300 kcal/day during pregnancy. This can be achieved by adding two milk servings and one serving of meat or alternative. Because of the varying caloric value, a woman needs to consider the advisability of using low-fat milk, lean cuts of meat, or fish broiled or baked instead of fried.	In planning the woman's diet to get optimum nutrition without too many additional calories, it is often helpful to ask her to plan and evaluate a sample menu.
Foods can be combined. For example, 1 cup spaghetti with a 2 oz meatball would count as 1 serving meat, 3/4 cup spaghetti = 1 grain, and 1/4 cup tomato sauce = 1/2 serving vegetable.	Provide handouts on which the woman can list the foods she has eaten and check off the corresponding nutrient categories. Have her bring her completed handouts to a subsequent visit.

Evaluation	Documentation
Evaluate the learning by providing time for discussion, questions, and practice using the calorie-counting guide. Teaching has been effective if all the identified goals are achieved and if the woman seems comfortable planning her diet to provide for the best nutrition possible.	Document the information given to the woman, including specifics on food groups, foods, and portion size. Specify if written instructions were provided in addition to verbal ones and describe the type of teaching method used. Document woman's verbalization of understanding and your clarification of any information.

See Patient Teaching: Helping the Pregnant Woman Add 300 kcal to Her Diet for basic nutritional information and suggestions for increasing caloric intake.

Carbohydrates

Carbohydrates provide the body's primary source of energy as well as fiber necessary for proper bowel functioning. If the carbohydrate intake is not adequate, the body uses protein for energy. Protein then becomes unavailable for growth needs. In addition, protein breakdown leads to ketosis. Ketosis can be a problem, especially in women with diabetes, because of glycosuria, reduced alkaline reserves, and lipidemia.

The carbohydrate and caloric needs of the pregnant woman increase, especially during the last two trimesters. Carbohydrate intake promotes weight gain and growth of the fetus, placenta, and other maternal tissues. Dairy products, fruits, vegetables, and whole grain cereals and breads all contain carbohydrates.

Protein

During pregnancy, the woman needs increased amounts of protein to provide amino acids for fetal development, blood volume expansion, and growth of other maternal tissues, such as the breasts and uterus. Protein also contributes to the body's overall energy metabolism. The recommendation for protein during pregnancy is 60 g, an increase of about 14 g over nonpregnant levels. The quality of dietary protein is as important as the total amount consumed. The quality is determined by the complex of amino acids that makes up the protein. Plant proteins can meet a woman's protein needs; however, more of a given protein may be needed as animal proteins are of higher quality (see later discussion of vegetarianism).

To obtain high-quality protein in the diet, it is best to eat a variety of foods. Animal products, such as lean meats, fish, poultry, and eggs, are sources of high-quality protein. Dairy products are also important protein sources. A quart of milk supplies 32 g of protein, more than half the average daily protein requirement. Milk can be incorporated into the diet in a variety of dishes, including soups, puddings, custards, sauces, yogurt, and beverages such as hot chocolate and fruited milk drinks. Various kinds of hard and soft cheeses and cottage cheese are also excellent protein sources, although cream cheese is categorized as a fat source only. Table 18-4 provides information on the protein content of common foods.

TABLE 18-4 Amount of Protein in Common Foods

FOOD	PROTEIN (G)
Dairy Products	
Milk, 8 oz	8
Cheese: cheddar, Swiss, and so forth, 1 oz	7
Cottage cheese, 1/4 cup	7
Meat and Meat Alternatives	
Meat, fish, poultry, 1 oz	7
Egg, 1	7
Cooked dry beans and peas, 1/2 cup	7
Cooked soybeans, 1/2 cup	11
Tofu, raw, 1/2 cup	10
Peanut butter, 2 tbsp	7
Peanuts (3 tbsp), cashews/almonds (5 tbsp)	7
Breads and Cereals	
Bread, 1 slice	2
Buns, biscuits, muffins, 1	2
Cooked cereals and grains, 1/2 cup	2
Breakfast cereal, 1 oz	2
Vegetables and Fruits	
Vegetables, 1/2 cup	0.5–1
Fruits and juices, 1/2 cup	0.5
Miscellaneous	
Soy milk, 8 oz	6.6

Women who have allergies to milk, who have lactose intolerance, or who practice vegetarianism may find soy milk acceptable. It can be used in cooked dishes or as a beverage. Soy cheeses are also available.

Fat

Fats are valuable sources of energy for the body. Fats are more completely absorbed during pregnancy, resulting in a marked increase in serum lipids, lipoproteins, and cholesterol and decreased elimination of fat through the bowel. Fat deposits in the fetus increase from about 2% at midpregnancy to almost 12% at term. The U.S. Dietary Guidelines recommend that about 25% to 30% of total daily caloric intake should be from dietary fat, of which only 10% of fat calories should be saturated fat (U.S. Department of Health and Human Services & U.S. Department of Agriculture, 2005).

Essential fatty acids are important for the development of the central nervous system of the fetus. Of particular interest are the omega-3 fatty acids and their derivative, docosahexaenoic acid (DHA). Maternal dietary intake of DHA during pregnancy may be beneficial to both the mother and the fetus by reducing the risk of preterm birth, preeclampsia, and low birth weight, as well as enhancing the development of the fetal and infant brain (Innis, 2007). Although there are no current recommendations, studies indicate pregnant women may benefit from including 200 mg/day of DHA (Koletzko, Cetin, & Brenna, 2007). Dietary sources of DHA are naturally occuring in oily fish (see information on fish consumption under "Mercury in Fish" later in this chapter) and are also found in fortified dairy products and even some fortified soymilk. Plant sources of omega-3 fatty acids include soybean oil, canola oil, flaxseeds and their oil, and walnuts.

Minerals

The woman can increase minerals needed for the growth of new tissue during pregnancy by improving mineral absorption and increasing mineral intake.

Calcium and Phosphorus

Calcium and phosphorus are involved in the mineralization of fetal bones and teeth, energy and cell production, and acid–base buffering. Calcium is absorbed and used more efficiently during pregnancy. Some additional calcium and phosphorus are required early in pregnancy, but most of the fetus's bone calcification occurs during the last 2 or 3 months. Teeth begin to form at about 8 weeks' gestation and are formed by birth. The 6-year molars begin to calcify just before birth. Additional calcium is stored in the maternal skeleton as a reserve for lactation.

The identified adequate intake for calcium for the pregnant or lactating woman 19 years of age or older is 1000 mg per day. It is 1300 mg/day for pregnant women under 19. If calcium intake is not adequate, fetal needs will be met at the mother's expense by demineralization of maternal bone. Food is the preferred source of calcium because food provides other nutrients as well. A diet that includes 4 cups of milk or an equivalent dairy alternative (see Table 18-5) and a variety of other foods will provide sufficient calcium. Smaller amounts of calcium are supplied by legumes, nuts, dried fruits, and dark green leafy vegetables (such as kale, broccoli,

TABLE 18-5 Foods That Provide Comparable Amounts of Calcium

FOOD	AMOUNT
Dairy Products	
Milk	8 oz
Cheese, cheddar	1 1/2 oz
Pudding, vanilla	1 cup
Dairy Alternatives	
Soy milk*	8 oz
Fruits	
Figs	10
Raisins	2 cups
Vegetables	
Broccoli	2 1/2 cups
Collards	1 cup
Kale	3 cups
Mustard greens	3 1/2 cups
Turnip greens	1 1/2 cups
Fish	
Salmon, canned, with bones	2/3 cup
Sardines	6
Nuts	
Almonds	4 oz
Brazil nuts	1/2 cup
Miscellaneous	
Molasses, blackstrap	2 tbsp

Source: Data from Pennington, J. A. T. (1989). Bowes and Church's food values of portions commonly used *(15th ed.). Philadelphia, PA: Lippincott.*

*Amounts may vary with brand; be sure to check label.

collard greens, and beet greens). It is important to remember that some of the calcium in beet greens, spinach, and Swiss chard is bound with oxalic acid, which makes it less available to the body. Larger amounts of these foods need to be consumed if they are substituted for dairy sources of calcium (Table 18-5).

The recommended dietary allowance (RDA) for phosphorus does not change from that of a nonpregnant woman age 19 or older: 700 mg per day. Similarly, for females age 18 and younger it remains stable at 1250 mg per day. Phosphorus is readily supplied through calcium- and protein-rich foods, especially milk, eggs, and meat.

Iodine

Iodine is an essential part of the thyroid hormone thyroxine. Inorganic iodine is excreted in the urine during pregnancy. Enlargement of the thyroid gland may occur if iodine is not replaced by adequate dietary intake or additional supplement. Iodine deficiency is the most widespread nutritional cause of impaired brain development. This can result in cretinism and lesser degrees of intellectual disability (mental retardation).

A woman can meet the iodine requirement of 220 mcg per day by using iodized salt. Seafood is also a good source of iodine. Plant sources vary because they reflect the iodine content of the soil in which they grow. When sodium is restricted, the physician may prescribe an iodine supplement.

Sodium

The sodium ion is essential for proper metabolism and the regulation of fluid balance. Sodium intake in the form of salt is never entirely curtailed during pregnancy, even when hypertension or preeclampsia is present. The woman can obtain moderate sodium intake (2 to 3 g) by using fresh food lightly seasoned to taste during cooking. The use of extra salt at the table should be avoided. Salty foods, such as potato chips, ham, sausages, and sodium-based seasonings, can be eliminated to avoid excessive intake.

Zinc

Zinc is a part of numerous enzymes and is involved in protein metabolism and the synthesis of deoxyribonucleic acid (DNA) and ribonucleic acid (RNA). It is essential for normal fetal growth and development as well as milk production during lactation. The RDA during pregnancy for women age 19 and older is 11 mg per day. This increases to 12 mg during lactation. Best sources of zinc are meats, shellfish, and poultry. Good sources include whole grains and legumes.

Magnesium

Magnesium is essential for cellular metabolism and structural growth. The RDA for pregnancy is 320 mg. Good sources include milk, whole grains, dark green vegetables, nuts, and legumes.

Iron

Iron requirements increase during pregnancy because of the growth of the fetus and placenta and the expansion of maternal blood volume. Anemia in pregnancy is mainly caused by low iron stores, although it may also result from inadequate intake of other nutrients, such as vitamins B_6 and B_{12}, folic acid, ascorbic acid, copper, and zinc. Women with poor diet histories, frequent conceptions, or records of prior iron depletion are particularly at risk.

Iron deficiency anemia is generally defined as a decrease in the oxygen-carrying capacity of the blood. This significantly reduces the hemoglobin per deciliter of blood, the volume of packed red cells per deciliter of blood (hematocrit), or the number of erythrocytes. Iron deficiency anemia is associated with a higher incidence of low-birth-weight infants and preterm birth (Cunningham et al., 2010).

The normal hematocrit in the nonpregnant woman is 38% to 47%. In the pregnant woman, the level may drop to as low as 34%, even when nutrition is adequate. This condition is called the *physiologic anemia of pregnancy* (see chapter 14 ∞). Fetal demands for iron further contribute to symptoms of anemia in the pregnant woman. The fetal liver stores iron, especially during the third trimester. The infant will need this stored iron during the first 4 months of life to compensate for the normally inadequate levels of iron in breast milk and non–iron-fortified formulas. To prevent anemia, the woman must balance iron requirements and intake. Doing so is a problem for nonpregnant women and a greater one for pregnant women. Although the rate of absorption increases during pregnancy, it is still important to select foods high in iron to increase the daily intake. Lean meats, dark green leafy vegetables, eggs, and whole grain and enriched breads and cereals are the foods usually depended on for their iron content. Other iron sources include dried fruits, legumes, shellfish, and molasses.

Iron absorption is generally higher for animal products than for vegetable products. However, the woman may enhance absorption of iron from nonmeat sources by combining them with meat or a food rich in vitamin C. In addition, the use of iron-fortified foods is a cost-effective and efficient way to increase iron intake.

The most iron that can reasonably be obtained from the average diet is about 15 to 18 mg per day. However, the recommended intake for iron during pregnancy is 27 mg per day. Thus during pregnancy a supplement of simple iron salt, such as ferrous gluconate, ferrous fumarate, or ferrous sulfate, is needed. This amount is available in most prenatal vitamins. Unfortunately iron supplements often cause gastrointestinal discomfort, especially if taken on an empty stomach. Consequently caregivers often begin iron supplementation in the second trimester after the incidence of nausea and vomiting subsides. Once the woman begins taking an iron supplement, absorption is increased if she takes it with a source of vitamin C such as orange juice. In addition, iron is often constipating, so it is important for the woman to consume sufficient fluids and roughage in her diet to combat this effect.

Vitamins

Vitamins are organic substances necessary for life and growth. They are found in small amounts in specific foods and generally cannot be synthesized by the body in adequate amounts.

Vitamins are grouped according to their solubility. Those that dissolve in fat are A, D, E, and K; those soluble in water include vitamin C and the B complex vitamins. An adequate intake of all vitamins is essential during pregnancy; however, several are required in larger than normal amounts to fulfill specific needs.

A balanced diet generally provides necessary vitamins without the need for supplementation. Despite this, many people who are concerned about nutrition have become involved in the practice of taking exceptionally large doses—megadoses—of vitamins. However, in vitamin therapy more is not necessarily better. Megadoses of vitamins, especially vitamins A, D, C, and B_6, have been documented to have a negative effect on the fetus. Furthermore, excessive intake of one vitamin may interfere with the body's use of another vitamin. For example, excessive intake of vitamin C may block the body's use of vitamin B_{12}. Consequently, although it is important to meet the recommended dietary allowances of vitamins during pregnancy, megadoses are best avoided.

Fat-Soluble Vitamins

The fat-soluble vitamins A, D, E, and K are stored in the liver and thus are available should the dietary intake become inadequate. They are not excreted in the urine, so excessive consumption of these vitamins, particularly vitamins A and D, can lead to toxicity. Symptoms of fat-soluble vitamin toxicity include nausea, gastrointestinal upset, dryness and cracking of the skin, and loss of hair.

VITAMIN A Vitamin A is involved in the growth of epithelial cells, which line the entire gastrointestinal tract and compose the skin. Vitamin A plays a role in the metabolism of carbohydrates and fats. The body cannot synthesize glycogen in the absence of vitamin A, and the body's ability to handle cholesterol is also affected. In addition, the protective layer of tissue surrounding nerve fibers does not form properly if vitamin A is lacking. Probably the best known function of vitamin A is its effect on vision in dim light. A person's ability to see in the dark depends on the eye's supply of retinol, a form of vitamin A. In this manner, vitamin A prevents night blindness. Vitamin A is associated with the formation and development of healthy eyes in the fetus.

If maternal stores of vitamin A are adequate, the overall effects of pregnancy on the woman's vitamin A requirements are not remarkable. The blood serum level of vitamin A decreases slightly in early pregnancy, rises in late pregnancy, and falls before the onset of labor. Thus the RDA for vitamin A is 770 mcg per day for pregnant women age 19 and older.

Deficiencies of vitamin A are not common in the United States. Among the poor of developing countries, vitamin A deficiency is a major cause of preventable childhood blindness and an important factor in morbidity and mortality from infection, especially among pregnant women and children (World Health Organizatioin, 2009). Although routine supplementation with vitamin A is not recommended, supplementation with 5000 international units is indicated for women whose dietary intake may be inadequate, specifically strict vegetarians and recent emigrants from countries where deficiency of vitamin A is endemic.

Rich plant sources of vitamin A include deep green and yellow or deep orange vegetables and some fruits; animal sources include liver, egg yolk, cream, butter, fortified margarine, and milk.

VITAMIN D Vitamin D is best known for its role in the absorption and utilization of calcium and phosphorus in skeletal development. To supply the needs of the developing fetus, the pregnant woman should have a vitamin D intake of 5 mcg per day.

Main food sources of vitamin D include fortified milk, margarine, butter, liver, and egg yolks. Drinking a quart of vitamin D–fortified milk daily provides the vitamin D needed during pregnancy. Vitamin D is also obtained through the synthesis of sunlight on the skin. During the winter months, however, women who live in northern latitudes are at risk for limited sun exposure. Foods that provide good sources of vitamin D should be encouraged.

Excessive intake of vitamin D is not usually a result of eating but of taking high-potency vitamin preparations. Overdoses during pregnancy can cause hypercalcemia or high blood calcium levels because of withdrawal of calcium from the skeletal tissue. Symptoms of toxicity include excessive thirst, loss of appetite, vomiting, weight loss, irritability, and high blood calcium levels.

VITAMIN E The major function of vitamin E, or tocopherol, is as an antioxidant. Vitamin E takes on oxygen, thus preventing other nutrients from undergoing chemical changes. For example, vitamin E helps spare vitamin A by preventing its oxidation in the intestinal tract and the tissues. It decreases the oxidation of polyunsaturated fats, thus helping to retain the flexibility and health of the cell membrane. In protecting the cell membrane, vitamin E affects the health of all cells in the body.

Vitamin E is also involved in certain enzymatic and metabolic reactions. It is an essential nutrient for the synthesis of nucleic acids required in the formation of red blood cells in the bone marrow. Vitamin E is beneficial in treating certain types of muscular pain and intermittent claudication, in surface healing of wounds and burns, and in protecting lung tissue from the damaging effects of smog. These functions may help explain the abundant claims and cures attributed to vitamin E, many of which have not been scientifically proved.

The newborn's need for vitamin E has been widely recognized. Human milk provides adequate vitamin E, whereas cow's milk is lower in vitamin E content. Deficiency symptoms of vitamin E are related to long-term inability to absorb fats. In humans, malabsorption problems exist in cases of cystic fibrosis, liver cirrhosis, postgastrectomy, obstructive jaundice, pancreatic problems, and sprue.

The recommended intake of vitamin E is unchanged at 15 mg per day. Vitamin E is widely distributed in foodstuffs, especially vegetable fats and oils, whole grains, greens, and eggs.

Some pregnant women massage vitamin E oil on the abdominal skin to make it supple and possibly prevent permanent stretch marks. It is questionable whether taking high doses orally will accomplish this goal or satisfy any other claims related to vitamin E's role in reproduction or virility. In addition, excessive intake of vitamin E has been associated with abnormal coagulation in the newborn.

VITAMIN K Vitamin K, or menadione as used synthetically in medicine, is an essential factor for the synthesis of prothrombin; its function is thus related to normal blood clotting. Synthesis occurs in the intestinal tract by the *Escherichia coli* normally inhabiting the large intestine. However, the body's need for vitamin K is not totally met through synthesis. Green leafy vegetables and liver are excellent sources. The requirement for vitamin K does not increase during pregnancy. It is 90 mcg per day.

Intake of vitamin K is usually adequate in a well-balanced prenatal diet. Secondary problems may arise if an illness results in malabsorption of fats or if antibiotics are used for an extended period. Antibiotics inhibit vitamin K synthesis by destroying intestinal *E. coli.*

Water-Soluble Vitamins

Water-soluble vitamins are excreted in the urine. Only small amounts are stored, so there is little protection from dietary inadequacies. Thus adequate amounts must be ingested daily. During pregnancy, the concentration of water-soluble vitamins in the maternal serum falls, whereas high concentrations are found in the fetus.

VITAMIN C The requirement for vitamin C (ascorbic acid) is increased in pregnancy from 75 to 85 mg per day. The major function of vitamin C is to aid the formation and development of connective tissue and the vascular system. Ascorbic acid is essential to the formation of collagen. Collagen is like cement that binds cells together, just as mortar holds bricks together. If the collagen begins to disintegrate because of lack of ascorbic acid, cell functioning is disturbed, and cell structure breaks down, causing muscular weakness, capillary hemorrhage, and eventual death. These are symptoms of scurvy, the disease caused by vitamin C deficiency. Newborns of women who have taken megadoses of vitamin C may experience a rebound form of scurvy.

Maternal plasma levels of vitamin C progressively decline throughout pregnancy, with values at term being about half those at midpregnancy. It appears that ascorbic acid concentrates in the placenta; levels in the fetus are 50% or more above maternal levels.

A nutritious diet should meet the pregnant woman's needs for vitamin C without additional supplementation. Common food sources of vitamin C include citrus fruit, tomatoes, cantaloupe, strawberries, potatoes, broccoli, and other leafy green vegetables. Ascorbic acid is readily destroyed by water and oxidation. Therefore, foods containing vitamin C should have limited exposure to air, heat, and water during storage and cooking.

THE B VITAMINS The B vitamins include thiamine (B_1), riboflavin (B_2), niacin, folic acid, pantothenic acid, vitamin B_6, and vitamin B_{12}. These vitamins serve as vital coenzyme factors in many reactions, such as cell respiration, glucose oxidation, and energy metabolism. Consequently, the quantities needed invariably increase as caloric intake increases to meet the metabolic and growth needs of the pregnant woman.

The *thiamine* requirement increases from the prepregnant level of 1.1 mg per day to 1.4 mg per day. Sources include pork, liver, milk, potatoes, enriched breads, and cereals.

Riboflavin deficiency is manifested by *cheilosis* (fissures and cracks of the lips and the corners of the mouth) and other skin lesions. During pregnancy, women may excrete less riboflavin and still require more because of increased energy and protein needs. Thus the recommended intake of riboflavin increases by 0.3 mg per day, to 1.4 mg per day for pregnant women age 19 and older. Sources include milk, liver, eggs, enriched breads, and cereals.

Niacin requirements increase by 4 mg per day during pregnancy to 18 mg. Sources of niacin include meat, fish, poultry, liver, whole grains, enriched breads, cereals, and peanuts.

Folic acid, or folate, is required for normal growth, reproduction, and lactation and prevents the macrocytic, megaloblastic anemia of pregnancy. Megaloblastic anemia due to folic acid deficiency is seldom found in the United States, but those caring for pregnant women must be aware that it does occur.

Even more significantly, an inadequate intake of folic acid has been associated with neural tube defects (NTDs) (spina bifida, anencephaly). Although these defects are considered multifactorial (see chapter 12 ∞), research indicates that 50% to 70% of spina bifida and anencephaly could be prevented by adequate intake of folic acid (Centers for Disease Control and Prevention [CDC], 2009). Consequently experts recommend that all women of childbearing age (15 to 45 years) consume 400 mcg

RESEARCH EVIDENCE IN PRACTICE Iron and Folic Acid Supplementation During Pregnancy

CLINICAL QUESTION

What is a safe, effective dosing regimen for iron and folic acid supplementation during pregnancy?

RESEARCH EVIDENCE

The effectiveness of iron supplementation in preventing maternal anemia has been well documented. Likewise, folic acid supplementation has been widely demonstrated to reduce the incidence of neural tube defects. However, there is a lack of clarity about the most effective dosage and regimen of both supplements.

The American College of Obstetricians and Gynecologists (ACOG) convened a study group to review the evidence and develop clinical guidelines for the use of folic acid supplements during pregnancy. Their recommendations are based on a systematic review of the literature and the opinions of an expert panel. The findings were confirmed by a large randomized controlled trial sponsored by the Canadian Society of Obstetricians and Gynaecologists.

Periconceptional folic acid supplementation is recommended because it has been shown to reduce the occurrence of neural tube defects. For low-risk women, the appropriate dosage is 400 mcg per day. For women at high risk or who have had a previous pregnancy that resulted in an infant with a neural tube defect, folic acid supplementation of 4 mg per day is recommended.

Two Cochrane Collaborative reviews of 89 trials involving more than 35,000 women support the safety and efficacy of iron supplementation during pregnancy. Daily iron supplementation was associated with increased maternal hemoglobin levels both pre- and post-birth. The risk of anemia was reduced in those mothers who took daily iron supplements. However, these benefits were seen both in women who took iron supplements daily and those who took the supplements intermittently. The women who took the iron supplements intermittently were less likely to have undesirable side effects and hemoconcentration. The risk of hemoconcentration among those women taking daily iron supplements was greater during the second and third trimesters.

While there are many foods that provide iron and folic acid naturally (spinach, lentils, broccoli, oranges, etc.) it is unlikely that diet alone can provide levels similar to folate-multivitamin supplementation.

WHAT QUESTIONS REMAIN UNANSWERED?

Intermittent folic acid therapy has not been tested. It is unclear whether the daily dosage of folic acid is required, but given the seriousness of neural tube defects, daily folic acid supplementation is recommended until further trials demonstrate the effectiveness of intermittent dosing.

WHAT IS BEST PRACTICE?

Universal prenatal supplementation with iron provided either daily or weekly is effective to prevent anemia at term. Women in the reproductive age group should be advised about the benefits of folic acid supplementation even before they become pregnant, during wellness visits, and especially if they are contemplating pregnancy. Daily dosages of 400 mcg of folic acid are effective for low-risk women; 4 mg should be taken by women in high-risk groups.

CRITICAL THINKING

For women who are contemplating pregnancy, what is the most effective way to ensure they will be compliant with a daily regimen of folic acid supplementation?

References

American College of Obstetricians and Gynecologists (ACOG). (2003). *Neural tube defects* (ACOG Practice Bulletin No. 44). Washington, DC: Author.

Pena-Rosas, J., & Biteri, F. (2009). Effects and safety of preventive oral iron or iron + folic acid supplementation for women during pregnancy. *Cochrane Database of Systematic Reviews,* Issue 4. Art. No.: CD004736. doi:10.1002/14651858

Wilson, R. D., Johnson, J. A., Wyatt, P., Allen, V., Gagnon, A., Langlois, S., . . . Kapur, B. (Genetics Committee of the Society of Obstetricians and Gynaecologists of Canada), (2007). Pre-conceptional vitamin/folic acid supplementation: The use of folic acid in combination with a multivitamin supplement for the prevention of neural tube defects and other congenital anomalies. *Journal of Obstetrics and Gynaecology (Canada), 29*(12), 1003–1013.

---

of folic acid daily, because half of all U.S. pregnancies are unplanned and NTDs occur very early in pregnancy (3 to 4 weeks after conception), before most women realize they are pregnant (CDC, 2009). See Research Evidence in Practice: Iron and Folic Acid Supplementation During Pregnancy.

The best food sources of folates are fresh green leafy vegetables, liver, peanuts, and whole-grain breads and cereals. Folic acid can be made inactive by oxidation, ultraviolet (UV) light, and heating. It can easily be lost during improper storage and cooking. To prevent unnecessary loss, foods should be stored covered to protect them from light, cooked with only a small amount of water, and not overcooked.

No allowance has been set for *pantothenic acid* in pregnancy but 5 mg per day is considered an adequate intake. Sources include meats, egg yolk, legumes, and whole grain cereals and breads.

Vitamin B_6 *(pyridoxine)* is associated with amino acid metabolism; thus a higher-than-average protein intake requires increased pyridoxine intake. The RDA for vitamin B_6 during pregnancy is 1.9 mg per day, an increase of 0.6 mg over the allowance for nonpregnant women. Generally the slightly increased need can be supplied by dietary sources, which include wheat germ, yeast, fish, liver, pork, potatoes, and lentils.

Vitamin B_{12}, or *cobalamin*, is the cobalt-containing vitamin found only in animal sources. Rarely is B_{12} deficiency found in women of reproductive age. Vegans (see later discussion of vegetarianism) can develop a deficiency, however, so it is essential that their dietary intake be supplemented with this vitamin. A deficiency may also be due to a congenital inability to absorb vitamin B_{12}, resulting in pernicious anemia; however, infertility is a complication of this type of anemia.

Occasionally, vitamin B_{12} levels decrease during pregnancy but increase again after birth. The RDA during pregnancy is 2.6 mcg per day, an increase of 0.2 mcg.

Folic acid and iron are the only nutritional supplements generally recommended during pregnancy. The increased need for other vitamins and minerals can usually be met with an adequate diet. To avoid possible deficiencies, however, many healthcare professionals still recommend a daily vitamin supplement.

CLINICAL TIP

In eliciting a pregnant woman's health history, keep in mind the fact that more women are consuming over-the-counter vitamin, mineral, and food supplements today than in the past. Thus it is important to ask about the use of any over-the-counter supplements to help avoid potentially harmful excess intakes.

Fluid

The nutrient water is essential for life and is found in all body tissues. It is necessary for many biochemical reactions. It also serves as a lubricant, acts as a medium of transport for carrying substances in and out of the body, and aids in the regulation of body temperature. A pregnant woman should consume at least 8 to 10 (8 oz) glasses of fluid each day, of which 4 to 6 glasses should be water. Other beverages such as juices and milk can contribute water as well as other nutrients to the diet. Sodas and diet sodas should be used in moderation because they do not contribute to the nutritional value of the diet.

Caffeine is found in beverages, foods, and medications. Its use during pregnancy remains controversial. High caffeine intake is associated with delayed conception, spontaneous miscarriage, and low birth weight but is not associated with birth defects (Higdon & Frei, 2006). Caffeinated beverages have a diuretic effect, which may be counterproductive to increasing fluid intake. In a position statement on maternal health, the American Dietetic Association states "pregnant women should avoid caffeine intakes above 300 mg" (ADA, 2008). The average 16 oz cup of coffee contains about 188 mg of caffeine, while carbonated sodas contain about 18–48 mg/12 oz, and energy drinks range from 33 to 75 mg per 8 oz (McCusker, Goldberger, & Cone, 2006).

Vegetarianism

Vegetarianism is the dietary choice of many people for religious, health, ethical, and economic reasons. Well-planned vegetarian diets are nutritionally adequate and appropriate for all stages of life, including pregnancy. Vegetarian diets are associated with many health benefits in the treatment and prevention of certain diseases (ADA, 2009). There are several types of vegetarians and dietary practices vary among the types. **Lacto-ovovegetarians** include milk, dairy products, and eggs in their diet. **Lacto-vegetarians** include dairy products but no eggs. **Vegans** are strict vegetarians who will not eat any food from animal sources.

The expectant woman who is lacto-ovovegetarian can obtain ample amounts of high-quality proteins from dairy products and eggs. Plant protein quality may be improved if consumed with these animal proteins. If the diet contains fewer than four servings of milk and dairy products, calcium supplementation may be necessary.

Appropriate meal planning for vegan diets ensures that a pregnant woman obtains necessary nutrients to promote the growth and development of the fetus. Protein needs increase slightly for vegans because of the lower quality protein sources ingested when animal proteins are excluded. Adequate dietary protein can be obtained by consuming a varied diet with adequate caloric intake and plant-based proteins. Consuming an assortment of plant proteins throughout the day such as beans and rice, peanut butter on whole grain bread, and whole grain cereal with soymilk, ensures the expectant mother obtains all essential amino acids. Protein and amino acid supplements are not recommended. Obtaining sufficient calories to achieve adequate weight gains can be difficult because vegan diets tend to be higher in fiber and, therefore, filling. Low prepregnancy weight and optimum pregnancy weight gains are often a problem. Supplementation with energy-dense foods helps provide increased energy intake to prevent the body from using protein for caloric needs.

Because vegans use no animal products, a daily supplement of 4 mg of vitamin B_{12} is necessary. If soy milk is used, only partial supplementation may be needed. If no soy milk is taken, daily supplements of 1200 mg of calcium and 10 mg of vitamin D are needed.

A vegan diet may be low in iron and zinc because the best sources of these minerals are found in animal products. In addition, a high-fiber intake may reduce mineral (calcium, iron, and zinc) bioavailability. The nurse should emphasize the use of foods containing these nutrients.

A guide to vegetarian food groups is provided in Table 18-6.

Practical Guide to Veganism During Pregnancy

Factors Influencing Nutrition

It is important to consider the many factors that affect a patient's nutrition. What are the age, lifestyle, dietary practices, and culture of the pregnant woman? What food beliefs and habits does she have? What a person eats is also determined by availability, economics, and symbolism. These and other factors influence the expectant mother's acceptance of the nurse's intervention.

Common Discomforts of Pregnancy

Gastrointestinal functioning can be altered at times during pregnancy, resulting in discomforts such as nausea, vomiting, heartburn, and constipation. Although these changes can be

TABLE 18-6 Vegetarian Food Groups

FOOD GROUP	MIXED DIET	LACTO-OVOVEGETARIAN	LACTO-VEGETARIAN	VEGAN
Grain	Bread, cereal, rice, pasta	Bread, cereal, rice, pasta	Bread, cereal, rice, pasta	Bread, cereal, rice, pasta
Fruit	Fruit, fruit juices	Fruit, fruit juices	Fruit, fruit juices	Fruit, fruit juices
Vegetable	Vegetables, vegetable juices	Vegetables, vegetable juices	Vegetables, vegetable juices	Vegetables, vegetable juices
Dairy and dairy alternatives	Milk, yogurt, cheese	Milk, yogurt, cheese	Milk, yogurt, cheese	Fortified soy milk, rice milk
Meat and meat alternatives	Meat, fish, poultry, eggs, legumes, tofu, nuts, nut butters	Eggs, legumes, tofu, nuts, nut butters	Legumes, tofu, nuts, nut butters	Legumes, tofu, nuts, nut butters

uncomfortable for the woman, they are seldom a major problem. These discomforts and dietary modifications that may provide relief are discussed in chapter 16 ∞.

Herbal, Botanical, and Alternative Therapies

While the use of some herbal, botanical, and alternative therapies may seem like a natural and safe alternative to some individuals, the pregnant consumer should take caution. Very few clinical trials exist that have examined the safety of supplements and herbs during pregnancy. Pregnant women should be advised to avoid alternative therapies until further research can determine their safety. Herbal and botanical supplements may potentially cause complications during the pregnancy and should be discontinued immediately when a woman determines she is pregnant. (ADA, 2009)

Use of Artificial Sweeteners

Foods and beverages that contain artificial sweeteners are increasingly available. Sweeteners classified as Generally Recognized as Safe (GRAS) by the Food and Drug Administration (FDA) are acceptable for use during pregnancy and include acesulfame potassium (Sweet One), aspartame (NutraSweet, Equal), saccharin (Sweet N Low, Sugar Twin), and sucralose (Splenda). As with other foods, moderation should be exercised in using artificial sweeteners.

Stevia sweeteners (Truvia, PureVia, SunCrystals) are the newest low-calorie sweeteners to become available. Derived from leaves of the Stevia rebaudiana Bertoni plant, Rebaudioside A is FDA approved for safe consumption as a sweetener. While Stevia sweeteners are marketed as natural, at this time the sweeteners offer no additional clinical advantages over any other non-nutritive sweetener (International Food Information Council, 2009).

Mercury in Fish

Fish and shellfish are important parts of a healthy diet but nearly all contain traces of mercury. Although this is not a concern for most people, some fish and shellfish contain higher levels of mercury than others, and mercury can pose a threat to the unborn baby or a young child. The developing fetal brain is quite susceptible to the neurotoxic effects of mercury, which crosses the placenta and the blood-brain barrier. Mercury exposure can have a negative effect on cognitive functioning, resulting in deficiencies in language, attention, motor function, memory, and visual-spatial abilities (Huffling, 2006). Because of this, the U.S. government has issued the following guidelines for women who are pregnant or who may become pregnant, breastfeeding mothers, and young children (FDA, 2004):

- Do not eat swordfish, shark, tilefish, or king mackerel, because these fish contain high levels of mercury.
- Eat up to 12 oz/week (two average meals) of a variety of shellfish and fish that are lower in mercury. (Commonly eaten fish that are lower in mercury include canned light tuna, shrimp, salmon, catfish, and pollack. Albacore [white] tuna has more mercury than canned light tuna, so only 6 ounces/week of albacore tuna is recommended.)
- Check local advisories about the mercury content of fish caught locally by family and friends. If no information is available, limit fish caught in local areas to 6 oz/week and avoid consuming additional fish that week.

Salmonella and Listeria Infection

The pregnant woman's immune system is somewhat weakened during pregnancy, As a result, pregnant women and their fetuses are at high risk for foodborne illnesses, which can cause miscarriage, serious health problems, or even maternal death.

Because of the risk of *Salmonella* contamination in raw eggs, pregnant women are advised to avoid eating or tasting foods that may contain raw or lightly cooked eggs. These foods include, for example, cake batter, cookie dough made with raw eggs, homemade eggnog, sauces made with raw eggs such as Caesar salad dressing and hollandaise sauce, and homemade ice cream (FDA, 2009).

Listeria monocytogenes is another bacterium that poses a threat to an expectant mother and her fetus. Listeria is especially challenging because the organism can be found in refrigerated, ready-to-eat foods such as unpasteurized milk and dairy products, meat, poultry, and seafood. To prevent listeriosis, pregnant women should be advised to do the following (FDA, 2009):

- Maintain refrigerator temperature at 40°F (4°C) or below and the freezer at 0°F (−18°C).
- Refrigerate or freeze prepared foods, leftovers, and perishables within 2 hours after eating or preparation.
- Do not eat hot dogs and luncheon meats unless they are reheated until they are steaming hot.
- Avoid soft cheeses such as feta, brie, Camembert, blue veined cheeses, queso fresco, or queso blanco (a soft cheese often used by Hispanic women in their cooking) unless the label clearly states that they are made with pasteurized milk.
- Do not eat refrigerated patés or meat spreads or foods that contain raw (unpasteurized) milk or drink unpasteurized milk.
- Avoid eating refrigerated smoked seafood such as salmon, trout, cod, tuna, or mackerel unless it is in a cooked dish such as a casserole. Canned or shelf-stable patés, meat spreads, and smoked seafood are considered safe to eat.

Lactase Deficiency (Lactose Intolerance)

Some individuals have difficulty digesting milk and dairy products. This condition, known as **lactase deficiency**, or **lactose intolerance**, results from an inadequate amount of the enzyme lactase, which breaks down the milk sugar lactose into smaller digestible substances.

Lactase deficiency is a common condition affecting millions in the United States. Some ethnic and racial populations are more affected than others and include African Americans, Hispanic Americans, American Indians, and Asian Americans (National Digestive Diseases Information Clearinghouse, 2009). People who are not affected are mainly of Northern European heritage. Symptoms may include abdominal distention, discomfort, nausea, vomiting, loose stools, and cramps.

When counseling pregnant women who might be intolerant of milk and milk products, the nurse should be aware that tolerances vary between individuals and even a partial serving of milk or dairy products can produce symptoms. Lactase deficiency need not be a problem for pregnant women, because the enzyme is available over the counter in tablets or drops. In addition, specially treated cow's milk is now available in most large grocery stores.

Cultural, Ethnic, and Religious Influences

Cultural, ethnic, and, occasionally, religious backgrounds determine one's experiences with food and influence food preferences and habits (Figure 18-3 ■). People of different nationalities are accustomed to eating foodstuffs available in their country of origin and prepared in a manner consistent with the customs and traditions of their ethnic and cultural group. In addition, the laws of certain religions allow particular foods, prohibit others, and direct the preparation and serving of meals. (See Developing Cultural Competence: The Kosher Diet.)

In each culture, certain foods have symbolic significance. Generally, these symbolic foods are related to major life experiences such as birth, death, or developmental milestones. Although generalizations have been made about the food practices of ethnic and religious groups, there are many variations. Food customs will differ among groups in various regions of the same country, among families within local regions, and among individuals within the same family. The extent to which the use of traditional ethnic foods and customs is continued is affected by the recency of immigration; the extent of exposure to other cultures; and the availability, quality, and cost of the traditional foods.

When working with a pregnant woman from any ethnic background, the nurse needs to understand the cultural influences on the woman's eating habits and to identify beliefs she may have about foods and pregnancy. Talking with the patient can enable the nurse to determine the level of influence that traditional food customs exert. Only then can the nurse provide dietary advice in a manner that is meaningful to the woman.

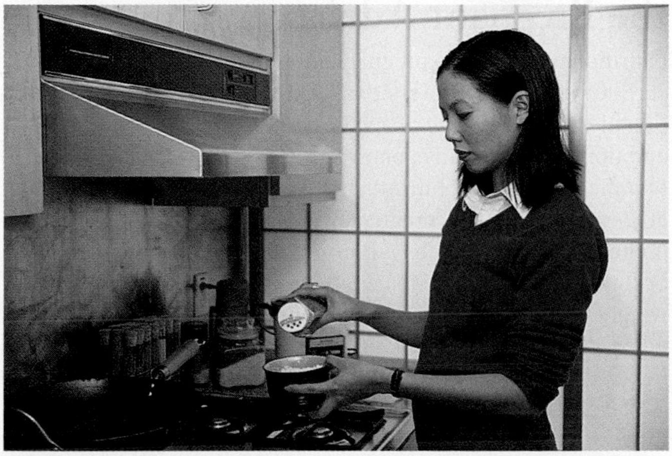

Figure 18-3 ■ Cultural factors affect food preferences and habits.

Source: Photographer, Elena Dorfman.

DEVELOPING CULTURAL COMPETENCE

The Kosher Diet

The kosher diet followed by many Jewish people forbids the eating of pig products and shellfish. Certain cuts of meat from sheep and cattle are allowed as are fish with fins and scales. In addition, many Jews believe that meat and dairy products should not be mixed or eaten at the same meal.

Psychosocial Factors

The sharing of food has long been a symbol of friendliness, warmth, and social acceptance in many cultures. Food is also symbolic of motherliness; that is, taking care of the family and feeding them well is a part of the traditional mothering role. Some foods and food-related practices are associated with status. Certain items may be prepared "just for company." Other foods are served only on special occasions—holidays such as Thanksgiving, for example.

Socioeconomic level may be a determinant of nutritional status. Poverty-level families are unable to afford the same foods that higher income families can. Thus, pregnant women with low incomes are frequently at risk for inadequate intake of nutrients.

Knowledge about the basic components of a balanced diet is essential. Often educational level is related to economic status, but even people on very limited incomes can prepare well-balanced meals if their knowledge of nutrition is adequate.

The expectant woman's attitudes and feelings about her pregnancy may influence her nutritional status. For example, food may be used as a substitute for the expression of emotions such as anger or frustration, or as a way of expressing feelings of joy. The woman who is depressed or who does not wish to be pregnant may manifest these feelings by loss of appetite or by an overindulgence of certain foods.

Eating Disorders

Millions of men and women are affected by eating disorders each year, but eating disorders are most common in adolescent girls and young women. These psychologic disorders can have a major impact on a pregnant patient's physiologic and emotional well-being.

Anorexia nervosa is an eating disorder that is characterized by an extreme fear of weight gain and fat. People with this problem have distorted body images and perceive themselves as fat even when they are extremely underweight. Their dietary intake is very restrictive in both variety and quantity. They may also engage in excessive exercise to prevent weight gain.

Bulimia nervosa, another eating disorder, is characterized by bingeing (secretly consuming large quantities of food in a short period) and purging. Self-induced vomiting is the most common method of purging; laxatives and/or diuretics may also be used. Individuals with bulimia often maintain normal or near-normal weight for their height, so it is often difficult to know whether bingeing and purging occur.

Although pregnancies occur most often in women of normal weight, the underweight woman can conceive. The presence of an eating disorder can be difficult to detect because of the secretive nature of the behaviors. Many women will decrease or

TABLE 18-7 Abnormalities That May Indicate an Undisclosed Eating Disorder

Somatic
- Arrested growth
- Marked change or frequent fluctuation in weight
- Inability to gain weight
- Fatigue
- Constipation or diarrhea
- Susceptibility to fractures
- Delayed menarche
- Hypokalemia, hyperphosphatemia, metabolic acidosis or alkalosis, or high serum amylase levels

Behavioral
- Change in eating habits
- Difficulty eating in social settings
- Reluctance to be weighed
- Depression
- Social withdrawal
- Absence from school or work
- Deceptive or secretive behavior
- Stealing (e.g., to obtain food)
- Substance abuse
- Excessive exercise

Source: Becker, A. E., Grinspoon, S. K., Klibanski, A., & Herzog, D. B. (1999). Eating disorders. New England Journal of Medicine, *340, 1092–1098. Copyright © 1999 Massachusetts Medical Society. All rights reserved.*

Application: Pica

discontinue their eating disorder behaviors during pregnancy, only to resume them postpartum. Table 18-7 identifies abnormalities that may indicate an eating disorder.

Women with eating disorders who become pregnant are at risk for a variety of complications. The consequences of the restricting, bingeing, and purging behaviors characteristic of eating disorders can result in a lack of nutrients available for the fetus. Women with eating disorders are at increased risk for miscarriage, low birth weight, premature birth, obstetric complications, perinatal mortality, and birth defects (Madsen, 2009). Pregnancy can be an especially difficult time for the woman with an eating disorder, even if she has long desired a child. For someone who already struggles with eating and body image, the consumption of additional food and the expectations that she will gain additional weight can result in feelings of fear, anxiety, depression, and guilt. Women with eating disorders also have high rates of depression postpartally (Astrachan-Fletcher, Veldhuis, Lively, et al., 2008). When working with a pregnant woman with an eating disorder, education and individualized meal plans can help the woman increase her dietary intake while maintaining a sense of control.

The treatment needs of a woman with an eating disorder can best be met by a team approach that includes medical, nutritional, and psychiatric practitioners who are familiar with eating disorders. The pregnant woman with an eating disorder needs to be closely monitored and supported throughout her pregnancy to help ensure the best possible outcome.

> “I developed anorexia during my sophomore year in college. My parents were shocked when they saw me at Thanksgiving and, fortunately, they got me some help. For the past several years I have maintained my weight in the low normal range and feel OK about it. Now I am expecting my first child. It is so hard to think of gaining 25 to 30 pounds, but I am working very hard to eat properly for my baby. I have reconnected with my therapist so that I can be sure I keep my head on straight about the importance of good nutrition. I don't think people realize how tough eating disorders are to overcome but I will NOT jeopardize my child, I just won't!”

Pica

Pica is the persistent craving and eating of substances such as ice, freezer frost, cornstarch, laundry starch, baby powder, clay, dirt, and other nonnutritive substances. Most women who eat such substances do so only during pregnancy.

Iron deficiency anemia is the most common concern with pica. The ingestion of laundry starch or certain types of clay may contribute to iron deficiency by replacing iron-containing foods from the diet or by interfering with iron absorption. Women with pica that involves eating ice or freezer frost often have poor weight gain because of lack of appetite, whereas the ingestion of starch may be associated with excessive weight gain. The ingestion of large quantities of clay could fill the intestine and cause fecal impaction.

Assessment for pica is an important part of a nutritional history. However, women may be embarrassed about their cravings or reluctant to discuss them for fear of criticism. It is helpful if the nurse uses a nonjudgmental approach and explains the possible harmful effects. Some women are able to switch to eating nonfat powdered milk instead of laundry starch and frozen fruit pops instead of ice. Others find that sucking on hard lemon or mint candies helps decrease the craving.

Nutritional Care of the Pregnant Adolescent

Nutritional care of the pregnant adolescent is of particular concern to healthcare professionals. Many adolescents are nutritionally at risk because of a variety of complex and interrelated emotional, social, and economic factors that may adversely affect dietary intake. Nutritional status is an important, modifiable variable in any pregnancy, but especially in adolescent pregnancy because teens are more likely than older women to be underweight at the onset of pregnancy and to gain less weight during pregnancy. For women who are underweight when they become pregnant, the greater the weight gain, the lower the incidence of perinatal mortality. Conversely, more adolescents are overweight or obese today than in the past. Overweight and obese teens are at increased risk for adult obesity and for developing diabetes and risk factors for coronary heart disease (Groth, 2006). Important nutrition-related factors to assess in pregnant adolescents include low prepregnant weight, low weight gain during pregnancy, younger age with regard to menarche, smoking, excessive prepregnant weight, anemia, unhealthy lifestyle (drugs, alcohol use), chronic disease, and history of an eating disorder.

Adolescent women generally are considered physiologically mature about 4 years after menarche because linear growth is usually completed by this time. Their nutritional needs would be similar to those of other "adult" women. Adolescents who become pregnant fewer than 4 years after menarche, however, are at a high biologic risk because of their physiologic and anatomic immaturity. They are most likely to be growing, which can impact the fetus's development. Nutritional needs for these young women will be higher than for those whose growth has been completed. Thus young adolescents (13 to 15 years) need to gain more weight than older adolescents (16 years or older) to produce babies of equal size. In determining the optimum weight gain for a pregnant adolescent, the nurse needs to add the recommended weight gain for a normal adult pregnancy to the amount of weight gain expected during the postmenarcheal year during which the pregnancy occurs. Young adolescents (2 years after menarche) should strive for a weight gain at the upper end of the range of weight gain for adults (see Table 18-2).

The nutritional needs of pregnant adolescents are generally estimated by using the dietary reference intake (DRI) for nonpregnant teenagers (ages 11 to 14 or 15 to 18) and adding nutrient amounts recommended for all pregnant women (see Table 18-1).

Specific Nutrient Concerns

Caloric needs of pregnant adolescents vary widely. Major factors in determining caloric needs include whether growth has been completed and the physical activity level of the individual. Figures as high as 50 kcal/kg have been suggested for young, growing teens who are very active physically. A satisfactory weight gain will confirm adequacy of caloric intake in most cases.

An inadequate iron intake is a major concern with the adolescent diet. Iron needs are high for the pregnant teen because of the requirement for iron by the enlarging maternal muscle mass and blood volume. Iron supplements—providing 30 to 60 mg of elemental iron—are indicated.

Calcium is another nutrient that demands special attention from pregnant adolescents. Inadequate intake of calcium is frequently a problem in this age group. Adequate calcium intake is needed to support normal growth and development of the fetus as well as growth and maintenance of calcium stores in the adolescent. Inadequate calcium has been associated with maternal hypertension and preeclampsia. Pregnant adolescents who consume adequate calcium have a lower incidence of hypertension, preterm birth, and low-birth-weight infants (Stang, Story, & Feldman, 2005). An extra serving of dairy products is usually recommended for teenagers. Calcium supplementation is indicated for teens with an aversion to or intolerance of milk unless other dairy products or significant calcium sources are consumed in sufficient amounts.

Because folic acid plays a role in cell reproduction, it is also an important nutrient for pregnant teens. As previously indicated, a supplement is often suggested for pregnant females, whether adult or adolescent.

Other nutrients and vitamins must be considered when evaluating the overall nutritional quality of the teenager's diet. Nutrients that have frequently been found to be deficient in this age group include zinc and vitamins A, D, E, and B_6. Eating a wide variety of foods—especially fresh and lightly processed foods—is helpful in obtaining adequate amounts of trace minerals, fiber, and other vitamins.

Dietary Patterns

Healthy adolescents often have irregular eating patterns. Many skip breakfast, and most tend to be frequent snackers. Teens rarely follow the traditional three-meals-a-day pattern; their day-to-day intake often varies drastically; and they eat food combinations that may seem bizarre to adults. Despite this, adolescents usually achieve a better nutritional balance than most adults would expect.

> “My mom is so cool. She has hung in with me throughout this pregnancy even though I know she feels bad about it—she thinks my life will be harder and I guess she is right. She is really working to make sure that I eat right so that I have a healthy baby but instead of nagging, she has turned this into something we are doing together. We have taken a couple of cooking classes and experimented with different recipes. Last week we made some great but healthy snacks and I brought them to my friend Cary's birthday party. Those snacks just disappeared!”

In assessing the diet of the pregnant adolescent, the nurse should consider the eating pattern over time, not simply a single day's intake. This pattern is critical because of the irregularity of most adolescent eating patterns. Once the pattern is identified, counseling can be directed toward correcting deficiencies.

Counseling Issues

A positive approach to nutritional counseling for the pregnant adolescent is more effective than a negative one. The nurse must be ready to suggest nutrient-dense foods that pregnant teens can choose in many places and at any time. If an adolescent's family member does most of the meal preparation, it may be useful to include that person in the discussion if the adolescent agrees. Involving the expectant father in counseling may be beneficial. The pregnant teenager will soon become a parent, and her understanding of nutrition will influence not only her well-being but also that of her child. However, teens tend to live in the present, and counseling that stresses long-term changes may be less effective than more concrete approaches. Messages should emphasize that the pregnant teen is eating for her own health and that of the baby and should focus on foods themselves rather than on nutrients. In many cases, classes with other teens are effective. In a group atmosphere, adolescents often work together to plan adequate meals including foods that are their special favorites.

Postpartum Nutrition

Nutritional needs will change following the birth. Nutrient requirements will vary depending on whether the mother decides to breastfeed. An assessment of postpartal nutritional status is necessary before the nurse provides nutritional guidance.

Postpartum Nutritional Status

Postpartum nutritional status is determined primarily by assessing the new mother's weight, hemoglobin and hematocrit levels, clinical signs, and dietary history.

As previously discussed, an ideal weight gain for the normal-weight woman during pregnancy is between 11.5 and 16 kg (25 and 35 lb). (See Table 18-2.) After birth, there is a weight loss of approximately 10 to 12 lb. Additional weight loss will be most rapid during the first few weeks after birth as the uterus returns to normal size, tissue fluids are released, and maternal blood volume returns to normal. The mother's weight will then begin to stabilize. Weight loss may also be affected by lactation. Individual weight loss of women who breastfeed will vary but tends to be greater than that of women who do not if breastfeeding continues for at least 6 months.

The rate of postpartum weight loss is influenced by many factors. Some women approach their prepregnancy weight several weeks after birth; most approach this weight about 6 months later. The amount of weight gained during pregnancy is a major determinant of weight loss after childbirth. Generally, women who gain excessive weight during pregnancy are more likely to sustain a weight gain 1 year following childbirth, putting them at increased risk of long-term overweight or obesity.

It is important to evaluate the mother's current weight, ideal weight for her height, weight before pregnancy, and weight before the birth. Women who are interested in weight reduction should be referred to a dietitian. Hemoglobin and erythrocyte values vary after birth, but they should return to normal levels within 2 to 6 weeks. Hematocrit levels should rise gradually because of hemoconcentration as extracellular fluid is excreted. The hematocrit is usually checked at the postpartum visit to detect any anemia. Mothers can be encouraged to eat a diet high in iron. Iron supplements are generally prescribed for 2 to 3 months following birth to replenish supplies depleted by pregnancy.

Care Plan Activity: Maternal Nutritional Requirements

The nurse assesses any clinical symptoms the new mother may be experiencing. Food cravings and aversions typically drop significantly during the postpartal period and do not usually pose a problem. However, constipation is a common problem following birth. The nurse can encourage the woman to maintain a high fluid intake to keep the stool soft. Dietary sources of fiber and physical exercise are also helpful in preventing constipation.

The nurse obtains specific information on diet and eating habits directly from the woman. Visiting the mother during mealtimes provides an opportunity for unobtrusive nutritional assessment. Which foods has a woman selected? Has she avoided fruits and vegetables? Is her diet nutritionally sound? A comment focusing on a positive aspect of her meal selection may initiate a discussion of nutrition.

The dietitian should be informed about any woman whose cultural or religious beliefs require specific foods. Appropriate meals can then be prepared for her. The nurse may also refer women with unusual eating habits or numerous questions about food or nutrition to a dietitian. In all cases, the nurse should provide literature on nutrition so that the woman will have a source of appropriate information at home.

Nutritional Care of Formula-Feeding Mothers

After birth, the formula-feeding mother's dietary requirements return to prepregnancy levels (see Table 18-1). If the mother has a good understanding of nutritional principles, it is sufficient to advise her to reduce her daily caloric intake by about 300 kcal and to return to prepregnancy levels for other nutrients.

If the mother has a poor understanding of nutrition, this is an opportunity to teach her the basic principles and the importance of a well-balanced diet. Her eating habits and dietary practices will eventually be reflected in the diet of her child.

If the mother has gained excessive weight during pregnancy (or perhaps was overweight before pregnancy), referral to a dietitian is appropriate. The dietitian can design weight reduction diets to meet nutritional needs and food preferences. Weight loss goals of 1 to 2 lb per week are usually suggested.

In addition to learning how to meet her own nutritional needs, the new mother will usually be interested in learning how to provide for her infant's nutritional needs. A discussion of infant feeding, which includes topics such as selecting infant formulas, formula preparation, and vitamin and mineral supplementation, is appropriate and generally well received.

Nutritional Care of Breastfeeding Mothers

Nutrient needs increase during breastfeeding. Table 18-1 lists the dietary reference intakes (DRIs) during breastfeeding for specific nutrients. Table 18-3 includes a daily food guide for lactating women. A few key nutrients need further discussion.

Calories

One of the most important factors in the breastfeeding woman's diet is calories. An inadequate caloric intake can reduce milk volume. However, milk quality generally remains unaffected. The breastfeeding mother should increase her caloric intake by 200 kcal over the pregnancy requirements (that is, a 500-kcal increase from her prepregnancy requirement). This results in a total of about 2500 to 2700 kcal per day for most women.

Depending on her own dietary preferences, the breastfeeding mother can use the MyPyramid for Moms food guide to assess her dietary intake. She should strive to include a variety of foods from each food group. Her caloric intake needs to provide enough energy to sustain lactation. After her weight stabilizes several weeks following childbirth, weight loss should not exceed more than 1 lb per week.

Protein
An adequate protein intake is essential while breastfeeding because protein is an important component of breast milk. An intake of 65 g per day during the first 6 months of breastfeeding and 62 g per day thereafter is recommended. As in pregnancy, it is important that the woman consume adequate nonprotein calories to prevent the use of protein as an energy source.

Calcium
Calcium is also an important nutrient in milk production, and increases over nonpregnancy needs are expected. Requirements during breastfeeding remain the same as requirements during pregnancy: 1000 mg per day. An inadequate intake of calcium from food sources necessitates the use of calcium supplements.

Iron
Iron needs during lactation are not substantially different from those of nonpregnant women because iron is not a principal component of breast milk. However, as previously mentioned, continued supplementation of the mother for 2 to 3 months after parturition is advisable to replenish maternal stores depleted by pregnancy.

Fluids
Liquids are especially important during lactation because inadequate fluid intake may decrease milk volume. The recommended fluid intake of 8 to 10 (8 oz) glasses daily can be met by the consumption of water, juices, milk, and soups.

> “For me, the hardest part of breastfeeding was drinking enough fluid. I am not a big water person and they told me to go easy on caffeine beverages. Once I started adding a slice of lemon to my water, I found it a lot easier. My baby is 13 months old now and I have stopped breastfeeding, but I still drink the water with lemon. I think I have developed a good new habit!”

Counseling Issues
In addition to counseling mothers on how to meet their increased nutrient needs during breastfeeding, nurses should discuss a few issues related to infant feeding. For example, many mothers are concerned about how specific foods they eat will affect their babies during breastfeeding. Generally, there are no foods the nursing mother must avoid except those to which she might be allergic. Occasionally, however, some breastfeeding mothers find that their babies are affected by certain foods. Onions, turnips, cabbage, chocolate, spices, and seasonings are commonly listed as offenders. The best advice to give the breastfeeding mother is to avoid those foods she suspects cause distress in her infant. For the most part, however, she should be able to eat any nourishing food she wants without fear that her baby will be affected. For further discussion of successful infant feeding, see chapter 32 ∞.

NURSING CARE MANAGEMENT

Nursing Assessment and Diagnosis
The nurse needs to assess nutritional status in order to plan an optimal diet with each woman. The nurse may gather data by consulting the woman's chart and by interviewing her. Information is obtained about the following:

- The woman's height and weight and her weight gain during pregnancy
- Pertinent laboratory values, especially hemoglobin and hematocrit
- Clinical signs that have possible nutritional implications, such as constipation, anorexia, or heartburn
- Diet history to determine the woman's views on nutrition as well as her specific nutrient intake

The nurse can obtain a diet history by asking the woman to complete a 24-hour diet recall, in which she lists everything consumed in the previous 24 hours, including foods, fluids, and any supplements. At least 3 days of diet recalls should be done to compensate for daily variations. Diet may also be evaluated using a food frequency questionnaire. The questionnaire lists common categories of foods and asks the woman how frequently in a day (or week) she consumes foods from the list. Common categories include vegetables, fruits, milk or cheese, meat or poultry, fish, desserts or sweets, coffee or tea, and alcoholic beverages. This method may be less reliable because it requires the individual to be accurate about her intake.

> **PROFESSIONALISM IN PRACTICE**
>
> ***Taking a Diet History***
>
> When completing a diet history, nurses who are effective communicators remember that it is as important to identify the foods a woman avoids as it is to determine which foods she eats.

During the data-gathering process, the nurse has an opportunity to discuss important aspects of nutrition in the context of the family's needs and lifestyle. The nurse also seeks information about psychologic, cultural, and socioeconomic factors that may influence food intake.

The nurse can use a nutritional questionnaire to gather and record important facts. This information provides a database that the nurse can use to develop an intervention plan to fit the woman's individual needs. The sample questionnaire shown in Figure 18-4 ■ has been filled in to demonstrate this process.

Once the data are obtained, the nurse begins to analyze the information, formulate appropriate nursing diagnoses, and develop patient goals. For a woman during the first trimester, for example, the diagnosis may be *Imbalanced Nutrition: Less than Body Requirements* related to nausea and vomiting. In many cases the diagnosis may be related to excessive weight gain. In such cases the diagnosis might be *Imbalanced Nutrition: More than Body Requirements* related to excessive calorie intake. Although these diagnoses are broad, the nurse must

NUTRITIONAL QUESTIONNAIRE

Name Susan Longmont Date 1-11-11

Age 20

Ethnic group Caucasian

Religion Protestant

Gravida i Para 0 EDB 9-8-11

Age of youngest child? NA

Birth weights of previous children? NA

Usual nonpregnant weight 115 Present weight 125

Weight gain during last pregnancy? NA

Vitamin supplements? none

Current medications? aspirin for headache

Do you smoke? yes How much per day? 1-1½ packs

Eating patterns:

1. How many meals per day? 2 when 12:30 pm 6:30 pm
2. How many snacks per day? 3 when 10:30 am 4:00 pm 10:00 pm
3. What other foods are important to your usual diet? chocolate and candy bars
4. Amount per day 4 bars/week
5. Do you have any different food preferences now? no
6. Do you eat nonfoods such as:

		Amount
laundry starch	no	NA
ice	yes	10 cubes/day
other (name)	no	NA

7. What foods do you dislike or do not eat? spinach and dried beans
8. For added information complete a typical daily intake (24-hour recall is suggested).

Do you have special problems in food preparation such as:

1. Physical disability yes ____ no ✔ Explain ____
2. Cooking appliances yes ____ no ✔ Explain ____
3. Refrigeration of food yes ____ no ✔ Explain ____

Who does the meal planning? I do. shopping? We both do.

cooking? I do most of the time but my husband likes to help.

Are there transportation problems? We have only one car but we go in the evening.

Financial situation: My husband is working and going to school. I am not working. Food stamps yes WIC no

Do you have any previous nutritional problems? No. I have never paid much attention to food before, but now I have lots of questions.

Are there any problems with this pregnancy? Nausea Yes, in the morning.

Constipation No Other NA

Assessment by the nurse following the completion of the questionnaire.

Basic estimated nutrient and caloric value of typical daily intake.

Please circle one of the following:

Protein intake was	low	(adequate)	high
Caloric intake was	low	adequate	(high)
Calcium intake was	(low)	adequate	high
Iron intake was	(low)	adequate	high
Vitamin C intake was	low	(adequate)	high

Figure 18-4 ■ Sample nutritional questionnaire used in nursing management of a pregnant woman.

be specific in addressing issues such as inadequate intake of nutrients such as iron, calcium, or folic acid; problems with nutrition because of a limited food budget; problems related to physiologic alterations, such as anorexia, heartburn, or nausea; and behavioral problems related to excessive dieting, anorexia nervosa, or bulimia. In some instances, the diagnosis *Readiness for Enhanced Knowledge* may seem most appropriate, especially if the woman asks for information about nutrition.

Nursing Plan and Implementation

After the nursing diagnosis is made, the nurse can plan an approach to correct any nutritional deficiencies or improve the overall quality of the diet.

Health Promotion Education

In counseling the pregnant woman, the nurse needs to avoid "talking down" to her or "preaching" to her. The nurse should present information in a clear, logical way, using appropriate language but avoiding jargon. Examples are often helpful in clarifying material. The nurse should also answer all questions appropriately and clearly.

When a person requires nutritional counseling, a dietary change usually is necessary. However, change is often difficult. Counseling will be more effective if the nurse understands the woman's values and explains the needed change in a way that is meaningful to the patient. Because the pregnant woman must follow the plan, it should be developed in cooperation with her; be suitable for her financial level and background; and be based on reasonable, achievable goals.

The following example demonstrates one way a nurse can implement a plan with a patient based on the nursing diagnosis.

Diagnosis: *Imbalanced Nutrition: Less than Body Requirements* related to low intake of calcium

Patient goal: The woman will increase her intake of calcium to the DRI level.

Implementation:

1. Plan with the woman additional milk or dairy products that she can reasonably add to the diet (specify amounts).
2. Encourage the use of other calcium sources, such as leafy green vegetables and legumes.
3. Plan for the addition of powdered milk in cooking and baking.
4. If none of the above is realistic or acceptable, consider the use of calcium supplements.

Most families can benefit from guidance about food purchasing and preparation. The nurse should advise women to plan food purchases thoughtfully by preparing menus and a grocery list before shopping. It is also helpful to advise patients to monitor sales, compare brands, and be selective when purchasing "convenience" foods, which tend to be expensive. Other techniques for keeping food costs down without jeopardizing quality include buying food in season, using bulk foods when appropriate, using whole grain or enriched products, buying lower grade eggs (grading has no relation to the egg's nutritional value but indicates color of the shell and delicacy of flavor), and avoiding fancy grades of food and foods in elaborate packaging.

Community-Based Nursing Care

Food is a significant portion of a family's budget, and meeting nutritional needs may be a challenge for families on limited incomes. Community-based services offered through clinics, local agencies, schools, and volunteer organizations are effective in addressing these needs. Increasingly, nurses play an important role in managing such community-based services, especially those services focusing on patient education. In addition, most communities offer special assistance to qualifying families to meet their nutritional needs. The Food Stamp Program provides stamps or coupons for participating households whose net monthly income is below a specified level. These stamps can be used to purchase food for the household each month.

The Special Supplemental Nutrition Program for Women, Infants, and Children (WIC) is designed to assist low-income pregnant, postpartum, or breastfeeding women and their children under 5 years of age. To be eligible, applicants must meet income guidelines (income at or below 185% of the U.S. poverty level), state residency requirements, and be individually determined to be nutritionally at risk by a healthcare professional (Food and Nutrition Service, 2009). The program provides food assistance, nutrition education, and referrals to healthcare providers. The food distributed, including dried beans and peas, peanut butter, eggs, cheese, milk, fortified adult and infant cereals, juice, and iron-fortified infant formula, is designed to provide good sources of iron, protein, and certain vitamins for individuals with an inadequate diet. Participation in the WIC program during pregnancy and infancy is associated with a reduced risk of infant death. In addition, the WIC program is credited with helping reduce the incidence of low birth weight in infants and in decreasing the incidence of anemia in the infants and young children of low-income families.

Evaluation

Once a plan has been developed and implemented, the nurse and patient may wish to identify ways of evaluating its effectiveness. Evaluation may involve keeping a food journal, writing out weekly menus, returning weekly for weighing, and the like. If anemia is a special problem, periodic hematocrit assessments are also indicated.

Women with serious nutritional deficiencies are referred to a dietitian. The nurse can then work closely with the dietitian and the patient to improve the pregnant woman's health by modifying her diet.

FOCUS YOUR STUDY

- Maternal weight gains averaging 11.5 to 16 kg (25 to 35 lb) for a normal-weight woman are associated with the best reproductive outcomes.
- If the diet is adequate, folic acid and iron are the only supplements generally recommended during pregnancy.
- Women should not restrict caloric intake to reduce weight during pregnancy.
- Pregnant women should be encouraged to eat regularly and to eat a wide variety of foods, especially fresh and lightly processed foods.
- Taking megadoses of vitamins during pregnancy is unnecessary and potentially dangerous.
- Pregnant women who eat vegetarian diets should place special emphasis on obtaining ample proteins, calories, calcium, iron, vitamin D, vitamin B_{12}, and zinc through food sources or supplementation if necessary.
- Pregnant women should avoid eating fish such as swordfish, shark, tilefish, or king mackerel, which contain high levels of mercury, and should limit their intake of fish that are lower in mercury.
- Food safety and sanitation should be a priority when preparing and storing food; foods that are known to cause foodborne illness should be avoided during pregnancy.
- Evaluation of physical, psychosocial, and cultural factors that affect food intake is essential before the nurse can determine nutritional status and plan nutritional counseling.
- Adolescents who become pregnant less than 4 years after menarche have higher nutritional needs and are considered to be at high biologic risk.
- Weight gains during adolescent pregnancy must accommodate recommended gains for a normal pregnancy plus necessary gains due to growth.
- After childbirth, the formula-feeding mother's dietary requirements return to prepregnancy levels.
- Breastfeeding mothers require an additional 200 calories above pregnancy intake and increased fluid intake to maintain ample milk volume.

Pearson Nursing Student Resources

Find additional review materials at
www.nursing.pearsonhighered.com

Prepare for success with additional NCLEX®-style practice questions, interactive assignments and activities, Web links, animations and videos, and more!

CRITICAL THINKING IN ACTION

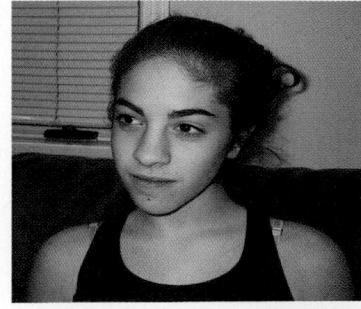

Sandra Hill is a 17-year-old at 19 weeks' gestation with her first pregnancy. She presents to you accompanied by her mother. Her mother tells you that Sandra is an active teenager who plays sports and has been taking dance lessons for 5 years. She maintains a B+ average in school. Sandra voices concern about potential weight gain during pregnancy. She tells you that this was not a planned pregnancy and she has ambivalent feelings about it. You become concerned as she tells you that she has reduced her caloric intake over the last few months to try to keep her weight down and camouflage her pregnancy. You do a nutritional assessment and find that she is deficient in calcium, iron, and protein. Sandra seems to have irregular eating patterns and she admits to skipping breakfast often. She asks why she has to gain so much weight when you explain the nutritional needs of her baby during the pregnancy.

1. Discuss weight distribution in pregnancy.
2. Discuss foods that will increase calcium, protein, and iron in her diet.
3. Explain why folate supplementation is important.
4. What criteria will measure adequate caloric intake during pregnancy?

See www.nursing.pearsonhighered.com for possible responses.

REFERENCES

American College of Obstetricians and Gynecologists (ACOG). (2009). *Nutrition during pregnancy.* Retrieved from http://www.acog.org/publications/patient_education/bp001.cfm

American Dietetic Association. (2008). Position of the American Dietetic Association: Nutrition and lifestyle for a healthy pregnancy outcome. *Journal of the American Dietetic Association, 108,* 553–561.

American Dietetic Association. (2009). Position of the American Dietetic Association: Vegetarian diets. *Journal of the American Dietetic Association, 109,* 1266–1282.

American Dietetic Association and the American Society for Nutrition. (2009). Position of the American Dietetic Association and the American Society for Nutrition: Obesity, reproduction, and pregnancy outcomes. *Journal of the American Dietetic Association, 109,* 918–927.

Astrachan-Fletcher, E., Veldhuis, C., Lively, N., Fowler, C., & Marcks, B. (2008). The reciprocal effects of eating disorders and the postpartum period: A review of the literature and recommendations for clinical care. *Journal of Women's Health, 17*(2), 227–239.

Centers for Disease Control and Prevention (CDC). (2009). *Preception care.* Retrieved from http://www.cdc.gov/ncbddd/preconception/default

Cunningham, F. G., Leveno, K. J., Bloom, S. L., Hauth, J. C., Rouse, D. J., & Spong, C. Y. (2010). *Williams obstetrics* (23rd ed.). New York, NY: McGraw-Hill.

Food and Drug Administration (FDA). (2004). *What you need to know about mercury in fish and shellfish* (Brochure). Retrieved from http://www.fda.gov/Food/ResourcesForYou/Consumers/ucm110591.htm

Food and Drug Administration (FDA). (2009). *Food safety for moms to be.* Retrieved from http://www.fda.gov/Food/ResourcesForYou/HealthEducators/ucm081785.htm

Food and Nutrition Service. (2009). *WIC: The special supplemental nutrition program for women, infants, and children.* Retrieved from http://www.fns.usda.gov/wic/default.htm

Groth, S. (2006). Adolescent gestational weight gain: Does it contribute to obesity? *American Journal of Maternal-Child Nursing, 31*(2), 101–105.

Higdon, J. V., & Frei, B. (2006). Coffee and health: A review of recent human research. *Critical Reviews in Food Science and Nutrition, 46,* 101–123.

Huffling, K. (2006). The effects of environmental contaminants in food on women's health. *Journal of Midwifery & Women's Health, 51*(1), 19–25.

Innis, S. M. (2007). Fatty acids and early human development. *Early Human Development, 83,* 761–766.

Institute of Medicine (IOM). (2009). *Weight gain during pregnancy: Reexamining the guidelines.* Retrieved from http://www.iom.edu/Reports/2009/Weight-Gain-During-Pregnancy-reexamining-the-Guidelines.aspx

Institute of Medicine, Subcommittee on Dietary Intake and Nutrient Supplements During Pregnancy, Committee on Nutrition Status During Pregnancy and Lactation, Food and Nutrition Board. (1990). *Nutrition during pregnancy: Weight gain and nutrient supplements.* Washington, DC: National Academy Press.

International Food Information Council. (2009). Stevia sweeteners: Another low-calorie option. *Food Insight.* Retrieved from http://www.foodinsight.org/Newsletter/Detail.aspx?topic=Stevia_Sweeteners_Anothr_Low_Calorie_Option

Koletzko, B., Cetin, I., & Brenna, J. T. (2007). Dietary fat intakes for pregnant and lactating women. *British Journal of Nutrition, 98,* 873–877.

Madsen, I. R. (2009). Remission of eating disorders during pregnancy: Five cases and brief clinical review. *Journal of psychosomatic obstetrics and gynaecology, 30*(2), 122–125.

McCusker, R. R., Goldberger, B. A., & Cone, E. J. (2006). Caffeine content of energy drinks, carbonated sodas, and other beverages. *Journal of Analytical Toxicology, 30,* 112–114.

National Digestive Diseases Information Clearinghouse. (2009). *Lactose intolerance.* Retrieved from http://www.digestive.niddk.nih.gov

Stang, J., Story, M., & Feldman, S. (2005). Nutrition in adolescent pregnancy. *International Journal of Childbirth Education, 20*(2), 4–11.

U.S. Department of Agriculture (USDA). (2009). *MyPyramid.gov.* Retrieved from http://www.mypyramid.gov

U.S. Department of Health and Human Services, U.S. Department of Agriculture. (2005). *Dietary guidelines for Americans, 2005.* Retrieved from http://www.health.gov/DietaryGuidelines/dga2005/document/default.htm

Waller, D. K., Shaw, G. M., Rasmussen, S. A., Hobbs, C. A., Canfield, M. A., Siega-Riz, A. M., . . . & Correa, A. (2007). Prepregnancy obesity as a risk factor for structural birth defects. *Archives of Pediatric and Adolescent Medicine, 161*(8), 745–750.

World Health Organization (WHO). (2009). Global prevalence of vitamin A deficiency in populations at risk 1995–2005. Retrieved from http://whqlibdoc.who.int/publications/2009/9789241598019–eng.pdf

CHAPTER 19

Pregnancy at Risk: Pregestational Problems

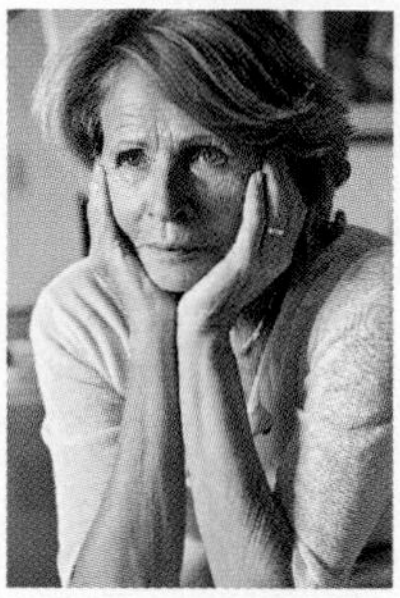

Today is the anniversary of my Julie's death. She died of a heroin overdose. During the years before her death, we tried everything to help her, but nothing worked. She would disappear, sometimes for weeks, and then reappear filled with good intentions to kick her habit—but she never could. She was 29 when I lost her, and 3 months pregnant with our grandchild. I miss her so. I don't know if my heart will ever mend.

LEARNING OUTCOMES

1. Summarize the effects of alcohol and illicit drugs on the childbearing woman and her fetus/newborn.
2. Discuss the pathology, treatment, and nursing care of pregnant women with diabetes.
3. Discriminate among the four major types of anemia associated with pregnancy with regard to signs, treatment, and implications for pregnancy.
4. Discuss AIDS, including care of the pregnant woman with HIV/AIDS, neonatal implications, and ramifications for the childbearing family.
5. Describe the effects of various heart disorders on pregnancy, including their implications for nursing care.
6. Compare the effects of selected gestational medical conditions on pregnancy.

KEY TERMS

AIDS *436*
Crack *419*
Gestational diabetes mellitus (GDM) *423*
HIV *436*
Macrosomia *424*

Pregnancy is biologically, physiologically, and psychologically stressful, even for healthy women. For women with preexisting (pregestational) conditions such as substance abuse, diabetes, HIV infection, and cardiac disease, it may be life threatening. For these women, pregestational counseling is especially important to identify early interventions designed to diminish the adverse effects of pregnancy on both the mother and fetus. In some cases, interventions before conception may be critical.

Prenatal care is aimed toward identification, assessment, and care management of women whose pregnancies are at risk because of potential or existing complications. This chapter focuses on women with pregestational medical disorders and their possible effects on the outcome of pregnancy. Chapter 20 ∞, in turn, focuses on medical disorders that develop during pregnancy.

Care of the Woman Practicing Substance Abuse

Substance abuse occurs when an individual experiences difficulties with work, family, social relations, and/or health as a result of alcohol or drug use. National survey data indicate that approximately 8% of people in the United States used illicit drugs in the month before the survey was taken (Substance Abuse and Mental Health Services Administration [SAMHSA], 2009). In general, the rate of illicit drug use among pregnant women is less than half the rate as among nonpregnant women (9.8%). Specifically, 5.1% of pregnant women reported using an illicit drug during pregnancy. However, illicit drug usage varies greatly by age, peaking at 21.6% of users in the 15- to 17-year-old age group for pregnant females, a much higher rate than nonpregnant females (12.9%) at the same age (SAMHSA, 2009). See Figure 19-1 ■.

Because women of childbearing age (15 to 44 years) make up a substantial proportion of the drug-using population, the problem has major significance for women and children. In testimony to these statistics is the increasing number of drug-exposed infants being born throughout the United States. Indiscriminate use of drugs during pregnancy, particularly in the first trimester, may adversely affect the health of the woman and the growth and development of her fetus. Drugs that are commonly misused include tobacco, alcohol, cocaine, marijuana, amphetamines, barbiturates, hallucinogens, club drugs, heroin, and other narcotics. Tobacco is discussed in chapter 16 ∞ as a teratogenic substance. Table 19-1 identifies common addictive drugs and their effects on the fetus and newborn.

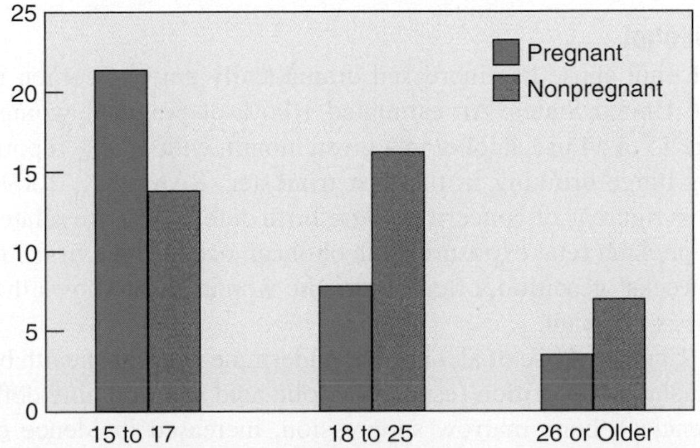

Figure 19-1 ■ Percentages of females ages 15 to 44 reporting past month use of any illicit drugs, by pregnancy status and age, 2008.

Source: Substance Abuse and Mental Health Services Administration. (2009). Results from the 2008 National Survey on Drug Use and Health: National Findings (Office of Applied Studies, NSDUH Series H-36, HHS Publication No. SMA 09-4434). Rockville, MD.

Drug use during pregnancy may be the most frequently missed diagnosis in all of maternity care. Substance-abusing women typically do not seek prenatal care until late in their pregnancy. They may be noncompliant or they may present in labor with no history of prenatal care. Even when they do seek care early, physicians and nurses may fail to ask the woman about drug and alcohol use because of their own lack of knowledge, discomfort, or biases. When asked, women may deny use of illegal substances out of fear, shame, or a reluctance to be confronted with the need to stop using the substance in question. Although some clinics perform routine or random drug screens, the patient should be informed that a drug screen is being performed and how the results will be provided to them.

CLINICAL TIP

Keep in mind that approximately 1 of 10 women in the United States, regardless of socioeconomic status or ethnic background, is currently abusing a substance. If you consider that possibility with every woman, you will ask the important questions about drug use and be alert for signs of substance abuse.

Providing prenatal care to chemically dependent women presents multiple dilemmas and challenges to clinicians. However, pregnancy represents a period in most women's lives when they recognize the need for and are receptive to caring and responsive interventions. By optimizing the prenatal experience of chemically dependent women, maternal-fetal outcomes can be improved and the groundwork laid for the ongoing therapeutic services that are needed to maintain the health and well-being of the mother and child (Amato et al., 2008).

The substance-abusing woman who seeks prenatal care may not voluntarily reveal her addiction, so caregivers should be alert for a history or physical signs that suggest substance abuse (Table 19-2). Because substance abuse has increased rapidly in the past decade, it is helpful to discuss the specific substances that are abused to increase understanding of this serious problem.

Substances Commonly Abused During Pregnancy

The substances most commonly abused during pregnancy are alcohol, nonmedical use of pain relievers and tranquilizers, inhalants, cocaine/crack, marijuana, phencyclidine (PCP),

TABLE 19-1 Possible Effects of Selected Drugs of Abuse/Addiction on Fetus and Newborn

MATERNAL DRUG	EFFECT ON FETUS/NEWBORN
Depressants	
Alcohol	Mental retardation, microcephaly, midfacial hypoplasia, cardiac anomalies, intrauterine growth restriction (IUGR), potential teratogenic effects, fetal alcohol syndrome (FAS), fetal alcohol effects (FAE).
Narcotics	
Heroin	Withdrawal symptoms, known as neonatal abstinence syndrome (NAS), include tremors, irritability, sneezing, vomiting, fever, diarrhea, abnormal respiratory function, and potential seizure activity.
Methadone	With abrupt maternal termination of the drug, severe withdrawal symptoms can include preterm labor, rapid labor, abruption, nonreassuring fetal status, and meconium aspiration. Neonates may present with NAS and be small for gestational age.
Barbiturates	Withdrawal symptoms.
Phenobarbital	Withdrawal symptoms. Fetal growth restriction.
Tranquilizers	
Diazepam (Valium)	Withdrawal symptoms (Gidai, Acs, Bánhidy, et al., 2008).
Antianxiety Drugs	
Lithium	Congenital anomalies.
Stimulants	
Amphetamines	
Amphetamines sulfate (Benzedrine)	Low birth weight, withdrawal symptoms (Thompson, Levitt, & Stanwood, 2009).
Cocaine	Cerebral infarctions, microcephaly, learning disabilities, poor state organization, decreased interactive behavior, central nervous system (CNS) anomalies, cardiac anomalies, genitourinary anomalies, sudden infant death syndrome (SIDS).
Nicotine (half to one pack cigarettes/day)	Increased rate of spontaneous abortion, increased incidence of placental abruption, small for gestational age (SGA), small head circumference, decreased length, SIDS, attention deficit hyperactivity disorder (ADHD) in school-age children.
Psychotropics	
PCP ("angel dust")	Withdrawal symptoms. Newborn behavioral and developmental abnormalities.
Marijuana	Possible association with structural and neurobehavioral defects (Hurt et al., 2009).

TABLE 19-2 Possible Signs of Substance Abuse

History
- History of vague or unusual medical complaints
- Family history of alcoholism or other addiction
- History of childhood physical, sexual, or emotional abuse
- History of cirrhosis, pancreatitis, hepatitis, gastritis, sexually transmitted infections, or unusual infections such as cellulitis or endocarditis
- History of high-risk sexual behavior
- Psychiatric history of treatment and/or hospitalization

Physical Signs
- Dilated or constricted pupils
- Inflamed nasal mucosa
- Evidence of needle "track marks" or abscesses
- Poor nutritional status
- Slurred speech or staggering gait
- Odor of alcohol on breath

Behavioral Signs
- Memory lapses, mood swings, hallucinations
- Pattern of frequently missed appointments
- Frequent accidents, falls
- Signs of depression, agitation, euphoria
- Suicidal gestures

MDMA (Ecstasy), and heroin (SAMHSA, 2009). For a discussion of the nonmedical abuse of pain relievers and tranquilizers, readers are referred to pharmacology textbooks. This chapter addresses alcohol use because of the profound, long-term effects it can have on a child and illicit substances to ensure that readers are aware of their implications.

Alcohol

Alcohol abuse has increased dramatically among women in the United States. An estimated 10.6% of pregnant women age 15 to 44 use alcohol in a given month, with 10.3% reporting binge drinking in the first trimester (SAMHSA, 2009). This figure is of concern because birth defects that are related to prenatal fetal exposure to alcohol can occur in the first 3 to 8 weeks' gestation, often before the woman even knows that she is pregnant.

Chronic abuse of alcohol can undermine maternal health by causing malnutrition (especially folic acid and thiamine deficiencies), bone marrow suppression, increased incidence of infections, and liver disease. As a result of alcohol dependence, the woman may have withdrawal seizures in the intrapartal period as early as 12 to 48 hours after she stops drinking. Delirium tremens may occur in the postpartal period, and the newborn may suffer withdrawal syndrome.

The effects of alcohol on the fetus may result in a group of signs referred to as fetal alcohol spectrum disorders (FASD). The syndrome has characteristic physical and mental abnormalities that vary in severity and combination. (See discussion in chapter 33 ∞.) There is no definitive answer as to how much alcohol a woman can safely consume during pregnancy. Consequently, the expectant woman should "play it safe" by avoiding alcohol completely. *Even low levels of alcohol should be avoided* (March of Dimes [MOD], 2008; O'Leary et al., 2009).

The nursing staff in the maternal-newborn unit must be aware of the manifestations of alcohol abuse so that they can prepare for the patient's special needs. The care regimen includes sedation to decrease irritability and tremors. Oral benzodiazepines such as lorazepam (Ativan) or diazepam (Valium) are most commonly used (Wisner et al., 2007). Seizure precautions, intravenous fluid therapy for hydration, and preparation for an addicted newborn are also part of care. Although high doses of sedatives and analgesics may be necessary for the woman, caution is advised because these can cause fetal depression.

Breastfeeding generally is not contraindicated, although alcohol is excreted in breast milk. Excessive alcohol consumption may intoxicate the infant and inhibit maternal let-down reflex. Discharge planning for the alcohol-addicted mother and newborn should be correlated with the social service department of the hospital.

Cocaine/Crack

Cocaine use appears to have reached its peak during the 1990s, but it continues to be of concern for the childbearing family (Bessaa et al., 2009). Cocaine acts at the nerve terminals to prevent the reuptake of dopamine and norepinephrine, which in turn results in vasoconstriction, tachycardia, and hypertension. Placental vasoconstriction decreases blood flow to the fetus.

Cocaine is usually taken in three ways: snorting, smoking, and intravenous (IV) injection. **Crack** is a form of freebase cocaine that is made up of baking soda, water, and cocaine mixed into a paste and microwaved to form a rock. The rock can then be smoked. Many women, especially those in low-income areas, favor this form of the drug over other forms because it is cheaper and readily available. In addition, smoking crack leads to a quicker, more intense high because the drug is absorbed through the large surface area of the lungs.

The onset of effects of cocaine occurs rapidly, but the euphoria lasts only about 30 minutes. Irritability, depression, pessimism, fatigue, and a strong desire for more cocaine usually follow this profound euphoria and excitement. This pattern often

RESEARCH EVIDENCE IN PRACTICE Nonpharmacologic Treatment for Alcoholism in Pregnancy

CLINICAL QUESTION

What are effective treatments for preexisting alcoholism in women who become pregnant?

RESEARCH EVIDENCE

Women who abuse alcohol during pregnancy increase the risk of problems for their children, both in the immediate postpartum period and in later childhood (e.g., fetal alcohol syndrome, developmental delays, and/or behavioral changes). Experts have long recommended that alcohol intake be avoided during pregnancy. However, pregnant women with acute alcohol addiction may find it difficult to abstain. Thus, women who are addicted to alcohol should have early treatment for their substance abuse to promote a normal pregnancy and birth.

Three randomized controlled trials involving more than 7000 women focused on nonpharmacologic treatments for alcoholism during pregnancy. A Cochrane Collaborative review summarized another four studies involving more than 700 women into a practice guideline for management of prenatal alcoholism.

The ideal treatment is to offer maternal abstinence and alcohol withdrawal programs when women are contemplating pregnancy but have not yet conceived. These programs may also be initiated during pregnancy with close medical monitoring. These studies showed that educational and counseling interventions initiated during pregnancy can be effective in supporting maternal abstinence from alcohol. The most effective is the provision of an educational session and a self-help manual, followed by reinforcement at each prenatal visit.

WHAT QUESTIONS REMAIN UNANSWERED?

There was substantial variation in the content and type of educational and psychosocial interventions in all of these studies. A standard approach to nonpharmacologic interventions for alcohol withdrawal and abstinence has yet to be developed and remains a question.

WHAT IS BEST PRACTICE?

Women who suffer alcohol addiction or abuse and who are contemplating pregnancy should be encouraged to undergo withdrawal prior to conception. However, alcohol withdrawal during pregnancy can still result in a normal pregnancy if abstinence is practiced. An initial educational session with educational materials, followed by periodic reinforcement and psychologic support, can help women remain alcohol-free during pregnancy.

CRITICAL THINKING

What elements of an educational intervention could form the basis for a standard approach? What psychologic support is needed by women who are withdrawing from alcohol addiction?

References

Bakker, R., Pluimgraaff, L., Steegers, E., Raat, H., Tiemeier, H., Hofman, A., & Jaddow, V. (2010). Associations of light and moderate maternal alcohol consumption with fetal growth characteristics in different periods of pregnancy: The generation R study. *International Journal of Epidemiology, 39*(3), 777–789.

Latino-Martel, P., Chan, D., Druesne-Pecollo, N., Barrandon, E., Hercberg, S., & Norat, T. (2010). Maternal alcohol consumption during pregnancy and risk of childhood leukemia: Systematic review and meta-analysis. *Cancer Epidemiology, Biomarkers, and Prevention, 19*(5), 1238–1260.

Michigan Quality Improvement Consortium. (2008). *Routine prenatal and postnatal care.* Southfield, MI: Author.

Ornoy, A., & Ergaz, Z. (2010). Alcohol abuse in pregnant women: Effects on the fetus and newborn, mode of action, and maternal treatment. *International Journal of Environmental Research and Public Health, 7*(2), 364–379.

Stade, B., Baily, C., Dzendoletas, D., Sgro, M., Dowswell, T., & Bennett, D. (2009). Psychological and/or educational interventions for reducing alcohol consumption in pregnant women and women planning pregnancy. *Cochrane Database of Systematic Reviews,* Issue 2. Art. No.: CD004228. doi:10.1002/14651858 leads the user to take repeated doses to sustain the effect. Cocaine metabolites may be present in the urine of a pregnant woman for up to 4 to 7 days following use.

The cocaine user is difficult to identify prenatally. Because cocaine is an illegal substance, many women are reluctant to volunteer information about their drug use. The nurse who is familiar with the woman may recognize subtle signs of cocaine use, including mood swings and appetite changes, and withdrawal symptoms such as depression, irritability, nausea, lack of motivation, and psychomotor changes.

Major adverse maternal effects of cocaine use include seizures and hallucinations, pulmonary edema, respiratory failure, and cardiac problems. Women who use cocaine have an increased incidence of spontaneous first trimester abortion, abruptio placentae, intrauterine growth restriction (IUGR), preterm birth, and stillbirth (Walton-Moss, McIntosh, Conrad, et al., 2009).

Exposure of the fetus to cocaine in utero seems to be associated with increased incidence of neonatal complications, especially decreased birth weight and head circumference (Singer et al., 2008). See chapter 33 ∞ for further discussion. A recent large, prospective randomized study demonstrated more autonomic nervous system dysfunction (irritability, jitteriness, tremors, high-pitched cry, and excessive suck) in exposed newborns (Richardson, Goldschmidt, & Willford, 2008). The study's authors note that often these women also use alcohol, tobacco, and marijuana as well as other drugs, so fetal exposure to multiple drugs may contribute to an increased incidence of congenital anomalies.

Exposed infants are found to have more feeding difficulties than nonexposed infants. These difficulties may be related to some extent to the infant's behaviors but have also been found to be related to maternal behaviors. Cocaine-using mothers were found to be less flexible, less engaged, and less responsive to their infants' feeding cues. Nursing interventions that help mothers interpret infant feeding cues and optimize the mother-infant relationship should be emphasized. In a longitudinal study of the effects of prenatal cocaine exposure, investigators continued to find changes in neurobehavioral function at 1 year and beyond (Richardson et al., 2008).

Cocaine does cross into the breast milk and may cause such symptoms in the breastfeeding infant as extreme irritability, vomiting, diarrhea, dilated pupils, and apnea. Thus women who continue to use cocaine following childbirth should avoid breastfeeding.

Marijuana

Typically, pregnant women use marijuana in conjunction with alcohol and tobacco. Men who smoke marijuana may have decreased sperm counts and may develop gynecomastia (enlarged breasts); women may experience menstrual cycle irregularities. To date, however, there is no evidence that marijuana has any teratogenic effects on the fetus (Cunningham et al., 2010; Wisner et al., 2007). The impact of heavy marijuana use on pregnancy is difficult to evaluate because of the variety of social factors that may influence the results. Nevertheless, smoking of any type—be it tobacco or marijuana—poses a risk during pregnancy and is best avoided (Wisner et al., 2007).

Phencyclidine (PCP)

Phencyclidine (PCP) is a popular hallucinogen that can be smoked, taken orally, or injected intravenously. The onset of effects occurs in 2 to 4 minutes and lasts about 4 to 6 hours with no withdrawal state. The drug causes confusion, delirium, and hallucinations and may produce feelings of euphoria. Signs of PCP use include constricted pupils, ataxia, nystagmus, double vision (diplopia), dizziness, and diaphoresis. The greatest risk for the pregnant woman is overdose or a psychotic response. Signs of overdose include hypertension, hyperthermia, diaphoresis, and possible coma, which may jeopardize fetal well-being (Rayburn & Bogenschutz, 2004).

MDMA (Ecstasy)

MDMA (methylenedioxymethamphetamine), a derivative of amphetamine better known as Ecstasy, is the most commonly used of a group of drugs referred to as *club drugs,* so called because they have become popular among adolescents and young adults who frequent dance clubs and "raves." Other club drugs include flunitrazepam (Rohypnol), gamma hydroxybutyrate (GHB), and ketamine hydrochloride. PCPs and lysergic acid diethylamide (LSD) are sometimes classified as club drugs as well. MDMA is the third most widely used illicit drug after marijuana and amphetamines.

Ecstasy has been widely perceived as "safe" because of a relatively low incidence of adverse reactions. However, adverse responses are very unpredictable and the incidence is growing (Gamma, Jerome, Liechti, et al., 2005). MDMA is taken by mouth usually in tablet form. Its effects last for about 4 to 6 hours. MDMA use is appealing because it produces euphoria and feelings of empathy for others (thus it is also called the "hug drug"). Short-term adverse effects include clouded thinking, agitation, disturbed behavior, sweating, dry mouth, increased heart rate, muscle spasms including jaw clenching, and hyperthermia (elevated temperature). The most common significant adverse effects occur when people take multiple doses in one night (called "stacking"). These effects include hyperthermia, hyponatremia (low blood sodium), hypertension, cardiac arrhythmias, and kidney failure (National Institute on Drug Abuse [NIDA], 2009). Deaths have occurred among users. Repeated use of Ecstasy is associated with mood, sleep, and anxiety disorders; memory deficits; increased impulsiveness; and attention problems, which may last for up to 2 years following cessation of use. In addition, because MDMA may deplete levels of serotonin, users may increase their risk of neurologic and psychiatric problems (O'Malley, 2005).

Little is yet known about the effects of MDMA on pregnancy. Preliminary research using rats suggests that prenatal use of MDMA may be associated with long-term impaired memory and learning in the child. However, the impact of the timing of Ecstasy exposure during brain development may be a critical issue (Thompson, Heiman, Chambers, et al., 2009).

Heroin

Heroin is an illicit central nervous system (CNS) depressant narcotic that alters perception and produces euphoria. It is an addictive drug that is generally administered intravenously although it may also be sniffed/snorted or smoked. Pregnancy in women who use heroin is considered high risk because of the associated increased incidence of poor nutrition, iron deficiency anemia, and preeclampsia-eclampsia (see chapter 20 ∞). There is also an increased rate of breech position, abnormal placental implantation, abruptio placentae, preterm labor, premature rupture of the membranes (PROM), and meconium staining. Heroin users also have a higher incidence of sexually transmitted infection because many must rely on prostitution to support their drug habits. They also are at increased risk of HIV infection because they may use nonsterile needles or share needles when administering the drug.

The fetus of a heroin-addicted woman is at increased risk for preterm birth, IUGR, and withdrawal symptoms after birth, such as restlessness; lack of habituation; shrill, high-pitched cry; irritability; fist sucking; vomiting; and seizures. Signs of withdrawal usually appear within 72 hours and may last for several days. These behaviors may interfere with successful maternal-infant attachment and increase the potential for parenting problems or abuse in an already high-risk mother (Vucinovic et al., 2009).

Methadone is the most commonly used drug in the treatment of women who are dependent on opioids such as heroin. Methadone blocks withdrawal symptoms and the craving for street drugs. Dosage should be individualized to achieve the most therapeutic level for the mother during pregnancy. Methadone does cross the placenta, and fetal exposure in utero may result in neonatal abstinence syndrome (NAS) in the newborn. Preliminary evidence indicates that buprenorphine, a partial opioid agonist, is safe and effective during pregnancy and may decrease the severity of NAS. Because it has been authorized for use in physician offices it provides addicted patients with another treatment option (NIDA, 2010). (See chapter 33 ∞ and Table 33-7 ∞, Neonatal Abstinence Score Sheet on page 932, for more information about NAS.) In either case, there currently does not seem to be a clear dose-related effect on the newborn (Jansson, Velez, & Harrow, 2009). The most important goal is to help the mother recover from illicit drug abuse to optimize the long-term health of both the mother and baby.

Clinical Therapy

Antepartum care of the substance-abusing woman involves medical, socioeconomic, and legal considerations. The use of a team approach allows for the comprehensive management necessary to provide safe labor and childbirth for the woman and her fetus.

The management of drug addiction may include hospitalization as necessary to initiate detoxification. "Cold turkey" withdrawal is not advisable during pregnancy because of potential risk to the fetus. Maintenance and support therapy are best individualized to the woman's history and condition.

Urine screening may also be done regularly throughout pregnancy if the woman is known or suspected to be abusing drugs. This testing is helpful in identifying the type and amount of drug being abused and in providing objective feedback to the woman. Screening strategies should include maternal informed consent before screening. Healthcare providers need to stay abreast of their state laws requiring consent for screening in pregnancy to ensure they are in compliance (Hulsey, 2005).

NURSING CARE MANAGEMENT

Nursing Assessment and Diagnosis

Nurses and other healthcare providers should make it a practice to screen all pregnant women for substance abuse. Because illicit drug users seldom use only one drug, it is necessary to complete a thorough drug and alcohol abuse history (Amato et al., 2008). Several simple screening tools are available. In addition, the nurse should be alert for clues in the history or appearance of the woman that suggest substance abuse (refer to Table 19-2). If abuse is suspected, the nurse needs to ask direct questions, beginning with less threatening questions about the use of tobacco, caffeine, and over-the-counter medications. The nurse can then progress to questions about alcohol consumption and finally to questions focusing on past and current use of illicit drugs. The nurse who is matter-of-fact and nonjudgmental in approach is more likely to elicit honest responses.

Nursing assessment of the woman who is known to abuse substances focuses on her general health status, with specific attention to nutritional status, susceptibility to infections, and evaluation of all body systems. The nurse also assesses the woman's understanding of the impact of substance abuse on herself and her pregnancy. Some women are reluctant to discuss their substance abuse; others are quite open about it. Once the nurse establishes a relationship of trust, the nurse can gain information to use in planning the woman's ongoing care.

Nursing diagnoses that may apply to the woman practicing substance abuse include the following:

- ***Imbalanced Nutrition: Less Than Body Requirements*** related to inadequate food intake secondary to substance abuse
- ***Risk for Infection*** related to use of inadequately cleaned syringes and needles secondary to IV drug use
- ***Ineffective Health Maintenance*** related to a lack of information about the impact of substance abuse on the fetus

Nursing Plan and Implementation

Preventing substance abuse during pregnancy is the ideal nursing goal and is best accomplished through education. Unfortunately, many women who abuse substances do not receive regular health care and may not seek care until far along in their pregnancies or at the onset of labor.

The nurse's role in providing prenatal care for the woman who is practicing substance abuse focuses on ongoing assessment and patient teaching. It is essential that nurses caring for childbearing families develop the knowledge and skill necessary to identify pregnant women who abuse substances. To provide care that is truly effective, it is equally important that nurses develop and maintain a nonjudgmental, nonpunitive, positive attitude when caring for these women. It is also useful for nurses to be aware of substances that are commonly abused in their communities and the signs and symptoms that characterize these substances.

When the nurse encounters a pregnant woman who screens positive for substance abuse, the nurse should review with the woman what the screen revealed and express concern for the health of the mother and infant. The nurse can then go on to state the belief that the mother is concerned about the baby's health and stress the need for the woman to stop using drugs or alcohol during pregnancy. The nurse can then discuss possible strategies to help the woman quit (addiction treatment programs, 12-step programs, individual counseling) and suggest a referral for more in-depth assessment by a specialist. If feasible, the nurse can make an appointment while the woman is in the office or clinic. Nurses should also be aware of treatment options available for women who lack financial resources. Finally the nurse should make a follow-up appointment to see the woman again after her drug or alcohol assessment. The knowledgeable nurse can provide information about the relationship between substance abuse and existing health problems and the implications for the woman's unborn child. By establishing a relationship of trust and support, the nurse may foster the woman's cooperation.

Preparation for labor and birth should be part of the prenatal planning. Fear, tension, or discomfort may be relieved through psychologic support and careful explanation of the labor process. If pain medication is necessary, it should not be withheld, however, because the notion that it will contribute to further addiction is not correct. Preferred methods of pain relief include the use of psychoprophylaxis and regional or local anesthetics, such as pudendal block and local infiltration. These techniques decrease the risk of additional fetal respiratory depression. Immediate intensive care should be available for the newborn who may have respiratory depression, be small for gestational age (SGA), and be premature. For care of the addicted newborn, see chapter 33 ∞.

Postpartum follow-up and referral is essential and may include home visits. Follow-up requires careful coordination with community agencies and may involve public health nurses and social workers.

Evaluation

Expected outcomes of nursing care include the following:

- The woman is able to describe the impact of substance abuse on herself and her unborn child.
- The woman successfully gives birth to a healthy infant.
- The woman agrees to cooperate with referral to social services (or other appropriate community agency) for follow-up care after discharge.

Care of the Woman with Diabetes Mellitus

Diabetes mellitus, an endocrine disorder of carbohydrate metabolism, results from inadequate production or utilization of insulin.

Normal Glucose Homeostasis

After consumption of a meal, the body metabolizes carbohydrates into glucose. Insulin, produced by the beta cells of the islets of Langerhans in the pancreas, lowers blood glucose levels by enabling the glucose to move from the blood into muscle and liver cells, where it is stored as glycogen. When several hours have passed since a meal, falling blood glucose levels stimulate the pancreas to release glucagon, which in turn stimulates breakdown of liver glycogen stores into glucose, which is returned to the bloodstream. Glucagon can also stimulate the synthesis of glucose directly from amino acids in stored body proteins.

Carbohydrate Metabolism in Normal Pregnancy

Carbohydrate metabolism is affected early in pregnancy by a rise in serum levels of estrogen, progesterone, and other hormones. These hormones stimulate maternal insulin production and increase tissue response to insulin; therefore, anabolism (building up) of glycogen stores in the liver and other tissues occurs.

In the second half of pregnancy, the woman demonstrates prolonged hyperglycemia and hyperinsulinemia (increased secretion of insulin) following a meal. Although the mother is producing more insulin, placental secretion of human placental lactogen (hPL) and prolactin (from the decidua), as well as elevated levels of cortisol (an adrenal hormone) and glycogen, cause increased maternal peripheral resistance to insulin. This resistance helps ensure that there is a sustained supply of glucose available for the fetus. This glucose is transported across the placenta to the fetus, who uses it as a major source of fuel. Maternal amino acids are also actively transported by the placenta from the mother to her fetus. These amino acids are used by the fetus for protein synthesis and as a source of energy. In addition to ensuring that glucose is available to the fetus, the increased maternal resistance to insulin also means that the pregnant woman has a lower peripheral uptake of glucose to meet her own needs. This results in a catabolic (destructive) state during fasting periods (e.g., during the night and after meal absorption). Because increasing amounts of circulating maternal glucose are being diverted to the fetus, maternal fat is metabolized (lipolysis) during fasting periods much more readily than in a nonpregnant person. This process is called *accelerated starvation.* Ketones may be present in the urine as a result of lipolysis.

The delicate system of checks and balances that exists between glucose production and glucose use is stressed by the growing fetus, who derives energy from glucose taken from the mother and by maternal resistance to the insulin her body produces. This stress is referred to as the diabetogenic effect of pregnancy. Thus any preexisting disruption in carbohydrate metabolism is augmented by pregnancy, and any diabetic potential may precipitate gestational diabetes mellitus.

Pathophysiology of Diabetes Mellitus

In diabetes mellitus, the pancreas does not produce sufficient amounts of insulin to allow necessary carbohydrate metabolism. With inadequate amounts of insulin, glucose cannot enter the cells but remains circulating in the blood. The body cells become energy depleted while the blood glucose level remains elevated. Fats and proteins in the body tissues are then oxidized by the cells as a source of energy. This results in wasting of fat and muscle tissue of the body, negative nitrogen balance due to protein breakdown, and ketosis due to fat metabolism. The strong osmotic force of the glucose concentration in the blood pulls water from the cells into the blood, which results in cellular dehydration. The high level of glucose in the blood eventually spills over into the urine, producing glycosuria. Osmotic pressure of the glucose in the urine prevents reabsorption of water into the kidney tubules, causing extracellular dehydration.

These pathologic developments cause the four cardinal signs and symptoms of diabetes mellitus: polyuria, polydipsia, weight loss, and polyphagia. *Polyuria* (frequent urination) results because water is not reabsorbed by the renal tubules because of the osmotic activity of glucose. *Polydipsia* (excessive thirst) is caused by dehydration from polyuria. *Weight loss* (seen in insulin-dependent diabetes, also called type 1 diabetes) is due to the use of fat and muscle tissue for energy. *Polyphagia* (excessive hunger) is caused by tissue loss and a state of starvation, which results from the inability of the cells to utilize the blood glucose. Diagnosis of diabetes is based on the presence of clinical symptoms and laboratory tests showing elevated glucose levels in the blood, glycosuria, and ketoacidosis.

Classification of Diabetes Mellitus

The primary classification of diabetes is based on cause and includes four main categories (ADA, 2010):

- Type 1 diabetes develops because of β-cell destruction and generally results in an absolute insulin deficiency.
- Type 2 diabetes, the most common form, results from a combination of an insulin secretory defect and insulin resistance.
- Other specific types, of which there are eight subcategories, including, for example, genetic defects, drug-induced diabetes, and endocrine disorders. (Note: the detailed list can be found in medical-surgical texts and through the ADA original source.)
- Gestational diabetes mellitus

Table 19-3 shows White's classification of diabetes in pregnancy. This classification is useful for describing the extent of the disease.

Gestational diabetes mellitus (GDM) is defined as carbohydrate intolerance of variable severity with onset or first recognition during pregnancy. It results from (1) an unidentified preexistent disease, (2) the unmasking of a compensated metabolic abnormality by the added stress of pregnancy, or (3) a direct consequence of the altered maternal metabolism stemming from changing hormonal levels. Diagnosis of GDM is important because even mild diabetes increases the risk of perinatal morbidity and mortality. (See discussion in Fetal-Neonatal Risks.) Although GDM incidence rates vary, it has been estimated that 15% to 50% of these individuals will progress to overt type 2 diabetes mellitus in the decades following the affected pregnancy (American College of Obstetricians and Gynecologists [ACOG], 2009).

Influence of Pregnancy on Diabetes

Pregnancy can affect diabetes significantly. First, the physiologic changes of pregnancy can drastically alter insulin requirements. Second, pregnancy may accelerate the progress of vascular disease secondary to diabetes.

TABLE 19-3 White's Classification of Diabetes in Pregnancy

CLASS	CRITERION
A	Chemical diabetes
B	Maturity onset (age over 20 years), duration under 10 years, no vascular lesions
C_1	Age 10 to 19 years at onset
C_2	10 to 19 years' duration
D_1	Under 10 years at onset
D_2	Over 20 years' duration
D_3	Benign retinopathy
D_4	Calcified vessels of legs
D_5	Hypertension
E	No longer sought
F	Nephropathy
G	Many failures
H	Cardiopathy
R	Proliferating retinopathy
T	Renal transplant (added by Tagatz and colleagues of the University of Minnesota)

Source: Reprinted from White, P. (1978). Classification of obstetric diabetes. American Journal of Obstetrics and Gynecology, 130, *228. Copyright © 1978, with permission from Elsevier.*

The disease may be more difficult to control during pregnancy because insulin requirements are changeable. Insulin need frequently decreases early in the first trimester. Levels of hPL, an insulin antagonist, are low; energy demands of the embryo are minimal; and the woman may be consuming less food because of nausea and vomiting. Nausea and vomiting may also cause dietary fluctuations, which can increase the risk of hypoglycemia or insulin shock. Insulin requirements usually begin to rise late in the first trimester as glucose use and glycogen storage by the woman and fetus increase. As a result of placental maturation and production of hPL and other hormones, insulin requirements may double or quadruple by the end of pregnancy.

Increased energy needs during labor may require more insulin to balance intravenous glucose. After delivery of the placenta, insulin requirements usually decrease abruptly with loss of hPL in the maternal circulation.

Other factors contribute to the difficulty in controlling the disease. As pregnancy progresses, the renal threshold for glucose decreases. There is an increased risk of ketoacidosis, which may occur at lower serum glucose levels in the pregnant woman with diabetes than in the nonpregnant woman with diabetes. The vascular disease that accompanies diabetes may progress during pregnancy. Hypertension may occur. Nephropathy may result from renal blood vessel impairment, and retinopathy may develop (from occlusion of the microscopic blood vessels of the eye).

The primary concern for the pregnant woman who has diabetes is control of circulating blood glucose levels. If control can be achieved and maintained, diabetes generally does not worsen during pregnancy. The woman's health status may even improve because of close medical supervision.

Influence of Diabetes on Pregnancy Outcome

The pregnancy of a woman who has diabetes carries a higher risk of complications, especially perinatal mortality and congenital anomalies. The risk has been reduced by the recent recognition of the importance of tight metabolic control (fasting blood glucose less than 95 mg/dl and 2-hour postprandial less than 120 mg/dl). New techniques for monitoring blood glucose, delivering insulin, and monitoring the fetus have also reduced perinatal mortality (ACOG, 2005).

Maternal Risks

Maternal health problems in diabetic pregnancy have been greatly reduced by the team approach to preconception planning and early prenatal care and by the increased emphasis on maintaining tight control of blood glucose levels. The prognosis for the pregnant woman with gestational, type 1, or type 2 diabetes that has not resulted in significant vascular damage is positive. However, diabetic pregnancy still carries higher risks for complications than normal pregnancy.

Hydramnios, or an increase in the volume of amniotic fluid, occurs in 10% to 20% of pregnant women with diabetes. It is thought to be a result of excessive fetal urination because of fetal hyperglycemia (Rinala, Dryfhout, & Lambers, 2009). *Preeclampsia-eclampsia* occurs more often in diabetic pregnancies, especially when diabetes-related vascular changes already exist.

Hyperglycemia due to insufficient amounts of insulin can lead to *ketoacidosis* as a result of the increase in ketone bodies (which are acidic) in the blood released when fatty acids are metabolized. Ketoacidosis usually develops slowly, but it may develop more rapidly in the pregnant woman because of the hyperketonemia associated with accelerated starvation in the fasting state. The tendency for higher postprandial glucose levels because of decreased gastric motility and the contrainsulin effects of hPL also predispose the woman to ketoacidosis. If the ketoacidosis is not treated, it can lead to coma and death of both mother and fetus.

Another risk to the pregnant woman with diabetes is a difficult labor (*dystocia*), caused by fetopelvic disproportion if fetal macrosomia exists. The pregnant woman with diabetes is also at increased risk for recurrent monilial vaginitis and urinary tract infections because of increased glycosuria, which contributes to a favorable environment for bacterial growth. If untreated, asymptomatic bacteriuria can lead to pyelonephritis, a serious kidney infection.

Several studies have demonstrated that pregnancy worsens *retinopathy* in women with diabetes. Most investigators agree that during a diabetic pregnancy, good control of blood glucose levels and the use of laser photocoagulation (a treatment used to prevent retinal hemorrhage when the retina shows changes in the blood vessels) when indicated minimize the risk of the negative effects of pregnancy. Hence, women with preexisting diabetes should be referred to an ophthalmologist for evaluation during pregnancy (ACOG, 2005).

Fetal-Neonatal Risks

Many of the problems of the newborn result directly from high maternal plasma glucose levels. In the presence of severe maternal ketoacidosis, the risk of fetal death has ranged from 35% to a decrease more recently of 10% (ACOG, 2005). Fetal enzyme systems cease functioning in an acidic environment.

The incidence of *congenital anomalies* in diabetic pregnancies is 5% to 10% and is the major cause of death for infants of mothers with diabetes. Research suggests that this increased incidence of congenital anomalies is related to multiple factors including high glucose levels in early pregnancy (Eriksson, 2009). The anomalies often involve the heart, central nervous system (CNS), and skeletal system. Septal defects, coarctation of the aorta, and transposition of the great vessels are the most common heart lesions seen. CNS anomalies include hydrocephalus, meningomyelocele, and anencephaly. One anomaly, *sacral agenesis,* appears only in infants of mothers with diabetes. In sacral agenesis, the sacrum and lumbar spine fail to develop and the lower extremities develop incompletely. To reduce the incidence of congenital anomalies, preconception counseling and strict diabetes control before conception and in the early weeks of pregnancy are indicated.

Characteristically, infants of mothers with diabetes in White's classes A, B, and C (see Table 19-3) are large for gestational age (LGA) as a result of high levels of fetal insulin production stimulated by the high levels of glucose crossing the placenta from the mother. Sustained fetal hyperinsulinism and hyperglycemia ultimately lead to excessive growth, called **macrosomia**, and deposition of fat. If born vaginally, the macrosomic infant is at increased risk for birth trauma such as fractured clavicle or brachial plexus injuries due to shoulder dystocia. To prevent such injuries, cesarean birth may be indicated if birth weight is expected to exceed 4500 g (ACOG, 2005).

After birth, the umbilical cord is severed, and, thus, the generous maternal blood glucose supply is eliminated. However, continued islet cell hyperactivity leads to excessive insulin levels and depleted blood glucose (hypoglycemia) in 2 to 4 hours in the neonate. Macrosomia can be significantly reduced by tight maternal blood glucose control.

Infants of mothers with diabetes with vascular involvement may demonstrate intrauterine growth restriction (IUGR). This occurs because vascular changes in the mother decrease the efficiency of placental perfusion, and the fetus is not as well sustained in utero.

Respiratory distress syndrome appears to result from inhibition, by high levels of fetal insulin, of some fetal enzymes necessary for surfactant production. Polycythemia in the newborn is due primarily to the diminished ability of glycosylated hemoglobin in the mother's blood to release oxygen. *Hyperbilirubinemia* is a result of the inability of immature liver enzymes to metabolize the increased bilirubin resulting from the polycythemia. Hypocalcemia, characterized by signs of irritability or even tetany, may occur. The cause of these low calcium levels in infants of mothers with diabetes is not known.

Clinical Therapy

Detection and Diagnosis of Gestational Diabetes

Gestational diabetes is more common than pregestational diabetes. It is estimated to range from 2% to 10% of pregnancies, depending on the population studied (ACOG, 2009). Therefore, screening for its detection is a standard part of prenatal care. If diabetes is suspected, further testing is undertaken for diagnosis.

All pregnant women should have their risk of diabetes assessed at the first prenatal visit. Women at high risk (prior history of GDM or birth of an LGA infant, marked obesity, diagnosis of polycystic ovarian syndrome, presence of glycosuria, or a strong family history of type 2 diabetes mellitus [DM]) should be screened for diabetes as soon as possible. Various screening approaches may be used. HA1c equal to or greater than 6.5% would be considered diagnostic as would a fasting plasma glucose level equal to or greater than 126 mg/dl (ADA, 2010a).

Differences of opinion exist about screening low-risk women. The ADA (2010a) identifies women at low risk as those who meet *all* of the following criteria:

- Age less than 25 years
- Normal weight prior to pregnancy
- Caucasian (i.e., member of an ethnic group with a low incidence of DM)
- No history of an abnormal glucose tolerance
- No known DM in a first-degree relative

In January 2010, it was the position of the ADA that women at low risk do not require screening. However, the ADA stated that it is planning to work with U.S. obstetric organizations to consider adopting a recommendation that "all women not known to have prior diabetes undergo a 75-g OGTT at 24-28 weeks of gestation" (2010a, p. S15) based on work being done by the International Association of Diabetes and Pregnancy Study Groups (IADPSG). In March 2010, the IADPSG recommended that at 24–28 weeks' gestation, a 2-hr 75-g oral glucose tolerance test (OGTT) be done for all women not previously diagnosed with overt diabetes. For the 75-g test the following values are used to diagnose GDM (IADPSG, 2010):

Fasting	92 mg/dl
1 hour	180 mg/dl
2 hours	153 mg/dl

It remains to be determined whether healthcare professionals in the United States will adopt the recommendations of the IADPSG.

Current practice dictates that women at average risk (those who meet any of the criteria identified as excluded for low-risk women) should be tested toward the end of the second trimester (24 to 28 weeks) using a 1-hour, 50-gram oral glucose challenge test (GCT).The oral glucose load is administered without regard to time of day or time of last meal, and venous plasma glucose is measured 1 hour later. A plasma level that is equal to or greater than 130 to 140 mg/dl (depending on the laboratory used) indicates a need for further diagnostic testing (ADA, 2010a). Because women who meet the low-risk criteria comprise only about 10% of the population, it is not unusual to find that some busy clinics and offices are using the 50-g GCT to screen all women who are not considered high risk (Landon, Catalano, & Gabbe, 2007).

During pregnancy, if the 1-hour oral glucose screen indicates that a woman might have gestational diabetes, diagnosis is made using a 100-gram 3-hour oral glucose tolerance test (OGTT). To do this test, the woman eats an unrestricted diet, consuming at least 150 grams of carbohydrates per day for at least 3 days before her scheduled test. She then ingests 100-gram oral glucose solution in the morning after an overnight fast. Plasma glucose is measured fasting and at 1, 2, and 3 hours. The woman should remain seated and not smoke throughout the test. Gestational diabetes is diagnosed if two or more of the following values are met or exceeded:

Fasting	95 mg/dl
1 hour	180 mg/dl
2 hours	155 mg/dl
3 hours	140 mg/dl

Laboratory Assessment of Long-Term Glucose Control

Glycosylated hemoglobin (HbA_{1c}) is a laboratory test that loosely reflects glucose control over the previous 4 to 8 weeks. It measures the percentage of glycohemoglobin in the blood. Glycohemoglobin, or HbA_{1c}, is the hemoglobin to which a glucose molecule is attached. The test is not reliable for screening for gestational diabetes and is not recommended at this time (Gandhia, Brown, Simmb, et al., 2008).

In women with known pregestational diabetes, however, abnormal HbA_{1c} values correlate directly with the frequency of spontaneous abortion and fetal congenital anomalies. A value greater than 10% is associated with a fetal anomaly rate of 20% to 25% (ACOG, 2005). Consequently, women with preexisting diabetes who plan to become pregnant should work to achieve HbA_{1c} levels at target levels (less than 6%) without significant hypoglycemia. Once pregnancy is achieved, HbA_{1c} levels should be tested at the initial prenatal visit and every 2 to 3 months if target levels have been achieved (Kitzmiller et al., 2008).

Antepartum Management of Diabetes

The major goals of medical care for a pregnant woman with diabetes—whether gestational or pregestational—are (1) to maintain a physiologic equilibrium of insulin availability and glucose utilization during pregnancy and (2) to ensure an optimally healthy mother and newborn. To achieve these goals, good prenatal care using a team approach is a top priority. The team consists of an obstetrician; an endocrinologist; a perinatologist; a diabetes nurse-educator; a perinatal nurse; a dietitian; a social worker; and, most important, the woman with diabetes and her partner if the partner is involved in the pregnancy. Education of the couple and their active involvement in managing her care are essential for a good outcome.

For the woman with gestational diabetes, the diagnosis may be a shock, leaving her frightened and anxious. This anxiety may lead to an inability to adhere to important treatment regimens. She needs clear explanation and teaching to enlist her participation in ensuring a good outcome. The diabetes

Case Study: Patient with Gestational Diabetes

nurse-educator plays a major role in this counseling (Jones, Roche, & Appel, 2009).

Diet therapy and regular exercise form the cornerstone of intervention for GDM. Insulin therapy is indicated when dietary management is unable to achieve a 1-hour postprandial blood glucose value less than 130 to 140 mg/dl, a 2-hour postprandial level less than 120 mg/dl, or a fasting glucose less than 95 mg/dl. In most instances, the overt diabetic manifestation disappears postpartum, though subtle manifestations of impaired insulin secretory capacity may remain.

Oral hypoglycemics are rarely used during pregnancy because they cross the placenta and have not been well studied. However, glyburide, a second-generation sulfonylurea, may not cross the placenta and has been found to be comparable to insulin without evidence of adverse effects in the mother or fetus. This oral agent is a viable alternative for treating women with gestational diabetes mellitus (Serlin & Lash, 2009).

The woman with pregestational diabetes needs to understand changes she can expect during pregnancy; thus she should receive such teaching in preconception counseling. At the initial prenatal visit, height, weight, and vital signs are assessed along with a thorough assessment of thyroid and cardiac function. Special attention is given to dating the pregnancy. Laboratory data are obtained, and the diabetes is classified using White's criteria. Women should be screened for diabetic neuropathy, and a funduscopic examination is done to detect any retinopathy. In some cases, the woman may be referred to an ophthalmologist for further evaluation (ACOG, 2005).

Care Plan Activity: Antepartum Patient at Risk

Dietary Regulation

The pregnant woman requires about 300 kilocalories (kcal) per day more than she does when she is not pregnant to meet increased metabolic demands. In general, women need approximately 30 kcal/kg of ideal body weight (IBW) during the first trimester and 35 to 36 kcal/kg IBW during the second and third trimesters. If ketonuria develops or the woman complains of hunger, the number of calories may be increased. Dietary guidelines are similar for women with gestational and pregestational diabetes. Approximately 40% to 50% of the kcal should come from complex carbohydrates, 15% to 20% from protein, and 20% to 30% from fats. This caloric intake is divided among three meals and three snacks. A prebedtime snack may be indicated to prevent hypoglycemia at night. Management should focus on food choices for appropriate weight gain, normoglycemia, and absence of ketones. Although weight loss is not recommended during pregnancy, modest carbohydrate and calorie restriction may be appropriate for overweight and obese woman to improve glycemic control and reduce weight gain (ADA, 2008).

Because it is so important that the pregnant woman follow these guidelines, a dietitian works out meal plans based on the woman's lifestyle, culture, and food preferences and teaches her food exchanges so she can vary and plan her own meals. Daily food records, weekly weight checks, and regular ketone testing can assist in identifying an individual's energy requirements in order to help avoid the need for insulin therapy (ADA, 2008).

Glucose Monitoring

Glucose monitoring is an essential part of diabetes management for determining the need for insulin and assessing glucose control. Many physicians have the woman come in for a weekly assessment of her fasting glucose levels and one or two postprandial levels. In addition, frequent self-monitoring of glucose levels is paramount in maintaining good glucose control. Self-monitoring is discussed beginning on page 428.

Insulin Administration

Whether the woman with gestational diabetes needs additional insulin (over her own body production) depends on how well her blood glucose levels can be maintained by diet alone. Individuals with pregestational diabetes usually have type 1 diabetes, requiring insulin administration. Whether the patient has gestational or pregestational diabetes, human insulin should be used because it is the least likely to cause an allergic response. If the woman has previously used bovine or porcine insulin, she may require smaller doses of human insulin to achieve the same pharmacologic effect. Insulin is given either in multiple injections or by continuous subcutaneous infusion. Multiple injections are used more commonly and with excellent results. Most women will need a mixture of intermediate and regular insulin. Some clinicians have moved away from the use of regular insulin, replacing it with a fast-acting human analog called lispro. Lispro is associated with better glucose control (ACOG, 2005). Often a 4-dose approach is used, with regular insulin or lispro taken before each meal and NPH or Lente insulin added at bedtime (ACOG, 2005). Other clinicians vary the NPH and regular insulin patterns slightly but still prefer a 4-dose approach. It is important to remember that the amount of insulin needed usually increases during each trimester of pregnancy.

Evaluation of Fetal Status

Information about the well-being, maturation, and size of the fetus is important for planning the course of the pregnancy and the timing of birth. Because pregnancies complicated by diabetes are at increased risk of neural tube defects, a quadruple screen, which includes testing for maternal serum *α-fetoprotein AFP*, is offered at weeks 16 to 20 of gestation (see chapter 15 and chapter 21).

Daily maternal evaluation of *fetal activity,* begun at about 28 weeks, is effective and simple to do. The woman is taught a particular method for counting fetal movements (see chapter 16). She records the results on a special card, and brings the card to each subsequent office visit.

Nonstress testing (NST) may be started at about 28 weeks. If evidence of IUGR, preeclampsia, oligohydramnios, or poorly controlled blood glucose exists, testing may begin as early as 26 weeks and may be done more often. NSTs are increased to twice weekly at 32 weeks' gestation. If the NST is nonreactive, a fetal biophysical profile or *contraction stress test* is performed. If the woman requires hospitalization (for example, to control glycemia or for complications), NSTs may be done daily. See chapter 21 for a further discussion of nonstress testing.

Ultrasound at 18 weeks confirms gestational age and diagnoses multiple pregnancy or congenital anomalies. It is repeated at 28 weeks to monitor fetal growth for IUGR or macrosomia. Some physicians order *fetal biophysical profiles* (ultrasound evaluation of fetal well-being in which fetal breathing movements, fetal activity, reactivity, muscle tone, and amniotic fluid volume are assessed) as part of an ongoing evaluation of fetal status.

Intrapartum Management of Diabetes Mellitus

During the intrapartum period, medical therapy includes the following:

- ***Timing of birth.*** Most diabetic pregnancies are allowed to go to term, with spontaneous labor, thereby decreasing the risk of respiratory distress in the newborn. Some clinicians do opt to induce labor in a woman at term to avoid problems related to decreased perfusion as the placenta ages. Cesarean birth may be indicated if evidence of nonreassuring fetal status exists. Birth before term may be indicated for women with diabetes who have vascular changes and worsening hypertension or if evidence of IUGR exists (ACOG, 2005). In pregnancies in which there is evidence of fetal macrosomia, fetal compromise, or elevated maternal HbA_{1c}, amniocentesis for fetal lung maturity may be indicated. Below is a list of available tests that help determine fetal lung maturity. No test has been proven to be superior, but recent modifications to performing the fluorescence polarization has increased its use in the clinical setting (ACOG, 2008c).

Test	Lung Maturity Value
Fluorescence Polarization (TDx-FLM II)	55 mg/g or greater of albumin
Lecithin/Sphingomyelin (L/S) ratio	2.0–3.5
Phosphatidylglycerol	Present or between 0.5–2.0

  Fetal lung maturity must be weighed against other considerations when deciding time of childbirth. If preterm labor occurs, tocolytic therapy (use of medications in an attempt to halt preterm labor) (see chapter 20 ∞) and β-sympathomimetic drugs should not be administered because they may worsen maternal glucose control (ACOG, 2003a).

- ***Labor management.*** The degree of prenatal maintenance of normal maternal glucose levels (euglycemia) and the maintenance of maternal euglycemia during labor are important in preventing neonatal hypoglycemia. Maternal insulin requirements often decrease dramatically during labor. Consequently, maternal glucose levels are measured hourly to determine insulin need (Figure 19-2 ■). The primary goal in controlling maternal glucose levels intrapartally is to prevent neonatal hypoglycemia (ACOG, 2005). During active labor, insulin may not be needed. Long-acting insulin should be reduced or stopped and regular insulin should be used to meet most or all of the woman's identified needs. Often two intravenous lines are used, one with a 5% dextrose solution and one with a saline solution. The saline solution is then available if a bolus is needed or for piggybacking insulin. Insulin clings to the plastic intravenous bag and tubing. To ensure that the woman receives the desired dose, the intravenous tubing must be flushed with insulin before the prescribed amount is added. During the second stage of labor and the immediate postpartum period, the woman may not need additional insulin. The intravenous insulin is discontinued with the completion of the third stage of labor.

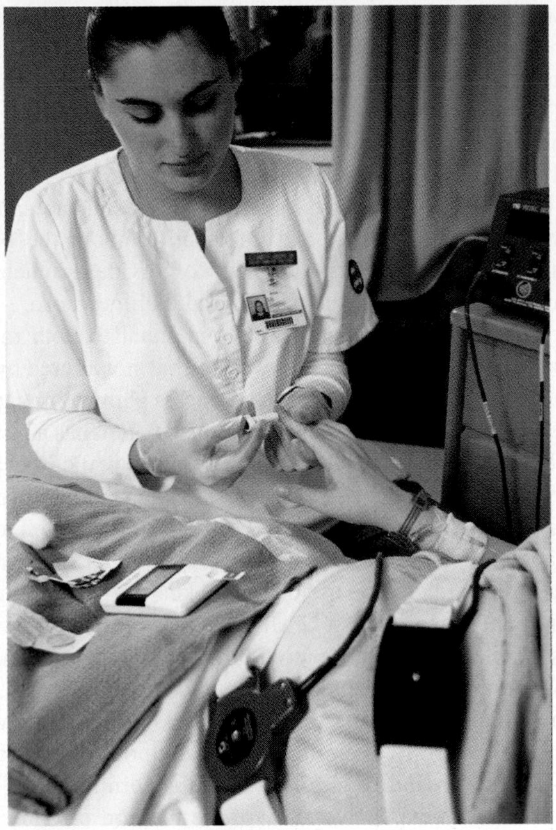

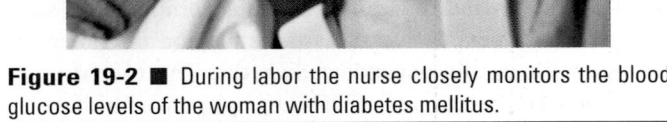

Figure 19-2 ■ During labor the nurse closely monitors the blood glucose levels of the woman with diabetes mellitus.

Source: Vicky Flanagan, RN, BSN/Pearson Education.

Application: Gestational Diabetes

Postpartum Management of Diabetes Mellitus

Maternal insulin requirements fall significantly postpartally because the levels of hPL, progesterone, and estrogen fall after placental separation, and their anti-insulin effect ceases, resulting in decreased blood glucose levels. The mother with diabetes may require no insulin for the first 24 hours or only one fourth to one half her previous dose. Then, reestablishment of insulin needs based on blood glucose testing is necessary. Diet and exercise levels must also be redetermined. Consequently, the woman with diabetes that is not controlled by diet alone may need insulin for a period of time (ACOG, 2005).

Women with GDM who did not require insulin during pregnancy generally do not need it during the postpartum period. Clinicians routinely discontinue insulin for women with GDM following childbirth and then monitor blood glucose levels. If elevated glucose levels develop, oral antihyperglycemic agents may be tried if the woman is not breastfeeding (ACOG, 2005). Antihyperglycemics are contraindicated during breastfeeding.

The woman should be reassessed 6 weeks postpartum to determine whether her glucose levels are normal. If her levels are normal, she should be reassessed at a minimum of 3-year intervals (ACOG, 2009).

Diabetic control and the establishment of parent-child relationships in light of neonatal needs are the priorities of this period. If her newborn must be cared for in a special care nursery, the mother needs support and information about the baby's condition. Every effort must be made to provide as much contact as possible between the parents and their newborn.

Breastfeeding is encouraged as beneficial to both mother and baby. The composition of breast milk is not altered by diabetes, and infants of mothers with diabetes gain weight appropriately. The lactating mother with diabetes often has a sense of well-being and diminished insulin needs even while increasing caloric intake. Blood glucose levels may be lower because glucose is transferred from serum to breast to be converted to lactose, and energy is expended in milk production. Caloric needs increase during lactation to 500 to 800 kcal above prepregnant requirements. Insulin must be adjusted according to individual needs. Home blood glucose monitoring should continue for the person with insulin-dependent diabetes.

The woman and her partner, if involved, should receive information on family planning. Barrier methods of contraception (diaphragm and condom) used with spermicide are safe, effective, and inexpensive and are the method of choice for women with insulin-dependent diabetes. The use of combined oral contraceptives (COCs) by women with diabetes is controversial because of the risk of vascular disease (Cunningham et al., 2010). Many physicians who prescribe low-dose COCs to women with diabetes restrict them to women who have no vascular disease and who do not smoke. The progesterone-only pill may also be used as may Depo-Provera. Many couples who have completed their families choose elective sterilization.

> “It's hard to realize that I have gestational diabetes and to know that it increases my chances of getting diabetes later. My grandmother had diabetes, so I always thought of it as an old person's disease. All the fingersticks, watching my diet, and keeping track has taken some getting used to. I'll be glad when our baby is born and I can put this behind me, at least for now.”

NURSING CARE MANAGEMENT

The Nursing Care Plan for a woman with diabetes mellitus summarizes nursing management.

Nursing Assessment and Diagnosis

Whether diabetes has been diagnosed before pregnancy occurs or the diagnosis is made during pregnancy (GDM), careful assessment of the disease process and the woman's understanding of diabetes is important. Thorough physical examination, including assessment for vascular complications, any signs of infectious conditions, and urine and blood testing for glucose, is essential at the first prenatal visit. Follow-up visits are usually scheduled twice a month during the first two trimesters and weekly during the last trimester.

Assessment also yields vital information about the woman's ability to cope with the combined stress of pregnancy and diabetes and her ability to follow a recommended regimen of care. It is necessary to determine the woman's knowledge about diabetes and self-care before formulating a teaching plan.

Nursing diagnoses that may apply to the pregnant woman with diabetes mellitus include the following:

- ***Risk for Imbalanced Nutrition: More Than Body Requirements*** related to imbalance between intake and available insulin
- ***Risk for Injury*** related to possible complications secondary to hypoglycemia or hyperglycemia
- ***Interrupted Family Processes*** related to the need for hospitalization secondary to GDM

Nursing Plan and Implementation

Prepregnancy counseling may be provided by a nurse and a physician, using a team approach. Ideally, the couple is seen before pregnancy so that the diabetes can be assessed by ophthalmologic evaluation, electrocardiographic study, and a 24-hour urine collection for creatinine clearance and protein excretion. Prepregnancy counseling about the importance of tight glucose control is cost effective in preventing congenital anomalies. If the diabetes is of recent onset without vascular complications, the outcome of pregnancy should be good, provided that glucose levels are controlled.

Community-Based Nursing Care

In many cases, women with GDM are stabilized in the hospital, and necessary teaching for self-care is begun. Women with preexisting diabetes may also require hospitalization for stabilization of their diabetes. In either case, the majority of ongoing teaching and supervision of pregnant women with diabetes is then carried out by nurses in clinics, community agencies, and the women's homes.

Effective Insulin Use

The nurse ensures that the couple understands the purpose of the insulin, the types of insulin the woman is to use, the number of doses she is to receive daily, and the correct procedure for its administration. The woman's partner is also instructed about insulin administration in case it should be necessary for the partner to give it. For some highly motivated women whose glucose levels are not well controlled with multiple injections, the continuous insulin infusion pump may improve glucose control.

The nurse teaches the patient how and when to monitor her blood sugar, the desired range of blood sugar levels, and the

NURSING CARE PLAN The Woman with Diabetes Mellitus

INTERVENTION	RATIONALE
1. Nursing Diagnosis: Imbalanced Nutrition: Less than body requirements related to poor carbohydrate metabolism **Goal:** Patient will maintain adequate nutrition throughout pregnancy.	
■ Emphasize importance of regular prenatal visits for assessment of *weight gain, controlled blood sugar,* heart tones, urine ketones, and fundal height measurement.	■ Regular follow-up and assessment of weight, blood sugar levels, fetal heart tones, urine ketones, and fundal height will promote a healthy pregnancy and outcome as well as allow for modifications in the treatment regimen if necessary.
■ Coordinate care with a dietitian to assist patient in meal planning and educate patient on the daily caloric needs of pregnancy.	■ A daily intake of high-quality foods promotes fetal growth and controls maternal glucose levels.
■ Instruct patient on signs and symptoms of hyperglycemia: polyphagia, nausea, hot flushes, polydipsia, polyuria, fruity breath, abdominal cramps, rapid deep breathing, headache, weakness, drowsiness, and general malaise. Instruct patient on signs and symptoms of hypoglycemia: hunger; clammy skin; irritability; slurred speech; seizures; tachycardia; headache; pallor; sweating; disorientation; shakiness; blurred vision; and, if untreated, coma or convulsions.	■ Maintaining a euglycemic state throughout pregnancy aids in preventing diabetic complications and promotes a positive pregnancy outcome.
■ Instruct patient on management of hyperglycemia and hypoglycemia.	
■ Include family members in meal.	■ Gives the family member a sense of involvement and an understanding of the importance of adequate nutrition in pregnancy.
EXPECTED OUTCOME:	The patient will maintain adequate nutrition as evidenced by adequate weight gain, normal blood sugar levels, fetal heart rate, verbalization of understanding of personal treatment regimen, and appropriate fetal growth and development during pregnancy.
2. Nursing Diagnosis: Risk for Injury to the fetus related to possible complications associated with altered tissue perfusion secondary to maternal diagnosis of diabetes mellitus **Goal:** Uncomplicated birth of a healthy newborn.	
■ Assess fetal heart tones for reassuring variability and accelerations.	■ Reassuring fetal heart rate variability and accelerations are interpreted as adequate placental oxygenation.
■ Instruct mother on how to lie in a left recumbent position after eating and record how many fetal movements she feels in an hour.	■ More than five fetal kicks in an hour are indicative of fetal well-being.
■ Collaborative: Perform oxytocin challenge test (OCT)/contraction stress test (CST) and nonstress tests as determined by physician.	■ Fetal surveillance testing assesses fetal well-being and adequate placental perfusion.
■ Prepare patient for frequent ultrasound assessments.	■ Ultrasonography is indicated at 7–9 weeks to confirm gestational age and then every 4–6 weeks to evaluate fetal well-being per physician's orders.
■ Prepare patient for possible amniocentesis procedure.	■ A sample of amniotic fluid that can be used to detect fetal lung maturity and enables medical personnel to prepare for a potential preterm birth.
■ Assist physician with biophysical profile assessment.	■ Helps ensure fetal well-being and a positive fetal outcome.
EXPECTED OUTCOME:	The fetus will not exhibit signs and symptoms of altered tissue perfusion as evidenced by positive fetal activity, reassuring fetal heart rate patterns, a biophysical profile score between 8 and 10, negative CST, L/S ratio indicating fetal lung maturity, and a reactive nonstress test.
3. Nursing Diagnosis: Readiness for Enhanced Knowledge about the effects of blood sugar on pregnancy related to an expressed desire to maintain stable blood glucose levels **Goal:** The patient and her family will verbalize the importance of maintaining blood sugar within prescribed ranges during pregnancy.	
■ Assess the patient and family's cognitive level and develop a teaching strategy that will facilitate learning at that level.	■ Behavior changes occur when teaching strategies are appropriate for the patient and family's cognitive level.

(continued)

NURSING CARE PLAN **The Woman with Diabetes Mellitus** continued

INTERVENTION	RATIONALE
■ Teach blood glucose monitoring, insulin administration, and predicted insulin needs throughout pregnancy, and then have patient and family members repeat the discussion.	■ Basic understanding of the relationship between blood sugar levels and how insulin needs change throughout pregnancy will foster compliance with prescribed regimen.
■ Emphasize the importance of maintaining a healthy diet and exercise program during pregnancy. Encourage patient and family to develop a sample diabetic diet and exercise regimen that is appropriate for pregnancy while present in the clinic or hospital and evaluate for appropriateness.	■ Involves the patient and her family members in the planning of her care, and the evaluation process promotes cooperation, positive reinforcement, and a time for modifications of regimen if necessary.
■ Emphasize the importance of prenatal care for the purpose of maternal and fetal surveillance.	■ Frequent prenatal visits allow for modifications in regimen and promote a healthy pregnancy outcome.

EXPECTED OUTCOME: The patient and family members will verbalize understanding of the effects of blood sugar fluctuations on pregnancy as evidenced by asking questions and seeking health information when necessary. The patient adheres to personal treatment regimen throughout pregnancy.

4. Nursing Diagnosis: Risk for Infection related to increased levels of glucose in urine
Goal: The patient will have no urinary tract infections (UTIs) during pregnancy.

INTERVENTION	RATIONALE
■ Encourage patient to utilize preventive measures to prevent UTIs: increasing intake of water and cranberry juice, wearing cotton underwear, wiping perineum from front to back, voiding frequently, and voiding before and immediately after sexual intercourse.	■ Utilizing preventive measures decreases the likelihood of patient acquiring a UTI.
■ Instruct patient on the signs and symptoms of UTIs: urinary frequency, dysuria, cloudy urine, hematuria, lower back pain, and foul-smelling urine.	■ Patient will be aware of signs and symptoms of UTIs and report to physician for immediate intervention.
Collaborative:	
■ Instruct patient on how to obtain a clean-catch urine sample and send to laboratory for culture and sensitivity per physician's orders.	■ A clean-catch urine sample will contain bacteria if a UTI is present.
■ Administer prescribed antibiotic therapy and teach patient about medication, adverse effects, and appropriate dosage.	■ Antibiotic therapy is the appropriate treatment for a UTI. Compliance increases when a patient fully understands medication regimen.
■ Encourage patient to drink 8–10 glasses of water each day.	■ Increased fluid intake assists in flushing bacteria out of the urinary tract system.

EXPECTED OUTCOME: Patient will remain free of UTIs during pregnancy as evidenced by verbalizing and complying with appropriate preventive measures, increasing fluid intake, and identifying negative urine samples during prenatal visits.

5. Nursing Diagnosis: Anxiety related to unfamiliarity with diagnosis
Goal: The patient expresses less anxiety.

INTERVENTION	RATIONALE
■ Assess patient's level of anxiety (mild-1, moderate-2, or severe-3) and have patient verbalize causes of anxiety.	■ Verbalization of anxiety provokers encourages expression of feelings and questions.
■ Share information on diabetes care such as nutrition, exercise, and glucose control in a clear and concise manner.	■ Accurate information gives the patient a sense of control and comfort.
■ Instruct patient on anxiety-reducing techniques such as imagery, breathing exercises, and massage used in pregnancy.	■ Gives patient the tools necessary for decreasing anxiety.
■ Refer patient to a diabetes support group.	■ A support group allows patients with similar problems to express concerns and share information with each other.

EXPECTED OUTCOME: The patient demonstrates appropriate coping strategies as evidenced by utilizing resources efficiently and verbalizing feelings of anxiety and the ways to deal with them.

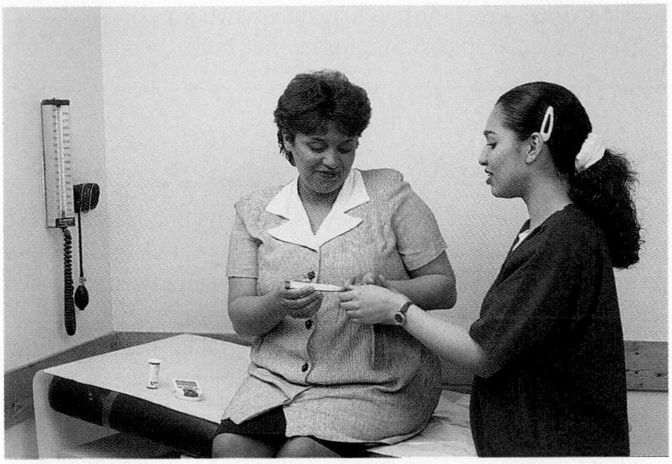

Figure 19-3 ■ The nurse teaches the pregnant woman with gestational diabetes mellitus how to do home glucose monitoring.

Source: Jenny Thomas Photography.

importance of good glycemic control (Figure 19-3 ■). Most women use a glucose meter because it provides a more accurate reading. The nurse teaches the patient to follow the manufacturer's directions exactly; to wash hands thoroughly before puncturing her finger; and to touch the blood droplet, not her finger, to the test pad on the strip.

With a blood glucose meter, an electronic eye measures the blood sugar, and a digital reading is given. The blood droplet should cover the test pad because uncovered portions are read as low sugar. The glucose meter is a portable pocket-sized device that is more accurate than the visual, color comparison method. Some meters are able to store and recall a specified number of readings, which helps ensure the accuracy of recorded results.

CLINICAL TIP

When teaching a pregnant woman to do her own blood glucose testing, have gloves available and put them on if it becomes necessary to help the woman obtain a blood sample. The woman does not need to wear gloves during the procedure.

Also be sure to wear gloves when doing fingersticks for blood glucose levels, when testing the urine for ketones, when starting an IV for insulin therapy, or when drawing blood for other laboratory tests.

The nurse may offer the patient the following tips about finger puncture:

- Various spring-loaded devices are available that make puncturing easier.
- Hanging the arm down for 30 seconds increases blood flow to the fingers.
- Warming the hands under running water increases blood flow to them.
- The sides of fingers should be punctured instead of the ends because the ends contain more pain-sensitive nerves.

Patients with diabetes need to keep a record of each blood sugar reading as a guide for management. Specific record sheets are available for this purpose and should be brought to each visit.

Planned Exercise Program

Exercise is encouraged for the woman's overall well-being. If she is used to a regular exercise program, she is encouraged to continue. She is advised to exercise after meals (when blood sugar levels are high), to wear diabetic identification, to carry a simple sugar such as hard candy (because of the possibility of exercise-induced hypoglycemia), to monitor her blood glucose levels regularly, and to avoid injecting insulin into an extremity that will soon be used during exercise.

If she has not been following a regular exercise plan, she is encouraged to begin gradually. Because exercise can alter metabolism, the woman's blood glucose should be well controlled before she begins an exercise program. Women with GDM should not use unusual, strenuous, and excessive exercise in an attempt to reduce glucose levels.

Health Promotion Education

Using the information gained during the nursing assessment of the pregnant woman with diabetes, the nurse provides appropriate teaching to the woman and her family so that the woman can meet her own healthcare needs as much as possible.

- ***Glucose monitoring.*** Home blood glucose monitoring is the most accurate and convenient way to determine insulin dose and assess control. It should be taught at the first visit after the diagnosis of gestational diabetes has been established. The woman with pregestational diabetes may already be monitoring her own blood sugar. Women with GDM typically measure their blood glucose 4 times a day (fasting and 1 to 2 hours after meals), while women with preexisting diabetes monitor their blood 5 to 7 times each day (Reece & Homko, 2008). Women are encouraged to maintain blood sugars in the normal ranges as follows: fasting (before eating or taking insulin), less than 95 mg/dl; 2 hours after each meal less than 120 mg/dl (Cleveland Clinic, 2007). New technology that is capable of automatically and painlessly monitoring blood glucose levels is currently being investigated and shows great promise.
- ***Symptoms of abnormal blood glucose levels.*** The pregnant woman with diabetes must recognize symptoms of changing glucose levels—whether hypoglycemia or hyperglycemia accompanied by ketoacidosis—and take appropriate action by immediately checking her capillary blood glucose level. Hypoglycemia may develop fairly rapidly. Symptoms include sweating, periodic tingling, disorientation, shakiness, pallor, clammy skin, irritability, hunger, headache, and blurred vision. If the pregnant woman is hypoglycemic with a mild blood glucose level less than 65 to 70 mg/dl, 1 cup of milk (8 oz, 14 grams of sugar) or 3–5 glucose tablets should be effective and prevent marked rebound hyperglycemia from excess glucose consumption. More severe hypoglycemia (less than 50 mg/dl) should be treated with 1 cup orange juice or 22 grams sugar (Kitzmiller et al., 2008). Many people overtreat their symptoms by continuing to eat, which can cause rebound hyperglycemia.

  The woman should carry a snack at all times and should have other fast sources of glucose (simple carbohydrates such as hard candy) at hand so that she can treat an insulin reaction when milk is not available. Family members are also taught how to inject glucagon in the event that food does not work or is not feasible, for instance, in the presence of severe morning sickness.

Hyperglycemia and ketoacidosis typically develop more slowly and tend to occur more commonly during the second half of pregnancy. Because most problems for the fetus are related to maternal hyperglycemia, this is a serious situation. Symptoms include polyuria, polydipsia, dry mouth, fatigue, nausea, hot flushed skin, rapid deep breathing, abdominal cramps, acetone breath, headache, drowsiness, depressed reflexes, oliguria or anuria, stupor, or coma. Hyperglycemia is treated with insulin.

- ***Smoking.*** Smoking has harmful effects on the maternal vascular system and the developing fetus and is contraindicated for both pregnancy and diabetes.
- ***Travel.*** Insulin can be kept at room temperature while traveling. Insulin supplies should be kept with the traveler and not packed in the baggage. Most airlines can supply special meals if notified a few days before departure. The woman should wear a diabetic identification bracelet or necklace. In addition, the woman should check with her physician for any instructions or advice before leaving.
- ***Support groups.*** Many communities have diabetes support groups or education classes, which can be helpful to women with newly diagnosed diabetes.
- ***Cesarean birth.*** Chances for a cesarean birth increase if the pregnant woman has diabetes because of the risk of fetal macrosomia and shoulder dystocia. This possibility should be anticipated—enrollment in cesarean birth preparation classes may be suggested. Many hospitals offer classes, and information is available through other organizations. The couple may prefer simply to discuss cesarean birth with the nurse and their obstetrician and read some books on the topic.

Hospital-Based Nursing Care

Hospitalization may become necessary during the pregnancy to evaluate blood glucose levels and adjust insulin dosages. In such cases, nurses monitor the woman's status and continue to provide teaching so that the woman is knowledgeable about her condition and its management. During the intrapartum period, the nurse must have a clear understanding about the impact of labor on the condition. The nurse carefully monitors the woman's status, maintains her intravenous fluids, is alert for signs of hypoglycemia, and provides the care indicated for any woman in labor. If a cesarean birth is indicated, the nurse provides appropriate care as described in chapter 28 ∞.

Evaluation

Expected outcomes of nursing care include the following:

- The woman is able to discuss her condition and its possible impact on her pregnancy, labor and birth, and postpartum period.
- The woman participates in developing a healthcare regimen to meet her needs and follows it throughout her pregnancy.
- The woman avoids developing hypoglycemia or hyperglycemia.
- The woman gives birth to a healthy newborn.
- The woman is able to care for her newborn.

Care of the Woman with Anemia

Anemia indicates inadequate levels of hemoglobin (Hb) in the blood. *Anemia* is defined as hemoglobin less than 12 g/dl in nonpregnant women and less than 11 g/dl in pregnant women (ACOG, 2008a). Race, altitude, smoking, nutrition, and medications can affect the normal limits of hemoglobin. The lower limit of normal tends to be higher for women who smoke and those who live at higher altitudes because their bodies require a greater quantity of red blood cells to maintain their tissue oxygen levels. For example, a pregnant woman who lives in Denver, Colorado (elevation 5280 feet), would be considered anemic if her hemoglobin dropped below 10.5 g/dl. Similarly, a pregnant African American woman or a smoker should be considered anemic at 10.2g/dl or below (ACOG, 2008a).

The common anemias of pregnancy are due either to insufficient hemoglobin production related to nutritional deficiency in iron or folic acid during pregnancy, or to hemoglobin destruction in inherited disorders, specifically sickle cell anemia and thalassemia.

Iron Deficiency Anemia

Dietary iron is needed to synthesize hemoglobin. Because hemoglobin is necessary to transport oxygen, a deficiency of iron may affect the body's transport of oxygen.

Iron deficiency anemia is the most common medical complication of pregnancy, primarily as a consequence of expansion of plasma volume without normal expansion of maternal hemoglobin mass (ACOG, 2008a). Approximately 200 mg of iron will be conserved because of the functional amenorrhea of pregnancy, but a pregnant woman needs approximately 1000 mg more iron intake during the pregnancy. Between 300 and 400 mg of iron is transferred to the fetus; 500 mg is needed for the increased red blood cell mass in the woman's own increased circulating blood volume; another 100 mg is needed for the placenta; and about 280 mg is needed to replace the 1 mg of iron lost daily through feces, urine, and sweat.

The greatest need for increased iron intake occurs in the second half of pregnancy. When the iron needs of pregnancy are not met, maternal hemoglobin falls below 11 g/dl. Serum ferritin levels, indicating iron stores, are below 12 mg/L.

Many women begin pregnancy in a slightly anemic state. In pregnancy, mild anemia can rapidly become more severe; therefore, it needs immediate treatment.

Maternal Risks

The woman with iron deficiency anemia may be asymptomatic, but she is more susceptible to infection, may tire easily, has an increased chance of preeclampsia and postpartal hemorrhage, and tolerates poorly even minimal blood loss during birth. Healing of an episiotomy or an incision may be delayed. If the anemia is severe (Hb less than 6 g/dl), cardiac failure may ensue.

Fetal-Neonatal Risks

There is evidence of increased risk of low birth weight, prematurity, stillbirth, and neonatal death in infants of women with severe iron deficiency (maternal Hb less than 6 g/dl). The infant is not iron deficient at birth because of active transport of iron across the placenta, even when maternal iron stores are low. However, these babies do have lower iron stores and are at increased risk for developing iron deficiency during infancy.

Clinical Therapy

The first goal of health care is to prevent iron deficiency anemia. If it occurs, the goal is to return low iron and hemoglobin levels to normal. To prevent anemia, the American Academy of Pediatrics (AAP) and ACOG (2008) recommend that pregnant women take at least 27 mg supplements of iron daily. This amount is contained in most prenatal vitamins. In addition, the woman should be encouraged to eat an iron-rich diet. To prevent constipation, the most common side effect of iron supplementation, a stool softener may be necessary.

If anemia is diagnosed, the dosage should be increased to 60 to 120 mg per day of iron. If the woman remains anemic after 1 month of therapy, further evaluation is indicated. With a twin pregnancy, a larger dose is needed. If a large dose of oral iron causes vomiting, diarrhea, or constipation, or if the anemia is discovered late in pregnancy, parenteral iron may be needed.

NURSING CARE MANAGEMENT

Nursing Assessment and Diagnosis

The main presenting symptom of iron deficiency anemia may be fatigue. Nutritional history usually gives evidence of poor dietary intake of iron. The nurse should also determine whether there was a history of anemia in a prior pregnancy. Physical examination reveals pallor of skin and conjunctiva. Laboratory studies show hemoglobin values below 10 g/dl, serum ferritin levels below 12 mg/L, and possibly microcytic and hypochromic red blood cells (a late finding).

Nursing diagnoses that may apply to a pregnant woman with iron deficiency anemia include the following:

- ***Risk for Imbalanced Nutrition: Less Than Body Requirements*** related to inadequate intake of iron-containing foods
- ***Constipation*** related to daily intake of iron supplements

Nursing Plan and Implementation

The nurse stresses the importance of an iron-rich diet and of iron supplements during pregnancy. Supplements are indicated because dietary sources cannot meet the extra requirements. The woman is taught to take iron tablets with vitamin C (e.g., orange juice) to increase absorption. Iron absorption is reduced by 40% to 50% if the tablets are taken with meals. However, gastrointestinal upset is more likely if they are taken on an empty stomach. The patient may tolerate the iron better if she starts with small doses and gradually increases the dosage over several days. She is informed that her stool will turn black and may be more formed. She is also advised to keep the tablets out of the reach of children because ingestion may be fatal to a young child.

Evaluation

Expected outcomes of nursing care include the following:

- The woman is able to identify the risks associated with iron deficiency anemia during pregnancy.
- The woman takes her iron supplements as recommended.
- The woman's Hb levels remain normal or return to normal during her pregnancy.

Application: Iron Deficiency Anemia

Folic Acid Deficiency Anemia

Folate deficiency is the most common cause of megaloblastic anemia during pregnancy, affecting between 1% and 4% of pregnant women in the United States. It is more prevalent with twin pregnancies.

Folic acid is needed for deoxyribonucleic acid (DNA) and ribonucleic acid (RNA) synthesis and cell duplication. In its absence, immature red blood cells fail to divide, become enlarged (megaloblastic), and are fewer in number. Even more significantly, an inadequate intake of folic acid has been associated with neural tube defects (NTDs) (spina bifida, anencephaly, meningomyelocele) in the fetus or newborn. With the tremendous cell multiplication that occurs in pregnancy, an adequate amount of folic acid is crucial. However, increased urinary excretion of folic acid and fetal uptake can rapidly result in folic acid deficiency.

Clinical Therapy

Diagnosis of folic acid deficiency anemia may be difficult, and it is usually not detected until late in pregnancy or the early puerperium. This is because serum folate levels normally fall as pregnancy progresses. Even though folate levels are lower with deficiency, they will fluctuate with diet. Measurement of erythrocyte folate status is more reliable but indicates folate status of several weeks previously. Women with true folic acid deficiency anemia often present with nausea, vomiting, and anorexia. Hemoglobin levels as low as 3 to 5 g/dl may be found. Typically the blood smear reveals that the newly formed erythrocytes are macrocytic.

Folic acid deficiency during pregnancy is prevented by a daily supplement of 0.4 mg of folate. Treatment of deficiency consists of 1-mg folic acid supplement. Because iron deficiency anemia almost always coexists with folic acid deficiency, the woman also needs iron supplements.

NURSING CARE MANAGEMENT

The nurse can help the pregnant woman avoid folate deficiency by teaching her food sources of folic acid and cooking methods for preserving folic acid. The best sources are fresh leafy green vegetables, orange juice, other citrus fruits and juices, red meats, fish, poultry, and legumes. As much as 50% to 90% of folic acid can be lost by cooking in large volumes of water. Microwave cooking destroys more folic acid than conventional cooking.

The Food and Drug Administration (FDA) requires the addition of folic acid for all foods labeled "enriched." Even with this addition, the U.S. Public Health Service recommends that all women of childbearing age (15 to 45 years) consume 0.4 mg of folic acid daily. This recommendation is important because half of all U.S. pregnancies are unplanned and NTDs occur very early in pregnancy (3 to 4 weeks after conception), before most women realize they are pregnant (AAP/ACOG, 2008). Nurses can play a crucial role in helping young women become aware of this important recommendation.

Sickle Cell Disease

Sickle cell disease (SCD) is a recessive autosomal disorder in which the normal adult hemoglobin, hemoglobin A (HbA), is abnormally formed. This abnormal hemoglobin is called hemoglobin S (HbS). It occurs primarily in people of African descent and occasionally in people of Southeast Asian or Mediterranean origin (i.e., Greeks, Italians, Arabs, and Turks) (ACOG, 2007). The abnormal red cells break down, causing anemia, which is characterized by acute, recurring episodes of tissue, abdominal, and joint pain. Individuals with the disorder are homozygous for the sickle cell gene. They inherit from each parent an allele causing an amino acid substitution in the two beta protein chains in the hemoglobin molecule. Heterozygous individuals are carriers for sickle cell trait (SCT) but are usually asymptomatic. One of the beta protein chains formed in their hemoglobin is normal; the other has the amino acid substitution. Approximately 1 in 12 African Americans has sickle cell trait and 1 in every 300 African American newborns has some form of sickle cell disease (ACOG, 2007).

Hemoglobin S (HbS) causes the red blood cells to be sickle or crescent shaped. In conditions of low oxygenation, normal hemoglobin is soluble, but HbS becomes semisolid and distorts the red blood cell shape. These erythrocytes easily interlock and clog capillaries, particularly in organs characterized by slow flow and high oxygen extraction, such as the spleen, bone marrow, and placenta. This phenomenon, called *sickling,* varies in frequency depending on the amount of the HbS in the red blood cells (there is seldom a crisis with levels below 40%) and other hemoglobin factors. Diagnosis is confirmed by hemoglobin electrophoresis or a test to induce sickling in a blood sample. Prenatal diagnosis and newborn screening for sickle cell disease are important components of perinatal care (ACOG, 2007).

Maternal Risks

Women with sickle cell trait have a good prognosis for pregnancy if they have adequate nutrition and prenatal care. They are, however, at increased risk for nephritis, bacteriuria, and hematuria, and tend to become anemic.

Women with sickle cell disease have considerably more risk during pregnancy. Low oxygen pressure—caused by high temperature, dehydration, infection, or acidosis, for example—may precipitate a vaso-occlusive crisis. The crisis produces sudden attacks of pain that may be general or localized in bones or joints, lungs, abdominal organs, or the spinal cord. The pain is due to ischemia in the tissues from occluded capillaries. Vaso-occlusive crises occur more often in the second half of pregnancy.

Maternal mortality due to sickle cell disease is rare. However, sickle cell crisis occurred in 47% of patients in one cohort study (Yu, Stasiowska, Stephens, et al., 2009). Other complications included anemia requiring blood transfusion (32%), infections (28%), and emergency cesarean sections (30%). Acute chest syndrome, congestive heart failure, or acute renal failure may also occur.

Fetal-Neonatal Risks

The incidence of fetal death during and immediately following an attack has decreased greatly in recent years (Creary, Williamson, & Kulkarni, 2007). Prematurity and intrauterine growth restriction (IUGR) are also associated with sickle cell disease. Fetal death is believed to be due to sickling attacks in the placenta.

Clinical Therapy

Because the woman with sickle cell disease maintains her hemoglobin levels by intense erythropoiesis, additional folic acid supplements (4 mg/day) are required. Maternal infection should be treated promptly because dehydration and fever can trigger sickling and crisis. Vaso-occlusive crisis is best treated by a perinatal team in a medical center. Proper management requires close observation and evaluation of all symptoms. The term *sickle cell crisis* should be applied only after all other possible causes for the pain are excluded (Creary et al., 2007).

Rehydration with intravenous fluids; administration of oxygen, antibiotics, and analgesics; and monitoring of fetal heart rate are important aspects of therapy. Antiembolism stockings may be used postpartum.

If vaso-occlusive crisis occurs during labor, the previous therapies are instituted and the woman is kept in a left lateral position. Oxytocics may be used if needed to promote labor. Episiotomy and outlet forceps may be recommended to shorten the second stage of labor.

Several antisickling agents are being researched, and in the future sickle cell crisis may be prevented.

NURSING CARE MANAGEMENT

Nursing Assessment and Diagnosis

The woman with sickle cell disease usually relates a history of frequent illnesses and recurrent abdominal and joint pains and is found to be extremely anemic. The woman may appear undernourished and have long, thin extremities. Ulcers are often present on her ankles. Anemia may be severe.

A diagnosis of sickle cell disease is confirmed by hemoglobin electrophoresis or a test to induce sickling in a blood sample. The woman is assessed for infection, which is associated with one third of sickle cell crises in adults. Infections most often seen during pregnancy or postpartum are pneumonia, urinary tract infections, puerperal endomyometritis, and osteomyelitis.

Fetal status is assessed during a crisis by electronic fetal monitoring. During labor, the woman's vital signs are assessed frequently and continuous fetal heart rate monitoring is initi-

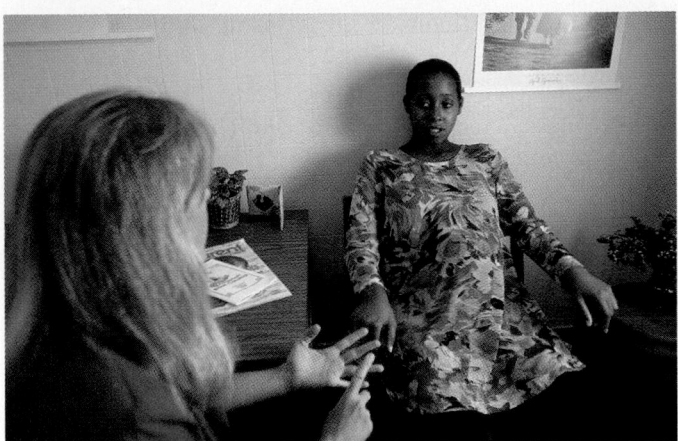

Figure 19-4 ■ Health teaching is an important part of nursing care for the pregnant woman with sickle cell anemia.

Source: Mark Richards/PhotoEdit, Inc.

ated. Compatible blood should be available for transfusion. Oxygen is administered if necessary. The woman is assessed for joint pains and other signs of sickle cell crisis.

Nursing diagnoses that might apply to the pregnant woman with sickle cell disease include the following:

- ***Acute Pain*** related to the effects of sickle cell crisis
- ***Readiness for Enhanced Knowledge*** about the need to avoid exposure to infection related to the risk of triggering a sickle cell crisis

Nursing Plan and Implementation

The nursing goal for a pregnant woman with sickle cell disease is to provide effective health teaching to help prevent a sickle cell crisis, improve the anemia, and prevent infection. The nurse teaches the woman to increase hydration, use good hygiene, avoid people with infections, seek immediate treatment for infection, and take folic acid supplements (Figure 19-4 ■). As stated earlier, folic acid is important because of its role in red blood cell production; therefore, folic acid supplements are essential. Bed rest is sometimes recommended to decrease the chance of preterm labor. Other nursing interventions are aimed at facilitating the medical therapy and alleviating anxiety through support and education.

Partners should be screened to evaluate their sickle cell status. If both partners have either sickle cell trait or sickle cell disease, genetic counseling is warranted.

Evaluation

Expected outcomes of nursing care include the following:

- The woman is able to describe her condition and identify its possible impact on her pregnancy, labor and childbirth, and postpartum period.
- The woman takes appropriate healthcare measures to avoid a sickle cell crisis.
- The woman gives birth to a healthy infant.
- The woman and her caregivers quickly identify and successfully manage any complications that arise.

Thalassemia

The thalassemias are a group of autosomal recessive disorders characterized by a defect in the synthesis of the alpha or beta chains in the hemoglobin molecule. The one most frequently encountered in the United States is β-thalassemia. Symptoms are caused by the shortened lifespan of the red blood cells, which result in active erythropoiesis in the liver, spleen, and bones. This produces hepatosplenomegaly and, sometimes, bony malformations. The thalassemias are seen most often in persons from Greece, Italy, or southern China and are also known as Mediterranean anemia and Cooley anemia. Early identification of thalassemia and preventive management avoids missed diagnosis and unnecessary treatment for iron deficiency anemia (ACOG, 2007). Prenatal genetic diagnosis is now available for this disorder.

If the woman is heterozygous for β-thalassemia, half of the beta chains are formed normally. This is β-thalassemia minor, or β-thalassemia trait. Mild anemia is usually the only symptom.

Persons born homozygous for the disease have β-thalassemia major. Because newborns have fetal hemoglobin (HbF), which does not have beta chains, no symptoms are present for several months. Once infants with β-thalassemia major start producing adult-type hemoglobin (HbA), they develop severe anemia and are dependent on transfusions from which they eventually develop iron overload. Iron chelation therapy must be instituted soon after chronic transfusions are begun because excess iron damages the liver and heart (Cunningham et al., 2010). Without chelation therapy, these children do not live past the second or third decade. Girls with the disorder are often amenorrheic and infertile.

Maternal-Fetal-Neonatal Risks

The woman with β-thalassemia minor has mild anemia with small (microcytic) red cells. This mild anemia must be distinguished from iron deficiency anemia because a woman with β-thalassemia minor should not receive iron therapy unless she is also deficient in iron. A woman with iron deficiency anemia typically has low serum iron and serum ferritin levels, whereas the woman with β-thalassemia minor has normal levels. β-thalassemia minor varies in degree of severity from extremely mild (minima) anemia, which results in a relatively smooth pregnancy, to a more symptomatic form (intermedia).

Pregnancy is rare in women with β-thalassemia major. If it does occur, the woman generally has severe anemia, needs transfusion therapy, and is at risk for congestive heart failure. These women are generally cared for by a perinatologist in a facility that can accommodate high-risk pregnancies.

Clinical Therapy

Folic acid supplements are indicated for women with thalassemia, but iron supplements are not given. Those with thalassemia intermedia and thalassemia major may need transfusion and chelation therapy. They should avoid exposure to infections and seek treatment promptly if an infection develops. Their care is similar to that of women with sickle cell anemia.

NURSING CARE MANAGEMENT

The woman with thalassemia needs to understand her disease and the possibility of transmitting it to her offspring. Thus genetic counseling may be helpful. These patients have lived with thalassemia since childhood but may have questions about its effect on pregnancy outcome and their own prognosis.

Care of the Woman with AIDS

AIDS (acquired immune deficiency syndrome), caused by the virus known as **HIV** (human immunodeficiency virus), is one of today's major health concerns. By the end of 2007, an estimated 551,932 persons in the United States were living with HIV/AIDS (Centers for Disease Control and Prevention [CDC], 2009). Male adults and adolescents are still the largest group of infected individuals (73%). Of this group, infection occurred as follows: male-to-male sexual contact (64%), intravenous (IV) drug use (16%), high-risk heterosexual contact (12%), and 7% through both male-to-male sexual contact and IV drug use. Among females with HIV/AIDS, 72% were infected through high-risk heterosexual contact and 26% were infected because of IV drug use (CDC, 2009).

Of the estimated 7181 children living with HIV/AIDS in the United States, 91% were exposed perinatally (CDC, 2009). Fortunately, the number of new pediatric AIDS cases is declining rapidly. The decline is associated with new CDC and ACOG guidelines (2008d) that emphasize:

1. Universal counseling about the risks of HIV transmission from mother to fetus
2. Recommended opt-out HIV screening of all pregnant women during each pregnancy
3. Repeat HIV testing in the third trimester in areas with high HIV prevalence rates; HIV negative individuals with high-risk behaviors; individuals with unknown HIV status at the time of labor
4. Immediate antiretroviral prophylaxis for HIV-positive pregnant women in labor and their infants following birth

In a review of the successes and challenges of preventing HIV transmission from mother-to-child internationally, Paintsil and Andiman (2009) highlight the disparities between resource-rich and poor countries. The authors maintain that prevention of transmission at a rate of less than 2% should be the goal and "resource-rich countries should be unrelenting in their efforts to provide access to HIV testing for all women . . . including antiretroviral treatment for HIV-infected women and children."

DEVELOPING CULTURAL COMPETENCE

Variations in the Prevalence Rates of New HIV Infections

The prevalence rates of individuals with HIV/AIDS infection vary significantly among races and ethnic groups: 83.7 per 100,000 in the black/African American population, 29.3 per 100,000 in the Hispanic/Latino population, and 11.5 per 100,000 in the white population (CDC, 2009).

Pathophysiology of HIV/AIDS

HIV found in blood, semen, vaginal fluid, and breast milk has been implicated in disease transmission, although the virus has been isolated in urine, tears, cerebrospinal fluid, lymph nodes, brain tissue, and bone marrow. HIV shedding has also been detected in the genital tract of women.

Once infected with the virus, the individual develops antibodies that can be detected with a reactive enzyme immunoassay (EIA) and confirmed with the Western blot test or immunofluorescence assay (IFA). A confirmed case is then categorized into one of four HIV infection stages for adults and adolescents over age 13. See Table 19-4.

TABLE 19-4 HIV Infection Stages for Adults and Adolescents over Age 13

STAGE	AIDS-DEFINING CONDITION	AND ONE OF THE FOLLOWING CD4+ T-LYMPHOCYTE FINDINGS
1	None	CD4+ T-lymphocyte count greater than or equal to 500 cells/mm^3 or CD4+ T-lymphocyte percentage of total lymphocytes greater than or equal to 29
2	None	CD4+ T-lymphocyte count 200–499 cells/mm^3 or CD4+ T-lymphocyte percentage of total lymphocytes of 14–28
3 (AIDS)	Documentation of an AIDS-defining condition supersedes CD4 count or %	CD4+ T-lymphocyte count less than 200 cells/mm^3 (without AIDS-defining condition) or CD4+ T-lymphocyte percentage of total lymphocytes of less than 14 (without AIDS-defining condition)
HIV test positive but other criteria unknown	No information available	No information available

Note: These infection stages are intended for public health surveillance only and not as a guide for clinical diagnosis. There are 24 AIDS-defining conditions ranging from multiple bacterial infections to HIV encephalopathy, Kaposi's sarcoma, and wasting syndrome.

Source: Adapted from Revised surveillance case definitions for HIV infection among adults, adolescents, and children aged less than 18 months and for HIV infection and AIDs among children aged 18 months to less than 13 years —United States, 2008. (2008, December 5). Morbidity and Weekly Report, 57*(RR10)*, 1–8.

For children aged 18 months to under 13 years, laboratory-confirmed evidence of HIV and AIDS is now required. Diagnostic confirmation of AIDS-defining conditions is no longer sufficient to confirm a case. A child less than18 months of age is categorized as definitively HIV infected if born to a mother who is HIV positive and if the child has two HIV-positive results from separate specimens (not including the umbilical cord) (Schneider et al., 2008).

Maternal Risks

Recent advances and availability of antiretroviral therapy (ART) have led HIV-positive women who adhere to their ART to consider pregnancy because of their increased life expectancy. If pregnancy is considered, priorities should focus on maintaining the health of the mother before, during, and after the pregnancy, preventing transmission to a potentially seronegative father, and preventing mother-to-child transmission. Reproductive assisted technology is one possibility along with further interventions including cesarean birth to reduce the risk of transmission to the fetus (Matthews & Mukherjee, 2009).

For women who have not had access to ART or who are noncompliant, AIDS-defining symptoms that are more common in women than men include wasting syndrome, esophageal candidiasis, and herpes simplex virus disease. Kaposi's sarcoma is rare in women. Non-AIDS-defining gynecologic conditions, such as vaginal *Candida* infections and cervical pathology, are prevalent among women at all stages of HIV infection.

Fetal-Neonatal Risks

HIV transmission can occur during pregnancy and through breast milk; however, it is believed that the majority of all infections occur during labor and birth. For HIV-infected pregnant women who receive no prophylactic medication, the rate of transmission to the newborn is about 25%. However, for HIV-infected pregnant women who receive prophylactic antiretroviral therapy, give birth by elective cesarean at 38 weeks, before rupture of membranes, and avoid breastfeeding, the rate of transmission drops to 2% or less (Panel on Treatment of HIV-Infected Pregnant Women and Prevention of Perinatal Transmission, 2010). These decreases in transmission are dramatic and impressive.

Clinical Therapy

Treatment of the HIV-Infected Mother

Early knowledge of a woman's HIV status is important for her well-being and that of her child. Thus the revised CDC screening guidelines for pregnant women state that HIV screening should be emphasized as a routine part of all prenatal care. To this end, the recommendation that all pregnant women should be tested for HIV has been strengthened while continuing to ensure that testing of pregnant women and their infants is voluntary and informed (Panel on Treatment of HIV-Infected Women, 2010). Initial testing is done using an enzyme-linked immunosorbent assay (ELISA) and confirmed with the Western blot test or immunofluorescence assay (IFA). A woman who tests positive should be counseled about the implications of the diagnosis for herself and her fetus to ensure an informed reproductive choice. The care of the woman who chooses to continue her pregnancy should focus on stabilizing the disease, preventing opportunistic infections and transmission of the virus from mother to fetus, and providing psychosocial and educational support.

Antiretroviral therapy should be recommended to all infected pregnant women regardless of whether they are symptomatic to reduce the rate of perinatal transmission. Women receiving highly active antiretroviral therapy (HAART) during pregnancy, whether for treatment or for prophylaxis, should be given a combination regimen that contains at least three drugs, and should include ZDV (Retrovir or zidovudine). Longer duration therapy is preferable to shorter duration approaches. Thus, it is best to start prophylaxis after the first trimester and no later than 28 weeks' gestation in women who do not require immediate therapy for their own health (Panel on Treatment of HIV-Infected Women, 2010). Treatment recommendations have also been developed for the mother and infant for the intrapartum and postpartum periods and take into account the therapeutic regimen they had been on prenatally. The decision about which regimen is most appropriate should be determined following discussion with the woman about the risks and benefits based on her individual HIV status.

HIV-infected women should be evaluated and treated for other sexually transmitted infections and for conditions occurring more commonly in women with HIV, such as tuberculosis, cytomegalovirus, toxoplasmosis, and cervical dysplasia. HIV-infected women with no history of hepatitis B should receive the hepatitis vaccine, which is not contraindicated prenatally, as well as the pneumococcal vaccine and an annual flu shot. In addition to routine prenatal laboratory tests, a platelet count and a complete blood count with differential should be obtained at the first prenatal visit and repeated each trimester to identify anemia, thrombocytopenia, and leukopenia, which are associated both with HIV infection and with antiviral therapy.

The woman with HIV also should be assessed regularly for serologic changes that indicate the disease is progressing. This is determined by the absolute $CD4^+$ T-lymphocyte count, which provides the number of helper T4 cells. When $CD4^+$ counts fall to $200/mm^3$ or lower, opportunistic infections such as *Pneumocystis carinii* pneumonia are more likely to develop, and prophylaxis may need to be instituted (Panel on Treatment of HIV-Infected Pregnant Women, 2010).

At each prenatal visit, asymptomatic HIV-infected women are monitored for early signs of complications, such as weight loss in the second or third trimester or fever. The woman is asked about signs of vaginal infection. Her mouth is inspected for signs of infections such as thrush (candidiasis) or hairy leukoplakia; her lungs are auscultated for signs of pneumonia; and her lymph nodes, liver, and spleen are palpated for signs of enlargement. Each trimester the woman should have a visual examination and a funduscopic examination to detect such complications as toxoplasmosis retinitis. Further discussion of therapy for the pregnant woman can be found at www.nursing.pearsonhighered.com.

AIDS in Pregnancy

A pregnancy complicated by HIV infection, even if asymptomatic, is considered high risk, and the fetus is monitored closely. Weekly nonstress testing (NST) is begun at 32 weeks' gestation, and serial ultrasounds are done to detect IUGR. Biophysical profiles are also indicated (see chapter 21 ∞). Invasive procedures such as amniocentesis are avoided when possible to prevent the contamination of a noninfected infant.

Scheduled cesarean birth is indicated for women with HIV RNA levels greater than 1000 copies/ml and for women with unknown HIV RNA levels near the time of birth whether they are on antiretroviral therapy or not. Data about the potential benefits of cesarean birth for women on combination antiretroviral therapy or prophylaxis and viral levels less than 1000 are not clear and women should be told about the risks associated with cesarean birth and the potential complications, especially because the use of combined antiretroviral therapy reduces the risk of vertical transmission of infection significantly (Panel on Treatment of HIV-Infected Women, 2010). The cesarean may be done as early as 38 weeks' gestation to decrease the risk of rupture of the membranes or onset of labor. Intrapartum care is similar to that for all pregnant women, although strict adherence to universal precautions is crucial to avoid nosocomial infection. To prevent exposure of an uninfected infant to HIV during labor and birth, invasive procedures such as vaginal examinations following rupture of the membranes, fetal scalp electrode monitoring, fetal scalp sampling, and vacuum extraction should be done only after carefully evaluating the risks and benefits.

Women who are HIV positive are at increased risk for complications such as intrapartal or postpartal hemorrhage, postpartal infection, poor wound healing, and infections of the genitourinary tract. Thus they need careful monitoring and appropriate therapy as indicated.

Following childbirth, the HIV-positive woman should be referred to a physician knowledgeable about treating individuals with HIV infection. Because of the profound implications of HIV infection for the woman, her family, the fetus/newborn, and her healthcare providers, screening is recommended for all pregnant women, and those at increased risk should be rescreened in the third trimester. These women include the following: prostitutes; women with multiple sexual partners; women whose current or previous sex partners have been bisexual, have abused IV drugs, had hemophilia, or tested positive for HIV; women who are or have been IV drug users; and women from countries where heterosexual transmission is common. In addition, clinics located in areas with a large HIV-positive population may require routine HIV screening of all prenatal patients.

Treatment of the Neonate

Following birth, all HIV-exposed infants should complete a 6-week regimen of oral zidovudine prophylactically (Panel on Treatment of HIV-Infected Pregnant Women, 2010). Testing for HIV in infants with known perinatal HIV exposure is best done at 14–21 days, 1–2 months, and 4–6 months using the HIV DNA polymerase chain reaction (PCR) or HIV RNA virologic assay. Some experts also test within 48 hours of birth because up to 30% to 40% of infected infants can be identified at that time (Working Group on Antiretroviral Therapy and Medical Management of HIV-Infected Children, 2009). If the results of the HIV DNA PCR are positive, prophylaxis should be discontinued and the newborn should be immediately referred to an HIV specialist for confirmation of the diagnosis and initiation of combination antiretroviral therapy (Panel on the Treatment of HIV-Infected Women, 2010).

In cases in which the woman does not begin antiretroviral therapy until she is in labor, prophylaxis for the newborn is provided by giving the mother an intravenous drug such as zidovudine, which crosses the placenta rapidly. The infant is also given zidovudine orally for 6 weeks to reduce the risk of transmission (Panel on the Treatment of HIV-Infected Pregnant Women, 2010). An HIV antibody positive test in the infant up to 18 months of age may indicate the presence of maternal antibodies, and so follow-up testing is required to confirm the infant's HIV status.

Progression of HIV to AIDS in infants and small children is associated with severe immune suppression (i.e., CD4 cell count less than 15%) and typically manifests as failure to thrive, hepatosplenomegaly, interstitial lymphocytic pneumonia, recurrent infections, cell-mediated immunodeficiency, evidence of Epstein-Barr virus, and neurologic abnormalities. Recurrent bacterial infections are common in children with AIDS; Kaposi's sarcoma is rare. Encephalopathy, characterized by delayed developmental milestones or the loss of acquired skills, including cognitive abilities, is found in 50% to 90% of children with AIDS. Treatments that prevent the central nervous system (CNS) effects of HIV have yet to be identified. The prognosis for an infected child remains poor (Working Group on Antiretroviral Therapy and Medical Management of HIV-Infected Children, 2009).

NURSING CARE MANAGEMENT

Nursing Assessment and Diagnosis

A woman who tests positive for HIV may be asymptomatic or may present with any of the following signs or symptoms: fatigue, anemia, malaise, progressive weight loss, lymphadenopathy, night sweats, diarrhea, fever, neurologic dysfunction, cell-mediated immunodeficiency, or evidence of Kaposi's sarcoma (purplish, reddish brown lesions, either externally or internally).

If a woman tests HIV positive or is involved in a relationship or an activity that places her at high risk, the nurse should assess the woman's knowledge level about the disease, its implications for her and her fetus, and self-care measures the woman can take.

Examples of nursing diagnoses that might apply for an HIV-positive pregnant woman include the following:

- ***Readiness for Enhanced Knowledge:*** Information About HIV/AIDS related to its long-term implications for the woman and her unborn child
- ***Risk for Infection*** related to altered immunity secondary to HIV/AIDS
- ***Compromised Family Coping*** related to the implications of a positive HIV test in one of the family members

> “I’ve been a nurse for 35 years now, and I’ve never seen anything change nursing practice more than HIV/AIDS has. Nursing students today will take universal precautions for granted because they won’t know any other way, but I can remember when we could touch more freely. I remember drying a newly born infant and stroking him—my hands warm against his skin. I remember a time when people didn’t think twice before trying to stop bleeding or give other first aid at an accident scene. I know this way is safer, but a part of me mourns what we have lost.”

Nursing Plan and Implementation

Community-Based Nursing Care

Nurses need to help women understand that HIV/AIDS is a fatal disease. HIV infection can be avoided if women avoid sharing IV drug needles and practice safe sex, including insisting that their sex partners wear a latex condom for each act of intercourse.

Women at risk for AIDS should be offered premarital and prepregnancy screening for HIV antibodies (ACOG, 2008d). They should be given clear information about the implications of a diagnosis of HIV and the importance of receiving and adhering to antiretroviral therapy, as well as living the healthiest lifestyle possible. Access to information about the disease and about the test results empowers women by enabling them to make informed decisions about their sexual activities and about becoming pregnant.

A detailed drug and sexual history of each prenatal patient is the first step in perinatal HIV/AIDS prevention. All women should be offered HIV counseling. The following are counseling guidelines for HIV testing:

- The nurse should discuss HIV testing during the normal prenatal assessment, explaining that HIV testing is recommended for all pregnant women and that they will receive an HIV test as part of the routine panel unless the woman declines (opt-out testing). No woman should be tested without her knowledge, but no written consent is required (ACOG 2008c).
- The nurse should assure the woman of confidentiality, explaining the difference between anonymity and confidentiality.
- The nurse should provide an environment that is private, comfortable, and nonjudgmental.
- The nurse should provide the woman with information about AIDS, including pathophysiology, mode of transmission of HIV, high-risk behaviors, and methods of decreasing transmission, such as practicing safe sex and not sharing needles.
- Post-test counseling should be provided. A negative test means that no HIV antibodies were found; it does not ensure that the woman has not been infected with the virus, because antibodies may not be detected for 6 weeks to 6 months after exposure.
- If test results are positive, supportive follow-up is necessary. This includes an explanation of the implications for the woman and her unborn child as well as the value of antiretroviral therapy, recommended medical therapy, follow-up of sex partners, transmission prevention, discussion of immediate posttest plans, and referral to appropriate psychologic and educational services. The nurse should tell the woman not to donate blood or blood products and not to share toothbrushes, razors, and other implements that could be contaminated with blood.

This information can be overwhelming to the woman who is HIV positive and should be provided orally and in writing. She will need more than one counseling session to absorb the information. The initial reaction may be one of shock or denial, so it is important for the nurse to allow her a little time to think and to give her empathy and support. The nurse needs to stress that being HIV positive does not mean that the woman has AIDS but that she can transmit the virus to others (by sexual contact, sharing IV drug needles, and donating blood) and to her fetus during pregnancy or childbirth or by breastfeeding. Antiretroviral therapy is now able to prolong life expectancy for HIV-positive individuals who adhere to their treatment plans and maintain as healthy a lifestyle as possible (CDC, 2008).

In monitoring the asymptomatic HIV-positive pregnant woman, the nurse should be alert for nonspecific symptoms such as fever, weight loss, fatigue, persistent candidiasis, diarrhea, cough, skin lesions, and behavior changes. Laboratory findings—such as decreased hemoglobin, hematocrit, and T4 lymphocytes; elevated erythrocyte sedimentation rate (ESR); and abnormal complete blood count, differential, and platelets—may indicate complications or progression of the disease.

Education about optimal nutrition and maintenance of wellness are important and should be reviewed frequently with the woman.

Hospital-Based Nursing Care

The Nursing Care Plan for the Woman with HIV Infection beginning on page 440 summarizes essential nursing management during the antepartum, intrapartum, and postpartum periods.

In community and hospital settings, the nurse faces the important task of taking the precautions necessary to protect staff, other patients, and families from exposure to HIV while meeting the needs of the childbearing woman with this infection.

In 1987 the CDC stated that the prevalence of AIDS and the risk of exposure faced by healthcare workers is significant enough that *precautions should be taken with all patients* (not only those with known HIV infection), especially in dealing with blood and body fluids. These practices are now called *standard precautions.*

Nurses who deal with childbearing families are exposed to blood and body fluids and should pay careful attention to the CDC guidelines, which are addressed in introductory nursing courses in preparation for clinical practice. Protocols have been established for postexposure treatment of caregivers who experience a needle stick or exposure to the body fluids of a person with HIV or a person whose HIV status is not known. The effectiveness of such therapy, using a combined drug approach, depends on starting therapy rapidly. Thus such exposure should be reported immediately.

NURSING CARE PLAN The Woman with HIV Infection

INTERVENTION	RATIONALE
1. Nursing Diagnosis: Risk for Infection related to inadequate defenses (leukopenia, suppressed inflammatory response) secondary to HIV-positive status **Goal:** Patient will remain free of opportunistic infection during the course of pregnancy.	
■ Obtain a complete health history and physical examination during first prenatal visit.	■ A complete health history will help determine risk factors for the development of opportunistic infections, and a physical examination will assist in identifying any underlying problem symptoms or illnesses that may compromise the pregnancy or complicate the treatment of HIV.
■ Educate the woman as to the signs and symptoms of infection.	■ Early recognition of signs and symptoms of infection will allow for immediate treatment, which may decrease the severity of the infection. Signs and symptoms of infections include fever, weight loss, fatigue, persistent candidiasis, diarrhea, cough, and skin lesions (Kaposi's sarcoma and hairy leukoplakia in the mouth).
■ Obtain nutritional history and monitor weight gain at each prenatal visit.	■ The HIV-infected woman needs to maintain optimal nutritional intake. A compromised nutritional status may affect maternal and fetal well-being. Depleted reserves of protein and iron may decrease the patient's ability to fight infection, thereby making her more susceptible to opportunistic infections.
Collaborative: Monitor the absolute $CD4^+$ T-lymphocyte count, erythrocyte sedimentation rate (ESR), complete blood count (CBC) with differential, and hemoglobin and hematocrit (H & H) at each prenatal visit.	■ Laboratory results provide information about the woman's immune system and the potential for disease progression. Opportunistic infections are more likely to occur when the $CD4^+$ T-lymphocyte count drops below a level of 200/mm^3. ESR can rise above 20 mm/hr with anemia and with acute and chronic inflammation. CBC with differential and platelet count helps identify anemia, thrombocytopenia, and leukopenia. H & H can also identify anemia.
EXPECTED OUTCOME:	Patient will remain free of opportunistic infection as evidenced by $CD4^+$ T-lymphocyte count within normal limits; no complaints of chills, fever, or sore throat; normal weight gain throughout pregnancy.
2. Nursing Diagnosis: Readiness for Enhanced Therapeutic Regimen Management related to an expressed desire for information a about HIV/AIDS and its long-term implications for the woman, her unborn child, and her family **Goal:** The patient and her family will verbalize the importance of following her medication regimen and of regular prenatal care.	
■ Assess the patient's and family's level of understanding of HIV infection, its modes of transmission, and the long-term implications.	■ Knowledge of the woman's (and her family's) level of understanding about her HIV infection forms a starting point for further health teaching.
■ Explain the risks of mother-to-child transmission of HIV infection.	■ In untreated women the risk of transmission is 25%. That risk can be reduced to less than 2% with the availability of antiretroviral therapy, the use of cesarean birth when indicated, and formula-feeding rather than breastfeeding.
■ Describe antiretroviral therapy (ART). Include the regimen prescribed, its purposes, and the procedures for taking it.	■ ART therapy approaches vary based on the health status of the individual woman and whether she is currently on ART therapy. Generally it includes oral Zidovudine (ZDV) daily, IV ZDV during labor and until birth, and ZDV therapy for the infant for 6 weeks following birth.
■ Discuss signs the woman should be alert for, including fever, fatigue, weight loss, cough, skin lesions, and behavior changes.	■ These symptoms may indicate that the woman is developing symptomatic loss, persistent candidiasis, diarrhea, HIV infection.
EXPECTED OUTCOME:	Woman will actively seek information about her condition, her treatment regimen, and her pregnancy and will cooperate with her caregivers.

NURSING CARE PLAN The Woman with HIV Infection continued

INTERVENTION	RATIONALE
3. Diagnosis: Compromised Family Coping related to the implications of positive maternal HIV status on fetal/neonatal well-being and long-term family functioning **Goal:** Family is able to manage stressors related to the maternal diagnosis.	
■ Assess ability and readiness of family to learn about HIV and its long-term implications.	■ Readiness is a key element in the teaching-learning process.
■ Provide woman and her family with accurate, reliable information about her diagnosis, its prognosis for her and for her baby, and the immediate and long-term implications for her care.	■ Fear and anxiety will lessen when the woman and her family understand her health status and the implications of the HIV diagnosis and can then plan for the future.
■ Assess interactions between the woman and her family. Be alert for potentially destructive behaviors.	■ If the HIV diagnosis was not expected, the couple may have to deal with issues of blame, concerns about mortality, and worries about the status of the baby. If the HIV diagnosis was known, concerns may focus on fetal/neonatal well-being. In either case, negative responses can lead to destructive behaviors.
■ Assist family in realistically identifying the needs of the woman and family unit.	■ Once needs are identified realistically, it is possible to plan interventions to meet the needs.
Collaborative: Explore available community resources and family support systems.	■ Because HIV is a long-term condition, the family may require ongoing assistance.

EXPECTED OUTCOME: Family members actively participate in the treatment plan, are involved in planning for labor and birth in light of a positive HIV status, and are able to express unresolved feelings about the diagnosis.

Health Promotion Education

The psychologic implications of HIV/AIDS for the childbearing family are staggering. The woman is faced with the knowledge that she and her newborn, if infected, may have a decreased life expectancy, although, as noted earlier, women who adhere to antiretroviral therapy are living longer, healthier lives. If her infant is not infected, the mother may face the possibility that others will raise her child. She may have feelings of fear, helplessness, anger, and isolation. If she shares her diagnosis with others, she may face rejection and condemnation. The couple must deal with the impact of the illness on the partner, who may or may not be infected, and on other children. Dealing with the tasks and responsibilities of a newborn may be especially difficult if the woman is physically depleted or if she is trying to come to grips with the long-term implications of her condition.

The nonjudgmental, supportive nurse plays an essential role in preserving confidentiality and the patient's right to privacy. In addition, the nurse can help ensure that the woman receives complete, accurate information about her condition and ways she might cope. This usually involves a referral to social services for follow-up care.

Evaluation

Expected outcomes of nursing care include the following:

- The woman discusses the implications of her positive HIV antibody screen (or diagnosis of AIDS), its implications for herself and her unborn child, the method of transmission, and treatment options.
- The woman uses information about referral to social services (or other agency) for follow-up assistance and counseling.
- The woman begins to verbalize her feelings about her condition and its implications in an atmosphere she finds supportive.

Care of the Woman with Heart Disease

A healthy woman with a normal heart has adequate cardiac reserve to adjust easily to the demands of pregnancy. The woman with heart disease, however, has decreased cardiac reserve, making it more difficult for her heart to accommodate the higher workload of pregnancy.

Heart disease ranks fourth after hypertension, hemorrhage, and infection as a cause of maternal mortality. Currently, cardiac disease complicates about 1% of pregnancies. Although rheumatic heart disease used to predominate, at least half of all cases of heart disease currently encountered during pregnancy are caused by congenital heart defects (Curry, Swan, & Steer, 2009). Other less common causes of heart disease in pregnancy include Marfan syndrome, peripartum cardiomyopathy, and Eisenmenger syndrome. All can cause significant maternal mortality. Mitral valve prolapse is usually asymptomatic but is addressed here because of its frequent occurrence during pregnancy.

Congenital Heart Defects

Congenital heart defects have become a more common finding in pregnant women as improved surgical techniques enable females born with heart defects to live to childbearing age. The exact pathology depends on the specific defect. Congenital defects most often seen in pregnant women include tetralogy of Fallot, atrial septal defect, ventricular septal defect, patent ductus arteriosus, and coarctation of the aorta. When surgical repair can be accomplished with no remaining evidence of organic heart disease, pregnancy may be undertaken with confidence. In such cases, antibiotic prophylaxis is recommended to prevent subacute bacterial endocarditis at the time of birth. When congenital heart disease is associated with cyanosis, whether the defect was originally uncorrected or the correction failed to relieve the cyanosis, the woman should be counseled that the risk to both her and the fetus would be higher than in the general population. She also needs to know that there is an increased risk that the baby will inherit the disorder.

Rheumatic Heart Disease

Rheumatic heart disease has declined rapidly in the last four decades because of prompt identification of pharyngeal infections caused by group A β-hemolytic streptococcus and the availability of penicillin for treatment. Rheumatic fever, which may develop in untreated streptococcal infections, is an inflammatory connective tissue disease that can involve the heart, joints, central nervous system (CNS), skin, and subcutaneous tissue. When the heart is affected, mitral valve stenosis is the most common and serious lesion. Aortic valve involvement, manifested by aortic insufficiency, is the second most common problem. The tricuspid and pulmonic valves are rarely affected.

The increased blood volume of pregnancy, coupled with the pregnant woman's need for increased cardiac output, stresses the heart of a woman with mitral valve stenosis. She may develop dyspnea, orthopnea, and pulmonary edema and is at increased risk for congestive heart failure (CHF). Even the woman who has no symptoms at the onset of pregnancy is at risk for CHF.

Marfan Syndrome

Marfan syndrome is an autosomal dominant disorder of connective tissue in which there may be serious cardiovascular involvement—usually dissection or rupture of the aorta. Because there may be a fivefold increase in morbidity during pregnancy, a pregnant woman with Marfan syndrome needs very careful cardiovascular assessment and counseling about her prognosis for pregnancy (Pacini et al., 2009). Because of its inheritance pattern, there is a 50% chance that the disease will be passed on to offspring.

Peripartum Cardiomyopathy

Peripartum cardiomyopathy is a dysfunction of the left ventricle that occurs in the last month of pregnancy or the first 5 months postpartum in a woman with no previous history of heart disease. This is a relatively rare but serious condition, which occurs in 1 in 3000 to 4000 live births. Early reports suggested a mortality rate of nearly 50%, but more recent studies indicate a 0%–5% rate in the United States (Ramaraj & Sorrell, 2009). The symptoms are related to CHF: dyspnea, orthopnea, chest pain, palpitations, weakness, and edema. The cause is unknown, although symptoms are often attributable to chronic hypertension, mitral stenosis, obesity, or viral myocarditis. The condition usually presents with anemia and infection; consequently, treatment focuses on underlying abnormalities. Digitalis, diuretics, vasodilators, anticoagulants, sodium restriction, and strict bed rest are often part of the treatment. Peripartum cardiomyopathy may resolve with bed rest as the heart gradually returns to normal size. Subsequent pregnancy is strongly discouraged because the disease tends to recur during pregnancy.

Eisenmenger Syndrome

Eisenmenger syndrome is not a single congenital defect, but a complication that can develop as a result of other cardiac lesions causing left-to-right shunting (as with atrial septal defects or ventricular septal defects). This shunting can result in progressive pulmonary hypertension. As pulmonary vascular resistance increases, the shunting becomes bidirectional or reverses to right-to-left shunting. This condition cannot be corrected surgically, and the maternal mortality rate remains as high as 40%, unchanged for the past 50 years (Makaryus, Forouzesh, & Johnson, 2006).

Mitral Valve Prolapse

Mitral valve prolapse (MVP) is a usually asymptomatic condition commonly found in women of childbearing age. The condition is more common in women than in men and seems to be inherited. In MVP, the mitral valve leaflets tend to prolapse into the left atrium during ventricular systole because the chordae tendineae that support them are long and thin. As a result, some mitral regurgitation may occur. On auscultation a midsystolic click and a late systolic murmur are heard.

Women with MVP usually tolerate pregnancy well, and the prognosis is excellent. Most women require assurance that they can continue with normal activities. A few women experience symptoms such as palpitations, chest pain, and dyspnea, which are usually due to arrhythmias. They are often treated with propranolol hydrochloride (Inderal). Limiting caffeine intake also helps decrease palpitations. Antibiotic prophylaxis is no longer recommended (Bonow et al., 2008).

Clinical Therapy

The primary goal of medical management is early diagnosis and ongoing treatment of the woman with cardiac disease. Auscultation of heart sounds along with a good history and physical are the first steps to diagnosis. Echocardiogram, chest x-ray, electrocardiogram, and sometimes cardiac catheterization may be necessary for establishing the type and severity of the heart disease. The severity of heart disease can also be determined by the individual's ability to perform ordinary physical activity. The following classification of functional capacity for those with cardiac disease has been standardized by the Criteria Committee of the New York Heart Association (1994):

- ***Class I.*** Individuals with cardiac disease but with no resulting limitation of physical activity and no symptoms of cardiac insufficiency. Ordinary physical activity causes no undue fatigue, dyspnea, or palpitations; anginal pain is not present.
- ***Class II.*** Individuals with cardiac disease that results in slight limitation of physical activity. They are comfortable at

rest but ordinary physical activity causes fatigue, dyspnea, palpitation, or anginal pain.

- *Class III.* Individuals with cardiac disease that results in marked limitation of physical activity. They are comfortable at rest but less than ordinary physical activity results in fatigue, dyspnea, palpitation, or anginal pain.
- *Class IV.* Individuals with cardiac disease that results in the inability to carry on any physical activity without experiencing discomfort. Even at rest, they may experience symptoms of cardiac insufficiency or anginal pain; discomfort increases with any physical activity.

Women in classes I and II usually experience a normal pregnancy and have few complications, whereas those in classes III and IV are at risk for more severe complications, which may affect both maternal and fetal outcomes. Preconception counseling is important for these women to optimize maternal and fetal outcomes.

Because anemia increases the work of the heart, it should be diagnosed early and treated. Infection also increases the cardiac workload, so even minor infections should be treated thoroughly. To reduce the risk of pyelonephritis, monthly screening for asymptomatic bacteriuria is indicated, with antibiotic therapy as needed.

As pregnancy progresses, it is important to minimize cardiac workload and promote tissue perfusion. Depending on the specific lesion, the woman's activity and weight gain may need to be limited (Bonow et al., 2008).

Drug Therapy

Besides the iron and vitamin supplements prescribed during pregnancy, the pregnant woman with heart disease may need additional drug therapy to maintain health. Antibiotic prophylaxis is not indicated for uncomplicated vaginal or cesarean birth unless infection is suspected. If the woman develops coagulation problems, the anticoagulant heparin may be used. Heparin offers the greatest safety to the fetus because it does not cross the placenta. The thiazide diuretics and furosemide (Lasix) may be used to treat congestive heart failure if it develops. Digitalis glycosides and common antiarrhythmic drugs may be used to treat cardiac failure and arrhythmias. These agents do cross the placenta but have no reported teratogenic effect; however, they have not been adequately studied to establish their safety in pregnancy (Bonow et al., 2008).

Labor and Childbirth

Spontaneous natural labor with adequate pain relief is usually recommended for patients in classes I and II. Special attention should be given to the prompt recognition and treatment of any signs of heart failure (Figure 19-5 ■). Those in classes III and IV may need to be hospitalized before onset of labor for cardiovascular stabilization. They may also require invasive cardiac monitoring during labor.

Vaginal birth with low-dose regional analgesia (epidural) is recommended with the use of forceps or vacuum assistance if necessary to limit maternal pushing. The regional analgesia helps decrease maternal cardiac output and oxygen demand by reducing pain and related maternal anxiety (Burt & Durbridge, 2009). Cesarean birth is usually used only if fetal or maternal indications exist, not on the basis of heart disease alone.

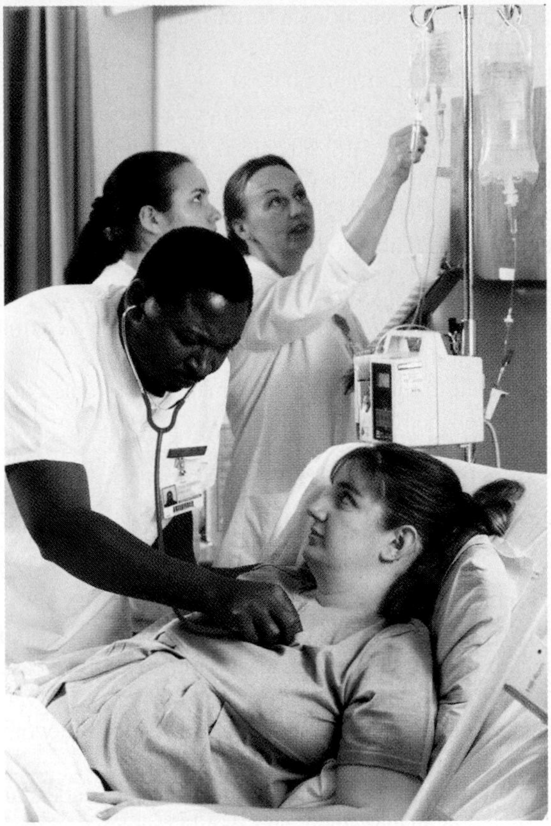

Figure 19-5 ■ When a woman with heart disease begins labor, the nursing students and instructor caring for her monitor her closely for signs of congestive heart failure.

Source: Vicky Flanagan, RN, BSN/Pearson Education.

NURSING CARE MANAGEMENT

Nursing Assessment and Diagnosis

The nurse assesses the stress of pregnancy on the functional capacity of the heart during every antepartal visit. The nurse notes the category of functional capacity assigned to the woman; takes the woman's pulse, respirations, and blood pressure; and compares them to the normal values expected during pregnancy and to the woman's previous values. The nurse then determines the woman's activity level, including rest, and any changes in the pulse and respirations that have occurred since previous visits. The nurse also identifies and evaluates other factors that would increase strain on the heart. These might include anemia, infection, anxiety, lack of support system, and household and career demands.

The following symptoms, if they are progressive, are indicative of CHF, the heart's signal of its decreased ability to meet the demands of pregnancy:

- Cough (frequent, with or without hemoptysis)
- Dyspnea (progressive, upon exertion)
- Edema (progressive, generalized, including extremities, face, eyelids)

- Heart murmurs (heard on auscultation)
- Palpitations
- Rales (auscultated in lung bases)

Progressiveness of the cycle is the critical factor, because some of these same symptoms are seen to a minor degree in a pregnancy without cardiac problems.

Nursing diagnoses that might apply to the pregnant woman with heart disease include the following:

- ***Decreased Cardiac Output:*** Easy fatigability
- ***Impaired Gas Exchange*** related to pulmonary edema secondary to cardiac decompensation
- ***Fear*** related to the effects of the maternal cardiac condition on fetal well-being

Nursing Plan and Implementation

Nursing care is directed toward maintaining a balance between cardiac reserve and cardiac workload.

Antepartum Period

Nursing actions are designed to meet the physiologic and psychosocial needs of the pregnant woman with heart disease. The priority of nursing actions varies according to the severity of the disease process and the individual needs of the woman as determined by nursing assessment.

The woman and her family should thoroughly understand her condition and its management and should recognize signs of potential complications. This will increase their understanding and decrease anxiety. When the nurse provides explanations, uses printed material, and offers frequent opportunities to ask questions and discuss concerns, the woman is better able to meet her own healthcare needs and seek assistance appropriately.

As part of health teaching, the nurse explains the purposes of the dietary and activity changes that are required. A diet is instituted that is high in iron, protein, and essential nutrients but low in sodium, with adequate calories to ensure normal weight gain. Such a diet best meets the nutrition needs of the patient with cardiac disease. Excessive weight gain is avoided because it taxes the heart. To help preserve her cardiac reserves, the woman may need to restrict her activities. In addition, 8 to 10 hours of sleep and frequent daily rest periods are essential. The nurse can encourage the woman to rest in the side-lying position to promote optimal placental perfusion. Because upper respiratory infections may tax the heart and lead to decompensation, the woman must avoid contact with sources of infection and report symptoms of infection immediately.

During the first half of pregnancy, the woman is seen approximately every 2 weeks to assess cardiac status. During the second half of pregnancy, the woman is seen weekly. These assessments are especially important between weeks 28 and 30, when the blood volume reaches maximum amounts. If symptoms of cardiac decompensation occur, prompt medical intervention is indicated to correct the cardiac problem.

Heart Disease and Pregnancy

Intrapartum Period

Labor and birth exert tremendous stress on the woman and her fetus. This stress could be fatal to the fetus of a woman with cardiac disease because the fetus may be receiving an inadequate oxygen and blood supply. Thus the intrapartum care of a woman with cardiac disease is aimed at reducing the amount of physical exertion and accompanying fatigue.

The nurse evaluates maternal vital signs frequently to determine the woman's response to labor. A pulse rate greater than 100 beats per minute or respirations greater than 24 per minute may indicate beginning cardiac decompensation, especially if accompanied by dyspnea, and require further evaluation. The nurse also auscultates the woman's lungs frequently for rales and carefully observes for other signs of developing decompensation.

To ensure cardiac emptying and adequate oxygenation, the nurse encourages the laboring woman to assume either a semi-Fowler's position with lateral tilt or side-lying position with her head and shoulders elevated. Oxygen by mask, diuretics to reduce fluid retention, sedatives and analgesics, prophylactic antibiotics, and digitalis may also be used as indicated by the woman's status.

The nurse remains with the woman to support her. It is essential that the nurse keep the woman and her family informed of labor progress and management plans, collaborating with them to fulfill their wishes for the birth experience as much as possible. The nurse needs to maintain an atmosphere of calm to lessen the anxiety of the woman and her family.

Continuous electronic fetal monitoring is used to provide ongoing assessment of the fetus's response to labor. To prevent overexertion and the accompanying fatigue, the nurse encourages the woman to sleep and relax between contractions and provides her with emotional support and encouragement. During pushing, the nurse encourages the woman to use shorter, more moderate open glottis pushing (see chapter 24 ∞), with complete relaxation between pushes. The nurse monitors vital signs closely during the second stage.

Postpartum Period

The postpartum period is a significant time for the woman with cardiac disease. After birth, the intra-abdominal pressure and the venous pressure are reduced, the splanchnic vessels engorge, and blood flow to the heart increases. As extravascular fluid returns to the bloodstream for excretion, cardiac output and blood volume increase. This physiologic adaptation places great strain on the heart and may lead to decompensation, especially in the first 48 hours postpartum.

So that the healthcare team can detect any possible problems, the woman may remain in the hospital longer than the low-risk woman postpartally. Her vital signs are monitored frequently, and she is assessed for signs of decompensation. She stays in the semi-Fowler's or side-lying position, with her head and shoulders elevated, and begins a gradual, progressive activity program. Appropriate diet and stool softeners facilitate bowel movement without undue strain.

The postpartum nurse gives the woman opportunities to discuss her birth experience and helps her deal with any feelings or concerns that cause her distress. The nurse also encourages maternal-infant attachment by providing frequent opportunities for the mother to interact with her child.

Because there is no evidence that cardiac output is compromised during lactation, the only concern about breastfeeding for women with cardiovascular disease is related to medications that the mother may be taking. These must be evaluated for their ability to pass into the milk and for any effect of the drug on lactation. The nurse can assist the breastfeeding mother to a comfortable side-lying position with her head moderately elevated or to a semi-Fowler's position. To conserve the mother's energy, the nurse should position the newborn at the breast and be available to burp the baby and reposition him or her at the other breast. The nurse can also encourage family members to provide the new mother with support and assistance as needed to help her avoid becoming fatigued.

In addition to providing the normal postpartum discharge teaching, the nurse stresses that follow-up for the new mother is imperative. Moreover, the nurse should ensure that the woman and her family understand the signs of possible problems resulting from her heart disease or from other postpartum complications. For women with heart disease, postpartum complications such as hemorrhage, thromboembolism, anemia, and infection pose a real threat and may even precipitate heart failure.

The nurse plans with the woman an activity schedule that is gradual, progressive, and appropriate to her needs and home environment. The nurse provides appropriate health teaching, including information about resumption of sexual activity and contraception. Visiting nurse or homemaker assistance referrals may be necessary, depending on the woman's status.

Evaluation

Expected outcomes of nursing care include the following:

- The woman is able to discuss her condition and its possible impact on her pregnancy, labor and birth, and the postpartum period.
- The woman participates in developing an appropriate health-care regimen and follows it throughout her pregnancy.
- The woman gives birth to a healthy infant.
- The woman does not develop congestive heart failure, thromboembolism, or infection.
- The woman is able to identify signs and symptoms of possible postpartum complications.
- The woman is able to care effectively for her newborn infant.

Other Medical Conditions and Pregnancy

A woman with a preexisting medical condition should be aware of the possible impact of pregnancy on her condition, as well as the impact of her condition on the outcome of her pregnancy. Table 19-5 discusses some of the less common medical conditions vis-à-vis pregnancy.

TABLE 19-5 Less Common Medical Conditions and Pregnancy

BRIEF DESCRIPTION	MATERNAL IMPLICATIONS	FETAL/NEONATAL IMPLICATIONS
Asthma		
Asthma, an obstructive lung condition, is the most common respiratory disease found in pregnancy, complicating approximately 8% of all pregnancies (Schatz & Dombrowski, 2009). Typical symptoms include wheezing, dyspnea, and episodic coughing. A severe asthmatic attack may require hospitalization. It is managed by long-term comprehensive drug therapy to prevent airway inflammation, combined with drug treatment to manage attacks or exacerbations. Patient education focuses on triggers (such as cold air, dust, smoke, exercise, food additives), methods of prevention, and treatment options.	The severity of asthma may improve, worsen, or remain unchanged during pregnancy. The mechanisms associated with these variations remain undefined; however, poor asthma control is associated with increased maternal and neonatal complications, most likely from poor adherence to the treatment regime. Maternal complications include preeclampsia, growth restriction, and preterm birth. Asthma management during labor and delivery focuses on maintenance of adequate hydration and analgesia as well as continuing asthma medications (ACOG, 2008b).	Prematurity and low birth weights are more common among the infants of women who have asthma (Schatz & Dombrowski, 2009). The goal of therapy is to prevent maternal exacerbations because even a mild exacerbation can cause severe hypoxia-related complications in the fetus. If an exacerbation occurs, it should be managed in the same way as for a nonpregnant woman because the asthma drugs used are less of a threat to the fetus than a serious asthma attack (ACOG, 2008b).
Epilepsy		
Chronic disorder characterized by seizures; may be idiopathic or secondary to other conditions, such as head injury, metabolic and nutritional disorders such as phenylketonuria (PKU) or vitamin B_6 deficiency, encephalitis, neoplasms, or circulatory interferences. Treated with anticonvulsants.	Vast majority of pregnancies in women with seizure disorders are uneventful and have an excellent outcome. Women with more frequent seizures before pregnancy may have exacerbations during pregnancy, but this may be related to nausea and vomiting, lack of cooperation with drug regimen, or sleep deprivation. During pregnancy the woman should continue to be treated with the medication that best controls her seizures. Folic acid therapy should be started prior to conception if possible. Folic acid and vitamin D are indicated throughout pregnancy (Tomson & Battino, 2009).	Certain anticonvulsant medications are associated with increased incidence of congenital anomalies, especially cleft lip and heart defects, although the incidence has decreased in recent years. The lowest dose of a single effective medication is the goal of treatment to decrease the potential for fetal anomalies. Multiple medications and valproic acid should also be avoided for women planning pregnancy when possible (Tomson & Battino, 2009).

(continued)

TABLE 19-5 Less Common Medical Conditions and Pregnancy continued

BRIEF DESCRIPTION	MATERNAL IMPLICATIONS	FETAL/NEONATAL IMPLICATIONS
Hepatitis B		
Hepatitis B, caused by the hepatitis B virus (HBV), is a major, growing health problem. Groups at risk include those from areas with a high incidence (primarily developing countries), illegal intravenous (IV) drug users, prostitutes, homosexuals, those with multiple sex partners, or occupational exposure to blood, although many infected people have no identifiable source of infection. HBV transmission is blood borne, primarily sexually and perinatally transmitted. Because of the dramatic increase and the difficulty of vaccinating high-risk individuals before they become infected, the CDC now recommends (1) testing all pregnant women for the presence of hepatitis B surface antigen and prophylactic treatment for all infants born to women who are HBsAG-positive or whose status is unknown; (2) routine infant vaccination; (3) vaccination of children and adolescents through age 18 years who have not been vaccinated; (4) vaccination of unvaccinated adults who are at risk for hepatitis B (Libbus & Phillips, 2009).	Hepatitis B does not usually affect the course of pregnancy. However, chronic HBV carriers have a great potential for infecting others when exposure to blood and body fluids occurs. In addition, chronic carriers may develop long-term sequelae, such as chronic liver disease and liver cancer. Approximately 4000 to 5000 deaths are caused annually by liver disease associated with chronic HBV infection. It is now recommended that all pregnant women be tested for the presence of hepatitis B surface antigen (HBsAg). A woman who is negative may be given the hepatitis vaccine.	Perinatal transmission most often occurs at or near the time of childbirth. More important, the risk of becoming a chronic carrier of the HBV is inversely related to the age of the individual at the time of initial infection. Therefore, infants infected perinatally have the highest risk of becoming chronically infected if not treated. Recommendations now include routine vaccination of all neonates born to HBsAg-negative women and immunoprophylaxis to all newborns of HBsAg-positive women (Libbus & Phillips, 2009).
Hyperthyroidism (thyrotoxicosis)		
Enlarged, overactive thyroid gland; increased T_4: thyroxine-binding globulin (TBG) ratio and increased basal metabolic rate (BMR). Symptoms include muscle wasting, tachycardia, excessive sweating, and exophthalmos. Treatment by antithyroid drug propylthiouracil (PTU) while monitoring free T_4 levels. Surgery used only if drug intolerance exists.	Mild hyperthyroidism is not dangerous. Increased incidence of preeclampsia and postpartum hemorrhage if not well controlled. Serious risk related to thyroid storm characterized by high fever, tachycardia, sweating, and congestive heart failure. Now occurs rarely. When diagnosed during pregnancy, may be transient or permanent.	Neonatal thyrotoxicosis is rare. Even low doses of antithyroid drug in mother may produce a mild fetal/neonatal hypothyroidism; higher dose may produce a goiter or mental deficiencies. Fetal loss not increased in euthyroid women. If untreated, rates of abortion, intrauterine death, and stillbirth increase. Breastfeeding contraindicated for women on antithyroid medication because it is excreted in the milk (may be tried by woman on low dose if neonatal T_4 levels are monitored).
Hypothyroidism		
Characterized by inadequate thyroid secretions (decreased T_4: TBG ratio), elevated thyroid-stimulating hormone (TSH), lowered BMR, and enlarged thyroid gland (goiter). Symptoms include lack of energy, excessive weight gain, cold intolerance, dry skin, and constipation. Treated by thyroxine replacement therapy.	Long-term replacement therapy usually continues at same dosage during pregnancy as before. Weekly nonstress test (NST) after 35 weeks' gestation.	If mother untreated, fetal loss 50%; high risk of congenital goiter or true cretinism. Therefore, newborns are screened for T_4 level. Mild TSH elevations present little risk because TSH does not cross the placenta.
Maternal Phenylketonuria (PKU) (hyperphenylalaninemia)		
Inherited recessive single gene anomaly causing a deficiency of the liver enzyme needed to convert the amino acid phenylalanine to tyrosine, resulting in high serum levels of phenylalanine. Brain damage and intellectual disability (mental retardation) occur if not treated early.	Low phenylalanine diet is mandatory before conception and during pregnancy. The woman should be counseled that her children will either inherit the disease or be carriers, depending on the zygosity of the father for the disease. Treatment at a PKU center is recommended.	Risk to fetus if maternal treatment not begun preconception. In untreated women increased incidence of fetal mental retardation, microcephaly, congenital heart defects, and growth retardation. Fetal phenylalanine levels are approximately 50% higher than maternal levels.
Multiple Sclerosis		
Neurologic disorder characterized by destruction of the myelin sheath of nerve fibers. The condition occurs primarily in young adults, more commonly in females, and is marked by periods of remission; progresses to marked physical disability in 10 to 20 years.	Exacerbation rate is reduced during the second and third trimester but increased during the 3 months following birth. Exclusive breastfeeding has recently been reported to reduce postpartum exacerbation (Franklin & Tremlett, 2009). Rest is important; help with child care should be planned. Uterine contraction strength is not diminished, but because sensation is frequently lessened, labor may be almost painless.	Some evidence for slightly lower birth weight infants (3%–4%). Increased evidence of a genetic predisposition. Therefore, reproductive counseling is recommended.
Rheumatoid Arthritis		
Chronic inflammatory disease believed to be caused by a genetically influenced antigen-antibody reaction. Symptoms include fatigue, low-grade fever, pain and swelling of joints, morning stiffness, pain on movement. Treated with salicylates, physical therapy, and rest. Corticosteroids used cautiously if not responsive to above.	Usually there is remission of rheumatoid arthritis symptoms during pregnancy, often with a relapse postpartum. Anemia may be present due to blood loss from salicylate therapy. Mother needs extra rest, particularly to relieve weight-bearing joints, but needs to continue range-of-motion exercises. If in remission, may stop medication during pregnancy.	Woman taking prednisone during pregnancy give birth slightly earlier (38 weeks vs. 39 weeks) and have corresponding lower birth weights (de Man et al., 2009).

TABLE 19-5 Less Common Medical Conditions and Pregnancy continued

BRIEF DESCRIPTION	MATERNAL IMPLICATIONS	FETAL/NEONATAL IMPLICATIONS
Systemic Lupus Erythematosus (SLE)		
Chronic autoimmune collagen disease, characterized by exacerbations and remissions; symptoms range from characteristic rash to inflammation and pain in joints, fever, nephritis, depression, cranial nerve disorders, and peripheral neuropathies.	SLE during pregnancy needs to be actively managed with careful surveillance of blood pressure, proteinuria, and placental blood flow. SLE medications may be necessary to control exacerbations and lupus flare. Preeclampsia, prematurity, and fetal growth restriction are common complications. Women with severe disease may be counseled to avoid pregnancy (Ruiz-Irastorza & Khamashta, 2009).	Increased incidence of spontaneous abortion, stillbirth, prematurity, intrauterine growth restriction (IUGR), and neonatal lupus. Neonatal lupus is characterized by a photosensitive skin rash, thrombocytopenia, neutropenia, or anemia, all of which resolve by about 6 months of age. Complete congenital heart block is the most serious complication of SLE, typically diagnosed in utero. When diagnosed, the mother is given corticosteroids that cross the placenta and decrease fetal heart inflammation. The prognosis for these infants varies based on the extent of the cardiac damage. An increased rate of learning disabilities is reported in these children (Tincani et al., 2006).
Tuberculosis (TB)		
Tuberculosis (TB) is a major health problem. Two billion people (approximately one third of the population of the world) carry the TB bacteria. Worldwide more women die from TB than from any other infection (Nhan-Chang & Jones, 2010). Infection is caused by *Mycobacterium tuberculosis;* inflammatory process causes destruction of lung tissue, increased sputum, and coughing. Associated primarily with poverty and malnutrition, 80% of new cases are found in developing countries primarily in Asia and Africa. In the United States the majority of cases occur in foreign-born people (Nhan-Chang & Jones, 2010).Treated with isoniazid and either ethambutol or rifampin, or both.	The incidence of pregnancy complications may be higher in women with TB. TB skin test screening is recommended for women in high-risk groups (healthcare workers; foreign-born women from countries with a high TB risk; women who have had known contact with infectious person, those who are HIV infected, alcoholics, or illicit drug users; women living or working in homeless shelters; prisoners and detainees [Cunningham et al., 2010]). If TB is inactive due to prior treatment, isoniazid therapy is delayed until the postpartum period unless the woman is HIV positive, has close contact with a person with active TB, or has had a skin test convert to positive within the last 2 years. For those women, isoniazid is started during pregnancy (Nhan-Chang & Jones, 2010). Women with active TB are treated with isoniazid, rifampin, and ethambutol during pregnancy (Cunningham et al., 2010). Extra rest and limited contact with others is required until disease becomes inactive.	If maternal TB is inactive, mother may breastfeed and care for her infant. If TB is active, newborn should not have direct contact with mother until she is noninfectious. Isoniazid crosses the placenta, but most studies show no teratogenic effects. Rifampin crosses the placenta. Possibility of harmful effects is still being studied.

FOCUS YOUR STUDY

- Almost any health problem that a person can have when not pregnant can coexist with pregnancy. Some problems, such as anemias, may be exacerbated by pregnancy. Others, such as collagen disease, may go into temporary remission with pregnancy. Regardless of the health problem, careful health care is needed throughout pregnancy to improve the outcome for mother and fetus.
- The diagnosis of high-risk pregnancy can shock an expectant couple. Providing emotional support, teaching about the condition and prognosis, and educating for self-care are important nursing measures that help the patient cope.
- Substance abuse (either drugs or alcohol) not only is detrimental to the mother's health but also may have profound lasting effects on the fetus.
- The key point in the care of the pregnant woman with diabetes is scrupulous maternal plasma glucose control. This is best achieved by home blood glucose monitoring, multiple daily insulin injections, regular exercise, and a

careful diet. To reduce incidence of congenital anomalies and other problems in the newborn, the woman should be euglycemic (have a normal blood glucose) throughout the pregnancy. Women with diabetes, even more than most other patients, need to be educated about their conditions and involved with their own care.

- Anemia indicates inadequate levels of hemoglobin (Hb) in the blood. Anemia is defined as hemoglobin less than 12 g/dl in nonpregnant women and less than 11 g/dl in pregnant and postpartum women. Iron deficiency anemia is the most common form of anemia. Other anemias include folic acid deficiency, sickle cell anemia, and thalassemia.
- HIV infection, which is transmitted via blood and body fluids, may also be transmitted transplacentally to the fetus. Currently, there is no definitive therapy for HIV/AIDS. Nurses should employ blood and body fluid precautions (standard precautions) in caring for all women to avoid potential spread of infection.
- Cardiac disease during pregnancy requires careful assessment, limitation of activity, and knowing and reporting signs of impending cardiac decompensation by both patient and nurse.
- Worldwide, more women die from TB than from any other infection. Most cases are concentrated in developing countries.

CRITICAL THINKING IN ACTION

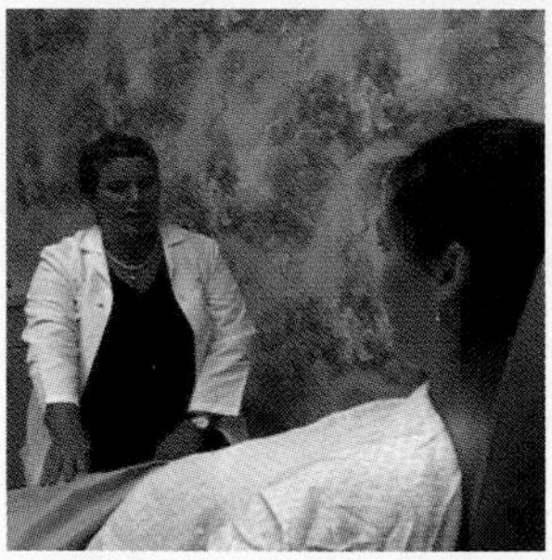

Jane Adams, a 23-year-old, G3 P2, at 37 weeks' gestation, presents to you in the birthing unit complaining of "vaginal pressure" but no contractions. You assess her and find that her history includes being HIV positive for 2 years, second-trimester cocaine and marijuana use, missed appointments, anemia (HCT 28%), and a positive syphilis serology. Jane tells you that she has other children and that they are being cared for by her mother, who has legal custody of them. You admit Jane and place her on the fetal monitor for evaluation of fetal well-being and contraction patterns. The monitor shows you that the fetal heart rate baseline is 120 to 130 with no decelerations; contractions are mild and irregular, lasting 20 to 30 seconds. You obtain vital signs of BP 130/88, temperature 97.0°F, P 88, R 14. A vaginal exam determines that Jane is 7 cm dilated at +1 station with intact membranes. She asks you if being HIV positive will affect her labor.

1. Discuss the prophylactic regimen for the prevention of HIV transmission to the fetus during labor.
2. Discuss the transmission of HIV to the fetus during pregnancy and birth.
3. Identify the emotional impact of HIV infection or other STIs on the woman.
4. On postpartum day 2 you inform Jane that her infant is HIV antibody positive. How would you clarify the results?

See www.nursing.pearsonhighered.com for possible responses.

Pearson Nursing Student Resources

Find additional review materials at
www.nursing.pearsonhighered.com

Prepare for success with additional NCLEX®-style practice questions, interactive assignments and activities, Web links, animations and videos, and more!

REFERENCES

Amato, L., Minozzi, S., Davoli, M., Vecchi, S., Ferri, M. M., & Mayet, S. (2008, July 16). Psychosocial and pharmacological treatments versus pharmacological treatments for opioid detoxification. *Cochrane Database Systematic Reviews*, Issue 3. Art. No.: CD005031.

American Academy of Pediatrics (AAP) & American College of Obstetricians and Gynecologists (ACOG). (2008). *Guidelines for prenatal care* (5th ed.). Elk Grove Village, IL: Author.

American College of Obstetricians and Gynecologists (ACOG). (2003a). *Management of preterm labor* (ACOG Practice Bulletin No. 43). Washington, DC: Author.

American College of Obstetricians and Gynecologists (ACOG). (2005). *Pregestational diabetes mellitus* (ACOG Practice Bulletin No. 60). Washington, DC: Author.

American College of Obstetricians and Gynecologists (ACOG). (2007). *Hemoglobinopathies in pregnancy* (ACOG Practice Bulletin No. 78). Washington, DC: Author.

American College of Obstetricians and Gynecologists (ACOG). (2008a). *Anemia in pregnancy* (ACOG Practice Bulletin No. 95). Washington, DC: Author.

American College of Obstetricians and Gynecologists (ACOG). (2008b). *Asthma in pregnancy* (ACOG Practice Bulletin No. 90). Washington, DC: Author.

American College of Obstetricians and Gynecologists (ACOG). (2008c). *Fetal lung maturity* (ACOG Practice Bulletin No. 97). Washington, DC: Author.

American College of Obstetricians and Gynecologists (ACOG). (2008d). *Prenatal and perinatal human immunodeficiency virus testing: Expanded recommendations* (ACOG Committee Opinion No. 418). Washington, DC: Author.

American College of Obstetricians and Gynecologists (ACOG). (2009). *Postpartum screening for abnormal glucose tolerance in women who had gestational diabetes mellitus.* (ACOG Committee Opinion No. 435). Washington, DC: Author.

American Diabetes Association (ADA). (2008). Nutrition recommendations and interventions for diabetes: A position statement of the American Diabetes Association. *Diabetes Care, 31*(Suppl. 1), S61–S78.

American Diabetes Association (ADA). (2010). Diagnosis and classification of diabetes mellitus. *Diabetes Care, 33*(Suppl.1), S62–S69.

Bessaa, M. A., Mitsuhiroa, S. S., Chalema, E., Barrosb, M. M., Guinsburg, R., & Laranjeira, R. (2009). Underreporting of use of cocaine and marijuana during the third trimester of gestation among pregnant adolescents. *Addictive Behaviors.* doi:10.1016/j.addbeh.2009.10.007

Bonow, R. O., Carabello, B. A., Chatterjee, K., de Leon, A. C., Faxton, D. C., Freed, M. D., & Shanewise, J. S. (2008). Focused update incorporated into the ACC/AHA 2006 guidelines for the management of patients with valvular heart disease: A report of the American College of Cardiology/American Heart Association Task Force on Practice Guidelines. *Circulation, 118*(15), e523.

Centers for Disease Control and Prevention. (2008, December 5). Revised surveillance case definitions for HIV infection among adults, adolescents, and children aged <18 months and for HIV infection and AIDS among children aged 18 months to <13 years—United States. *Morbidity and Mortality Weekly Report. Recommendations and Reports, 57*(RR-10), 1–12.

Centers for Disease Control and Prevention. (2009). *HIV/AIDS surveillance report, 2007, 19.* Retrieved from http://www.cdc.gov/hiv/topics/surveillance/resources/reports/2007report/pdf/2007SurveillanceReport.pdf

Cleveland Clinic. (2007). *Gestational diabetes.* Retrieved from http://my.clevelandclinic.org/disorders/diabetes_gestational/hic_gestational_diabetes.aspx

Creary, M., Williamson, D., & Kulkarni, R. A, (2007). Sickle cell disease: Current activities, public health implications, and future directions. *Women's Health, 16*(5), 575–582.

Criteria Committee of the New York Heart Association. (1994). *Nomenclature and criteria for diagnosis of diseases of the heart and great vessels* (9th ed.). Dallas, TX: American Heart Association.

Cunningham, F. G., Leveno, K. J., Bloom, S. L., Hauth, J. C., Rouse, D. J., & Spong, C. Y. (2010). *Williams obstetrics* (23rd ed.). New York, NY: McGraw-Hill.

Curry, R., Swan, L., & Steer, P. J. (2009). Cardiac disease in pregnancy. *Current Opinion in Obstetrics and Gynecology, 21,* 508–513.

de Man, Y. A., Hazes, J. M., van der Heide, H., Willemsen, S. P., de Groot, C. J., Steegers, E. A., & Dolhain, R. J. (2009). Association of higher rheumatoid arthritis disease activity during pregnancy with lower birth weight: Results of a national prospective study. *Arthritis Rheumatology, 60*(11), 3196–3206.

Eriksson, U. J. (2009). Congenital anomalies in diabetic pregnancy. *Seminars Fetal Neonatal Medicine, 14*(2), 85–93.

Franklin G. M., & Tremlett, H. (2009). Multiple sclerosis and pregnancy: What should we be telling our patients? *Neurology, 73*(22), 1820–1822.

Gamma, A., Jerome, L., Liechti, M. E., & Sumnall, H. R. (2005). Is ecstasy perceived to be safe? A critical survey. *Drug and Alcohol Dependence, 77*(2), 185–193.

Gandhia, R. A., Brown, J., Simmb, A., Pagea, R. C., & Idris, I. (2008). HbA1c during pregnancy: Its relationship to meal related glycaemia and neonatal birth weight in patients with diabetes. *European Journal of Obstetrics & Gynecology and Reproductive Biology, 138*(1), 45–48.

Gidai, J., Acs, N., Bánhidy, F., & Czeizel, A. E. (2008). No association found between use of very large doses of diazepam by 112 pregnant women for a suicide attempt and congenital abnormalities in their offspring. *Toxicology and Industrial Health, 24*(1-2), 29–39.

Hulsey, T. (2005). Prenatal drug use: The ethics of testing and incarcerating pregnant women. *Newborn and Infant Nursing Reviews, 5*(2), 93–96.

Hurt, H., Betancourt, L. M., Malmud, E. K., Shera, D. M., Giannetta, J. M., Brodsky, N. L., & Farah, M. J. (2009). Children with and without gestational cocaine exposure: A neurocognitive systems analysis. *Neurotoxicology Teratology, 31*(6), 334–341.

International Association of Diabetes and Pregnancy Study Groups Consensus Panel (IADPSG). (2010). International Association of Diabetes and Pregnancy Study Groups recommendations on the diagnosis and classification of hyperglycemia in pregnancy. *Diabetes Care, 33*(3), 676–683.

Jansson, L. M., Velez, M., & Harrow, C. (2009). The opioid exposed newborn: Assessment and pharmacologic management. *Journal of Opioid Management, 5*(1), 47–55.

Jones, E. J., Roche, C. C., & Appel, S. J. (2009). A review of the health beliefs and lifestyle behaviors of women with previous gestational diabetes. *Journal Obstetric, Gynecologic, and Neonatal Nursing, 38*(5), 516–526.

Kitzmiller, J. L., Block, J. M., Brown, F. M., Catalano, P. M., Conway, D. L., Coustan, D. R., Gunderson, E. P., . . . Kirkman, M. S. (2008). Managing preexisting diabetes for pregnancy: Summary of evidence and consensus recommendations for care. *Diabetes Care, 31*(5), 1060–1079.

Landon, M. B., Catalano, P. M., & Gabbe, S. (2007). Diabetes mellitus complicating pregnancy. In Gabbe, S. G., Niebyl, J. R., & Simpson, J. L. (Eds.), *Obstetrics: Normal and problem pregnancies.* Philadelphia, PA: Churchill Livingstone Elsevier.

Libbus, M. K., & Phillips, L. M. (2009, July–August). Public health management of perinatal hepatitis B virus. *Public Health Nursing, 26*(4), 353–361.

Makaryus, A. N., Forouzesh, A., & Johnson, M. (2006). Pregnancy in the patient with Eisenmenger's syndrome. *Mt Sinai Journal of Medicine, 73*(7), 1033–1036.

March of Dimes (MOD). (2008). *Drinking alcohol during pregnancy.* Retrieved from http://www.marchofdimes.com/professionals/19695_1170.asp

Matthews L. T., & Mukherjee J. S. (2009). Strategies for harm reduction among HIV-affected couples who want to conceive. *AIDS and Behavior, 13*(Suppl. 1), 5–11.

National Institute on Drug Abuse (NIDA). (2009). *The neurobiology of Ecstasy (MDMA).* Retrieved from http://www.drugabuse.gov/pubs/teaching/teaching4/teaching4.html

National Institute on Drug Abuse (NIDA). (2010). *NIDA InfoFacts: Heroin.* Retrieved from http://www.drugabuse.gov/Infofacts/heroin.html

Nhan-Chang, C., & Jones, T. B. (2010). Tuberculosis in pregnancy. *Clinical Obstetrics and Gynecology, 53*(2), 311–321.

O'Leary, C. M., Nassar, N., Zubrick, S. R., Kurinczuk, J. J., Stanley, F., & Bower, C. (2009). Evidence of a complex association between dose, pattern and timing of prenatal alcohol exposure and child behaviour problems. *Addiction.* doi:10.1111/j.1360-0443.2009.02756.x

O'Malley, P. (2005). Ecstasy for intimacy: Potentially fatal choices for adolescents and young adults: Update for the clinical nurse specialist. *Clinical Nurse Specialist, 19*(2), 63–64.

Ondersma, S. J., Winhusen, T., & Lewis, D. F. (2010). External pressure, motivation, and treatment outcome among pregnant substance-using women. *Drug and Alcohol Dependence, 107*(2–3), 149–153.

Pacini, L., Digne, F., Boumendil, A., Muti, C., Detaint, D., Boileau, C., & Jondeau, G. (2009). Maternal complication of pregnancy in Marfan syndrome. *International Journal of Cardiology, 136*(2), 156–161.

Paintsil, E., & Andiman, W. A. (2009). Update on successes and challenges regarding mother-to-child transmission of HIV. *Current Opinion in Pediatrics, 21*(1), 94–101.

Panel on Treatment of HIV-Infected Pregnant Women and Prevention of Perinatal Transmission. (2010, May 24). *Recommendations for the use of antiretroviral drugs in pregnant HIV-1-infected women for maternal health and interventions to reduce perinatal HIV transmission in the United States* (pp. 1–117). Retrieved from http://aidsinfo.nih.gov/ContentFiles/PerinatalGL.pdf

Rayburn, W. F., & Bogenschutz, M. P. (2004). Pharmacotherapy for pregnant women with addictions. *American Journal of Obstetrics & Gynecology, 191*(6), 1885–1897.

Ramaraj, R., & Sorrell, V. L. (2009). Peripartum cardiomyopathy: Causes, diagnosis, and treatment. *Cleveland Clinic Journal of Medicine, 76*(5), 289–296.

Reece, E. A., & Homko, C. J. (2008). Diabetes mellitus and pregnancy. In R. S. Gibbs, B. Y. Karlan, A. F. Haney, & I. E. Nygaard (Eds.), *Danforth's obstetrics and gynecology* (10th ed.). Philadelphia, PA: Wolters Kluwer/Lippincott, Williams & Wilkins.

Richardson, G. A., Goldschmidt L., & Willford, J. (2008). The effects of prenatal cocaine use on infant development, *Neurotoxicology and Teratology, 30*(2), 96–106.

Rinala, S. G., Dryfhout, V. L., & Lambers, D. S. (2009). Correlation of glucose concentrations in maternal serum and amniotic fluid in high-risk pregnancies. *American Journal of Obstetrics & Gynecology, 200*(5), e43–44.

Ruiz-Irastorza, G., & Khamashta, M. A. (2009). Managing lupus patients during pregnancy. *Best Practice and Research. Clinical Rheumatology, 23*(4), 575–582.

Schatz, M., & Dombrowski, M. P. (2009). Clinical practice. Asthma in pregnancy. *New England Journal of Medicine, 360*(18), 1862–1869.

Schneider, E., Whitmore, S., Glynn, K. M., Dominguez, K., Mitsch, A., & McKenna, M. T. (2008). Revised surveillance case definitions for HIV infection among adults, adolescents, and children aged <18 months and for HIV infection and AIDS among children aged 18 months to <13 years—United States, *Morbidity and Mortality Weekly Report. Recommendations and Reports, 57,* 1–12.

Serlin, D. C., & Lash, R. W. (2009). Diagnosis and management of gestational diabetes mellitus. *American Family Physician, 80*(1), 57–62.

Singer, L. T., Nelson, S., Short, E., Min, M. O., Lewis, B., Russ, S., & Minnes. S. (2008). Prenatal cocaine exposure: Drug and environmental effects at 9 years. *Journal of Pediatrics, 153*(1), 105–111.

Substance Abuse and Mental Health Services Administration (SAMHSA). (2009). *Results from the 2008 National Survey on Drug Use and Health: National Findings* (Office of Applied Studies, NSDUH Series H-36, HHS Publication No. SMA 09-4434). Rockville, MD: Author.

Thompson, B. L., Levitt, P., & Stanwood, G. D. (2009). Prenatal exposure to drugs: Effects on brain development and implications for policy and education. *Nature Reviews Neuroscience, 10*(4), 303–312.

Thompson, V. B., Heiman, J., Chambers, J. B., Benoit, S. C., Buesing, W. R., Norman, M. K., . . . Lipton, J. W. (2009). Long-term behavioral consequences of prenatal MDMA exposure. *Physiology & Behavior, 96*(4-5), 593–601.

Tincani, A., Danieli, E., Nuzzo, M., Scarsil, M., Motta, M., Cimaz, R., & Meroni, P. (2006). Impact of in utero environment on the offspring of lupus patients. *Lupus, 15*(11), 801–807.

Tomson, T., & Battino, D. (2009). Teratogenic effects of antiepileptic medications. *Neurology Clinics, 27*(4), 993–1002.

Vucinovic, M., Roje, D., Vucinovic, Z., Capkun, V., Bucat, M., & Banovic, I. (2009). Maternal and neonatal effects of substance abuse during pregnancy: Our ten-year experience. *Yonsei Medical Journal, 49*(5), 705–713.

Walton-Moss, B. J., McIntosh, L. C., Conrad, J., & Kiefer, E. (2009). Health status and birth outcomes among pregnant women in substance abuse treatment. *Women's Health Issues,19*(3), 167–175.

Wisner, K. L., Sit, D. K. Y., Reynolds, S. K., Altemus, M., Bogen, D. L., Sunder, K. R., & Perel, J. M. (2007). Psychiatric disorders. In Gabbe, S. G., Niebyl, J. R., & Simpson, J. L. (Eds.), *Obstetrics: Normal and problem pregnancies.* Philadelphia, PA: Churchill Livingstone Elsevier.

Working Group on Antiretroviral Therapy and Medical Management of HIV-Infected Children. (2009, February 23). *Guidelines for the use of antiretroviral agents in pediatric HIV infection* (pp. 1–139). Retrieved from http://aidsinfo.nih.gov/contentfiles/PediatricGuidelines.pdf

Yu, C. K., Stasiowska, E., Stephens, A., Awogbade, M., & Davies, A. (2009). Outcome of pregnancy in sickle cell disease patients attending a combined obstetric and haematology clinic. *Journal of Obstetrics and Gynaecology, 29*(6), 512–516.

CHAPTER 20

Pregnancy at Risk: Gestational Onset

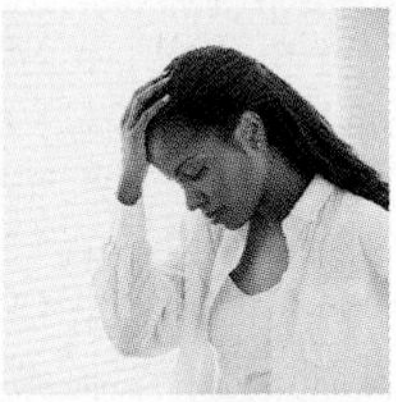

I had taken more than a year to conceive and was so excited when my home pregnancy test turned positive. My husband was with me when I called my family. I could hardly breathe with the excitement of the moment. Five weeks later, I was in an ambulance speeding to a medical center equipped to save my life. My ectopic pregnancy had not yet been diagnosed when it ruptured at home. I underwent surgery to remove my tube and the pregnancy that was contained within. Afterward, I was dazed and debilitated. For weeks I focused on my recovery rather than my loss. How ironic that I was fully confronted with the reality of my loss on what would have been my due date when in the mail I received a package of samples congratulating me on the birth of my new baby.

—Kristin, R.N.

LEARNING OUTCOMES

1. Delineate the bleeding problems associated with pregnancy.
2. Contrast the etiology, medical therapy, and nursing interventions for the various bleeding problems associated with pregnancy.
3. Discuss the medical therapy and nursing care of a woman with hyperemesis gravidarum.
4. Describe the development and course of hypertensive disorders associated with pregnancy.
5. Explain the cause and prevention of hemolytic disease of the newborn secondary to Rh incompatibility.
6. Compare Rh incompatibility to ABO incompatibility with regard to occurrence, treatment, and implications for the fetus/newborn.
7. Summarize the effects of surgical procedures on pregnancy, and explain ways in which pregnancy may complicate diagnosis of conditions that require surgery.
8. Discuss the implications of trauma due to accidents or battering for the pregnant woman and her fetus.
9. Describe the effects of infections on the woman and her unborn child.

KEY TERMS

Abortion *451*
Eclampsia *460*
Ectopic pregnancy *454*
Erythroblastosis fetalis *478*
Gestational trophoblastic disease (GTD) *456*
HELLP syndrome *463*
Hydatidiform mole *456*
Hydrops fetalis *478*
Hyperemesis gravidarum *459*
Miscarriage *451*
Preeclampsia *460*
Rh immune globulin *476*

Pregnancy is usually a normal, uncomplicated experience. In some cases, however, problems arise during the pregnancy that place the woman and her unborn child at risk. Regular prenatal care serves to detect these potential complications quickly so that effective care can be provided. This chapter focuses on problems that primarily occur during pregnancy, those with a gestational onset.

Care of the Woman at Risk Because of Bleeding During Pregnancy

During the first and second trimesters of pregnancy the major cause of bleeding is abortion. Broadly, this is the expulsion of the fetus before viability. This definition is imprecise, however, because the definition of viability changes. **Abortion** is often defined as "pregnancy termination prior to 20 weeks' gestation or with a fetus weighing less than 500 g" (Cunningham et al., 2010, p. 215). Abortions are either spontaneous, occurring naturally, or induced, occurring as a result of medical or surgical interruption. **Miscarriage** is a lay term applied to spontaneous abortion.

Other complications that can cause bleeding in the first half of pregnancy are ectopic pregnancy and gestational trophoblastic disease. In the second half of pregnancy, particularly in the third trimester, the two major causes of bleeding are placenta previa and abruptio placentae.

General Principles of Nursing Intervention

Vaginal bleeding is relatively common during pregnancy. Bleeding can arise following sexual intercourse or exercise as a result of trauma to the highly vascular cervix, from cervical or vaginal lesions, implantation of the pregnancy, or threatened or impending miscarriage. However, the woman is advised to report any spotting or bleeding that occurs during pregnancy so that it can be evaluated.

It is often the nurse's responsibility to make the initial assessment of bleeding. In general, the following nursing measures should be implemented for pregnant women being evaluated for bleeding during pregnancy:

- Monitor blood pressure and pulse frequently. The frequency is determined by the extent of the bleeding and the stability of the woman's condition.
- Observe the woman for indications of shock, such as pallor, clammy skin, perspiration, dyspnea, or restlessness.
- Count and weigh pads to assess amount of bleeding over a given time period; save any tissue or clots expelled.
- If pregnancy is of 12 weeks' gestation or beyond, assess fetal heart tones with a Doppler.
- Prepare for intravenous (IV) therapy. There may be standing orders to start IV therapy on bleeding patients.
- Prepare equipment for examination.
- Have oxygen therapy available.
- Collect and organize all data, including antepartum history, onset of bleeding episode, any associated pain, laboratory studies (hemoglobin, hematocrit, Rh status, and hormonal assays).
- Obtain an order to type and cross-match for blood if there is evidence of significant blood loss.
- Assess coping mechanisms and support system of the woman in crisis. Give emotional support to enhance her coping abilities by continuous, sustained presence, by clear explanation of procedures, and by communicating her status to her family. Most important, prepare the woman for possible fetal loss. Assess her expressions of anger, denial, guilt, depression, or self-blame.
- Assess the family's response to the situation.

Spontaneous Abortion (Miscarriage)

Many pregnancies end in the first trimester as a result of spontaneous abortion. Pregnancy loss during the early weeks of gestation, when the pregnancy may not yet be recognized, may be seen as a heavy menstrual period. However, when only clinically recognized pregnancies are considered, the incidence is at least 15% (Porter, Branch, & Scott, 2008). In healthy women, advanced maternal age is the most significant risk factor for spontaneous miscarriage. Women younger than age 20 have a 12% risk while the risk is greater than 50% for women over age 45 (Porter et al., 2008).

Over half of first trimester spontaneous abortions are related to chromosomal abnormalities (Calleja-Agius, 2008; Cunningham et al., 2010). Other causes include teratogenic drugs, faulty implantation due to abnormalities of the female reproductive tract, a weakened cervix, placental abnormalities, chronic maternal diseases, endocrine imbalances, and maternal infections. Women who use hot tubs or jacuzzis are twice as likely to have miscarriages as nonusers (Centers for Disease Control and Prevention [CDC], 2005). Fever may also increase the risk of miscarriage although research results about this hypothesis are contradictory. The major malformations most commonly associated with febrile illnesses in women are neural tube defects (American Academy of Pediatrics [AAP] & American College of Obstetricians and Gynecologists [ACOG], 2007a).

The pathophysiology of spontaneous abortion differs according to the cause. Chromosomal defects are generally seen as spontaneous abortions during weeks 4 to 8. Insufficient or excessive hormonal levels usually will result in loss by 10 weeks' gestation. Infectious and environmental factors may also be seen in first trimester pregnancy loss. In late spontaneous abortion, the cause is usually a maternal factor, for example, cervical insufficiency or maternal disease, and fetal death may not precede the onset of abortion (Valley, Jackson-Williams, & Fly, 2006). See chapter 26 ∞ for discussion of cervical insufficiency.

Spontaneous abortion can be extremely distressing to the couple desiring a child. Chances for carrying the next pregnancy to term after one spontaneous abortion are as good as they are for the general population. Thereafter, however, chances of successful pregnancy decrease with each succeeding abortion. Following two to three consecutive losses, a

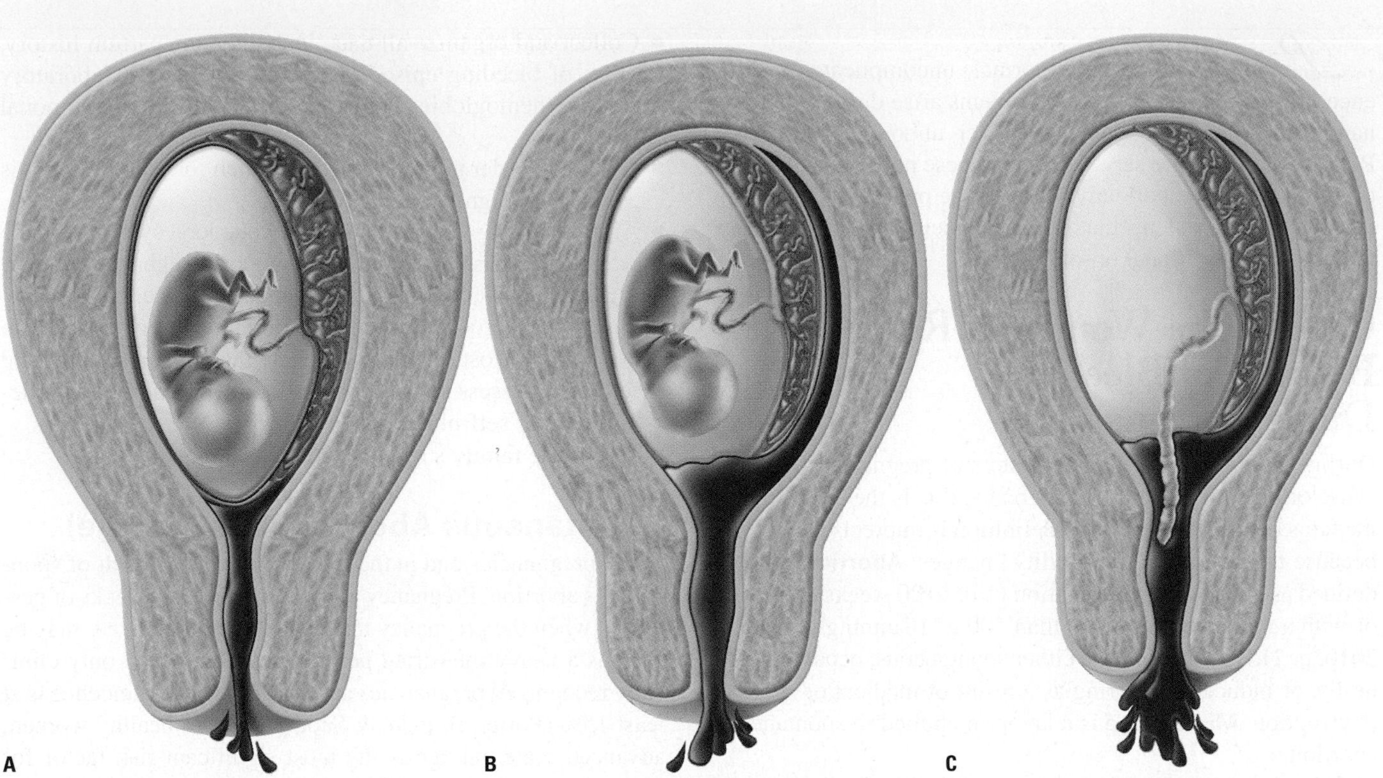

Figure 20-1 ■ Types of spontaneous abortion. A. Threatened. The cervix is not dilated, and the placenta is still attached to the uterine wall, but some bleeding occurs. B. Imminent. The placenta has separated from the uterine wall, the cervix has dilated, and the amount of bleeding has increased. C. Incomplete. The embryo/fetus has passed out of the uterus; however, the placenta remains.

woman and her partner should be evaluated and are candidates for genetic counseling.

Classification

Spontaneous abortions are subdivided into the following categories so that they can be differentiated clinically:

- *Threatened abortion* (Figure 20-1A ■). Unexplained bleeding, cramping, or backache indicate that the fetus may be in jeopardy. Bleeding may persist for days. The cervix is closed. It may be followed by partial or complete expulsion of pregnancy, or it may resolve without threatening the fetus. Evaluation for hydatidiform mole or ectopic pregnancy (discussed shortly) is advisable.
- *Imminent abortion* (Figure 20-1B ■). Bleeding and cramping increase. The internal cervical os dilates. Membranes may rupture. The term *inevitable abortion* also applies.
- *Incomplete abortion* (Figure 20-1C ■). Part of the products of conception are retained, most often the placenta. The internal cervical os is dilated.
- *Complete abortion.* All the products of conception are expelled. The uterus is contracted and the cervical os may be closed.
- *Missed abortion.* The fetus dies in utero but is not expelled. Uterine growth ceases, breast changes regress, and the woman may report a brownish vaginal discharge. The cervix is closed. Diagnosis is made based on history, pelvic examination, and a drop in hCG levels or a negative pregnancy test and may be confirmed by ultrasound if necessary. If the fetus is retained beyond 4 weeks, fetal autolysis (breakdown of cells or tissue) results in the release of thromboplastin, and disseminated intravascular coagulation (DIC) may develop.
- *Recurrent pregnancy loss, formerly called habitual abortion.* Abortion occurs consecutively in three or more pregnancies.
- *Septic abortion.* There is presence of infection; may occur with prolonged, unrecognized rupture of the membranes, pregnancy with intrauterine device (IUD) in utero, or attempts by inadequately prepared individuals to terminate a pregnancy. Septic abortion is less common since the availability of legal abortion.

Clinical Therapy

One of the more reliable indicators of potential spontaneous abortion is the presence of pelvic cramping and backache. These symptoms are usually absent in bleeding caused by polyps, ruptured cervical blood vessels, or cervical erosion.

Vaginal bleeding occurs in 20% to 25% of first trimester pregnancies. Of these, approximately half will result in subsequent miscarriage (Cunningham et al., 2010). Several days of spotting or light bleeding associated with pain may also increase the chance of miscarriage. Painless spotting or light bleeding for a day or two did not increase the risk of miscarriage above the risk for women with no bleeding.

Evaluations to help determine the cause of vaginal bleeding include speculum examination to determine the presence of cervical polyps or cervical erosion, ultrasound scanning for the presence of cardiac activity and a gestational sac, or crown-rump length that is small for gestational age. Presence of a fetal heartbeat on ultrasound provides a high likelihood of the pregnancy continuing. Laboratory determination of hCG level can confirm a pregnancy, but because the hCG level falls slowly after fetal death, it cannot confirm a live embryo/fetus. Hemoglobin and hematocrit levels are obtained to assess blood loss. Blood is typed and cross-matched for possible replacement needs.

Although there is no evidence that supports the value of restricting physical activity, the therapy prescribed for the pregnant woman with bleeding often includes bed rest, abstinence from coitus, and, perhaps, sedation. If bleeding persists and abortion is imminent or incomplete, the woman may be hospitalized, IV therapy or blood transfusions may be started to replace fluid, and dilation and curettage (D&C) or suction evacuation is performed to remove the remainder of the products of conception. If the woman is Rh negative and not sensitized, and there has been prior ultrasound documentation of fetal cardiac activity, Rh immune globulin (RhoGAM) is given within 72 hours (Moise, 2008a). (See discussion of Rh sensitization later in this chapter.)

In missed abortions, the products of conception eventually are expelled spontaneously. If this does not occur within 1 month to 6 weeks after fetal death, hospitalization is necessary. Suction evacuation, or D&C, is done if the pregnancy is in the first trimester. Beyond 12 weeks' gestation, induction of labor by IV oxytocin and intra-amniotic prostaglandin $F_{2\alpha}$, intravaginal prostaglandin E_2, or intravaginal misoprostol (a synthetic prostaglandin E_1 analog) may be used to expel the dead fetus.

NURSING CARE MANAGEMENT

Nursing Assessment and Diagnosis

The nurse assesses the amount and appearance of any vaginal bleeding and monitors the woman's vital signs and degree of discomfort. The woman's blood type and antibody status should be identified to determine the need for Rh immune globulin (see page 482). If the pregnancy is 10 to 12 weeks or more, fetal heart rate should be assessed by Doppler. The nurse also assesses the responses of the woman and her family to this crisis and evaluates their coping mechanisms and ability to comfort each other.

Nursing diagnoses that may apply include the following:

- ***Fear*** related to the risk of pregnancy loss
- ***Acute Pain*** related to abdominal cramping secondary to threatened abortion
- ***Grieving*** related to expected loss of unborn child

Nursing Plan and Implementation

Community-Based Nursing Care

If a woman in her first trimester of pregnancy begins cramping or spotting, she may be evaluated on an outpatient basis if the bleeding is not heavy. Providing emotional support is an important task for nurses caring for women who have spontaneously aborted. Couples who approached the pregnancy with feelings of joy and a sense of expectancy now feel grief, sadness, and possibly anger.

Because many women, even with planned pregnancies, feel some ambivalence initially, guilt is a common emotion. The woman may harbor negative feelings about herself, ranging from lowered self-esteem resulting from a belief that she is lacking or abnormal in some way, to a notion that the abortion may be a punishment for some wrongdoing.

The nurse can offer invaluable psychologic support to the woman and her family by encouraging them to verbalize their feelings. Reflective listening gives the woman an opportunity to express and explore her feelings. The nurse can take cues from questions the woman asks, discuss the grief cycle, and provide resources. Referrals can help the woman and her family find ways to deal with their loss. If the woman has older children, she may need guidance in how to help them understand and cope with what has occurred. Commemorating the pregnancy and baby is helpful in validating the significance of the loss. The grieving period following a spontaneous abortion usually lasts 6 to 24 months. Many couples can be helped during this period by an organization or support group established for parents who have lost a fetus or newborn. Nurses may benefit from education to help them understand the impact of early pregnancy loss through programs such as those available through Bereavement Services of LaCrosse, WI. See chapter 37 ∞ for further discussion.

DEVELOPING CULTURAL COMPETENCE

Culture and Response to Fetal Loss

Remember that individual responses to fetal loss following miscarriage may vary greatly and may be influenced by ethnic or cultural norms.

- Miscarriage may be viewed in many ways. For example, it may be seen as a punishment from God, as the result of the evil eye or of a hex or curse by an enemy, or as a natural part of life.
- When grieving over a pregnancy loss, women from some cultures and ethnic groups may show their emotions freely, crying and wailing, whereas other women may hide their feelings behind a mask of stoicism.
- In some cultures the woman's partner is her primary source of support and comfort. In others, the woman turns to her mother or close female relatives for comfort.
- Avoid stereotyping women according to culture. Individual responses are influenced by many factors, including the degree of assimilation into the dominant culture.

> **"I was stunned by the depth of loss I felt following my miscarriage when I was 2 1/2 months along. It didn't seem possible that I had already become so emotionally attached to the baby I carried. Afterward I was surprised by the number of women I knew who shared stories of their own miscarriages and confirmed that the emotions I was feeling were normal, if painful."**

The physical pain of the cramps and the amount of bleeding may be more severe than a couple anticipates, even when they are prepared for the possibility of an abortion. Nurses need to be aware that couples feel unprepared for their first experience of spontaneous abortion. Nurses should offer support in dealing with the physical experience by explaining why the discomfort is occurring and by offering analgesics for pain relief.

Hospital-Based Nursing Care

A suction D&C is performed if the woman experiences an incomplete or missed abortion. This can be performed on an outpatient basis, and, barring any complications, the woman can return home a few hours after the procedure with instructions for self-care. An Rh-negative woman with a negative antibody screen should be given Rh immune globulin before discharge.

Throughout the procedure the nurse monitors the woman's physical status and provides emotional support. The nurse also answers any questions the woman or her partner may have and provides referrals to community agencies as needed.

Health Promotion Education

If the woman had a D&C, someone should remain with her for the first 12 to 24 hours. The woman is instructed to report all episodes of heavy bleeding, fever, chills, foul-smelling vaginal discharge, or abdominal tenderness to her healthcare provider. The woman who experiences a pregnancy loss requires information about possible causes of the loss and the chances of recurrence with a future pregnancy. She may also require information about the grief process so she is prepared for it when she goes home. In addition, she should receive information about available resources, including support groups to help her cope with her feelings related to the loss of the pregnancy. The woman's partner or a family member should be included in the educational process when possible to assist him or her in personal grief work as well as to provide tools to help support the woman through the loss.

Evaluation

Expected outcomes of nursing care include the following:

- The woman is able to explain spontaneous abortion, the treatment measures employed in her care, and long-term implications for future pregnancies.
- The woman suffers no complications.
- The woman and her partner are able to begin verbalizing their grief and to recognize that the grieving process usually lasts several months.

Ectopic Pregnancy

Ectopic pregnancy is an implantation of a fertilized ovum in a site other than the endometrial lining of the uterus. It may result from a number of different causes. Risk factors for ectopic pregnancy include tubal damage caused by pelvic inflammatory disease; previous pelvic or tubal surgery; endometriosis; previous ectopic pregnancy; presence of an IUD; high levels of progesterone, which can alter the motility of the egg in the fallopian tube; congenital anomalies of the tube; use of ovulation-inducing drugs; primary infertility; smoking; and advanced maternal age.

Ectopic pregnancy occurs in 1.5% to 2.0% of pregnancies. In recent years, the mortality rate has declined to 0.5 deaths per 1000 in the United States. This decrease can be credited to improved recognition of early signs and symptoms and better diagnostic methods, which allow detection before tubal rupture. Nevertheless, ectopic pregnancy accounts for 6% of all maternal deaths in the United States. The recurrence risk of ectopic pregnancy in a woman with one previous ectopic pregnancy is 10% and in women with two or more, the risk is at least 25% (Barnhart, 2009).

The actual pathogenesis of ectopic pregnancy occurs when the fertilized ovum is prevented or slowed in its progress down the tube. The fertilized ovum implants in either the fallopian tube or the ovary, peritoneal cavity, cervix, or uterine cornua (Figure 20-2 ■). The most common location for implantation of an ectopic pregnancy is the ampulla of the tube. The occurrence of ectopic pregnancy in women who have used assisted reproductive technology is 4%. A heterotopic pregnancy (one conceptus is ectopic and one is intrauterine) is extremely rare

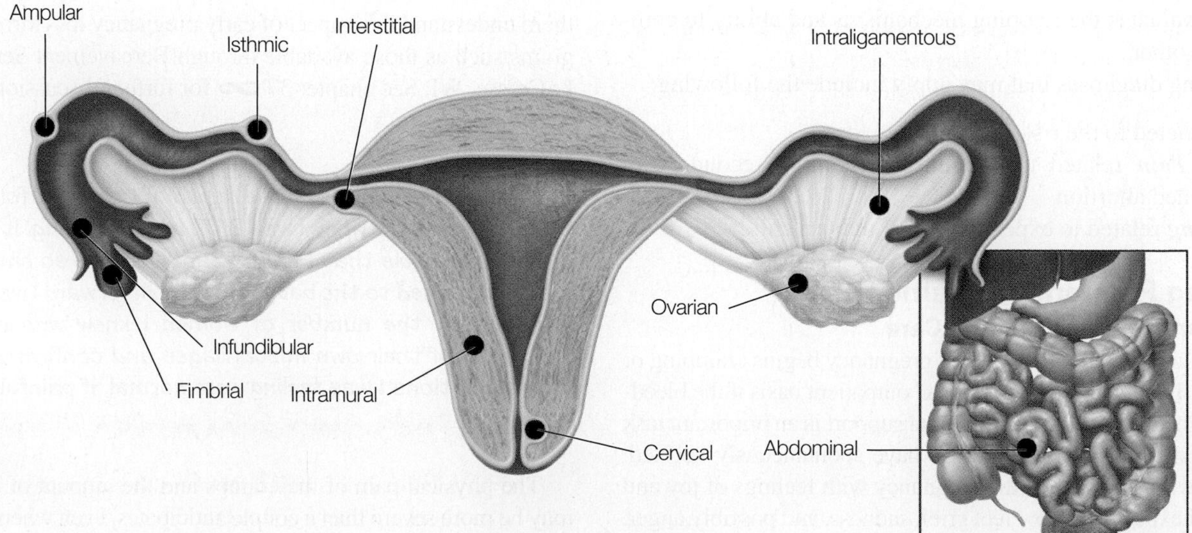

Figure 20-2 ■ Various implantation sites in ectopic pregnancy. The most common site is within the fallopian tube, hence the name "tubal pregnancy."

in spontaneously occurring pregnancies but may be as high as 1% in assisted conception (Barnhart, 2009).

Initially, the normal symptoms of pregnancy may be present, specifically, amenorrhea, breast tenderness, and nausea. The normal clinical signs of early pregnancy such as the bluish discoloration of the cervix (Chadwick's sign) and the softening of the isthmus (Hegar's sign) may be noted on physical exam. The hormone hCG is present in the blood and urine. With an ectopic implantation, the trophoblastic cells grow into the adjacent tissue, often the tubal wall, and arterial vessels. This results in internal hemorrhage. The faulty implantation of the placenta causes fluctuation of hormone levels. Hormones first stimulate the endometrial lining of the uterus to grow, but fluctuation in levels cannot support the endometrium, and vaginal bleeding ensues. The implanted ovum quickly begins to rupture the fallopian tube if it is implanted there. The woman may experience one-sided lower abdominal pain or diffuse lower abdominal pain and vasomotor disturbances such as fainting or dizziness. In about 50% of cases, referred right shoulder pain occurs from blood irritating the subdiaphragmatic phrenic nerve.

In many instances, the symptoms are not obvious. One fourth of ectopic pregnancies may involve uterine enlargement. Physical examination usually reveals adnexal tenderness; an adnexal mass is palpable in approximately one half of the cases.

If internal hemorrhage is profuse, the woman rapidly develops signs of hypovolemic shock. More commonly, the bleeding is slow (chronic), and the abdomen gradually becomes rigid and very tender. If bleeding into the pelvic cavity has been extensive, vaginal examination causes extreme pain, and a mass of blood may be palpated in the cul-de-sac of Douglas.

Laboratory tests may reveal low hemoglobin and hematocrit levels and rising leukocyte levels. In a normal pregnancy β-hCG titers double every 48 hours from 3 to 6 weeks' gestation. Ectopic pregnancies are associated with β-hCG titers that increase more slowly.

Clinical Therapy

It is important to differentiate an ectopic pregnancy from other disorders with similar clinical presenting pictures. Consideration must be given to possible spontaneous abortion, ruptured corpus luteum cyst, appendicitis, salpingitis, torsion of the ovary, ovarian cysts, and urinary tract infection.

The following measures are used to establish the diagnosis of ectopic pregnancy and assess the woman's status:

- A careful assessment of menstrual history, particularly the last menstrual period (LMP).
- Careful pelvic exam to identify any abnormal pelvic masses and tenderness.
- Laboratory testing as described previously.
- Ultrasonography. In a normal pregnancy, transvaginal ultrasound should detect an intrauterine pregnancy with almost 100% accuracy at greater than 5.5 weeks gestation and an intrauterine gestational sac when the β-hCG is greater than 1500 milli–International Unit/ml. If there is failure to determine the location of a pregnancy on the initial ultrasound, repeat ultrasound examination 2 to 7 days later may provide a diagnosis (Barnhart, 2009). Confirming an intrauterine pregnancy nearly eliminates the diagnosis of ectopic pregnancy.
- Serial measurements of serum hCG values should increase a minimum of 53% in 2 days. Seventy-one percent of women with an ectopic pregnancy have serial serum hCG values that increase more slowly than expected with a viable intrauterine pregnancy (Barnhart, 2009).
- Laparoscopy. If the presence or absence of an ectopic pregnancy cannot be confirmed by other measures, laparoscopic intervention may be necessary for both diagnosis and treatment.

Once an ectopic pregnancy is confirmed, therapy options are reviewed with the woman. Medical management using methotrexate is indicated for the woman who desires future pregnancy if her ectopic pregnancy is unruptured and of 3.5 cm size or less and if her condition is stable. In addition, there must be no fetal cardiac motion and no evidence of maternal thrombocytopenia, leukopenia, kidney disease, or liver disease.

Methotrexate is a folic acid antagonist that interferes with the proliferation of trophoblastic cells. The medication is administered intramuscularly using either a single-dose, two-dose, or multiple-dose regimen. As an outpatient, the woman is monitored for increasing abdominal pain. β-hCG titers are monitored regularly. β-hCG titers increase for 1 to 4 days and then decrease. If hCG levels do not decrease by at least 15% from day 4 to day 7 after the initial injection but the patient is clinically stable, an additional dose of methotrexate on day 7 is generally recommended (Thurman, Cornelius, Korte, et al., 2010). If the patient is not clinically stable, surgical intervention may be required. The single-dose regimen is useful in patients with a low initial hCG level and requires fewer patient visits, but is associated with higher treatment failures. The multidose regimen, which includes methotrexate and leucovorin administered on alternate days, is preferred for women with presenting hCG levels greater than 5000 miU/ml. The two-dose regimen was designed to address the failure rate associated with the single dose approach but has not yet been well studied (Barnhart, 2009).

If surgery is indicated and the woman desires future pregnancies, a laparoscopic linear salpingostomy will be performed to gently evacuate the ectopic pregnancy and preserve the tube. If the tube is ruptured or if future childbearing is not an issue, laparoscopic salpingectomy (removal of the tube) is performed. If the woman is in shock and unstable, an abdominal incision will be made. During surgery, the most important risk to be considered is potential hemorrhage. Bleeding must be controlled, and replacement therapy should be on hand. The Rh-negative nonsensitized woman is given Rh immune globulin to prevent sensitization.

NURSING CARE MANAGEMENT

Nursing Assessment and Diagnosis

When the woman with a suspected ectopic pregnancy is admitted to the hospital, the nurse assesses the appearance and amount of vaginal bleeding. The nurse monitors vital signs, particularly blood pressure and pulse, for evidence of developing shock.

It is also the nurse's responsibility to assess the woman's emotional status and coping abilities and to evaluate the couple's informational needs. If surgery is necessary, the nurse performs the ongoing assessments appropriate for any patient postoperatively.

Nursing diagnoses that may apply for a woman with an ectopic pregnancy include the following:

- ***Grieving*** related to the loss of the pregnancy
- ***Acute Pain*** related to abdominal bleeding secondary to tubal rupture
- ***Deficient Fluid Volume*** related to hypovolemia secondary to maternal blood loss
- ***Readiness for Enhanced Knowledge (Treatment of Ectopic Pregnancy)*** related to an expressed desire to gain better understanding of the condition and its long-term implications

Nursing Plan and Implementation

Community-Based Nursing Care

Women with ectopic pregnancy are often seen initially in a clinic or office setting. Nurses need to be alert to the possibility of ectopic pregnancy if a woman presents with complaints of abdominal pain and lack of menses for 1 to 2 months. Once an initial evaluation is complete, if no ultrasound is available, the woman should be referred to another facility where ultrasound is available. The nurse plays an important role in monitoring the woman's condition and in providing her with information.

A woman with a confirmed ectopic pregnancy who meets the criteria for methotrexate administration is followed as an outpatient. The nurse should advise the woman that some abdominal pain is common following the injection but it is generally mild and lasts only 24 to 48 hours. More severe pain might indicate treatment failure and should be evaluated. The woman should also report heavy vaginal bleeding, dizziness, or tachycardia. In addition, the nurse should stress the need to return for follow-up β-hCG testing.

For all women treated for ectopic pregnancy, a follow-up phone call by the nurse may be especially welcome. It gives the woman the opportunity to ask any questions she may have. In addition, the nurse can use the opportunity to assist the woman in dealing with her grief.

Hospital-Based Nursing Care

Once a diagnosis of ectopic pregnancy is made and surgery is scheduled, the nurse starts an IV as ordered and begins preoperative teaching. The nurse should report signs of developing shock to the physician immediately and initiate interventions. If the woman is experiencing severe abdominal pain, the nurse can administer appropriate analgesics and evaluate their effectiveness.

Health Promotion Education

Teaching is an important part of nursing care. The woman may want her condition and various procedures explained. She may need instruction about measures to prevent infection, symptoms to report (pain, bleeding, fever, chills), and her follow-up visit. The woman needs to understand that she is at increased risk of ectopic pregnancy with a subsequent pregnancy. Thus it is important for her to seek early pregnancy confirmation and access to prenatal care.

The woman and her family will need emotional support during this difficult time. Their feelings and responses to this crisis will probably be similar to those that occur in cases of spontaneous abortion. As a result, similar nursing actions are required.

Evaluation

Expected outcomes of nursing care include the following:

- The woman is able to explain ectopic pregnancy, treatment alternatives, and implications for future childbearing.
- The woman and her caregivers detect possible complications early and manage them appropriately.
- The woman and her partner are able to begin verbalizing their loss and recognize that the grieving process usually lasts several months.

Gestational Trophoblastic Disease

As discussed in chapter 11 ∞, the trophoblast is the outermost layer of embryonic cells and gives rise to the chorion. **Gestational trophoblastic disease (GTD)** is the pathologic proliferation of trophoblastic cells, and includes partial or complete hydatidiform mole, invasive mole (chorioadenoma destruens), and choriocarcinoma.

Hydatidiform mole (molar pregnancy) is a condition in which a proliferation of trophoblastic cells results in the formation of a placenta characterized by *hydropic* (fluid-filled) grapelike clusters. The significance of this disease for the woman who has it is the loss of the pregnancy and the possibility, though remote, of developing choriocarcinoma, a form of cancer, from the trophoblastic tissue. Molar pregnancies are classified into two types, complete and partial, both of which meet the preceding criteria. Little is known about the cause of either type, but some of the pathophysiology has been clarified. The *complete mole* develops from an anuclear ovum that contains no maternal genetic material, an "empty" egg. In most cases, a haploid sperm, 23X, fertilizes this anuclear egg and duplicates before the first cell division (diploidy). The conceptus then contains in its cells a 46XX chromosomal set of totally paternal origin (Berkowitz & Goldstein, 2009). A 46XY chromosomal set is far less common and occurs when an empty egg is fertilized by two sperm. The hydropic vesicles that form from the chorionic villi are avascular in the complete mole. No embryonic or fetal tissue or membranes are found. Choriocarcinoma seems to be associated primarily with the complete mole (ACOG, 2008c).

In contrast to the complete mole, the *partial mole* usually has a triploid karyotype, that is, 69 chromosomes. Most often, a normal ovum with 23 chromosomes is fertilized by two sperm (dispermy) or by a sperm that has failed to undergo the first meiosis and therefore contains 46 chromosomes (Berkowitz & Goldstein, 2009). In partial molar pregnancy, the villi are often vascularized and may be hydropic only in sections of the placenta rather than universally as with a complete mole. Often partial moles are recognized only after sponta-

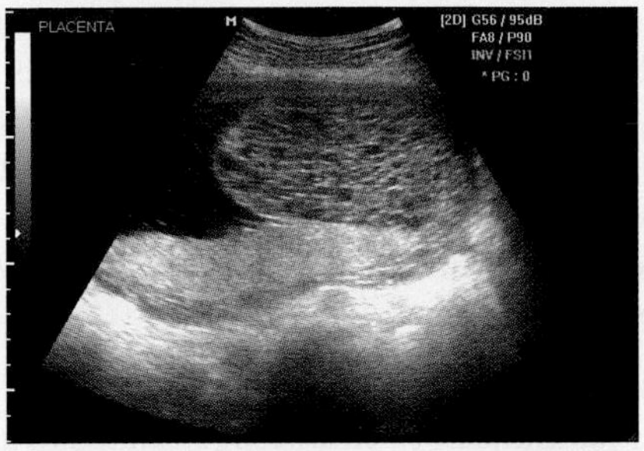

Figure 20-3 ■ Ultrasound image of the placenta in a twin gestation. Molar changes can be seen in one, thickened placenta while the placenta of the normal co-twin has the expected appearance.

Source: Courtesy of Angela Gray, MD. Obstetrix Medical Group of Colorado.

neous abortion, or they may go unnoticed. Unlike the complete mole, identifiable fetal parts may be present. Twin pregnancies in which a normal fetus coexists with a molar pregnancy have been reported. Because fetal development is not seen in complete moles, this can present a diagnostic pitfall leading to an erroneous diagnosis of a partial mole. (See Figure 20-3 ■).

Hydatidiform mole occurs in about 1 in 1500 pregnancies in the United States (ACOG, 2008c). The incidence of molar pregnancy increases with extremes in maternal age and has higher rates in certain populations, including Asia and Latin America.

Invasive mole (chorioadenoma destruens) is similar to a complete mole but involves the uterine myometrium. Treatment is the same as for a complete mole.

Choriocarcinoma is invasive, malignant trophoblastic disease that is usually metastatic and can be fatal. It is discussed in more detail shortly.

Clinical Therapy

Diagnosis of hydatidiform mole is often suspected in the presence of the following signs:

- Vaginal bleeding is almost universal with molar pregnancies and may occur as early as the fourth week or as late as the second trimester. It is often brownish, "like prune juice," because of liquefaction of the uterine clot, but it may be bright red.
- Anemia occurs frequently because of the loss of blood.
- Hydropic vesicles may be passed and, if so, are diagnostic (Figure 20-4 ■). With a partial mole, the vesicles are often smaller and may not be noticed by the woman.
- Uterine enlargement greater than expected for gestational age is a classic sign with complete moles, present in about 50% of cases. In the remainder of cases, the uterus is appropriate or small for the gestational stage. Enlargement is due to the proliferating trophoblastic tissue and to a large amount of clotted blood.
- Absence of fetal heart sounds in the presence of other signs of pregnancy is a classic sign of molar pregnancy. (Only rarely has a viable fetus been born in a partial molar pregnancy.)
- Markedly elevated serum hCG may be present because of continued secretion by the proliferating trophoblastic tissue. (Normally hCG levels increase from the time of implantation, peak at 60 to 70 days, and then decline slowly, reaching a low point at 100 to 130 days.)

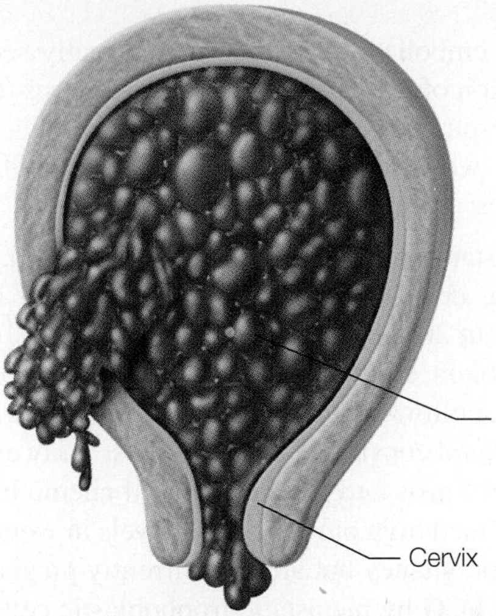

Figure 20-4 ■ Hydatidiform mole. A common sign is vaginal bleeding, often brownish (the characteristic "prune juice" appearance) but sometimes bright red. In this figure, some of the hydropic vessels are being passed. This occurrence is diagnostic for hydatidiform mole.

- Very low levels of maternal serum α-fetoprotein (MSAFP) are found.
- Hyperemesis gravidarum may occur, probably as a result of the high levels of hCG.
- Preeclampsia (discussed shortly) may be seen, especially if the molar pregnancy continues into the second trimester. Because preeclampsia is a disease of late pregnancy, if symptoms occur in the first half of pregnancy, molar pregnancy must be considered as the first diagnosis.
- Rarely, hyperthyroidism results from production of thyrotropin by molar tissue. It produces thyrotoxicosis, which may precipitate a clinical emergency.

Ultrasound is the primary means of diagnosing a molar pregnancy, usually after 6 to 8 weeks, when the vesicular enlargement of the villi can be identified.

Therapy begins with suction evacuation of the molar pregnancy and curettage of the uterus to remove all fragments of the placenta. Early evacuation decreases the possibility of other complications. If the woman is older and has completed her childbearing, or if there is excessive bleeding, hysterectomy may be the treatment of choice to reduce the incidence of malignant sequelae. Uterine contractions can cause trophoblastic tissue to be engulfed in the large venous sinusoids of the uterus. Therefore, stimulation of uterine contractions is avoided until the uterus is evacuated to prevent embolization of trophoblastic tissue to the lungs. The RhD antigen is contained in trophoblasts, therefore, at the time of evacuation of the uterus, Rh immune globulin must be administered to women with an Rh negative blood type (Berkowitz & Goldstein, 2009).

Complications associated with hydatidiform mole that require medical recognition and therapy include the following:

- Anemia
- Hyperthyroidism
- Infection, usually seen with late diagnosis and spontaneous abortion of the mole

- DIC
- Trophoblastic embolization of the lung, usually seen after molar evacuation of a significantly enlarged uterus (this creates a cardiorespiratory emergency)
- Ovarian cysts, which may be small or large enough to displace the uterus

Malignant gestational trophoblastic disease (GTD), usually choriocarcinoma, develops following evacuation of a molar pregnancy in about 20% of women (ACOG, 2008c). To detect this serious problem early and initiate treatment, follow-up care is essential. Follow-up for women who have had a molar pregnancy evacuated consists of baseline chest x-ray examination to detect metastasis and a repeat x-ray if chemotherapy is necessary. Continued high or rising hCG levels in women who have had molar pregnancy but are not currently pregnant suggest secretion of hCG by metastatic trophoblastic cells. Thus, radioimmunoassay hCG values should be determined weekly until negative three consecutive times, then should be monitored monthly for 6 months (Berkowitz & Goldstein, 2009). Effective contraception, preferably using hormonal contraceptives, is needed during this time to prevent pregnancy and the resulting confusion about the cause of changes in hCG level. In addition, pregnancy could mask an hCG rise associated with malignant GTD (Cunningham et al., 2010; Li, 2008).

If hCG plateaus or rises during this time or metastases are detected, chemotherapy is started immediately. Treatment at a center specializing in GTD is advised. Once pregnancy has been ruled out, a complete physical and pelvic examination, baseline hCG level, complete blood count and baseline blood chemistries, pelvic ultrasound, chest x-ray, and computed tomography (CT) of the brain, chest, abdomen and pelvis are done to stage the cancer and rule out metastatic spread. Chemotherapy is then begun using methotrexate alone or in combination with other chemotherapy agents (Li, 2008).

After treatment, careful follow-up monitoring of hCG levels is important. Malignant GTD is curable if diagnosed early and treated appropriately. The risk of a molar pregnancy in subsequent pregnancies is about 1% after the first one; after two molar pregnancies, the risk is 15% to 18% (Berkowitz & Goldstein, 2009).

Currently research is under way to identify risk factors for GTD and to examine the role of genetics in its development. In addition, efforts are under way to develop better, more sensitive ways to detect minimal levels of hCG and clinical trials are focusing on the effectiveness of established chemotherapy approaches in treating malignant GTD (Bess & Wood, 2006).

NURSING CARE MANAGEMENT

Nursing Assessment and Diagnosis

It is important for nurses involved in antepartum care to be aware of symptoms of hydatidiform mole and observe for them at each antepartal visit. The classic symptoms used to diagnose molar pregnancy are found more frequently with the complete than with the partial mole. The partial mole may be difficult to distinguish from a missed abortion before evacuation.

When the woman is hospitalized for evacuation of the molar pregnancy, the nurse should monitor vital signs and vaginal bleeding for evidence of hemorrhage. In addition, the nurse determines whether abdominal pain is present and assesses the woman's emotional state and coping ability.

Nursing diagnoses that may apply to a woman with a hydatidiform mole include the following:

- ***Fear*** related to the possible development of choriocarcinoma
- ***Readiness for Enhanced Knowledge*** related to an expressed desire to understand the need for regular monitoring of hCG levels and the long-term implications of the disease
- ***Grieving*** related to the loss of the pregnancy

Nursing Plan and Implementation

Community-Based Nursing Care

When molar pregnancy is suspected, the woman needs emotional support. The nurse can relieve some of the woman's anxiety by answering questions about the disease process and explaining what ultrasound and other diagnostic procedures will entail. If a molar pregnancy is diagnosed, the nurse supports the childbearing family as they deal with their grief about the lost pregnancy. Healthcare counselors, the hospital chaplain, or their own clergy may be of assistance in helping them deal with this loss.

Hospital-Based Nursing Care

When the woman is hospitalized for evacuation of the molar pregnancy, explanation of the curettage procedure is necessary. Although the physician is responsible for providing this explanation, the woman and her partner may have many questions and concerns that the nurse can discuss with them. The nurse may also clarify areas of confusion or misunderstanding.

Typed and cross-matched blood must be available for surgery because of previous blood loss and the potential for hemorrhage. Oxytocin is administered to keep the uterus contracted and prevent hemorrhage. In addition, acute renal failure, a syndrome of rapid onset, may occur when significant hemorrhage results in absolute loss of fluid volume. Following surgery, the nurse carefully observes the woman's urinary output, watches for further signs of bleeding, and assesses for any signs of infection.

If the woman is Rh negative and not sensitized, she is given Rh immune globulin to prevent antibody formation. (See discussion on Rh sensitization later in this chapter.)

Health Promotion Education

The woman needs to know the importance of the follow-up visits. She is advised to use contraception to delay becoming pregnant again until after the follow-up program is completed.

Evaluation

Expected outcomes of nursing care include the following:

- The woman has a smooth recovery following successful evacuation of the molar pregnancy.
- The woman is able to explain GTD, its treatment, follow-up, and long-term implications for pregnancy.
- The woman and her partner are able to begin verbalizing their grief at the loss of their anticipated child.

- The woman is able to discuss the importance of follow-up assessment and indicates her willingness to cooperate with the regimen.

Care of the Woman with Hyperemesis Gravidarum

Nausea and vomiting of mild to moderate intensity are common during early pregnancy, occurring most commonly in the first trimester (see chapter 16). **Hyperemesis gravidarum** is a relatively rare condition, occurring in about 0.3% to 2% of all pregnancies, in which nausea and vomiting are so severe that they affect hydration and nutritional status (Goldberg, Szilagyi, & Graves, 2007; Holmgren, Aagaard-Tillery, Silver, et al., 2008). Dehydration, electrolyte imbalances, acidosis, weight loss, ketonuria, and, possibly, hepatic and renal damage are attributable to hyperemesis.

Hyperemesis can be a temporarily disabling condition in which affected women may need multiple hospitalizations and face disruption of work, family, or social routines. In rare instances, the psychologic impact is so extreme that a woman may request pregnancy termination. It occurs more frequently in nulliparous women, adolescents, women with a multiple gestation, women with increased body weight, certain ethnic groups, pregnancies complicated by gestational trophoblastic disease (GTD) or fetal abnormalities, women with a mother or sister who experienced hyperemesis, or women with a history of hyperemesis in a previous pregnancy (ACOG, 2009b).

The cause of hyperemesis during pregnancy is still unclear, but it has been suggested that hCG plays a role (Holmgren et al., 2008). An argument against this mechanism is that nausea and vomiting are not common in women with choriocarcinoma, which is characterized by high levels of hCG. Higher levels of estradiol as well as lower levels of prolactin have been implicated as well. Other mechanisms that may relate to hyperemesis are displacement of the gastrointestinal tract, hypofunction of the anterior pituitary gland and adrenal cortex, abnormalities of the corpus luteum, and psychologic factors. Hyperemesis is rare in populations of developing countries.

In severe cases, the pathology of hyperemesis begins with dehydration. This leads to fluid-electrolyte imbalance and alkalosis from the loss of hydrochloric acid. More prolonged vomiting can result in loss of predominantly alkaline intestinal juices and the occurrence of acidosis. Hypovolemia from dehydration leads to hypotension and increased pulse rate, with increased hematocrit and blood urea nitrogen levels and decreased urine output. Severe potassium loss (hypokalemia) interferes with the ability of the kidneys to concentrate urine and disrupts cardiac functioning. Starvation causes muscle wasting and severe protein and vitamin deficiencies. Jaundice, hyperpyrexia, and peripheral neuritis may develop. If inadequately or incorrectly treated, complications such as Wernicke encephalopathy, esophageal rupture, or even maternal death may occur.

The diagnostic criteria for hyperemesis include a history of intractable vomiting in the first half of pregnancy, dehydration, ketonuria, and a weight loss of 5% of prepregnancy weight.

Clinical Therapy

The goals of treatment include controlling vomiting, correcting dehydration, restoring electrolyte balance, and maintaining adequate nutrition. It may be beneficial to avoid environmental triggers such as odors (perfume, chemicals, food, smoke), stuffy rooms, heat, humidity, noise, and visual or physical motion, brushing teeth after a meal, and not getting enough rest. Frequent small meals of high-carbohydrate, low-fat content may be helpful. Carbonated or sour beverages taken in small quantities between meals also appear to help.

Complementary and alternative therapies have also been tried in treating hyperemesis because they may offer relief for nausea and vomiting of pregnancy. Ginger has been used for its beneficial effects on motion sickness and nausea. The use of acupuncture or acupressure may also cause a reduction in the severity of symptoms (ACOG, 2009a). Hypnosis has been helpful in some women.

Pyridoxine (vitamin B_6) is a reasonable first-line pharmacologic treatment for nausea and vomiting of pregnancy. It has a good safety profile and minimal side effects. It can be administered alone or with doxylamine succinate, an antihistamine that improves efficacy. This was the formulation of Bendectin, which was voluntarily withdrawn from the market in 1983 because of a lawsuit alleging teratogenicity. Scientific evidence supports its safety and efficacy in the reduction of symptoms. Typical dosing is pyroxidine 10 to 25 mg orally three times daily and one 25 mg over-the-counter tablet (sold as Unisom Sleep Tabs) at bedtime (Yankowitz, 2008). If this is not effective, other pharmacologic options include promethazine (Phenergan), metoclopramide (Reglan), and ondansetron (Zofran).

If the woman with intractable nausea and vomiting does not respond to frequent small meals of simple carbohydrates and the occasional use of antiemetics, she may require IV fluids on an outpatient basis. If the woman's symptoms do not improve, hospitalization may be necessary.

The initial workup should include an ultrasound to exclude the possibility of molar pregnancy. Initially the woman is given nothing by mouth; IV fluids are administered to correct dehydration. Potassium chloride is typically added to the IV infusion to prevent hypokalemia. Replacement of thiamine (vitamin B_1) and pyroxidine (vitamin B_6) is important to correct deficiencies of these vitamins and prevent peripheral neuropathy. Administration of dextrose solution before the correction of thiamine deficiency could lead to Wernicke encephalopathy (loss of memory, confusion). Desired urine output is a minimum of 1000 ml/24 hours.

If the woman does not respond to this management, total parenteral nutrition may be used to meet the caloric and nutritional needs of the woman and her fetus. When the woman's condition has improved, oral feedings are started. Six small dry feedings followed by clear liquids is one suggested treatment. Another method is 1 oz of water offered each hour, followed as tolerated by clear, then nourishing liquids, progressing on succeeding days to low-fat soft and regular diets.

NURSING CARE MANAGEMENT

Nursing Assessment and Diagnosis

When a woman is hospitalized for control of vomiting, the nurse must regularly assess the amount and character of further emesis, intake and output, fetal heart rate, maternal vital signs, initial weight, evidence of jaundice or bleeding, and the woman's emotional state.

Nursing diagnoses that may apply to the woman with hyperemesis gravidarum include the following:

- ***Imbalanced Nutrition: Less Than Body Requirements*** related to persistent vomiting secondary to hyperemesis
- ***Fear*** related to the effects of hyperemesis or its treatment on fetal well-being

Nursing Plan and Implementation

Community-Based Nursing Care

The initial evaluation of the woman is designed to distinguish between morning sickness, which is amenable to self-care, and real nutritional risk. The nurse should take this opportunity to evaluate possible family and lifestyle stressors. It is wise to include both the woman and her family in the discussion of strategies to reduce nausea and vomiting she can try at home, including such tactics as small carbohydrate meals, high-protein snacks, total avoidance of fatty foods, resting with her feet up and head elevated, or slowly sipping carbonated beverages when nauseated. Herbal tea, such as spearmint, peppermint, raspberry, chamomile, or ginger root, may be helpful. Odors, very hot or cold liquids, ice, and straws should be avoided. If the nausea and vomiting progress to a point where oral intake is not tolerated and dehydration is evident, medical intervention is required.

Home Care

Parenteral therapy provided at home in collaboration with a physician and registered dietitian is sometimes used to allow the woman to remain in her home and help decrease healthcare costs. It also gives the nurse an opportunity to observe family interactions and evaluate the home environment. This assessment is often useful in determining the pregnant woman's level of support, any significant stressors in her life, her understanding of nutrition and self-care measures, and so forth.

Hospital-Based Care

Nursing care should be supportive and directed at maintaining a relaxed, quiet environment away from food odors or offensive smells. Once oral feedings are started, food should be attractively served. Oral hygiene is important because the mouth is dry and may be irritated from vomitus. Weight gain or loss should be monitored regularly. Because emotional factors have been found to play a major role in this condition, psychotherapy may be recommended. With proper treatment, the prognosis is favorable.

Health Promotion Education

As part of patient teaching, the nurse should review actions the woman can take to prevent or decrease nausea. These are discussed in chapter 16 ∞.

Evaluation

Expected outcomes of nursing care include the following:

- The woman is able to explain hyperemesis gravidarum, its therapy, and its possible effects on her pregnancy.
- The woman's condition is corrected, and possible complications are avoided.

Care of the Woman with a Hypertensive Disorder

Hypertension is the most common medical disorder in pregnancy, accounting for up to 15% of prenatal hospitalizations. The incidence of hypertension among pregnant women ranges from 12% to 22%, and hypertension is directly responsible for 17.6% of maternal deaths in the United States (ACOG, 2008b).

The classification of hypertension in pregnancy is as follows (ACOG, 2008b):

- Preeclampsia-eclampsia
- Chronic hypertension
- Chronic hypertension with superimposed preeclampsia
- Gestational hypertension

The pathophysiology and collaborative care of women with these disorders are quite different; thus, each is discussed separately.

Preeclampsia and Eclampsia

Preeclampsia occurs in 5% to 8% of all pregnancies in the United States and 3% to 14% of all pregnancies worldwide; it is the most common hypertensive disorder in pregnancy (Kuklina, Ayala, & Callaghan, 2009; Lim, Kim, Park, et al., 2008). It is estimated that 50,000 women die from preeclampsia each year worldwide. In the United States, it is the second leading cause of maternal death. Among women with chronic hypertension, 22% to 25% will develop this complication (Chappellee et al., 2008).

Preeclampsia, a syndrome that affects both mother and fetus, is clinically defined as an increase in blood pressure after 20 weeks' gestation accompanied by proteinuria in a previously normotensive woman. Edema is not included in the definition because it is a common feature in normal pregnancy (Martin, 2009). However, sudden onset of severe edema warrants close evaluation to rule out preeclampsia or other pathologic processes such as renal disease. It is important to remember that severe preeclampsia can occur without edema.

Eclampsia is the occurrence of a seizure in a woman with preeclampsia who has no other cause for seizure. Women who are going to develop preeclampsia usually become hypertensive before they develop proteinuria. In any event, the onset of hypertension in pregnancy warrants close observation.

Pathophysiology of Preeclampsia

Preeclampsia has been called a "disease of theories" because the true mechanisms behind the pathogenesis remain unclear. It has been suggested that mechanisms leading to the development of preeclampsia include impaired trophoblast differentiation and invasion, placental and endothelial dysfunction, an immune reaction to paternal antigens, and an exaggerated systemic inflammatory response (Barton & Sibai, 2008). Alterations in the rennin-angiotensin system and insulin resistance may be involved in pathogenesis as well (Thadhani & Solomon, 2008).

Some pieces of the puzzle may be coming together as new research has suggested that the pathogenesis of preeclampsia may be related to an imbalance between circulating angiogenesis-related factors (Karumanchi & Lindheimer, 2008; Lim et al., 2008; Thadhani & Solomon, 2008). Angiogenesis, the process of neovascularization from preexisting blood vessels and vasculogenesis, the process of blood vessel generation from angioblast precursor cells, occurs in the placenta causing impaired placentation associated with preeclampsia (Kopcow & Karumanchi, 2007). Widespread systemic vascular dysfunction and microangiopathy is demonstrated in the mother, but not in the fetus (Kopcow & Karumanchi 2007). The placenta plays a central role in the development of the disease, for which the only known cure is birth of the fetus and removal of the placenta.

Key features of preeclampsia involve the failure of the uterine spiral arteries to transform from thick-walled muscular vessels to saclike flaccid vessels, exaggerated inflammatory response, and inappropriate endothelial-cell activation (Barton & Sibai, 2008). Characteristics of preeclampsia include maternal vasospasm resulting in decreased perfusion to virtually all organs, including the placenta (Figure 20-5 ■), a decrease in plasma volume, activation of the coagulation cascade, and

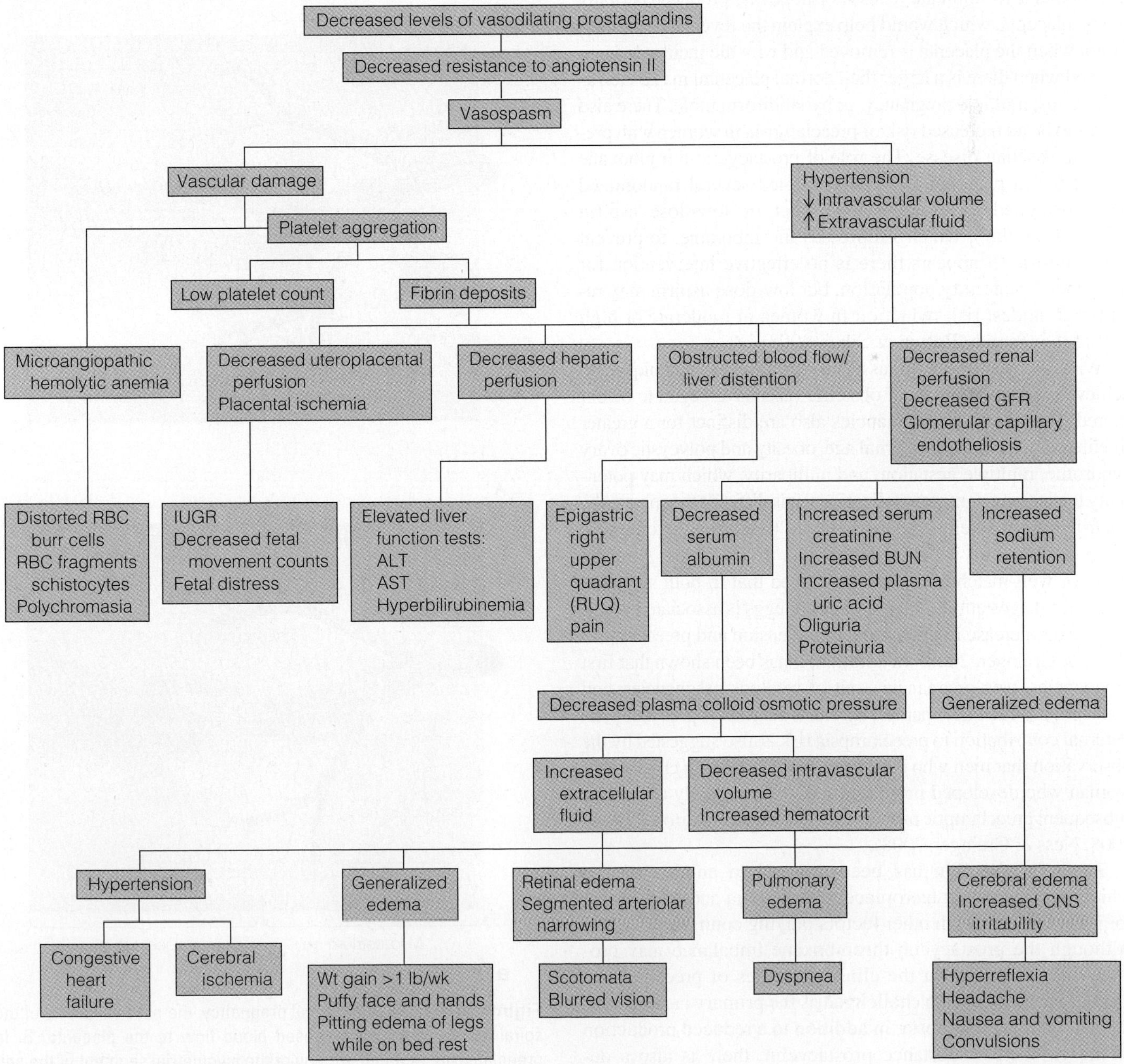

Figure 20-5 ■ Clinical manifestations and possible pathophysiology of preeclampsia-eclampsia.

alterations in glomerular capillary endothelium. The increased platelet activation and markers of endothelial activation can predate clinically evident preeclampsia by weeks or even months. In preeclampsia, a greater degree of placental infarction may be seen than occurs in normal pregnancy.

Women who develop preeclampsia become more sensitive to pressor agents (substances that increase blood pressure) rather than less sensitive to them, as in normal pregnancy. This response has been linked to the ratio between the prostaglandins prostacyclin and thromboxane. Prostacyclin, a vasodilator produced by endothelial cells, decreases blood pressure, prevents platelet aggregation, and promotes uterine blood flow. Thromboxane, produced by platelets, causes vessels to constrict and platelets to clump together. Prostacyclin is decreased in preeclampsia, allowing the potent vasoconstrictor and platelet-aggregating effects of thromboxane to dominate. These hormones are produced partially by the placenta, which would help explain the reversal of the condition when the placenta is removed and why the incidence is increased when there is a larger than normal placental mass, such as in hydrops, multiple pregnancy, or hydatidiform mole. There also seems to be an increased risk of preeclampsia in women with preexisting vascular disease. The role of prostacyclin-thromboxane imbalance in preeclampsia has prompted several randomized trials designed to evaluate the effect of low-dose aspirin (50–150 mg/day), which suppresses thromboxane, to prevent preeclampsia. It appears there is no effective intervention for the general maternity population, but low-dose aspirin may result in a modest risk reduction in women at moderate or high risk of the disease (Barton & Sibai, 2008).

With increasing use of assisted reproductive techniques to achieve pregnancy, potential obstetric risks have begun to be explored. Because these pregnancies also are distinct for a greater likelihood of advanced maternal age, obesity and polycystic ovary syndrome, multiple gestation, and nulliparity, which may potentially lead to pregnancy complications, it is difficult to separate the contribution of foreign genetic material (donor egg) from these other confounding variables (Barton & Sibai, 2008). A recent study of well-matched women concluded that in both singleton and multiple gestations, the use of donor eggs is associated with a significant increase in gestational hypertension and preeclampsia (Ness & Grainger, 2008). In addition, it has been shown that first pregnancies, teen pregnancies, out-of-wedlock pregnancies, and conception with a new partner increase the risk of preeclampsia. Paternal contribution to preeclampsia risk is also suggested by the observation that men who have previously fathered a child with a woman who developed preeclampsia are more likely to father a subsequent preeclamptic birth with a new partner (Barton & Sibai, 2008; Ness & Grainger, 2008).

Recently, attention has been directed to another theory, which postulates that uteroplacental ischemia acts as a trigger for preeclampsia, with other factors playing contributory roles. Although the prostacyclin-thromboxane imbalance may provide an explanation for the clinical features of preeclampsia, this theory is now being challenged as the primary cause. In the woman with preeclampsia, in addition to a reduced production of the vasoactive substance prostacyclin, there is also a decreased production of nitric oxide. Nitric oxide is a potent vasodilator and important regulator of maternal blood pressure. Nitric oxide synthesis in the placenta may play a meaningful role in maintaining a low-pressure, high-flow placental system and also may prevent intervillous thrombosis. The loss of normal vasodilatation of uterine arterioles results in decreased placental perfusion (Figure 20-6 ■), potentially leading to fetal growth restriction and chronic hypoxia or distress.

Hyperhomocysteinemia may play a role in the etiology or pathophysiology of preeclampsia through oxidative stress and endothelial dysfunction. Mild elevations of homocysteine have been found in normotensive women who go on to develop preeclampsia. Once preeclampsia is established, homocysteine levels are considerably increased. It is unclear whether the circulating levels of homocysteine have caused preeclampsia or if they reflect metabolic alterations resulting from the disease

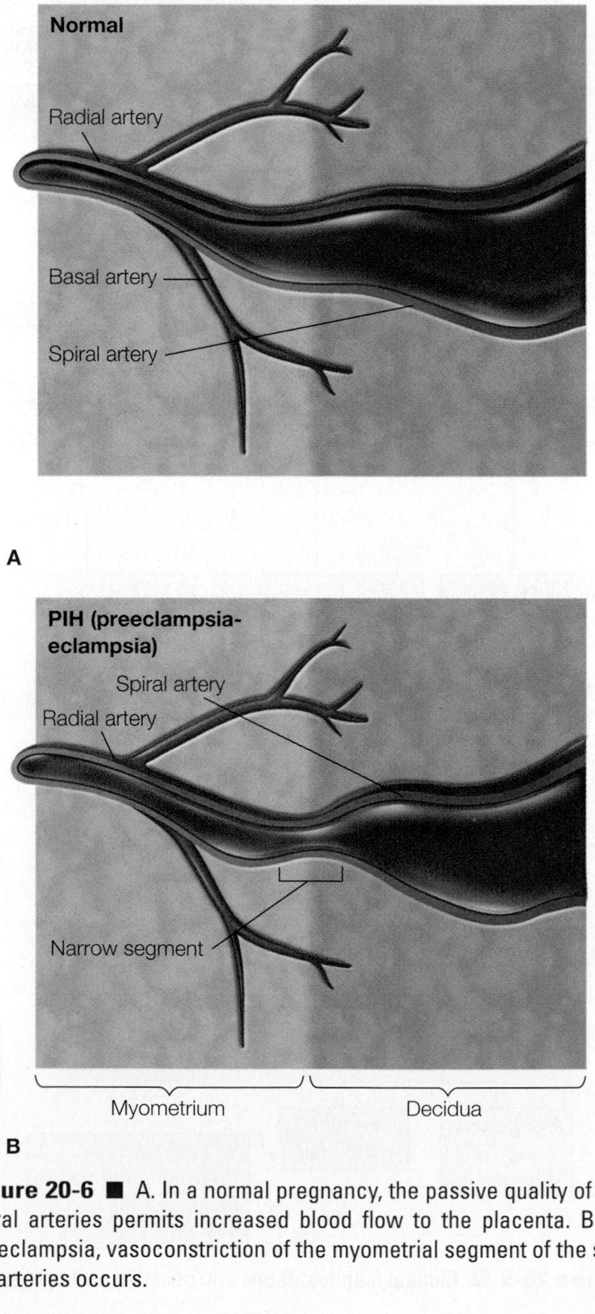

Figure 20-6 ■ A. In a normal pregnancy, the passive quality of the spiral arteries permits increased blood flow to the placenta. B. In preeclampsia, vasoconstriction of the myometrial segment of the spiral arteries occurs.

process. In the presence of regulatory gene mutations, deficiencies of vitamins B_6, B_{12}, or folic acid may cause a rise in homocysteine. If a causal link can be demonstrated, this might lead to strategies for preventing preeclampsia. In a study of approximately 4000 women who received folic acid supplementation, it was found that folic acid supplementation was associated with a decrease in plasma homocysteine and a reduced risk of preeclampsia (Wen et al., 2008).

Decreased renal perfusion is associated with preeclampsia. With a reduction in glomerular filtration rate (GFR), serum levels of creatinine, blood urea nitrogen (BUN), and uric acid begin to rise from normal pregnant levels, whereas urine output diminishes. For each 50% decrease in GFR, serum creatinine and BUN plasma levels double, whereas sodium is retained in increased amounts. Sodium retention results in increased extracellular volume and increased sensitivity to angiotensin II. The typical kidney lesion of preeclampsia involves swollen glomerular capillary endothelial cells containing fibrin deposits. Stretching of the capillary walls allows the large protein molecules, primarily albumin, to escape into the urine, decreasing serum albumin.

Edema is usually more profound in preeclampsia than in normal pregnancy although some of the most severe forms of the disease may occur without edema. The pathologic basis of edema is twofold:

1. The higher salt retention draws out intravascular fluid.
2. Plasma colloid osmotic pressure decreases because of serum albumin loss through edematous renal glomeruli and damaged vascular endothelium. This causes fluid movement to extracellular spaces.

The decreased intravascular volume causes increased viscosity of the blood and a corresponding rise in hematocrit.

HELLP Syndrome

HELLP syndrome (*h*emolysis, *e*levated *l*iver enzymes, and *l*ow *p*latelet count) is associated with severe preeclampsia, although it may occur in women with normal or minimally elevated blood pressure and no proteinuria. Hypertension or proteinuria may be absent in 10% to 15% of women with HELLP syndrome (Airoldi & Weinstein, 2007; Sibai, 2007). Ninety percent of women with HELLP syndrome present with symptoms before 36 weeks' gestation. In women with severe preeclampsia-eclampsia, the incidence of HELLP syndrome is 2% to 20% (ACOG, 2008b; Hay, 2008). Twenty-five percent first demonstrate the disease in the postpartum period (Hay, 2008).

The hemolysis that occurs is termed *microangiopathic hemolytic anemia.* It is thought that red blood cells are distorted or fragmented during passage through small, damaged blood vessels. Vascular damage is associated with vasospasm, and platelets aggregate at sites of damage, resulting in low platelet count (less than $100{,}000/mm^3$). Elevated liver enzymes occur from blood flow that is obstructed because of fibrin deposits. Deposits of fibrin-like material found in the hepatic sinusoids cause obstruction and hepatocellular injury. This necrosis is the classic hepatic lesion associated with HELLP. Increase in intrahepatic pressure causes swelling of the liver. Liver distention causes epigastric pain and may ultimately result in rupture. Hyperbilirubinemia and jaundice may also be seen.

Symptoms can include nausea, vomiting, malaise, flulike symptoms, or epigastric pain. This can lead to misdiagnoses of gastroenteritis, hepatitis, gallbladder disease, pyelonephritis, renal disease, or thrombocytopenia purpura. Regardless of their blood pressure or the presence of protein in their urine, women presenting with the preceding symptoms should have a CBC with platelet count and liver enzymes drawn. Perinatal morbidity and mortality with HELLP syndrome are high; therefore, the possibility of HELLP should be considered carefully.

Women with HELLP syndrome are best cared for in a tertiary care center. Initially, the mother's condition should be assessed and stabilized, especially if her platelets are very low. The fetus is also assessed using a nonstress test and biophysical profile. All women with true HELLP syndrome should give birth regardless of gestational age.

Maternal Risks

Hypertensive disorders account for 16% of maternal mortality in developed countries (Cunningham et al., 2010). Preeclampsia can impact most organ systems, causing serious complications. Central nervous system (CNS) changes include hyperreflexia, headache, and eclamptic seizure. The underlying cause of the seizures is not known. Once thought to be from cerebral edema, there is some controversy as to whether cerebral edema is a feature of eclampsia or a postmortem phenomenon.

Application: Preeclampsia and HELLP

Intracerebral hemorrhage is a rare complication, but it is the most common cause of death in women with severe preeclampsia and eclampsia, being fatal in 50% to 65% of cases; those who survive may suffer permanent disability (Mihu, Costin, Mihu, et al., 2007). Risk factors for pregnancy-related stroke include hypertension, cardiac disease, infection, hyperemesis gravidarum, fluid and electrolyte imbalances, anemia/hemorrhage, sickle cell anemia, history of migraine headaches, smoking, drug abuse, thrombocytopenia, age greater than 35, and African American race (ACOG, 2008a).

Increased intraocular pressure can cause retinal detachment, but spontaneous reattachment usually occurs with reduction in blood pressure and diuresis.

Acute tubular necrosis may result from underperfusion of the kidneys. This is associated with hypovolemia and renal vasoconstriction. Although many women with preeclampsia will have oliguria, most do not develop acute tubular necrosis. One of the more common problems related to preeclampsia is pulmonary edema due to increased capillary permeability.

Thrombocytopenia complicates severe preeclampsia in about 7% to 11% of women (Ghulmiyyah & Sabai, 2006). The exact mechanism is not fully understood, but platelet consumption is believed to be related to endothelial damage and activation of thrombin. Abruptio placentae is a risk associated with preeclampsia. The release of procoagulants, such as thromboplastin, can result in acute disseminated intravascular coagulation (DIC).

Subcapsular hematoma of the liver is a rare but important occurrence in women with preeclampsia and HELLP syndrome. In addition to the signs of preeclampsia, physical examination may reveal hepatomegaly and peritoneal irritation.

Rupture of a subcapsular hematoma is a life-threatening event. The woman may complain of right shoulder pain or severe epigastric pain persisting for several hours before circulatory collapse is evident. This is a surgical emergency requiring a multidisciplinary approach to management. Maternal and fetal mortality is over 50%, and women who survive are at risk for adult pulmonary distress syndrome, pulmonary edema, and acute renal failure in the postoperative period.

Vaginal birth is preferable to cesarean birth in women with preeclampsia or HELLP syndrome. Aggressive induction of labor should take place regardless of the favorability of the cervix. Cesarean birth is considered if vaginal birth does not take place within a reasonable amount of time, usually 24 hours, or for the usual obstetric indications.

Fetal-Neonatal Risks

Preeclampsia is a primary cause of placental insufficiency and premature birth. In addition, it has numerous effects on the neonate.

Infants of women with preeclampsia during pregnancy tend to be small for gestational age (SGA) because of intrauterine growth restriction. The cause is related specifically to maternal vasospasm and hypovolemia, which result in fetal hypoxia and malnutrition. Placental abruption secondary to hypertension may result in fetal hypoxia or even death. In addition, the newborn may be premature because the treatment for the maternal condition may require early childbirth.

At birth, the newborn may be oversedated because of medications administered to the woman. The newborn may also have hypermagnesemia caused by treatment of the woman with large doses of magnesium sulfate.

Clinical Manifestations and Diagnosis

The most commonly occurring clinical manifestations and diagnoses are discussed here.

MILD PREECLAMPSIA The diagnosis of preeclampsia is made based on the presence of new onset hypertension and proteinuria. After 20 weeks' gestation, a blood pressure of 140 mm Hg systolic or 90 mm Hg diastolic on at least two occasions 6 hours apart in a woman who was previously normotensive before pregnancy is used for diagnosis. The blood pressure measurements should be no more than 7 days apart (Habli & Sibai, 2008).

With mild preeclampsia, proteinuria is generally between 300 mg/L (1+ dipstick) and 1 g/L (2+ dipstick). This is measured in a midstream clean-catch or catheter-derived urine specimen.

The gold standard for the measurement of proteinuria is the 24-hour urine. Excretion of more than 300 mg of protein in a 24-hour period is considered abnormal (Airoldi & Weinstein, 2007). This correlates approximately with a dipstick protein reading of 1+ (30 mg/dl) or greater if specific gravity is between 1.010 and 1.030. Protein measurement may vary throughout the 24-hour period, partly related to urine concentration. This can be adjusted for with the use of a protein/creatinine ratio rather than the simple protein concentration alone. Although edema is no longer considered a diagnostic criterion, generalized edema, seen as puffy face, hands, and dependent areas such as the ankles and lower legs, may be present. Edema is identified by a weight gain of more than 1.5 kg/month (3.3 lb) in the second trimester or more than 0.5 kg/week (1.1 lb) in the third trimester. Edema is assessed on a 1+ to 4+ scale.

SEVERE PREECLAMPSIA Severe preeclampsia may develop suddenly. The following clinical signs are often present (ACOG, 2008b):

- Blood pressure of 160/110 mm Hg or higher on two occasions at least 6 hours apart while the woman is on bed rest
- Proteinuria 5 g/L or higher in 24 hours or 3+ or greater on two random urine samples collected at least 4 hours apart
- Oliguria: urine output less than or equal to 500 ml in 24 hours
- Cerebral or visual disturbances
- Pulmonary edema or cyanosis
- Epigastric or right upper quadrant pain
- Impaired liver function (elevated hepatic enzymes–alanine aminotransferase (ALT) or aspartate aminotransferase (AST) to at least twice normal
- Thrombocytopenia (less than 100,000 platelets per cubic millimeter)
- Fetal growth restriction

Other signs or symptoms that may be present include severe headache or one that persists despite analgesic therapy, blurred vision or scotomata (spots before the eyes), narrowed segments on the retinal arterioles when examined with an ophthalmoscope, retinal edema (retinas appear wet and glistening) on funduscopy, dyspnea due to pulmonary edema, moist breath sounds on auscultation, pitting edema of lower extremities while on bed rest, epigastric pain, hyperreflexia, nausea and vomiting, irritability, and emotional tension.

ECLAMPSIA Eclampsia, characterized by convulsion or coma, may occur before the onset of labor, during labor, or early in the postpartum period. Late postpartum eclampsia (convulsions occurring more than 48 hours following birth) occurs rarely but has been documented. Some women experience only one convulsion, especially if it occurs late in labor or during the postpartum period. Others may have from 2 to 20 or more. Unless they occur extremely frequently, the woman often regains consciousness between convulsions.

Clinical Therapy

The goals of medical management are prevention of cerebral hemorrhage, convulsion, hematologic complications, and renal and hepatic diseases, and birth of an uncompromised newborn as close to term as possible. Reduction of elevated blood pressure is essential in accomplishing these goals.

ANTEPARTUM MANAGEMENT The only known cure for preeclampsia is birth of the infant. As mentioned earlier, recent research has focused on preventing preeclampsia in at-risk women through the use of low-dose (50 to 150 mg daily) aspirin begun between 12 and 18 weeks' gestation. Aspirin is known to block the action of an enzyme, cyclooxygenase, essential to the production of prostaglandins. This results in lowered levels of thromboxane, the vasoconstrictor. At the same time, levels of the vasodilator prostacyclin are not significantly affected.

Several dietary approaches have been suggested, including supplementation with zinc, magnesium, and fish oil. Results of trials have either been conflicting or have revealed minimal or no benefit from nutritional supplementation. Recent studies have examined Vitamin D supplementation and report a protective effect on preeclampsia development (Haugen et al., 2009). Supplementation with calcium may be effective for the mother, but the impact on the fetus is not clear (Meads, Cnossen, Meher, et al., 2008). Antioxidants (Vitamin C and E) have been advanced as potential protective mechanisms, but research does not support their effectiveness in reducing the risk of preeclampsia. One large, international study showed that antioxidants may actually increase adverse events, including fetal loss and premature rupture of the membranes (Xu, Perez-Cuevas, Xiong, et al., 2010). Based on available data, neither vitamin supplementation nor low-dose aspirin should be prescribed routinely for prevention of preeclampsia in nulliparous women (ACOG, 2008b; Barton & Sibai, 2008).

Home Care of Gestational Hypertension and Mild Preeclampsia In general, women with proteinuric preeclampsia should be admitted to the hospital. However, with changes in health care, more attention has been given to decreasing inpatient hospital days for women whose symptoms allow. Close maternal monitoring is essential to establish the severity and progression of the disease. The woman must be able to comply with frequent maternal/fetal evaluations and have ready access to medical care.

A woman should be considered for management at home if she meets the following criteria: blood pressure less than or equal to 150/100 mm Hg, proteinuria less than 1 g/24 hours or 3+ dipstick, platelet count greater than 120,000 mm^3, and normal fetal growth if not at term or showing signs of complicating factors such as vaginal bleeding. She must have a basic understanding of her condition, be able to recognize the signs and symptoms of worsening preeclampsia (Table 20-1), be able to accurately count fetal movements, be cooperative, and know when to call the doctor. Although decreased activity is generally recommended, she is not restricted to bed rest but is encouraged to rest frequently, especially in the left lateral position.

The woman monitors her blood pressure, weight, and urine protein daily. Weight gains of 1.4 kg (3 lb) in 24 hours or 1.8 kg (4 lb) in a 3-day period are generally causes for concern. Remote NSTs are performed on a daily to biweekly basis. Companies that provide this service have equipment that allows phone transmission of blood pressure readings as well as fetal monitor tracings. This eliminates concerns about inaccurate reporting on the part of the woman. Nursing contact varies from daily to weekly, depending on physician request. Laboratory testing regularly evaluates platelet counts, uric acid and BUN, liver enzymes, and 24-hour urine specimens for creatinine clearance and total protein. Estimates of fetal growth and amniotic fluid volume should be made at the time preeclampsia is diagnosed and repeated every 3 weeks if normal. Any woman with worsening symptoms or severe preeclampsia should be hospitalized.

TABLE 20-1 Signs and Symptoms of Worsening Preeclampsia

- Increasing edema, especially of hands and face (If on bed rest, observe for sacral edema.)
- Worsening headache
- Epigastric pain
- Visual disturbances
- Decreasing urinary output
- Nausea/vomiting
- Bleeding gums
- Disorientation
- Generalized complaints of not feeling well

RESEARCH EVIDENCE IN PRACTICE Preventing Preeclampsia

CLINICAL QUESTION

What role can rest play in helping decrease the risk of preeclampsia?

RESEARCH EVIDENCE

The most cost-effective and widely tested measure to prevent the development of preeclampsia is periodic rest periods for the mother during pregnancy. Rest is effective in preventing hypertension and proteinuria in women who began their pregnancy with normal blood pressure.

WHAT QUESTIONS REMAIN UNANSWERED?

How much rest is needed to gain the benefits of preeclampsia prevention without causing the adverse effects of lack of exercise?

WHAT IS BEST PRACTICE?

The most cost-effective preventative method without detectable adverse effects for mother and baby is rest periods of between 30 minutes and 4 hours, lying in the left lateral position.

CRITICAL THINKING

How can the nurse incorporate this evidence into prenatal teaching plans? What adverse events from excessive rest should be included in the routine prenatal assessment?

References

Meads, C., Cnossen, J., Meher, S., Juarez-Garcia, A., terRiet, G., Duley, L., . . . Khan, K. S. (2008). Methods of prediction and prevention of preeclampsia: Systematic reviews of accuracy and effectiveness literature with economic modeling. *Health Technology Assessment, 12*(6), iii–iv, 1–270.

Meher, S. & Duley, L. (2006). Rest during pregnancy for preventing preeclampsia and its complications in women with normal blood pressure. *Cochrane Database of Systematic Reviews.* Issue 2. Article No.: CD005939. doi:10.1002/14651858.Cd005939

Hospital Care of Mild Preeclampsia The woman is placed on bed rest, primarily in the left lateral recumbent position, to decrease pressure on the vena cava, thereby increasing venous return, circulatory volume, and placental and renal perfusion. Improved renal blood flow helps decrease angiotensin II levels, promotes diuresis, and lowers blood pressure.

Her diet should be well balanced and nutritious. Sodium intake should be moderate, not to exceed 6 g/day. Excessively salty foods should be avoided, but strict sodium restriction and diuretics are no longer used in treating preeclampsia.

Tests to evaluate fetal status are done more frequently as a pregnant woman's preeclampsia progresses. These tests are described in detail in chapter 21 ∞. Monitoring fetal well-being is essential to achieving a safe outcome for the fetus. The following tests are used:

- Fetal movement record
- NST
- Ultrasonography at least every 3 to 4 weeks for serial determination of growth
- Biophysical profile
- Amniocentesis to determine fetal lung maturity
- Doppler velocimetry beginning at 30 to 32 weeks to screen for fetal compromise

Maternal well-being is monitored by the following:

- Blood pressure four times daily
- Daily weight and daily evaluation for worsening edema, persistent headache, visual changes, or epigastric pain
- Daily urine dipstick for protein
- Periodic assessment of laboratory values to include CBC with platelet count, liver function tests (AST, ALT), lactic dehydrogenase (LDH), uric acid, serum creatinine, bilirubin, and 24-hour urine for protein and creatinine clearance

Hospital Care of Severe Preeclampsia Any patient with severe preeclampsia is hospitalized immediately. It is widely accepted that childbirth should be considered in all pregnant women who develop preeclampsia after 34 weeks' gestation because the risks of prolonging the pregnancy are so severe for the mother. Expectant management may be used in selected women who are less than 34 weeks because the approach significantly improves neonatal outcomes (Cunningham et al., 2010; Habli & Sibai, 2008). Fetal well-being is assessed daily and birth is indicated regardless of gestational age if maternal or fetal condition worsens (Habli & Sibai, 2008). Other medical therapies for severe preeclampsia include the following:

- ***Bed rest.*** Bed rest must be complete. Stimuli that may bring on a convulsion should be reduced.
- ***Diet.*** A high-protein, moderate-sodium diet is given as long as the woman is alert and has no nausea or indication of impending convulsion.
- ***Anticonvulsants.*** Magnesium sulfate is the treatment of choice for seizure prophylaxis in preeclampsia and treatment of eclamptic convulsions and has been used for more than 60 years because of its CNS-depressant action (Costantine & Weiner, 2009; Pryde & Mittendorf, 2009). Blood levels of magnesium sulfate should be maintained at therapeutic levels (levels vary according to laboratory). Excessive blood levels may produce respiratory paralysis or cardiac arrest. (See Drug Guide: Magnesium Sulfate on page 468.) Anticonvulsant therapy may prevent seizures, but does not prevent the ultimate progression of the disease.
- ***Corticosteroids.*** Betamethasone or dexamethasone is often administered to the woman whose fetus has an immature lung profile to promote fetal lung maturation. Dexamethasone, which has the potency 1.25 times that of betamethasone, is often chosen for use with HELLP syndrome. Dexamethasone may be administered intravascularly, which may also influence its effectiveness. The benefits of corticosteroids in women with HELLP syndrome were first recognized when the drugs were given for fetal lung maturity enhancement to women with preterm gestations. Antepartum platelet counts stabilized or increased, whereas hepatic enzymes and LDH stabilized or decreased and mean arterial pressure and urinary output improved. The use of intravenous dexamethasone to improve maternal outcome in women with HELLP syndrome remains controversial (Katz, de Amorim, Figueiroa, et al., 2008; Sibai & Stella, 2009).
- ***Fluid and electrolyte replacement.*** The goal of fluid intake is to achieve a balance between correcting hypovolemia and preventing circulatory overload. Fluid intake may be oral or supplemented with IV therapy. IV fluids may be started "to keep lines open" in case they are needed for drug therapy, even when oral intake is adequate. Criteria vary for determining appropriate fluid intake. Electrolytes are replaced as indicated by daily serum electrolyte levels. Women with preeclampsia are at risk for hyponatremia (low blood sodium), which is indicative of low serum osmolality. A rapid decrease in serum osmolality can cause seizures as a result of cerebral dysfunction. It is imperative that serum sodium levels be evaluated to assess the need for fluid restriction and the switch from IV administration to an isotonic sodium chloride administration.
- ***Antihypertensives.*** The major indication for antihypertensive therapy is the prevention of stroke. In general, antihypertensive therapy is given for sustained systolic blood pressure of at least 160 mm Hg or diastolic blood pressures of 105 to 110 mm Hg or above (Habli & Sibai, 2008).

The therapeutic goal is to maintain the diastolic blood pressure between 90 and 100 mm Hg. Decreasing the diastolic below 90 mm Hg may decrease uterine blood flow, causing fetal compromise. Methyldopa is often used for long-term control of mild to moderate hypertension in pregnancy because it is effective and has a well-documented fetal and maternal safety record. However, its slow onset of action does not make it an option for treatment of elevated blood pressure in severe preeclampsia. Labetalol and hydralazine are commonly used drugs for the treatment of acute hypertension in pregnancy and are generally administered by IV boluses (McCoy & Baldwin, 2009). Labetalol should be avoided in women with asthma or congestive heart failure. Oral nifedipine acts rapidly and has favorable hemodynamic effects and fewer side effects than IV hydralazine. Some guidelines recommend against using any calcium channel blocker with magnesium sulfate because of a potential drug interaction resulting in a neuromuscular blockade and hypotension. Based on the Magnesium Sulfate for Prevention of Preeclampsia Trial as well as a retrospective look at concurrent use of nifedipine and magnesium sulfate, there appears to be no clinically significant interaction between the two drugs (McCoy & Baldwin, 2009). If these medications are not successful in controlling blood pressure, sodium nitroprusside may be indicated for an acute emergency (McCoy & Baldwin, 2009; NIH, 2000).

Hospital Care of Eclampsia Eclampsia is defined as the occurrence of either seizure or coma associated with pregnancy and not caused by other neurologic disease. The overall incidence is about 1 in 2000 to 1 in 3448 (Cunningham et al., 2010). Seizures may be focal, multifocal, or generalized. The possible etiology of the seizure is likely related to cerebral vasospasm, edema, hemorrhage, ischemia, or loss of autoregulation of cerebral blood flow due to high systemic pressure (hypertensive encephalopathy) but no mechanism has been proven conclusively. Many women experience an increase in deep tendon reflexes (DTRs) before seizure, but seizures may also occur without hyperreflexia. The woman with preeclampsia should be monitored for signs and symptoms of impending eclampsia: scotomata, which can appear as dark spots or flashing lights in the field of vision; blurred vision; epigastric pain; vomiting; persistent or severe headache, generally frontal in location; neurologic hyperactivity; pulmonary edema; and cyanosis. Eclamptic seizures are almost always self limiting and generally last no more than 3 to 4 minutes.

If a seizure occurs, nursing assessment should include time of onset, progress of the seizure, body involvement, duration, presence of incontinence, status of the fetus, and signs of placental abruption. The airway should be maintained and oxygen administered during the seizure. The woman is positioned on her side to avoid aspiration. Suctioning may be necessary to keep the airway clear; a tongue blade should not be inserted into the back of the throat because it may stimulate the gag reflex. To prevent injury, side rails should be up and padded, but the woman should not be restrained.

Magnesium sulfate has long been used in the treatment of preeclampsia. A bolus of 6 g magnesium sulfate is administered intravenously over 20 to 30 minutes followed by 2–3 g/hour IV infusion (Habli & Sibai, 2008). In 10% of cases, an eclamptic woman will experience a second seizure. An additional bolus of 2 g of magnesium sulfate can be administered intravenously over 5 to 10 minutes. If convulsions continue, sodium amobarbitol is administered intravenously (Habli & Sibai, 2008).

Side effects with the loading dose may include flushing, a feeling of warmth, headache, nystagmus, nausea, dry mouth, and dizziness. Other side effects include lethargy and sluggishness and a risk of pulmonary edema if the woman has predisposing conditions such as multiple gestation or infection; has had excessive IV fluid administration; or has concurrent β-sympathomimetic therapy. See Drug Guide: Magnesium Sulfate for other side effects. Fetal side effects may include hypotonia and lethargy that persist for 1 or 2 days following birth, hypoglycemia, and hypocalcemia. (See chapter 26 ∞ for a discussion of magnesium sulfate and preterm labor.)

> **CLINICAL TIP**
>
> When caring for a woman with preeclampsia who is receiving IV magnesium sulfate, it is imperative to follow protocols for monitoring blood levels of magnesium. It is imperative to provide close surveillance of a woman receiving magnesium sulfate rather than relying only on blood levels to guide dosing. You are probably already aware of the common signs of increasing magnesium levels, such as diminished reflexes and decreased respiratory rate. However, there are some subtle clues you can also watch for that may suggest either the therapeutic or toxic range. When a woman's magnesium level is in the therapeutic range, she usually has some slurring of speech, awkwardness of movement, and decreased appetite. If the woman is slow to arouse, has slow/shallow respirations, or begins to have difficulty swallowing and begins to drool, she may be approaching the toxic range.

Antihypertensive agents are used to keep the diastolic blood pressure between 90 and 100 mm Hg, thus avoiding a potential reduction in uteroplacental blood flow or cerebral perfusion. The drugs used to achieve this goal are 5 to 10 mg bolus of hydralazine hydrochloride every 15 minutes to a maximum of 20 mg IV or 20 mg bolus of labetalol intravenously, followed by 20 to 80 mg every 10 minutes as needed to a maximum dose of 300 mg. An IV infusion of 1–2 mg/minute can be used in lieu of intermittent therapy. Nifedipine and nicardipine are oral options (McCoy & Baldwin, 2009).

During a seizure, fetal bradycardia, transient late decelerations, decreased variability, or compensatory tachycardia may occur. Stabilizing the mother can help the fetus recover in utero. If the fetal heart tracing remains nonreassuring for more than 10 to15 minutes despite maternal and fetal resuscitative efforts, emergency birth should be considered. An eclamptic seizure increases uterine irritability and may cause a precipitous birth. Therefore a minimum ratio of one nurse to one patient is imperative to assess fetal and maternal status. Although she may still be unconscious, the woman should be observed for onset of labor. The woman is also observed for signs of placental separation (see chapter 26 ∞). She should be checked every 15 minutes for vaginal bleeding, which may or may not be present with abruptio placentae. The abdomen is palpated for uterine rigidity.

Following a seizure, frequent auscultation of maternal lungs is required to assess for complications from aspiration and to rule out pulmonary edema, which is common in eclamptic patients. The woman is watched for circulatory and renal failure and for signs of cerebral hemorrhage. Furosemide (Lasix) may be given in low doses for pulmonary edema; digitalis may be given for circulatory failure. An indwelling Foley catheter is often inserted and intake and output are monitored hourly.

A woman may have a single convulsion or many convulsions, usually followed by a period of unresponsiveness. She may be combative and confused as she awakens, but having a

DRUG GUIDE Magnesium Sulfate

PREGNANCY RISK CATEGORY: B

OVERVIEW OF OBSTETRIC ACTION

Magnesium sulfate acts as a CNS depressant by decreasing the quantity of acetylcholine released by motor nerve impulses and thereby blocking neuromuscular transmission. This action reduces the possibility of convulsion, which is why magnesium sulfate is used in the treatment of preeclampsia. Because magnesium sulfate secondarily relaxes smooth muscle, it may decrease the blood pressure, although it is not considered an antihypertensive. Magnesium sulfate may also decrease the frequency and intensity of uterine contractions; as a result it is also used as a tocolytic in the treatment of preterm labor.

ROUTE, DOSAGE, FREQUENCY

Magnesium sulfate is generally given intravenously to control dosage more accurately and prevent overdosage. An occasional physician still prescribes intramuscular administration. However, it is painful and irritating to the tissues and does not permit the close control that IV administration does. The IV route allows for immediate onset of action. It must be given by infusion pump for accurate dosage.

FOR TREATMENT OF PREECLAMPSIA

Loading dose: 4–6 g magnesium sulfate is administered over a 20- to 30-minute period.

Maintenance dose: 2–3 g/hour via infusion pump (Habli & Sibai, 2008).

NOTE: Magnesium sulfate is excreted via the kidneys. Because women in preterm labor typically have normal renal function, they generally require higher levels of magnesium to achieve a therapeutic range than women who have preeclampsia and may have compromised renal function. Maintenance dose may need to be adjusted based on serum magnesium levels.

MATERNAL CONTRAINDICATIONS

Diagnosed maternal myasthenia gravis is the only absolute contraindication to the administration of magnesium sulfate (ACOG, 2008b). A history of myocardial damage or heart block is a relative contraindication to use of the drug because of the effects on nerve transmission and muscle contractility. Extreme care is necessary in administration to women with impaired renal function because the drug is eliminated by the kidneys, and toxic magnesium levels may develop quickly.

MATERNAL SIDE EFFECTS

Most maternal side effects are dose related. Lethargy and weakness related to neuromuscular blockade are common. Sweating, a feeling of warmth, flushing, and nasal congestion may be related to peripheral vasodilation. Other side effects include nausea and vomiting, constipation, visual blurring, headache, slurred speech, palpitations, and pulmonary edema. Signs of developing toxicity include depression or absence of reflexes, oliguria, confusion, respiratory depression, circulatory collapse, and respiratory paralysis. Rapid administration of large doses may cause cardiac arrest. A potential for uterine atony and postpartum hemorrhage may occur from magnesium's tocolytic effect. Magnesium can cause a rapid suppression of parathyroid hormone release which may cause a transient hypocalcemia. If symptoms of myoclonus, delirium, or EKG abnormalities are present, calcium gluconate should be administered.

EFFECTS ON FETUS/NEWBORN

The drug readily crosses the placenta. A transient decrease in fetal heart rate (FHR) baseline and variability may occur. In general, magnesium sulfate therapy does not pose a risk to the fetus. Ill effects in the newborn may actually be related to fetal growth retardation, prematurity, or perinatal asphyxia.

NURSING CONSIDERATIONS

1. Monitor the blood pressure closely during administration.
2. Monitor maternal serum magnesium levels as ordered (usually every 6–8 hours). Therapeutic levels are in the range of 4–8 mg/dl. Reflexes often disappear at serum magnesium levels of 9–12 mg/dl; respiratory depression may occur at levels of 14 mg/dl; cardiac arrest occurs at levels above 24–30 mg/dl.
3. Monitor respirations closely. If the rate is less than 12/minute, magnesium toxicity may be developing, and further assessments are indicated. Many protocols require stopping the medication if the respiratory rate falls below 12/minute.
4. Assess knee jerk (patellar tendon reflex) for evidence of diminished or absent reflexes. Loss of reflexes is often the first sign of developing toxicity. Also note marked lethargy or decreased level of consciousness and hypotension.
5. Determine urinary output. Output less than 30 ml/hour may result in the accumulation of toxic levels of magnesium.
6. If the respirations or urinary output fall below specified levels or if the reflexes are diminished or absent, no further magnesium should be administered until these factors return to normal.
7. The antagonist of magnesium sulfate is calcium. Consequently, an ampule of calcium gluconate should be available at the bedside. For respiratory paralysis or cardiac arrest, the usual dose is 1 g given IV over a period of about 3 minutes.
8. Monitor fetal heart tones continuously with IV administration.
9. Continue magnesium sulfate infusion for approximately 24 hours after birth as prophylaxis against postpartum seizures if given for preeclampsia.
10. If the mother has received magnesium sulfate close to birth, the newborn should be closely observed for signs of magnesium toxicity for 24–48 hours.

Note: Protocols for magnesium sulfate administration may vary somewhat according to agency policy. Consequently, individuals are referred to their own agency protocols for specific guidelines.

family member at her side helps to reduce her agitation. Also, it is important to avoid bright light, noises, and frequent disturbances. The most serious complication, cerebral hemorrhage, arises from uncontrolled hypertension. Loss of vision, which is usually temporary, is a sign of impending hemorrhage. IV options for the treatment of hypertension are hydralazine, labetalol, or nitroprusside. Nitroprusside has been restricted to hypertensive crises when childbirth is imminent and other medications have not worked. Fetal cyanide poisoning may occur if the drug is continued and birth is delayed. Use of nitroprusside requires an arterial line because of its quick action and profound effects on blood pressure.

INTRAPARTUM MANAGEMENT

Preeclampsia Labor may be induced by IV oxytocin when there is evidence of fetal maturity and cervical readiness. In very severe cases, cesarean birth may be necessary regardless of fetal maturity.

The woman may receive both IV oxytocin and magnesium sulfate simultaneously. Because magnesium sulfate has a depressant action on smooth muscle, uterine contractions may diminish, and labor may be augmented with oxytocin. Equipment and IV lines for both fluids must be checked frequently to ensure that they are being administered at the proper rate. Infusion pumps should be used to guarantee accuracy. Bags and tubing must be labeled carefully.

Narcotics may be given intravenously for pain relief in labor. An epidural, spinal, or combined spinal-epidural can be safely administered to the woman with preeclampsia in the absence of thrombocytopenia. Hypotension is a major concern and can be avoided by careful attention to technique and careful volume expansion. The woman with preeclampsia is in total body fluid overload but has a depleted intravascular volume, making her prone to hypotension when the vascular bed dilates in response to epidural/spinal administration.

Childbirth in the Sims' position should be considered. If the lithotomy position is used, a wedge should be placed under the right buttock to displace the uterus. The wedge should also be used if birth is by cesarean. Oxygen is administered to the woman during labor if the need is indicated by fetal response to the contractions.

Eclampsia If not in a tertiary care center, the woman with eclampsia is cared for in an intensive care unit until labor begins or is induced. Invasive hemodynamic monitoring of either central venous pressure (CVP) or pulmonary artery wedge pressure (PAWP) may be instituted using a Swan-Ganz catheter. Both these procedures carry risk to the woman, and the decision to use them should be made judiciously. Invasive hemodynamic monitoring may be indicated for the woman with the following (ACOG, 2008b):

- Oliguria
- Severe cardiac disease
- Severe renal disease
- Pulmonary edema resulting in impaired maternal oxygenation
- Refractory hypertension with administration of a vasoactive drug, such as nitroprusside or dopamine

When the woman's vital signs have stabilized, urinary output is good, and the maternal and fetal hypoxic and acidotic states are alleviated, birth of the fetus should be considered. Birth is the only known cure for preeclampsia-eclampsia. If the newborn will be preterm, it may be necessary to transfer the woman to a tertiary center for childbirth. The woman and her partner deserve careful explanation about the status of the fetus and woman and the treatment they are receiving. Plans for childbirth and further treatment must be discussed with them.

A pediatrician, neonatologist, or neonatal nurse practitioner must be available to care for the newborn at birth. This caregiver must be aware of all amounts and times of medication the woman has received during labor.

POSTPARTUM MANAGEMENT The woman with preeclampsia usually improves rapidly after childbirth, although seizures can still occur during the first 48 hours postpartum. A woman who has required magnesium sulfate antepartally will continue to receive the infusion for about 24 hours postpartum. Antihypertensive medication may also be required for a period of time.

Postpartum nurses should be acutely aware of the possibility of a worsening of the maternal condition in the immediate postpartum period. The potential for HELLP syndrome, liver rupture, or seizure continues. Some women may develop late postpartum eclampsia (seizures occurring more than 48 hours but less than 4 weeks postpartum). Thus it is important to provide education as to the warning signs of worsening disease prior to discharge.

When a woman's blood pressure remains above 150/100 mm Hg for 2 to 3 days postpartum, antihypertensive therapy should be used. Blood pressure should then be monitored at least weekly during the postpartum period. If blood pressure fails to return to normal by 12 weeks' postpartum, further evaluation is indicated to rule out underlying causes for hypertension.

In general, the recurrence rate of preeclampsia is approximately 18% in subsequent pregnancies, but the risk of recurrence depends upon several factors (Habli & Sibai, 2008). The rate is substantially higher in women with multiple gestations, early-onset preeclampsia-eclampsia, previous HELLP syndrome, preexisting hypertension, renal disease, or underlying vascular disease. Women who were normotensive in a previous pregnancy are at increased risk when they conceive with a new partner. Also, in vitro fertilization using donor eggs and/or donor sperm has a higher incidence of preeclampsia (Wiggins & Elliott, 2005).

Selective screening should be done for inherited coagulopathies (clotting disorders) in women who have had early-onset preeclampsia or a poor pregnancy history related to repeated miscarriages, intrauterine growth restriction, fetal demise, or prior history of a thrombotic event. An association between hyperhomocysteinemia and preeclampsia has been found. There is controversy surrounding the association of other hereditary thrombophilias and preeclampsia (Lockwood & Bauer, 2009). However, this information is important in patient counseling and management not only related to future pregnancies, but also to assess the woman's risk for thrombotic episodes outside of pregnancy.

NURSING CARE MANAGEMENT

See the Nursing Care Plan: The Woman with Preeclampsia for information on nursing care.

Nursing Assessment and Diagnosis

An essential part of nursing assessment is to obtain a baseline blood pressure early in pregnancy. Arterial blood pressure varies with position and is highest when the woman is sitting, intermediate when she is supine, and lowest when she is in the left lateral recumbent position. Therefore it is important that the woman be in the same position when the blood pressure is measured each visit.

Blood pressure is taken and recorded at each antepartal visit. If the blood pressure rises or if the normal slight decrease in blood pressure expected between 8 and 28 weeks of pregnancy does not occur, the woman should be followed closely.

Blood pressure elevations should be based on at least two determinations not more than 1 week apart. To minimize errors in blood pressure measurements and improve reproducibility, the following precautions should be taken when measuring blood pressure:

- Take blood pressure measurements while the woman is seated, with feet supported and her arm at the level of the heart.
- Use Korotkoff phase V (sound disappearance) to measure the diastolic pressure.
- Calibrate the mercury sphygmomanometer and use the nearest 2 mm measurement.
- If using an electronic device, use one that has been validated for pregnancy.

When blood pressure and other signs indicate that the preeclampsia is worsening, hospitalization is necessary to monitor the woman's condition closely. The nurse then assesses the following:

- ***Blood pressure.*** Blood pressure should be determined every 1 to 4 hours, more frequently if indicated by medication or other changes in the woman's status.
- ***Temperature.*** Temperature should be determined every 4 hours, every 2 hours if elevated or if premature rupture of the membranes (PROM) has occurred.
- ***Pulse and respirations.*** Pulse rate and respirations should be determined along with blood pressure.
- ***Fetal heart rate.*** The FHR should be determined with the blood pressure or monitored continuously with the electronic fetal monitor if the situation indicates.
- ***Urinary output.*** Every voiding should be measured. Frequently, the woman will have an indwelling catheter. In this case, hourly urine output can be assessed. Output should be 700 ml or greater in 24 hours or at least 30 ml per hour.
- ***Urine protein.*** Urinary protein is determined hourly if an indwelling catheter is in place or with each voiding. Readings of 3+ or 4+ indicate loss of 5 g or more protein in 24 hours.
- ***Urine specific gravity.*** Specific gravity of the urine should be determined hourly or with each voiding. Readings over 1.040 correlate with oliguria and proteinuria.
- ***Edema.*** The face (especially eyelids and cheekbone area), fingers, hands, arms (ulnar surface and wrist), legs (tibial surface), ankles, feet, and sacral area are inspected and palpated for edema. The degree of pitting is determined by pressing over bony areas.
- ***Weight.*** The woman is weighed daily at the same time, wearing the same robe or gown and slippers. Weighing may be omitted if the woman is to maintain strict bed rest, or a bed scale may be used.
- ***Pulmonary edema.*** The woman is observed for coughing, shortness of breath, or difficult breathing. The lungs are auscultated for moist respirations.
- ***Deep tendon reflexes.*** The woman is assessed for evidence of hyperreflexia in the brachial, wrist, patellar, or Achilles tendons (Table 20-2). The patellar reflex is the easiest to assess. (See Procedure 20-1: Assessing Deep Tendon Reflexes and Clonus.)
- ***Clonus.*** Clonus should also be assessed by vigorously dorsiflexing the woman's foot while her knee is held in a flexed position. Normally no clonus is present. If it is present, it is measured as one to four beats, or sustained, and is recorded as such.
- ***Placental separation.*** The woman should be assessed hourly for vaginal bleeding and/or uterine rigidity.
- ***Headache.*** The woman should be questioned about the existence and location of any headache.
- ***Visual disturbance.*** The woman should be questioned about any visual blurring or changes, including scotomata. The results of the daily funduscopic exam should be recorded on the chart.
- ***Epigastric pain.*** The woman should be asked about any epigastric pain. It is important to differentiate it from simple heartburn, which tends to be familiar and less intense. *Nausea and vomiting or right upper quadrant pain,* occasionally radiating to the back, are also of concern.
- ***Laboratory blood tests.*** Daily tests of hematocrit to measure hemoconcentration; BUN, creatinine, and uric acid levels to assess kidney function; clotting studies for any indication of thrombocytopenia or disseminated intravascular coagulation (DIC); liver enzymes; and electrolyte levels for deficiencies are all indicated.
- ***Level of consciousness.*** The woman is observed for alertness, mood changes, and any signs of impending convulsion or coma.
- ***Emotional response and level of understanding.*** The woman's emotional response should be carefully assessed so that support and teaching can be planned accordingly.

TABLE 20-2 Deep Tendon Reflex Rating Scale

RATING	ASSESSMENT
4+	Hyperactive; very brisk, jerky, or clonic response; abnormal
3+	Brisker than average; may not be abnormal
2+	Average response; normal
1+	Diminished response; low normal
0	No response; abnormal

NURSING CARE PLAN The Woman with Preeclampsia

INTERVENTION	RATIONALE
1. Nursing Diagnosis: Deficient Fluid Volume related to fluid shift from intravascular to extravascular space secondary to vasospasm	
Goal: Patient is restored to normal fluid volume levels.	
■ Encourage woman to lie in the left lateral recumbent position.	■ The left lateral recumbent position decreases pressure on the vena cava, thereby increasing venous return, circulatory volume, and placental and renal perfusion. Angiotensin II levels are decreased when there is improved renal blood flow, which helps to promote diuresis and lower blood pressure.
■ Assess blood pressure every 1 to 4 hours as necessary.	■ Frequent monitoring will assess for progression of the disorder and allow for early intervention to ensure maternal and fetal health and well-being.
■ Monitor urine for volume and proteinuria every shift or every hour per agency protocol.	■ Monitoring provides information to assess renal perfusion. Proteinuria is the last cardinal sign of preeclampsia to appear. As the disorder worsens, the capillary walls of the glomerular endothelial cells stretch, allowing protein molecules to pass into the urine. Normally urine does not contain protein. Reading of 3+ and 4+ indicate loss of 5 g or more protein in 24 hours. Urinary output decreases when there is a reduction of the glomerular filtration rate. Urinary output that falls below 30 ml per hour or less than 700 ml in a 24-hour period should be reported.
■ Assess deep tendon reflexes and clonus.	■ Hyperreflexia may occur as preeclampsia worsens. Eliciting deep tendon reflexes provides information about CNS status and is also used to assess for magnesium sulfate toxicity. Reflexes are graded on a scale of 0 to 4+ using the Deep Tendon Reflex Rating Scale. A rating of 4+ is abnormal and indicates hyperreflexia. A rating of 0 or no response is also abnormal and is seen with high maternal serum magnesium levels. Clonus, an abnormal finding, is present if the foot "jerks" or taps the examiner's hand, at which time the examiner counts the number of taps or beats. The presence of clonus indicates a more pronounced hyperreflexia and is indicative of CNS irritability.
■ Assess for edema.	■ Edema develops as fluid shifts from the intravascular to the extravascular spaces. Edema is assessed either by weight gain (more than 3.3 lb/month in the second trimester or more than 1.1 lb/week in the third trimester) or by assessing for pitting edema (assessed by using finger pressure to a swollen area, usually the lower extremities, and grading on a scale of 1+ to 4+).
■ Administer magnesium sulfate per infusion pump as ordered.	■ As preeclampsia worsens, the risk of an eclamptic seizure increases. Magnesium sulfate is the treatment of choice for seizures because of its CNS depressant action. As a secondary effect, magnesium sulfate relaxes smooth muscles and may therefore decrease the blood pressure. Magnesium sulfate is contraindicated in women with myasthenia gravis.
■ Assess for magnesium sulfate toxicity.	■ Side effects of magnesium sulfate are dose related. Therapeutic levels are in the range of 4.8–8.4 mg/dl. As maternal serum magnesium levels increase, toxicity may occur. Signs of toxicity include decreased or absent DTRs, urine output below 30 ml/hr, respirations below 12, and confusion.
■ Provide a balanced diet that includes 80–100 g/day or 1.5 g/kg/day of protein.	■ A diet rich in protein is necessary to replace protein that is excreted in the urine.

EXPECTED OUTCOME: The signs and symptoms of preeclampsia will diminish as evidenced by decreased blood pressure, urine protein levels of zero, and a return of the deep tendon reflexes to normal.

(continued)

NURSING CARE PLAN The Woman with Preeclampsia continued

INTERVENTION	RATIONALE
2. Nursing Diagnosis: Risk for Injury (to the Fetus) related to uteroplacental insufficiency secondary to vasospasm **Goal:** The fetus avoids complications related to uteroplacental insufficiency.	
■ Instruct patient to count fetal movements 3 times a day for 20 to 30 minutes.	■ Fetal activity provides reassurance of fetal well-being. Decrease in fetal movement or cessation of movement may indicate fetal compromise.
■ Encourage patient to rest in the left lateral recumbent position.	■ Lying in the left lateral recumbent position decreases pressure on the vena cava, which increases venous return, circulatory volume, and placental and renal perfusion. Blood flow to the fetus is increased, thereby reducing the risk of fetal hypoxia and malnutrition.
Collaborative: Assist with serial ultrasounds.	■ Maternal vasospasm and hypovolemia result from preeclampsia, which may lead to intrauterine growth restriction and oligohydramnios. Ultrasound provides assessment of fetal growth and fluid levels.
■ Perform nonstress test as ordered.	■ A nonstress test is performed to assess the fetal heart rate in response to fetal movement. Accelerations of fetal heart rate with fetal movement may indicate the fetus has adequate oxygenation and an intact central nervous system. (Refer to chapter 21 ∞ for interpretation of NST results.)
■ Describe for the woman the purposes of a biophysical profile (BPP).	■ Preeclampsia or eclampsia places the woman at risk for uteroplacental insufficiency due to the loss of normal vasodilation of uterine arterioles and maternal vasospasm. This results in decreased uteroplacental perfusion, which may lead to fetal hypoxia. A BPP is one assessment tool used to evaluate fetal well-being. Providing explanation of the diagnostic test helps relieve anxiety and ensures the woman understands what the test evaluates and what the results mean.
■ Assist with amniocentesis to obtain lecithin/sphingomyelin (L/S) ratio.	■ Women with preeclampsia may give birth before term. Amniotic fluid may be analyzed to determine the maturity of the fetal lungs. An L/S ratio of 2:1 or greater indicates fetal lung maturity and is usually achieved by 35–36 weeks' gestation.
■ Explain the purpose of Doppler flow studies.	■ Doppler flow studies (umbilical velocimetry) help to assess placental function and sufficiency. Uteroplacental insufficiency is a risk for a woman with preeclampsia. If fetal growth restriction is present, Doppler velocimetry of the umbilical artery is useful for fetal surveillance.
EXPECTED OUTCOME:	The fetus will have an adequate supply of oxygen and nutrients as evidenced by absence of signs of nonreassuring fetal status and fetal diagnostic test results within normal limits.
3. Nursing Diagnosis: Ineffective Health Maintenance related to deficient knowledge about new diagnosis (preeclampsia) **Goal:** The woman will describe the condition and treatment regimen.	
■ Assess the woman and the family's understanding of preeclampsia and its implications for pregnancy.	■ This assessment provides information about the woman's cognitive level and her understanding of her diagnosis. Behavior changes occur when teaching strategies are appropriate for the woman and family's cognitive level.
■ Provide information about the disease process, impact on maternal well-being, risks of progression, implications for the fetus, and dangers of eclampsia.	■ Basic understanding of the condition and its implications is necessary for the woman to understand the treatment plan. A woman who shows signs of early preeclampsia often feels well and may have difficulty accepting the need to rest.
■ Emphasize the importance of self-monitoring for signs that her condition is worsening and the importance of regular prenatal care for the purpose of maternal and fetal surveillance.	■ The woman should be able to identify signs of disease progression, including evidence of increasing edema, decreased urine output, signs of cerebral disturbance (frontal headache, blurred vision, scotomata), epigastric or right upper quadrant pain, nausea or vomiting, and increased irritability.
EXPECTED OUTCOME:	Woman will demonstrate understanding of preeclampsia and its implications as evidenced by verbalization of basic condition, signs and symptoms of progression, importance of sufficient rest in side-lying position, and need to follow prescribed diet.

PROCEDURE 20-1 Assessing Deep Tendon Reflexes and Clonus

NURSING ACTION

Preparation

- Explain the procedure, indications for its use, and information that will be obtained.
- Check the patellar reflex and one other such as the biceps, triceps, or brachioradialis.

  Rationale: *DTRs are assessed to gain information about CNS irritability secondary to preeclampsia and to assess the effects of magnesium sulfate if the woman is receiving it.*

Equipment and Supplies

- Percussion hammer

> **CLINICAL TIP**
> If a percussion hammer is not available, you may use the side of your stethoscope or the side of your hand or the tips of the index and middle fingers to elicit DTRs.

Procedure

1. Elicit reflexes.
   - Patellar reflex. Position the woman with her legs hanging over the edge of the bed (feet should not be touching the floor). (See Figure 20-7 ■.) Briskly strike the patellar tendon, which is located just below the patella. Normal response is extension or a thrusting forward of the foot.

   Note: In an inpatient setting the patellar reflex is often assessed while the woman lies supine. Flex her knees slightly and support them.

   Rationale: *The correct position causes the muscle to be slightly stretched. Then when the tendon is stretched, with a tap the muscle should contract. Correct positioning and technique are essential to elicit the reflex.*

   - Biceps reflex. Flex the woman's arm 45 degrees at the elbow and place your thumb on the biceps tendon. Allow your fingers to hold the biceps muscle. Strike your thumb in a slightly downward motion and assess the response. Normal response is flexion of the arm.
   - Triceps reflex. Flex the woman's arm up to 90 degrees and allow her hand to hang against the side of her body. Using the percussion hammer, strike the triceps tendon just above the elbow. Normal response is contraction of the muscle, which causes extension of the arm.
   - Brachioradialis reflex. Flex the woman's arm slightly and lay it on your forearm with her hand slightly pronated. Using the percussion hammer, strike the brachioradialis tendon, which is found about 1 to 2 inches above the wrist. Normal response is pronation of the forearm and flexion of the elbow.
2. Grade reflexes. Reflexes are graded on a scale of 0 to 4+, as follows:

   4+ Hyperactive; very brisk, jerky, or clonic response; abnormal

   3+ Brisker than average; may not be abnormal

   2+ Average response; normal

   1+ Diminished response; low normal

   0 No response; abnormal

   Rationale: *Normally reflexes are 1+ or 2+. With CNS irritation, hyperreflexia may be present; with high magnesium levels, reflexes may be diminished or absent.*
3. Assess for clonus. With the woman's knee flexed and the leg supported, vigorously dorsiflex the foot, maintain the dorsiflexion momentarily, and then release (Figure 20-8 ■). With a normal response, the foot returns to its normal position of plantar flexion. Clonus is present if the foot "jerks" or taps against the examiner's hand. If so, record the number of taps or beats of clonus.

   Rationale: *Clonus occurs with more pronounced hyperreflexia and indicates CNS irritability.*
4. Report and record findings. For example: DTRs 2+, no clonus or DTRs 4+, 2 beats clonus.

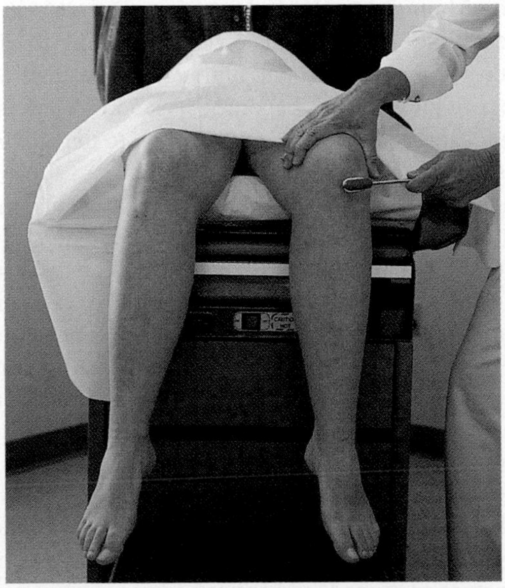

Figure 20-7 ■ Correct position for eliciting patellar reflex: sitting.

Source: Photographer, Elena Dorfman.

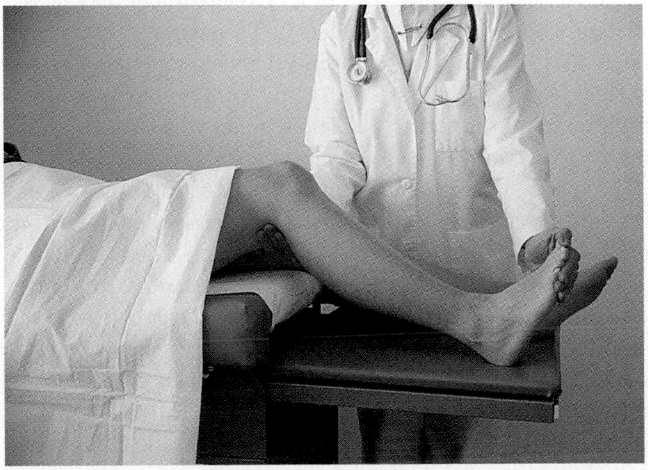

Figure 20-8 ■ To elicit clonus, sharply dorsiflex the foot.

Source: Photographer, Elena Dorfman.

PROFESSIONALISM IN PRACTICE

Measuring Blood Pressure

Common errors in measuring blood pressure include the following:

- Incorrect cuff size—a cuff that is too small results in a falsely elevated BP, whereas one that is too large falsely lowers BP.
- Elevating the arm above the level of the heart, such as occurs when a woman lies on her left side using her right arm for a BP measurement, will falsely lower the BP 10 to 20 mm Hg.
- Korotkoff's phase—when BP is checked during pregnancy, the disappearance of the sound (phase V) is the preferred indicator rather than the muffling of the sound (phase IV).
- Anxiety, exercise, and smoking can elevate BP. Wait 10 minutes after the woman's arrival to check a resting BP.

In addition, the nurse continues to assess the effects of any medications administered. Because the administration of prescribed medications is an important aspect of care, the nurse is, of course, familiar with the more commonly used medications, their purpose, implications, and associated untoward or toxic effects.

Examples of nursing diagnoses that may apply for the pregnant woman with preeclampsia-eclampsia include the following:

- ***Deficient Fluid Volume*** related to fluid shift from the intravascular to extravascular space secondary to vasospasm and endothelial injury
- ***Risk of Injury*** related to convulsion secondary to cerebral edema
- ***Anxiety*** related to uncertain maternal and fetal status

Nursing Plan and Implementation

Community-Based Nursing Care

Case Study: Patient with Preeclampsia

A woman with preeclampsia has several major concerns. She may fear losing the fetus. She may worry about the impact of separation on her relationships with her husband and children should she be hospitalized. She may be concerned about finances—health insurance does not always cover all the tests, prolonged hospitalization, and other expenses that may be associated with complications during pregnancy. Finally, the woman may be depressed or resentful about being left alone or may feel bored. If she has small children, she may have difficulty providing for their care. The woman who does not have children may worry that she never will.

The nurse should identify and discuss each of these areas with the woman and her partner. It is necessary to explain to them the reasons for bed rest. A woman with mild preeclampsia may feel very well and be unable to see the need for resting even a few hours a day. The nurse can refer the couple to many community resources, such as homemaking services, a support group for the partner, or a hotline. Arrangements may be made for the partner to attend childbirth classes alone if the mother is not able to, or a nurse may be found to teach the classes privately. In addition, childbirth classes can be accessed over the Internet, thereby enabling the couple to participate together even if the woman is limited to bed rest at home.

The woman needs to know which symptoms are significant and should be reported at once. Usually, the woman with mild preeclampsia is seen once or twice a week, but she may need to come in earlier if symptoms indicate the condition is progressing. She must understand her diet plan, which must match her culture, finances, and lifestyle.

Hospital-Based Nursing Care

The development of worsening preeclampsia is a cause for increased concern to the woman and her family. The most immediate concerns of the woman and her partner usually are about the prognosis for herself and the fetus. The nurse can offer honest, hopeful information. The nurse can also explain the plan of therapy and the reasons for procedures to the extent that the woman or her partner is interested. The nurse should keep the couple informed of the fetal status and should also take the time to discuss other concerns the couple may express. The nurse provides as much information as possible and seeks other sources of information or aid for the family as needed. Nurses can offer to contact a member of the clergy or counselor for additional support if the couple so chooses. In addition, the nurse can provide educational videos that help address the couple's educational needs and access other support services including social services, a nutritionist, and even a lactation consultant if the woman is hospitalized for an extended period of time.

The nurse should maintain a quiet, low-stimulus environment for the woman. The woman should be placed in a private room in a quiet location where she can be watched closely. Visitors are limited to close family or main support persons. The woman should maintain the left lateral recumbent position most of the time, with side rails up for her protection. Unlimited phone calls are avoided because the phone ringing unexpectedly may be too jarring. To avoid a sense of isolation, however, some women find it preferable to limit calls to a certain time of the day rather than refusing all calls.

Nursing Management of Eclampsia

The occurrence of a convulsion is frightening to any family member who may be present, although the woman will not be able to recall it when she becomes conscious. Therefore, offering explanations to family members, and to the woman herself later, is essential.

When the tonic phase of the convulsion begins, the woman should be turned to her side (if she is not already in that position) to aid circulation to the placenta. Her head should be turned face down to allow saliva to drain from her mouth. Attempting to insert a padded tongue blade has been questioned, and in many facilities it is no longer advocated. In others, it is used if it can be done without force because it may prevent injury to the woman's mouth. The side rails should be padded or a pillow put between the woman and each side rail. After 15 to 20 seconds, the clonic phase starts. In approximately 30 to 90 seconds, when the thrashing subsides, intensive monitoring and therapy begin. An oral airway is inserted, the woman's nasopharynx is suctioned, and oxygen administration is begun by nasal catheter. The attending physician and the anesthesiologist should be notified immediately. Fetal heart tones are monitored continuously. Maternal vital signs are monitored every 5 minutes until they are stable, then every 15 minutes.

Nursing Management During Labor and Birth
The plan of care for the woman with preeclampsia in labor depends on both maternal and fetal condition. The woman may have mild or severe preeclampsia, may become eclamptic during labor, or may have been eclamptic before the onset of labor. Therefore, careful monitoring of blood pressure and checking for edema and proteinuria are necessary for all women in labor. The prenatal record should be obtained so that current blood pressure readings may be compared with the baseline reading from early in her pregnancy.

The woman with preeclampsia in labor is kept positioned on her side as much as possible. Both woman and fetus are monitored carefully throughout labor. Signs of progressing labor are noted. In addition, the nurse must be alert for indications of worsening preeclampsia, placental separation, pulmonary edema, circulatory renal failure, and nonreassuring fetal status.

During the second stage of labor the woman is encouraged to push while lying on her side or with a wedge under her hip. If she is unable to do so comfortably or effectively, she can be helped to a semisitting position for pushing and resume the lateral position between each contraction. Birth is in the side-lying position if possible. If the lithotomy position is used, a wedge is placed under the woman's hip.

A family member is encouraged to stay with the woman as long as possible throughout labor and childbirth. This is especially needed if the woman has been transferred to a high-risk center from another facility. The woman in labor and the family member or support person should be oriented to the new surroundings and kept informed of progress and plan of care. When possible the woman should be cared for by the same nurses throughout her hospital stay.

Nursing Management During the Postpartum Period
The amount of postpartum vaginal bleeding should be noted carefully. Because the woman with preeclampsia is hypovolemic, even normal blood loss can be serious. Rising pulse rate and falling urine output are late indications of excessive blood loss. The uterus should be palpated frequently and massaged when needed to keep it contracted.

Blood pressure and pulse are checked every 4 hours for 48 hours. Hematocrit, platelets, uric acid, AST, and ALT may be measured daily. The woman is instructed to report any headache, visual disturbance, or epigastric pain. No ergot preparations, such as Methergine, are given because they have a hypertensive effect. Intake and output recordings are continued for 48 hours postpartum. Increased urinary output within 48 hours after birth is a highly favorable sign. With the diuresis, edema recedes and blood pressure returns to normal.

Postpartum depression can develop after the long ordeal of a difficult pregnancy. Family members are urged to visit, and as much mother-infant contact as possible should be allowed. There may be fears about a future pregnancy. The couple needs information about the chance of preeclampsia occurring again. They also should be given family-planning information. Combined oral contraceptives may be used if the woman's blood pressure has returned to normal by the time they are prescribed (usually 4 to 6 weeks postpartum). Progesterone-only pills may be prescribed regardless of hypertension and may be a good alternative for women with chronic hypertension or for those women who are breastfeeding.

Evaluation

Expected outcomes of nursing care include the following:

- The woman is able to explain preeclampsia, its implications for her pregnancy, the treatment regimen, and possible complications.
- The woman suffers no eclamptic seizures.
- The woman and her caregivers detect signs of increasing severity of the preeclampsia or possible complications early so that appropriate treatment measures can be instituted.
- The woman gives birth to a healthy newborn.

Chronic Hypertension

Chronic hypertension exists when the blood pressure is 140/90 or higher before pregnancy or before the 20th week of gestation or persists 42 days following childbirth. If the diastolic blood pressure is greater than 80 mm Hg during the second trimester, chronic hypertension should be suspected. For the majority of chronic hypertensive women, the disease is mild. One of the challenges the healthcare team faces is differentiating chronic hypertension from preeclampsia. This is even more difficult if a woman arrives for her first prenatal visit during the second trimester when blood pressure is generally lower and preexisting hypertension is more difficult to recognize.

Early prenatal care is important to determine accurately the gestational age and the severity of hypertension. Adverse maternal and neonatal outcomes are increased in women with chronic hypertension, even if they do not develop superimposed preeclampsia. (Catov, Nohr, Olsen, et al., 2009; Chappell et al., 2008). These risks include fetal growth restriction, preterm birth, and cesarean birth, as well as the associated economic burden of longer maternal hospitalization and neonatal intensive care admission.

At the time of the first visit, the woman should be counseled on several aspects of her pregnancy:

- ***Nutrition.*** Sodium is limited to about 2.4 g per day; the woman is advised about recommended weight gain and healthy food choices.
- ***Bed rest.*** Frequent rest periods are advisable. At a minimum, the woman should rest twice a day for 1-hour periods of time.
- ***Medication.*** Studies have shown that women with mild chronic hypertension have outcomes similar to the general maternity population. Therefore, unless the blood pressure is over 150–160/100–110 mm Hg, antihypertensive medications are not used during pregnancy. Methyldopa or Labetalol are generally the first choice for use in pregnancy when medication is required. Angiotensin-converting enzyme (ACE) inhibitors are contraindicated during the 2nd and 3rd trimesters due to fetal risks of renal failure, IUGR, and death (ACOG, 2008a).

- ***Prenatal visits.*** Counseling regarding the importance of frequent prenatal visits to reduce the incidence of adverse outcomes for mother or fetus is stressed.
- ***Blood pressure monitoring.*** The woman and her partner can be taught how to monitor blood pressure at home and maintain a record to be brought to each prenatal visit. Home monitoring is often more accurate because the woman is in a familiar environment and relaxed.
- ***Fetal surveillance.*** Starting at about 24 weeks, the woman should begin to keep fetal movement records and notify her care provider of any significant decrease in fetal movement. Serial ultrasonography to assess fetal growth and amniotic fluid volume is indicated. Antepartum fetal testing may begin as early as 26 weeks.

During the first prenatal visit, the woman should have a thorough physical examination, which includes a funduscopic examination, blood pressure and pulses in all four extremities, and auscultation of chest and flanks. Laboratory work includes a urinalysis and culture; 24-hour urine for protein, creatinine clearance, sodium, and potassium; CBC; serum electrolytes; and a glucose tolerance test. The usual prenatal laboratory assessments and an ultrasound for confirming gestational age are also done if the woman is currently pregnant. Although essential hypertension is the most likely explanation for hypertension in early pregnancy, a thorough evaluation can rule out rare but serious causes of secondary hypertension such as pheochromocytoma or coarctation of the aorta.

A woman with chronic hypertension generally has more frequent prenatal visits. She should be seen every 2 to 3 weeks in the first two trimesters and then more frequently in the third trimester, depending on how she and the fetus are progressing. Twenty-four-hour urines, serum creatinine, uric acid, hematocrit, and ultrasound examinations are repeated at least once in the second and third trimesters.

Chronic Hypertension with Superimposed Preeclampsia

Preeclampsia develops in approximately 22% of women previously found to have chronic hypertension (Chappell et al., 2008). The development of superimposed preeclampsia can be difficult to diagnose. After 20 weeks' gestation the onset of proteinuria and worsening hypertension is suggestive of superimposed preeclampsia (ACOG, 2008a). If the woman has underlying renal disease, it may be very difficult to confirm the diagnosis of superimposed preeclampsia. A rise in serum uric acid is helpful in identifying preeclampsia, which frequently occurs late in the second trimester or early in the third.

Gestational Hypertension

Gestational hypertension exists when transient elevation of blood pressure occurs for the first time after midpregnancy without proteinuria or other signs of preeclampsia. The final determination that the woman has gestational hypertension is made in the postpartum period. If preeclampsia does not develop and blood pressure returns to normal by 12 weeks' postpartum, the diagnosis of gestational hypertension may be assigned. If the blood pressure elevation persists after 12 weeks' postpartum, the woman is diagnosed with chronic hypertension.

> **CLINICAL JUDGMENT**
>
> **Case Study: Jillian Rundus**
>
> Jillian Rundus is a 31-year-old G1P0 who is 35 weeks' pregnant. She presents for a routine office visit with complaints of nausea and abdominal pain rating 7/10. She has had a headache and general malaise for 2 days. She denies visual changes. Upon examination, you find her to be alert and oriented and her physical exam is unremarkable with the exception of abdominal tenderness and a blood pressure of 170/110. She has had no previous history of hypertension. Fetal heart rate ranges from 140–150 beats per minute.
>
> **Critical Thinking**
>
> What should the nurse do at this time?
>
> *See www.nursing.pearsonhighered.com for possible responses.*

Care of the Woman at Risk for Rh Alloimmunization

The Rh blood group is present on the surface of erythrocytes of most of the population. When it is present a person is said to be Rh positive. Those without the factor are Rh negative. If an Rh-negative person is exposed to Rh-positive blood, an antigen-antibody response occurs, antibodies are formed, and the person is said to be *sensitized.* Subsequent exposure to Rh-positive blood can then cause a serious reaction that results in agglutination and hemolysis of red blood cells (RBCs). Rh *alloimmunization* (sensitization), also called *isoimmunization,* most often occurs when an Rh-negative woman carries an Rh-positive fetus either to term or to termination by miscarriage or induced abortion. It can also occur if an Rh-negative nonpregnant woman receives an Rh-positive blood transfusion, experiences an Rh-positive tubal pregnancy, has an amniocentesis, or experiences any traumatic event that might allow Rh-positive fetal cells to enter the circulation of the Rh-negative woman.

A number of known RBC antigens are involved in the Rh system, all of which are controlled by three pairs of genes: Cc, Dd, and Ee. Antigens in the D group are usually involved with incompatibility between the mother and fetus, although there are more than 400 other "atypical" RBC antigens, and at least 43 have the potential to cause hemolytic disease of the fetus or newborn (Lobo, Nardozza, & Camano, 2006).

In the United States, only about 6 of every 1000 live births is complicated by maternal sensitization to the D red cell antigen (Moise, 2008a). Approximately 85% of white Americans, 92% to 95% of African Americans, and 98% to 99% of Asian and Native Americans are Rh positive (ACOG, 2006a). Screening of the Rh negative woman for D antibodies is widely accepted. The use of **Rh immune globulin** has resulted in a marked decrease in the prevalence of alloimmunization to the RhD antigen in pregnancy. However, some "atypical" antibodies can also cause fetal hemolysis. No prophylaxis is available to prevent the formation of other red cell antigens. Kell (anti-K1) antibody is an irregular (non-RhD) antibody in which the incidence is increasing (Moise, 2008a). It has been calculated that alloimmunization associated with Kell occurs in approximately one of every 1000 pregnancies (Santiago, Ramos-Corpas, Oyonarte, et al., 2008). The Kell (K-1) antigen is found on the red cells of 9% of Caucasians and 2% of those of African descent. In the United States, current transfusion practices do not include the use of Kell negative blood. Two-thirds of the women sensitized to Kell have a history of previous blood transfusion that can be attributed to the etiology of their sensitization. In the case of Kell alloimmunization, unlike the pathogenesis of other antibodies, the mechanism that contributes to fetal and neonatal disease is the depression of fetal bone marrow. It appears that Kell alloimmunization can occur at lower maternal titers than the titers for D alloimmunization (critical titer 1:8 versus 1:16 for anti-D antibody) (Moise, 2008a).

Pathophysiology of RhD Alloimmunization

During a normal pregnancy, small amounts of fetal blood may cross the placenta. An Rh-negative mother whose fetus is Rh positive may develop anti-D antibodies in response to this exposure. During delivery of the placenta or as a result of trauma, even larger quantities of fetal blood can enter maternal circulation. After exposure to the Rh-positive antigen, the primary immune response is development of immunoglobulin M (IgM) antibodies. This primary response develops slowly over several weeks or months with a detectable titer developing 5 to 16 weeks after the sensitizing event. IgM antibodies are large and do not cross the placenta. Once a woman develops these antibodies, she is immunized for life.

Fetal RBCs express the RhD antigen at 38 days after conception. Although the risk is very low, in theory it is possible for RhD sensitization to occur during the first trimester. Fetal-maternal hemorrhage can occur with elective pregnancy termination, hemorrhage from an early threatened or spontaneous abortion, chorionic villus sampling, or ectopic pregnancy. Although the risk of sensitization is low and the evidence to support the use of Rh immune globulin in the first trimester is sparse, the reproductive implications of sensitization and the safety of Rh immune globulin makes it reasonable to treat Rh-negative women if the partner's blood type is not confirmed to be Rh negative. Following the primary response, a subsequent exposure to the RhD cells results in a more rapid production of immunoglobulin G (IgG) anti-D antibodies, developing as quickly as a few days after exposure. IgG is capable of crossing the placenta and coating the fetal RhD positive red cells, causing hemolysis. This secondary immune response may occur with exposure to a very small amount of RhD positive cells and produce a response stronger than the primary response (Figure 20-9 ■). Thus, although hemolysis is not generally a

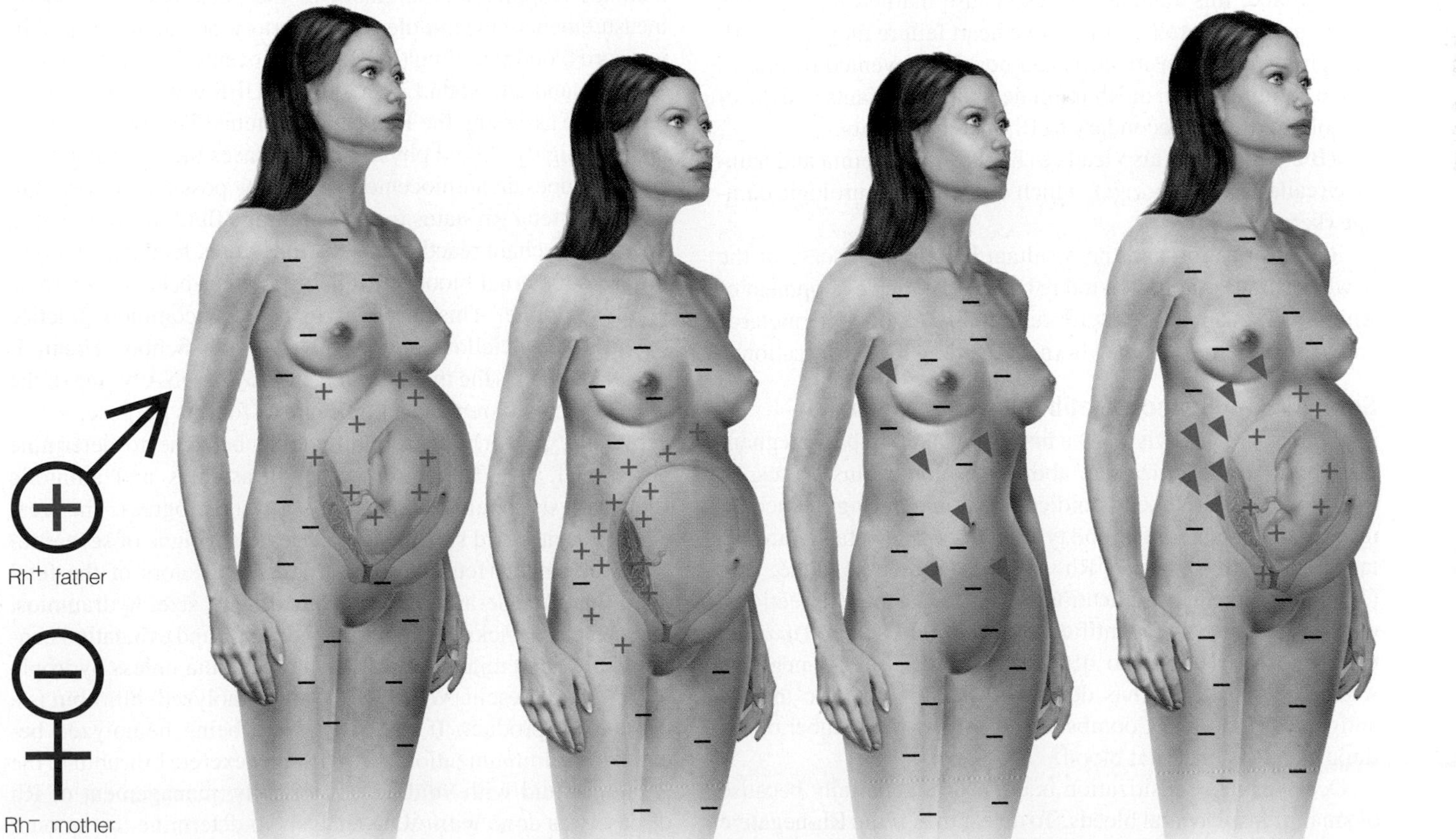

Figure 20-9 ■ Rh alloimmunization sequence. A. Rh-positive father and Rh-negative mother. B. Pregnancy with Rh-positive fetus. Some Rh-positive blood enters the mother's blood. C. As the placenta separates, the mother is further exposed to the Rh-positive blood. D. The mother is sensitized to the Rh-positive blood; anti-Rh-positive antibodies (triangles) are formed. E. In subsequent pregnancies with an Rh-positive fetus, Rh-positive red blood cells are attacked by the anti-Rh-positive maternal antibodies, causing hemolysis of red blood cells in the fetus.

problem for the fetus during a first pregnancy, it may create problems during subsequent pregnancies. There also may be an increased risk for fetal anemia when multiple maternal antibodies to other red cell antigen groups (collectively referred to as "irregular antibodies") are present as compared with anti-D antibodies alone. Specifically, the presence of anti-C, anti-E, and anti-e have an additive effect to that of the anti-D antibody on the fetus (Moise, 2008a).

The possibility also exists that an Rh-negative female fetus carried by an Rh-positive mother may become sensitized in utero. This female would not demonstrate signs of hemolytic disease, but because she would be sensitized before even becoming pregnant, she would have a positive antibody screen when receiving prenatal care with her first Rh-positive fetus. Mismatched blood transfusion of Rh-positive blood to an Rh-negative person can also result in sensitization. To prevent sensitization after exposure to Rh-positive blood, Rh immune globulin is administered.

Fetal-Neonatal Risks

The hemolysis caused by the maternal IgG antibodies in the fetus creates fetal anemia. The fetus responds by increasing RBC production. The presence of nucleated RBCs (erythroblasts) is why the term **erythroblastosis fetalis** was coined for this severe hemolytic disease of the fetus and newborn. If treatment is not initiated, this anemia can also cause marked fetal edema, called **hydrops fetalis**. Congestive heart failure may result. Although maternal sensitization can now be prevented by appropriate administration of Rh immune globulin, infants still die of hemolytic disease secondary to Rh incompatibility.

RBC destruction also leads to hyperbilirubinemia and jaundice (called *icterus gravis*), which can lead to neurologic damage (kernicterus).

Rh sensitization and the resultant hemolytic disease of the newborn are less common today because of the development of RhIgG. See chapter 34 ∞ for further discussion of kernicterus and of treatment of the newborn affected by Rh sensitization.

Screening for Rh Incompatibility and Sensitization

At the first prenatal visit, (1) a history is taken of past pregnancies, previous sensitization, abortions, blood transfusions, or children who developed jaundice or anemia during the neonatal period; (2) maternal blood type (ABO) and Rh factor are determined, and a routine Rh antibody screen is done; and (3) other medical complications, such as diabetes, infections, or hypertension, are identified. An antibody screen (*indirect Coombs' test*) is done to determine whether an Rh-negative woman is sensitized (has developed isoimmunity) to the Rh antigen. The indirect Coombs' test measures the number of antibodies in the maternal blood.

Occasionally, sensitization may occur antepartally because of small transplacental bleeds. To detect this, if the Rh-negative woman is not D-isoimmunized, a repeat D antibody determination should be made at 28 weeks' gestation. If it is negative, 300 mcg Rh immune globulin are administered prophylactically.

If the woman is Rh negative (dd), the father of the unborn child is asked to come into the clinic or physician's office to be assessed for his Rh factor and blood type. If he is homozygous for Rh positive (DD), all his offspring will be Rh positive. If he is heterozygous (Dd), 50% of his offspring will be Rh negative and 50% heterozygous for Rh positive. If the father is Rh negative, all their children will be Rh negative, and no Rh incompatibility with the mother will occur. If the father is Rh positive or the mother is known to have previously carried an Rh-positive fetus, further testing and careful management are needed.

In women who are alloimmunized, anti-D antibody titers should be determined every 2 to 4 weeks beginning at 16 to 18 weeks, biweekly during the third trimester, and the week before the due date. Traditionally, if the test shows a maternal antibody titer of 1:16 or greater, a delta optical density (ΔOD) analysis of the amniotic fluid is performed. (See later discussion.) If the titer is 1:16 or less late in pregnancy, birth at 38 weeks or spontaneous labor at term can be anticipated.

Negative antibody titers can consistently identify the fetus not at risk. However, the titers cannot reliably point out the fetus in danger because the level of the titer does not correlate with the severity of the disease. For instance, in a severely sensitized woman antibody titers may be moderately high and remain at the same level although the fetus is being more and more severely affected. Conversely, a woman sensitized by previous Rh-positive fetuses may show a high fixed antibody titer during a pregnancy in which the fetus is Rh negative. Fetal assessment includes Doppler measurement of the peak systolic velocity measurement of the middle cerebral artery, percutaneous umbilical cord blood sampling (PUBS), amniocentesis, amniotic fluid analysis, and ultrasound. Previously, PUBS was the only direct method of assessing the Rh status of a fetus. This procedure requires a highly skilled physician and places the fetus at greater risk than does an amniocentesis. It is now possible, however, to determine fetal Rh status from an amniotic fluid specimen using polymerase chain reaction (PCR). In Europe, fetal Rh genotyping from maternal blood is available and has been shown to be highly accurate. This is about to become common practice (Rouillac-Le Sciellour et al., 2007; Van der Schoot, Hahn, & Chitty, 2008). As the methodology improves, DNA typing of the fetus will clearly replace amniocentesis for this purpose.

Ideally, an early ultrasound should be done to determine gestational age. Thereafter serial ultrasounds and amniotic fluid analysis should be done to follow fetal progress. The presence of ascites and subcutaneous edema are signs of severe fetal involvement (fetal hydrops). Other indicators of the fetal condition include an increase in fetal heart size, hydramnios, and placental thickness and texture. Ultrasound evaluation cannot distinguish mild from severe fetal anemia unless hydropic changes are present. When RBCs are hemolyzed, bilirubin is a breakdown product. If fetal RBCs are being hemolyzed because of isoimmunization, the fetus may excrete bilirubin in the amniotic fluid with voiding. Historically, management of Rh disease was done with ΔOD analysis to determine the amount of bilirubin pigment found in the amniotic fluid. Normally the concentration of bilirubin pigments in the amniotic fluid declines during pregnancy. Elevated bilirubin levels are significant. Because the amount of bilirubin found in the amniotic fluid correlates roughly with the extent of the hemolysis, the

ΔOD analysis serves as an indirect predictor of the severity of the fetal anemia. To determine the ΔOD level, amniotic fluid, obtained by transabdominal amniocentesis, is separated from its cellular components by centrifuge. The amount of bilirubin pigment from the degradation of RBCs can then be measured by spectrophotometric analysis and plotted on a special chart called a Liley graph.

Readings within zone III (the highest zone) indicate a severely affected fetus who may require intrauterine transfusion every 1 to 2 weeks between weeks 26 and 32 until viability is reached, followed by birth, usually by cesarean. Neonatal exchange transfusion is anticipated. Prognosis is guarded. Fetal monitoring may identify the very ill fetus by documenting less movement or lack of movement. The appearance of sinusoidal pattern suggests fetal anemia and a deteriorating fetal condition (see chapter 23 ∞).

A new approach has replaced the use of the traditional technique of serial amniocentesis and ΔOD in the management of alloimmunized pregnancies. It is the use of velocimetry of the fetal middle cerebral artery (MCA) to monitor affected pregnancies for the detection of fetal anemia (ACOG, 2006a). It is believed that the decreasing fetal red cell mass and concurrent decrease in blood viscosity will result in an increase in fetal cardiac output. This, in turn, increases the velocity of the flow through the middle cerebral artery, which is demonstrated by an increase in the peak systolic velocities of the middle cerebral artery (PSV of MCA) (Pickelsimer et al., 2007). The noninvasive method of using Doppler ultrasonography to monitor fetal anemia via the measurement of the PSV of the MCA has been shown to be accurate and much safer than amniocentesis for detecting fetal anemia. PSVs correlate well with increasing levels of bilirubin in the amniotic fluid and should be monitored weekly (Moise, 2008b) (Figure 20-10 ■).

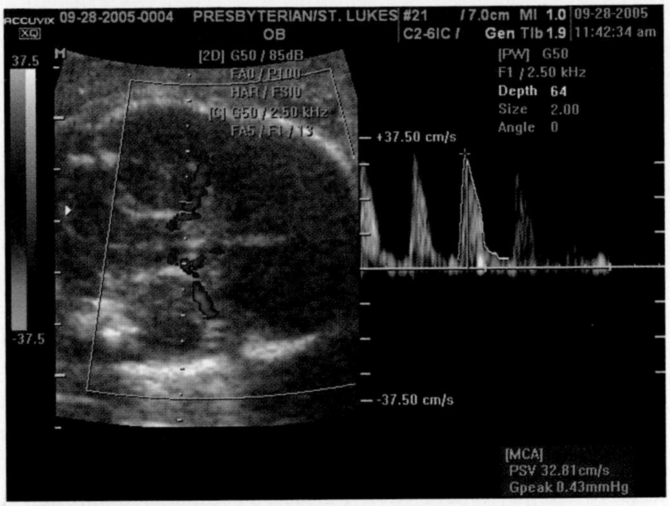

Figure 20-10 ■ Ultrasound measurement of peak systolic velocity (PSV) of the middle cerebral artery. The fetal middle cerebral arteries can be seen as major lateral branches of the circle of Willis and may be used during pregnancy to detect either fetal anemia or a fetal response to hypoxia as redistribution of cardiac output in favor of the brain, myocardium, and adrenal glands. This image demonstrates a flow velocity wave form and displays the normal continuous forward blood flow in the fetal cerebral arteries throughout the cardiac cycle. Normal peak systolic velocity values change throughout gestation, increasing with advancing gestational age. In the case of fetal anemia, the velocity of blood will be increased above the norms for gestational age. The PSV in the middle cerebral artery of this fetus is 32.81 cm/s, which is appropriate for this gestational age.

Source: Courtesy of Debbie McGee, MSN, PNNP, RDMS.

Clinical Therapy

The goal of medical management is the birth of a mature fetus who has not developed severe hemolysis in utero. This requires early identification and treatment of maternal conditions that predispose the infant to hemolytic disease, coordinated obstetric-pediatric treatment for the seriously affected newborn, and prevention of Rh sensitization if none is present.

Antepartum Management

Four Rh immune globulin products are now available: RhoGAM (the first approved for clinical use) and HyperRHO, which are administered intramuscularly, and Rhophlac and WinRho-SDF, which can be administered intramuscularly or intravenously. When the woman is Rh negative and not sensitized and the father is Rh positive or unknown, Rh immune globulin is given prophylactically at 28 weeks' gestation. It is also given after each spontaneous or induced abortion, ectopic pregnancy, chorionic villus sampling, multifetal pregnancy reduction, partial molar pregnancy, amniocentesis, PUBS, antepartum hemorrhage, fetal death in the second or third trimester, blunt trauma to the maternal abdomen, or external cephalic version.

Whether sensitization is the result of a blood transfusion or maternal-fetal hemorrhage for any reason, a Kleihauer-Betke or rosette test can be performed to determine the amount of Rh(D) positive blood present in the maternal circulation and to calculate the amount of Rh immune globulin needed. The standard dose of Rh immune globulin (300 mcg) can prevent sensitization after exposure of up to 30 ml of Rh(D) positive fetal whole blood or 15 ml of red cells. Up to five doses of Rh immune globulin can be administered in a 24-hour period. Should a large dose be required, it may be preferable to use one of the intravenous forms to avoid multiple injections (Moise, 2007).

Two primary interventions are used by the physician to aid the fetus whose blood cells are being destroyed by maternal antibodies: early birth of the fetus and intrauterine transfusion, both of which carry risks. Ideally, birth should be delayed until fetal pulmonary maturity is confirmed at about 36 to 37 weeks. Severely sensitized fetuses may require birth at 32 to 34 weeks. The use of Doppler ultrasonography of the PSV of the MCA, when properly performed, is an accurate predictor of fetal anemia. After 35 weeks' gestation, the false positive rate for the prediction of anemia increases, but in the presence of normal PSV of the MCA, weekly measurements can continue until the induction of labor is scheduled (Moise, 2008b).

Intrauterine transfusion is done to correct the anemia produced by the RBC hemolysis and thereby improve fetal oxygenation. This may be done either intravascularly through PUBS or intraperitoneally as early as 18 weeks. In a fetus who shows no signs of hydrops, a fetal blood sample should be used to check for significant anemia (hematocrit greater than 30%) before starting transfusion therapy.

Intravascular transfusion has greatly improved the outcome for severely affected fetuses. Under ultrasound visualization, the umbilical vein is entered, and the fetus is temporarily paralyzed with 0.1 mg/kg estimated fetal weight of pancuronium bromide. A fetal hematocrit is obtained; then leukocyte-poor Rh-negative packed red blood cells (PRBCs) are transfused. The volume of PRBCs is determined by a formula based on estimated normal blood volume, the pretransfusion hematocrit, the hematocrit of the blood to be transfused, and the desired hematocrit. Repeat transfusions can be scheduled as necessary until the fetus is sufficiently mature to tolerate birth. If access to the umbilical vein is problematic, intrauterine transfusions can be performed by introducing the needle into the fetal abdomen and peritoneal cavity. Blood is transfused through a catheter into the peritoneal cavity, where diaphragmatic lymphatics absorb the RBCs into fetal circulation.

About 80% to 90% of transfused fetuses survive. The procedure poses risks for the fetus, however. Complications include nonreassuring fetal status, fetal hematoma, fetal-maternal hemorrhage, fetal death, and chorioamnionitis. Birth is delayed until at least 32 weeks' gestation if possible. Premature newborns are generally more susceptible to damage from hemolytic disease. They often require exchange transfusion and usually require intensive nursery care.

Postpartum Management

The goals of postpartum care are to prevent sensitization in the as-yet-unsensitized pregnant woman and to treat the isoimmune hemolytic disease in the newborn.

The Rh-negative mother who has no titer (indirect Coombs' negative, nonsensitized) and who has given birth to an Rh-positive fetus (direct Coombs' negative) is given an intramuscular injection of 300 mcg Rh immune globulin within 72 hours so that she does not have time to produce antibodies to fetal cells that entered her bloodstream when the placenta separated. This protocol reduces the incidence of antenatal sensitization dramatically. Rh immune globulin works to destroy the fetal cells in the maternal circulation before sensitization occurs, thereby blocking maternal antibody production. This provides temporary passive immunity for the mother, which prevents the development of permanent active immunity (antibody formation). The normal dose of Rh immune globulin should suppress the immune response to approximately 30 ml Rh-positive whole blood. As discussed previously, if a larger fetomaternal bleed might have occurred, a Kleihauer-Betke test can be performed to obtain an estimate of the extent of the bleed and the dose of Rh immune globulin can be increased as necessary.

Rh immune globulin is not given to the newborn or the father. It is not effective for and should not be given to a previously sensitized woman. However, sometimes after childbirth or an abortion, the results of the blood test do not clearly show whether the mother is already sensitized to the Rh antigen. In such cases, Rh immune globulin should be given because it will cause no harm.

NURSING CARE MANAGEMENT

Nursing Assessment and Diagnosis

As part of the initial prenatal history the nurse asks the mother whether she knows her blood type and Rh factor. Many women are aware that they are Rh negative and that this status has implications for pregnancy. If the woman knows she is Rh negative, the nurse can assess the woman's knowledge of what that means. The nurse can also ask the woman whether she ever received Rh immune globulin, whether she has had any previous pregnancies and their outcome, and whether she knows her partner's Rh factor. Should the partner be Rh negative, there is no risk to the fetus, who will also be Rh negative. Uncertain paternity is an awkward situation; nevertheless, it is essential for the physician to have this information. Nurses often have a more intimate relationship with pregnant women, allowing them to obtain sensitive information that is vital in the management of pregnancy. When paternity is uncertain or the father is unavailable for testing, the fetus is assumed to be antigen positive until proven otherwise.

If the woman does not know what Rh immune type she is, intervention cannot begin until the initial laboratory data are obtained. If the woman is Rh negative, the father's blood type and zygosity, if he is Rh positive, are obtained. Once that is complete, the nurse plans intervention based on the findings.

If the woman becomes sensitized during her pregnancy, nursing assessment focuses on the knowledge level and coping skills of the woman and her family. The nurse also provides ongoing assessment during procedures to evaluate fetal well-being, such as ultrasound and amniocentesis.

Postpartally, the nurse reviews data about the Rh type of the fetus. If the fetus is Rh positive, the mother is Rh negative, and no sensitization has occurred, nursing assessment reveals the need to administer Rh immune globulin within 72 hours of birth. If inadvertently the dose of RhIgG is not given within the 72-hour window, some protection has been documented with administration within 13 days. The recommendation is to administer the dose up to 28 days after birth. Nursing diagnoses that might apply to the pregnant woman at risk for Rh sensitization include the following:

- *Readiness for Enhanced Knowledge (Information About the Purpose of RhIgG)* related to an expressed desire to understand the treatment of Rh incompatibility
- *Ineffective Coping* related to depression secondary to the development of indications of the need for fetal exchange transfusion

Nursing Plan and Implementation

During the antepartum period, the nurse explains the mechanisms involved in isoimmunization and answers any questions the woman and her partner may have. It is imperative that the woman understand the importance of receiving Rh immune globulin after every spontaneous or therapeutic abortion or ectopic pregnancy if she is not already sensitized. The nurse also

> “I've been a nurse for almost 40 years now. I remember when RhoGAM first started to be used—what a difference it made in the lives of so many women. Young women who are Rh negative today will hopefully never know the pain and tragedy the simple absence of a blood factor can mean. It is nothing short of miraculous!”

explains the purpose of the Rh immune globulin administered at 28 weeks if the woman is not sensitized.

If the woman is sensitized to the Rh factor, it poses a threat to any Rh-positive fetus she carries. The nurse provides emotional support to the family to help them deal with their grief and any feelings of guilt about the infant's condition. Should an intrauterine transfusion become necessary, the nurse continues to provide emotional support while also assuming responsibilities as part of the healthcare team.

During labor, the nurse caring for an Rh-negative woman who has not been sensitized ensures that the woman's blood is assessed for any antibodies and also has been cross-matched for Rh immune globulin. On the postpartum unit, the nurse generally is responsible for administering the Rh immune globulin (see Procedure 20-2: Administration of Rh Immune Globulin [RhoGAM, HyperRHO, Rhophlac, and WinRho-SDF]).

Table 20-3 summarizes the major considerations in caring for an Rh-negative woman. The treatment of the newborn with isoimmune hemolytic disease is discussed in chapter 34 ∞.

TABLE 20-3 Rh Sensitization

When trying to work through Rh problems, the nurse should remember the following:

- A potential problem exists when an Rh-negative mother and an Rh-positive father conceive a child who is Rh positive.
- In this situation, the mother may become sensitized or produce antibodies to her fetus's Rh-positive blood.

The following tests are used to detect sensitization:

- Indirect Coombs' tests—done on the mother's blood to measure the number of Rh-positive antibodies.
- Direct Coombs' test—done on the infant's blood to detect antibody-coated Rh-positive RBCs.

Based on the results of these tests, the following may be done:

- If the mother's indirect Coombs' test is negative and the infant's direct Coombs' test is negative (confirming that sensitization has not occurred), the mother is given Rh immune globulin within 72 hours of birth.
- If the mother's indirect Coombs' test is positive and her Rh-positive infant has a positive direct Coombs' test, Rh immune globulin is *not* given; in this case, the infant is carefully monitored for hemolytic disease.
- It is recommended that Rh immune globulin be given at 28 weeks antenatally to decrease possible transplacental bleeding concerns.
- Rh immune globulin is also administered after each abortion (spontaneous or therapeutic), antepartum hemorrhage mismatched blood transfusion, ectopic pregnancy, amniocentesis, chorionic villus sampling (CVS), percutaneous umbilical blood sampling (PUBS), fetal cephalic version, or maternal trauma.

Evaluation

Expected outcomes of nursing care include the following:

- The woman is able to explain the process of Rh sensitization and its implications for her unborn child and for subsequent pregnancies.
- If the woman has not been sensitized, she is able to explain the importance of receiving Rh immune globulin when necessary and cooperates with the recommended dosage schedule.
- The woman gives birth to a healthy newborn.
- If complications develop for the fetus (or newborn), they are detected quickly, and therapy is instituted.

Care of the Woman at Risk Due to ABO Incompatibility

ABO incompatibility is somewhat common (occurring in 15% to 25% of pregnancies) but rarely causes significant hemolysis (Black & Maheshwari, 2009). In most cases, ABO incompatibility is limited to type O mothers with a type A or B fetus. The group B fetus of a group A mother and the group A fetus of a group B mother are only occasionally affected. Group O infants, because they have no antigenic sites on the RBCs, are never affected regardless of the mother's blood type. The incompatibility occurs as a result of the maternal antibodies present in her serum and interaction between the antigen sites on the fetal RBCs.

Anti-A and anti-B antibodies are naturally occurring; that is, women are naturally exposed to the A and B antigens through the foods they eat and through exposure to infection by gram-negative bacteria. As a result, some women have high serum anti-A and anti-B titers before they become pregnant. Once the woman becomes pregnant, the maternal serum anti-A and anti-B antibodies cross the placenta and produce hemolysis of the fetal RBCs. With ABO incompatibility, the first infant is frequently involved, and no relationship exists between the appearance of the disease and repeated sensitization from one pregnancy to the next.

Unlike the case of Rh incompatibility, treatment is never warranted antepartally. As part of the initial assessment, however, the nurse should note whether the potential for an ABO incompatibility exists. This alerts caregivers so that following birth the newborn can be assessed carefully for the development of hyperbilirubinemia (see chapter 34 ∞). Affected neonates usually have only mild anemia and the severity of the disease demonstrated with the first-born infant is generally similar in all subsequent pregnancies (Black & Maheshwari, 2009).

Care of the Woman Requiring Surgery During Pregnancy

Although elective surgery should be delayed until the postpartum period, essential surgery can generally be undertaken during pregnancy. Approximately 1 in 500 pregnant women requires general surgery (Dietrich, Hill, & Hueman, 2008. Surgery does pose some risks. The incidence of spontaneous

PROCEDURE 20-2 Intramuscular Administration of Rh Immune Globulin (RhoGAM, HyperRHO, Rhophlac, WinRho-SDF)

NURSING ACTION

Preparation

- Confirm that Rh immune globulin is indicated by checking the woman's prenatal or intrapartal record to verify that she is Rh negative. Then confirm that sensitization has not occurred—maternal indirect Coombs' negative. Postpartally, confirm that the baby is Rh positive but not sensitized (direct Coombs' negative) and that the mother's indirect Coombs' is negative. Rh immune globulin is *not* indicated if the infant is Rh negative, too.

  Rationale: *Rh immune globulin is only indicated for Rh-negative, unsensitized women.*

- Confirm that the woman does not have a history of allergies to immune globulin preparations by checking entries on medication allergies in her chart and by asking her whether she has ever had any allergic reactions to medications, globulins, or blood products.

  Rationale: *Rh immune globulin is made from the plasma portion of blood. Allergic reactions are possible.*

- Explain purpose and procedure. Have consent form signed if required by agency policy.

  Rationale: *Many agencies require separate consent for the administration of Rh immune globulin because it is a blood product. The woman should clearly understand the purpose of the Rh immune globulin, its rationale, the administration procedure, and any related risks. Generally the primary side effects are redness and tenderness at the injection site and allergic responses.*

Equipment and Supplies

- Rh immune globulin, which is obtained from the blood bank or pharmacy according to agency protocol. Lot numbers for the drug and the cross-match should be the same.
- Syringe and IM needle

Procedure

1. Confirm the woman's identity and administer one vial of 300 mcg Rh immune globulin IM in the deltoid muscle.

   Rationale: *The normal 300-mcg dose provides passive immunity following exposure to 15 ml of transfused RBCs or 30 ml of fetal blood.*

2. An immune globulin microdose is used after miscarriage, elective abortion, ectopic pregnancy, or molar pregnancy occurring within the first 12 weeks' gestation. Antepartally, the Rh immune globulin is generally given within 3 hours but not longer than 72 hours of the event.
3. If a larger bleed is suspected at birth (as in cases of severe abruptio placentae), additional doses may be administered at one time using multiple sites at regular intervals as long as all doses are given within 72 hours of childbirth.
4. Provide opportunities for the woman to ask questions and express concerns.

   Rationale: *Many women, especially primigravidas, are not aware of the risks for an Rh-positive fetus of a sensitized Rh-negative mother. They need to understand the importance of receiving Rh immune globulin for each pregnancy to ensure continued protection.*

5. Chart according to agency policy. Most agencies chart lot number, route, dose, and patient education.

CLINICAL TIP

In most cases, Rh immune globulin is administered in the deltoid muscle. However, in an extremely thin woman, or in the cases of a larger-than-normal dose, consider administering the medication in the ventrogluteal or posterior gluteal site. You may also divide the dose into multiple injections. Both Rhophlac and WinRho-SFD may be administered intravenously.

abortion is increased for women who have surgery in the first trimester. The risks to the pregnancy can be significantly reduced when surgery can be delayed until the second trimester or to the postpartum period. Surgery during the third trimester is difficult because of the enlarging uterus and an increased risk of preterm labor.

The most common nonpregnancy-related indications for surgical treatment are appendicitis, cholecystitis, bowel obstruction, melanoma, ovarian disorders, breast or cervical disease, or trauma (Dietrich, Hill, & Hueman, 2008). Although general preoperative and postoperative care are similar for pregnant and nonpregnant women, special considerations must be kept in mind whenever the surgical patient is pregnant. The early second trimester is the best time to operate because there is less risk of causing spontaneous abortion or early labor, and the uterus is not so large as to impinge on the abdominal field.

The preoperative chest radiograph and electrocardiogram, which are routine for persons over age 40, should be done on the same basis for the pregnant woman. If a chest radiograph is done, the fetus should be shielded from the radiation. Because of decreased intestinal motility and decreased free gastric acid secretion during pregnancy, stomach emptying time is delayed, which increases risk of vomiting during induction of anesthesia and during the postoperative period. Therefore, a nasogastric tube may be recommended before major surgery. An indwelling urinary catheter prevents bladder distention, decreases risk of injury to the bladder, and promotes ease of monitoring output. Sequential compression devices (SCDs) or support stockings during and after surgery help prevent venous stasis and the development of thrombophlebitis. Fetal heart tones must be monitored before, during, and after surgery.

Pregnancy causes increased secretions of the respiratory tract and engorgement of the nasal mucous membrane, often making breathing through the nose difficult. Because of this, pregnant women often need an endotracheal tube for respiratory support during surgery. Caregivers must guard against maternal hypoxia during surgery because uterine circulation will be decreased and fetal oxygenation can decline very quickly.

During surgery and the recovery period, the woman is positioned to allow optimal uteroplacental-fetal circulation. A wedge is placed under her hip to tip the uterus and thereby avoid pressure by the fetus on the maternal vena cava.

Spinal or epidural anesthesia is preferred because local anesthetics are not associated with birth defects. Caution must be exercised because this type of anesthesia may produce hypotension and respiratory apnea in the pregnant woman. The frequency and degree of the hypotension increase with higher anesthetic levels. This can be prevented in many cases with a preanesthetic infusion of 900 to 1000 ml of fluid.

Blood loss during surgery is monitored carefully. Measurement of fetal heart tones gives the best indication of blood loss. Because of the normal increased blood volume of pregnancy, uterine blood flow may be reduced significantly before the maternal blood pressure begins to fall. Fluid replacement should be done with balanced electrolyte solution and, if needed, with whole blood.

NURSING CARE MANAGEMENT

Nursing Assessment and Diagnosis

During the preoperative period, the nurse assesses the pregnant woman's health status in the same way that any preoperative patient is assessed. Is there any sign of respiratory infection, fever, urinary tract infection, or anemia? Are laboratory values all within normal limits for surgery (except in the case of emergency surgery, which may, of necessity, be done even with abnormal laboratory values)? Do the woman and her family understand the surgical procedure? Do they know what to expect postoperatively? Do they have any questions or concerns?

The nurse also considers the impact of surgery on the woman's pregnancy. Is the fetal heart rate normal? Does the woman understand the implications of surgery with regard to her pregnancy? How is she coping?

Intraoperatively, fetal heart rate is assessed if at all possible. Postoperatively, the nurse completes all necessary postoperative assessments and also continues to assess fetal status, primarily by monitoring the fetal heart rate.

Nursing diagnoses that might apply to the pregnant woman who requires surgery include the following:

- ***Anxiety*** related to lack of knowledge of preoperative and postoperative procedures
- ***Fear*** related to the possible effect of surgery on fetal outcome

Nursing Plan and Implementation

Much of the nurse's care during the preoperative period is directed toward the educational needs of the woman and her family. The nurse plans time to review the procedure and answer any questions the family may have. The nurse recognizes that the need for surgery during the woman's pregnancy is probably very distressing for the family. The nurse works to help decrease their anxiety by providing information and emotional support.

Postoperatively, the nurse is caring for two patients: the mother and her unborn child. In addition to monitoring the status of both, the nurse considers both in providing care. If surgery is done in the first trimester, the nurse should be aware of the potential teratogenic effect of any medications prescribed and should discuss the implications with the surgeon and obstetrician. During the third trimester, the nurse, recognizing the potential for vena caval syndrome if the woman lies flat on her back, helps the woman maintain a side-lying position. To avoid inadequate oxygenation, the nurse encourages the woman to turn, breathe deeply, and cough regularly and also to use any ventilation therapy, such as incentive spirometry, to avoid developing pneumonia. The pregnant woman is also at increased risk for thrombophlebitis, so the nurse applies SCDs or antiembolism stockings, encourages leg exercises while the woman is confined to bed, and begins ambulation as soon as possible. In addition, the nurse encourages the woman to maintain or resume an adequate diet as soon as possible. If cultural factors influence the woman's dietary practices, the nurse and dietitian should work together to meet the woman's needs.

Discharge teaching is especially important. The woman and her family should have a clear understanding of what to expect regarding activity level, discomfort, diet, medications, and any special considerations. In addition, they ought to know any warning signs that they should report to their physician immediately.

Evaluation

Expected outcomes of nursing care include the following:

- The woman is able to explain the surgical procedure, its risks and benefits, and its implications for her pregnancy.
- Caregivers maintain adequate maternal oxygenation throughout surgery and postoperatively.
- Potential complications are avoided or detected early and treated successfully.
- The woman is able to describe any necessary postdischarge activities, limitations, and follow-up and agrees to cooperate with the recommended regimen.
- The woman maintains her pregnancy successfully.

Care of the Woman Suffering Trauma from an Accident

Accidents and injury are the leading causes of death in women of reproductive age. Major trauma complicates 3% to 8% of all pregnancies (Brown, 2009). When the woman is critically injured, fetal death occurs at least 40% of the time (ACOG, 2006b). Approximately 66% to 75% of all traumas during pregnancy are the result of motor vehicle accidents, and these accidents are the leading cause of fetal and maternal death (ACOG, 2006b; Brown, 2009). Falls and assaults—including domestic violence—are the next most common causes of injury.

In early pregnancy, body changes increase the potential for injury through fatigue, fainting spells, and hyperventilation. Late in pregnancy, the woman has less balance and coordination and may fall. Her protruding abdomen is vulnerable to a variety of minor injuries. The fetus is usually well protected by the amniotic fluid, which distributes the force of a blow equally in all directions, and by the muscle layers of the uterus and abdominal wall. In early pregnancy, while the uterus is still in the pelvis, it is shielded from blows by the surrounding pelvic organs, muscles, and bony structures. Trauma that causes concern includes blunt trauma, from an automobile accident, for example; penetrating abdominal injuries, such as knife or gunshot wounds; and the complications that commonly accompany maternal trauma, such as shock, premature labor, and spontaneous abortion.

The normal physiologic changes of pregnancy have clinical implications for victims of trauma. Blood volume increases by 40% to 50% and cardiac output increases 30% to 50% above prepregnant levels (Gordon, 2007). Generally, the pregnant woman has a greater volume of blood loss compared with a nonpregnant woman before evidence of shock is seen. The pregnant woman with significant volume loss is able to maintain hemodynamic stability temporarily by decreasing uteroplacental perfusion, thereby compromising fetal status. In the second and third trimesters, supine positioning can decrease blood return to the heart and cause overt hypotension and even loss of consciousness. During pregnancy, minute ventilation and oxygen consumption increase. This makes the gravid woman more susceptible to hypoxemia with apnea. Clotting factors normally increase in pregnancy, making it a hypercoagulable state. Thus, the risk of thrombosis after injury is increased. Disseminated intravascular coagulation (DIC) occurs commonly with severe trauma. Because the normal fibrinogen level in pregnancy is increased to between 350 and 400 mg/dl, normal nonpregnant values may indicate early DIC.

Maternal mortality most often occurs from head trauma or hemorrhage. Uterine rupture results from strong deceleration forces in an automobile accident in only 0.1% to 1% of pregnant women (ACOG, 2006b). All automobile passengers should wear seat belts. The small risk of uterine or placental injury from seat belt use is far outweighed by the fact that maternal death is the most common cause of fetal death. The use of seat belts by pregnant women has been shown to decrease morbidity and mortality of the mother. The National Highway Transportation Safety Administration recommends that pregnant women place the shoulder harness portion of the seatbelt over the collarbone between the breasts and the lap portion under the pregnant abdomen as low as possible on the hips and across the upper thighs (Brown, 2009). Traumatic separation of the placenta can occur even if the site of injury is remote from the abdomen. It results in a high rate of fetal mortality. Premature labor is another serious hazard to the fetus, often following rupture of membranes during an accident. Premature labor can ensue even if the woman is not injured.

Fractures of the pelvis can result in significant retroperitoneal hemorrhage. If there is an unstable or dislocated fracture of the pelvis, cesarean birth will probably be necessary, but with a slightly displaced pelvic fracture, vaginal birth may be attempted. Hematuria or difficulty placing a urinary catheter may be associated with injuries to the bladder or urethra.

Penetrating trauma includes gunshot wounds and stab wounds. The mother generally fares better than the fetus if the penetrating trauma involves the abdomen as the enlarged uterus is likely to protect the mother's bowel from injury. Unfortunately, the fetal injury rate is as high as 71% with gunshot wounds and 42% with stabbings (Brown, 2009).

Clinical Therapy

The goals of clinical therapy are to stabilize the injury and promote well-being for both mother and fetus. Thus clinical therapy initially focuses on ensuring airway adequacy, maintaining ventilation and adequate circulatory volume, controlling acute bleeding, and splinting fractures to prevent vascular or tissue injury. The Glascow Coma Scale is useful in evaluating for neurologic deficit. Once the mother is stabilized, fetal status is assessed.

Care must be taken at the scene of the injury to avoid the development of supine hypotensive syndrome. At approximately 20 weeks of gestation, compression of the inferior vena cava can result in a reduction of cardiac output when the woman is in a supine position. A wedge placed under the woman's right hip displacing the uterus to the left is critical in restoring cardiac output. A neck brace is used if a neck injury is suspected, or the woman is placed on a backboard and the entire board is tilted to displace the uterus. Prompt treatment of maternal hypotension or hypovolemia also averts poor fetal oxygenation. Obstetric consultation is necessary to ensure that the needs of both mother and fetus are met.

In cases of noncatastrophic trauma, that is, where the mother's life is not directly threatened, fetal monitoring for 4 hours should be sufficient if there is no vaginal bleeding, uterine tenderness, contractions, or leaking amniotic fluid. Abruptio placentae may occur following a blow to the abdomen as the flexible myometrium of the uterus sustains a contour-changing impact that the relatively inelastic placenta cannot match. The increased intrauterine pressure during the blow further shears the placenta from the underlying decidua basalis. Abruptio placentae may occur in up to 5% of women who sustain minor injuries and in up to 35% of women who sustain major abdominal trauma. Increased uterine irritability in the first few hours following trauma helps identify women who may be at high risk for this potentially catastrophic complication. Of those women who contract every 10 minutes or more, 20% will have placental abruption. Ultrasonography does not seem to be as sensitive as fetal monitoring for diagnosing abruptio placentae. In women who have experienced significant maternal trauma, most cases of placental abruption evolve within 24 hours. Placental abruption occurs in 40% or more of women who have sustained severe blunt abdominal trauma and in 3% of those who have sustained minor trauma (Brown, 2009). If the woman is bleeding, contracting, or has uterine tenderness or a nonreassuring fetal heart rate tracing, a 24- to 48-hour observation is recommended. If uterine contractions are fewer than every 10 minutes and bleeding is not present, with a reassuring fetal heart rate tracing, monitoring for 4 to 6 hours is probably sufficient (Brown, 2009).

Fetomaternal hemorrhage may occur and is more likely in women whose placenta is located on the anterior wall of her uterus (Brown, 2009). Fetal jeopardy from significant fetal hemorrhage is generally accompanied by fetal tachycardia, loss of variability, or a sinusoidal fetal heart rate pattern. A Kleihauer-Betke test may be useful in helping identify unsensitized Rh-negative women who have experienced fetal-maternal bleeds due to trauma. Rh immune globulin should be given to any unsensitized Rh-negative woman to be certain she is covered for small fetal hemorrhages that may be below the sensitivity of the Kleihauer-Betke test.

There has been controversy about the use of beta-adrenergic tocolytics in pregnant women following trauma because of the concerns regarding hemodynamic instability and the potential for masking uterine irritability or contractions that forewarn of abruptio placentae. Radiographic studies should be performed as needed to evaluate injuries regardless of fetal exposure.

When cardiopulmonary resuscitation (CPR) is performed on the pregnant woman late in gestation, perimortem cesarean birth is advocated if CPR is unsuccessful in the first 4 minutes. Chest compressions are less effective in the third trimester because of compression of the inferior vena cava by the gravid uterus. Cesarean birth alleviates this compression and improves resuscitation efforts in both the fetus and the mother (Brown, 2009).

NURSING CARE MANAGEMENT

Nursing Assessment and Diagnosis

Each individual must be assessed according to the type and extent of her injuries. As with all trauma victims, initial assessments focus on adequacy of the airway, evidence of breathing, existence of cardiovascular stability, extent of injury, and a brief neurologic assessment. When an injured woman is pregnant, it is necessary to assess fetal status as well to avoid fetal hypoxia. Frequent maternal blood gas determinations are indicated if respiratory function is compromised.

Ongoing assessments include evaluation of uterine tone, contractions and tenderness, fundal height, fetal heart rate, intake and output and other indicators of shock, normal postoperative evaluation in those women requiring surgery, determination of neurologic status, and assessment of mental outlook and anxiety level.

Nursing diagnoses that might apply to the pregnant woman suffering trauma include the following:

- ***Acute Pain*** related to the effects of the trauma experienced
- ***Constipation*** related to immobility secondary to the effects of the accident
- ***Fear*** related to the effects of the trauma on fetal well-being

Nursing Plan and Implementation

As a member of the healthcare team the nurse is actively involved in the ongoing assessment of the status of the woman and fetus. The nurse also has a primary responsibility to assess the childbearing woman's emotional state. The trauma victim must be oriented to her situation and receive explanation and reinforcement as necessary to help her understand any interventions. Family members should be involved as appropriate. The nurse also gives the pregnant woman an opportunity to discuss her feelings and concerns.

Evaluation

Expected outcomes of nursing care include the following:

- The woman and her family are able to understand the effects of the trauma on her and on her unborn child.
- Adequate maternal oxygenation is maintained to ensure fetal well-being.
- The woman's pain is adequately relieved, and her trauma is treated.
- Potential complications are quickly identified, and appropriate interventions are instituted.
- The woman gives birth to a healthy newborn.
- If the trauma results in fetal demise, the woman is able to verbalize her feelings and begin working through the grief process.

Care of the Battered Pregnant Woman

The true extent of domestic violence during pregnancy is difficult to determine. Estimates suggest that violence during pregnancy affects up to 23% of women (AAP & ACOG, 2007b; Lutgendorf et al., 2009); however, these statistics are most likely understated because many victims are unwilling to disclose their experiences. In addition, child abuse occurs in 33% to 77% of families in which there is abuse of adults (AAP & ACOG, 2007b).

Domestic violence frequently has its onset during pregnancy, or increases if already present. Battering may result in psychologic distress, loss of pregnancy, preterm labor, low-birth-weight infants, injury to the fetus, and fetal death. Complications such as poor maternal weight gain, infection, anemia, and second and third trimester bleeding are also seen more frequently among pregnant women who are abused. Women who are battered may also experience sexual abuse and are at increased risk of contracting sexually transmitted infections from their partner. This pattern of violence may escalate during pregnancy and may occur even more frequently in the postpartum period. In some instances, abuse may decrease during pregnancy, and the woman feels safe while she is pregnant only to have the abuse resume shortly after childbirth. These women may repeatedly become pregnant to escape abuse (ACOG, 2009a). The first step toward helping the battered woman is to identify her. Regularly scheduled prenatal visits are a window of opportunity for domestic violence screening and intervention. The woman needs support, confidence in her decision making, and the recognition that she can help herself.

Chronic psychosomatic symptoms can be an indicator of abuse. The woman may have nonspecific or vague complaints. It is important to assess old scars around the head, chest, arms, abdomen, and genitalia. Any bruising or evidence of pain is also evaluated. The nurse should be especially alert for signs of bruising or injury to the woman's breasts, abdomen, or genitals because these areas are common targets of violence during pregnancy. Other indicators include a decrease in eye contact, silence when the partner is in the room, and a history of nervousness, insomnia, drug overdose, or alcohol problems. Frequent visits to the emergency department and a history of accidents without understandable causes are possible indicators of abuse.

The goals of treatment are to identify the woman at risk, increase her decision-making abilities to decrease the potential for further abuse, and provide a safe environment for her and her unborn child. In a prospective observational study, investigators found that women who declined to be interviewed about domestic violence were found to be at greater risk for adverse pregnancy outcomes when compared with women who reported experiencing verbal or physical abuse. Twenty-seven percent of women who are abused and living in a violent environment will demonstrate abusive behaviors toward the children in that home (AAP & ACOG, 2007b).

Screening must be done in a private setting and by using direct questions. ACOG recommends that *all* women be screened for intimate partner violence. During pregnancy, women should be screened multiple times because they may not disclose abuse if they are asked only one time, or the abuse may begin later in pregnancy. The suggested schedule for screening is at the first prenatal visit, at least once per trimester, and at the postpartum visit. See chapter 9 for discussion of specific screening questions.

Once domestic violence is identified, the next step is to determine the immediate safety of the woman. She needs to be aware of community resources available to her, such as emergency shelters; police, legal, and social services; and counseling. It is important to establish an exit plan in situations of ongoing violence. Pocket cards and resource materials can be handed to women or left in restrooms for them to pick up. Nurses need to recognize that, ultimately, it is the woman's decision either to seek assistance or to return to old patterns. For further information, see chapter 9.

Care of the Woman with a Perinatal Infection Affecting the Fetus

Fetal infection may develop at any time during pregnancy. In general, perinatal infections are most likely to cause harm when the embryo is exposed during first trimester organ development. Infections later in pregnancy create various concerns such as growth restriction, nonimmune hydrops, and neurologic disturbances. The most commonly occurring viral and parasitic infections that may have an impact on the fetus if acquired during pregnancy include toxoplasmosis, rubella, cytomegalovirus, herpes simplex virus, group B streptococcus, and parvovirus B19.

Toxoplasmosis

Toxoplasmosis is caused by the protozoan *Toxoplasma gondii (T. gondii)*. The domestic cat is the only definitive host for toxoplasmosis and the infective oocysts are passed in its feces. In the United States, there are between 400 and 4000 cases of congenital toxoplasmosis annually or 0.8 per 10,000 live births; in Europe it is estimated to be 10 cases per 10,000 live births (Cunningham et al., 2010).

T. gondii is acquired through ingestion of undercooked meat, contact with feline feces either in the soil or through the cat litter box, and rarely through transplantation of an infected organ (Pappas, Roussos, & Falagas, 2009). It is innocuous in most adults, resembling a minor viral illness, but can be devastating to the immunosuppressed person. For example, in a woman with systemic lupus erythematosus or AIDS who has had a previous infection with *T. gondii,* the latent infection may reactivate, increasing the risk of perinatal transmission (Pappas et al., 2009). A primary infection contracted shortly before or during pregnancy can profoundly affect the fetus and create long-term sequelae for those children and adults.

Fetal-Neonatal Risks

Maternal infection during the first trimester is associated with the lowest incidence of fetal infection, but when it occurs, first trimester infection typically results in more severe fetal damage and often ends in a spontaneous abortion. The highest rate of fetal infection (72%) occurs when the mother contracts the infection in the last month of pregnancy, but most infants are born without clinical signs of infection (Cunningham et al., 2010). Up to 50% of these infants will develop signs and symptoms if left untreated (Johnson, 2009).

In very mild cases, retinochoroiditis (inflammation of the retina and choroid layer of the eye) may be the only recognizable damage, and it and other manifestations may not appear until adolescence or young adulthood. Severe neonatal disorders associated with congenital infection include convulsions, coma, microcephaly, and hydrocephalus. The infant with a severe infection may die soon after birth. Survivors are often blind, deaf, and severely retarded. Treatment of the mother can reduce the incidence of fetal infection by 60% (ACOG, 2008f).

Clinical Therapy

The goal of medical treatment is to identify the woman at risk for toxoplasmosis and to treat the disease promptly if diagnosed. Diagnosis can be made by serologic testing, including the IgM and IgG fluorescent antibody tests. Elevated IgM titers are detectable 5 days after infection and may remain elevated for 1 year or more (ACOG, 2008f). Therefore, it is not a reliable test for diagnosing recent infection; a positive IgG and negative IgM in the third trimester or any positive IgM result should be followed by confirmatory testing. Polymerase chain reaction (PCR) for *T. gondii* DNA in amniotic fluid is the best way to diagnose fetal infection. Ultrasound can reveal findings suggestive of severe fetal infection such as ascites, ventriculomegaly, microcephaly, and growth restriction (ACOG, 2008f).

Women in whom maternal infection is established should receive spiramycin to decrease the frequency of fetal transmission, particularly in the first trimester. Spiramycin does not reliably cross the placenta; thus, while it can reduce the risk of congenital infection, it does not treat an established infection. If fetal infection is suspected, spiramycin should be replaced with pyrimethamine/sulfadiazine/folinic acid after the 18th week of pregnancy. Spiramycin is not commercially available in the United States, but can be obtained if an Investigational New Drug number is procured from the Food and Drug Administration (FDA) (Cunningham et al., 2010).

NURSING CARE MANAGEMENT

Nursing Assessment and Diagnosis

The incubation period for the disease is 10 days. The woman with acute toxoplasmosis may be asymptomatic, or she may develop myalgia, malaise, rash, splenomegaly, fever, headache, and enlarged posterior cervical lymph nodes. Symptoms usually disappear in a few days or weeks.

Nursing diagnoses that might apply to the pregnant woman with toxoplasmosis include the following:

- ***Readiness for Enhanced Knowledge (Toxoplasmosis)*** related to a desire to understand the ways in which a pregnant woman can contract the disease
- ***Grieving*** related to potential effects on infant of maternal toxoplasmosis

Nursing Plan and Implementation

The nurse caring for women during the antepartal period has the primary opportunity to discuss methods of prevention of toxoplasmosis with the childbearing woman. The woman must understand the importance of avoiding poorly cooked or raw meat, especially pork, beef, lamb, and, in the arctic region, caribou. Ten percent to 70% of lamb, 25% of pork, and 10% of beef samples have been reported to have *T. gondii* cysts. Fruits and vegetables should be washed. She should avoid contact with the cat litter box by having someone else clean it. In addition, because it takes approximately 48 hours for a cat's feces to become infectious, the litter should be cleaned frequently. The nurse should also discuss the importance of the woman wearing gloves when gardening and of avoiding garden areas frequented by cats.

Evaluation

Expected outcomes of nursing care include the following:

- The woman is able to discuss toxoplasmosis, its method of transmission, the implications for her fetus, and measures she can take to avoid contracting it.
- The woman implements health measures to avoid contracting toxoplasmosis.
- The woman gives birth to a healthy newborn.

Rubella

Rubella is a mild illness in children and adults. In fact, up to 60% of the cases are subclinical. On the other hand, rubella infection in the fetus can have overwhelming consequences. In the United States, large epidemics of rubella are rare because of immunization. Still, today there are pockets of unvaccinated people and cases continue to occur among infants born to women who emigrate from countries without rubella vaccination programs, or where programs have recently been put into place (Johnson, 2009). Estimates suggest that in the United States up to 10% of women are susceptible to rubella (Cunningham et al., 2010). Prepubertal girls and nonpregnant women of childbearing age who do not have antirubella antibodies should be immunized with the live, attenuated rubella vaccine. Although no fetal infection has resulted from immunization of a pregnant woman, pregnancy should be avoided for 1 month after immunization. Nurses need to be aware of the importance of postpartum immunization of the nonimmune woman to decrease unnecessary perinatal transmission.

Fetal-Neonatal Risks

The period of greatest risk for the teratogenic effects of rubella on the fetus is during the first trimester when maternal-fetal transmission occurs in up to 80% of cases of maternal rubella infection (Cunningham et al., 2010). Defects are rare when infection develops after 20 weeks' gestation (AAP & ACOG, 2007a). The most common clinical signs of rubella syndrome are congenital cataracts, sensorineural deafness, and congenital heart defects (particularly patent ductus arteriosus). Other abnormalities, such as mental retardation or cerebral palsy, may become evident in infancy. Diagnosis in the newborn can be conclusively made in the presence of these conditions and with an elevated rubella IgM antibody titer at birth.

Infants born with congenital rubella syndrome are infectious and should be isolated. These infants may continue to shed the virus for up to 12 months and, unless nasopharyngeal and urine cultures done after 3 months of age are negative for the rubella virus, should be considered contagious (AAP & ACOG, 2007a).

Clinical Therapy

The best therapy for rubella is prevention. Live, attenuated vaccine is available and should be given to all children. Women of childbearing age should be tested for immunity and vaccinated if susceptible and if it is established that they are not pregnant. Health counseling in high school and in premarital clinic visits can stress the importance of screening before planning a pregnancy. As part of the prenatal laboratory screen the woman is evaluated for rubella using hemagglutination inhibition (HAI), a serology test. The presence of a 1:18 titer or greater is evidence of immunity. A titer less than 1:8 indicates susceptibility to rubella.

Because the vaccine is made with attenuated virus, pregnant women are not vaccinated. However, it is considered safe for newly vaccinated children to have contact with pregnant women. Children should be given a single dose of the rubella vaccine at 1 year of age or at 15 months as part of the measles, mumps, and rubella (MMR) vaccine. All rubella-susceptible women should receive the MMR vaccine in the postpartum period.

If a woman who is pregnant becomes infected during the first trimester, therapeutic abortion may be an alternative.

NURSING CARE MANAGEMENT

Nursing Assessment and Diagnosis

A woman who develops rubella during pregnancy may be asymptomatic or may show signs of a mild infection, including a maculopapular rash, lymphadenopathy, muscular achiness, and joint pain. The presence of IgM antirubella antibody is diagnostic of a recent infection. These titers remain elevated for approximately 1 month following infection.

Nursing diagnoses that may apply to the woman who develops rubella early in her pregnancy include:

- ***Ineffective Coping*** due to an inability to accept the possibility of fetal anomalies secondary to maternal rubella exposure
- ***Risk for Ineffective Health Maintenance*** related to lack of knowledge about the importance of rubella immunization before becoming pregnant

Nursing Plan and Implementation

Nursing support and understanding are vital for the couple contemplating abortion because of a diagnosis of rubella. Such a decision may initiate a crisis for the couple who have planned their pregnancy. They need objective data to understand the possible effects on their fetus and the prognosis for the offspring.

Evaluation

Expected outcomes of nursing care include the following:

- The woman is able to describe the implications of rubella exposure during the first trimester of pregnancy.
- If exposure occurs in a woman who is not immune, she is able to identify her options and make a decision about continuing her pregnancy that is acceptable to her and her partner.
- The nonimmune woman receives the rubella vaccine during the early postpartum period.
- The woman gives birth to a healthy infant.

Cytomegalovirus

Cytomegalovirus (CMV) belongs to the herpes simplex virus group and causes both congenital and acquired disorders. The significance of this virus in pregnancy is related to its ability to be transmitted by asymptomatic women across the placenta to the fetus or by the cervical route during birth.

The virus can be found in urine, saliva, cervical mucus, semen, and breast milk (Tremblay, 2009). It can be passed between humans by any close contact such as kissing, breastfeeding, and sexual intercourse. Asymptomatic CMV infection is particularly common in children and gravid women. Transmission is common in day care centers, where excretion rate is as high as 70%, especially among children between 1 and 3 years of age (Tremblay, 2009). It is a chronic, persistent infection in that the individual may shed the virus continually over many years. The cervix can harbor the virus, and an ascending infection can develop after birth. Although the virus is usually innocuous in adults and children, it may be fatal to the fetus.

Accurate diagnosis in the pregnant woman is best documented by seroconversion. Shedding of the virus in urine and saliva can be intermittent and does not distinguish primary infection from recurrent infection. Identification of the virus in amniotic fluid by PCR or culture is the most sensitive and specific way of diagnosing congenital infection. This is even superior to fetal blood sampling and can be done earlier in pregnancy and with less risk to the fetus. Ultrasound findings may include fetal hydrops, growth restriction, hydramnios, cardiomegaly, and fetal ascites. At present no treatment exists for maternal CMV or for the congenital disease in the newborn.

Fetal-Neonatal Risks

CMV is the most common viral cause of infection in the human fetus. It infects 0.5% to 2% of newborns. Although 85% to 90% of infected fetuses will be asymptomatic at birth, the remaining 10% to 15% will have abnormalities of varying severity (Johnson, 2009). There is a 20% to 30% mortality rate among the symptomatic infants, and 90% of the survivors have significant neurologic complications. Subclinical infections in the newborn are capable of producing intellectual disability (mental retardation) and auditory deficits, sometimes not recognized for several months, or learning disabilities not seen until childhood. CMV may be the most common cause of intellectual disability.

For the fetus, this infection can result in extensive intrauterine tissue damage that leads to fetal death; it can result in fetal survival but with microcephaly, hydrocephaly, cerebral palsy, or intellectual disability; or it can result in fetal survival with no damage at all.

The infected newborn is often SGA. The principal tissues and organs affected are the blood, brain, and liver. However, virtually all organs are potentially at risk. Hemolysis leads to anemia and hyperbilirubinemia. Thrombocytopenia and hepatosplenomegaly may also develop.

Currently no effective therapy exists to manage this infection. A recent placebo-controlled, randomized, double-blind trial evaluated a CMV vaccine and has shown that it has the potential to decrease cases of maternal and congenital CMV infection (Pass et al., 2009).

Herpes Simplex Virus

It has been estimated that 1 in 6 people between the ages of 14 and 49 (16.2%) is infected with genital herpes in the United States (Centers for Disease Control and Prevention [CDC], 2010a). Herpes simplex virus (HSV-I or HSV-II) infection can cause painful lesions in the genital area. Lesions may also develop on the cervix. This condition and its implications for nonpregnant women are discussed in chapter 6 ∞. However, because the presence of herpes lesions in the genital tract may profoundly affect the fetus, herpes infection as it relates to a pregnant woman is discussed here.

Fetal-Neonatal Risks

According to data from the United States, the incidence of neonatal herpes infection is 1:3500 live births (Society of Obstetricians & Gynaecologists of Canada [SOGC], 2008). A primary herpes simplex infection can increase the risk of spontaneous abortion when infection occurs in the first trimester. Preterm labor (PTL), intrauterine growth restriction, and neonatal infection are greater risks if the primary infection occurs late in the second trimester or early in the third trimester. Recurrent infections during pregnancy do not appear to increase the risk for abortion or low-birth-weight infants.

Up to 80% of new cases of genital HSV may be caused by HSV-1, especially in adolescents and young adults (Hollier, 2009a). The risk to the fetus varies with the route of birth and whether the lesion that is present at the time of birth is primary or recurrent. If HSV-1 or HSV-2 is acquired close to the time of labor, the risk of transmission is 30% to 60% for a vaginal birth (AAP & ACOG, 2007a). Exposure of the newborn to a *recurrent* lesion drops the risk of transmission to between 2% and 5% (SOGC, 2008). For a woman with either a primary or a secondary outbreak of genital herpes during labor, or symptoms that may indicate an impending outbreak, the preferred method of childbirth is cesarean birth. Although fetal transmission with recurrent outbreaks is low, a cesarean birth is warranted because of the serious nature of the disease in the newborn. An estimated number of 1500 to 2000 newborns contract herpes each year, with 85% of neonatal herpes resulting from viral transmission near the time of birth. Most newborns infected with HSV are born to women who have unrecognized or asymptomatic infections (AAP & ACOG, 2007a). Despite the small risk of asymptomatic shedding, vaginal birth is appropriate for women with a history of HSV but no evidence of active genital disease at the time of childbirth (SOGC, 2008).

The infected infant is often asymptomatic at birth but symptoms can occur anytime after birth and up to 4 weeks of age (Johnson, 2009). Symptoms include fever (or hypothermia), jaundice, seizures, and poor feeding. Approximately one half of infected infants develop the characteristic vesicular skin lesions. Infants with disseminated disease present the earliest, usually within the first week after delivery. CNS symptoms generally occur during the second or third week. All infants who have neonatal herpes should be evaluated promptly and treated with acyclovir (CDC, 2009).

Clinical Therapy

A woman planning pregnancy who has no history of HSV but who has had a partner with genital HSV should have type-specific serology testing to determine her risk of acquiring HSV. If she is already pregnant, this should be done as early in pregnancy as possible.

Antiviral therapy is recommended after 36 weeks' gestation for women who experience recurrent outbreaks during pregnancy (SOGC, 2008). Oral antiviral therapies are available, including acyclovir (Zovirax), famciclovir, and valacyclovir. Famciclovir and valacyclovir have an advantage of better absorption and a longer half-life than acyclovir. Currently, there is no evidence that there are any adverse fetal effects related to exposure to any of these drugs during any trimester (Kriebs, 2008). Acyclovir, valacyclovir, and famciclovir have a Category B_m pregnancy classification (Briggs, Freeman, & Yaffee, 2008a). The CDC (2009) does not recommend the routine use of antivirals for recurrent infection during pregnancy but recognizes that the use of acyclovir near term may reduce the need for cesarean birth. The dosage is unchanged during pregnancy.

NURSING CARE MANAGEMENT

Nursing Assessment and Diagnosis

During the initial prenatal visit, it is important to learn whether the woman or her partner have had previous herpes infections. If so, ongoing assessment is indicated as pregnancy progresses.

Nursing diagnoses that may apply to the pregnant woman with HSV include the following:

- ***Acute Pain*** related to the presence of lesions secondary to herpes infection
- ***Ineffective Coping*** related to depression secondary to the risk to the fetus if herpes lesions are present at birth

Nursing Plan and Implementation

Nurses need to be particularly concerned with patient education about this fast-spreading disease. Women should be informed about what herpes is, how it is spread, and preventive measures. Condoms do not afford complete protection (approximately 50% effective); therefore, couples should be advised to abstain from sexual contact while prodromal symptoms or lesions are present (APP & ACOG, 2007a; Kriebs, 2008). Women should also receive information about the association of genital herpes with spontaneous abortion, neonatal mortality and morbidity, and the possibility of cesarean birth. A woman needs to inform her future healthcare providers of her infection. She also should know of the possible association of genital herpes with cervical cancer and the importance of a yearly Pap smear.

The woman who acquired HSV as an adolescent may be concerned by the possible risks as a mature young adult who wants to have a family. Patients may be helped by counseling that allows expression of the anger, shame, and depression so often experienced by women with herpes. Literature may be helpful and is available from many public health agencies.

Evaluation

Expected outcomes of nursing care include the following:

- The woman is able to describe her infection with regard to its method of spread, expected medical therapy, comfort measures, implications for her pregnancy, and long-term implications.
- The woman has appropriate cultures done as recommended throughout her pregnancy.
- The woman gives birth to a healthy infant.

Group B Streptococcus Infection

Group B streptococcus (GBS) infection is a bacterial infection found in the lower GI or urogenital tract. Women may transmit GBS to their fetus in utero or during childbirth. During the 1970s, GBS was recognized as the leading infectious cause of neonatal sepsis and mortality and remains so today (Hollier, 2009b). Fortunately, improved recognition and rapid treatment of infected infants has reduced morbidity and mortality rates considerably. Currently fewer than 10% of neonatal cases of GBS are fatal.

An estimated 10% to 30% of pregnant women are carriers of GBS. Rates of colonization vary by ethnicity, with African American women being colonized at twice the rate of Caucasian women (AAP & ACOG, 2007a; Hollier, 2009b). Colonization may be intermittent, transient, or chronic, and it is likely that nearly every woman is GBS colonized at some time. The reservoir for GBS is thought to be the gastrointestinal tract. In symptomatic women, GBS is responsible for considerable maternal morbidity from infections such as pyelonephritis, chorioamnionitis, postpartum endometritis, sepsis, wound infections, and in rare instances, meningitis (Hollier, 2009b).

Fetal-Neonatal Risks

GBS may result in unexpected intrapartum stillbirths (Cunningham et al., 2010). Newborns become infected either by vertical transmission from the mother as the fetus passes through the birth canal, resulting in early onset GBS in the first week of life, or from horizontal transmission from colonized nursery personnel or colonized infants, which may result in late onset GBS (Hollier, 2009b). Although most newborns who are born to colonized mothers will be born healthy, the transmission rate is influenced by how heavily the mother is colonized, whether or not she is persistently culture positive, the site of colonization (rectal versus vaginal), as well as other risk factors.

Risk factors for GBS neonatal sepsis include the following:

- Prematurity
- Maternal intrapartum fever
- Membranes ruptured for longer than 18 hours
- A previously infected infant with GBS disease
- GBS bacteriuria in the current pregnancy
- Young maternal age
- African American or Hispanic race

GBS causes severe, invasive disease in affected infants. In newborns, the majority of cases occur within the first week of life and are thus designated as early-onset disease. Late-onset disease occurs 1 week or more after birth. Early-onset GBS is often characterized by signs of serious illness including respiratory distress or pneumonia, apnea, and shock. Infants with late-onset GBS often develop meningitis. Long-term neurologic complications are common in survivors of both types of GBS.

Clinical Therapy

Guidelines for the detection of carriers and preventive treatment of newborns at risk include the following (AAP & ACOG, 2007a; Hollier 2009b):

- All pregnant women should be screened for both vaginal and rectal GBS colonization at 35 to 37 weeks' gestation. Treatment should be based on these results, even if cultures were done earlier in pregnancy.
- Women identified as GBS carriers should receive antibiotic prophylaxis at the onset of labor or the rupture of membranes.
- Women with GBS in their urine in any concentration should receive antibiotic prophylaxis intrapartally because such women typically have heavy colonization with GBS and thus have an increased risk of giving birth to a newborn with early-onset disease. These women do not need vaginal and rectal cultures at 35 to 37 weeks because therapy is already indicated.
- Women who have already given birth to a newborn with invasive GBS disease should receive intrapartum antibiotic prophylaxis. Culture-based screening is not necessary for them.
- If the results of GBS screening are not known when labor begins, prophylaxis is indicated for women with any of the following risk factors: gestation less than 37 weeks, membranes ruptured equal to or longer than 18 hours, temperature greater than 100.4°F (38°C).

Intrapartum prophylaxis is not indicated in the following circumstances:

- Women who undergo a cesarean birth and have not been in labor and have intact membranes do not require GBS prophylaxis regardless of their GBS status.
- Positive GBS culture in a previous pregnancy with a negative culture result in the current pregnancy.
- Negative vaginal and rectal GBS screening results done at the appropriate gestational age regardless of intrapartum risk factors.

Figure 20-11 ■ provides an algorithm for assessing the need for intrapartum antibiotic prophylaxis.

Intrapartum antibiotic therapy is recommended as follows: initial dose of penicillin G 5 million units IV followed by

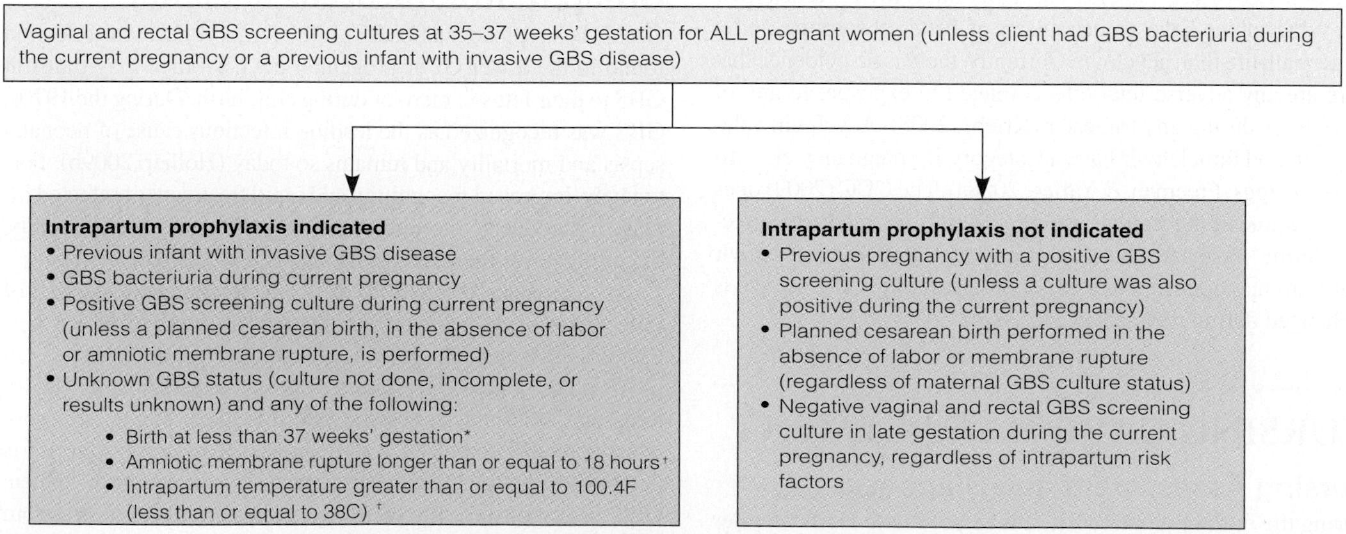

Vaginal and rectal GBS screening cultures at 35–37 weeks' gestation for ALL pregnant women (unless client had GBS bacteriuria during the current pregnancy or a previous infant with invasive GBS disease)
Intrapartum prophylaxis indicated
• Previous infant with invasive GBS disease
• GBS bacteriuria during current pregnancy
• Positive GBS screening culture during current pregnancy (unless a planned cesarean birth, in the absence of labor or amniotic membrane rupture, is performed)
• Unknown GBS status (culture not done, incomplete, or results unknown) and any of the following:
• Birth at less than 37 weeks' gestation*
• Amniotic membrane rupture longer than or equal to 18 hours†
• Intrapartum temperature greater than or equal to 100.4F (less than or equal to 38C) †
Intrapartum prophylaxis not indicated
• Previous pregnancy with a positive GBS screening culture (unless a culture was also positive during the current pregnancy)
• Planned cesarean birth performed in the absence of labor or membrane rupture (regardless of maternal GBS culture status)
• Negative vaginal and rectal GBS screening culture in late gestation during the current pregnancy, regardless of intrapartum risk factors

* If onset of labor or rupture of amniotic membrane occurs at less than 37 weeks' gestation and there is a significant risk for preterm birth (as assessed by the clinician).

† If amnionitis is suspected, broad-spectrum antibiotic therapy that includes an agent known to be active against GBS should replace GBS prophylaxis.

Figure 20-11 ■ Indications for intrapartum antibiotic prophylaxis to prevent perinatal GBS disease under a universal prenatal screening strategy based on combined vaginal and rectal cultures collected at 35 to 37 weeks' gestation from all pregnant women.

Source: Centers for Disease Control and Prevention (CDC).

2.5 million units IV every 4 hours until childbirth. Alternately, ampicillin 2 g initial dose IV followed by 1 g IV every 4 hours until childbirth may be used. Women at high risk for an anaphylactic reaction to penicillin because of marked allergy may be treated with clindamycin or erythromycin if the GBS is sensitive to those agents. When GBS resistance is an issue or susceptibility is unknown, vancomycin is an alternative (Hollier, 2009b; Matteson, Lievense, & Catanzaro, 2008).

Human B19 Parvovirus

Human B19 parvovirus causes erythema infectiosum or fifth disease in children. It is a mild disease in adults that produces a characteristic "slapped cheek" rash. More than one half of pregnant women are immune to parvovirus B19 (AAP & ACOG, 2007a). Incubation period to maternal symptoms, when they occur, is 4 to 14 days. Symptoms in adults include myalgia; coryza (inflammation of the nasal membranes with profuse nasal discharge); and headache, fever, and nausea, which coincides with contagiousness. In some cases, a week later this phase may be followed by an erythematous maculopapular rash on the trunk and limbs. Arthropathy (any disease or condition affecting a joint) is a common manifestation in women and adolescents and may be the only clinical symptom of the infection (Tolfvenstam & Broliden, 2009). Nonimmune women with school-aged children are more likely to acquire parvovirus, and serologic evaluation should be performed if the pregnant woman has been exposed to a child diagnosed with fifth disease. Epidemics are noted about every 3 to 4 years (Tolfvenstam & Broliden, 2009).

Although there is a low risk of fetal morbidity, transplacental (vertical) transmission is reported to be as high as 33% with a fetal loss rate of less than 10%. Fetal infection is associated with spontaneous abortion, fetal hydrops, and stillbirth. Severe effects occur most frequently with maternal infection before 20 weeks' gestation (AAP & ACOG, 2007a). The major fetal concern is nonimmune hydrops and fetal anemia, which, if left untreated, may result in death. Asymptomatic infections can resolve spontaneously with a mean time span between maternal infection and fetal symptoms of 6 weeks (Tolfvenstam & Broliden, 2009).

Weekly measurements of peak systolic velocity of the MCA (middle cerebral artery) are indicated. Values of greater than 1.5 multiples of the median (MoM) for gestational age have been associated with fetal anemia. Hydrops may be seen up to 8 weeks after maternal infection; however, they may not always occur even in the face of marked anemia. In up to one third of fetuses, there may be spontaneous resolution of hydrops. If hydrops and fetal anemia are diagnosed, intrauterine fetal transfusion may reduce the mortality from about 50% to 18% (Tolfvenstam & Broliden, 2009).

Fetal death may occur at 4 to 12 weeks' postinfection; therefore, fetal surveillance should be maintained for 8 to 12 weeks. The risk of fetal death remains several months post maternal infection even when fetal hydrops is not evident. In fetuses who survive the infection, long-term development appears to be normal.

Other Infections in Pregnancy

Table 20-4 summarizes other urinary tract, vaginal, and sexually transmitted infections that put pregnancy at risk. (These are described in detail in chapter 6 ∞). Spontaneous abortion is frequently the result of a severe maternal infection, and research links infection with prematurity. In addition, if the pregnancy is carried to term in the presence of infection, the risk of maternal and fetal morbidity and mortality increases. Thus it is essential to maternal and fetal health that infection be diagnosed and treated promptly.

TABLE 20-4 Infections That Put Pregnancy at Risk

CONDITION AND CAUSATIVE ORGANISM	SIGNS AND SYMPTOMS	TREATMENT	IMPLICATIONS FOR PREGNANCY
Urinary Tract Infections (UTI)			
Asymptomatic bacteriuria (ASB): *Escherichia coli, Klebsiella, Proteus* most common	Bacteria present in urine on culture with no accompanying symptoms.	Oral sulfonamides early in pregnancy, ampicillin and nitrofurantoin (Furadantin) in late pregnancy. Antibody sensitivity results will guide the selection of an appropriate antibiotic.	Women with ASB in early pregnancy may go on to develop cystitis or acute pyelonephritis by third trimester if not treated. Oral sulfonamides taken in the last few weeks of pregnancy may lead to neonatal hyperbilirubinemia and kernicterus.
Cystitis (lower UTI): Causative organisms same as for ASB	Dysuria, urgency, frequency, low-grade fever, and hematuria may occur. Urine culture (clean catch) shows ≠ leukocytes. Presence of 10^5 (100,000) or more colonies bacteria per ml urine.	Same	If not treated, infection may ascend and lead to acute pyelonephritis. Suppressive therapy is recommended for bacteriuria that persists after 2 or more courses of therapy during pregnancy. Nitrofurantoin 50–100 mg at bedtime for the duration of pregnancy is a common choice (Eckert, 2009).
Acute pyelonephritis: Causative organisms same as for ASB	Sudden onset. Chills, high fever, flank pain. Nausea, vomiting, malaise. May have decreased urine output, severe colicky pain, dehydration. Increased diastolic BP, positive fluorescent antibody (FA) test, low creatinine clearance. Marked bacteremia in urine culture, pyuria, WBC casts.	Hospitalization; IV antibiotic therapy. Other antibiotics safe during pregnancy include carbenicillin, methenamine, cephalosporins. Catheterization if there is no urine output. Supportive therapy for comfort. Follow-up urine cultures are necessary.	Increased risk of premature birth and intrauterine growth restriction (IUGR). These antibiotics interfere with urinary estriol levels and can cause false interpretations of estriol levels during pregnancy.

(continued)

TABLE 20-4 Infections That Put Pregnancy at Risk continued

CONDITION AND CAUSATIVE ORGANISM	SIGNS AND SYMPTOMS	TREATMENT	IMPLICATIONS FOR PREGNANCY
Vaginal Infections			
Vulvovaginal candidiasis (yeast infections): *Candida albicans*	Often thick, white, curdy discharge, severe itching, dysuria, dyspareunia. Diagnosis based on presence of hyphae and spores in a wet-mount preparation of vaginal secretions.	Intravaginal insertion of miconazole butoconazole, or other topical azole preparation, or clotrimazol vaginal tablets at bedtime for 1 week. Cream may be prescribed for topical application to the vulva if necessary (CDC, 2006).	If the infection is present at birth and the fetus is born vaginally, the fetus may contract thrush.
Bacterial vaginosis: *Gardnerella vaginalis*	Thin, watery, yellow gray discharge with foul odor often described as "fishy." Wet-mount preparation reveals "clue cells." Application of potassium hydroxide (KOH) to a specimen of vaginal secretions produces a pronounced fishy odor.	Metronidazole 250 mg PO TID × 7 days or metronidazole 500 mg PO BID × 7 days or clindamycin 300 mg PO BID × 7 days (CDC, 2010b).	CDC (2006) reports that multiple studies have failed to demonstrate a teratogenic effect from metronidazole. BV during pregnancy is associated with PROM, PTL, intra-amniotic infection, and endometritis postpartally (CDC, 2006).
Trichomoniasis: *Trichomonas vaginalis*	Occasionally asymptomatic. May have frothy greenish gray vaginal discharge, pruritus, urinary symptoms. Strawberry patches may be visible on vaginal walls or cervix. Wet-mount preparation of vaginal secretions shows motile flagellated trichomonads.	Single 2-g dose of metronidazole orally (CDC, 2006).	Increased risk for PROM, preterm birth, and low birth weight.
Chlamydial infection: *Chlamydia trachomatis*	Women are often asymptomatic. Symptoms may include thin or purulent discharge, urinary burning and frequency, or lower abdominal pain. Lab test available to detect monoclonal antibodies specific for *Chlamydia*.	Doxycycline, ofloxacin, and levofloxacin are contraindicated during pregnancy. Thus, pregnant women are treated with azithromycin or amoxicillin followed by repeat culture in 3 weeks (CDC, 2006).	Infant of woman with untreated chlamydial infection may develop newborn conjunctivitis, which can be treated with erythromycin eye ointment (but not silver nitrate). Infant may also develop chlamydial pneumonia. May be responsible for premature labor and fetal death.
Syphilis: *Treponema pallidum*, a spirochete	Primary stage: chancre, slight fever, malaise. Chancre lasts about 4 weeks, then disappears. Secondary stage occurs 6 weeks to 6 months after infection. Skin eruptions (condyloma latal), also symptoms of acute arthritis, liver enlargement, iritis, chronic sore throat with hoarseness. Diagnosed by blood tests such as VDRL, RPR, FTA, ABS. Dark-field examination for spirochetes may also be done.	Treatment for pregnant women follows the regimen recommended for the general population and is based on the stage of syphilis. For early latent syphilis (less than 1 year duration), 2.4 million units benzathine penicillin G IM. For late latent syphilis (more than 1 year duration) or latent syphilis of unknown duration, 2.4 million units benzathine penicillin G IM once a week for 3 weeks. Pregnant women who are allergic to penicillin should be desensitized and then treated with penicillin. Sexual partners should also be screened and treated (CDC, 2006).	Syphilis can be passed transplacentally to the fetus. If untreated, one of the following can occur: second trimester abortion, stillborn infant at term, congenitally infected infant, uninfected live infant.
Gonorrhea: *Neisseria gonorrhoeae*	Majority of women asymptomatic; disease often diagnosed during routine prenatal cervical culture. If symptoms are present they may include purulent vaginal discharge, dysuria, urinary frequency, inflammation, and swelling of the vulva. Cervix may appear eroded.	Nonpregnant women are treated with a single dose of ceftriaxone IM or a single dose of cefixime orally plus treatment for chlamydia if not ruled out. Fluoroquinolones (ciprofloxacin, ofloxacin, or levofloxacin) are no longer recommended for the treatment of gonorrhea because of the prevalence of fluoroquinolone-resistant gonorrhea (CDC, 2007). Pregnant women should be treated with a cephalosporin (ceftriaxone, cefixime); if they cannot tolerate a cephalosporin, they should receive spectinomycin (CDC, 2006).	Infection at time of birth may cause ophthalmia neonatorum in the newborn.
Condylomata acuminata: caused by a papilloma virus	Soft, grayish pink lesions on the vulva, vagina, cervix, or anus.	Podophyllin, podofilox, and imiquimod are contraindicated during pregnancy. Some caregivers recommend removing warts by surgical methods or laser because the warts can proliferate and become friable (bleed easily) during pregnancy.	Possible teratogenic effect of podophyllin. Large doses have been associated with fetal death. The HPV vaccine is not recommended during pregnancy; however, it is safe to administer during breastfeeding (AAP & ACOG, 2007a).

FOCUS YOUR STUDY

- Several health problems associated with bleeding arise from the pregnancy itself, such as spontaneous abortion, ectopic pregnancy, and gestational trophoblastic disease. The nurse needs to be alert to early signs of these situations, to guard the woman against heavy bleeding and shock, to facilitate the medical treatment, and to provide educational and emotional support.
- Hyperemesis gravidarum, excessive vomiting during pregnancy, may cause fluid and electrolyte imbalance, dehydration, and signs of starvation in the mother and, if severe enough, death of the fetus. Treatment is aimed at controlling the vomiting, correcting fluid and electrolyte imbalance, correcting dehydration, and improving nutritional status.
- Hypertension may exist before pregnancy or, more often, may develop during pregnancy. Preeclampsia can lead to growth retardation for the fetus and, if untreated, may lead to convulsions (eclampsia) and even death for the mother and fetus. A woman's understanding of the disease process helps motivate her to maintain the required rest periods in the left lateral position. Antihypertensive or anticonvulsive drugs may be part of the therapy.
- Rh incompatibility can exist when an Rh-negative woman and an Rh-positive partner conceive a child who is Rh positive. The use of Rh immune globulin has greatly decreased the incidence of severe sequelae due to Rh incompatibility because the drug "tricks" the body into thinking antibodies have been produced in response to the Rh antigen.
- The impact of surgery or trauma on the pregnant woman and her fetus is related to timing in the pregnancy, seriousness of the situation, and other factors influencing the situation.
- Physical violence often begins or continues during pregnancy. The nurse needs to be alert for signs of abuse, including bruising or injury to the breasts, abdomen, and genitals. The nurse should provide the woman information about violence and about community resources available to assist her.
- Toxoplasmosis, rubella, cytomegalovirus, parvovirus B19, herpes, group B streptococcus (GBS) infection, and other perinatal infections all pose a grave threat to the fetus. Prevention is the best therapy. There is no known treatment for rubella or parvovirus B19, but antimicrobial drugs are available for toxoplasmosis, herpes, and GBS. A vaccine for CMV may be available in the near future.
- Universal screening for GBS is now recommended for all pregnant women at 35 to 37 weeks' gestation.

CRITICAL THINKING IN ACTION

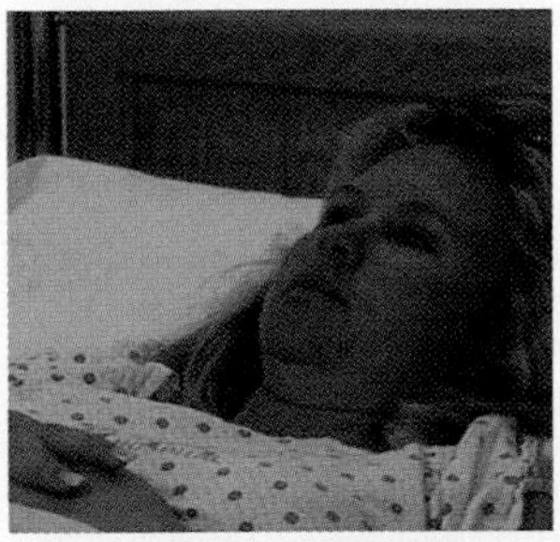
Source: George Dodson/Pearson Education.

Carol Smith, a 40-year-old, single, G2, P0010, presents to you at 32 weeks' gestation while you are working in the birthing unit. Her chief complaint is severe headache, nausea, and trouble seeing. She describes "blackened areas" in her visual fields bilaterally. Her prenatal record reveals long-term substance abuse, depression, and hypertension currently treated with nifedipine 60 mg by mouth once in the morning. You note that she has had two prenatal visits with this pregnancy. You determine her blood pressure to be 170/110; deep tendon reflexes are 3+, clonus negative. She has general edema and 3+ protein uria. You place Carol on the external fetal monitor to observe for fetal well-being and any contractions. You position her on her left side with her head elevated and use pillows for comfort. You observe that the fetal heart rate is 143–148 with decreased long-term variability. No fetal heart rate decelerations or accelerations are noted. The uterus is soft, and no contractions are palpated or noted on the fetal monitor.

Carol asks you why she should stay on her left side.

1. How would you explain the importance of the left side-lying position when on bed rest?
2. You administer nifedipine 10 mg sublingual and a loading dose of magnesium sulfate 4 gm IV piggyback to the main IV line of Ringer's lactate. What findings would indicate that Carol has therapeutic levels of magnesium?
3. What signs of magnesium toxicity should you monitor Carol for?
4. Carol asks if magnesium sulfate will affect her infant. How would you answer her?
5. Which signs of premature labor would you ask Carol to notify you of if she experiences?

See www.nursing.pearsonhighered.com for possible responses.

REFERENCES

Airoldi, J., & Weinstein, L. (2007). Clinical significance of proteinuria in pregnancy. *Obstetrical & Gynecological Survey, 62*(2), 117–124.

American Academy of Pediatrics (AAP) & American College of Obstetricians and Gynecologists (ACOG). (2007a). Antepartum care. In *Guidelines for perinatal care.* Elk Grove Village, IL: Author.

American Academy of Pediatrics (AAP) & American College of Obstetricians and Gynecologists (ACOG). (2007b). Domestic violence. In *Guidelines for perinatal care.* Elk Grove Village, IL: Author.

American College of Obstetricians and Gynecologists (ACOG). (2006a). *Management of alloimmunization during pregnancy* (ACOG Practice Bulletin No. 75). Washington, DC: Author.

American College of Obstetricians and Gynecologists (ACOG). (2006b). *Obstetric aspects of trauma management* (ACOG Educational Bulletin No. 251). Washington, DC: Author.

American College of Obstetricians and Gynecologists (ACOG). (2008a). Chronic hypertension in pregnancy. (ACOG Practice Bulletin No. 29). Washington, DC: Author.

American College of Obstetricians and Gynecologists (ACOG). (2008b). *Diagnosis and management of preeclampsia and eclampsia* (ACOG Practice Bulletin No. 33). Washington, DC: Author.

American College of Obstetricians and Gynecologists (ACOG). (2008c). *Diagnosis and treatment of gestational trophoblastic disease* (ACOG Practice Bulletin No. 53). Washington, DC: Author.

American College of Obstetricians and Gynecologists (ACOG). (2008f). *Perinatal viral and parasitic infections* (ACOG Practice Bulletin No. 20). Washington, DC: Author.

American College of Obstetricians and Gynecologists (ACOG). (2009a). *Domestic violence* (Educational Pamphlet AP083). Washington, DC: Author.

American College of Obstetricians and Gynecologists (ACOG). (2004. Reaffirmed 2009b). *Nausea and vomiting of pregnancy* (ACOG Practice Bulletin No. 52). Washington, DC: Author.

Barnhart, K. T. (2009). Ectopic pregnancy. *The New England Journal of Medicine, 361*(4), 379–387.

Barton, J. R., & Sibai, B. M. (2008). Prediction and prevention of recurrent preeclampsia. *Obstetrics & Gynecology, 112*(2 Part 1), 359–372.

Berkowitz, R. S., & Goldstein, D. P. (2009). Molar pregnancy. *The New England Journal of Medicine, 360*(16), 1639–1645.

Bess, K. A., & Wood, T. L. (2006). Understanding gestational trophoblastic disease: How nurses can help those dealing with a diagnosis. *AWHONN Lifelines, 10*(4), 321–326.

Black, V. L., & Maheshwari, A. (2009). Disorders of the fetomaternal unit: Hematologic manifestations in the fetus and neonate. *Seminars in Perinatology, 33,* 12–19.

Briggs, G. G., Freeman, R. K., & Yaffee, S. J. (2008a). Acyclovir. In G. G. Briggs, R. K. Freeman, & S. J. Yaffee (Eds.), *Drugs in pregnancy and lactation* (7th ed.). Philadelphia, PA: Lippincott Williams & Wilkins.

Brown, H. L. (2009). Trauma in pregnancy. *Obstetrics & Gynecology, 114*(1), 147–160.

Calleja-Agius, J. (2008, October). Vaginal bleeding in the first trimester. *British Journal of Midwifery, 16*(10), 656–661.

Catov, J. M., Nohr, E. A., Olsen, J., & Ness, R. B. (2009). Chronic hypertension related to risk for preterm and term small for gestational age births. *Obstetrics & Gynecology, 112*(2 Part 1), 290–296.

Centers for Disease Control and Prevention [CDC]. (2005). Having a healthy pregnancy. Retrieved from http://www.cdc.gov/ncbddd/bd/abc.htm

Centers for Disease Control and Prevention (CDC). (2006). Sexually transmitted diseases treatment guidelines, 2006. *Morbidity and Mortality Weekly Report, 55*(RR-11), 1–93.

Centers for Disease Control and Prevention (CDC). (2007, April 13). Update to CDC's *Sexually transmitted diseases treatment guidelines, 2006:* Fluoroquinolones no longer recommended for treatment of gonococcal infections. *MMWR Weekly, 56*(14), 332–336.

Centers for Disease Control and Prevention (CDC). (2009). Genital herpes simplex (HSV) Module. Retrieved June 14, 2010 from www2a.cdc.gov/stdtraining/ready-to-use/Manuals/HSV/hsv-notes-2009.pdf

Centers for Disease Control and Prevention (CDC). (2010a). CDC analysis of national herpes prevalence. Retrieved from www.cdc.gov/std/Herpes/herpes-NHANES-2010.htm

Centers for Disease Control and Prevention (CDC). (2010b). Self-study STD module—vaginitis: Bacterial vaginosis. Retrieved from www.2a.cdc.gov/stdtraining/self-study/default.asp

Chappell, L. C., Enye, S., Seed, P., Briley, A., Poston, L, & Shennan, A. H. (2008). Adverse perinatal outcomes and risk factors for preeclampsia in women with chronic hypertension: A prospective study. *Hypertension, 51*(4 Part 2), 1002–1009.

Costantine, M. M., & Weiner, S. J. (2009). Effects of antenatal exposure to magnesium sulfate on neuroprotection and mortality in preterm infants. *Obstetrics & Gynecology, 14*(2 part 1), 354–364.

Cunningham, F. G., Leveno, K. J., Bloom, S. L., Hauth, J. C., Rouse, D. J., & Spong, C. Y. (2010). *Williams obstetrics* (23rd ed.). New York, NY: McGraw-Hill.

Dietrich, C. S., Hill, C. C., & Hueman, M. (2008). Surgical diseases presenting in pregnancy. *Surgical Clinics of North America, 88,* 403–419.

Eckert, L. O. (2009). Urinary tract infections. (ACOG, *Infectious Disease in Obstetrics and Gynecology: A Systematic Approach to Management).* Washington, D.C.

Ghulmiyyah, L. M., & Sabai, B. M. (2006). Managing an eclamptic seizure and its aftermath. *Contemporary OB/GYN, 51*(3), 54–66.

Goldberg, D., Szilagyi, A., & Graves, L. (2007). Hyperemesis gravidarum and helicobacter pylori infection: A symptomatic review. *Obstetrics & Gynecology, 10*(3), 695–703.

Gordon, M. C. (2007). Maternal physiology in pregnancy. In S. G. Gabbe, J. R. Niebyl, & J. L. Simpson (Eds.), *Obstetrics: Normal and problem pregnancies* (5th ed.). Philadelphia, PA: Churchill Livingstone Elsevier.

Habli, M., & Sibai, B. M. (2008). Hypertensive disorders of pregnancy. In R. S. Gibbs, B. Y. Karlan, A. F. Haney, & I. E. Nygaard (Eds.), *Danforth's obstetrics and gynecology* (10th ed.). Philadelphia, PA: Wolters Kluwer/Lippincott Williams & Wilkins.

Haugen, M., Brantsaeter, A. L., Trogstad, L., Alexander, J., Roth, C., Mangus, P., & Meltzer, H. M. (2009). Vitamin D supplementation and reduced risk of preeclampsia in nulliparous women. *Epidemiology, 20*(5), 720–726.

Hay, J. E. (2008). Liver disease in pregnancy. *Hepatology,* 47(3), 1067–1076.

Hollier, L. (2009a). Genital Herpes. (ACOG, *Infectious Disease in Obstetrics and Gynecology: A Systematic Approach to Management).* Washington, D.C.

Hollier, L. (2009b). Group B streptococcus. (ACOG, *Infectious Disease in Obstetrics and Gynecology: A Systematic Approach to Management).* Washington, D.C.

Holmgren, C., Aagaard-Tillery, K. M., Silver, R. M., Porter, T. F., & Varner, M. (2008). Hyperemesis in pregnancy: An evaluation of treatment strategies with maternal and neonatal outcomes. *American Journal of Obstetrics and Gynecology, 198*(1), 56, e1–4.

Johnson, K. E. (2009). Overview of TORCH infections. Retrieved 9/23/2009 at UpToDate.com.

Karumanchi, S. A., & Lindheimer, M. D. (2008). Preeclampsia pathogenesis: "Triple A rating – Autoantibodies and antiangiogenic factors. *Hypertension, 51*(4 part 2), 991–992.

Katz, L., de Amorim, M. M., Figueiroa, J. N., & Pinto e Silva, J. L. (2008).Postpartum dexamethasone for women with hemolysis, elevated liver enzymes, and low platelets (HELLP) syndrome: a double-blind, placebo-controlled, randomized clinical trial. *American Journal of Obstetrics & Gynecology 198*(3), 283.e1–8.

Kopcow, H. D., & Karumanchi, S. A. (2007). Angiogenic factors and natural killer (NK) cells in the pathogenesis of preeclampsia. *Journal of Reproductive Immunology, 76*(1–2) 23–29.

Kriebs, J. M. (2008). Understanding Herpes simplex virus: Transmission diagnosis, and considerations in pregnancy management. *Journal of Midwifery and Women's Health, 53*(3), 202–208.

Kuklina, E. V., Ayala, C., Callaghan, W. M. (2009). Hypertensive disorders and severe obstetric morbidity in the United States. *Obstetrics & Gynecology, 113*(6), 1299–1306.

Li, A. J. (2008). Gestational trophoblastic neoplasms. In R. S. Gibbs, B. Y. Karlan, A. F. Haney, & I. Nygaard (Eds.), *Danforth's obstetrics and gynecology* (10th ed). Philadelphia, PA: Wolters Kluwer/Lippincott Williams & Wilkins.

Lim, J. H., Kim, S. Y., Park, S. Y., Kim, M. Y., & Ryu, H. M. (2008). Effective prediction of preeclampsia by a combined ratio of angiogenesis-related factors. *Obstetrics & Gynecology 111*(6), 1403–1409.

Lobo, G. A. R., Nardozza, L. M. M., & Camano, L. (2006). Non-anti-D antibodies in red-cell alloimmunization. *International Journal of Gynecology & Obsteterics, 94,* 139–140.

Lockwood, C. J., & Bauer, K. A. (2009). Inherited thrombophilias in pregnancy. Retrieved from www.UpToDate.com.

Lutgendorf, M. A., Busch, J. M., Doherty, D. A., Conza, L. A., Moone, S. O., & Magann, E. F. (2009). Prevalence of domestic violence in a pregnant military population. *Obstetrics & Gynecology, 113*(4), 866–872.

Martin, D. (2009). HELLP syndrome A-Z: Facing an obstetric emergency. *Air Medical Journal, 28*(5), 229–256.

Matteson, K. A., Lievense, S. P., & Catanzaro, B. (2008). Intrapartum group B streptococci prophylaxis in patients reporting a penicillin allergy. *Obstetrics & Gynecology, 111*(2 Part 1), 356–364.

McCoy, S., & Baldwin, K. (2009). Pharmacotherapeutics options for the treatment of preeclampsia. *American Journal of Health-System Pharmacy, 66*(4), 337–344.

Meads, C., Cnossen, J., Meher, S., Juarez-Garcia, A., terRiet, G., Duley, L. . . Khan, K. S. (2008). Methods of prediction and prevention of pre-eclampsia: systematic reviews of accuracy and effectiveness literature with economic modeling. *Health Technology Assessment, 12*(6):iii–iv,1–270.

Mihu, D., Costin, N., Mihu, C. M., Seicean, A., & Ciortea, R. (2007). HELLP syndrome – A multisystemic disorder.

Journal of Gastrointestinal and Liver Disease, 16(4), 419–424.

Moise, K. J. (2007). Red cell alloimmunization. In S. G. Gabbe, J. R. Niebyl, & J. L. Simpson (Eds), *Obstetrics: Normal and problem pregnancies* (5th ed.). Philadelphia, PA: Churchill Livingstone Elsevier.

Moise, K. J. (2008a). Management of Rhesus alloimmunization in pregnancy. *Obstetrics & Gynecology, 112*(1), 164–176.

Moise, K. J. (2008b). The usefulness of middle cerebral artery Doppler assessment in the treatment of the fetus at risk for anemia. *American Journal of Obstetrics and Gynecology, 198*, 161.e1–161.e4.

National Institutes of Health (NIH). (2000). *Working group report on high blood pressure in pregnancy.* Retrieved from www.nhibi.nih.gov/health/prof/heart/hbp/hbp-preg.htm

Ness, R. B., & Grainger, D. A. (2008). Male reproductive proteins and reproductive outcomes. *American Journal of Obstetrics and Gynecology 198*(6), 620.e1–620.e4. Retrieved from www.ajog.org.

Pappas, G., Roussos, N., & Falagas, M. E. (2009). Toxoplasmosis snapshots: Global status of Toxoplasmosis gondii seroprevalence and implications for pregnancy and congenital toxoplasmosis (2009). *International Journal for Parasitology, 39*(12), 1385–1394.

Pass, R. F., Zhang, C., Evans, A., Simpson, T., Andrews, W., Huang, M-L., ..., Cloud, G. (2009). Vaccine prevention of maternal cytomegalovirus infection. *The New England Journal of Medicine, 360*(12), 1191–1199.

Pickelsimer, A. H., Oepkes, D., Moise, K. J., Kush, M. L., Weiner, C. P., Harman, C. R., & Baschat, A. A. (2007). Determinants of the middle cerebral artery peak systolic velocity in the human fetus. *The American Journal of Obstetrics & Gynecology, 197*, 526e.1–526e.4.

Porter, T. F., Branch, D. W., & Scott, J. R. (2008). Early pregnancy loss. In R. S., Gibbs, B. Y. Karlan, A. F. Haney, & I. Nygaard (Eds.). *Danforth's obstetrics and gynecology* (10th ed.). Philadelphia, PA: Wolters Kluwer/Lippincott Williams & Wilkins.

Pryde, P. G., & Mittendorf, R. (2009). Contemporary usage of obstetric magnesium sulfate. *Obstetrics & Gynecology 114*(3), 669–673.

Rouillac-Le Sciellour, C., Serazin, V., Brossard, Y., Oudin, O., Le Van Kim, S., Colin, Y., ..., Cartron, J.-P. (2007). Noninvasive fetal RHD genotyping from maternal plasma. Use of a new developed Free DNA Fetal Kit RhD. *Transfusion Clinique et Biologique, 14*, 572–577.

Santiago, J. C., Ramos-Corpas, D., Oyonarte, S., & Montoya, F. (2008). Current clinical management of anti-Kell alloimmunization in pregnancy. *European Journal of Obstetrics & Gynecology and Reproductive Biology, 136*, 151–154.

Sibai, B. M. (2007). Caring for women with hypertension in pregnancy. *The Journal of the American Medical Association, 298*, 1566–1568.

Sibai, B. M. & Stella, C. L. (2009). Diagnosis and management of atypical preeclampsia-eclampsia. *American Journal of Obstetrics, and Gynecology, 200*(5), 481.e1–481.e7.

Society of Obstetricians & Gynaecologists of Canada (SOGC). (2008). Guidelines for the management of herpes simplex virus in pregnancy, No. 208. *International Journal of Gynecology and Obstetrics, 104*, 167–171.

Thadhani, R., & Solomon, C. G. (2008). Preeclampsia—a glimpse into the future? *The New England Journal of Medicine, 359*(8), 858–860.

Thurman, A. R., Cornelius, M., Korte, J. E., & Fylstra,, D. L. (2010). An alternative monitoring protocol for single-dose methotrexate therapy in ectopic pregnancy. *American Journal of Obstetrics and Gynecology, 202*(2), 139.e1–139.e6.

Tolfvenstam, T., & Broliden, K. (2009). Parvovirus B19 infection. *Seminars in Fetal & Neonatal Medicine, 14*, 218–221.

Tremblay, C. (2009). Cytomegalovirus infection in pregnancy. Retrieved at UpToDate.com.

Valley, V. T., Jackson-Williams, L., & Fly, C. A. (2006). Abortion, Complete. Retrieved from http://emedicine.medscape.com/article/794918-overview

Van der Schoot, C. E., Hahn, S., & Chitty, L. S. (2008). Non-invasive prenatal diagnosis and determination of fetal Rh status. *Seminars in Fetal and Neonatal Medicine, 13*(2), 63–68.

Wen, S. W., Chen X-K., Rodgers, M., White, R. R., Yang, Q., Smith, G. N., ..., Walker, M. C. (2008). Folic acid supplementation in early second trimester and the risk of preeclampsia. *American Journal of Obstetrics & Gynecology, 198*(1), 45.e1–45.e7.

Wiggins, D. A., & Elliott, M. (2005). Outcomes of pregnancies achieved by donor egg in vitro fertilization—a comparison with standard in vitro fertilization pregnancies. *American Journal of Obstetrics and Gynecology, 192*(6): 2002–2008.

Xu, H., Perez-Cuevas, R., Xiong, S., Reyes, H., Roy, C., Julien, P. . . Audibert, F. (2010). An international trial of anti-oxidants in the prevention of pre-eclampsia. *American Journal of Obstetrics and Gynecology*, 202(3):239.e1–239.e10.

Yankowitz, J. (2008). Drugs in pregnancy. In R. S. Gibbs, B. Y. Karlan, A. F. Haney, & I. Nygaard (Eds.). *Danforth's obstetrics and gynecology* 10th ed. Philadelphia, PA: Wolters Kluwer/Lippincott Williams & Wilkins.

CHAPTER 21

Assessment of Fetal Well-Being

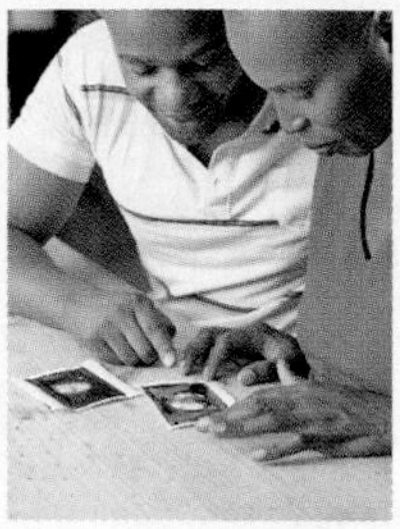

My first pregnancy was very complicated and I hoped for a healthy baby throughout, but my baby did not survive. This experience made us very reserved and anxious through our next pregnancy as we could only do so much to ensure the well-being of our baby. We enjoyed seeing our baby's heartbeat on ultrasound and feeling it move inside me. We were happy to have certain tests and technology to assist us in tracking the health of our baby.

LEARNING OUTCOMES

1. Describe the various psychologic responses to antenatal testing.
2. Identify indications and interpret findings for ultrasound examinations performed in the first trimester.
3. Describe the procedures used in the first trimester to confirm fetal viability.
4. Delineate the use of ultrasound in the second trimester to assess fetal life, number, presentation, anatomy, age, and growth.
5. Identify the indications and procedures for fetal movement awareness, the nonstress test, and vibroacoustic stimulation.
6. Compare the indications and procedures for contraction stress test, biophysical profile, and amniotic fluid index.
7. Explain the purpose of sequential and contingent testing and quadruple testing and the implications of abnormal values.
8. Contrast the use of amniocentesis and chorionic villus sampling in detecting a fetus with a chromosomal disorder.
9. Discuss fetal fibronectin and transvaginal measurement of cervical length as predictors of preterm labor.
10. Discuss how the lecithin/sphingomyelin ratio of the amniotic fluid and phosphatidylglycerol (PG) can be used to assess fetal lung maturity.

KEY TERMS

Alpha-fetoprotein (AFP) *518*
Amniocentesis *519*
Amniotic fluid index (AFI) *505*
Beta human chorionic gonadotropin (beta hCG) *501*
Biophysical profile (BPP) *514*
Birth defects *518*
Cervical funneling *500*
Chorionic villus sampling (CVS) *522*
Contraction stress test (CST) *511*
Cordocentesis *524*
Fetal fibronectin (fFN) *524*
Intrauterine growth restriction (IUGR) *517*
Late decelerations *513*
Lecithin/sphingomyelin (L/S) ratio *525*
Macrosomia *517*
Maternal serum alpha-fetoprotein (MSAFP) *518*
Nonstress test (NST) *508*
Nuchal folds *503*
Nuchal translucency testing *503*
Oligohydramnios *514*
Phosphatidylglycerol (PG) *525*
Surfactant *525*
Ultrasound *498*
Viability *501*
Vibroacoustic stimulation (VAS) *510*

Every parent dreams of a perfectly healthy baby and indeed the vast majority of babies are born healthy. However, maternal conditions, genetics, and environmental influences continue to adversely affect a small percentage of babies. Although the antenatal fetal assessment techniques discussed in this chapter are designed to maximize the chances of identifying a fetus at risk, a perfect pregnancy outcome can never be predicted or guaranteed.

Although the United States spends a greater percentage of its gross national product on health care than any other country, it continues to have a higher infant mortality rate than many other industrialized countries (American Public Health Association, 2009). Reproductive technologies significantly raise the cost of health care. These technologic advances are not without risks; therefore, prevention of perinatal morbidity must always be a primary goal. The decision to use the tests discussed in this chapter is made by the childbearing family only after a careful analysis of their risks and costs compared with their possible benefit to the mother or her fetus. The nurse communicates the value of various antenatal testing options in relationship to the patient's gestational age. In addition, limitations of the testing options should be discussed.

Psychologic Reactions to Antenatal Testing

Little has been written about the psychologic impact of antenatal diagnostic testing on childbearing families; however, several studies indicate that the need for testing usually provokes fear (Harpel, 2008). Nurses often play a key role not only in teaching families about various testing options, but also in providing clarity and emotional support to the woman and her family undergoing antenatal testing. To decrease anxiety and alleviate fear for the woman and her family, the nurse provides clear, concise explanations of possible results from testing and management options after the testing has been completed. See Table 21-1 for sample nursing approaches to pretest teaching. Although the family may approach antenatal testing with a great deal of anxiety, normal results may reassure parents; however, distress may persist with false-positive screening results, equivocal results, and positive results that indicate additional testing needs.

Some tests, such as ultrasound, have become almost routine, and many couples view this antepartum test as an expected part of the prenatal care. However, the American College of Obstetricians and Gynecologists (ACOG), the American Institute for Ultrasound in Medicine (AIUM), and the American College of Radiology (ACR) advise against use of ultrasonography during pregnancy without an identified medical indication (ACOG, 2009; ACR, 2007; AIUM, 2008a,b). Its use in improving pregnancy outcomes is controversial. It has been found to be effective in identifying multiple gestation, fetal anomalies, placental disorders, and fetal malposition (Cunningham et al., 2010). All women should be counseled appropriately prior to undergoing any antenatal testing, including ultrasonography, in order to minimize shock and confusion with adverse findings. When more invasive testing is recommended, it may evoke fear and anxiety in the woman and her partner as they consider the reason for the test, the risk to the fetus and woman during the test, and the implications of the test results. All testing should be presented as optional and only performed when the woman so desires.

TABLE 21-1 Sample Nursing Approaches to Pretest Teaching

Assess whether the woman knows the reason the screening or diagnostic test is being offered or recommended.
Examples:
"What has your doctor/nurse-midwife told you about this test?"
"Sometimes tests are done for many different reasons. Can you tell me why you are having this test?"
"What is your understanding about what the test will show?"
Provide an opportunity for questions.
Examples:
"What questions do you have about the test?"
"What things about the test are unclear to you?"
Explain the test procedure, paying particular attention to any preparation the woman needs to do prior to the test.
Example:
"The test that has been ordered for you is designed to . . . " (Add specific information about the particular test. Give the explanation in simple language.)
Validate the woman's understanding of the preparation.
Example:
"Tell me what you will have to do to get ready for this test."
Give permission for the woman to continue to ask questions if needed.
Example:
"I'll be with you during the test. If you have any questions at any time, please don't hesitate to ask."

NURSING CARE MANAGEMENT

Nurses in a variety of settings have an opportunity to provide care to families undergoing antenatal testing. Antenatal assessment tests are performed by perinatal nurse practitioners and/or nurses who have received additional specialized perinatal education and practice. The nurse, whatever the role, is a vital link between the woman and the physician or certified nurse-midwife. Nurses also need to provide easy to understand information to the mother and family. The nurse should encourage the family to ask questions, voice concerns and fears, and become actively involved in the antenatal testing process. Nurses are often responsible for the follow-up care that is needed as a result of test findings, such as arranging for additional testing and interpreting results. Nurses also need to answer questions the family or woman may have and provide emotional support.

Nursing Assessment and Diagnosis

Nursing assessment begins with a history of the present prenatal course and identifying possible indications for a particular diagnostic test. Examples may include identifying possible testing related to advanced maternal age, previous history of a child with a birth defect, or the presence of a particular maternal medical condition. The nurse assesses the woman and her partner's knowledge about the reason the test is being offered or advised, the information that the woman and her support person have about the test, their questions and concerns, and the presence of any psychosociocultural factors that may influence the teaching or learning process. During the test and afterward, the nurse completes needed assessments to monitor the status of the woman and her fetus.

The primary nursing diagnoses are directed toward providing information about the screening or diagnostic test and minimizing any risks to the woman and her unborn child. Examples of nursing diagnoses that may be applicable include:

- ***Health-Seeking Behavior: Health Education*** related to fetal assessment testing due to an expressed desire to understand its purpose, benefits, risks, and alternatives
- ***Fear*** related to the risks of a specific test or possible unfavorable test results
- ***Risk for Impaired Attachment*** because of high-risk label attached to the pregnancy
- ***Anxiety*** related to the potential outcomes or unfavorable test results

Ultrasound in Obstetrics

Nursing Plan and Implementation

The nursing plan of care is directed toward each specific nursing diagnosis. The nurse generally plays a vital role in providing needed and desired information about the screening or diagnostic test. The nurse also functions as an advocate for the expectant woman by helping her clarify question areas and obtain needed information. The nurse frequently knows the areas of greatest concern for women and can anticipate many of their fears. When the woman is not able to verbalize questions, the nurse can assist by providing information that answers questions that other women have had. For example, many women undergoing an amniocentesis fear pain during the procedure. The nurse can inform the woman that she will feel pressure during the insertion of the needle and may feel subsequent cramping, which can last for several hours. The nurse can provide information about the procedure itself and follow-up monitoring to evaluate fetal well-being.

It is important for the nurse to realize that women react differently to pregnancy and testing. The nurse's role is to remain nonjudgmental and to offer support when needed. Establishing a trusting relationship increases the possibility that a woman will talk to the nurse and share her concerns and emotional needs. The nurse is often the one to coordinate services the woman may need, such as community resources for financial, psychologic, or social support.

Nurses working in community clinics have an integral role in performing fetal surveillance tests throughout the antepartum period. Nurses may find themselves not only performing some of these tests, such as nonstress tests, but also performing comprehensive assessments of the woman's health, her family dynamics, and her living situation. Community health nurses often have a more accurate understanding of the woman's physical resources, such as the adequacy of living conditions, proximity to healthcare resources, and availability of public transportation. It is often the nurse who has the most contact with the pregnant woman. Because of this, the nurse is in an excellent position to provide anticipatory guidance, reiterate teaching provided by the woman's healthcare provider, and monitor her current plan of care. The nurse should approach each encounter with calmness, compassion, and honesty.

Evaluation

The nurse evaluates the woman and her family's understanding of antepartum testing procedures. Determining if the family understands the indication for follow-up testing is imperative. The nurse should also assess whether the teaching methods used are effective for that family. Evaluation should include both physical and psychologic factors. In addition, the nurse determines if adequate resources, such as social support and physical resources, are available for the pregnant woman. Women from different cultures may need additional support because they may encounter language and other cultural barriers.

Ultrasound

Ultrasound has become one of the most commonly used diagnostic and screening tools in pregnancy (Cunningham et al., 2010). For the last 20 years, it has played a critical role in the practice of obstetrics. Because ultrasound is used widely to assess fetal well-being in all 3 trimesters, it also is discussed within this framework later in the chapter.

Ultrasound is a diagnostic procedure that uses high-frequency sound waves exceeding 20,000 cycles per second, greater than what the human ear can hear, to produce an image that varies based on the density of the structure under the transducer. The reflected energy creates a small electrical voltage that is displayed on the screen. Very dense components, such as bone, appear white on the screen, whereas soft tissues appear gray and fluid appears black (Cunningham et al., 2010). Instruments used in ultrasonography operate at 2 to 10 megahertz (MHz). The higher the frequency of the sound, the shallower the depth of penetration but the better the resolution of the image produced. Ultrasound uses a device called a *transducer* to turn the sound waves into electrical signals. Transducers can be used either transabdominally (Figure 21-1 ■), operating at 3 to 5 MHz,

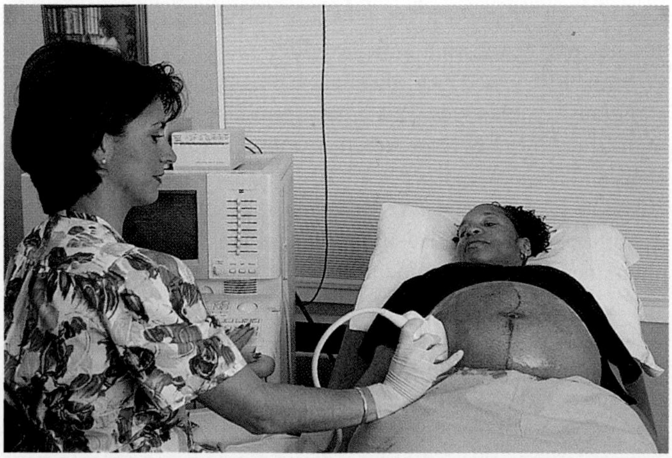

Figure 21-1 ■ Ultrasound scanning permits visualization of the fetus in utero.

Source: Photographer, Elena Dorfman.

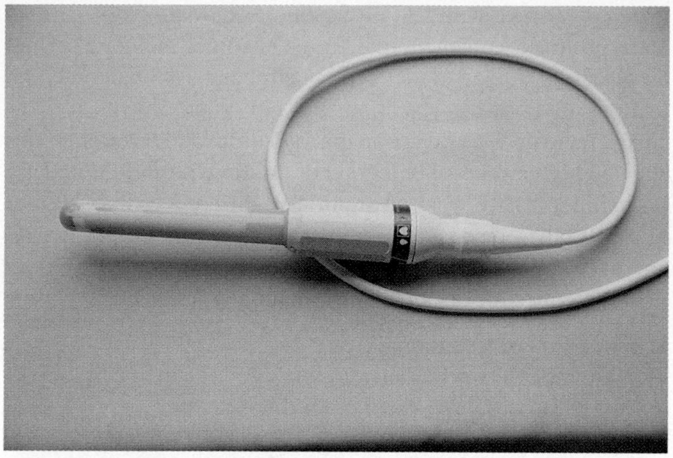

Figure 21-2 ■ Transvaginal ultrasound transducer.

Source: Photographer, Elena Dorfman.

or transvaginally (Figure 21-2 ■), operating at 5 to 10 MHz (ACOG, 2009). These transducers and their use are described fully later in the chapter.

Ultrasound can be used to produce images called *sonograms* in several different ways. In motion mode (M mode), the reflected echo generates a moving display. This is how fetal cardiac activity is seen. Brightness modulation (B mode) converts the signals into varying degrees of brightness and produces a two-dimensional image. Three-dimensional ultrasound uses algorithms to vary opacity, transparency, and depth to project an image. This allows curved structures such as the fetal face to be viewed (Figure 21-3 ■).

Extent of Ultrasound Exams

According to the American College of Obstetricians and Gynecologists (ACOG), ultrasound examinations are classified as standard or basic, limited (identifying only certain components), or specialized (sometimes referred to as detailed) (2009). A *limited ultrasound* may be used to address a specific question, or determine specific information. A limited ultrasound should not take the place of a standard ultrasound evaluation (ACOG, 2009). Following are examples of information that can be obtained by a limited ultrasound:

- Determine fetal presentation before or during labor.
- Locate the placenta.
- Confirm fetal heart activity.
- Estimate amniotic fluid volume.
- Diagnose multiple gestation.
- Evaluate interval growth.
- Evaluate the cervix.
- Guide amniocentesis.

A *standard ultrasound examination* is performed during the second or third trimester. It includes an evaluation of fetal presentation, fetal number, amniotic fluid volume, placental position, cardiac activity, fetal biometry, and anatomic survey. A standard ultrasound should also attempt to evaluate the maternal cervix and the uterus and ovaries when feasible. A specialized, or detailed, examination is performed when an anomaly is suspected, and the components of the exam are determined by the expert conducting the examination. These components may include fetal Doppler, biophysical profile, fetal echocardiogram, amniotic fluid assessment, or additional biometric studies (ACOG, 2009).

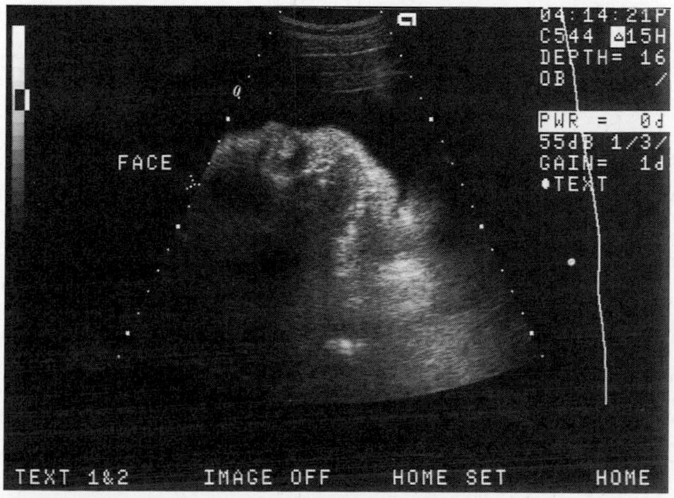

Figure 21-3 ■ Ultrasound of the fetal face.

Methods of Ultrasound Scanning

The two most common methods of ultrasound scanning are *transabdominal* and *transvaginal* scanning.

Transabdominal Ultrasound

In the transabdominal approach, a transducer is moved across the abdomen (see Figure 21-1). The woman is usually scanned with a full bladder, except when ultrasound is used to localize the placenta before amniocentesis. When the bladder is full, the examiner can assess other structures, especially the vagina and cervix, in relation to the bladder. This is particularly important when vaginal bleeding is noted and placenta previa is the suspected cause. It can also determine if vaginal bleeding is being caused by premature dilatation of the cervix. The woman is advised to drink 1 to 1.5 quarts of water approximately 2 hours before the examination, and she is asked to refrain from emptying her bladder. If the bladder is not sufficiently filled, she is asked to drink 3 to 4 (8 oz) glasses of water and is rescanned 30 to 45 minutes later (Hobbins, 2007).

Transmission gel is generously spread over the woman's abdomen, and the sonographer slowly moves a transducer over the abdomen to obtain a picture of the contents of the uterus. Testing takes 20 to 30 minutes. The woman may feel discomfort from pressure applied over a full bladder. In some instances, the sonographer may advise the woman to urinate a small amount to relieve the discomfort. In addition, if the woman lies on her back during the test, shortness of breath can develop. This may be relieved by elevating her upper body during the test. The woman may also develop dizziness or postural hypotension related to compression of the inferior vena cava by the uterus.

Transvaginal Ultrasound

The transvaginal (or endovaginal) method uses a probe inserted into the vagina (see Figure 21-2). Once inserted, the transvaginal probe is close to the structures being imaged and so produces a better, clearer image. The improved images obtained by transvaginal ultrasound have enabled sonographers to identify structures and fetal characteristics earlier in pregnancy (McAuliffe et al., 2005). Transvaginal ultrasound is used to assess the gestational sac, the presence or absence of a yolk sac or embryo, the crown rump length to most accurately determine gestational age, the presence of cardiac motion, and fetal number. The uterus, cervix, and adnexal structures are also examined and recorded. Transvaginal ultrasound can most accurately identify shortened cervical length and **cervical funneling** (a cone-shaped indentation in the cervical os), indicating cervical incompetence or risk of preterm labor (ACOG, 2009).

After the procedure is fully explained to the woman, she is prepared in the same manner as for a pelvic examination: in lithotomy position, with appropriate drapes to provide privacy, and a female attendant in the room. It is important that the woman's buttocks are at the end of the table so that, once inserted, the probe can be moved in various directions. The small, lightweight vaginal transducer is covered with a specially fitted sterile sheath, a condom, or one finger of a latex or vinyl glove. Ultrasound coupling gel is then applied to the covering, making insertion into the vagina easier and providing a medium for enhancing the ultrasound image. In addition to providing a clearer image than the transabdominal method, the transvaginal procedure can be accomplished with an empty bladder. Most women do not feel discomfort during the exam. The probe is smaller than a speculum, so insertion is usually completed with ease. The woman may feel some movement of the probe during the exam as various structures are imaged. Some women may want to insert the probe themselves to enhance their comfort; others may feel embarrassed even to be asked. The certified nurse-midwife, physician, or ultrasonographer offers the choice based on the clinician's comfort level and the rapport the clinician has established with the woman.

Safety of Ultrasound

In the last 20 years, the use of ultrasound as a diagnostic tool in pregnancy has increased exponentially, and there is no evidence of physical harm to the fetus (Abramowicz, 2007; ACOG, 2009). The World Health Organization (WHO) concludes ultrasonography in pregnancy is not associated with increased risk of childhood malignancy, impaired physical or neurological development, cognitive ability, or mental disease. In fact, no adverse maternal, fetal, or neonatal outcomes have been identified (Torloni et al., 2009). The Food and Drug Administration (FDA) has stated that obstetric sonograms fall within an acceptable level of safety because they use low-intensity ultrasound, however they do not approve of nonmedical uses such as videos and pictures for "keepsakes" (AIUM, 2008a).

Is there such a category as "routine ultrasound" in pregnancy? Not necessarily, according to ACOG (2009). In large studies, researchers compared several outcomes between a group of women who had ultrasound examinations performed and a group of women who did not. Outcomes included perinatal mortality, Apgar score, birth weight, maternal outcome, detections of multiple gestation and abnormalities, as well as cost-effectiveness. The group that had ultrasound examinations showed higher rates of detection of multiple gestations and abnormalities. There were no significant differences in outcomes related to the other factors (Cunningham et al., 2010). ACOG endorses American College of Radiology (ACR) (2007) practice guidelines for obstetric ultrasound indications:

- Estimation of gestational age
- Evaluation of cervical insufficiency
- Evaluation of fetal growth or fetal well-being
- Evaluation of vaginal bleeding
- Determination of fetal presentation
- Evaluation of abdominal or pelvic pain
- Suspected multiple gestation
- Significant discrepancy between uterine size and clinical date
- Evaluation of pelvic mass or uterine abnormality
- Examination of suspected hydatidiform mole
- Adjunct to special procedures including amniocentesis, cervical cerclage placement, or external cephalic version
- Evaluation for premature rupture of membranes or premature labor
- Evaluation of suspected fetal death
- Evaluation of suspected ectopic pregnancy
- Evaluation of suspected amniotic fluid abnormalities
- Evaluation of suspected placental abruption
- Evaluation of abnormal biochemical markers
- Follow-up evaluation of fetal anomaly
- Follow-up evaluation of placental location for suspected placenta previa
- Evaluation of those with history of previous congenital anomaly
- Evaluation of fetal condition in late presentation for prenatal care
- To assess findings that may increase the risk of chromosomal abnormalities
- To screen for fetal anomalies

Who Should Perform Ultrasound Examinations?

The accuracy of ultrasound as a diagnostic tool is highly dependent on the knowledge, skills, and judgment of the person performing the exam. Licensed medical practitioners, following published standards and guidelines, perform ultrasound examinations. The practitioner's training includes indications as well as limitation of obstetrical ultrasound (ACOG, 2009). The Association of Women's Health, Obstetric and Neonatal Nurses (AWHONN) has set guidelines and nursing practice competencies for experienced maternal-newborn nurses to perform limited ultrasound exams. The guidelines indicate that the nurse must complete an educational program that includes didactic presentations and a clinical practicum (Simpson & Creehan, 2008). All ultrasound examinations and interpretations should be recorded and documented.

NURSING CARE MANAGEMENT

The nurse plays a key role in providing the mother and family with information related to the ultrasound procedure itself and expected outcomes. The nurse answers questions and helps clarify ultrasound findings. Some women, especially those who lack insurance coverage, may worry about the cost of the test itself. The nurse can discuss the rationale for obtaining an ultrasound and what will be done with the information once it is obtained. The nurse provides support for the woman and her family, recognizing that some women may feel anxious or fearful.

Assessment of Fetal Well-Being in the First Trimester

The first trimester represents a crucial time for establishing fetal viability and determining an accurate gestational age. Ultrasound can be used during the first trimester to help determine certain characteristics, including some chromosomal disorders. There are a variety of methods that the practitioner can use to determine fetal well-being in early pregnancy.

Viability

Viability, or the potential for the pregnancy to result in a live infant, is the first issue to consider in pregnancy. A positive urine pregnancy test does not confirm viability, but represents the presence of beta human chorionic gonadotropin (hCG) hormone. This hormone becomes present in the bloodstream when the developing embryo implants into the uterus at approximately 10 to 14 days after conception has occurred (Cunningham et al., 2010). Bleeding is the most common symptom causing a woman to question the viability of her pregnancy. One in four women will experience bleeding in her pregnancy; nevertheless, half of such women will continue to have viable pregnancies (Cunningham et al., 2010). Bleeding can also be associated with a nonviable pregnancy in cases of spontaneous abortion (miscarriage) or ectopic (tubal) pregnancy. Serial quantitative beta hCG testing, progesterone-level testing, and ultrasound can be used to distinguish a normally developing fetus from an ectopic pregnancy, which, if undiagnosed, carries a high rate of maternal morbidity.

Quantitative Beta hCG Testing

Beta human chorionic gonadotropin (beta hCG) is a product of the trophoblast or placenta and is a very accurate marker of the presence of pregnancy and placental health. Beta hCG is detectable in the blood serum of approximately 5% of pregnant women by 8 days after conception, and in virtually all pregnancies by 11 days. The level in the serum approximately doubles every 2 days in the first 10 days of pregnancy, peaking at 60 to 90 days after conception (Cunningham et al., 2010) (Table 21-2). In early pregnancy, two quantitative beta hCG levels drawn 48 hours apart serve as an excellent test of the viability of the pregnancy. Conversely, if the beta hCG level remains stable or falls over 48 hours, a miscarriage or ectopic pregnancy should be suspected. See chapter 20 for a discussion of beta hCG testing in ectopic pregnancy.

TABLE 21-2 Approximate Beta hCG Values in Pregnancy

GESTATIONAL AGE (WEEKS)	BETA HCG VALUES (MILLI–INTERNATIONAL UNITS/ML)
1–2	16–156
2–3	101–4870
3–4	1110–31,500
4–5	2560–82,300
5–6	23,100–151,000
6–7	27,300–233,000
7–11	20,900–291,000
11–16	6140–103,000
16–21	4720–80,100
21–39	2700–78,100

Although not routine in all pregnancies, serologic evaluation is indicated in women with a history of spontaneous abortion, ectopic pregnancy, or risk of ectopic pregnancy (intrauterine device in place, previous pelvic inflammatory disease, or reversal of a tubal sterilization). Women who are spotting should also have a beta hCG level drawn to ensure adequate levels. Many women who have conceived through assisted reproductive methods also have their beta hCG levels monitored to ensure the pregnancy is developing normally.

The 48 hours between the beta hCG tests can be an extremely anxious time for the couple. To offer effective counseling, the nurse must understand the information these tests provide, as well as their limitations. For example, the woman may not know why she must wait 48 hours for a repeat blood test. The nurse needs to allow time for the woman and her partner, if present, to express their anxiety and fears. False reassurances should not be offered. Instead, attention is directed toward helping them cope with the inherent uncertainty that occurs while the exams are being completed and until a definitive diagnosis can be made.

Progesterone Level Testing

Progesterone is secreted in early pregnancy by the corpus luteum until approximately 8 weeks' gestation at which point the placenta begins to manufacture its own progesterone. Low levels of progesterone are associated with spontaneous abortions and ectopic pregnancies (Cunningham et al., 2010). Although progesterone levels are not routinely tested in early pregnancy, they can be assessed by performing a simple blood test when there is a history of spontaneous abortions or spotting in early pregnancy. Progesterone levels above 25 ng/ml are typically associated with normally developing intrauterine pregnancies. Progesterone levels that are below 5 ng/ml typically indicate a nonviable fetus. Levels between 5 ng/ml and 25 ng/ml are inconclusive. Approximately 10% of women have progesterone levels below 25 ng/ml (Cunningham et al., 2010). The nurse notifies the physician or certified nurse-midwife if levels are low. The physician or certified nurse-midwife, in conjunction with the woman's desires, bases the decision of whether or not to supplement progesterone during early pregnancy on current progesterone levels, past history of spontaneous abortions, and/or presence of spotting or vaginal bleeding. However, supplementing with progesterone also has the potential of prolonging an inevitable nonviable pregnancy. Low progesterone levels can be treated by giving the woman progesterone either orally or via vaginal suppositories. This supplementation is warranted throughout the first trimester. After 12 gestational weeks, supplements are not needed because the placenta will make adequate progesterone levels (Cunningham et al., 2010).

Ultrasound

The sonographic landmarks (presence of gestational sac, cardiac motion, embryo development) of normal early pregnancy, detected by transvaginal ultrasound, are very predictable. Up to about 4 1/2 to 5 weeks of gestation, before the appearance of a gestational sac, only the endometrial stripe can be seen in the uterus. The gestational sac at first appears empty and may be confused with the pseudogestational sac of ectopic pregnancy. A true gestational sac is associated with beta hCG levels of 1800 milli–International Units/ml if the sonogram is being done transvaginally and 6500 milli–International Units/ml if the sonogram is being done transabdominally. At approximately 5 1/2 weeks the yolk sac, a small round structure sometimes resembling a "double ring," is visible within the gestational sac. It is an embryonic structure, so its appearance provides strong evidence supporting the presence of an intrauterine pregnancy (Seungdamrong et al., 2008). At 6 to 6 1/2 weeks, the embryo itself becomes visible, and shortly thereafter cardiac activity is detectable (Creasy, Resnik, Iams, et al., 2008). During the ultrasound examination, the gestational sac and embryo (crown rump length) are measured to determine gestational age (Figure 21-4 ■).

Gestational Age

Determination of an accurate expected date of birth (EDB) early in pregnancy is essential for evaluating well-being throughout the pregnancy. Labor contractions that may be perfectly normal at 37 weeks could be a problem if they occur prior to 34 weeks. Conversely, a 40-week pregnancy inadvertently thought to be 42 weeks may result in an unnecessary and risk-laden induction of labor. Much of the physician's or midwife's efforts are aimed at determining the most accurate EDB possible. Traditional means of establishing an EDB are documenting a reliable last menstrual period (LMP) from the woman, measuring uterine size, noting the date of the first audible fetal heart tones, and noting the date of quickening (the first recognized fetal movement). A definite and normal LMP established early in pregnancy is considered the most reliable indicator of an EDB (Hoffman et al., 2008). Problems occur if the woman cannot recall her LMP, if her menstrual cycles were extremely irregular, if she was lactating, if she was using hormonal contraception, or if she had bleeding in early pregnancy.

An early transvaginal or abdominal sonogram is indicated when there is a need to establish an accurate gestational age. The crown-rump length is considered the most accurate sonographic measurement for gestational age if performed between 6 and 12 weeks' gestation. It is accurate to within plus or minus 3 to 5 days of the EDB based on the crown-rump length (Cunningham et al., 2010) (Figure 21-5 ■). This means that an ultrasound performed at 6 weeks would be accurate in predicting the EDB within either 3 to 5 days before or 3 to 5 days after the predicted EDB by LMP. Beyond 12 weeks, the fetus begins to curve and the crown-rump length loses its accuracy (Cunningham et al., 2010). For example, if an EDB based on a 10-week sonogram is September 9, it is reasonable to expect that date determined by LMP is accurate from September 4 through September 14. After the first trimester, gestational age is obtained by a combination of measurements of femur length, abdominal circumference, and biparietal diameter (Figure 21-6 ■). Gestational age by sonogram is reliable in the second trimester to plus or minus 7 to 14 days. For example, if a due date of October 1 is given by a second trimester sonogram, the reasonable date of birth can be from September 16 through October 14. Although practice may vary, most physicians and midwives do not change a due date based on the second trimester sonogram unless there is a discrepancy of greater than 11 to 14 days from the LMP. After 26 weeks, fetal growth rates are less uniform, making ultrasound an inappropriate means of determining gestational age. Specifically, during the third trimester, ultrasound can estimate an EDB with plus or minus 14 to 21 days of accuracy. See Table 21-3.

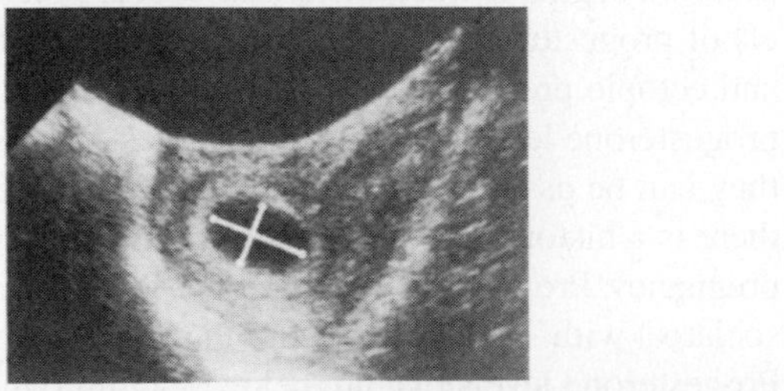

Figure 21-4 ■ Measurement of the gestational sac. The ultrasound shows the uterus; the blackened oval area is the gestational sac. The fluid in the gestational sac does not generate echoes from the ultrasound and thus appears dark in contrast to the uterine tissue surrounding it. The lines through the gestational sac represent measurements that are taken.

Source: Reprinted from Ultrasonography in obstetrics and gynecology, *2nd ed., by P. W. Cullen, p. 49. Copyright © 1998, with permission from Elsevier.*

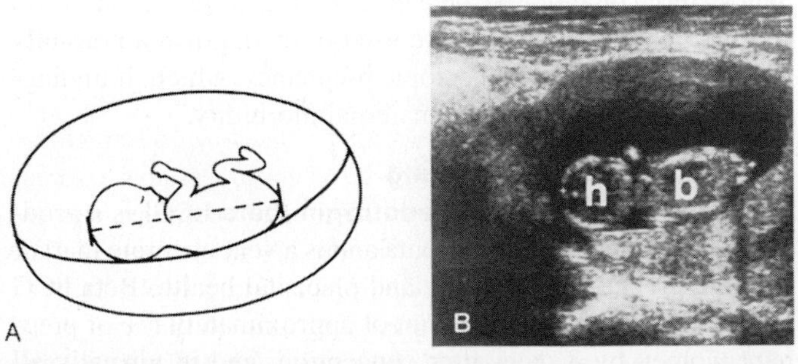

Figure 21-5 ■ Measurement of the crown-rump length. A. Schematic diagram. Dotted line shows the measurement from the top of the fetal crown (head) to the bottom of the rump (buttocks). B. Ultrasound scan of the pregnant uterus, showing the longest length of a 9-week fetus. The head (h) can be differentiated from the body (b), but the internal anatomy cannot be clearly distinguished.

Source: Reprinted from Ultrasonography in obstetrics and gynecology, *2nd ed., by P. W. Cullen, p. 50. Copyright © 1998, with permission from Elsevier.*

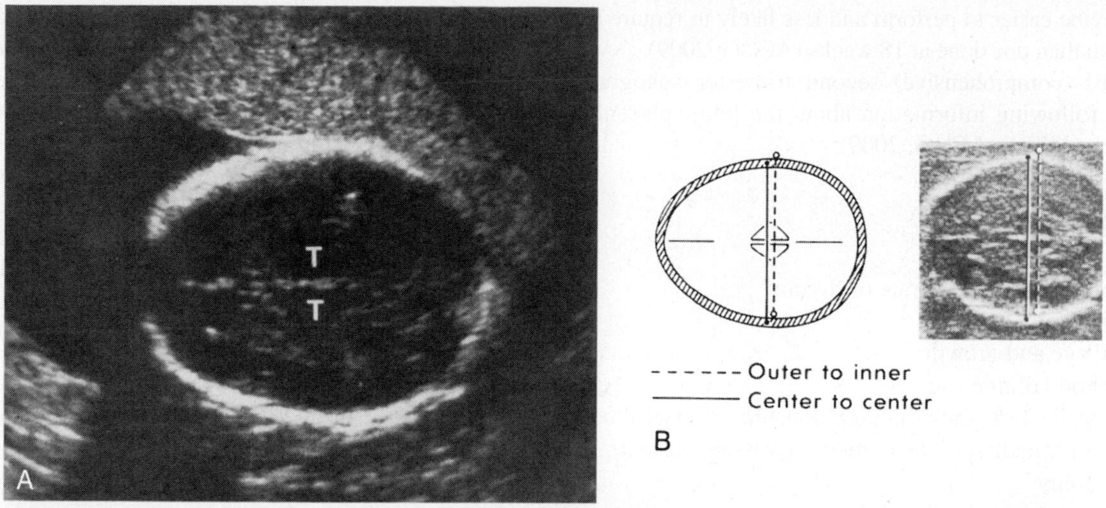

Figure 21-6 ■ Measurement of the biparietal diameter. A. Ultrasound transaxial image of the fetal head, taken with the thalami (T) imaged in the midline, equidistant from the temporoparietal tables of the calvarium. B. Diagram and image showing the leading edge (outer) to the leading edge (inner) measurements of the fetal head, taken at the level of the thalami.

Source: Reproduced with permission from Ultrasonography in obstetrics and gynecology, *2nd ed., by P. W. Cullen, p. 51. Copyright © 1998, with permission from Elsevier.*

TABLE 21-3 Parameters for Estimating Gestational Age

SOURCE OF EVIDENCE	WHEN OBTAINED	ESTIMATED ACCURACY
In vitro fertilization	At conception	Less than 1 day
Ultrasound measurement of crown-rump length	6–10 weeks	3 days
Clinical measurement of normal uterus	Less than 12 weeks	7 days
Ultrasound measurement of biparietal diameter	Less than 20 weeks	7 days
Ultrasound measurement of biparietal diameter	20–26 weeks	10 days
Ultrasound measurement of biparietal diameter	26–30 weeks	14–21 days
Ultrasound measurement of biparietal diameter	Greater than 30 weeks	21–28 days

Determining an accurate EDB early in pregnancy can be extremely important later in pregnancy if there is inadequate uterine or fetal growth. An accurate EDB based on a first trimester ultrasound can assist the physician or certified nurse-midwife in diagnosing intrauterine growth restriction (to be discussed later in this chapter).

Nuchal Translucency Testing

Nuchal translucency testing is a combination of an ultrasound and a maternal serum test that is used to screen fetuses between 11 weeks and 1 day and 13 weeks and 6 days to determine if a fetus is at risk for a chromosomal disorder, such as Down syndrome (trisomy 21), trisomy 13, and trisomy18. The ultrasound assesses the accumulation of fluid between the posterior cervical spine and the overlying skin in the fetal neck, known as **nuchal folds**. If the nuchal folds are greater than 3 mm, the incidence of Down syndrome is increased (ACOG, 2007b). The test is performed in conjunction with a maternal serum blood test in which biochemical markers PAPP-A and free beta hCG are obtained to calculate the risk of having an affected fetus. The combination of blood testing and the ultrasound screening test is 82% to 87% accurate for detecting Down syndrome (ACOG, 2007b). Because the screening is noninvasive, there are no maternal or fetal risks. If an abnormal test result is obtained, the mother is referred for diagnostic testing, such as a chorionic villus sampling (CVS) or amniocentesis. During nuchal translucency testing, the presence or absence of a nasal bone may be examined because three European studies have found the absence of the fetal nasal bone in 66.7% to 80% of Down syndrome fetuses. However, a study in the United States found this to be less accurate because of ethnic variations within the population (ACOG, 2007a).

Assessment of Fetal Well-Being in the Second Trimester

The second trimester is considered by many to be the most advantageous time for basic obstetric ultrasound for several reasons. First, the relative uniformity of fetal growth during the first 20 weeks allows biometric measurements that continue to provide an accurate estimation of gestational age. Second, the large volume of amniotic fluid relative to the fetal size allows for excellent images of fetal anatomy. Finally, fetal anatomy can be visualized in extreme detail, allowing confirmation of normal anatomy. The ideal time for the second trimester basic sonogram is 18 to 24 weeks. There is some evidence that sonograms done at 20 to

22 weeks may be easier to perform and less likely to require an additional scan than one done at 18 weeks (ACOG, 2009).

A standard (comprehensive) second trimester sonogram provides the following information about the fetus, placenta, and uterine conditions (ACOG, 2009):

- Fetal life
- Fetal number
- Fetal presentation
- Presence of abnormal heart rate or rhythm
- Evaluation of fetal anatomy
- Gestational age and growth
- Amniotic fluid volume
- Placental localization, including relationship to cervical os
- Umbilical cord, including the number of vessels present
- Uterine anatomy

In addition, multiple gestations should be assessed for chorionicity, amnionicity, comparison of fetal sizes, the amount of amniotic fluid on each side of the membrane, and fetal genitalia if visible (ACOG, 2009).

Fetal Life

Presence of cardiac motion confirms fetal life. If gestational age has already been established and fetal heart tones have been visualized with an ultrasound or heard with a Doppler in the first trimester, then absence of cardiac motion in the second trimester is consistent with fetal demise.

Fetal Number

The second trimester is an ideal time to identify multiple gestation or the number of fetuses in the uterus. The number of placentas and their location can also be noted at this point.

Fetal Presentation

Although an ultrasound in the second trimester can determine whether a fetus is in the breech, transverse, or vertex position, the large amount of amniotic fluid relative to the fetal size along with the lack of fetal engagement makes it highly likely that the noted presentation will change repeatedly before birth (Cunningham et al., 2010). Fetal presentation is commonly documented on a second trimester ultrasound, but it is not usually of any clinical significance.

Fetal Anatomy Survey

A systematic examination of the fetal parts is conducted to identify possible abnormalities. Components of this examination include the fetal parts discussed in the following sections.

Head

The skull should be symmetrical with the cranium ossified and intact. The ventricular system (passageways within the brain) is evaluated. The choroids should appear symmetrical. The choroid plexuses are found within the ventricles of the brain and in the subarachnoid space around the brain and spinal cord. They produce cerebral spinal fluid. Choroid cysts, if noted, are usually benign but have been associated with chromosomal abnormalities in 1% of fetuses (Creasy et al., 2008). The nuchal fold thickness should be measured because thickening of the nuchal fold, the skin at the base of the fetal skull, has also been associated with certain chromosomal abnormalities.

The most dramatic abnormality diagnosed by ultrasound is anencephaly (a neural tube defect in which a portion of the fetal brain is missing). It is abnormal not to see the bony structures of the skull above the orbits of the eye after 14 weeks' gestation. The skull is brightly echogenic (appearing white because of its increased density) and is easily visualized. Failure to see the skull should alert the experienced examiner to the possibility of anencephaly (Cunningham et al., 2010).

Spine

The spine is examined both sagittally and coronally for the presence of a sac or an outward splaying of the vertebrae laminae. Either of these conditions may suggest a possible spinal cord defect such as spina bifida.

Thorax and Heart

A transverse plane of the fetal thorax provides valuable information about the size, shape, and symmetry of the chest. The size, location, and axis of the heart are also evaluated. A four-chambered view of the heart should demonstrate ventricles and atria of approximately equal size and an intact intraventricular septum. The heart occupies one quarter to one third of the chest cavity on transverse image. The lungs should have a homogenous appearance. The diaphragm should be imaged. Chest size is correlated with lung size.

Abdomen

The bladder, stomach, and kidneys should all be visualized. The fetal stomach and bladder can be seen on ultrasound by 14 weeks. Persistent failure to visualize the fetal stomach can be due to various fetal abnormalities, the most common being esophageal atresia. Mild dilation of the renal pelvis of less than 10 mm is rarely progressive and usually physiologic (Creasy et al., 2008). The abdominal wall should be visualized to be intact. A transverse image of the umbilical cord should reveal a three-vessel cord. Insertion site of the umbilical cord is also carefully inspected.

Extremities

The femur is the only bone routinely measured on the basic ultrasound. If the length seems abnormal, a more comprehensive exam is performed to compare it with the lengths of the other long bones. The upper extremities and the presence of hands and feet are also documented.

Gestational Age and Growth

The Hadlock method uses an average of measures of the biparietal diameter, head circumference, abdominal circumference, and femur length to estimate gestational age (Figures 21-7 to 21-10 ■). Comparison of measures made at intervals to standardized measures can be used to estimate fetal growth (Creasy et al., 2008).

Amniotic Fluid Volume

Amniotic fluid volume changes with gestational age. In general, a subjective assessment of amniotic fluid volume as

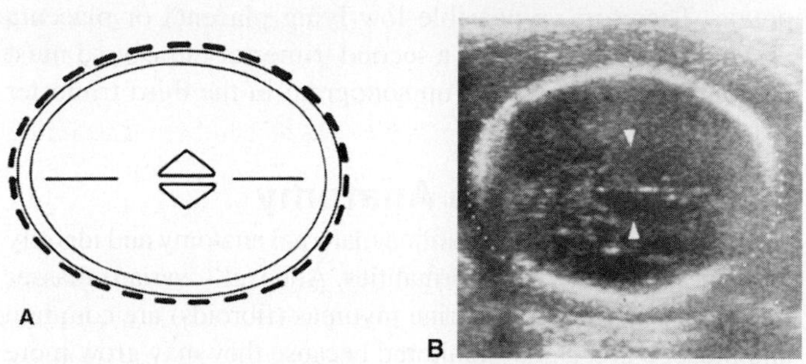

Figure 21-7 ■ Measurement of the head circumference. A. Diagram showing a dotted line outlining the head, which indicates the correct place to make a circumference measurement. B. Ultrasound transaxial scan showing the thalami (arrowheads), positioned in midline. A dotted line created by the digitizer outlines the correct parameter, just outside of the hyperechoic calvarium to obtain a circumference measurement.

Source: Reproduced with permission from Ultrasonography in obstetrics and gynecology, *2nd ed., by P. W. Cullen, p. 55. Copyright © 1998, with permission from Elsevier.*

decreased, normal, or increased is adequate during the second trimester examination. However, the **amniotic fluid index (AFI)** is another method of reporting fluid volume (Cunningham et al., 2010). The AFI is calculated by dividing the maternal abdomen into four quadrants with the umbilicus as the reference point. The deepest vertical pocket of fluid in each quadrant is then measured, and these four measurements are summed to calculate the AFI.

Placenta Location

The placenta's appearance, location, and relationship to the cervical os should be evaluated to assess for the possible complication of a placenta previa. Placental positions that are noted by sonogram in early pregnancy may not correlate well with the location at the time of birth. Factors such as the woman's position during the assessment or overdistention of the bladder may give a false-positive diagnosis of placenta

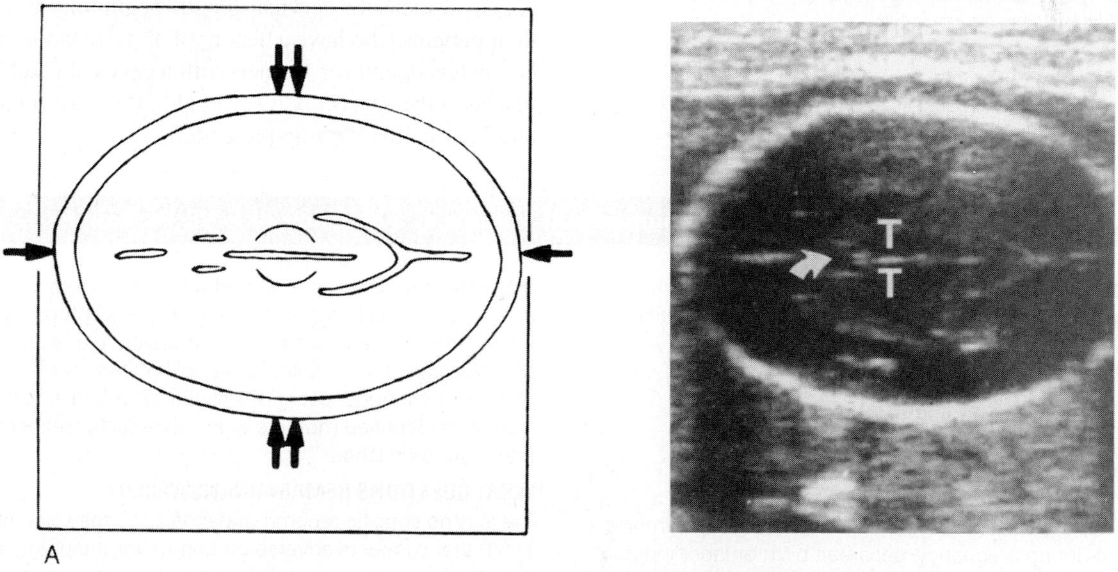

Figure 21-8 ■ Measurement of the cephalic index. A. The biparietal diameter (double arrows) and fronto-occipital diameter (single arrows) are both taken outer edge to outer edge. A ratio of the two gives the cephalic index. B. Ultrasound transaxial scan of the fetal head of the thalami (T) and cavum septi pellucidi (curved arrow).

Source: Reprinted from Ultrasonography in obstetrics and gynecology, *2nd ed., by P. W. Cullen, p. 53. Copyright © 1998, with permission from Elsevier.*

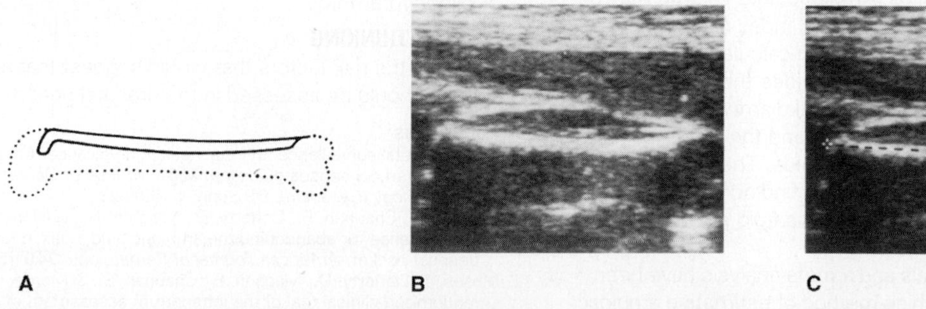

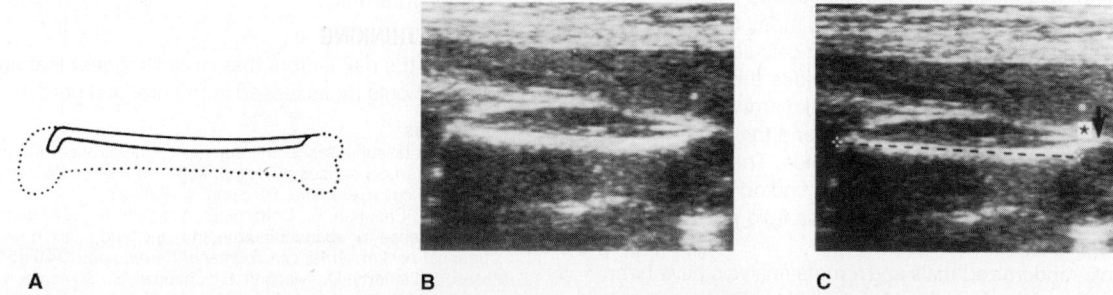

Figure 21-9 ■ Measurement of the femur length. A. Schematic diagram. B. Ultrasound image. The hyperechoic line is in the ossified lateral margin of the femoral diaphysis. The ends of the bone are the epiphyseal cartilages that have not yet calcified and are therefore hypoechoic. C. The hyperechoic diaphysis is measured from one end to the other, denoted by the cursors and a dotted line. The "distal femoral point" (* and arrow) is a nonossified extension of the distal epiphyseal cartilage. It should be included in the measurement.

Source: Reprinted from Ultrasonography in obstetrics and gynecology, *2nd ed., by P. W. Cullen, p. 58. Copyright © 1998, with permission from Elsevier.*

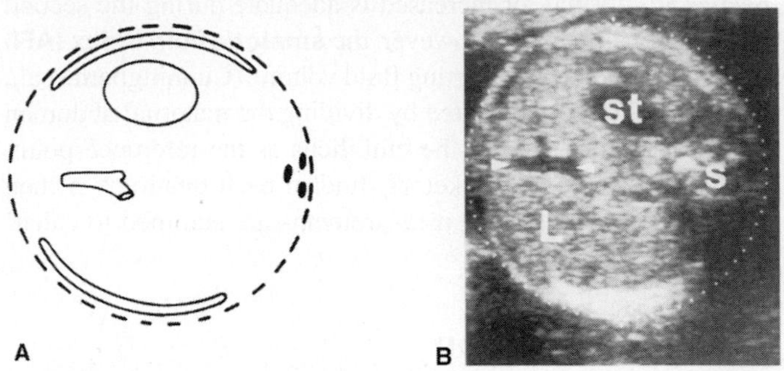

Figure 21-10 ■ Measurement of the abdominal circumference. A. Diagram showing the abdominal circumference as a dotted line traced at the outer margin of the abdomen. B. Ultrasound transaxial image showing the umbilical portion of the left portal vein (arrowheads) correctly positioned within the liver and equidistant from the lateral walls. (S, spine; L, liver; ST, stomach.) A dotted line, created by a digitizer, outlines the outer margins of the abdomen, the correct place to obtain an abdominal circumference measurement.

Source: Reprinted from Ultrasonography in obstetrics and gynecology, *2nd ed., by P. W. Cullen, p. 57. Copyright © 1998, with permission from Elsevier.*

previa. Therefore, a possible low-lying placenta or placenta previa that is identified on a second trimester ultrasound must be confirmed by a follow-up sonogram in the third trimester (Creasy et al., 2008).

Survey of Uterine Anatomy

The uterus is assessed to examine maternal anatomy and identify any uterine defects or abnormalities. Adnexal (ovarian) masses or cysts may be noted. Uterine myomas (fibroids) are common and must be noted and monitored because they may grow more quickly in pregnancy, affecting the growth and well-being of the fetus or causing overdistention of the uterus, leading to preterm labor or birth (Cunningham et al., 2010). Ultrasound may also be used to measure both cervical length and dilatation of the internal cervical os. A shortened cervix and a dilated internal os noted by ultrasound have been used to predict preterm birth. However, false-positive results using this technique may be common since the degree of effacement or dilatation may be inaccurate. Some obstetricians will schedule weekly transvaginal ultrasound to measure cervical length beginning at 20 weeks for their patients who have a history of preterm labor or cervical incompetence, and for women with a cervical cerclage (a suture placed in the cervix) (Creasy et al., 2008) (see chapter 26 ∞ and Figure 26-1 ∞ on page 663).

RESEARCH EVIDENCE IN PRACTICE Assessing Amniotic Fluid Volume as a Measure of Fetal Well-Being

CLINICAL QUESTION

What intrapartum estimate of amniotic fluid volume identifies a pregnancy that is at risk for an adverse outcome?

RESEARCH EVIDENCE

Amniotic fluid supports and protects the fetus during development. A decreased amount of amniotic fluid (oligohydramnios) can occur for a variety of reasons, including fetal abnormalities, intrauterine growth problems, preeclampsia, or postterm pregnancy. When oligohydramnios is diagnosed during pregnancy, cesarean birth or labor induction may be recommended to prevent adverse pregnancy outcomes. The estimation of amniotic fluid volume, then, becomes an important diagnostic test during late pregnancy.

The American College of Obstetricians and Gynecologists (ACOG) recommends an ultrasound with evaluation of amniotic fluid volume when there is any suspicion of fetal growth restriction or oligohydramnios. Amniotic fluid volume may be assessed using either an amniotic fluid index (AFI) or a measure of an amniotic fluid pocket. In calculating the amniotic fluid index, the ultrasound operator divides the uterine cavity into four quadrants. The largest vertical diameter of a fluid pocket is measured in each quadrant, and the four measures are summed to provide a single AFI value. The single deepest vertical pocket (SDVP) is measured by finding the length, width, and depth of the largest amniotic fluid pocket in the uterus, regardless of its quadrant.

Multiple randomized trials and a meta-analysis have been conducted to determine which method of estimating amniotic fluid volume is associated with the best outcomes. More than 4000 women were included in these studies and reviews.

Both measures are effective in identifying oligohydramnios, although the AFI was more sensitive than the SDVP. While AFI may appear to be a superior method for this reason, it resulted in more cesarean births and labor inductions without significant improvement in fetal outcomes (admission to a neonatal intensive care unit; umbilical artery pH of less than 7.1; presence of meconium; Apgar score of less than 7 at 5 minutes). Neither technique identified mothers who subsequently experienced fetal distress in labor.

WHAT QUESTIONS REMAIN UNANSWERED?

There is no specific recommendation as to the value of the SDVP that suggests adverse outcomes for the pregnancy. A threshold has yet to be developed that is associated with a reduction in adverse perinatal outcomes.

WHAT IS BEST PRACTICE?

An estimate of amniotic fluid volume using the single deepest vertical pocket technique is an effective diagnostic tool for mothers at risk of intrauterine growth restriction or oligohydramnios.

CRITICAL THINKING

What are the risk factors that would suggest that amniotic fluid volume should be assessed in the prenatal period?

References

Antenatal fetal surveillance. In Fetal health surveillance: Antepartum and intrapartum consensus guideline. 2007. *Journal of Obstetrics & Gynaecology (Canadian), 9*(9 Suppl 4), S9–S23.

Magann, E., Chauhan, P., Doherty, D., Magann, M., & Morrison, J. (2007). The evidence for abandoning the amniotic fluid index in favor of the single deepest pocket. *American Journal of Pernatology, 24*(9), 549–555.

Moses, J., Doherty, D., Magann, E., Chauhan, S., & Morrison, J. (2004). A randomized clinical trial of the intrapartum assessment of amniotic fluid volume: Amniotic fluid index versus the single deepest pocket technique. *American Journal of Obstetrics and Gynecology, 190*(6), 1564–1569.

Nabhan, A., & Abdelmoula, Y. (2009). Amniotic fluid index versus single deepest vertical pocket: A meta-analysis of randomized controlled trials. *International Journal of Gynaecology and Obstetrics, 104*(3), 184–188.

Assessment of Fetal Well-Being in the Third Trimester

Various maternal and prenatal conditions warrant antenatal testing during the third trimester. The type of testing performed is determined by the specific condition and the choice of the physician or certified nurse-midwife.

Conditions Warranting Fetal Surveillance

There are several indications for surveillance of fetal well-being in the third trimester. The following maternal and prenatal conditions require regular assessment (Cunningham et al., 2010):

Maternal Conditions

- Hypertensive disorders
- Type 1 diabetes mellitus
- Chronic renal disease
- Cyanotic heart disease
- Systemic lupus erythematosus
- Hyperthyroidism (poorly controlled)
- Antiphospholipid syndrome
- Hemoglobinopathies

Prenatal Conditions

- Preeclampsia
- Decreased fetal movement
- Oligohydramnios
- Hydramnios
- Intrauterine growth restriction
- Postterm pregnancy
- Isoimmunization (moderate to severe)
- Previous fetal demise
- Multiple gestation
- Known fetal anomaly
- Abnormal biochemical test results

Fetal Movement Assessment

Fetal movement assessment is considered an acceptable, noninvasive, cost-effective method of fetal surveillance in both high- and low-risk pregnancies. Monitoring fetal movement serves as an indirect measure of fetal central nervous system integrity and function. The coordination of whole-body movement in the fetus requires complex neurologic control. For this reason, clinicians generally agree that vigorous fetal movement provides reassurance of fetal well-being and oxygenation. A reduction in activity is often associated with complications of chronic rather than acute nonreassuring fetal status as the compromised fetus decreases its oxygen requirements by reducing activity. Documented cessation of activity warns of the possibility of preterm birth, asphyxia, intrauterine growth restriction, and fetal death (Flenady et al., 2009). It is these observations that provide the rationale for utilizing fetal movement counting as a means of antepartum fetal surveillance.

There is considerable variation in fetal movement that depends on the individual and the gestational age of the fetus. Fetal movement first begins to occur as early as 7 weeks, although the movements are too fine to be perceived until approximately 16 weeks for a multiparous woman and up to 20 weeks for those who are primiparous. Muscle tone is limited before 28 weeks (Blackburn, 2007). Certain substances such as tobacco smoke, drugs, alcohol, and caffeine have been shown to affect fetal movements. Altered fetal movements will usually reverse after drug clearance. There have been conflicting reports on whether carbohydrate intake increases fetal movement. Some studies suggest a decrease in fetal movements with maternal fasting (Cunningham et al., 2010).

Several methods are used to assess fetal movement perceived by the pregnant woman. The woman should be clearly instructed regarding the specific technique used and the importance of recognizing decreased fetal activity. Instruction is usually started at 28 weeks' gestation. Fetal movements peak at 26 to 32 weeks and then start to decrease because of the constraints of the uterine environment (Blackburn, 2007). Continued encouragement, education, and support by nurses within the office of the physician, midwife, or community clinic is important. The expectant woman should also be instructed to call the office if at any time she is concerned about a decrease in fetal movement from the fetus's usual daily pattern. The procedure for fetal movement assessment is discussed in chapter 16 ∞.

Pregnant women need to understand that fetal movements are significant and that they change during pregnancy, both in number and strength. The expectant woman should be reassured that there are fetal rest-sleep cycles during which minimal or no movement may occur for up to 40 minutes. After 28 weeks, if less than the expected movements are perceived by the pregnant woman, further fetal surveillance tests, such as the nonstress test, may be used to assess fetal well-being. See Patient Teaching: What to Tell the Pregnant Woman About Assessing Fetal Activity in chapter 16 ∞.

> "In 1981, I visited the First International Peace Hospital in Shanghai. At the prenatal clinic, the mothers and fathers were given a jar that contained many small black stones. The couple was instructed to complete a fetal movement count each day by starting at a similar time and then placing a stone in the jar each time they felt the baby move. Toward the end of the pregnancy, the father was encouraged to place his hand on the expectant mother's abdomen and feel the movements. Then he was responsible for placing the stones in the jar. The mothers and fathers seemed so proud when they brought their recording of the movements back to the clinic for review.
>
> Since that visit, I have often wondered what it would have been like to hold my newborn in my arms and look at the jar of stones. A simple jar but so special."
>
> —*Sally*

Nonstress Test

The **nonstress test (NST)** has become a widely accepted method of evaluating fetal status. (See Procedure 21-1.) This test involves using an external electronic fetal monitor to obtain a tracing of the fetal heart rate (FHR) and observation of acceleration of the FHR with fetal movement. The test is based on the knowledge that the fetus is normally active throughout pregnancy and that fetal activity will result in acceleration of the FHR when the normal fetus moves. Accelerations of the FHR imply an intact central and autonomic nervous system that is not being affected by intrauterine hypoxia. FHR acceleration in response to fetal movement is, therefore, an accepted sign of fetal health. It must be noted, however, that a nonreactive NST is not diagnostic of fetal compromise. In other words, failure to provide evidence of fetal health does not indicate that the fetus is in trouble.

The advantages of the NST are that it is relatively quick, inexpensive, and easy to interpret; it can be done in an outpatient setting and there are no known side effects. The disadvantages are that it is sometimes difficult to obtain a suitable tracing because the woman has to recline and be relatively still for 20 to 30 minutes, and the fetus may be in a sleep cycle at the time the test is performed, resulting in a nonreactive test result or need for extended monitoring (Cunningham et al., 2010).

Fetal age must be considered in the use and evaluation of NSTs. The central nervous system (parasympathetic and sym-

PROCEDURE 21-1 Performing a Nonstress Test (NST)

NURSING ACTION

Preparation

- Explain the procedure, the information it provides, and the process for completing the test.
- Ask the woman if she has recently eaten or smoked cigarettes.

  Rationale: *The test should be performed after the woman has eaten. Cigarette smoking can adversely affect the test results, so the woman should be counseled to avoid smoking prior to testing.*
- Ask the woman to void.

  Rationale: *The procedure will take at least 20 minutes to complete and the woman will need to remain in semi-Fowler's or a side-lying position and will be unable to void without interrupting the testing procedure.*

Equipment and Supplies

External fetal monitor with a monitoring strip

Blood pressure cuff

Procedure

1. Place the woman in a semi-Fowler's position with a small pillow or towel placed under her right hip after she has voided.
2. Place the ultrasound transducer from the external fetal monitor on the woman's abdomen over the FHR (typically over the fetal back or chest) so a tracing can be obtained on the monitoring strip.
3. If the FHR is not consistently recorded on the monitoring strip, adjust the ultrasound transducer until an adequate reading is obtained.

   Rationale: *Fetal or maternal movement can cause an inconsistency in the FHR on the monitoring strip. Multiple adjustments may be needed to obtain consistency in recording the FHR.*
4. Place the tocodynamometer (pressure transducer) on the woman's abdomen over the uterine fundus.

   Rationale: *Contractions are best detected when the device is directly placed on the uterine fundus.*
5. Obtain baseline measurements, including blood pressure, fetal activity, variations in the FHR during fetal movement, and contractions, for 20 minutes.

   Rationale: *Baseline measurements provide a reference for normal maternal and fetal assessment parameters.*
6. Perform the test for 20 minutes but it may be extended up to 40 minutes.

   Rationale: *Testing may be extended for the additional 20 minutes if the fetus is in a sleep cycle.*
7. Give the woman a handheld marker to indicate when she feels fetal movement.

   Rationale: *Fetal movement is accompanied by an increase in the FHR in the healthy fetus. Lack of FHR accelerations may be an indication of uteroplacental perfusion problems.*
8. Interpret the results as reactive or nonreactive.

   Rationale: *A reactive NST has two or more fetal heart accelerations within a 20-minute period. The FHR acceleration must be at least 15 beats per minute above baseline for at least 15 seconds from baseline to baseline. A nonreactive NST is one that lacks sufficient FHR accelerations over a 40-minute period (Cunningham et al., 2010).*
9. Explain the results to the woman and relate information from the healthcare provider regarding further management needs or additional follow-up that is needed.

   Rationale: *The nurse is the key communicator in providing information regarding the test results and their meaning to the woman.*

Documentation

Document baseline maternal and fetal assessment information that was obtained before and during the test. The results of the test should be documented along with information regarding how the information was reported to the healthcare provider. The specific name of the healthcare provider and date and time should be recorded. Any additional orders and instructions to the client should be documented. Verbalization of understanding of the test results by the woman should be documented along with her understanding of follow-up instructions and future appointments.

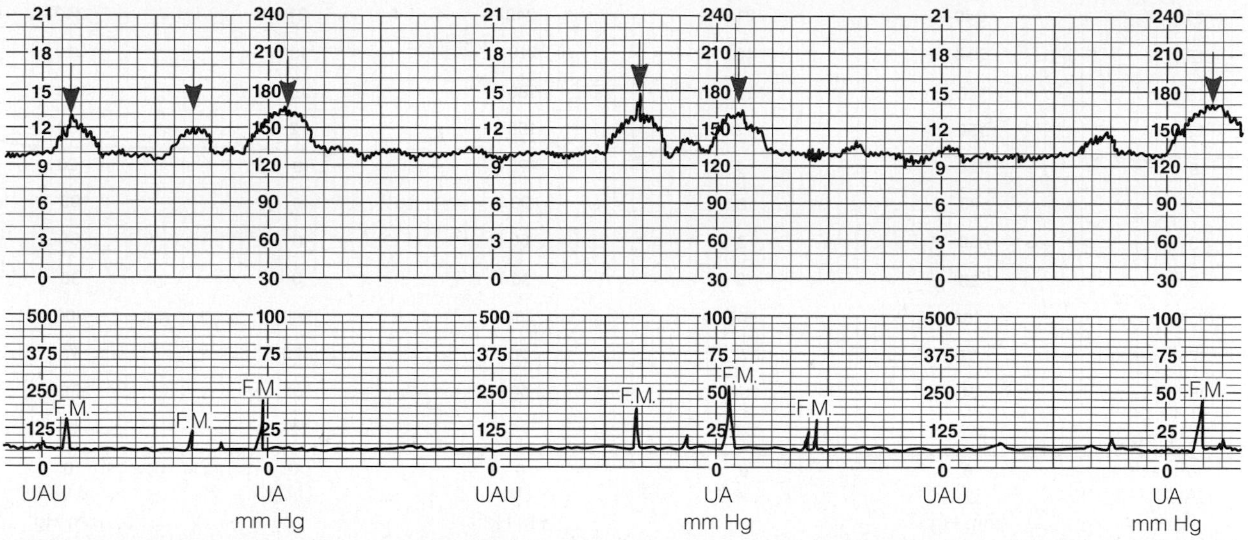

Figure 21-11 ■ Example of a reactive nonstress test (NST). Accelerations of 15 beats/min lasting 15 seconds with each fetal movement (FM). Top of strip shows fetal heart rate (FHR); bottom of strip shows uterine activity tracing. Note that FHR increases (above the baseline) at least 15 beats and remains at that rate for at least 15 seconds before returning to the former baseline.

pathetic nervous systems) of the fetus is not sufficiently mature to allow frequent accelerations of the heart rate when fetal movement occurs until 30 to 32 weeks of gestation. Acceleration patterns are directly affected by gestational age. The acme of acceleration is 15 beats per minute or more above the baseline rate. The acceleration lasts 15 seconds or longer for less than 2 minutes in fetuses at or beyond 32 weeks (Figure 21-11 ■). There must be at least two accelerations within a 20-minute period. Before 32 weeks, accelerations are defined as having an acme of 10 beats per minute or more for 10 seconds or longer (Cunningham et al., 2010). One study examined FHR pattern changes that occurred with advancing gestational age. Mean baseline FHR, signal loss, and fetal movement all decreased in advancing gestational age (Cunningham et al., 2010).

The NST can be used as an assessment tool in any pregnancy but is especially useful in the presence of diabetes, preeclampsia, intrauterine growth restriction, spontaneous rupture of membranes, multiple gestation, postdates, and other high-risk pregnancy conditions. These conditions can lead to a decline in uteroplacental functioning, which can result in decreased oxygenation to the fetus and eventual asphyxia. Testing intervals may vary, depending on the condition of the mother and fetus and recommendations of various experts. Most clinicians test twice weekly for high-risk patients and once a week for other conditions (Cunningham et al., 2010).

Procedure for Performing an NST

The NST is usually scheduled during daytime hours. It may be performed either in the office or hospital setting. Women are requested to be nonfasting and to have refrained from recent cigarette smoking because this can adversely affect test results. The NST is typically performed with the woman in the semi-Fowler's position with a small pillow or blanket under the right hip to displace the uterus to the left. The FHR is monitored by the placement of an electronic fetal monitor (see discussion in chapter 23 ∞). Either one or two belts are placed around the woman's abdomen. One belt holds the ultrasound transducer to record the FHR and the other holds a tocodynamometer that detects uterine or fetal movement. The FHR is usually monitored for 20 minutes, but monitoring may be extended to 40 minutes if it appears the fetus is in a sleep cycle. The woman is often requested to record each fetal movement by the use of self-operated markers. Under ideal conditions, a correlation of more than 90% between maternal perceived and actual fetal movements can be achieved; however, typically more than 40% of actual movements remain undetected by pregnant women (Flenady et al., 2009). Recent studies have examined NST administration in alternative positions, such as walking or in a sitting position. These studies found maternal perceptions of fetal movements was highest in the reclining position, but the walking and sitting positions resulted in a shortened time period to obtain two accelerations (Flenady et al., 2009).

Interpretation of the NST

NSTs are categorized as either reactive or nonreactive. The most common definition of a reactive (normal) test is that there are two or more fetal heart accelerations within a 20-minute period, with or without fetal movement discernible by the woman. The FHR acceleration must be at least 15 beats per minute above the baseline and last 15 seconds from baseline to baseline. A nonreactive (abnormal) NST is one that lacks sufficient FHR accelerations over a 40-minute period (Figure 21-12 ■) (Cunningham et al., 2010). Again, it is important to take into account the gestational age of the fetus. Both fetal movement and the amplitude of the FHR accelerations increase with gestational age.

Spontaneous decelerations of the FHR, known as variable decelerations, that occur during the testing period must also be noted. Variable decelerations may be observed in up to 50% of NSTs. Variable decelerations, if nonrepetitive and brief (less than 30 seconds), do not indicate fetal compromise nor the need for obstetric intervention (Cunningham et al., 2010). In contrast, repetitive variable decelerations (at least 3 in 20 minutes),

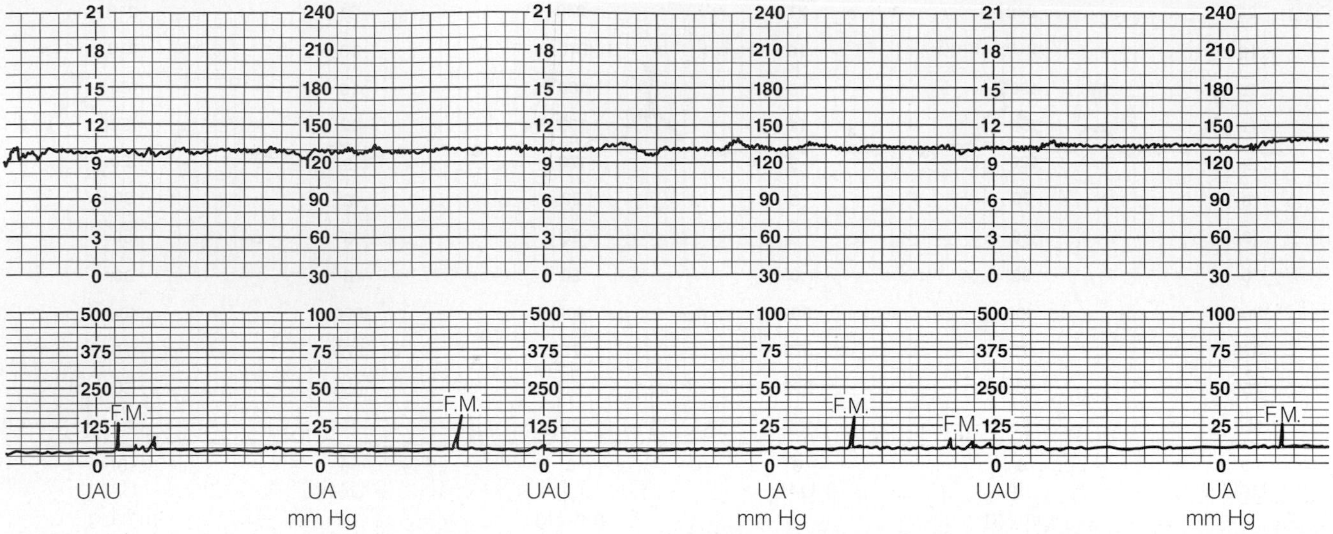

Figure 21-12 ■ Example of a nonreactive NST. There are no accelerations of FHR with fetal movement (FM). Baseline FHR is 130 beats/min. The tracing of uterine activity is on the bottom of the strip.

even if mild, have been associated with an increased risk of cesarean birth for nonreassuring intrapartum FHR pattern. The prognosis for decelerations lasting 1 minute or longer is even more ominous (Cunningham et al., 2010). It is the responsibility of the nurse performing this test to consult the physician or nurse-midwife for further evaluation of fetal status if there is any question concerning the reactivity of the test or the presence of repetitive decelerations.

Clinical Management

The clinical management of a woman following an NST may vary. If the NST is reactive after 20 minutes, the test is concluded and the woman is rescheduled for further testing as indicated by the condition of, or risk factors present for, the mother and/or fetus. The interval between testing is typically 1 week if the maternal medical condition is stable. Testing may be performed twice weekly if warranted by maternal or fetal risk factors. Any significant deterioration in the maternal medical status requires fetal reevaluation regardless of the amount of time that has elapsed since the last test (Cunningham et al., 2010).

NURSING CARE MANAGEMENT

The nurse first must ascertain the woman's understanding of the NST. The nurse then reviews the indications for the NST, the equipment being used, and the procedure before beginning the test. The nurse positions the woman and applies the electronic fetal monitor. Maternal blood pressure is monitored during the NST to determine whether hypotension is present. The nurse administers the NST, may or may not interpret the results, and reports the findings to the family physician/obstetrician or certified nurse-midwife and the patient. The nurse uses this opportunity to assess learning needs concerning the importance of fetal movement and provides information and teaching.

Vibroacoustic Stimulation

Vibroacoustic stimulation (VAS), also called *FAST* for *fetal acoustic stimulation test* or *VST* for *vibroacoustic stimulation test*, is an application of sound and vibration to the mother's abdomen to stimulate movement in the fetus (Figure 21-13 ■). A device is used that delivers 90 dB of sound for 1 to 3 seconds to the fetus with the purpose of changing the fetal sleep cycle, thereby accelerating the FHR (Cunningham et al., 2010).

NSTs that are interpreted as nonreactive often depict the normal state of quiet sleep by the fetus, which can last for up to 40 minutes. In these cases, VAS can be used to facilitate the timely interpretation of the NST. The typical VAS response of a healthy term fetus shows a rise of at least 10 beats per minute in baseline, occurring within 10 seconds and lasting from 5 to 10 minutes. Gestational age influences the reliability and reproducibility of the fetal response. The purpose of the VAS is to improve the specificity and efficiency of interpretation of FHR monitoring patterns. Although many obstetricians and certified nurse-

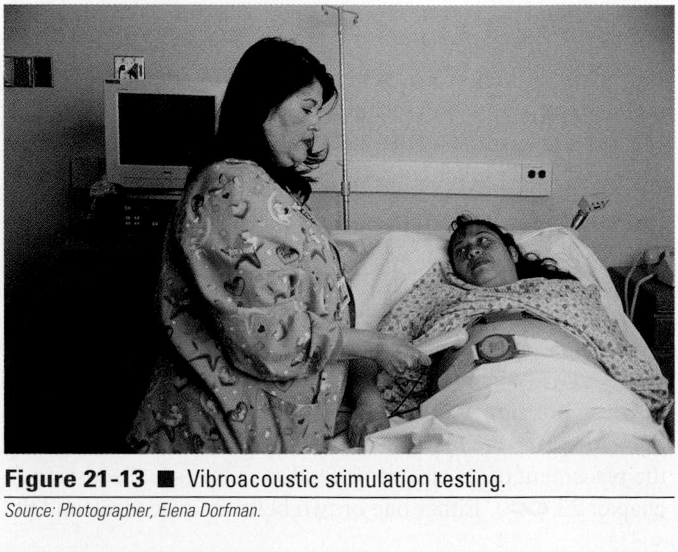

Figure 21-13 ■ Vibroacoustic stimulation testing.

Source: Photographer, Elena Dorfman.

midwives are enthusiastic about the VAS test because of its potential to minimize the need for more invasive follow-up testing, concerns for fetal hearing loss prevent universal use of this exam. Hearing loss has been demonstrated in newborns whose mothers were exposed to chronic levels of sound at 90 dB or more (Creasy et al., 2008). Although there are no documented cases of newborn hearing loss related to VAS, some advocate judicious use of this exam. Others have advocated simply rescheduling the NST in 1 to 2 hours when the fetus is likely to have moved from the quiet sleep state that may have resulted in the first nonreactive test as an alternative to VAS.

Contraction Stress Test

The **contraction stress test (CST)** is a means of evaluating the respiratory function (oxygen and carbon dioxide exchange) of the placenta (i.e., uteroplacental function). (See Procedure 21-2.) It enables the healthcare team to identify the fetus at risk for intrauterine asphyxia by observing the response of the FHR to the stress of uterine contractions (spontaneous or induced). During contractions, intrauterine pressure increases. Blood flow to the intervillous space of the placenta is reduced momentarily, thereby decreasing oxygen transport to the fetus. A healthy fetus usually tolerates this reduction well. If the placental reserve is insufficient, fetal hypoxia, depression of the myocardium, and a decrease in FHR occur (Blackburn, 2007).

Indications and Contraindications

The CST is indicated for pregnancies at risk for placental insufficiency or fetal compromise because of any of the following (Cunningham et al., 2010):

- Intrauterine growth restriction
- Diabetes mellitus
- Postdates (42 or more weeks' gestation)
- Nonreactive NST
- Abnormal or suspicious biophysical profile

Contraindications for the CST are the following:

- Third trimester bleeding (placenta previa, marginal abruptio placentae, or unexplained vaginal bleeding)
- Previous cesarean birth with classical uterine incision
- Instances in which the risk of possible preterm labor outweighs the advantage of the CST, including:
  a. Premature rupture of the membranes
  b. Incompetent cervix or Shirodkar-Barter operation (cerclage—surgical procedure in which an incompetent cervix is encircled with a suture to prevent it from dilating before term) (See chapter 26 ∞.)
  c. Multiple gestation

CST Procedure

A necessary component of the CST is the presence of three uterine contractions of at least 40 seconds' duration in 10 minutes. The response of the FHR when contractions occur provides data on the fetal status. The contractions may occur spontaneously, or they may be induced by oxytocin (Pitocin) or nipple stimulation. The most common method of stimulating uterine contractions for a CST has been intravenous administration of oxytocin, but many facilities now use breast self-stimulation to obtain a CST (see later discussion) (Cunningham et al., 2010). This method is based on the fact that endogenous oxytocin is produced in response to stimulation of the breasts or nipples.

The CST is performed on an outpatient basis by qualified maternity nurses well acquainted with fetal monitoring and the interpretation of various FHR patterns. Most facilities require that the test be administered in or near the labor and birth unit so that treatment is available in the event that adverse reactions to oxytocin stimulation occur. The procedure, reasons for administering the test, equipment, and normal variations in monitoring that occur during the test should be clearly explained before the test to alleviate the woman's apprehension. A consent form may be signed.

During the test, the woman assumes a semi-Fowler's or side-lying position to avoid supine hypotension. The ultrasonic transducer (from the electronic fetal monitor) is placed on the woman's abdomen over the area of the fetal back or chest so that the FHR can be accurately recorded on the monitoring strip. (See chapter 23 ∞ for further discussion of fetal monitoring.) To record uterine contractions, the tocodynamometer (pressure transducer) is placed over the area of the uterine fundus. For the first 15 to 20 minutes, the nurse records baseline measurements, including blood pressure, fetal activity, variations of the FHR during fetal movement, and spontaneous contractions. In addition, pertinent medical and obstetric information may be obtained from the woman to aid in her further management.

After the baseline recording is done, an intravenous oxytocin contraction stress test or breast self-stimulation test (BSST) is done.

> **CLINICAL TIP**
> When performing a contraction stress test (CST), provide comfort measures to the woman who may experience discomfort during the procedure.

INTRAVENOUS OXYTOCIN CST In a CST using intravenous oxytocin, an electrolyte solution such as lactated Ringer's solution is started as a primary infusion. A piggyback infusion of oxytocin in a similar solution is attached. An infusion pump is used so that the amount of oxytocin being infused can be measured accurately. The administration procedure is the same as that for inducing labor through oxytocin administration (see chapter 28 ∞). Oxytocin is administered until three uterine contractions lasting 40 to 60 seconds occur in a 10-minute period (called the 10-minute window). If late decelerations occur with all three contractions, the oxytocin infusion is discontinued. The woman's blood pressure and pulse are assessed every 15 minutes and recorded on the tracing.

CST WITH BREAST SELF-STIMULATION TEST (BSST) A woman receiving a BSST is instructed to stimulate her nipples with her fingers, palms, or a warm, moist face cloth, either directly or through her clothing, for 2 minutes or until a contraction begins. Stimulation may also be done mechanically by the use of a breast pump. Once the contraction begins, the woman

PROCEDURE 21-2 Performing a Contraction Stress Test (CST)

NURSING ACTION

Preparation

- Explain the procedure, the information it provides, and the process for completing the test.
- Ask the woman to void.

  Rationale: *The procedure will take at least 10 minutes to complete and the woman will need to remain in semi-Fowler's or a side-lying position and will be unable to void without interrupting the testing procedure.*
- Advise the woman that if uterine contractions are not occurring spontaneously, intravenous oxytocin or breast stimulation may be needed to perform the test.

  Rationale: *The test requires three contractions lasting at least 40 seconds in duration in a 10-minute period in order to be performed.*

Equipment and Supplies

External fetal monitor with a monitoring strip

Blood pressure cuff

Procedure

1. Place the woman in a semi-Fowler's or side-lying position after she has voided.
2. Place the ultrasound transducer from the external fetal monitor on the woman's abdomen over the FHR (typically over the fetal back or chest) so a tracing can be obtained on the monitoring strip.
3. If the FHR is not consistently recorded on the monitoring strip, adjust the ultrasound transducer until an adequate reading is obtained.

   Rationale: *Fetal or maternal movement can cause an inconsistency in the FHR on the monitoring strip. Multiple adjustments may be needed to obtain consistency in recording the FHR.*
4. Place the tocodynamometer (pressure transducer) on the woman's abdomen over the uterine fundus.

   Rationale: *Contractions are best detected when the device is directly placed on the uterine fundus.*
5. Obtain baseline measurements, including blood pressure, fetal activity, variations in the FHR during fetal movement, and contractions, for 15 to 20 minutes.

   Rationale: *Baseline measurements provide a reference for normal maternal and fetal assessment parameters.*
6. If less than three contractions lasting at least 40 seconds are occurring within a 10-minute period, administer intravenous oxytocin or instruct the woman in the breast stimulation technique until three contractions in a 10-minute period are occurring. The method chosen is based on the healthcare provider's orders and the woman's preference.

   Rationale: *If the woman has a preference over one method or another, the healthcare provider should be made aware of that preference.*
7. If using intravenous oxytocin, start an electrolyte solution as a primary infusion and attach a piggyback infusion of oxytocin in a similar solution using an infusion pump.

   Rationale: *Intravenous oxytocin is always infused using a piggyback line because a small quantity is infusing. An infusion pump should be used to ensure accuracy.*
8. Administer oxytocin and increase at regular intervals per agency protocol until three contractions lasting 40 to 60 seconds occur in a 10-minute period.

   Rationale: *Because there are several formulas used to mix oxytocin and several different protocols to increase the dosage, specific agency protocol should be consulted regarding the preparation of the oxytocin solution and the dosage and interval increases used within the facility.*
9. If using breast self-stimulation (BSST), instruct the woman to stimulate her breasts with her fingers, palms, or a warm, moist washcloth, either directly or through her clothing for 2 minutes or until a contraction begins.

   Rationale: *Breast stimulation will facilitate the natural release of oxytocin by the woman's body. Some women may prefer a more natural method of testing and may prefer BSST over intravenous oxytocin.*
10. Instruct the woman to stop the stimulation once the contraction occurs and to restart the stimulation if a contraction has not occurred within 5 minutes (Creasy et al., 2008).

    Rationale: *Continuous breast stimulation can result in uterine hyperstimulation, which can lead to a uterine rupture.*
11. Advise the woman to increase the frequency of stimulation as needed to obtain three contractions within a 10-minute period.
12. Interpret the test as negative, positive, equivocal-suspicious, equivocal-hyperstimulatory, or unsatisfactory and report the findings to the healthcare provider immediately.

    Rationale: *The CST interpretations are based on specific criteria and should be reported to the healthcare provider as soon as the results are obtained. The results provide data regarding uteroplacental perfusion and indicate whether the fetus can withstand the stress of uterine contractions.*
13. Explain the results to the woman and relate information from the healthcare provider regarding further management needs or additional follow-up that is needed.

Documentation

Document baseline maternal and fetal assessment information that was obtained before and during the test. The results of the test should be documented along with information regarding how the information was reported to the healthcare provider. The specific name of the healthcare provider and date and time should be recorded. Any additional orders and instructions to the client should be documented. Verbalization of understanding of the test results by the woman should be documented along with her understanding of follow-up instructions and future appointments.

is instructed to stop the stimulation, waiting to restart if another contraction has not followed by 5 minutes. It is important to monitor the frequency of contractions to avoid uterine hyperstimulation.

Interpretation and Clinical Management

A CST is usually not done before 28 weeks' gestation, primarily for two reasons. First, in light of a positive test, birth and extrauterine survival would be questionable at such an early gestational age. Second, sufficient research has not been done to determine whether the same test results apply to a fetus of this gestation. CST is usually done no earlier than 32 to 34 weeks' gestation and typically in preparation for induction of labor.

INTERPRETATION OF CST RESULTS A CST can be interpreted once three moderately strong contractions of 40 to 60 seconds' duration have been noted in a 10-minute window of time. A CST can be interpreted as negative, positive, equivocal, or unsatisfactory (Table 21-4). Cunningham et al. (2010) offered the following CST interpretations:

Negative—The absence of late or significant variable decelerations (the most common deceleration pattern noted during labor; attributed to umbilical cord compression or occlusion) is considered a reassuring sign that the fetus is receiving sufficient transfer of oxygen through the placenta (Figure 21-14 ■).

Positive—The presence of **late decelerations** (a symmetrical decrease in FHR beginning at or after the peak of the contraction and returning to baseline only after the contraction has ended following 50% or more of contractions, even if the contraction frequency is fewer than three in 10 minutes) is a sign of uteroplacental insufficiency and may indicate that the fetus is not receiving adequate oxygenation (Figure 21-15 ■).

Equivocal-suspicious—The presence of intermittent late decelerations or significant variable decelerations should be viewed as a suspicious finding that merits follow-up testing.

TABLE 21-4 Interpretation of the Contraction Stress Test

RESULT	INTERPRETATION
Negative	No late or significant variable decelerations.
Positive	Late decelerations following 50% or more of contractions (even if the contraction frequency is fewer than three in 10 minutes).
Equivocal	
Suspicious	Intermittent late decelerations or significant variable decelerations.
Hyperstimulatory	Fetal heart rate decelerations that occur in the presence of contractions more frequent than every 2 minutes or lasting longer than 90 seconds.
Unsatisfactory	Fewer than three contractions in 10 minutes or an uninterpretable tracing.

Source: ACOG Practice Bulletin No. 9, October 1999. Clinical Management Guidelines for Obstetrician-Gynecologists, *pp. 2–3.*

Equivocal-hyperstimulatory—FHR decelerations may occur in the presence of contractions that occur more frequently than every 2 minutes or that last longer than 90 seconds. This test should be repeated after hyperstimulation has been rectified and the patient has been hydrated and allowed to rest.

Unsatisfactory—The CST cannot be interpreted if fewer than three contractions lasting 40 to 60 seconds occur in a 10-minute window of time.

CST results are also evaluated for the presence of accelerations that would meet the criteria of the NST. Combining the CST assessment with NST results showing characteristics such as variability of the FHR baseline and the presence of other types of decelerations helps the clinician determine the best management plan for the fetus.

Case Study: Patient Undergoing Contraction Stress Test

CLINICAL MANAGEMENT BASED ON CST RESULTS In most cases, a negative CST with a reactive NST is the desired result. The uteroplacental perfusion is sufficient at present to allow the fetus to withstand the stress of uterine contractions. Retesting

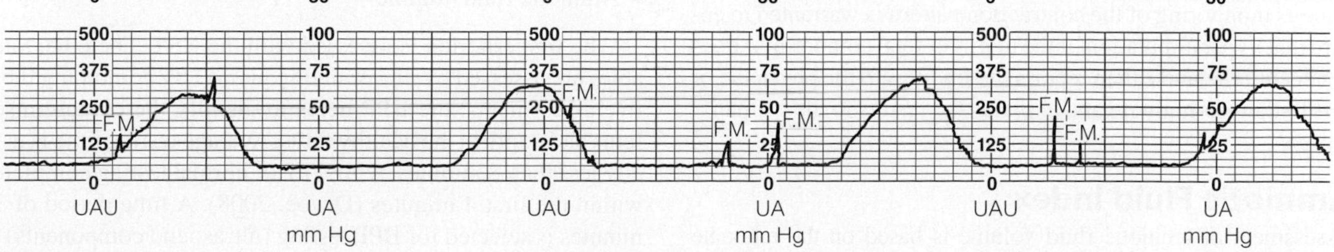

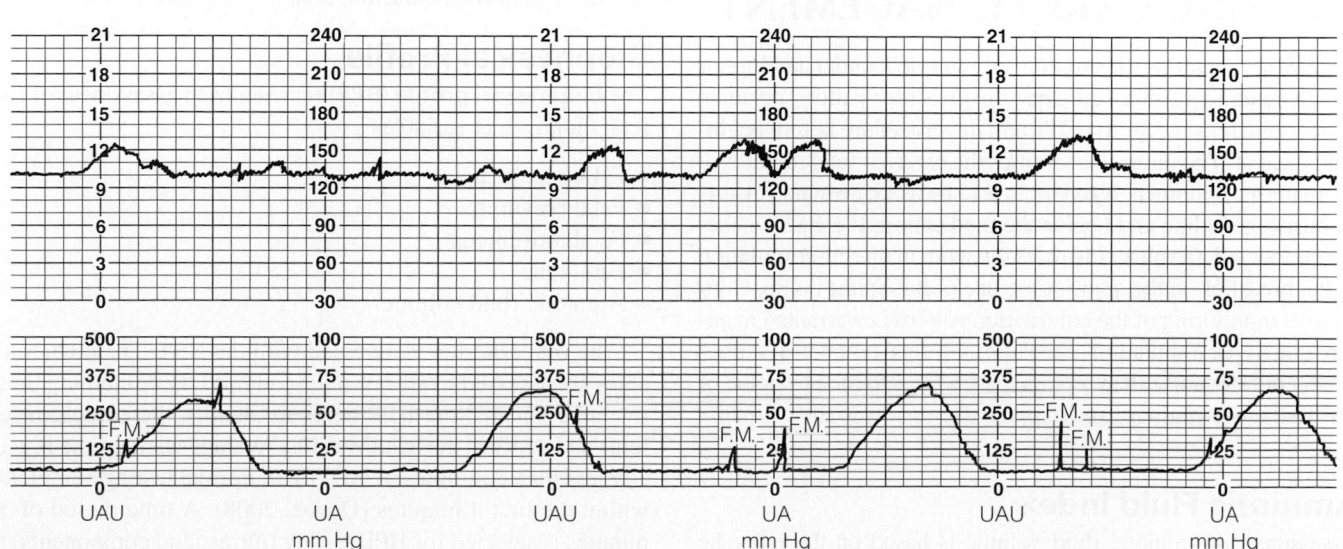

Figure 21-14 ■ Example of a negative CST (and reactive NST). The baseline FHR is 130 beats/min with acceleration of FHR of at least 15 beats/min lasting 15 seconds with each fetal movement (FM). Uterine contractions recorded on the bottom half of the strip indicate three contractions in 8 minutes.

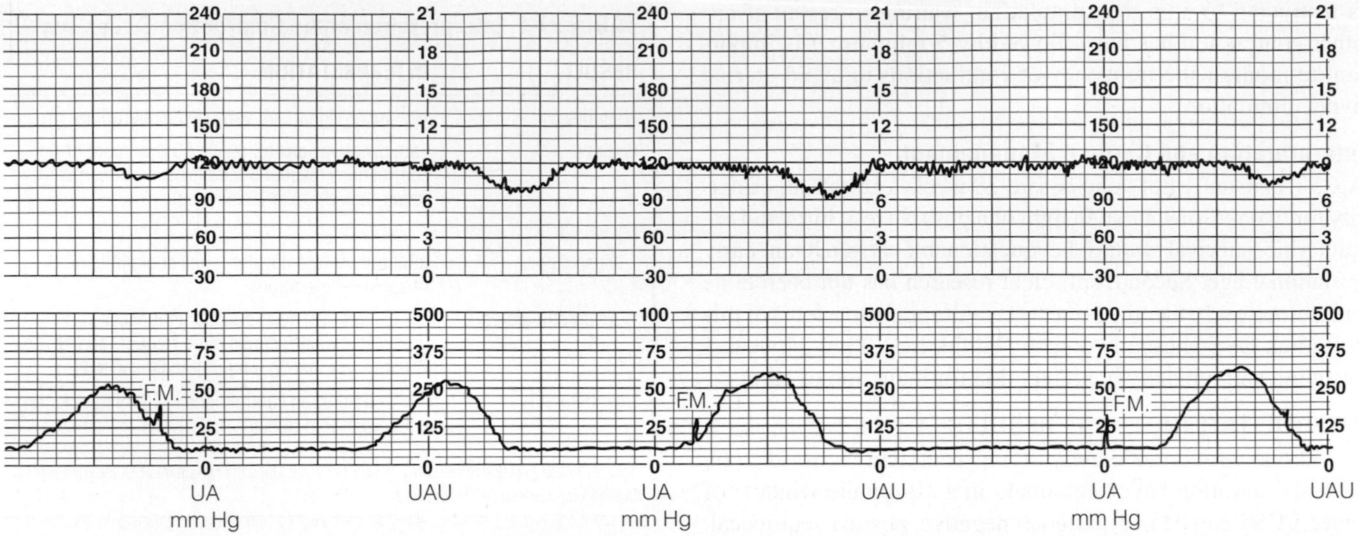

Figure 21-15 ■ Example of a positive contraction stress test (CST). Repetitive late decelerations occur with each contraction. Note that there are no accelerations of FHR with three fetal movements (FM). The baseline FHR is 120 beats/min. Uterine contractions (bottom half of strip) occurred four times in 12 minutes.

would most likely be scheduled in 7 days. If the pregnant woman is diabetic, the CST schedule would remain the same, except an NST would be done in 3 to 4 days (Creasy et al., 2008). A negative CST with a nonreactive NST is more difficult. It should be assessed very carefully for subtle late decelerations. If there are none, a CST would be repeated in 7 days.

All equivocal tests should be repeated in 24 hours, especially in the presence of a postterm pregnancy (Creasy et al., 2008). If the gestation is less than 37 weeks, then other surveillance methods should be added.

A positive CST with a nonreactive NST presents evidence that the fetus would probably not withstand the stress of labor. If the gestation is 32 weeks or over, a cesarean birth should be scheduled (Creasy et al., 2008).

NURSING CARE MANAGEMENT

Biophysical Profile

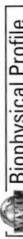

The nurse ascertains the woman's or couple's understanding of the CST before the procedure and the possible results. The nurse reviews the reasons for the CST and the procedure before beginning the test. The nurse then applies the external fetal monitor to the maternal abdomen. If oxytocin is to be used, the nurse inserts an intravenous line and begins the medication. If a BSST is being conducted, the nurse instructs the woman on self-stimulation of the breast or on the appropriate use of the breast pump. Continuous monitoring of the contraction pattern is warranted to ensure that hyperstimulation of the uterus or fetal compromise does not occur. The nurse then reports the findings to the physician or certified nurse-midwife and explains the results to the woman.

Amniotic Fluid Index

Assessment of amniotic fluid volume is based on the rationale that decreased uteroplacental perfusion may lead to diminished fetal renal blood flow, decreased urination, and, ultimately, **oligohydramnios** (decreased amniotic fluid volume). Fetal urine output and fetal swallowing are the major determinants of amniotic fluid volume. Oligohydramnios may be the result of diminished urinary output caused by fetal hypoxemia. The resulting placental insufficiency may cause hypoxia and hence oligohydramnios. Therefore, assessment of long-term uteroplacental function may be performed by evaluating amniotic fluid volume (Gabbe et al., 2007). Some poor pregnancy outcomes, such as intrauterine growth restriction, postterm pregnancy, and nonreassuring fetal status in labor, have been associated with abnormalities of amniotic fluid volume. The procedure for performing an amniotic fluid index (AFI) was discussed previously on page 505.

An AFI value of 5 or less serves as a red flag that requires some type of further assessment or management decision (Cunningham et al., 2010). The gestational age of the fetus and the composite maternal condition may influence management decisions, leading to additional testing, induction of labor, or cesarean birth.

Biophysical Profile

The **biophysical profile (BPP)** represents an assessment of five fetal biophysical variables:

- FHR acceleration
- Fetal breathing
- Fetal movements
- Fetal tone
- Amniotic fluid volume

The first criterion is assessed with the NST. The other variables are assessed by ultrasound scanning. By combining these five assessments, the BPP helps to identify the compromised fetus and confirm the healthy fetus. Average testing time is usually less than 8 minutes, with 90% of normal testing completed within the first 4 minutes (Devoe, 2008). A time period of 30 minutes is selected for BPP testing (ultrasound components) to account for the average duration of sleep-wake cycles in the normal fetus, which are approximately 20 minutes.

TABLE 21-5 Criteria for Normal and Abnormal Assessments of the BPP

COMPONENT	NORMAL (SCORE = 2)	ABNORMAL (SCORE = 0)
Fetal breathing movements	Greater than or equal to 1 episode of rhythmic breathing lasting greater than or equal to 30 sec within 30 min	Less than 30 sec of breathing in 30 min
Gross body movements	Greater than or equal to 3 discrete body or limb movements in 30 min (episodes of active continuous movement considered as single movement)	Less than or equal to 2 movements in 30 min
Fetal tone	Greater than or equal to 1 episode of extension of a fetal extremity with return to flexion, or opening or closing of hand	No movements or extension/flexion
Reactive fetal heart rate Nonstress test	Greater than or equal to 2 accelerations of greater than or equal to 15 beats/min for greater than or equal to 15 sec in 20–40 min	0 or 1 acceleration in 20–40 min
Amniotic fluid volume	At least 1 pocket of anmiotic fluid of at least 2 cm AFI >5	Less than 1 pocket of amniotic fluid measuring less than 2 cm

Indications for the biophysical profile include those situations in which the NST and CST would be done. Assessment of these fetal biophysical activities is most useful in the evaluation of women who experience decreased fetal movement (who might subsequently have a nonreactive NST) and in the management of intrauterine growth restriction, preterm labor, gestational diabetes, postterm pregnancies, and premature rupture of the membranes (PROM) (Devoe, 2008).

The two most important components of the BPP are the NST and the amniotic fluid volume index. The NST reflects the intactness of the nervous system and the AFI reflects kidney perfusion. A normal AFI indicates that shunting has not occurred and that the fetal kidneys are adequately functioning. Reactive NST and normal fluid therefore reflect fetal well-being.

Specific criteria for normal and abnormal assessments are delineated in Table 21-5. Normal variables are assigned a score of 2 each and abnormal variables a score of 0 (zero). Thus, the highest score possible for a normal fetus is 10.

Clinicians suggest that management not be based solely on BPP scores. Biophysical activities of the fetus that develop first are the last to disappear when all activities are arrested because of asphyxia (Devoe, 2008). Those that are the last to develop are the most sensitive to hypoxia, and their disappearance can be noted first. For example, fetal tone (exhibited by flexion of the extremities) is the first to develop and the last activity to cease during asphyxia. Other activities in the normal developmental sequence are fetal movement, followed by fetal breathing, and then reactivity of the FHR. Therefore, FHR reactivity is the most sensitive to hypoxia (Cunningham et al., 2010). One of the first indications of fetal compromise is a nonreactive NST. Table 21-6 outlines BPP test interpretation and the recommended management (Cunningham et al., 2010).

Modified Biophysical Profile

The biophysical profile is labor intensive and expensive. It requires a trained person in ultrasonic visualization of the fetus. In addition, studies have shown that when the four dynamic ultrasound variables are normal, the probability of encountering an abnormal (nonreactive) NST is exceedingly small (Devoe, 2008). For these reasons, a modified biophysical profile (BPP) has been developed. This test consists of an NST and a measurement of the AFI, both of which reflect long-term uteroplacental function. The

TABLE 21-6 BPP Test Interpretation and Recommended Management

TEST SCORE	INTERPRETATION	PERINATAL MORTALITY WITHIN 1 WEEK WITHOUT INTERVENTION	MANAGEMENT
10/10	Normal nonasphyxiated fetus	Less than 1/1000	No fetal indication for intervention; repeat test weekly except in patient with diabetes and pregnancies that are postterm (twice weekly)
8/10 (normal fluid) 8/8 if no NST done	Risk of fetal asphyxia extremely rare	Less than 1/1000	Same as above
8/10 (abnormal fluid)	Chronic fetal asphyxia suspected	89/1000	Induce birth
6/10	Possible fetal asphyxia	89/1000	If amniotic fluid volume abnormal, induce birth If normal fluid at greater than 36 weeks with favorable cervix, induce birth If repeat test less than or equal to 6, induce birth If repeat test greater than 6, observe and repeat per protocol
4/10	Probable fetal asphyxia	91/1000	Repeat testing same day; if BPP score less than or equal to 6, induce birth
2/10	Almost certain fetal asphyxia	125/1000	Induce birth
0/10	Certain fetal asphyxia	600/1000	Induce birth

functioning of the placenta is important because a poorly functioning placenta (placental dysfunction) may result in diminished fetal renal perfusion, leading to oligohydramnios. The amniotic fluid volume assessment can therefore be used to evaluate long-term uteroplacental function. A modified BPP is considered normal if the amniotic fluid volume is greater than 5 cm and if the NST is reactive. The test is abnormal if either the NST is nonreactive or the AFI is 5 or less. The frequency of this test is the same as with the standard BPP.

Doppler Flow Studies

Recent advances in ultrasound technology have made it possible to study noninvasively the blood flow changes that occur in maternal and fetal circulations in order to assess placental function. An ultrasound beam, like that provided by the pocket Doppler (a handheld ultrasound device), is directed at the umbilical artery. The signal is reflected off the red blood cells moving within the vessels, and the subsequent "picture" (waveform) that is received looks like a series of waves. The highest velocity peak of the waves is the systolic measurement, and the lowest point is the diastolic velocity. The umbilical artery waveform can then be analyzed to provide information about velocity of blood flow in the vessel (Kiserud, Ebbing, Kessler, et al., 2007). Examples of these waveforms are displayed in Figures 21-16 ■ and 21-17 ■.

The most common evaluation of blood flow velocity is the systolic to diastolic (S/D) ratio. The S/D ratio normally decreases as the fetus nears term. This phenomenon reflects the decreasing resistance of placental and umbilical vasculature to allow for greater umbilical blood flow to meet the needs of a growing fetus. The S/D ratio is considered abnormal if it is elevated above the 95th percentile for gestational age or reversed after 18 to 20 weeks of gestation (Peterson, Wong, Urs, et al., 2009). Absent or reversed end-diastolic flow signifies increased impedance and is uniquely associated with intrauterine growth restriction. It is also associated with a high perinatal mortality rate (Peterson et al., 2009).

A decrease in fetal cardiac output or an increase in resistance of placental vessels will reduce umbilical artery blood flow. Doppler velocimetry is best used when intrauterine growth restriction is diagnosed, whether it occurs as an idiopathic process (cause unknown) or in the presence of hypertension or preeclampsia (Peterson et al., 2009). No benefit has been demonstrated for umbilical artery velocimetry for other conditions such as postterm pregnancy, diabetes, systemic lupus erythematosus, or antiphospholipid antibody syndrome. Also, it has not been shown to be of value as a screening test for detecting fetal compromise in the general obstetric population (Cunningham et al., 2010).

Evaluation of Placental Maturity

Placental maturity is evaluated by a grading process that uses ultrasound to measure the changes in the basal layer, chorionic plate, and intervening placental substance. A grade of 0 through III is assigned (grade III is the most mature, showing extensive calcifications) (Figure 21-18 ■). Placentas with multiple calcifications are less likely to function as adequately as those with lower grades. Certain factors can cause a placenta to mature, including maternal smoking, postterm pregnancy, and certain

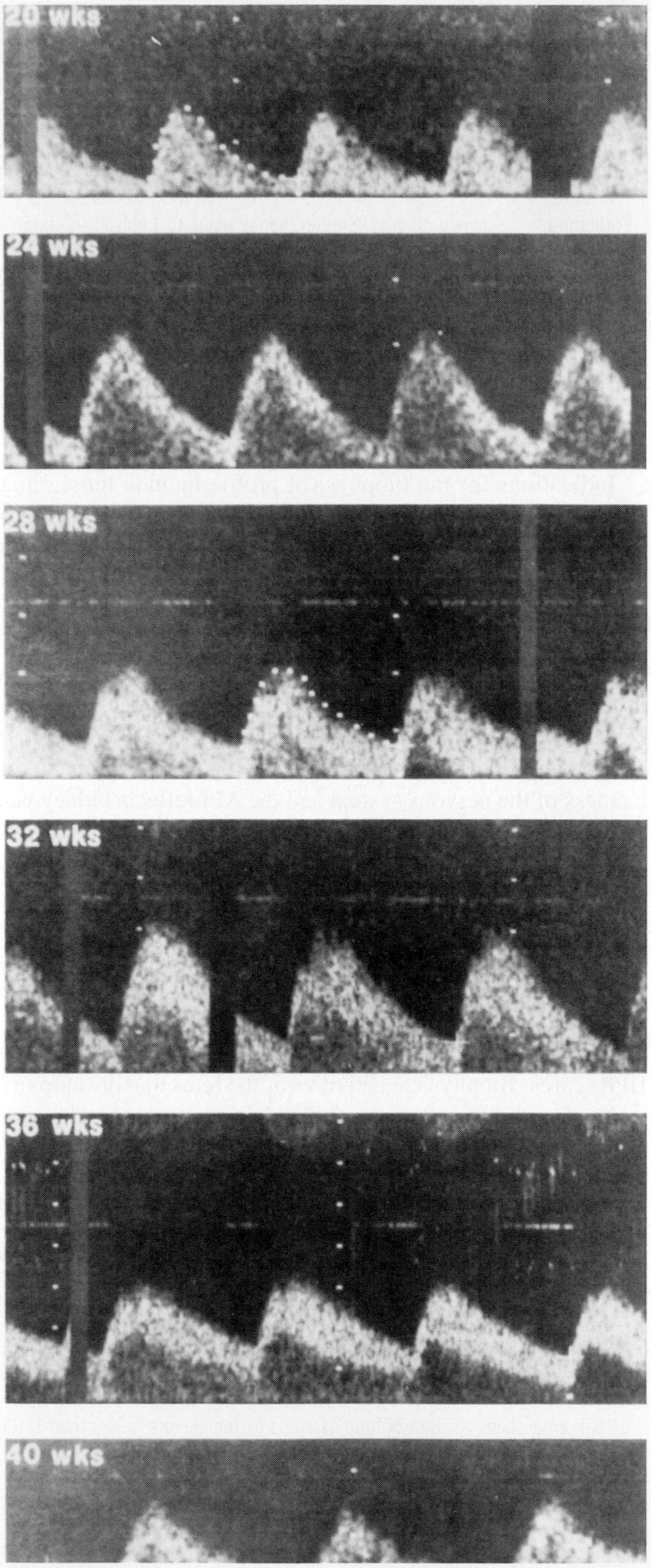

Figure 21-16 ■ Serial studies of the umbilical artery velocity waveforms in a normal pregnancy from one patient.

Source: AWHONN. (1990). Cundiff, J. L., Haybrich, K. L., & Hinzman, N. G. Umbilical artery Doppler flow studies during pregnancy. Journal of Obstetric, Gynecologic, & Neonatal Nursing, *19(4), 475–481 (Figure 3, p. 478). Washington, DC: Author. ©1990 by the Association of Women's Health, Obstetric and Neonatal Nurses. All rights reserved.*

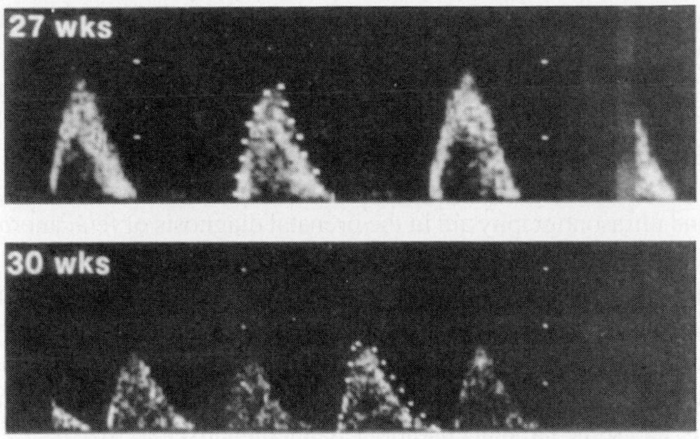

Figure 21-17 ■ Two examples of abnormal umbilical artery velocity waveforms taken from a patient with intrauterine growth restriction.

Source: AWHONN. (1990). Cundiff, J. L., Haybrich, K. L., & Hinzman, N. G. Umbilical artery Doppler flow studies during pregnancy. Journal of Obstetric, Gynecologic, & Neonatal Nursing, *19(4), 475–481 (Figure 4, p. 478). Washington, DC: Author. ©1990 by the Association of Women's Health, Obstetric and Neonatal Nurses. All rights reserved.*

maternal conditions, such as preeclampsia and gestational diabetes. Placental grade may be used to correlate with other findings; however, placental grade alone does not dictate management of a pregnancy (Cunningham et al., 2010).

Estimation of Fetal Weight

Estimating the fetal weight in the third trimester of pregnancy is an important aspect of fetal assessment. Particularly, findings of the fetal weight at either end of the spectrum—inadequate fetal growth or excessive fetal growth—are critical risk factors for alterations in fetal well-being.

Intrauterine growth restriction (IUGR), also known as *inadequate fetal growth,* is a term used to describe any fetus that falls below the 10th percentile in ultrasonic estimation of weight at a given gestational age. Other terms to describe the small fetus include *low birth weight, small for gestational age,* and *intrauterine growth retardation (IUGR).* IUGR may or may not be associated with prematurity.

The etiology of IUGR can be separated into either fetoplacental or maternal origin. Fetoplacental etiologies would include infections, genetic abnormalities, and placental abnormalities. Maternal etiologies stem from reduced uteroplacental blood flow associated with hypertension, poor maternal weight gain, poor nutrition, substance use such as tobacco or medications, anemia, or chronic illness (Cunningham et al., 2010).

If a fetus is suspected to have IUGR, the management includes careful surveillance of the fetus with NSTs and BPPs and continuous assessment of growth through sonographic assessment. In addition to regular fetal surveillance, women with IUGR are instructed to do daily fetal movement assessments (previously discussed in this chapter) and to maintain bed rest. If growth ceases altogether or if other nonreassuring fetal factors occur (nonreassuring FHR patterns), delivery may be warranted.

Macrosomia (excessive fetal growth) is defined by ACOG (2009) as weight greater than 4000 to 4500 g (8 lb 13 oz to 9 lb 4 oz). If a fetus is suspected to be macrosomic, the management of the labor and birth is carefully evaluated to prevent birth-related

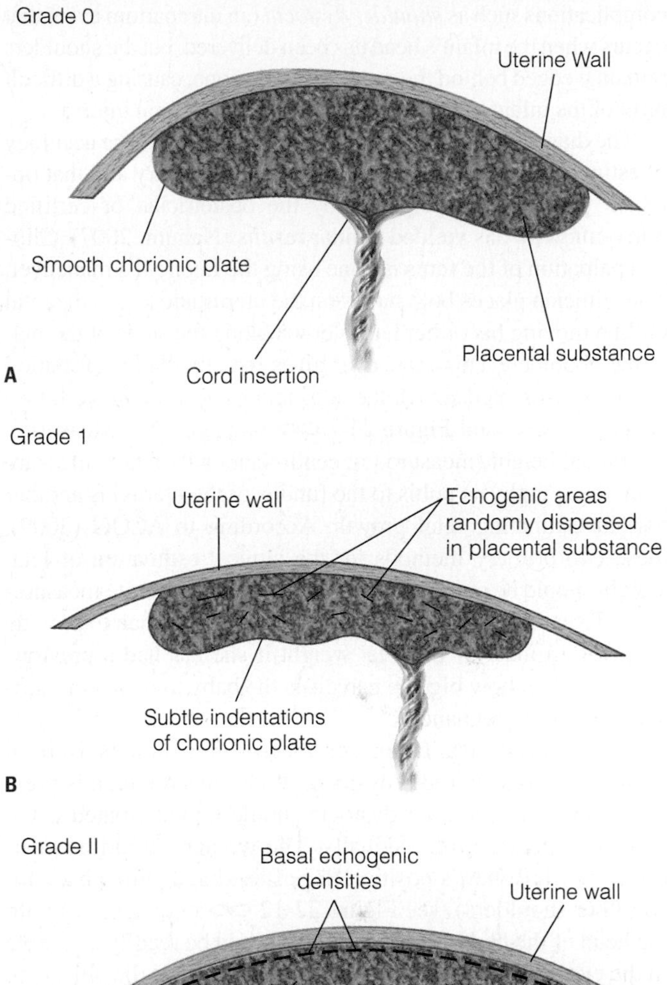

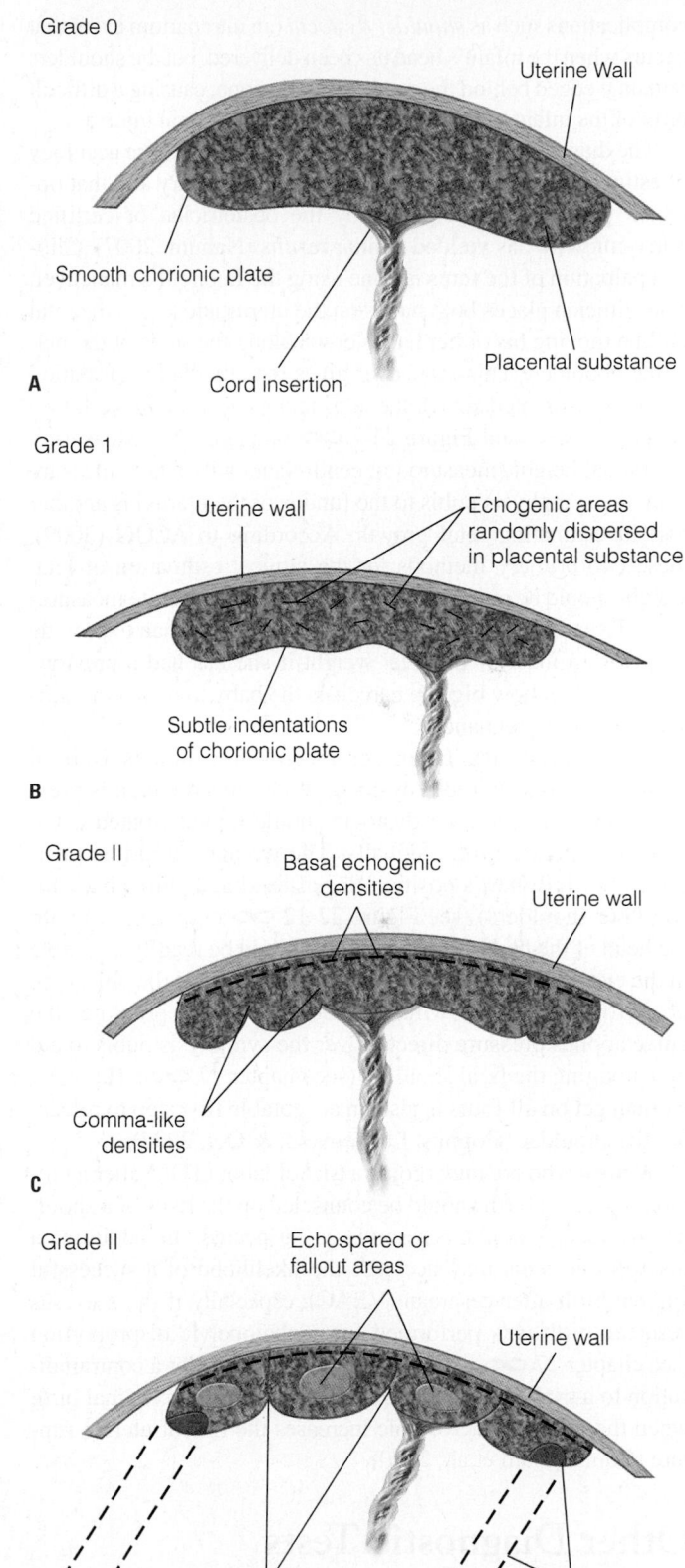

Figure 21-18 ■ Placental grading. A. Diagram showing the ultrasonic appearance of a grade 0 placenta. B. Diagram showing the ultrasonic appearance of a grade I placenta. C. Diagram showing the ultrasonic appearance of a grade II placenta. D. Diagram showing the ultrasonic appearance of a grade III placenta.

complications such as *shoulder dystocia* (an intrapartum event that occurs when the infant's head has been delivered, but the shoulders remain wedged behind the mother's pubic bone, causing a difficult birth of the infant with potential for maternal or fetal injury).

The diagnosis of fetal macrosomia is imprecise. The accuracy of estimated fetal weight using ultrasound biometry and that obtained with clinical palpation by the obstetrician or certified nurse-midwife has yielded similar results (Nahum, 2007). Clinical palpation of the fetus is done using the Leopold's maneuver. The clinician places both hands on the uterus and traces the fetal outline moving his or her hands down along the sides of the maternal abdomen. This maneuver gives the clinician information about the estimated size of the fetus and its position in utero (see chapter 23 ∞ and Figure 23-7 ∞ on page 571). Measuring the fundal height (measured in centimeters with a tape measure from the symphysis pubis to the fundus of the uterus) is another tool in estimating fetal growth. According to ACOG (2009), these two primary methods for the clinical estimation of fetal weight should be combined to produce a more accurate measurement. Experienced providers may also ask the woman to provide her own estimate of the fetal weight if she has had a previous birth based on how big she perceives the baby to be in comparison to her last pregnancy.

Alpha-Fetoprotein

The greatest risk factor for macrosomic infants is birth trauma due to a shoulder dystocia. When macrosomia is present, a potential shoulder dystocia should be anticipated if the woman is giving birth vaginally. The woman should be positioned in McRobert's position (legs flexed and pulled back toward her shoulders) (see Figure 27-12 ∞ on page 712) with the head of the bed lowered. A stool should be readily available in the event that suprapubic pressure is needed. If the physician or certified nurse-midwife requests suprapubic pressure, the nurse applies pressure directly over the symphysis pubis to aid in dislodging the fetal shoulder (see chapter 27 ∞). Having a woman get on all fours is also an acceptable first step to releasing the shoulder (Coppus, Langenveld, & Oei, 2007).

Women who are undergoing a trial of labor (TOL) after a previous cesarean birth should be counseled on the risks of a shoulder dystocia when macrosomia is suspected. In addition, a macrosomic fetus may decrease the likelihood of a successful vaginal birth after cesarean (VBAC), especially if the previous cesarean birth was performed for cephalopelvic disproportion (see chapter 27 ∞). Although macrosomia is not a contraindication to a trial of labor, a TOL without a previous vaginal birth when the fetus is macrosomic increases the risk of uterine rupture (Cunningham et al., 2010).

Other Diagnostic Tests

Birth defects, defined as structural abnormalities present at birth, are the leading cause of infant mortality and a major contributor to infant morbidity in the United States. Birth defects account for 1 in 5 infant deaths in the United States annually (March of Dimes, 2009). Birth defects affect 8 million children worldwide and affect 6% of all infants born each year (March of Dimes, 2009). In the United States, 1 in 33 infants are born with a birth defect (March of Dimes, 2009). Infant mortality due to birth defects has not declined as rapidly as overall infant mortality. It has been estimated that approximately 20% of all birth defects are due to gene mutations, and 5% to 10% are due to exposure to a teratogen such as drugs, chemicals, or radiation. About half of all birth defects remain unexplained (March of Dimes, 2009).

Rapidly developing technologies of biochemical markers and ultrasonography aid in the prenatal diagnosis of fetal anomalies and genetic disorders. Some of the better known genetic tests include the screening test for alpha-fetoprotein and the amniocentesis or chorionic villi diagnostic tests. As discussed in chapter 12 ∞, conditions that can be diagnosed prenatally include trisomies 21, 18, and 13, spina bifida and anencephaly, cystic fibrosis, and some familial conditions (Cunningham et al., 2010).

Maternal Serum Alpha-Fetoprotein (MSAFP)

Alpha-fetoprotein (AFP) is a fetal protein that is excreted from the fetal yolk sac during the first 6 weeks of pregnancy. The production of AFP is then taken over by the fetal liver as the pregnancy progresses. AFP levels can be high or low, each with different implications to the fetus. If the fetus has a neural tube defect (NTD), the AFP levels will be elevated. The incidence of NTDs is 1 per 2000 births and is the most commonly occurring birth defect in the United States (March of Dimes, 2009). NTDs can range from *anencephaly* (absence of a portion of the fetal brain that is incompatible with extrauterine life) to *spina bifida* (an incomplete closure of the vertebral arch that may allow protrusion of the meningeal tissue, spinal cord, or nerve roots through the opening on the spinal cord, and which is associated with lower extremity paralysis, incontinence, and developmental delay).

Quadruple Check

Maternal serum alpha-fetoprotein (MSAFP) is a component of the screening test, the "quadruple check" that utilizes the multiple markers, including AFP, hCG, diameric inhibin-A, and estriol to screen pregnancies for NTD, trisomy 21 (Down syndrome), and trisomy 18. Screening can be performed between 15 and 22 weeks' gestation (15 to 16 yields the most accurate results) (Cunningham et al., 2010). ACOG (2009) recommends that all pregnant women be offered aneuploidy screening. See chapter 12 ∞ for a discussion of chromosomal testing and analysis. Recent studies have shown that using a second trimester ultrasound along with MSAFP testing had a higher detection rate than this quadruple marker screening test alone. Even higher detection rates can be achieved by looking for nuchal translucency. For that reason, many practitioners perform both ultrasound testing and serologic screening (ACOG, 2007a,b).

Universal screening should be offered to all women, because 90% of NTD cases occur in women with no risk factors. MSAFP screening detects approximately 85% of open neural tube defects. Most causes of NTDs are unknown; however, risk factors include a previous fetus with an NTD, maternal age less than 20 or greater than 35 years, primiparity or grandmultiparity, low socioeconomic status with nutritional deficiencies, English or Irish ancestry, and inadequate folic acid intake (Cunningham et al., 2010).

The MSAFP is the first marker used in the quadruple check. Most laboratories use a cutoff of 2 to 2.5 multiples of the mean (MoM) of AFP to define a test as abnormally high. The lower the cutoff, the greater the detection rate but also the higher the false-positive rate. Levels of 2.5 to 3.5 MoM are considered indiscriminate because both normal and abnormal fetuses typically test within this zone. Levels greater than 3.5 MoM are outside the normal distribution and are at high risk for a neural tube defect. Using a cutoff of 2 to 2.5 MoM would yield a 90% detection rate, resulting in 3% to 5% of positive screens with a 2% to 6% false-positive rate (Creasy et al., 2008). The majority of women with an elevated MSAFP do not have affected fetuses. In 90% to 95% of the group with an elevated MSAFP, the elevation is caused from other variables, such as incorrect gestational age, more than one fetus, other fetal anomalies such as gastroschisis (a hole in the abdominal wall that allows the abdominal contents to protrude outside the body), and fetal death (Cunningham et al., 2010).

The quadruple screen has also been used to screen for trisomy 21 (Down syndrome), which is the most common chromosomal abnormality found in live births, and for trisomy 18, which is less common, but usually results in death of the infant within the first year of life (see chapter 12 ∞). Unlike NTDs, the risk of Down syndrome and trisomy 18 increases with increasing maternal age; thus genetic counseling and diagnostic testing are usually offered to women who will be 35 years of age or older at their estimated date of birth (EDB).

Abnormal test results are generally defined as a calculated Down syndrome risk of 1 in 270 or 1 in 200 (depending on the laboratory). Women who have abnormal results are counseled about these risks and offered a diagnostic test such as amniocentesis, which is considered to be greater than 99% accurate in the diagnosis of chromosomal anomalies.

Screening tests require patient education and counseling to avoid confusion and undue stress. A key point for the nurse to understand and reinforce to the patient is that the MSAFP and the quadruple check are screening tests, and are ***not*** diagnostic. The nurse has an important role in educating the woman about various aspects of these tests. The importance of an accurate gestational age determination before taking the test cannot be overstated. A miscalculated gestational age may result in the incorrect interpretation of the MSAFP level, causing extreme stress to the woman and her family. In addition, further testing is required. An elevation of the MSAFP requires recalculation with an accurate gestational age and repeat test, and a low MSAFP may require an amniocentesis. The nurse also educates the patient on the importance of proper timing of the MSAFP. As stated earlier, the ideal time for screening is between 15 and 18 weeks. False-positives can occur with tests done either before or after this window in the gestation.

All healthcare providers should be sensitive to the ethical issues these screening tests present to the childbearing family. What benefit would knowing the results of an abnormal MSAFP provide? If the fetus has an NTD, the family and healthcare provider can use this information before the birth to choose the appropriate birth site or birth type. (An infant with an NTD would need to be born in a tertiary care center where immediate care could be given to the infant if needed.) Knowing an infant has Down syndrome would not necessarily change an obstetric decision about birth method or site, but it would give the family time for psychologic preparation, a chance to talk with social services and support groups, or the opportunity to opt for termination of the pregnancy.

Amniocentesis

Amniocentesis is a procedure used for genetic diagnosis. A sterile needle (under ultrasound guidance) is inserted into the uterine cavity through the maternal abdomen so a small amount of amniotic fluid can be removed, and genetic testing is performed. Amniocentesis is performed between 15 and 20 weeks' gestation. Two large studies in the United States and Canada have confirmed the safety and the 99% diagnostic accuracy of this procedure (Cunningham et al., 2010).

Amniocentesis

Amniocentesis can make chromosomal and biochemical determinations (enzyme analysis, AFP measurement for neural tube defects, blood typing, or cytogenetic, metabolic, or other DNA testing) and can validate abnormalities detected by ultrasound. Later in pregnancy, from about 30 to 39 weeks' gestation, amniocentesis may be done for lung maturity studies, such as lecithin/sphingomyelin ratio and the presence of phosphatidylglycerol and phosphatidylcholine (see discussion on p. 525) (Cunningham et al., 2010).

Indications for Amniocentesis

The following conditions are commonly considered indications for amniocentesis:

- Pregnant women who will be 35 or older on their due date. The risk of having an infant with a chromosomal problem such as Down syndrome increases with the age of the woman (see chapter 12 ∞).
- Couples who already have had a child with a birth defect or have a family history of certain birth defects.
- Pregnant women with other abnormal screening or genetic test results.

Procedure for Performing Amniocentesis

Amniocentesis is done on an outpatient basis but needs to be performed near a birthing area in case acute nonreassuring fetal status is encountered. The pregnant woman should be placed in a left lateral tilt position by placing a wedge under her right hip to prevent hypotension during the procedure.

The abdomen is scanned by ultrasound to locate the placenta, the fetus, and an adequate pocket of fluid. The needle insertion site is of the utmost importance because the fetus, placenta, umbilical cord, bladder, and uterine arteries must all be avoided (Figure 21-19 ■). The importance of locating the placenta cannot be stressed enough, especially in cases of Rh isoimmunization, in which trauma to the placenta increases fetal–maternal transfusion and worsens the isoimmunization (see chapter 20 ∞). If the amniocentesis is being performed in the last few weeks of pregnancy, the fetus may occupy what appears to be all the available space in the uterus, and there is a normal decrease in the amount of amniotic fluid; however, with the aid of ultrasound, fluid can be located. The amniocentesis is then done before the fetus has the opportunity to move.

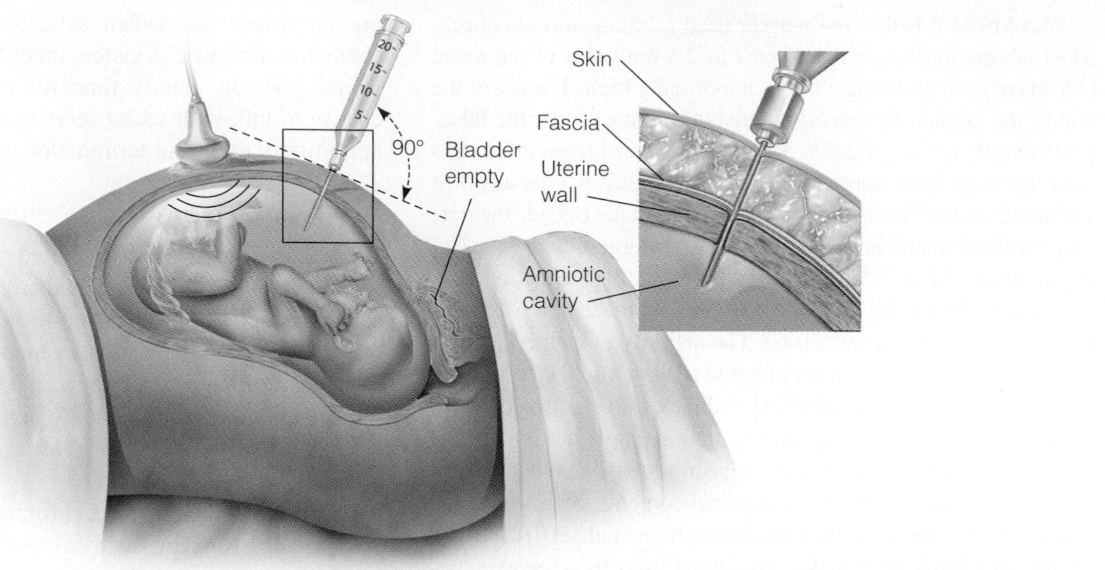

Figure 21-19 ■ Amniocentesis. The woman is usually scanned by ultrasound to determine the placental site and to locate a pocket of fluid. As the needle is inserted, three levels of resistance are felt when the needle penetrates the skin, fascia, and uterine wall. When the needle is placed within the amniotic cavity, amniotic fluid is withdrawn.

After the abdomen is scanned, the abdominal skin is cleansed with povidone-iodine (Betadine). The woman is given the option of a local anesthetic for the insertion site. A 22-gauge spinal needle is inserted into the uterine cavity. Generally, fluid immediately flows into the needle. The first few drops are discarded; a syringe is then attached to the needle, and the fluid is aspirated (Figure 21-20 ■). From 15 to 20 ml of amniotic fluid are withdrawn, placed in brown-tinted test tubes (to shield the fluid from light to prevent breakdown of bilirubin and other pigments), and sent to the laboratory for analysis. The needle is withdrawn using ultrasound, and the insertion site is evaluated for streaming (movement of fluid), which would indicate bleeding into the amniotic fluid. The FHR is monitored to assess fetal well-being. If the woman's vital signs and the FHR are normal, she is allowed to leave (see Procedure 21-3) (Cunningham et al., 2010).

If the collected amniotic fluid is contaminated with blood, the fluid should be centrifuged immediately. The woman is observed for alterations in the FHR. The blood should be tested to determine whether it is maternal or fetal.

Rh-negative women are given Rh immune globulin after amniocentesis, provided that they are not already sensitized.

Risks/Side Effects

Minor complications are infrequent and may include transient vaginal spotting, cramping, or amniotic fluid leakage in 1% to 2% of cases performed. Chorioamnionitis may occur in fewer than 1 in 1000 cases. Needle injuries to the fetus are rare when ultrasound guidance is used. Fetal loss rate is less than 0.5% (1 in 200) (Creasy et al., 2008). When early amniocentesis is performed (11 to 14 weeks) there is a higher pregnancy loss and complication rate than with traditional amniocentesis (Cunningham et al., 2010). This is due to the lack of membrane fusion to the uterine wall, which makes the puncture of the sac difficult, and to the fact that there is less fluid to withdraw (ACOG, 2007b).

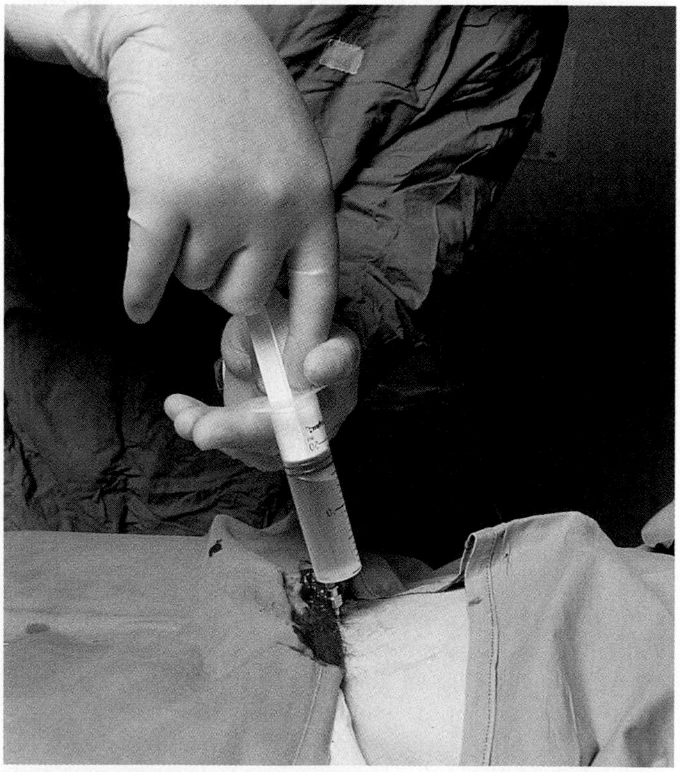

Figure 21-20 ■ During amniocentesis, amniotic fluid is aspirated into a syringe.

Source: © John Watney/Photo Researchers, Inc.

CLINICAL TIP

Have the woman lie on her left side to ensure adequate placental perfusion.

PROCEDURE 21-3 Assisting During Amniocentesis

NURSING ACTION

Preparation

- Explain the procedure and the indications for it and reassure the woman.
- Determine whether an informed consent form has been signed. If not, verify that the woman's doctor has explained the procedure and ask her to sign a consent form.

  Rationale: *It is the physician's responsibility to obtain informed consent. The woman's signature indicates her awareness of the risks and gives her consent to the procedure.*

Equipment and Supplies

22-gauge spinal needle with stylet

10- and 20-ml syringes

1% lidocaine (Xylocaine)

Povidone-iodine (Betadine)

Three 10-ml test tubes with tops (amber colored or covered with tape)

Rationale: *Amniotic fluid must be protected from light to prevent breakdown of bilirubin.*

Procedure: Sterile Gloves

1. Obtain baseline vital signs including maternal blood pressure (BP), pulse, respirations, temperature, and fetal heart rate (FHR) before procedure begins.
2. Monitor BP, pulse, respirations, and FHR every 15 minutes during procedure.

   Rationale: *Baseline information is essential to detect any changes in maternal or fetal status that might be related to the procedure.*
3. The physician uses real-time ultrasound to determine the location of the placenta and to locate a pocket of amniotic fluid. Provide gel for the ultrasound and assist with the procedure as needed.
4. Cleanse the woman's abdomen.

   Rationale: *Cleansing the abdomen before needle insertion helps decrease the risk of infection.*
5. The physician dons gloves, inserts the needle into the identified pocket of fluid (see Figure 21-19), and withdraws a sample.
6. Obtain the test tubes from the physician. Label the tubes with the woman's correct identification and send to the lab with the appropriate lab slips.
7. Monitor the woman and reassess her vital signs.
   - Determine the woman's BP, pulse, respirations, and the FHR.
   - Palpate the woman's fundus to assess for uterine contractions.
   - Monitor her using an external fetal monitor for 20 to 30 minutes after the amniocentesis.
   - Determine a treatment course to counteract any supine hypotension and to increase venous return and cardiac output.

   Rationale: *Monitoring maternal and fetal status postprocedure provides information about response to the procedure and helps detect any complications such as inadvertent fetal puncture.*
8. Assess the woman's blood type and determine any need for Rh immune globulin.
9. Administer Rh immune globulin if indicated (see Procedure 20.2 on page 482).

   Rationale: *To prevent Rh sensitization in an Rh-negative woman, Rh immune globulin is administered prophylactically involving amniocentesis.*
10. Instruct the woman to report any of the following changes or symptoms to her primary caregiver:
    - Unusual fetal hyperactivity or, conversely, any lack of fetal movement
    - Vaginal discharge—either clear drainage or bleeding
    - Uterine contractions or abdominal pain
    - Fever or chills

    Rationale: *These are signs of potential complications and require further evaluation.*
11. Encourage the woman to engage only in light activities for 24 hours and to increase her fluid intake.

    Rationale: *Decreased maternal activity helps decrease uterine irritability and increase uteroplacental circulation. Increased fluid intake helps replace amniotic fluid through the uteroplacental circulation.*
12. Complete the client record. Record the type of procedure, the date and time, and the name of the physician who performed the procedure. Also record the maternal-fetal response, disposition of the specimen, and discharge teaching.

Documentation

The nurse documents maternal and fetal responses to the procedure. Maternal vital signs, including level of discomfort, should be recorded. The FHR, presence of contractions, bleeding, and fluid leakage should be documented. Discharge instructions and abnormal symptoms that need to be reported to the physician should also be documented.

NURSING CARE MANAGEMENT

The nurse assists the physician during the amniocentesis (see Procedure 21-3: Assisting During Amniocentesis). In addition, the nurse supports the woman undergoing amniocentesis. Women are usually apprehensive about the procedure as well as about the information that will be obtained. The physician explains the procedure before the woman signs the consent form. As it is being performed, the woman may need additional emotional support. She may become anxious during the procedure. She may also become lightheaded, nauseated, and diaphoretic from lying on her back with a heavy uterus compressing the abdominal vessels, so it is important to have her in a lateral tilt with a wedge placed under her right hip. The nurse can provide support to the woman by further clarifying the physician's instructions or explanations, by relieving the woman's physical discomfort when possible, and by responding verbally and physically to the woman's need for reassurance.

Chorionic Villus Sampling

Much like amniocentesis, **chorionic villus sampling (CVS)** is a procedure that is used to detect genetic, metabolic, and DNA abnormalities. CVS involves obtaining a small sample (5 to 40 mg) of chorionic villi from the edge of the developing placenta. CVS is performed in some medical centers for first trimester diagnosis after 9 completed weeks (ACOG, 2007b). Villi in the chorion frondosum, present from 8 to 12 weeks' gestation, are believed to reflect fetal chromosome, enzyme, and DNA content, thereby permitting earlier diagnosis than can be obtained by amniocentesis. CVS cannot detect neural tube defects, however, and the MSAFP test should still be performed at 16 weeks.

Risks and Benefits of CVS

The woman should be aware of the risks and benefits of CVS. There is a spontaneous abortion risk of 0.3% in cases. This rate is only slightly higher than the 0.1% in cases of a second-trimester amniocentesis (Cunningham et al., 2010). Other references cite 0.5% to 1.0% of CVS procedures and 0.25% to 0.50% of amniocentesis procedures. There is also an incidence of 1 in 3000 births of fetal limb reduction defects (a portion of a finger or a toe is missing), especially when the CVS is performed before 9 1/2 weeks' gestation. Therefore, it is not recommended that CVS be performed before 10 weeks' gestation (ACOG, 2007b).

Additional risks of CVS include failure to obtain tissue, rupture of membranes, leakage of amniotic fluid, vaginal spotting or bleeding, chorioamnionitis (0.5% of cases), intrauterine infection, maternal tissue contamination of the specimen, oromandibular defects, and Rh isoimmunization. Rh-negative women are given Rh immune globulin to cover the risk of immunization from the procedure (Cunningham et al., 2010).

Like amniocentesis, CVS can detect fetal karyotype, hemoglobinopathies (e.g., sickle cell anemia and alpha and some beta thalassemias), phenylketonuria, alpha antitrypsin deficiency, Down syndrome, Duchenne muscular dystrophy, and factor IX deficiency. Early sex determination can be made so that pregnancies with a male fetus who would be affected in X-linked disorders can be identified (Creasy et al., 2008). Because NTDs are not diagnosed by this test, all mothers undergoing CVS should be offered MSAFP screening at 15 to 20 weeks' gestation. A major disadvantage of the earlier testing (CVS) is that if a woman later has an abnormal MSAFP test indicating an increased risk of NTDs, she may then have to undergo an amniocentesis, thus again putting the fetus at risk with an additional invasive procedure.

One of the greatest advantages to a woman undergoing this procedure is earlier diagnosis and decreased waiting time for results. Whereas amniocentesis is not done until at least 16 weeks' gestation, CVS is performed between 10 and 12 weeks. The CVS results are obtained in 24 hours if the direct preparation method is used and in 7 to 10 days when tissue culture is used. Earlier diagnosis may relieve many of the personal, social, and psychologic concerns of families, particularly if therapeutic abortion is being considered. There may be less emotional stress involved with having an abortion at an earlier stage of gestation. First trimester abortions are also easier to perform, require less time, and are less costly.

Procedure for CVS

Before CVS, an ultrasound is done to determine placental location, uterine position (retroverted or anteverted), and presence of intervening structures (i.e., bowel, blood vessels). Various equipment can be used to aspirate chorionic villi from the placenta.

After counseling regarding diagnosis and procedure techniques, preliminary blood work may be obtained. The morning of the procedure, the woman is asked to drink fluids to fill her bladder because displacement of an anteverted uterus by a full bladder may aid in positioning the uterus for catheter insertion. Ultrasound is used to determine uterine position, cervical position, gestational sac size, and crown-rump length measurement and to identify the area of placental formation and cord insertion.

For the transcervical CVS the woman is placed in lithotomy position, the vulva is cleansed with povidone-iodine solution (Betadine), and a sterile speculum is inserted into the vagina. The vaginal vault and cervix are cleansed with the same solution to decrease contamination from the vagina into the uterus. The anterior lip of the cervix is sometimes grasped with a tenaculum to aid in straightening anteflexion of the uterus. The catheter (or cannula) is slowly inserted under ultrasound guidance through the endocervix to the sampling site at the extra-amniotic placental edge (outside the gestational sac). The obturator is withdrawn from the catheter. A 30-ml syringe, containing 3 to 4 ml of tissue culture medium with heparin, is attached, and a sample of villi is aspirated by using a pressure of 20 to 30 ml. The contents of the syringe are flushed into a petri dish containing nutrient medium, and the villi are inspected microscopically and prepared for cell culture.

For the transabdominal sampling, the woman is placed in the supine position. After the skin is cleansed with Betadine and local anesthesia is given, an 18- or 20-gauge needle is inserted percutaneously through the maternal abdominal wall and uterine myometrium. The tip of the needle is advanced into the long axis of the chorion frondosum under ultrasound guidance. Chorionic villi are obtained by repeated, rapid aspirations of the syringe containing tissue culture medium and heparin.

A normal CVS result indicating normal chromosomal configuration in the first trimester does not ensure a healthy infant. Routine prenatal care and appropriate follow-up are needed. Follow-up ultrasound and lab evaluation of each pregnancy must be done after performance of this procedure to evaluate fetal status. Further neonatal follow-up studies are necessary to evaluate the long-term effects of this technique.

Through the Eyes of a Nurse Genetic Testing Options in Pregnancy

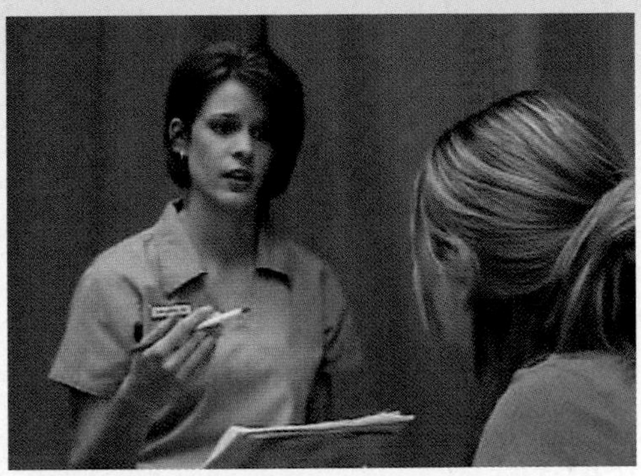

Family's Experience

"There seems like there are so many tests available, we are really confused about what to do. We don't feel like we have any risk factors, but we want to make sure our baby is healthy. What tests should we get? Which ones do we really need?"

Nurse's Response

"There are various testing options. I can explain your options and help you weigh the pros and cons of each test. Because of your age and the fact that you do not have any risk factors identified in your medical or family history, you would not be a candidate for the amniocentesis or chorionic villus sampling tests. You may want to consider the other optional tests though, such as the quadruple screen, nuchal translucency test, and cystic fibrosis testing.

"The quadruple screen is a test that screens for neural tube defects and trisomy 18 and 21. This test is only a screening tool, which means it does not tell you if your baby *definitely* has one of these problems. It could help us know if your baby is at risk though. The test is not perfect and you can get false-positives or false-negatives. If the test did come back abnormal, you have other testing options such as a more detailed sonogram or an amniocentesis.

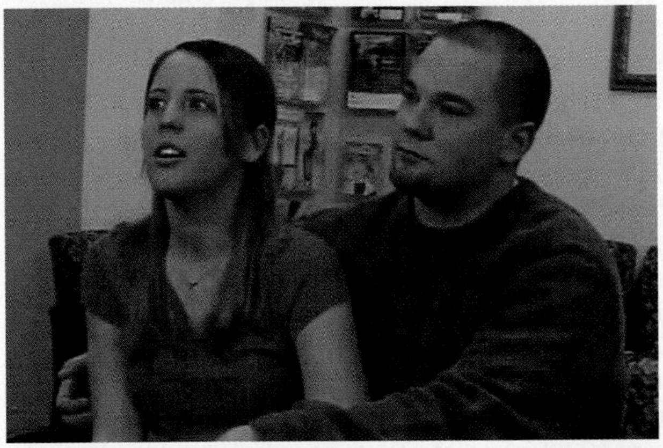

"The nuchal translucency test is a blood test and sonogram combined that screens for trisomy 18 and 21. The test is more accurate than the quadruple screen and is done earlier. Some insurance may not cover the test though, so you will need to call your insurance company to see if it is covered.

"The cystic fibrosis test screens for known gene mutations that cause cystic fibrosis. If your screen is positive, we will then have the father of the baby tested to determine if he is also a carrier. If you are both carriers, there is a 25% chance that the baby could have the disease. If only one of you is a carrier, there would be a chance the baby would also be a carrier, but the baby could not inherit the disease."

Nurse's Actions and Rationale

The nurse's role is to explain all testing options and to answer questions related to the various tests. The nurse presents the information in an objective manner without expressing a personal opinion. The couple must weigh each choice carefully and determine what tests are right for them. The nurse can also provide written resource material to the couple. The couple should be allowed to discuss the information and make an informed decision.

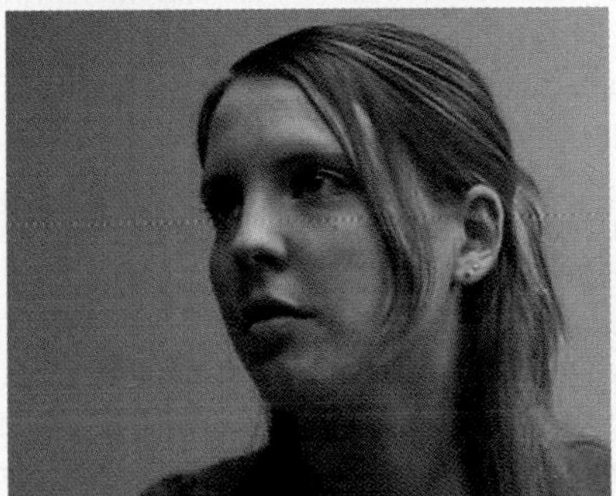

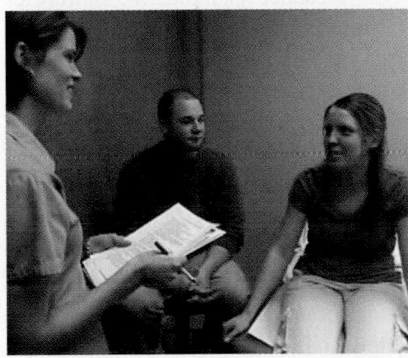

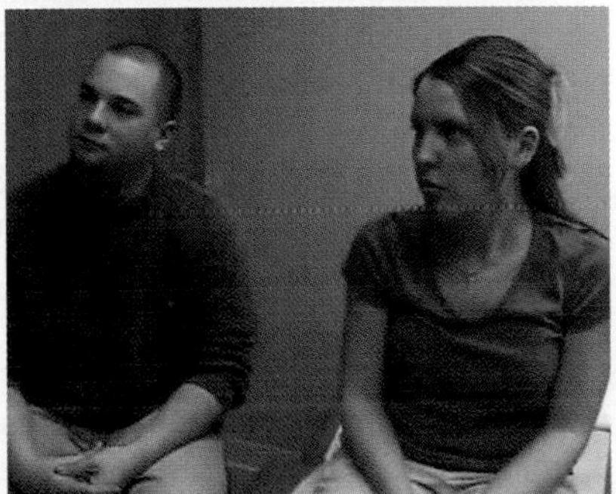

NURSING CARE MANAGEMENT

Before the test, the nurse ascertains the woman's understanding of CVS, its uses, the procedure, and the possible results. The nurse provides opportunities for questions and acts as an advocate when additional questions or concerns are raised. The nurse completes assessments following the procedure, including monitoring for vaginal bleeding or fluid leakage, excessive cramping, and basic maternal vital signs.

The nurse supports the woman or couple and encourages them to express any feelings and fears regarding the procedure and also regarding the decision-making process if abortion is being considered. That supportive role continues if abortion is chosen, even though the nurse may not be present for the procedure. It is important that support be provided following the procedure by the nurse who established a relationship with the couple previously.

Cordocentesis

Cordocentesis (also called *percutaneous umbilical blood sampling [PUBS]*) is a technique used to obtain pure fetal blood from the umbilical cord while the fetus is in utero. This procedure has been used for diagnosis of hemophilias, hemoglobinopathies, fetal infections, chromosome abnormalities, nonimmune hydrops, and isoimmune hemolytic disorders, as well as assessment of fetal hemoglobin and hematocrit for calculation of transfusion requirements in the second and third trimesters (Acar et al., 2007). During the 1990s, PUBS was used more frequently; however, its use is now more limited to the diagnosis of anemia and for treatment of fetal anemia when hemoglobin levels fall below 10 g/dl or hematocrit is less than 30%. Although now less commonly used, cordocentesis can also be used for the following (Creasy et al., 2008):

- Rapid fetal karyotyping and genotyping
- Diagnosis of fetal infection (cytomegalovirus, toxoplasmosis, parvovirus, rubella)
- Platelet disorders
- Fetal blood grouping
- Diagnosis and treatment of isoimmunization
- Assessment of fetal well-being (pH, Po_2)
- Fetal metabolic disorders

The woman is scanned with an ultrasound transducer with sterile probe cover. A 25-gauge spinal needle is inserted into her abdomen through the skin alongside the transducer and into the fetal umbilical vein approximately 1 to 2 cm from the insertion of the cord into the placenta. The stylet is removed from the needle, and fetal blood is aspirated into a syringe containing an anticoagulant. Red blood cell size is determined to distinguish fetal from maternal cells. A paralytic agent, such as pancuronium bromide (Pavulon), may be given to prevent fetal movement during the procedure. If the mother is given a medication to help her relax, care must be taken to avoid oversedating her and causing deep breathing. Deep chest/diaphragmatic respirations can interfere with accurate puncture of the umbilical vein (Creasy et al., 2008).

Application: Fetal Lung Maturity

Within the last 10 years, improvements in ultrasonographic technique have made PUBS a relatively safe procedure with overall fetal loss rate less than 2%. The complication rate after PUBS is less than 0.5%. Complications include failure to obtain a sample, bleeding from the sampling site, premature rupture of membranes, chorioamnionitis, and fetal bradycardia (Acar et al., 2007). PUBS is used with less and less frequency because newer tests have replaced the need for a direct fetal sample.

NURSING CARE MANAGEMENT

The nurse collaborates with other members of the healthcare team to provide care for the woman for whom PUBS is recommended. Although a genetic counselor and/or obstetrician will have explained the risk for genetic defects and other disorders, the woman and her partner may need help to understand the procedure and its risks. They may need anticipatory guidance to help lessen their anxiety, as well as emotional support during the procedure and follow-up evaluation and testing. Support can come in many forms, including encouraging relaxation, providing reassurance, and giving the woman information throughout the procedure. The nurse may need to assist with coordination of financial and social service resources. The nurse can help promote relaxation during the procedure by instructing the woman in shallow breathing techniques. The nurse completes assessments during and immediately following the procedure and in some cases performs an NST test following the procedure.

Fetal Fibronectin

Fetal fibronectin (fFN) is a glycoprotein produced by the trophoblast and other fetal tissues. The absence of cervicovaginal fFN between 20 and 34 weeks' gestation has been shown to be a strong predictor of a woman not experiencing preterm birth due to spontaneous preterm labor or premature rupture of membranes. Positive findings indicate a 99% probability of birth within the next 2 weeks (Cunningham et al., 2010). Positive findings should lead to follow-up including a sterile speculum exam, nitrazine testing, and an evaluation of a slide of cervico-vaginal secretions to assess for the presence of ferning, which would indicate the prescence of amniotic fluid. Levels of fFN can be measured with an enzyme immunoassay. Its presence is indicative of further evaluation, such as an ultrasound for cervical length, funneling, dilatation, and cultures to rule out an infectious process. Because vaginal examinations, sexual intercourse within the previous 24 hours, some vaginal creams, and medications can cause false findings, these should be avoided prior to fFN testing.

Evaluation of Fetal Lung Maturity

In managing the woman and fetus at risk, the physician is constantly faced with the possibility of having to induce the birth of an infant before term and before the onset of labor. There are many indications for early termination of pregnancy, including repeat cesarean birth, premature rupture of membranes, diabetes, hypertensive conditions in the pregnant woman, and placental insufficiency. Unfortunately, the most common cause of perinatal mortality is prematurity, especially in infants weighing 1500 g or less and with particular complications arising from pulmonary immaturity (Cunningham et al., 2010). Birth of an infant with immature pulmonary function frequently results in respiratory distress syndrome (RDS), also known as *hyaline membrane disease* (see chapter 34 ∞).

Because gestational age, birth weight, and the rate of development of organ systems do not necessarily correspond, it may be necessary to determine the lung maturation of the fetus by amniotic fluid analysis before elective childbirth. In these cases, amniocentesis is performed, and concentrations of certain phospholipids in the amniotic fluid are measured. In many cases, birth of the infant can be delayed until the lungs show maturity.

Lecithin/Sphingomyelin Ratio

The alveoli of the lungs are lined by a substance called **surfactant**, which is composed of phospholipids. Surfactant lowers the surface tension of the alveoli during extrauterine respiratory exhalation. By lowering the alveolar surface tension, surfactant stabilizes the alveoli, and a certain amount of air always remains in the alveoli during expiration (Cunningham et al., 2010). When a newborn with mature pulmonary function takes his or her first breath, a tremendously high pressure is needed to open the lungs. Upon breathing out, the lungs do not collapse, and about half the air in the alveoli is retained. An infant born too early, when synthesis of surfactant is incomplete, is unable to maintain lung stability, resulting in underinflation of the lungs and development of RDS.

Fetal lung maturity can be assessed by determining the ratio of two components of surfactant—lecithin and sphingomyelin. Early in pregnancy the lecithin concentration in amniotic fluid is less than that of sphingomyelin (0.5:1 at 20 weeks), resulting in a low **lecithin/sphingomyelin (L/S) ratio**. At about 30 to 32 weeks' gestation, the amounts of the two substances become equal (1:1). The concentration of lecithin begins to exceed that of sphingomyelin, and at 35 weeks the L/S ratio is 2:1. When at least two times as much lecithin as sphingomyelin is found in the amniotic fluid, RDS is very unlikely (Creasy et al., 2008). Clinical outcomes, including respiratory distress and other respiratory disorders, should be correlated in individual institutions before specific ratios indicating pulmonary maturity are accepted. Infants of diabetic mothers (IDMs) are an exception to this finding and have a high incidence of false-positive results (i.e., the L/S ratio is thought to indicate lung maturity, but after birth the baby develops RDS). Although the same ratios are used, it is important to remember that even when IDMs are term (greater than 37 weeks' gestational age), delayed lung maturation can occur because the high blood sugars interfere with biochemical development. A delay in lung maturation has also been found in babies whose mothers have nonhypertensive renal disease and isoimmunization (Creasy et al., 2008).

Some types of chronic intrauterine fetal stress cause an acceleration of lung maturation in the fetus. Prolonged rupture of membranes (over 24 hours) results in acceleration of lung maturation by approximately 1 week and therefore has a protective effect. Although the L/S ratio is the most universally used test for evaluating pulmonary maturity, the results are not accurate when blood or meconium contaminates the amniotic fluid (ACOG, 2008).

The L/S ratio remains a cumbersome and labor-intensive test despite numerous changes to the original technique. Moreover, improper handling can affect results. For these reasons, many institutions are looking to other fetal lung maturity tests that are being developed.

Phosphatidylglycerol

Phosphatidylglycerol (PG) is the second most abundant phospholipid in surfactant. PG appears at about 36 weeks' gestation and increases in amount until term. In instances of diabetes complicated by premature rupture of membranes, vascular disease, or severe preeclampsia, PG may be present before 35 weeks' gestation. PG is not measured in specific concentrations; rather, the mere presence of this substance is associated with very low risk of RDS, and the absence of PG is associated with the development of RDS (Creasy et al., 2008).

PG determination is also useful in blood-contaminated specimens. Because PG is not present in blood or vaginal fluids, its presence in a vaginal specimen is reliable for indicating lung maturity.

In recent years lung maturity has been most frequently assessed by a combination of L/S ratio and PG. Lung maturity apparently can be confirmed in most pregnancies if PG is present in conjunction with an L/S ratio of 2:1.

Fluorescence Polarization

The fluorescence polarization (TDx-FLM II) test was developed in the 1990s and utilizes fluorescence polarization to measure the ratio of surfactant to albumin (S/A) in uncentrifuged amniotic fluid. The results are reported quantitatively in mg/g. The test has been used as a predictive indicator for predicting RDS in preterm infants. Values greater than 55 mg/g in a non-diabetic woman (or greater than 70 mg/g in a diabetic woman) indicate fetal lung maturity. The test can be conducted in 1 hour or less. Although blood and amniotic fluid can interfere with the findings, it should not result in immature results being reported as mature findings. Amniotic fluid collected vaginally that indicates fetal lung maturity should be considered accurate (Cunningham et al., 2010).

Care Plan Activity: Monitoring Well-Being of a Slow-Developing Fetus

NURSING CARE MANAGEMENT

In women whose amniotic membranes are prematurely ruptured, a vaginal specimen is obtained for analysis. The nurse assists the certified nurse-midwife or physician by gathering appropriate supplies. Typically, a sterile speculum, a light source, a sterile syringe or a nasogastric tube, and appropriate collection tubes are needed. The nurse positions the woman for the speculum exam while providing information about the collection process. The nurse places the woman in a lithotomy position and places her legs in stirrups. If stirrups are not available, the nurse can place a bedpan upside down and position the woman with her buttocks on the bedpan to facilitate collection of the vaginal fluid. The certified nurse-midwife or physician gathers vaginal secretions with a syringe and places the specimen in a collection tube (Cunningham et al., 2010).

In women undergoing early birth for medical indications (uncontrolled preeclampsia or eclampsia or uncontrolled diabetes) when the amniotic membranes are intact, evaluation of fetal lung maturity may be obtained through amniocentesis. See previous discussion on page 521 regarding nursing care management for the woman undergoing amniocentesis.

FOCUS YOUR STUDY

- Nurses often play a key role not only in teaching families about various testing procedures, but also in providing clarity and emotional support to the woman and her family undergoing antenatal testing.
- Ultrasound offers a valuable means of assessing intrauterine fetal growth because the growth can be followed over a period of time. It is noninvasive and painless, allows the physician to study the gestation serially, is nonradiating to both the woman and her fetus, and to date has shown no known harmful effects.
- Using ultrasound, the gestational sac may be detected as early as 5 or 6 weeks after the last menstrual period. Measurement of the crown-rump length in early pregnancy is most useful for accurate dating of a pregnancy. The most important and frequently used ultrasound measurements in the second trimester are biparietal diameter, head circumference, abdominal circumference, and femur length.
- Maternal assessment of fetal activity is very useful as a screening procedure in evaluation of fetal status.
- A nonstress test (NST) measures fetal heart rate (FHR) during fetal activity; FHR normally increases in response to fetal activity. The desired result is a reactive test.
- A contraction stress test (CST) provides a method for observing the response of the FHR to the stress of uterine contractions. The desired result is a negative test.
- A fetal biophysical profile (BPP) includes five fetal variables (breathing movement, body movement, tone, amniotic fluid volume, and FHR reactivity). It assesses the fetus at risk for intrauterine compromise.
- Aneuploidy screening includes nuchal translucency and PAPP-A and Beta hCG or quadruple screening of AFP, hCG, diameric inhibin-A, and estriol.
- Amniocentesis can be used to obtain amniotic fluid for testing. A variety of tests is available to evaluate the presence of disease, genetic conditions, and fetal maturity.
- Chorionic villus sampling is a procedure that obtains fetal karyotype in the first trimester. It is used to diagnose hemoglobinopathies (e.g., sickle cell anemia and alpha and some beta thalassemias), phenylketonuria, alpha antitrypsin deficiency, Down syndrome, Duchenne muscular dystrophy, and factor IX deficiency.
- Percutaneous umbilical blood sampling (PUBS) is a technique used in the second and third trimesters for fetal diagnosis, assessment, and therapy.
- The lecithin/sphingomyelin (L/S) ratio of the amniotic fluid can be used to assess fetal lung maturity. The presence of phosphatidylglycerol may also provide information about fetal lung maturity. The fluorescence polarization (TDx-FLM II) test can be used as a predictive indicator for predicting RDS in preterm infants.

CRITICAL THINKING IN ACTION

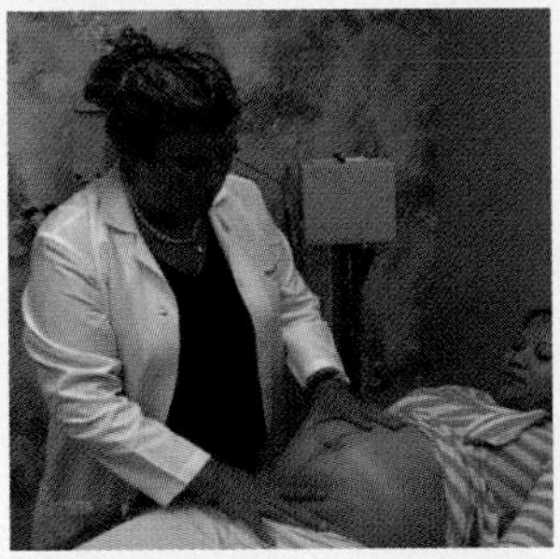

Patricia Adams is a 20-year-old, married, G2, P0010 at 36 weeks' gestation with gestational diabetes. She presents to you during her prenatal visit with a complaint of decreased fetal movement for the "last day or so." Her OB history includes a 13 lb weight gain, hematocrit of 29%, diastolic BP ranging 80–96 mm Hg, and 1+ proteinuria. A 19-week ultrasound demonstrated no fetal anatomic defects. A hemoglobin A_1c at 23 weeks was 5.8%. Patricia has had weekly NST since 28 weeks' gestation. You place Patricia on the fetal monitor for an NST. You obtain vital signs of T 97°F, P 88, R 14, BP 130/88. After 30 minutes you observe that the fetal heart rate baseline is 160–165, long-term variability is decreased, and repetitive variable decelerations are occurring. No contractions are noted. The fetus is very active. You notify the physician of the fetal heart rate baseline and unsatisfactory NST. The physician orders a biophysical profile (BPP) for fetal well-being. You describe and explain the biophysical profile test to Patricia.

1. How would you describe and explain the biophysical profile test?
2. To heighten Patricia's awareness of fetal movement, how would you instruct her to do a daily fetal movement record (FMR)?
3. Explain when Patricia should contact her care provider.
4. Discuss the significance of fetal movement.
5. Explore factors that decrease fetal movements.

See www.nursing.pearsonhighered.com for possible responses.

Pearson Nursing Student Resources

Find additional review materials at
www.nursing.pearsonhighered.com

Prepare for success with additional NCLEX®-style practice questions, interactive assignments and activities, Web links, animations and videos, and more!

REFERENCES

Abramowicz, J. S. (2007). Prenatal exposure to ultarasound waves: Is there a risk? *Ultrasound in Obstetrics & Gynecology, 29,* 363.

Acar, A., Balci, O., Gezginc, K., Onder, C., Capar, M., Zamani, A., & Acar, A. (2007). Evaluation of the results of cordocentesis. *Taiwanese Journal of Obstetrics & Gynecology, 46*(4), 405–409.

American College of Obstetricians and Gynecologists (ACOG). (2007a). *Invasive prenatal testing for aneuploidy* (ACOG Practice Bulletin No 88). Washington, DC: Author.

American College of Obstetricians and Gynecologists (ACOG). (2007b). *Screening for fetal chromosomal abnormalities* (ACOG Practice Bulletin No. 77). Washington, DC: Author.

American College of Obstetricians and Gynecologists (ACOG). (2008). *Fetal lung maturity* (ACOG Practice Bulletin No 97). Washington, DC: Author.

American College of Obstetricians and Gynecologists (ACOG). (2009). *Ultrasonography in pregnancy* (ACOG Practice Bulletin No. 101). Washington, DC: Author.

American College of Radiology (ACR). (2007). Practice guideline for the performance of obstetrical ultrasound. Retrieved from http://www.acr.org/SecondaryMainMenuCategories%2fquality_safety%2fguidelines%2fus%2fus_obstetrical.aspx

American Institute for Ultrasound in Medicine (AIUM). (2008a). Prudent use of ultrasound in obstetrics. Retrieved from http://www.aium.org/publications/viewStatement.aspX?id=33

American Institute for Ultrasound in Medicine (AIUM). (2008b). Ultrasonography in pregnancy. *Obstetrics & Gynecology, 112,* 951.

American Public Health Association. (2009). U.S. lagging behind many other nations on infant mortality rates: Healthy behavior, healthier babies. Retrieved from http://www.apha.org/publications/tnh/archives/2009/February09/Nation/BabiesNAT.htm

Blackburn, S. T. (2007). *Maternal, fetal, & neonatal physiology: A clinical perspective* (3rd ed.). St. Louis, MO: Saunders.

Coppus, S. F., Langenveld, J., & Oei, S. G. (2007). An underestimated technique for the management of shoulder dystocia: The all-fours manoeuvre. *Nederlands Tijdschrift Voor Geneeskunde 151*(27), 1493–1497.

Creasy, R. K., Resnik, R., Iams, J. D., Lockwood, C. J., & Moore, T. R. (2008). Creasy & Resnik's *Maternal fetal medicine: Principles and practice* (6th ed.). Philadelphia, PA: Saunders.

Cunningham, F. G., Leveno, K. J., Bloom, S. L., Hauth, J. C., Gilstrap, L. C., & Wenstrom, K. D. (2010). *Williams obstetrics* (23rd ed.). New York, NY: McGraw-Hill.

Devoe, L. D. (2008). Antenatal fetal assessment: Contraction stress test, nonstress test, vibroacoustic stimulation, amniotic fluid volume, biophysical profile, and modified biophysical profile—an overview. *Seminars In Perinatology, 32*(4), 247–252.

Flenady, V., MacPhail, J., Gardener, G., Chadha, Y., Mahomed, K., Heazell, A., . . . , Frøen, F. (2009). Detection and management of decreased fetal movements in Australia and New Zealand: A survey of obstetric practice. *The Australian & New Zealand Journal of Obstetrics & Gynaecology, 49*(4), 358–363.

Gabbe, S. G., Simpson, J. L. , Niebyl, J. R., Galan, H., Goetzl, L., Jauniaux, E. R. M., & Landon, M. (2007). *Normal and problem pregnancies* (5th ed.). Philadelphia, PA: Churchill Livingstone.

Harpel, T. S. (2008). Fear of the unknown: Ultrasound and anxiety about fetal health. *Health, 12*(3), 295–312.

Hobbins, J. C. (2007). *Obstetric ultrasound: Artistry in practice.* San Francisco, CA: Wiley-Blackwell.

Hoffman, C. S., Messer, L. C., Mendola, P., Savitz, D. A., Herring, A. H., & Hartmann, K. E. (2008). Comparison of gestational age at birth based on last menstrual period and ultrasound during the first trimester. *Paediatric and Perinatal Epidemiology, 22*(6), 587–596.

Kiserud, T., Ebbing, C., Kessler, J., & Rasmussen, S. (2007). Fetal cardiac output, distribution to the placenta and impact of placental compromise. *Ultrasound In Obstetrics & Gynecology, 28*(2), 126–136.

March of Dimes. (2009). Birth defects. Retrieved from http://www.marchofdimes.com/pnhec/4439_1206.asp

McAuliffe, F. M., Fong, K. W., Toi, A., Chitayat, D., Keating, S., & Johnson, J. (2005, September). Ultrasound detection of fetal anomalies in conjunction with first-trimester nuchal translucency screening: A feasibility study. *American Journal of Obstetrics & Gynecology, 193*(3, Pt. 2), 1260–1265.

Nahum, G. G. (2007). Estimation of fetal weight. Retrieved from http://emedicine.medscape.com/article/262865-overview

Peterson, S. G., Wong, S. F., Urs, P., Gray, P. H., & Gardner, G. J. (2009). Early onset, severe fetal growth restriction with absent or reversed end-diastolic flow velocity waveform in the umbilical artery: Perinatal and long-term outcomes. *Australian and New Zealand Journal of Obstetrics and Gynaecology, 49*(1), 45–51.

Seungdamrong, A., Purohit, M., McCulloh, D. H., Howland, R. D., Colon, J. M., & McGovern, P. G. (2008). Fetal cardiac activity at 4 weeks after in vitro fertilization predicts successful completion of the first trimester of pregnancy. *Fertility and Sterility, 90*(5), 1711–1715.

Simpson, K. R., & Creehan, P. A. (2008). *AWHONN's perinatal nursing* (4th ed.). Washington, D.C.: AWHONN.

Torloni, M. R., Vedmedovska, N., & Merialdi, M., et al. (2009). Safety of ultrasonography in pregnancy: WHO systematic review of the literature and meta-analysis. *Ultrasound in Obstetrics & Gynecology, 33,* 502.

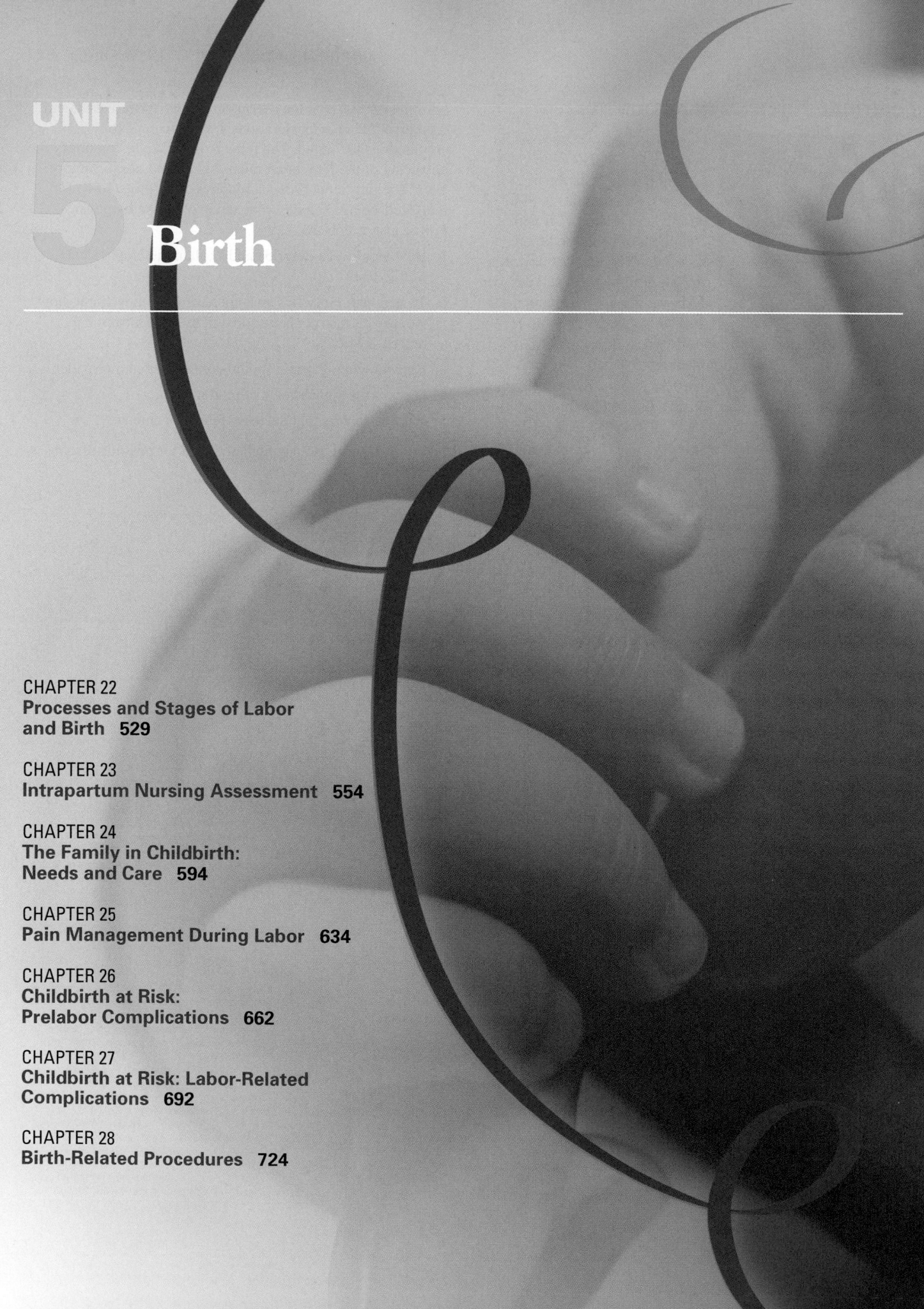

UNIT 5

Birth

CHAPTER 22

Processes and Stages of Labor and Birth

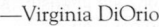

Just as a woman's heart knows how and when to pump, her lungs to inhale, and her hand to pull back from fire, so she knows when and how to give birth.

—Virginia DiOrio

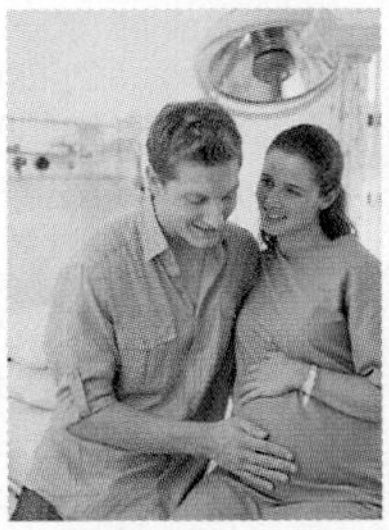

LEARNING OUTCOMES

1. Examine the five critical factors that affect the labor process.
2. Describe the physiology of labor.
3. Discuss premonitory signs of labor.
4. Differentiate between false and true labor.
5. Describe the characteristics of the four stages of labor and their accompanying phases.
6. Describe the physiologic and psychosocial changes that are indicative of the maternal progress during each of the stages of labor.
7. Summarize maternal systemic responses to labor.
8. Describe fetal adaptations to labor.

KEY TERMS

Bloody show *540*
Cardinal movements *543*
Cervical dilatation *539*
Crowning *543*
Duration *537*
Effacement *539*
Engagement *534*
Fetal attitude *531*
Fetal lie *532*
Fetal position *534*
Fetal presentation *533*
Fontanelle *531*
Frequency *537*
Intensity *537*
Lightening *540*
Malpresentations *533*
Molding *531*
Presenting part *533*
Rupture of membranes (ROM) *540*
Spontaneous rupture of membranes (SROM) *540*
Station *534*
Sutures *531*

In the final weeks of pregnancy, both mother and baby begin to prepare for birth. The fetus develops and grows in readiness for life outside the womb. The expectant woman undergoes various physiologic and psychosocial changes that gradually prepare her for childbirth and for the role of mother. The onset of labor begins a remarkable change in the relationship between the woman and her baby. During labor, particularly at the end, a woman instinctively knows she is engaging in one of the most important tasks she will ever do. A precious life is about to emerge. In those hours and moments the birth process may seem to carry all the power in the universe. The mother-to-be and her partner may be stretched beyond all of their normal limits of concentration, purpose, endurance, and pain. The dynamic nature of this experience is what makes the birth of a baby both a physiologic and a psychosocial transition into parenthood.

Critical Factors in Labor

Five factors are important in the process of labor and birth: the birth passageway (birth canal), the passenger (fetus), the physiologic forces of labor, the position of the mother, and the woman's psychosocial considerations (Table 22-1). The progress of labor is critically dependent on the complementary relationship of these five factors. Abnormalities that affect any component of these critical forces can alter the outcome of labor and jeopardize both the expectant woman and her baby. Complications during labor and birth are discussed in chapter 27 ∞.

TABLE 22-1 Critical Factors in Labor

1. **Birth passage**
   - Size of the maternal pelvis (diameters of the pelvic inlet, midpelvis, and outlet)
   - Type of maternal pelvis (gynecoid, android, anthropoid, platypelloid, or a combination)
   - Ability of the cervix to dilate and efface and ability of the vaginal canal and the external opening of the vagina (the introitus) to distend
2. **Fetus**
   - Fetal head (size and presence of molding)
   - Fetal attitude (flexion or extension of the fetal body and extremities)
   - Fetal lie
   - Fetal presentation (the body part of the fetus entering the pelvis in a single or multiple pregnancy)
3. **The relationship between the passage and the fetus**
   - Engagement of the fetal presenting part
   - Station (location of fetal presenting part in the maternal pelvis)
   - Fetal position (relationship of the presenting part to one of the four quadrants of the maternal pelvis)
4. **Physiologic forces of labor**
   - Frequency, duration, and intensity of uterine contractions as the fetus moves through the passage
   - Effectiveness of the maternal pushing effort
5. **Psychosocial considerations**
   - Mental and physical preparation for childbirth
   - Sociocultural values and beliefs
   - Previous childbirth experience
   - Support from significant others
   - Emotional status

Birth Passageway

The true pelvis and soft tissues of the cervix, vagina, and the pelvic floor form the birth passageway. The true pelvis is the critical factor of the passageway because the fetus must progress through this bony canal during the vaginal birth process. The true pelvis is divided into three sections: the inlet, the pelvic cavity (midpelvis), and the outlet. The four classic types of pelvises are *gynecoid, android, anthropoid,* and *platypelloid* (see Figure 10-15 ∞ on page 203). Implications of each type for childbirth are described in Table 22-2. The ability of the cervix to dilate and efface and the ability of the vaginal canal and the external opening of the vagina (the introitus) to distend are additional factors of the birth passageway. See chapter 10 ∞ for a discussion of each part of the pelvis, and chapter 15 ∞ for techniques to assess the size and shape of the pelvis.

Birth Passenger (Fetus)

Several aspects of the fetus's body and the way the fetus moves through the mother's birth canal are considered critical factors of the passenger that affect the outcome of labor. These inter-

TABLE 22-2 Implications of Pelvic Type for Labor and Birth

PELVIC TYPE	PERTINENT CHARACTERISTICS	IMPLICATIONS FOR BIRTH
Gynecoid	Inlet rounded with all inlet diameters adequate Midpelvis diameters adequate with parallel side walls Outlet adequate	Favorable for vaginal birth
Android	Inlet heart-shaped with short posterior sagittal diameter Midpelvis diameters reduced Outlet capacity reduced	Not favorable for vaginal birth Descent into pelvis is slow Fetal head enters pelvis in transverse or posterior position with arrest of labor frequent
Anthropoid	Inlet oval in shape, with long anteroposterior diameter Midpelvis diameters adequate Outlet adequate	Favorable for vaginal birth
Platypelloid	Inlet oval in shape, with long transverse diameters Midpelvis diameters reduced Outlet capacity inadequate	Not favorable for vaginal birth Fetal head engages in transverse position Difficult descent through midpelvis Frequent delay of progress at outlet of pelvis

Note: Description of pelvic shape is exaggerated for easier comprehension.

acting factors are: the fetal head, fetal attitude, fetal lie, fetal presentation, and fetal position. The placenta must also pass through the birth canal but rarely impedes the labor process, except in cases of placenta previa (see chapter 26 ∞ for placental complications).

Fetal Head

The fetal head is composed of bony parts, which can either hinder childbirth or make it easier. Once the head (the least compressible and largest part of the fetus) has been born, the birth of the rest of the body is rarely delayed.

The fetal skull has three major parts: the face, the base of the skull (cranium), and the vault of the cranium (roof). The bones of the face and cranial base are well fused and essentially fixed. The base of the cranium is composed of the two temporal bones, each with a sphenoid bone and an ethmoid bone. The bones composing the vault are the two frontal bones, the two parietal bones, and the occipital bone (Figure 22-1 ■). These bones are not fused, allowing this portion of the head to adjust as it passes through the narrow portions of the maternal pelvis. The cranial bones overlap under pressure of the powers of labor and the demands of the unyielding pelvis. This overlapping is called **molding**.

The **sutures** of the fetal skull are membranous joints that unite the cranial bones. Sutures allow for molding of the fetal head and help the clinician identify the position of the fetal head during vaginal examination. The important sutures of the cranial vault are as follows (see Figure 22-1).

- ***Frontal (mitotic) suture.*** Located between the two frontal bones; becomes the anterior continuation of the sagittal suture
- ***Sagittal suture.*** Located between the parietal bones; divides the skull into left and right halves; runs anteroposteriorly, connecting the two fontanelles
- ***Coronal sutures.*** Located between the frontal and parietal bones; extend transversely left and right from the anterior fontanelle (bregma)

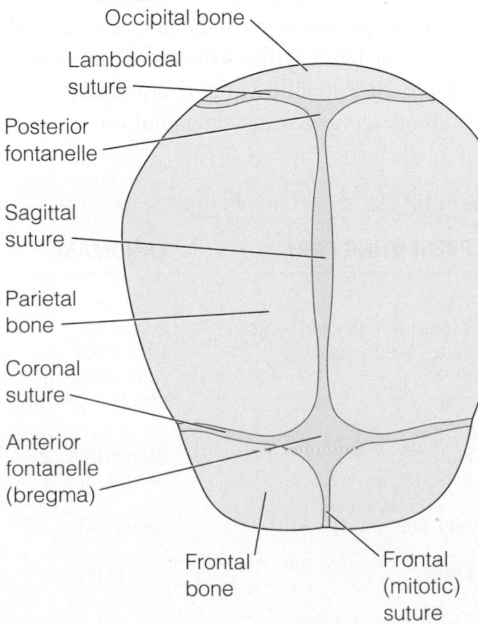

Figure 22-1 ■ Superior view of the fetal skull.

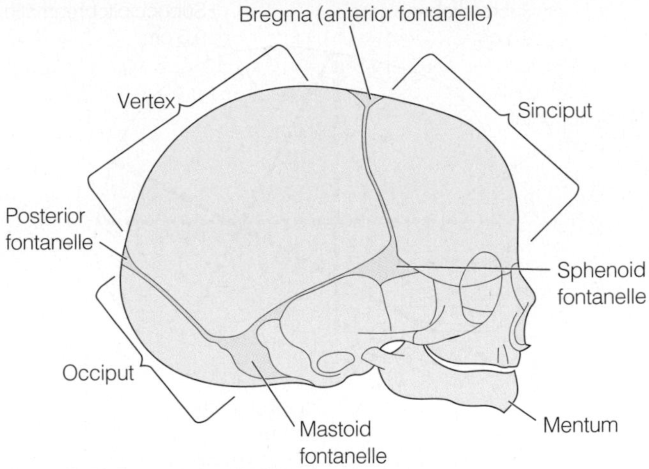

Figure 22-2 ■ Lateral view of the fetal skull identifying the landmarks that have significance during birth.

- ***Lambdoidal suture.*** Located between the two parietal bones and the occipital bone; extends transversely left and right from the posterior fontanelle

The intersection of several cranial sutures forms an irregular space that is enclosed by a membrane and called a **fontanelle**. The anterior and posterior fontanelles are clinically useful in identifying the position of the fetal head in the pelvis and in assessing the status of the newborn after birth. The greater, or anterior, fontanelle (bregma) is diamond shaped, measures 2 to 3 cm, and is situated at the junction of the sagittal, coronal, and frontal sutures. It permits growth of the brain by remaining unossified for as long as 18 months. The lesser, or posterior, fontanelle is shaped like a small triangle, measures about 1 to 2 cm, and is situated at the intersection of the sagittal and lambdoidal sutures. It closes within 8 to 12 weeks after birth.

Following are several other important landmarks of the fetal skull (Figure 22-2 ■):

- ***Mentum.*** The fetal chin
- ***Sinciput.*** The anterior area known as the brow
- ***Vertex.*** The area between the anterior and posterior fontanelles
- ***Occiput.*** The area of the fetal skull occupied by the occipital bone, beneath the posterior fontanelle

The diameters of the fetal skull vary considerably within normal limits. Some diameters shorten and others lengthen as the head is molded during labor. Fetal head diameters are measured between the various landmarks on the skull (Figure 22-3A ■). For example, the suboccipitobregmatic diameter is the distance from the undersurface of the occiput to the center of the bregma (anterior fontanelle). The biparietal diameter is the largest part of the fetal head (Figure 22-3B ■).

Fetal Attitude

Fetal attitude refers to the relation of the fetal body parts to one another. Fetal attitude describes the posture the fetus assumes as it conforms to the shape of the uterine cavity. The normal attitude of the fetus is termed *general flexion,* where the head is flexed so that the chin is on the chest with the arms

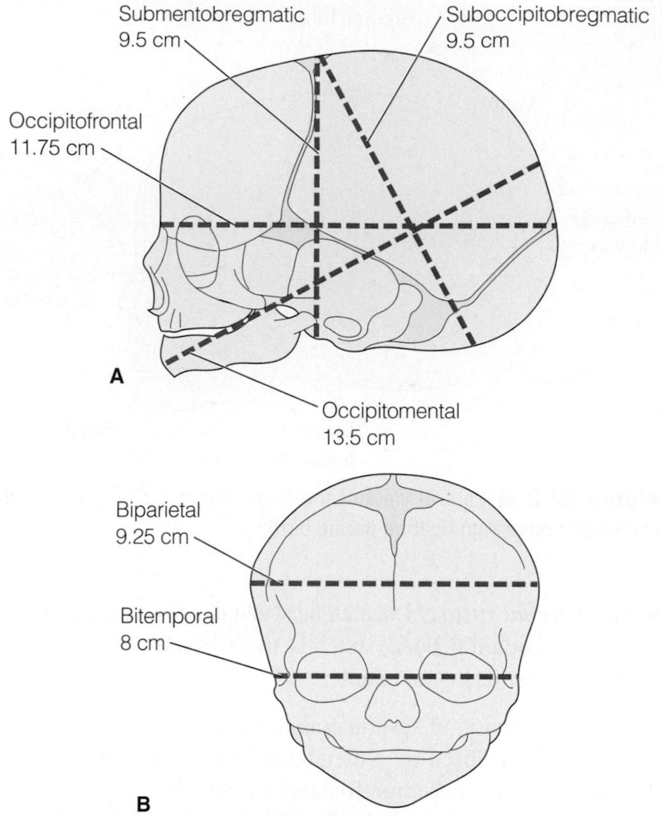

Figure 22-3 ■ A. Anteroposterior diameters of the fetal skull. When the vertex of the fetus presents and the fetal head is flexed with the chin on the chest, the smallest anteroposterior diameter (suboccipitobregmatic) enters the birth canal. B. Transverse diameters of the fetal skull.

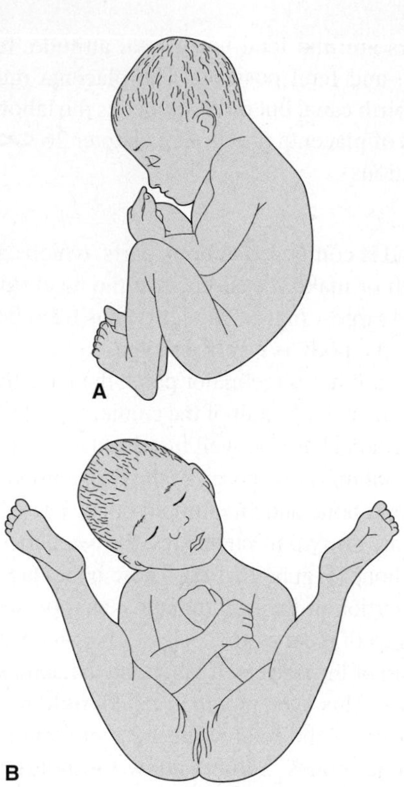

Figure 22-4 ■ Fetal attitude. A. The attitude (or relationship of body parts) of this fetus is normal. The head is flexed forward with the chin almost resting on the chest. The arms and legs are flexed. B. In this view, the head is tilted to the right. Although the arms are flexed, the legs are extended.

crossed over the chest, and the legs flexed at the knees with the thighs on the abdomen (Figure 22-4A ■).

Changes in fetal attitude, particularly in the position of the head, cause the fetus to present larger diameters of the fetal head to the maternal pelvis. These deviations from a normal fetal attitude often contribute to a longer, more difficult labor (Figure 22-4B ■).

Fetal Lie

Fetal Lie

Fetal lie refers to the relationship of the long, or cephalocaudal, axis (spinal column) of the fetus to the long, or cephalocaudal, axis of the mother. The fetus may assume either a longitudinal (vertical) or a transverse (horizontal) lie. A *longitudinal lie* occurs when the cephalocaudal axis of the fetus is parallel to the woman's spine. A *transverse lie* occurs when the cephalocaudal axis of the fetal spine is at a right angle to the woman's spine (see Figure 27-11 ∞) on page 710. A transverse lie is associated with a shoulder presentation and can lead to complications in the later stages of labor. This is discussed in detail in chapter 27 ∞. Table 22-3 identifies the characteristics associated with a longitudinal versus a transverse fetal lie.

TABLE 22-3 Characteristics Associated with Longitudinal Versus Transverse Fetal Lie

FETAL LIE	ATTITUDE	PRESENTING PART	LANDMARK
Longitudinal Lie (99.5%)			
Cephalic presentation (96% to 97%)	Flexion of fetal head onto chest	Vertex (posterior part—occiput)	Occiput (O)
	Military (no flexion, no extension)	Vertex (median part)	Occiput (O)
	Partial extension	Brow	Forehead (frontum) (Fr)
	Complete extension of the head	Face	Chin (mentum) (M)
Breech presentation (Approximately 3%)			
Complete breech	Flexed hips and knees	Buttocks	Sacrum (S)
Frank breech	Flexed hips, extended knees with legs against abdomen and chest	Buttocks	Sacrum (S)
Footling breech: single, double	Extended hips and at least one knee extended with foot in cervical canal	Feet (one or two)	Sacrum (S)
Kneeling breech: single, double	Extended hips, flexed knees	Knees	Sacrum (S)
Transverse or Oblique Lie (Approximately 0.5%)			
Shoulder presentation	Variable	Shoulder, arm	Scapula (Sc or A)

Fetal Presentation

Fetal presentation is determined by fetal lie and refers to the body part of the fetus that enters the maternal pelvis first and leads through the birth canal during labor. The **presenting part** or the portion of the fetus that is felt through the cervix on vaginal examination determines the presentation. Fetal presentation may be cephalic (head first), breech (buttocks or feet first), or shoulder.

The most common presentation is cephalic. When this presentation occurs, labor and birth are more likely to proceed normally. Breech and shoulder presentations are associated with difficulties during labor and do not proceed as normal; therefore, they are called **malpresentations**. (See chapter 27 ∞ for discussion of malpresentations.)

CEPHALIC PRESENTATION The fetal head presents to the birth passage in approximately 97% of term births. The cephalic presentation can be further classified into vertex, sinciput, brow, or face presentation according to the degree of flexion or extension of the fetal head (attitude).

Vertex Presentation When the presenting part is the occiput, the presentation is noted as vertex.

- Vertex is the most common type of presentation.
- The fetal head is completely flexed onto the chest.
- The smallest diameter of the fetal head (suboccipitobregmatic) presents to the maternal pelvis (Figure 22-5A ■).

Sinciput Presentation

- The fetal head is partially flexed.
- The occipitofrontal diameter presents to the maternal pelvis (Figure 22-5B ■).
- The top of the head is the presenting part.

Brow Presentation

- The fetal head is partially extended.
- The occipitomental diameter, the largest anteroposterior diameter, is presented to the maternal pelvis (Figure 22-5C ■).

Face Presentation

- The fetal head is hyperextended (complete extension).
- The submentobregmatic diameter presents to the maternal pelvis (Figure 22-5D ■).

Application: Breech Presentation

BREECH PRESENTATION A breech presentation indicates that the presenting part is the lower extremities or buttocks. Breech presentations occur in approximately 3% of all term births (Cunningham et al., 2010). These presentations are classified according to the attitude of the fetus's hips and knees. In all variations of the breech presentation (complete, frank, or footling breech), the sacrum (the bone on the buttocks that is felt when palpating) is the landmark.

Complete Breech

- The fetal knees and hips are both flexed, the thighs are on the abdomen, and the calves are on the posterior aspect of the thighs.
- The buttocks and feet of the fetus present to the maternal pelvis.

Frank Breech

- The fetal hips are flexed, and the knees are extended.
- The buttocks of the fetus present to the maternal pelvis.

Footling Breech

- The fetal hips and legs are extended.
- The feet of the fetus present to the maternal pelvis.
- In a single footling one foot presents; in a double footling both feet present.

SHOULDER PRESENTATION When the fetal shoulder is the presenting part, the fetus is in a transverse lie and the acromion process of the scapula is the landmark. This type of presentation occurs less than 1% of the time (Cunningham et al., 2010).

Relationship of Maternal Pelvis and Presenting Part

The third critical factor, in addition to the birth passage and fetus, is the relationship between these two factors. When assessing the relationship of the maternal pelvis and the presenting

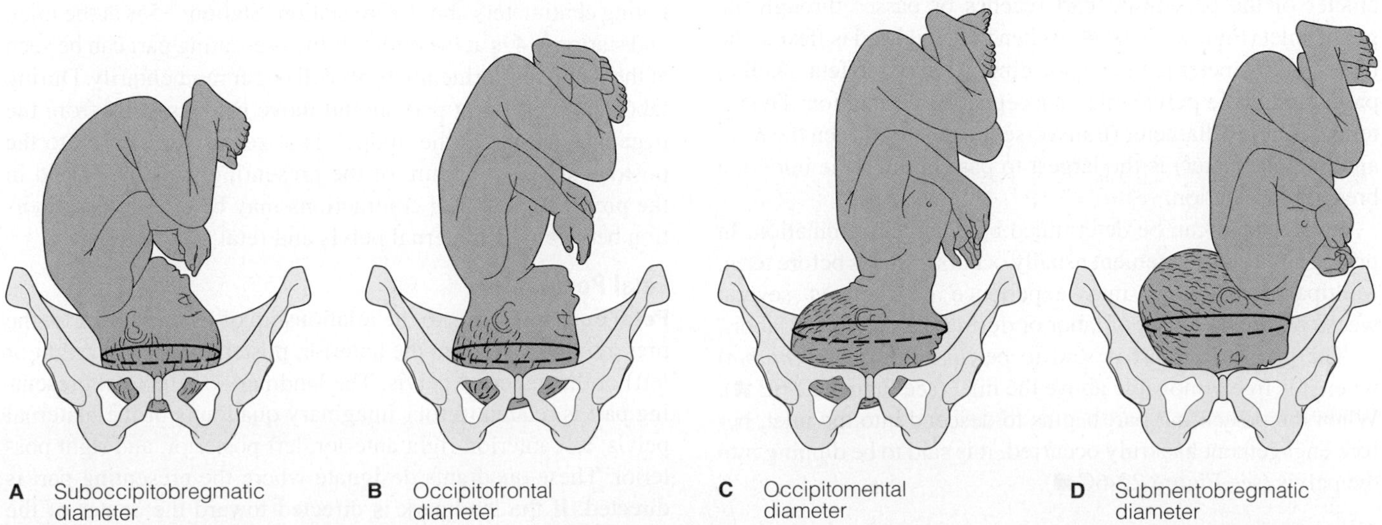

Figure 22-5 ■ Cephalic presentation. A. Vertex presentation. Complete flexion of the head allows the suboccipitobregmatic diameter to pre-sent to the pelvis. B. Sinciput (median vertex) presentation (also called *military presentation*) with no flexion or extension. The occipitofrontal diameter presents to the pelvis. C. Brow presentation. The fetal head is in partial (halfway) extension. The occipitomental diameter, which is the largest diameter of the fetal head, pre-sents to the pelvis. D. Face presentation. The fetal head is in complete extension, and the submentobregmatic diameter presents to the pelvis.

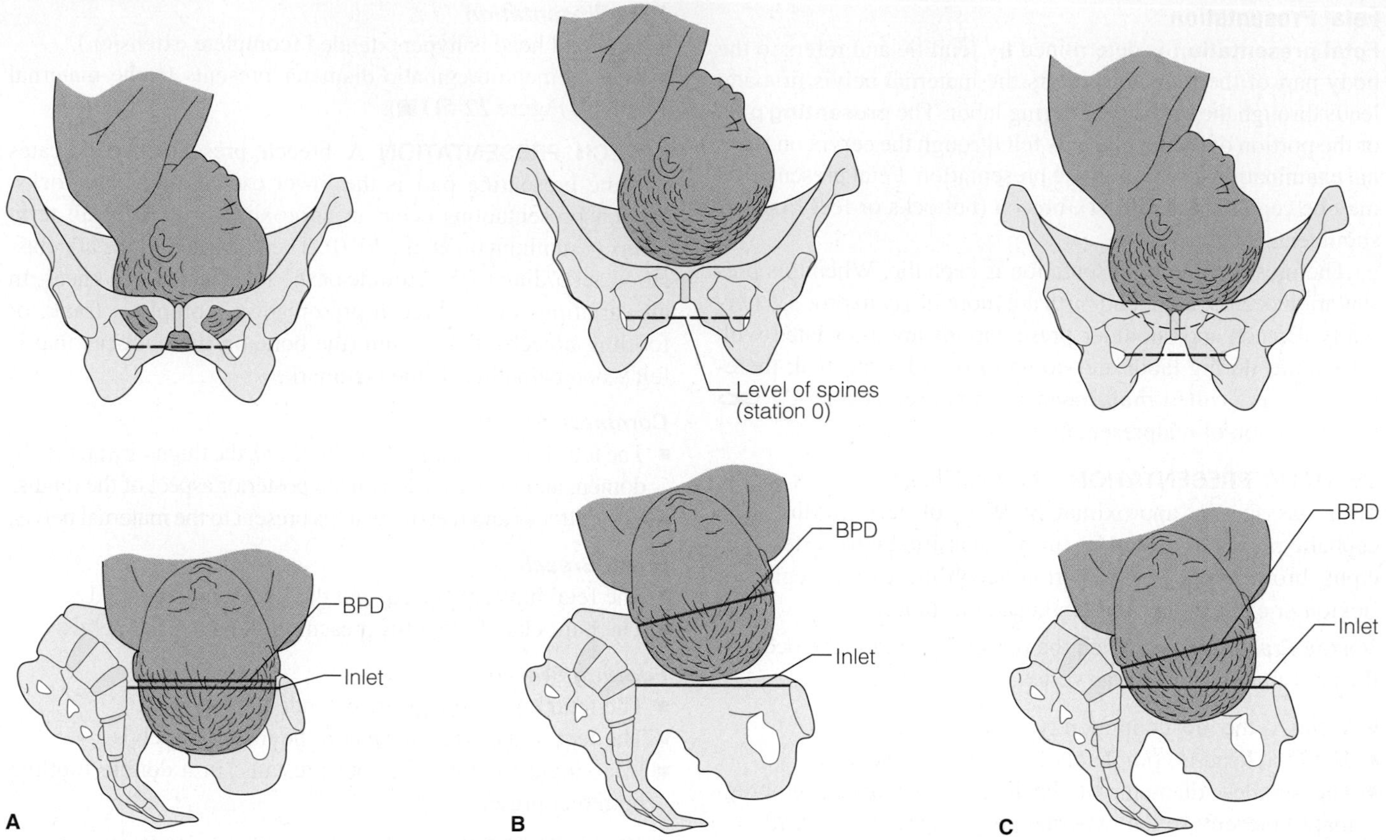

Figure 22-6 ■ Process of engagement in cephalic presentation. A. Engaged. The biparietal diameter (BPD) of the fetal head is in the inlet of the pelvis. In most instances, the presenting part (occiput) will be at the level of the ischial spines (0 station). B. Floating. The fetal head is directed down toward the pelvis but can still easily move away from the inlet. C. Dipping. The fetal head dips into the inlet but can be moved away by exerting pressure on the fetus.

part of the fetal body, the nurse considers engagement, station, and fetal position.

Engagement

Engagement of the presenting part occurs when the largest diameter of the presenting part reaches or passes through the pelvic inlet (Figure 22-6A ■). When the fetal head is flexed, the biparietal diameter is the largest dimension of the fetal skull to pass through the pelvic inlet in a cephalic presentation. The intertrochanteric diameter (transverse diameter between the right and left trochanter) is the largest to pass through the inlet in a breech presentation.

Engagement can be determined by vaginal examination. In primigravidas, engagement usually occurs 2 weeks before term. Multiparas, however, may experience engagement several weeks before the onset of labor or during the process of labor.

The presenting part is said to be *floating* (or *ballottable*) when it is freely movable above the inlet (see Figure 22-6B ■). When the presenting part begins to descend into the inlet, before engagement has truly occurred, it is said to be dipping into the pelvis (see Figure 22-6C ■).

Station

Station refers to the relationship of the presenting part to an imaginary line drawn between the ischial spines of the maternal pelvis. In a normal pelvis the ischial spines mark the narrowest diameter through which the fetus must pass. These spines are not sharp protrusions but rather blunted prominences at the midpelvis. The ischial spines as a landmark have been designated as zero station (Figure 22-7 ■). If the presenting part is higher than the ischial spines, a negative number is assigned, noting centimeters above zero station. Station −5 is at the inlet, and station +4 is at the outlet. If the presenting part can be seen at the woman's perineum, birth will occur momentarily. During labor the presenting part should move progressively from the negative stations to the midpelvis at zero station and into the positive stations. Failure of the presenting part to descend in the presence of strong contractions may be due to disproportion between the maternal pelvis and fetal presenting part.

Fetal Position

Fetal position refers to the relationship of the landmark on the presenting fetal part to the anterior, posterior, or sides (right or left) of the maternal pelvis. The landmark on the fetal presenting part is related to four imaginary quadrants of the maternal pelvis: left anterior, right anterior, left posterior, and right posterior. These quadrants designate where the presenting part is directed. If the landmark is directed toward the center of the side of the pelvis, fetal position is designated as transverse, rather than anterior or posterior.

The landmark chosen for vertex presentations is the occiput, and the landmark for face presentations is the mentum. In

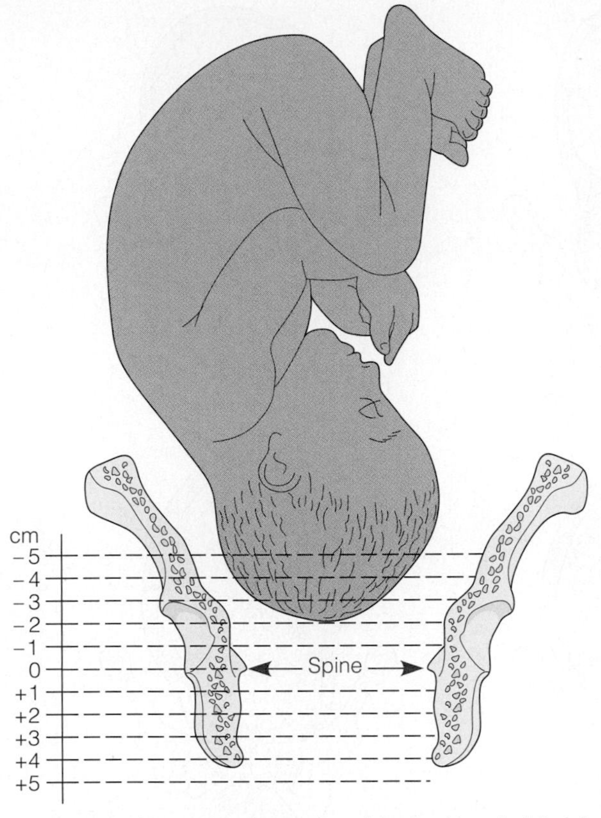

Figure 22-7 ■ Measuring the station of the fetal head while it is descending. In this view the station is −2.

breech presentations the sacrum is the designated landmark, and the acromion process on the scapula is the landmark in shoulder presentations.

In summary, three notations are used to describe the fetal position:

1. Right (R) or left (L) side of the maternal pelvis
2. The landmark of the fetal presenting part: occiput (O), mentum (M), sacrum (S), or acromion (scapula [Sc]) process (A)
3. Anterior (A), posterior (P), or transverse (T), depending on whether the landmark is in the front, back, or side of the pelvis

The abbreviations of these notations help the healthcare team communicate the fetal position. Thus, when the fetal occiput is directed toward the back and to the left of the passage, the abbreviation used is LOP (left-occiput-posterior). The following is a list of positions for various fetal presentations, some of which are illustrated in Figure 22-8 ■.

Positions in Vertex Presentation

ROA Right-occiput-anterior
ROT Right-occiput-transverse
ROP Right-occiput-posterior
LOA Left-occiput-anterior
LOT Left-occiput-transverse
LOP Left-occiput-posterior

Positions in Face Presentation

RMA Right-mentum-anterior
RMT Right-mentum-transverse
RMP Right-mentum-posterior
LMA Left-mentum-anterior
LMT Left-mentum-transverse
LMP Left-mentum-posterior

Positions in Breech Presentation

RSA Right-sacrum-anterior
RST Right-sacrum-transverse
RSP Right-sacrum-posterior
LSA Left-sacrum-anterior
LST Left-sacrum-transverse
LSP Left-sacrum-posterior

The term *dorsal (D)* is added when denoting the fetal position in a shoulder presentation; it refers to the fetal back. Thus the abbreviation RADA indicates that the acromion process of the scapula is directed toward the woman's right, and the fetus's back is anterior.

Positions in Shoulder Presentation

RADA Right-acromion-dorsal-anterior
RADP Right-acromion-dorsal-posterior
LADA Left-acromion-dorsal-anterior
LADP Left-acromion-dorsal-posterior

The fetal position influences labor and birth. For example, the fetal head presents a larger diameter in a posterior position than in an anterior position. A posterior position increases the pressure on the maternal sacral nerves, causing the laboring woman to experience backache and pelvic pressure. As a result, the woman may bear down or feel the urge to push earlier than needed. In addition, the second stage of labor may be prolonged when the fetal head remains in a posterior position.

The most common fetal position is occiput anterior. When this position occurs, the labor and birth are more likely to proceed normally. Positions other than occiput anterior are more frequently associated with problems during labor; therefore, they are called malpositions. (See chapter 27 ∞ for discussion of malpositions and their management.)

Assessment techniques to determine fetal position include inspection and palpation of the maternal abdomen and vaginal examination. (See chapter 23 ∞ for further discussion of assessment of fetal position.)

Physiologic Forces of Labor

Primary and secondary forces work together to deliver the fetus, the fetal membranes, and the placenta from the uterus into the external environment. The *primary force* is uterine muscular contractions, which cause the changes of the first stage of labor—complete effacement and dilatation of the cervix. The *secondary force* is the use of abdominal muscles to push during the second stage of labor. The pushing adds to the primary power after full dilatation.

Contractions

Uterine contractions are rhythmic tightenings and shortenings of the uterine muscles during labor. Each contraction has three phases: (1) *increment,* the "building up" of the contraction (the longest phase); (2) *acme,* or the peak of the contraction; and

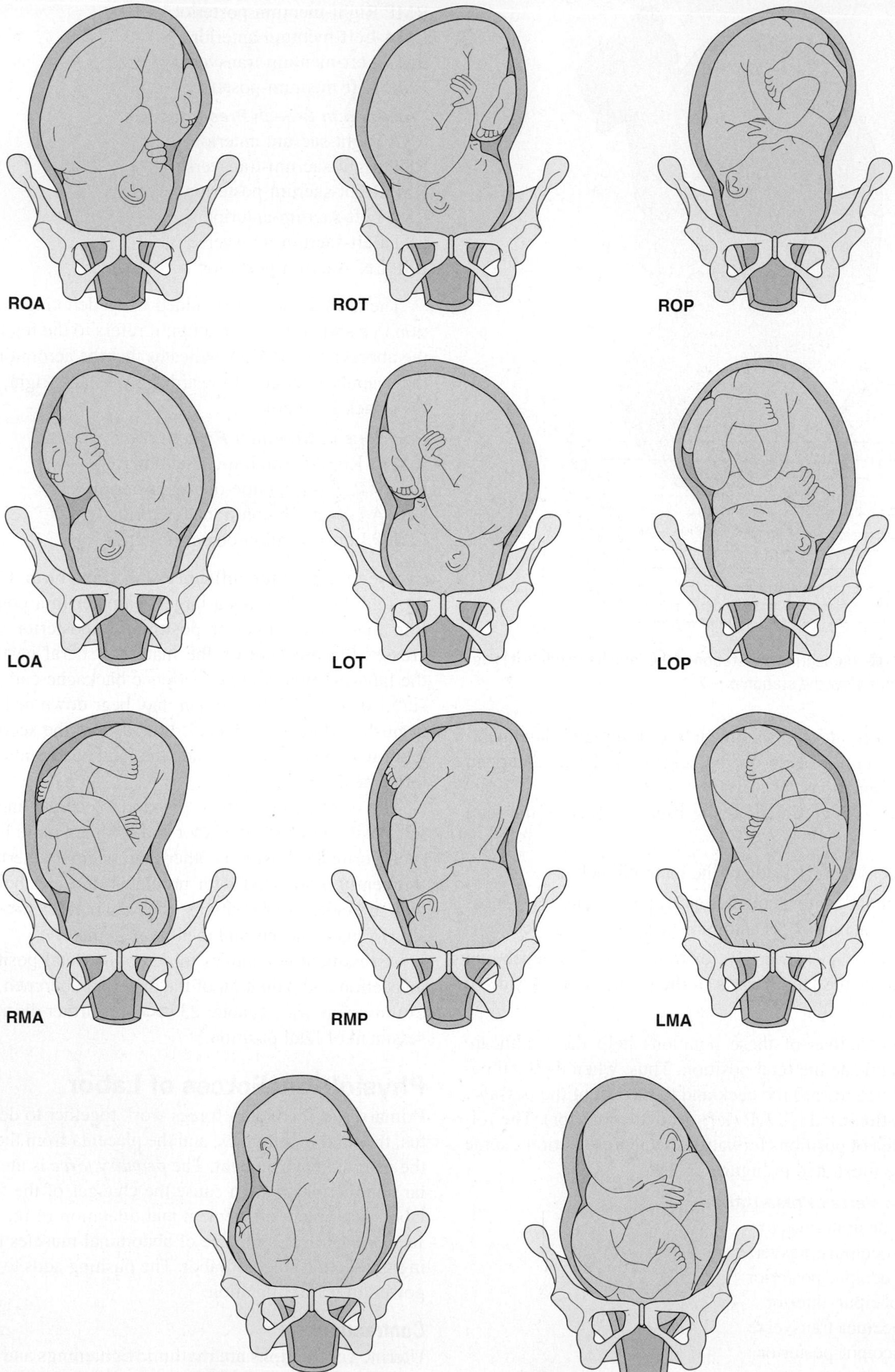

Figure 22-8 ■ Categories of presentation.

Source: Courtesy of Ross Laboratories, Columbus, OH.

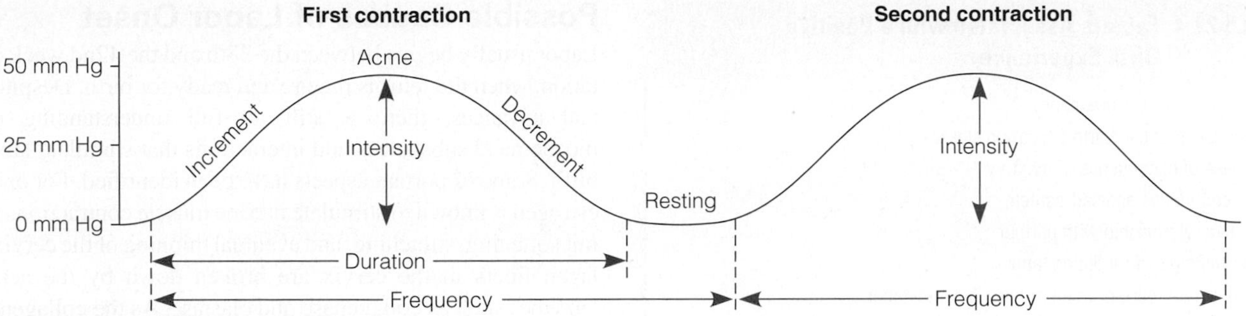

Figure 22-9 ■ Characteristics of uterine contractions.

(3) *decrement,* or the "letting up" of the contraction. Between contractions is a period of relaxation. This period of relaxation allows uterine muscles to rest and provides respite for the laboring woman. It also restores uteroplacental circulation, which is important to fetal oxygenation and adequate circulation in the uterine blood vessels.

When describing uterine contractions during labor, caregivers use the terms *frequency, duration,* and *intensity.*

Frequency refers to the time between the beginning of one contraction and the beginning of the next contraction. The **duration** of each contraction is measured from the beginning of the contraction to the completion of the contraction (Figure 22-9 ■). In beginning labor, the duration is 30 to 40 seconds. As labor continues, duration increases to 30 to 90 seconds (Cunningham et al., 2010).

Intensity refers to the strength of the uterine contraction during acme. In most instances the intensity is estimated by palpating the contraction, but it may be measured directly with an intrauterine catheter attached to an electronic fetal monitor. Intensity of uterine contractions cannot be accurately measured by external monitoring with an electronic fetal monitor, because several variables affect the external monitor, including maternal weight, specifically the amount of adipose tissue, and positioning of the monitor on the maternal abdomen. When estimating intensity by palpation, the nurse determines whether it is mild, moderate, or strong by judging the amount of indentability of the uterine wall during the acme of a contraction. If the uterine wall can be indented easily, the contraction is considered mild. Strong intensity exists when the uterine wall cannot be indented. Moderate intensity falls between these two ranges. When intensity is measured with an intrauterine catheter, the normal resting tonus (between contractions) is about 10 to 12 mm Hg of pressure. During acme the intensity ranges from 25 to 40 mm Hg in early labor, 50 to 70 mm Hg in active labor, 80 to 100 mm Hg during transition, and greater than 100 mm Hg while the woman is pushing in the second stage (Cunningham et al., 2010). (See chapter 23 ∞ for further discussion of assessment techniques.)

At the beginning of labor the contractions are usually mild, of short duration, and relatively infrequent. As labor progresses, duration and intensity increase, and the frequency is every 2 to 3 minutes. Because the contractions are involuntary, the laboring woman cannot control their duration, frequency, or intensity.

Bearing Down

After the cervix is completely dilated, the maternal abdominal musculature contracts as the woman pushes. This pushing is called *bearing down.* The pushing aids in the expulsion of the fetus and the placenta. If the cervix is not completely dilated, bearing down can cause cervical edema (which retards dilatation), possible tearing and bruising of the cervix, and maternal exhaustion. The combined involuntary pressure of the uterine contractions and the voluntary muscle contractions of the abdomen force the fetus toward the outlet so birth can occur.

Psychosocial Considerations

Thus far, the discussion has focused on physical influences on labor outcomes. But the final critical factor is the parents' psychosocial readiness, including their fears, anxieties, birth fantasies, and level of social support. Similar psychosocial factors affect both parents. Both are making a transition into a new role, and both have expectations of themselves and their partner during the labor and birth experience. Although many prospective parents attend childbirth preparation classes, they still tend to be concerned about what labor will be like. Concerns include whether they will each be able to perform the way they expect, whether the discomfort and pain will be more than the mother expects or is able to cope with, whether the father or partner can provide helpful support, and whether they can maintain a sense of control and be advocates for themselves (McKellar, Pincombe, & Henderson, 2008). In addition, both partners face an irrevocable event—the birth of a new family member—and, consequently, disruption of lifestyle, relationships, and self-image.

Many women have preconceived ideas about what birth should be like and some fear "losing control" of their body functions, emotions, or ability to handle the pain associated with labor. Women whose birth experiences do not meet their preconceived ideas may feel loss and disappointment. They may also feel that they have failed to live up to the expectations of friends, family, and peers.

Various factors influence a woman's reaction to labor and contribute to a positive birth experience (Table 22-4). Her accomplishment of the tasks of pregnancy, usual coping mechanisms in response to stressful life events, previous experiences, support system, preparation for childbirth, and cultural influences are all significant factors (Goldbort, 2009).

Many women have dreams about their birthing experience, their infant, and their early parenting experiences. Dreaming

TABLE 22-4 Factors Associated with a Positive Birth Experience

- Motivation for the pregnancy
- Attendance at childbirth education classes
- A sense of competence or mastery
- Self-confidence and self-esteem
- Positive relationship with partner
- Maintaining control during labor
- Support from partner or other person during labor
- Not being left alone in labor
- Trust in the medical/nursing staff
- Having personal control of breathing patterns, comfort measures
- Choosing a physician/certified nurse-midwife who has a similar philosophy of care
- Receiving clear information regarding procedures

and fantasizing about the unborn baby is a developmental process of pregnancy (Alhusen, 2008). The nurse can encourage the woman to share her dreams and fantasies and use them as a tool to examine the woman's expectations, fears, and coping mechanisms. This can assist the woman in forming a maternal role and facilitate bonding with her fetus.

When a woman is facing labor, especially for the first time, she may worry about her ability to withstand the pain of contractions. Some women may place great emphasis on withstanding the pain of childbirth stoically—without medication, crying, moaning, or making other sounds. The nurse's role is to help childbearing families explore options and identify interventions to help each woman cope with the discomfort of labor in a way that is acceptable to her.

The laboring woman's support system may also influence the course of labor and birth. Although some women may prefer not to have a support person or family member with them, for many women the presence of her partner and other significant persons (especially the nurse) tends to have a positive effect. A labor partner's presence at the bedside provides a means to enhance communication and to demonstrate feelings of love. Communication needs may include talking and the use of affectionate and understanding words from the partner. Showing love may take the form of holding hands, hugging, or touching (McKellar, Pincombe, & Henderson, 2008).

How the woman views the birth experience in hindsight may have implications for mothering behaviors. A significant relationship exists between the birth experience and mothering behaviors. It appears that any activities by the expectant woman or by healthcare providers that enhance the birth experience will be beneficial to the mother-baby connection. The father's experience of childbirth and his opportunities for bonding may have important implications for fathering as well (Goldbort, 2009).

Physiology of Labor

Physiology of Labor

In addition to considering the five critical factors affecting the progress of labor and birth, it is essential to explore the physiology of the normal labor experience.

Possible Causes of Labor Onset

Labor usually begins between the 38th and the 42nd week of gestation, when the fetus is mature and ready for birth. Despite medical advances, there is still no full understanding of the biochemical substances and interactions that stimulate labor and birth. Some important aspects have been identified. For example, estrogen is known to stimulate uterine muscle contractions to permit softening, stretching, and eventual thinning of the cervix. Collagen fibers in the cervix are broken down by the action of enzymes such as collagenase and elastase. As the collagen fibers change, their ability to bind is decreased because of increasing amounts of hyaluronic acid (which loosely binds collagen fibrils) and decreasing amounts of dermatan sulfate (which tightly binds collagen fibrils). There is also an increase in the water content of the cervix. All these changes result in a weakening and softening of the cervix, which facilitates cervical stretching and effacement.

Hypotheses have also been formed about the roles of progesterone withdrawal, of prostaglandin, and of corticotropin-releasing hormone.

Progesterone Withdrawal Hypothesis

Progesterone produced by the placenta relaxes uterine smooth muscle by interfering with conduction of impulses from one cell to the next. For this reason, the uterus is usually without coordinated contractions during pregnancy. Biochemical changes toward the end of gestation result in decreased availability of progesterone to myometrial cells. The decrease in availability may be associated with a yet-unknown antiprogestin that inhibits the relaxant effect on the uterus but allows other progesterone actions such as lactogenesis (Challis, 2008).

Prostaglandin Hypothesis

Although the exact relationship between prostaglandin and the onset of labor is not yet established, the effect is clinically demonstrated by the successful induction of labor after vaginal application of prostaglandin E. In addition, preterm labor may be stopped by using an inhibitor of prostaglandin synthesis such as indomethacin (Challis, 2008).

The amnion and decidua are the focus of research on the source of prostaglandins. Once prostaglandin is produced, stimuli for its synthesis may include rising levels of estrogen, decreased availability of progesterone, increased levels of oxytocin or response to oxytocin, platelet-activating factor, and endothelin-1 (Challis, 2008).

Corticotropin-Releasing Hormone Hypothesis

Corticotropin-releasing hormone (CRH) is also a focus for researchers. Its possible role in onset of labor is suggested by the fact that CRH concentration increases throughout pregnancy, with a sharp increase at term. Also, CRH may play a role in increased risk for preterm birth, and CRH levels are elevated in multiple gestations. Finally, CRH is known to stimulate the synthesis of prostaglandin F and prostaglandin E by amnion cells (Goldenberg, Culhane, Iams, et al., 2009).

Myometrial Activity

In true labor the uterus divides into two portions. This division is known as the *physiologic retraction ring*. The upper portion,

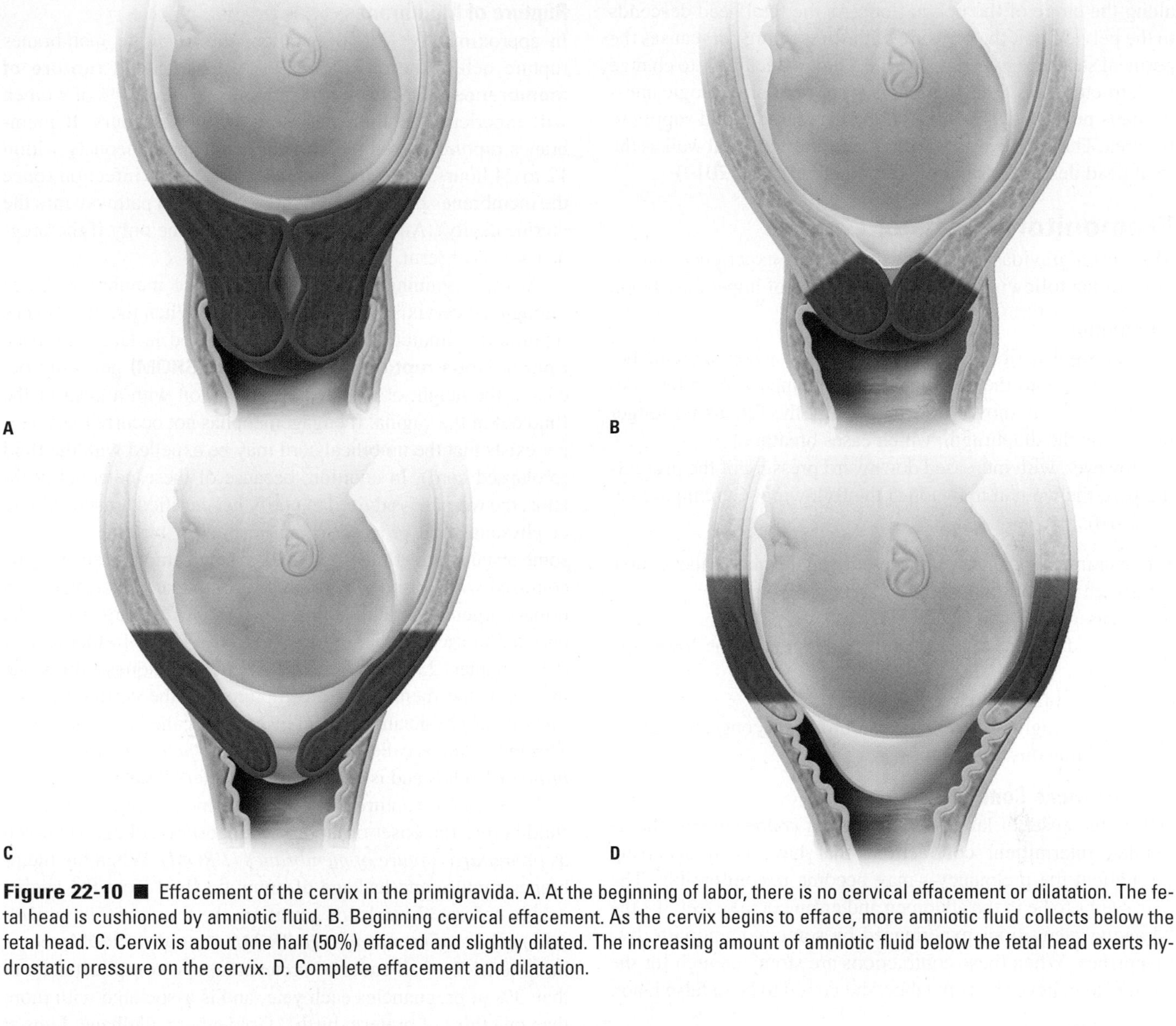

Figure 22-10 ■ Effacement of the cervix in the primigravida. A. At the beginning of labor, there is no cervical effacement or dilatation. The fetal head is cushioned by amniotic fluid. B. Beginning cervical effacement. As the cervix begins to efface, more amniotic fluid collects below the fetal head. C. Cervix is about one half (50%) effaced and slightly dilated. The increasing amount of amniotic fluid below the fetal head exerts hydrostatic pressure on the cervix. D. Complete effacement and dilatation.

which is the contractile segment, becomes progressively thicker as labor advances. The lower portion, which includes the lower uterine segment and cervix, is passive. As labor continues, the lower uterine segment expands and thins out.

With each contraction, the muscles of the upper uterine segment shorten and exert a longitudinal traction on the cervix, causing effacement. **Effacement** is the taking up (or drawing up) of the internal os and the cervical canal into the uterine side walls. The cervix changes progressively from a long, thick structure to a structure that is tissue-paper thin (Figure 22-10 ■). In primigravidas effacement usually precedes dilatation. The uterine muscle remains shorter and thicker and does not return to its original length. This phenomenon is known as *brachystasis.* The space in the uterine cavity decreases as a result of brachystasis, and this places downward pressure on the fetus (Cunningham et al., 2010).

The uterus elongates with each contraction, decreasing the horizontal diameter. This elongation causes a straightening of the fetal body, pressing the part of the fetus in the upper portion of the uterus against the fundus and thrusting the presenting part down toward the lower uterine segment and the cervix. The pressure exerted by the fetus is called *fetal axis pressure.* As the uterus elongates, the longitudinal muscle fibers are pulled upward over the presenting part. This action and the hydrostatic pressure of the fetal membranes cause **cervical dilatation**. The cervical os and cervical canal widen from less than 1 cm to approximately 10 cm, allowing birth of the fetus. When the cervix is completely dilated and retracted up into the lower uterine segment, it can no longer be palpated.

The round ligament pulls the fundus forward, aligning the fetus with the bony pelvis. This facilitates engagement of the presenting part. Pressure exerted on the cervix by the presenting part aids in both effacement and cervical dilatation (Gabbe et al., 2007).

Musculature Changes in the Pelvic Floor

The levator ani muscle and fascia of the pelvic floor draw the rectum and vagina upward and forward with each contraction,

Rupturing Membranes

along the curve of the pelvic floor. As the fetal head descends to the pelvic floor, the pressure of the presenting part causes the perineal structure, which was once 5 cm in thickness, to change to a structure less than 1 cm thick. A normal physiologic anesthesia is produced as a result of the decreased blood supply to the area. The anus everts, exposing the interior rectal wall as the fetal head descends forward (Cunningham et al., 2010).

Premonitory Signs of Labor

Most primigravidas and many multiparas experience one or more of the following signs and symptoms of impending labor.

Lightening

Lightening describes the effects that occur when the fetus begins to settle into the pelvic inlet (engagement). With fetal descent, the uterus moves downward, and the fundus no longer presses on the diaphragm, which eases breathing.

However, with increased downward pressure of the presenting part, the woman may notice the following (Cunningham et al., 2010):

- Leg cramps or pains due to pressure on the nerves that course through the obturator foramen in the pelvis
- Increased pelvic pressure
- Increased venous stasis, leading to edema in the lower extremities
- Increased urinary frequency
- Increased vaginal secretions resulting from congestion of the vaginal mucous membranes

Braxton Hicks Contractions

Before the onset of labor, *Braxton Hicks contractions*—the irregular, intermittent contractions that have been occurring throughout the pregnancy—may become uncomfortable. The pain seems to be in the abdomen and groin but may feel like the "drawing" sensations experienced by some women with dysmenorrhea. When these contractions are strong enough for the woman to believe she is in labor, she is said to be in false labor.

Cervical Changes

Considerable change occurs in the cervix during the prenatal and intrapartal period. At the beginning of pregnancy the cervix is rigid and firm, and it must soften so that it can stretch and dilate to allow fetal passage. This softening of the cervix, called *ripening,* is under the influence of hormonal factors discussed shortly.

Bloody Show

During pregnancy, cervical secretions accumulate in the cervical canal to form a barrier called a *mucous plug.* With softening and effacement of the cervix, the mucous plug is often expelled, resulting in a small amount of blood loss from the exposed cervical capillaries. The resulting pink-tinged secretions are called **bloody show**.

Bloody show is considered a sign of impending labor, usually within 24 to 48 hours. Vaginal examination that includes manipulation of the cervix may also result in a blood-tinged discharge, which is sometimes confused with bloody show. However, this discharge is typically brownish in color and is not accompanied by the mucous plug.

Rupture of Membranes

In approximately 12% of women, the amniotic membranes rupture before the onset of labor. This is called **rupture of membranes (ROM)**. After membranes rupture, 80% of women will experience spontaneous labor within 24 hours. If membranes rupture and labor does not begin spontaneously within 12 to 24 hours, labor may be induced to avoid infection (once the membranes have ruptured there is an open pathway into the uterine cavity). An induction of labor is done only if the pregnancy is near term.

At the beginning of labor, the amniotic membranes bulge through the cervix in the shape of a cone. When the membranes rupture, the amniotic fluid may be expelled in large amounts. **Spontaneous rupture of membranes (SROM)** generally occurs at the height of an intense contraction with a gush of the fluid out of the vagina. If engagement has not occurred, the danger exists that the umbilical cord may be expelled with the fluid (prolapsed cord). In addition, because of these potential problems, the woman is advised to notify her certified nurse-midwife or physician and proceed to the hospital or birthing center. In some instances the fluid is expelled in small amounts and may be confused with episodes of urinary incontinence associated with urinary urgency, coughing, or sneezing. The discharge should be checked to ascertain its source and to determine further action. (See chapter 23 ∞ for assessment techniques.) In some instances, the membranes are ruptured by the certified nurse-midwife or physician, using an instrument called an amniohook. This procedure is called *amniotomy* or *artificial rupture of membranes (AROM)* and is discussed in chapter 28 ∞.

Spontaneous rupture of membranes and leakage of amniotic fluid before the onset of labor at any gestational age is known as *premature rupture of membranes (PROM).* When the membranes rupture and leakage of amniotic fluid from the vagina occurs before 37 weeks of gestation, the term *preterm premature rupture of membranes (PPROM)* is used. PPROM occurs in up to 25% of all cases of preterm labors, complicates more than 3% of pregnancies each year, and is associated with more than one third of preterm births (Goldenberg, Culhane, Iams et al., 2009). Infection often precedes PPROM. When PPROM is suspected, strict sterile technique should be used in any vaginal examination. (For a complete discussion of PROM and PPROM, see chapter 26 ∞.)

Sudden Burst of Energy

Some women report a sudden burst of energy approximately 24 to 48 hours before labor. The cause of the energy spurt is unknown. In prenatal teaching the nurse should warn prospective mothers not to overexert themselves during this energy burst so that they will not be excessively tired when labor begins.

Other Signs

Other premonitory signs include the following:

- Weight loss of 2.2 to 6.6 kg (1 to 3 lb) resulting from fluid loss and electrolyte shifts produced by changes in estrogen and progesterone levels
- Increased backache and sacroiliac pressure from the influence of relaxin hormone on the pelvic joints

- Diarrhea, indigestion, or nausea and vomiting just before the onset of labor (the causes of these signs are unknown)

Differences Between True Labor and False Labor

The contractions of true labor produce progressive dilatation and effacement of the cervix. They occur regularly and increase in frequency, duration, and intensity. The discomfort of true labor contractions usually starts in the back and radiates around to the abdomen. The pain is not relieved by ambulation (in fact, walking may intensify the pain) or by resting.

The contractions of false labor do not produce progressive cervical effacement and dilatation. Classically, they are irregular and do not increase in frequency, duration, and intensity. The contractions may be perceived as a hardening or "balling up" without discomfort, or discomfort may occur mainly in the lower abdomen and groin. The discomfort may be relieved by ambulation, changes of position, resting, or a hot bath or shower (Cunningham et al., 2010). A comparison of true labor and false labor is provided in Table 22-5.

Nurse's Response to False Labor

During the third trimester, the woman will find it helpful to learn the characteristics of true labor contractions as well as the premonitory signs of ensuing labor. The nurse informs the woman that false labor is common and many times cannot be distinguished from true labor except by vaginal examination. She must feel free to come in for accurate assessment of labor and should be counseled not to feel foolish if the labor is false.

In addition, false labor can last for several hours and can be exhausting. The nurse can suggest interventions to decrease the anxiety and physical discomforts associated with false labor such as walking, changing position, or a warm tub bath.

TABLE 22-5 Comparison of True Labor and False Labor

TRUE LABOR	FALSE LABOR
Contractions are at regular intervals.	Contractions are irregular.
Intervals between contractions gradually shorten.	Usually no change.
Contractions increase in duration and intensity.	Usually no change.
Discomfort begins in back and radiates around to abdomen.	Discomfort is usually in abdomen.
Intensity usually increases with walking.	Walking has no effect on or lessens contractions.
Cervical dilatation and effacement are progressive.	No change.
Contractions do not decrease with rest or warm tub bath.	Rest and warm tub baths lessen contractions.

Stages of Labor and Birth

To assist caregivers, common terms have been developed as benchmarks to subdivide the process of labor into *stages* and *phases* of labor. It is important to note, however, that these represent theoretic separations in the process. A laboring woman will not usually experience distinct differences from one to the other. The first stage begins with the beginning of true labor and ends when the cervix is completely dilated at 10 cm. The second stage begins with complete dilatation and ends with the birth of the infant. The third stage begins with the birth of the infant and ends with the expulsion of the placenta.

Some clinicians identify a fourth stage of labor. During this stage, which lasts 1 to 4 hours after expulsion of the placenta, the uterus effectively contracts to control bleeding at the placental site (Cunningham et al., 2010). Nursing care of the laboring woman is discussed in chapter 24 ∞.

The following discussion characterizes the four stages and their accompanying phases.

Case Study: Patient in First Stage of Labor

First Stage

The first stage of labor is divided into the latent or early, active, and transition phases (Table 22-6). Each phase of labor is characterized by physical and psychologic changes.

Latent or Early Phase

The latent or early phase begins with the onset of regular contractions. As the cervix begins to dilate it also effaces, although little or no fetal descent is evident. For a woman in her first labor (nullipara), the latent or early phase averages 8.6 hours but should not exceed 20 hours. This early phase in

TABLE 22-6 Characteristics of Labor

			FIRST STAGE	SECOND STAGE
	LATENT (EARLY) PHASE	ACTIVE PHASE	TRANSITION PHASE	
Nullipara	8.6 hr	4.6 hr	3.6 hr	Up to 3 hr
Multipara	5.3 hr	2.4 hr	Variable	0–30 min
Cervical dilatation	0–3 cm	4–7 cm	8–10 cm	
Contractions				
Frequency	Every 3–30 min	Every 2–5 min	Every 1 1/2–2 min	Every 1 1/2–2 min
Duration	20–40 sec	40–60 sec	60–90 sec	60–90 sec
Intensity	Begin as mild and progress to moderate; 25–40 mm Hg by intrauterine pressure catheter (IUPC)	Begin as moderate and progress to strong, 50–70 mm Hg by IUPC	Strong by palpation; 70–100 mm Hg by IUPC	Strong by palpation; 70–90 mm Hg by IUPC

Care Plan Activity: Labor Progress in the First Stage of Labor

multiparas averages 5.3 hours but should not exceed 14 hours (Cunningham et al., 2010).

Uterine contractions become established during the latent phase and increase in frequency, duration, and intensity. They may start as mild contractions lasting 20 to 40 seconds with a frequency of 3 to 30 minutes. They average 25 to 50 mm Hg by intrauterine pressure catheter (IUPC) at acme (Cunningham et al., 2010).

In the early or latent phase of the first stage of labor, contractions are usually mild. The woman feels able to cope with the discomfort. She may be relieved that labor has finally started. Although she may be anxious, she is able to recognize and express those feelings of anxiety. The woman is often talkative and smiling and is eager to talk about herself and answer questions. Excitement is high, and her partner or other support person is often as elated as she is.

Active Phase

When the woman enters the early *active phase,* her anxiety tends to increase as she senses the intensification of contractions and pain. She begins to fear a loss of control and may use a variety of coping mechanisms. Some women exhibit a decreased ability to cope and a sense of helplessness. Women who have support persons and family available may experience greater satisfaction and less anxiety than those without support. During this phase the cervix dilates from about 4 to 7 cm. Fetal descent is progressive. The cervical dilatation should be at least 1.2 cm per hour in nulliparas and 1.5 cm per hour in multiparas (Cunningham et al., 2010).

First Stage of Labor and Transition

Transition Phase

The transition phase is the last part of the first stage. When the woman enters the transition phase, she may demonstrate significant anxiety. She becomes acutely aware of the increasing force and intensity of the contractions. She may become restless, frequently changing position. By the time the woman enters the transition phase, she is often inner directed and tired. She may fear being left alone at the same time the support person may be feeling the need for a break. The nurse should reassure the woman that she will not be left alone. It is crucial that the nurse be available as a relief support at this time and keep the woman informed about where her labor support people are, if they leave the room.

Cervical dilatation slows as it progresses from 8 to 10 cm and the rate of fetal descent increases. The average rate of descent is at least 1 cm per hour in nulliparas and 2 cm per hour in multiparas. The transition phase should not be longer than 3 hours for nulliparas and 1 hour for multiparas (Cunningham et al., 2010). The total duration of the first stage may be increased by approximately 1 hour if epidural anesthesia is used.

Second Stage of Labor

During the active and transition phases, contractions become more frequent, are longer in duration, and increase in intensity. At the beginning of the active phase, the contractions have a frequency of 2 to 5 minutes, a duration of 40 to 60 seconds, and are strong in intensity. During transition, contractions have a frequency of 1 1/2 to 2 minutes, a duration of 60 to 90 seconds, and are strong in intensity (Cunningham et al., 2010).

As dilatation approaches 10 cm, there may be increased rectal pressure and an uncontrollable urge to bear down, an increase in bloody show, and ROM (if this has not already occurred). The woman may also fear that she will be "torn open" or "split apart" by the force of the contractions. The woman may experience a sensation of pressure so great with the peak of a contraction that it seems to her that her abdomen will burst open. The woman should be informed that this is a normal sensation and reassured that such bursting will not happen.

During transition the woman will most likely withdraw into herself. Increasingly she may doubt her ability to cope with labor. The woman may become apprehensive and irritable. Although she may be terrified of being left alone, she may not want anyone to talk to her or touch her. However, with the next contraction she may ask for verbal and physical support. She may need help regaining focus. Other characteristics that may accompany this phase include the following:

- Hyperventilation, as the woman increases her breathing rate
- Restlessness
- Difficulty understanding directions
- A sense of bewilderment and anger at the contractions
- Generalized discomfort, including low back pain, shaking, and cramping in the legs
- Increased sensitivity to touch
- Increased need for partner's and/or nurse's presence or support
- Increased apprehension and irritability
- Statements that she "can't take it anymore"
- Requests for medication
- Hiccupping, belching, nausea, or vomiting
- Beads of perspiration on the upper lip
- Increasing rectal pressure
- Curling of her toes
- Loss of control
- Crying or yelling

The woman in this phase is anxious to "get it over with." She may be amnesic and sleep between her now-frequent contractions. Her support persons may start to feel helpless and may turn to the nurse for increased participation as their efforts to alleviate her discomfort seem less effective.

Second Stage

The second stage of labor begins when the cervix is completely dilated (10 cm) and ends with birth of the infant. The second stage is typically completed within 2 hours after the cervix becomes fully dilated for primigravidas (multiparas average 15 minutes). The use of epidural anesthesia may extend the duration of the second stage an additional hour. Contractions continue with a frequency of 1 1/2 to 2 minutes, a duration of 60 to 90 seconds, and strong intensity. Descent of the fetal presenting part continues until it reaches the perineal floor.

As the fetal head descends, the woman has the urge to push because of pressure of the fetal head on the sacral and obturator nerves. As she pushes, intra-abdominal pressure is exerted from contraction of the maternal abdominal muscles. As the fetal head continues its descent, the perineum begins to bulge, flatten, and move anteriorly. The amount of bloody show may increase. The labia begin to part with each contraction. Between contractions, the fetal head appears to recede. With succeeding contractions and maternal pushing effort, the fetal head descends farther.

RESEARCH EVIDENCE IN PRACTICE — Passive Descent Versus Immediate Pushing in Women with Epidural Analgesia

CLINICAL QUESTION

Which method of pushing—passive descent or active pushing upon full cervical dilatation—most benefits women with epidural analgesia?

RESEARCH EVIDENCE

Epidural analgesia has become a common method of pain management for laboring women, yet one of its side effects is a decrease in a woman's lower body sensations. This may inhibit the natural urge to push upon full cervical dilatation. Traditionally, active management of labor meant that women were directed to push immediately upon full cervical dilatation, whether they felt the urge or not. The chief concern leading to this practice was that an extended second stage of labor was deleterious for both mother and baby, leading to acidosis, maternal exhaustion, and neonatal morbidity.

The natural second stage of labor includes a period of rest and descent, often described as passive descent. This practice involves allowing the woman to delay pushing until she feels the urge to push, or the head is visible vaginally.

A group of obstetric and gynecologic nurse experts conducted a meta-analysis of studies comparing the effects and outcomes of immediate pushing versus passive descent in women with epidural analgesia. The results demonstrated that immediate pushing did not reduce the incidence of acidosis or shorten the second stage of labor. Indeed, prolonged active pushing was shown to increase the incidence of fetal and maternal acidosis, increased the risk of having an instrument-assisted birth, and decreased the chance a woman would have a spontaneous vaginal birth. Pushing time was lengthened with immediate pushing as compared to passive descent.

Furthermore, passive descent had additional benefits in that it allowed for further fetal descent and rotation, better situating the fetus in the woman's pelvis. It also caused further release of oxytocin that augmented the progress of labor. These findings suggest that the duration of active pushing should be limited, not the duration of the second stage of labor.

No differences were found between immediate pushing and passive descent in terms of the rate of cesarean birth, lacerations, or episiotomies.

WHAT QUESTIONS REMAIN UNANSWERED?

Are there any conditions under which active pushing should be used? Are there differences in these findings when women do not use epidural analgesia?

WHAT IS BEST PRACTICE?

Passive descent should be used during birth to safely and effectively increase spontaneous vaginal births, decrease instrument-assisted birth, and shorten pushing time.

CRITICAL THINKING

How can the nurse help the mother recognize the urge to push at an effective time when epidural analgesia is in place?

References

Brancato, R., Church, S., & Stone, P. (2008). A meta-analysis of passive descent versus immediate pushing in nulliparous women with epidural analgesia in the second stage of labor. *Journal of Gynecological and Neonatal Nursing, 37,* 4–12. doi:10.1111/J.1552-6909.2007.00205.x

---

Crowning occurs when the fetal head is encircled by the external opening of the vagina (introitus) and means birth is imminent. Some women feel acute, increasingly severe pain and a burning sensation as the perineum distends. The woman may continue to fear that she will tear apart. The nurse needs to instruct the woman to "push through the pain and burning."

Usually, a childbirth-prepared woman feels relieved that the acute pain she felt during the transition phase is over. She also may be relieved that the birth is near and she can now push. Some women feel a sense of control now that they can be actively involved. Others, particularly those without childbirth preparation, may become frightened. They tend to fight each contraction and any attempt of others to persuade them to push with contractions. The woman may feel she has lost control and become embarrassed and apologetic, or she may demonstrate extreme irritability toward the staff or her supporters in an attempt to regain control over external forces against which she feels helpless. Such behavior may be frightening and disconcerting to her support persons. The nurse needs to provide reassurance to the support person(s) that this is a common reaction.

Spontaneous Birth (Vertex Presentation)

As the head distends the vulva with each contraction, the perineum becomes extremely thin, and the anus stretches and protrudes. As extension occurs under the symphysis pubis, the head is born. When the anterior shoulder meets the underside of the symphysis pubis, a gentle push by the mother aids in birth of the shoulders. The body then follows (Figure 22-11 ■).

Positional Changes of the Fetus

For the fetus to pass through the birth canal, the fetal head and body must adjust to the maternal pelvis by certain positional changes. These changes, called **cardinal movements** or mechanisms of labor, are described in the order in which they occur (Figure 22-12 ■).

DESCENT Descent is thought to occur because of four forces: (1) pressure of the amniotic fluid, (2) direct pressure of the fundus of the uterus on the breech of the fetus, (3) contraction of the abdominal muscles, and (4) extension and straightening of the fetal body. The head enters the inlet in the occiput transverse or oblique position because the pelvic inlet is widest from side to side. The sagittal suture is an equal distance from the maternal symphysis pubis and sacral promontory.

FLEXION Flexion occurs as the fetal head descends and meets resistance from the soft tissues of the pelvis, the musculature of the pelvic floor, and the cervix. As a result of the resistance, the fetal chin flexes downward onto the chest.

INTERNAL ROTATION The fetal head must rotate to fit the diameter of the pelvic cavity, which is widest in the anteroposterior diameter. As the occiput of the fetal head meets resistance from the levator ani muscles and their fascia, the occiput rotates from left to right, and the sagittal suture aligns in the anteroposterior pelvic diameter.

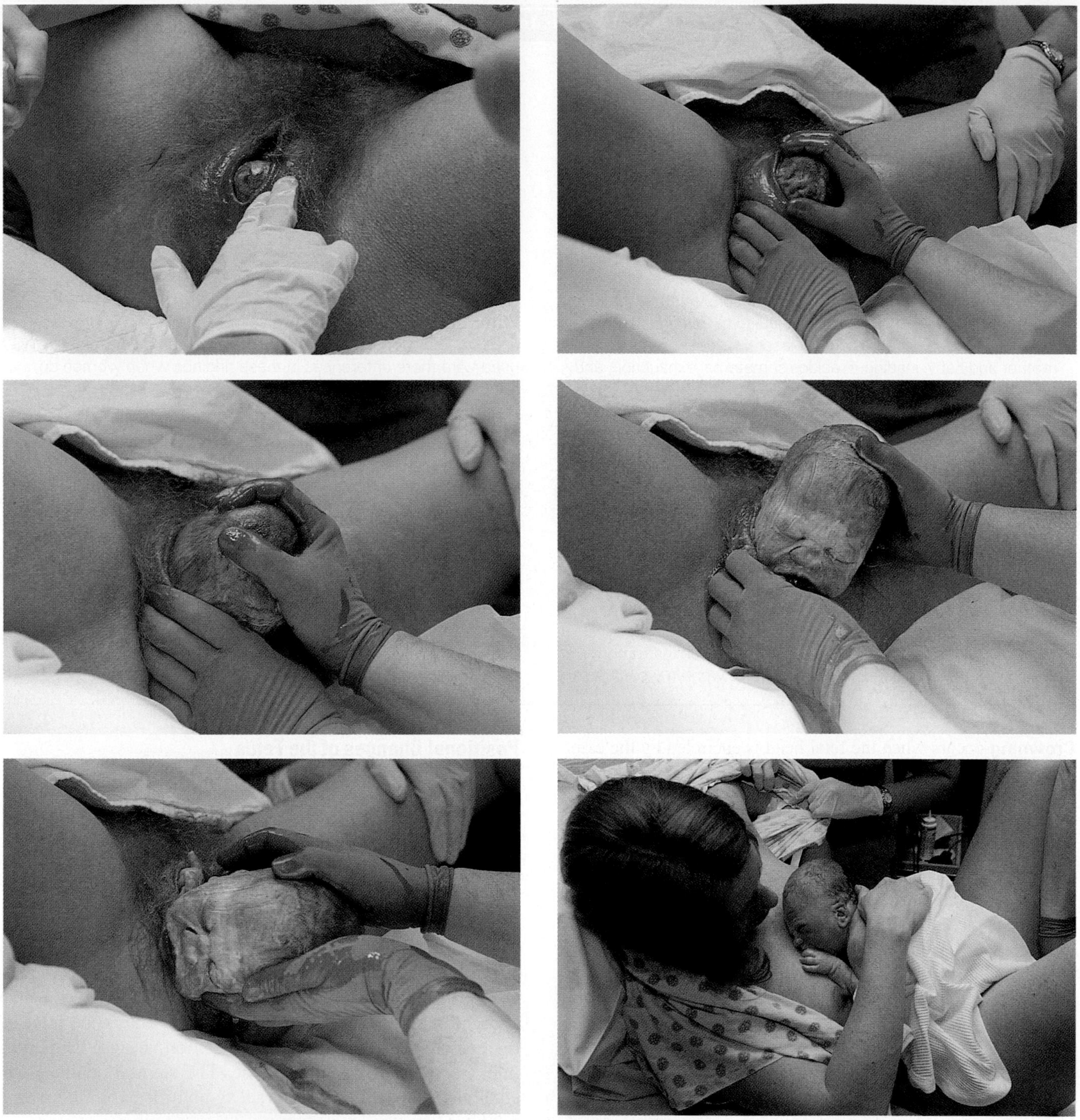

Figure 22-11 ■ The birth sequence.

Source: © Stella Johnson (www.stellajohnson.com).

EXTENSION The resistance of the pelvic floor and the mechanical movement of the vulva opening anteriorly and forward assist with extension of the fetal head as it passes under the symphysis pubis. With this positional change the occiput, then brow and face, emerge from the vagina.

RESTITUTION The shoulders of the infant enter the pelvis obliquely and remain oblique when the head rotates to the anteroposterior diameter through internal rotation. Because of this rotation the neck becomes twisted. Once the head emerges and is free of pelvic resistance the neck untwists, turning the head to one side (restitution), and aligns with the position of the back in the birth canal.

EXTERNAL ROTATION As the shoulders rotate to the anteroposterior position in the pelvis, the head is turned farther to one side (external rotation).

EXPULSION After the external rotation and through expulsive efforts of the laboring woman, the anterior shoulder meets the

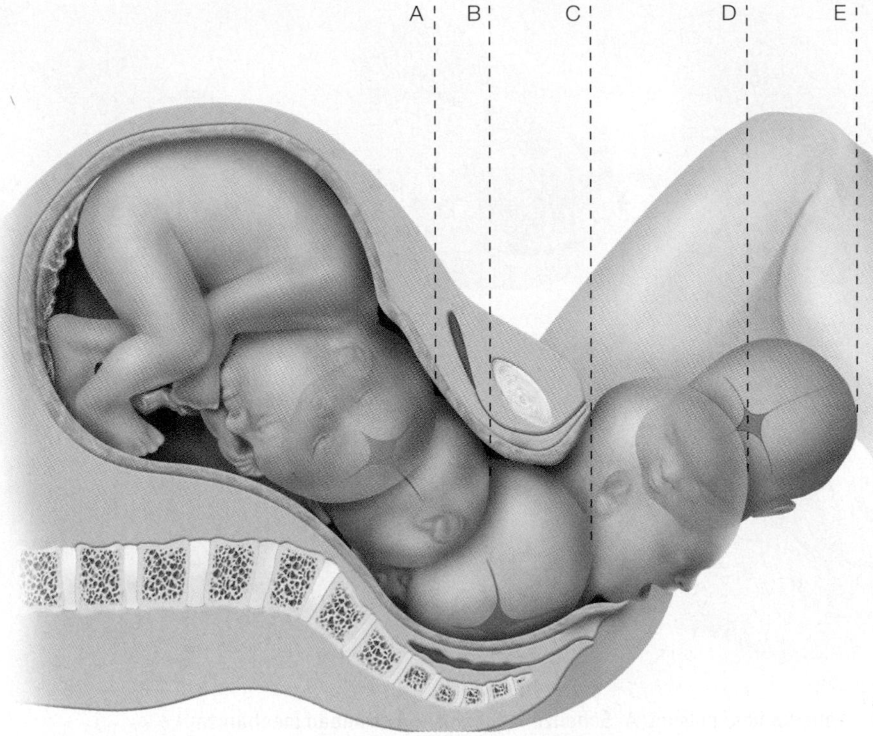

Figure 22-12 ■ Mechanisms of labor. A. and B. Descent. C. Internal rotation. D. Extension. E. External rotation.

undersurface of the symphysis pubis and slips under it. As lateral flexion of the shoulder and head occurs, the anterior shoulder is born before the posterior shoulder. The body follows quickly.

Third Stage

The third stage of labor is defined as the period of time from the birth of the infant until the completed delivery of the placenta.

Placental Separation

After the infant is born, the uterus contracts firmly, diminishing its capacity and the surface area of placental attachment. The placenta begins to separate because of this decrease in surface area. This separation is accompanied by bleeding, leading to the formation of a hematoma between the placental tissue and the remaining decidua. This hematoma accelerates the separation process. The membranes are the last to separate. They are peeled off the uterine wall as the placenta descends into the vagina.

Signs of placental separation usually appear around 5 minutes after birth of the infant, but can take up to 30 minutes to manifest. These signs are (1) a globular-shaped uterus, (2) a rise of the fundus in the abdomen, (3) a sudden gush or trickle of blood, and (4) further protrusion of the umbilical cord out of the vagina.

Placental Delivery

When the signs of placental separation appear, the woman may bear down to aid in placental expulsion. If this fails and the certified nurse-midwife or physician has ascertained that the fundus is firm, gentle traction may be applied to the cord while pressure is exerted on the fundus. The weight of the placenta as it is guided into the placental pan (a basin that holds the placenta once it is expelled) aids in the removal of the membranes from the uterine wall. A placenta is considered to be *retained* if more than 30 minutes have elapsed from completion of the second stage of labor.

If the placenta separates from the inside to the outer margins, it is expelled with the fetal (shiny) side presenting (Figure 22-13A ■). This is known as the *Schultze mechanism* of placental delivery or, more commonly, *shiny Schultze.* If the placenta separates from the outer margins inward, it will roll up and present sideways with the maternal surface delivering first. This is known as the *Duncan mechanism* of placental delivery and is commonly called *dirty Duncan* because the placental surface is rough (Figure 22-13B ■). Also see Figures 11-11 and 11-12 ∞ on page 228.

Nursing and medical interventions during the third stage of labor are discussed in chapter 24 ∞.

Third Stage of Labor

Fourth Stage

The fourth stage of labor is the time from 1 to 4 hours after birth in which physiologic readjustment of the mother's body begins. With the birth, hemodynamic changes occur. Blood loss at birth ranges from 250 to 500 ml. With this blood loss and the easing of pressure exerted by the pregnant uterus on the surrounding vessels, blood is redistributed into venous beds. This results in a moderate drop in both systolic and diastolic blood pressure, increased pulse pressure, and moderate tachycardia (Cunningham et al., 2010).

The uterus remains contracted and is in the midline of the abdomen. The fundus is usually midway between the symphysis pubis and umbilicus. Its contracted state constricts the vessels at the site of placental implantation. Immediately after birth of the placenta, the cervix is widely spread and thick.

Nausea and vomiting experienced during transition usually cease. The woman may be thirsty and hungry. She may

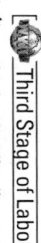

Placental Delivery

A

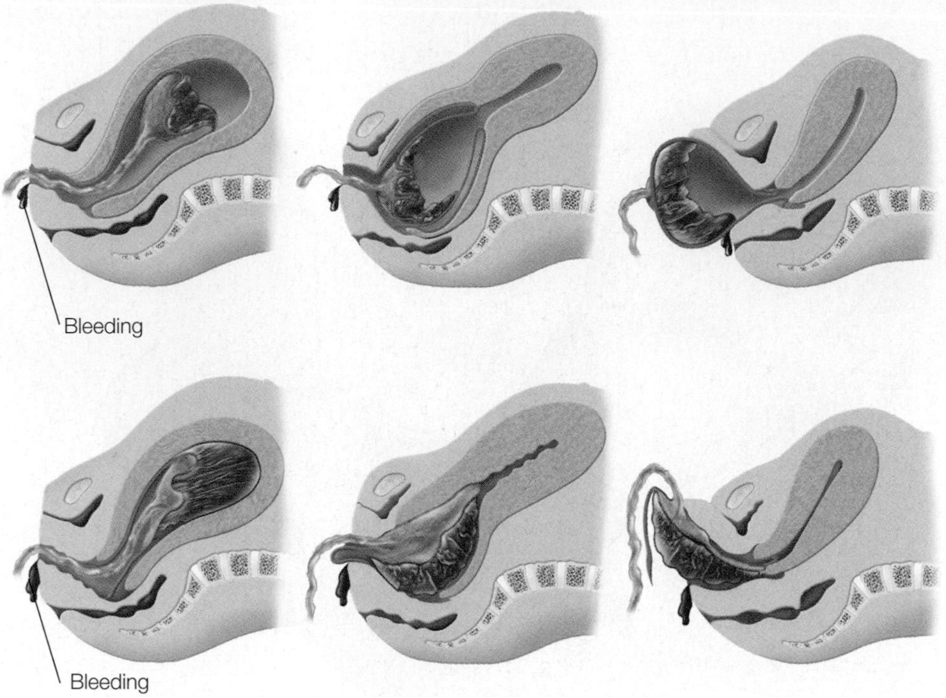

B

Figure 22-13 ■ Placental separation and expulsion. A. Schultze mechanism. B. Duncan mechanism.

experience a shaking chill, which is thought to be associated with the ending of the physical exertion of labor. The bladder is often hypotonic due to trauma during the second stage and/or the administration of anesthetics that may decrease sensations. Hypotonic bladder leads to urinary retention. Nursing care during this stage is discussed in chapter 24 ∞.

> “I have had the privilege of practicing nursing in the birthing area for many years. In my head I know all the factors that must work together to bring this new life into the world. But it is in my heart and in working with and watching the laboring woman (and her partner if she has one) that I truly believe each labor and birth is a miracle. I, along with these parents, get to participate in a moment of time that will never occur again for any of us. I will never tire of this and will never get enough.”

Care Plan Activity: Teenage Patient in Uncomplicated Labor

Maternal Systemic Response to Labor

The labor process affects nearly every major body system. Each system adapts to these changes through various compensation mechanisms.

Cardiovascular System

The woman's cardiovascular system is stressed both by the uterine contractions and by the pain, anxiety, and apprehension the woman experiences. In pregnancy, the resting pulse rate increases by 10 to 18 beats per minute (Gabbe et al., 2007). During labor there is a significant increase in cardiac output. Each strong contraction greatly decreases or completely stops the blood flow in the branches of the uterine artery that supply the intervillous space (in the placenta). This leads to a redistribution of about 300 to 500 ml of blood into the peripheral circulation and an increase in peripheral resistance, resulting in increased systolic and diastolic blood pressure, a slowing of the pulse rate, and an increase of about 30% in cardiac output (Cunningham et al., 2010).

Maternal position also affects cardiac output, blood pressure, and pulse. When the laboring woman turns to a side-lying position, cardiac output increases by about 22%, the pulse rate decreases by about 6 beats per minute, and stroke volume increases by 27%. When the woman is supine, cardiac output increases 25%, stroke volume increases 33%, pulse pressure increases more than 26%, blood pressure rises significantly, and pulse rate decreases by 15%.

There is an additional effect on hemodynamics during the bearing-down efforts in the second stage. When the laboring woman holds her breath and pushes against a closed glottis (Valsalva maneuver), intrathoracic pressure rises. As intrathoracic pressure increases, the venous return is interrupted, increasing venous pressure. In addition the blood in the lungs is forced into the left atrium, which leads to a transient increase in cardiac output, blood pressure, and pulse pressure, and causes bradycardia. As venous return to the lungs continues to be diminished while the breath is held, a decrease in blood pressure, pulse pressure, and cardiac output occurs.

When the next breath is taken (Valsalva maneuver is interrupted), the intrathoracic pressure is decreased. Venous return increases, refilling the pulmonary bed and resulting in recovery of the cardiac output and stroke volume. This process is repeated with each pushing effort.

Immediately after birth, cardiac output peaks with an 80% increase over prelabor values. Then in the first 10 minutes it decreases 20% to 25%. Cardiac output further decreases in the first hour after the birth. However, these decreases still leave the woman with an elevated cardiac output for at least 24 hours after the birth (Cunningham et al., 2010).

Blood Pressure

As a result of increased cardiac output, systolic blood pressure rises during uterine contractions. In the first stage, systolic pressure may increase by 35 mm Hg, and there may be further increases in the second stage during pushing efforts. Diastolic pressure also increases by about 25 mm Hg in the first stage and 65 mm Hg in the second stage. These increases begin just before the uterine contraction, with a return to baseline as soon as the contraction ends (Cunningham et al., 2010). Blood pressure may also rise as a result of fear, apprehension, and pain (Gabbe et al., 2007).

Blood pressure may drop precipitously when the woman lies in a supine position and experiences aortocaval compression. In addition to hypotension there is an increase in the pulse rate, diaphoresis, nausea, weakness, and air hunger. These changes are attributed to the decreased cardiac output and a subsequent drop in stroke volume.

Women with hydramnios, women with multiple gestation, and obese women have the highest risk of developing aortocaval compression. Other predisposing factors include hypovolemia, dehydration, hemorrhage, metabolic acidosis, administration of narcotics (which results in vasodilation and inhibits compensatory mechanisms), and administration of epidural anesthesia, which results in *sympathetic blockade* (blocking of the sympathetic nervous system, leading to vasodilation and hypotension).

Fluid and Electrolyte Balance

Profuse perspiration (diaphoresis) occurs during labor. Hyperventilation also occurs, altering electrolyte and fluid balance from insensible water loss. The muscle activity elevates the body temperature, which increases sweating and evaporation from the skin. As the woman responds to the work of labor, the rise in the respiratory rate increases the evaporative water volume because each breath of air must be warmed to the body temperature and humidified. With the increased evaporative water volume, maintaining adequate oral fluids/hydration is important. Parenteral intravenous fluids may be used to maintain fluid and electrolyte balance.

Respiratory System

Oxygen demand and consumption increase at the onset of labor because of the presence of uterine contractions. Approximately 50% of the increased oxygen is used by the placenta, the uterus, and the fetus (Gabbe et al., 2007). As anxiety and pain from uterine contractions increase, hyperventilation frequently occurs. With hyperventilation there is a fall in $PaCO_2$, and respiratory alkalosis results (Cunningham et al., 2010).

As labor progresses and contractions become more frequent, stronger, and prolonged, the workload, tension, and anxiety of the woman continue to change. A mild increase in the respiratory rate is normal in labor and is related to the increase in metabolism (Gabbe et al., 2007).

By the end of the first stage most women have developed a mild metabolic acidosis compensated by respiratory alkalosis. As she pushes in the second stage of labor, the woman's $PaCO_2$ levels may rise along with blood lactate levels (due to muscular activity), and mild respiratory acidosis occurs. By the time the baby is born (end of second stage), there is metabolic acidosis uncompensated by respiratory alkalosis (Cunningham et al., 2010).

The changes in acid–base status that occur in labor are quickly reversed in the fourth stage because of changes in the woman's respiratory rate. Acid–base levels return to pregnancy levels by 24 hours after birth, and nonpregnant values are attained a few weeks after birth.

Renal System

During labor there is an increase in maternal renin, plasma renin activity, and angiotensinogen. This elevation is thought to be important in the control of uteroplacental blood flow during birth and the early postpartal period (Cunningham et al., 2010).

Polyuria is common during labor. This results from the increase in cardiac output, which causes an increase in the glomerular filtration rate and renal plasma flow. Slight proteinuria occurs in one half to one third of women in labor (Gibbs, Karlan, Haney, et al., 2008).

Structurally, the base of the bladder is pushed forward and upward when engagement occurs. The pressure from the presenting part may impair blood and lymph drainage from the base of the bladder, leading to edema of the tissues (Cunningham et al., 2010). Hematuria may be present as a result of trauma to the lower urinary tract.

Gastrointestinal System

During labor, gastric motility and absorption of solid food are reduced. Gastric emptying time is prolonged, and gastric volume (amount of contents that remain in the stomach) remains over 25 ml, regardless of the time the last meal was taken. This is even more marked in women who have received analgesia agents (Cunningham et al., 2010). These women may be at risk for aspiration should general anesthesia need to be used. During labor, anaerobic and aerobic carbohydrate metabolism rise due to an increase in skeletal muscle activity and maternal anxiety (Gabbe et al., 2007).

The fluid requirements of women in labor have not been clearly established. In some instances oral hydration is the primary goal. In other situations a saline lock may be inserted so that intravenous access is available if needed. If intravenous fluids are used, it is important to remember that when hypertonic glucose infusions are used, there is an increase in maternal blood glucose; this can lead to fetal hyperglycemia and hyperinsulinemia and to hypoglycemia in the newborn.

Immune System and Other Blood Values

The white blood cell (WBC) count increases to 25,000/mm^3 to 30,000/mm^3 during labor and early postpartum (Gibbs et al., 2008). The change in WBC count is due mostly to increased neutrophils resulting from a physiologic response to stress. The increased WBC count makes it difficult to identify the presence of an infectious process.

Maternal blood glucose levels decrease because glucose is used as an energy source during uterine contractions. The decreased blood glucose levels lead to a decrease in insulin requirements (Cunningham et al., 2010). Glucose levels can drop significantly during a prolonged or difficult labor.

Pain

Pain during labor comes from a complexity of physical causes. Each woman will experience and cope with pain differently. Multiple factors affect a woman's reaction to labor pain.

Pain During Labor

The pain associated with the first stage of labor is unique in that it accompanies a normal physiologic process. Even though perception of the pain is determined to some extent by cultural patterning, there is unquestionably a physiologic basis for pain during labor. Pain during the first stage of labor arises from (1) dilatation of the cervix, (2) hypoxia of the uterine muscle cells during contraction, (3) stretching of the lower uterine segment, and (4) pressure on adjacent structures. The primary source of pain is dilatation or stretching of the cervix. Nerve impulses travel through the uterine plexus, to the pelvis through hypogastric plexuses, and then into the lumbar sympathetic chain (Figure 22-14 ■). They enter the spinal cord through the posterior roots of the 10th through 12th thoracic and 1st lumbar nerves.

As with other visceral pain, pain from the uterus is also directly referred to the dermatomes supplied by the 10th through 12th thoracic nerves. The areas of referred pain include the lower abdominal wall and the areas over the lower lumbar region and the upper sacrum (Figure 22-15 ■).

During the second stage of labor, pain is due to (1) hypoxia of the contracting uterine muscle cells, (2) distention of the vagina and perineum, and (3) pressure on adjacent structures including the lower back, buttocks, and thighs. The nerve impulses from the vagina and perineum are transmitted by way of

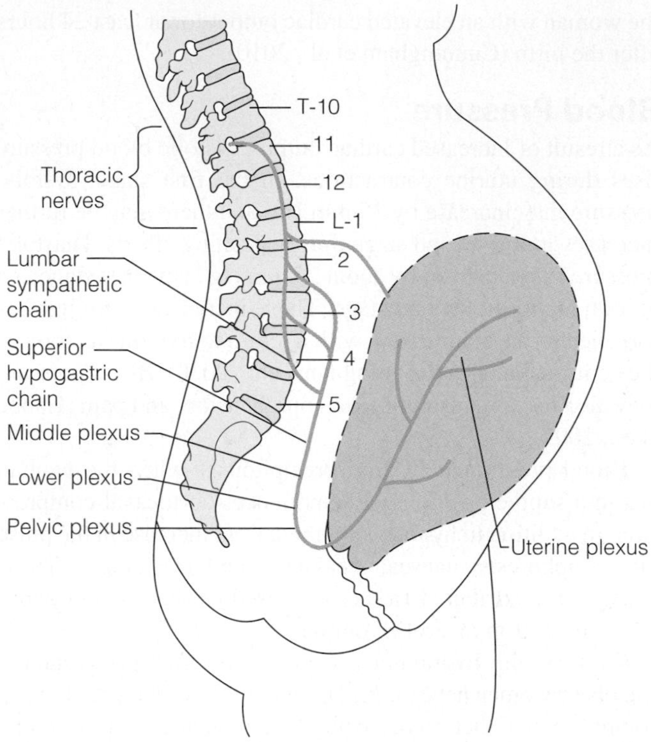

Figure 22-14 ■ Pain pathway from uterus to spinal cord. Nerve impulses travel through the uterine plexus; pelvic plexus; lower, middle, and superior hypogastric plexuses; and lumbar sympathetic chain. They enter the neuroaxis through the 10th, 11th, and 12th thoracic and 1st lumbar spinal segments.

Source: Modified from Bonica, J. J. (1972). Principles and practice of obstetric analgesia and anesthesia *(p. 492). Copyright © 1972 F. A. Davis Company.*

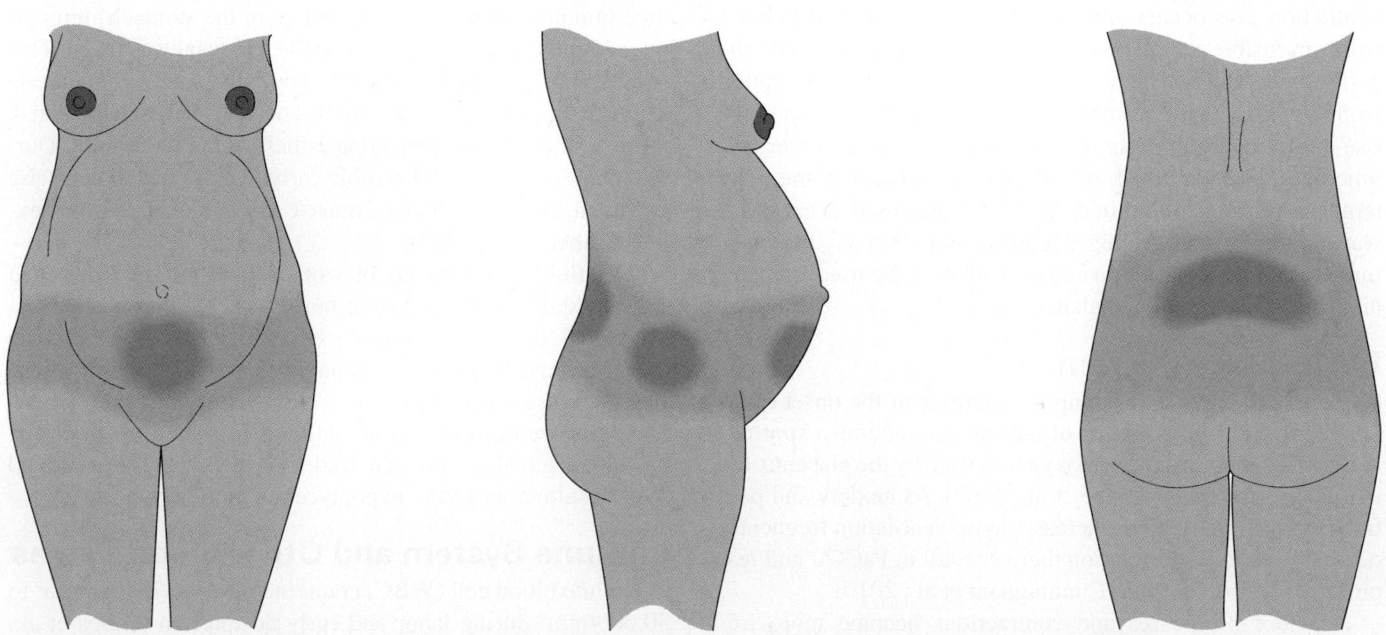

Figure 22-15 ■ Area of reference of labor pain during the first stage. Pain is most intense in the darker colored areas.

Source: Reprinted with permission from Bonica, J. J. (1972). Principles and practice of obstetric analgesia and anesthesia *(p. 108). Copyright © 1972 F. A. Davis Company.*

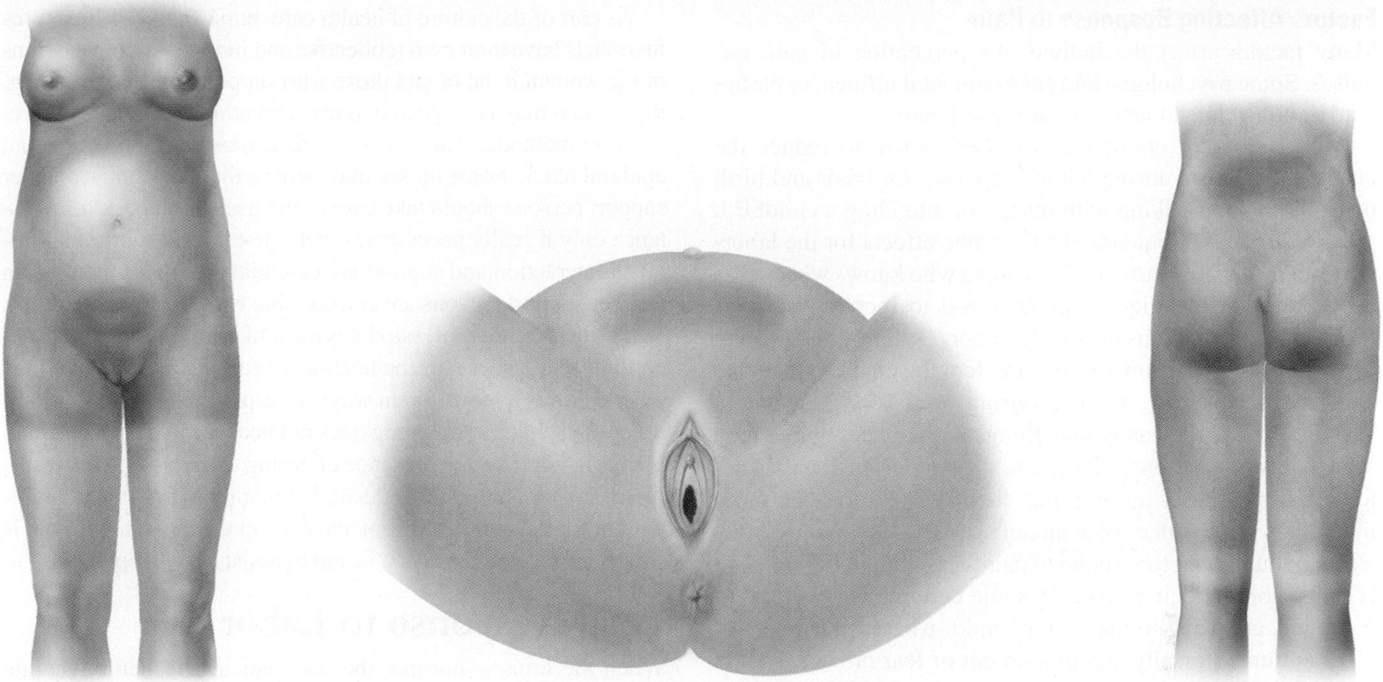

Figure 22-16 ■ Distribution of labor pain during the later phase of the first stage and early phase of the second stage. The darkest colored areas indicate the location of the most intense pain; moderate color, moderate pain; and light color, mild pain. The uterine contractions, which at this stage are very strong, produce intense pain.

Source: Reprinted with permission from Bonica, J. J. (1972). Principles and practice of obstetric analgesia and anesthesia *(p. 109). Copyright © 1972 F. A. Davis Company.*

the pudendal nerve plexus and enter the spinal cord through the posterior roots of the 2nd through 4th sacral nerves. The area of pain increases as shown in Figure 22-16 ■.

Pain during the third stage results from uterine contractions and cervical dilatation as the placenta is expelled. Sensations of pain are felt above the symphysis pubis bone in the perineal area and in the lower back (Figure 22-17 ■). The mechanism for the transmission of nerve impulses is the same as for the first stage of labor. The third stage of labor is short, and after this phase anesthesia is needed primarily for episiotomy repair.

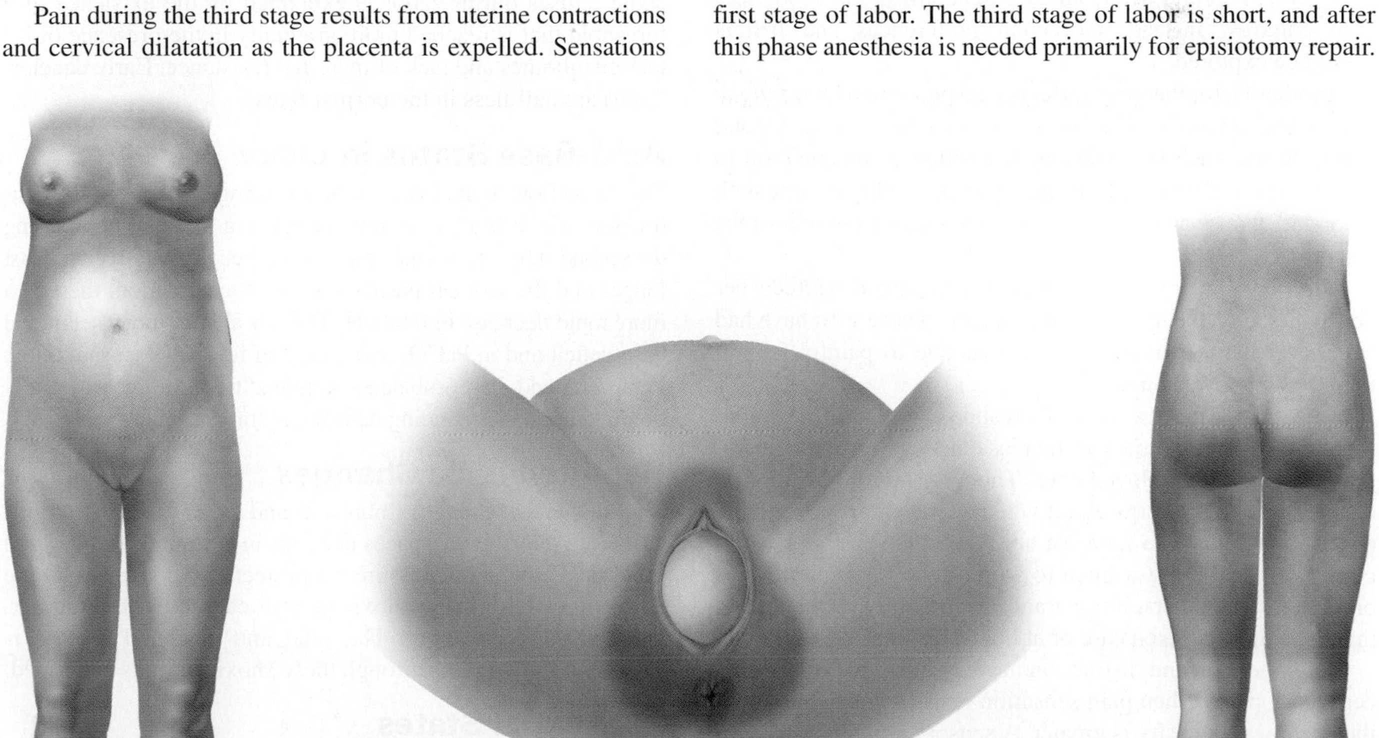

Figure 22-17 ■ Distribution of labor pain during the later phase of the second stage and actual birth. The perineal component is the primary cause of discomfort. Uterine contractions contribute much less.

Source: Reprinted with permission from Bonica, J. J. (1972). Principles and practice of obstetric analgesia and anesthesia *(p. 109). Copyright © 1972 F. A. Davis Company.*

Factors Affecting Response to Pain

Many factors affect the individual's perception of pain impulses. Some psychologic and environmental influences particularly appropriate to labor are discussed here.

Preparation for childbirth has been shown to reduce the need for analgesia during labor. Preparing for labor and birth through reading, talking with others, or attending a childbirth preparation class frequently has positive effects for the laboring woman and her partner. The woman who knows what to expect and what techniques she may use to increase comfort tends to be less anxious during the labor. A tour of the birthing center and an opportunity to see and feel the environment also help reduce anxiety, because during admission (especially with the first child) many new things are happening and they seem to occur all at once. The more the woman and her partner learn during classes and through their own efforts, the more likely they will reduce some anxiety.

Individuals tend to respond to painful stimuli in the way that is acceptable in their culture. In some cultures, it is natural to communicate pain, no matter how mild, whereas members of other cultures stoically accept pain out of fear or because it is expected. Nurses need to be aware of cultural norms and demonstrate culturally sensitive care to women and their families in the intrapartum setting (Vedam, Goff, & Marnin, 2007).

Families will react to the healthcare system based on their own cultural beliefs. Nurses need to identify specific cultural norms with each individual family so appropriate care can be provided. Whenever possible, requests that include the family's cultural preferences should be incorporated into the woman's care. Nurses should avoid making generalizations about specific cultures. Instead, individual preferences and beliefs should be explored.

Another factor that may influence response to pain is *fatigue* and *sleep deprivation.* The fatigued woman has less energy and ability to use such strategies as distraction or imagination to deal with pain. As a result, she may lose her ability to cope with labor and choose analgesics or other medications to relieve the discomfort.

The woman's *previous experience* with pain also affects her ability to manage current and future pain. Those who have had experience with pain seem more sensitive to painful stimuli than those who have not.

Anxiety can affect a woman's response to pain. Unfamiliar surroundings and events can increase anxiety, as does separation from family and loved ones. The woman's anticipation of discomfort and concerns about whether she can cope with the contractions may also increase her anxiety level. It is not uncommon for laboring women to worry about their partners or other family members. Reassurance from family members that things are being "taken care of at home" can help.

Both attention and distraction have an influence on the perception of pain. When pain sensation is the focus of attention, the perceived intensity is greater. A sensory stimulus such as a backrub can be a distraction that focuses the woman's attention on the stimulus rather than the pain. The nurse can offer suggestions to support persons on interventions to initiate physical distractions for the laboring woman.

As part of the culture of health care, nursing and medical professionals have their own (collective and individual) expectations of the woman in labor and those who support her. In one setting, the woman may be expected to use a breathing technique and relaxation methods, whereas in another, most women receive an epidural block. Some nurses may believe that the woman and her support persons should take care of themselves and ask for assistance only if really necessary; other nurses may believe that frequent interaction and support are essential as long as the woman and her support persons are comfortable with the interaction.

The healthcare professional is most likely to interpret pain according to the norms of the healthcare culture, although various other cultures have different ways of responding to pain. The absence of crying and moaning does not necessarily mean that pain is absent, nor does the presence of crying and moaning necessarily mean that pain relief is desired at that moment. It is very important for the nurse to accept and respect the fact that the pain is whatever the woman says it is and to assist her in coping with it.

Fetal Response to Labor

When the fetus is normal, the mechanical and hemodynamic changes of normal labor have no adverse effects.

Heart Rate Changes

Fetal heart rate decelerations can occur with intracranial pressures of 40 to 55 mm Hg. The currently accepted explanation of this early deceleration is hypoxic depression of the central nervous system, which is under vagal control. The absence of these head compression decelerations (early decelerations) in some fetuses during labor is explained by the existence of a threshold that is reached more gradually in the presence of intact membranes and lack of maternal resistance. Early decelerations are harmless in the normal fetus.

Acid–Base Status in Labor

The blood flow to the fetus is slowed during the acme of the contraction, which leads to a slow decrease in the fetal pH. During the second stage, as uterine contractions become stronger and last longer and the woman pushes with each contraction, there is a more rapid decrease in fetal pH. There is also an increase in fetal base deficit and in $PaCO_2$ and a drop in fetal oxygen saturation. Persistent acid–base imbalance can lead to multiorgan dysfunction in the infant, including neurologic impairment.

Hemodynamic Changes

The adequate exchange of nutrients and gases in the fetal capillaries and intervillous spaces depends in part on the fetal blood pressure. Fetal blood pressure is a protective mechanism for the normal fetus during the anoxic periods caused by the contracting uterus during labor. The fetal and placental reserve is enough to see the fetus through these anoxic periods unharmed.

Behavioral States

The human fetus develops behavioral states between 36 and 38 weeks of gestation. The behavioral states seem to continue during labor even in the presence of uterine contractions. Two sleep states (quiet and active) are most prevalent, although quiet and active awake states are occasionally observed. A decrease in fetal heart rate variability accompanies the quiet sleep state, and there is also a decrease in fetal breathing movements and other general body activity. The quiet sleep state generally lasts less than 40 minutes.

Fetal Sensation

Beginning at about 37 or 38 weeks' gestation (full term), the fetus is able to experience sensations of light, sound, and touch. Fetal hearing begins to develop at 23 to 24 weeks but is not considered reliable until 28 weeks (Blackburn, 2007). Even in utero, the fetus is sensitive to light and will move away from a bright light source. Additionally, the term baby is aware of pressure sensations during labor such as the touch of the caregiver during a vaginal exam or pressure on the head as a contraction occurs. Although the fetus may not be able to process this input, as the woman labors the fetus is experiencing the labor as well.

FOCUS YOUR STUDY

- Five factors that continually interact during labor and birth are the birth passage, the birth passenger (fetus), the relationship between the birth passage and the fetus, the physiologic forces of labor, and factors associated with the woman's psychosocial status.
- Four types of pelves have been identified, and each has a different effect on labor. The diameters of gynecoid and anthropoid pelves are usually large enough for labor and birth to progress normally. In the android and platypelloid types, the pelvic diameters are diminished (smaller than in gynecoid and anthropoid). Labor is more likely to be difficult (longer) and a cesarean birth is more likely.
- Important dimensions of the maternal pelvis include the diameters of the pelvic inlet, pelvic cavity, and pelvic outlet.
- The fetal head contains bones in the top portion (cranial vault) that are not fused. This allows them to overlap somewhat in response to the pressures on the fetal head during labor. The pressure and overlapping of the sutures, which are membranous spaces between the cranial bones, result in a change in the shape of the head called molding.
- Fetal attitude refers to the relation of the fetal parts to one another. The head is usually held in midline and not to one side or the other, and the extremities are usually flexed and held close to the body because there is little extra room within the uterine cavity.
- Fetal lie refers to the relationship of the cephalocaudal (head to sacral area) axis of the fetus to the maternal spine. The fetal lie is either longitudinal (both the maternal and fetal spines are vertical) or transverse (the fetal spine is at a right angle to the maternal spine).
- Fetal presentation is determined by the body part lying closest to the inlet of the maternal pelvis. In a longitudinal lie the fetal presentation is usually cephalic (head first) but may also be breech (buttocks or one or both feet first). In a transverse lie the fetal shoulder is usually closest to the pelvic inlet.
- Engagement of the presenting part occurs when the largest diameter of the fetal presenting part reaches or passes through the pelvic inlet.
- Station refers to the relationship of the presenting part to an imaginary line drawn between the maternal ischial spines, which are in the midpoint of the pelvic cavity. The fetal presenting part enters the pelvic inlet at what is termed about a −5 and descends toward the ischial spines, where it is called a 0 (zero) station. Further descent from 0 to +4 occurs as the presenting part descends below the ischial spines toward the vaginal opening.
- Fetal position is the relationship of a specified landmark on the presenting fetal part to the sides, front, or back of the maternal pelvis. Once the position is known, the positions of the fetal head and back can be determined.
- Each uterine contraction has an increment, acme, and decrement.
- Contraction frequency is the time from the beginning of one contraction to the beginning of the next contraction.

- Duration of contractions refers to the period of time from the beginning to the end of one contraction.
- Intensity of contractions refers to the strength of the contraction during acme. Intensity of contractions is termed mild, moderate, or strong.
- Labor stresses the coping skills of women. Women with prenatal education about childbirth usually report more positive responses to labor.
- Women with support persons tend to use their coping skills more effectively than those who lack support.
- Premonitory signs of labor include lightening, Braxton Hicks contractions, cervical softening and effacement, bloody show, sudden burst of energy, weight loss, and, sometimes, rupture of membranes.
- True labor contractions occur regularly with an increase in frequency, duration, and intensity. The contractions usually start in the back and radiate around the abdomen. The discomfort is not relieved by ambulation, rest, or warm tub baths. False labor contractions do not produce progressive cervical effacement and dilatation. They are irregular and do not increase in intensity. The discomfort may be relieved by ambulation, rest, or warm tub baths.
- Possible causes of labor onset include the progesterone withdrawal hypothesis, the prostaglandin hypothesis, and the corticotropin-releasing hormone hypothesis.
- There are four stages of labor and birth. The first stage is from beginning of true labor to complete dilatation of the cervix. The second stage is from complete dilatation of the cervix to birth. The third stage is from birth to expulsion of the placenta. The fourth stage is from expulsion of the placenta to a period of 1 to 4 hours after.
- The fetus accommodates to the maternal pelvis in a series of movements called the cardinal movements of labor, which include descent, flexion, internal rotation, extension, restitution, external rotation, and expulsion.
- Placental separation is indicated by lengthening of the umbilical cord, a small spurt of blood, change in uterine shape, and a rise of the fundus in the abdomen.
- The placenta is expelled by Schultze or Duncan mechanism. This is determined by the way it separates from the uterine wall.
- Maternal systemic responses to labor involve the cardiovascular, respiratory, renal, gastrointestinal, and immune systems. Cardiac output and blood pressure increase, as do oxygen demand and consumption. Polyuria is common, and gastric motility and absorption are reduced. The white blood cell count increases, and blood glucose levels decrease.
- Factors that affect the response to labor pain include education, cultural beliefs, fatigue and sleep deprivation, personal significance of pain, previous experience, anxiety, and the availability of coping techniques.
- The fetus is usually able to tolerate the labor process with no untoward changes.

CRITICAL THINKING IN ACTION

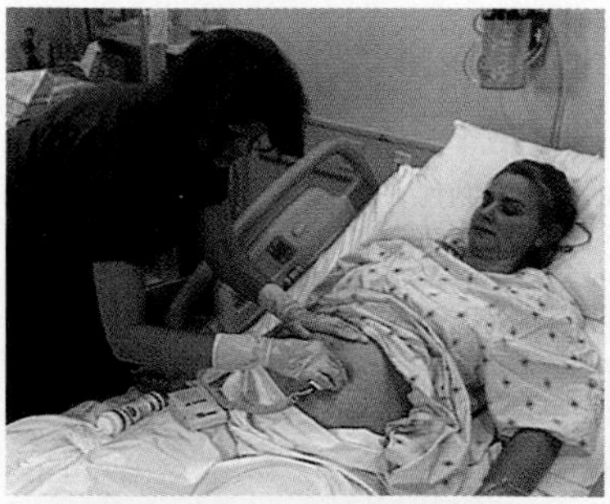

Source: George Dodson/Pearson Education.

Ann Nelson, a 28-year-old, G2, P0010 at 41 weeks' gestation, is admitted to the birthing unit where you are working. She is here for cervical ripening and induction of labor due to postdate pregnancy and decreased amniotic fluid volume. A review of her prenatal chart reveals a pertinent history of infertility (Clomid-induced pregnancy) and asthma (treated with inhalers on a PRN basis). The Doppler picks up a fetal heart rate of 120 beats/min. You place Ann on the electronic fetal monitor and obtain the following data: BP 126/76, T 98°F, P 82, R 16; vaginal exam reveals a 20% effaced cervix, 1 cm dilatation in the posterior position, and vertex at −2 station. The fetal monitor shows a fetal heart rate baseline of 120 to 128 with occasional variable decelerations, accelerations to 140 with fetal activity. No contractions are noted on the monitor or palpated. Ann asks you what to expect with "cervical ripening" using prostaglandin gel.

1. Discuss the action of prostaglandin gel.
2. Ann asks you why cervical ripening and induction of labor are recommended for her and her baby. How would you best respond to her?
3. Ann asks how she will know if she is getting contractions. How would you answer her?
4. Discuss the difference between mild, moderate, and strong contractions.
5. Describe the latent phase of labor.

See www.nursing.pearsonhighered.com for possible responses.

REFERENCES

Alhusen, J. L. (2008). A literature update on maternal-fetal attachment. *Journal of Obstetric, Gynecologic, and Neonatal Nursing: (JOGNN), 37*(3), 315–328.

Blackburn, S. (2007). *Maternal, fetal and neonatal physiology: A clinical perspective* (3rd ed.). Philadelphia, PA: Saunders.

Challis, J. R. G. (2008) Characteristics of Parturition. In *Creasy & Resnik's Maternal-fetal medicine* (6th ed.). Philadelphia, PA: Saunders.

Cunningham, F. G., Leveno, K. J., Bloom, S. L., Hauth, J. C., Rouse, D. J., & Spong, C. (2010). *Williams obstetrics* (23rd ed.). New York, NY: McGraw-Hill.

Gabbe, S. G., Niebyl, J. R., Simpson, J. L., Galan, H., Goetzl, L., Landan, M., & Jauniaux, E. R. (2007). *Obstetrics: Normal and problem pregnancies* (5th ed.). Philadelphia, PA: Churchill Livingstone.

Gibbs, R. S., Karlan, B. Y., Haney, A. F., & Nygaard, I., (2008). *Danforth's obstetrics and gynecology* (10th ed.). Philadelphia, PA: Lippincott Williams & Wilkins.

Goldbort, J. G. (2009). Women's lived experience of their unexpected birthing process. MCN. *The American Journal of Maternal Child Nursing, 34*(1), 57–62.

Goldenberg, R., Culhane, J., Iams, J., & Romero, R. (2009). Epidemiology and causes of preterm birth. *The Lancet, 371*(9606), 75–84.

McKellar L., Pincombe J., & Henderson A. (2008). Enhancing fathers' educational experiences during the early postnatal period. *The Journal of Perinatal Education, 17*(4), 12–20.

Vedam, S., Goff, M., & Marnin, V. N. (2007). Closing the theory-practice gap: Intrapartum midwifery management of planned homebirths. *Journal of Midwifery & Women's Health, 52*(3), 291–300.

CHAPTER 23

Intrapartum Nursing Assessment

Birth is the sudden opening of a window, through which you look out upon a stupendous prospect. For what has happened? A miracle. You have exchanged nothing for the possibility of everything.

—William MacNeile Dixon

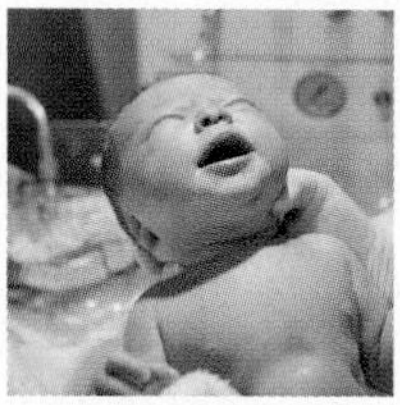

LEARNING OUTCOMES

1. Summarize intrapartum physical, psychosocial, and cultural assessments necessary for optimum maternal-fetal outcome.
2. Discuss the outer limits of normal progress of each of the phases and stages of labor.
3. Compare the various methods of monitoring fetal heart rate and contractions, giving advantages and disadvantages of each.
4. Describe the procedure for performing Leopold's maneuvers and the information that can be obtained.
5. Differentiate between baseline and periodic changes in the fetal heart rate.
6. Examine the differences between fetal tachycardia and fetal bradycardia.
7. Discuss fetal heart rates and patterns using National Institute of Child Health and Human Development (NICHD) terminology.
8. Explain the steps to be performed in the systematic evaluation of fetal heart rate tracings.
9. Evaluate abnormal findings on a fetal heart rate tracing.
10. Explain the interventions that are indicated when a nonreassuring fetal heart rate pattern is identified.
11. Describe the steps used to perform fetal scalp stimulation.

KEY TERMS

The labor process is a period of increased physiologic stress for the pregnant woman and her fetus. The physiologic events that occur during the intrapartum period require many changes and rapid adaptations; thus accurate and frequent assessment is crucial. The primary purpose of the intrapartum assessment is to collect the essential data needed to evaluate the response of the mother and fetus to the changes in labor and the well-being of the "maternal-fetal unit" throughout those changes. The nurse in the birth setting uses a wide variety of assessment skills, including observation, palpation, and auscultation, to provide care for two primary patients, the mother and her child. The expectant mother's partner or support person is also an important member of the birthing team, and assessments of the couple's coping, interactions, and teamwork are integral to the nurse's knowledge base. The nurse's physical presence with the laboring woman provides the best opportunity for ongoing assessment, even as the nurse quietly provides comfort measures and gently assists the "coach" in offering support.

In current practice, "hands-on" techniques can be augmented by the use of technology. For example, the nurse or clinician can use Doppler ultrasound (US) to listen to the fetal heart rate (FHR) or an electronic fetal monitor to assist in recording contractions and the FHR. No matter what technology is used, however, it is important that the nurse remember that "the machine" or "the test" only provides information; it cannot replace the human interaction and support that are provided by the nurse. In the birth setting that provides "high-touch" nursing care, the "high-tech" assessments are easily integrated to provide comprehensive, high-quality care.

This chapter discusses the assessments that are an important part of nursing care in the birth setting.

Maternal Assessment

The goal of a maternal assessment is to create an accurate database of information from which healthcare providers best formulate an optimal plan of care for a patient given her current clinical situation. Assessment of the intrapartal woman begins with a patient history and screening for intrapartal risk factors. Data collection includes a variety of data assessment methods: the prenatal record, admission interviews of the patient and family members to obtain historical data, a psychologic assessment, and the initial and ongoing assessments of the mother and fetus throughout labor.

Assessment and evaluation of the potential intrapartum patient may vary from patient to patient depending on the woman's condition and stage of labor. The professional guidelines for perinatal care state that pregnant women who present to the acute care setting should be evaluated in a timely manner. Women may often need to be triaged upon presentation to the obstetrical unit; thus, nursing staff may be required to perform intrapartal assessments in various phases to facilitate prompt and efficient care for all patients. For instance, initial evaluation of a pregnant woman who presents for admission may minimally include only the assessment of her vital signs, fetal heart rate (FHR), status of uterine contractions, and any abnormal symptoms or signs of distress such as vaginal bleeding, acute abdominal pain, temperature above 100.4°F, premature labor, premature rupture of membranes (PROM), hypertension, or nonreassuring fetal patterns (American Academy of Pediatrics [AAP] & American College of Obstetricians and Gynecologists [ACOG], 2007).

If a pregnant woman is suspected of being in labor or has ruptured membranes or vaginal bleeding, the nurse should promptly continue to assess and evaluate the mother and initiate appropriate treatment. If a woman is in early labor and presents without complications, the nurse may defer the complete physical assessment and admission of the mother once fetal well-being has been determined. Assessment and evaluation may be limited to the interval between the points of care of a woman who has received prenatal care, has recently been evaluated, and presents with no risk factors to the present admission. On the other hand, a woman who has received no prenatal care may require a complete assessment including history and physical, obstetrical evaluation, laboratory tests, ultrasound, and other indicated procedures as her condition warrants (AAP & ACOG, 2007). Regardless of status, the well-being of the mother and fetus are of primary concern, and it is the responsibility of the nursing and medical staff to obtain accurate and appropriate data regarding the patient and to provide appropriate services as needed.

Prenatal Record

According to perinatal guidelines, when a pregnant woman approaches approximately 36 weeks' gestation, a copy of the prenatal record should be available at the acute care facility so that the medical record is accessible to members of the healthcare delivery team. If the prenatal record is available, it can provide the foundation for the intrapartum assessment. Health conditions, risk factors, abnormal test results, and ongoing assessments that have been completed during the course of the pregnancy are often useful information in determining patient care needs. Information contained in the prenatal record should be verified if possible to avoid the possibility of conflicts during subsequent patient interviews.

Historical Data

During assessment interviews, the pregnant patient is likely to be the primary source of information. Often her partner or another family member may be present and capable of providing information in the event that the mother cannot concentrate or participate in the interview because of her physical state or stage of labor. The patient's privacy must still remain a concern for the nurse in every circumstance, and every measure must be taken to safeguard it and the patient's right to confidentiality.

The historical data is the foundation for the intrapartum assessment. The historical or background data include the patient's demographic and socioeconomic information; medical, surgical, family, obstetrical, and gynecological histories; psychosociocultural assessments; and physical examination

Through the Eyes of a Nurse
Signs and Symptoms of Labor

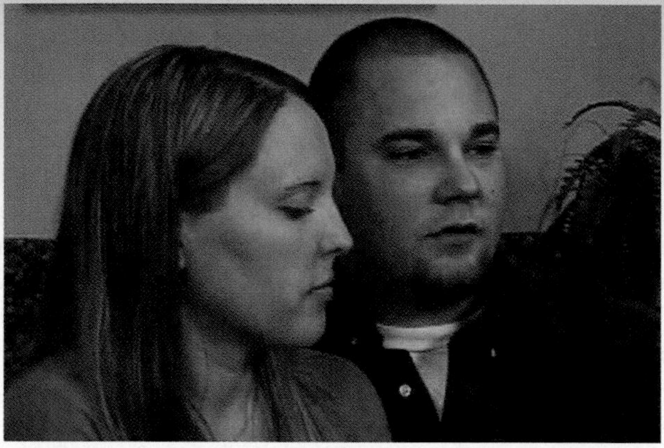

Family's Experience

At the prenatal visit, the father of the baby expresses concerns about recognizing true labor signs. "She has been having so many of these Braxton Hicks contractions, I am afraid we won't know if it is really labor and she will have the baby at home! Is it that different? I keep having a reoccurring dream that she has the baby at home and we're all alone!"

Nurse's Response

"Many couples worry that the baby will come quickly and will be born at home, but this is quite rare. The contractions (Braxton Hicks) that she is having now are for the most part painless tightening although they can be more uncomfortable when you get closer to the due date. They are common and do not have any particular pattern to them.

"True labor is marked by regular contractions that result in cervical change. The only way to know if you are having cervical change is to be examined. Once your contractions become regular and painful, you will come to the hospital where we will monitor your contraction pattern and examine your cervix.

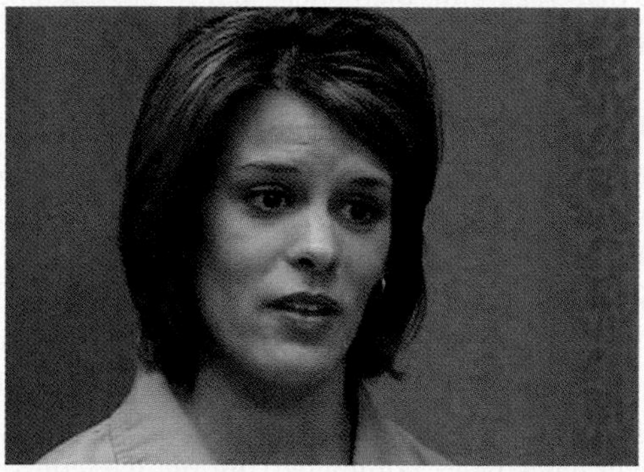

"You will also need to come in to the birth setting if your water breaks or if you have any vaginal bleeding or a decrease in the baby's movement patterns."

Nurse's Actions and Rationale

The nurse reassures the couple that labor is usually recognized and that there usually is adequate time to get to the birth setting. The nurse should review the signs of labor and danger signs and advise the couple when they should come to the birth setting. A written information sheet is helpful and allows the couple to review the information at home.

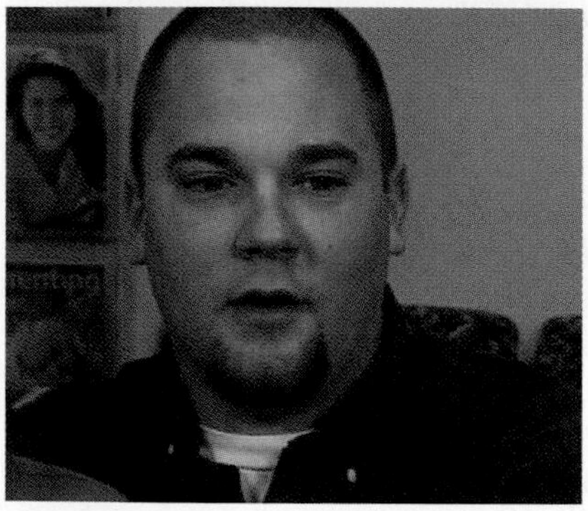

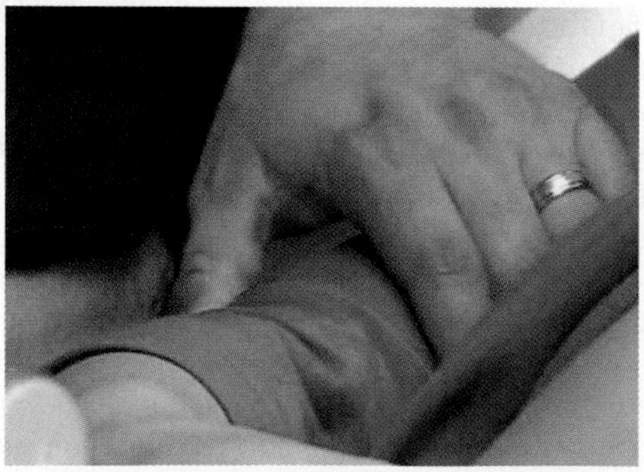

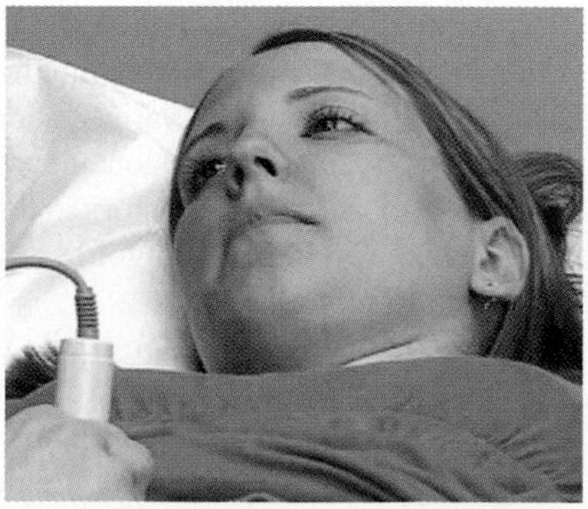

(Simpson & Creehan, 2007). Relevant data include the following (Cunningham et al., 2010):

- Demographic information
  - Name and age
  - Attending obstetrician or certified nurse-midwife (CNM)
  - Pediatrician/family physician
- Socioeconomic factors
  - Housing, transportation
  - Ability to provide for the new baby
  - Support system
- Psychosocial assessment
  - Cultural factors
  - Resources and support systems
  - Domestic violence screening
  - Substance abuse/exposure
- Medical and surgical histories
  - History of previous illness, such as tuberculosis, heart disease, diabetes, convulsive disorders, immune system abnormalities, hematologic disorders, thyroid disorders, gastrointestinal abnormalities, asthma, sickle cell anemia, Tay-Sachs disease, psychologic disorders, and other inherited disorders
  - Surgeries
- Family history
  - Genetic disorders, medical conditions, psychiatric conditions
- Obstetrical history
  - Past pregnancies
    - Complications during pregnancy (e.g., preeclampsia/eclampsia, gestational diabetes, anemia, hyperemesis, hydramnios or oligohydramnios, placenta previa)
    - Labor complications (e.g., dystocia [malpresentation, cephalopelvic disproportion (CPD), macrosomia, failure to progress], precipitous or prolonged labor, prolonged pushing, hemorrhage, placenta abruption or accreta, cord prolapse, embolism, mechanical delivery [forceps or vacuum], pain management [epidural or medications], episiotomy/laceration)
    - Postpartum complications (e.g., hemorrhage, infection, thrombus, postpartum depression, difficulty breastfeeding)
    - High-risk factors
    - Previous abortions, term and preterm infants, number of living children, neonatal deaths
    - Mode of birth
  - Current pregnancy
    - Gravidity, parity
    - High-risk factors
    - Blood type; Rh factor; results of serology testing; complete blood count (CBC); glucose testing; screens for hepatitis, syphilis, rubella, chlamydia, gonorrhea, and group beta strep; quadruple screen, and results of any genetic diagnostic (nuchal translucency testing, chorionic villus sampling, amniocentesis), and specialized testing (Tay-Sachs, cystic fibrosis, sickle cell)
    - Allergies to medications, foods, or substances
    - Drug and alcohol consumption and smoking during pregnancy
    - Elevated blood pressure, bleeding problems, recurrent urinary tract infection
    - Medications used during the pregnancy, including prescription medication, over-the-counter medications, and herbal supplements
    - Method chosen for infant feeding
    - Type of prenatal education (childbirth preparation classes)
    - Woman's preferences regarding labor and birth, such as no episiotomy, no analgesics or anesthetics, or the presence/participation of the father or others at the birth
  - Gestational age assessment
  - Fetal activity
  - Leopold's maneuvers
  - Fetal positioning
- Clinical assessment
  - Maternal vital signs
  - Maternal weight, height, and weight gain this pregnancy
  - Nutritional status
  - Uterine activity
    - Contraction assessment
      - Onset, duration, frequency of uterine contractions
    - Fetal response to uterine contractions
  - Membrane status
    - Status of membranes, color of amniotic fluid
    - Date and time of rupture
  - Vaginal examination
    - Vaginal bleeding and discharge
    - Cervical exam
- Biochemical examinations during pregnancy
  - Laboratory studies
    - CBC, blood type, and Rh and antibody screen
    - Toxicology screening (if ordered)
    - Blood glucose screening
    - Urine for protein and sugar
  - Infectious disease evaluation
    - Chlamydia, gonorrhea, group beta strep, hepatitis B, rubella, syphilis
    - Optional infectious disease evaluation: cytomegalovirus, tuberculosis, trichomonas, HIV, hepatitis A and C, herpes simplex virus
- Fetal assessment
  - Gestational age assessment
    - Last menstrual period (LMP)
    - Fetal movement
    - Ultrasound exams for dating
  - Fetal activity
    - Fetal movement by maternal report
    - Fetal movement by palpation
  - Antenatal assessments
    - Nonstress tests (NSTs)
    - Contraction stress tests (CSTs)
    - Biophysical profiles
    - Ultrasounds
    - Amniotic fluid index (AFI)

- Method of monitoring
  - Auscultation
  - External
    - Ultrasound
    - Tocodynamometer
  - Internal
    - Fetal spiral electrode
    - Intrauterine pressure catheter

Intrapartum High-Risk Screening

Screening for intrapartum high-risk factors is an integral part of assessment of the normal laboring woman. While obtaining the history, the nurse notes the presence of any factors that may be associated with a high-risk condition (Simpson & Creehan, 2007). For example, the woman who reports a physical symptom such as intermittent bleeding needs further assessment to rule out abruptio placentae or placenta previa before the admission process continues. In addition to identifying the presence of a high-risk condition, the nurse must recognize the implications of the condition for the laboring woman and her fetus. For example, in the case of an abnormal fetal presentation, the nurse understands that the labor may be prolonged, prolapse of the umbilical cord may be more likely, and there is a greater possibility of a cesarean birth.

Although physical conditions are frequently listed as the major factors that increase risk in the intrapartum period, psychosocial and cultural variables such as poverty, nutrition, the amount of prenatal care, and cultural beliefs regarding pregnancy can also precipitate a high-risk situation in the intrapartum period. Women who suffer from post-traumatic stress disorder (PTSD) or depression may be at increased risk for some intrapartal complications (Lev-Wiesel, Chen, Daphna-Tekoah, & Hod, 2009). The nurse should begin gathering data about these psychosocial and cultural factors as the woman enters the birthing area.

Communication problems can also affect the course of labor, as well as the nurse's ability to provide support and education. Thus, the nurse observes the communication pattern between the woman and her support person(s) and their responses to admission questions and initial teaching. If the nurse or other birthing room staff does not speak the primary language of the woman and her support person(s) or if the woman is hearing impaired, an appropriate interpreter should be obtained so that the patient can make informed decisions. (See further discussion in appendices C ∞, D ∞, and E ∞.) Communication may also be affected by cultural standards regarding when it is acceptable to speak, who should ask questions, or whether it is acceptable for the woman to let others know if she is experiencing discomfort (Spector, 2009).

An intimate partner violence (IPV) assessment should be performed on all women throughout the pregnancy and at admission to the intrapartum unit. Since women with a history of IPV are at greater risk for certain adverse events, such as preterm labor, low birth weight, neonatal admissions, and infant death, an assessment of IPV is essential (New York City Department of Health and Mental Hygiene, 2010). Victims of IPV are also more likely to experience an unintended pregnancy and are more at risk for depression and postpartum depression (New York City Department of Health and Mental Hygiene, 2010).

A partial list of intrapartum risk factors appears in Table 23-1. The factors precede the Intrapartum Assessment Guide because they must be kept in mind during the assessment.

Intrapartum Physical and Psychosociocultural Assessment

A physical examination is part of the admission procedure and part of the ongoing care of the patient. Although the intrapartum physical assessment is not as complete and thorough as the initial prenatal physical examination (see chapter 15 ∞), it does involve assessment of some body systems and the actual labor process. The Intrapartum Assessment Guide on pages 560–563 provides a framework that the maternity nurse can use when examining the laboring woman.

The physical assessment includes assessments performed immediately on admission as well as ongoing assessments. When labor is progressing very quickly, the nurse may not have time for a complete assessment. In this case, the critical physical assessments would include maternal vital signs, labor status, fetal status, and laboratory findings. Psychologic disorders can also affect the intrapartum course. For example, the woman suffering from clinical depression may exhibit apathy, lack of energy, fear or hopelessness about the outcome of labor, or increased physical symptoms (Kamysheva, Skouteris, Wertheim, et al., 2009). The woman with a panic disorder may have short-lived, unpredictable episodes of intense anxiety, whereas the woman with a generalized anxiety disorder may experience continual and excessive anxiety or worrying. The woman with obsessive-compulsive disorder may have irrational impulses that are relieved only with performing a ritualistic behavior, such as repetitive hand washing. Psychosis is one of the most disabling psychiatric disorders, and the woman may experience hallucinations and delusions. Women with acute psychosis typically require inpatient hospitalization.

Pregnancy further complicates psychiatric disorders because many of the medications used to treat the symptoms are contraindicated in pregnancy (ACOG, 2008). For these reasons, the woman with a psychologic disorder may require additional support from the nurse.

Assessment of psychosocial history is a critical component of intrapartum nursing assessment. Because of the prevalence of physical and sexual assault against women in our society (see chapter 9 ∞), the nurse needs to consider the possibility that the woman may have experienced such violence at some point in her life. If this is the case, she may be anxious about the labor process, or anxiety may arise during labor. Therefore, it is essential to review the woman's prenatal record and any other available records for information that may indicate abuse.

The cultural assessment provides a starting point for a plan that honors the values and beliefs of the laboring woman (Spector, 2009). Frequently, however, the nurse feels uncertain about what to ask or consider, perhaps because there has been no personal opportunity to become aware of varying cultural values and beliefs. It is important to remember that despite one's cultural background, variations in different individuals and families can vary dramatically. Some individuals may not embrace cultural beliefs that are inherent in their culture. The cultural assessment section of the assessment guide (see pages 562–563) helps to encourage cultural sensitivity in the nurse (Spector, 2009).

TABLE 23-1 Intrapartum High-Risk Factors

FACTOR	MATERNAL IMPLICATION	FETAL-NEONATAL IMPLICATION
Abnormal presentation	↑ Incidence of cesarean birth ↑ Incidence of prolonged labor ↑ Incidence of fibroids	↑ Incidence of placenta previa Prematurity ↑ Risk of congenital abnormality Neonatal physical trauma ↑ Risk of intrauterine growth restriction (IUGR)
Multiple gestation	↑ Uterine distention → ↑ risk of postpartum hemorrhage ↑ Risk of cesarean birth ↑ Risk of preterm labor	Low birth weight Prematurity ↑ Risk of congenital anomalies Feto-fetal transfusion
Hydramnios	↑ Discomfort ↑ Dyspnea ↑ Risk of preterm labor Edema of lower extremities/varicosities	↑ Risk of esophageal or other high alimentary tract atresias ↑ Risk of central nervous system (CNS) anomalies (myelocele) ↑ Risk of TORCH (toxoplasmosis, rubella, cytomegalovirus, herpes virus hominis type 2) infections ↑ Risk of prolapse cord
Oligohydramnios	Maternal fear of "dry birth"	↑ Incidence of congenital anomalies ↑ Incidence of renal lesions ↑ Risk of intrauterine growth restriction (IUGR) ↑ Risk of fetal acidosis ↑ Risk of cord compression Postmaturity
Meconium staining of amniotic fluid	↑ Psychologic stress due to fear for baby	↑ Risk of fetal asphyxia ↑ Risk of meconium aspiration ↑ Risk of pneumonia due to aspiration of meconium
Premature rupture of membranes (PROM)	↑ Risk of infection (chorioamnionitis) ↑ Risk of preterm labor ↑ Anxiety/fear for the baby Prolonged hospitalization ↑ Incidence of tocolytic therapy	↑ Perinatal morbidity Prematurity ↓ Birth weight ↑ Risk of respiratory distress syndrome (RDS) Prolonged hospitalization
Induction of labor	↑ Risk of uterine rupture ↑ Length of labor if cervix not ready ↑ Anxiety	Prematurity if gestational age not assessed correctly ↑ Risk of hypoxia
Abruptio placentae/placenta previa	Hemorrhage Uterine atony ↑ Incidence of cesarean birth ↑ Maternal morbidity	Fetal hypoxia/acidosis Fetal exsanguination ↑ Perinatal mortality
Failure to progress in labor	Maternal exhaustion ↑ Incidence of augmentation of labor ↑ Incidence of cesarean birth	Fetal hypoxia/acidosis Intracranial birth injury
Precipitous labor (less than 3 hours)	Perineal, vaginal, cervical lacerations ↑ Risk of postpartum hemorrhage	Neonatal tentorial (brain) tears Trauma—neural or tissue, cephalohematoma
Prolapse of umbilical cord	↑ Fear for baby Cesarean birth → emergent	Acute fetal hypoxia/acidosis
Fetal heart decelerations	↑ Fear for baby ↑ Risk of cesarean birth, forceps, vacuum Continuous electronic monitoring and intervention in labor	Tachycardia, chronic asphyxic insult, bradycardia Acute asphyxic insult Chronic hypoxia Congenital heart block
Uterine rupture	Hemorrhage Cesarean birth/hysterectomy ↑ Risk of morbidity/mortality	Fetal anoxia Fetal hemorrhage ↑ Neonatal morbidity and mortality
Postdates (greater than 42 weeks)	↑ Anxiety ↑ Incidence of induction of labor ↑ Incidence of cesarean birth ↑ Use of technology to monitor fetus ↑ Risk of shoulder dystocia	Postmaturity syndrome ↑ Risk of fetal-neonatal mortality and morbidity ↑ Risk of antepartum fetal death ↑ Incidence/risk of large baby ↑ Hypoglycemia
Diabetes	↑ Risk of hydramnios ↑ Risk of hypoglycemia or hyperglycemia ↑ Risk of preeclampsia	↑ Risk of malpresentation ↑ Risk of macrosomia ↑ Risk of intrauterine growth restriction (IUGR) ↑ Risk of respiratory distress syndrome (RDS) ↑ Hypoglycemia, polycythemia ↑ Birth trauma ↑ Risk of congenital anomalies
Preeclampsia	↑ Abruptio placentae ↑ Risk of seizures ↑ Risk of stroke ↑ Risk of HELLP	↑ Risk of small-for-gestational-age (SGA) baby ↑ Risk of preterm birth ↑ Risk of mortality
AIDS/STD	↑ Risk of additional infections	↑ Risk of transplacental transmission

ASSESSMENT GUIDE Intrapartum—First Stage of Labor

Physical Assessment/Normal Findings	Alterations and Possible Causes*	Nursing Responses to Data[†]
VITAL SIGNS		
Blood Pressure (BP): less than or equal to 135 systolic and less than or equal to 85 diastolic in adult 18 years of age or older or no more than 15–20 mm Hg rise in systolic pressure over baseline BP during early pregnancy	High blood pressure (essential hypertension, gestational hypertension, preeclampsia, renal disease, apprehension, anxiety or pain) Low blood pressure (supine hypotension) Hemorrhage/hypovolemia Shock Drugs	Evaluate history of preexisting disorders and check for presence of other signs of preeclampsia. Do not assess during contractions; implement measures to decrease anxiety and reassess. Turn woman on her side and recheck BP. Provide quiet environment. Have oxygen (O_2) available.
Pulse: 60–90 beats/min	Increased pulse rate (excitement or anxiety, cardiac disorders, early shock, drug use)	Evaluate cause, reassess to see if rate continues; report to physician/CNM.
Respirations: 12–24/min (or pulse rate divided by 4)	Marked tachypnea (respiratory disease), hyperventilation in transition phase Decreased respirations (Narcotics)	Assess between contractions; if marked tachypnea continues, assess for signs of respiratory disease or respiratory distress.
	Hyperventilation (anxiety/pain)	Encourage slow breaths if woman is hyperventilating.
Pulse oximetry 95% or greater	Less than 90%: hypoxia, hypotension, hemorrhage	Apply O_2; notify physician/CNM.
Temperature: 36.2–37.6°C (98–99.6°F)	Elevated temperature (infection, dehydration, prolonged rupture of membranes, epidural regional block)	Assess for other signs of infection or dehydration.
WEIGHT		
25–35 lb greater than prepregnant weight if BMI is 18.5–24.9; 28–40 lb greater if BMI is below 18.5; 15–25 lb greater if BMI is 25–29.9; 37–54 lb greater if multiple gestation	Weight gain greater than 35 lb (fluid retention, obesity, large infant, diabetes mellitus, preeclampsia); weight gain less than 15 lb (small for gestational age [SGA], substance abuse, psychosocial problems)	Assess for signs of edema. Evaluate dietary patterns. Assess for substance abuse and eating disorders.
LUNGS		
Normal breath sounds, clear and equal	Rales, rhonchi, friction rub (infection), pulmonary edema, asthma	Reassess; refer to physician/CNM
FUNDUS		
At 40 weeks' gestation located just below xiphoid process	Uterine size not compatible with estimated date of birth (small [SGA] or large [LGA] for gestational age, molar pregnancy, hydramnios, multiple pregnancy, placental/fetal anomalies, malpresentation)	Reevaluate history regarding pregnancy dating. Refer to physician for additional assessment.
EDEMA		
Slight amount of dependent edema	Pitting edema of face, hands, legs, abdomen, sacral area (preeclampsia)	Check deep tendon reflexes for hyperactivity; check for clonus; refer to physician.
HYDRATION		
Normal skin turgor, elastic	Poor skin turgor (dehydration)	Assess skin turgor; refer to physician for deviations. Provide fluids per physician/CNM orders.
PERINEUM		
Tissues smooth, pink color (see Prenatal Initial Physical Assessment Guide, chapter 15 ∞)	Varicose veins of vulva, herpes lesions/genital warts	Note on patient record need for follow-up in postpartum period; reassess after birth; refer to physician/CNM.
Clear mucus; may be blood tinged with earthy or human odor.	Profuse, purulent, foul-smelling drainage	Suspected gonorrhea or chorioamnionitis; report to physician; initiate care to newborn's eyes; notify neonatal nursing staff and pediatrician.
Presence of small amount of bloody show that gradually increases with further cervical dilatation	Hemorrhage	Assess BP and pulse, pallor, diaphoresis; report any marked changes. Standard precautions.
LABOR STATUS		
Uterine Contractions (UC): regular pattern	Failure to establish a regular pattern, prolonged latent phase Hypertonicity Hypotonicity Dehydration	Evaluate whether woman is in true labor; ambulate if in early labor. Evaluate patient status and contractile pattern; oxygen, stop pitocin; terbutaline. Obtain a 30-minute electronic fetal monitoring (EFM) strip. Notify physician or CNM. Provide hydration.
Cervical Dilatation: progressive cervical dilatation from size of fingertip to 10 cm (see Procedure 23-1)	Rigidity of cervix (frequent cervical infections, scar tissue, failure of presenting part to descend)	Evaluate contractions, fetal engagement, position, and cervical dilatation. Inform patient of progress.
	*Possible causes of alterations are identified in parentheses.	[†]This column provides guidelines for further assessment and initial nursing intervention.

ASSESSMENT GUIDE Intrapartum—First Stage of Labor continued

Physical Assessment/Normal Findings	Alterations and Possible Causes*	Nursing Responses to Data†
LABOR STATUS (continued)		
Cervical Effacement: progressive thinning of cervix (see Procedure 23-1)	Failure to efface (rigidity of cervix, failure of presenting part to engage); cervical edema (pushing effort by woman before cervix is fully dilated and effaced, trapped cervix)	Evaluate contractions, fetal engagement and position. Notify physician/CNM if cervix is becoming edematous; work with woman to prevent pushing until cervix is completely dilated. Keep vaginal exams to a minimum.
Fetal Descent: progressive descent of fetal presenting part from station −5 to +4 (see Figure 23-4 in Procedure 23-1)	Failure of descent (abnormal fetal position or presentation, macrosomic fetus, inadequate pelvic measurements)	Evaluate fetal position, presentation, and size.
Membranes: may rupture before or during labor	Rupture of membranes more than 12–24 hours before initiation of labor	Assess for ruptured membranes using Nitrazine test tape before doing vaginal exam. Follow standard precautions. Instruct woman with ruptured membranes to remain on bed rest if presenting part is not engaged and firmly down against the cervix. Keep vaginal exams to a minimum to prevent infection. When membranes rupture in the birth setting **immediately assess FHR** to detect changes associated with prolapse of umbilical cord (FHR slows).
Findings on Nitrazine Test Tape: Membranes probably intact yellow pH 5.0 olive pH 5.5 olive green pH 6.0	False-positive results may be obtained if large amount of bloody show is present, previous vaginal examination has been done using lubricant, infection is present, or tape is touched by nurse's fingers.	Assess fluid for consistency, amount, odor; assess FHR frequently. Assess fluid at regular intervals for presence of meconium staining. Follow standard precautions while assessing amniotic fluid.
Membranes probably ruptured blue-green pH 6.5 blue-gray pH 7.0 deep blue pH 7.5		Teach woman that amniotic fluid is continually produced (to allay fear of "dry birth"). Teach woman that she may feel amniotic fluid trickle or gush with contractions. Change Chux pads often.
Amniotic fluid clear, with earthy or human odor, no foul-smelling odor	Greenish amniotic fluid (nonreassuring fetal status) Bloody fluid (vasoprevia, abruptio placentae)	Assess FHR; do vaginal exam to evaluate for prolapsed cord; apply fetal monitor for continuous data; report to physician/CNM.
	Strong or foul odor (amnionitis)	Take woman's temperature and report to physician/CNM.
FETAL STATUS		
FHR: 110–160 beats/min Tachycardia Bradycardia	Less than 110 or greater than 160 beats/min (nonreassuring fetal status); abnormal patterns on fetal monitor: decreased variability, late decelerations, variable decelerations, absence of accelerations with fetal movement	Initiate interventions based on particular FHR pattern.
Presentation: Cephalic, 97% Breech, <3% Shoulder, <1%	Face, brow, breech, or shoulder presentation	Report to physician; after presentation is confirmed as face, brow, breech, or shoulder, woman may be prepared for cesarean birth.
Position: left-occiput-anterior (LOA) most common	Persistent occipital-posterior (OP) position; transverse arrest	Carefully monitor maternal and fetal status. Reposition mother side-lying or hands/knee to promote rotation of fetal head.
Activity: fetal movement	Tachysystole (more than 5 contractions in 10 minutes) (may precede fetal hypoxia)	Carefully evaluate FHR; apply fetal monitor.
	Complete lack of movement (nonreassuring fetal status or fetal demise)	Carefully evaluate FHR; apply fetal monitor. Report to physician/CNM.
LABORATORY EVALUATION		
Hematologic Tests ***Hemoglobin:*** 12–16 g/dl	Less than 11 g/dl (anemia, hemorrhage, sickle cell disorders, pernicious anemia)	Evaluate woman for problems due to decreased oxygen-carrying capacity caused by lowered hemoglobin.
CBC *Hematocrit:* 38%–47% *RBC:* 4.2–5.4 million/mm^3 *WBC:* 4500–11,000/mm^3, although leukocytosis to 20,000/mm^3 is not unusual *Platelets* 150,000–400,000/mm^3	Presence of infection or blood dyscrasias, loss of blood (hemorrhage, disseminated intravascular coagulation [DIC])	Evaluate for other signs of infection or for petechiae, bruising, or unusual bleeding.
	*Possible causes of alterations are identified in parentheses.	†This column provides guidelines for further assessment and initial nursing intervention.

(continued)

ASSESSMENT GUIDE Intrapartum—First Stage of Labor continued

Physical Assessment/Normal Findings	Alterations and Possible Causes*	Nursing Responses to Data†
LABORATORY EVALUATION (continued)		
Serologic Testing Serologic test for syphilis (STS) or Rapid Plasma Reagent (RPR) test: nonreactive Rh	Positive reaction (see chapter 15 ∞, Initial Prenatal Physical Assessment Guide)	For reactive test notify newborn nursery and pediatrician.
Rh negative	Rh-positive fetus in Rh-negative woman or O+ woman	Assess prenatal record for titer levels during pregnancy. Obtain cord blood for direct Coombs' at birth.
Urinalysis: Glucose: negative	Glycosuria (low renal threshold for glucose, diabetes mellitus)	Assess blood glucose; test urine for ketones; ketonuria and glycosuria require further assessment of blood sugars.‡
Ketones: negative	Ketonuria (starvation ketosis)	Assess nutritional status.
Proteins: negative	Proteinuria (urine specimen contaminated with vaginal secretions, fever, infection, kidney disease); proteinuria of 2+ or greater found in uncontaminated urine may be a sign of ensuing preeclampsia	Instruct woman in collection technique; incidence of contamination from vaginal discharge is common. Report any increase in proteinuria to physician/CNM.
Red blood cells: negative	Blood in urine (calculi, cystitis, glomerulonephritis, neoplasm)	Assess collection technique (may be bloody show).
White blood cells: negative	Presence of white blood cells (infection in genitourinary tract)	Assess for signs of urinary tract infection.
Casts: none	Presence of casts (nephrotic syndrome)	
Nitrites	Infection	Assess for signs of urinary tract infection.
Cultural Assessment§	**Variations to Consider**	**Nursing Responses to Data†**
Cultural influences determine customs and practices regarding intrapartal care.	Individual preferences may vary.	
Ask the following questions: Who would you like to remain with you during your labor and birth?	She may prefer only her coach to remain or may also want family and/or friends.	Provide support for her wishes by encouraging desired people to stay. Provide information to others (with the woman's permission) who are not in the room.
What would you like to wear during labor?	She may be more comfortable in her own clothes.	Offer supportive materials such as Chux if needed to protect her own clothing. Avoid subtle signals to the woman that she should not have chosen to remain in her own clothes. Have other clothing available if the woman desires. If her clothing becomes contaminated, it will be simple to place it in a plastic bag.
What activity would you like during labor?	She may want to ambulate most of the time, stand in the shower, sit in the whirlpool bath, sit on a chair/stool/birthing ball, remain on the bed, and so forth.	Support the woman's wishes; provide encouragement and complete assessments in a manner so her activity and positional wishes are disturbed as little as possible.
What position would you like for the birth?	She may feel more comfortable in lithotomy with stirrups and her upper body elevated, or side-lying or sitting in birthing bed, or standing, or squatting, or on hands and knees.	Collect any supplies and equipment needed to support her in her chosen birthing position. Provide information to the coach regarding any changes that may be needed based on the chosen position.
Is there anything special you would like?	She may want the room darkened or to have curtains and windows open, music playing, a Leboyer birth, her coach to cut the umbilical cord, to save a portion of the umbilical cord, to save the placenta, to videotape the birth, and so forth.	Support requests, and communicate requests to any other nursing or medical personnel (so requests can continue to be supported and not questioned). If another nurse or physician does not honor the request, act as advocate for the woman by continuing to support her unless her desire is truly unsafe.
Ask the woman if she would like fluids, and ask what temperature she prefers.	She may prefer clear fluids other than water (tea, clear juice). She may prefer iced, room-temperature, or warmed fluids. See institution policy regarding oral intake in labor.	Provide fluids as desired.
Observe the woman's response when privacy is difficult to maintain and her body is exposed.	Some women do not seem to mind being exposed during an exam or procedure; others feel acute discomfort.	Maintain privacy and respect the woman's sense of privacy. If the woman is unable to provide specific information, the nurse may draw from general information regarding cultural variation: Southeast Asian women may not want any family member in the room during exam or procedures. Her partner may not be involved with coaching activities during labor or birth. Muslim women may need to remain covered during the labor and birth and avoid exposure of any body part. The husband may need to be in the room but remain behind a curtain or screen so he does not view his wife at this time.
If the woman is to breastfeed, ask if she would like to feed her baby immediately after birth.	She may want to feed her baby right away or she may want to wait a little while.	

§These are only a few suggestions. We do not mean to imply that this is a comprehensive cultural assessment; rather, it is a tool to encourage cultural sensitivity.

*Possible causes of alterations are identified in parentheses.

†This column provides guidelines for further assessment and initial nursing intervention.

‡Glycosuria should not be discounted. The presence of glycosuria necessitates follow-up.

ASSESSMENT GUIDE Intrapartum—First Stage of Labor continued

Psychosocial Assessment	Variations to Consider	Nursing Responses to Data[†]
PREPARATION FOR CHILDBIRTH		
Woman has some information regarding process of normal labor and birth.	Some women do not have any information regarding childbirth.	Add to present information base.
Woman has breathing and/or relaxation techniques to use during labor.	Some women do not have any method of relaxation or breathing to use, and some do not desire them.	Support breathing and relaxation techniques that patient is using; provide information if needed.
Woman and support person have done extensive preparation for childbirth (Bradley Classes, Lamaze).	Some women have strong opinions regarding labor and birth preparation.	Support woman's wishes to participate in her birth experience; support birth plan.
RESPONSE TO LABOR		
Early or Latent Phase: (0–3 cm) relaxed, excited, anxious for labor to be well established	May cope well or feel unable to cope with contractions because of fear, anxiety, or lack of information.	Provide support and encouragement; establish trusting relationship.
Active Phase: (4–7 cm) becomes more intense, begins to tire	May remain quiet and without any sign of discomfort or anxiety, may insist that she is unable to continue with the birthing process.	Provide support and coaching if needed.
Transitional Phase: (8–10 cm) feels tired, may feel unable to cope, needs frequent coaching to maintain breathing patterns		
Coping Mechanisms: Ability to cope with labor through use of support system, breathing, relaxation techniques, and comfort measures including frequent position changes in labor, warm water immersion, and massage	May feel marked anxiety and apprehension, may not have coping mechanisms that can be brought into this experience, or may be unable to use them at this time.	Support coping mechanisms if they are working for the woman; provide information and support if she exhibits anxiety or needs alternative to present coping methods.
	Survivors of sexual abuse may demonstrate fear of IVs or needles, may recoil when touched, may insist on a female caregiver, may be very sensitive to body fluids and cleanliness, and may be unable to labor lying down. May show extreme distress with vaginal examinations.	Encourage participation of coach/significant other if a supportive relationship seems apparent. Establish rapport and a trusting relationship. Provide information that is true and offer your presence.
ANXIETY		
Some anxiety and apprehension is within normal limits.	May show anxiety through rapid breathing, nervous tremors, frowning, grimacing, clenching of teeth, thrashing movements, crying, increased pulse and blood pressure.	Provide support, encouragement, and information. Teach relaxation techniques; support controlled breathing efforts. May need to provide a paper bag to breathe into if woman says her lips are tingling. Note FHR.
SOUNDS DURING LABOR		
	Some women are very quiet; others moan or make a variety of noises.	Provide a supportive environment. Encourage woman to do what feels right for her.
SUPPORT SYSTEM		
Physical intimacy between mother and father (or mother and support person/doula): caretaking activities such as soothing conversation, touching	Some women would prefer no contact, others may show clinging behaviors.	Encourage caretaking activities that appear to comfort the woman; encourage support for the woman; if support is limited, the nurse may take a more active role.
Support person stays in close proximity	Limited interaction may come from a desire for quiet.	Encourage support person to stay close (if this seems appropriate).
Relationship between mother and father (or support person): involved interaction	The support person may seem to be detached and maintain little support, attention, or conversation.	Support interactions; if interaction is limited, the nurse may provide more information and support. Ensure that coach/significant other has short breaks, especially/prior to transition.

[†]This column provides guidelines for further assessment and initial nursing intervention.

The final section of the guide addresses psychosocial factors. The laboring woman's psychosocial status is an important part of the total assessment. The woman has previous ideas, knowledge, and fears about childbearing. The adequacy of resources, such as housing, transportation, utilities, and access to social services, should also be questioned. By assessing her psychosocial status, the nurse can meet the woman's needs for information and support. The nurse can then support the woman and her partner; in the absence of a partner, the nurse may become the support person.

Evaluating Labor Progress

Intrapartum nursing care requires competent assessment and clinical skills and a comprehensive knowledge of maternal-fetal anatomy and the physiology of the labor process. An ongoing, accurate assessment of both the mother and fetus and their responses to labor is necessary to provide the data required to make sound clinical judgments and provide appropriate care. Labor can be monitored in a number of ways, each having its own benefits and limitations. If a "low technology" approach is desired, a nurse can monitor uterine contractions and the FHR intermittently using techniques such as palpation and auscultation. However, if the clinical situation demands, as in the case of a high-risk pregnancy, the laboring woman may be monitored electronically. External devices (tocodynanometer and ultrasound) or internal devices (intrauterine pressure catheter and fetal scalp electrode) may be used when a continuous graphic data record is needed to evaluate the mother and fetus during labor.

The method of monitoring during labor may vary, depending on the presence of risk factors at admission, the preferences of the woman and healthcare provider, and the institution's policies (AAP & ACOG, 2007; ACOG, 2005). If intermittent monitoring is used, the nurse must perform a "hands-on" assessment, including auscultation of fetal heart tones (FHT) and palpation of uterine contractions (UC). If continuous **electronic fetal monitoring (EFM)** is used, the amount of physical "hands-on" care may vary depending on whether an internal or external mode of monitoring is used. EFM provides a continuous tracing of the FHR.

Professional associations, such as American College of Obstetricians and Gynecologists (ACOG) and Association of Women's Health, Obstetric and Neonatal Nurses (AWHONN), and individual healthcare institutions generally set the guidelines for the level of intrapartum monitoring. The frequency of the maternal-fetal assessment and documentation depends on the mother's stage of labor and the presence of risk factors. When EFM is used, ACOG recommends that the nurse or physician review EFM data frequently. For low-risk pregnancies, FHR tracings can be reviewed every 30 minutes in first stage labor and every 15 minutes in second stage labor. The FHR tracings of high-risk pregnancies should be reviewed more frequently—every 15 minutes in first stage labor and every 5 minutes in second stage labor. Periodic documentation should accompany each review of the FHR tracing. See Table 23-2 for the frequency of recommended assessments and documentations.

The recommended frequency of FHR tracing assessment and documentation is only a guideline for practice. At times, the nurse may find it necessary to monitor the FHR more frequently. Certain clinical events such as vaginal exams, rupture of membranes, abnormal uterine activity patterns, administration of medications, or procedures such as epidurals, amniocentesis, external versions, and other events have the potential to adversely affect the FHR tracing. It is beneficial to assess the FHR tracing before and after such events or anytime a nonreassuring FHR tracing is detected (Simpson & Creehan, 2007).

TABLE 23-2 Frequency of Maternal-Fetal Assessment and Documentation

	FIRST STAGE	SECOND STAGE
Low risk	Every 30 minutes	Every 15 minutes
High risk	Every 15 minutes	Every 5 minutes

Sources: Data from AAP & ACOG, 2007; Macones, Hankins, Spong, Hauth, & Moore, 2008.

Since its introduction into clinical practice in the late 1960s, EFM has continuously been researched and evaluated in regard to its ability to improve fetal outcomes and reduce morbidity and mortality. In the beginning, EFM was used in high-risk pregnancies, because it was thought that electronic assessment was far more accurate and valuable for diagnosing nonreassuring fetal status in labor. It was believed that continuous fetal monitoring could identify nonreassuring fetal status earlier, facilitate earlier interventions, and prevent fetal morbidity and mortality. Researchers originally thought EFM could prevent cerebral palsy, which was thought to be caused by neurologic damage from nonreassuring fetal status (Cunningham et al., 2010). Today's research does not support these earlier suppositions.

In 2002, 85% of all labors were monitored electronically, making EFM the most prevalent assessment procedure in maternal-fetal health care (Janet, 2009). However, despite its widespread use, research has failed to show that it has significantly improved the outcomes at birth. Multiple controlled random trials have failed to show that EFM is beneficial over intermittent auscultation in preventing neonatal morbidity and mortality (ACOG, 2005; AWHONN, 2008a; Cunningham et al., 2010). Intermittent assessment of the maternal-fetal couplet labor is generally considered to be as appropriate an assessment technique as electronic monitoring, especially for low-risk pregnancies when proper technique and 1:1 nurse-to-patient ratio are used (AWHONN, 2008b).

Uterine Activity Assessment

Monitoring uterine activity throughout labor is essential and provides data regarding the labor progress and fetal well-being. Numerous internal and external factors affect maternal and fetal well-being. Uterine contractions (UCs) interrupt the flow of blood to the placenta and reduce the amount of oxygen immediately available to the fetus. Decreased oxygen and blood flow directly affect the FHR. The pattern and intensity of contractions have a direct effect on the duration and progress of labor and the ability of the fetus to adapt to the intrapartal process.

UCs occur in wavelike patterns. Beginning at the fundus (top or apex of the uterus), the UC progresses downward through the lower segments of the uterus and is then followed by a similar wave of relaxation. The contraction of the upper uterine segment increases intrauterine pressure and leads to cervical dilatation and effacement and the descent of the fetus. During and between UCs, the fundus changes shape and firmness, reflecting the intensity of the UC. By monitoring the changes in the fundus, the nurse can determine the timing and intensity of the UC and the resting tone of the uterus between contractions (AWHONN, 2008a). The intensity and frequency of the UC varies from woman to woman and labor to labor. Three methods of monitoring UCs are currently used: palpation, external electronic monitoring with a tocodynanometer, and internal electronic monitoring with an intrauterine pressure catheter. Each method is discussed in the following sections.

PALPATION **Palpation** is the technique of assessing a UC by touch. To assess UCs, the nurse places the fingertips of one hand on the top of the uterus. Hand placement is usually on the fundus, but the location may vary based on maternal or fetal position, uterine size and shape, or maternal body composition. Gentle pressure is applied to the abdomen until the firmness of the underlying uterine wall is felt.

The *frequency* of the contractions is measured from the beginning of one contraction to the beginning of the next. The length of the contraction, referred to as the *duration,* is measured from the beginning of the contraction, when the muscle begins to tense, to the end of the same contraction, when the muscle is completely relaxed. Uterine resting tone is determined between UCs, when optimum uterine relaxation is achieved (Cunningham et al., 2010).

During the acme (peak) of the contraction, intensity can be evaluated subjectively by estimating the firmness of the fundus. It can be useful to compare the contraction to the firmness of a nose, chin, or forehead. A tense fundus that is easily indented (tip of the nose) is considered mild intensity. When the fundus becomes firm and difficult to indent with the fingertips (chin), the strength of the UC is considered moderate. The fundus that is hard and cannot be indented (forehead) is classified as strong (Cunningham et al., 2010). The nurse should assess successive contractions to provide reliable data. Table 23-3 compares contraction characteristics in different phases of labor. Direct uterine palpation is used with intermittent auscultation of the fetal heart or in conjunction with continuous EFM. The frequency of palpation depends on the risk status of the mother and fetus and the stage of labor along with the quality of contraction tracing from an internal or external monitor (Cunningham et al., 2010).

Palpation has its capabilities, benefits, and limitations. Palpation allows the nurse to assess relative frequency, duration, and subjective strength of the contraction and uterine resting tone. UC assessment by palpation is beneficial over electronic monitoring because it (1) is noninvasive and does not increase the risk for infection or patient injury; (2) is readily accessible, requiring no equipment; (3) increases the "hands-on" care of the patient that can be reassuring to her; and (4) allows the mother freedom from restricting and sometimes uncomfortable abdominal belts, thus permitting her to move freely and ambulate if her condition permits. Palpation is limited because it does not provide actual quantitative measure of uterine pressure; thus subjective differences between nurses and nurse-to-patient interpretations may exist. Palpation offers no permanent record, which can hinder interpretation by others. Maternal size and increased adipose tissue from obesity and maternal positioning may prevent direct palpation of the fundus. The limitations of palpation may outweigh the benefits in some clinical situations, and electronic monitoring may be a more appropriate choice for uterine assessment (Cunningham et al., 2010).

TABLE 23-3 Contraction and Labor Progress Characteristics

Contraction Characteristics	
Early/Latent phase:	Every 10–30 min × 20–40 sec; mild, progressing to moderate
	Every 3–7 min × 30–40 sec; moderate
Active phase:	Every 2–5 min × 40–60 sec; moderate to strong
Transition phase:	Every 1 1/2–2 min × 60–90 sec; strong
Labor Progress Characteristics	
Primipara:	1.2 cm/hr dilatation 1 cm/hr descent At least 2 hr in second stage if progress is made; up to 3 hr
Multipara:	1.5 cm/hr dilatation 2 cm/hr descent Less than 30 minutes in second stage

Source: Cunningham et al., 2010.

ELECTRONIC MONITORING WITH EXTERNAL TOCODYNAMOMETER Electronic monitoring of uterine contractions can be done externally by using a tocodynamometer or tocotransducer (toco). A toco is a pressure-monitoring device that is placed on the maternal abdomen at or near the fundus (the area of greatest contractility) and held in place with an elastic belt, belly band, or other adhesive material (Figure 23-1 ■). By placing the toco over a fetal part in the fundus rather than a pocket of amniotic fluid, a better contraction tracing can be obtained (Cunningham et al., 2010). As the uterus contracts, pressure exerted against the toco is amplified and transmitted to the EFM and recorded on graph paper.

The procedure for applying the tocotransducer begins with palpation of the uterus to locate the fundus. The toco monitors uterine activity transabdominally by detecting changes in the abdominal wall and converting the fundal movement into electronic impulses. The toco can be used to assess UCs for *frequency* (timing) and *duration* (length). However, it cannot determine UC intensity (strength). The displayed numbers and graph tracing for UC intensity are arbitrary and are influenced by how tightly the belt is applied around the maternal abdomen and/or the maternal position. Palpation must be used to assess UC intensity when the external toco monitor is used. When the belt is tight enough, the nurse should be able to note the beginning of contractions on the monitor just before or at the same time the woman begins to feel them (Cunningham et al., 2010).

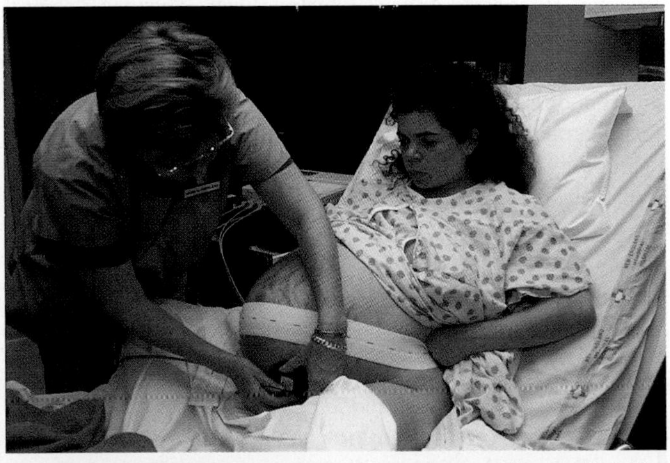

Figure 23-1 ■ Woman in labor with external monitor applied. The tocodynamometer placed on the uterine fundus is recording uterine contractions. The lower belt holds the ultrasonic device that monitors the fetal heart rate. The belts can be adjusted for comfort.

Source: © Stella Johnson (www.stellajohnson.com).

Case Study: Maternal Assessment During Labor

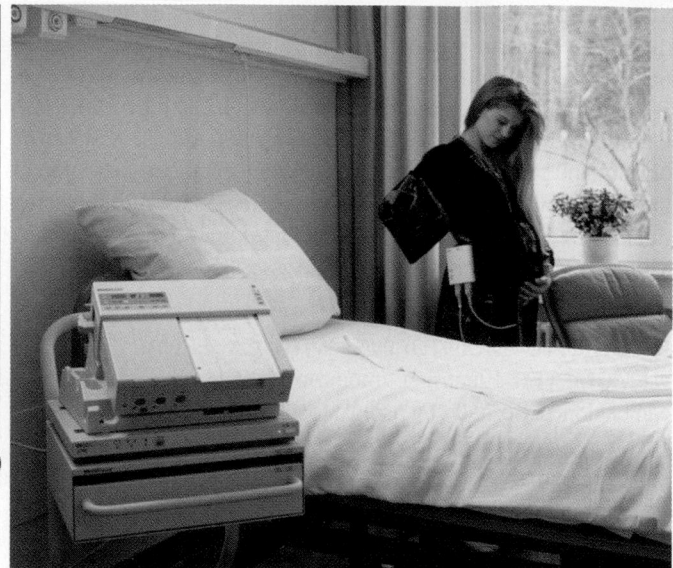

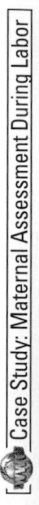

Figure 23-2 ■ The beltless tocodynamometer system features remote telemetry.

Source: Courtesy of Hewlett-Packard Company.

A beltless tocodynamometer system featuring remote telemetry is available. This system consists of an adhesive transducer that is applied to the most prominent part of the woman's abdomen with a double-sided adhesive film. The nonbelted tocodynamometer tends to be preferred by the laboring woman because it allows more freedom of movement, is easily applied, needs readjustment only infrequently, and generally is more convenient (Figure 23-2 ■). It enables upright positions, which promote fetal descent by gravity, as well as ambulation, which can shorten the labor course and increase comfort for the laboring woman (Cunningham et al., 2010).

The advantages to using a toco for assessing uterine contractions are that it is noninvasive, easy to place, and may be used both before and following rupture of membranes. Because it is noninvasive, it can be used intermittently to allow the woman to ambulate, shower, or use a whirlpool bath. The toco also provides a permanent, continuous recording of the duration and frequency of contractions for future evaluation. Placement of the tocotransducer influences the accuracy of the uterine graphic tracing (Cunningham et al., 2010). As with any type of technology, no toco is flawless, and the monitor cannot fill the role of the nurse. The nurse should routinely palpate the intensity of the contractions and the relaxation of the uterus between contractions and compare the assessment with data recorded by the monitor. Another disadvantage is that sometimes the belt may become uncomfortable because it must be worn snugly to monitor UCs accurately. The belt may require frequent readjustment as the mother changes position. The mother may also feel inhibited to move or as though she needs to remain in one position so as not to disturb the belt.

> “Trying to figure out if I was in labor was quite a task. Here I was, a birthing room nurse, and I couldn't decide if my contractions were the real thing. I timed them, and about the time I decided this was it, they would slow down. How exasperating not to know! It was so hard on me. But now I see that all women are in this spot. They want so much to be right, and we often treat them as if they should be able to sense when it's the real thing. I'd like the birthing room nurses to remember this.”

ELECTRONIC MONITORING BY INTERNAL PRESSURE CATHETER Electronic monitoring of UCs can be done internally by using an **intrauterine pressure catheter (IUPC)**. The IUPC is a catheter that is inserted into the uterine cavity through the cervical os. With correct placement in the uterus, usually in the area of the fetal small parts (arms or legs), the catheter reflects the pressure inside the uterine cavity. As the pressure changes in the uterus, the changes are relayed through a transducer to the fetal monitor, producing a tracing on the graph paper. The IUPC can measure the resting tone of the uterus between contractions and the actual amount of intrauterine pressure during contractions, referred to as UC intensity (Cunningham et al., 2010).

IUPCs can be one of two types: fluid-filled catheters and solid-tipped catheters. Fluid-filled catheters are a single-lumen catheter connected to a pressure-sensitive diaphragm outside the uterus. As intrauterine pressure changes, the column of fluid in the catheter fluctuates and exerts pressure on the diaphragm, sending signals to the transducer and fetal monitor. The solid-tipped catheter uses more recent technology in that the catheter contains a solid-state micropressure transducer (electronic sensor) at its tip, and the catheter that is inserted directly into the uterine cavity through the cervical os. The catheter is then connected by a cable to the EFM. The catheter also incorporates a second lumen, permitting amnioinfusion while simultaneously providing accurate monitoring of intrauterine pressure (Figure 23-3 ■) (Cunningham et al., 2010). Regardless of the type of catheter, fluid filled or solid tipped, the IUPC can be used only after membranes are ruptured and the patient has adequate cervical dilation, usually 3 centimeters or more (Cunningham et al., 2010).

The IUPC has several benefits over an external tocotransducer or palpation. Because the IUPC is inserted directly into the uterus, it provides near-exact pressure measurements for contraction intensity and uterine resting tone. The increased sensitivity of the IUPC allows for very accurate timing of UCs, thus making it extremely useful in cases when the provider needs closer uterine monitoring. The IUPC may be the preferred method of monitoring when it is particularly important to avoid tachysystole and possible uterine rupture in women with a previous history of cesarean birth who are attempting a vaginal birth after cesarean (VBAC) and are receiving oxytocin. If the woman's labor is prolonged, internal monitoring can be used to accurately assess the frequency and strength of contractions. If a nonreassuring FHR tracing is present, internal monitoring with IUPC and fetal scalp electrode may be essential to correlate UC timing and FHR pattern response. IUPCs are also preferred when amnioinfusion is indicated, such as in cases with meconium-stained amniotic fluid (Wiederman, Saugstad, Branes-Powell, et al., 2008). The IUPC provides a permanent record of the uterine

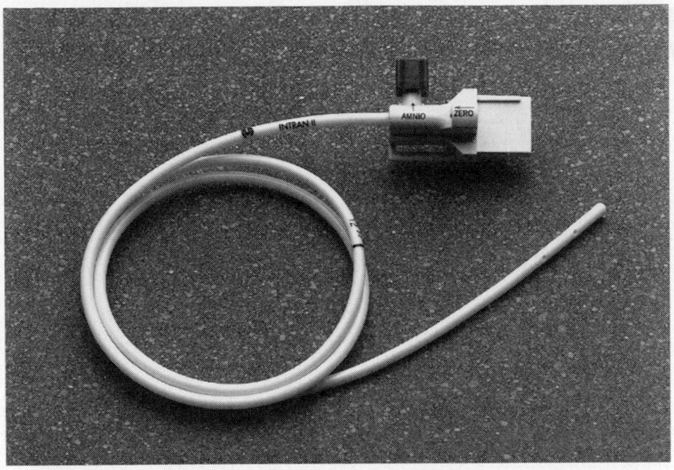

Figure 23-3 ■ INTRAN Plus intrauterine pressure catheter. There is a micropressure transducer (electronic sensor) located at the tip of the catheter and a port for amnioinfusion at the distal end of the catheter.

Source: Photographer, Elena Dorfman.

activity for future analysis and documentation, making it useful in patient care decision making.

However, with all of its benefits, the IUPC has its limitations and risks. Use of IUPCs is limited by the clinical situation. Membranes must be ruptured and adequate cervical dilation must be achieved for insertion. The procedure is invasive and increases the risk of uterine infection or uterine perforation or trauma. When an intrauterine catheter is used, there is a 1% risk of infection, but this seems to depend on the duration of ruptured membranes and length of labor (Cheng & Caughley, 2009). Invasive equipment like the IUPC is contraindicated in cases when active infections can be transmitted vertically through the cervix into the uterus to the fetus. Insertion of an IUPC with a low-lying placenta can result in placenta puncture, which can cause hemorrhage and nonreassuring fetal status (Cunningham et al., 2010). IUPCs also require proper insertion and zeroing procedures; thus, competency in insertion technique and equipment maintenance and troubleshooting is essential.

Cervical Assessment

Cervical dilatation and effacement are evaluated directly by vaginal examination (see Procedure 23-1: Performing an Intrapartum Vaginal Examination). The vaginal examination can also provide information regarding fetal position, station of the presenting part, and membrane status (intact or ruptured). To assist in evaluating membrane status, the nurse assesses for the presence of amniotic fluid (Procedure 23-2: Assessing for Amniotic Fluid).

PROCEDURE 23-1 Performing an Intrapartum Vaginal Examination

NURSING ACTION

Preparation

- Explain the procedure, the indications for the exam, what the exam may feel like, and that it may cause discomfort.
- Assess for latex allergies.
- Position the woman with her thighs flexed and abducted. Instruct her to put the heels of her feet together. Drape the woman with a sheet, leaving a flap to access the perineum.

  Rationale: *This position provides access to the woman's perineum. The drape ensures privacy.*
- Encourage the woman to relax her muscles and legs.
- Inform the woman before touching her. Be gentle.

  Rationale: *Relaxation decreases muscle tension and increases comfort.*

> **CLINICAL TIP**
> Use nonlatex gloves if the woman has a latex allergy.

EQUIPMENT AND SUPPLIES

Clean disposable gloves if membranes not ruptured
Sterile gloves if membranes ruptured
Lubricant
Nitrazine test tape
Slide
Sterile cotton-tipped swab (Q-tip)

Before the Procedure: Test for Fluid Leakage

If fluid leakage has been reported or noted, use Nitrazine test tape and Q-tip with slide for fern test before performing the exam (see Procedure 23-2).

Procedure: Clean Gloves (Sterile if membranes ruptured)

> **CLINICAL TIP**
> Digital examination may be deferred if the woman has ruptured membranes but is not in active labor (AAP & ACOG, 2007).

1. Pull glove onto dominant hand.

   Rationale: *Single glove is worn when membranes are intact. If a sterile exam is needed, both hands will be gloved with sterile gloves.*
2. Using your gloved hand, position the hand with the wrist straight and the elbow tilted downward. Insert your well-lubricated second and index fingers of the gloved hand gently into the vagina until they touch the cervix. Use care when positioning your hand.

   Rationale: *This position allows the fingertips to point toward the umbilicus and find the cervix.*
3. If the woman verbalizes discomfort, acknowledge it and apologize. Pause for a moment and allow her to relax before progressing.

   Rationale: *This validates the woman's discomfort and helps her feel more in control.*

(continued)

PROCEDURE 23-1 Performing an Intrapartum Vaginal Examination continued

4. To determine the status of labor progress, perform the vaginal examination during and between contractions.

   Rationale: *Cervical effacement, dilatation, and fetal station are affected by the presence of a contraction.*

5. Palpate for the opening, or a depression, in the cervix. Estimate the diameter of the depression to identify the amount of dilatation (Figure 23-4 ■).

   Rationale: *Allows determination of effacement and dilatation.*

6. Determine the status of the fetal membranes by observing for leakage of amniotic fluid. If fluid is expressed, test for amniotic fluid.

   Rationale: *Determine the presenting part is necessary to assess the position of the fetus and to evaluate fetal descent.*

7. Palpate the presenting part (Figure 23-5 ■).
8. Assess the fetal descent (Figure 23-6 ■) and station by identifying the position of the posterior fontanelle in relation to the ischial spines.
9. Record findings on woman's chart and on fetal monitor strip if fetal monitor is being used.

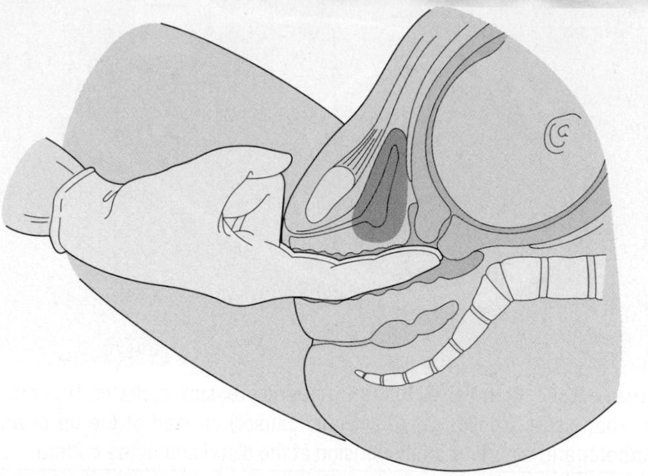

Figure 23-4 ■ To gauge cervical dilatation, the nurse places the index and middle fingers against the cervix and determines the size of the opening. Before labor begins, the cervix is long (approximately 2–5 cm), the sides feel thick, and the cervical canal is closed, so an examining finger cannot be inserted. During labor, the cervix begins to dilate, and the size of the opening progresses from 1 cm to 10 cm in diameter.

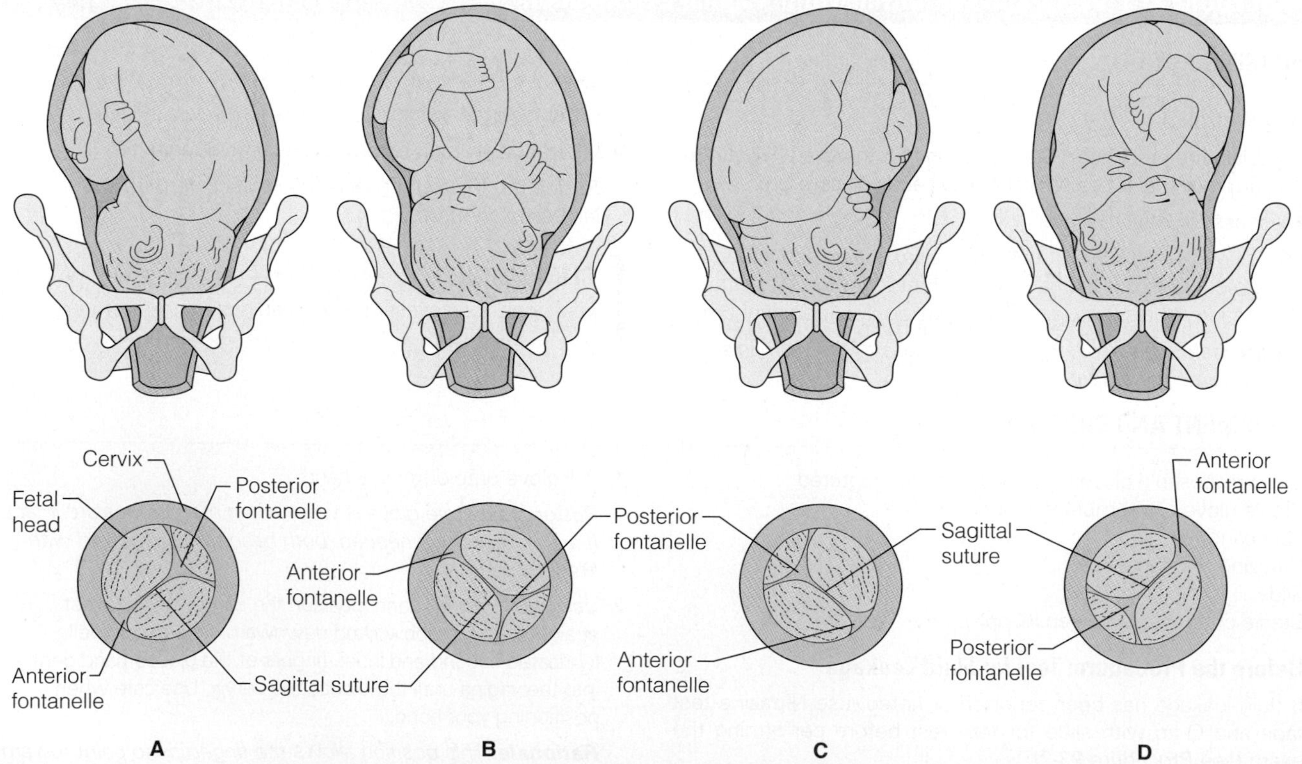

Figure 23-5 ■ Palpation of the presenting part (the portion of the fetus that enters the pelvis first). A. Left occiput anterior (LOA). The occiput (area over the occipital bone on the posterior part of the fetal head) is in the left anterior quadrant of the woman's pelvis. When the fetus is in LOA, the posterior fontanelles (located just above the occipital bone and triangular in shape) are in the upper left quadrant of the maternal pelvis. B. Left occiput posterior (LOP). The posterior fontanelle is in the lower left quadrant of the maternal pelvis. C. Right occiput anterior (ROA). The posterior fontanelle is in the upper right quadrant of the maternal pelvis. D. Right occiput posterior (ROP). The posterior fontanelle is in the lower right quadrant of the maternal pelvis.

Note: The anterior fontanelle is diamond shaped. Because of the roundness of the fetal head, only a portion of the anterior fontanelle can be seen in each of the views, so it appears to be triangular in shape.

PROCEDURE 23-1 Performing an Intrapartum Vaginal Examination continued

Documentation	Document that the procedure was explained to the patient, and that the woman verbalized understanding and provided consent before the vaginal examination. The woman's reaction and how the procedure was tolerated should be documented. The findings of the examination should be clearly documented using a facility-appropriate documentation form.

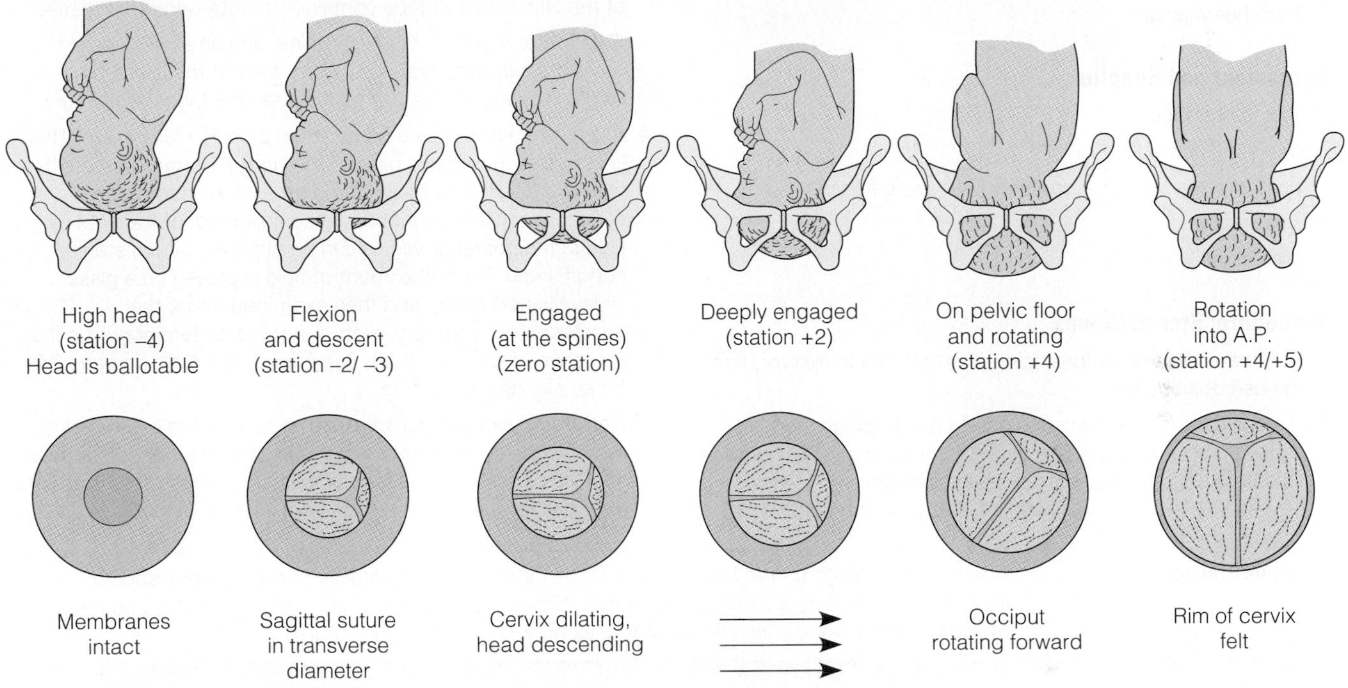

Figure 23-6 ■ Descent of the fetus through the maternal pelvis can be assessed by determining station (the relationship of the presenting part to an imaginary line between the maternal ischial spines). As the fetus moves downward, cardinal movements occur (see chapter 22 ∞). The nurse assesses the station and identifies the cardinal movements by determining the position of the posterior fontanelle. The upper panels depict the fetal head progressing downward through the pelvis. From left to right, the first four views depict descent and flexion of the fetal chin onto the fetal chest. In the last two views, internal rotation occurs. Each view also depicts downward movement of the fetal head through the maternal pelvis as measured by the change in station. The lower panels depict the cervix, which is still rather thick (little effacement has occurred). The amniotic membranes are still intact over the fetal head. When the fetus is at –4 station, the fetal head is ballotable (when it is touched by the examining nurse's finger, the head floats upward and resettles downward). In the second view, note the thinner cervix (which indicates that more effacement has occurred). The sagittal suture and posterior fontanelle can be palpated. The next two views depict further effacement and descent of the fetal head from 0 station to +2. The last two views depict continuing effacement and position that would be felt on vaginal examination of the presenting part while the fetal head is completing internal rotation.

Fetal Assessment

A complete intrapartum fetal assessment requires determination of the fetal position and presentation and evaluation of the fetal status.

Determination of Fetal Position and Presentation

Fetal position is determined in several ways, including the following:

- Inspection of the woman's abdomen
- Palpation of the woman's abdomen (Leopold's maneuvers)
- Vaginal examination to determine the presenting part
- Ultrasound (US)

Inspection

The nurse should observe the woman's abdomen for size and shape. The lie of the fetus should be assessed by noting whether the uterus projects up and down (longitudinal lie) or left to right (transverse lie) (Cunningham et al., 2010).

Palpation: Leopold's Maneuvers

Leopold's maneuvers are a systematic way to evaluate the maternal abdomen (Figure 23-7 ■). Frequent practice increases the examiner's skill in determining fetal position by palpation. Leopold's maneuvers may be difficult to perform on an obese woman or on a woman who has excessive amniotic fluid (hydramnios) (Cunningham et al., 2010).

Care should be taken to ensure the woman's comfort during Leopold's maneuvers. The woman should have recently emptied

PROCEDURE 23-2 Assessing for Amniotic Fluid

NURSING ACTION

Preparation

- Explain the procedure, indications for the procedure, what the woman will feel, and information that may be obtained.
- Determine whether she has noted the escape of any fluid from her vagina.

Equipment and Supplies

Nitrazine test tape

Sterile speculum

A glass slide and a sterile cotton-tipped swab (Q-tip)

Sterile syringe

Microscope

Procedure: Sterile Gloves

1. Complete this test before doing an examination that requires the use of lubricant.
2. Put on sterile gloves. With one gloved hand, spread the labia, and with the other gloved hand place a small section of Nitrazine tape (approx. 2 in. long) against the vaginal opening. Take care not to touch the tape with bare fingers before the test.

   Rationale: *Contamination of the Nitrazine test tape with lubricant can make the test unreliable. Enough fluid needs to be placed on the test tape to make it wet.*
3. Compare the color on the test tape to the guide on the back of the Nitrazine test tape container to determine test results.

   Rationale: *Amniotic fluid is alkaline, and an alkaline fluid turns the Nitrazine test tape a dark blue. If the test tape remains a beige color, the test is negative for amniotic fluid.*
4. Amniotic fluid may also be obtained by speculum exam. This is indicated in preterm premature rupture of membranes. If fluid is present in sufficient amount to draw some into a syringe, a small amount should be collected, or the pool of fluid in the posterior vagina can be obtained with a sterile cotton swab. A small amount of fluid is placed on a glass slide, allowed to dry, and then examined under the microscope or sent to the lab. A ferning pattern confirms the presence of amniotic fluid. See Figure 12-4 ∞ on page 249 for an example of ferning.

   Rationale: *Obtaining a specimen by speculum examination reduces the contamination of the fluid with other substances such as blood and cervical mucus and reduces the chance of infection for the woman who is not actively laboring.*

Documentation Record the findings on the labor record. Documentation of the status of membranes should include whether they are intact or ruptured. Other characteristics, such as color, odor, and amount of fluid present, should also be recorded, along with the time of rupture.

her bladder and should lie on her back with her abdomen uncovered. To aid in relaxation of the abdominal wall, the shoulders should be raised slightly on a pillow and the knees drawn up a little. The procedure should be completed between contractions. The examiner's hands should be warm. The order in which Leopold's maneuvers are performed may vary from one clinician to another.

While inspecting and palpating the maternal abdomen, the nurse should consider the following questions:

- Is the fetal lie longitudinal or transverse?
- What is in the fundus? Am I feeling buttocks or head?
- Where is the fetal back?
- Where are the small parts or extremities?
- What is in the inlet? Does it confirm what I found in the fundus?
- Is the presenting part engaged, floating, or dipping into the inlet? (See Figure 22-6 ∞ on page 534).
- Is there fetal movement?
- How large is the fetus (appropriate, large, or small for gestational age)?
- Is there one fetus or more than one?
- Is fundal height proportionate to the estimated gestational age?

Leopold's Maneuvers

FIRST MANEUVER While facing the woman, the nurse palpates the upper abdomen with both hands (see Figure 23-7A). The nurse determines the shape, size, consistency, and mobility of the form that is found. The fetal head is firm, hard, and round and moves independently of the trunk. The breech feels softer and symmetric and has small bony prominences; it moves with the trunk.

SECOND MANEUVER After ascertaining whether the head or the buttocks occupies the fundus, the nurse tries to determine the location of the fetal back and notes whether it is on the right or left side of the maternal abdomen. Still facing the woman, the nurse palpates the abdomen with deep but gentle pressure, using the palms (see Figure 23-7B). The right hand should be steady while the left hand explores the right side of the uterus. The nurse then repeats the maneuver, probing with the right hand and steadying the uterus with the left hand. The fetal back should feel firm and smooth and should connect what was found in the fundus with a mass in the inlet. Once the back is located, the nurse validates the finding by palpating the fetal extremities (small irregularities and protrusions) on the opposite side of the abdomen.

THIRD MANEUVER Next, the nurse should determine what fetal part is lying above the inlet by gently grasping the lower portion of the abdomen just above the symphysis pubis with the thumb and fingers of the right hand (see Figure 23-7C). This maneuver yields the opposite information from what was found in the fundus and validates the presenting part. If the head is presenting and is not engaged, it may be gently pushed back and forth.

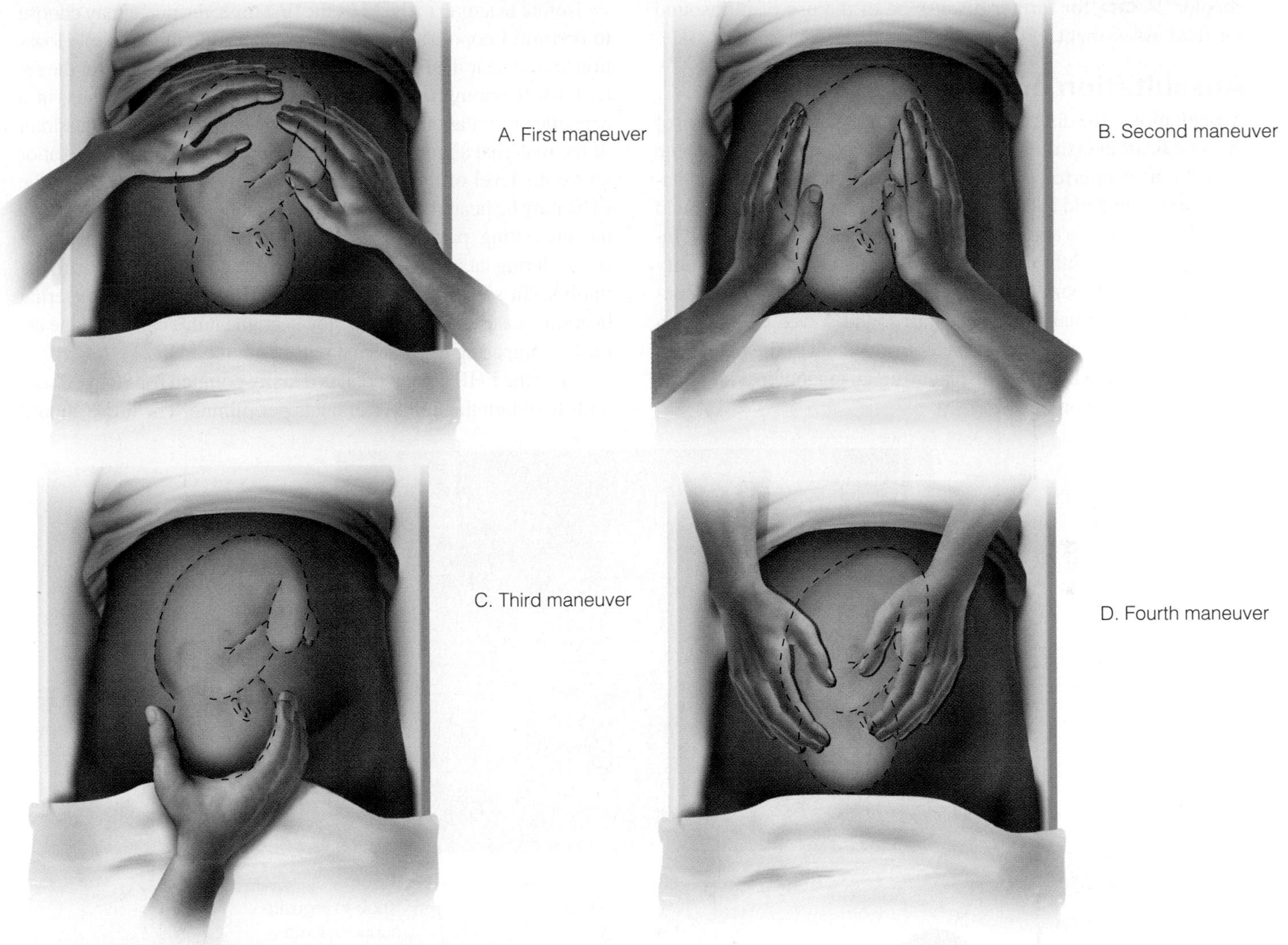

Figure 23-7 ■ Leopold's maneuvers for determining fetal head position, presentation, and lie.

Note: Some practitioners may perform the sequence differently. Many nurses do the fourth maneuver first to identify the part of the fetus in the pelvic inlet.

FOURTH MANEUVER For this portion of the examination, the nurse faces the woman's feet and attempts to locate the cephalic prominence or brow. Location of this landmark assists in assessing the descent of the presenting part into the pelvis. The fingers of both hands are moved gently down the sides of the uterus toward the pubis (see Figure 23-7D). The cephalic prominence (brow) is located on the side where there is greatest resistance to the descent of the fingers toward the pubis. It is located on the opposite side from the fetal back if the head is well flexed. However, when the fetal head is extended, the occiput is the first cephalic prominence felt, and it is located on the same side as the back. Therefore, when completing the fourth maneuver, if the nurse finds that the first cephalic prominence palpated is on the same side as the back, the head is not flexed. If the first prominence found is opposite the back, the head is well flexed (Cunningham et al., 2010).

Vaginal Examination

The vaginal examination reveals information regarding the fetus such as presentation, position, station, degree of flexion of the fetal head, and any swelling that may be present on the fetal scalp (caput succedaneum).

> **CLINICAL TIP**
>
> If you are having difficulty reaching the posterior cervix, ask the woman to place her fists under her buttocks or use a bedpan to facilitate a pelvic tilt, which will make the cervix more accessible.

Ultrasound

Real-time ultrasound (US) is frequently available in the birth setting. It may be used to assess fetal lie, presentation, and position; obtain measurements of biparietal diameter to estimate gestational age; assess for anomalies when a vaginal examination reveals suspicious findings; and assess placement of the placenta. Ultrasound is often helpful to pinpoint the fetal heart location when the nurse is having difficulty finding it, such as in cases where there are multiple fetuses. It can also be used to diagnose a fetal demise (Cunningham et al., 2010). (See chapter 21 ∞ for further discussion of the use of ultrasound for fetal assessment.)

Auscultation of Fetal Heart Rate

Auscultation is the direct auditory monitoring and interpretation of the fetal heart in utero. The number of fetal heart beats per minute (beats/min) is referred to as the fetal heart rate (FHR). Auscultation uses a handheld instrument, such as a fetoscope or ultrasound Doppler, to listen to and count the FHR (Figure 23-8 ■). Each instrument uses slightly different technology. Fetoscopes magnify actual fetal heart sounds, whereas Dopplers use ultrasound to convert fetal myocardial movement into sound waves that are then amplified and sent through a speaker from which the heart rate can be counted. Some Dopplers display a digital readout in addition to the audible sound produced.

Before listening to the FHR the first time, the nurse may choose to perform Leopold's maneuvers to determine the probable location to best hear the FHR. The FHR is heard most clearly at the fetal back (Cunningham et al., 2010) (Figure 23-9 ■). Thus, in a cephalic presentation, the FHR is best heard in the lower quadrant of the maternal abdomen. In a breech presentation it is heard at or above the level of the maternal umbilicus. In a transverse lie the FHR may be heard best just above or just below the umbilicus. As the presenting part descends and rotates through the maternal pelvis during labor, the FHR tends to descend and move toward the midline. In some instances, the monitor may track the maternal heart rate instead of the FHR. However, the nurse can avoid the error by comparing the maternal pulse with the FHR.

After the FHR is located, it is usually counted for 30 to 60 seconds to obtain the number of beats per minute. The nurse should

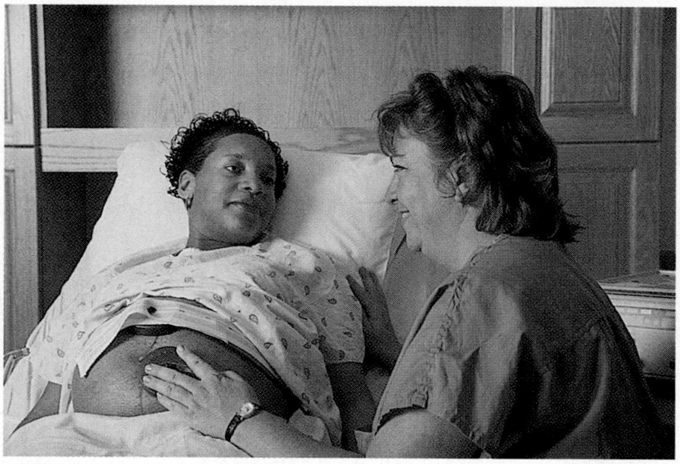

A

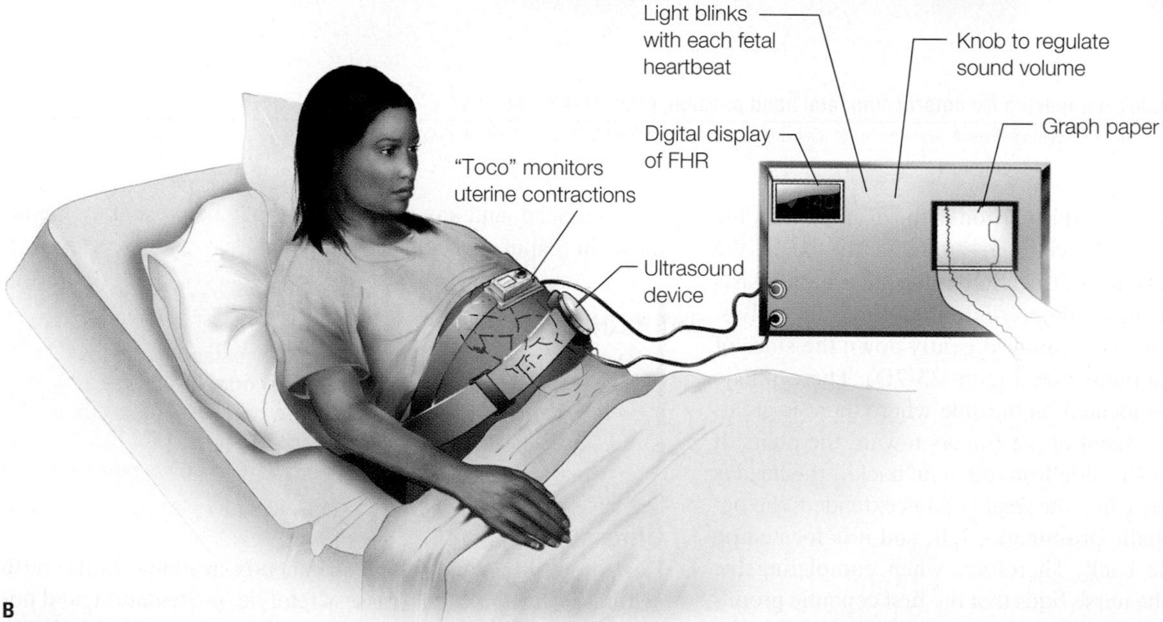

B

Figure 23-8 ■ A. The nurse uses a Doppler to assess the fetal heart rate. Doppler monitors can be used for intermittent labor monitoring or in the outpatient or community setting. When the fetal heart rate is picked up by the electronic monitor, the sound of the heartbeat can be heard by all persons in the room. B. Electronic monitoring by external technique. The ultrasound device is placed over the area of the fetal back and transmits information about the FHR. The tocodynamometer ("toco") is placed over the uterine fundus to provide information used to monitor uterine contractions. Information from both devices is transmitted to the electronic fetal monitor. The FHR is shown in a digital display (as a blinking light), on the special monitor paper, and audibly (by ajdusting a knob on the monitor). The uterine cotnractions are displayed on the special monitor paper as well.

Source: (A) Photographer, Elena Dorfman.

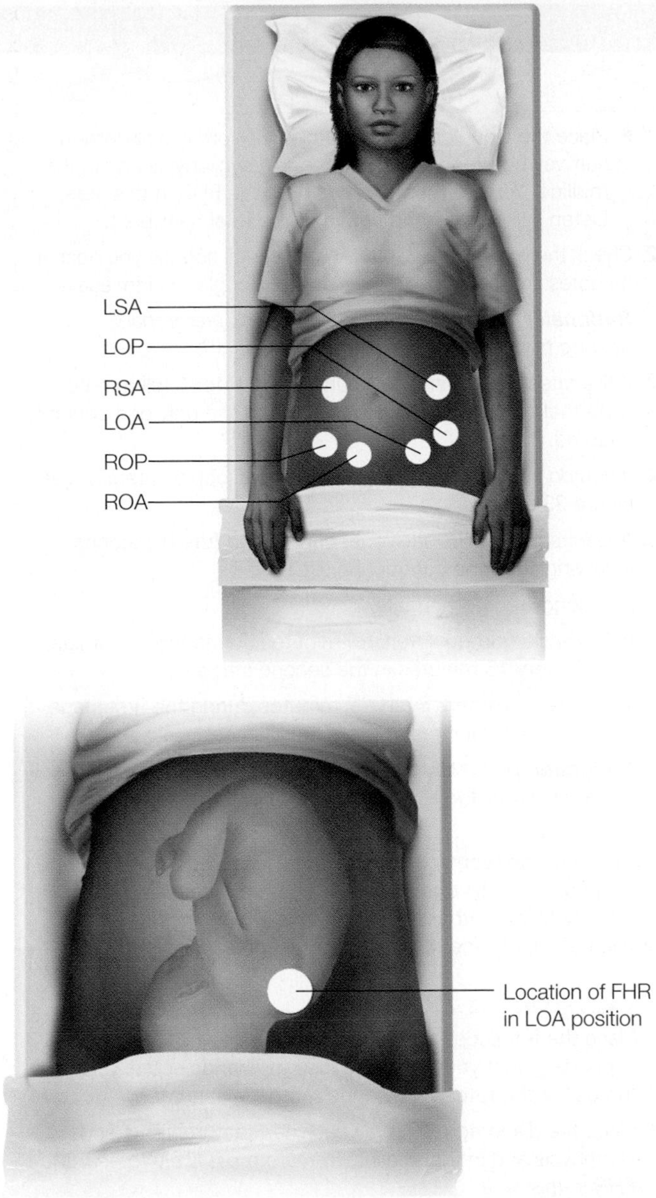

Figure 23-9 ■ Location of FHR in relation to the more commonly seen fetal positions. The FHR is heard more clearly over the fetal back.

TABLE 23-4 Frequency of Auscultation: Assessment and Documentation

LOW-RISK PATIENTS	HIGH-RISK PATIENTS
First stage of labor every 30 min	First stage of labor every 15 min
Second stage of labor every 15 min	Second stage of labor every 5 min

Labor Events

Assess FHR before:
Initiation of labor-enhancing procedures (e.g., artificial rupture of membranes)
Periods of ambulation
Administration of medications
Administration or initiation of analgesia/anesthesia

Assess FHR following:
Rupture of membranes
Recognition of abnormal uterine activity patterns, such as increased basal tone or tachysystole
Evaluation of oxytocin (maintenance, increase, or decrease of dosage)
Administration of medications (at time of peak action)
Expulsion of enema
Urinary catheterization
Vaginal examination
Periods of ambulation
Evaluation of analgesia and/or anesthesia (maintenance, increase, or decrease of dosage)

listen before, during, and just after a contraction to detect any abnormal heart rate, especially if the FHR is over 160 (tachycardia), under 110 (bradycardia), or if irregular beats (such as a deceleration) are heard (Cunningham et al., 2010). Listening through a contraction may be difficult because of maternal movement or a muffling of the FHR sounds. It is especially important to listen during and after the contraction to detect any deceleration that might occur. It is also important to listen immediately after each contraction when the woman is pushing during second stage, because fetal bradycardia frequently occurs as pressure is exerted on the fetal head during descent. See Procedure 23-3: Auscultation of Fetal Heart Rate and Table 23-4 for guidelines regarding how often to auscultate FHR.

Auscultation has been used for many years and remains a very valuable assessment technique even though it uses less technology than electronic fetal monitoring (EFM). Research and standards have shown that intermittent auscultation is equally effective for monitoring the FHR as EFM when a 1:1 nurse-to-patient ratio is maintained and the pregnant patient remains low risk. Low-risk status has been defined as "no pregnancy risk factors, no meconium stained fluid, normal labor patterns, and labor without augmentation or induction" (Cunningham et al., 2010). Outside these parameters, intermittent auscultation may not be appropriate and should not be used to assess high-risk pregnancies (Cunningham et al., 2010).

Auscultation is a learned skill and requires practice and knowledge of its benefits and limitations as an assessment tool. It has many advantages that make it a preferred method of monitoring by both mothers and nurses. Auscultation uses minimum instrumentation, is portable, and allows for maximum maternal movement; thus it is convenient and economical. Its disadvantages include the limited data this technique can provide compared with EFM. Only the baseline FHR (BL or BL FHR), rhythms of the FHR, and obvious increases and decreases can be monitored. Auscultation also does not provide a permanent record, thus making interpretation of the FHR impossible in the future or by another care provider. Identifying patterns and nonreassuring FHR is difficult and requires training. Auscultation must be practiced to ensure accurate interpretation of data.

Identifying UCs and the FHR simultaneously is necessary to determine patterns in the FHR and the relationship between the FHR and the UC. Auscultation does not allow for the detection of small changes in the FHR and cannot determine baseline variability (BL VAR). It may also be limited by maternal obesity and movement by the mother and fetus (Simpson & Creehan, 2007). In such instances, it may be essential to monitor using electronic means, regardless of the patient's risk status.

PROCEDURE 23-3 Auscultation of Fetal Heart Rate

NURSING ACTION

Preparation

- Explain the procedure, the indications for it, and the information that will be obtained.
- Uncover the woman's abdomen.

Equipment and Supplies

Doppler device

Ultrasonic gel

Procedure

> **CLINICAL TIP**
> The fetal heart rate (FHR) is heard most clearly through the fetal back. Locate the fetal back using Leopold's maneuvers.

1. To use the Doppler:
   - Place ultrasonic gel on the diaphragm of the Doppler. Gel is used to maintain contact with the maternal abdomen and enhances conduction of sound.
   - The diaphragm should be warmed prior to using the Doppler.
   - Place the Doppler diaphragm on the woman's abdomen halfway between the umbilicus and symphysis and in the midline. You are most likely to hear the FHR in this area. Listen carefully for the sound of the fetal heartbeat.
2. Check the woman's pulse against the fetal sounds you hear. If the rates are the same, reposition the Doppler and try again.

   Rationale: *If the rates are the same, you are probably hearing the maternal pulse and not the FHR.*
3. If the rates are not similar, count the FHR for 1 full minute. Note that the FHR has a double rhythm and only one sound is counted.
4. If you do not locate the FHR, move the Doppler laterally (see Figure 23-8A).
5. Auscultate the FHR between, during, and for 30 seconds following a uterine contraction (UC).
6. Frequency recommendations:
   - Low-risk women: Every 30 minutes during the first stage, and every 15 minutes in the second stage.
   - High-risk women: Every 15 minutes during the first stage, and every 5 minutes in the second stage.

   Rationale: *This evaluation provides the opportunity to assess the fetal status and response to labor.*

Documentation Document that the procedure was explained to the woman and that she verbalized understanding. The location of the FHR, FHR baseline, changes in FHR that occur with contractions, and presence of accelerations or decelerations should be included. Other characteristics should include variability, maternal position, type of device used, uterine activity, maternal pulse, and nursing interventions that were performed.

The Fetoscope

The fetoscope is an older assessment tool; however, some clinicians prefer it because it is "natural" and does not rely on ultrasound.

To use the fetoscope:

- The bell should be warmed prior to using the fetoscope.
- Place the fetoscope earpieces in your ears and the device support against your forehead; use the handpiece to position the bell of the fetoscope on the mother's abdomen.
- Place the diaphragm halfway between the umbilicus and symphysis and in the midline. *You are most likely to hear the FHR in this area.*
- Without touching the fetoscope, listen carefully for the FHR.

Electronic Fetal Monitoring

Monitoring a Fetal Heart Rate

Electronic fetal monitoring (EFM) provides a continuous tracing of the fetal heart rate (FHR), allowing characteristics of the FHR to be observed and evaluated (see Procedure 23-4: Electronic Fetal Monitoring and Figure 23-8B). EFM requires advanced assessment and clinical judgment skills, regardless of the setting in which it is used. Therefore, a licensed, experienced healthcare professional should perform each aspect of fetal heart monitoring (FHM), consistent with their state or provincial scope of practice. AWHONN (2008b) maintains that fetal heart monitoring includes: (1) application of fetal monitoring components; (2) intermittent auscultation; (3) ongoing monitoring and interpretation of FHR data; (4) initial assessment of the laboring woman and fetus; and (5) ongoing clinical interventions and evaluations of the woman and fetus.

Initiation of monitoring and ongoing clinical evaluation should only be performed by healthcare professionals who have education and skills validation in FHM and in the care of the laboring woman. AWHONN regards these healthcare professionals with expertise in fetal monitoring as: (1) registered nurses; (2) certified nurse midwives (CNMs), certified midwives (CMs), and registered midwives (RMs [Canada]); (3) other advanced practice nurses such as nurse practitioners and clinical nurse specialists; (4) physicians; and (5) physician assistants (PAs) (2008b).

In the late 1990s, standardized definitions for FHR tracings were proposed (National Institute of Child Health and Human Development [NICHD], 1997) in an effort to resolve controversy surrounding the benefits of EFM, the primary interpretation of FHR patterns, and appropriate interventions for nonreassuring tracings (Cunningham et al., 2010). In 2004, the

PROCEDURE 23-4 Electronic Fetal Monitoring

NURSING ACTION

Preparation

- Explain the procedure, the indications for it, and the information that will be obtained.

Equipment and Supplies

Monitor

Two elastic monitor belts

Tocodynamometer ("toco")

Ultrasound transducer

Ultrasound gel

Procedure

CLINICAL TIP

Evaluating the FHR tracing provides information about fetal status and response to the stress of labor. The presence of reassuring characteristics is associated with good fetal outcomes. Rapid identification of nonreassuring characteristics allows prompt interventions and the opportunity to determine the fetal response to the interventions.

1. Turn on the monitor.
2. Place the two elastic belts around the woman's abdomen.
3. Place the "toco" over the uterine fundus off the midline on the area palpated to be most firm during contractions. Secure it with one of the elastic belts.

   Rationale: *The uterine fundus is the area of greatest contractility.*
4. Note the uterine contraction (UC) tracing. The resting tone tracing (that is, without a UC) should be recording on the 10 or 15 mm Hg pressure line. Adjust the line to reflect that reading.

   Rationale: *If the resting tone is set on the zero line, there often is a constant grinding noise.*
5. Apply the ultrasonic gel to the diaphragm of the ultrasound transducer.

   Rationale: *Ultrasonic gel is used to maintain contact with the maternal abdomen. The ultrasonic beam is directed toward the fetal heart.*
6. Place the diaphragm on the maternal abdomen in the midline between the umbilicus and the symphysis pubis.
7. Listen for the FHR, which will have a whiplike or galloping sound. Move the diaphragm laterally if necessary to obtain a stronger sound (see Figure 23-9).
8. When the FHR is located, attach the second elastic belt snugly to the transducer.

   Rationale: *Firm contact is necessary to maintain a steady tracing.*
9. Place the following information on the beginning of the fetal monitor paper: date, time, woman's name, gravida, para, membrane status, and name of physician or certified nurse-midwife.

Note: *Each birthing unit may have specific guidelines about additional information to include.*

Documentation

Document that the procedure was explained to the woman and that she verbalized understanding. In addition, document the maternal position, the type of device used and location of the FHR. The record of both the FHR and uterine activity should be of adequate quality for visual interpretation. A full description of the electronic fetal monitor tracing requires a qualitative and quantitative description of: (1) uterine contraction characteristics (duration, frequency, strength), (2) baseline FHR, (3) baseline FHR variability, (4) presence of accelerations, (5) periodic or episodic decelerations, and (6) changes or a trend of FHR patterns over time (Macones, Hankins, Spong, Hauth, & Moore, 2008).

Further documentation should include maternal pulse and blood pressure, presence of fetal movement, and any interventions and/or procedures performed including fetal response to the interventions.

> Example: 8-3-10 BL FHR 135–140. Minimal FHR baseline variability noted. Late decelerations noted with decrease of FHR to 130 beats/min for 20 sec with each UC. UC every 3 min × 50–60 sec of moderate intensity by palpation. Patient turned to left side. No further deceleration with three subsequent UCs. Two accelerations of 20 beats/min × 20 sec noted with fetal movement. Patient instructed to remain on left side. B. Burch, RNC

Joint Commission on Accreditation of Healthcare Organizations (JCAHO) recommended standardized and consistent use of fetal monitoring terminology among all healthcare professionals and the development of clear guidelines for fetal monitoring of potential high-risk patients. In response, in May 2005, ACOG issued a bulletin that reviewed FHR assessment terminology and described the management of nonreassuring FHR patterns (ACOG, 2005). At the same time, AWHONN revised its fetal monitoring courses to incorporate the standardized terminology. In December 2005, ACOG modified its May bulletin to match AWHONN guidelines and NICHD terminology.

Subsequently, the Royal College of Obstetricians and Gynaecologists (RCOG) of the United Kingdom and the Society of Obstetricians and Gynaecologists of Canada (SOGC) convened expert groups to assess the evidence-based use of electronic fetal monitoring (EFM) (Liston, Sawchuck, & Young, 2007).

These groups produced consensus documents with more specific recommendations for FHR pattern classification and intrapartum management actions (Liston et al., 2007; RCOG, 2008). In addition, new interpretations and definitions have been proposed, including terminology and new interpretative systems using three and five tiers (Liston et al., 2007; Parer & Ikeda, 2007; RCOG, 2008). Recently, NICHD, ACOG, and the Society for Maternal-Fetal Medicine (SMFM) jointly sponsored a workshop focused on EFM. The goals of this workshop were to (1) review and update the definitions for FHR pattern categorization, (2) assess existing classification systems for interpreting specific FHR patterns and to make recommendations about a system for use in the United States, and (3) make recommendations for research priorities for EFM. This chapter reflects the most recent guidelines at the time of this book's publication instituted by ACOG, AWHONN, and NICHD for FHR tracings.

Indications for Electronic Fetal Monitoring

ACOG states that the frequency of FHR monitoring used during labor should be based on risk factors (Barclay, 2009). Although there is as yet no standardized list, Table 23-5 identifies some common indications for EFM.

TABLE 23-5 Possible Indications for Electronic Fetal Monitoring

Fetal Factors
Decreased fetal movement
Abnormal auscultatory FHR
Meconium passage
Abnormal presentations/positions
Intrauterine growth restriction (IUGR) or small-for-gestational-age (SGA) fetus
Postdates (greater than 41 weeks)
Multiple gestation
Maternal Factors
Fever
Infections
Preeclampsia
Disease conditions (e.g., hypertension, diabetes)
Anemia
Rh alloimmunization
Previous perinatal death
Grand multiparity
Previous cesarean birth
Borderline/contracted pelvis
Uterine Factors
Dysfunctional labor
Failure to progress in labor
Oxytocin induction/augmentation
Uterine anomalies
Complications of Pregnancy
Prolonged rupture of membranes
Premature rupture of membranes
Preterm labor
Marginal abruptio placentae
Partial placenta previa
Occult/frank prolapse of cord
Amnionitis
Regional Anesthesia
Elective Monitoring

External Monitoring

Application: Fetal Monitoring

Electronic monitoring of the FHR can be done externally by using an ultrasound (US) transducer. The US transducer is a Doppler device with computerized logic to interpret and count the Doppler signals (Cunningham et al., 2010). The US transducer is placed on the maternal abdomen over the fetal back (as determined by Leopold's maneuvers), where the FHR is usually the loudest, and is held in place with an elastic belt. A water-soluble gel is applied to the underside of the transducer to aid in conduction of the fetal heart sounds. The US transducer then emits ultrasonic beams that reflect off the moving fetal myocardium and return to the transducer. The transducer receives the signal and interprets it before amplifying it in the fetal monitor and recording it on graph paper. The US image can be influenced by other moving structures in the maternal abdomen, such as maternal arterial blood flow and maternal or fetal movement. Interference is generally filtered out; however, on occasion the maternal heart rate is detected by the US transducer and must be distinguished from the FHR by comparing the signal with the maternal pulse.

The external US transducer can be more beneficial than auscultating the FHR because it produces a continuous graphic recording. The US transducer can show the baseline (BL), baseline variability (BL VAR), and changes in the FHR. It is noninvasive and does not require rupture of membranes or minimal cervical dilation. FHR monitoring by US transducer is limited because it is susceptible to interference from maternal and fetal movement, as discussed earlier, and may produce a weak signal (Simpson & Creehan, 2007). The tracing may become sketchy and difficult to interpret. Repeating the procedure for US placement usually remedies the weak signal and tracing.

Internal Monitoring

Internal fetal monitoring is accomplished with a fetal scalp electrode (FSE), a fine surgical spiral wire, attached to the fetal scalp. The FSE is the most precise method of monitoring because it is a direct electrocardiogram (ECG) of the FHR and produces the most accurate FHR tracing. The FSE is attached to the fetus during a vaginal exam. Once in place, the electrode is connected to the fetal monitor. The monitor determines the time between fetal "R" waves in the "QRS" complex and calculates the findings into a FHR. The FHR is then recorded on graph paper.

For the spiral electrode to be inserted, the cervix must be dilated at least 2 cm, the presenting fetal part must be accessible by vaginal examination, and the membranes must be ruptured. Even though it is not possible to apply the electrode and catheter under strict sterile conditions, the procedure should be performed as aseptically as possible. After determining fetal position by vaginal examination, the examiner (physician or nurse) inserts the electrode, which is encased in a plastic guide, to the level of the internal cervical os and attaches it to the presenting part, being careful not to apply it to the face, suture

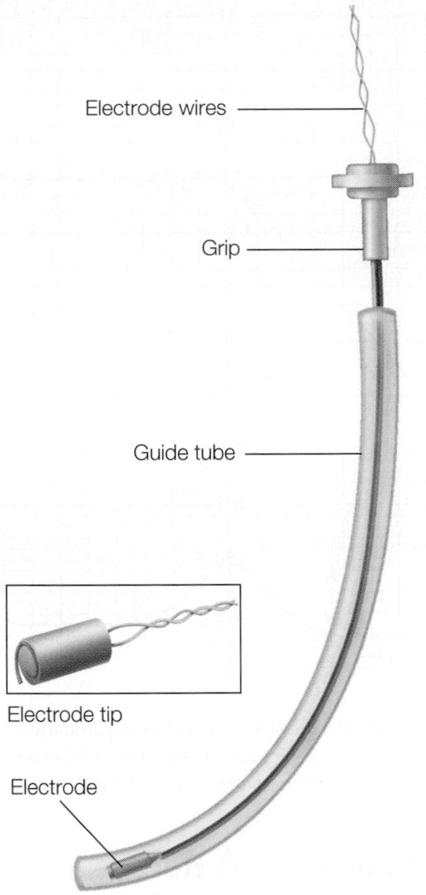

A

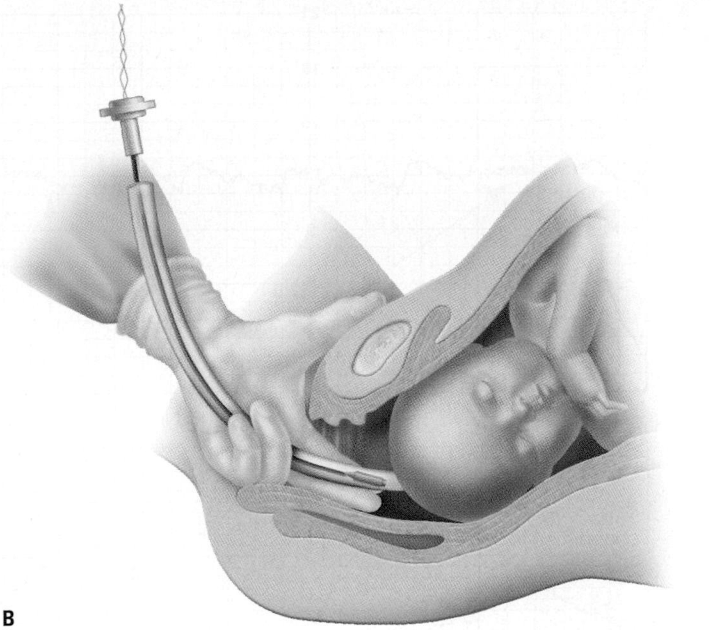
B

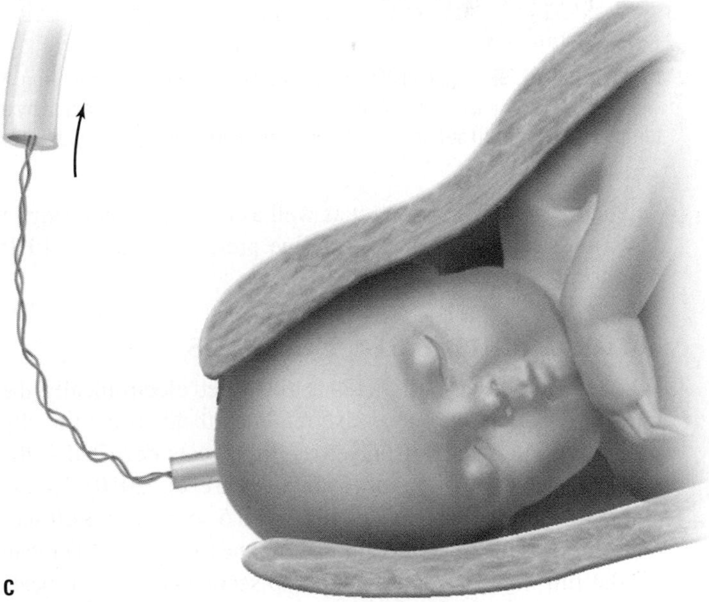
C

Figure 23-10 ■ Techniques for internal, direct fetal monitoring. A. Spiral electrode. B. Attaching the spiral electrode to the scalp. C. Attached spiral electrode with guide tube removed.

lines, fontanelles, cervix, or perineum if the fetus is in a breech presentation (Cunningham et al., 2010). The electrode is rotated clockwise until it is attached to the presenting part and is then disengaged from the guide tube (Figure 23-10 ■). The guide tube is removed, and the end wires are connected to a leg plate that is attached to the woman's thigh. The cable from the leg plate is connected to the monitor. Infections and injuries from internal electrodes and catheters are a small but actual risk. Although nurses in some facilities apply internal monitors, in many settings their application is limited to the physician or certified nurse-midwife (CNM).

Because the risk of transmission to the fetus is increased by the small puncture in the fetal scalp, use of internal scalp electrodes should be avoided if at all possible in the presence of known maternal infections such as HIV, hepatitis, or group B streptococcus. Also, women who have had internal monitors and subsequently given birth by cesarean are more likely to have postpartum infections (Chan & Johnson, 2008). The fetal scalp electrode is removed prior to birth. Fetal scalp monitors are also avoided in preterm infants because of the increased risk of ventricular hemorrhage (Cunningham et al., 2010).

The FHR tracing at the top of Figure 23-11 ■ was obtained by internal monitoring, and the uterine contraction tracing at the bottom was obtained by external monitoring. A comparison shows that the spiral electrode provides an instantaneous and continuous recording of FHR that is clearer than the data provided by external monitoring. Notice that the FHR shows variability (the tracing moves up and down instead of in a straight line), ranging between about 140 and 155 beats/min.

Telemetry

As discussed previously, FHR and uterine activity may also be monitored by a telemetry system. Equipment consists of US along with external uterine pressure transducers connected to a small battery-operated transmitter. Signals are transmitted to a receiver connected to a monitor that displays FHR and uterine activity data. A printout provides documentation. This system, which can be worn on a shoulder strap, allows the woman to ambulate, helping her to feel more comfortable and less confined during labor, yet provides for continuous monitoring.

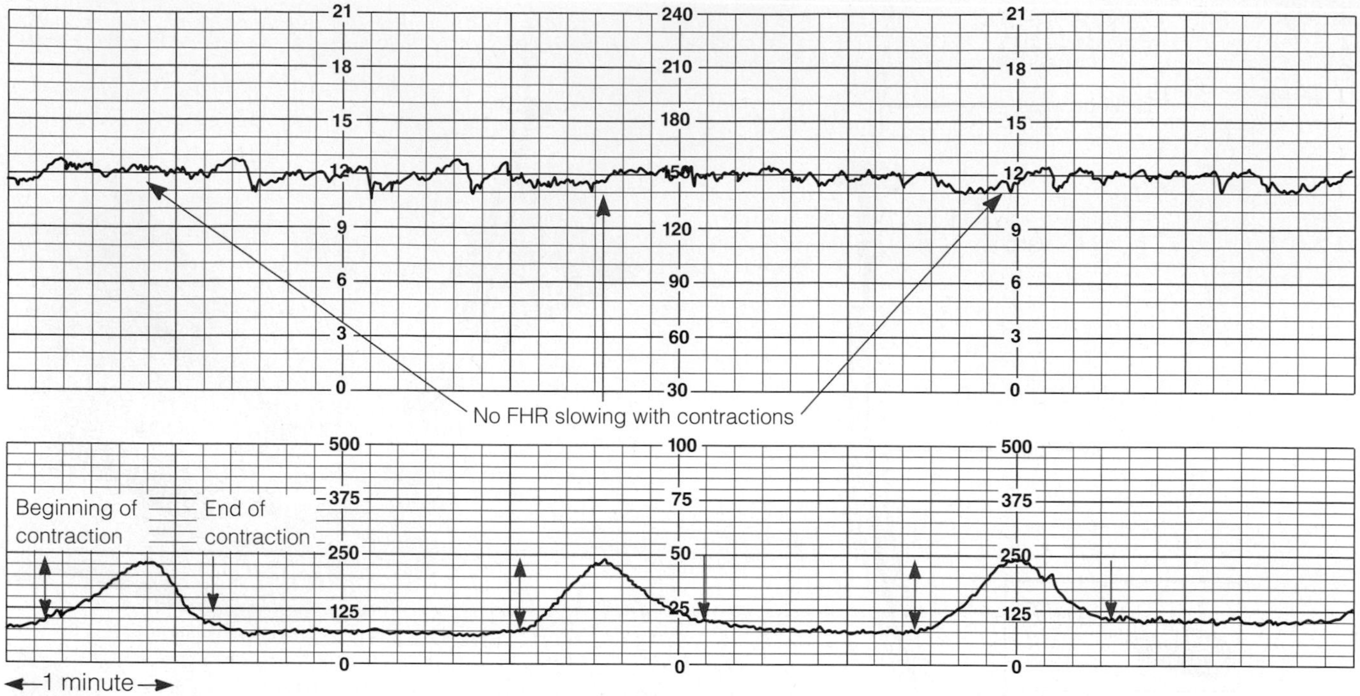

Figure 23-11 ■ Top: A FHR tracing obtained by internal monitoring. Normal FHR range is 110 to 160 beats/min. This tracing indicates a FHR range of 140 to 155 beats/min. Bottom: A uterine contraction tracing obtained by external monitoring. Each dark vertical line marks 1 minute, and each small rectangle represents 10 seconds. The contraction frequency is about every 3 minutes, and the duration of the contractions is 50 to 60 seconds.

Telemetry provides for direct as well as indirect monitoring of FHR, indirect monitoring of uterine pressure, and dual FHR monitoring of twins.

Fetal Heart Rate Patterns

When the fetal heart rate (FHR) is monitored electronically, the interval between two successive fetal heartbeats is continually measured. The rate is displayed as if the beats occurred at the same interval for 60 seconds (Cunningham et al., 2010). For example, if the interval between beats is 0.5 seconds per 60 seconds, then divide the interval time into the time frame. The rate for the full minute would then be 60 seconds/0.5 = 120 beats per minute (beats/min).

Fetal heart rate patterns are defined by the characteristics of baseline, variability, accelerations, and decelerations. The features of the FHR patterns are categorized as either baseline, periodic, or episodic. Periodic patterns are those associated with uterine contractions, and episodic patterns are those not associated with uterine contractions (Macones et al., 2008).

The definitions for FHR pattern categorization, jointly developed by NICHD, ACOG, and SMFM mentioned previously, have potential benefits. Standardized terminology minimizes variation among care providers and allows for accurate documentation of the fetal status in medical records. If everyone on the perinatal team communicates clearly, treatment can be initiated promptly and there may be a decreased risk of adverse outcomes (AWHONN, 2005). The FHR definitions and interpretive system was developed for consistent use by perinatal care providers in clinical practice and research (Macones et al., 2008).

Baseline Fetal Heart Rate

The **baseline fetal heart rate (BL FHR)** is determined by approximating the mean (average) FHR during a 10-minute period, rounded to increments of 5 beats/min (e.g., 125, 130, 135, 140). Accelerations, decelerations, and periods of marked FHR variability (>25 beats/min) are excluded. There must be at least 2 minutes of identifiable baseline segments (not necessarily contiguous) in any 10-minute window, or the baseline for that period is indeterminate, and the preceding 10-minute window must be used to determine the baseline (Macones et al., 2008). For example, if FHR over a period of 10 minutes fluctuates between 142 beats/min and 156 beats/min, the BL FHR would be documented as 150 beats/min with moderate variability.

The normal baseline (BL) rate ranges from 110 to 160 beats/min, depending on gestational age. As the gestational age of the fetus increases, the FHR decreases. The FHR decreases an average of 16 beats/min between 16 weeks' gestation and term. The slowing of the FHR occurs as the parasympathetic nervous system (PNS) matures and exerts control over the fetal heart activity (Cunningham et al., 2010).

Tachycardia

Fetal tachycardia is a BL FHR greater than 160 beats/min for at least a 10-minute period. The possible causes of tachycardia may be idiopathic, maternal, fetal, or a combination of maternal and fetal. Some of the most common causes are the following (Cunningham et al., 2010):

Maternal

- Fever (Metabolism of the fetus accelerates because of increased maternal temperature.)

RESEARCH EVIDENCE IN PRACTICE Fetal Monitoring During Labor

CLINICAL QUESTION

What is the most effective method for monitoring fetal status during labor?

RESEARCH EVIDENCE

During labor, there are multiple ways to monitor fetal status as labor progresses. The fetus can be monitored externally using a special stethoscope or hand-held monitor, or the baby can be continuously assessed using cardiotocography (CTG) and assessing the baby's condition with an electrocardiogram (ECG). Also available is fetal pulse oximetry, which measures how much oxygen the baby's blood is carrying via a probe that sits inside the vagina during labor.

Several Cochrane Collaborative reviews critically appraised research related to these methods—continuous CTG, ECG, and fetal pulse oximetry—to determine the method that is most effective in producing desirable outcomes for mother and baby. The Cochrane Collaborative is a highly rigorous source of research evidence. Among these three reviews, randomized trials involving more than 54,000 women in labor were reviewed.

From an acceptability standpoint, CTG restricts movement of the mother and requires insertion of an internal electrode in the baby's head after rupture of the membranes. The fetal oximetry probe does not limit the mother's mobility.

Monitoring the baby's heart using an ECG plus CTG during labor helps mothers and babies when continuous electronic fetal heart rate monitoring is indicated. In other words, these monitoring methods are useful if monitoring is needed based on heart rate or rhythm irregularities in the fetus. The application of this type of monitoring must be considered in light of the limitations on the mother's mobility and the need for an invasive procedure during labor.

There was limited support for the use of fetal pulse oximetry when used in the presence of a nonreassuring ECG. The data revealed only a small reduction in the cesarean birth rate under these conditions. In general, continuous CTG and ECG were associated with increased cesarean birthrates and instrument-assisted births. None of the monitoring methods was associated with a reduction in cerebral palsy, infant mortality, or other measures of neonatal well-being.

WHAT QUESTIONS REMAIN UNANSWERED?

It is unclear whether any type of internal monitoring is needed when the mother and baby are low risk and no problems arise during labor. It does appear that monitoring is associated with a higher rate of instrumental or cesarean births, but this may be due to the risks that are associated with applying internal monitoring in the first place.

WHAT IS BEST PRACTICE?

Internal monitoring of fetal heart rate and rhythm using CTG is indicated for high-risk pregnancies or those in which fetal condition must be continuously assessed.

CRITICAL THINKING

What are the conditions under which the nurse should recommend internal monitoring methods? How is the assessment plan altered when internal monitoring is applied?

References

Alfirevic, A., Devane, D., & Gyte, G. 2008. Continuous cardiotocography (CTG) as a form of electronic fetal monitoring (EFM) for fetal assessment during labour. *Cochrane Database of Systematic Reviews,* Issue 3. Art. No.: CD006066. doi:10.1002/14651858

East, C., Chan, F., Colditz, P., & Begg, L. 2010. Fetal pulse oximetry for fetal assessment in labour. *Cochrane Database of Systematic Reviews,* Issue 2. Art. No.: CD004075. doi:10.1002/104651858

Neilson, J. 2009. Fetal electrocardiogram (ECG) for fetal monitoring during labour. *Cochrane Database of Systematic Reviews,* Issue 3. Art. No.: CD000116. doi:10.1002/14651858

- Dehydration
- Anxiety
- Betasympathomimetic or sympathetic drugs, such as ritodrine, terbutaline, atropine, and isoxsuprine (These drugs have a cardiac stimulant effect.)
- Maternal hyperthyroidism (Thyroid-stimulating hormones may cross the placenta and stimulate the FHR.)
- Supraventricular tachycardia

Fetal

- Early fetal hypoxia (This leads to stimulation of the sympathetic nervous system (SNS) as the fetus compensates for reduced blood flow.)
- Asphyxia
- Fetal anemia (The heart rate increases as a compensatory mechanism to improve tissue perfusion.)
- Infection
- Prematurity
- Prolonged fetal stimulation

Tachycardia is considered a nonreassuring sign if it is accompanied by other FHR patterns such as late decelerations, severe variable decelerations, or decreased or absent variability. If tachycardia is associated with maternal fever, treatment may consist of antipyretics, cooling measures, and antibiotics (Cunningham et al., 2010). Fetal arrhythmia or dysrhythmia needs to be ruled out. The pediatrician should be notified, because tachycardia may cause heart failure in the newborn.

Intervention for tachycardia usually requires treatment of the underlying cause. Additional testing and monitoring may be used to further determine fetal well-being.

Bradycardia

Fetal bradycardia is by definition a FHR baseline less than 110 beats/min for at least a 10-minute period. The lower limits of the FHR have been debated in the past. A FHR as low as 90 beats/min with good variability has been classified as benign and reassuring. When bradycardia is accompanied by decreased variability or late decelerations, or both, it is considered ominous and a sign of advanced fetal compromise (Cunningham et al., 2010). The possible causes of bradycardia include the following (Cunningham et al., 2010):

Application: Fetal Bradycardia

- Stimulation of the vagus nerve (prolonged head compression as in early decelerations, application of the forceps or vacuum extractor, or prolonged scalp stimulation)
- Drugs that stimulate the PNS or block the SNS (anesthesia and regional analgesia)

- Maternal hypotension (Maternal hypotension results in decreased blood flow to the fetus.)
- Prolonged umbilical cord compression (Fetal baroreceptors are activated by cord compression, which produces vagal stimulation, and in turn decreases FHR.)
- Fetal dysrhythmia (This is associated with complete heart block in the fetus.)
- Hypoxemia or late fetal asphyxia (There is depression of myocardial activity.)
- Accidental monitoring of maternal pulse

Wandering Baseline

A *wandering baseline* is a smooth, meandering, unsteady BL that fluctuates in the normal BL range without variability (Cunningham et al., 2010). The possible causes of this type of BL may be a congenital defect or metabolic acidosis. Immediate interventions should be taken to enhance fetal oxygenation, and delivery should be anticipated (AWHONN, 2006).

Sinusoidal Fetal Heart Rate Pattern

A sinusoidal FHR pattern is defined as having a visually apparent, smooth, wavelike, undulating sine pattern in FHR baseline (Macones et al., 2008). The pattern has a series of cycles that are extremely smooth and regular (not necessarily identical) in amplitude and duration. It resembles a perfect letter "S" lying on its side. The FHR undulates in a sine pattern between 120 and 160 beats/min with variability amplitude of 5 to 15 beats/min. The pattern has a cycle frequency of 3–5/minute that persists for 20 minutes or more (Macones et al., 2008). Accelerations do not occur spontaneously, nor can they be induced (Figure 23-12 ■).

Sinusoidal patterns may be benign (pseudosinusoidal) or pathological (true sinusoidal) patterns. Pathologic sinusoidal patterns are indicative of nonreassuring fetal status and require immediate attention (Cunningham et al., 2010). The possible causes of a true sinusoidal pattern include the following (Cunningham et al., 2010):

- Fetal anemia
- Chronic fetal bleeding
- Fetal isoimmunization
- Twin-to-twin transfusion
- Umbilical cord occlusion
- Central nervous system (CNS) malformations

If the sinusoidal pattern is uncorrectable, interventions include immediate notification of the healthcare provider and expeditious delivery.

Arrhythmias and Dysrhythmias

Arrhythmias, a term often used interchangeably with *dysrhythmias,* are disturbances in the FHR pattern that are not associated with abnormal electrical impulse formation or conduction in the fetal cardiac tissue. An arrhythmic pattern demonstrates a normal P wave and QRS complexes (Tucker, Miller, & Miller, 2008). However, dysrhythmic FHR patterns may exhibit abnormal electrical impulse formation and/or conduction in the fetal cardiac tissues, resulting in abnormal P waves or QRS complexes, or both. Arrhythmic and dysrhythmic patterns get their names from the origin of the pattern, for example, sinus node variants, atrial node patterns, or ventricular patterns (Tucker, Miller, & Miller, 2008).

FHR dysrhythmias are estimated to occur in 2% to 14% of all pregnancies. Whereas 90% of dysrhythmias are benign, 10% can be life threatening and require the consultation of a neonatal or pediatric cardiology expert (Tucker, Miller, & Miller,

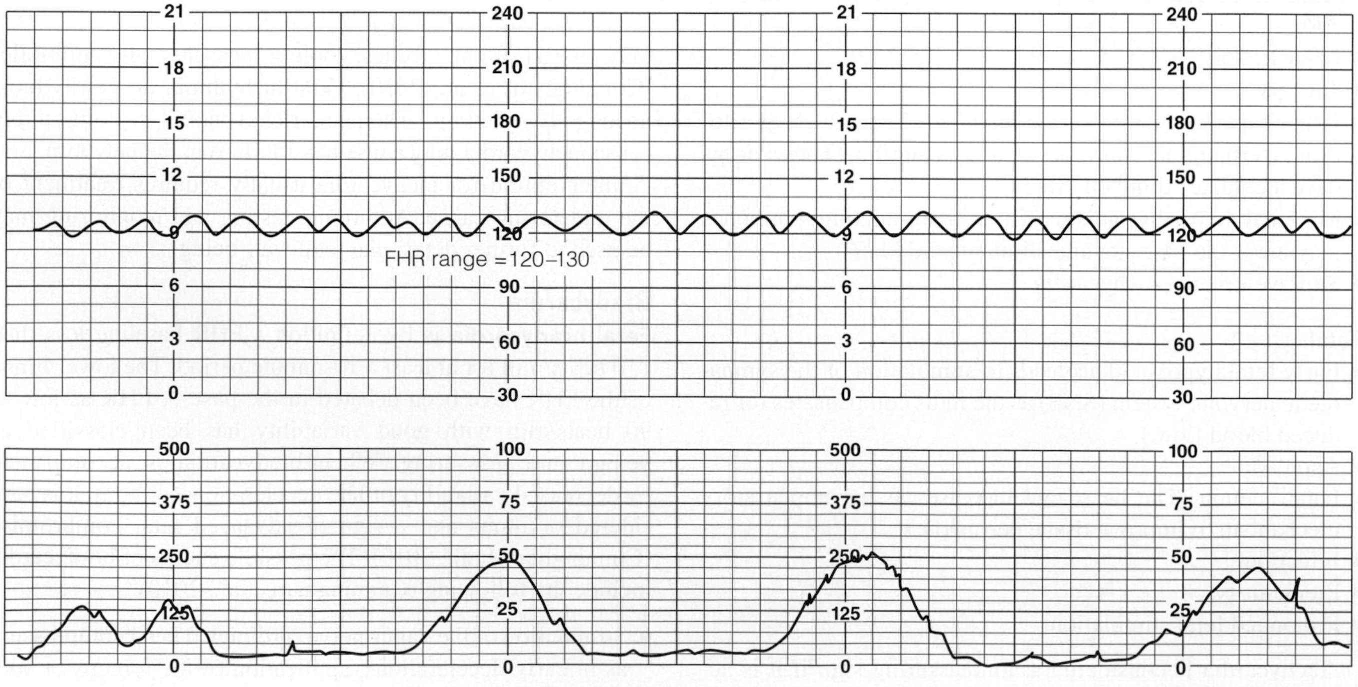

Figure 23-12 ■ Sinusoidal pattern. Note the undulating waveform evenly distributed between the 120 and 130 beats/min baseline. There is minimal variability.

TABLE 23-6 Common Causes of Various Types of Fetal Dysrhythmias

SINUS NODE VARIANTS	ATRIAL DYSRHYTHMIAS	VENTRICULAR DYSRHYTHMIAS
• Bradycardia	• Parasympathetic response to fetal hypoxemia	• Beta-blocker drugs
• Tachycardia	• Maternal ingestion of stimulants (e.g., caffeine, tobacco, alcohol, cocaine)	• Complete heart blocks (AV malformation)
• Marked sinus arrhythmia	• Abnormal reentry conduction	• Congenital heart disease
• Infections	• Cardiomyopathy	• Autoimmune disease (AV malformation)
• CNS disturbances	• Fetal-maternal placental hemorrhage	• Maternal collagen disorders (AV malformation)
	• Nonimmune hydrops fetalis	
	• Wolf-Parkinson White syndrome	
	• Cardiac structural abnormalities (e.g., atrial septal defect (ASD), ventricular septal defect (VSD), valve malformation)	

Sources: Data from AWHONN, 2004; Cunningham et al., 2010; Tucker, Miller, & Miller, 2008).

2008). For this reason, it is important to accurately diagnose abnormal FHR patterns and distinguish fetal arrhythmias from artifact and electrical interference. Fetal dysrhythmias can be difficult to diagnose, because detection of the fetal cardiac electrical activity is best accomplished by invasive or advanced monitoring techniques such as fetal scalp electrode, real-time ultrasound, Doppler velocimetry, fetal echocardiogram, and echocardiogram monitoring (e.g., M-Mode EchoCG, and Pulsed Doppler EchoCG) (Tucker, Miller, & Miller, 2008). With the exception of the fetal scalp electrode, more advanced and expensive diagnostic testing may not be readily available.

The most common causes of FHR dysrhythmias are discussed in Table 23-6.

Baseline Variability

Baseline variability (BL VAR) is a reliable indicator of fetal cardiac and neurological function and well-being. The opposing "push-pull" balancing between the sympathetic nervous system and the parasympathetic nervous system directly affects the FHR. ACOG, AWHONN, and NICHD define baseline variability (BL VAR) as baseline (BL) fluctuations in the baseline FHR that are irregular in amplitude and frequency. The fluctuations are visually quantified as the amplitude of the peak-to-trough in beats/min (Macones et al., 2008). Evaluation of BL VAR is based on visual assessment of the amplitude of the BL cycles (AWHONN, 2005). Variability is classified by ACOG, AWHONN, and NICHD as follows (Macones et al., 2008):

- Absent FHR variability—amplitude range undetected
- Minimal FHR variability—amplitude range detectable but 5 beats/min or less
- Moderate FHR variability—amplitude range of 6 to 25 beats/min
- Marked FHR variability—amplitude range greater than 25 beats/min

Figures 23-13 ■ and 23-14 ■ illustrate examples of each of these categories.

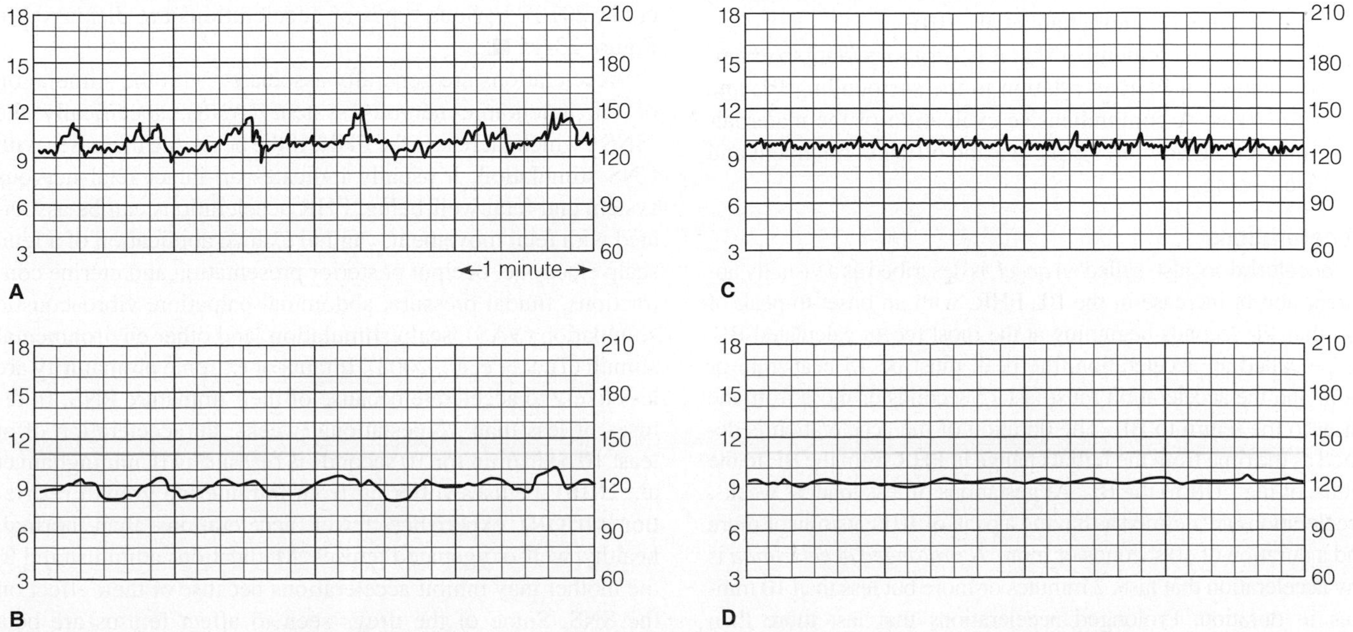

Figure 23-13 ■ A. and B. Moderate variability. C. Minimal variability. D. Absent variability.

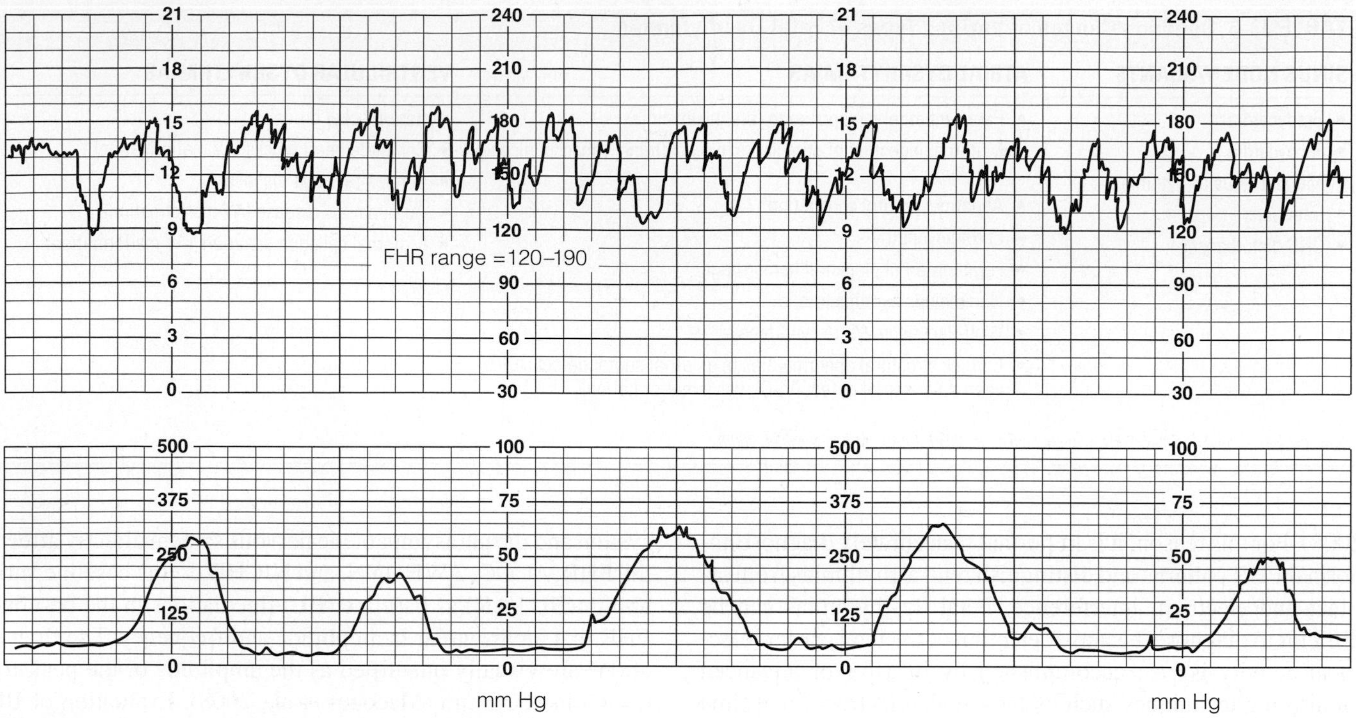

Figure 23-14 ■ Marked variability. FHR varies markedly between 120 and 190 beats/min. With this type of pattern, it is not possible to determine average baseline FHR because of the wide, marked variations.

Fetal Heart Rate Changes

In addition to changes in the average BL FHR range, the FHR may also exhibit intermittent or transient deviations or changes from the BL that are commonly referred to as accelerations and decelerations. These transient deviations or changes in BL are categorized as episodic or periodic. Episodic changes (formerly referred to as nonperiodic changes) are not associated with uterine contractions (UCs). Periodic changes occur with UCs. If a periodic change occurs with 50% or more of UCs in a 20-minute period, it is further categorized as a recurrent change or pattern (Cunningham et al., 2010).

The nurse must remember that it is very important to examine all changes in FHR in relation to the surrounding BL and uterine activity. A comprehensive evaluation of the maternal-fetal interaction facilitates effective and efficient treatment and fetal well-being.

Accelerations

An **acceleration**, also called an *accel*, is described as a visually apparent abrupt increase in the BL FHR, with an onset-to-peak of less than 30 seconds beginning at the most recent calculated BL. To be called an acceleration, the peak must be 15 beats/min or more and the acceleration must last 15 seconds or more from the onset to the return to BL. The duration of the acceleration is defined as the time from the initial change in FHR from the BL to the return of the FHR to the BL. At gestations of less than 32 weeks, accelerations are defined as having a peak of 10 beats/min or more and a duration of 10 seconds or more. A *prolonged acceleration* is any acceleration that lasts 2 minutes or more but less than 10 minutes in duration. Prolonged accelerations that last more than 10 minutes are defined as a baseline change (Macones et al., 2008).

As discussed earlier in this chapter, accelerations can be either episodic or periodic. *Episodic accelerations* are not associated with contractions and tend to be more peaked and abrupt. They are often associated with fetal movement, stimulation, or an environmental stimulus. Episodic accelerations are reassuring FHR patterns, whether or not they are accompanied by fetal movement. *Periodic accelerations* are associated with uterine contractions. When they occur on a repetitive basis, they may be smooth in configuration, multiphasic, and may precede variable decelerations (Cunningham et al., 2010). Various types of accelerations are displayed in Figure 23-15 ■.

Accelerations are generally associated with the stimulation of the autonomic nervous system (ANS), specifically the (SNS), which increases the FHR. If the heart rate increases with CNS stimulation, it usually indicates an intact fetal nervous system and fetal well-being. FHR accelerations can be associated with fetal movement, vaginal exams, application of a fetal scalp electrode, occiput posterior presentation and uterine contractions, fundal pressure, abdominal palpation, vibroacoustic stimulation (VAS), scalp stimulation, and other environmental stimuli (Tucker et al., 2008). Infants of extreme prematurity are less likely to accelerate because of their immature PNS. In fetuses of less than 32 gestational weeks, an acceleration of at least 10 beats/min for 10 seconds is reassuring (Cunningham et al., 2010). Fetuses suffering from intrauterine growth restriction (IUGR) experience fewer accelerations than normal, healthy, well-oxygenated fetuses. Medications administered to the mother may inhibit accelerations because of their effect on the SNS. Some of the drugs seen to affect fetuses are beta blockers and CNS depressants. Hypoxia is also a large con-

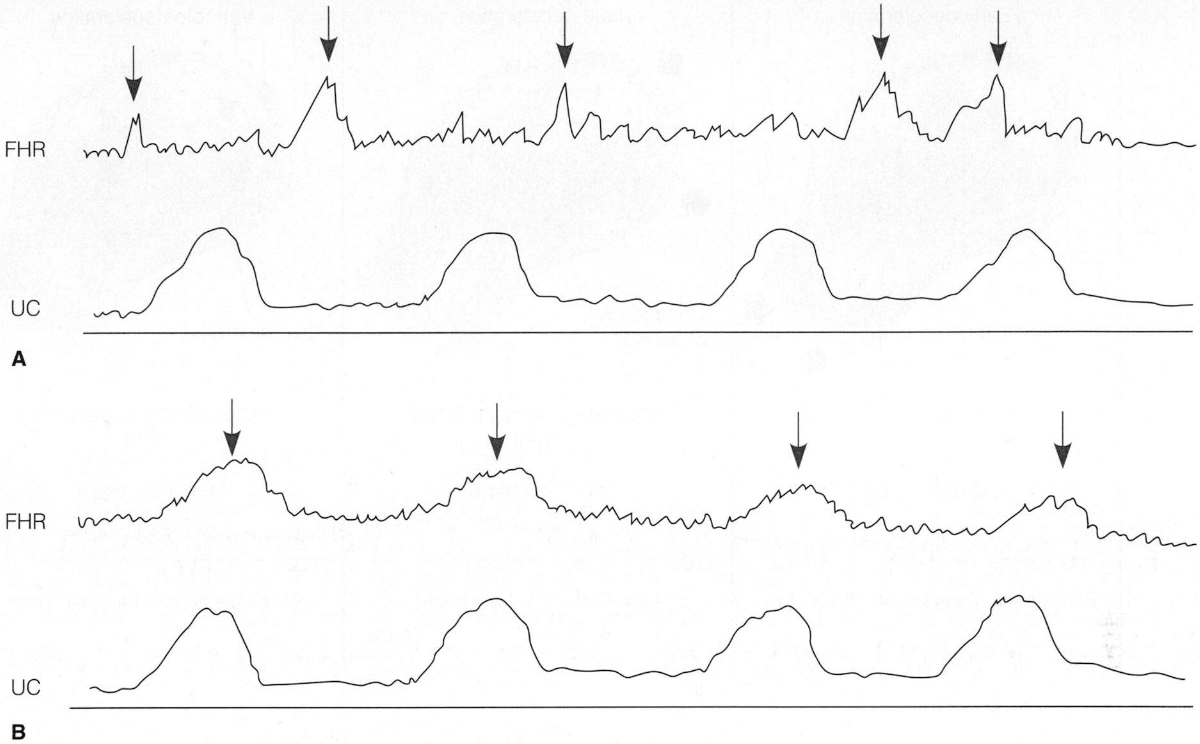

Figure 23-15 ■ Types of accelerations. A. Episodic accelerations. B. Periodic accelerations.

tributing factor to lack of accelerations and may be the first sign of a nonreassuring FHR tracing (Cunningham et al., 2010).

Accelerations are generally benign because they are associated with an intact fetal nervous system, lack of fetal hypoxia, and acidosis. The patterns are considered reassuring, thus no intervention is required (Cunningham et al., 2010; Tucker et al., 2008).

Decelerations

Decelerations, often referred to as *decels,* are generally defined as decreases in the FHR below the BL. Each deceleration has its own unique characteristics, etiology, and significance. Each deceleration consists of several components:

- *Onset:* point at which the deceleration leaves the BL FHR
- *Descent:* time from onset to nadir
- *Nadir:* lowest point of the deceleration
- *Depth:* the level (in beats per minute) a deceleration reaches its nadir
- *Recovery:* time from nadir to return to BL
- *Duration:* the total length of time from onset to return to BL

Decelerations are identified and classified as late, early, or variable based on specific characteristics of their shape, appearance, rate of descent, and timing in relationship to uterine contractions (Figure 23-16 ■). Variable decelerations may be accompanied by other characteristics, the clinical significance of which requires further research investigation. Macones et al. (2008) provide some examples of these characteristics including a slow return of the FHR after the end of the contraction, biphasic decelerations, tachycardia after variable deceleration(s), accelerations preceding and/or following a deceleration (sometimes called "shoulders" or "overshoots"), and fluctuations in the FHR in the trough of the deceleration. See Figure 23-17 ■.

Macones et al. (2008) describe characteristics of decelerations according to the 2008 NICHD Workshop Report on Electronic Fetal Monitoring: Update on Definitions, Interpretation, and Research Guidelines as follows:

Early Deceleration

- Visually apparent, usually symmetrical, gradual decrease and return of the FHR associated with a uterine contraction.
- A gradual FHR decrease is defined as one from the onset to the FHR nadir of 30 seconds or more.
- The decrease in FHR is calculated from the onset to the nadir of the deceleration.
- The nadir of the deceleration occurs at the same time as the peak of the contraction.
- In most cases the onset, nadir, and recovery of the deceleration are coincident with the beginning, peak, and ending of the contraction, respectively.

Late Deceleration

- Visually apparent, usually symmetrical, a gradual decrease and return of the FHR to BL, associated with a uterine contraction.
- A gradual FHR decrease is defined as from the onset to the FHR nadir of 30 seconds or more.
- The decrease in FHR is calculated from the onset to the nadir of the deceleration.
- The deceleration is delayed in timing, with the nadir of the deceleration occurring after the peak of the contraction.
- In most cases, the onset, nadir, and recovery of the deceleration occurs after the beginning, peak, and ending of the contraction, respectively.

Care Plan Activity: Patient with Decelerations

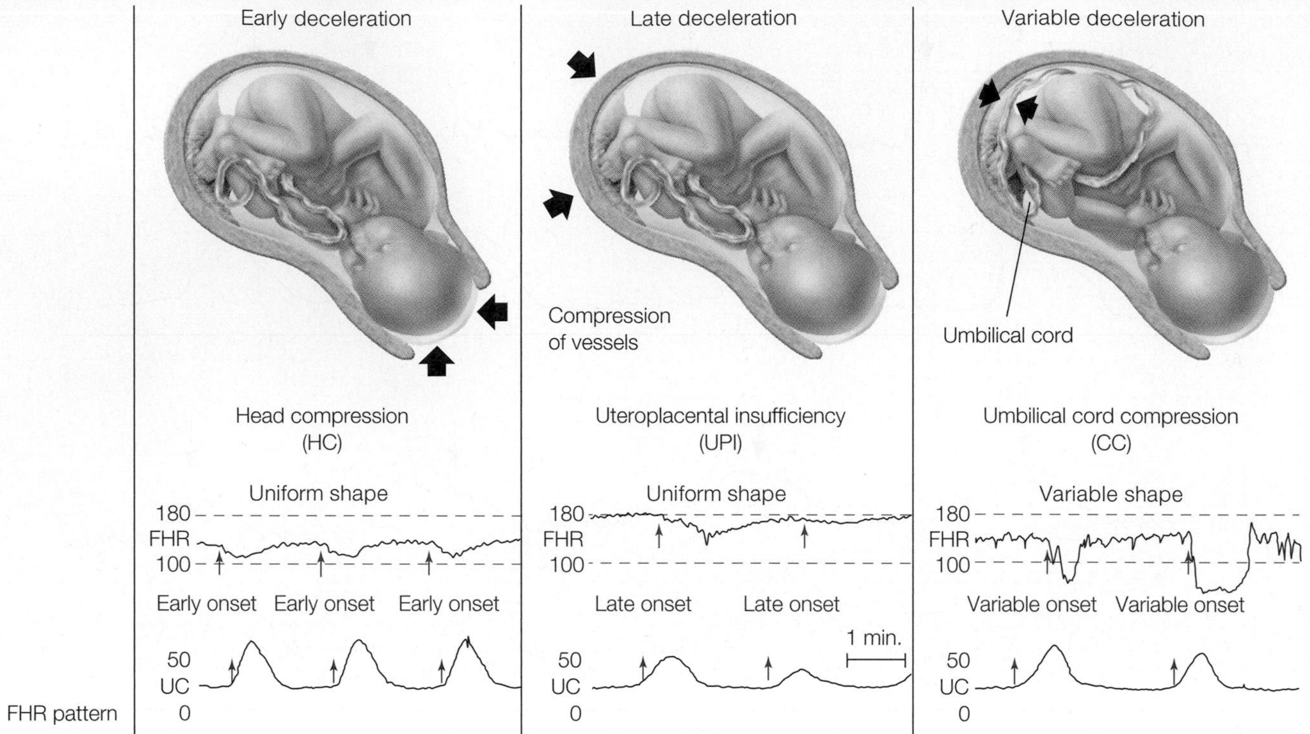

	Early deceleration	Late deceleration	Variable deceleration
Shape	Waveform consistently uniform; inversely mirrors contraction	Waveform uniform; shape reflects contraction	Waveform variable; generally sharp drops and returns
Onset	Just prior to or early in contraction	Late in contraction	Abrupt with fetal insult; not related to contraction
Lowest level	Consistently at or before midpoint of contraction	Consistently after the midpoint of the contraction	Variable around midpoint
Range	Usually within normal range of 120–160 beats/min	Usually within normal range of 120–130 beats/min	Not usually within normal range
Ensemble	Can be single or repetitive	Occasional, consistent, gradual increase—repetitive	Variable—single or repetitive

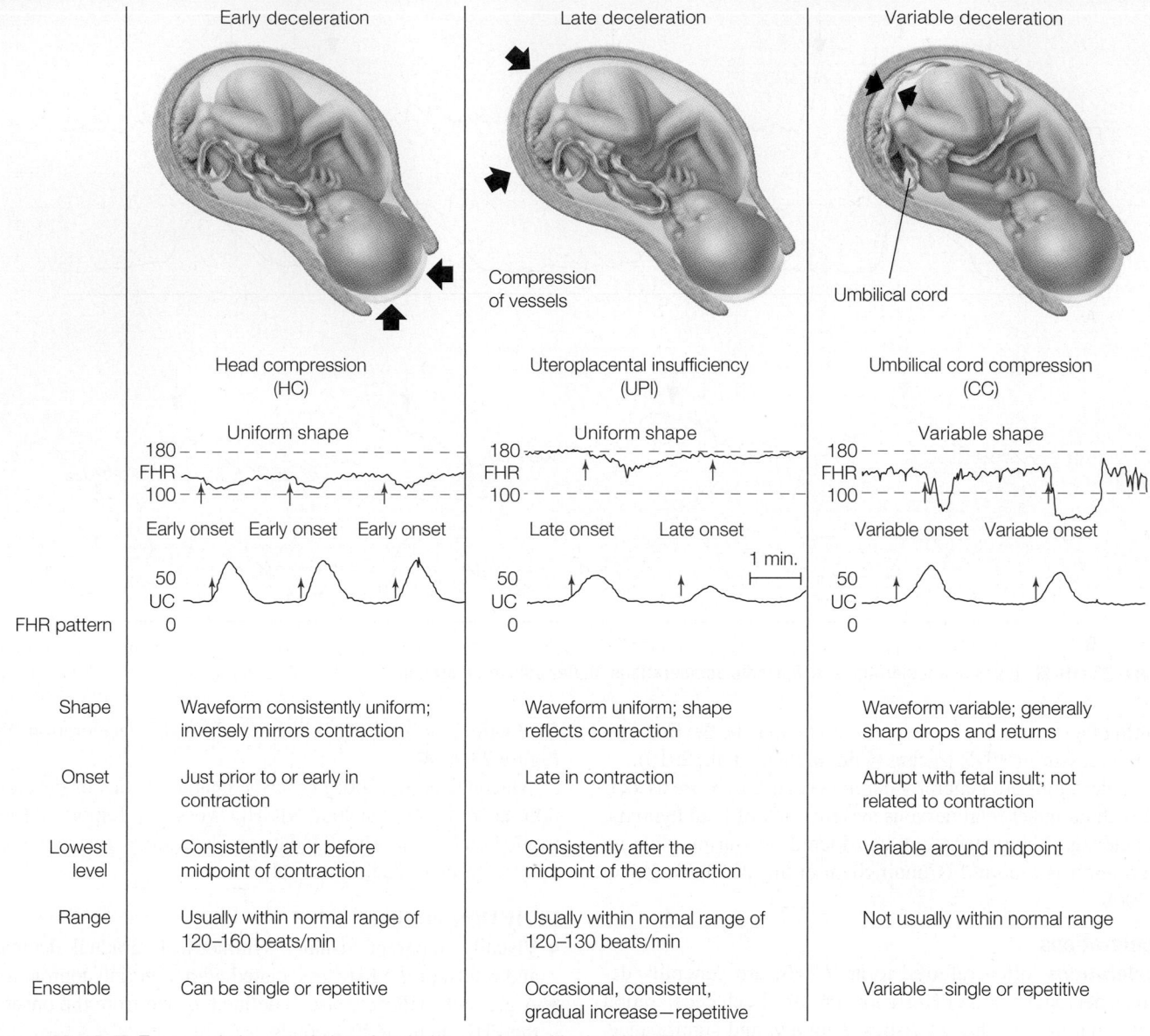

Figure 23-16 ■ Types and characteristics of early, late, and variable decelerations.

Source: Hon, E. (1976). An introduction to fetal heart rate monitoring *(2nd ed., p. 29). Los Angeles: University of Southern California School of Medicine.*

Variable Deceleration

- Visually apparent abrupt decrease in FHR.

An abrupt FHR decrease is defined as from the onset of the deceleration to the beginning of the FHR nadir of 30 seconds or less. The decrease in FHR is calculated from the onset to the nadir of the deceleration.

- The decrease in FHR is 15 beats/min or more, lasting 15 seconds or more but less than 2 minutes in duration.
- When variable decelerations are associated with uterine contractions, their onset, depth, and duration commonly vary with successive uterine contractions.

Early decelerations are a result of vagal nerve stimulation caused by fetal head compression that occurs during UCs (Figure 23-18 ■). They are usually uniform in shape and mirror the shape of the UC. The depth of the deceleration is rarely more than 30 to 40 beats/min (Cunningham et al., 2010) (Figure 23-19 ■). Early decels are not associated with loss of variability, tachycardia, or other FHR changes that are associated with fetal hypoxia, acidosis, or low Apgar scores. They are viewed as reassuring unless they are seen with the lack of descent of the fetal head into the pelvis (Cunningham et al., 2010).

Late decelerations, often referred to as *lates* or *late decels,* are due to uteroplacental insufficiency and are a result of decreased blood flow and/or oxygen transfer to the fetus through the intervillous space during contractions. Late decels may be one of two types: reflexive or myocardial. The pathophysiology of late decels is complicated and is not always understood (Cunningham et al., 2010).

When uteroplacental reserve is adequate, the fetus normally tolerates the transient stress of repetitive contractions. If a decrease in uteroplacental blood flow (for example, from maternal hypotension or excessive uterine activity) lowers the

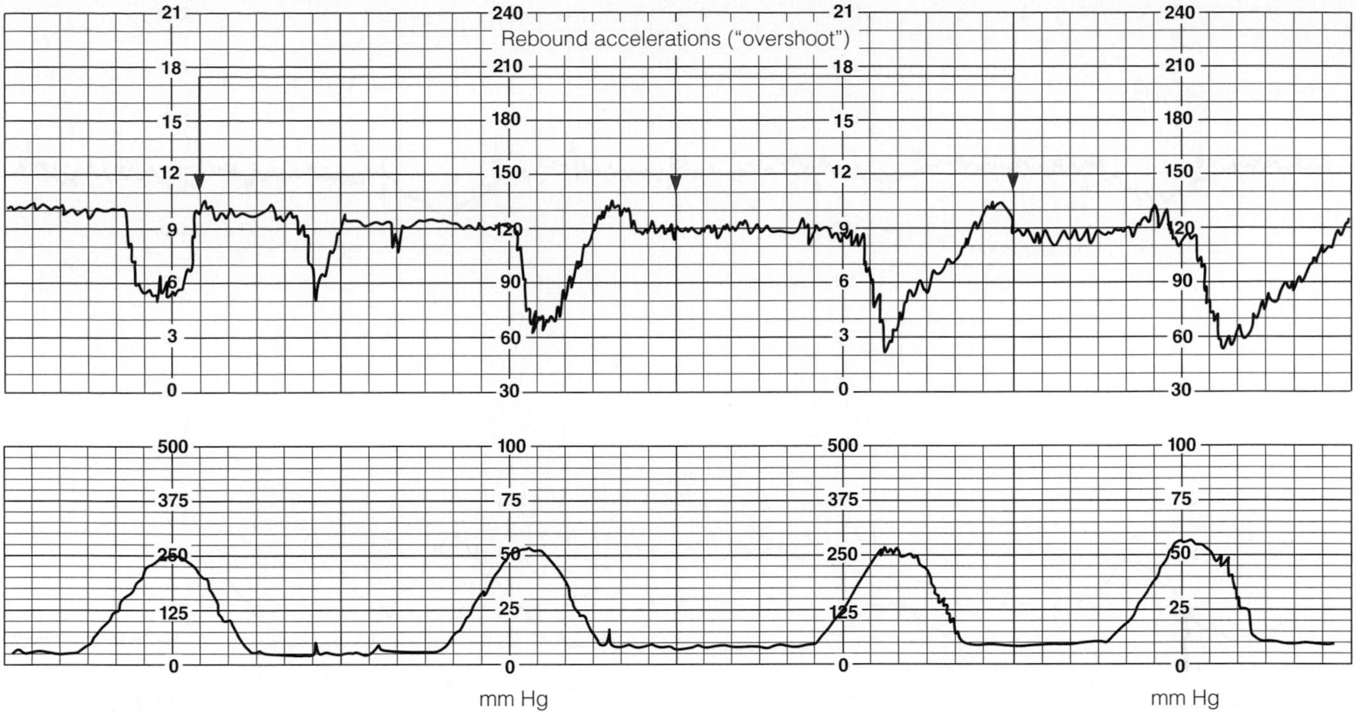

Figure 23-17 ■ Variable decelerations with overshoot. The timing of the decelerations is variable, and most have a sharp decline. A rebound acceleration (overshoot) occurs after most of the decelerations. Baseline FHR is 115 to 130 beats/min. Nadir of decelerations is 55 to 80 beats/min. Variability is minimal.

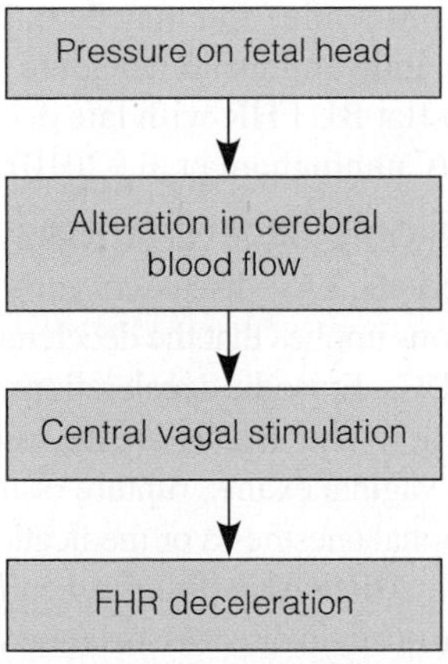

Figure 23-18 ■ Mechanism of early deceleration (head compression).

Source: Adapted with permission from Freeman, R. K., & Garite, T. J. (1981). The physiologic basis of fetal monitoring. In Fetal heart rate monitoring *(p. 13). Copyright © 1981 Lippincott, Williams & Wilkins.*

oxygen level in the intervillous space to a level lower than the oxygen level in the fetus, fetal chemoreceptors are stimulated and FHR decreases. This response to the lowered oxygen level is reflexive, because it is a normal physiologic chemical response to low oxygen levels in the blood. The delay in the FHR deceleration is due to the time it takes for the normal physiologic response of the neurologic system to respond to the lowered oxygen environment. This type of late decels is generally considered nonacidemic and is associated with moderate BL VAR. The BL VAR is the key to determining an intact fetal CNS and should always be considered when evaluating late decelerations and the level of intervention required (Cunningham et al., 2010).

In some cases, repetitive or chronic episodes of decreased oxygen in the intervillous space exist and the fetus experiences a chronic state of hypoxia that leads to metabolic acidosis. The fetal CNS is affected by the metabolic acidosis and progresses to myocardial depression. Late decelerations are produced by the myocardial depression (Tucker et al., 2008) (Figure 23-20 ■).

The decrease in heart rate resulting from late decelerations is usually shallow, typically 10 to 20 beats/min; however, it may approach 30 to 40 beats/min below the BL (Cunningham et al., 2010) (Figure 23-21 ■). The depth of the late deceleration is usually proportional to the strength of the UC; late decelerations are considered a nonreassuring sign. When they are repetitive and uncorrectable and associated with minimal or absent BL VAR and/or BL rate changes, they indicate fetal hypoxia and acidemia and require prompt attention and intervention. The objective of intervention is to improve fetal oxygenation and uteroplacental perfusion while assessing and eliminating the stressor as reflected by the deceleration (Cunningham et al., 2010). If this is not possible, immediate birth may be indicated.

Sometimes late or variable decelerations are due to the supine position of the laboring woman. In this case, the decrease in uterine blood flow to the fetus may be alleviated by raising the woman's upper trunk or turning her to the side to displace pressure of the gravid uterus on the inferior vena cava. If the woman remains flat on her back, the fetus will continue to have decelerations because of oxygen compromise. Immediate nursing interventions include changing the maternal position and increasing the administration of intravenous fluids. Oxygen should be provided to the mother via face mask if hypoxia is suspected, such as when there is absent or minimal variability. If oxytocin (Pitocin) is being administered, the infusion

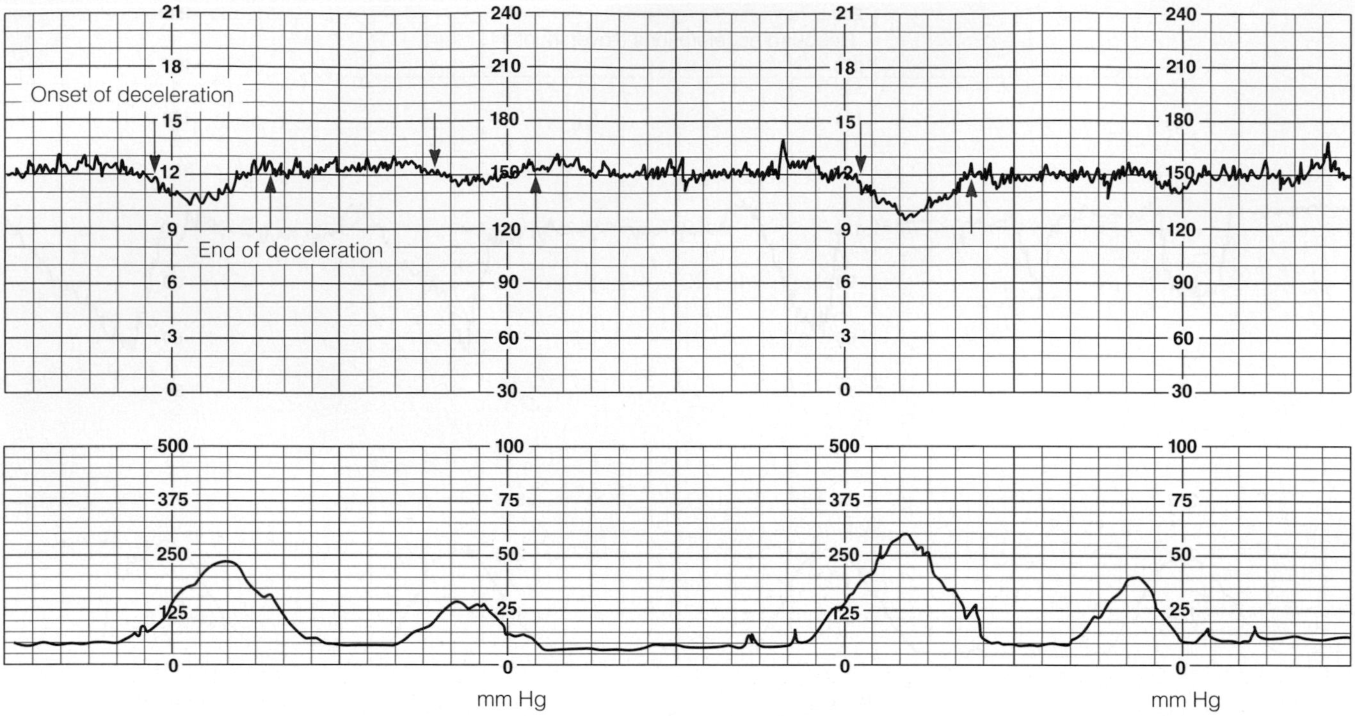

Figure 23-19 ■ Early decelerations. Baseline FHR is 150 to 155 beats/min. Nadir (lowest point) of decelerations is 130 to 145 beats/min.

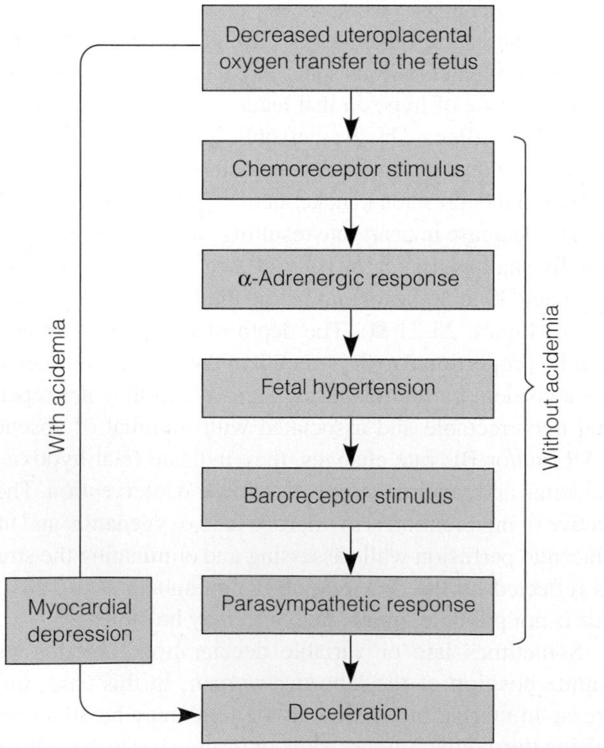

Figure 23-20 ■ Mechanism of late deceleration.

Source: Reprinted with permission from Freeman, R. K., & Garite, T. J. (1981). The physiologic basis of fetal monitoring. In Fetal heart rate monitoring *(p. 15). Copyright © 1981 Lippincott, Williams & Wilkins.*

should be stopped immediately until the FHR recovers or the physician or certified nurse-midwife (CNM) has instructed that the infusion be resumed. The physician or CNM should be notified immediately in the event that late decelerations occur.

Late decelerations normally occur within the normal heart range (110 to 160 beats/min) and may be quite obvious or very subtle and almost indistinguishable. Some fetuses at highest risk demonstrate a flat BL FHR with late decelerations that are barely noticeable (Cunningham et al., 2010).

EPISODIC OR PERIODIC DECELERATIONS Decelerations can be episodic or periodic. As discussed earlier in this chapter, episodic decelerations implies that the deceleration occurred without relationship to UCs. Episodic decelerations may occur without or between contractions and usually are the result of environmental stimuli, such as vaginal exams, rupture of membranes, the administration of regional anesthesia or medications, or other events (Cunningham et al., 2010). Also discussed earlier, periodic refers to decelerations that occur in direct association with UCs. Episodic or periodic decelerations are considered *repetitive* if they occur with 50% or more of UCs (Tucker et al., 2008).

EARLY OR LATE DECELERATIONS Periodic decelerations associated with UCs are also classified by their timing in respect to them. The etiology and clinical significance of each type of deceleration are unique. Clinical interventions and treatments are based on the systematic assessment of the FHR tracing and the overall evaluation of the mother, the fetus, and labor status. Deceleration characteristics and the discussion of their clinical significance and interventions are included in the following sections.

PROLONGED DECELERATIONS A **prolonged deceleration** is a visually apparent decrease in the FHR of 15 beats/min or more below the BL that lasts more than 2 minutes and less than 10 minutes from onset to return to BL (Figure 23-22 ■).

VARIABLE DECELERATIONS **Variable decelerations** are those that have a U or V shape and are typically associated with

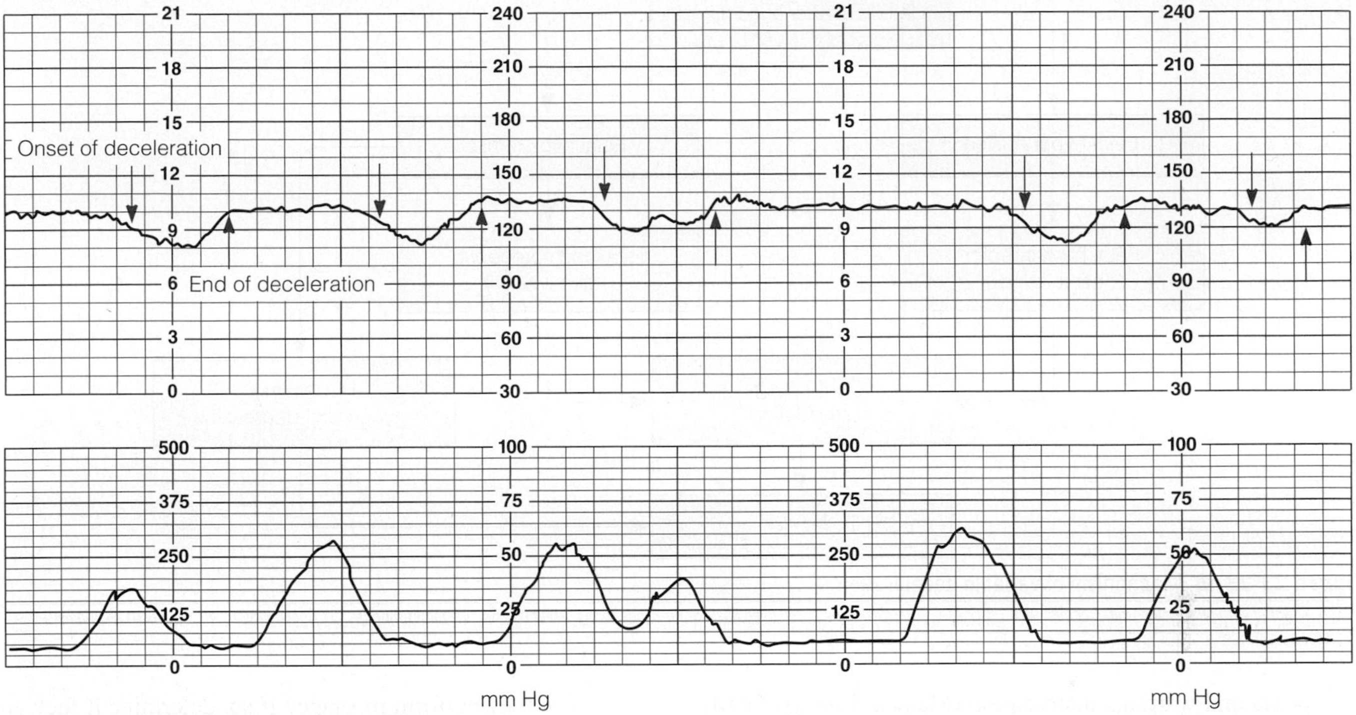

Figure 23-21 ■ Late decelerations. Baseline FHR is 130 to 148 beats/min. Nadir (lowest point) of decelerations is 110 to 120 beats/min. Absent variability.

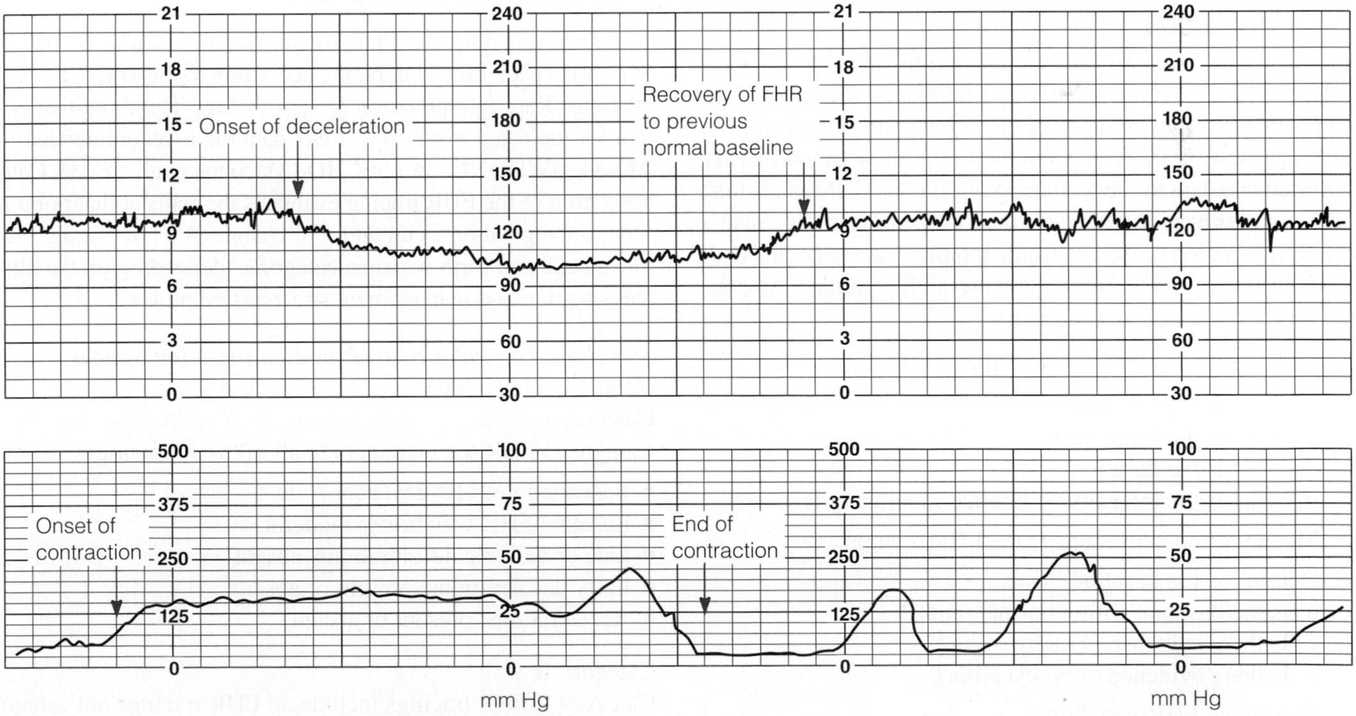

Figure 23-22 ■ The prolonged deceleration depicted lasts approximately 160 seconds.

Note: the prolonged contraction of 120 seconds. The deceleration begins after 80 seconds of uterine contraction. Note the beginning return of FHR 30 seconds after uterine tone returns to normal resting tone (contraction ends). Minimal variability is present despite the deceleration.

cord compression. They may vary somewhat in shape but have an abrupt onset and return to normal abruptly as well. They vary in intensity and duration and usually correlate to uterine contractions. They are thought to result from vagus nerve firing resulting from umbilical cord compression that occurs. They are usually not concerning unless the deceleration is less than 70 beats/min and lasts more than 60 seconds. In addition, if the variable is slow to return to baseline, it could be an indication

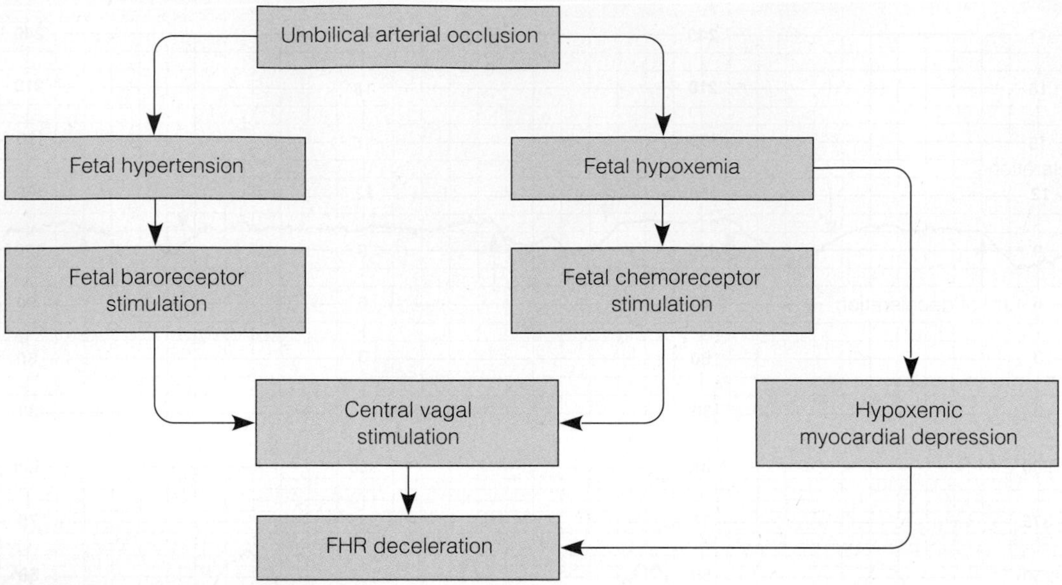

Figure 23-23 ■ Mechanism of variable deceleration.

Source: Adapted with permission from Freeman, R. K., & Garite, T. J. (1981). The physiologic basis of fetal monitoring. In Fetal heart rate monitoring *(p. 13). Copyright © 1981 Lippincott, Williams & Wilkins.*

of hypoxia and warrants intervention (Medical Library, 2010) (Figures 23-23 ■ and 23-24 ■).

Interpretation of Fetal Heart Rate Patterns

The effective nurse uses a systematic approach in evaluating FHR tracings to avoid interpreting findings on the basis of inadequate or erroneous data. With a systematic approach, the nurse can make a more accurate and rapid assessment; easily communicate data to the woman, physician or CNM, and staff; and have a universal language for documenting the woman's record. Evaluation of the electronic monitor tracing begins with a look at the uterine contraction pattern. To evaluate the contraction pattern, the nurse should:

1. Determine the uterine resting tone.
2. Assess the contractions:
   a. What is the frequency?
   b. What is the duration?
   c. What is the intensity (if internal monitoring)?

   The next step is to evaluate the FHR tracing.

1. Determine the baseline:
   a. Is the baseline within normal range?
   b. Is there evidence of tachycardia?
   c. Is there evidence of bradycardia?
2. Determine FHR variability:
   a. Is variability absent, minimal, or moderate? Is variability minimal or marked?
3. Determine whether a sinusoidal pattern is present.
4. Determine whether there are periodic changes.
   a. Are accelerations present?
   b. Is there a reassuring tracing or FHR pattern?
   c. Are decelerations present?
   d. Are they uniform in shape? If so, determine if they are early or late decelerations.
   e. Are they nonuniform in shape? If so, determine if they are variable decelerations.

After evaluating the FHR tracing for the factors listed, the nurse may categorize the tracing according to the Three-Tier Fetal Heart Rate Interpretation System below. The three-tier system for the categorization of FHR patterns is recommended by ACOG, AWHONN, and NICHD (Macones et al., 2008). Categorization of the FHR tracing evaluates the fetus at that point in time; tracing patterns can and will change. A FHR tracing may move back and forth between categories depending on the clinical situation and management strategies employed.

The Three-Tier Fetal Heart Rate Interpretation System (Macones et al., 2008).

Category I

Category I FHR tracings include <u>all</u> of the following:

- Baseline rate: 110–160 beats/min
- Baseline FHR variability: moderate
- Late or variable decelerations: absent
- Early decelerations: present or absent
- Accelerations: present or absent

Category II

Category II FHR tracings include all FHR tracings not categorized as Category I or Category III. Category II tracings may represent an appreciable fraction of those encountered in clinical care. Examples of Category II FHR tracings include any of the following:

- Baseline rate
  - Bradycardia not accompanied by absent baseline variability
  - Tachycardia

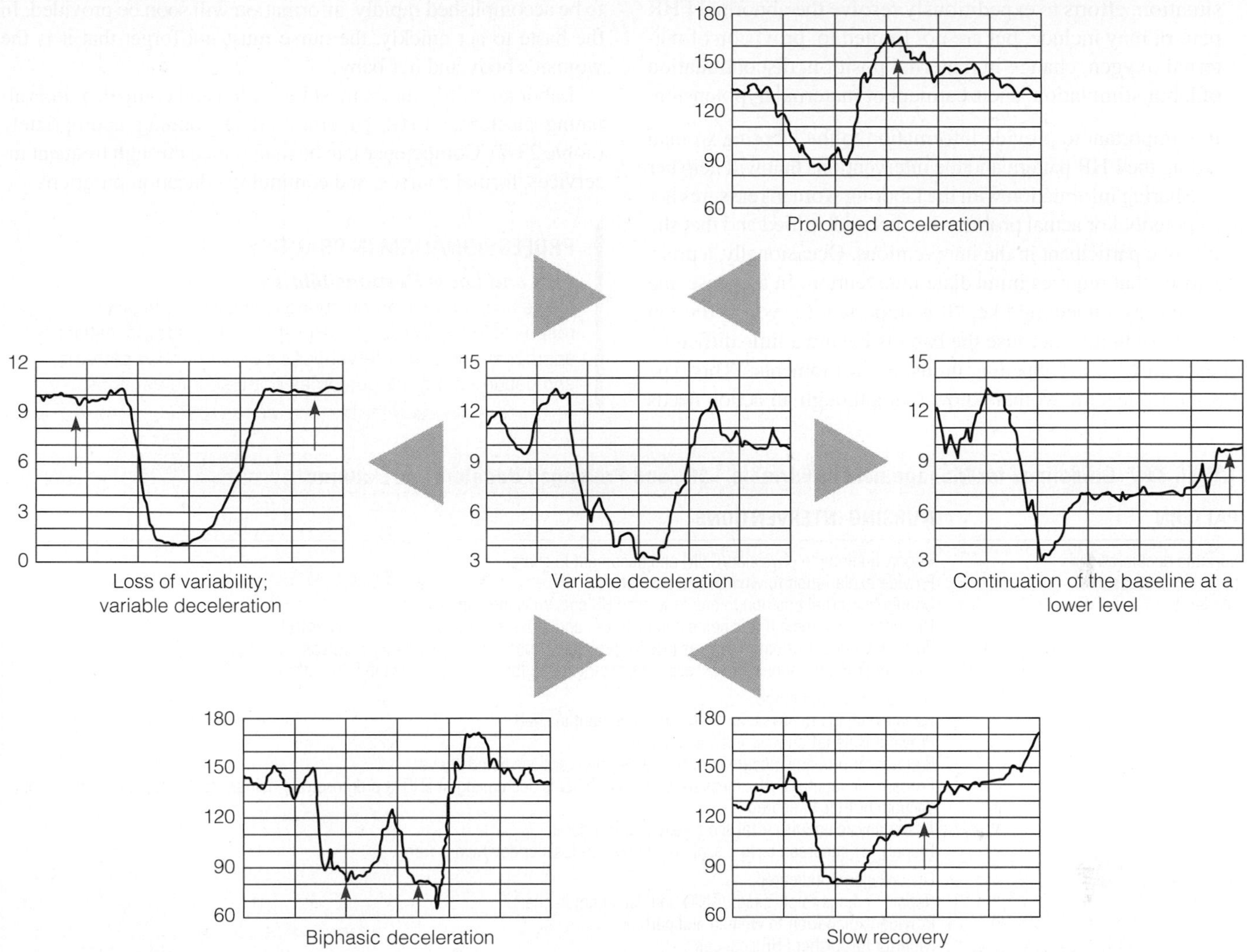

Figure 23-24 ■ Atypical variable decelerations. The presence of any of these types of variable decelerations strongly suggests fetal hypoxia, especially when variability is decreased.

Source: Reprinted with permission from Krebs, H. B., Petrie, R. E., & Dunn, L. J. (1983). Atypical variable decelerations. American Journal of Obstetrics & Gynecology, 145*(3), 298. Copyright © Elsevier, 1983.*

- Baseline FHR variability
  - Minimal baseline variability
  - Absent baseline variability not accompanied by recurrent decelerations
  - Marked baseline variability
- Accelerations
  - Absence of induced accelerations after fetal stimulation
- Periodic or episodic decelerations
  - Recurrent variable decelerations accompanied by minimal or moderate baseline variability
  - Prolonged deceleration of 2 minutes or more but less than 10 minutes
  - Recurrent late decelerations with moderate baseline variability
  - Variable decelerations with other characteristics, such as slow return to baseline, "overshoots," or "shoulders"

Category III

Category III FHR tracings include either:

- Absent baseline FHR variability and any of the following:
  - Recurrent late decelerations
  - Recurrent variable decelerations
  - Bradycardia
- Sinusoidal pattern

Category I FHR tracings are normal. They are strongly predictive of normal fetal acid–base status at the time of observation. The FHR tracings may be followed in a routine manner, and no specific action is required.

Category II FHR tracings are indeterminate. They are not predictive of abnormal fetal acid–base status, yet we do not have adequate evidence at present to classify these as Category I or Category III. Category II tracings require evaluation and continued surveillance and reevaluation, taking into account the entire associated clinical circumstances.

Category III FHR tracings are abnormal. They are predictive of abnormal fetal acid–base status at the time of observation. They require prompt evaluation. Depending on the clinical situation, efforts to expeditiously resolve the abnormal FHR pattern may include, but are not limited to, provision of maternal oxygen, change in maternal position, discontinuation of labor stimulation, and treatment of maternal hypotension.

It is important to provide information to the laboring woman regarding the FHR pattern and the interventions that will help her fetus. Sharing information with the laboring woman reassures her that a potential or actual problem has been identified and that she is an active participant in the interventions. Occasionally, a problem arises that requires immediate intervention. In that case, the nurse can say something like, "It is important for you to turn on your side right now because the baby is having a little difficulty. I'll explain what is happening in just a few moments." This type of response lets the woman know that although an action needs to be accomplished rapidly, information will soon be provided. In the haste to act quickly, the nurse must not forget that it is the woman's body and her baby.

Labor and birth nurses must be skilled and competent in evaluating electronic FHR patterns and responding appropriately (Table 23-7). Competence can be maintained through frequent inservices, formal courses, and continuing education programs.

PROFESSIONALISM IN PRACTICE

FHR and Legal Responsibilities

Nurses caring for women during childbirth are legally responsible for correctly interpreting FHR patterns, initiating appropriate nursing interventions based on those patterns, and documenting the outcomes of those interventions.

TABLE 23-7 Guidelines for Management of Variable, Late, and Prolonged Deceleration Patterns

PATTERN	NURSING INTERVENTIONS
Variable decelerations Isolated or occasional Moderate	Report findings to physician/CNM and document in chart. Provide explanation to woman and partner. Change maternal position to one in which FHR pattern is most improved. Discontinue oxytocin if it is being administered and other interventions are unsuccessful. Perform vaginal examination to assess for prolapsed cord or change in labor progress. Monitor FHR continuously to assess current status and for further changes in FHR pattern.
Variable decelerations Severe and uncorrectable	Give oxygen if indicated. Report findings to physician/CNM and document in chart. Provide explanation to woman and partner. Prepare for probable cesarean birth. Follow interventions listed above. Prepare for vaginal birth unless baseline variability is decreasing or FHR is progressively rising—then cesarean, forceps, or vacuum birth is indicated. Assist physician with fetal scalp sampling if ordered. Prepare for cesarean birth if scalp pH shows acidosis or downward trend.
Late decelerations	Give oxygen if indicated. Report findings to physician/CNM and document in chart. Provide explanation to woman and partner. Monitor for further FHR changes. Maintain maternal position on left side. Maintain good hydration with intravenous (IV) fluids (normal saline or lactated Ringer's). Discontinue oxytocin if it is being administered and late decelerations persist despite other interventions. Administer oxygen by face mask at 7–10 L/min. Monitor maternal blood pressure and pulse for signs of hypotension; possibly increase flow rate of IV fluids to treat hypotension. Follow physician's orders for treatment for hypotension if present. Increase IV fluids to maintain volume and hydration (normal saline or lactated Ringer's). Assess labor progress (dilatation and station). Assist physician with fetal blood sampling: If pH stays above 7.25, physician will continue monitoring and resample; if pH shows downward trend (between 7.25 and 7.20) or is below 7.20, prepare for birth by most expeditious means.
Late decelerations with tachycardia or variability decreasing	Report findings to physician/CNM and document in chart. Maintain maternal position on left side. Administer oxygen by face mask at 7–10 L/min. Discontinue oxytocin if it is being administered. Assess maternal blood pressure and pulse. Increase IV fluids (normal saline or lactated Ringer's). Assess labor progress (dilatation and station). Prepare for immediate cesarean birth. Explain plan of treatment to woman and partner. Assist physician with fetal blood sampling (if ordered).
Prolonged decelerations	Perform vaginal examination to rule out prolapsed cord or to determine progress in labor status. Change maternal position as needed to try to alleviate decelerations. Discontinue oxytocin if it is being administered. Notify physician/CNM of findings/initial interventions and document in chart. Provide explanation to woman and partner. Increase IV fluids (normal saline or lactated Ringer's). Administer tocolytic if hypertonus noted and ordered by physician/CNM. Anticipate normal FHR recovery following deceleration if FHR previously normal. Anticipate intervention if FHR previously abnormal or deceleration lasts greater than 3 minutes.

Indirect Methods of Fetal Assessment

When there is a question regarding fetal status, indirect methods such as **scalp stimulation** (pressing on the fetal scalp with the examining fingers during a vaginal exam to elicit an acceleration of fetal heart rate [FHR]), *acoustic stimulation* (using a sound device placed against the maternal abdomen to elicit an acceleration in FHR), or stimulation by maternal abdominal palpation (patting or shaking the abdomen) can be used to assess the fetus. Ongoing scalp stimulation is not recommended and should not be used by nurses (Tucker, Miller, & Miller, 2008). When one of the indirect methods is used, the fetus who is not in any stress responds with an acceleration of the FHR, described as a reactive response (acceleration of 15 beats per minute (beats/min) amplitude with a duration of 15 seconds). Whereas reactivity is associated with fetal well-being, the absence of acceleration does not diagnose acidemia or predict fetal compromise (Tucker et al., 2008). Further observation and assessment measures are indicated.

Cord Blood Analysis at Birth

In cases in which significant abnormal FHR patterns have been noted before birth, amniotic fluid is meconium stained, or the infant is depressed at birth, umbilical cord blood may be analyzed immediately after birth to assess the infant's respiratory status. The cord is usually clamped before the infant takes his or her first breath to provide an evaluation of blood gas status before the infant interacts with the extrauterine environment, because values can change after only a few seconds of neonatal breathing.

An 8- to 10-inch segment of the umbilical cord is double-clamped and cut, and a small amount of blood is aspirated from one of the umbilical arteries (arterial blood seems to provide the most reliable indication of blood gas status and fetal tissue pH). Blood is collected in a heparinized syringe unless it is to be analyzed immediately; it should not be allowed to remain in the segment of cord longer than 30 minutes. Some clinicians may collect a segment of cord and send blood samples only if the Apgar score is below 7 at 5 minutes, as recommended by AAP and ACOG (2007). In this instance, values might be used to clarify the cause of a low Apgar score while minimizing any medical-legal exposure and expense. Determination of pH and base deficit values can differentiate whether fetal acidemia is due to hypoperfusion of the placenta or to cord compression.

FOCUS YOUR STUDY

- Intrapartum assessment includes attention to both physical and psychosociocultural parameters of the laboring woman, assessment of the fetus, and ongoing assessment for conditions that place the woman and her fetus at an increased risk.
- Birthing room nurses have responsibilities for recognizing and interrupting fetal monitoring patterns, notifying the physician or certified nurse-midwife (CNM) of problems, and initiating corrective and supportive measures when needed.
- Uterine contractions (UCs) may be assessed externally through palpation or by an electronic monitor. An intrauterine pressure catheter can be placed internally to measure uterine activity more accurately.
- A vaginal examination determines the status of cervical dilatation, effacement, and fetal presentation, position, and station.
- Fetal presentation can also be assessed by inspection, vaginal examination, or ultrasound (US).
- Leopold's maneuvers provide a systematic evaluation of fetal presentation and position.
- Indications for electronic fetal monitoring (EFM) include fetal, maternal, and uterine factors; presence of pregnancy complications; regional anesthesia; and elective monitoring.
- The fetal heart rate (FHR) may be assessed by auscultation or electronic fetal monitoring.
- Electronic fetal monitoring (EFM) is accomplished by indirect ultrasound or by direct methods that require the placement of a spiral electrode on the fetal presenting part.
- Variability refers to baseline (BL) fluctuations of 2 cycles per minute or greater in the FHR and it is classified by the

visually quantified amplitude of peak-to-trough in beats per minute.

- The normal range of FHR is 110 to 160 beats per minute.
- Baseline changes in the FHR include tachycardia, bradycardia, and variability.
- Tachycardia is defined as a rate of 160 beats per minute or more for at least a 10-minute segment of time.
- Bradycardia is defined as a rate of 110 beats per minute or less for at least a 10-minute segment of time.
- Baseline variability is an important parameter of fetal well-being.
- Periodic changes in the FHR from baseline include decelerations and accelerations. Accelerations are normally caused by fetal movement.
- Decelerations are categorized as early, late, or variable according to NICHD categories.
- Early decelerations are due to compression of the fetal head during contractions and are generally considered benign when they occur with ongoing fetal descent. They typically do not require intervention.
- Late decelerations are associated with uteroplacental insufficiency.
- Variable decelerations are associated with compression of the umbilical cord.
- Sinusoidal patterns are characterized by an undulant sine wave.

CRITICAL THINKING IN ACTION

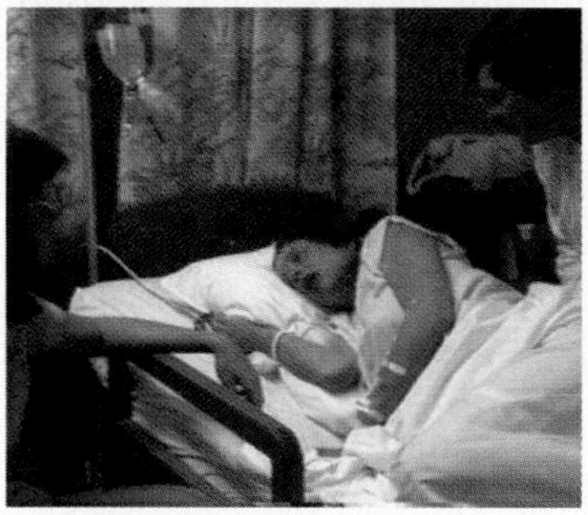
Source: George Dodson/Pearson Education.

Cindy Bell, a 20-year-old gravida 2, para 1 at 40 weeks' gestation, presents to you in the birthing unit with contractions every 5 to 7 minutes. She is accompanied by her husband. Spontaneous rupture of membranes occurred 2 hours prior to admission. Cindy tells you that the fluid was colorless and clear. You orient Cindy and her family to the birthing room and perform a physical assessment, documenting the following data: vital signs are normal. A vaginal exam demonstrates the cervix is 75% effaced, 4 cm dilated with a vertex at –1 station in the LOP position. You place Cindy on an external fetal monitor. The fetal heart rate baseline is 140–147 with accelerations to 156; no decelerations are noted. Contractions are 5–6 minutes apart, moderate intensity and lasting 40–50 seconds. Cindy states she would like to stay out of bed as long as possible because lying down seems to make the contractions more painful, especially in her back.

1. Discuss the benefits of ambulation in labor.
2. Cindy would like her daughter to be present for the baby's birth. What would you discuss with her about the impact of having a young sibling present during labor and birth?
3. What fetal heart rate assessment will best ensure fetal well-being during the period Cindy is ambulating?
4. When a nonreassuring fetal heart pattern is detected, what remedial nursing intervention is carried out?
5. What are indications for continuous fetal monitoring in labor?

See www.nursing.pearsonhighered.com for possible responses.

Pearson Nursing Student Resources

Find additional review materials at
www.nursing.pearsonhighered.com

Prepare for success with additional NCLEX®-style practice questions, interactive assignments and activities, Web links, animations and videos, and more!

REFERENCES

American Academy of Pediatrics (AAP) & American College of Obstetricians and Gynecologists (ACOG). (2007). *Guidelines for perinatal care* (6th ed.). Washington, DC: Author.

American College of Obstetricians and Gynecologists (ACOG). (2005). Intrapartum fetal heart rate monitoring. ACOG Practice Bulletin No. 70. Washington, DC: Author.

American College of Obstetricians and Gynecologists (ACOG). (2008). Use of psychiatric medications during pregnancy and lactation. ACOG Practice Bulletin No. 92. Washington, DC: Author.

Association of Women's Health, Obstetric, and Neonatal Nurses (AWHONN). (2005). *Foundations of fetal heart monitoring: An introduction to the AWHONN fetal heart monitoring principles and practices program.* Baltimore, MD: Lippincott Williams & Wilkins.

Association of Women's Health, Obstetric, and Neonatal Nurses (AWHONN). (2006). In J. Poole (Ed.), *Foundations of fetal heart rate monitoring: An introduction to AWHONN's fetal heart rate monitoring principles and practices program.* Baltimore, MD: Lippincott Williams & Wilkins.

Association of Women's Health, Obstetric, and Neonatal Nurses (AWHONN). (2008a). *Nursing care and management of the second stage of labor* (2nd ed.). Washington, DC: Author.

Association of Women's Health, Obstetric, and Neonatal Nurses (AWHONN). (2008b). *Fetal heart monitoring.* Washington, DC: Author.

Barclay, L. (2009). Fetal heart rate monitoring guidelines updated. Retrieved from http://www.medscape.com/viewarticle/705210

Chan, P. D., & Johnson, S. M. (2008). *Gynecology and obstetrics.* Laguna Hills, CA: Current Clinical Strategies.

Cheng, Y., & Caughley, A. B. (2009). Normal labor and delivery. Retrieved from http://emedicine.medscape.com/article/260036-overview

Cunningham, F. G., Leveno, K. J., Bloom, S. L., Hauth, J. C., Rouse, D. J., & Spong, C. (2010). *Williams obstetrics* (23rd ed.). New York, NY: McGraw-Hill.

Janet, H. A. (2009). How electronic fetal monitoring can prevent cerebral palsy. Retrieved from http://myadvocates.com/practice-areas/cerebral-palsy/how-electronic-fetal-monitoring-can-prevent-cerebral-palsy/

Joint Commission on Accreditation of Healthcare Organizations. (2004, July 21). *Preventing infant death and injury during delivery.* Retrieved from http://www.jointcommission.org/SentinelEvents/SentinelEventAlert/sea_30.htm

Kamysheva, E., Skouteris, H., Wertheim, E. H., Paxton, S. J., & Milgrom, J. (2009) A prospective investigation of the relationships among sleep quality, physical symptoms, and depressive symptoms during pregnancy. *Journal of Affective Disorders, 123*(1–3), 317–320.

Lev-Wiesel, R., Chen, R., Daphna-Tekoah, S., & Hod, M. (2009). Past traumatic events: Are they a risk factor for high-risk pregnancy, delivery complications, and postpartum posttraumatic symptoms? *Journal of Womens Health,* 18(1), 119–125.

Liston, R., Sawchuck, D., & Young, D. (2007). Society of Obstetrics and Gyneacologists of Canada, British Columbia Perinatal Health Program, Fetal health surveillance: Antepartum and intrapartum consensus guidelines. In *Journal of Obstetrics and Gynaecology Canada* 2007; 29–909.

Macones, G. A., Hankins, G. D. V., Spong, C. Y., Hauth, J., & Moore, T. (2008). The 2008 National Institute of Child Health and Human Development workshop report on electronic fetal monitoring: Update on definitions, interpretation, and research guidelines. In *Journal of Obstetrics, Gynecology & Neonatal Nursing (JOGNN), 37*(5), 510–515. doi: 10.1111/j.1552-6909.2008.00284

Medical Library. (2010). Fetal heart rate monitoring. Retrieved from http://www.medical-library.org/journals2a/fetal_heart_monitoring.htm

National Institute of Child Health and Human Development (NICHD). (1997). *NICHD fetal monitoring workshop.* Bethesda, MD: Author.

New York City Department of Health and Mental Hygiene. (2010). Intimate partner violence. Retrieved from http://www.nyc.gov/html/doh/html/epi/domviol.shtml

Parer, J. T., & Ikeda, T. (2007). A framework for standardized management of intrapartum fetal heart rate patterns. *American Journal of Obstetrics and Gynecology, 197,* e1–e6.

Royal College of Obstetricians and Gynaecologists (RCOG). (2008). Intrapartum care: Management and delivery of care to women in labour. Evidence-based NICE guideline. National Collaborating Center for Women's and Children's Health. London, UK: Royal College of Obstetricians and Gynecologists Press. Retrieved from http://www.rcog.org.uk/womens-health/clinical-guidance/use-electronic-fetal-monitoring

Simpson, K. R., & Creehan, P. A. (2007). *AWHONN's perinatal nursing* (3rd ed.). Washington, D.C.: AWHONN.

Spector, R. E. (2009). *Cultural diversity in health and illness* (7th ed.). Upper Saddle River, NJ: Pearson-Prentice Hall.

Tucker, S. M., Miller, L. A., & Miller, A. (2008). *Mosby's pocket guide to fetal monitoring: A multidisciplinary approach.* St. Louis, MO: Mosby.

Wiederman, J. R., Saugstad, A. M., Branes-Powell, L., & Duran, K. (2008). Meconium aspiration syndrome. *Neonatal Network, 27*(2), 81–87.

CHAPTER 24

The Family in Childbirth: Needs and Care

The moment our daughter was born, time seemed to stand still. We couldn't keep our eyes off of her. I remember vividly the first time I touched her tiny finger and stroked her cheek. Those moments together as a family are forever engraved in my memory.

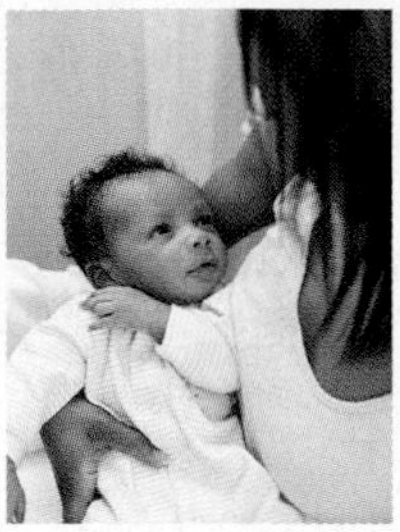

LEARNING OUTCOMES

1. Identify nursing diagnoses specific to the first, second, third, and fourth stages of labor.
2. Describe factors that are assessed in the laboring woman during the admission process.
3. Discuss the components of a social history and its role in caring for the laboring woman.
4. Summarize the importance of incorporating family expectations and cultural beliefs into the nursing care plan.
5. Discuss nursing interventions to meet the care needs of the laboring woman and her partner during each stage of labor.
6. Describe nursing interventions for promoting the woman's comfort during each stage of labor.
7. Summarize immediate nursing care of the newborn following birth.
8. Discuss the components of care for the woman during the third stage of labor.
9. Discuss initial measures to help the woman and family integrate the newborn into family life.
10. Explore the nurse's role in providing sensitive care to adolescent parents.
11. Delineate management of a nurse-managed precipitous birth.

KEY TERMS

Apgar score *620*
Hyperventilation *611*
Precipitous birth *630*

It is time for a child to be born. The waiting is over; labor has begun. The dreams and wishes of the past months fade as the expectant family faces the reality of the tasks of childbearing and childrearing that are ahead.

The couple is about to undergo one of the most meaningful and stressful events in their life together. Physical and psychologic resources, coping mechanisms, and support systems will all be challenged. Despite months of childbirth education classes, the laboring woman may question her ability to cope with labor and to meet her own expectations of herself. The partner may wonder whether he will be able to provide the support his partner and newborn will need. They may worry about the baby's health. Although they look forward to the birth of their baby, they are entering an unfamiliar landscape where, even with prenatal preparation, unknown possibilities await them.

Some childbearing families may worry that they will not be provided with adequate care during labor due to lack of medical insurance or healthcare coverage. In 1986, the Emergency Medical Treatment and Labor Act (EMTLA) was passed by Congress to ensure that patients requiring emergency medical services, including women in labor, had access to medical services regardless of their ability to pay for services (U.S. Department of Health and Human Services, 2010).

Many childbearing families look to the nurse for support and guidance. Indeed, for laboring women who are admitted alone, the nurse may be their sole support. It is essential, therefore, to provide holistic care that addresses the patient's or couple's physiologic, psychologic, and comfort needs throughout the challenging and emotional process of labor and birth.

The previous two chapters present information that lays the foundation for this chapter. Chapter 22 ∞ presents a database of information regarding physiologic and psychologic changes during labor and birth, and chapter 23 ∞ discusses intrapartum assessment. This chapter discusses nursing care during labor and birth. The Clinical Pathway on pages 596–598 summarizes nursing care of the childbearing family in the first through fourth stages of labor and birth.

Nursing Diagnosis During Labor and Birth

In devising a plan of care for the intrapartum period, the nurse can develop a general plan that encompasses the whole process, from the beginning of labor through the fourth stage, or the nurse can develop a plan for each stage of labor and birth. The nurse's plan and actions are based on current findings from nursing and medical research. By providing evidence-based guided care, the nurse ensures that the woman and her family are appropriately cared for during their labor and birth. An overall plan presents an overview of the whole process, but it is usually general in nature. A plan of care that identifies nursing diagnoses for (at least) each stage provides an opportunity to identify more specific nursing interventions.

In the first stage of labor, nursing diagnoses that may apply include the following:

- ***Fear/Anxiety*** related to discomfort of labor and unknown labor outcome
- ***Health-Seeking Behaviors: Health Education Regarding Information About the Fetal Monitor*** related to an expressed desire to understand equipment used
- ***Compromised Family Coping*** related to labor process
- ***Acute Pain*** related to uterine contractions, cervical dilatation, and fetal descent
- ***Deficient Knowledge*** related to lack of information about normal labor process and comfort measures
- ***Fear/Anxiety*** related to unknown birth outcome and anticipated discomfort

Nursing diagnoses for the second and third stages may include the following:

- ***Acute Pain*** related to uterine contractions, birth process, and/or perineal trauma from birth
- ***Deficient Knowledge*** related to lack of information about pushing methods
- ***Ineffective Coping*** related to birth process
- ***Fear/Anxiety*** related to outcome of birth process

In the fourth stage, possible nursing diagnoses include the following:

- ***Acute Pain*** related to perineal trauma
- ***Deficient Knowledge*** related to lack of information about involutional process and self-care needs
- ***Readiness for Enhanced Family Processes*** related to incorporation of the newborn into the family

Nursing Care During Admission

Many families worry that they will not reach the birthing center in time for the birth or that cues indicating the onset of labor will be missed. Sometimes labor occurs so rapidly that birth is imminent upon admission. Usually, the family is advised to arrive at the birth setting at the beginning of the active phase of labor or when the following occur:

- Rupture of membranes (ROM)
- Decreased fetal movement
- Regular, frequent uterine contractions (UCs) (nulliparas, about 5 minutes apart for 1 hour; multiparas, 6 to 8 minutes apart for 1 hour)
- Any vaginal bleeding

If time permits and the family is not familiar with what will occur during labor, the nurse can provide information on admission. (See Patient Teaching: What to Expect During Labor.)

The family may be facing a number of unfamiliar procedures that are routine for healthcare providers. It is important to remember that each woman has the right to determine what happens to her body. Informed consent should be obtained before any procedure that involves touching the body.

Establishing a Positive Relationship

The initial interaction with the nurse and how it is perceived by the woman and her partner greatly influences the course

CLINICAL PATHWAY For Intrapartum Stages

Category	First Stage	Second and Third Stage	Fourth Stage Birth to 1 Hour Past Birth
Referral	Review prenatal record Advise CNM/physician of admission	Labor record for first stage	Report to recovery room nurse ■ ***Expected Outcomes*** Appropriate resources identified and utilized
Assessments	Admission assessments: Ask about problems since last prenatal visit; labor status (contraction frequency and duration), membrane status (intact or ruptured); coping level; support; woman's desires during labor and birth; ability to verbalize needs; laboratory testing (blood and UA) Intrapartal assessments: Cervical assessment: from 1 to 10 cm dilatation; nullipara (1.2 cm/h), multipara (1.5 cm/h) Cervical effacement: from 0% to 100%, multiparas may not fully efface prior to birth. Fetal descent: progressive descent from −4 to +4 Membrane assessment: intact or ruptured; when ruptured, Nitrazine positive, fluid clear, no foul odor Comfort level: woman states is able to cope with contractions Behavioral characteristics: facial expressions, tone of voice, and verbal expressions are consistent with comfort level and ability to cope Latent Phase: • BP, P, R q30min for low-risk women and q15min for high-risk women if in normal range (BP 90–135/60–85 or not greater than 30 mm Hg systolic or 15 mm Hg diastolic over baseline; pulse 60–90; respirations 12–24/min, quiet, easy) • Temp every 4h unless greater than 37.6°C (99.6°F) or membranes ruptured then q1h • Uterine contractions q30min for low-risk women and q15min for high-risk women (contractions q5–10min, 15–40 sec, mild intensity) • FHR q30min (for low-risk women) and q15min (for high-risk women) if reassuring (reassuring FHR has: baseline 110–160, variability present, average, accelerations with fetal movement, no late decelerations); if nonreassuring, position on side, start O_2, assess for hypotension, monitor continuously, discontinue Pitocin if infusing, notify CNM/physician Active Phase: • BP, P, R, q30min if WNL for low-risk women and q15min for high-risk women • Temp as above • Uterine contractions q15–30min: contractions q2–3min, 60 sec, moderate to strong • FHR q30min (for low-risk women) and q15min (for high-risk women) if reassuring; if nonreassuring institute interventions Transition: • BP, P, R, q30min • Uterine contractions q30min for low-risk women and q15min for high-risk women; contractions q2min, 60–75 sec, strong • FHR q30min for low-risk women and every 15 minutes for high-risk women if reassuring; if nonreassuring, see above	Second stage assessments: • BP, P, R q5–15min • Uterine contractions palpated continuously • FHR q15min (for low-risk women) and q5min (for high-risk women) if reassuring; if nonreassuring, monitor continuously Fetal descent: descent continues to birth Comfort level: woman states is able to cope with contractions and pushing Behavioral characteristics: response to pushing, facial expressions, verbalization Third stage assessments: • BP, P, R q5min • Uterine contractions, palpate occasionally until placenta is delivered, fundus maintains tone and contraction pattern continues to birth of placenta Newborn assessments: • Assess Apgar score of newborn • Respirations: 30–60, irregular • Apical pulse: 110–160 and somewhat irregular • Temperature: Skin temp above 36.5°C (97.8°F) • Umbilical cord: two arteries, one vein (if one artery, assess for anomalies and urine output) • Gestational age: 38–42 weeks	Immediate postbirth assessments of mother q15min for 1h: • BP: 90–135/60–85; should return to prelabor level • Pulse: slightly lower than in labor; range is 60–90 • Respirations: 12–24/min; easy; quiet • Temperature: 36.2–37.6°C (98–99.6°F) • Fundus firm, in midline, at the umbilicus • Lochia rubra; moderate amount; less than 2 pad/h; no free flow or passage of clots with massage • Perineum: sutures intact; no bulging or marked swelling; minimal bruising may be present; no c/o severe pain nor rectal pain • Bladder nondistended; spontaneous void of greater than 100 ml clear, straw-colored urine; bladder nondistended following voiding • If hemorrhoids present, no tenseness or marked engorgement; less than 2 cm diameter Comfort level: less than 3 on scale of 1 to 10 Energy level: awake and able to hold newborn Newborn assessments if newborn remains with parents: • Respirations: 30–60; irregular • Apical pulse: 110–160 and somewhat irregular • Temperature: skin temp above 36.5°C (97.8°F); skin feels warm to touch • Skin color noncyanotic • Mucus: small amount, clear, easily suctioned with bulb syringe without skin color change • Behavioral: newborn opens eyes widely if room is slightly darkened • Movements rhythmic; no hand tremors present ■ ***Expected Outcomes*** Findings indicate normal progression with absence of complications

CLINICAL PATHWAY For Intrapartum Stages continued

Category	First Stage	Second and Third Stage	Fourth Stage Birth to 1 Hour Past Birth
Teaching/ psychosocial	Establish rapport Orient to environment, expected assessments, and procedures Answer questions and provide information Orient to EFM if used Teach relaxation, visualization, and breathing pattern if needed Explain comfort measures available Assume advocacy role for woman/family during labor and birth	Orient to expected assessments and procedures Answer questions and provide information Explain comfort measures available Continue advocacy role	Explain immediate assessments and care after this first hour Teach self-massage of fundus and expected findings Instruct to call for assistance if mother desires to get OOB Begin newborn teaching; bulb syringe, positioning; maintaining warmth Assist parents in exploring their newborn Assist with first breastfeeding experience ■ ***Expected Outcomes*** Patient and partner verbalize/demonstrate understanding of teaching
Nursing care management and report	Straight cath prn if bladder distended If regional block administered monitor BP, FHR, sensation per protocol Provide continuing status reports to CNM/physician Perform sterile vaginal examination as indicated	Indwelling catheter or straight cath prn if bladder distended Continue monitoring VS, FHR, and sensation if regional block has been given	Straight cath if bladder distended Monitor return of motor ability and sensation if regional block has been given Weigh perineal pads if lochia flow greater than 1 saturated pad in 15 min, presence of boggy uterus and clots; ↓ BP, ↑ P ■ ***Expected Outcomes*** • Maternal/fetal well-being maintained and supported • Mother and newborn experience safe labor and birth • Family participates in process as desired
Activity	Encourage ambulation unless contraindicated Maintain bed rest immediately after administration of IV pain medication, or following regional block Woman rests comfortably between contractions	Position comfortably for birth Woman rests comfortably between pushing efforts and while awaiting birth of placenta	Position of comfort ■ ***Expected Outcomes*** • Activity maintained as desired unless contraindicated • Comfort enhanced by positioning/ movement
Comfort	Institute comfort measures: ambulation, frequent position change, effleurage, focal point, patterned paced breathing, visualization, therapeutic touch, backrub, moist cloths to face, holding hand, words of encouragement, changing underpad, shower, whirlpool, staying with the woman/family, warmed blanket at back, sacral pressure Offer pain medication or administer if requested Assist with administration of regional block	Institute comfort measures: • Second stage: cool cloth to forehead, encouragement, coaching, help support legs while pushing, position of comfort for pushing and birth • Third stage: cool cloth to forehead, assist parents to see newborn, position mother to hold newborn, provide encouragement	Institute comfort measures: • Perineal discomfort: gently cleanse and apply ice pack; position to decrease pressure on perineum • Uterine discomfort; palpate fundus gently • Hemorrhoids: ice pack • General fatigue: position of comfort, encourage rest • Administer pain medication PRN ■ ***Expected Outcomes*** Optimal comfort level maintained Active reduction of pain/discomfort achieved
Nutrition	Ice chips and clear fluids Evaluate for signs of dehydration	Ice chips and clear fluids	Regular diet if assessments are WNL Encourage fluids ■ ***Expected Outcomes*** Nutritional needs met
Elimination	Voids at least q2h; urine clear, straw-colored, negative for protein Bladder nondistended May have bowel movement Monitor I&O with IVs	May void spontaneously with pushing May pass stool with pushing	Voids spontaneously ■ ***Expected Outcomes*** Urinary bladder and bowel function unimpaired

(continued)

CLINICAL PATHWAY For Intrapartum Stages continued

Category	First Stage	Second and Third Stage	Fourth Stage Birth to 1 Hour Past Birth
Medications	Administer pain medication per woman's request	Local infiltration of anesthetic agent for birth by CNM/physician Pitocin 10–20 units IM, IVP per IV, tubing, or added to IV fluids	Continue Pitocin infusion Administer pain medication PRN ■ ***Expected Outcomes*** Comfort enhanced by pain-relieving techniques, administration of analgesia agent or an analgesic or anesthetic block
Discharge planning	Evaluate knowledge of labor and birth process Evaluate support system and need for referral after birth		Provide information if mother to be moved from LDR room Provide opportunity for parents to ask questions regarding newborn Evaluate knowledge of normal postpartum, newborn care ■ ***Expected Outcomes*** Mother and newborn transferred to low-risk postpartal and newborn care
Family involvement	Identify available support person(s) Recognize possible impact of culture on responses Observe interaction between woman and partner Create moment alone with woman to identify possible abuse Assess current parenting skills	Provide opportunities for woman and support person(s) to watch newborn assessments Perform newborn assessment on mother's abdomen/chest if possible	Provide opportunity for parents to be with baby Encourage skin-to-skin contact Darken room to encourage eye-to-eye contact Provide quiet time for new family Parenting: demonstrates early culturally expected parenting behaviors ■ ***Expected Outcomes*** • Incorporation of newborn into family • Family verbalizes comfort with newborn care
Date			

Abbreviations: CNM, certified nurse-midwife; BP, blood pressure; FHR, fetal heart rate; LTV long-term variability; WNL, within normal limits; VS, vital signs; EFM, electronic fetal monitoring; IV, intravenous; I&O, intake and output; IM, intramuscularly; IVP, intravenous push; LDR, labor, delivery, and recovery; OOB, out of bed; UA, urinary analysis; PRN, as needed

of her hospital stay. For some women, the hospital environment itself can be perceived as cold, impersonal, and technical and can produce anxiety or emotional stress. If the family is greeted in a brusque, harried manner, they are less likely to look to the nurse for support. A calm, pleasant manner, in contrast, indicates to the family that they are important. It helps instill in the couple a sense of confidence in the staff's ability to provide quality care and ensure safety during this critical time.

It is important to establish rapport and to create an environment in which the family feels free to ask questions. The support and encouragement of the nurse in maintaining a caring environment begins with the initial admission but needs to be attended to with all subsequent actions. Before completing assessments, the nurse may provide the opportunity for questions and may explain the environment and the procedures that will be a part of the labor and birthing care. In many hospitals, the admission process also includes signing an informed consent for treatment, and the patient is given information on arranging advance directives or instructions about her wishes if she were to become critically ill. In all cases, an identification bracelet and a bracelet that lists all known drug allergies are attached to her wrist.

Another important aspect of the initial contact is communicating in the woman and family's primary language. In addition to having interpreters available for Hispanic, Korean, Vietnamese, and other patients who do not speak English fluently, the nurse must consider the special needs of the deaf woman or family. There are more than 400,000 Americans who have a bilateral hearing loss, so there is a good chance that the nurse will work with a deaf expectant mother, father, grandparents, or siblings at some point. Table 24-1 provides suggestions for communicating more effectively with a woman or support person who is deaf.

Culture plays a major role in how a woman and her family view the labor and birth process. Trends in American culture are moving toward a shared partnership model between the woman and her partner in which the partner is actively involved in the birth process and often stays with the mother throughout the labor and birth. In contrast, Iranian and Turkish women are less likely to have their partner with them in the labor and birth setting. Instead, this is primarily the role of elder women family members and female friends (Ozsoy & Katabi, 2008).

PATIENT TEACHING What to Expect During Labor

ASSESSMENT As the woman is admitted into the birthing area, assess the woman's knowledge regarding the childbirth experience. Her knowledge base will be affected by previous births, attendance at childbirth education classes, and the amount of information she has been able to gather during her pregnancy by asking questions or reading. You may also assess the factors that affect communication and anxiety level. Assess labor progress to determine what to teach and the time available for teaching. If the woman is in early labor and she needs additional information, proceed with teaching.

NURSING DIAGNOSIS The key nursing diagnosis will probably be ***Deficient Knowledge*** related to lack of information about nursing care during labor.

NURSING PLAN AND IMPLEMENTATION The teaching plan will focus on the assessments and support the woman will receive during labor.

PATIENT GOALS At the completion of teaching, the woman will be able to:

- Verbalize the assessments the nurse will complete during labor
- Discuss the support and comfort measures that are available

TEACHING PLAN

Content	Teaching Method
■ Describe aspects of the admission process, including: ■ Taking an abbreviated history ■ Physical assessment (maternal vital signs [VS], fetal heart rate [FHR], contraction status, status of membranes) ■ Assessment of uterine contractions (frequency, duration, intensity) ■ Orientation to surroundings ■ Introductions to other support staff ■ Determination of woman's and family support person's expectations of the nurse	Provide information on the basic assessment and care activities. Allow time for questions and discussion as labor progress permits.
■ Present aspects of ongoing physical care, such as when to expect assessment of material VS, FHR, and contractions.	
■ If the electronic fetal monitor is used, describe how it works and the information it provides. Orient the woman to the sights and sounds of the monitor. Explain what "normal" data will look like and what characteristics are being watched for.	Demonstrate the fetal monitor.
■ Be sure to note that assessments will increase as the labor progresses, especially during the transition phase (usually the time the woman would like to be left alone) to help keep the mother and baby safe by noting deviations from normal course.	
■ Describe the vaginal examination and the information it elicits.	Use a cervical dilatation chart to illustrate the amount of dilatation.
■ Review comfort techniques that may be used in labor and ascertain what the woman thinks will promote comfort.	Focus on open discussion.
■ Review the breathing techniques the woman has learned so that you will be able to support her technique.	Ask the woman to demonstrate the techniques she has learned.
■ Review comfort and support measures, such as positioning, backrub, effleurage, touch, distraction techniques, and ambulation.	Focus on open discussion.
■ If the woman is in early labor, offer her a tour of the birthing area.	Provide a tour of birthing area, explaining equipment and routines. Include the woman's partner.

Evaluation

At the end of this teaching session, the woman will be able to describe the assessments that will occur during her labor and to discuss comfort and support measures that may be used.

Documentation

Documentation of patient teaching should include the teaching information discussed, the patient's verbalization of understanding, and specific interventions or warning signs that were given, along with the patient's understanding of follow-up, if needed in the future.

TABLE 24-1 Improving Communication with a Deaf Woman or Support Person

- Determine how the deaf individual prefers to communicate: speech reading (lip reading), sign language, pantomime, writing, or a combination of methods.
- If speech reading is used, face the person directly, speak with a natural tone and rhythm (exaggerated pronunciation may distort lip movements), and keep your hands away from your face. Do not chew gum.
- Use gestures and pantomime if necessary to enhance your speech.
- Do not assume written communication is the most effective approach. Writing carries a great potential for miscommunication and should not be forced unless the deaf person requests it.
- Most deaf individuals in the United States use American Sign Language (ASL) (see appendix E ∞). If the woman signs, call a professional ASL interpreter.
- Use a family member as an interpreter only until the professional interpreter arrives. Family members may not interpret all that is said or may add additional information. Professional ASL interpreters are bound by a code of ethics to maintain strict confidentiality, to transmit accurate messages, and to refrain from editing or adding information.
- Keep the woman's dominant hand and arm free for signing.
- Explain any procedures before they are needed.
- Look at the deaf individual, not the interpreter, when speaking.
- Speak in first person to the patient.
- Be alert for signs of "smiling and nodding." Often, when a deaf person does not understand something, the person will simply smile and nod. If that occurs, assess the person's understanding by asking the person to repeat the information to you.

Source: Adapted from Shelp, S. G. (1997). Your patient is deaf, now what? RN, 60*(2), 37–38, 40. Reprinted by permission of Medical Economics. Montvale, NJ.*

Labor Assessment

Following the initial greeting, the woman may either be taken into a labor assessment area (sometimes called a *triage area*) for evaluation or admitted directly into a birthing room. Some couples prefer to remain together during the admission process, and others prefer to have the partner or support person wait outside. The nurse should ask the woman's preference whenever possible. As the nurse helps the woman undress and get into a hospital gown, the nurse can begin to develop rapport and establish the nursing database. The labor and birth nurse can obtain essential information regarding the woman and her pregnancy. By doing an admission history, the nurse can initiate any immediate interventions needed and establish individualized priorities. The nurse is then able to make effective nursing decisions regarding intrapartal care:

- Is the woman in labor or is she a candidate to be sent home with a clear understanding of when to return?
- Are there factors that put the laboring woman or the fetus at risk?
- Should ambulation or bed rest be encouraged?
- Is more frequent monitoring needed?
- What does the woman or couple want during labor and birth?
- Who will be with the laboring woman for social support?

The woman is made comfortable. If she wants to rest in bed, a side-lying or semi-Fowler's position rather than a supine position is most comfortable and avoids supine hypotensive syndrome (vena caval syndrome).

After obtaining the essential information from the woman and her prenatal records from her certified nurse-midwife (CNM) or physician, the nurse begins the intrapartal assessment (chapter 23 ∞ discusses intrapartal assessment in depth).

As the assessments begin, the nurse auscultates the fetal heart rate (FHR). (Detailed information on monitoring FHR is presented in chapter 21 ∞.) The woman's blood pressure, pulse, respirations, and oral temperature are assessed. Contraction status (frequency, duration, and intensity), cervical dilatation and effacement, and fetal presentation and station are determined. If the woman is a nullipara in the early latent phase (for example, contractions are 10 to 30 minutes apart, with mild intensity and very little discomfort; cervix is long and thick, with dilatation of 1 to 2 cm; membranes are intact) she may be sent home to ambulate and rest in her own surroundings or directed to remain in a birthing center area and ambulate. When further progress is documented, she is admitted. Women who are admitted in the latent phase are more likely to have a longer duration of labor, increased use of epidural analgesia for pain, and increased use of oxytocin to augment labor than women who are clearly in the active phase at admission.

After the vaginal examination, the nurse shares the findings with the couple. If there are signs of advanced labor (frequent contractions, advanced cervical dilatation, and/or an urge to bear down), the physician or CNM is notified immediately, and actions are taken to prepare for the birth. If there are signs of excessive bleeding upon admission or if the woman reports episodes of painless bleeding in the last trimester, placenta previa may be present; in such cases, vaginal examination is not performed because it may stimulate copious bleeding.

Results of FHR assessment, uterine contraction evaluation, and the vaginal examination help determine whether the rest of the admission process can proceed at a more leisurely pace or whether additional interventions have higher priority. For example, an FHR of 110 beats per minute (beats/min) on auscultation indicates that an electronic fetal monitor (EFM) should be applied immediately to obtain additional data. The woman's vital signs will then be assessed immediately (Table 24-2).

Depending on how rapidly labor is progressing, the nurse notifies the CNM or physician before or after completing the admission procedures. If high-risk or emergency data are identified, the nurse immediately reports the findings to the CNM or physician; otherwise all assessment data should be gathered before initiating contact with the healthcare provider (Carolan, 2009). The report should include the following information: cervical dilatation and effacement, station, presenting part, status of the membranes, contraction pattern, FHR, vital signs that are not in the normal range, the woman's wishes, and her response to labor.

Collecting Laboratory Data

After admission data are obtained, multiple laboratory tests are performed to provide more extensive physiologic data that are

TABLE 24-2 Indicators of Normal Labor Process on Admission

INDICATOR	NORMAL CHARACTERISTICS
Uterine contractions	Frequency of not less than 2 minutes Duration of less than 75 seconds Uterine relaxation between contractions Most intense discomfort only with contractions (Some women, especially those with occiput posterior position, complain of less intense lower abdominal and/or back pain between contractions.)
Fetal heart rate	Rate 110–160 with average variability Absence of late decelerations
Maternal vital signs	BP below +140/90 or less than +30/+15 above prepregnancy readings Pulse 60–100 Temperature between 97.8°F and 99.6°F (36.5°C and 37.5°C)
If membranes ruptured	Fluid clear without odor

used to determine appropriate care for the woman and her fetus. A clean-voided midstream urine specimen is usually collected. The woman with intact membranes may collect her specimen in the bathroom. The nurse can test the woman's urine for the presence of protein, ketones, glucose, and leukocytes by using a dipstick before sending the sample to the laboratory. This procedure is especially important if nondependent edema or elevated blood pressure is noted on admission. Proteinuria of +1 or more may be a sign of preeclampsia. Glycosuria is found frequently in pregnant women because of the increased glomerular filtration rate in the proximal tubules and the inability of these tubules to increase glucose reabsorption. However, it may also be associated with gestational diabetes and should not be discounted. Leukocytes can be found in the urine when bacteria are present. The presence of a urinary tract infection can contribute to uterine irritability, pelvic pressure, and back pain, all symptoms that can be mistaken for labor.

Laboratory tests can be performed in the outpatient setting before admission but are most commonly done at the time of admission in the birthing center. Hemoglobin and hematocrit values help determine the oxygen-carrying capacity of the circulatory system and the ability of the woman to withstand blood loss at birth. Elevation of the hematocrit indicates hemoconcentration of blood, which occurs with edema or dehydration. A low hemoglobin, in the absence of other evidence of bleeding, suggests anemia. Blood may be typed and cross-matched if the woman is in a high-risk category, has active bleeding, or has a history of blood disorders. A serology test for syphilis is obtained if one has not been done in the last 3 months or if an antepartal serology result was positive. The Centers for Disease Control and Prevention (CDC) recommends that all women undergo voluntary screening for HIV during pregnancy. Women who have not been screened during the pregnancy should be screened for HIV in the intrapartum setting once consent has been obtained (Udeh, Udeh, & Graves, 2008).

Social Assessment

Once initial physical assessments are performed, the nurse can then take a detailed social history that provides a comprehensive view of both the woman's social habits and psychologic factors that may affect her birth experience. The presence of certain risk factors—including family violence or sexual assault (see chapter 9 ∞); use of drugs, alcohol, or tobacco; and presence of sexually transmitted infections—can influence a

RESEARCH EVIDENCE IN PRACTICE: Routine Perineal Shaving on Admission in Labor

CLINICAL QUESTION

Does routine perineal shaving on admission in labor provide any benefit for the mother?

RESEARCH EVIDENCE

In some parts of the world, women may have their pubic hair shaved with a razor when they are admitted to the hospital to give birth. This is based on the belief that shaving reduces the risk of infection if the perineum tears or if an episiotomy is necessary. It is thought that shaving may make suturing of lacerations easier and may help with instrument-assisted births.

The Cochrane Collaborative sponsored a review of the research evidence regarding the effects of perineal shaving. The Cochrane Database of Systematic Reviews is a source of high quality, research-based evidence.

The review found no benefit from routine perineal shaving. Controlled trials involving more than 1000 women were reported in this review. Each used antiseptic skin preparation and compared perineal shaving with simply cutting hairs on the vulva to less than a centimeter. No differences were found between the women who were shaved and those who were not. While there were no differences in wound infection, the incidence of open wounds, and ease of suturing, there were differences in complaints in the weeks following the birth. Women who had their perineum shaved complained of irritation, redness, multiple superficial scratches from the razor, and burning and itching of the vulva.

WHAT QUESTIONS REMAIN UNANSWERED?

Does it remain necessary to clip the hair of the vulva and perineum? Is the simple application of antiseptic as effective as clipping the hair? Is shaving effective in developing countries where antiseptic may not be available?

WHAT IS BEST PRACTICE?

The application of antiseptic and clipping of longer hairs in the perineum is as effective as shaving, without the complaints that accompany regrowth of pubic hair.

CRITICAL THINKING

How can the mother be reassured that perineal shaving is unnecessary?

References

Basevi, V., & Lavender. T. 2009. Routine perineal shaving on admission to labor. *Cochrane Database of Systematic Reviews,* Issue 4. Art. No.: CD001236. doi:10.1002/14651858

Care Plan Activity: Presence of Extended Family

woman's labor, birth, and future childrearing choices. With the prevalence of domestic violence, it is imperative to ask the woman about family violence and sexual assault (Chambliss, 2008). Because many women find questions about psychosocial risk factors embarrassing, the nurse should always ask such questions when the woman is alone and should use a straightforward, nonjudgmental approach. For example, a question such as "How many times per week do you drink alcohol?" prompts the woman to be specific in her answer. If the woman reports that she does drink alcohol on a daily basis, the nurse then asks about the amount. Drug use can be assessed in a similar manner.

A social assessment should also include data about the woman's current living situation, availability of resources, preparedness for the infant, community resources, and the woman's social support network. This dialog provides an opportunity for the nurse to continue to build support, to provide information when requested, and to be direct yet supportive. Referrals to social services, the Special Supplemental Food Program for Women, Infants, and Children (WIC), and new parent support programs can be initiated. It is important to begin this dialog early in the admission process so that adequate resources can be obtained for the family.

Documentation of Admission

A nursing admission note is entered into the computer or the charting system. The admission note should include the reason for admission; the date, time, and method of the woman's arrival; notification of the CNM or physician; the condition of the woman and her baby; labor and membrane status; and pertinent social assessment information (Simpson & Creehan, 2008). Her comfort level and support system should also be addressed. For a woman who speaks a different language, an interpreter should be provided, and documentation should include that the interpreter was used and that the woman verbalized understanding.

Nursing Care During the First Stage of Labor

After completing the nursing assessment and diagnosis steps, the nurse creates a plan of care to achieve nursing goals (Simpson & Creehan, 2008). During the first stage of labor, the nurse is concerned about the physical safety of the laboring woman and her child, as well as the emotional well-being of the laboring couple and their support system. Therefore, the nurse continually assesses the effects of uterine contractions (UCs) on the course of labor and the well-being of the fetus, and monitors the woman's vital signs (VS), contraction pattern, cervical changes, and intake and output. Additionally, the nurse monitors the couple's and support system's responses to labor.

Developing a Birth Plan

Labor support is a primary role for nurses who are caring for couples during the first stage of labor. Couples look to their nurse for information about labor progress, pain management, procedures, and examinations, and for assistance with pain management techniques such as breathing and relaxation. Couples need reassurance that labor is progressing in normal trajectory and explanations when it is not within normal limits. They also need praise for their accomplishments and support during labor. For most couples, the nurse's presence in the room is highly valued as labor advances; however, the nurse should assess the woman's individual preferences, because some women may prefer privacy. Clinical research has established that laboring women have fewer complications and shorter labors when they perceive support from their nurse, doula, and/or friends and family members (Barnett, 2008; McGrath & Kennell, 2008).

Integration of Family Expectations

Laboring families have certain expectations of the experience, of themselves, of the nurse, and of the physician or certified nurse-midwife (CNM). Some of these expectations may not be realistic. Unrealistic expectations can increase the anxiety level of both the laboring woman and her partner. The labor nurse should assess the family's expectations to integrate them into the labor plan and/or assist the family in reestablishing expectations that are realistic. Some families may present to the facility with a birth plan (discussed in chapter 13 ∞). The plan should be reviewed and requests should be incorporated into the woman's nursing care plan whenever possible. Requests that cannot be met should be discussed and a clear rationale should be provided.

Laboring families' expectations of the nurse can range from wanting the nurse to be highly involved in the labor, to wanting the nurse to be minimally involved (Barnett, 2008). The couple who desires high involvement expects the labor nurse to be in the room continuously and to provide direct labor support. The couple may view the labor nurse as the woman's primary labor coach, providing guidance and emotional support. The couple who desires minimal involvement of the labor nurse prefers that the nurse is present only when assessments and interventions need to be done and when the couple requests the nurse's presence.

With the variety of expectations patients have of nurses, it becomes a challenge to provide individualized care. The nurse needs to assess and respond to the couple's needs and desires. To determine preferences, the nurse can look for cues. When the woman and her coach are admitted, do they seem to take control and know what is going to happen? Do they have a birth plan that they have already worked out, or do they seem hesitant and unsure of the process?

Although these two ends of the spectrum are obvious, they are a starting point. It would be fairly safe to assume that the "situation-is-in-control" couple would want a little less involvement, and the couple who is hesitant and asking questions will want more extensive involvement. The nurse can also gain more information by asking questions such as, "Other than the assessments that I will be making, what kind of involvement would you like from me? Would you like to call me when you need something or have me come in now and then, or would you be more comfortable if I stay in the room most of the time?" This gives the couple an opportunity to make their wishes known. This approach also provides the couple with the opportunity to ask questions and seek advice as needed. It is also important that the couple knows that the nurse understands that their wishes may change during labor and that the nurse will be available for them throughout the process.

During the labor process, the nurse also serves as an advocate for the woman and her partner. The partner may need support, guidance, or an opportunity for rest periods. The nurse models behavior to family members who may feel uncomfortable or uneasy in the labor and birth setting (Sauls, 2007).

Integration of Cultural Beliefs

Values, customs, and practices of different cultures are as important during labor as they are in the prenatal period. Research indicates that an individual's experiences in labor are highly dependent upon social and cultural norms (Reitmanova & Gustafson, 2008). Without this knowledge, a nurse is less likely to understand a family's behavior and may impose personal values and beliefs upon them. As cultural sensitivity increases, so does the likelihood of providing high-quality care (Spector, 2008).

The following sections briefly present a few possible cultural responses to labor. Additional information on culturally sensitive care is provided in chapter 2 ∞. It is difficult to present such a limited discussion without appearing to advance stereotypes. No statement of a specific behavior can accurately reflect the preference of all people in a group. Within every culture, each person develops his or her own beliefs and value system. Nurses must regard general information about any culture or belief system as background information to help them determine the person's own needs and desires.

CLINICAL TIP

It is best not to assume that women of any culture have the information they desire regarding birth, self-care, and newborn care, regardless of the number of children they have had. An important aspect of nursing is to teach, so always offer culturally sensitive information. Most nurses are not knowledgeable regarding all cultural practices. So be sensitive, and ask what is important to the mother. For example, is there special clothing she wants the newborn to wear, or does she have any preference about how she wants the umbilical stump cared for? Remain aware that the information you learned in class or a text reflects primarily the nursing culture and the Western, chiefly European, culture. To believe that the healthcare practices of these two cultures are relevant to all people is an example of ethnocentrism. Strive to increase your understanding of other cultures as your clinical practice base grows.

Modesty

Modesty is an important consideration for women, regardless of the culture to which they belong. However, some women may be more uncomfortable than others with the degree of exposure needed for some procedures during the labor and birth processes. Some women may be particularly uncomfortable when men are present and feel more comfortable with women; others may be uncomfortable with exposure of personal body parts regardless of the gender of the examiner or person who assists them. The nurse needs to be observant of the woman's responses to examinations and procedures and to provide appropriate draping and privacy (Spector, 2008). It is more prudent to assume that embarrassment will occur with exposure and take measures to provide privacy than to assume that it will not matter to the woman.

CLINICAL JUDGMENT

Case Study: Fatima Al Ahala

Fatima Al Ahala is a 22-year-old G1 who presents in labor. Fatima and her husband, Samir, are from Pakistan. The couple has stated that they can only accept care from female providers. The couple is being attended by a female nurse-midwife and the back-up physician is also a female. When her labor intensifies, Fatima requests an epidural. The only anesthesiologist available is a male physician.

Critical Thinking

What actions can you take to help this family meet their cultural preferences?

See www.nursing.pearsonhighered.com for possible responses.

For example, many Hispanic women may fear loss of privacy, so they labor at home as long as possible. Maintaining dignity for the couple is important (Spector, 2008). Some Asian women are not accustomed to male physicians and attendants, and some Muslims forbid any male (other than the husband) to see a woman who is uncovered. The nurse should be aware that in the Muslim culture, the man is the primary source of information. It may be necessary to speak to the man before interacting with the woman. This communicates respect and shows cultural sensitivity. The nurse should ensure coverage of the woman whenever possible, even during vaginal exams and the second stage (Spector, 2008).

Pain Expression

Women's reactions to the discomfort of labor vary greatly. Some turn inward and remain very quiet during the whole process, whereas others may be very vocal, with behaviors such as counting out loud, moaning quietly or loudly, crying, or cursing. They may also turn from side to side or change positions frequently. The nurse supports a woman's individual expression of pain, whatever it may be, to enhance the birthing experience for mother, baby, and family.

In the Korean culture it used to be important for the laboring woman to be silent so she would not bring shame on her family. However, today women are encouraged to be less passive. Vocalization is more common, although older in-laws or other family members may discourage shouting or outcries as aggressive behavior. Hmong women are frequently quiet during labor, although behavior varies from one individual to the next. European Americans demonstrate a wide variety of behaviors in response to pain. Especially in the transitional phase, some women want to squeeze their partner's (or the nurse's) hand, and some may be tempted to bite during the most intense part of the contraction. Vietnamese women tend to report more pain, use less pain medication, and regard labor as a negative experience (Fisher, Tran, & Tran, 2007).

Examples of Cultural Beliefs

Some differences between cultures are apparent with regard to specific practices related to position and food and drink during labor. In most non-European societies uninfluenced by Westernization, women assume an upright position in childbirth. For example, during birth some Native American women use meditation, self-control, or indigenous plants, and the father may be expected to avoid certain rituals such as eating meat. Some Native Americans may ask to take the placenta home for a ritualistic ceremony that involves returning the placenta to the earth.

For Hmong women from Laos, the beginning of labor signifies the beginning of a transition and entails certain dietary restrictions. The woman usually prefers only "hot" foods, tea made with loose tea leaves, and warm water to drink. The woman usually maintains self-control, and may wish to move about freely during the first stage of labor. She may smile even throughout intense contractions. The husband is frequently present and actively involved in providing comfort. Traditionally, the woman prefers that the amniotic membranes not be ruptured until just before birth. It is thought that the escape of fluid at this time makes the birth easier. She may choose to kneel or squat for the birth of her baby. As soon as the baby is born, a soft-boiled egg must be given to the mother to restore her energy. During the postpartum period, the mother prefers "warm" foods, such as chicken prepared with warm water and warm rice (Hoang, Le, & Kilpatrick, 2009). The newborn is protected from praise to prevent jealousy from individuals outside of the family.

Latina women often want their partners to stay with them during labor and birth and to reassure them that everything will be all right. The women want their partners to show caring and love as they labor and to speak to them using affectionate words. Standing close to the woman and using touch are important roles for the partner (Spector, 2008).

Muslim women may have their husband, a female friend or relative, or a male relative with them during childbirth. Family support may be particularly important but does not preclude the importance of the nurse's presence. The woman may want to retain her head covering (*khimar*), and two long-sleeved gowns can be offered. Examinations should be done by a female nurse, physician, or CNM whenever possible. Some Muslim women are not comfortable in the presence of a male physician or nurse. If male physicians are involved with their care, they may wish for their husbands to remain in the room during all care by the physicians. Male providers should only enter the room after receiving permission from the husband. Modesty needs vary, and each individual will need to be assessed. After the birth, Muslim fathers traditionally call praise to Allah (*adhan*) in the newborn's right ear and clean the newborn. It is helpful if the birthing room personnel are aware of these practices so that the family's expectations and wishes can be incorporated into care. Many Middle-Eastern patients also believe that compliments addressed to the parents about their new baby will bring on the evil eye. The "evil eye" is the name given for the passage of sickness from one person to another, either intentionally or unintentionally, as a result of being jealous or envious (Spector, 2008). Thus, the nurse should avoid directly complimenting the couple, but instead direct compliments to God (*Allah*).

> "I am in an area with a very small Muslim population, and one of the nursing students with me had the opportunity to work with a Muslim couple during labor, birth, and then in the postpartum area the following day. During labor, the woman's sister remained at her side, and her husband sat on the other side of a drawn curtain inside the labor room and close to the door. He requested that a sign be placed on the door indicating that no males were to enter the room. We took care to ensure that we asked for a female lab tech for blood drawing, and a female physician attended the birth. The labor and birth went smoothly, and the woman did not utter any sound, even during pushing. After the birth, the father was shown the child before his wife held the newborn boy. The father was very pleased and talked quietly to his son, with his head down beside the newborn's ear. The next day, the student was once again assigned to this family. The sign remained on the door, and at all times that day, the sister and father remained in the room, the father always sitting away from the bed, close to the door. This was the woman's fifth child, so at first the student thought that she would not want much self-care, newborn, or breastfeeding information. But she began to talk to the woman, with her husband interpreting all questions and giving answers, and as each topic was brought up, the mother indicated that she wanted more information. Building on the trust that they had established the previous day in labor, the father told the student to "give the instruction," and he left the room. The mother and sister were full of questions about their health and their bodies—questions they had had for years! The student was proud that she did not make assumptions and was able to share so much information with them. It was an experience that the student and I will always remember with great joy."

Sometimes cultural norms are passed down from one generation to the next. African Americans, especially those whose ancestors are from Western Africa, may have beliefs rooted in traditional folk healing. Some African Americans have strong beliefs in healers and faith healers (Edgar, 2009). Some of these beliefs are centered on labor and childrearing. For example, it is widely believed that an infant born with a caul (a piece of the amniotic membrane covering the head at birth) will have the ability to communicate with spirits. This is viewed as a sign of good luck and is widely embraced within this culture.

In working with women from another culture, the nurse needs an awareness of their beliefs, values, and practices to understand their needs. The maternity nurse would do well to make it a priority to become acquainted with the beliefs and practices of the various cultures in the community. In the birthing situation, the nurse supports the family's cultural practices as long as it is safe to do so.

Provision of Care in the First Stage

Throughout the first stage, the nurse needs to evaluate physical parameters of the woman and her fetus. Maternal temperature is monitored every 4 hours unless the temperature is over 37.5°C (99.6°F); in such cases, it must be taken every hour. Once the amniotic fluid has ruptured, temperature should be monitored every 2 hours.

The nurse monitors blood pressure, pulse, and respirations every hour. If the woman's blood pressure is over 140/90 mm Hg or her pulse is more than 100, the CNM or physician must be notified. The blood pressure and pulse are then reevaluated more frequently. The nurse palpates uterine contractions for frequency, intensity, and duration.

Intrapartal vaginal exams are done to assess cervical changes, status of membranes, fetal position, and station. However, frequent vaginal exams increase the risk of infection and should be performed only when needed. Some providers advocate performing vaginal examinations only when a change of management will occur, such as before an epidural or to provide scalp stimulation.

The fetal heart rate (FHR) is auscultated every 30 minutes as long as it remains between 110 and 160 beats per minute (beats/min) without the presence of decelerations (Association of Women's Health, Obstetric, and Neonatal Nurses [AWHONN], 2009b; Tucker, Miller, & Miller, 2008). The FHR should be auscultated throughout one contraction and for about 15 seconds after the contraction to ensure that there are no decelerations. If the FHR is not in the 110 to 160 range and/or decelerations are heard, continuous electronic monitoring is recommended. Table 24-3 summarizes nursing assessments in the first stage of labor. The nurse documents labor progress, status of fetus, and interventions in the woman's chart.

CLINICAL TIP

If the monitor is no longer recording the fetal heart tracing, check that there is adequate gel under the transducer and reposition it before you assume there is a problem with the baby.

Latent Phase

If the laboring woman has not had childbirth education classes, the latent phase is a time when the nurse can give anticipatory guidance. Most women are not too uncomfortable with contractions at this time and are responsive to teaching about breathing and other techniques for coping with labor contractions. In fact, many women in the latent phase seek information about what to expect. The unprepared woman may hesitate to ask questions and thus can benefit even more from anticipatory guidance by the nurse.

As long as there are no contraindications (such as vaginal bleeding or rupture of membranes [ROM] with the fetus unengaged), the woman may be encouraged to ambulate, because upright positions shorten labor (Hansen, 2009). A tour of the birthing facility can help decrease anxiety and distract her from her discomfort. Many women feel much more at ease and comfortable if they can move around and do not have to remain in bed. Ambulation also aids in fetal descent, increases the frequency and intensity of contractions, and provides the woman with a sense of control (Figure 24-1 ■).

The nurse should offer fluids in the form of clear liquids or ice chips at frequent intervals. Because gastric emptying time is prolonged during labor, solid foods are usually avoided. Fasting during labor is the subject of some controversy. Some providers believe that eating and drinking in labor should be an option for women. Research has shown that oral intake during labor does not result in adverse maternal or fetal outcomes (American College of Obstetricians and Gynecologists [ACOG], 2009). Although women are still advised to avoid solid foods for 6 to 8 hours before elective cesarean birth, modest amounts of clear liquids are recommended for women experiencing a normal labor (ACOG, 2009). Vomiting during labor occurs frequently because of the decreased gastric emptying time. It is not uncommon for women to vomit during the first stage, especially during the transition phase. The nurse should reassure the woman and provide oral care.

Active Phase

During the active phase, the contractions have a frequency of 2 to 3 minutes, a duration of 50 to 60 seconds, and moderate intensity. Contractions need to be palpated every 15 to 30 minutes. As the contractions become more frequent and

TABLE 24-3 Nursing Assessments in the First Stage

PHASE	MOTHER	FETUS
Latent	Blood pressure, respirations each hour if in normal range Temperature every 4 hours unless over 37.5°C (99.6°F) or membranes ruptured, then every hour Uterine contractions every 15–30 minutes	FHR every 30 minutes for low-risk women and every 15 minutes for high-risk women if normal characteristics present (presence of variability, baseline (BL) in the 110–160 beats/min range, without late decelerations). Note fetal activity. If electronic fetal monitor in place, assess for reactive nonstress test (NST).
Active	Blood pressure, pulse, respirations every hour if in normal range Uterine contractions palpated every 15–30 minutes	FHR every 30 minutes for low-risk women and every 15 minutes for high-risk women if normal characteristics are present (AWHONN, 2009a).
Transition	Blood pressure, pulse, respirations every 15–30 minutes Contractions palpated at least every 15–30 minutes	FHR every 15–30 minutes if normal characteristics are present.

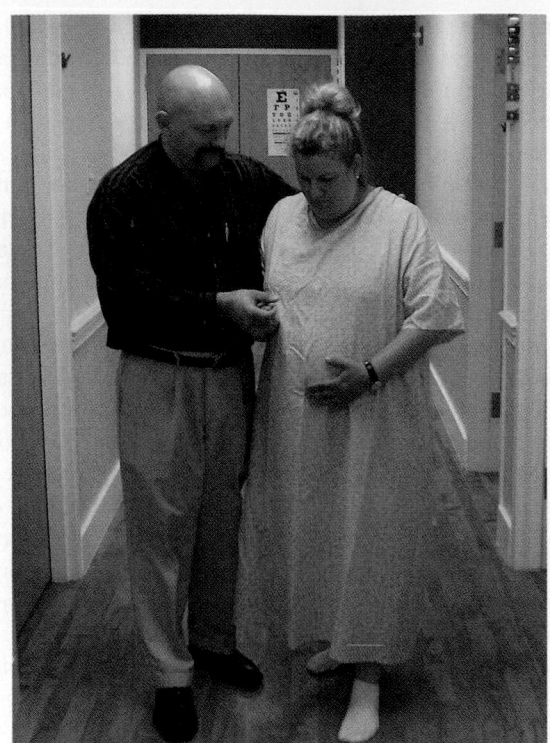

Figure 24-1 ■ Woman and her partner walking in the hospital during labor.

intense, intrapartal vaginal examination may be performed to assess cervical dilatation and effacement and fetal station and position. During the active phase, the cervix dilates from 4 to 7 cm, and vaginal discharge and bloody show increase. The woman should be encouraged to void because a full bladder can interfere with fetal descent. If the woman is unable to void, catheterization may be necessary. Maternal vital signs, including blood pressure, pulse, and respirations, should be assessed every hour for low-risk women (unless previously elevated), and every 30 minutes for high-risk women. The FHR is auscultated every 30 minutes for women without complications and more frequently (every 15 minutes) for women with complications (AWHONN, 2009a; Tucker, Miller, & Miller, 2008).

For the woman experiencing slow progress of labor or the inability to tolerate fluids, an intravenous (IV) electrolyte solution may be started to provide energy and prevent dehydration. If an IV is started, it becomes even more important to encourage voiding every 1 to 2 hours to prevent bladder distention.

CLINICAL TIP

Catheterizing a woman during a contraction is uncomfortable for her and difficult to do because of the increased downward pressure. To avoid these problems, pass the catheter between contractions. If the baby's head is low in the pelvis, you will have to change the direction of the catheter. Visualize passing it up and over the baby's head rather than straight into the urethra.

If the amniotic membranes have not ruptured previously, the CNM or physician may do so during this phase. When the membranes rupture, the nurse notes the color and odor of the amniotic fluid and the time of rupture and immediately auscultates the FHR. The fluid should be clear with no odor. Meconium-stained amniotic fluid may be a sign of a compromised fetus or may be present when the fetus is in a breech presentation. In the case of a breech fetus, meconium staining may not indicate a compromised fetus. In a cephalic presentation, however, meconium staining may indicate a compromised fetal state. When the fetus is compromised, the intestines and anal sphincter relax, leading to the release of meconium into the amniotic fluid. Meconium turns the fluid greenish brown (AWHONN, 2009b; Verklan & Walden, 2009). Whenever the nurse notes meconium-stained fluid, an electronic monitor is applied to continuously assess the FHR (AWHONN, 2009a; Tucker, Miller, & Miller, 2008). The time of rupture is noted because the incidence of amnionitis increases with rupture over 24 hours. An additional concern is prolapse of the umbilical cord, which occurs when membranes rupture and the fetus is not engaged. The concern is that the amniotic fluid coming through the cervix will propel the umbilical cord through the cervix (prolapsed cord). Prolapsed cord is assessed by monitoring for signs of nonreassuring fetal status and performing a vaginal examination with a sterile glove. The FHR is auscultated because a drop in the rate might indicate an undetected prolapsed cord. Immediate intervention is necessary to remove pressure on a prolapsed umbilical cord until a cesarean birth can be performed (see chapter 28). (See Table 24-4 for additional deviations from normal.)

See the section, Promotion of Comfort in the First Stage, later in the chapter for comfort management for the patient.

Transition Phase

During transition, the contraction frequency is every 2 to 3 minutes, duration is 60 to 90 seconds, and intensity is strong. Cervical dilatation increases from 8 to 10 cm, effacement is complete (100%), and a heavy amount of bloody show is usually present. Some multiparous women may not completely efface prior to the birth. Nulliparous women should completely efface prior to the birth of the infant. Contractions are palpated at least every 15 minutes. Sterile vaginal examination can be done during this stage of labor to assess rapid changes in status. Maternal blood pressure, pulse, and respirations are taken at least every 30 minutes, and FHR is auscultated every 30 minutes for low-risk women and every 15 minutes for high-risk women (AWHONN, 2009a; Tucker, Miller, & Miller, 2008).

Throughout labor the woman's center of focus gradually turns inward. She becomes less aware of what is going on around her and intensely aware of her uterine contractions. She experiences body boundary diffusion, which hampers her ability to know where her body ends and her external environment begins. Women during this time will reach out to others but may be uncomfortable with others touching them.

The woman's ability to speak in coherent sentences can be impaired during the transitional phase. This makes it difficult for the woman to communicate her needs to healthcare providers

TABLE 24-4 Deviations from Normal Labor Process Requiring Immediate Intervention

PROBLEM	IMMEDIATE ACTION
Women admitted with vaginal bleeding or history of painless vaginal bleeding	• Do not perform vaginal examination. • Assess FHR. • Evaluate amount of blood loss. • Evaluate labor pattern. • Notify physician/CNM immediately.
Presence of greenish or brownish amniotic fluid	• Continuously monitor FHR. • Evaluate dilatation of cervix and determine if umbilical cord is prolapsed. • Evaluate presentation (vertex or breech). • Maintain woman on complete bed rest on left side. • Notify physician/CNM immediately. • Have suction equipment and laryngoscope at the bedside to provide immediate suctioning upon delivery.
Decrease in FHR below 110 beats/min	• Perform vaginal examination to assess for prolapsed cord. • Turn woman to a side-lying or hands and knees position. • Administer oxygen by face mask. • Discontinue pitocin. • Call the CNM/physician. • Continue continuous external monitoring or place internal fetal monitor if hospital protocol allows and ROM has occurred. • Provide fetal scalp stimulation.
Absence of FHR and fetal movement	• Notify physician/CNM. • Provide truthful information and emotional support to laboring couple. • Remain with the couple.
Prolapse of umbilical cord	• Relieve pressure on cord manually. • Continuously monitor FHR; watch for changes in FHR pattern. • Notify physician/CNM. • Assist woman into knee-chest position or place in Trendelenburg position. • Administer oxygen.

Woman admitted in advanced labor; birth imminent	• Prepare for immediate birth.
	• Obtain critical information:
	  • Estimated date of birth (EDB)
	  • History of bleeding problems
	  • History of medical or obstetric problems
	  • Past and/or present use/abuse of prescription/OTC/illicit drugs
	  • Problems with this pregnancy
	  • FHR and maternal vital signs
	  • Whether membranes are ruptured and how long since rupture
	  • Blood type and Rh
	• Direct another person to contact physician/CNM.
	• Do not leave woman alone.
	• Provide support to couple.
	• Put on gloves.

and her support team. The support person(s) and nurse need to follow the woman's cues and change interventions as needed.

The nurse should encourage the woman to rest between contractions by instructing the woman at the end of her contraction to take a deep breath and to let it out slowly while she relaxes her muscles. Helping to maintain a quiet room between contractions can also enhance the woman's ability to rest. The woman during this phase is present focused; thus, providing instruction between contractions should be kept to a minimum.

Some women have difficulty coping with the intensity of labor during this time and need assistance in performing breathing techniques. Either the support person or the nurse can breathe along with the woman during each contraction to help her maintain her pattern. It is helpful to encourage her and assure her that she is doing a good job. The woman will begin to feel increased rectal pressure as the fetal presenting part moves down the birth canal and sometimes a burning sensation as the tissues begin to stretch. The nurse encourages the woman to refrain from pushing until the cervix is completely dilated. For the woman who is unmedicated, the urge to push may seem unbearable. Specific instructions, such as encouraging the woman to "blow in short breaths like you are blowing out a candle" or "pant like a puppy," can help prevent the woman from involuntarily pushing. This measure also helps prevent cervical edema or lacerations.

The end of transition and beginning of the second stage may be indicated by involuntary passage of flatus or stool and the movement of the fetus from the side of the maternal abdomen to the midline. Other indications include a change in the woman's voice or the sounds she is making. As the fetus moves down and she feels increased pressure and a bearing-down sensation, her voice tends to deepen. A moan during a contraction takes on a more guttural quality. Labor nurses recognize this sound as a sign that the woman may have entered the second stage.

Promotion of Comfort in the First Stage

The first step in planning care for the laboring woman is to talk with the woman and her partner or support person to identify their goals. Usually the couple is concerned with discomfort, so it is important to identify factors that may contribute to discomfort. These factors include uncomfortable positions, diaphoresis, continual leaking of amniotic fluid, a full bladder, dry mouth, anxiety, and fear. Nursing interventions can minimize the effects of these factors. These interventions are discussed later in this section.

There are many responses to pain. As the intensity of the contraction increases with the progression of labor, the woman becomes less aware of the environment and may have difficulty hearing and understanding verbal instructions. The pattern of coping with labor contractions varies from the use of highly structured breathing techniques to turning inward.

In labor, the more common pain reactions, such as increased pulse and respiratory rates, dilated pupils, increased blood pressure, and muscle tension, are transitory because the pain is intermittent. However, increased muscle tension may impede the progress of labor; therefore, the nurse encourages the woman to relax her skeletal muscles and avoid holding her breath.

Sounds are an important part of the labor and birthing process. Some women naturally make sounds such as moans and grunts and feel that it helps them cope and do the work of labor; they are responding to what their body tells them to do. Others begin to make loud sounds (screams) only as they lose their ability to cope and feel they do not have any other options.

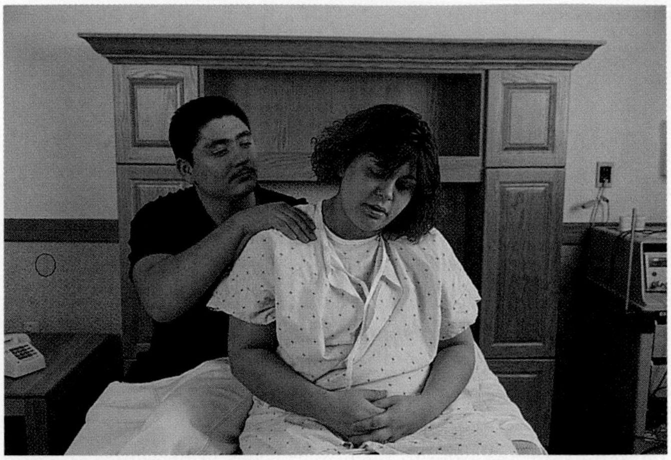

Figure 24-2 ■ The woman's partner provides support and encouragement during labor.

Source: Photographer, Elena Dorfman.

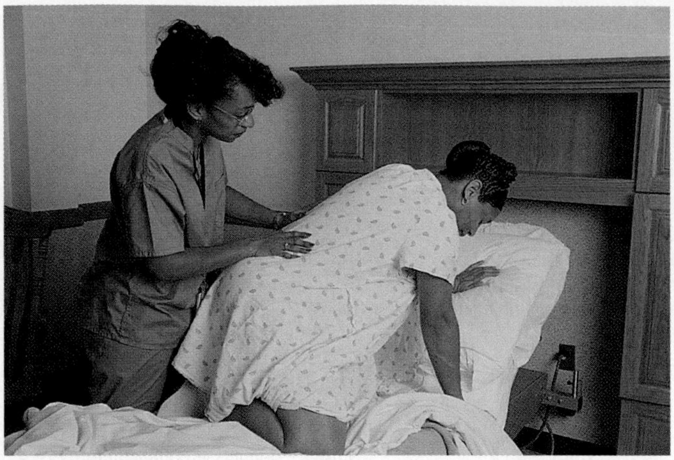

Figure 24-3 ■ The laboring woman is encouraged to choose a position of comfort. The nurse modifies assessments and interventions as necessary.

Source: Photographer, Elena Dorfman.

Some women may want physical contact during contractions. They may provide verbal and nonverbal signs, such as crying, moaning, and beseeching the coach or nurse to hold their hand or rub their back. They may look at the support person or reach out for help to indicate their anxiety. Touch may be used to convey support and enhance comfort for the woman (Figure 24-2 ■). She may be soothed by a neck or back rub or by holding the hand of her partner or the nurse. A woman generally wants touching and physical contact during the first part of labor, but when she moves into the transition phase, she may rebuff all efforts and pull away. Other women do not want to be touched at all, regardless of the phase of labor.

A decrease in the intensity of discomfort is one of the goals of nursing support during labor. Nursing measures to decrease pain include the following:

- Encouraging position changes
- Assisting with personal comfort measures
- Decreasing anxiety
- Providing information
- Using specific supportive relaxation techniques
- Encouraging paced breathing
- Administering pharmacologic agents as desired by the woman

Position Changes

Laboring Positions

Women in labor may wish to remain ambulatory to promote comfort and aid in labor progression (Roberts & Hanson, 2007). Some women who have been ambulatory up to this point may wish to sit in a chair or on a bed. The woman may also need to take periodic rest periods as contractions intensify.

The woman is encouraged to ambulate if the fetal head is engaged and the electronic fetal monitoring (EFM) has shown a reassuring FHR pattern. However, to avoid the risk of umbilical cord prolapse, the woman is generally instructed to remain in bed if membranes are ruptured and the presenting part is not engaged.

If she stays in bed, the woman is encouraged to assume any position that she finds comfortable (Figure 24-3 ■). A side-lying position is generally the most advantageous for the laboring woman. Care should be taken that all body parts are supported, with the joints slightly flexed. Pillows may be placed against her chest and under the uppermost arm. A pillow or folded bath blanket is placed between her knees to support the uppermost leg and relieve tension or muscle strain. A pillow (or warmed rolled blanket) placed at the woman's midback also helps provide support. If the woman is more comfortable on her back, the head of the bed should be elevated to relieve the pressure of the uterus on the vena cava, and the uterus should be tilted by placing a towel or blanket under the woman's back. Pillows may be placed under each arm and under the knees to provide support. Because a pregnant woman is at increased risk for thrombophlebitis, excessive pressure behind the knee and calf should be avoided, and frequent assessment of pressure points needs to be made.

> **CLINICAL TIP**
>
> When assisting with position changes, provide the woman with a sheet to provide continued coverage and assist with modesty and maintaining dignity throughout labor.

Frequent position changes (at least every hour) seem to achieve more efficient contractions, and contribute to comfort and relaxation. It is also helpful for the woman to sit up in a rocking chair or other comfortable chair, or in the shower.

Personal Comfort Measures

Because vaginal discharge increases, the nurse needs to change the underpads frequently. Washing the perineum with warm soap and water removes secretions and increases comfort. The nurse needs to use standard precautions to avoid exposure to vaginal secretions.

Diaphoresis and the constant leaking of amniotic fluid can dampen the woman's gown and bed linen. Fresh, smooth, dry bed linen promotes comfort. To avoid having to change the bottom sheet following ROM, the nurse may replace the underpads at frequent intervals (standard precautions need to be followed). The perineal area should be kept as clean and dry as possible to promote comfort. The woman may also find comfort in applying a cool washcloth to her forehead or behind the back of her neck.

CLINICAL TIP

To promote maternal comfort, dampen a washcloth with cool water and wring it out thoroughly. Hold one corner of the washcloth and swing the cloth in a circular motion for a cooling fanlike effect.

A full bladder adds to the discomfort during a contraction and may prolong labor by interfering with the descent of the fetus. Even though the woman is voiding, urine may be retained because of the pressure of the fetal presenting part. A full bladder can be detected by palpation directly over the symphysis pubis. Some of the procedures for regional analgesia during labor contribute to the inability to void, and catheterization may be necessary. The woman should be encouraged to empty her bladder about every 1 to 2 hours. The nurse should offer the woman a bedpan before catheterization because some women are able to void despite anesthesia, and spontaneous voiding decreases the risk of infection that is associated with repeated catheterizations.

The woman may experience dryness of her mouth because her breathing is more rapid. The woman can be instructed to breathe in through her nose and out through her mouth. Clear fluids and ice chips are usually offered unless a complication exists that makes cesarean birth a possibility. The nurse can also apply A and D ointment or a lip emollient to the dry lips. Some prepared childbirth programs advise the woman to bring lollipops to suck on to help combat the dryness that occurs with some of the breathing patterns. If the woman vomits, the nurse should wipe her mouth and offer water to rinse her mouth.

Some women feel discomfort from cold feet. Wearing socks or slippers may increase their comfort. Some women may wish to wear their own nightgown, although they need to know that the gown will most likely be soiled and may be more difficult to move around in.

Birthing balls—large, heavy plastic balls that accommodate an adult's weight—are used by some laboring women to increase comfort (Figure 24-4 ■). The woman sits on the ball and can roll it back and forth gently. The slow rock is thought to widen the pelvis and enhance fetal descent, while leaning forward on the knees with the head, arms, and chest over the ball simulates a hands-and-knees position and may facilitate rotation of an occiput-posterior. When a birthing ball is used, the nurse should remain close by the woman to help provide balance. Many balls come with aluminum frames to prevent falls.

Some family members or support persons can assist the woman with comfort measures. They may help with position changes, provide ice chips, walk with the laboring woman, and give effleurage or back rubs. If the family is not already involved in providing comfort measures and seems to want to be,

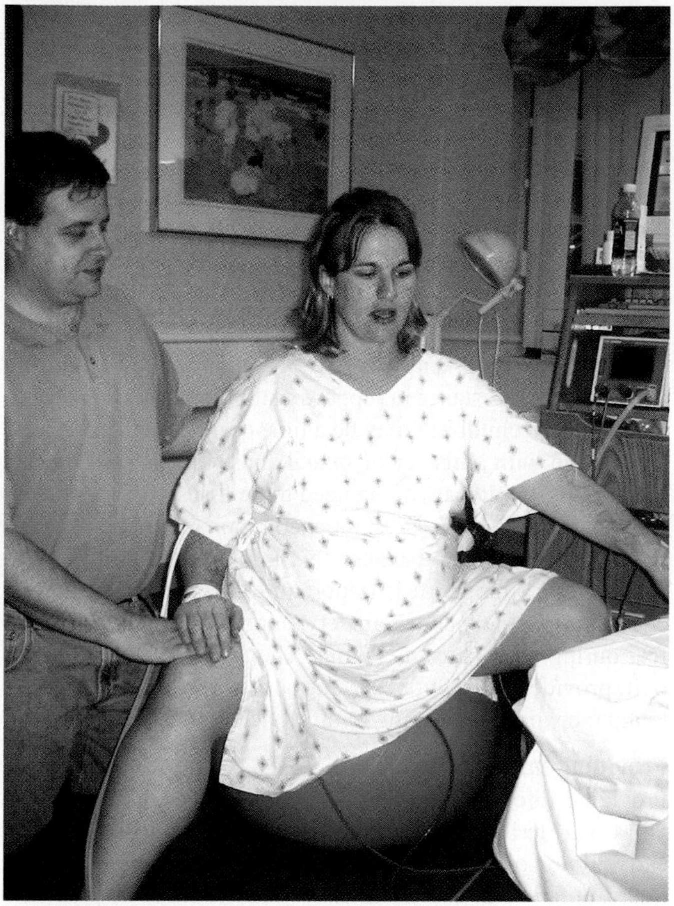

Figure 24-4 ■ A birthing ball is used to promote maternal comfort during labor. The birthing ball facilitates fetal descent and fetal rotation and helps increase the diameter of the pelvis.

the nurse can act as a role model while providing comfort measures and then invite the support person(s) to join in if they like.

Family members also need to be encouraged to maintain their own comfort. As their attention is directed toward the laboring woman, they may forget their own needs. The nurse may have to encourage them to take breaks, maintain food and fluid intake, and rest.

Reducing Anxiety

The anxiety experienced by women entering labor is related to a combination of factors inherent to the process. A moderate amount of anxiety enhances the ability to deal with the pain. But an excessive degree of anxiety decreases the woman's ability to cope with the pain.

To decrease anxiety that is not related to pain, the nurse can give information (which eases fear of the unknown), establish rapport with the couple (which helps them preserve their personal integrity), express confidence in the couple's ability to work with the labor process, and assist with breathing and relaxation techniques. In addition to being a good listener, the nurse needs to demonstrate genuine concern for the laboring woman. Remaining with the woman as much as possible conveys a caring attitude and dispels fear of abandonment. Praise for correct breathing, relaxation efforts, and pushing efforts not only encourages repetition of the behavior but also decreases anxiety about the ability to cope with labor.

The woman's partner and other members of her support team may also experience increasing anxiety as the woman advances through labor. Their anxiety can stem from watching their loved one in pain, feeling helpless about their ability to assist her in reducing the pain, a lack of knowledge or information about the labor experience, and lack of support from the labor nurse. Their anxiety may be reduced or kept at a minimum by keeping them informed about the progress of labor, reassuring them that the sounds and behaviors of the woman in labor are normal, explaining procedures and the use of equipment, and praising them for their assistance in supporting the woman through labor.

Labor and childbirth may be a time of increased anxiety for the woman with a history of sexual abuse or rape. All women entering the healthcare arena need to be assessed for a history of sexual abuse or rape. It is not uncommon for women to deny sexual abuse or rape, because this information is difficult to share with a stranger. It is important to be alert for nonverbal cues, such as unexplained anxiety, unrelenting pain, or intense fear during vaginal examinations. The nurse should offer support, provide information, and introduce relaxation techniques to aid the woman in coping to offset her anxiety.

Providing Information

Providing information about the nature of the discomfort that will occur during labor is important and is best achieved in the early portion of labor. Stressing the intermittent nature and maximum duration of the contractions can be most helpful. The woman can cope with pain better when she knows how far she has progressed and that a period of relief will follow. Describing the type of discomfort and specific sensations that will occur as labor progresses helps the woman recognize these sensations as normal and expected when she does experience them.

A thorough explanation of surroundings, procedures, and equipment being used also decreases anxiety, thereby reducing pain. For some patients, attachment to an electronic monitor can produce fear because equipment of this type is associated with critically ill people. For others, hearing the infant's heartbeat is reassuring. The nurse should explain the purpose of the monitor and the monitor strip, and show the woman and her support persons how the monitor can help them use controlled breathing techniques to relieve pain. The monitor may indicate the beginning of a contraction just seconds before the woman feels it. The woman and coach can learn how to read the tracing to identify the beginning of the contraction.

Supportive Relaxation Techniques

Tense muscles increase resistance to the descent of the fetus and contribute to maternal fatigue and anxiety. This fatigue increases pain perception and decreases the woman's ability to cope with the pain. Comfort measures, massage, techniques for decreasing anxiety, and patient teaching can conserve energy. The laboring woman needs to be encouraged to use the periods between contractions to rest and relax her muscles.

Distraction is a method of increasing relaxation and coping with discomfort. During early labor, conversation or activities such as light reading, cards, or other games serve as distractions.

Touch is another type of distraction. Although some women regard touching as an invasion of privacy or threat to their independence, others want to touch and be touched during a painful experience. Nurses can make themselves available to the woman who desires touch. The nurse can place a hand on the side of the bed within the woman's reach. The person who needs touch will reach out for contact, and the nurse can pick up and follow through with this behavioral cue.

Mild to moderate abdominal discomfort during contractions may be relieved or lessened by effleurage. Back pain associated with labor may be relieved more effectively by firm pressure on the lower back or sacral area. To apply firm pressure, the nurse or a support person places a hand or a rolled, warmed towel or blanket in the small of the woman's back. Warm compresses can also provide relief.

Visualization techniques also enhance relaxation. For example, the nurse might encourage the woman to imagine herself floating in a warm pool of water, fully supported; to imagine the birth canal slowly opening up as the baby descends; or to visualize a rose opening its petals. Or the woman may simply wish to recall and concentrate on a pleasant experience she has had in the past. Table 24-5 describes a simple visualization method.

In addition to these measures, the nurse can enhance the woman's relaxation by providing encouragement and support for controlled breathing techniques.

Breathing Techniques

Breathing techniques may help the laboring woman. Breathing techniques increase the woman's pain threshold, encourage relaxation, provide distraction, enhance the ability to cope with uterine contractions, and allow the uterus to function more efficiently.

Many women learn breathing techniques during prenatal education classes. Patterned-paced breathing, which is commonly used in the Lamaze method, has three levels. The woman tends to begin with the first level and then proceed to the next when she feels the need. Regardless of the level of breathing used, a cleansing breath begins and ends each pattern. A cleansing

TABLE 24-5 Simple Visualization Method

- Direct a visualization by saying something like the following: "Think about a place you have been that has pleasant memories and feelings around it. A place that was relaxing, where all your stress disappeared. As you think about this place, take in a breath and remember the smells around it. If it was outside, feel the warmth of the sun or the way the breeze felt on your face. Sit in the place again in your mind. Let all your tension and tiredness leave your body as you feel the warmth and breezes."
- Give the woman a few moments to think about her special place: Ask if she would like to share information about the setting. If the woman chooses to do this, add the information to help her with the visualization (for example, "Think about the mountain cabin and the warmth of the sun on your face as you sit in the rocking chair on the front porch").
- After the woman has a visualization set up, suggest thinking about it during contractions as a means of increasing relaxation and focusing concentration. You could say, "As each contraction begins, think about this special place for a moment, and let your body relax. Keep a picture of your place in your mind as you breathe with the contraction. When the contraction is over, let your body stay relaxed. Feel the comfort of this room and support of those around you."

breath involves only the chest. It consists of inhaling through the nose and exhaling through pursed lips (as if blowing on a spoonful of hot food). See Table 24-6 for information regarding nursing support of patterned-paced breathing.

Other childbirth education models encourage different types of breathing exercises. Abdominal breathing, which is commonly used in the Bradley method, encourages the woman to move the abdominal wall upward as she inhales and downward as she exhales (see Table 24-6). This method tends to lift the abdominal wall off the contracting uterus and thus may provide some pain relief. The breathing is deep and rhythmic. If the woman has not been trained in a particular technique, teaching her the "quick method," which uses a pant-pant-blow breathing pattern, may help her from breathing too rapidly (see Table 24-6).

Hyperventilation may occur when a woman breathes very rapidly over a prolonged period of time. Hyperventilation is the result of an imbalance of oxygen and carbon dioxide (that is, too much carbon dioxide is exhaled, and too much oxygen remains in the body). The signs and symptoms of hyperventilation are tingling or numbness in the tip of nose, lips, fingers, or toes; dizziness; spots before the eyes; or spasms of the hands or feet (carpal-pedal spasms). If hyperventilation occurs, the woman should be encouraged to slow her breathing rate and to take shallow breaths. With instruction and encouragement, many women are able to change their breathing to correct the problem. Encouraging the woman to relax and counting out loud for her so she can pace her breathing during contractions are also helpful. If the signs and symptoms continue or become more severe (that is, if they progress from numbness to spasms), the woman can breathe into a paper surgical mask or into her hands until symptoms abate. Breathing into a mask or her hands causes rebreathing of carbon dioxide. The nurse should remain with the woman to reassure her.

As the woman uses her breathing technique, the nurse can assess and support the interaction between the woman and her coach or support person. In the absence of a coach, the nurse supports the laboring woman by helping to identify the beginning of each contraction and encouraging her as she breathes through it.

TABLE 24-6 Nursing Support of Patterned-Paced Breathing

Determine which breathing method the woman (couple) has learned. Provide encouragement as needed in maintaining breathing pattern. Provide support to the labor coach and assist as needed.

Lamaze Breathing Pattern Levels

First Level (slow paced)

Pattern begins and ends with a cleansing breath (in through the nose and out through pursed lips as if cooling a spoonful of hot food). While inhaling through the nose and exhaling through pursed lips, slow breaths are taken, moving only the chest. The rate should be approximately 6–9 breaths/minute or 2 breaths/15 seconds. The coach or nurse may assist by reminding the woman to take a cleansing breath, and then the breaths could be counted out if needed to maintain pacing. The woman inhales as someone counts "one one thousand, two one thousand, three one thousand, four one thousand." Exhalation begins and continues through the same count.

Second Level (modified paced)

Pattern begins and ends with a cleansing breath. Breaths are then taken in and out silently through the mouth at approximately 4 breaths/5 seconds. The jaw and entire body need to be relaxed. The rate can be accelerated to 2–2 1/2 breaths/second. The rhythm for the breaths can be counted out as "one and two and one and two and . . ." with the woman exhaling on the numbers and inhaling on "and."

Third Level (pattern paced)

Pattern begins and ends with a cleansing breath. All breaths are rhythmical, in and out through the mouth. Exhalations are accompanied by a "hee" or "hoo" sound in a varying pattern, 2:1, which begins as 3:1 (hee hee hee hoo) and can change to 2:1 (hee hee hoo) or 1:1 (hee hoo) as the intensity of the contraction changes. The rate should not be more rapid than 2–2 1/2 breaths/second. The rhythm of the breaths would match a "one and two and . . ." count.

Abdominal Breathing Pattern Cues

The abdomen moves outward during inhalation and downward during exhalation. The rate remains slow with approximately 6–9 breaths/minute.

Quick Method

When the woman has not learned a particular method and is in active phase of labor, the nurse may teach her a combination of two patterns. Abdominal breathing may be used until labor is more advanced. Then a more rapid pattern consisting of two short blows from the mouth followed by a longer blow can be used. (This pattern is called "pant-pant-blow" even though all exhalations are a blowing motion.)

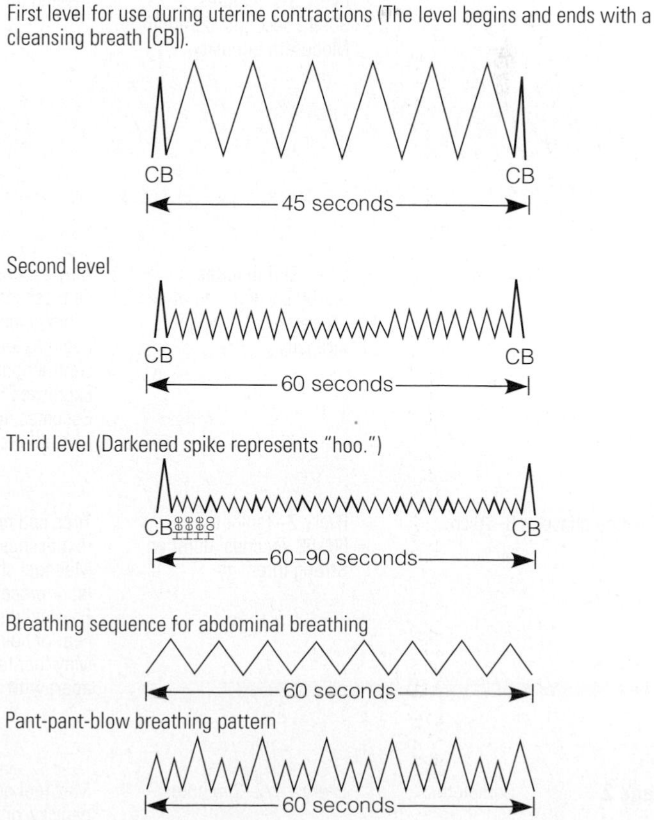

Continued encouragement and support with each contraction through labor yield immeasurable benefits.

COMPLEMENTARY AND ALTERNATIVE THERAPIES

The use of hydrotherapy during labor promotes maternal relaxation and pain management and decreases the length of labor. Thus women can be encouraged to use a warm bath, shower, or whirlpool to increase comfort during labor. Centuries-old water immersion in hot springs, and more recently in hot tubs and whirlpools, is used all over the world to promote relaxation and relax muscles. Current evidence supports the use of hydrotherapy in labor as an effective method of pain management in the first stage of labor. Women who use hydrotherapy report less pain and use less analgesia during the first stage of labor. Use of hydrotherapy also facilitates upright positioning, which facilitates labor and coping (Stark, Rudell, & Haus, 2008). Water immersion has both physical and psychologic benefits, including counterpressure and support of stretching tissues.

Other Comfort Measures

In some instances, analgesic agents or regional anesthetic blocks may be used to enhance comfort and relaxation during labor. See chapter 25 for a discussion of analgesia and anesthesia.

Table 24-7 summarizes labor progress, possible responses of the laboring woman, and nursing care during the first and second stages of labor.

Nursing Care During the Second Stage of Labor

Nursing care in the second stage entails both physical and psychologic support, continual encouragement, and appropriate patient teaching to facilitate birth.

Provision of Care in the Second Stage

The second stage begins when the cervix is completely dilated (10 cm). The uterine contractions continue as in the transition

TABLE 24-7 Normal Progress, Psychologic Characteristics, and Nursing Support During First and Second Stages of Labor

PHASE	CERVICAL DILATATION	UTERINE CONTRACTIONS	WOMAN'S RESPONSE	SUPPORT MEASURES
Stage 1				
Latent phase	1–3 cm	Every 10–20 minutes, 15–20 seconds' duration Mild intensity *progressing to* Every 5–7 minutes, 30–40 seconds' duration Moderate intensity	Usually happy, talkative, and eager to be in labor Exhibits need for independence by taking care of own bodily needs and seeking information	Establish rapport on admission and continue to build during care. Assess information base and learning needs. Be available to consult regarding breathing technique if needed; teach breathing technique if needed and in early labor. Orient family to room, equipment, monitors, and procedures. Encourage woman and partner to participate in care as desired. Provide needed information. Assist woman into position of comfort; encourage frequent change of position; encourage ambulation during early labor. Offer fluids/ice chips. Keep couple informed of progress. Encourage woman to void every 1 to 2 hours. Assess need for an interest in using visualization to enhance relaxation and teach if appropriate.
Active phase	4–7 cm	Every 2–3 minutes, 50–60 seconds' duration Moderate to strong intensity	May experience feelings of helplessness Exhibits increased fatigue and may begin to feel restless and anxious as contractions become stronger Expresses fear of abandonment Becomes more dependent as she is less able to meet her needs	Encourage woman to maintain breathing patterns. Provide quiet environment to reduce external stimuli. Provide reassurance, encouragement, support; keep couple informed of progress. Promote comfort by giving back rubs, sacral pressure, cool cloth on forehead, assistance with position changes, support with pillows, effleurage. Provide ice chips, ointment for dry mouth and lips. Encourage to void every 1 to 2 hours. Offer shower/whirlpool/warm bath if available.
Transition phase	8–10 cm	Every 2–3 minutes, 60–90 seconds' duration Strong intensity	Tires and may exhibit increased restlessness and irritability May feel she cannot keep up with labor process and is out of control Physical discomforts Fear of being left alone May fear tearing open or splitting apart with contractions	Encourage woman to rest between contractions. If she sleeps between contractions, wake her at beginning of contraction so she can begin breathing pattern (increases feeling of control). Provide support, encouragement, and praise for efforts. Keep couple informed of progress; encourage continued participation of support persons. Promote comfort as listed above but recognize many women do not want to be touched when in transition. Provide privacy. Provide ice chips, ointment for lips. Encourage to void every 1 to 2 hours.
Stage 2	Complete	Every 1 1/2–2 minutes	May feel out of control, helpless, panicky, or may be happy that she can take a more active role in pushing	Assist woman in pushing efforts. Encourage woman to assume position of comfort. Provide encouragement and praise for efforts. Keep couple informed of progress. Provide ice chips. Maintain privacy as woman desires.

TABLE 24-8 Nursing Assessments in the Second Stage

MOTHER	FETUS
Blood pressure, pulse, respiration every 5–15 minutes.	FHR every 5 minutes.
Uterine contraction palpated continuously.	

phase. Sterile vaginal examinations are performed to assess fetal descent. Maternal pulse, blood pressure, and fetal heart rate (FHR) are assessed every 5 minutes; some protocols recommend assessment after each contraction (Cunningham et al., 2010). Table 24-8 summarizes nursing assessments in the second stage of labor.

As the woman pushes during the second stage, she may make a variety of sounds. At times, these sounds are disturbing for nurses and physicians, and they feel the need to help her or encourage her to be more quiet. Other nurses feel more comfortable with maternal sounds and use them as cues. For example, if the woman begins to feel she is losing control, her sound may change to a high-pitched cry or whimper, or she may even shriek in pain. The nurse stays sensitive to changes in the sounds for clues that the woman needs help coping with her pain. The nurse may encourage her to push harder and not let any breath out, or to put all her effort into the push and not into making noise. But the nurse needs to be aware that maternal sounds may be a coping mechanism for some women and may assist in their pain management.

Several nursing research studies have been conducted focusing on when a woman should push during the second stage of labor. A review article on research focusing on pushing during the second stage recommends that the woman be allowed to rest at the beginning of the second stage and to begin pushing when she feels the natural urge to bear down. There is a decrease in maternal fatigue levels and an increase in fetal oxygenation with fewer decelerations noted when women delay pushing until they feel the urge to push. Furthermore, women who delayed pushing pushed for a shorter period of time and experienced less postpartum fatigue (Lin, Lin, Li, et al., 2009).

When the woman reports feeling an uncontrollable urge to push (bear down), the nurse can help her greatly by letting her know that these new sensations are normal. This is because some women interpret the increased rectal pressure as a need to move her bowels. The instinctive response is to tighten muscles rather than bear down. The woman may also report that she fears she is "splitting apart" or that she feels a "ring of fire." The woman who expects these sensations and understands that bearing down contributes to progress at this stage is more likely to do so.

> **"When I tried to push with the contractions, I felt as if I would tear apart. It hurt so badly that I was shaking. I knew it was time to push and my body was telling me, too, but it hurt so much. The nurse kept saying, "Just push and you will feel better." I wanted to scream at her. She had no idea what was happening to me."**

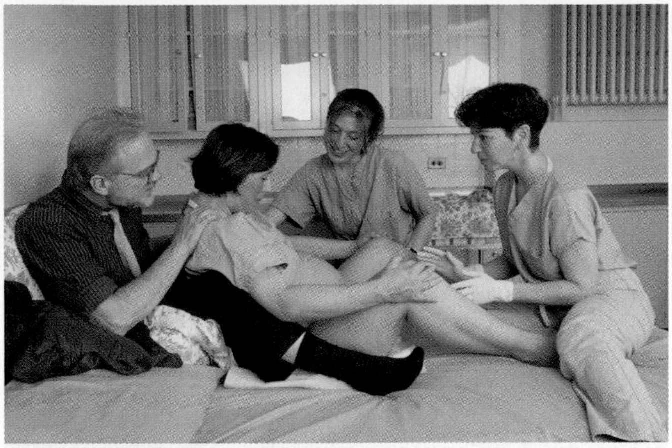

Figure 24-5 ■ The nurse provides encouragement and support during pushing efforts.

Source: Margaret Miller/Photo Researchers, Inc.

When the contraction begins, the nurse tells the woman to take two short breaths, then to take a third breath and hold it while pulling back on her knees and pushing down with her abdominal muscles (Figure 24-5 ■). Some women prefer to exhale slightly (exhale breathing) while pushing to avoid the physiologic effects of the Valsalva maneuver. With this method the woman takes several deep breaths and then holds her breath for 5 to 6 seconds. Then, through slightly pursed lips, she exhales slowly every 5 to 6 seconds while continuing to hold her breath. The woman takes another breath and continues exhale breathing and pushing during the contraction.

> **" I knew when I was completely dilated. I knew when to push and I did it without tearing. My body told me to listen. I knew what to do.**
>
> **When I began pushing, I felt in control because I could do something . . . I could push the baby out. I knew he was ready to be born. "**
>
> —*Harriette Hartigan, Women in Birth*

The woman is encouraged to rest between contractions. Although the laboring woman may appear exhausted at this time, most experience relief at being able to push with contractions. Perspiration increases with the pushing efforts, and a cold washcloth for the forehead and face is most soothing. The birthing woman may also appreciate sips of fluid or ice chips at this time.

The nurse and/or support person can assist the woman into a comfortable position for pushing. Maternal positions, such as standing, squatting while leaning back on a partner or leaning forward on a birthing bar (Figure 24-6 ■), lying in a lateral or Sims' position, or crouching on hands and knees, may increase comfort and effectiveness of pushing. Some women feel that sitting on a toilet seat is a comfortable position that assists their pushing efforts. This position may cause anxiety in the caregivers, however, for fear that the birth may occur quickly in this most inopportune place. Some women benefit from gripping

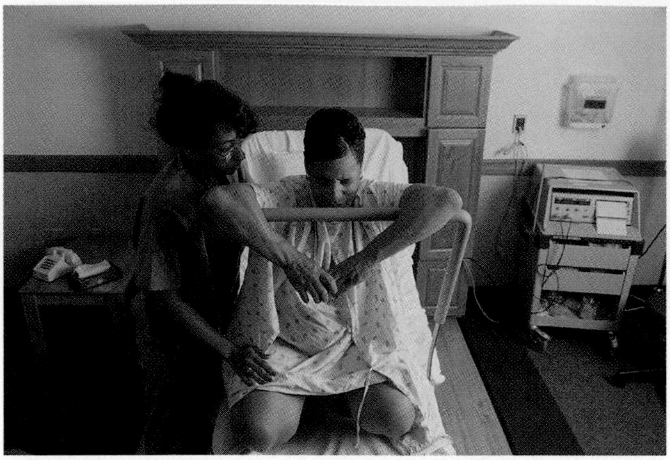

Figure 24-6 ■ Using a birthing bar.

Source: Photographer, Elena Dorfman.

the hands of the support person or nurse. This technique increases intra-abdominal pressure, which aids in the expulsion effort. Another variation of this technique, which can be quite effective, is to have the woman grip a towel while the support person or nurse pulls the towel in the opposite direction. Care should be taken that the nurse or support person does not suffer a back injury. Pushing efforts should be maximized by having the woman place her chin to her chest and avoid hyperextension of the neck by having her "curl around the baby" to facilitate descent into the pelvis.

If anticipated progress is not made or the laboring woman wants to try other positions for pushing, the nurse should support her. Some nurses have their own preferences and may be more comfortable directing the laboring woman to use these preferred positions; however, it is important to remember that the nurse is there to support the birth, and that frequent changes in position may assist in the descent of the baby.

If the maternal pushing effort diminishes because of frustration or fatigue, many women benefit from short rest periods. Rest periods are appropriate if maternal and fetal assessments are stable. In addition, the physician or certified nurse-midwife (CNM) should be informed of the actual time that has been spent pushing and not the time that has elapsed since the beginning of the second stage. If the maternal vital signs are stable and the FHR is reassuring, rest periods can be used to prevent maternal exhaustion (Cunningham et al., 2010).

Throughout the second stage, it remains important to provide information regarding progress and what is happening in the labor. It is also imperative to address the woman's questions honestly, to acknowledge her concerns, and to continue to provide support.

A nullipara is usually prepared for birth when the perineum begins to bulge. A multipara usually progresses much more quickly, so she may be prepared for the birth when the cervix is dilated 7 to 8 cm.

The woman's blood pressure and the FHR are monitored between contractions, and the contractions are palpated until the birth. The nurse continues to assist the woman in her pushing efforts. Both the woman and the coach are kept informed of procedures and of progress, and both are supported throughout the birth.

In addition to assisting the woman and her partner, the nurse assists the physician or CNM in preparing for the birth. The physician or CNM usually dons a sterile gown and gloves and may place sterile drapes over the woman's abdomen and legs. Some providers may perform a sterile preparation before birth; others may not do so as part of their normal routine. Although some physicians and CNMs may place the woman in stirrups for birth, others may opt to drop the foot of the bed lower than the upper portion and let the woman rest her feet on the bed to facilitate maternal comfort. An episiotomy may be done just before birth if there is a need for one or if the provider performs them on a routine basis. See the discussion of episiotomy in chapter 28 ∞.

Promotion of Comfort in the Second Stage

Most of the comfort measures that have been used during the first stage remain appropriate at this time. Cool cloths to the face and forehead may help provide cooling as the woman is involved in the intense physical exertion of pushing. If she has been diaphoretic, a dry gown may be comforting. The woman may feel hot and want to remove some of the covering. Care still needs to be taken to provide privacy even though covers are removed. Some women may want to remove all of their clothing. Healthcare providers should allow the woman to give birth in a way that will promote her comfort.

Additional comfort measures may be used during this stage. Warm perineal, abdominal, and back compresses may be used to increase muscle relaxation. Perineal massage and stretching with a lubricant (Lubafax) may relieve the tearing and burning sensation as the perineal tissue distends. Providing perineal massage before imminent crowning can result in considerable perineal edema. For this reason, some institutions may limit perineal massage to physicians and CNMs.

The woman can be encouraged to rest and "let all muscles go" during the period between contractions. The nurse and support person(s) can assist the woman into a pushing position with each contraction to further conserve energy. Sips of fluid or ice chips may be used to provide moisture and relieve dryness of the mouth. Constant reassurance is imperative.

Visualization techniques may be helpful. The woman can be encouraged to envision the infant descending the birth canal and the vagina opening up. Phrases such as "Open to your baby" and "Let the baby come; don't try to hold back" can be useful and calming. Many women benefit from visualizing the descent of the fetus in a mirror. The nurse should ask the woman if she would like to watch in the mirror.

Assisting the Couple and Physician or CNM During Birth

Shortly before the birth, the birthing room or delivery room is prepared with equipment and materials that may be needed. Family members do not need to change into other clothing if the birth occurs in a birthing room; they don a disposable scrub suit if the birth is to occur in a delivery room or surgery suite. Meticulous handwashing is required of the nurses and CNM or physician. Nurses who will be in direct contact with the mother at the time of birth need to wear protective clothing, such as an apron or gown with a splash apron, disposable gloves, and eye covering. The CNM or physician will also need to wear a gown with a splash apron or a plastic apron, eye covering, and sterile gloves.

Most facilities now use one room for labor, delivery, and recovery (LDR) rooms. Use of a separate birthing room is rare. If the laboring woman is to give birth in a separate birthing room, she will be moved shortly before birth on her bed or a cart. It is important to preserve her privacy during the transfer, and safety must be provided by raising the side rails into a locked position. In the birthing room, the labor bed or transfer cart must be carefully supported against the delivery table; this ensures the woman's safety during the transfer.

If the woman is to be moved from one bed to another, it should be done between contractions. During the contraction, the woman feels increased discomfort and may be involved in pushing efforts. Perineal bulging may be occurring, which adds to the discomfort and difficulty in moving. All of these factors make moving the woman very uncomfortable. If birth seems imminent (within the next minute), it is safer for the woman to give birth in her labor bed or on the cart. Transfer to the delivery table is then delayed until after the baby is born and the cord has been clamped and cut.

Even though there are differences in the birthing room setting, the family can still be together during the birth. It is important to provide encouragement for family members to participate because the delivery room environment may be unfamiliar and seem less relaxed. The family member may be hesitant to continue to provide support for fear of interfering or being in the way. The nurse can ensure that family members are included throughout the birthing process by giving them simple directions about how they can assist and be involved in the process.

Maternal Birthing Positions

The woman is usually positioned for birth on a bed, birthing chair, or delivery table. In some instances, she may give birth standing at the side of the bed or on her hands and knees on the floor. The position the woman assumes is determined not only by her individual wishes but also by the CNM or physician.

If stirrups are used, they should be padded to alleviate pressure, and both legs should be lifted simultaneously to avoid strain on abdominal, back, and perineal muscles. The stirrups should be adjusted to fit the woman's legs. The feet are supported in the stirrup holders. The height and angle of the stirrups are adjusted so there is no pressure on the back of the knees or the calf, which might cause discomfort and postpartal vascular problems. This is particularly true of women with epidural anesthesia. The birthing bed is elevated 30 to 60 degrees to help the woman bear down, and handles are provided so she may pull back on them.

The upright posture for birth was considered normal in most societies until modern times. Alternatively, women selected squatting, kneeling, standing, and sitting for birth. Only within the last 200 years has the recumbent position become the norm in the Western world. Its use in this century has been reinforced because of the convenience it offers in applying new technology, and it has thus become the conventional manner in which North American women give birth in hospitals. In searching for alternative positions, consumers and professionals alike continue to refocus on the comfort of the laboring woman and the advantages of alternative positions rather than on the convenience of the CNM or physician (Table 24-9).

RECUMBENT POSITION The recumbent (lithotomy) position for birth is used sometimes to enhance the maintenance of asepsis, assessment of FHR, and performance of episiotomy and repair. In contrast, when the comfort and well-being of the woman and fetus are considered, the following disadvantages have been noted (Blackburn, 2007):

- There is a decrease of as much as 30% in the blood pressure of 10% of women.
- Many women experience difficulty breathing because of pressure of the uterus on the diaphragm.
- The uterine axis is directed toward the symphysis pubis instead of the pelvic inlet, thus interfering with fetal alignment.
- Aspiration of vomit is more likely.
- The woman may feel resentment at being forced to assume an "embarrassing" position.
- Supine hypotension syndrome may occur.
- The labor may be prolonged and may lead to the use of medications to augment labor.
- The contractions may seem more uncomfortable, making coping more difficult.
- Tightening of the vagina and perineum as the thighs are flexed may increase the likelihood of an episiotomy or laceration.
- The position may interfere with the frequency and intensity of contractions.
- Stirrups cause excessive pressure on the legs.
- The woman works against gravity.

These disadvantages may be lessened slightly if the woman has her back elevated 30 to 40 degrees.

LEFT LATERAL SIMS' POSITION A common position favored by some women and birth attendants is the left lateral Sims' or side-lying position (Figure 24-7A ■). In assuming this position for birth, the woman lies on her left side with her left leg extended and her right knee drawn against her abdomen or flexed by her side or with both legs bent at the knees. Although the frequency of contractions may decrease in this position, the intensity increases, yielding greater uterine efficiency (Blackburn, 2007). Those who favor this position find that it increases overall comfort, does not compromise venous return from the lower extremities, puts less stress and pressure on the maternal neck, and diminishes the chances of aspiration should vomiting occur. Women also perceive the lateral Sims' as a more natural and comfortable position and less intrusive with no stirrups or overhead lights required. Birth attendants have found that the position has a positive effect on the management of fetal shoulder dystocias. Side-lying positions are also helpful in labors in which the fetus is in a posterior position, because this position allows the uterine weight and the fetus to tip away from the maternal back (Blackburn, 2007). Fewer episiotomies are required in this position because the perineum tends to be more relaxed.

Application: Positioning Options During Labor and Delivery

TABLE 24-9 Comparison of Birthing Positions

POSITION	ADVANTAGES	DISADVANTAGES	NURSING ACTIONS
Recumbent	Enhances ability to maintain sterile field. May be easier to monitor FHR. Easier to perform episiotomy or laceration repair.	May decrease blood pressure. It is difficult for the woman to breathe due to pressure on the diaphragm. There is an increased risk of aspiration. May increase perineal pressure making laceration more likely. May interfere with uterine contractions.	Ensure that stirrups do not cause excess pressure on the legs. Assess legs for adequate circulation and support.
Left lateral Sims'	Does not compromise venous return from lower extremities. Increases perineal relaxation and decreases need for episiotomy. Appears to prevent rapid descent.	It is difficult for the woman to see the birth.	Adjust position so that the upper leg lies on the bed (scissor fashion) or is supported by the partner or on pillows.
Squatting	Size of pelvic outlet is increased. Gravity aids descent and expulsion of newborn. Second stage may be shortened (Cunningham et al., 2010).	It may be difficult to maintain balance while squatting.	Help woman maintain balance. Use a birthing bar if available.
Semi-Fowler's	Does not compromise venous return from lower extremities. Women can view birth process.	If legs are positioned wide apart, relaxation of perineal tissues is decreased.	Assess that upper torso is evenly supported. Increase support of body by changing position of bed or using pillows as props.
Sitting in birthing bed	Gravity aids descent and expulsion of the fetus. Does not compromise venous return from lower extremities. Woman can view the birth process. Leg position may be changed at will.		Ensure that legs and feet have adequate support.
Sitting on birthing stool	Gravity aids descent and expulsion of infant. Does not compromise venous return from lower extremities. Woman can view birth process.	It is difficult to provide support for the woman's back.	Encourage woman to sit in a position that increases her comfort.
Hands and knees	Increases perineal relaxation and decreases need for episiotomy. Increases placental and umbilical blood flow and decreases nonreassuring fetal status. Improves fetal rotation. Better able to assess perineum. Better access to fetal nose and mouth for suctioning at birth. Facilitates birth of infant with shoulder dystocia.	Woman cannot view birth. There is decreased contact with birth attendant. Caregivers cannot use instruments. There may be increased maternal fatigue.	Adjust birthing bed by dropping the foot down. Supply extra pillows for increased support.

The disadvantages cited relate to the difficulty of cutting and repairing large episiotomies and problems with difficult forceps births. These disadvantages, however, can be rectified by repositioning the woman if forceps are needed or if a repair is needed after the birth.

SQUATTING POSITION Squatting is favored by some women primarily for the positive use it makes of gravity, which allows the abdominal wall to relax (Blackburn, 2007). Squatting is thought to facilitate the entrance of the presenting part into the pelvic inlet, thus hastening engagement. This engagement facilitates pressure being applied to the cervix, which aids in stretching it. This in turn can stimulate the myometrium to produce more intense uterine contractions and shorten the length of labor. A squatting bar (birthing bar) may be used across a bed or on the floor to increase the woman's balance and provide some support (see Figure 24-6). During the second stage of labor, squatting increases the size of the pelvic outlet by 28% and helps in the woman's pushing efforts. The pressure from the thighs against the uterus can also aid in fetal descent and help facilitate a favorable fetal position (Blackburn, 2007). Some birth attendants object to this position because the perineum is relatively inaccessible, and it is difficult for them to control the birth process. Squatting also increases the difficulty of administering analgesia, using instruments, and monitoring fetal status. Perineal edema can also occur from prolonged squatting. Ice may be applied intermittently to lessen perineal edema. Women with epidural anesthesia may be unable to assume this position because of the heaviness in their lower extremities.

SEMI-FOWLER'S POSITION Some care providers advocate a semi-Fowler's position as an appropriate middle ground between the recumbent and upright positions. This position has also been associated with shorter first and second stages of labor than the traditional lithotomy position (Blackburn, 2007). This position enhances the effectiveness of the abdominal mus-

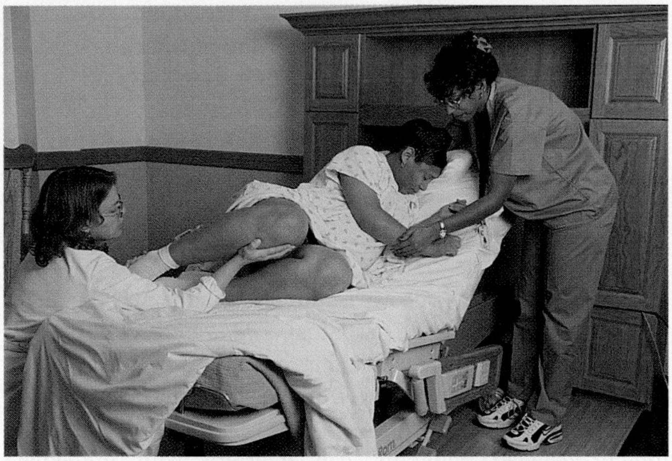

A

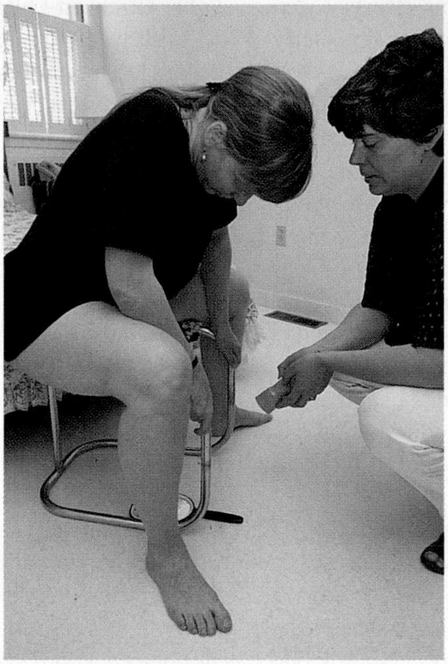

B

Figure 24-7 ■ Birthing positions. A. Side-lying (also known as left lateral Sims') position. B. Using a birthing stool.

Source: A. Photographer, Elena Dorfman. B. © Stella Johnson (www.stellajohnson.com).

cle efforts while the woman is pushing and thereby shortens the second stage of labor. Raising and supporting the torso helps the woman view the birth process. At the same time the birth attendant has access to the perineum. Supporting a woman in this position is not difficult with most birthing beds.

SITTING POSITION The sitting position is becoming an option for more women with the increased availability of birthing chairs. The use of birthing chairs or stools can be traced back to ancient Egypt, and they were widely used in ancient Greek, Roman, and Incan civilizations. In the wake of the 19th-century battle against puerperal fever, birthing chairs began to vanish on hygienic grounds. Birthing chairs are being used again during the second stage of labor and are perceived by some women as a positive way to participate in the birth process (see Figure 24-7B ■). A supported sitting position may also be achieved in a birthing bed.

The upright sitting position offers advantages similar to squatting. It has been associated with stronger, more effective uterine contractions. It has been postulated that the weight of a term fetus is sufficient force in itself to supply much of what is needed to bring the newborn into the world. Proponents of the birthing chair state that it makes possible spontaneous births that would have required operative assistance in the recumbent position. Women experiencing severe back pain have found that use of the chair can diminish or eliminate the pain. The woman can curl forward and grasp her knees and ankles during pushing efforts. She can usually see the birth without aid of mirrors, and following birth she can lift the baby up toward her face.

Duration of the second stage and fetal outcome are not significantly affected by use of the birthing chair. However, it may carry a potential for increased blood loss.

HANDS AND KNEES POSITION The hands and knees position is more comfortable for a woman experiencing back labor because there is less pressure on the maternal back from the fetus, and the fetus may be able to rotate more easily from the posterior position. The mother can be well supported by dropping the foot of the birthing bed and supplying extra pillows upon which she can rest her forearms. Because there is less pressure on the perineum, there is less need for an episiotomy, and the incidence of lacerations is less. The birth attendant is better able to assess the perineum for stretching and has good access to the fetal nose and mouth for suctioning at the time of birth. This position may also increase placental and umbilical blood flow during episodes of nonreassuring fetal status. This position also increases the intensity of the uterine contractions. Lastly, the hands and knees position may increase the pelvic diameter and facilitate birth of the infant with shoulder dystocia. Disadvantages of this position include decreased eye contact between the mother and birth attendant, the inability to use instruments, and the potential necessity of repositioning the mother for perineal repair. Women may also become easily fatigued in this position.

Cleansing the Perineum

If a perineal prep is to be performed, the woman is positioned for the birth, and her vulvar and perineal area is cleansed to increase her comfort and to remove the bloody discharge that is present before the actual birth. An aseptic technique such as the one that follows is recommended.

After thorough handwashing, the nurse opens the sterile prep tray, dons sterile gloves, and cleans the vulva and perineum with the cleansing solution. Beginning with the mons pubis, the area is cleansed up to the lower abdomen. A second sponge is used to clean the inner groin and thigh of one leg, and a third is used to clean the other leg, moving outward to avoid carrying material from surrounding areas to the vaginal outlet. The last three sponges are used to clean the labia and vestibule with one downward sweep each. The used sponges are discarded. Once the cleansing is completed, the woman returns to the desired birthing position. Not all birthing facilities use such formalized cleansing procedures. Some facilities use

Case Study: Labor and Birth of Patient Who Received No Prenatal Care

a spray bottle with povidone-iodine (Betadine) or other cleansing agent and simply spray the perineal area. Because birth is not truly a "sterile procedure" some providers do not perform perineal cleansing techniques.

Supporting the Couple

The nurse assesses the woman's partner or other support person for comfort and knowledge and assists him or her in activities that will support the woman during the second stage. Some support persons will want to take an active role in coaching the woman through the birth process, whereas others will prefer simply to observe the birth process. The nurse assesses the roles the members of the support team desire and provides interventions that enhance these roles. It is important to keep the support team informed of the woman's progress, provide explanations of what is happening, and praise them for their supportive activities. A nurse who provides calm reassurance can help promote a positive experience.

Assisting with the Birth of the Infant

When the fetal head has distended the perineum, the clinician may perform a hand maneuver, such as supporting the perineum between the thumb and four fingers, which is believed to prevent undue trauma to the fetal head and maternal soft tissues. The woman may be asked to breathe rapidly, pant, or blow to avoid too rapid birth of the fetal head. The woman may also be instructed to push and take a breath intermittently to avoid rapid expulsion.

After the infant's head is born, the clinician palpates the neck for the presence of a cord, which can be slipped over the fetal head if it is loose. If the cord is tight, it is double-clamped and cut.

Restitution and external rotation occur after the head is born. The only assistance needed during this time is support of the maternal perineum. While awaiting completion of external rotation, the clinician suctions the newborn's nose and mouth to remove mucus. When the newborn's shoulder appears at the symphysis pubis, the clinician may use both hands to grasp the newborn's head gently and pull downward for release of the anterior shoulder. Gentle upward traction facilitates release of the posterior shoulder.

Application: Cord Blood Banking

Birth of the newborn's body may be controlled by grasping the posterior shoulder with one hand, palm turned toward the perineum. The left hand may be used for this if the newborn is left occiput anterior (LOA). The right hand then follows along the infant's back, and the feet are grasped as they are expelled. The newborn's head is kept down and to the side as the feet, legs, and body are tucked under the clinician's left arm in a football hold. The clinician's right hand is then free for further care of the newborn, and the newborn is securely held. CNMs often place the newborn directly on the mother's abdomen. The nose and mouth are suctioned with a bulb syringe, and respiratory passages are cleared. Figure 24-8 ■ depicts an entire birthing experience.

Assisting with Clamping the Cord

There is controversy about when to clamp and cut the cord. If the newborn is held at or below the vagina as cord clamping is delayed, as much as 50 to 100 ml of blood may be shifted from the placenta to the newborn. If the newborn is held 50 to 60 cm above the vagina, blood may be transferred from the newborn to the placenta. The extra amount of blood added to the newborn's circulation by holding the newborn below the vagina may reduce the frequency of iron deficiency anemia, which can occur later in infancy. However, in some cases the circulatory overload may produce polycythemia and favor hyperbilirubinemia.

Some parents may specify a preference in their birth plan regarding exactly when the umbilical cord is to be cut. There is some evidence that suggests that delayed cord clamping in preterm infants results in fewer transfusions, lower rates of intraventricular hemorrhage, and a lower incidence of sepsis, although delayed clamping can interfere with immediate resuscitation efforts (Mercer, Vohr, Erickson-Owens, et al., 2009). Infants in one study of low birth weight males who had undergone delayed cord clamping had less motor disabilities at 7 months of age (Mercer et al., 2009). Delayed cord clamping may also benefit infants with a nuchal cord. One study that compared cutting the umbilical cord before the birth of the shoulders versus delayed cord cutting by reducing the cord around the fetal neck showed a reduction in hypovolemia, anemia, shock, hypoxic-ischemic encephalopathy, and cerebral palsy when the delayed approach was used (Mercer et al., 2009). The pros and cons of early and late cord clamping can be discussed before the birth.

The cord is usually clamped with two Kelly clamps and cut between them. The father, other support person, or the mother may wish to cut the cord after it has been clamped by the physician or CNM.

The physician or CNM may double-clamp the cord so that a section can be made available for the collection of cord blood gases. After the cord has been cut, cord blood is collected and sent to the lab as needed.

If the physician or CNM has not placed a cord clamp on the newborn's umbilical stump, it is the responsibility of the nurse to do so. Before applying the cord clamp, the nurse examines the cut end for the presence of two arteries and one vein. The umbilical vein is the largest vessel, and the arteries are smaller vessels. The presence of only one artery in the umbilical cord is associated with genitourinary abnormalities. The number of vessels is recorded on the birth and newborn records.

The cord is clamped approximately 1/2 to 1 inch from the abdomen to allow room between the abdomen and clamp as the cord dries (Figure 24-9 ■). Abdominal skin must not be clamped because this will cause necrosis of the tissue. The clamp is removed in the newborn nursery approximately 24 hours after birth if the cord has dried.

Cord Blood Collection for Banking

Growing numbers of parents are arranging for cord blood banking (see discussion in chapter 1 ∞). Immediately after the newborn's umbilical cord is clamped and cut and before the placenta is expelled, the physician or CNM withdraws blood from the umbilical cord. The blood is placed in a spe-

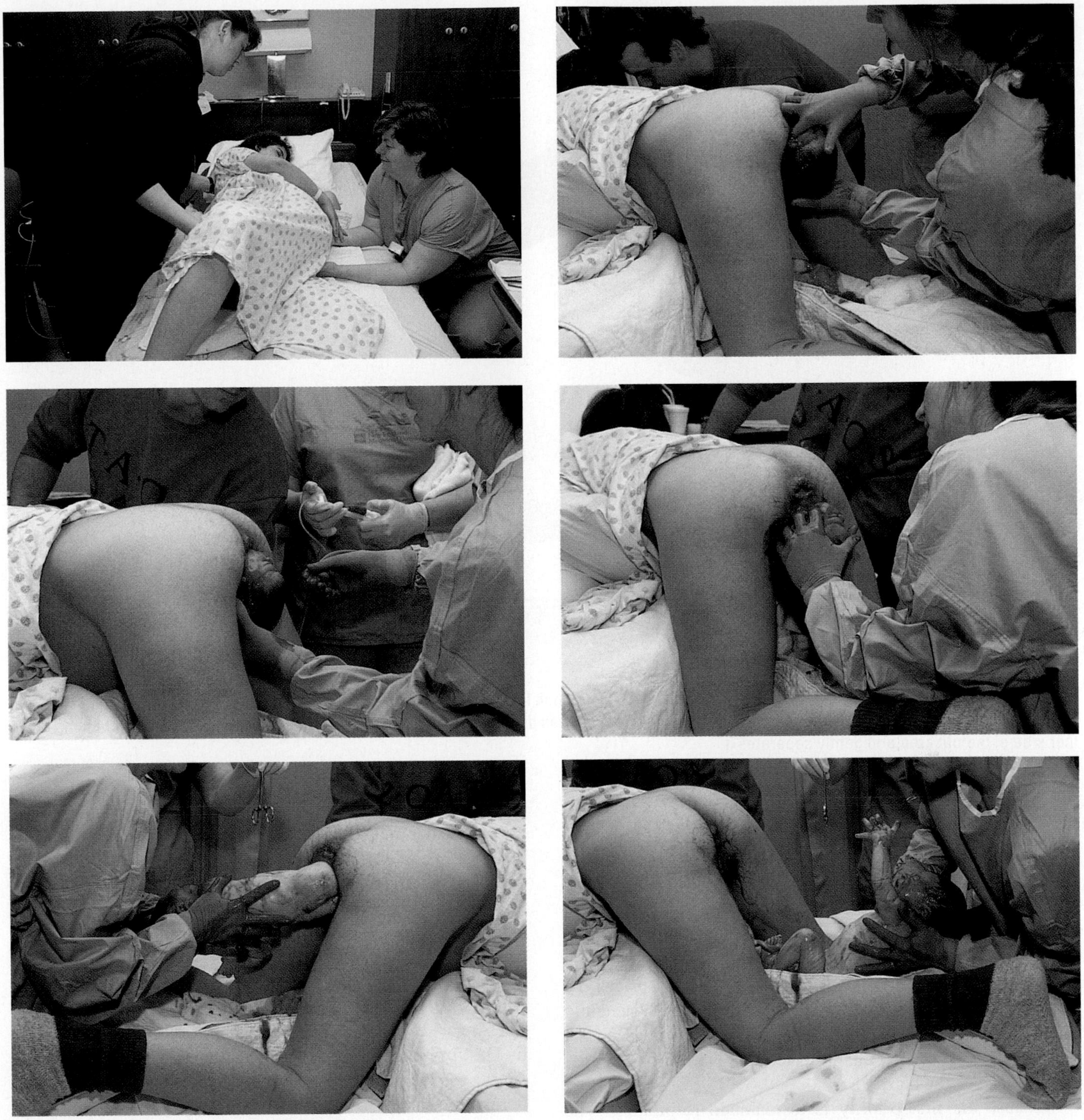

Figure 24-8 ■ A birthing sequence.

Source: © Stella Johnson (www.stellajohnson.com).

cial container that parents receive from the Cord Blood Registry and bring with them for the birth. The parents will have any special directions that are required for storage and care of the container. Although current recommendations for cord blood banking include a family history of an illness that can be treated with fetal cells and children whose parents are from a nontraditional lineage, such as mixed race backgrounds or other ethnic combinations that are uncommon, many families are choosing to bank their infants' cord blood. Stem cell transplants are now used to treat many different types of diseases (Table 24-10). The future of stem cell transplantation is promising, with rapid expansion of uses (Lanfranchi, Porta, & Chirico, 2009).

Table 24-7 on page 612 summarizes labor progress, possible responses of the laboring woman, and nursing care during the first and second stages of labor.

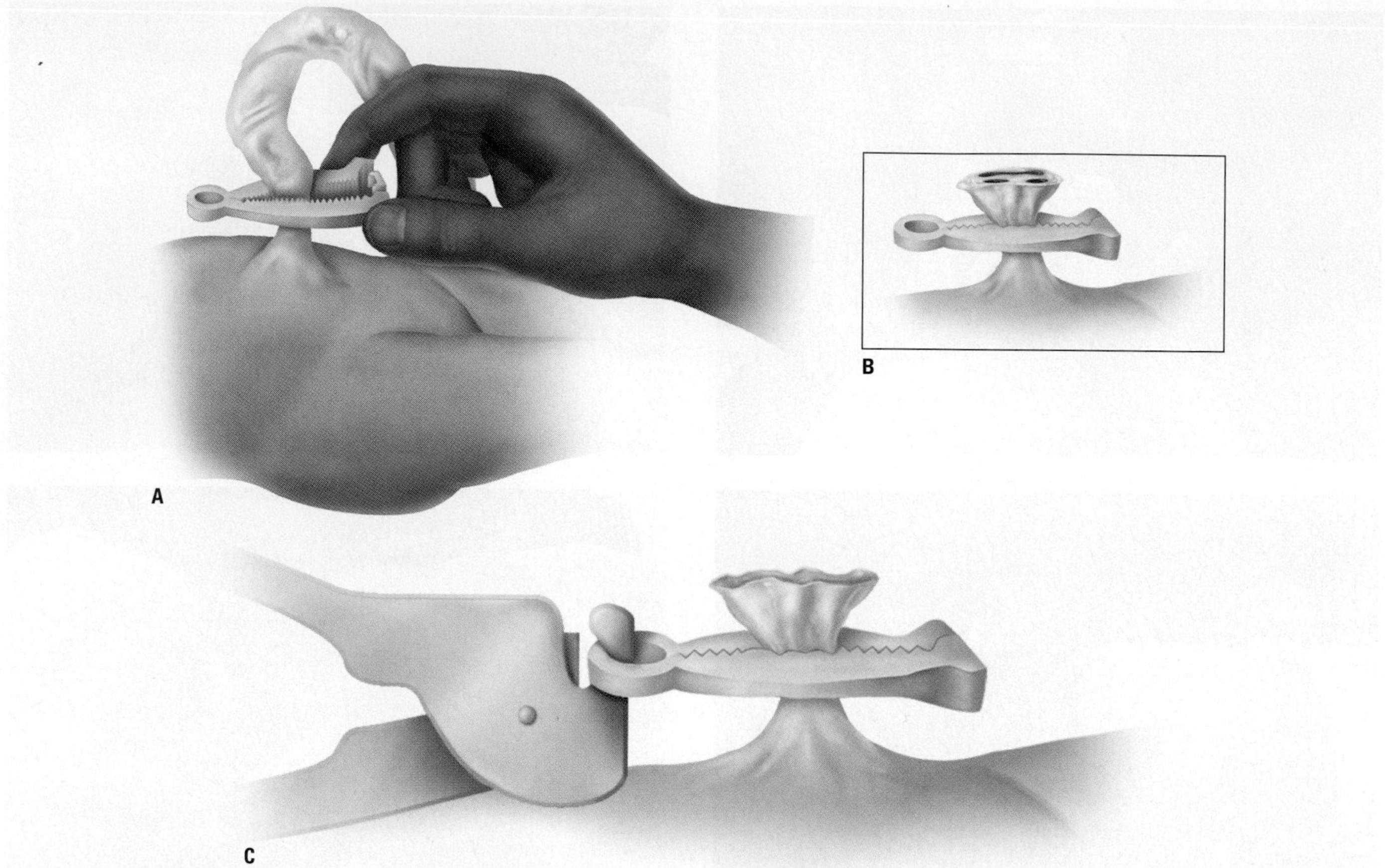

Figure 24-9 ■ Hollister cord clamp. A. Clamp is positioned 1/2 to 1 inch from the abdomen and then secured. B. Cut cord. The one vein and two arteries can be seen. C. Plastic device for removing clamp after cord has dried. After the cord is dried, the nurse grasps the Hollister clamp on either side of the cut area and gently separates it.

Nursing Care During the Third Stage of Labor

Nursing care in the third stage focuses on providing initial newborn care and assisting with birth of the placenta.

Provision of Initial Newborn Care

The physician or certified nurse-midwife (CNM) places the newborn on the mother's abdomen or in the radiant-heated unit to begin the initial care. If the newborn is not placed on the mother's abdomen, the radiant-heated unit is positioned so the parents can see the baby.

Because the first priority is to maintain respirations, the newborn is placed in a modified Trendelenburg position to aid drainage of mucus from the nasopharynx and trachea. The newborn is also suctioned with a bulb syringe or DeLee mucus trap as needed (see Procedure 24-1: Performing Nasal Pharyngeal Suctioning).

The second priority is to provide and maintain warmth, so the newborn is dried immediately with warmed, soft infant blankets. Wet blankets should be immediately removed to prevent heat loss. The nurse dries the newborn's head first to minimize heat loss. Warmth can be maintained by putting the newborn in skin-to-skin contact with the mother and placing warmed blankets over both of them. If the newborn is placed in a radiant-heated unit, he or she is dried, laid on a dry blanket, and left uncovered under the radiant heat. Because radiant heat warms the outer surface of objects, a newborn wrapped in blankets will receive no benefit. In many settings a stocking cap is placed on the newborn's head to conserve heat. See chapter 29 ∞ and chapter 31 ∞ for more information on infant heat loss and keeping infants warm.

Apgar Scoring System

The Apgar scoring system (Table 24-11) was designed in 1952 by Dr. Virginia Apgar, an anesthesiologist. The purpose of the **Apgar score** is to evaluate the physical condition of the newborn at birth. The newborn is rated 1 minute after birth and again at 5 minutes and receives a total score ranging from 0 to 10 based on the following criteria:

1. The heart rate is auscultated or palpated at the junction of the umbilical cord and skin. This is the most important assessment. A newborn heart rate of less than 100 beats/min indicates the need for immediate resuscitation.
2. The respiratory effort is the second most important Apgar assessment. Complete absence of respirations is termed *apnea.* A vigorous cry indicates good respirations.
3. The muscle tone is determined by evaluating the degree of flexion and resistance to straightening of the extremities.

TABLE 24-10 Diseases That May Be Treated with Stem Cell Transplants

Arthritis
- Rheumatoid Arthritis
- Osteoarthritis

Blood Disorders and Cancers
- Aplastic Anemia
- Thrombocytopenia
- Leukemias
- Lymphomas
- Immune Deficiencies
- Marrow Failure
- Sickle Cell Disease
- Thalassemia
- Inherited Disorders Caused by Defective Monocytes

Other Cancers
- Brain Tumors
- Ewing Sarcoma
- Neuroblastoma
- Ovarian Cancer
- Renal Cell Carcinoma
- Rhabdomyosarcoma
- Small Cell Lung Cancer
- Testicular Cancer
- Thymoma (Thymic Carcinoma)

Chronic Pain Disorders

Diabetes and Diabetic Complications
- Type 1 Diabetes Mellitus
- Type 2 Diabetes Mellitus
- Diabetic Ulcers

Inflammatory Bowel Disorders
- Crohn's Disease
- Ulcerative Colitis

Diseases and Disorders of the Eye
- Macular Degeneration
- Diabetic Retinopathy

Heart & Circulatory Diseases
- Hypertension
- Coronary Artery Disease
- Congestive Heart Failure

Liver Diseases
- Hepatitis
- Liver cirrhosis

Nervous System Disorders & Spinal Cord Injuries
- Stroke
- Multiple Sclerosis
- Amyotrophic Lateral Sclerosis (Lou Gehrig's disease)
- Parkinson's Disease
- Alzheimer's Disease
- Epileptiform (or trigeminal) neuralgia
- Muscular Dystrophy (Duchenne's Disease)

Myelodysplastic/Myeloproliferative Disorders

Inherited Immune System Disorders

Inherited Metabolic Disorders

TABLE 24-11 The Apgar Scoring System

	SCORE		
SIGN	**0**	**1**	**2**
Heart rate	Absent	Slow—below 100	Above 100
Respiratory effort	Absent	Slow—irregular	Good crying
Muscle tone	Flaccid	Some flexion of extremities	Active motion
Reflex irritability	None	Grimace	Vigorous cry
Color	Pale blue	Body pink, blue extremities	Completely pink

Source: Reprinted from Pediatric Clinics of North America, 13, *V. Apgar,* The Newborn (Apgar) Scoring System, Reflections and Advice, *p. 645. Copyright © 1966, with permission from Elsevier.*

A normal term newborn's elbows and hips are flexed, with the knees positioned up toward the abdomen.

4. The reflex irritability is evaluated as the newborn is dried or by lightly rubbing the soles of the feet. A cry is a score of 2. A grimace is 1 point, and no response is 0.
5. The skin color is inspected for cyanosis and pallor. Newborns generally have blue extremities, and the rest of the body is pink, which merits a score of 1. This condition, termed *acrocyanosis,* is present in 85% of normal newborns at 1 minute after birth. A completely pink newborn scores a 2, and a totally cyanotic, pale infant is scored 0. Newborns with darker skin pigmentation will not be pink. Their skin color is assessed for pallor and acrocyanosis, and a score is selected based on the assessment.

A score of 7 to 10 indicates a newborn in good condition and requires only nasopharyngeal suctioning. An Apgar score between 4 and 7 indicates the need for stimulation; a score under 4 indicates the need for resuscitation (ACOG, 2006). See further discussion in chapter 34.

Newborn Physical Assessment by the Nurse

An abbreviated systematic physical assessment is performed by the nurse in the birthing area to detect any abnormalities (Table 24-12). First, the nurse notes the size of the newborn and the contour and size of the head in relationship to the rest of the body. The newborn's posture and movements indicate tone and neurologic functioning. The appearance of the head is noted

PROCEDURE 24-1 Performing Nasal Pharyngeal Suctioning

NURSING ACTION

Preparation

- Suction equipment is always available in the birthing area to clear secretions from the newborn's nose or oropharnyx if respirations are depressed or if amniotic fluid was meconium stained.
- Tighten the lid on the DeLee mucus trap or other suction device collection bottle.

  Rationale: *This avoids spillage of secretions and prevents air from leaking out of the lid.*
- Connect one end of the DeLee tubing to low suction.

Equipment and Supplies

DeLee mucus trap or other suction device

Procedure: Clean Gloves

1. Don gloves.
2. Without applying suction, insert the free end of the DeLee tubing 3 to 5 inches into the newborn's nose or mouth (Figure 24-10 ■).

   Rationale: *Applying suction while passing the tube would interfere with smooth passage of the tube.*
3. Place your thumb over the suction control and begin to apply suction. Continue to suction as you slowly remove the tube, rotating it slightly.

   Rationale: *Suctioning during withdrawal removes fluid and avoids redepositing secretions in the newborn's nasopharynx.*
4. Continue to reinsert the tube and provide suction for as long as fluid is aspirated.

Note: *Excessive suctioning can cause vagal stimulation, which decreases the heart rate.*

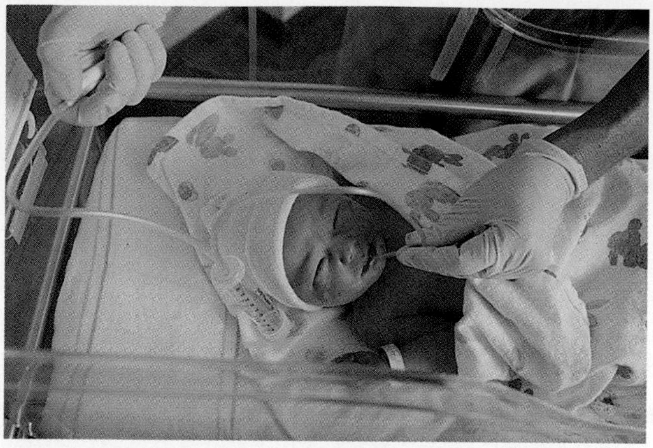

Figure 24-10 ■ A newborn infant being suctioned with a DeLee mucus trap to remove excess secretions from the mouth and nares.

Source: Photographer, Elena Dorfman.

5. If it is necessary to pass the tube into the newborn's stomach to remove meconium secretions that the newborn swallowed before birth, insert the tube through the newborn's mouth into the stomach. Apply suction and continue to suction as you withdraw the tube.

   Rationale: *Because the newborn's nares are small and delicate, it is easier and faster to pass the suction tube through the mouth.*
6. Document the completion of the procedure and the amount and type of secretions.

   Rationale: *This documentation provides a record of the intervention and the status of the infant at birth.*

along with palpation of the fontanelles. The face should be inspected along with the ears and neck.

The skin is inspected for discoloration, presence of vernix caseosa and lanugo, and evidence of trauma and desquamation (peeling of skin). *Vernix caseosa* is a white, cheesy substance normally found on newborns. It is absorbed within 24 hours after birth. Vernix is abundant on preterm infants and absent on postterm newborns. A large quantity of fine hair *(lanugo)* is often seen on preterm newborns, especially on their shoulders, foreheads, backs, and cheeks. Desquamation of the skin is seen in postterm newborns.

The nares are observed for flaring. As the newborn cries, the palate can be inspected for cleft palate. Mucus in the nose and mouth can be assessed and removed with the bulb syringe as needed. The chest is inspected for respiratory rate and the presence of retractions. If retractions are present, the newborn is assessed for grunting or stridor. A normal respiratory rate is 30 to 60 per minute. The lungs may be auscultated bilaterally for breath sounds. Absence of breath sounds on one side may indicate pneumothorax. Rales may be heard immediately after birth because a small amount of fluid may remain in the lungs; this fluid will be absorbed. Rhonchi indicate aspiration of oral secretions. The abdomen is inspected and palpated for masses. The heart is assessed for heart rate, rhythm, and the presence of any murmurs. The normal newborn heart rate is 110 to 160 beats/min. The umbilical cord is inspected, and the number of vessels is recorded.

The genital area, buttocks, and anus are inspected. The elimination of urine or meconium is noted and recorded on the newborn record. The extremities are inspected and compared for symmetry. Reflexes are assessed to determine central nervous system maturity. A complete newborn assessment can be found in chapter 30 ∞.

Newborn Identification

To ensure correct identification, the nurse gives the mother and the newborn identification bands with identical codes in the

TABLE 24-12 Initial Newborn Evaluation

ASSESS	NORMAL FINDINGS
Respirations	Rate 30–60 irregular No retractions, no grunting
Apical pulse	Rate 110–160 and somewhat irregular
Temperature	Skin temp above 36.5°C (97.8°F)
Skin color	Body pink with bluish extremities
Umbilical cord	Two arteries and one vein
Gestational age	Should be 38–42 weeks to remain with parents for extended time
Sole creases	Sole creases that involve the heel

In general, expect scant amount of vernix on upper back, axilla, groin, lanugo only on upper back; ears with incurving of upper 2/3 of pinnae and thin cartilage that springs back from folding; male genitals—testes palpated in upper or lower scrotum; female genitals—labia majora larger; clitoris nearly covered.

In the following situations, newborns should generally be stabilized rather than remaining with parents in the birth area for an extended period of time.

Apgar less than 8 at 1 minute and less than 9 at 5 minutes or baby requires resuscitation measures (other than whiffs of oxygen)

Respirations below 30 or above 60, with retractions and/or grunting

Apical pulse below 110 or above 160 with marked irregularities

Skin temperature below 36.5°C (97.8°F)

Skin color pale blue or circumoral pallor

Baby less than 38 or more than 42 weeks' gestation

Baby very small or very large for gestational age

Congenital anomalies involving open areas in the skin (meningomyelocele)

birthing or delivery room. One bracelet is placed on the mother's wrist and sometimes on the wrist of her partner or a support person whom she designates. Two bracelets are placed on the newborn—one on the wrist and one on the ankle. The newborn bands must be applied snugly to prevent their loss. Infants should not be removed from the room until these identification bands have been placed. The bands should remain in place until the mother and infant are discharged home.

Some facilities now use security devices that are placed on the umbilical cord clamp or the identification bracelet of the infant (Figure 24-11 ■). The alarm is left in place until discharge. The alarm sounds if the infant is removed from the hospital unit or if the alarm is cut or disengaged. Some systems activate a "lockdown" of the birthing unit, thus making abduction of an infant more difficult.

Additional security measures are now commonplace in many maternity settings. Staff must wear appropriate identification at all times. Parents are advised not to allow individuals without proper identification to remove their infant under any circumstances. The nurse also advises the parents to keep the infant on the side of the bed furthest from the door. The infant should be returned to the nursery if the mother plans to nap or shower if no other family member is present.

Although infants were once footprinted for security reasons, the practice is now performed to provide a souvenir for parents and is no longer considered a safety measure. To prepare the newborn for footprinting, the nurse wipes the soles of both the newborn's feet to remove any vernix caseosa. The footprint can be placed on a card or in the parents' baby book.

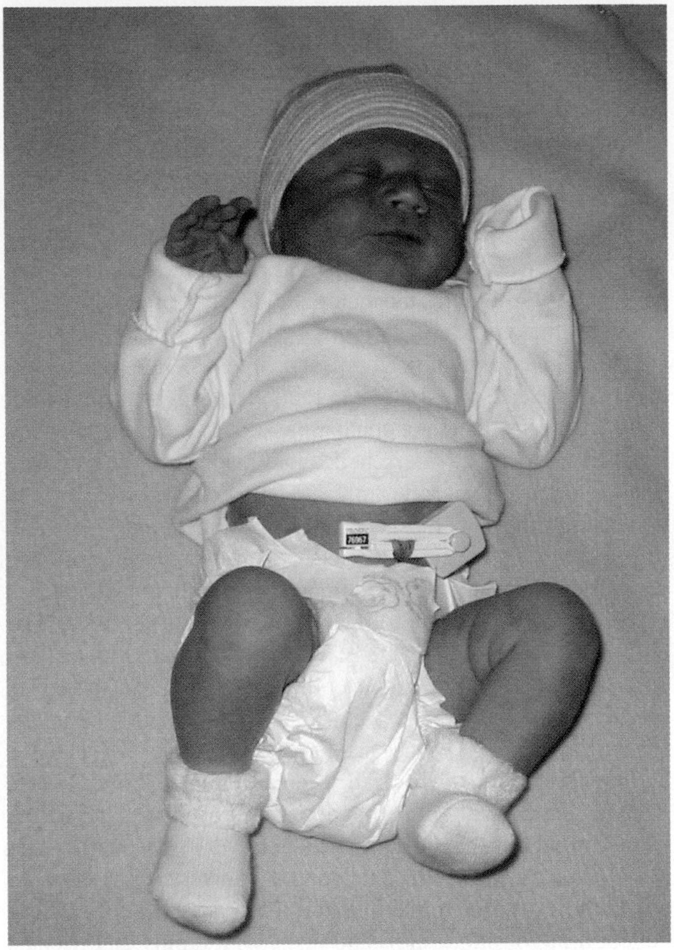

Figure 24-11 ■ Umbilical alarm in place on a newborn infant.

Initiation of Attachment

The birth of the baby is usually an emotionally charged time for all members of the family. The sight of the new baby and the sounds of the first cry may fill the parents with utter amazement. As the baby is placed on the mother's abdomen or chest, she frequently reaches out to touch and stroke her baby. When the newborn is placed in this position, the father also has a very clear, close view and can also reach out to touch his baby.

When the parents feel comfortable in the environment, they may talk to the newborn, and some mothers talk to their babies in a high-pitched voice, which seems to soothe newborns. Some couples verbally express amazement and pride when they see they have produced a beautiful, healthy baby. Their verbalization enhances feelings of accomplishment and profound happiness.

If lights in the birthing area can be dimmed, the newborn will probably open his or her eyes wide and gaze at the surroundings. In this first hour after birth, the newborn is usually quiet and continues to gaze. This is a wonderful opportunity for eye contact with the parents, and many parents are content to gaze quietly at their newborn.

Even though the baby is on the mother's abdomen or chest, the nurse can complete any needed assessments or interventions such as footprinting and applying an identification bracelet to the child. As soon as possible the nurse can assist the mother to a more comfortable position for holding the newborn. Breastfeeding can be encouraged if the mother and baby desire. When the baby is held close to the breast, the baby will seek out the nipple. Even if the newborn does not actively nurse, she or he can lick, taste, and smell the mother's skin. This activity stimulates the maternal release of prolactin, which promotes the onset of lactation.

The initial parental-newborn attachment period can be enhanced if the care providers keep routine investigations to a minimum, delay instillation of ophthalmic antibiotic for the first hour, keep the room slightly darkened, avoid loud noises, talk in quiet tones, and provide privacy. Both parents need to be encouraged to do whatever they feel most comfortable doing. Parents may have differing wishes concerning contact with their newborn. Some want immediate and unlimited time; some prefer to wait until all birth-related activities are completed (the placenta is expelled and episiotomy repair is completed); others prefer limited contact immediately after birth and quiet time later. Although immediate contact may be important for attachment and initiation of breastfeeding, the parents' wishes need to be supported.

Parents can be encouraged to delay phone calls and visits from friends until after the first hour of birth because it is a time when the baby is the most alert. Most facilities have policies in place where the newborn is taken to the nursery for assessment and bathing after an initial visit with the parents. This is an excellent time for phone calls and visits with family and friends. It enables the new family to spend valuable time together and facilitates bonding.

> **"I was hungry for the baby as he was born. I wanted to see, hold him. It was hours before I realized or even thought love in relation to him."**
>
> —Harriette Hartigan, *Women in Birth*

Delivery of the Placenta

Placental Delivery

Delivery of Placenta

After the cord has been clamped and cut, the physician or CNM observes for the following signs of placental separation:

1. The uterus rises upward in the abdomen because the placenta settles downward into the lower uterine segment.
2. As the placenta proceeds downward, the umbilical cord lengthens.
3. A sudden trickle or spurt of blood appears.
4. The uterus changes from a discoid to a globular shape.

While waiting for these signs, the nurse gently palpates the uterus to check for ballooning caused by uterine relaxation and subsequent bleeding into the uterine cavity.

After the placenta has separated, it may be expelled by various techniques such as maternal bearing-down effort, controlled cord traction, and fundal pressure. Maternal effort allows the placenta to be expelled spontaneously and is best accomplished in an upright position. When the mother is in a dorsal recumbent or lithotomy position, she or the nurse can help the process by splinting or supporting her abdominal muscles. The mother or nurse can place her palms over the lower abdomen, or the mother can flex her thighs over her abdomen. The mother then bears down to expel the placenta.

> **DEVELOPING CULTURAL COMPETENCE**
> **Midwife-Attended Births: Malaysia**
>
> In Malaysia, 75% of all births are attended by a *dukun* (midwife). In many parts of the country, especially in rural areas, a home setting is preferred over a hospital setting for birth. It is believed that the baby's first cry is symbolic of loyalty to the parents and should be heard at home. The birth itself is a social event in which many women sit with the laboring woman. It is customary for the woman in labor and her female company to chew red-staining betel nuts. At the time of birth, either the mother or a female relative is given the honor of cutting the umbilical cord.

To help the woman expel her placenta, the physician or CNM first ensures that separation has occurred and then places one hand above the symphysis pubis with the palm against the anterior surface of the uterus. The uterus is displaced upward and backward as the mother is asked to relax her abdominal muscles and breathe through an open mouth. The elevation of the uterus straightens out the birth canal and facilitates expulsion of the placenta, as well as protecting the uterus from inversion. Gentle traction is exerted on the umbilical cord. Excessive pulling may increase the risk of uterine inversion, snapping off of the cord, and subsequent hemorrhage. During this procedure, the nurse encourages the mother to continue breathing through an open mouth and to relax her abdominal muscles.

Fundal pressure is not a method of choice because it is very uncomfortable for the mother, may damage uterine supports, and may invert the uterus. If this method is needed, the mother is asked to relax her abdominal muscles, and then the hand of the physician or CNM is placed behind the uterus with the fingers directed downward toward the maternal spine. With a quick "scooping" motion, the contracted uterus is pressed downward in an arc. This motion is different from direct downward pressure, which folds the uterus over the lower segment and does not enhance movement of the placenta. During the procedure, the nurse provides continued encouragement to maintain abdominal relaxation. This is very difficult because of the discomfort of the procedure.

After expulsion of the placenta, the physician or CNM inspects the placental membranes to make sure they are intact and that all cotyledons are present. This inspection is especially important with placentas expelled via the Duncan mechanism (the chance of tearing off a portion of a cotyledon is greatest with this mechanism of placental separation). If there is a defect or a part missing from the placenta, a digital uterine examination is done. The time and mechanism (Schultze or Duncan) of expulsion of the placenta are noted on the birth record (see chapter 22 and Figures 11-11 ■ and 11-12 ■ on page 228). The vagina and cervix are inspected for lacerations, and any necessary repairs are made. An episiotomy or laceration may be repaired now if it has not been done previously. (See further discussion of episiotomy in chapter 28 ∞.) The fundus of the uterus is palpated; normal position is at the midline and below the umbilicus. If the fundus is displaced, it may be because of a full bladder or a collection of blood in the uterus.

The medical-nursing culture tends to refer to the placenta as the "afterbirth" and considers that its value is fulfilled once it is expelled and examined. Disposal of the placenta is prescribed by the hospital or birth center, and no more thought is given to it. However, many cultures have other beliefs regarding the placenta. Some patients will have specific beliefs about disposal of the placenta and will ask to take it home with them. Labor nurses will need to review hospital policies for disposal of the placenta before giving the placenta to the woman or family members.

Use of Oxytocics

Some CNMs and physicians advocate the use of an oxytocic drug (Pitocin) to stimulate uterine contractions after birth and to reduce the incidence of third-stage hemorrhage.

The physician or CNM may request that 10 units of oxytocin be given intramuscularly to the woman when the anterior shoulder of the infant appears at the vaginal opening. Some practitioners believe that this procedure facilitates the expulsion of the placenta. Others question whether this method increases the incidence of neonatal hyperviscosity because an additional bolus of blood may be infused into the fetus when the uterus contracts in response to the oxytocin. At other times 10 units of oxytocin may be administered intramuscularly at the time of placental expulsion. Both techniques are thought to prevent uterine atony and excessive bleeding. Some prefer to add 10 to 20 units of oxytocin to IV fluids administered over a period of hours. Additional information and associated nursing implications are presented in the Drug Guide: Oxytocin (Pitocin) in chapter 28 ∞. Methylergonovine maleate (Methergine), 0.2 mg can be administered intramuscularly. Methergine should not be given if preeclampsia is present. Carboprost tromethamine (Hemabate) 250 mcg/ml can also be administered intramuscularly (See Drug Guide: Carboprost Tromethamine [Hemabate]). Although the use of misoprostol (Cytotec) in treating postpartum hemorrhage is an off-label use, it is used in some settings with favorable results; however, it does have undesirable side effects including shivering, pyrexia, and diarrhea (Anderson & Etches, 2007).

Nursing Care During the Fourth Stage of Labor

The period immediately following expulsion of the placenta is referred to as the fourth stage of labor and birth. Actually, the label is misleading because labor and birth are completed with delivery of the placenta, and the next few hours are actually the immediate recovery phase. The fourth stage is usually defined as lasting from 1 to 4 hours after the birth or until vital signs are stable. Nursing care in this phase involves the basics of postpartum nursing care.

Immediately after the placenta is expelled, the episiotomy or vaginal lacerations are repaired. The uterus is palpated at frequent intervals, usually every 15 minutes for an hour until bleeding is within normal limits, to ensure that it remains

DRUG GUIDE Carboprost Tromethamine (Hemabate)

PREGNANCY RISK CATEGORY: D

OVERVIEW OF ACTION

Carboprost tromethamine (Hemabate) is used to reduce blood loss secondary to uterine atony. It stimulates myometrial contractions to control postpartum hemorrhaging that is unresponsive to usual techniques. Carboprost tromethamine can also be used to induce labor in women desiring an elective termination of a pregnancy. The drug is also used to induce labor in cases of intrauterine fetal death and hydatidiform mole (Wilson, Shannon, & Stang, 2010).

ROUTE, DOSAGE, FREQUENCY

In cases of immediate postpartum hemorrhage, the usual intramuscular dose is 250 mcg (1 ml) which can be repeated every 1 1/2 to 3 1/2 hours if uterine atony persists. The dosage can be increased to 500 mcg (2 ml) if uterine contractility is inadequate after several doses of 250 mcg. The total dosage should not exceed 12 mg. The maximum duration of use is 48 hours (Wilson et al., 2010).

CONTRAINDICATIONS

The drug is contraindicated in women with active cardiac, pulmonary, or renal disease. It should not be administered during pregnancy or in women with acute pelvic inflammatory disease. It should be used with caution in women with asthma, adrenal disease, hypotension, hypertension, diabetes mellitus, epilepsy, fibroids, cervical stenosis, or previous uterine surgery (Wilson et al., 2010).

SIDE EFFECTS

The most common side effects are nausea and diarrhea. Fever, chills, and flushing can occur. Headache, muscle, joint, abdominal, or eye pain can also occur (Wilson et al., 2010).

NURSING CONSIDERATIONS

1. The injection should be given in a large muscle. Aspiration should be performed to avoid injection into a blood vessel which can result in bronchospasm, tetanic contractions, and shock.
2. After administration, monitor uterine status and bleeding carefully.
3. Report excess bleeding to the physician/CNM.
4. Check vital signs routinely, observing for an increase in temperature, elevated pulse, and decreased blood pressure.
5. Breastfeeding should be delayed for 24 hours after administration (Wilson et al., 2010).

firmly contracted. Although labor is completed, the uterus is sensitive to touch. Palpation of the uterine fundus will be uncomfortable for the woman. If the mother has not held her baby, immediate newborn care should be completed at her side and within her reach so that she can touch her baby during this time. As soon as immediate care is completed, the new mother is usually eager to cuddle and explore her baby. If she plans to breastfeed and the baby is interested, she should be encouraged and helped to do so right after birth while the baby is awake and alert. Care should be taken not to try to force an uninterested baby to breastfeed because it will just lead to frustration for both mother and baby.

Behavioral characteristics of the mother vary, according to such factors as the length of labor, level of fatigue, extent of interruption in normal sleep patterns, and cultural norms. After the initial excitement of becoming acquainted with their new baby and notifying others of the birth, many new mothers are very tired and want to rest. Others are wide awake, eager to talk about their labor, and satisfy basic body needs, such as hunger and thirst.

Provision of Care in the Fourth Stage

As soon as the certified nurse-midwife (CNM) or physician completes the repair of any perineal lacerations or an episiotomy, drapes (if used) are removed. If the mother is to remain in the birthing bed, the nurse places clean absorbent pads beneath her and applies maternity pads. A cold pack may be placed directly on the perineum if perineal edema is present or an episiotomy has been done. If a mother prefers to shower immediately after birth, the nurse can assist her as needed and change the bed linens while the mother is up.

If stirrups were used, her perineum is cleansed and maternity pads applied before her legs are removed from the stirrups. To avoid muscle strain, both legs are removed from the stirrups at the same time. The legs may be held together and gently pushed toward the woman's abdomen, back to a neutral position and then gently lowered toward her right side and then the left side to promote circulation return. If the woman has given birth on a delivery table, she is transferred to a recovery room bed. If the mother has not had a chance to hold her infant, she may do so before she is transferred from the birthing room. The nurse ensures that the mother and father or support person and newborn are given time to begin the attachment process.

In addition to encouraging family celebration of the birth, the immediate recovery period involves assessing both maternal bleeding and newborn stabilization. The most significant source of bleeding is from the site where the placenta was implanted and where uterine vessels previously provided pooling of maternal blood to nourish the fetus. It is therefore critical that the fundus stay well contracted to clamp off these uterine vessels and prevent hemorrhage. It is the nurse's responsibility to assess the mother's blood pressure, pulse, firmness and position of fundus, and amount and character of vaginal blood flow every 15 minutes for the first 1 or 2 hours. Deviations from the normal ranges require more frequent checking.

Blood pressure should return to the prelabor level, and pulse rate should be slightly lower than it was in labor. The maternal blood pressure should be monitored at 5- to 15-minute intervals. The return of the blood pressure is due to an increased volume of blood returning to the maternal circulation from the uteroplacental shunt. Baroreceptors cause a vagal response, which slows the pulse. The physiologic slowing may be offset by excitement, increased temperature, or dehydration. A rise in the blood pressure may be a response to oxytocic drugs or may be caused by preeclampsia. Blood loss may be reflected by a lowered blood pressure and a rising pulse rate. Table 24-13 summarizes maternal changes following birth.

TABLE 24-13 Maternal Adaptations Following Birth

CHARACTERISTIC	NORMAL FINDING
Blood pressure	Returns to prelabor level
Pulse	Slightly lower than in labor
Uterine fundus	In the midline at the umbilicus or 1–2 fingerbreadths below the umbilicus
Lochia	Red (rubra), small to moderate amount (from spotting on pads to 1/4–1/2 of pad covered in 15 minutes) Doesn't exceed saturation of one pad in first hour
Bladder	Nonpalpable
Perineum	Smooth, pink, without bruising or edema
Emotional state	Wide variation, including excited, exhilarated, smiling, crying, fatigued, verbal, quiet, pensive, and sleepy

The fundus should be firm at the umbilicus or lower and in the midline. The uterus should be palpated but not massaged unless boggy (atonic) (Procedure 24-2). When the uterus becomes boggy, pooling of blood occurs within it, resulting in the formation of clots. Anything left in the uterus prevents it from contracting effectively. Thus if it becomes boggy or appears to rise in the abdomen, the fundus should be massaged until firm. The uterus at this time is very tender, and palpation and massage cause discomfort. All palpation and massage should be done as gently as possible.

A boggy uterus feels very soft instead of firm and hard. The uterus may have relaxed so much that it cannot be found when the nurse attempts to palpate it. In this case the nurse places a hand in the midline of the abdomen at the level of the umbilicus and begins to make kneading motions. This motion stimulates the uterine fundus to contract, and the nurse will feel the fundus tighten to a firm, hard object.

CLINICAL TIP

Teach the woman to gently massage her own uterus by feeling for the uterus at the level of the umbilicus. Describe the uterus as a commonly known identifiable object, such as a grapefruit or a softball, to provide a visual cue for the woman. Once she identifies her uterus, she can gently massage it to increase uterine contractions.

The nurse inspects the bloody vaginal discharge, called *lochia,* for amount and charts it as minimal, moderate, or heavy (see chapter 35 ∞). It should be bright red. Because different brands of maternity pads absorb varying amounts of blood, it may be necessary to weigh the maternity pad to determine actual blood loss. A gram scale is used, and 1 g is equivalent to

PROCEDURE 24-2 Assessing the Uterine Fundus Following Vaginal Birth

NURSING ACTION

Preparation

- Explain the procedure, the information it provides, and what it might feel like.
- Ask the woman to void.

  Rationale: *A full bladder can cause uterine atony.*
- Have the woman lie flat in bed with her head on a pillow. If the procedure is uncomfortable, she may find that it helps to flex her legs.

  Rationale: *The supine position prevents falsely high assessment of fundal height. Flexing the legs relaxes the abdominal muscles.*

Equipment and Supplies

A clean perineal pad

Procedure

1. Gently place one hand on the lower segment of the uterus. Using the side of the other hand, palpate the abdomen until you locate the top of the fundus.

   Rationale: *One hand stabilizes the uterus while the other hand locates the top of the fundus.*

> **CLINICAL TIP**
> Gloves may be put on before assessing the abdomen and fundus or when you are ready to assess the perineum and lochia.

2. Determine whether the fundus is firm. If it is, it will feel like a hard round object in the abdomen. If it is not firm, massage the abdomen lightly until the fundus is firm.

   Rationale: *A firm fundus indicates that the uterine muscles are contracted and bleeding will not occur.*
3. Measure the top of the fundus in fingerbreadths above, below, or at the fundus. See Figure 24-12 ■.

   Rationale: *Fundal height gives information about the progress of involution.*
4. Determine the position of the fundus in relation to the midline of the body. If it is not in the midline, locate it and then evaluate the bladder for distention.

   Rationale: *The fundus may deviate from the midline when the bladder is full because the enlarged bladder pushes the uterus aside.*
5. If the bladder is distended, use nursing measures to help the woman void. If she is not able to void after a specified period of time, catheterization may be necessary.
6. Measure urine output for the next few hours until normal elimination is established.

   Rationale: *During the postpartum as diuresis occurs, the bladder may fill far more rapidly than normal, putting the woman at risk for uterine atony and hemorrhage.*
7. Assess the lochia.

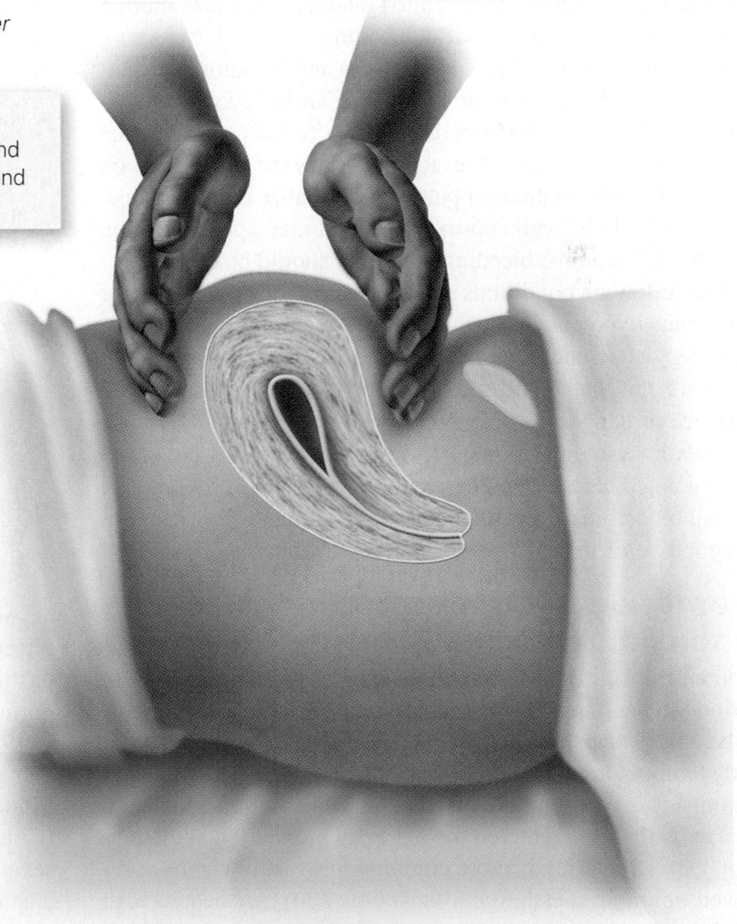

Figure 24-12 ■ Suggested method of palpating the fundus of the uterus during the fourth stage. The left hand is placed just above the symphysis pubis, and gentle downward pressure is exerted. The right hand is cupped around the uterine fundus.

Documentation

The nurse documents the position (midline, deviated to the left or right), fundal height in relation to the umbilicus (F @ U or F @ U ↑ 1 or F @ U ↓ 1), and consistency (firm, boggy). The bladder status should also be recorded (distended, appears empty), along with the time of the last void.

approximately 1 ml of blood. If the perineal pad becomes soaked in a 15-minute period or if blood pools under the buttocks, continuous observation is necessary. As long as the woman remains in bed during the first hour, bleeding should not exceed saturation of one pad. Laceration of the vagina, cervix, or an unligated vessel in the episiotomy may be indicated by a continuous trickle of blood even though the fundus remains firm. (See Procedure 35-2: Evaluating Lochia, on page 1011 ∞).

If the fundus rises and displaces to the right, the nurse palpates the bladder to determine whether it is distended. All measures should be taken to enable the mother to void. If she is unable to void, catheterization is necessary. Postpartal women have decreased sensations to void as a result of the decreased tone of the bladder caused by the trauma imposed on the bladder and urethra during childbirth. The bladder fills rapidly as the body attempts to rid itself of the extra fluid volume returned from the uteroplacental circulation and of IV fluid that may have been received during labor and birth. If the mother is unable to void, a warm towel placed across the lower abdomen, warm water poured over the perineum, or spirits of peppermint poured into a bedpan may help the urinary sphincter relax and thus facilitate voiding. A distended bladder can cause uterine atony, thus increasing postpartal bleeding.

The perineum is inspected for edema and hematoma formation. With an episiotomy or laceration, an ice pack often reduces swelling and alleviates discomfort. To fully visualize the episiotomy or laceration site, the nurse has the woman lie on her side and lifts her anterior buttock to visualize the suture line. The site should be well approximated and may appear swollen or bruised. No active bleeding at the site should be observed.

The following conditions should be reported to the CNM or physician: hypotension, tachycardia, uterine atony, excessive bleeding, or a temperature over 38°C (100°F). The nurse should be aware that the blood pressure may not fall rapidly in the presence of dangerous bleeding in postpartal mothers because of the extra systemic volume. However, an increasing pulse rate may be noted before a decrease in blood pressure is detected. A normal blood pressure with the mother in the Fowler's position is a good confirmation of a normotensive woman.

Promotion of Comfort in the Fourth Stage

Women frequently have tremors in the immediate postpartum period. It has been proposed that this shivering response is caused by exhaustion or a difference in internal and external body temperatures (higher temperature inside the body than on the outside). Another theory is that the woman is reacting to the fetal cells that have entered the maternal circulation at the placental site. Shivering is more common in women who have received epidural anesthesia (Blackburn, 2007). A heated bath blanket placed next to the woman and perhaps a warm drink tend to alleviate the problem.

The couple may be tired, hungry, and thirsty. Some hospitals serve the couple a meal. The tired mother may initially have a period of excitement but may then drift off into a welcome sleep because of exhaustion from the energy that was exerted during labor. The partner should also be encouraged to rest because his supporting role is physically and mentally tiring. The mother is usually transferred from the birthing unit to the postpartum unit after 2 hours or more, depending on agency policy and whether the following criteria are met: stable vital signs, stable lochia, nondistended bladder, firm fundus, and sensations fully recovered from any anesthetic agent received during childbirth.

Nursing Care of the Adolescent

Adolescent pregnancy rates have declined by 28% since 1990, although in 2006 the teenage pregnancy rates began slowly climbing after a 15-year decline (National Campaign to Prevent Teen and Unplanned Pregnancy [NCPTUP], 2010). The United States continues to have the highest adolescent pregnancy rate of any Western industrialized nation. Factors associated with teen pregnancy include early puberty, substance abuse, alcohol abuse, childhood sexual abuse, Latino ethnicity, teenage girls with live-in boyfriends, lack of community-based contraceptive clinics, and lack of an adult role model with whom a teen can discuss sexuality issues (Baker, Guthrie, Hutchinson, et al., 2007).

Adolescent patients need ongoing support throughout labor and the birth process. Each adolescent in labor is different. The nurse must assess what each patient brings to the experience by asking the following questions:

- Has the young woman received prenatal care?
- What are her attitudes and feelings about the pregnancy?
- How does her developmental stage influence her behavior, and how are her specific needs different?
- Who will support her during the birth, and what is the person's relationship to her?
- What preparation has she had for the experience?
- What are her expectations and fears regarding labor and birth?
- How has her culture influenced her?
- What are her usual coping mechanisms?
- Does she have adequate social support?
- Does she plan to keep the newborn? If so, does she need to learn parenting skills?
- Will the father of the baby be involved in the labor and birth experience?

Adolescents are at highest risk for pregnancy and labor complications and must be assessed carefully. Any adolescent who has not had prenatal care requires especially close observation during labor. The status of the fetus is monitored to ensure its well-being. The young woman's prenatal record is carefully reviewed for risks. The adolescent is more likely to have poor nutritional intake, preeclampsia, cephalopelvic disproportion (CPD), anemia, prematurity, drugs ingested during pregnancy, sexually transmitted infections, fetal death, and size-date discrepancies (gestation appears to be less than dates indicate because of minimal weight gain) (Baker et al., 2007; March of Dimes, 2009). Infants born to teenage mothers are more likely to have lower birth weights. They are also more likely to be exposed to alcohol, drugs, and tobacco in utero and in early childhood.

The nurse's support role depends on the young woman's support system during labor. When the patient is not accompanied by someone who will stay with her during childbirth, it is even more important for the nurse to establish a trusting relationship with her. In this way, the nurse can help her cope with labor and understand what is happening to her. Establishing rapport without recrimination will provide emotional support and encouragement. The adolescent who is given positive reinforcement for "work well done" will leave the experience with increased self-esteem, despite the emotional stress and difficulty of giving birth at such a young age.

The adolescent who has taken childbirth education classes is generally better prepared than the adolescent who has had no preparation. The nurse must keep in mind, however, that the younger the adolescent, the less she may be able to participate actively in the process.

Age-Related Responses to Labor and Birth

The very young adolescent (under age 14) has fewer coping mechanisms and less experience to draw on than her older counterparts have. Because her cognitive development is incomplete, the younger adolescent may have fewer problem-solving capabilities. Her ego integrity may be more threatened by the experience, and she may be more vulnerable to stress and discomfort.

The very young woman needs someone to rely on at all times during labor. She may be more childlike and dependent than older teens. The nurse must be sure that instructions and explanations are simple and concrete. During the transition phase, the young teenager may become withdrawn and unable to express her need to be nurtured. Touch, soothing encouragement, and measures to promote her comfort help her maintain control and meet her needs for dependence. During the second stage of labor, the young adolescent may feel as if she is losing control and may reach out to those around her. By remaining calm and giving directions, the nurse helps her control feelings of helplessness.

> “One of the most memorable expectant mothers I cared for during my nursing course was Cara, a 13-year-old. I met her each week as she came into the OB clinic at our hospital and stayed with her as she waited for her appointment and was then seen by the medical student. I noticed that with each passing visit, she became more and more anxious. I did my best to determine the source of her anxiety, provide general teaching, and try to answer all of her questions. I consulted with my professor, and she sat in with me during some visits. But Cara became more and more anxious. Near term, she began asking if she could just have the baby cut out. Whatever was she afraid of? Finally, in the 38th week, after 2 1/2 months of building trust, she told me she was afraid because her baby had gotten too big, and it would never be able to come out through her belly button. I was speechless for a moment. For 2 1/2 months, I had answered questions and felt so proud of my support and teaching, and for all this time, she had not been able to ask the most important question of all—the question that paralyzed her with fear. I was finally able to provide specific information, made drawings on a paper towel, had the medical student talk with her, and best of all, was able to be on call and be with her in labor and during birth. The beautiful smile on her face as her baby daughter was born was unbelievable. Cara wasn't afraid! It's been 39 years since then, and I still remember her.”

The middle adolescent (ages 14 to 16 years) often attempts to remain calm and unflinching during labor. If unable to break through the teenager's stoic barrier, the nurse needs to rise above frustration and realize that a caring attitude will still positively affect the young woman.

Many older adolescents (ages 16 to 19 years) feel that they "know it all," but they may be no more prepared for childbirth than their younger counterparts. The nurse's reinforcement and nonjudgmental manner will help them save face. If the adolescent has not taken classes, she may require preparation and explanations. The older teenager's response to the stresses of labor is similar to that of the adult woman.

The Adolescent Father

Consideration of the adolescent father is a very important aspect of labor and birthing care. Nurses need to be aware that this is a stressful time for the young father. There are some specific interventions that increase comfort, enhance education, and perhaps decrease stress. In the early part of labor, the nurse can talk with the father about his expectations for parenting the newborn and what resources are available in the community. Many adolescents are reluctant to ask questions, but an accepting attitude may help in establishing rapport and gaining trust.

The teen father may need encouragement to provide supportive care and to know what actions are acceptable in the birthing area. He may be encouraged to hold the mother's hand, to sit on the bed beside her, to give a back massage, or to stroke her forehead. He may need assistance in how to give a shoulder rub or back rub; he can watch the nurse first and then perform the action himself with the encouragement of the nurse. He may need more encouragement than the older father to share a Jacuzzi or shower or to support the mother in changing positions and ambulating. It is important for the nurse to speak in lay terms and to anticipate questions, to answer all vocalized questions honestly, and to provide opportunities for the parents to ask for further information.

Other Members of the Support Team

In addition to the adolescent's partner, the mother may want her parents or friends with her as members of her support team. Some teens may want their mothers as their primary support person, whereas others may strive to prove their independence and "do this on their own." Still other young women may look to friends for advice and support. The nurse includes parents and friends of the adolescent mother in the patient teaching and other aspects of the mother's care. It is important to respect the young woman's privacy and honor her wishes regarding whom she wants in the room for the birth. The nurse may have to advocate for the young woman in certain circumstances.

Teaching the Adolescent Mother

During the latent phase of labor, the nurse can explain to the young woman what changes in body sensations and emotional reactions she might anticipate as labor and birth progress. The adolescent also needs teaching about what possible medical procedures (such as electronic fetal monitoring [EFM], etc.) might be used, as well as what nursing care measures are available. Some adolescents might not realize that they can request the nurse's presence, touch, or advice, unless the nurse specifically informs them that these options are available.

Adolescents are oriented to the present time and may not adequately predict future needs for themselves or their infant. The nurse should assess to make sure adequate resources are available, including infant and postpartum supplies, transportation to and from follow-up visits, and child care, if the adolescent mother is planning on returning to school or work.

Young mothers may need more information on infant care and feeding choices than older women. Some adolescents may be reluctant to breastfeed because of embarrassment or lack of information. The nurse can assist the young woman to explore her feelings related to breastfeeding and provide information (Figure 24-13 ■). The nurse should provide encouragement and support the young mother's decision. Sometimes, young women feel "pressured" to breastfeed their infants when they truly do not feel comfortable with this feeding choice. The nurse should give the young mother permission to make her own decision. Young women who choose to use formula should be given clear instructions on the importance of mixing the formula per the manufacturer's directions because overdiluting or underdiluting can cause adverse side effects for the baby.

Although rarer than in previous decades, some adolescents may choose to relinquish their newborns. In these situations, the nurse informs the adolescent that seeing the infant can facilitate the grieving process but lets her know that seeing the newborn is her choice. (See chapter 36 ∞ for further discussion of the relinquishing mother and the adolescent parent.)

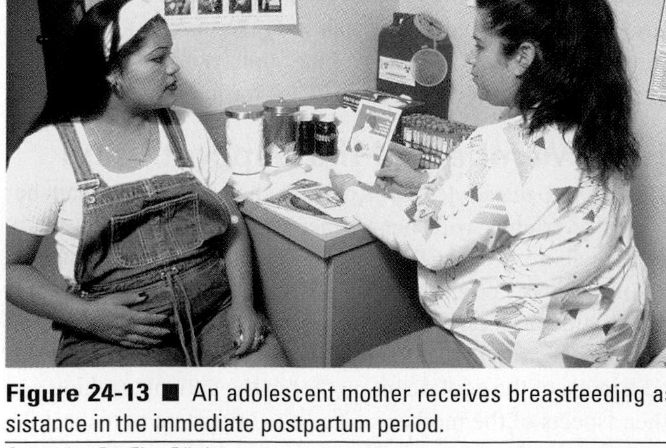

Figure 24-13 ■ An adolescent mother receives breastfeeding assistance in the immediate postpartum period.

Source: Amy Etra/PhotoEdit, Inc.

Nursing Care During Precipitous Birth

Occasionally, labor progresses so rapidly that the nurse is faced with the task of managing the birth of the baby. This is called a **precipitous birth**. The attending nurse has the primary responsibility for providing a physically and psychologically safe experience for the woman and her baby.

A woman whose physician or certified nurse-midwife (CNM) is not present may feel disappointed, frightened, cheated, and abandoned, especially if she is not prepared through childbirth education. The nurse can support the woman by keeping her informed about the labor progress and assuring her that the nurse will stay with her. If birth is imminent, the nurse must not leave the mother alone. Auxiliary personnel can be directed to contact the attending physician or CNM, or other physicians or CNMs who are in the facility. The auxiliary personnel should also retrieve the emergency pack ("precip pack"), which should be readily accessible to the birthing/labor rooms. A typical pack contains the following items: a small drape that can be placed under the woman's buttocks to provide a sterile field, a bulb syringe to clear mucus from the newborn's mouth, two sterile clamps (Kelly or Rochester) to clamp the umbilical cord before applying a cord clamp, sterile scissors to cut the umbilical cord, a sterile umbilical cord clamp, a baby blanket to wrap the newborn in after birth, and a package of sterile gloves.

As the materials are being gathered, the nurse must remain calm. The woman is reassured by the nurse's composure and feels that the nurse is competent. The primary goal of nursing care is the safe birth of the infant.

Birth of the Infant

The nurse manages precipitous birth in the hospital by encouraging the woman to assume a comfortable position. If time permits, the nurse scrubs both hands with soap and water and puts on sterile gloves. Sterile drapes are placed under the woman's buttocks.

At all times during the birth, the nurse gives clear instructions to the woman, supports her efforts, and provides reassurance. The nurse needs to remain calm and proceed in a slow, confident manner.

Most infants will be born in vertex presentation. When the infant's head crowns, the nurse instructs the woman to either blow or pant, which decreases her urge to push. The nurse checks whether the amniotic sac is intact. If it is, the nurse tears the sac with a clamp so that the newborn will not breathe in amniotic fluid with the first breath.

The nurse may place an index finger inside the lower portion of the vagina and the thumb on the outer portion of the perineum and gently massage the area to aid in stretching of perineal tissues and to help prevent perineal lacerations. This is called "ironing the perineum."

With one hand, the nurse applies gentle pressure against the fetal head to maintain flexion and prevent it from popping out rapidly. The nurse does not hold the head back forcibly. Rapid birth of the head may tear the woman's perineal tissues. The rapid change in pressure within the fetal head may cause subdural or dural tears. The nurse supports the perineum with the other hand and allows the head to be delivered between contractions.

As the woman continues to blow or pant, the nurse inserts one or two fingers along the back of the fetal head to check for the umbilical cord. If the cord is around the neck, the nurse bends her fingers like a fish hook, grasps the cord, and pulls it over the baby's head, loosens it, or slips it down over the shoulders. It is important to check that the cord is not wrapped around more than one time. If the cord is tightly looped and cannot be slipped over the baby's head, the nurse places two clamps on the cord, cuts it between the clamps, and unwinds the cord. Because this ceases oxygenation to the baby, all efforts should be made to reduce (remove) the cord over the head whenever possible. The head typically rotates (restitutes) to the left or right. The nurse needs to let the head rotate (restitute) to the side before attempting delivery of the head.

Immediately after birth of the head, the nurse suctions first the mouth, throat, and then the nasal passages. The nurse places a hand on each side of the head and instructs the woman to push gently so that the rest of the body can be expelled quickly. The newborn must be supported as it emerges.

Breech vaginal births are quite rare. Because the incidence of breech presentations is only 3%, most breech presentations are scheduled for cesarean births, and women are advised to come to the hospital immediately if labor does begin spontaneously. Because the primary concern in a breech birth is to prevent the entrapment of the head in the cervix, intervention is avoided until the buttocks are born. The nurse then pulls down a loop of cord (to avoid stress on its point of insertion) and supports the breech in both hands. The infant's body is lifted slightly upward for birth of the posterior shoulder and arm. The newborn may then be lowered, and the anterior shoulder and arm will pass under the symphysis pubis. Suprapubic pressure should be applied to maintain the normal flexion of the baby's head and should be continued until the baby is born. The nape of the neck pivots under the symphysis, and the rest of the head is born over the perineum by a movement of flexion.

Regardless of the presentation at birth, the newborn is held at the level of the uterus to facilitate blood flow through the umbilical cord immediately after birth. The combination of amniotic fluid and vernix makes the newborn very slippery, so the nurse must be careful to avoid dropping the baby. Placing the woman in stirrups is not recommended for this reason; instead, the foot of the bed can be lowered. The nurse suctions the nose and mouth of the newborn again, using a bulb syringe. The nurse then dries the newborn quickly to prevent heat loss. Wet blankets should be removed and replaced with warmed, dry blankets.

As soon as the nurse determines that the newborn's respirations are adequate, the infant can be placed on the mother's abdomen. The newborn's head should be slightly lower than the body to aid drainage of fluid and mucus. The weight of the newborn on the mother's abdomen stimulates uterine contractions, which aid in placental separation. The umbilical cord should not be pulled. The Apgar score is assessed at 1 and 5 minutes.

The nurse is alert for signs of placental separation. When these signs are present, the nurse places one hand just above the symphysis pubis to guard the uterus and uses the other hand to maintain gentle downward traction on the cord while instructing the mother to push so that the placenta can be expelled. In some instances the mother can squat, and this usually helps expel the placenta. The nurse inspects the placenta to determine whether it is intact. Because the physician or CNM is usually en route, delivery of the placenta can be delayed until the practitioner arrives. Traction should not be applied because this can result in hemorrhage or detaching the umbilical cord from the placenta.

The nurse checks the firmness of the uterus. Palpation of the uterus should not be performed before separation of the placenta. The fundus may be gently massaged to stimulate contractions and decrease bleeding. Putting the newborn to breast also stimulates uterine contractions through release of oxytocin from the pituitary gland.

The umbilical cord may now be cut. Two sterile clamps are placed approximately 2 to 4 inches from the newborn's abdomen. The cord is cut between them with sterile scissors. A sterile cord clamp (Hollister or Hesseltine) can be placed adjacent to the clamp on the newborn's cord, between the clamp and the newborn's abdomen. The clamp must not be placed snugly against the abdomen because the cord will dry and shrink.

The area under the mother's buttocks is cleaned, and her perineum is inspected for lacerations. Bleeding from lacerations may be controlled by pressing a clean perineal pad against the perineum and instructing the woman to keep her thighs together. Further evaluation by the CNM or physician will be needed to determine if lacerations are present that need to be repaired.

If the arrival of the physician or CNM is delayed or if the newborn is having respiratory distress, the newborn should be transported immediately to the nursery. The newborn must be properly identified before he or she leaves the birthing area.

Record Keeping

The nurse notes and places on the record the following information:

1. Position of fetus at birth.
2. Presence of cord around neck or shoulder (nuchal cord).
3. Time of birth.
4. Apgar scores at 1 and 5 minutes after birth.
5. Gender of newborn.
6. Time of expulsion of placenta.
7. Method of placental expulsion.
8. Appearance and intactness of placenta.
9. Mother's condition.
10. Any medications that were given to mother or newborn (per agency protocol).

CLINICAL TIP

Since time is typically very limited and rushed in a precipitous birth, the nurse can write interventions and birth outcomes on the fetal heart rate (FHR) monitoring strip so that times and details are more precise and exact.

Postbirth Interventions

Postbirth interventions are the same as those discussed in the Nursing Care During the Third Stage of Labor section.

Evaluation

Evaluation provides an opportunity to determine the effectiveness of nursing care. As a result of comprehensive nursing care during the intrapartum period, the following outcomes may be anticipated:

- The mother's physical needs and the psychologic well-being of the family have been maintained and supported.
- The baby's physical and psychologic well-being has been protected and supported.
- The family has had input into the birth process, and members have participated as much as they desired.
- The birth was safe and promoted family cohesiveness.

FOCUS YOUR STUDY

- Admission to the birth setting involves assessment of many physiologic, psychologic, and social factors. The information gained helps the nurse establish priorities of care.
- Before initiating care, the nurse explains what will be done, the reasons, potential benefits and risks, and possible alternatives if appropriate. This helps the woman determine what happens to her body and is a critical element in the process of obtaining informed consent.
- Behavioral responses to labor vary with the phase of labor, the woman's preparation and previous experience, cultural beliefs, and developmental level.
- Each woman's cultural beliefs affect her need for privacy, her expression of discomfort, her expectations for the birth, and the role she wishes the father to play in the birth event.
- The laboring woman's comfort may be increased by general comfort measures, supportive relaxation techniques, methods of handling anxiety, controlled breathing, and support by a caring person.
- The laboring woman fears being alone during labor. Even though there is a support person available, the woman's anxiety may be decreased when the nurse remains with her.
- Maternal birthing positions include a wide variety of possibilities, such as recumbent, side-lying, sitting, squatting, and crouching on hands and knees.
- Immediate assessments of the newborn include evaluation of the Apgar score and an abbreviated physical assessment. These early assessments help determine whether there is a need for resuscitation and whether the newborn's adaptation to extrauterine life is progressing normally. The newborn who is not experiencing problems may remain with the parents for an extended period of time following birth.
- Immediate care of the newborn following birth also includes maintaining respirations, promoting warmth, preventing infection, and providing accurate identification.
- The new parents and their baby are given time together as soon as possible after birth.
- Nursing assessments continue after the birth and are important to ensure that normal physiologic adaptations are taking place.
- The adolescent has special needs in the birth setting. Her developmental needs require specialized nursing care.
- Nurse-assisted births are sometimes performed in the absence of the CNM or physician when birth is imminent.

CRITICAL THINKING IN ACTION

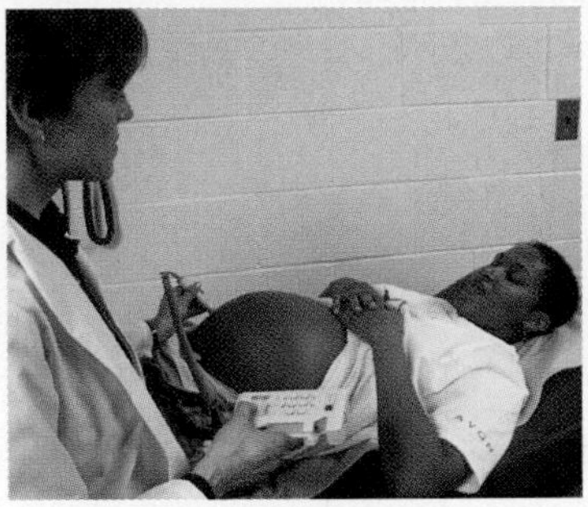

Anita Grey, a 22-year-old primigravida at 40 weeks' gestation, is admitted by you to the birthing center in labor. Anita was sent from her physician's office after being evaluated at her prenatal visit. While in the office, she was assessed to be 4 cm dilated, 100% effaced, vertex at 0 station with bulging membranes. She tells you that her husband is on his way to the birthing center and that she is anxious for him to arrive. A review of her prenatal record shows no complications affecting this pregnancy. Anita's vital signs are within normal limits. You assess the fetal heart rate and contraction pattern with the fetal monitor and observe a fetal heart rate of 140 to 150 beats/min with acceleration to 160s. Contractions are every 3 to 4 minutes $\times$ 30 seconds of moderate intensity by palpation. Anita seems to be tolerating the contractions well, but still seems anxious about her husband's arrival.

1. What steps can you take to reduce the stress and anxiety of the laboring woman and her family?
2. When you notify the physician/midwife, what pertinent information should the report contain?
3. What support measures can you give in the active phase of labor?
4. What measures can be used to decrease discomfort/pain as labor progresses?
5. What observations reflect the physiologic manifestations of pain?

See www.nursing.pearsonhighered.com for possible responses.

Pearson Nursing Student Resources

Find additional review materials at
www.nursing.pearsonhighered.com

Prepare for success with additional NCLEX®-style practice questions, interactive assignments and activities, Web links, animations and videos, and more!

REFERENCES

American College of Obstetricians and Gynecologists (ACOG). (2006). *The Apgar score* (ACOG Committee Opinion No. 333). Washington, DC: Author.

American College of Obstetricians and Gynecologists (ACOG). (2009). *Oral intake during labor.* (ACOG Committee Opinion, No. 441). Washington, DC: Author.

Anderson, J. M., & Etches, D. (15 March, 2007). Prevention and management of postpartum hemorrhage. *American Family Physician,* 875–895.

Association of Women's Health, Obstetric, and Neonatal Nurses (AWHONN). (2009a). *Fetal heart monitoring principles and practices* (4th ed.). Washington, DC: Author.

Association of Women's Health, Obstetric, and Neonatal Nurses (AWHONN). (2009b). M. T. Verklan & M. Walden (Eds.), *Core curriculum for neonatal intensive care nursing.* Washington, DC: AWHONN.

Baker, P., Guthrie, K., Hutchinson, C., Kane, R., & Wellings, K. (2007). *Teenage pregnancy and reproductive health.* London, England: Royal College of Obstetricians & Gynecologists.

Barnett, G. V. (2008). A new way to measure nursing: Computer timing of nursing time and support of labor-ing patients. *Computers, Informatics, Nursing, 26*(4), 199–206.

Blackburn, S. T. (2007). *Maternal, fetal, and neonatal physiology: A clinical perspective* (3rd ed.). Philadelphia, PA: Saunders.

Carolan, M. C. (2009). Towards understanding the concept of risk for pregnant women: Some nursing and midwifery implications. *Journal of Clinical Nursing, 18*(5), 652–658.

Chambliss, L. R. (2008). Intimate partner violence and its implication for pregnancy. *Clinical Obstetrics and Gynecology, 51*(2), 385–397.

Cunningham, F. G., Gant, N. F., Leveno, K. J., Gilstrap, L. C., Hauth, J. C., & Wenstrom, K. C. (2010). *William's obstetrics.* (22nd ed.). Philadelphia, PA: McGraw-Hill.

Edgar, H. J. (2009). Biohistorical approaches to "race" in the United States: Biological distances among African Americans, European Americans, and their ancestors. *American Journal of Physical Anthropology, 139*(1), 58–67.

Fisher, J. R., Tran, H. T., & Tran, T. (2007). Relative socio-economic advantage and mood during advanced pregnancy in women in Vietnam. *International Journal of Mental Health Systems, 1*(1), 3.

Hansen, L. (2009). Second-stage labor care: Challenges in spontaneous bearing down. *Journal of Perinatal & Neonatal Nursing, 23*(1), 31–41.

Hoang, H. T., Le, Q., & Kilpatrick, S. (2009). Having a baby in the new land: A qualitative exploration of the experiences of Asian migrants in rural Tasmania, Australia. *Rural and Remote Health, 9*(1), 1084–1092.

Lanfranchi A., Porta, F., & Chirico, G. (2009). Stem cells and the frontiers of neonatology. *Early Human Development, 85*(10 Suppl): S15–S18.

Lin, M. L., Lin, K. C., Li, H. Y., Shey, K. S., & Gau, M. L. (2009). Effects of delayed pushing during the second stage of labor on postpartum fatigue and birth outcomes in nulliparous women. *Journal of Nursing Research, 17*(1), 62–72.

March of Dimes. (2009). Quick reference: Fact Sheets: Teenage pregnancy. Retrieved from http://www.marchofdimes.com/professionals/14332_1159.asp

McGrath, S. K., & Kennell, J. H. (2008). A randomized controlled trial of continuous labor support for middle-class couples: Effect on cesarean delivery rates. *Birth, 35*(2), 92–97.

Mercer, J. S., Vohr, B. R., Erickson-Owens, D. A., Padbury, J. F., & Oh, W. (2009). Seven-month developmental outcomes of very low birth weight infants enrolled in a randomized controlled trial of delayed versus immediate cord clamping. *Journal of Perinatology, 30*(1), 11.

National Campaign to Prevent Teen and Unplanned Pregnancy (NCPTUP). (2010). *Our mission: Goal.* Retrieved from http://www.thenationalcampaign.org/about-us/our-mission.aspx

Ozsoy, S. A., & Katabi, V. (2008). A comparison of traditional practices used in pregnancy, labour and the postpartum period among women in Turkey and Iran. *Midwifery, 24*(3), 291–300.

Reitmanova, S., & Gustafson, D. L. (2008). "They can't understand it": Maternity health and care needs of immigrant Muslim women in St. John's, Newfoundland. *Maternal and Child Health Journal, 12*(1), 101–111.

Roberts, J., & Hanson, L. (2007). Best practices in second stage labor care: Maternal bearing down and positioning. *Journal of Midwifery & Women's Health, 52*(3), 238–245.

Sauls, D. J. (2007). Nurses' attitudes toward provision of care and related health outcomes. *Nursing Research, 56*(2),117–123.

Simpson K. R., & Creehan, P. A. (2008). *AWHONN's perinatal nursing care.* (4th ed.). Washington, DC: AWHONN.

Spector, R. E. (2008). *Cultural diversity in health and illness* (7th ed.). Upper Saddle River, NJ: Prentice Hall.

Stark, M. A., Rudell, B., & Haus, G. (2008). Observing position and movements in hydrotherapy: A pilot study. *Journal of Obstetric, Gynecologic, and Neonatal Nursing: JOGNN / NAACOG, 37*(1), 116–122.

Tucker, S. M., Miller, L. A., & Miller, D. A. (2008). *Mosby's pocket guide to fetal monitoring: A multidisciplinary approach.* St. Louis, MO: Mosby.

Udeh, B., Udeh, C., & Graves, N. (2008). Perinatal HIV transmission and the cost-effectiveness of screening at 14 weeks gestation, at the onset of labour and the rapid testing of infants. *BMC Infectious Diseases, 8,* 174–182.

U.S. Department of Health and Human Services. (2010). Overview of EMTALA. Retrieved from http://www.cms.gov/EMTALA/

Verklan, M.T., & Walden, M. (2009). Core curriculum for neonatal intensive care nursing. Philadelphia, PA: Saunders.

Wilson, B. A., Shannon, M. T., & Stang, C. L. (2010). *Nurse's drug guide: 2010.* Upper Saddle River, NJ: Prentice Hall.

CHAPTER 25

Pain Management During Labor

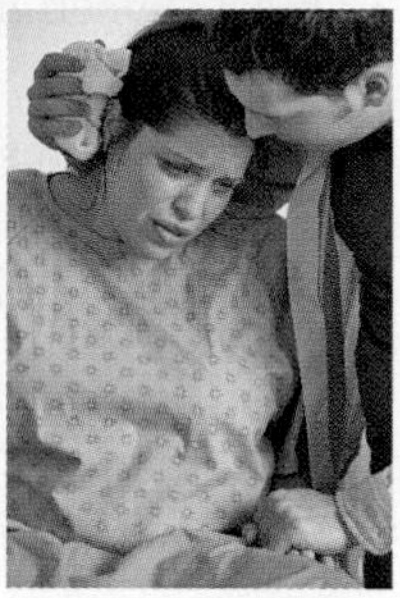

We had attended childbirth classes and practiced through the last few weeks, and I had hoped to go through all of labor and birth without medication. But when the contractions really came on strong, I just wasn't ready for the amount and the kind of pain that I felt. I've always been able to tolerate pain well, but this was different. My husband and I talked about it and he reassured me that, if I felt I needed something, it was okay with him. My nurse was also very supportive. She helped me feel I was making a good decision and wasn't failing somehow.

LEARNING OUTCOMES

1. Discuss the nurse's role in supporting pharmaceutical pain relief measures in labor.
2. Describe the use of systemic analgesics to promote pain relief during labor.
3. Compare the major types of regional analgesia and anesthesia, including the area affected, advantages, disadvantages, techniques, and nursing implications.
4. Summarize possible complications of regional anesthesia.
5. Describe the three methods used to provide general anesthesia.
6. Delineate the major complications of general anesthesia.
7. Identify contraindications to specific types of analgesia and anesthesia for high-risk mothers.

KEY TERMS

Epidural block *645*
General anesthesia *656*
Local anesthesia *655*
Pudendal block *655*
Regional analgesia *641*
Regional anesthesia *641*
Spinal block *652*

When a childbearing woman experiences discomfort during labor and birth, the nurse can assist her to have a positive birth experience by providing effective comfort measures. Nursing interventions directed toward pain relief begin with the nonpharmacologic measures described in chapter 24 ∞, such as providing information, encouragement, back rubs, and clean linens. Many women need no further interventions.

For other women, the progression of labor brings increasing levels of pain that interfere with their ability to cope effectively. For these women, pharmacologic agents may be used to decrease discomfort, increase relaxation, and reestablish the ability to participate more actively in the labor and birth experience. In addition to systemic analgesics, regional nerve blocks (epidural, spinal, and combined epidural-spinal) and local anesthetic blocks (pudendal and perineal) are available. The methods are not mutually exclusive and may be used in combination with nonpharmacologic comfort measures.

Nurses need to recognize that the decision to have an unmedicated or a medicated birth involves many factors and reflects a great deal of thought and planning for most women and their families. Some of these factors include patient and caregiver preferences, availability of anesthesia and analgesia, fear of risks and complications, past life experiences, previous experiences with pain, and cultural influences. Other factors, such as the amount of sleep the woman has had or the length of labor, can also influence the need or desire for pharmacologic pain relief measures. The woman should be supported regardless of her decision even if it changes during the course of labor.

Each year in the United States, over 4 million infants are born. Of these births, 50% of all women will receive epidural anesthesia (Gibbs, Karlan, Haney, et al., 2008). Many couples who have had childbirth education approach their birth experience confident that the techniques they have learned will enable them to cope with the pain of labor. Nurses should respect these couples' choices and provide support to help them meet their goals. Analgesics and anesthetics do affect the fetus and can be accompanied by maternal side effects. Following an unmedicated birth, many women report a quicker postpartum recovery. Many are able to ambulate, urinate, shower, and eat within an hour of giving birth. Additionally, many women feel an enormous sense of empowerment after successfully having an unmedicated birth.

For the woman who has advised the nursing staff that she wants no pharmacologic remedies, the nurse should offer alternative comfort measures. All nurses in the intrapartum setting need to be familiar with various nonpharmacologic techniques available to help women cope with the pain they may experience. The nurse should avoid offering these women pain medications unless they specifically ask for them or for information about pharmacologic options.

On the other hand, many women are simply unprepared for the intense pain of active labor and may request medication. They may begin labor undecided about whether to use medication, then request pain relief as contractions intensify. Frequently, feelings of inadequacy and guilt accompany such decisions. The nurse plays a special role in assisting the woman and her partner to explore their options for pain relief realistically. The nurse can explain to the couple that, although pharmacologic agents do affect the fetus, so do the pain and stress experienced by the laboring mother. In response to stress, the woman's ventilation and oxygen consumption increase, thus decreasing the amount of oxygen available to the fetus. In addition, pain and stress can lead to metabolic acidosis and the release of catecholamines, causing the maternal blood vessels to constrict. This in turn decreases oxygen and nutrient supply to the fetus (Blackburn, 2007). Thus, if the woman's pain and anxiety are more than she can cope with, the adverse physiologic effects on the fetus may be as great as would occur with the administration of a small amount of an analgesic agent. The nurse should reassure the woman and her partner that accepting medication for pain is not a failure. The emphasis should be on the goal of a healthy, satisfying outcome for the family.

> **“I felt really prepared for labor! We went through all of the classes and had envisioned the “perfect birth.” After 16 hours of labor and no progress, I was exhausted and frustrated; sobbing, I totally broke down. I felt like a failure for getting an epidural. My nurse, Madison, was great! She comforted me and reinforced that I was not a failure. She reassured me that in the end the most important thing would be holding my daughter in my arms. She was right, my despair was forgotten when I was able to enjoy the rest of labor, rest, and get some much needed sleep before Katherine was born. As I gazed at my newborn daughter, I learned what was really important that day and in my life!”**

Systemic Analgesia

The goal of systemic analgesia during labor is to provide maximal pain relief with minimal risk for the woman and fetus.

Multiple factors must be considered in the use of analgesic agents:

- Effects on the woman
- Effects on the fetus
- Effects on the labor contractions
- Medical status of the woman
- Progress of labor

The effects on the mother are of primary importance, because the well-being of the fetus depends on adequate functioning of the maternal cardiopulmonary system. Any alteration of function that disturbs the woman's homeostatic mechanism affects the fetal environment. Maintaining the maternal respiratory rate and blood pressure within normal range is thus of prime importance. The use of electronic fetal monitoring (EFM) provides a means of accurately assessing the effects of pharmacologic agents on uterine contractions.

All systemic analgesics can cross the placental barrier by simple diffusion, with some agents crossing more readily than others. Drug action in the body depends on the rate at which the substance is metabolized by liver enzymes and excreted by the kidneys. The fetal liver enzymes and renal systems are inadequate to metabolize analgesic agents, so high doses remain active in fetal circulation for a prolonged period of time. The percentage of blood volume flowing to the fetal brain increases during intrauterine stress, so the hypoxic fetus receives an even larger amount of a depressant drug. The blood-brain barrier is more permeable at the time of birth, a factor that also increases the amount of drug carried to the central nervous system (Blackburn, 2007).

Administration of Analgesic Agents

The optimal time for administering analgesia is determined after a complete assessment of many factors. In the past, an analgesic agent was administered to nulliparas when the active phase of labor was well established (cervix had dilated to 5 or 6 cm) and to multiparas when the cervix had reached 3 or 4 cm dilatation. There is debate on the ideal timing of medication administration; however, both the American College of Obstetricians and Gynecologists (ACOG) and the American Society of Anesthesiologists (ASA) agree that a woman's request for pain medications is ample reason to administer them (Gibbs et al., 2008). In general, the woman should receive pain medication when she is uncomfortable and in a well-established labor pattern with contractions occurring regularly and of significant duration with moderate to strong intensity. Analgesia given too early may prolong labor and depress the fetus. Analgesia given too late is of no value to the woman and may cause neonatal respiratory depression. In many institutions, the nurse decides when to give the analgesic agent prescribed by the physician, certified nurse-midwife (CNM), or certified registered nurse anesthetist (CRNA). The nurse observes the woman for cues that indicate she would benefit from the administration of analgesics. The nurse performs needed assessments of both the mother and fetus and then notifies the CNM or physician. The decision to administer pain medication is based on a complete assessment of the woman and fetus and the progress of labor. The CNM or physician may evaluate the woman at the bedside or may rely on the nurse's assessment and instruct the nurse to administer the medications. In most institutions, the CRNA is available to monitor analgesia-related complications and provide ongoing monitoring for women who later receive an epidural. The American Society for Anesthesiologists practice guidelines mandate that all women undergo a history and physical examination prior to the initiation of anesthesia (ASA Task Force, 2007). Facilities may have anesthesiologists (physicians who specialize in administering anesthesia) or certified nurse anesthetists provide these services.

Maternal Assessment

The following maternal assessments are critical before administering systemic analgesics:

- The woman is willing to receive medication after being advised about it (Table 25-1).
- Vital signs are stable.
- Contraindications (such as drug allergies, respiratory compromise, or current drug dependence) are not present.
- Knowledge of other medications being administered, such as magnesium sulfate or tocolytics.

TABLE 25-1 What Women Need to Know About Pain Relief Medications

Before receiving medications, the woman should understand the following:
- Type of medication administered
- Route of administration
- Expected effects of medication
- Implications for fetus/newborn
- Safety measures needed (for example, remain in bed with side rails up)
- Side effects/complications

Fetal Assessment

The following assessments of the fetus are also required:

- Fetal heart rate (FHR) is between 110 and 160 beats per minute.
- Reactive nonstress test (NST) (accelerations of FHR are present with fetal movement).
- Variability is present.
- Periodic late decelerations or nonperiodic (variable) decelerations are absent.

Assessment of Labor

The following assessment parameters must also be evaluated:

- Contraction pattern
- Cervical dilatation
- Cervical effacement
- Fetal presenting part
- Station of the fetal presenting part

If normal parameters are absent or if nonreassuring maternal or fetal factors are present, the nurse may need to complete further assessments with the physician or CNM. In addition, no complications that would preclude administering an analgesic agent should be present, such as drug allergies or drug-specific contraindications.

Routes of Administration

Oral analgesics are not used because they are poorly absorbed and gastric emptying time is prolonged during labor. The intramuscular (IM), intravenous (IV), or subcutaneous (SC) routes are used instead. For IM administration, the needle must be of sufficient length to penetrate the muscle and the subcutaneous fat. The IV route is preferred because it results in prompt, smooth, and more predictable action with a smaller total dose required than the IM route. When an agent is given intravenously, it is suggested that the injection be given with the onset of a contraction, when the blood flow to the uterus and the fetus is normally decreased (Blackburn, 2007).

When an analgesic medication is administered by IM or SC route, it takes a few minutes for the effect to be felt. The nurse can continue with other supportive measures to enhance comfort until the effect of the medication is perceived. When the medication begins to take effect, the woman may be able to sleep between contractions. This short period of rest can restore her energy. When an IV route is prescribed, the woman feels the effect of the drug within a minute or two, so if any change of position is necessary or if the woman needs to void, the nurse may suggest that these activities be completed before the drug is administered

(Cunningham et al., 2010). As in all cases when there is a possibility of coming into contact with body fluids, Standard Precautions should be used. Consistent hand washing before and after procedures along with wearing disposable gloves can reduce the risk of blood or body fluid exposure. Sometimes analgesics are administered via IV and IM routes simultaneously. The benefit of this technique is that the woman receives a rapid onset from the IV route as well as the longer duration of pain control that is achieved with the IM route (Gibbs et al., 2008).

Before administering the medication, the nurse once again ascertains whether the woman has a history of any drug reactions or allergies and provides information regarding the medication (see Table 25-1). After giving the medication, the nurse records the drug name, dose, route, site, and the woman's blood pressure and pulse (before and after) on the EFM strip and on the woman's record. If the woman is alone, the nurse raises the side rails to provide safety and assesses the FHR for possible side effects of the medication.

CLINICAL TIP

The anesthesiologists should be notified of any complications or unexpected outcomes that occur as the result of medication administration.

Sedatives

In current labor and birth practice, sedatives are used primarily in the early latent phase of labor, when the cervix is long, closed, and thick, and rest is prescribed for the expectant woman. Sedatives promote relaxation and allow the woman to sleep for a few hours. Upon the woman's awakening, contractions have either ceased (i.e., the woman was in false labor) or contractions return and take on a regular pattern that promotes changes in cervical dilatation and effacement. Sedatives should not be given when a woman is in active labor because they can cause respiratory depression in the infant. Sedatives have minimal analgesic properties and can actually increase the reaction to painful stimuli. They should be administered only to decrease anxiety and promote sleep, because they cross the placenta and can cause depression in the newborn (Creasy, Resnik, Iams, et al., 2009).

Barbiturates

The most common barbiturates used in labor are secobarbital (Seconal) and zolpidem tartrate (Ambien). Seconal is fast acting, usually providing effects in 10 to 15 minutes with a duration of 3 to 4 hours. It is administered orally and is well tolerated. Its primary role is to treat false labor and produce a sedation effect. Both Seconal and Ambien can be used in latent labor to promote rest and relaxation and thereby prevent maternal exhaustion. Hypnotic effects also occur with many drugs in this category. Seconal has a long half-life and can remain in the maternal and fetal blood for up to 40 hours after administration, whereas Ambien has a half-life of 4.5 hours (Wilson, Shannon, & Shields, 2010). For this reason, Ambien may be more desirable for women in early labor. A barbiturate should not be administered to women in active labor because it can cause fetal depression and, in fact, is rarely used at anytime during true labor.

Benzodiazepines

Benzodiazepines, such as diazepam (Valium), are similar to barbiturates in their mechanism of action. They are primarily used to treat anxiety. They can also be used for their anticonvulsant action. They have a rapid onset of action and are absorbed quite easily when ingested orally. Although this class of drugs can be used to decrease anxiety, some have an amnesic effect, which may not be desirable for childbearing women. Fetal side effects have been reported but are usually mild. These include a decrease in variability of the FHR, hypotonicity, hypoactivity, impaired temperature regulation, and metabolic response to cold stress (Gibbs et al., 2008). Midazolam (Versed), which is commonly used during operative procedures, has been associated with low Apgar scores when administered 5 minutes or less before birth. Because of this side effect, it is not advisable to use midazolam for childbearing women (Gibbs et al., 2008). It is primarily used for maternal anxiety during cesarean births and is given after the fetus is born when the surgical procedure is being completed. Many practitioners are hesitant to use Versed because of its amnestic properties, which are unfavorable in the obstetrical setting (Gibbs et al., 2008). Flumazenil, the drug used to reverse benzodiazepine sedative effects, should be kept on hand in case of accidental overdose.

H_1-Receptor Antagonists

H_1-receptor antagonists block the action of histamines at the receptor sites. These drugs cross the blood-brain barrier and inhibit N-methyltransferase, which is a by-product of histamine. It is this mechanism that leads to the sedative effects of this class of drugs. In addition, these drugs also have anti-Parkinson and antiemetic effects. There are seven subtypes of H_1-receptor antagonists. These drugs cause drowsiness and are frequently used in early labor to promote sleep and decrease anxiety. The degree of drowsiness experienced depends on which drug is administered. Common H_1-receptor antagonists used in labor include promethazine (Phenergan), hydroxyzine (Vistaril), and diphenhydramine (Benadryl).

Promethazine (Phenergan), which is a phenothiazine, results in marked sedation and is often combined with opiates because it potentiates their effects. It also has strong antiemetic effects and can be combined with opiates to relieve nausea and vomiting, which can be a side effect of certain drugs, such as meperidine (Demerol). All phenothiazines cross the placental barrier and can result in decreased beat-to-beat variability. Promethazine has not, however, resulted in lower Apgar scores. Promethazine injections are typically painful and should be avoided if possible in laboring women (Gibbs et al., 2008). Phenothiazines can also bind to bilirubin binding sites in newborns whose mothers are exposed to the drug at term. This can result in an increased incidence of neonatal hyperbilirubinemia and jaundice (Wilson et al., 2010).

Hydroxyzine (Vistaril) is a piperazine subtype. It can be given in early or prodromal labor to decrease anxiety and nausea. It also results in sedation so the mother can rest. This drug is administered intramuscularly in a large muscle. Women in false labor are able to rest and frequently will awaken to find that their uterine contractions have dissipated. Commonly, women who receive this drug in early or prodromal labor are able to rest and may enter active labor.

Diphenhydramine (Benadryl) is an ethanolamine subtype of the H_1 antagonists. Most commonly, this over-the-counter medication is used to treat allergic rhinitis and urticaria; however, it also possesses sedative and antiemetic properties that can be used to treat women in early labor. The drug has a relatively short half-life (1 to 4 hours) and can last up to 6 to 8 hours (Wilson et al., 2010). Nurses can advise women to use this drug at home if medically indicated, because it is readily available. It should be noted that this drug causes agitation in some women. If this side effect occurs, women should discontinue the medication (Wilson, et al., 2010).

NURSING CARE MANAGEMENT

The nurse should carefully assess the woman before administration of analgesic agents. Common indications for various medications are summarized in Table 25-2. Because they are not indicated for women in active labor, the nurse needs to determine the stage of labor. The nurse should evaluate the woman to determine the frequency, duration, and intensity of her contractions (Simpson & Creehan, 2008). A vaginal exam is performed to determine if cervical change has occurred. Fetal well-being is established by obtaining electronic fetal monitoring and ensuring a reactive fetal heart tracing. The nurse should explain the desired effects of the medication and possible side effects. If the woman is not in active labor, she can be given the medication and be advised to return home and rest. Since drowsiness can occur, however, the nurse needs to ensure the woman has a safe form of transportation home. Nurses need to review the symptoms of active labor and warning signs and advise the woman to call her healthcare provider should they occur.

Narcotic Analgesics

Narcotic analgesic agents that are injected into the circulation have their primary action at sites in the brain. Specifically, a narcotic that diffuses out of cerebral capillaries and reaches the periventricular/periaqueductal gray matter of the brain activates the neurons that descend to the spinal cord and inhibits the transmission of pain impulses in the substantia gelatinosa. Nausea and vomiting are produced by stimulation of the medullary chemoreceptor trigger zone.

A brief discussion of some selected narcotic analgesic agents follows. Both narcotic and non-narcotic analgesic drugs are summarized in Table 25-3.

Butorphanol Tartrate (Stadol)

Butorphanol tartrate (Stadol) is a mixed agonist-antagonist agent. The analgesic potency is 30 to 40 times that of meperidine and 7 times that of morphine (Wilson et al., 2010). Administration of butorphanol reverses the analgesic effect of other opioids or narcotics in the woman's body and precipitates withdrawal in drug-dependent individuals. For this reason, it is important to assess each woman's history of narcotic drug use during the admission assessment; if she has been using drugs, she should not receive butorphanol.

For the woman in labor, butorphanol is most frequently given by the IV route; however, it can also be given by IM injection. When administered intravenously, the recommended dose is 1 to 2 mg (the smaller dose is most frequently used). The onset of action is rapid, peak analgesia occurs in 30 to 60 minutes and duration is 3 to 4 hours (Wilson et al., 2010). If given by IM route, the recommended dose is 1 to 2 mg, although 2 mg is the most usual dose. Onset of action occurs in 10 to 15 minutes, peak analgesia occurs in 30 to 60 minutes, and duration is 3 to 4 hours (Wilson et al., 2010).

Respiratory depression of both the mother and fetus/newborn can occur. The effects of butorphanol (Stadol) can be reversed with naloxone (Narcan). Although not a common side effect, urinary retention can occur. The nurse should frequently assess the woman's bladder for distention. The nurse may need to perform an in-and-out catheterization using sterile technique to alleviate bladder distention. Major side effects include somnolence, dizziness, and feelings of dysphoria (Cunningham et al., 2010).

Fentanyl (Sublimaze)

Fentanyl (Sublimaze) is a short-acting synthetic opioid with moderate analgesia and mild sedation properties. The main advantage of fentanyl (Sublimaze) is that it has a rapid onset. In addition, the drug has limited placental transfer and thus has a lower incidence of reduced fetal heart rate variability. Women who receive fentanyl (Sublimaze) are less likely to require naloxone (Narcan) for neonatal respiratory depression. Be-

TABLE 25-2 Common Indications for Medications in Labor

DRUG	PAIN RELIEF	ANXIETY OR APPREHENSION	SEDATION	ANTIEMETIC
Demerol (meperidine)	X		X	
Nubain (nalbuphine)	X		X	
Phenergan (promethazine)		X	X	X
Stadol (butorphanol)	X		X	
Vistaril (hydroxyzine)		X	X	
Seconal (secobarbital)		X	X	X
Benadryl (diphenhydramine hydrochloride)		X	X	X

TABLE 25-3 Analgesics Used in Labor

DRUG/CLASS	DOSAGE, ROUTE, FREQUENCY	COMMON SIDE EFFECTS	LIFE-THREATENING REACTIONS	CONTRAINDICATIONS
Stadol (butorphanol tartrate): central nervous system (CNS) agent, analgesic, narcotic agonist/antagonist	IM 1–4 mg every 3–4 hours IV 0.5–2 mg every 6–8 hours Intranasal: 1 mg (1 puff) may repeat in 90 seconds (max dose every 3–4 hours)	Sedation	Respiratory depression	Narcotic dependency, breastfeeding
Nubain (nalbuphine hydrochloride): CNS agent, analgesic, narcotic agonist, antagonist	10–20 mg every 3–6 hours prn SC/IM/IV	Sedation; sweaty, clammy skin; nausea and vomiting	Respiratory depression	Hypersensitivity to the drug
Demerol (meperidine hydrochloride): CNS agent, analgesic, narcotic agonist	50–100 mg IM or SC every 3–4 hours 25–50 mg IV every 3–4 hours	Nausea, vomiting, itching, urinary retention, sedation, respiratory depression, dizziness	Respiratory depression in mother and/or newborn, seizures, cardiovascular collapse, cardiac arrest, bronchoconstriction	Narcotic dependency, epilepsy, hypersensitivity to the drug
Morphine (morphine sulfate): CNS agent, analgesic, narcotic, agonist	IV 2.5–15 mg every 4 hours IM/SC 5–20 mg every 4 hours	Pruritus (itching), constipation, nausea	Anaphylactic reaction, respiratory depression; overdose; respiratory arrest, cardiac arrest	Hypersensitivity to opiates, increased intracranial pressure, convulsive disorders, acute alcoholism, acute asthma, chronic pulmonary diseases, decreased respirations, pulmonary edema, biliary tract surgery, anastomosis, pancreatitis, acute ulcerative colitis, liver/renal insufficiency, Addison's disease, hypothyroidism
Phenergan (promethazine hydrochloride): gastrointestinal (GI) agent, antiemetic, antivertigo agent, phenothiazine	25–50 mg every 3–4 hours po/pr/IM/IV	Sedation, drowsiness, dry mouth, blurred vision	Respiratory depression, agranulocytosis	Hypersensitivity to phenothiazines, glaucoma, peptic ulcer, pyloroduodenal obstruction, bladder neck obstruction, epilepsy, bone marrow depression, and breastfeeding
Vistaril (hydroxyzine pamoate): antihistamine, antianxiety, sedative, antipruritic, antiemetic	25–100 mg po/IM every 6 hours	Sedation, dizziness, dry mouth, nausea, headache	Seizures	Hypersensitivity to drug. Can be used with caution in glaucoma, urinary retention
Benadryl (diphenhydramine hydrochloride): antihistamine, antiemetic, antivertigo, antitussive, sedative-hypnotic	25–50 mg every 6 hours po/IM/IV	Drowsiness, sedation, dry mouth, hypotension, nausea and vomiting, GI symptoms	Anaphylaxis, seizures, coma, respiratory depression	Hypersensitivity to drug. Can be used during an acute asthma attack; use with caution in glaucoma, bladder obstruction, hypertension, hypothyroidism, renal disease

cause of its short half-life, repeated doses are required. The usual dosage is 50 to 100 μg every 1 hour (Gibbs et al., 2008).

NURSING CARE MANAGEMENT

Administering butorphanol or fentanyl with other central nervous system depressants, such as sedatives, phenothiazides, other tranquilizers, hypnotic agents, and general anesthetics, can exacerbate respiratory depression and cause other effects. For this reason, the nurse should evaluate the woman's respiratory and cardiac status by careful observation of vital signs and pulse oximetry. The woman's level of consciousness is also checked frequently. Continuous electronic monitoring of the FHR pattern is recommended. Respiratory depression in the mother or fetus/newborn can be reversed by naloxone (Narcan), which is a specific antagonist for this agent. The nurse ensures that naloxone is readily available should respiratory depression occur. A slightly depressed newborn is not likely to experience prolonged drowsiness or sluggishness, however, because the metabolites of butorphanol are inactive.

Nalbuphine Hydrochloride (Nubain)

Like butorphanol, nalbuphine hydrochloride (Nubain) is a synthetic agonist-antagonist narcotic analgesic and may precipitate drug withdrawal if the woman is physically dependent on narcotics (Cunningham et al., 2010). Nalbuphine crosses the placenta to the fetus and can cause nonreassuring fetal status and neonatal respiratory depression (Gibbs et al., 2008). Nalbuphine may be given by the IM, SC, or IV route. It is most frequently given by the IV route in the birth setting. The usual dose for adults is 10 mg/70 kg. If given intravenously, onset of action occurs in 2 to 3 minutes, peak of action occurs in 15 to 20 minutes, and duration is 3 to 6 hours. When given by the IM or SC route, the onset

DRUG GUIDE Nalbuphine Hydrochloride (Nubain)

OVERVIEW OF ACTION

Nubain is a synthetic narcotic analgesic with agonist and weak antagonist properties. Analgesic properties are equal to that produced by morphine. Nubain's potency is 3 to 4 times greater than pentazocine. The incidence of respiratory depression that occurs is equivalent to morphine.

DOSAGE ROUTE

Nubain is indicated for moderate to severe pain. Adults: 10–20 mg every 3–6 hours prn SC/IM/IV.

MATERNAL CONTRAINDICATIONS

Hypersensitivity or allergy to nalbuphine hydrochloride.

MATERNAL SIDE EFFECTS

Sedation; clammy, sweaty skin; dry mouth; bitter taste in mouth; nausea and vomiting; dizziness; vertigo; nervousness; restlessness; depression; crying; euphoria; dysphoria; confusion; hallucinations; unusual dreams; distortion of body image; numbness; tingling sensations; headache; miosis; hypertension; hypotension; bradycardia; tachycardia; flushing; abdominal cramps; dyspnea; asthma; speech difficulty; and urinary urgency.

NURSING CONSIDERATIONS

- Assess patient's sensitivity to narcotics on admission.
- Inform patient of potential side effects.
- Monitor and evaluate analgesic effect. Ask patient about comfort level and notify anesthesiologist of inadequate pain relief.
- Observe for symptoms of hypersensitivity: pruritus, urticaria, and/or burning sensation.
- May produce an allergic response in patients with sulfite sensitivity. If allergic reaction (urticaria, edema, or respiratory difficulties) occurs, administer naloxone or diphenhydramine per physician order.
- Assess respiratory rate before administration. Notify health-care provider if respirations less than 12 per minute.
- Monitor urinary output and assess bladder for distention. Assist patient to void.
- Assist patient with ambulation after administration.
- Counsel patient that use with alcohol or other central nervous system depressants may increase medication effects.
- Counsel patient that prolonged use with abrupt discontinuation can result in symptoms consistent with narcotic withdrawal.

of action occurs in less than 15 minutes, peak of action occurs in 30 to 60 minutes, and duration is 3 to 6 hours. When given by the IV route, nalbuphine may be given directly into the tubing of a running IV infusion; 10 mg should be administered over 3 to 5 minutes (Wilson et al., 2010). Adverse maternal effects include respiratory depression, drowsiness, dizziness, crying, blurred vision, nausea, diaphoresis, and urinary urgency (Wilson et al., 2010). See Drug Guide: Nalbuphine Hydrochloride (Nubain).

NURSING CARE MANAGEMENT

The nurse assesses the woman's history to identify contraindications to use of nalbuphine, such as the possibility of current narcotic drug dependence, sensitivity to sulfites, and history of asthma (Wilson et al., 2010). If no contraindications exist, the IV route is frequently used during labor. The woman's respiratory rate, quality of respirations, and characteristics of the FHR must be carefully assessed. Anticipation of urinary urgency is important. Because the woman may experience dizziness and sedation, use of a bedpan may be necessary.

Meperidine Hydrochloride (Demerol)

Meperidine hydrochloride is also a synthetic agonist-antagonist narcotic analgesic. Like Nubain, it may also precipitate drug withdrawal if the woman is physically dependent on narcotics (Cunningham et al., 2010). Meperidine crosses the placenta within 90 seconds of maternal administration, with maternal and fetal concentrations achieving equilibrium at 6 minutes (Blackburn, 2007). Meperidine can be administered IM or IV in labor. The subcutaneous and oral routes are not routinely used for laboring women. The typical dose is 50 to 100 milligrams IM or 25 to 50 milligrams IV (Wilson et al., 2010). Whereas IM administration can take up to 40 to 50 minutes to be effective, IV administration can provide pain relief within 5 to 10 minutes after administration (Wilson et al., 2010). Adverse maternal effects include nausea, vomiting, itching, urinary retention, sedation, respiratory depression, and dizziness (Wilson et al., 2010). Since meperidine can cause convulsions, it should not be given to women with known convulsive disorders, such as epilepsy (Wilson et al., 2010).

Meperidine has multiple fetal side effects, including alteration in fetal electroencephalogram, decreased or absent respiratory movements, a decrease in fetal movements, and decreased variability with the FHR (Blackburn, 2007). In addition, newborns who have received meperidine take longer to sustain respirations after birth, have lower Apgar scores, lower oxygen saturation, a higher incidence of respiratory acidosis, and a higher incidence of abnormal neurologic examinations at birth (Blackburn, 2007). Meperidine has also been associated with delays in initiation of successful breastfeeding. Newborns whose mothers had received meperidine during labor had more sucking problems, including lack of sucking and incorrect sucking technique (Blackburn, 2007).

NURSING CARE MANAGEMENT

The nurse assesses the woman's history to identify if contraindications exist, such as the possibility of current narcotic drug dependence or convulsive disorders (Wilson et al., 2010). If no contraindications exist, the IV or IM route is frequently used during labor. Because respiratory depression can occur, the woman's respiratory rate and quality of respirations are routinely assessed. Characteristics of the FHR must be carefully assessed. Although meperidine can cause a decrease in variability, the FHR should be continuously assessed for signs of late decelerations. Anticipation of urinary retention is important. The woman is offered a bedpan, and bladder distention is routinely assessed. If her bladder becomes distended and she is unable to void, catheterization may be necessary. Because the woman may experience dizziness and sedation, the woman typically remains on bed rest and does not ambulate after the medication is administered. The nurse assesses the woman for side effects and reports undesired side effects to the physician or CNM.

Opiate Antagonist: Naloxone (Narcan)

Because naloxone (Narcan) is an antagonist with little or no agonistic effect, it exhibits little pharmacologic activity in the absence of narcotic agents. Naloxone can be used to reverse the mild respiratory depression, sedation, and hypotension following small doses of opiates (Creasy et al., 2009). Naloxone exerts its effect by competing for opiate receptors and taking the place of the opiate on the receptor. In this manner, naloxone blocks or reverses the action of the narcotic analgesic (Cunningham et al., 2010). The drug is useful for respiratory depression caused by butorphanol (Stadol), nalbuphine (Nubain), and meperidine hydrochloride (Demerol) (Cunningham et al., 2010). *Naloxone is the drug of choice when the depressant is unknown because it will cause no further depression.* Naloxone's duration of action is less than that of most narcotic analgesics; however, respiratory depression may return as the antagonistic effect of naloxone wears off. Withdrawal symptoms may occur when Narcan is given to a woman or a newborn who is physically dependent on narcotics. A careful assessment that includes opiate drug use is imperative.

> **CLINICAL TIP**
> Each patient birthing room should be stocked with Naloxone (Narcan) at the bedside. Upon admission of a new patient, check the room to ensure the medication is supplied.

NURSING CARE MANAGEMENT

When naloxone is administered to the laboring mother or to the newborn just after birth, resuscitative measures and trained personnel should be readily available in the event that additional respiratory support is needed. When administered to the laboring mother, naloxone may be injected undiluted at a rate of 0.4 mg over 15 seconds into the tubing of a running IV infusion. Naloxone may also be diluted in an IV infusion of 5% dextrose or normal saline for a titrated dose. Titrated doses of naloxone are more likely to be used in a postoperative setting, when epidural analgesia has been given with a cesarean birth. After the direct IV administration, maternal vital signs should be obtained at 5-minute intervals until the respiratory rate has been stabilized and then every 30 minutes (Balestrieri-Martinez, 2009). Neonatal administration can be administered via IV, IM, or endotracheal (ET) routes. The standard neonatal dosage is 0.01 mg/kg (Wilson et al., 2010).

The duration of naloxone is shorter (minutes to hours) than the analgesic drug it is acting as an antagonist for, so the nurse must be alert to the return of respiratory depression and the need for repeated doses. Naloxone should be given with caution in women with known or suspected opiate dependence, because it may precipitate severe withdrawal symptoms in the mother and the newborn.

Regional Analgesia and Anesthesia

Regional anesthesia is the temporary and reversible loss of sensation produced by injecting an anesthetic agent (called a local anesthetic) into an area that will bring the agent into direct contact with nervous tissue. Loss of sensation occurs because the local agents stabilize the cell membrane, which prevents initiation and transmission of nerve impulses. The regional anesthetic blocks most commonly used in childbearing include epidural, spinal, or combined epidural-spinal. Epidural blocks may be used for analgesia during labor and vaginal birth and for anesthesia during cesarean birth. A combined epidural-spinal block may also be used. With this approach, the epidural is used to provide analgesia for labor, and the spinal provides anesthesia for birth or analgesia following birth.

An epidural relieves pain associated with the first stage of labor by blocking the sensory nerves supplying the uterus. Pain associated with the second stage of labor and with birth can be alleviated with epidural, combined epidural-spinal, and pudendal blocks (Figure 25-1 ■ and Table 25-4).

Regional anesthesia carries considerably less risk than general anesthesia. Risk of maternal death with general anesthesia during a cesarean birth is primarily related to intubation difficulties and hypovolemia. Other risk factors include obesity, African American race, and faulty monitoring during general anesthesia (Mhyre, Riesner, Polley, & Naughton, 2007).

> **PROFESSIONALISM IN PRACTICE**
> ***Timing Epidural Anesthesia***
> If the laboring woman has voiced a desire to have epidural anesthesia, advise her to tell you ahead of time when she might want it so the anesthesiologist has ample time to arrive before the woman's pain level becomes too intense.

Until fairly recently, the same anesthetic agents used for regional epidural anesthesia were also used to produce **regional analgesia** (pain relief) during labor. This approach was somewhat problematic because anesthetic agents alter the transmission of impulses to the bladder, making voiding difficult. The agents also interfere with the woman's ability to maintain her blood pressure and move her lower extremities. In addition, the descent of

Through the Eyes of a Nurse
Epidural for Pain Management

Family's Experience

"I know I really want to have the option of having something for pain, but I learned in our (childbirth) class that some of the medications can affect the baby's heart rate. I don't want anything that will hurt the baby! What is the safest choice for me and the baby?"

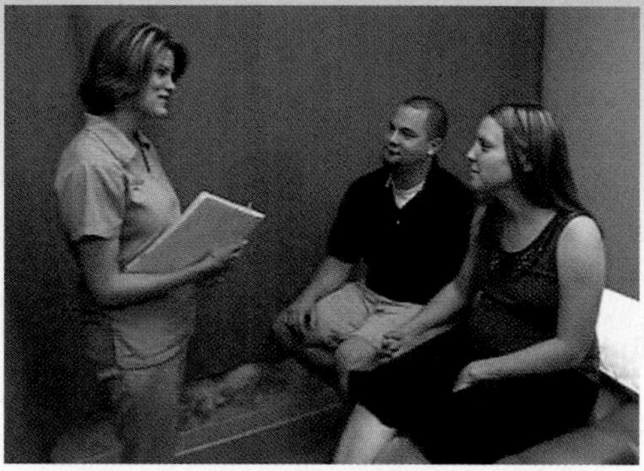

Nurse's Response

"Typically, the intravenous medications, such as Demerol or Nubain, can cause some changes in the baby's heartbeat and can cause respiratory problems at birth. For this reason, those medications are not given when birth will occur within a few hours.

"The epidural is another option and gives better pain relief. It can be given throughout labor. It can affect the heartbeat when it is first given if the mother's blood pressure drops immediately after it is administered. This is prevented by giving intravenous fluids to the mother before administering the epidural."

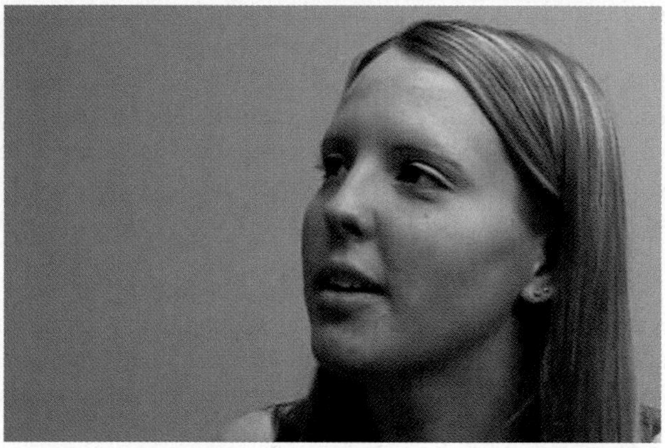

Nurse's Actions and Rationale

There are many types of analgesic and anesthesia options to the laboring woman. Analgesics commonly used in labor are summarized in Table 25-3. The nurse reviews the pros and cons of each option. Epidural anesthesia can also have risks and benefits. The medications should be reviewed with the woman before administration. Although complications are rare, the nurse explains possible complications that can occur. The nurse gives clear objective information based on evidence-based practice. All questions should be answered before the onset of labor so the woman can make informed choices when labor occurs.

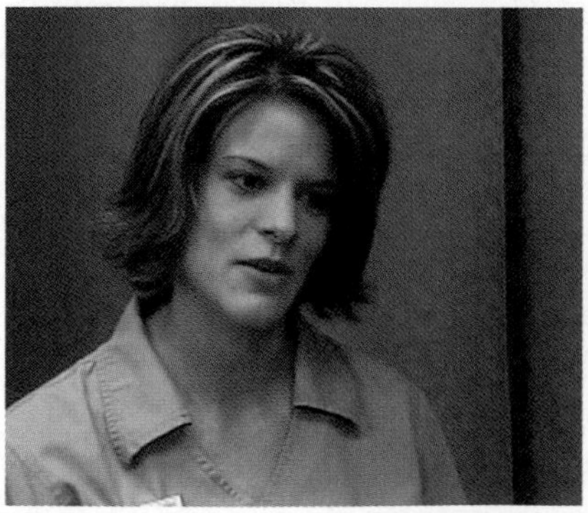

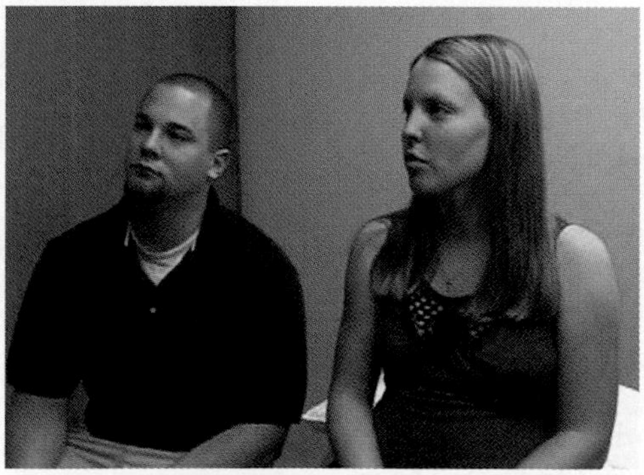

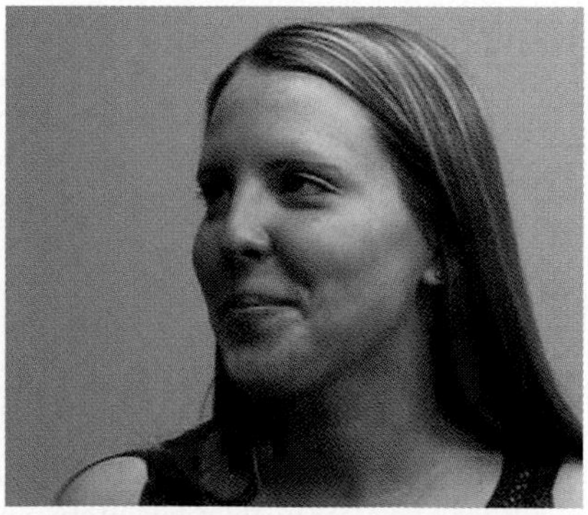

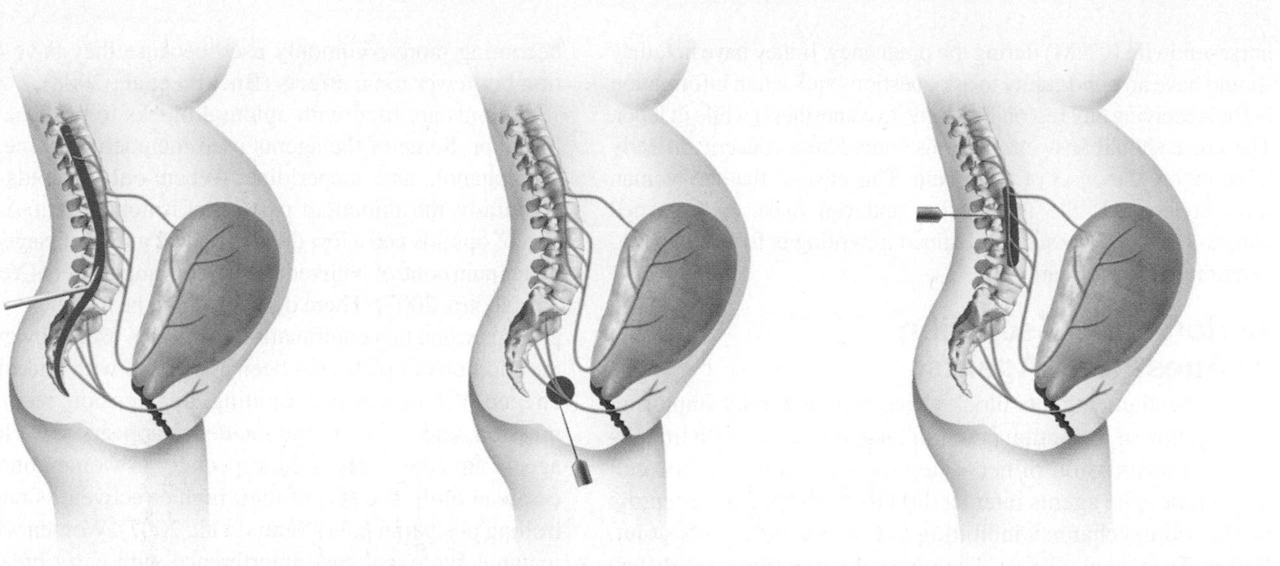

Figure 25-1 ■ Schematic diagram showing pain pathways and sites of interruption. A. Lumbar sympathetic (spinal) block: relief of uterine pain only. B. Pudendal block: relief of perineal pain. C. Lumbar epidural block: Dark area demonstrates peridural (epidural) space and nerves affected, and the gray tube represents a continuous plastic catheter.

Source: Bonica, J. J. (1972). Principles and practice of obstetric analgesia and anesthesia *(pp. 492, 512, 521, 614). Philadelphia, PA: Davis.*

the fetus may be slowed, because the agents also decrease the woman's ability to push effectively during the second stage of labor (Cunningham et al., 2010). To address these problems, regional analgesia is now obtained by injecting a narcotic agent such as fentanyl along with only a small amount of a local anesthetic agent. This approach yields effective pain relief without the troubling side effects of epidural anesthesia. The woman's pain is relieved, her blood pressure remains stable, and, because there is no motor blockage, she may be able to move about freely and ambulate. Urinary retention can still occur, but it can be treated with the placement of an indwelling Foley catheter or an in-and-out catheter (Cunningham et al., 2010). Urinary retention is usually a short-term complication that resolves on its own after the anesthesia has completely worn off.

The intrathecal injection of narcotics results in another type of regional analgesia. In this case, the narcotic is injected into the subarachnoid (spinal) space. Fentanyl citrate and preservative-free morphine are the most frequently used narcotic agents. The woman's pain is usually relieved; however, she may experience urinary retention. Delayed respiratory depression may also occur and seems to be more frequent with the use of morphine (Wilson et al., 2010).

It is important for the laboring woman to have information about the regional analgesia or anesthesia that is to be administered. As with other procedures, the woman needs to know how the block is given, the expected effect on her and the fetus, advantages and disadvantages, and possible risks. Many women discuss possible analgesic and anesthetic blocks with their physician or certified

TABLE 25-4 Summary of Commonly Used Regional Blocks

TYPE OF BLOCK	AREAS AFFECTED	USE DURING LABOR AND BIRTH	NURSING ACTIONS
Lumbar epidural	Uterus, cervix, vagina, and perineum	Given in first stage and second stage of labor.	Assess woman's knowledge regarding the block. Act as advocate to help her obtain further information if needed. Monitor maternal blood pressure to detect the major side effect, which is hypotension. Provide support and comfort. See Nursing Care Plan: For Epidural Anesthesia on page 651 for further nursing actions.
Combined spinal-epidural	Uterus, cervix, vagina, and perineum	Spinal analgesia may be given in latent phase for pain relief. Epidural is given when active labor begins.	Assess woman's knowledge regarding the block. Monitor maternal vital signs and fetal heart rate (FHR) status. Provide comfort measures.
Pudendal	Perineum and lower vagina	Given in the second stage just before birth to provide anesthesia for episiotomy or for low forceps birth.	Assess woman's knowledge regarding the block. Act as advocate to help her obtain further information if needed.
Local infiltration	Perineum	Administered just before birth to provide anesthesia for episiotomy or after birth for repair of a laceration.	Assess woman's knowledge regarding the block. Provide information as needed. Provide comfort and support. Observe perineum for bruising or other discoloration in the recovery period.
Spinal	Uterus, cervix, vagina, and perineum	Given during first stage for pain relief. Provides immediate onset of anesthesia.	Assess woman's knowledge regarding the block. Monitor maternal vital signs and FHR status.

nurse-midwife (CNM) during the pregnancy. If they have not, they should have an opportunity to ask questions and obtain information before receiving any regional analgesia or anesthesia while in labor. The nurse should answer questions and address concerns in early labor before the onset of acute pain. This ensures that the woman fully understands the information and can make an informed choice. Informed consent is obtained in writing before the administration of the medication.

Action and Absorption of Anesthetic Agents

Local anesthetic agents block nerve conduction by impairing propagation of the action potential in axons along with impairing the transmission of nerve impulses by stabilizing the cell membrane. The agents interact directly with specific receptors on the sodium channel, inhibiting sodium ion influx (Chestnut, Polley, Tsen, et al., 2009). The types of nerve fibers are differentially sensitive to the various anesthetic agents. In general, the smaller the fiber, the more sensitive it is to local agents. For example, it is possible to block the small C and A delta fibers, which transmit pain, touch, and temperature, without blocking the larger A alpha, A beta, and A gamma fibers, which continue to maintain a sense of pressure, muscle tone, position sense, and motor function (Chestnut et al., 2009).

Absorption of local anesthetic agents depends primarily on the vascularity of the area of injection. The agents also increase blood flow by causing vasodilatation (Chestnut et al., 2009). Higher concentrations cause greater vasodilatation. Good maternal physical condition or a high metabolic rate aids absorption. Malnutrition, dehydration, electrolyte imbalance, and cardiovascular and pulmonary problems increase the potential for toxic effects. The pH of tissues affects the rate of absorption, which has implications for fetal complications, such as acidosis (Blackburn, 2007). The addition of vasoconstrictors, such as epinephrine, delays absorption and prolongs the anesthetic effect. Epinephrine decreases uteroplacental blood flow, making it an undesirable additive in many situations. The breakdown of local anesthetics in the body is accomplished by the liver and plasma esterase, and the resulting substance is eliminated by the kidneys. It is important to use the weakest concentration and the smallest amount necessary to produce the desired results (Bucklin, Gambling, & Wlody, 2008).

Local Anesthesia

Types of Local Anesthetic Agents

Three types of local anesthetic agents are currently available—esters, amides, and opiates. The ester type includes procaine hydrochloride (Novocain), chloroprocaine hydrochloride (Nesacaine), and tetracaine hydrochloride (Pontocaine). Esters are rapidly metabolized; therefore, toxic maternal levels are not as likely to be reached, and placental transfer to the fetus is prevented.

Amide types include bupivacaine hydrochloride (Marcaine), mepivacaine hydrochloride (Carbocaine), and lidocaine hydrochloride (Xylocaine). Amide types are more powerful and longer-acting agents than ester types. They readily cross the placenta, can be measured in the fetal circulation, and affect the fetus for a prolonged period. Newer amide types of local anesthetic agents, such as ropivacaine and levobupivacaine, are becoming more commonly used because they have a long action but fewer toxic effects (Bucklin et al., 2008).

Opioids are used with epidural blocks to produce analgesia for labor. Some of the agents used include morphine, fentanyl, butorphanol, and meperidine. When only opioids are used epidurally, the amount of pain relief is not as great. A combination of opioids and a low dose of a local anesthetic agent achieve better pain control with reduced motor impairment (Yentis, May, & Mahotra, 2007). There does appear to be a higher incidence of pruritus when this combination method is used, however. While the addition of opiates has been associated with undesirable side effects, such as nausea, vomiting, hypotension, respiratory depression, and sedation, the incidence appears to be low. These agents are commonly used, especially in women undergoing a cesarean birth, because of their high effectiveness rates in controlling postpartal pain (Yentis et al., 2007). Women who receive fentanyl can experience interference with early breastfeeding, with higher dosages having more negative impact than lower dosages (Gambling, Douglas, & McKay, 2008). Other evidence supports the use of fentanyl and butorphanol for administration in labor. There are no differences in cesarean and operative birth rates between women who received epidural opiates and those who received systemic analgesia. In fact, women who receive epidural opiates sometimes have a shorter first stage than those who receive systemic analgesic agents (Yentis et al., 2007).

A variety of anesthetic agents and a wide range of doses have been used for epidural anesthesia with varying results. The most commonly used agents are lidocaine 2% with epinephrine 1:200,000, bupivacaine 0.25%, and 2-chloroprocaine 3%. Each agent provides adequate anesthesia with 15 to 20 ml of the solution, but each has been associated with side effects. The pharmacology of each drug must be understood before it is used (Balestrieri-Martinez, 2009).

Adverse Maternal Reactions to Anesthetic Agents

Reactions to local anesthetic agents range from mild symptoms to cardiovascular collapse. Mild reactions include palpitations, vertigo, tinnitus, apprehension, confusion, headache, and a metallic taste in the mouth. Common side effects include pruritus, vertigo, dizziness, and urinary retention (Macksey, 2009). Moderate reactions include more severe degrees of the mild symptoms plus nausea and vomiting, hypotension, and muscle twitching, which may progress to convulsions and loss of consciousness. Severe reactions are sudden loss of consciousness, coma, severe hypotension, bradycardia, respiratory depression, and cardiac arrest (Macksey, 2009). High concentrations of the agents may also cause local toxic effects on tissues. It is important to remember that when the mother experiences an adverse reaction, the fetus is also affected.

Systemic toxic reactions most commonly occur with an excessive dose because of too great a concentration or too large a volume. Pregnant women in labor generally require less medication because of hormonal factors, uterine compression, an increase in cardiac output, and an increased sensitivity of the neural axons (Barash, Cullen, Stoelting et al., 2009). Accidental intravenous (IV) injection that suddenly increases the amount of the drug in maternal circulation results in depression of vasomotor, respiratory, and other medullary centers of the brain (Blackburn, 2007). It also depresses the heart and peripheral vascular bed. A massive intravascular dose can result in sudden circulatory collapse within 1 minute. Reactions to subcutaneous and extradural injection occur in 5 to 40 minutes. The short-acting agent procaine can produce toxic reactions in 10 to 15 minutes, and the long-acting agent mepivacaine in 20 to 40 minutes (Chestnut et al., 2009). It is imperative that the woman is under close supervision by knowledgeable personnel throughout the time that an agent is being used and that an IV line is in place.

If epinephrine has been added to the anesthetic agent to prolong the anesthesia, it is necessary to differentiate between reaction to the anesthetic agent and to the epinephrine. Reaction to epinephrine is characterized by pallor, perspiration, dyspnea, and a greater increase in blood pressure and pulse than occurs with reactions to anesthetic agents.

Psychogenic reactions such as severe anxiety, hallucinations, inability to move or speak, or catatonic appearance can also occur, with symptoms similar to those occurring with systemic toxic reactions (Chestnut et al., 2009). This phenomenon may occur as the procedure is begun and before the injection of the anesthetic agent. Regardless of the cause, the symptoms must be treated.

Allergic reactions to anesthetic agents may also occur. The manifestations of the antigen-antibody reaction include urticaria, laryngeal edema, joint pain, swelling of the tongue, and bronchospasm.

Treatment of Systemic Toxicity

Preferred treatment of mild toxicity involves the administration of oxygen by mask and IV injection of a short-acting barbiturate to decrease anxiety (Gambling et al., 2008). The clinician should anticipate the possibility of convulsions or cardiovascular collapse and make appropriate preparations to treat them.

Treatment of Convulsions

The best treatment for convulsions is to establish the airway and administer 100% oxygen. Thiopental or diazepam may be administered to stop convulsions (Chestnut et al., 2009). Small doses are adequate and help avoid cardiorespiratory depression.

Treatment of Sudden Cardiovascular Collapse

In sudden cardiovascular collapse, an airway must be established as cardiopulmonary resuscitation begins. IV fluids are increased, and emergency cesarean birth may be started immediately (Chestnut et al., 2009).

Lumbar Epidural Block

A lumbar **epidural block** involves injection of a local anesthetic agent into the epidural space. The epidural space is a potential space between the dura mater and the ligamentum flavum, extending from the base of the skull to the end of the sacral canal (Figure 25-2 ■). It contains areolar tissue, fat, lymphatics, and the internal vertebral venous plexus (Blackburn, 2007). This space is accessed through the lumbar area. The technique is most often used as a continuous block to provide analgesia and anesthesia from active labor through the birth and episiotomy repair. Complete pain relief is achieved for 85% of women; 12% experience partial relief; and only 3% of women report no relief at all (Cunningham et al., 2010).

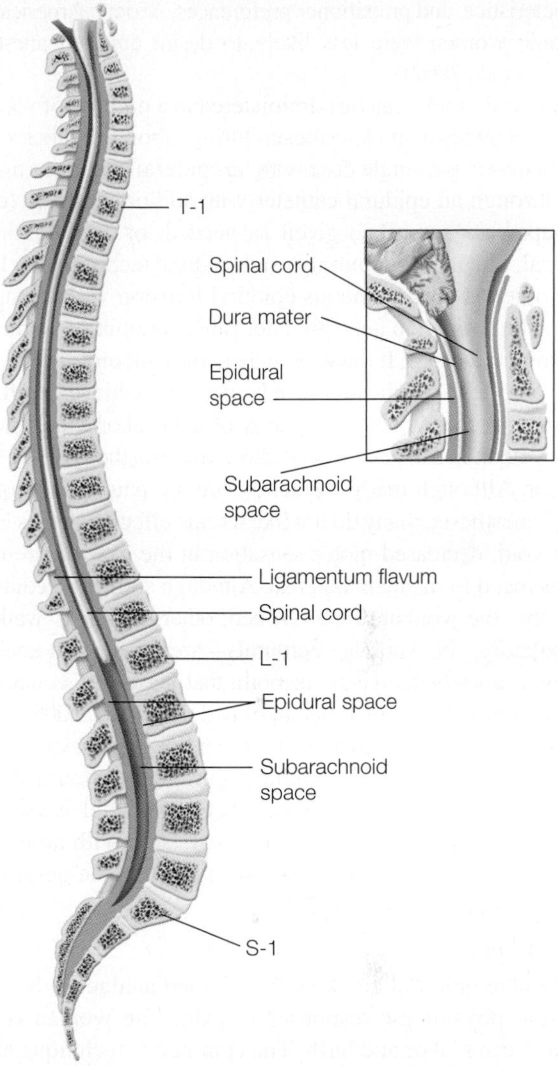

Figure 25-2 ■ The epidural space lies between the dura mater and the ligamentum flavum, extending from the base of the skull to the end of the sacral canal.

Lumbar epidural block has become fairly common during labor and birth. In the United States, epidural blocks are used by more than 60% of all women giving birth (Wolf, 2009). Moreover, recent studies have shown that the use of epidural anesthesia is the preferred method of pain relief for laboring women.

In the United States, epidural rates have continued to rise because of an increase in 24-hour availability of anesthesia services, the rise in cesarean birth rates, and a decline in the number of women who attempt a vaginal birth after a previous cesarean section (VBAC) (Wolf, 2009). In the past, it was thought that epidural availability might be linked to socioeconomic status. Recent research has shown that women in lower socioeconomic groups and those of African American race are less likely to accept epidural anesthesia than those in higher socioeconomic groups (Ochroch, Troxel, & Farrer, 2007). Women who were employed, had a college degree, and had previous experiences with epidural anesthesia were more likely to desire an epidural placement (Ochroch et al., 2007). Another study examining racial differences in epidural preference found that even when controlling for insurance coverage, clinical characteristics, and practitioner preferences, African American and Hispanic women were less likely to desire epidural anesthesia (Glance et al., 2007).

Epidural blocks can be administered in a number of ways. To provide analgesia and anesthesia during labor, the block can be administered as a single dose with an epidural needle, as a single dose through an epidural catheter with additional doses (called "top-ups" or "top-offs") given as needed, or as a continuous epidural. The most commonly used epidural technique for laboring women is the continuous epidural infusion via a pump that allows the woman to get a predetermined amount of medication on a continual basis. If the woman becomes uncomfortable, a bolus of additional medication can be given to achieve comfort.

Many women equate the quality of their labor experience directly with their satisfaction with the anesthesia they receive while in labor. Although many women desire the pain relief from regional anesthesia, many do not like its side effects, such as inability to void, decreased motor sensation in the lower extremities, and the need to maintain bed rest. Although some procedures require that the woman remain in bed, others—called "walking," "ambulatory," or "mobile" epidurals—are given with analgesic agents or anesthetic agents, or both, that leave the woman with sufficient motor control to be out of bed (Macksey, 2009).

Current guidelines by the American Society of Anesthesiologists (ASA) states that epidural placement should be performed when the woman experiences pain and asks for an epidural. Early epidural use is not associated with an increase in operative or cesarean births and improves analgesia effectiveness (ASA Task Force, 2007).

Epidurals: Risks and Benefits

Advantages

The lumbar epidural block produces good analgesia that alters maternal physiologic responses to pain. The woman is fully awake during labor and birth. The continuous technique allows different blocking for each stage of labor so that internal rotation of the fetus can be accomplished. In many cases, the dose of anesthetic agent can be adjusted to preserve the woman's reflex urge to bear down.

Disadvantages

The most common complication of an epidural block is maternal hypotension. Hypotension commonly occurs as a result of peripheral vasodilatation (Braveman, 2006). This is increased by the blockade of the sympathetic nerve supply to the adrenal glands, which prevents the release of catecholamines (Blackburn, 2007). This is generally prevented by preloading with a rapid infusion of IV fluids, then providing IV fluids continuously. Although hypotension can occur, the incidence of hypotension requiring ephedrine is relatively low, less than 2% (Cunningham et al., 2010). Other serious complications, although rare, have been reported, including postdural puncture seizures, meningitis, cardiorespiratory arrest, and vertigo (vestibulocochlear dysfunction) (Barash et al., 2009).

There are multiple regional anesthesia approaches for women undergoing cesarean birth. When an epidural block is used for cesarean birth, an epidural catheter is inserted and a single dose can be given. This approach allows for a more gradual onset and requires less medication to be administered. This reduces the risk of hypotension (Gambling et al., 2008). The catheter provides access to the epidural space, so that additional anesthetic agents and opioids may be administered if needed and so that opioids may be given to provide pain relief for the 24 hours following birth.

Another disadvantage of an epidural block is that the onset of analgesia may not occur for up to 30 minutes. In addition, an epidural block requires skilled personnel for administration and close observation of the woman and her fetus. The anesthesia provider must be careful while administering the block to avoid perforating the dura mater, which would place the needle in the subarachnoid space; if the error is not recognized, the anesthetic agent would be injected into the spinal canal. Skilled nurses are also required to maintain close observation of the laboring woman and her fetus. Variability of the fetal heart rate (FHR) may decrease, and late decelerations can occur if maternal hypotension develops. Finally, epidural anesthesia is more costly than systemic agents. This may be a crucial factor for women and families without insurance who are paying out of pocket for their birthing costs.

Some women with epidurals may have decreased sensation and movement, or they may have essentially no control over movement in the anesthetized region. Some studies have demonstrated that epidural use prolonged the first stage of labor and contributed to the need to augment labors with oxytocin (Chestnut et al., 2009). On the other hand, other clinical studies, along with healthcare providers, assert that epidural analgesia may shorten the active and transition phases because of the pain relief (Wolf, 2009). A meta-analysis showed that women who had received continuous infusion epidural anesthesia had a longer second stage (24 minutes) compared to women who received parenteral opioids (ASA Task Force, 2007). Women with epidurals experienced greater pain relief than those who received opioids by intramuscular or intravenous routes (ASA Task Force, 2007).

Contraindications

Absolute contraindications for epidural block are (New York School of Regional Anesthesia, 2009):

- Maternal refusal
- Local or systemic infection
- Uncorrected hypovolemia
- Coagulation disorders
- Actual or anticipated maternal hemorrhage
- Increased intracranial pressure
- Allergy to a specific class of local anesthetic agents

Relative contraindications include (New York School of Regional Anesthesia, 2009):

- Platelet count less than 100,000/mm^3
- Severe anatomic abnormalities of the spine
- Uncooperative patient
- Sepsis
- Hypertension

Patients with previous back surgery, suspicion of neurologic disease, long-term use of aspirin or anti-inflammatory agents, abruptio placentae, acute infection at the epidural site, and the lack of trained staff at the facility are also causes for concern that need to be evaluated on an individual basis (New York School of Regional Anesthesia, 2009).

Epidurals can be used in women with heart failure or aortic stenosis although invasive monitoring may be needed to evaluate blood pressure variations (Ioscovich, Goldszmidt, Fadeev, et al., 2009). Often a cesarean birth is indicated to prevent the stress associated with the second stage and maternal pushing efforts (Ioscovich et al., 2009).

Technique for Continuous Lumbar Epidural Block

In administering a continuous lumbar epidural block, the following actions are taken (Barash et al., 2009; Chestnut et al., 2009):

1. Maternal and fetal status and labor progress are assessed. Because maternal blood pressure and pulse will be taken frequently, an automatic blood pressure device may be useful. FHR is continuously monitored by electronic fetal monitoring (EFM) by the nurse.
2. Oxygen and resuscitative equipment is readied. The nurse ensures all equipment is in the room and properly functioning.
3. An IV infusion is begun, and a preload of 500 to 2000 ml of IV fluid (e.g., 0.45% normal saline or lactated Ringer's) is given over approximately 15 to 30 minutes by the nurse.
4. The woman is positioned on her left or right side, at the edge of the bed (the mattress is firmer and provides more support) with the assistance of the nurse, with her legs slightly flexed, or she is asked to sit on the edge of the bed. She is advised to drop her shoulders, round out the small of her back, and place her chin on her chest. It may be helpful to advise the woman to "arch her back like a cat" to achieve the proper position. This position is especially effective for positioning obese women. The spinal column is not kept convex, as it is for a spinal block, because the convex position reduces the peridural space to a greater degree and stretches the dura mater, making it more susceptible to puncture. The epidural space is decreased during pregnancy because of venous engorgement. It is also smaller in obese and short individuals (Cunningham et al., 2010). A small pillow may be placed under the woman's head and in front of her chest to provide support for her arms. The nurse typically stands beside the woman, offering support and assisting her in maintaining this position. The nurse assists the woman with breathing techniques and alerts the anesthesia provider when a contraction occurs. See Figure 25-3 ■ for incorrect and correct positions for lumbar epidural block.

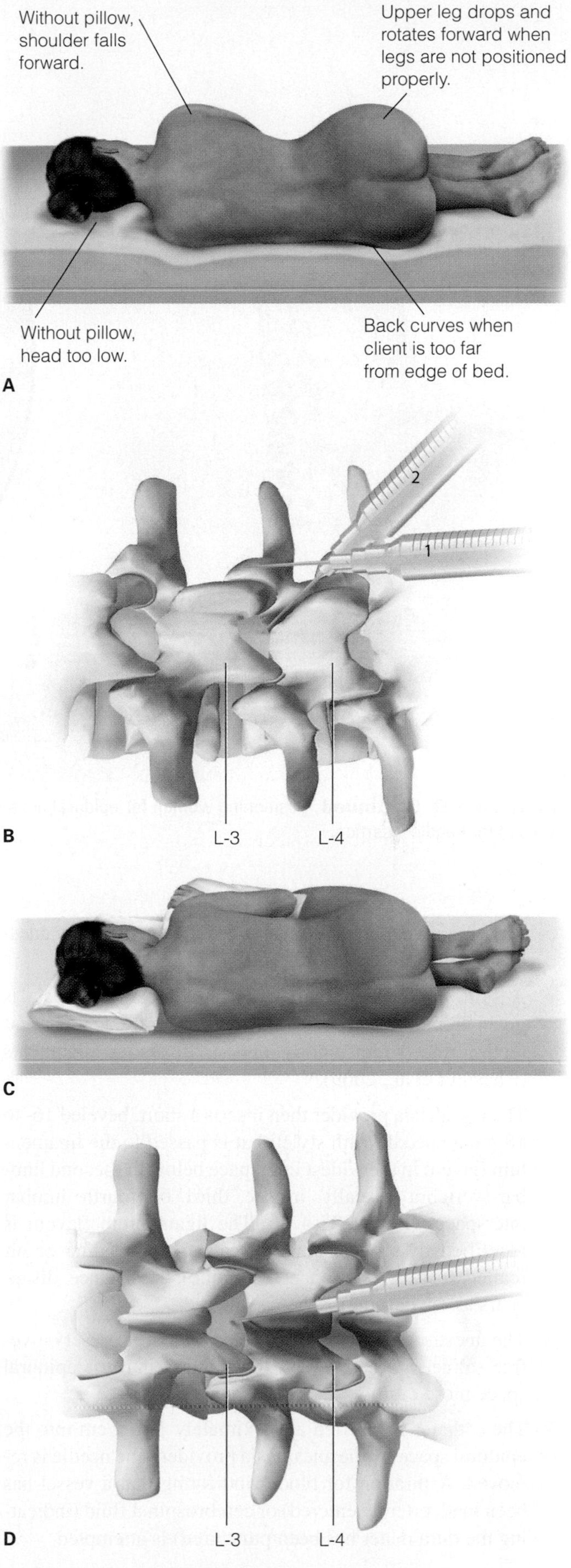
Without pillow, shoulder falls forward.
Upper leg drops and rotates forward when legs are not positioned properly.
Without pillow, head too low.
Back curves when client is too far from edge of bed.
A
2
1
B
L-3
L-4
C
D
L-3
L-4

Figure 25-3 ■ Positioning woman for epidural anesthesia block. A. Incorrect maternal positioning for placing subarachnoid or epidural block. The upper shoulder has fallen forward, upper leg has rotated forward, and the patient is positioned on the center of the bed so that there is no support from the edge and the back can curve. B. Vertebral position with patient in incorrect position. The vertebrae rotate forward and, if the needle is inserted in the usual way (needle 1), the apophyseal joints are encountered. Needle 2 shows the proper insertion of the needle entering the epidural space. C. Correct maternal positioning. The back is straight and vertical, the shoulders are square, and the upper leg is prevented from rolling forward. D. Vertebral position with the woman correctly positioned.

Source: A–D adapted from S. M. Shnider & G. Levinson, Anesthesia for obstetrics, *3rd ed., Copyright © Lippincott Williams & Wilkins, 1993. Reprinted with permission.*

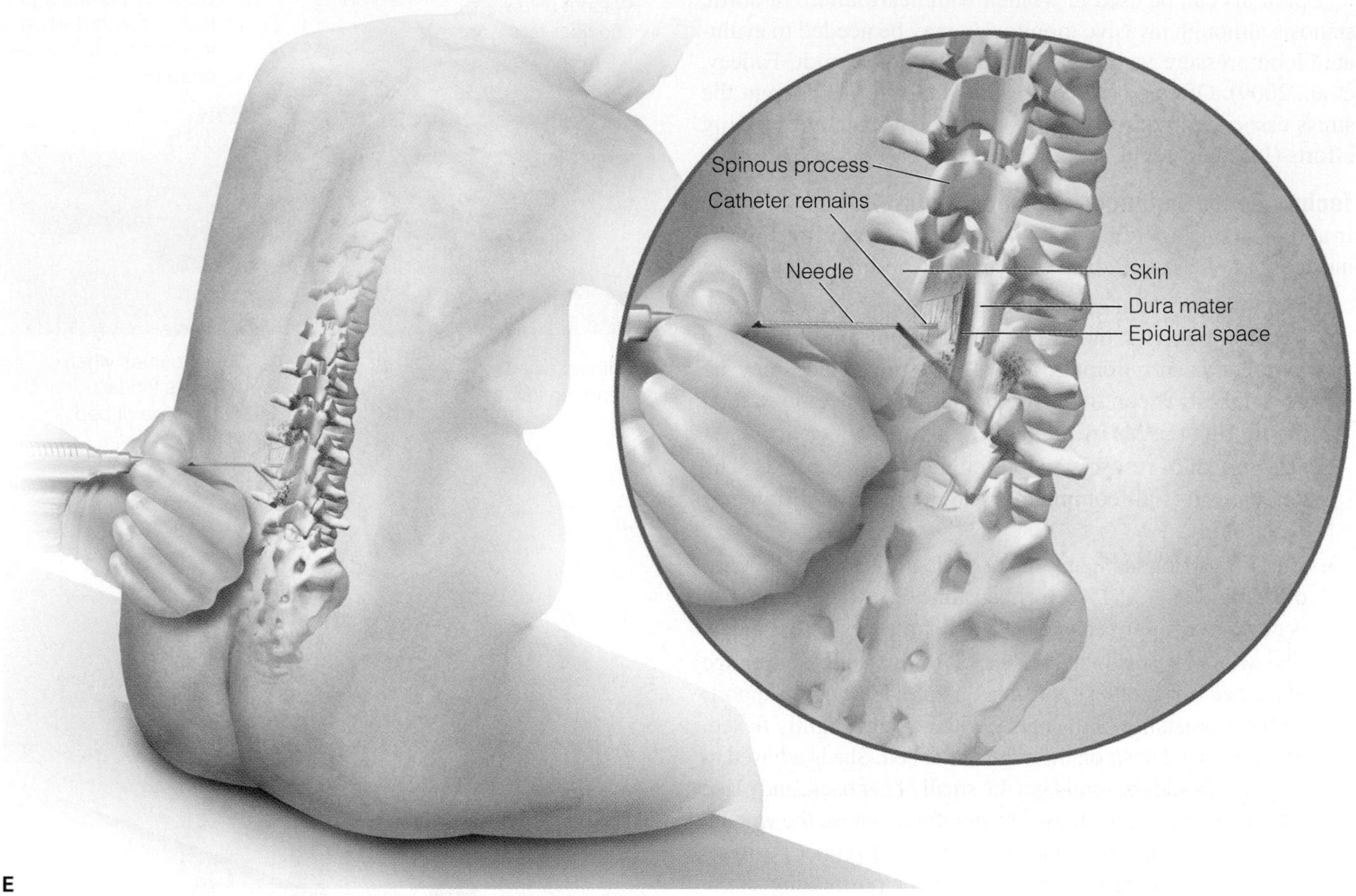

E

Figure 25-3 ■ Continued. Positioning woman for epidural anesthesia block. E. Sitting position with the shoulders rolled forward and back exposed for needle insertion.

Epidural Placement

5. The skin is prepared with an antiseptic agent by the anesthesia provider.
6. A skin wheal of a small amount of local anesthesia is given intradermally by the anesthesia provider to anesthetize the supraspinous and interspinous ligaments (Chestnut et al., 2009).
7. The anesthesia provider then inserts a short, beveled 16- to 18-gauge needle with stylet that is passed to the ligamentum flavum in the widest interspace below the second lumbar vertebra (usually in the third or fourth lumbar interspace) (Figure 25-4 ■). The ligamentum flavum is identified by its resistance to injection of saline or air (called loss of resistance technique). Resistance disappears as the peridural space is entered.
8. The anesthesia provider then injects 5 ml of preservative-free saline in order to pass the catheter into the epidural space more easily.
9. The catheter is inserted approximately 1 to 2 cm into the epidural space by the anesthesia provider. The needle is removed. Aspiration for blood (indicating that a vessel has been inadvertently entered) or cerebrospinal fluid (indicating the dura mater has been punctured) is attempted.
10. If aspiration tests are negative, a test dose of local anesthetic agent containing 1.5% lidocaine with epinephrine 1:200,000 concentration or 3 ml of 0.25% bupivacaine with 1:200,000 concentration of epinephrine is injected. The anesthesiologist usually injects the medication after aspiration and after a uterine contraction to minimize the risk of tachycardia that can occur if the drug is directly injected into a vessel (Cunningham et al., 2010). If the subarachnoid space has been entered, sensory and motor changes occur in the woman's extremities. If there are no untoward effects, additional anesthetic agent is injected. The catheter is securely taped so that its placement will not be disturbed. Pain relief should occur within 15 to 20 minutes after administration (Cunningham et al., 2010).
11. The nurse then assists the woman into a semireclining position with a lateral tilt of her uterus for 10 minutes to allow for distribution of the block. This also prevents aortocaval compression (see chapter 14 ∞). She is then maintained in a side-lying position to maximize uteroplacental perfusion. If she needs to be turned to a supine position for fetal blood sampling or other procedures, the nurse turns the woman as quickly as possible and repositions her on her side.

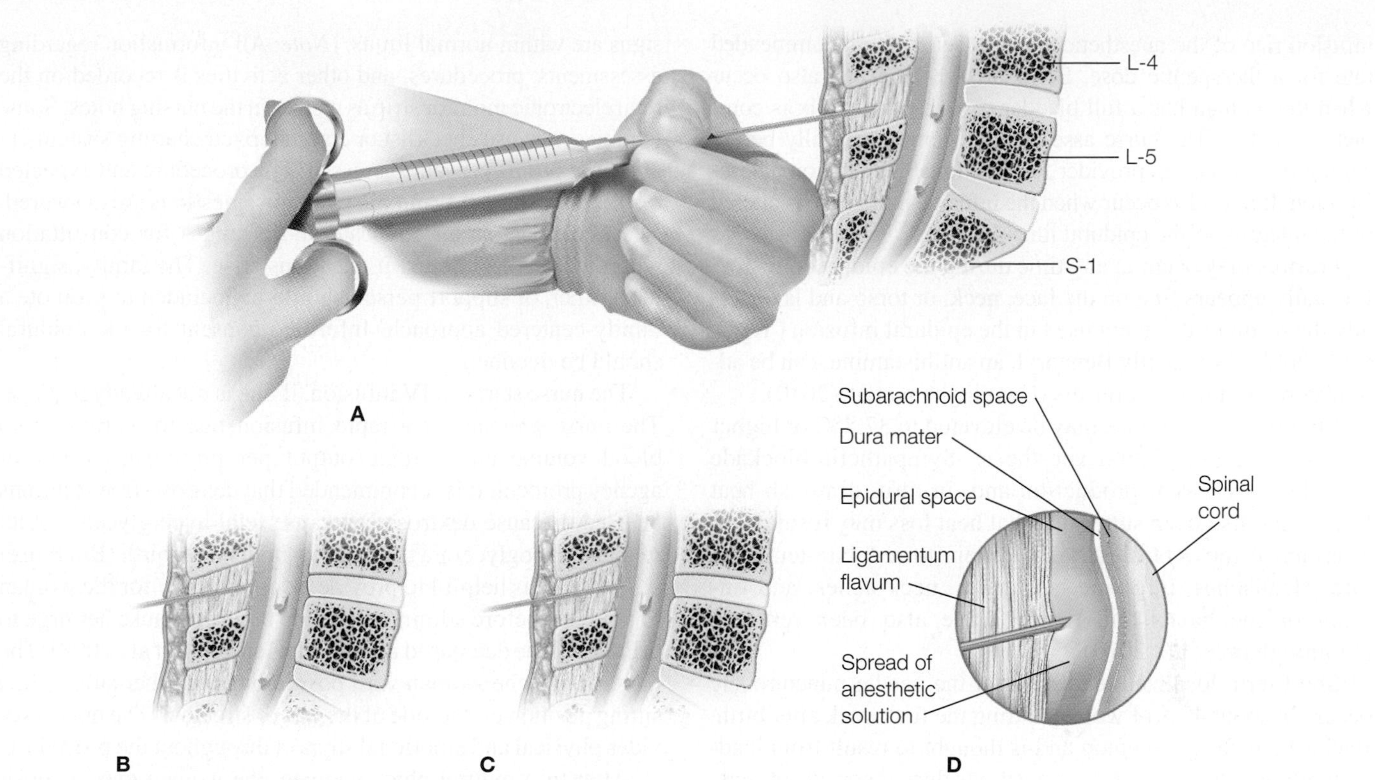

Figure 25-4 ■ Technique for lumbar epidural block. A. Proper position of insertion. B. Needle in the ligamentum flavum. C. Tip of needle in epidural space. D. Force of injection pushing dura away from tip of needle.

Source: Reprinted with permission from Bonica, J. J. (1972). Principles and practice of obstetric analgesia and anesthesia *(p. 631). Copyright © 1972 F. A. Davis Company.*

12. The anesthesia provider or the nurse then monitors the maternal blood pressure every 1 to 2 minutes for the first 10 minutes past the injection and then every 5 to 15 minutes until the block wears off. Maternal vital signs are evaluated by either the nurse or the anesthesia provider against baseline readings obtained just before the beginning of the procedure. The nurse is responsible for documentation of assessment data that are obtained throughout the procedure.
13. The woman must be attended by a nurse, nurse anesthetist, or an anesthesiologist for the first 20 minutes following the initial dose and after administration of any additional dose.
14. If hypotension (a 20% to 30% fall in systolic pressure or a drop to below 100 mm Hg) occurs, the nurse ensures that left lateral displacement of the uterus is maintained, and the IV fluids are infused more rapidly. Oxygen is delivered by a face mask to ensure proper oxygenation of the fetus. A 10- to 20-degree Trendelenburg position may be used. If the blood pressure is not restored within 1 to 2 minutes, a vasopressor such as ephedrine, 5 to 15 mg, may be administered IV.
15. The maternal blood pressure and pulse and the FHR continue to be monitored by the nurse.
16. If the epidural is not being administered by continuous pump, the anesthesiologist aspirates the catheter before administering subsequent doses.

Technique for Single-Dose Lumbar Epidural Block

The procedure for a single-dose lumbar epidural block is the same as for the lumbar block just described, except that instead of injecting 5 ml of saline, the anesthesiologist injects a test dose of 2 to 3 ml of anesthetic agent to make sure the dura mater has not been penetrated. After checking again to confirm that the dura mater has not been perforated, the clinician injects a single dose of 10 to 12 ml to provide anesthesia for birth. Subsequent care continues as for the procedure just described, from step 11 (Chestnut et al., 2009).

Problems and Adverse Effects

The major adverse effect of epidural anesthesia is maternal hypotension caused by a spinal blockade, which lowers peripheral resistance, decreases venous return to the heart, and subsequently lessens cardiac output and lowers blood pressure. Maternal hypotension results in uteroplacental insufficiency in the fetus, which is manifested as late decelerations on the fetal monitoring strip. The risk of hypotension can be minimized by hydrating the vascular system with 500 to 1000 ml of IV solution (Balestrieri-Martinez, 2009) before the procedure and changing the woman's position and/or increasing the IV rate afterward.

Application: Epidural Analgesia

A potentially distressing maternal problem is an inadequate block, unilateral block, or block failure. Epidural anesthesia has a higher failure rate than spinal anesthesia because the catheter must be properly placed to produce adequate anesthesia (Mackey, 2009). A one-sided block is fairly common and can be overcome by having the woman lie on the unanesthetized side and injecting more of the local anesthetic agent. If the woman has a continuous epidural block, she should turn from side to side every hour to avoid a one-sided block. A block may be effective except for a "spot" ("hot spot") or "window" of pain in the inguinal or suprapubic area. Breakthrough pain may occur at any time during the epidural infusion. It usually occurs when the continuous

Case Study: Patient Requesting an Epidural

Care Plan Activity: Managing Side Effects of an Epidural

infusion rate of the anesthetic agent is below the recommended rate for a therapeutic dose. Breakthrough pain can also occur when the woman has a full bladder or when the cervix is completely dilated. The nurse assesses the woman carefully before calling the anesthesia provider for additional medication administration. It may also occur when the infusion pump rate is altered or the integrity of the epidural line is broken.

Pruritus may occur at any time during the epidural infusion. It usually appears first on the face, neck, or torso and is generally the result of the agent used in the epidural infusion (Yentis et al., 2007). Frequently Benadryl, an antihistamine, can be administered to manage pruritus (Cunningham et al., 2010).

Maternal temperature may be elevated to 37.8°C or higher with the use of epidural anesthesia. Sympathetic blockade may decrease sweat production and, in turn, diminish heat loss. It has also been suggested that heat loss may result from a failure of the central nervous system to regulate temperature. Headaches, migraine headaches, neck aches, and tingling of the hands and fingers have also been reported (Cunningham et al., 2010).

Short-term localized tenderness at the needle puncture site occurs in about 40% of women during the first week after birth. Backache is fairly common and is thought to result from inadvertently maintaining stressed positions during periods of muscle relaxation and pain relief from the epidural block. Long-term back pain is uncommon. Other problems or adverse effects include urinary retention, shivering, nausea, and vomiting.

Complications

One of the most serious complications of regional anesthesia, systemic toxic reaction, has been discussed in "Adverse Maternal Reactions to Anesthetic Agents" on p. 644. Toxic reactions following a lumbar epidural block may be caused by unintentional placement of the drug in the arachnoid or subarachnoid space, excessive amount of the drug in the epidural space (massive epidural), or accidental intravascular injection (Chestnut et al., 2009). Because large quantities of anesthetic agent are used for epidural block, the likelihood of toxic reactions is higher than with some of the other regional procedures. The incidence of drug reactions is relatively low, but the possibility is always present.

Pain during cesarean birth with epidural anesthesia has been reported by a growing number of women. In light of this, some anesthesiologists use both temperature and pinprick tests to assess sensory loss. Dermatomes from T_4 to S_3 should be tested for sensory loss before beginning a cesarean (Chestnut et al., 2009). The method of assessment and the results should be documented in the anesthesia record.

Spinal headaches can also be a complication that occurs with epidural anesthesia. Spinal headaches occur when the dura is accidently punctured during epidural placement (Bucklin et al., 2008).

NURSING CARE MANAGEMENT

The nurse assesses the maternal vital signs and the FHR for baseline information and to ensure that both maternal and fetal vital signs are within normal limits. (*Note*: All information regarding assessments, procedures, and other activities is recorded on the fetal electronic monitor strip as well as in the nursing notes. Some facilities may use checklist or computerized charting systems.)

Labor progress is also assessed. The procedure and expected results are explained, and the woman's questions are answered. The nurse acts as an advocate and arranges for consultation with the anesthesiologist if questions arise. The family, significant other, or support person should be included to promote a family-centered approach. Informed consent for the epidural should be obtained.

The nurse starts an IV infusion, if one is not already in place. The nurse preloads at a rapid infusion rate to increase both blood volume and cardiac output per physician's order or agency protocol. It is recommended that dextrose-free solutions be used, because dextrose can cause fetal hyperglycemia with rebound hypoglycemia the first few hours after birth (Bucklin et al., 2008). It is helpful to provide an opportunity for the woman to void just before administering the block, because her urge to urinate will be decreased afterward (Gambling et al., 2008). The nurse assists the woman with positioning on either side or in a sitting position on the side of the bed or stretcher. The nurse provides physical and emotional support throughout the procedure.

After the epidural block is given, the woman may be positioned in a semireclining position (head at 25 degrees) with lateral uterine tilt to provide equal distribution of the block; then she is turned to a side-lying position (Yentis et al., 2007). If she is supine for procedures such as sterile vaginal examinations or fetal scalp blood sampling, the nurse places a wedge under her hip to help eliminate aortocaval compression. The nurse takes maternal blood pressure and pulse every 5 minutes for at least 30 minutes and then at least every 30 minutes thereafter while the block is present (Macksey, 2009). The FHR is monitored and assessed by continuous EFM.

If hypotension (systolic blood pressure below 100 mm Hg) occurs, the nurse assists with corrective measures such as positioning the woman in a left side-lying position, increasing the flow rate of the IV infusion, and placing the bed in a 10- to 20-degree Trendelenburg position (Balestrieri-Martinez, 2009). If maternal blood pressure does not increase within 1 to 2 minutes, 5 to 15 mg of ephedrine may be administered IV per physician or protocol order. These measures are usually sufficient; however, if hypotension persists, oxygen by mask at 7 to 10 L/min and additional vasopressors may be needed (Cunningham et al., 2010). During episodes of maternal hypotension, the nurse observes the FHR for signs of late decelerations related to uteroplacental insufficiency. Nausea and vomiting may be associated with hypotension. An antiemetic may be ordered to increase the woman's comfort. With severe or prolonged hypotension, added treatment includes elevating the woman's legs for 2 or 3 minutes to increase blood return from the extremities (Macksey, 2009). See Nursing Care Plan For Epidural Anesthesia for more information about maternal hypotension associated with epidural anesthesia.

If additional local anesthetic agents are injected, the regimen of assessing maternal blood pressure and initial surveillance should be repeated each time the epidural catheter is reinjected. If the woman's legs have been in stirrups during a

NURSING CARE PLAN For Epidural Anesthesia

1. Nursing Diagnosis: Risk for Injury related to maternal hypotension associated with epidural anesthesia secondary to vasodilation and venous pooling

Goal: Maternal and fetal effects associated with hypotension will be minimized.

INTERVENTION	RATIONALE
■ Obtain baseline maternal vital signs and fetal heart rate.	■ Normal ranges include temperature 98 to 99.6°F/36.6 to 37.5°C, pulse 60 to 90, respirations 14 to 22/min, blood pressure 90–140/60–90, fetal heart rate 110 to 160 beats/min.
■ Insert IV with large gauge catheter.	■ Allows for IV fluid to be administered quickly if hypotension occurs.
■ Provide hydration with 500 to 1000 ml of intravenous solution (e.g., lactated Ringer's) 15 to 30 min before procedure. Dextrose-free solution is recommended.	■ Increases intravascular volume and maintains cardiac output by preloading the patient before epidural anesthesia. Rapid infusion of dextrose solution can cause fetal hyperglycemia and rebound neonatal hypoglycemia.
■ Educate the patient about treatment measures to expect if unwanted side effects from the epidural occur.	■ Advance preparation will decrease anxiety and the patient will be more compliant. Treatment measures include oxygen administration, increase of IV fluids, possible administration of a vasopressor such as ephedrine, and repositioning the patient.
■ Assist the patient into position for the procedure.	■ Place patient in a supine position for 5 to 10 min following administration of block to allow medication to diffuse bilaterally. After 5 to 10 min, position patient on side.
■ Monitor blood pressure every 1 to 2 min for the first 10 min then every 5 to 15 min until the block wears off.	■ Hypotension is the most common side effect of epidural anesthesia. Close monitoring will allow for quick assessment and treatment of any changes from baseline blood pressure before the procedure.
EXPECTED OUTCOMES: Decrease in blood pressure is identified and treated successfully.	
■ Observe, record, and report symptoms of hypotension, including systolic pressure <100 mm Hg or a 20% to 30% fall in systolic pressure, apprehension, restlessness, dizziness, tinnitus, and headache.	■ These signs are related to hypotension and must be treated immediately to avoid health risk to mother and fetus.
EXPECTED OUTCOMES: Hypotension is identified and treatment measures started.	
■ Initiate treatment measures to reverse hypotension.	■ Treatment measures include placing patient in left lateral position as directed, increase IV rate, administer oxygen by face mask at 7 to 10 L/min as needed, administer vasopressors as ordered (usually ephedrine 5 to 10 mg IV), manually displace uterus laterally to left using a wedge or pillow. Notify analgesia provider or certified nurse anesthetist immediately.
EXPECTED OUTCOMES: Hypotension is treated successfully, and blood pressure returns to normal limits.	
■ Observe, record, and report fetal bradycardia (FHR less than 110 beats/min) and loss of beat-to-beat variability.	■ Maternal hypotension results in decreased blood flow to the fetus. Normal fetal heart rate ranges between 110 and 160 beats/min. Fetal bradycardia occurs when the fetal heart rate falls below 110 beats/min during a 10-min period of continuous monitoring. When fetal bradycardia is accompanied by decreased beat-to-beat variability, it is considered ominous and could be a sign of advanced fetal compromise.
EXPECTED OUTCOMES: Treatment of maternal hypotension increases blood flow to the fetus, reversing fetal bradycardia. Fetal heart rate stays within normal limits with good beat-to-beat variability.	

vaginal birth, her blood pressure should be assessed as soon as her legs are taken out of the stirrups. While the legs were elevated, circulating blood volume in the trunk increased. Restoring circulation to the legs decreases the overall blood volume and may precipitate hypotension.

Additional nursing care following the block includes frequent assessment of the bladder to avoid bladder distention. Catheterization may be necessary, because most women are unable to void; however, the nurse should first offer the woman a bedpan, because catheterization increases the risk of urinary tract infections (Berman, Synder, Kozier, & Erb, 2008).

Shivering may be caused by heat loss from increased peripheral blood flow or alteration of thermal input to the central nervous system when warm but not cold sensations have been suppressed. New studies suggest the maternal temperature in the lower extremities is lower than in the upper extremities and thus stimulates a shivering reaction (Doufas, Morioka, Maghoub, et al., 2008). Although warming intravenous fluids enhances maternal comfort, it does not reduce shivering (Woolnough, Allam, Hemingway, et al., 2009). Applying warmed blankets and reassuring the woman may make her feel more comfortable.

The nurse assesses the woman's level of pain relief. The nurse can promote equal distribution of the anesthetic agent by assessing the temperature of the woman's feet. If one foot warms more quickly than the other, the woman should be positioned with the cooler side dependent (Doufas et al., 2008). It is important for the woman to turn from side to side every hour to promote equal distribution of the anesthetic agent. Again, the woman should be assessed for advanced cervical dilatation and bladder distention. If positioning changes and emptying the bladder do not help and the woman has inadequate pain relief, the anesthesia provider needs to be notified. During a continuous epidural block, the anesthesiologist should titrate the infusion to maintain a sensory level of T_{10}, and the presence of motor block and height of sensory block should be documented at least hourly (Chestnut et al., 2009).

Respiratory rate and quality of the respirations should be assessed at least every 15 to 30 minutes. The nurse should notify the anesthetist of any significant decreases in respiratory rate or respiratory pattern changes. If the respiratory rate falls below 14 respirations per minute, naloxone (Narcan) may be given to remove the effect of the anesthetic agent; respirations will then return to a normal rate (Bucklin et al., 2008).

The nurse asks the woman if she is experiencing pruritus and is alert for signs of scratching, especially on the face, neck, and torso. If present, pruritus is usually treated with diphenhydramine (Benadryl), 25 mg administered IV or 50 mg IM per physician's or CNM's order (Cunningham et al., 2010).

During the second stage of labor, the woman may require assistance with pushing, because she may not feel her contractions or experience the urge to push. If the woman does not feel the urge to push, the nurse may collaborate with the anesthesia provider so that the block can be turned down or temporarily turned off until the urge to push returns. She may also need assistance holding or controlling her legs in order to push. After birth, return of complete sensation and the ability to control the legs are essential before ambulation is attempted. This may take several hours, depending on the agent and the total dose. The woman must also be able to maintain blood pressure in a sitting and then standing position.

Epidural Analgesia After Birth

To provide analgesia for approximately 24 hours after the birth, the anesthesiologist may inject an opioid, such as morphine (Duramorph) 5 mg or 7.5 mg, into the epidural space immediately following the birth. These agents are typically reserved for women who have had a cesarean birth. The analgesic effect of Duramorph begins approximately 30 to 60 minutes after the injection. The side effects include pruritus, nausea and vomiting, and urinary retention (Wilson et al., 2010). See Drug Guide: Postbirth Epidural Morphine in chapter 36 ∞.

Other agents are being examined that offer equal or better pain control with fewer side effects. Meperidine (Demerol) may be injected during an epidural block for birth, and then continued through use of patient-controlled epidural analgesia (PCEA). Epidural meperidine is associated with fewer side effects than epidural morphine and does not cause hemodynamic changes (Chestnut et al., 2009). Epidural fentanyl and lidocaine have also been used. The addition of lidocaine has been associated with a more rapid onset of sensory block without the increased side effects (Chestnut et al., 2009).

Spinal Block

In a **spinal block**, a local anesthetic agent is injected directly into the spinal fluid in the subarachnoid space to provide anesthesia for cesarean birth. The subarachnoid space is the fluid-filled area between the dura mater and the spinal cord. During pregnancy, the space decreases because of the distention of the epidural veins. Thus a specific dose of anesthetic produces a much higher level of anesthesia in the pregnant woman than in the nonpregnant woman. When a spinal block is properly administered, failure rate is low. Unlike epidural anesthesia, spinal blocks allow the anesthesia to mix directly with the cerebrospinal fluid, which eliminates "windows" where anesthesia coverage is not obtained (Chestnut et al., 2009). Cesarean birth requires anesthetic blockade to the T_4 dermatome (Figure 25-5 ■).

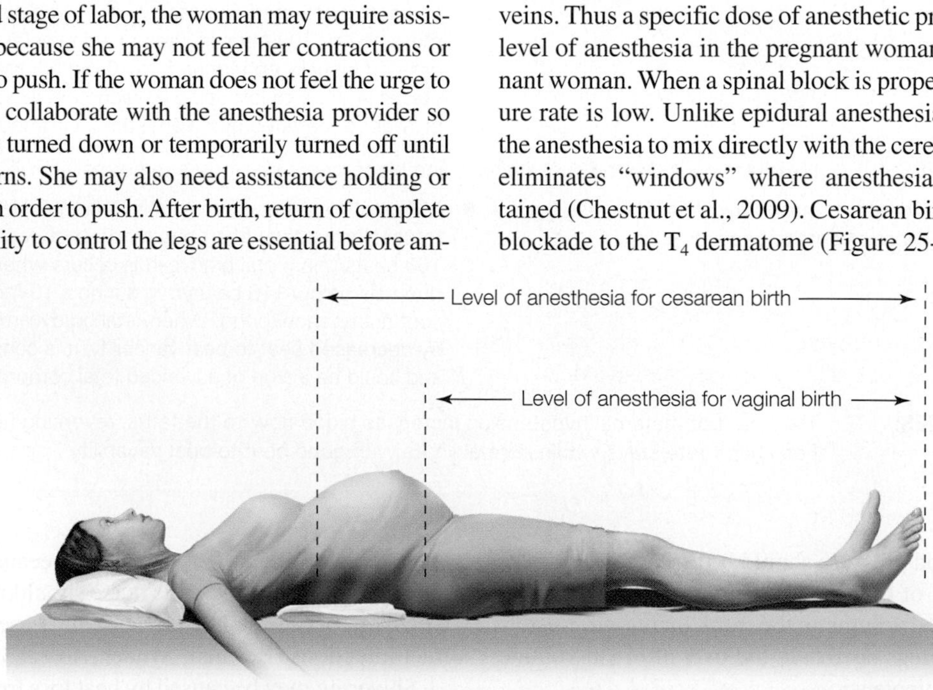

Figure 25-5 ■ Levels of anesthesia for vaginal and cesarean births.

Source: Reprinted with permission of Ross Laboratories, Columbus, OH. From Clinical Education Aid No. 17.

Advantages

The advantages of spinal block are immediate onset of anesthesia, relative ease of administration, a smaller drug volume, and maternal compartmentalization of the drug. Spinal anesthesia is frequently the regional block of choice in acute obstetrical emergencies because it is the safest and fastest anesthesia technique (Chestnut et al., 2009).

Disadvantages

The primary disadvantage of spinal block is intense blockade of sympathetic fibers, resulting in a high incidence of hypotension. This leads to a greater potential for fetal hypoxia. In addition, uterine tone is maintained, which makes intrauterine manipulation difficult. Spinal anesthesia is traditionally short acting, and it is difficult to maintain adequate anesthesia coverage for prolonged procedures (Chestnut et al., 2009).

Contraindications

Spinal anesthesia is contraindicated for women with severe hypovolemia, regardless of cause; central nervous system disease; infection over the site of puncture; maternal coagulation problems; and allergy to local anesthetic agents (Chestnut et al., 2009). Sepsis and active genital herpes may be considered relative rather than absolute contraindications. Spinal block is also contraindicated for women who do not wish to have spinal procedures or are unable to appropriately consent (Cunningham et al., 2010).

Technique

The following steps are followed in administering a subarachnoid block (Chestnut et al., 2009):

1. The nurse assists the woman into a sitting or left lateral position.
2. Intravenous infusion is checked for patency.
3. The woman places her arms between her knees, bows her head, and arches her back to widen the intervertebral space.
4. The anesthesiologist or nurse anesthetist prepares the skin carefully, maintaining sterility before initiating the procedure.
5. A skin wheal is made over L_3 or L_4.
6. An 18- or 19-gauge needle is introduced through the skin and into the interspinous ligament. Then, a 24- to 27-gauge pencil-point needle is introduced inside the larger needle and inserted into the ligamentum flavum, the epidural space through the dura mater, and into the subarachnoid space (Figure 25-6 ■).
7. The appropriate amount of anesthetic agent is injected slowly, and both needles are removed.
8. Upon removal, a drop of cerebrospinal fluid can be seen in the hub of the needle if the subarachnoid space has been entered.
9. With hyperbaric solutions, the woman remains sitting up for 45 seconds.
10. The nurse assists the woman onto her back with a pillow under her head. Position changes can alter the dermatome level if done within 3 to 5 minutes. After 10 minutes, a position change will not affect the level of anesthesia.

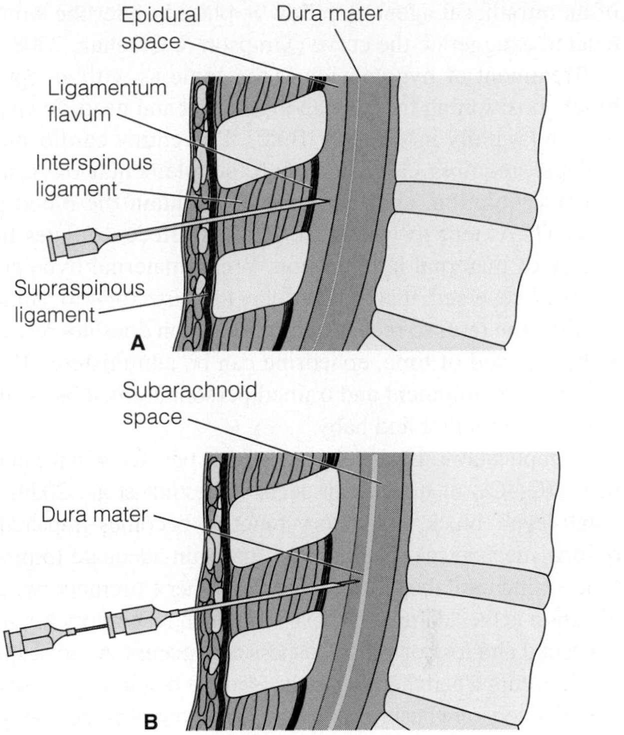

Figure 25-6 ■ Double-needle technique for spinal injection. A. Large needle in epidural space. B. 25-gauge needle in larger needle entering the subarachnoid space.

Source: Reprinted with permission from Bonica, J. J. (1972). Principles and practice of obstetric analgesia and anesthesia *(p. 563). Copyright © 1972 F. A. Davis Company.*

11. The nurse monitors blood pressure, pulse, and respirations every 1 to 2 minutes for the first 10 minutes, then every 5 to 10 minutes.

The nurse provides encouragement and support during the procedure. The nurse informs the physician when a contraction is beginning so the anesthetic agent will not be injected at that time.

In the absence of maternal hypotension or toxic reaction, a spinal block exerts no direct effect on the fetus. The amount of anesthetic used is too small to reach fetal circulation in a quantity that might cause fetal depression. Spinal anesthesia has been shown to be well tolerated by a healthy fetus when a maternal IV fluid preload in excess of 500 to 1000 ml precedes the administration of the spinal.

Complications

The complications of spinal anesthesia include hypotension, drug reaction, total spinal neurologic sequelae, and spinal headache. The side effects include nausea, shivering, and urinary retention.

Hypotension can be minimized by prehydrating with 500 to 2000 ml of non–dextrose-containing fluids and displacing the uterus to a lateral position. The practice of placing an already hypotensive woman in a sitting position following injection to prevent upward spread of hyperbaric solution is dangerous because it will cause venous pooling in the lower extremities, further decreasing the maternal blood pressure (Blackburn, 2007). The normal curve of the thoracic spine prevents cranial spread of an intrathecal agent. A pillow is placed under the woman's head to exaggerate the curve (Simpson & Creehan, 2008).

Treatment of hypotension is the same as with an epidural block: positioning the woman in a lateral and head-down position and rapidly infusing IV fluids. Preventing cardiovascular collapse requires early detection, supplemental oxygen, assisted ventilation, and measures to maintain the blood pressure. The extent to which the fetus is affected relates to the degree of maternal hypotension. When maternal hypotension has been reversed, it is best to delay the birth for 4 to 5 minutes to allow the fetus to recover. If hypotension does not resolve in a short period of time, ephedrine can be administered IV. Resuscitative equipment and trained personnel must be available to treat the mother and baby.

Complications that involve anesthesia occurring in the phrenic nerve (C_3–C_5) or higher can occur (Chestnut et al., 2009). In a "high-level" block, respiratory function becomes impaired, requiring mechanical ventilation to maintain adequate respiratory functioning until the block recedes. Another extremely rare complication is the "complete spinal" in which respiratory assistance is needed and loss of consciousness also occurs. A "total spinal" block occurs when there is paralysis of the respiratory muscles. It is a relatively rare but critical event. The symptoms include apnea, dilation of pupils, loss of consciousness, and absence of blood pressure. The onset of symptoms usually occurs within minutes of the injection but can occur in a span of time ranging from 30 seconds to 45 minutes. Resuscitative treatment, airway control, and support of blood pressure must begin immediately. If this complication occurs, it is important to remember that the woman is not asleep; although she may be paralyzed, she may be aware of everything going on around her. She requires assurance that her respiratory status will be maintained until she can breathe on her own again (Chestnut et al., 2009).

On the other hand, a spinal block can render inadequate anesthesia coverage (in which the anesthesia does not reach the T_4 level) and discomfort can occur. During intraoperative procedures, this may warrant the need for a repeat insertion or the need for general anesthesia (Chestnut et al., 2009).

Neurologic complications may occur coincidentally with spinal anesthesia, for example, with preexisting disease or faulty positioning of the woman. Hypotension and apnea can occur, requiring prompt treatment to prevent cardiac arrest. The woman should be positioned with a left tilt, and fluids should be administered to treat hypotension (Cunningham et al., 2010). Genuine neurologic sequelae, such as paralysis, are extremely rare.

Although much less serious than other complications, headache may be an unpleasant aftermath of spinal anesthesia. It is the most frequent complication with an incidence of about 1% to 3% (Cunningham et al., 2010). Leakage of spinal fluid at the site of dural puncture is thought to be the cause. Several techniques have been suggested to decrease the possibility of headache. The use of a narrow-gauge pencil-point anesthesia needle (24- to 27-gauge) reduces the incidence of spinal headache (ASA Task Force, 2007). Conservative treatments, such as hyperhydration and keeping the woman flat in bed after birth, have been used with minimal success. An abdominal binder may provide some relief. Postdural headaches can last up to 7 days and not only are painful but can also interfere with maternal-infant interactions and breastfeeding success. In severe cases, a blood patch can be performed. A few milliliters of the woman's blood is drawn and, before coagulation occurs, injected into the epidural space at the site of the puncture, which generally results in immediate pain relief.

NURSING CARE MANAGEMENT

The nurse should assist in positioning the woman, provide oxygen via nasal cannula or mask, assess and record baseline vital signs of the mother and fetus, and start an IV infusion before the block. A bolus of fluid should be given before initiation of the block whenever possible (Bucklin et al., 2008). After the block is instilled, the nurse should continue to monitor maternal blood pressure, pulse, and respiration until the anesthesiologist takes over. The nurse monitors the FHR at least every 5 minutes until it is no longer accessible because the abdominal surgical prep is begun. The anesthesiologist is responsible for assessing and recording the level of the spinal block.

The nurse positions the woman as described earlier and supports her in this position. The nurse palpates the woman's uterus to detect the beginning of a contraction. Intrathecal agents are not administered during a contraction because the increased pressure could cause a higher level of anesthesia than desired. After the agent has been administered, the woman is supported upright for the length of time determined by the anesthesiologist and is then assisted to the supine position with a wedge under her right hip to displace the uterus; a pillow is placed under her head. In the surgical setting, a safety belt is placed across the woman's thighs to prevent injury. The nurse regularly monitors blood pressure, pulse, and respirations every 5 minutes until the birth. Oxygen may be given as a prophylactic measure. The woman should be kept informed of everything that is going on in the birthing area, particularly if she is receiving mask oxygen. Raising her legs facilitates venous return from the extremities. If using stirrups, both legs should be raised at the same time to avoid undue tension and possible injury to back muscles.

If hypotension should occur, the IV fluids should be increased and the uterus displaced manually to the left (Barash et al., 2009). If the woman reports that she is having difficulty breathing, she needs to be assessed very carefully. Total spinal block rarely occurs, but the possibility must always be kept in mind. The woman should be observed for apnea, unconsciousness, pupil dilation, and unobtainable blood pressure. Prompt treatment, which may include the use of a vasopressor (such as ephedrine), may avert maternal or fetal death. It is essential to establish an airway and give oxygen with positive pressure until the woman can be intubated and other emergency measures instituted.

Following the birth, the woman may be kept flat. Although the effectiveness of the supine position to avoid headache following a spinal is controversial, the physician's orders may include lying flat for 6 to 12 hours.

Combined Spinal-Epidural Block

Spinal anesthesia may be combined with an epidural block. The combined spinal-epidural (CSE) can be used for labor analgesia and for cesarean birth. The anesthetic and analgesic agents used differ according to the purpose of the CSE. A CSE is accomplished by inserting an epidural needle into the epidural space. A narrow-gauge pencil-point anesthesia needle (24- to 27-gauge) is inserted through the epidural needle, through the dura, and into the cerebrospinal fluid. A small amount of local anesthetic agent, opioid, or both, is injected, and the needle is withdrawn. An epidural catheter is then threaded through the epidural needle into the epidural space. The epidural needle is removed and the epidural catheter is securely placed against the woman with tape.

An advantage of CSE is that the spinal agent will have a faster onset than medications that are injected into the epidural space. A CSE is versatile in that medication can be added to increase the effectiveness. Maternal satisfaction is high when a CSE is used because there is a quick onset of pain relief. Additional medication can also be added if an instrument-assisted birth or cesarean is needed (Okutomi, Saito, Mochizuki, et al., 2009). Studies show that the optimal timing of an epidural with the CSE is within 30 minutes of the spinal placement (Okutomi et al., 2009). CSE also preserves motor functioning. Most drugs are used in low dose, so spinal analgesia may be given in early labor to assist with labor pain. The nurse assesses the woman's strength and motor functioning before ambulation occurs. If ambulation is desired, a continuous assessment of the FHR and the maternal blood pressure is needed. Close supervision is needed to prevent falls or other injuries. When CSE is used, there does appear to be a higher incidence of nausea and pruritus. There are no reports of increased risks of fetal or neonatal complications.

Pudendal Block

The **pudendal block** technique provides perineal anesthesia for the second stage of labor, birth, and episiotomy repair. An anesthetic agent is injected below the pudendal plexus, as shown in Figure 25-1. The pudendal plexus arises from the anterior division of the second and third sacral nerves and the entire fourth sacral nerve. Below the plexus, the branches converge into the pudendal nerve, which crosses the sacrosciatic notch and passes the tip of the ischial spine, where it divides into the perineal, dorsal, and inferior hemorrhoidal nerves of the pudendal plexus. The perineal nerve, which is the largest branch of the pudendal plexus, supplies the skin of the vulvar area, the perineal muscles, and the urethral sphincter. The dorsal nerve supplies the clitoris, and the inferior hemorrhoidal nerve supplies the skin and muscles of the perineal region as well as the internal anal sphincter. Pudendal block provides relief of pain from perineal distention but does not relieve pain of uterine contractions (Figure 25-7 ■).

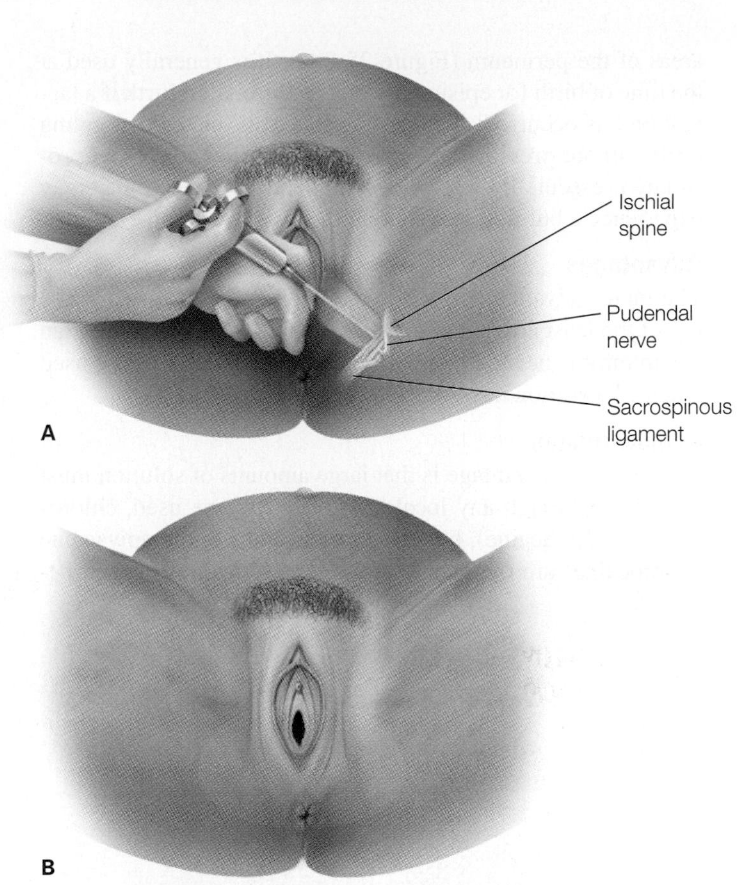

Figure 25-7 ■ A. Pudendal block by the transvaginal approach. B. Area of perineum affected by pudendal block.

Advantages and Disadvantages

The advantages of pudendal block are ease of administration and absence of maternal hypotension. It also allows the use of low forceps or vacuum extraction for birth.

A moderate dose of anesthetic agent (10 ml per side) has minimal ill effects on the woman and the course of labor. The urge to bear down during the second stage of labor may be decreased, but the woman is able to do so with appropriate coaching. There is usually little effect on the uncompromised fetus unless overly rapid or intravascular injection occurs. The block may be done by a transvaginal or transperineal approach. The woman may experience a burning sensation when the block is administered. Transvaginal injection is simpler, safer, and more direct, making it the procedure of choice.

Complications

A systemic toxic reaction can occur from accidental vascular injection. Other possible maternal complications specific to pudendal block include broad ligament hematoma, perforation of the rectum, and trauma to the sciatic nerve.

NURSING CARE MANAGEMENT

The nurse explains the procedure and the expected effect and answers any questions. Pudendal block does not alter maternal vital signs or FHR, so assessments in addition to the expected ones are not necessary.

Local Infiltration Anesthesia

Local anesthesia is accomplished by injecting an anesthetic agent into the intracutaneous, subcutaneous, and intramuscular areas of the perineum (Figure 25-8 ■). It is generally used at the time of birth for episiotomy and repair or after birth if a laceration has occurred; it is especially useful for women giving birth without previous pharmacologic interventions. The procedure is essentially free from complications. The woman may experience a burning sensation at the time of administration.

Advantages

The major advantage of the local block is that it involves the use of the least amount of anesthetic agent. It can be done if an episiotomy is needed just before the birth. It can also be used when a laceration has occurred and a repair is needed.

Disadvantages

The major disadvantage is that large amounts of solution must be used. Although any local anesthetic may be used, chloroprocaine (Nesacaine), lidocaine (Xylocaine), and mepivacaine (Carbocaine) are the agents of choice in local infiltration because of their capacity for diffusion. A burning sensation at the time of injection is common.

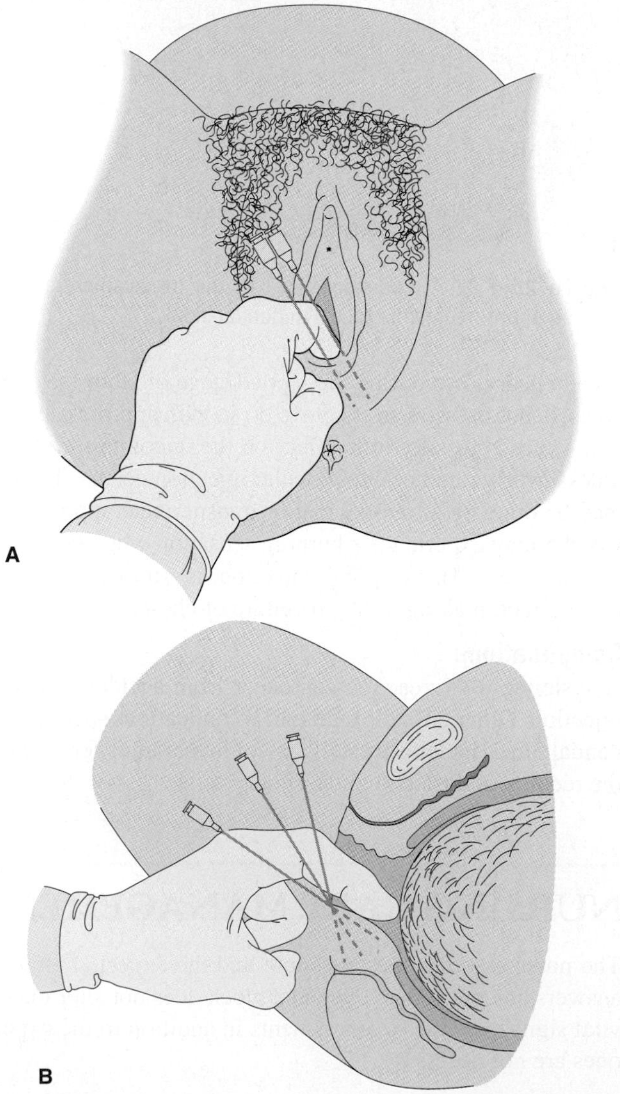

Figure 25-8 ■ Local infiltration anesthesia. A. Technique of local infiltration for episiotomy and repair. B. Technique of local infiltration showing fan pattern for the fascial planes.

Source: Reprinted with permission from Bonica, J. J. (1972). Principles and practice of obstetric analgesia and anesthesia *(p. 505). Copyright © 1972 F. A. Davis Company.*

Application: Risks and Benefits of Using IV Medications for Pain Relief During Labor

NURSING CARE MANAGEMENT

The nurse explains the procedure and the expected effect and answers any questions. Local anesthetic agents have no effect on maternal vital signs or FHR, so additional assessments are unnecessary.

General Anesthesia

General anesthesia (induced unconsciousness) may be needed for cesarean birth and surgical intervention with some obstetric complications. The method used to achieve general anesthesia may be intravenous (IV) injection, inhalation of anesthetic agents, or a combination of both methods. The use of general anesthesia in the obstetrical setting continues to decline because of adverse fetal effects and the increase in maternal risks. The most common indications for general anesthesia include perceived lack of time for regional anesthesia, contraindications to regional anesthesia, failure to successfully insert regional anesthesia, and patient refusal (Chestnut et al., 2009).

Intravenous Anesthetics

Sodium thiopental (Pentothal) is an ultra-short-acting barbiturate, which means that it exerts its effect rapidly and has a brief duration of action. Sodium thiopental produces narcosis within 30 seconds after IV administration. Introduction and emergence from its effects are smooth and pleasant, with little incidence of nausea and vomiting. Sodium thiopental is most frequently used for initiating unconsciousness and as an adjunct to other more potent anesthetics. Ketamine is an intermediate-acting barbiturate that is used for anesthesia induction. The effects typically last 20 to 60 minutes. Hypersalivation can occur but can be treated with an anticholinergic drug to decrease this side effect. The drug is contraindicated in women with preeclampsia or chronic hypertension.

Inhaled Anesthesia Agents

The most commonly used inhaled anesthesia agent is nitrous oxide. Nitrous oxide does not produce significant uterine relaxation. Although it crosses the placenta immediately after administration, fetal tissue uptake occurs 20 minutes after administration, which results in a lower fetal arterial concentration and less neonatal depression. In recent years, the recommended dosage has been decreased to 50% (down from 70%) and the time from administration until birth has been shortened as much as possible. In order to decrease the length of fetal exposure and tetrogenic effects, it is recommended that the woman be fully prepped and the obstetrician be fully prepared to make the initial incision when nitrous oxide is introduced (Yentis et al., 2007).

The use of other low-dose halogenated agents, such as isoflurane, halothane, sevoflurane, desflurane, and enflurane, are also used, often in combination with nitrous oxide. These agents have been used commonly and have been found to increase maternal inspired oxygen levels and may increase uterine blood flow (Yentis et al., 2007). The use of sevoflurane has been associated with uterine relaxation when administered in high dosages, suggesting that the lowest dose possible should be used (Yentis et al., 2007).

Inhaled anesthetic agents have also been used in combination with spinal or epidural techniques when the epidural anesthesia was ineffective or severe maternal anxiety was present. Inhaled agents may also be used for women with aortic stenosis instead of regional anesthesia if advised by the cardiologist. Inhaled anesthetic agents have been associated with cardiovascular stability throughout surgery without adverse fetal outcomes (Gambling et al., 2008).

Complications of General Anesthesia

A primary danger of general anesthesia is fetal depression. Most general anesthetic agents reach the fetus in about 2 minutes. The depression of the fetus is directly proportional to the depth and duration of the anesthesia. The long-term significance of fetal depression in a normal birth has not been determined. The poor fetal metabolism of general anesthetic agents is similar to that of analgesic agents administered during labor. General anesthesia is not advocated when the fetus is considered to be at high risk, particularly in preterm birth.

Most general anesthetic agents cause some degree of uterine relaxation although the inhalation agents effect uterine relaxation to a lesser degree than the IV agents. They may also cause vomiting and aspiration.

Pregnancy results in decreased gastric motility, and the onset of labor halts the process almost entirely. Food eaten hours earlier may remain undigested in the stomach. Even when food and fluids have been withheld, the gastric juice produced during fasting is highly acidic and can produce chemical pneumonitis if aspirated. This pneumonitis is known as Mendelson syndrome. The signs and symptoms are chest pain, respiratory distress, cyanosis, fever, and tachycardia. Women undergoing emergency cesarean births appear to be at considerable risk for adverse events. The leading cause of maternal deaths in women who have had general anesthesia is the failure to establish a patent airway (Bucklin et al., 2008).

Care During General Anesthesia

Prophylactic antacid therapy is given to reduce the acidic content of the stomach before general anesthesia. Administration of a nonparticulate antacid (such as Bicitra) may be used. Cimetidine (Tagamet) may also be used (Cunningham et al., 2010).

Before the induction to anesthesia, the woman should have a wedge placed under her hip to displace the uterus and avoid vena caval compression in the supine position. She should also be preoxygenated with 3 to 5 minutes of 100% oxygen. IV fluids should be started so that access to the intravascular space is immediately available.

During the process of rapid induction of anesthesia, the nurse applies cricoid pressure. This is accomplished by depressing the cricoid cartilage 2 to 3 cm posteriorly so that the esophagus is occluded. Cricoid pressure is continued until the anesthesiologist has placed the cuffed endotracheal tube and indicates that the pressure can be released. Figure 25-9 ■ shows the appropriate technique. The woman's neck should be supported by the nurse's other hand.

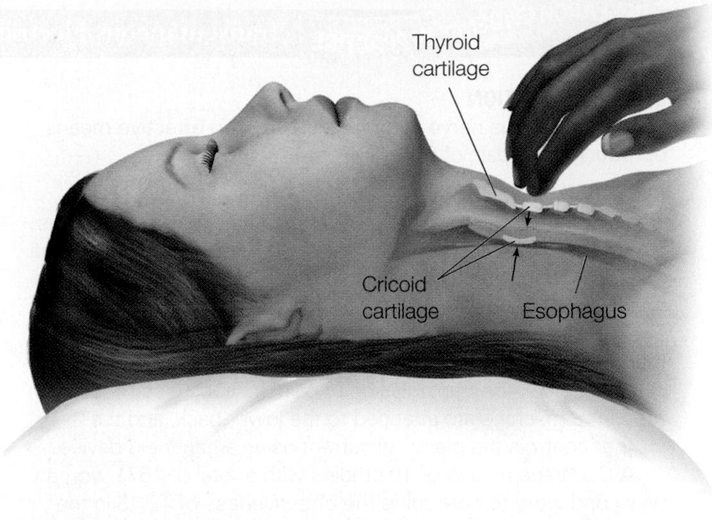

Figure 25-9 ■ Proper position for fingers in applying cricoid pressure until a cuffed endotracheal tube is placed by the anesthesiologist or certified nurse anesthetist. The cricoid cartilage is depressed 2 to 3 cm so that the esophagus is occluded.

Neonatal Neurobehavioral Effects of Anesthesia and Analgesia

Studies have focused on the neurobehavioral effects on the newborn of pharmacologic agents used during labor and birth. Although analgesic and anesthetic agents may alter the behavioral and adaptive function of the newborn, physiologic factors such as hunger, degree of hydration, time within the sleep-wake cycle, gestational age, and birth weight may also exert an influence (Nabhan, El-Din, Rabie, & Fahmy, 2009).

Women who receive general anesthesia are also slower to initiate breastfeeding in the immediate postpartum period, which could have long-term effects on breastfeeding success. Women who receive general anesthesia and undergo a cesarean birth need more assistance with breastfeeding than women who deliver vaginally (Cakmak & Kuguoglu, 2007).

Analgesic and Anesthetic Considerations for the High-Risk Mother and Fetus

Up to this point the discussion of obstetric analgesia and anesthesia has dealt with the healthy woman and healthy fetus. Pain relief for high-risk women during labor and birth requires skill in decision making, close observation, and awareness of potential threats to the woman and fetus. Safety for all involved requires the close cooperation of the obstetrician, anesthesiologist, pediatrician, and labor nurse. The pathophysiologic changes that accompany maternal disorders have a direct influence on the choice of agent or technique. It is difficult to separate maternal and fetal complications because whatever alters the woman's response will also affect the fetus. The effects on the woman cannot be considered without the potential effects on the fetus.

RESEARCH EVIDENCE IN PRACTICE Transcutaneous Electrical Nerve Stimulation for Pain Relief in Labor

CLINICAL QUESTION

Is transcutaneous nerve stimulation (TENS) an effective means of reducing the pain of labor?

RESEARCH EVIDENCE

Transcutaneous nerve stimulation (TENS) has been proposed as a means of reducing pain in labor. A TENS unit emits low-voltage electrical impulses that vary in frequency and intensity, and have been shown to be effective for a variety of painful conditions. The mechanism of action is not well understood. It is thought that the electrical pulses stimulate nerve pathways in the spinal cord that block the transmission of pain. In labor, electrodes from the TENS machine are attached to the lower back, and the mother controls the electrical current using a handheld device.

A Cochrane review of 19 studies with a total of 1671 women was conducted to determine the effectiveness of TENS in the control of labor pain. In addition, a group of nurse midwife-researchers conducted a national survey of the use of TENS in labor in Great Britain, where the National Health Service has issued recommendations against the use of TENS machines, based on a reported lack of documented effectiveness.

The Cochrane review did in fact identify that there was little difference in pain control between women using TENS and control groups. There was some evidence that women using TENS were less likely to rate their pain as severe, but the results were not consistent nor widespread among the studies. TENS did not seem to have an effect on length of labor or the well-being of mothers or babies. However, the British survey did find that women who used TENS believed it helped their pain and reported they would use it again given the chance.

Given the perceptual nature of pain, it may be that TENS exerts a placebo effect that is helpful to some women. The device may offer a useful distraction, and the fact that the woman operates the device may enhance her sense of control. However, it cannot be demonstrated that TENS has a predictable or consistent effect in reducing the pain of labor.

WHAT QUESTIONS REMAIN UNANSWERED?

The treatments were inconsistently described in these trials. Could the consistent application of a standard TENS device help reduce the severity of pain?

WHAT IS BEST PRACTICE?

While TENS may offer a distraction from the pain of labor and may help women feel more in control of their labor, there is no conclusive evidence that TENS offers better pain relief than placebo.

CRITICAL THINKING

Are there other ways to help mothers achieve the sense of control that may be the source of the placebo effect in these trials? Are there other distractions that could help mothers manage the pain of labor better?

References

Blincoe, A. 2007. TENS machines and their use in managing labour pain. *British Journal of Midwifery, 15*(8), 516–519.

Dowswell, T., Bedwell, C., Lavender, T., & Neilson, J. 2009. Transcutaneous electrical nerve stimulation for pain relief in labor. *Cochrane Database of Systematic Reviews,* Issue 2. Art. No.: CD007214. doi:10.1002/14651858

McMunn, V., Bedwell, C., Neilson, J., Jones, A., Dowswell, T., & Lavender, T. 2009. A national survey of the use of TENS in labour. *British Journal of Midwifery, 17*(8), 492–495.

Preterm Labor

The preterm fetus has special risks and requirements. An immature fetus is more susceptible to depressant drugs because he or she has less protein available for binding; has a poorly developed blood-brain barrier, which increases the likelihood that pharmacologic agents will attain a higher concentration in the central nervous system; and has a decreased ability to metabolize and excrete drugs after birth (Blackburn, 2007). Analgesia during labor should be avoided whenever possible. If it becomes necessary, the smallest dose that will provide relief should be administered. General anesthesia should be avoided in premature gestations (Creasy et al., 2009). Emotional support will be very valuable to the woman in this situation.

Preeclampsia

Pregnancies complicated by preeclampsia are high-risk situations, as indicated in chapter 20 ∞. The potential for chronic placental insufficiency or preterm birth is also present. The woman with mild preeclampsia usually may have the analgesia or anesthesia of choice, although the incidence of hypotension with epidural anesthesia is increased (Creasy et al., 2009). If hypotension occurs with the epidural block, it provides further stress on an already compromised cardiovascular system. Hypotension can usually be managed with judicious fluid increase and positioning.

The woman with severe preeclampsia poses a real challenge. Regional anesthesia seems to be the preferred method as long as hypotension can be avoided. Raising the central venous pressure by 3 to 4 cm H_2O with IV fluids helps avoid hypotension, but it must be remembered that this woman is already threatened with heart failure (Creasy et al., 2009). The effect of fluid intake can be monitored with a pulmonary artery occlusion pressure monitoring catheter. Pulmonary artery catheterization is used to correct volume deficits and appears more accurate than central pressure catheters in monitoring left- and right-side cardiac filling pressures, cardiac output, and systemic vascular resistance (Creasy et al., 2009). Although invasive monitoring is indicated, it is not associated with better maternal or neonatal outcomes (ASA Task Force, 2007). It is important to monitor and record the fluid intake and output. Some physicians use vasopressors; others avoid them because of the possible decrease in uterine blood flow to an already compromised fetus and the threat of a maternal cerebral vascular accident (Creasy et al., 2009). Spinal anesthesia is rarely used because of the greater potential for hypotension.

The use of general anesthesia poses a risk of aggravating maternal hypertension. In general, the safest method for general anesthesia is intubation, but because it may cause a hypertensive episode, it is avoided if possible. Another important consideration is that women with preeclampsia are more prone to have mucosal edema in the oral cavity and glottis, making intubation more difficult (Creasy et al., 2009).

Diabetes Mellitus

The fetus of a mother with diabetes mellitus may have a reduction in placental blood flow. Hypotension, which can result during regional anesthesia, can deplete this blood flow even further. If the fetus is tolerating labor well without an indication of nonreassuring fetal status, the continuous epidural technique may be undertaken. If nonreassuring fetal status occurs, cesarean birth may be necessary.

Anesthesia for cesarean birth requires special consideration in this case. The diabetic woman is more likely to experience cardiovascular depression during a regional block because of higher sympathetic blockade (Chestnut et al., 2009). If a regional block is selected, it is recommended that acute hydration (preload) be provided by administering dextrose-free solution. In addition, left uterine displacement is initiated before the administration of the block and maintained throughout the surgery. Hypotension is treated promptly.

Cardiac Disease

Pregnancy imposes significant risks for the woman with cardiac disease. With mild mitral stenosis, the preferred anesthetic is continual epidural anesthesia with low forceps birth. This method avoids the cardiovascular changes associated with contractions and the Valsalva maneuver during bearing down in the second stage of labor. Hypotension can be avoided with carefully controlled IV fluids and by measuring central venous pressure to avoid overload. Epidural block or general anesthesia may be used in cesarean birth. Ketamine should be avoided because it produces tachycardia (Creasy et al., 2009). Women at risk for congestive heart failure require invasive pulmonary artery occlusion pressure monitoring (Creasy et al., 2009).

Bleeding Complications

The current trend in treating bleeding complications during labor is to schedule cesarean birth when possible. When the maternal cardiovascular system is stable and there is no evidence of nonreassuring fetal status, an epidural may be given for birth. However, when either of these conditions results in active bleeding, the threat of hypovolemia must be treated immediately. Maternal hypovolemia and shock produce fetal hypoxia, acidosis, and possible fetal death (Creasy et al., 2009).

Regional blocks are contraindicated during active bleeding because the sympathetic block causes vasodilatation and further reduction of the vascular volume. Women with thrombocytopenia should also avoid regional blocks. Platelet status is an important consideration when choosing the best approach for anesthesia and, when at all possible, hematologic conditions should be corrected before initiating birth (Creasy et al., 2009). General anesthesia is recommended for these cases. Sodium thiopental may be used, but it is a cardiac depressant and vasodilator, and ketamine may be a more appropriate choice for induction. Following birth of the infant and placenta, oxytocin should not be given as an intravenous (IV) bolus to contract the uterus because it causes vasodilatation, which in turn causes a decrease in blood pressure and in total peripheral resistance. Oxytocin should be given as a dilute infusion to gain an oxytocic effect to treat uterine atony (relaxation) and to control postpartum bleeding. Resources that should be on hand to handle hemorrhagic emergencies include large-bore IV catheters, a fluid warmer, a forced-air body warmer, the woman's specific blood type or O negative blood, trained personnel, and equipment to infuse blood products rapidly (Chestnut et al., 2009).

FOCUS YOUR STUDY

- Pain relief during labor may be enhanced by nonpharmacologic methods and administration of analgesic agents and regional anesthesia blocks. The nurse can offer alternative comfort measures, avoid offering pain medication to women who do not desire pain medication, provide the woman who does desire pain medication with the opportunity to explore available options, and provide education and reassurance to the expectant woman and her support person.
- The goal of pharmacologic analgesia during labor is to provide maximal pain relief with minimal risk for the woman and fetus.
- The optimal time for administering analgesia is determined after a complete assessment of vital factors, including maternal, fetal, and labor assessments and the woman's perception of her pain level and her need and desire for pain medication.

- Two common analgesic agents are butorphanol (Stadol) and nalbuphine (Nubain).
- Opiate antagonists, such as naloxone (Narcan), counteract the respiratory depressant effect of the opiate narcotics by acting at specific receptor sites in the central nervous system.
- Sedatives, including barbiturates, benzodiazepines, and H_1-receptor antagonists, are primarily used in latent or early labor to promote rest and allow the woman to sleep.
- Regional anesthesia is achieved by injecting local anesthetic agents into an area that will bring the agent into direct contact with nerve tissue. Methods most commonly used in childbearing include lumbar epidural, spinal block, combined spinal-epidural block, pudendal block, and local infiltration.
- Three types of local anesthetic agents used in regional blocks are amides, esters, and opiates. The amides are absorbed quickly and can be found in maternal blood within minutes after administration. The esters are metabolized more rapidly and have only limited placental transfer. Opiates act on specific opiate receptors in the spinal cord and have a greater analgesic effect when combined with a low dose of local anesthetic.
- Possible maternal complications of regional anesthesia, although rare, include systemic toxicity, convulsions, and sudden cardiovascular collapse.
- Agents in use for epidural and spinal routes include the opioids morphine and fentanyl. Adverse reactions of the woman to local anesthetic agents range from mild symptoms, such as palpitations, to cardiovascular collapse. The newer amides, including ropivacaine and levobupivacaine, are longer acting and have fewer side effects.
- Pudendal blocks provide perineal anesthesia during the second stage of labor, birth, episiotomies, or laceration repair.
- General anesthesia can be achieved by intravenous injection, inhalation of anesthetic agents, or a combination of both methods.
- The goal of general anesthesia is to provide maximal pain relief with minimal side effects to the woman and her fetus.
- Complications of general anesthesia include fetal depression, uterine relaxation, vomiting, and aspiration.
- The choice of analgesia and anesthesia for the high-risk woman and fetus requires careful evaluation.

CRITICAL THINKING IN ACTION

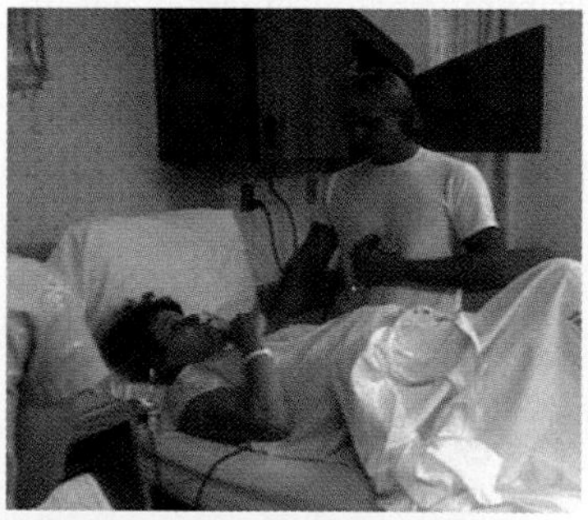

Source: George Dodson/Pearson Education.

Sandra, a 26-year-old G1 P0000, is in active labor when she presents to you at the birthing center. She has been in labor for 5 hours and is clearly tired and seems to be having difficulty coping with the pain. Her contractions are occurring every 2 to 4 minutes lasting 50 to 60 seconds, and are moderate to strong in intensity. You assess the fetal heart rate of 120 to 130 with early decelerations; moderate long-term variability is present. Sandra's vital signs are stable and her laboratory results are within normal limits. She is requesting an epidural analgesia for pain control. A vaginal exam demonstrates the cervix is 100% effaced, 6 cm dilated with the vertex at 0 station in the LOT position. You notify the physician of Sandra's wish for pain relief and labor progress. You review the client's record for written consent for regional analgesia and assist the anesthesiologist with the procedure.

1. Discuss the advantages of regional analgesia.
2. Describe the nursing responsibility during the administration of regional analgesia.
3. Discuss the side effects of regional analgesia.
4. What are the absolute contraindications for an epidural block?
5. How do you assist Sandra with the second stage of labor when she cannot feel her contractions?

See www.nursing.pearsonhighered.com for possible responses.

REFERENCES

American Society of Anesthesiologists (ASA) Task Force. (2007). Practice guidelines for obstetric anesthesia: An update report by the American Society of Anesthesiologists Task Force on obstetric anesthesia. *Anesthesiology, 106*(4), 843–863.

Balestrieri-Martinez, B. (2009). Complications in obstetric anesthesia: Nursing's role to anticipate, recognize, and respond. *Journal of Perinatal & Neonatal Nursing, 23*(1), 23–30.

Barash, P. G., Cullen, B. F., Stoelting, R. K., & Cahalan, M. (2009). *Clinical anesthesia.* Philadelphia, PA: Lippincott Williams & Wilkins.

Berman, A., Synder, S. J., Kozier, B., & Erb, G. (2008). *Kozier & Erb's fundamentals of nursing: Concepts, process, and practice.* (10th ed.). Upper Saddle River, NJ: Pearson.

Blackburn, S. T. (2007). *Maternal, fetal, and neonatal physiology: A clinical perspective.* (3rd ed.). Philadelphia, PA: Saunders.

Braveman, F. R. (2006). *Obstetric and gynecologic requisites.* Philadelphia, PA: Maryland Heights, MO: Elsevier.

Bucklin, B., Gambling, D., & Wlody, D. (2008). *A practical approach to obstetric anesthesia.* Philadelphia, PA: Lippincott Williams & Wilkins.

Cakmak, H., & Kuguoglu, S. (2007). Comparison of the breastfeeding patterns of mothers who delivered their babies per vagina and via cesarean section: An observational study using the LATCH breastfeeding charting system. *International Journal of Nursing Studies, 44*(7), 1128–1137.

Chestnut, D. H., Polley, L. S., Tsen, L. C., & Wong, C. A. (2009). *Chestnut's obstetrical anesthesia: Principles and practice.* St. Louis, MO: Mosby.

Creasy, R. K., Resnik, R., Iams, J. D., Lockwood, C. J., & Moore, T. R. (2009). *Creasy & Resnik's maternal-fetal medicine: Principles and practice* (6th ed.). Philadelphia, PA: Saunders.

Cunningham, F. G., Leveno, K. J., Bloom, S. L., Hauth, J. C., Rouse, D. J., & Spong, C. Y. (2010). *William's obstetrics* (23rd ed.). New York, NY: McGraw-Hill.

Doufas, A. G., Morioka, N., Maghoub, A. N., Mascha, E., & Sessler, D. I. (2008). Lower-body warming mimics the normal epidural-induced reduction in the shivering threshold. *Anesthesia and Analgesia, 106*(1), 252–256.

Gambling, D. R., Douglas, M. J., & McKay, R. S. F. (2008). *Obstetric anesthesia and uncommon disorders.* London, England: Cambridge Press.

Gibbs, R. S., Karlan, B. Y., Haney, A. F., & Nygaard, I. (2008). *Danforth's obstetrics and gynecology* (10th ed.). Philadelphia, PA: Lippincott Williams & Wilkins.

Glance, L. G., Wissler, R., Glantz, C., Osler, T. M., Mukamel, D. B., & Dick, A. W. (2007). Racial differences in the use of epidural analgesia for labor. *Anesthesiology, 106*(1), 19–25.

Ioscovich, A. M., Goldszmidt. E., Fadeev, A. V., Grisaru-Granovsky, S., & Halpern, S. H. (2009). Peripartum anesthetic management of patients with aortic valve stenosis: A retrospective study and literature review. *International Journal of Obstetric Anesthesia, 18*(4), 379–386.

Macksey, L. F. (2009). *Nurse anesthesia pocket guide: A resource for students and clinicians.* Sudbury, MA: Jones & Bartlett.

Mhyre, J. M., Riesner, M. N., Polley, L. S., & Naughton, N. N. (2007). A series of anesthesia-related maternal deaths in Michigan, 1985–2003. *Anesthesiology, 106*(6), 1096–1104.

Nabhan, A. F., El-Din, L. B., Rabie, A. H., & Fahmy, G. M. (2009). Impact of intrapartum factors on oxidative stress in newborns. *Journal of Maternal-Fetal & Neonatal Medicine, 22*(10) 867–872.

New York School of Regional Anesthesia. (2009). Epidural blockade. Retrieved from http:/www.nysora.com/.../3026-Epidural-Blockade.html

Ochroch, E. A., Troxel, A. B., & Farrer, J. T. (2007). The influence of race and socioeconomic factors on patient acceptance of perioperative epidural analgesia. *Anesthesia and Analgesia, 105*(6), 1787–1792.

Okutomi, T., Salto, M., Mochizuki, J., & Kuczkowski, K. M. (2009). Combined spinal-epidural analgesia for labor pain: Best timing of epidural infusion following spinal dose. *Archives of Gynecology and Obstetrics, 279*(3), 329–334.

Simpson, K. R., & Creehan, P. A. (2008). *AWHONN's perinatal nursing.* Washington, DC: AWHONN.

Wilson, B. A., Shannon, M. T., & Shields, K. (2010). *Pearson's drug guide: 2010.* Upper Saddle River, NJ: Pearson.

Wolf, J. H. (2009). Deliver me from pain: Anesthesia and birth in America. Baltimore, MD: Johns Hopkins University Press.

Woolnough, M., Allam, J., Hemingway, C., Cox, M., & Yentis, S. M. (2009). Intra-operative fluid warming in elective caesarean section: A blinded randomised controlled trial. *International Journal of Obstetric Anesthesia, 18*(4), 346–51.

Yentis, S., May, A., & Malhotra, S. (2007). *Analgesia, anesthesia, and pregnancy: A practical guide.* London, England: Cambridge University Press.

CHAPTER 26

Childbirth at Risk: Prelabor Complications

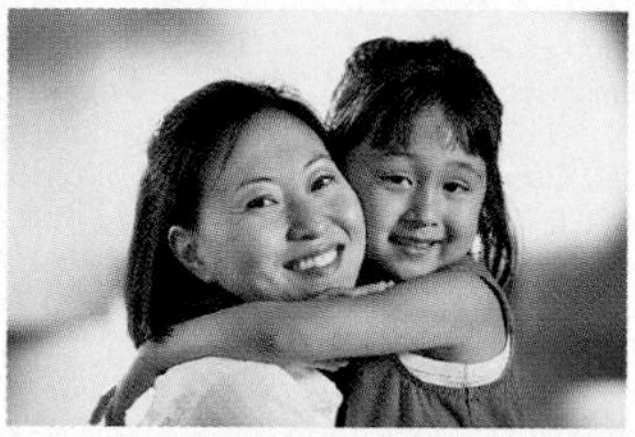

As a fourth time mother, I was unprepared to deal with the hardship of 6 months of bed rest after having three uncomplicated pregnancies. Each day brought me closer to a safe delivery, but the stress and strain of three active young children and the worry of the condition of my unborn baby made each day a struggle.

LEARNING OUTCOMES

1. Identify the causes and risk factors of cervical insufficiency.
2. Describe the clinical therapies and appropriate nursing interventions for the mother with cervical insufficiency and her unborn fetus.
3. Identify the causes and risk factors for premature rupture of membranes.
4. Describe the clinical therapy for premature rupture of membranes and preterm labor in determining hospital-based and community-based nursing care management of the woman and her fetus-newborn.
5. Analyze the implications and maternal and fetal risks of preterm labor.
6. Compare placenta previa and abruptio placentae, including implications for the mother and fetus, and their nursing care.
7. Discuss the differences between developmental and degenerative placental problems.
8. Analyze the maternal and fetal-newborn implications and clinical therapy in determining community-based and hospital-based nursing care of the woman with a multiple gestation.
9. Describe the identification of the woman with hydramnios and the maternal and fetal-neonatal implications.
10. Describe the identification of the woman with oligohydramnios and the maternal and fetal-neonatal implications.
11. Compare the clinical therapy and nursing care management of the woman with hydramnios and the woman with oligohydramnios.

KEY TERMS

Abruptio placentae *675*
Cerclage *663*
Cervical insufficiency *663*
Hydramnios *688*
Incompetent cervix *663*
Oligohydramnios *688*
Placenta previa *680*
Premature rupture of membranes (PROM) *664*
Preterm labor (PTL) *668*
Tocolysis *671*
Vasa previa *681*

After the first trimester, the majority of pregnancies progress smoothly to term. In some cases, however, complications can occur before the onset of labor that significantly impact the outcome of pregnancy. This chapter presents information related to the most common of these conditions. It also serves as a prelude to the labor-related complications discussed in chapter 27 ∞.

Care of the Woman with Cervical Insufficiency

Many questions remain unanswered about cervical insufficiency (formerly termed **incompetent cervix**). The classic definition presents **cervical insufficiency** or *cervical incompetence* as painless dilatation of the cervix without contractions because of a structural or functional defect of the cervix. The woman is usually unaware of contractions and presents with advanced effacement and dilatation and, possibly, bulging membranes. It is difficult to determine the incidence because of the inconsistency in definition and lack of clear diagnostic criteria (American College of Obstetricians and Gynecologists [ACOG], 2008).

The origin of cervical insufficiency is multifactorial; the etiology may be either congenital or acquired (Johnson & Iams, 2009). Factors that may contribute to the tendency for the cervix to dilate prematurely can be divided into three categories: congenital factors, acquired factors, and biochemical (hormonal) factors. Congenitally incompetent cervix may be found in women exposed to diethylstilbestrol (DES) or those with a bicornuate uterus. Acquired cervical incompetence may be related to inflammation, infection, subclinical uterine activity, cervical trauma, cone biopsy, late second trimester elective abortions, or increased uterine volume (as with a multiple gestation). Loop electrosurgical excision procedure (LEEP) of the cervix has been found to significantly increase the risk of preterm births in both singleton and twin gestations (Noehr, Jensen, Frederiksen, et al., 2009). The hormone relaxin may be an endocrine cause of cervical incompetence.

A woman's obstetric history may give her healthcare provider an indication of increased risk for incompetent cervix. Factors include multiple gestations, repetitive second trimester losses, previous preterm birth, progressively earlier births with each subsequent pregnancy, short labors, previous elective abortion or cervical manipulation, DES exposure, or other uterine anomaly. These women will benefit from close surveillance of cervical length with transvaginal ultrasound beginning between 16 and 24 weeks' gestation. Cervical effacement occurs from the internal os out and can be seen on ultrasound as "funneling." Alteration is apparent in transvaginal scan when fundal pressure is applied or the woman assumes a standing position. In addition, women at risk for incompetent cervix need to be informed early in pregnancy of warning signs of impending birth, such as lower back pain, pelvic pressure, and changes in vaginal discharge.

A number of contemporary studies have concluded that endovaginal ultrasound measurements of cervical length between 15 and 28 weeks' gestation identify groups at risk for preterm birth. However, the placement of a cervical cerclage (see the following discussion) does not substantially reduce the risk of prematurity (Johnson & Iams, 2009). This has led to a reconsideration of both medical and surgical treatment options for women with a history of midtrimester losses. Medical therapies used are serial cervical ultrasound assessments, bed rest, progesterone supplementation, antibiotics, and anti-inflammatory drugs (Berghella, Roman, Daskalakis, et al., 2007; Mancuso & Owen, 2009).

Cerclage Procedures

A **cerclage** is a surgical procedure in which a stitch is placed in the cervix to prevent a spontaneous abortion or premature birth (Encyclopedia of Surgery, 2010). See Figure 26-1 ■. Surgical options include the various types of cerclage procedures. An elective cervical cerclage may be placed late in the first trimester or early in the second trimester with an 80% to 90% success rate in preventing fetal loss and premature labor and birth (Encyclopedia of Surgery, 2010). A cerclage placed for emergent reasons, when dilatation and effacement have already occurred, is successful in 40% to 60% of cases (Encyclopedia of Surgery, 2010). A cervical cerclage involves using a heavy suture to reinforce the cervix at the level of the internal os. The McDonald cerclage utilizes a purse-string technique high up on the cervix to tie it closed. The Shirodkar method uses a submucosal band placed at the level of the internal os.

An abdominal cerclage approach may be required for women with a congenitally short or amputated cervix, cervical defects, a cervix previously scarred, or unhealed lacerations or subacute cervicitis (ACOG, 2008). Figure 26-2 ■ compares a cervix of normal length with one indicative of cervical shortening. A cerclage is in place.

In cases in which cervical dilatation is discovered unexpectedly, an attempt may be made to "rescue" the pregnancy by

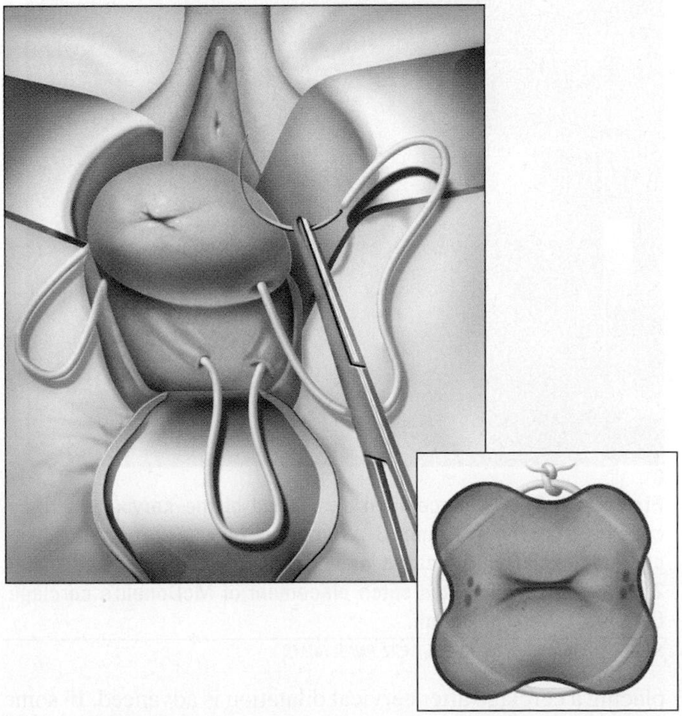

Figure 26-1 ■ A cerclage or purse-string suture is inserted in the cervix to prevent preterm cervical dilatation and pregnancy loss. After placement, the string is tightened and secured anteriorly.

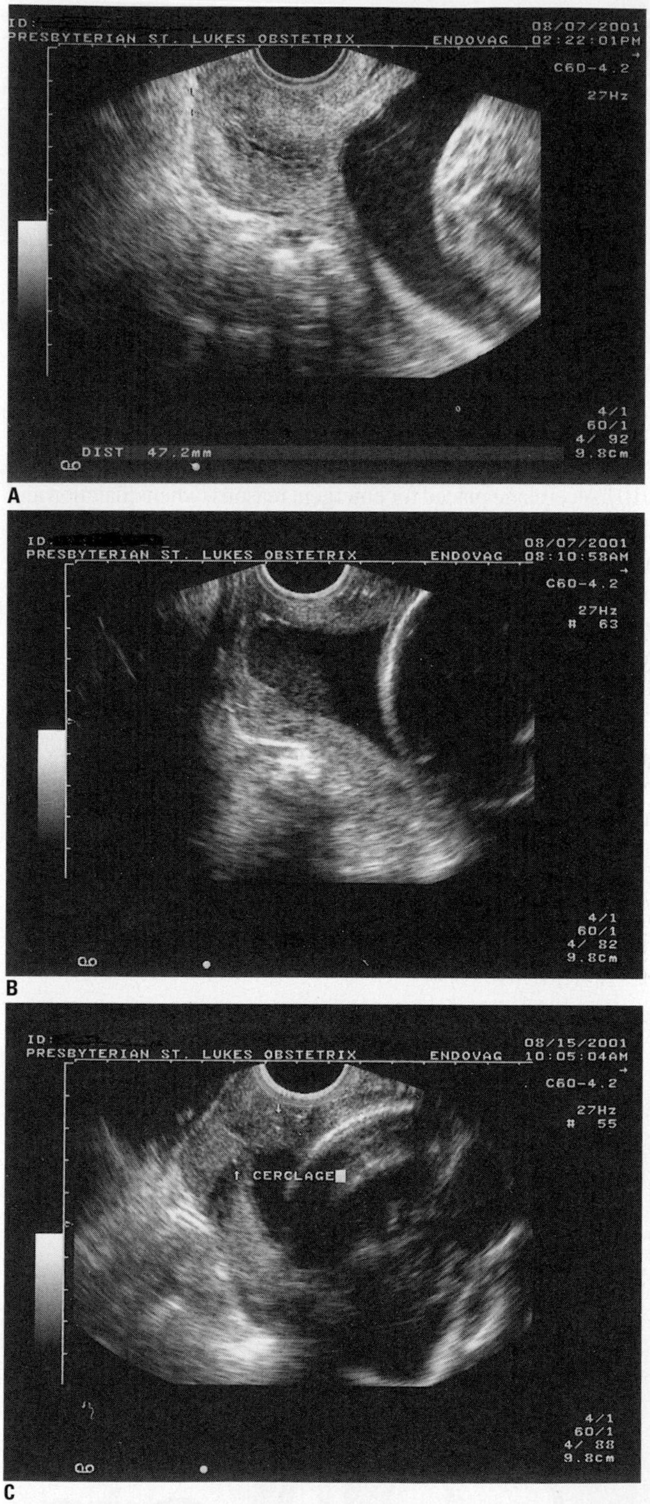

Figure 26-2 ■ Endocervical ultrasound of the cervix. A. Normal cervix measuring 47.2 mm. B. Woman at 24 weeks' gestation with chorioamnionitis and preterm labor. Cervix is fully effaced and dilated 2 cm. C. Arrow indicates stitch placement of McDonald's cerclage. Cervix is 18.5 mm in length.

Source: Courtesy of Debbie McGee, MSN, PNNP, RDMS.

placing a cerclage after cervical dilatation is advanced. In some instances, decompression of a bulging amniotic sac must be accomplished immediately before the cerclage placement. In this situation, a preoperative evaluation for infection, ruptured membranes, and uterine activity may be prudent. Tocolytics (drugs that stop labor), broad-spectrum antibiotics, and anti-inflammatory agents are given perioperatively and for ongoing treatment. Exposure of the amniotic membranes increases the chance of cerclage failure when compared with an elective placement of a cerclage.

An uncomplicated elective cerclage may be done on an outpatient basis or the woman may be hospitalized and discharged after 24 to 48 hours. An emergency cerclage, however, requires hospitalization for 5 to 7 days or longer. After 37 completed weeks' gestation, the suture may be cut and vaginal birth permitted, or the suture may be left in place and a cesarean birth performed to avoid repeating the procedure in subsequent pregnancies.

Care of the Woman with Premature Rupture of Membranes

Spontaneous rupture of the membranes before the onset of labor is known as **premature rupture of membranes (PROM)**. Some authorities define PROM as the rupture of the bag of waters any time after 37 completed weeks but before the onset of labor (Jazayeri, 2008); some have further defined PROM as a specific period elapse without labor, generally between 1 and 12 hours. Preterm PROM (PPROM) has been described as rupture before 37 weeks' gestation. Prolonged rupture of the membranes is rupture more than 24 hours before birth. In the United States, PPROM complicates more than 3% (or 150,000) of pregnancies each year and is associated with more than 30% to 40% of the preterm births (Jazayeri, 2008).

Whereas preterm labor tends to be the cause of preterm birth in more educated and affluent women, PPROM is seen more frequently in less educated women of lower economic status. Although the cause of PPROM is unknown, it is thought that PPROM occurs because of multiple, interrelated factors. The most significant risk factors for PPROM are previous preterm birth and previous PPROM; hence, incompetent cervix may be the cause of second trimester PPROM. Cervicitis, urinary tract infection (UTI), asymptomatic bacteriuria, amniocentesis, placenta previa, abruptio placentae, hydramnios, history of laser conization or loop electrosurgical excision procedure (LEEP) of the cervix, multiple pregnancy, and maternal genital tract anomalies may also result in PPROM. It has been suggested that nulliparous women who work outside the home are at increased risk as well. Other risk factors include smoking, substance abuse, connective tissue disorders, fetal anomalies, and lower socioeconomic status; however, in most cases the cause is undefined (Gibbs, Karlan, Haney, et al., 2010). Once membranes have ruptured, labor may occur within a relatively short time. The latency period, the period of time between rupture of membranes and the onset of labor, decreases with increasing gestational age. Shorter latency periods are associated with oligohydramnios, cervical dilatation more than 1 centimeter, fetal growth restriction, and nulliparity (Melamed, Hadar, Ben-Haroush, et al., 2009). With appropriate and conservative therapy, 50% of those women who rupture membranes between 28 and 34 weeks will give birth within 7 days (Jazayeri, 2008).

Maternal Risks

Maternal risk is related to infection, specifically *chorioamnionitis* (intra-amniotic infection resulting from bacterial invasion and inflammation of the membranes before birth) and *endometritis* (infection of the endometrium postpartally that may be related to chorioamnionitis or may occur independently).

Chorioamnionitis occurs in about 3% to 15% of all cases of PROM but in 13% to 60% of cases of preterm PROM (Jazayeri, 2008). Collection of amniotic fluid by amniocentesis permits analysis of the fluid for subclinical chorioamnionitis. Gram stain, white cell count, glucose concentration, and culture of the fluid are useful in determining treatment; however, the results of the amniotic fluid culture could take as long as 48 hours. Interleukin-6 concentrations appear to be the best biomarker for infection but most hospitals do not yet have the ability to measure them (Gibbs et al., 2010). In addition, fluid gathered either by amniocentesis or from fluid that has pooled in the vagina can be analyzed for fetal lung maturity. The lecithin/surfactant ratio is the biochemical marker associated with fetal lung maturity. A ratio greater than 2.0 is associated with fetal lung maturity. When the fetal lungs are mature, the risk of serious pulmonary complication in newborns is minimal and labor is allowed to progress naturally.

Abruptio placentae occur more frequently in women with PPROM. It is not clear whether infection causes inflammation of the decidua, which facilitates premature separation, or whether the bleeding episode contributes to a weakening of the membranes, which eventually leads to rupture. Childbirth may be complicated by malpresentation and reduced amniotic fluid volume (Jazayeri, 2008).

Fetal-Neonatal Risks

The most significant cause of neonatal morbidity and mortality is prematurity and its associated complications such as respiratory distress syndrome, necrotizing enterocolitis, and intraventricular hemorrhage (see chapter 33 ∞). Neonatal infection (sepsis) occurs in 2% to 4% of newborns, but the preterm infant is much more likely to develop sepsis and die than a baby born at term. Fetal hypoxia may occur from cord prolapse or cord compression. In cases of early, prolonged PPROM, the oligohydramnios that occurs may result in fetal pulmonary hypoplasia, facial anomalies, limb position defects, and fetal growth restriction (Hutzal et al., 2008).

Clinical Therapy

Any time a woman complains of watery vaginal discharge or a sudden gush of fluid, rupture of the membranes must be considered. The woman should be questioned about the time of initial loss of fluid; if continuous leaking is occurring; the color, consistency, and amount of the fluid; and any odor noted. These questions not only help to determine whether there is blood, meconium, or vernix present but also may help to differentiate PROM/PPROM from increased vaginal secretions associated with infection or preterm labor, urinary incontinence, normal leukorrhea of pregnancy, or the passage of the mucous plug.

During the initial physical inspection, any fluid leaking from the vaginal introitus can be checked with nitrazine paper or nitrazine swabs. This test relies on the fact that amniotic fluid is more alkaline (pH 7 to 7.5) than normal vaginal secretions (pH 4.5 to 5.5). A color change in the paper to blue-green or blue is highly suggestive of ruptured membranes. Factors that can yield a false-positive result are contamination of the fluid with semen, urine, 50% or more blood in the specimen, or antiseptic cleansers and soap. The elevated pH associated with bacterial vaginosis can also lead to misleading results. If there is copious fluid leaking from the vaginal introitus, the diagnosis of PROM/PPROM is considered confirmed.

If further evaluation is required, a sterile speculum exam is done. Unless the woman is in active labor, direct digital exam of the cervix or vagina is avoided until PPROM is ruled out or a management plan has been determined. Speculum exam relies on gross pooling of amniotic fluid in the vaginal vault. The woman can be asked to "bear down," performing a Valsalva maneuver, if fluid is not visualized in the vagina. The woman may also remain in a supine position for several hours to allow collection of fluid to occur; the exam is then repeated. In addition to performing a nitrazine test on the fluid, a fern test can be performed by applying a thin sample of secretions onto a clean slide and looking for microscopic evidence of a fernlike pattern (see chapter 12 ∞). When combined with patient history, positive nitrazine testing and positive ferning have been shown to have an accuracy rate of 93.1% (Cunningham et al., 2010). Vaginal cultures for group B streptococcus, chlamydia, and gonorrhea may be obtained at this time. Ultrasound can be used in conjunction with other tests to look for reduced amniotic fluid.

In situations in which the diagnosis of PPROM cannot be made with any certainty, an amniocentesis may be performed to instill either indigo carmine or Evan's blue dye. A tampon is inserted in the vagina for several hours and then is inspected for blue tinged fluid. The woman should be warned that as the dye is absorbed, it will temporarily change her urine to a green color.

Concurrently, fetal well-being should be assessed through a fetal heart rate tracing or biophysical profile. In addition, the gestational age of the fetus must be calculated to decide on a management plan (Table 26-1). At greater than 36 weeks' gestation, labor will begin in 50% of women within 12 hours. Labor induction may be delayed for 12 to 24 hours unless a situation exists that would preclude expectant management.

Management of PPROM in the absence of infection and gestation of less than 37 weeks is usually conservative. Amniocentesis may be done to evaluate for intra-amniotic infection. Fetal lung maturity studies will also be done if the fetus is nearing 34 weeks' gestation. The woman is hospitalized on bed rest. An admission, complete blood count (CBC), and urinalysis are obtained. Nonstress tests (NSTs) or biophysical profiles are used to monitor fetal well-being. Typically, NSTs are performed every shift (8–12 orders per policy) or the frequency is determined by physician/certified nurse-midwife (CNM) order. Biophysical profiles should be performed every 24 hours (Gjoni, 2010). Maternal blood pressure, pulse, and temperature are assessed every 4 hours. Regular laboratory evaluations should be performed to detect maternal infection. After initial treatment and observation, if the fetus has not reached viability or if leaking of fluid ceases, some women may be followed at home; however, careful screening is warranted (Ellestad et al., 2008). The woman is advised to continue bed rest (with bathroom privileges); monitor her temperature

TABLE 26-1 Currently Used Plans for Women with Premature Rupture of Membranes

Preterm

- Expectant management (observation); birth when labor or clinical infection develops
- Fetal pulmonary status determined by amniotic fluid testing; birth if fetus is mature
- Risk of infection determined by amniotic fluid Gram stain; white cell count, glucose and culture; maternal white cell count and assessment for maternal fever or uterine tenderness; assessment for fetal well-being through electronic fetal monitoring or ultrasound for biophysical profile scoring; birth if infection develops
- Penicillin G or ampicillin for treatment of group B streptococcus (GBS), or antibiotic prophylaxis if GBS status unknown
- Adjunctive antibiotic therapy with erythromycin or azithromycin for 7 days to increase latency period from PPROM to birth
- Administration of corticosteroids, with or without birth in 48 hours after first dose; tocolytics as needed to delay birth for 48 hours to promote fetal lung maturity
- Birth after an arbitrary latent period (e.g., 16–72 hours)
- Assess for group B streptococci, chlamydia, or *Neisseria gonorrhoeae;* treatment indicated if positive
- Combinations of the above

Term

- Induction if spontaneous labor does not begin in approximately 12 hours, or if cervix is ripe, or if there are other complications (e.g., preeclampsia)
- Expectant management for women with uncomplicated pregnancies and cervix unfavorable for induction

RESEARCH EVIDENCE IN PRACTICE Antibiotics for Premature Rupture of Membranes

CLINICAL QUESTION

Do antibiotics reduce the risk of complications following the premature rupture of membranes?

RESEARCH EVIDENCE

Premature rupture of the membranes (PROM) is an important problem, placing both mother and child at risk of infection, preterm delivery, and the complications of prematurity. There are multiple causes of PROM. Infection appears to play a central role, both as a cause and as a result of PROM. Some organisms weaken the amnion and chorion and lead to PROM; other infections may occur secondary to membrane rupture. Infections may also be linked to preterm labor, because it is thought that some bacteria may stimulate the biosynthesis of prostaglandins that subsequently stimulate labor. Antibiotic therapy has been advanced as a treatment to reduce maternal and fetal infections and to delay the progression to preterm birth.

A large number of trials have focused on the effectiveness of antibiotic therapy and its sequelae for mother and baby. Twenty-two randomized trials involving more than 6000 women were summarized in a Cochrane review, one of the most rigorous sources of evidence. Additional studies have focused on the length of time needed for optimal antibiotic therapy and the most effective type of antibiotic to use. A meta-analysis was also conducted, which focused on whether antibiotics were effective in preventing preterm labor following PROM.

All of the reviews and trials showed that routine antibiotic administration to women with PROM reduced maternal and neonatal morbidity. The evidence supported the effectiveness of antibiotic therapy in postponing preterm labor in women with PROM. Chorioamnionitis and neonatal infections were also reduced by antibiotic use. Other complications—including babies requiring oxygen therapy, time in neonatal intensive care, abnormal cerebral ultrasound, intraventricular hemorrhage, and low birthweight—were also lower when antibiotic therapy was used following PROM.

Relative to the length of antibiotic therapy, both 3- and 7-day regimens were tested, and there was no advantage detected for the longer length of therapy. While any penicillin and macrolide antibiotics (clindamycin or erythromycin) were effective and unrelated to complications, the use of co-amoxiclav antibiotics, while effective, were associated with higher rates of necrotizing enterocolitis.

WHAT QUESTIONS REMAIN UNANSWERED?

What is the long-term consequence of the abnormal cerebral ultrasounds in the neonates whose mothers were not treated with antibiotics? Are there overall effects on perinatal mortality?

WHAT IS BEST PRACTICE?

A 3-day course of either a penicillin or a macrolide antibiotic should be routinely administered to mothers with premature rupture of membranes. Neither antibiotic causes untoward complications for mother or baby, and effective use will prevent many complications associated with PROM.

CRITICAL THINKING

How can the nurse incorporate this information into the teaching and treatment plan of the mother with premature rupture of the membranes? Premature rupture of the membranes is often a traumatic experience, but mothers are often resistant to using medications during pregnancy. How can she be reassured that antibiotic use will prevent subsequent complications and will have no untoward effects?

References

Alvarez, J., Williams, S., Ganesh, V., & Apuzzio, J. (2007). Duration of antimicrobial prophylaxis for group B streptococcus in patients with preterm premature rupture of membranes who are not in labor. *American Journal of Obstetrics & Gynecology, 197*(4), 390.e1–4.

Hutzal, C., Boyle, E., Kenyon, S., Nash, J., Winsor, S., Taylor, D., & Kirpalani, H. (2008). Use of antibiotics for the treatment of preterm parturition and prevention of neonatal morbidity: A meta-analysis. *American Journal of Obstetrics & Gynecology, 199*(6), 620.e1–8.

Kenyon, S., Boulvain, M., & Neilson, J. (2009). Antibiotics for preterm rupture of membranes. *Cochrane Database of Systematic Reviews* (2), Art. No.: CD001058. doi: 10.1002/14651858

Marowitz, A., & Jordan, R. (2007). Midwifery management of prelabor rupture of membranes at term. *Journal of Midwifery & Women's Health, 52*(3), 199–206.

4 times a day; keep a fetal movement record; and avoid intercourse, douches, and tampons ("pelvic rest"). The woman is advised to contact her physician and return to the hospital if she has fever, uterine tenderness or contractions, increased leakage of fluid, decreased fetal movement, or a foul vaginal discharge. During this time, twice weekly NSTs and CBCs and weekly ultrasound and cervical visualization may be completed. Research indicates no significant difference in latency periods, gestational age at birth, infection, or perinatal outcomes between home care and hospitalization when this regimen is followed (Gjoni, 2010).

Authorities disagree regarding the ideal management of PPROM. Prophylactic antibiotics are administered to any woman with an unknown group B streptococcal (GBS) status or a history of a positive culture during the present pregnancy (Hutzal et al., 2008). The goal of antibiotic use for preterm PROM is to treat or prevent ascending infection to prolong the interval from rupture of membranes to childbirth. Antibiotic use also may allow sufficient time for corticosteroids used to enhance fetal lung maturity to take effect. In addition, the neonatal mortality rate is significantly lower in newborns whose mothers received antibiotics (Hutzal et al., 2008). If vaginal cultures are positive, antibiotics will be continued for at least 7 days. If amniotic fluid studies indicate a low glucose level, high white blood cell (WBC) count, a positive Gram stain, or organisms in the fluid, immediate birth is indicated. Results of studies about the potential benefits versus the risks of cervical cerclage retention after PPROM are conflicting. Current practice includes early cerclage removal after PPROM; a multicentered randomized trial to answer this question is needed.

Betamethasone, a corticosteroid, decreases the likelihood of neonatal respiratory distress syndrome, necrotizing enterocolitis, intraventricular hemorrhage, and perinatal death in infants who are born prematurely. Administration of single-course betamethasone (12 mg intramuscularly [IM] with a second dose in 24 hours or dexamethasone 6 mg im every 12 hours for 2 doses) is the current recommendation (Abbasi, Oxford, Gerdes, et al., 2009; Simpson & Creehan, 2008). Corticosteroids have been associated with increased maternal and neonatal infection, decreased neonatal birth weight, reduction of brain size, maternal and fetal adrenal suppression, and psychomotor delay and behavioral problems. Data on these effects are not conclusive, but until there are additional data from clinical trials, the recommendation is that repeat courses of corticosteroids should not be used routinely (Mazumder, Sarkar, & Khatun, 2009). See Drug Guide: Betamethasone.

Use of tocolytics is generally not indicated in the woman who has ruptured membranes. Short-term use of tocolytics may be considered, however, to allow a course of steroids to be given.

NURSING CARE MANAGEMENT

Nursing Assessment and Diagnosis

Determining the time, amount, color, odor, and duration of the rupture of membranes is a significant component of the antepartal assessment. The nurse asks the woman when her membranes ruptured and when contractions began because the risk of infection may be directly related to the time involved. The color and odor are important variables that can indicate possible infection or meconium passage. Gestational age is determined to prepare for the possibility of a preterm birth. The nurse observes the mother for signs and symptoms of infection, especially by reviewing her WBC count, temperature, and pulse rate, and the character of her amniotic fluid. If the mother has a fever, the nurse checks hydration status. Fetal heart rate tracings should be watched for tachycardia, loss of variability, or decelerations. When a preterm or cesarean birth is anticipated, the nurse evaluates the childbirth preparation and coping abilities of the woman and her partner.

Nursing diagnoses that may be used for the woman with PPROM include the following:

- ***Risk for Infection*** related to premature preterm rupture of membranes
- ***Risk for Impaired Gas Exchange (Fetus)*** related to compression of the umbilical cord secondary to prolapse of the cord
- ***Ineffective Coping*** related to unknown outcome of the pregnancy

Nursing Plan and Implementation

Nursing actions should focus on the woman, her partner, and the fetus. Uterine activity and fetal response to the labor are evaluated, but vaginal exams are not done unless absolutely necessary. The woman is encouraged to rest on her right or left side to promote optimal uteroplacental perfusion. Comfort measures may help promote rest and relaxation. The nurse must also ensure that hydration is maintained, particularly if the woman's temperature is elevated.

Health Promotion Education

Education is another important aspect of nursing care. The couple needs to understand the implications of PROM and all treatment methods. It is important to address side effects and alternative treatments. The couple needs to know that although the membranes are ruptured, amniotic fluid continues to be produced. Accurate information about neonatal outcomes for the given gestational age will help the woman and those she looks to for support have a more realistic view of the situation. This is often done by a care provider experienced in the care of high-risk newborns such as a neonatologist or a neonatal nurse practitioner. Providing psychologic support for the couple is critical. The nurse may reduce anxiety by listening empathetically, relaying accurate information, and providing explanations of procedures. It may be necessary to prepare the couple for a cesarean birth, a preterm newborn, and the possibility of fetal or neonatal demise.

Evaluation

Expected outcomes of nursing care include the following:

- The woman's risk of infection and cord prolapse are decreased.
- The couple is able to discuss the implications of PPROM and all treatment options.
- The pregnancy is maintained without trauma to the mother or fetus.

DRUG GUIDE Betamethasone (Celestone Soluspan)

OVERVIEW OF MATERNAL-FETAL ACTION

Studies have provided ample evidence that glucocorticoids such as betamethasone are capable of inducing pulmonary maturation and decreasing the incidence of respiratory distress syndrome in preterm infants. The mechanism by which corticosteroids accelerate fetal lung maturity is unclear, but it is related to the stimulation of enzyme activity by the drug. The enzyme is required for biosynthesis of surfactant by the type II pneumocytes. Surfactant is of major importance to the proper functioning of the lung in that it decreases the surface tension of the alveoli. Glucocorticoids also increase the rate of glycogen depletion, which leads to thinning of the interalveolar septa and increases the size of the alveoli. The thinning of the epithelium brings the capillaries into closer proximity with the air spaces and improves oxygen exchange.

ROUTE, DOSAGE, FREQUENCY

Prenatal maternal intramuscular injections of 12 mg of betamethasone are given once a day for 2 days. Dexamethasone may also be given in doses of 6 mg every 12 hours for 2 doses (Simpson & Creehan, 2008). To obtain maximum results, birth should be delayed for at least 24 hours after completing the first round of treatment. The effect of corticosteroids may be transient. Currently, it is suggested that repeat courses of corticosteroids should not be used routinely.

CONTRAINDICATIONS

- Inability to delay birth
- Adequate lecithin/sphingomyelin L/S ratio
- Presence of a condition that necessitates immediate birth (e.g., maternal bleeding)
- Presence of maternal infection, diabetes mellitus (relative contraindication)
- Gestational age greater than 34 completed weeks
- Cushing's syndrome

MATERNAL SIDE EFFECTS

Increased risk for infection has not been supported in large studies. There may, however, be some increase in the incidence of infection in women with premature rupture of the membranes. Maternal hyperglycemia may occur during corticosteroid administration. Women with insulin-dependent diabetes may require insulin infusions for several days to prevent ketoacidosis. Corticosteroids possibly may increase the risk of pulmonary edema, especially when used concurrently with tocolytics, which may cause sodium and fluid retention, nausea, and impaired wound healing (Wilson, Shannon, & Shields, 2010).

EFFECTS ON FETUS/NEWBORN

- Lowered cortisol levels at birth, but rebound occurs by 2 hours of age
- Hypoglycemia
- Increased risk of neonatal sepsis

Animal studies have shown serious fetal side effects such as reduced head circumference, reduced weight of the fetal adrenal and thymus glands, and decreased placental weight. Human studies have not shown these effects, however (Wilson et al., 2010).

NURSING CONSIDERATIONS

1. Assess for presence of contraindications.
2. Provide education regarding possible side effects.
3. Administer betamethasone deep into the gluteal muscle, avoiding injection into the deltoid (high incidence of local atrophy). (Dexamethasone may be administered IM or IV.)
4. Periodically evaluate blood pressure (BP), pulse, weight, and edema.
5. Assess laboratory data for electrolytes and blood glucose.

Although concomitant use of betamethasone and tocolytic agents has been implicated in increased risk of pulmonary edema, the betamethasone has little mineral corticoid activity; therefore, it probably does not add significantly to the salt and water retention effects of beta-adrenergic agonists. Other causes of noncardiogenic pulmonary edema should also be investigated if pulmonary edema develops during administration of betamethasone to a woman in preterm labor.

Early Preterm Labor

Care of the Woman at Risk Due to Preterm Labor

Labor that occurs between 20 and 37 completed weeks of pregnancy is referred to as **preterm labor (PTL)**. Prematurity continues to be the number one cause of neonatal mortality in the United States today—preterm births are preceded by preterm labor 50% of the time (Ross & Eden, 2009). Preterm birth has risen by more than 20% since 1990 (March of Dimes, 2007).

In the United States, preterm birth occurs in 12.8% of births and is the leading cause of neonatal mortality in the United States (Hamilton, Martin, & Ventura, 2007). Preterm birth accounts for 70% of neonatal morbidity. Most healthcare dollars spent on preterm births are due to the 2% of premature births that occur prior to 32 gestational weeks (Ross & Eden, 2009). In the United States, African American women experience preterm birth and have low-birth-weight infants at twice the rate of white women (Ross & Eden, 2009). Regardless of gestational age or birth weight, black infants are less likely than white infants to survive. Despite new diagnostic and therapeutic technologies, efforts to prevent preterm birth have been largely ineffective. Table 26-2 presents a list of risk factors for spontaneous preterm birth.

Maternal Risks

The initial cause of preterm labor—for example, antepartum hemorrhage, trauma, or maternal infection—may pose a risk to the pregnant woman. In addition, the treatment itself is another area of significant risk. Certain medications are needed to manage preterm labor and prevent premature birth. Beta-sympathomimetic drugs cause a myriad of maternal side effects, including pulmonary edema, especially in women with multiple gestations, overdistention of the uterus, or chorioamnionitis. Diabetes, cardiac disease,

TABLE 26-2 Risk Factors for Spontaneous Preterm Labor

Abdominal surgery during the second or third trimester	Insulin-dependent diabetes
Abdominal trauma	Known cervical incompetence
Age (less than 18 or more than 35)	Low maternal weight
Alcohol consumption	Low socioeconomic status
Anemia	More than two first trimester abortions
Asymptomatic bacteriuria	Multiple gestation
Bacterial vaginosis, *E. coli* (ascending intrauterine infection)	Non-white race
Bleeding after 12 weeks	Periodontal disease
Cervical cerclage in situ	Polyhydramnios
Cervical incompetence	Poor weight gain
Cervix dilated more than 1 cm at 32 weeks	Previous preterm birth
Cigarettes—more than 10/day	Previous preterm labor with term birth
Diethylstilbestrol (DES) exposure	Second trimester abortion
Domestic violence	Sexually transmitted infection (STI) (trichomoniasis, chlamydia)
Drug abuse	Smoking
Febrile illness	Stress
Fetal abnormality	Substance abuse
Foreign body (intrauterine device [IUD])	Uterine anomaly
History of cone biopsy	Uterine fibroids
History of pyelonephritis or other maternal infection	Uterine irritability
In vitro fertilization (singleton or multiple gestation)	Uteroplacental ischemia
Inadequate prenatal care	

and thyrotoxicosis may contribute to maternal risk with the administration of this class of drugs. Magnesium sulfate is a drug used to displace intracellular calcium, which inhibits uterine contractions. Prostaglandin synthesis inhibitors inhibit contractions by interfering with prostaglandin synthesis. Calcium channel blockers antagonize the action of calcium within the myometrial cells, which reduces contractions. These agents may have adverse maternal consequences and require close monitoring during administration (El-Mowafi, 2010).

Bed rest is frequently prescribed for women having preterm contractions, although there is no evidence to support or refute its use to prevent PTL (Denney, Culhane, & Goldenberg, 2008). Bed rest in general is associated with adverse physiologic effects, including maternal thromboembolism and decreased muscle mass. It is also linked with psychologic effects that extend to the entire family. Financial loss, child care issues, disruption of routines, depression, anxiety, and family/marital stress are among the problems that the woman and her family face. Hospitalization of those women with threatened preterm birth for enforced bed rest has an even greater impact on these issues. The social and financial blow to families who face a long-term hospitalization far from home, either because they had traveled away from their usual site of residence on holiday or have been transported to a hospital that provides a higher level of care, adds to the stress of a high-risk pregnancy and the ability of the patient and her partner to cope.

Fetal-Neonatal Risks

Mortality increases for newborns born before 37 weeks' gestation. In fact, preterm birth accounts for 75% of neonatal morbidity and mortality in infants who are born without congenital anomalies (Ross & Eden, 2009). Although the preterm infant is faced with many maturational deficiencies (fat storage, heat regulation, immaturity of organ systems), the most critical factor is the lack of development of the respiratory system—to the extent that life cannot be supported. Infants born at 24 gestational weeks have a 70% chance of acquiring respiratory distress syndrome (RDS) and a 40% survival rate, whereas a 32-week infant has a 95% survival rate with only a 28% chance of developing RDS. The greater the gestational age, the lower the incidence of RDS and the higher the survival rate (Ross & Eden, 2009). In some instances, such as severe maternal diabetes or serious isoimmunization, continuation of the pregnancy may be more life threatening to the fetus than the hazards of prematurity. See chapter 33 for in-depth consideration of the preterm newborn.

Clinical Therapy

The prevention and treatment of PTL has been widely studied. In the 1970s, the focus on prevention of preterm birth was on the use of tocolytic drug therapy. It has been found that these agents have limited effectiveness. The primary goal of tocolytic therapy should be to delay birth by 48 hours so the maximum benefit of glucocorticoids can occur and decrease the incidence of RDS (Whitworth & Quenby, 2008). Preterm birth prevention programs, which were implemented in the 1980s and early 1990s, focused on identifying women who were at high risk for PTL. Once identified, those women were educated about signs and symptoms of PTL and had weekly contact with a nurse or other healthcare provider. However, these educational programs did not significantly prevent preterm birth. One contributing factor is that risk assessment screenings have poor ability to predict those women who will eventually develop PTL and give birth early. Up to 60% of preterm births occur in women who would initially be scored at low risk. Nevertheless, the screening tests currently used, such as fetal fibronectin (fFN), cervical length, screening for bacterial vaginosis, and Bishop's score, a prelabor status evaluation scoring system (see chapter 28 ∞ and Table 28-3 on page 732), have not been recommended for use in asymptomatic, low-risk women. Screening might be helpful in women with a history of preterm birth and those with symptoms of PTL. Screening can also be done at well woman gynecology exam visits since 30% of those women will become pregnant in the next 2 years (Ross & Eden, 2009).

Nonpharmacologic treatments that historically have been used to prevent preterm births, specifically bed rest, pelvic rest, and hydration, do not appear to aid in PTL prevention and should not be routinely recommended (Ross & Eden, 2009).

Prompt diagnosis of PTL is difficult because many of its symptoms are also common in normal pregnancy. These include the following:

- Abdominal pain
- Back pain
- Pelvic pain
- Menstrual-like cramps
- Vaginal bleeding
- Increased vaginal discharge (may be pinkish stained or mucus-like in consistency)
- Pelvic pressure
- Urinary frequency
- Diarrhea

Some women have frequent contractions without changes in the cervix. In these women, a clinical assay for fFN obtained between 22 weeks' and 34 weeks' gestation may aid in diagnosis. fFN is an extracellular matrix protein that is an adhesive "glue" produced by the fetal membranes and binds the membranes and placenta to the decidua.

The presence of fFN in the cervicovaginal fluid is normal in the first half of pregnancy as the gestational sac attaches to the inside of the uterus. After 20 weeks' gestation, its presence is abnormal and can signal inflammatory or mechanical disruption of the fused membranes. fFN is also found in the amniotic fluid, and a positive test can indicate ruptured membranes. Near term, it is normal for fFN to once again appear in vaginal secretions (Pelaez, Fox, & Chasen, 2008). The negative predictive value of the fFN test is 99.2%. This means that a negative fFN in a woman with preterm contractions is associated with a very low risk (less than 1 in 100 chances) of birth within 14 days (Berghella, Hayes, Vistintine, et al., 2008). A positive test is associated with recent sexual intercourse, vaginal examination, bacterial vaginosis, and vaginal bleeding. With a positive predictive value of 15% to 25%, fFN does not give a good indication of those women who will give birth in the next 14 days. Although conducting fFN testing is associated with a lower preterm birth rate, a Cochrane review of 474 women did not recommend routine screening for all women in preterm labor but did encourage more extensive study (Berghella et al., 2008).

Contraction frequency alone is not enough to establish a diagnosis of preterm labor. A woman suspected of being in PTL should have a digital cervical examination once rupture of the membranes has been ruled out. If she is a candidate for fFN testing, this should be performed before a digital or endovaginal ultrasound exam. Electronic fetal monitoring should take place for a minimum of 1 to 2 hours to detect uterine contractions.

Although assessing cervical length by endovaginal ultrasonography is another diagnostic tool that has been used, a Cochrane review found that there was no statistical difference in women who had undergone a transvaginal ultrasound of the cervix and those who had not (Berghella, Baxter, & Hendrix, 2009). Studies have shown that in symptomatic women, a cervical length of at least 30 mm (3 cm) is good evidence that the woman is not in PTL (Berghella et al., 2009). However, only 30% to 40% of women with a shortened cervix will give birth prematurely (Chao, Chao, & Hsieh, 2008). Care should be taken when performing an endovaginal ultrasound for cervical length, as excessive pressure on the vaginal probe or a full maternal bladder are associated with falsely long measurements. A cervical length of less than 25 mm in the presence of regular contractions, or a digital exam that identifies the cervix to be 3 cm or more dilated or 80% or more effaced in the presence of regular contractions, establishes the diagnosis of PTL (Chao et al., 2008). fFN testing is useful when the digital or ultrasound information is equivocal (Duhig, Chandiramani, Seed, et al., 2009).

Intervention to reduce preterm birth can be divided into primary prevention and secondary prevention. Primary prevention includes diagnosis and treatment of infections, cervical cerclage, and progesterone administration. Secondary prevention strategies are antibiotic treatment and tocolysis.

Maternal bacterial infection has been implicated as a causative factor of PTL with microbial invasion of the amniotic cavity being present in approximately 10% of women with PTL (Jones, Harris, Azizia, et al., 2009). The microbial colonization may even precede conception and ascend from the cervix and vagina into the uterus. A woman who is diagnosed with an STI has a 25% risk of becoming reinfected within the next 12 months (Ross & Eden, 2009). Lower genital tract infections that are associated with preterm birth include bacterial vaginosis (BV), *Trichomonas vaginalis, Chlamydia trachomatis,* urinary group B streptococcus (GBS), mycoplasmas, gonorrhea, high concentration of anaerobes, or aerobic gram-negative rods. It is hypothesized that there may be an association with the ability of a species of bacteria to stimulate prostaglandin production. Hydrogen peroxide–producing lactobacilli, which help to maintain an acidic vaginal environment, are associated with a significant decrease in preterm birth (Yeganegi et al., 2009).

BV is the most common lower genital tract infection among women of reproductive age and has consistently been associated with increased risks of PTL, preterm premature rupture of membranes (PPROM), miscarriage, chorioamnionitis, endometritis, and cesarean section wound infections. In spite of this, it remains unclear whether screening and treatment of BV will reduce the frequency of these complications (Denney & Culhane, 2009). Treatment of BV in low-risk populations has not been shown to improve obstetric outcomes, but some studies have shown that women with a history of preterm birth who received oral treatment with metronidazole or clindamycin had a reduction in preterm birth or premature rupture of membranes (PROM).

An estimated 20% to 30% of all women are GBS carriers. Neonatal infection from GBS is a potentially severe consequence of maternal GBS infection; nevertheless, there is no association of preterm birth and vaginal GBS colonization (Ohlsson & Shah, 2009). GBS is discussed more fully in chapter 20 ∞.

PTL is also associated with urinary tract infections (UTIs), so it is prudent to obtain a clean-catch or catheterized urine specimen to identify and treat the infection. If untreated, asymptomatic bacteriuria is associated with a 30% incidence of pyelonephritis later in pregnancy and an up to 50% increase in preterm birth (Mazor-Dray, Levy, Schlaeffer, et al., 2009). Even asymptomatic bacteriuria alone increases the risk of preterm birth; therefore, screening and treatment of all pregnant women at the first prenatal visit are important components of care. Women with a positive culture should be retested following therapy to ensure that the infection is resolved. Because asymptomatic bacteriuria is common during pregnancy, women with frequent UTIs can be given low-dose suppression therapy with daily antibiotics.

A link has been identified between preterm, low-birth-weight infants, and gum disease, and it suggests that periodontal treatment during pregnancy reduces preterm birth (Marakoglu, Gursoy, Marakoglu, et al., 2008).

As early as the 1950s, progesterone had been investigated for its ability to improve pregnancy outcome. Progesterone's importance related to pregnancy lies in its ability to promote uterine relaxation, suppressing contractions, and to prevent gestational immune tolerance or immune tolerance in pregnancy (Blackburn, 2007). It is produced by the corpus luteum and the placenta and is essential for the maintenance of early pregnancy.

When given to women at high risk for preterm births, studies have shown a significant improvement in preterm birth rates (Anderson, Martin, Higgins, et al., 2009). Trials examining the use of progesterone for the treatment of PTL have not demonstrated effectiveness in halting labor or as an adjunct to the use of other tocolytic drugs to halt labor (Anderson et al., 2009).

If the efficacy of progesterone is a result of immune suppression, this may explain why progestogins can be effective if given prophylactically but not once labor has started. Currently the evidence points to treatment for prevention of preterm birth in women with singleton pregnancies at high risk for labor with 17-alpha-hydroxyprogesterone caproate (17P) 250 mg/week. This is administered intramuscularly beginning at 16 weeks and continuing to 36 weeks (Anderson et al., 2009). At this time, 17P has not been approved by the Food and Drug Administration (FDA) for use in the prevention of preterm birth. Moreover, the drug is not readily available and must be obtained from a compounding pharmacy. Table 26-3 summarizes common criteria for diagnosing PTL.

No attempt is made to stop labor if any of the following conditions exists (Ross & Eden, 2009):

- Fetal demise
- Lethal fetal anomaly
- Severe preeclampsia/eclampsia
- Hemorrhage/abruptio placentae
- Chorioamnionitis
- Severe fetal growth restriction
- Fetal maturity
- Acute nonreassuring fetal status

Tocolysis is the use of medications in an attempt to stop labor. These medications may delay birth for 24 to 48 hours (Simpson & Creehan, 2008). Although the delay of childbirth in itself may not improve neonatal outcome, it may permit the administration of betamethasone for fetal surfactant induction or allow for the transport of the mother to a tertiary care facility. Such a facility can generally provide better equipment and services and more experienced, highly trained staff. If labor cannot be arrested, the priority becomes successful preterm birth and management of its psychologic effect on the woman and her partner.

Ritodrine hydrochloride (Yutopar) remains the only drug approved by the FDA for use as a tocolytic (Simpson & Creehan, 2008). However, drugs currently used for tocolysis include beta-adrenergic agonists (also called β-mimetics or β-agonists), magnesium sulfate, calcium channel blockers (nifedipine), and prostaglandin synthetase inhibitors (celecoxib, sulindac, indomethacin, ketorolac). There is no clear choice for a tocolytic; instead a pharmacologic agent is chosen on an individual basis based on the presentation of labor and maternal history. The use of β-mimetics does pose a significant risk to the mother in PTL. β-mimetics, which may be administered intravenously, intramuscularly, subcutaneously, or orally, can significantly affect maternal cardiovascular and metabolic physiology. The most serious effects include hypotension, cardiac arrhythmia, tachycardia, palpitations, myocardial ischemia, pulmonary edema, and maternal hyperglycemia.

Magnesium sulfate, long used in the treatment of preeclampsia, is the most commonly prescribed pharmacologic agent in the United States because it is effective and has fewer side effects than beta-adrenergic agonists. The usual recommended loading dose is 4 to 6 g intravenously in 100 ml of intravenous (IV) fluid over 20 minutes. The maintenance dose is then 1 to 4 g/hr titrated to deep tendon reflexes and serum magnesium levels. The therapy is maintained for 12 hours at the lowest rate to significantly diminish contractions (Simpson & Creehan, 2008). The maternal

TABLE 26-3 Criteria for Diagnosis of Preterm Labor in Gestations 20–37 weeks

Uterine contractions very 5 minutes for 20 minutes
or
8 contractions in a 60 minute period
and
Documented cervical change or cervical effacement of 80% or more
or
Cervical dilation greater than 1 centimeter

serum level that is usually necessary for tocolysis seems to be 5.5 to 7.5 mg/dl.

Side effects with the loading dose may include flushing, a feeling of warmth, headache, nystagmus, nausea, dry mouth, and dizziness. Other side effects include lethargy and sluggishness and a risk of pulmonary edema if the woman has predisposing conditions such as multiple gestation or infection; has had excessive IV fluid administration; or has concurrent β-sympathomimetic therapy (Simpson & Creehan, 2008). Fetal side effects may include hypotonia and lethargy that persist for 1 or 2 days following birth, hypoglycemia, and hypocalcemia. See Drug Guide: Magnesium Sulfate in chapter 20 ∞ for other side effects.

Of the calcium channel blockers approved for use in the United States, nifedipine is frequently used as a tocolytic. Nifedipine acts by reducing the flow of extracellular calcium ions into the intracellular space of the myometrial smooth muscle cells, thereby inhibiting contractile activity. Nifedipine is well absorbed either orally or sublingually, has fewer side effects than comparative agents, and is at least as effective (Simpson & Creehan, 2008). The most common side effects are related to arterial vasodilation, that is, hypotension, tachycardia, facial flushing, and headache. Because the mechanism of action of nifedipine is different from the beta-adrenergic drugs, coadministration of nifedipine and terbutaline or ritodrine may prove beneficial in the treatment of PTL. Because both magnesium sulfate and nifedipine block calcium, however, coadministration of them has been implicated in serious maternal side effects related to low calcium levels and has resulted in maternal cardiovascular collapse (Simpson & Creehan, 2008). Nifedipine is contraindicated in women with heart disease, cardiovascular compromise, intrauterine infection, multiple pregnancy, and maternal hypertension (Simpson & Creehan, 2008).

Prostaglandins enhance the formation of myometrial gap junctions and stimulate the influx of intracellular calcium ions needed for muscle contraction. Prostaglandin synthetase inhibitors, therefore, are a logical choice for tocolysis. Indomethacin, sulindac, or celecoxib are the prostaglandin synthetase inhibitors most often used to suppress labor. Maternal side effects are few. Dyspepsia, nausea, vomiting, depression, and dizzy spells may occur. On rare occasions, psychosis or renal failure may result. These drugs are best administered with an antacid or taken with meals to reduce the chance of gastrointestinal (GI) upset. Prostaglandin synthetase inhibitors are generally not used in women with drug-induced asthma, coagulation disorders, hepatic or renal insufficiency, or peptic ulcer disease.

Indomethacin crosses the placenta readily, and oligohydramnios and premature closure of the fetal ductus arteriosus may occur with long-term use. Consequently the drug, which is no longer widely used, is not recommended after 34 weeks' gestation or for a course of therapy longer than 48 hours (Simpson & Creehan, 2008). Indomethacin has been associated with necrotizing enterocolitis and grades III and IV intravascular hemorrhage (IVH) in the newborn. The risk for IVH increases with decreasing gestational age at birth. Chorioamnionitis is associated with an increased risk of intraventricular hemorrhage in the newborn and may be the cause of IVH rather than the therapy itself.

The National Institute of Child Health and Human Development (NICHD) recommends that corticosteroids (typically betamethasone or dexamethasone) be administered antenatally to women at risk of preterm birth because of their beneficial effect on fetal lung maturation (Simpson & Creehan, 2008). Any women who are candidates for tocolysis are candidates for antenatal corticosteroids, regardless of fetal gender, race, or availability of surfactant therapy for the newborn, especially between 24 and 34 weeks' gestation.

NURSING CARE MANAGEMENT

Nursing Assessment and Diagnosis

During the antepartal period, the nurse identifies the woman at risk for PTL by noting the presence of predisposing factors. The primary areas for ongoing assessment are change in risk status for PTL, educational needs of the woman and her loved ones, and the woman's responses to medical and nursing interventions.

Nursing diagnoses that may apply to the woman with PTL include the following:

- ***Readiness for Enhanced Knowledge*** related to an expressed desire to understand the causes, identification, and treatment of PTL and its implications
- ***Fear*** related to early labor and birth
- ***Ineffective Coping*** related to need for constant attention to pregnancy
- ***Anxiety*** related to the possibility of a preterm birth (PTB)

Nursing Plan and Implementation

Community-Based Nursing Care

Once uterine activity stops, the woman is sometimes placed on continued pharmacologic therapy. She may then be discharged and followed by home care nurses or as part of a specialized prematurity prevention program.

Home Care

Once thought to be a potentially effective tool for home management of PTL, more recent studies have cast doubt on the value of home uterine activity monitoring (Simpson & Creehan, 2008). The only exception is the woman who is paralyzed and cannot feel any uterine contractions (Ross & Eden, 2009). Outpatient management of a woman at risk for preterm birth includes frequent office visits to assess symptoms and cervical length and in-depth patient education about the signs and symptoms of PTL.

Consideration of the woman's ability to care for herself, the impact of the changes in relationships that will occur, and care of any young children in the home are among the issues that affect the woman's ability to cope effectively with this situation. Care providers need to be alert to any signs that the woman is failing to achieve the emotional and developmental tasks of pregnancy, such as lack of maternal attachment. An individualized nursing management plan helps focus on each woman's specific needs. Although current evidence does not show that increased social support or home uterine activity monitoring are effective in preventing preterm birth (Ross & Eden, 2009), these therapies continue to be used.

Health Promotion Education

Once the woman at risk for PTL has been identified, she needs to be taught about the importance of recognizing the onset of labor. Increasing the woman's awareness of the subtle symptoms of PTL is one of the most important teaching objectives of the nurse (see Patient Teaching: Preterm Labor).

Signs and symptoms of preterm labor include the following:

- Uterine contractions that occur every 10 minutes or less with or without pain.
- Mild menstrual-like cramps felt low in the abdomen.
- Constant or intermittent feelings of pelvic pressure that may feel like the baby pressing down.
- Rupture of membranes.
- Low, dull backache, which may be constant or intermittent.
- A change in the vaginal discharge (an increase in amount, a change to more clear and watery, or a pinkish tinge).
- Abdominal cramping with or without diarrhea.

The woman is also taught to evaluate contraction activity once or twice a day. She does so by lying down tilted to one side with a pillow behind her back for support. The woman places her fingertips on the fundus of the uterus (which is above the umbilicus after 20 weeks' gestation). She checks for contractions (hardening or tightening in the uterus) for about 1 hour. It is important for the pregnant woman to know that uterine contractions occur occasionally throughout the pregnancy. If they occur every 10 minutes for 1 hour, however, the cervix could begin to dilate, and labor could continue.

The nurse ensures that the woman knows when to report signs and symptoms. If contractions occur every 10 minutes (or less) for 1 hour, if any of the other signs and symptoms is present for 1 hour, or if clear fluid begins leaking from the vagina, she should telephone her physician or nurse-midwife, clinic, or hospital birthing unit and make arrangements to be checked for ongoing labor. If the woman experiences any PTL symptoms for more than 15 minutes while physically active, she should be instructed to do the following:

- Empty her bladder.
- Lie down tilted toward her side.
- Drink 3 to 4 (8 oz) cups of fluid.
- Palpate for uterine contractions, and if contractions occur 10 minutes apart or less for 1 hour, notify the healthcare provider.
- Soak in a warm tub bath with the uterus completely submerged.
- Rest for 30 minutes after the symptoms have subsided, and gradually resume activity.
- Call her healthcare provider if symptoms persist, even if uterine contractions are not palpable.

Caregivers need to be aware that the woman is knowledgeable and attuned to changes in her body and to take her call seriously. When a woman is at risk for PTL, she may have many episodes of contractions and other signs or symptoms. If she is treated positively, she will feel freer to report problems as they arise. Other preventive measures the woman might follow are presented in Table 26-4.

Care Plan Activity: Patient at Risk for Preterm Labor

Hospital-Based Nursing Care

Providing supportive nursing care to the woman in PTL is important during hospitalization. This care consists of promoting bed rest, monitoring vital signs, measuring intake and output, and continuously monitoring fetal heart rate (FHR) and uterine contractions. Placing the woman on her left side facilitates maternal-fetal circulation. Vaginal examinations are kept to a minimum. If tocolytic agents are being administered, the mother and fetus are monitored closely for any adverse effects.

Whether PTL is arrested or proceeds, the woman and her partner, if one is involved, experience intense psychologic stress. Decreasing the anxiety associated with the unknown and the risk of a preterm newborn is a primary aim of the nurse. The nurse also recognizes the stress of prolonged bed rest and of lack of sexual contact and helps the couple find satisfactory ways of dealing with these stresses. With empathetic communication, the nurse can facilitate the couple's expression of their feelings, which commonly include guilt and anxiety, thereby helping the couple identify and implement coping mechanisms. The nurse also keeps the couple informed about the labor progress, the treatment regimen, and the status of the fetus so that their full cooperation can be elicited. In the event of imminent vaginal or cesarean birth, the couple should be offered brief but ongoing explanations to prepare them for the actual birth process and the events following the birth. The nurse may also offer to arrange consultations for the woman and her support person with the neonatologist, social worker, or hospital chaplain if requested.

TABLE 26-4 Self-Care Measures to Prevent Preterm Labor

- Rest 2 or 3 times a day, lying on your left side.
- Drink 2 to 3 quarts of water or fruit juice each day. Avoid caffeine drinks. Filling a quart container and drinking from it will eliminate the need to keep track of numerous glasses of fluid.
- Empty your bladder at least every 2 hours during waking hours.
- Avoid lifting heavy objects. If small children are in the home, work out alternatives for picking them up, such as sitting on a chair and having them climb on your lap.
- Pace necessary activities to avoid overexertion.
- Sexual activity may need to be curtailed or eliminated.
- Find pleasurable ways to help compensate for limitations of activities and boost the spirits.
- Try to focus on 1 day or 1 week at a time rather than on longer periods of time.
- If on bed rest, get dressed each day and rest on a couch rather than becoming isolated in the bedroom.

Source: Prepared in consultation with Susan Bennett, RN, ACCE, Coordinator of the Prematurity Prevention Program.

Through the Eyes of a Nurse
Preterm Labor

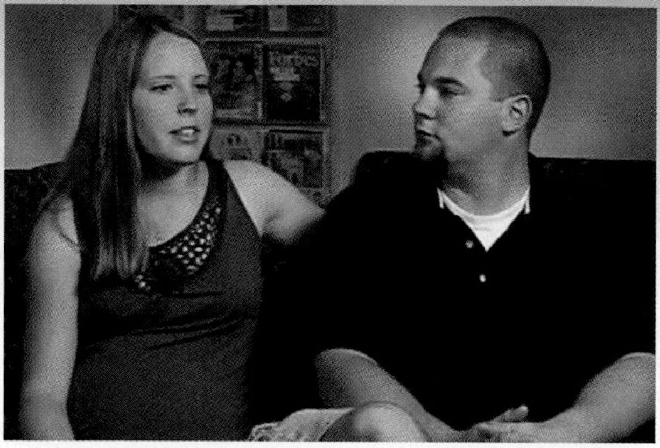

Family's Experience

"I am getting some contractions throughout the day. I am not sure if I should be concerned or not. I wouldn't say they are painful, but I can definitely feel them. I don't want to be overly concerned, but I don't want to ignore them and end up having the baby early. I read the signs on the sheet the other nurse gave me at my last appointment, but I am still unsure if this is normal or something to be worried about."

Her husband is also concerned about her. "She seems to feel them more at the end of the day. When I get home and see her having contractions, I don't know whether to panic or assume it is normal."

Nurse's Response

"Many women experience Braxton-Hicks contractions during the third trimester. This type of contraction is normal. It feels like tightening but is not really painful. Typically, they are irregular, not in a regular pattern. They also occur infrequently compared with preterm labor contractions. It is not uncommon to get them at the end of the day when you have been on your feet all day. When you feel them, get off your feet, rest, and drink several glasses of water. If they continue, you need to time them and call us if they are occurring regularly or if there are more than eight contractions in 1 hour.

"Preterm labor is diagnosed when there are at least eight contractions in 1 hour and cervical change occurs. In order to diagnose preterm labor, you need to call us if you are having frequent contractions and come to the hospital for an examination to see if your cervix has changed."

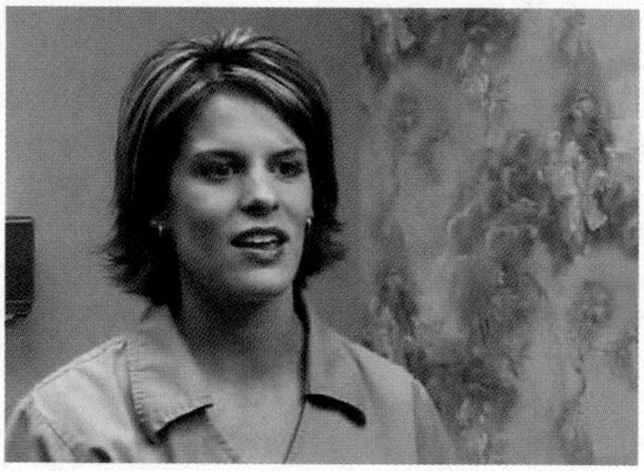

Nurse's Actions and Rationale

The nurse reviews preterm labor symptoms with the couple. The woman should be assessed for possible risk factors. Risk factors are included in Table 26-2. Since Braxton-Hicks contractions are quite common, the differences between preterm labor and these types of contractions should be thoroughly explained. The nurse provides written instructions and provides the couple with a telephone number to call should preterm labor occur.

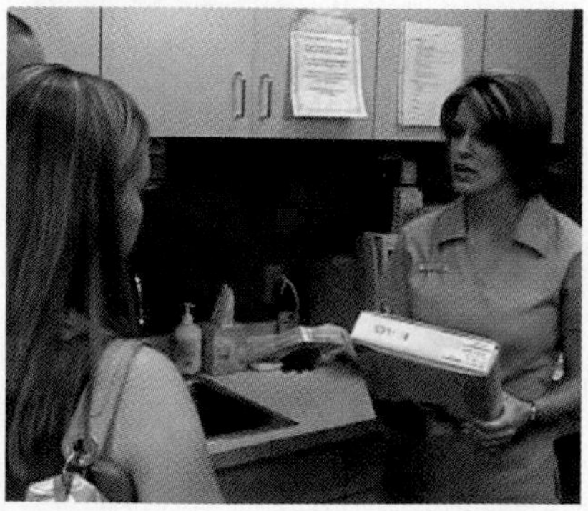

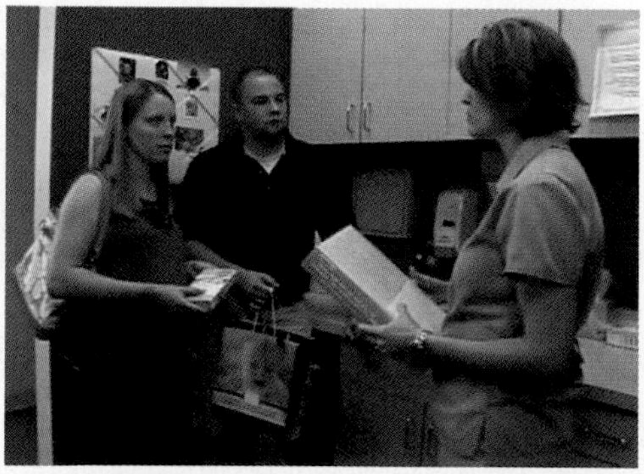

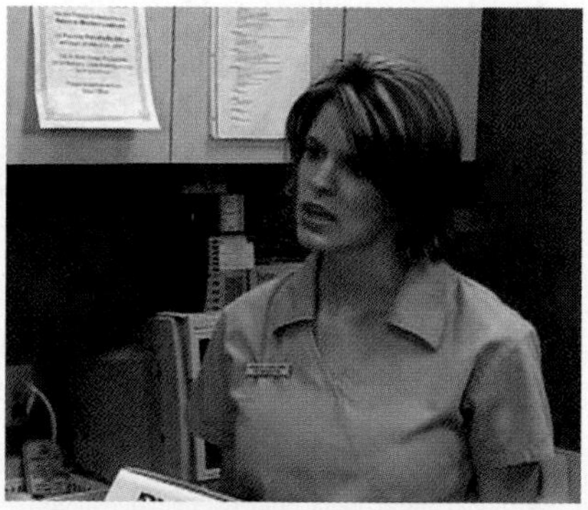

PATIENT TEACHING Preterm Labor

PATIENT GOALS At the completion of teaching the woman will be able to:

1. Discuss the risks of preterm labor.
2. Describe the purpose of home monitoring.
3. Demonstrate the correct procedures for doing home monitoring.
4. Explain self-care measures that help decrease the risk of preterm labor.

TEACHING PLAN

Content	Teaching Method
■ Describe the dangers of preterm labor, especially the risk of prematurity in the infant, and all the potential problems.	Discuss the risks specifically. Many people understand in a general way that prematurity can be dangerous, but they fail to understand how the baby is affected.
■ Emphasize that many of the early symptoms of labor, such as backache and increased bloody show, may be subtle initially.	Use handouts during the discussion. Help the woman clearly understand the value of the program because, to be successful, it requires a real commitment on her part.
■ Be prepared to reinforce the information provided and answer questions that may arise.	Teach the woman how to palpate for uterine contractions. Do a demonstration and ask for a return demonstration.
■ Summarize self-care measures, such as maintaining generous fluid intake (2 to 3 quarts daily), voiding every 2 hours, avoiding lifting and overexertion, avoiding nipple stimulation or orgasm, limiting sexual activity, and cooperating with activity restrictions and bed rest requirements. (See Table 26-4.)	Use a handout during the discussion. Provide opportunities for discussion. If the woman has concerns about certain recommendations, try to modify the approach to best meet her needs.

Evaluation	Documentation
At the end of the teaching session the woman will be able to discuss the risks of preterm labor, demonstrate home monitoring techniques and explain their rationale, and implement self-care activities to decrease the risks of preterm labor.	Document the information given to the woman, including specifics on risk factors, early symptoms, and self-care measures. Specify if written instructions were provided in addition to verbal ones and describe the type of teaching method used. Document the woman's verbalization of understanding and your clarification of any information.

Evaluation

Expected outcomes of nursing care include the following:

- The woman can discuss the cause, diagnosis, and treatment of PTL.
- The woman affirms that her fears about early labor are decreased.
- The woman states that she feels comfortable in her ability to cope with her situation and has resources to call on if needed.
- The woman can identify signs and symptoms of PTL that need to be reported to her caregiver.
- The woman can describe appropriate self-care measures to initiate in the event that she experiences any symptoms of PTL.
- The woman successfully gives birth to a healthy infant.

Care of the Woman and Fetus at Risk Because of Placental Problems

Maintaining placental function is paramount to ensuring fetal well-being and continuation of the pregnancy. Because the placenta is highly vascular, problems that develop are usually associated with maternal and possibly fetal hemorrhage. Causes and sources of hemorrhage are reviewed in Table 26-5. Other placental problems are discussed in chapter 27 ∞.

Abruptio Placentae

Abruptio placentae is the premature separation of a normally implanted placenta from the uterine wall. The incidence of abruptio placentae requiring delivery is 1% of all pregnancies, but it accounts for 15% of perinatal mortality (Beckmann et al., 2010). It is more frequent in pregnancies complicated by smoking, premature rupture of membranes, multiple gestation, advanced maternal age, cocaine use, chorioamnionitis, and hypertension (Beckmann et al., 2010). The risk of recurrence is 10 times higher if a previous abruption has occurred (Beckmann et al., 2010).

The cause of abruptio placentae is largely unknown. Theories have been proposed relating its occurrence to decreased blood flow to the placenta through the sinuses during the last trimester. It is estimated that maternal hypertension is the most common cause (44%) with maternal trauma accounting for 2% to 10% of the cases. Domestic violence, abdominal trauma, presence of fibroids, uterine overdistention, fetal growth restriction, alcohol consumption, a short umbilical cord, and high parity also contribute (Beckmann et al., 2010). Abruptions also appear to be more common in certain ethnic groups. Caucasian and African American women have higher incidences of abruptions than Asian and Latin American women (Cunningham et al., 2010). Classification of abruption is based on the extent of separation (Table 26-6).

TABLE 26-5 Causes and Sources of Hemorrhage

CAUSES AND SOURCES	SIGNS AND SYMPTOMS
Antepartum Period	
Abortion	Vaginal bleeding Intermittent uterine contractions Rupture of membranes
Placenta previa	Painless vaginal bleeding after seventh month
Abruptio placentae	
Partial	Vaginal bleeding: no increase in uterine pain
Severe	Vaginal bleeding may or may not be present Extreme tenderness of abdominal area Rigid, boardlike abdomen Increase in size of abdomen
Intrapartum Period	
Placenta previa	Bright red vaginal bleeding
Abruptio placentae	Same signs and symptoms listed above
Uterine atony in Stage III	Bright red vaginal bleeding Ineffectual contractility
Postpartum Period	
Uterine atony	Boggy uterus Dark vaginal bleeding Presence of clots
Retained placental fragments	Boggy uterus Dark vaginal bleeding Presence of clots
Lacerations of cervix or vagina	Firm uterus Bright red blood

TABLE 26-6 Classification of Abruption

Class 0	Asymptomatic; diagnosed after birth
Class I	Mild; most common, occurring in 48% of cases
Class II	Moderate; both mother and fetus show signs of distress; 27% of cases
Class III	Severe; maternal shock and fetal death likely; 24% of cases

Source: Used with permission from Gaufberg, S. A. (2008). "Abruptio Placenta." eMedicine Journal *(series online). Available at: http:www.emedicine.com/emerg/topic12.htm*

Pathophysiology

Premature separation of the placenta may be divided into three types (Figure 26-3 ■):

1. *Marginal:* The blood passes between the fetal membranes and the uterine wall and escapes vaginally. Separation begins at the periphery of the placenta; this marginal sinus rupture may or may not become more severe.
2. *Central:* The placenta separates centrally, and the blood is trapped between the placenta and the uterine wall. Entrapment of the blood results in concealed bleeding.
3. *Complete:* Massive vaginal bleeding is seen in the presence of almost total separation.

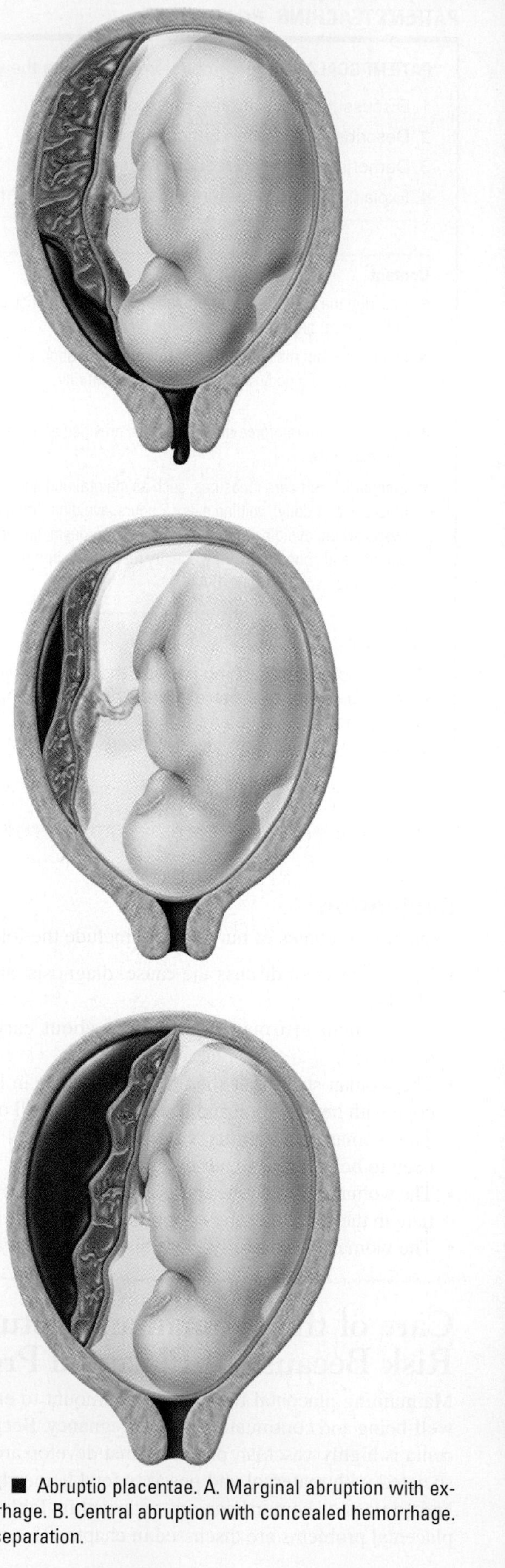

A

B

C

Figure 26-3 ■ Abruptio placentae. A. Marginal abruption with external hemorrhage. B. Central abruption with concealed hemorrhage. C. Complete separation.

In severe cases of central abruptio placentae, a blood clot forms behind the placenta. With no place to escape, the blood invades the myometrial tissues between the muscle fibers. This occurrence accounts for the uterine irritability that is a significant sign of premature separation of the placenta. If hemorrhage continues, eventually the uterus turns entirely blue in color. After the baby is born, the uterus contracts only with difficulty. This syndrome is known as a *Couvelaire uterus* and frequently necessitates hysterectomy.

As a result of the damage to the uterine wall and the retroplacental clotting with covert abruption, large amounts of thromboplastin are released into the maternal blood supply, which in turn triggers the development of disseminated intravascular coagulation (DIC) and the resultant hypofibrinogenemia. Fibrinogen levels, which are ordinarily elevated in pregnancy, may drop to incoagulable amounts within a matter of minutes as a result of rapidly developing premature separation of the placenta. Additional information on DIC may be found in a medical–surgical nursing textbook.

Maternal Risks

Maternal mortality is now uncommon, although maternal morbidity is still common (Beckmann et al., 2010). Problems following the birth depend in large part on the severity of the intrapartal bleeding, coagulation defects (DIC), hypofibrinogenemia, and length of time between separation and the birth. Moderate to severe hemorrhage results in hemorrhagic shock, which ultimately may prove fatal to the mother if not reversed. In the postpartal period, women who have suffered this disorder are at risk for hemorrhage and renal failure due to shock, vascular spasm, intravascular clotting, or a combination of the three. Another cause of renal failure is incompatible emergency blood transfusion. Failure is directly proportional to the number of units transfused. In some cases, hysterectomy is performed if bleeding cannot be controlled.

Fetal-Neonatal Risks

Perinatal mortality associated with abruptio placentae is approximately 25% (Cunningham et al., 2010). In severe cases in which separation occurs to approximately 50% of the placenta, infant mortality is 100%. In less severe separation, fetal outcome depends on the level of maturity. The most serious complications in the newborn arise from preterm labor, anemia, and hypoxia. If fetal hypoxia progresses unchecked, irreversible brain damage or fetal demise may result. Neurologic defects within the first year of life occur in approximately 14% of infants who survive (Cunningham et al., 2010). With thorough assessment and prompt action on the part of the healthcare team, fetal and maternal outcome can be optimized.

Clinical Therapy

Because of the risk of DIC, evaluating the results of coagulation tests is imperative. DIC occurs as a complication secondary to a major medical complication. In DIC, fibrinogen levels and platelet counts are usually decreased; prothrombin times (PT) and partial thromboplastin times (PTT) are normal to prolonged (Creasy, Resnik, Iams, et al., 2009). If the values are not markedly abnormal, serial testing may be helpful in establishing an abnormal trend that is indicative of coagulopathy. Another very sensitive test determines fibrin degradation products; these levels rise with DIC.

After the diagnosis is established, emphasis is placed on maintaining the cardiovascular status of the mother and developing a plan for effecting the birth of the fetus. Intravenous access with a large-gauge cannula is warranted along with continuous electronic fetal monitoring (EFM). Which birth method is selected depends on the condition of the woman and fetus; in many circumstances cesarean birth may be the safest option (Creasy et al., 2009).

If the separation is mild and gestation is near term, labor may be induced, and the fetus may be born vaginally with as little trauma as possible. If rupture of membranes and oxytocin infusion by pump do not initiate labor within a short time, a cesarean birth is usually done. A longer delay would increase the risk of hemorrhage, with resulting hypofibrinogenemia. Supportive treatment to decrease risk of DIC includes typing and cross-matching for blood transfusions (at least three units), clotting mechanism evaluation, and intravenous fluids (Creasy et al., 2009).

In cases of moderate to severe placental separation, a cesarean birth is done after hypofibrinogenemia has been treated by intravenous infusion of cryoprecipitate or fresh frozen plasma (FFP). Vaginal birth is impossible in the event of a Couvelaire uterus because it could not contract properly in labor. Cesarean birth is necessary in the face of severe hemorrhage to allow an immediate hysterectomy to save both woman and fetus.

The hypovolemia that accompanies severe abruptio placentae is life threatening and must be combated with whole blood. If the fetus is alive but experiencing stress, emergency cesarean birth is the method of choice. With a stillborn fetus, vaginal birth is preferable unless shock from hemorrhage is uncontrollable. Intravenous fluids of a balanced salt solution such as lactated Ringer's solution are given through a 16- or 18-gauge cannula (Cunningham et al., 2010). Central venous pressure (CVP) monitoring may be needed to evaluate intravenous fluid replacement. Hemodynamic monitoring is an essential aspect of nursing care for the woman with abruption. If there is any evidence of hypovolemia, two venous lines should be started. Urine output should be monitored with an indwelling catheter. If the output drops below 30 ml per hour with adequate fluid replacement, CVP should be used to assess for hypovolemia. CVP will be the guide to fluid replacement. An absolute level is not as significant as the response to fluid replacement. Pulmonary artery catheter measurement, such as with a Swan-Ganz catheter, may be necessary to manage the hemodynamic changes. However, a significant abruption may preclude placing a catheter in the jugular or subclavian vein because the DIC is causing bleeding from multiple sites. The CVP is evaluated hourly, and results are communicated to the physician. Elevations of CVP may indicate fluid overload and pulmonary edema. The hematocrit is maintained at 30% through the administration of packed red cells or whole blood, or both (Cunningham et al., 2010).

Laboratory testing is ordered to provide ongoing data regarding hemoglobin, hematocrit, and coagulation status. A clot observation test may be done at the bedside to evaluate coagulation status. A red top glass tube containing 5 ml of maternal blood is inverted 4 to 5 times. If a clot fails to form in 6 minutes, a fibrinogen level of less than 150 mg/dl is suspected. If a clot is not formed in 30 minutes, the fibrinogen level may well be less than 100 mg/dl. A clot observation test may be completed by a physician or a nurse.

Measures are taken to stimulate labor to effect vaginal birth as indicated by the condition of the mother and fetus. The birth may be hastened by performing an amniotomy and by oxytocin stimulation. Previously, birth within 6 hours of the diagnosis of severe placental abruption was recommended to reduce maternal mortality and morbidity. Currently, changing medical practice directed to ensuring adequate fluid replacement, especially blood, appears to accomplish the same outcome (Cunningham et al., 2010). These interventions should be started immediately as birth is to be facilitated without delay.

A Kleihauer-Betke is also needed to determine the amount of fetal maternal hemorrhage in Rh negative women. The appropriate amount of Rh D immunoglobulin is calculated based on the test results and number of units of blood that is given (Beckmann et al., 2010).

NURSING CARE MANAGEMENT

Nursing Assessment and Diagnosis

Electronic monitoring of the uterine contractions and resting tone between contractions provides information regarding the labor pattern and effectiveness of the oxytocin induction. Because uterine resting tone is frequently increased with abruptio placentae, it must be evaluated frequently for further increase. Abdominal girth measurements may be ordered hourly and are obtained by placing a tape measure around the maternal abdomen at the level of the umbilicus. Another method of evaluating uterine size, which increases as more bleeding occurs at the site of abruption, is to place a mark at the top of the uterine fundus. The distance from the symphysis pubis to the mark may be evaluated hourly.

Nursing diagnoses that may apply to the woman with abruptio placentae include the following:

- ***Risk for Deficient Fluid Volume*** related to hypovolemia secondary to excessive blood loss
- ***Ineffective Peripheral Tissue Perfusion*** related to blood loss secondary to uterine atony following birth
- ***Anxiety*** related to concern for personal status and the baby's safety
- ***Impaired Gas Exchange (Fetus)*** related to decreased blood volume and hypotension

Nursing Plan and Implementation

The psychologic aspects of nursing care are very important. Maternal apprehension increases as the clinical picture changes. Factual reassurance and an explanation of the procedures and what is happening are essential for the emotional well-being of the expectant couple. The nurse can reinforce positive aspects of the woman's condition, such as normal fetal heart rate (FHR), normal vital signs, and decreased evidence of bleeding.

Other nursing care measures are addressed in the Nursing Care Plan: Hemorrhage in the Third Trimester on pages 678–680.

Evaluation

Expected outcomes of nursing care include the following:

- The woman and her baby have a safe labor and birth without further complications for the mother or child.
- The woman and family verbalize understanding of reasons for medical therapy and risks.

NURSING CARE PLAN Hemorrhage in the Third Trimester

INTERVENTION	RATIONALE
1. Nursing Diagnosis: Risk for Deficient Fluid Volume related to excessive vascular loss during pregnancy **Goal:** Woman will not experience significant fluid volume deficit during the third trimester of pregnancy.	
■ Monitor vital signs (i.e., temperature—normal range is 96.8°–100.4°F, pulse—normal is 60–90, respirations—normal is 12–22, blood pressure—normal range is 110/70 to 135/85, central venous pressure—normal range is 5–10 mm H_2O). Compare present blood pressure with woman's baseline blood pressure. Note pulse pressure.	■ Any deviations in a woman's baseline vital signs could indicate intravascular fluctuations.
■ Weigh pads and chux. If the woman has bathroom privileges, instruct her on initiating pad counts. Teach the woman how to weigh pads and chux, with each gram equal to approximately 1 ml of blood loss. ■ Report amount of blood loss within a specific period (e.g., 50 ml of bright-red blood on pad in 20 minutes).	■ The combination of weighing and counting pads and chux assists medical personnel in determining the woman's blood loss.
■ Monitor urinary output hourly and measure urine specific gravity (normal: 1.010–1.025).	■ A decrease in urinary output (less than 30 ml/hr) and an increase in specific gravity suggest dehydration and a need for an increase in fluid intake.

NURSING CARE PLAN Hemorrhage in the Third Trimester continued

INTERVENTION	RATIONALE
■ Palpate bilateral peripheral pulses (normal: equal and strong) and note capillary refill (normal: less than 3 seconds). Also, assess skin color and temperature (normal: pink, warm, dry, and intact).	■ Helps determine signs of circulatory loss or hypovolemic shock that include weak pulses, capillary refill greater than 3 seconds, skin color that is cyanotic or pallor, and skin temperature that is cool and clammy.
■ Assess mental status at frequent intervals.	■ Excessive blood loss can lead to changes in mentation.
■ Assess the woman for signs and symptoms of disseminated intravascular coagulation.	■ Provides vital information on maternal status.
■ Instruct the woman on the importance of strict bed rest and avoidance of any sexual activity that involves nipple stimulation or that might lead to orgasm.	■ Bleeding may cease with limited activity. Pressure on the abdomen and orgasms can stimulate uterine activity, thereby causing bleeding. Nipple stimulation may result in uterine contractions, as can orgasm.
■ Monitor fetal status and uterine activity by continuous fetal monitoring.	■ May determine the origin of bleeding and fetal well-being.
Collaborative:	
■ Collect and review blood work: complete blood count (CBC), type and cross-match, Rh titer, fibrinogen levels, platelet count, activated partial thromboplastin time (APTT), prothrombin time (PT), and human chorionic gonadotropin (hCG) levels.	■ Determines blood loss and need for intervention if blood work is abnormal.
■ Administer appropriate isotonic IV solutions and blood products (e.g., plasma expanders, whole blood, serum albumin, or packed red blood cells) as ordered by the physician.	■ Reverses shock symptoms by increasing blood volume.
■ Insert Foley catheter.	■ Close monitoring of urinary output will aid in determining adequate renal perfusion.

EXPECTED OUTCOME: The woman will show signs of adequate fluid volume during pregnancy as evidenced by vital signs within normal limits, capillary refill in less than 3 seconds, adequate sensorium, and urine output greater than 30 ml/hr.

2. Nursing Diagnosis: Ineffective Peripheral Tissue Perfusion (Uteroplacental) related to hypovolemia secondary to excessive maternal blood loss
Goal: The fetus will have no evidence of hypoxia during pregnancy.

INTERVENTION	RATIONALE
■ Assess maternal vital signs.	■ Closely monitoring maternal physiologic status and circulatory status will assist in determining if an episode of bleeding has occurred and allow for interventions to protect maternal and fetal well-being.
■ Monitor fetal heart tones continuously, assessing for variability, accelerations, and decelerations, and record.	■ Continuous electronic fetal monitoring will aid in detecting signs of fetal hypoxia and allow time for appropriate intervention.
■ Assess fundal height.	■ Determines an approximate gestational age.
■ Assess labor progression by determining cervical dilatation and effacement if contractions are present.	■ This provides information on maternal labor status.
Collaborative:	
■ Perform scalp stimulation to assess fetal accelerations.	■ FHR acceleration is considered 15 beats above the baseline lasting for 15 seconds and is indicative of fetal well-being.
■ Assess amniotic fluid for meconium.	■ Impaired gas exchange relaxes fetal intestinal motility, causing expulsion of meconium into amniotic fluid.
■ Assist the physician during ultrasonography and amniocentesis for lecithin/sphingomyelin (L/S) ratio sample.	■ Determines viability and alerts appropriate medical personnel of fetal age if birth is imminent.

EXPECTED OUTCOME: Fetus will demonstrate adequate tissue perfusion as evidenced by fetal heart tones that remain within 110–160 beats/min, long-term variability and short-term variability present, positive periodic changes (no variable or late decelerations), and fetal scalp blood pH greater than 7.25.

(continued)

NURSING CARE PLAN Hemorrhage in the Third Trimester continued

INTERVENTION	RATIONALE
3. Nursing Diagnosis: Fear/Anxiety related to personal and fetal well-being secondary to third-trimester hemorrhage **Goal:** The woman will verbalize a decrease in fear and anxiety.	
■ Maintain frequent contact with the woman and family members.	■ Establishes trust with the woman and her family members, so the patient will not feel alone or abandoned.
■ Provide the woman with accurate, reliable information concerning diagnosis and prognosis.	■ Fear and anxiety will lessen when the woman is informed of health status and is allowed to make decisions based on present situation.
EXPECTED OUTCOME: The woman will actively seek information about diagnosis and prognosis.	
■ Allow the woman and family members to verbalize the origin of fears.	■ Recognizing the origin of fear gives the woman and her family the appropriate tool to begin the process of developing coping strategies for dealing with the fears.
■ Explain all procedures in an easy-to-understand, nonthreatening manner, and allow the woman and family members to ask questions.	■ Accurate information prepares the woman and family members for the impending procedures, thereby reducing fear of the unknown.
EXPECTED OUTCOME: The woman and her family members develop appropriate coping strategies that decrease fear and anxiety.	

Placenta Previa

Application: Placenta Previa

In **placenta previa**, the placenta is improperly implanted in the lower uterine segment. This implantation may be on a portion of the lower segment or over the internal os (Figure 26-4 ■). As the lower uterine segment contracts and dilates in the later weeks of pregnancy, the placental villi are torn from the uterine wall, thus exposing the uterine sinuses at the placental site. Bleeding begins, but because the amount depends on the number of sinuses exposed, it may initially be either scanty or profuse.

The cause of placenta previa is unknown. Statistically, it occurs in about 1 in 200 pregnancies (Beckmann et al., 2010). Factors associated with placenta previa are previous placenta previa, multiparity, increasing age, placenta accreta (discussed in a following section), defective development of blood vessels in the decidua, prior cesarean birth or other uterine surgery, cocaine use, smoking, a recent spontaneous or induced abortion, and a large placenta (Beckmann et al., 2010).

Placenta previa is classified in four degrees:

1. ***Total placenta previa:*** Internal os is covered completely by the placenta.
2. ***Partial placenta previa:*** Internal os is partially covered by the placenta.
3. ***Marginal placenta previa:*** Edge of the placenta is at the margin of the internal os.
4. ***Low-lying placenta:*** Placenta is implanted in the lower segment but does not reach the os although it is in close proximity of it.

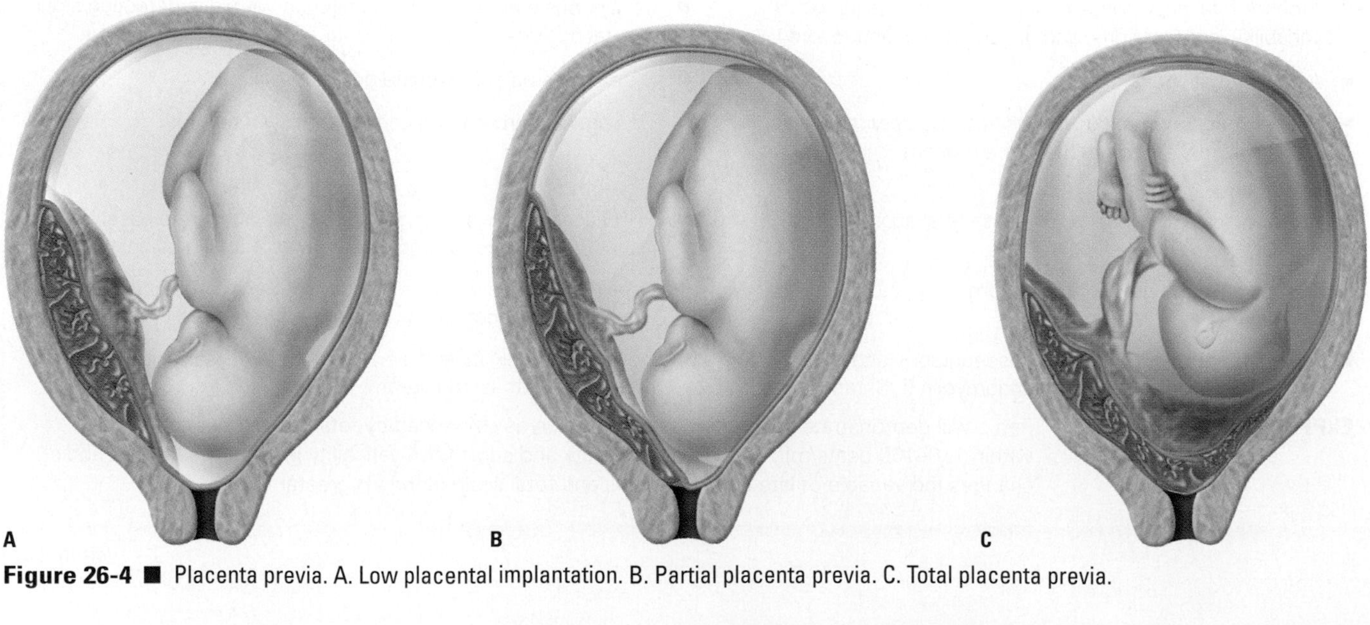

A B C

Figure 26-4 ■ Placenta previa. A. Low placental implantation. B. Partial placenta previa. C. Total placenta previa.

Another condition, **vasa previa**, occurs when the fetal vessels course through the amniotic membranes and are present at the cervical os. Vasa previa occurs in 1 in 2500 pregnancies. Although this is a rare cause of antepartum bleeding, it is associated with a high rate of fetal death (Beckmann et al., 2010).

Clinical Therapy

Women who present with vaginal bleeding should be questioned regarding any history of abnormal placenta placement that was diagnosed during the pregnancy. When possible, prenatal records should be reviewed. Women who have not had a routine ultrasound examination and have no history of bleeding during the pregnancy may have an undiagnosed placenta previa. The goal of medical care is to identify the cause of bleeding and to provide treatment that will ensure birth of a mature newborn. It must be determined whether the cause of the bleeding is placenta previa or advanced labor with copious bloody show (which is normal). Indirect diagnosis is made by localizing the placenta via tests that require no vaginal examination. The most commonly employed diagnostic test is the transabdominal ultrasound scan. Abdominal or transvaginal sonography is used to identify the presence of placenta previa. If placenta previa is ruled out, a vaginal examination can be performed with a speculum to determine the cause of bleeding (such as cervical lesions or polyps).

Direct diagnosis of placenta previa can be made only by feeling the placenta inside the cervical os. However, such an examination may cause profuse bleeding because of tearing of tissue in the cotyledons of the placenta. Because of the danger of bleeding, a vaginal examination is generally contraindicated and is performed only if ultrasound is not available, the pregnancy is near term, and there is already profuse vaginal bleeding. The examination is done by a physician using a double setup procedure; that is, the delivery room is set up for the vaginal examination and normal vaginal birth and for a cesarean birth should placenta previa be present and the examination precipitate brisk bleeding. Adequate personnel must be present to respond to treatment decisions.

CLINICAL TIP

When assessing a woman for vaginal bleeding, make sure to have the woman lift her bottom completely off the bed so you can observe for blood loss beneath the buttocks.

The differential diagnosis of placental or cervical bleeding takes careful consideration. Table 26-7 provides a comparison of the signs and symptoms of placenta previa and abruptio placentae. Partial separation of the placenta may also present with painless bleeding, and a true placenta previa may not demonstrate overt bleeding until labor begins, thus confusing the diagnosis. In fact, the causes of slight to moderate antepartal bleeding episodes in 20% to 25% of women are never accurately diagnosed.

Care of the woman with painless late gestational bleeding depends on (1) the week of gestation during which the first bleeding episode occurs and (2) the amount of bleeding (Figure 26-5 ■). If the pregnancy is less than 37 weeks' gestation, expectant management is employed to delay birth until about 37 weeks' gestation to allow the fetus to mature. Expectant management involves stringent compliance with the following:

1. Bed rest with bathroom privileges only as long as the woman is not bleeding.
2. No vaginal examinations.
3. Monitoring of blood loss, pain, and uterine contractility.
4. Evaluation of FHR with external monitor.
5. Monitoring of maternal vital signs.
6. Complete laboratory evaluation: hemoglobin, hematocrit, Rh factor, and urinalysis.
7. Administration of intravenous fluid (lactated Ringer's solution) with drip rate monitored.
8. Availability of two units of cross-matched blood for possible transfusion.
9. Administration of betamethasone to facilitate fetal lung maturity.

TABLE 26-7 Differential Signs and Symptoms of Placenta Previa and Abruptio Placentae

	PLACENTA PREVIA	ABRUPTIO PLACENTAE
Onset	Quiet and sneaky	Sudden and stormy
Bleeding	External	External or concealed
Color of blood	Bright red	Dark venous
Anemia	= Blood loss	Greater than apparent blood loss
Shock	= Blood loss	Greater than apparent blood loss
Toxemia	Absent	May be present
Pain	Only labor	Severe and steady
Uterine tenderness	Absent	Present
Uterine tone	Soft and relaxed	Firm to stony hard
Uterine contour	Normal	May enlarge and change shape
Fetal heart tones	Usually present	Present or absent
Engagement	Absent	May be present
Presentation	May be abnormal	No relationship

Source: Reprinted with permission from Oxorn, H., & Foote, W. (1986). Human labor and birth *(5th ed., p. 507). Copyright © 1986 The McGraw-Hill Companies, Inc.*

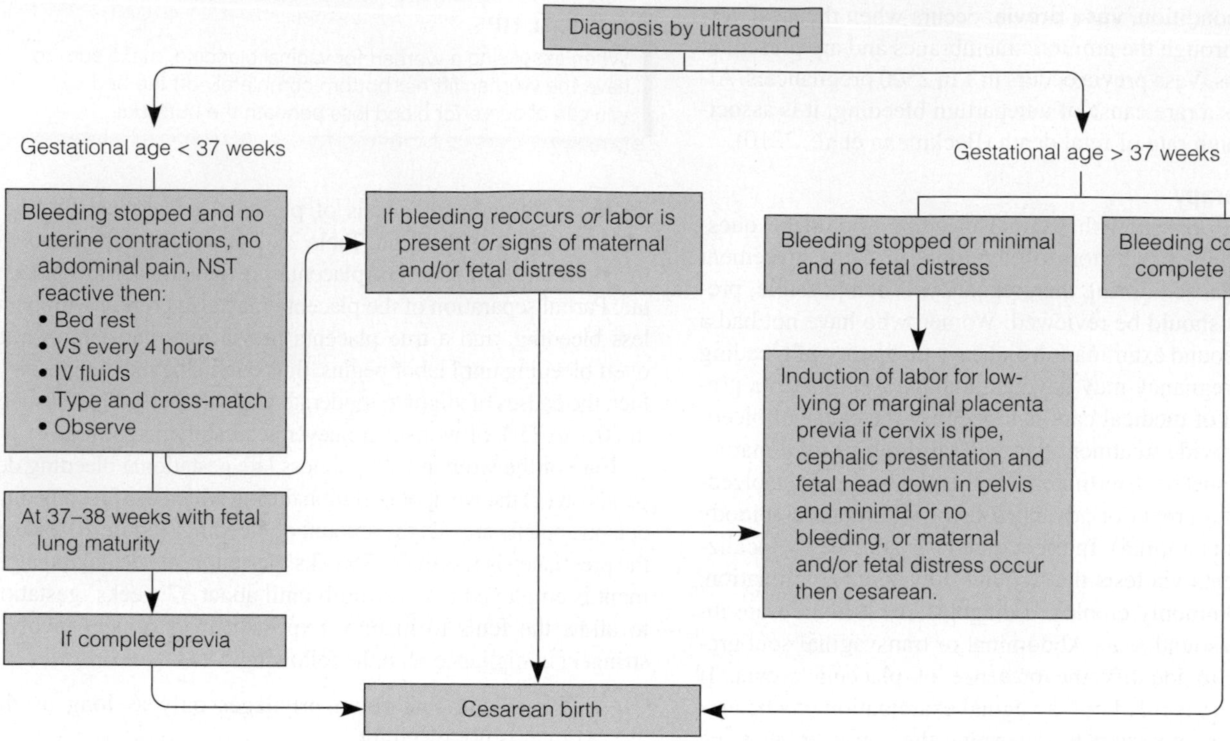

Figure 26-5 ■ Management of placenta previa.

Source: Reprinted from Handbook of Obstetrics, Gynecology, and Primary Care, *F. P. Zuspan & E. J. Quilligan. Copyright © 1998, with permission from Elsevier.*

10. Administration of Rh D immunoglobulin in Rh D negative women.

If frequent, recurrent, or profuse bleeding persists or if fetal well-being appears threatened, a cesarean birth needs to be performed.

NURSING CARE MANAGEMENT

Nursing Assessment and Diagnosis

Assessment of the woman with placenta previa must be ongoing to prevent or treat complications that are potentially lethal to the mother and fetus. Painless, bright red vaginal bleeding is the best diagnostic sign of placenta previa. If this sign should develop during the last 3 months of a pregnancy, placenta previa should always be considered until ruled out by ultrasound examination. The first bleeding episode is generally scanty. If no vaginal examinations are performed, it often subsides spontaneously. However, each subsequent hemorrhage is more profuse.

The uterus remains soft, and if labor begins, it relaxes fully between contractions. The FHR usually remains stable unless profuse hemorrhage and maternal shock occur. As a result of the placement of the placenta, the fetal presenting part is often unengaged, and transverse lie is common.

The nurse appraises blood loss, pain, and uterine contractility from both subjective and objective perspectives. Maternal vital signs and the results of blood and urine tests provide the nurse with additional data about the woman's condition. FHR is evaluated with an external fetal monitor. Another nursing responsibility is observing and verifying the family's ability to cope with the anxiety associated with an unknown outcome.

Nursing diagnoses that may apply to the woman experiencing placenta previa are as follows:

- ***Deficient Fluid Volume*** related to hypovolemia secondary to excessive blood loss
- ***Ineffective Peripheral Tissue Perfusion*** related to blood loss secondary to uterine atony following birth
- ***Anxiety*** related to concern for own personal status and the baby's safety
- ***Impaired Gas Exchange*** related to decreased blood volume and hypotension
- ***Fear*** related to concern for safety of the baby

Nursing Plan and Implementation

The nurse continues to monitor the woman and her fetus to determine the status of the bleeding and to determine the mother's and baby's responses. Vital signs, intake and output, and other pertinent assessments must be made frequently. The nurse evaluates the electronic monitor tracing to evaluate the fetal status.

Emotional support for the family is an important nursing care goal. When active bleeding is occurring, the assessments and management must be directed toward physical support. However, emotional aspects need to be addressed simultaneously. The nurse can explain the assessments being completed and the treatment measures that need to be done. Time can be provided for questions, and the nurse can act as an advocate in obtaining information for the family. The nurse can also offer emotional support by staying with the family and by the use of touch.

Case Study: Patient with Placental Problems

The newborn's hemoglobin, cell volume, and erythrocyte count should be checked immediately after birth and then monitored closely. The newborn may require oxygen and administration of blood and admission into a neonatal intensive care unit.

Additional information regarding nursing care is addressed in the Nursing Care Plan: Hemorrhage in the Third Trimester.

Evaluation

Expected outcomes of nursing care include the following:

- The cause of hemorrhage is recognized promptly, and corrective measures are taken.
- The woman's vital signs remain in the normal range.
- The woman and her baby have a safe labor and birth.
- The family understands what has happened and the implications and associated problems of placenta previa.

CLINICAL TIP

When faced with an emergent situation, tell the woman she needs to follow your instructions quickly and that you will explain what is happening as soon as possible once you take the necessary measures to ensure that she and the baby are safely cared for.

Care of the Woman with a Multiple Gestation

The incidence of twins in the United States accounts for 3% of all pregnancies; however, with advances in reproductive technologies, the incidence is increasing (Gibbs et al., 2010). It is estimated that triplets and higher order multiples account for 1.8% of all births. The incidence of these higher order births is declining because of recent recommendations from the American College of Obstetricians and Gynecologists (ACOG) to reduce the number of fetuses transferred during in vitro fertilization procedures. Because twin birth is by far the most common multiple birth, the discussion focuses on this type. The chapter also identifies specific variations for triplets and higher order multiple gestations as appropriate.

Embryology of Multiple Gestation

Terminology related to various types of twins is presented in Table 26-8. Twins can develop from either the fertilization of two separate ova or from the division of one fertilized ovum. Twins that occur from two separate ova are called *dizygotic* (two zygotes, also referred to as fraternal twins). In this type, the fetuses may be the same sex or different sexes and there are two complete amnions and two chorions. The fetuses are no more closely related genetically than any other siblings. The majority of twins conceived through in-vitro fertilization are fraternal since multiple fertilized ova are inserted into the uterus (Gibbs et al., 2010).

In contrast, 33% of twins are *monozygotic* (also referred to as identical twins); that is, they develop from one fertilized ovum (Blackburn, 2007). These twins are genetically identical, and thus always of the same sex (see Table 26-8). If the zygote divides within the first 72 hours past fertilization, the twins will be diamniotic and dichorionic. If the division occurs from the fourth to the eighth day past fertilization, the embryos will develop with two separate amnions and one chorion. If the division happens after the eighth day, the two fetuses will share both a common amniotic sac and chorion. The terminology is important because the perinatal morbidity and mortality rates differ greatly among different types of twins (Blackburn, 2007). For example, monozygotic twins have a high incidence of cord entrapment, twin-to-twin transfusion, and fetal demise (Blackburn, 2007).

Pregnancy Loss in Multiple Gestation

The development of sensitive human chorionic gonadotropin (hCG) assays and increasingly sensitive ultrasound techniques

TABLE 26-8 Characteristics of Twin Pregnancy

TYPE	TIME OF DIVISION	CHARACTERISTICS	FREQUENCY
Dizygotic			
(Two separate ova) Fraternal twins Dichorionic-diamniotic twins	Develop from two ova released at the same time.	Each twin has own placenta, chorion, amnion. Dizygotic twins are called fraternal twins. They may be the same or different sex. Increases with maternal age up to 35 years, then falls abruptly. Increases with parity.	67% of all twins
Monozygotic			
(Single ovum identical twins)			33% of all twins
Dichorionic-diamniotic twins	Division occurs within 72 hours past fertilization. Inner cell mass not yet developed.	Each twin has own chorion, amnion, placenta.	30% of monozygotic twins
Monochorionic-diamniotic twins	Division occurs at blastocyst stage, 4 to 8 days after fertilization. Inner cell mass divides in two.	Placenta has one chorion and two amnions. Each twin lies in own sac.	70% of monozygotic twins
Monochorionic-monoamniotic twins	Division occurs in primitive germ disk, 9 to 13 days past fertilization.	Twins lie in the same amniotic sac. Increased risk of umbilical cords becoming tangled or knotted.	2% of monozygotic twins

Source: Adapted from Creasy, R. K., Resnik, R., Iams, J. D., Lockwood, C. J., & Moore, T. R. (2009). Creasy & Resnik's maternal-fetal medicine: Principles and practices *(6th ed.). Philadelphia, PA: Saunders.*

has made it possible to determine more accurately the early pregnancy loss rate of twins, including both complete pregnancy loss and spontaneous resorption of one twin (called the "vanishing twin" phenomenon). Of all twin pregnancies, approximately 25% are lost before the end of the first trimester (Blackburn, 2007). Causative factors in the loss of both twins in the first trimester include environmental factors, infectious organisms, trophoblast dysfunction, poor embryo quality, or a lower concentration of placentally produced substances. Although loss of one twin can occur at any time during the pregnancy, it more commonly occurs in the first trimester. Marginal and velamentous cord insertions (discussed in chapter 27 ∞) are more likely to be present when there is a vanishing twin, and the presence of a monochorionic placenta is more likely to result in either a singleton gestation (because of a vanishing twin) or complete pregnancy loss (Blackburn, 2007).

Pregnancy loss of twins in the second trimester is associated with congenital anomalies, growth restriction, chromosomal abnormalities, and cervical incompetence. Congenital anomalies are twice as likely to occur in twin gestations (Gibbs et al., 2010). In a monochorionic placenta, there may be a vascular anastomosis that leads to twin-to-twin transfusion syndrome. When this syndrome is present, blood is chronically drained from one fetus to the other. The donor fetus becomes growth restricted, and oligohydramnios develops. The recipient fetus becomes polycythemic and hydropic, and hydramnios develops. If the fetuses become severely affected during the second trimester, untreated mortality may be 100% (Cunningham et al., 2010).

The incidence of preterm birth is also higher in multiple gestations. Preterm birth occurs in 50% of twins, 76% of triplets, and 90% of quadruplets (Simpson & Creehan, 2008). In singletons, the perinatal mortality is at the lowest point at 40 weeks' gestation; for twins, the perinatal mortality rate decreases until 37 weeks and then increases steadily from 38 to 42 weeks. The optimal delivery time for triplet pregnancies is 35 weeks (Gibbs et al., 2010). A woman pregnant with twins who has not spontaneously begun labor by 38 gestational weeks is typically induced.

Implications

Women with a multiple gestation are more likely to develop complications, which include the following (Simpson & Creehan, 2008):

- Spontaneous abortions are more common, as previously discussed.
- Gestational diabetes occurs more often in multiple gestations. Three percent to six percent of twin pregnancies and 22% to 39% of triplet pregnancies are complicated by gestational diabetes.
- Hypertension is the major maternal complication. The risk of developing severe hypertension or preeclampsia is 2.6 times higher in twins and significantly higher in triplets.
- Multiple gestations are more likely to acquire HELLP (hemolytic anemia, elevated liver enzymes, and low platelet count) syndrome, a complication resulting from eclampsia or preeclampsia (discussed in chapter 20 ∞).
- Women with multiple gestations are more likely to develop acute fatty liver, which is manifested by severe coagulopathy, hypoglycemia, and hyperammonemia, which can lead to maternal and fetal death.
- Pulmonary embolism is 6 times more likely to develop during pregnancy with multiple gestations.
- Maternal anemia occurs because of demands of the multiple gestation. The hemoglobin averages 10 g/dl from the 20th week on. Anemia is indicated by hemoglobin levels below 11 g/dl in the first or third trimester or below 10.5 g/dl in the second trimester. When decreased hemoglobin is accompanied by serum ferritin concentration of less than 12 mg/dl, iron deficiency anemia is diagnosed.
- Hydramnios may be due to increased renal perfusion from cross-vessel anastomosis of monozygotic twins.
- Premature rupture of membranes, incompetent cervix, and intrauterine growth restriction occur more commonly.
- Rare complications associated with twins include twin-to-twin transfusion (previously discussed), conjoined (Siamese) twins, and *acardia* (twin reversed arterial perfusion sequence).
- Complications during labor include preterm labor, uterine dysfunction due to an overstretched myometrium, abnormal fetal presentations, instrumental or cesarean birth, and postpartum hemorrhage.
- Due to cardiovascular changes, pulmonary edema is more common in multiple gestations.
- Dermatologic complications, such as pruritic urticarial papules and plagues of pregnancy (PUPP), occur in 2.9% of twin and 14% of triplet pregnancies.
- Multiple births account for 21% of low-birth-weight infants, 19% to 24% of very low-birth-weight infants, 20% of neonatal intensive care unit (NICU) admissions, and 26% of neonatal deaths.

The woman with a multiple gestation may experience more physical discomfort during her pregnancy, such as shortness of breath, dyspnea on exertion, backaches, round ligament pain, heartburn, pelvic or suprapubic pressure, and pedal edema because of the oversized uterus.

Clinical Therapy

The goals of medical care are to promote normal fetal development, to prevent maternal complications, to prevent preterm birth, and to diminish fetal trauma during labor.

Ultrasound examinations play a crucial role in the care and treatment of multiple gestations. Ultrasound assists with identifying the presence of more than one fetus early in the pregnancy, providing accurate dating of the pregnancy, and detecting fetal anomalies. Because the incidence of perinatal mortality and morbidity is increased in twins, use of ultrasound in the first and second trimesters can be particularly helpful. Evidence supports the use of ultrasound for accurately determining chorionicity and amnionicity in multiple pregnancies (Beckmann et al., 2010).

Knowledge of chorionicity is essential in differentiating twin-to-twin transfusion from fetal growth restriction secondary to abnormal placental blood flow. Knowledge of chorionicity is also important in determining the management of a multiple pregnancy in which one twin is sonographically abnormal. If the twins are dichorionic/diamniotic (DC/DA), then selective termination could be considered.

Determination of amnionicity is based on ultrasound visualization or the lack of visualization of an intertwin membrane. Visualization of this membrane becomes more difficult as the gestation advances because of progressive thinning of the intertwin membrane, fetal crowding, and an increasing incidence of oligohydramnios. Knowledge regarding the presence of one amnion is crucial, because management of monochorionic/monoamniotic (MC/MA) twins requires more intensive surveillance and earlier birth, usually by cesarean (Beckmann et al., 2010; Gibbs et al., 2010). Women with (MC/MA) twins are frequently cared for by perinatologists in a facility that has high-risk services available.

Preventing preterm labor is a major goal. Prenatal care should begin early, and more frequent visits are usually scheduled. Many practitioners perform vaginal examinations at each visit after 28 weeks to identify cervical changes, such as cervical shortening, effacement, or dilatation, or the beginning of bulging membranes. Assessing cervical length via ultrasound has been predictive in identifying women at risk for preterm birth (PTB). A cervical length of less than 25 mm between 14 and 20 weeks is associated with PTB prior to 32 weeks. Cervical length less than 25 mm for triplets between 15 and 20 weeks is associated with a 100% delivery rate by 28 weeks (Simpson & Creehan, 2008). Digital examinations are often helpful as well but to be accurate they should be performed by the same examiner at each prenatal visit (Simpson & Creehan, 2008). Fetal fibronectin (fFN) as a predictor of preterm labor has been well established in singleton pregnancies. A study of 147 twin gestations revealed that a negative fFN test is associated with a less than 3% risk of PTB in the following 2-week period. This test can be beneficial since women with multiple gestations are often symptomatic (Gibbs et al., 2010). Further research is needed to determine if this test results in fewer PTBs.

There is insufficient evidence to support policies for routine cervical cerclage, reduced activity and work, and prophylactic bed rest (Gibbs et al., 2010). A systematic review of studies of hospitalization and bed rest for multiple gestation showed insufficient evidence to support routine bed rest (Gibbs et al., 2010). Although home monitoring was commonly used in the 1990s, the effectiveness of this intervention has been disputed by large randomized studies and is no longer endorsed for preterm labor monitoring (Gibbs et al., 2010).

Some areas offer twin clinics, which provide many advantages for the woman with a multiple gestation. These advantages include consistent evaluation, intensive prenatal education, counseling, and support from the same healthcare providers.

Intrapartal management and assessment require careful attention to maternal and fetal status. The mother should have an intravenous infusion in place with a large-bore needle. Anesthesia and cross-matched blood should be readily available. The twins are monitored by dual electronic fetal monitoring (EFM). The labor may progress very slowly or very quickly.

The decision about method of birth may not be made until labor occurs, and the method depends on a variety of factors. The presence of maternal complications such as placenta previa, abruptio placentae, or severe preeclampsia usually indicates the need for cesarean birth. Fetal factors such as severe intrauterine growth restriction (IUGR), preterm birth, fetal anomalies, nonreassuring fetal status, or unfavorable fetal position or presentation also require cesarean birth. Typically, a cesarean birth is performed if the presenting twin is in a presenting position other than vertex and cannot be turned to a vertex presentation.

Birth of three or more fetuses is best accomplished by cesarean because of the risk of fetal insult due to decreased placental perfusion and hemorrhage from the separating placenta during the intrapartal period (Cunningham et al., 2010). Complicated obstetric maneuvers such as breech extraction and podalic version, the risk of prolapse of the cord, and an increase in fetal collision provide additional reasons for cesarean birth.

Any combination of presentations and positions can occur with twins (Figure 26-6 ■). Approximately 40% of twins present in a vertex/vertex presentation. More than 80% of twins in vertex/vertex presentation are born vaginally. Another 40% of twins present in vertex/nonvertex presentation. Although research shows no differences in infant mortality or morbidity when the second twin is born via breech delivery, many practitioners choose to deliver any nonvertex presentation via cesarean birth (Gibbs et al., 2010). In 20% of cases, twin A is nonvertex and requires a cesarean birth (Gibbs et al., 2010).

The placentas are examined after the birth. If the twins are of the same sex, the placentas are sent to the pathology laboratory for examination to determine whether they are monozygotic or dizygotic twins.

NURSING CARE MANAGEMENT

Nursing Assessment and Diagnosis

When obtaining a maternal history at the beginning of antenatal care, the nurse should identify any family history of twinning. Equally important is a history of medication taken to enhance fertility or artificial reproductive technology that may have been used to conceive. These facts should be noted on the antepartal record.

At each antepartal clinic visit, the nurse should measure the fundal height. During the prenatal period, a fundal height greater than expected for the weeks of gestation and auscultation of two heartbeats that differ by at least 10 beats per minute are the most likely clues of twin pregnancy. Some women experience severe nausea and vomiting and develop severe anemia despite the intake of multiple-vitamin therapy.

Any growth, fetal movement, or heart tone auscultation out of proportion to gestational age by dates is indicative of twins. During palpation, the nurse may feel many small parts on all

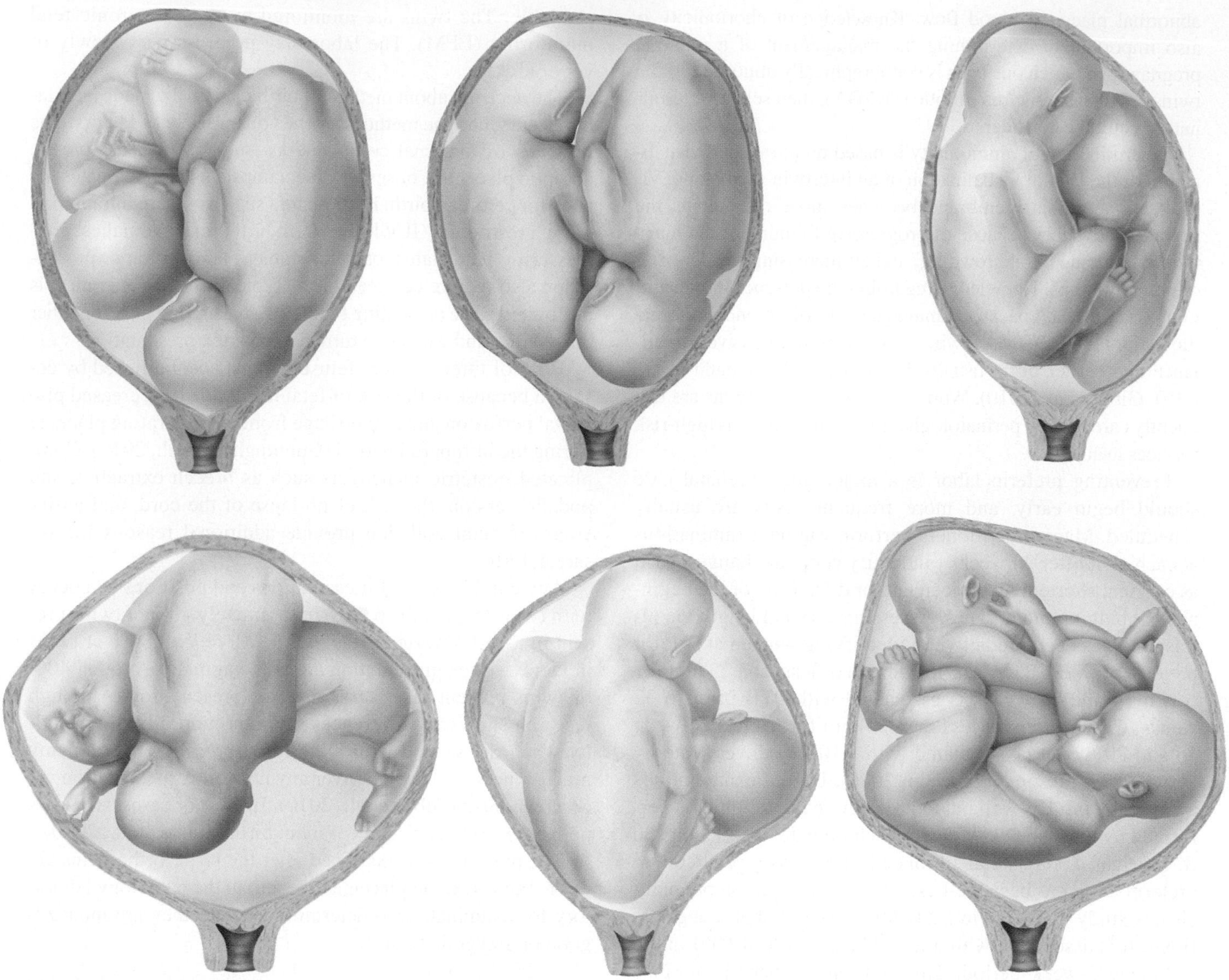

Figure 26-6 ■ Twins may be in any of these presentations in utero.

sides of the abdomen (Figure 26-7 ■). If twins are suspected, the nurse should attempt to auscultate two separate heartbeats in different quadrants of the maternal abdomen. Use of the Doppler device may be helpful. Conclusive evidence of twins is found on sonography.

During the prenatal visits the nurse should determine the family's level of preparation for integrating more than one new member. Although the thought of having twins can be very exciting, the reality of attaching to two infants and adapting to the parental role may be trying.

During labor it is important to monitor each fetus. In the case of twins, an external electronic monitor can be applied to both, or if conditions permit, the internal monitor can be applied to twin A and the external monitor to twin B. The heart rates may be auscultated on different quadrants of the maternal abdomen, but continuous monitoring is more beneficial. Signs of nonreassuring heart rate patterns should be reported to the certified nurse-midwife (CNM) or obstetrician.

After a multiple birth, the mother is closely monitored for postpartal hemorrhage. Nursing diagnoses that may apply to a woman with a multiple gestation include the following:

- ***Fear*** related to unknown outcome of the birth process
- ***Ineffective Coping*** related to uncertainty about the labor and birth plan
- ***Deficient Knowledge*** related to lack of information about the problems associated with multiple gestation
- ***Impaired Gas Exchange (Fetuses)*** related to decreased oxygenation secondary to cord compression

Nursing Plan and Implementation

Community-Based Nursing Care

Antepartally, the woman may need counseling about diet and daily activities. The nurse can help her plan meals to meet her increased needs. A daily intake of 4000 kcal (minimum) and 135 g of protein are recommended for optimal weight gain and fetal

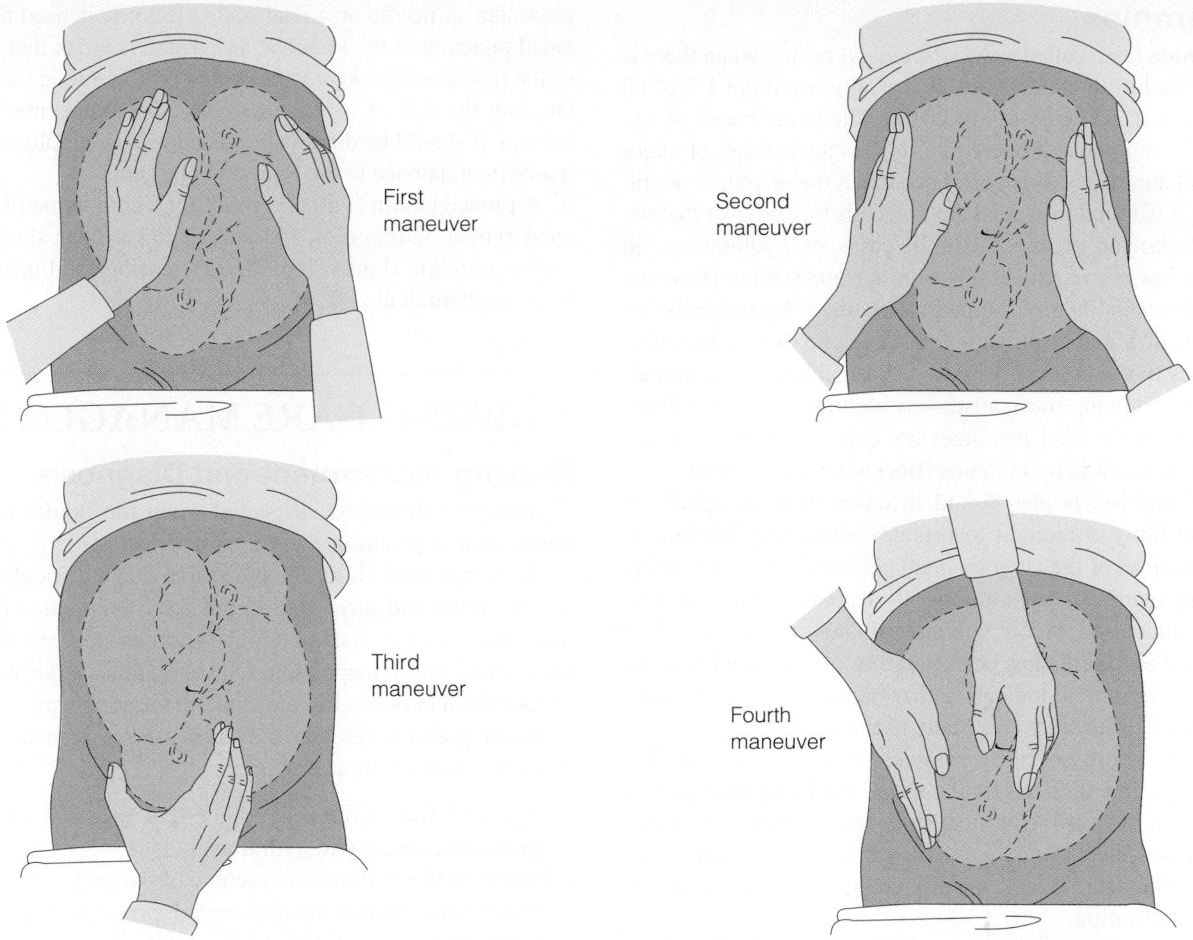

Figure 26-7 ■ Leopold's maneuvers in twin pregnancy for determing the fetuses' head positions, presentations, and lie. The fetus on the mother's right side is in cephalic presentation, and the fetus on the left is in breech presentation. Leopold's maneuvers may be done in a different sequence.

growth. A prenatal vitamin and 1 mg of folic acid and iron should also be taken daily. A weight gain of 35 to 45 lb is recommended.

Maternal hypertension is treated with bed rest in the lateral position to increase uterine and kidney perfusion. Back discomfort can be alleviated by pelvic rocking, good posture, and good body mechanics. The nurse can help the woman schedule frequent periods of rest during the day. Family members or friends may be willing to care for the woman's other children periodically to allow her time to get rest. Community support systems, such as neighbors or church members, may be available to assist the family with meals, grocery shopping, and household chores. Many communities now have support groups specifically designed for mothers of multiples. Members provide invaluable peer support throughout pregnancy and the postpartum period. Teaching regarding prevention and recognition of preterm labor is very important.

Hospital-Based Nursing Care

The nurse needs to prepare to receive multiple newborns. This means a multiplication of resuscitation equipment and newborn identification papers and bracelets. The newborns may be placed in individual radiant warmers or in the same one once identification bands have been applied. Additional staff members should be available for newborn resuscitation, monitoring, and newborn care. Special precautions should be observed to ensure correct identification of the newborns. The first born is usually tagged Baby A; the second, Baby B; and so on.

Evaluation

Expected outcomes of nursing care include the following:

- The woman is able to discuss the implications and problems associated with a multiple gestation.
- The woman feels she is able to cope with the pregnancy and birth.
- The woman understands the treatment plan and how to gain further information.
- The mother, father, and babies have a safe prenatal course, labor, and birth and a safe postpartal and newborn course.

Care of the Woman and Fetus at Risk Because of Amniotic Fluid-Related Complications

Complications related to amniotic fluid include hydramnios and oligohydramnios.

Hydramnios

Hydramnios (also called *polyhydramnios*) occurs when there is over 2000 ml of amniotic fluid. It typically occurs in 1% of all pregnancies (Beckmann et al., 2010). The exact cause of hydramnios is unknown; however, it often occurs in cases of major congenital anomalies. It is postulated that a major source of amniotic fluid is found in special amnion cells that lie over the placenta (Beckmann et al., 2010). In cases of hydramnios, no pathology has been found in this amniotic epithelium. However, during the second half of the pregnancy, the fetus normally begins to swallow and inspire amniotic fluid and to urinate, which contributes to the amount present. Fetal malformations that affect this swallowing mechanism—as well as neurologic disorders in which the fetal meninges are exposed in the amniotic cavity—can result in hydramnios (Beckmann et al., 2010).

This condition is also found in cases of anencephaly in which the fetus is thought to urinate excessively because of overstimulation of the cerebrospinal centers. When a monozygotic twin manifests hydramnios, it is possible that the twin with the increased blood volume urinates excessively. The weight of the placenta has been found to be increased in some cases of hydramnios, indicating that increased functioning of the placental tissue may contribute to the problem.

There are two types of hydramnios: chronic and acute. The chronic type, in which the fluid volume gradually increases, is a problem of the third trimester. Most cases are of this variety. In acute cases, the volume increases rapidly over a period of a few days. The acute type is usually diagnosed between 20 and 24 weeks' gestation.

When the amount of amniotic fluid is over 3000 ml, the woman experiences shortness of breath and edema in the lower extremities from compression of the vena cava. If hydramnios is severe enough, she can experience intense pain. The acute form of hydramnios tends to be more severe. Milder forms of hydramnios occur more frequently and are associated with minimal symptoms. Hydramnios is associated with such maternal disorders as diabetes and Rh sensitization. It can also occur as a result of infections such as syphilis, toxoplasmosis, cytomegalovirus, herpes, and rubella (Beckmann et al., 2010).

Fetal malformations and preterm birth are common with hydramnios; thus there is a fairly high rate of perinatal mortality. Prolapsed umbilical cord can occur when the membranes rupture, which adds a further complication for the fetus. The incidence of malpresentations is also increased (Beckmann et al., 2010).

Clinical Therapy

Hydramnios is managed with supportive treatment unless the intensity of the woman's distress and symptoms dictate otherwise.

If the accumulation of amniotic fluid is severe enough to cause maternal dyspnea and pain, hospitalization and removal of the excessive fluid are required. This can be done vaginally by artificial rupture of membranes (AROM) or by amniocentesis. The dangers of performing AROM vaginally are prolapsed cord and the inability to remove the fluid slowly. A *needle amniotomy* may be preferred because this releases the fluid at a slower rate and allows the presenting part to descend gradually. A needle amniotomy is performed by the certified nurse-midwife (CNM) or physician. A needle or a fetal scalp electrode is used to make a small puncture in the amniotic sac. There is a risk that the force of the fluid could make a larger hole in the amniotic sac, thus increasing the risk of a prolapsed cord. If amniocentesis is performed, it should be done with the aid of sonography to prevent inadvertent damage to the fetus and placenta.

A prostaglandin synthesis inhibitor (indomethacin) is often used to treat hydramnios. Indomethacin has been shown to decrease amniotic fluid volume by decreasing fetal urine output (Cunningham et al., 2010).

NURSING CARE MANAGEMENT

Nursing Assessment and Diagnosis

Hydramnios should be suspected when the fundal height increases out of proportion to the gestational age.

With increased fluid, the nurse may have difficulty palpating the fetus and auscultating the fetal heart rate (FHR). In more severe cases the maternal abdomen appears extremely tense and tight on inspection. On sonography large spaces can be identified between the fetus and the uterine wall.

Nursing diagnoses that may apply for a woman with hydramnios include the following:

- ***Impaired Gas Exchange*** related to pressure on the diaphragm secondary to hydramnios
- ***Fear*** related to unknown outcome of the pregnancy
- ***Acute Pain*** related to abdominal pressure secondary to hydramnios

Nursing Plan and Implementation

When amniocentesis is performed, sterile technique is used to prevent infection. The nurse can offer support to the couple by explaining the procedure to them.

If the fetus has been diagnosed with a congenital defect in utero or is born with the defect, psychologic support is needed to assist the family. Often the nurse collaborates with social services to offer the family this additional help. The nurse can also offer to contact chaplain services at the family's request.

Evaluation

Expected outcomes of nursing care include the following:

- The woman and her partner can discuss the procedure, implications, risks, and characteristics that need to be reported to the caregiver.

Oligohydramnios

Oligohydramnios is defined as a less than normal amount of amniotic fluid (approximately 500 ml is considered normal). Although no exact amount of fluid has been definitively identified as diagnostic of this condition, oligohydramnios is diagnosed when the largest vertical pocket of amniotic fluid visible on ultrasound examination is 5 cm or less (Beckmann et al., 2010). The exact cause of oligohydramnios is unknown. It is found in cases of postmaturity, with intrauterine growth restriction

(IUGR) secondary to placental insufficiency, and in fetal conditions associated with major renal malformations, including renal aplasia with dysplastic kidneys and obstructive lesions of the lower urinary tract. If oligohydramnios occurs in the first part of pregnancy, there is a danger of fetal adhesions (one part of the fetus may adhere to another part).

During the gestational period, fetal skin and skeletal abnormalities may occur because fetal movement is impaired as a result of inadequate amniotic fluid volume. Because there is less fluid available for the fetus to use during fetal breathing movements, pulmonary hypoplasia may develop. During the labor and birth, the lessened amounts of fluid reduce the cushioning effect for the umbilical cord, and cord compression is more likely to occur.

Clinical Therapy

During the antepartum period, oligohydramnios may be suspected when the uterus does not increase in size in accordance with established gestational dating, the fetus is easily palpated and outlined by the examiner, and the fetus is not ballottable. The fetus can be assessed by biophysical profile (BPP), nonstress tests (NSTs), and serial ultrasounds. During labor the fetus will be monitored by continuous electronic fetal monitoring (EFM) to detect cord compression, which will be indicated by nonperiodic decelerations. Amnioinfusion can replace some fluid volume and remove pressure on the umbilical cord (see chapter 28 ∞).

NURSING CARE MANAGEMENT

Nursing Assessment and Diagnosis

Oligohydramnios should be suspected when the fundal height is less than the gestational age and the fetal parts are easily palpated through the fundal wall. Continuous EFM is an important part of assessment during the labor and birth. The nurse evaluates the EFM tracing for the presence of nonperiodic decelerations or other nonreassuring signs (such as increasing or decreasing baseline, decreased variability, or presence of periodic decelerations). If nonperiodic decelerations are noted, the nurse can change the woman's position (to relieve pressure on the umbilical cord) and must then notify the physician or CNM. If position changes are insufficient to relieve the pattern, an amnioinfusion may be performed. After the birth, the newborn is evaluated for signs of congenital anomalies, pulmonary hypoplasia, or postmaturity.

On sonography there is a lack of amniotic fluid. An amniotic fluid index is typically performed to determine the amount of amniotic fluid. Less than 5 cm of amniotic fluid is considered low and the diagnosis of oligohydramnios is made (Simpson & Creehan, 2008).

Nursing diagnoses that may apply for a woman with hydramnios include the following:

- ***Impaired Gas Exchange*** related to cord compression secondary to oligohydramnios
- ***Fear*** related to unknown outcome of the pregnancy

Nursing Plan and Implementation

The fetus is continually monitored during labor and birth. An amnioinfusion (discussed in chapter 28 ∞) is often performed to increase the amount of fluid surrounding the fetus and to decrease the incidence of variable decelerations. In the event that the fetal heart rate tracing is nonreassuring, late decelerations occur, and birth is not imminent, a cesarean birth may be performed.

Evaluation

Expected outcomes of nursing care include the following:

- The woman and her partner can discuss the diagnosis, implications, and risks to the caregiver.
- The fetus remains uncompromised during labor and birth.

FOCUS YOUR STUDY

- Cervical insufficiency (incompetent cervix), the premature dilatation of the cervix, is the most common cause of second-trimester abortion. It is treated surgically with a cerclage, which involves placing a suture in the cervix to keep it from opening.
- Both premature rupture of membranes and preterm labor place the fetus at risk. Women with preterm premature rupture of membranes (PPROM) and no signs of infection are managed conservatively with bed rest and careful monitoring of fetal well-being.
- Preterm labor is often treated with tocolytics, which can be effective in stopping labor; however, they do have side effects.
- Abruptio placentae is the separation of the placenta from the uterine wall before the birth of the infant that often results in painful vaginal bleeding. Abruptio placentae may be central, marginal, or complete.

- Placenta previa occurs when the placenta implants low in the uterus or over the cervix. A low-lying or marginal placenta is one that lies near the cervix. In a partial placenta previa, part of the placenta lies over the cervix. In a complete placenta previa, the entire placenta covers the cervix. Bleeding associated with placenta previa is typically painless.
- Placental problems can be either developmental or degenerative.
- Multiple gestation is associated with both maternal and fetal/neonatal complications.
- Hydramnios, also known as polyhydramnios, occurs when there is more than 2000 ml of amniotic fluid contained within the amniotic membranes.
- Oligohydramnios occurs when there is a severely reduced volume of amniotic fluid. Oligohydramnios is associated with intrauterine growth restriction (IUGR), postmaturity, and fetal renal and urinary malformations. The fetus is more likely to experience variable decelerations because the amniotic fluid is insufficient to keep pressure off the umbilical cord.

CRITICAL THINKING IN ACTION

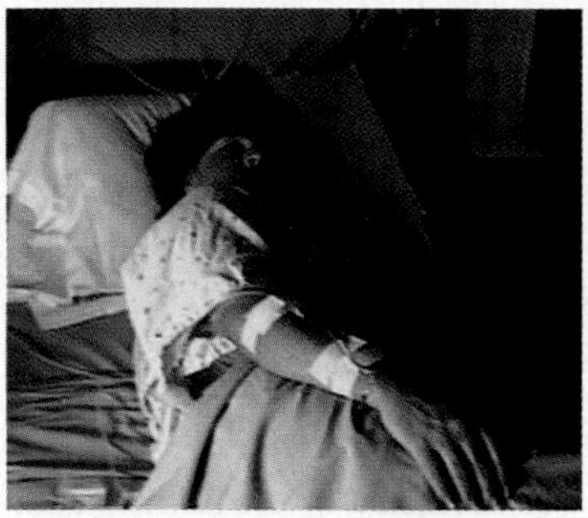
Source: George Dodson/Pearson Education.

Monique Waleski, a 34-year-old G1 P0000, at 32 weeks' gestation, contacts her physician's office because she has been experiencing labor contractions that have gradually increased in frequency. She reports that she has been having about 8 contractions an hour for the past 2 hours. She is instructed to meet her doctor at the birthing unit for further evaluation.

At the birthing unit a vaginal examination reveals that Monique's cervix is dilated 3 cm and 80% effaced. Contractions continue to occur every 7 to 8 minutes. Her fFN test is positive. She is diagnosed with preterm labor.

You position her on her left side and start an IV infusion. Her physician tells Monique that she wants to begin tocolysis using magnesium sulfate and then prescribes 2 doses of betamethasone. You explain to Monique and her partner that you will be giving her the magnesium sulfate by infusion pump and the betamethasone by IM injection once a day today and tomorrow. She asks you about the two medications, including their specific purposes.

1. Explain the concept of tocolysis and the purpose of magnesium sulfate.
2. Describe the concept of a loading dose and maintenance dose.
3. How will you know if Monique is developing toxic levels of magnesium?
4. Describe the role of corticosteroids used during preterm labor.

See www.nursing.pearsonhighered.com for possible responses.

Pearson Nursing Student Resources

Find additional review materials at
www.nursing.pearsonhighered.com

Prepare for success with additional NCLEX®-style practice questions, interactive assignments and activities, Web links, animations and videos, and more!

REFERENCES

Abbasi, S., Oxford, C., Gerdes, J., Sehdev, H., & Ludmir, J. (2009). Antenatal corticosteroids prior to 24 weeks gestation and neonatal outcome of extremely low birth weight infants. *American Journal of Perinatology, 27*(1), 61–66. doi: 00001833-201027010-00011

American College of Obstetricians and Gynecologists (ACOG). (2003; Reaffirmed 2008). *Cervical insufficiency* (ACOG Practice Bulletin No. 48). Washington, DC: Author.

Anderson, L., Martin, W., Higgins, C., Nelson, S., & Norman, J. (2009). The effect of progesterone on myometrial contractility, potassium channels, and efficacy. *Reproductive Science. 16*(11), 1052–1061. doi: 10.1177/1933719109340926

Beckmann, C. R. B., Ling, F. W., Barzansky, B. M., Herbert, W. N. P., Laube, D. W., & Smith, R. P. (2010). *ACOG Obstetrics and Gynecology* (6th ed.). Philadelphia, PA: Lippincott, Williams & Wilkins.

Berghella, V., Baxter, J. K., & Hendrix, N. W. (2009). Cervical assessment by ultrasound for preventing preterm delivery. *Cochrane Database of Systematic Review, 8*(3), CD007235.

Berghella, V., Hayes, E., Vistintine, J., & Baxter, J. K. (2008). Fetal fibronectin testing for reducing the risk of preterm birth. *Cochrane Database of Systematic Reviews* (4), Art No: CD006843. doi: 10.1002/14651858.CD006843. pub2

Berghella, V., Roman, A., Daskalakis, C., Ness, A., & Baxter, J. K. (2007). Gestational age at cervical length measurement and incidence of preterm birth. *Obstetrics & Gynecology, (110)*2 (Pt. 1), 311–317.

Blackburn, S. (2007). *Maternal, fetal, and neonatal physiology: A clinical perspective* (3rd ed.). Philadelphia, PA: Saunders.

Chao, A. S., Chao, A., & Hsieh, P. C. (2008). Ultrasound assessment of cervical length in pregnancy. *Taiwan Journal of Obstetrics & Gynecology, 47*(3), 291–295.

Creasy, R. K., Resnik, R., Iams, J. D., Lockwood, C. J., & Moore, T. R. (2009). *Creasy & Resnik's maternal-fetal medicine: Principles and practice* (6th ed.). Philadelphia, PA: Saunders.

Cunningham, F. G., Leveno, S. L., Gant, N. F., Gilstrap, L. C., Hauth, J. C., & Wenstrom, K. D. (2010). *Williams obstetrics* (23rd ed.). New York, NY: McGraw-Hill.

Denney, J. M., & Culhane, J. F. (2009). Bacterial vaginosis: A problematic infection from both a perinatal and neonatal perspective. *Seminars in Fetal Neonatal Medicine, 14*(4), 200–203.

Denney, J. M., Culhane, J. F., & Goldenberg, R. L. (2008). *Prevention of premature birth.* Retrieved from http://www.medscape.com/viewarticle/582761

Duhig, K. E., Chandiramani, M., Seed, P. T., Briley, A. L., & Kenyon, A. P. (2009). Fetal fibronectin as a predictor of spontaneous labor. *American Journal of Obstetrics & Gynaecology, 116*(6), 799–803.

Ellestad, S. C., Swamy, G. K., Sinclair, T., James, A. H., Heine, R. P., & Murtha, A. P. (2008). Preterm premature rupture of membrane management-inpatient verses outpatient: A retrospective study. *American Journal of Perinatology, 25*(1), 69–73.

El-Mowafi, D. M. (2010). *Tocolytics*. Retrieved from http://www.gfmer.ch/Obstetrics_simplified/tocolytic_drugs.htm

Encyclopedia of Surgery. (2010). *Cervical cerclage*. Retrieved from http://www.surgeryencyclopedia.com/Ce-Fi/Cervical-Cerclage.html

Gibbs, R. S., Karlan, B. Y., Haney, A. F., & Nygaard, I. (2010). *Danforth's obstetrics & gynecology* (10th ed.). Philadelphia, PA: Lippincott, Williams & Wilkins.

Gjoni, M. (2010). *Premature rupture of membranes*. Retrieved from http://www.gfmer.ch/Endo/PGC_network/Preterm_premature_rupture_Gjoni.htm

Hamilton, B. E., Martin, J. A., & Ventura, S. J. (2007). Births: Preliminary data for 2006. *National Vital Statistics Reports, 56*(7), 1–8.

Hutzal, C. E., Boyle, E. M., Kenyon, S. L., Nash, J. V., Winsor, S., Taylor, D. J., & Kirpalani, H. (2008). Use of antibiotics for the treatment of preterm parturition and prevention of neonatal morbidity: A meta-analysis. *American Journal of Obstetrics & Gynecology, 199*(6), 620.e1–8.

Jazayeri, A. (2008). *Premature rupture of membranes*. Retrieved from http://www.emedicine.medscape.com/article/261137-overview

Johnson, J. R., & Iams, J. D. (2009). *Cervical insufficiency*. Retrieved from http://www.UpToDate.com

Jones, H. E., Harris, K. A., Azizia, M., Bank, L., Carpenter, B., Hartley, J. C., . . . Middleton, P. (2009). Differing prevalence and diversity of bacterial species in fetal membranes from very preterm and term labor. *PLoS ONE, 4*(12), e8205. doi:10.1371/journal.pone.0008205

Mancuso, M. S., & Owen, J. (2009). Prevention of preterm birth based on a short cervix: Cerclage. *Seminars in Perinatology* (33), 325–333.

Marakoglu, I., Gursoy, U. K., Marakoglu, K., Cakmak, H., & Ataoglu, T. (2008). Peridonititis as a risk factor for preterm low birth weight. *Yonsei Medical Journal, 49*(2), 200–203.

March of Dimes. (2007). *March of Dimes Peristats: More babies born prematurely new report shows*. Retrieved from http://www.marchofdimes.com

Mazor-Dray, E., Levy, A., Schlaeffer, E., & Sheiner, E. (2009). Maternal urinary tract infection: Is it independently associated with adverse pregnancy outcome? *Journal of Maternal Fetal Neonatal Medicine, 22*(2), 124–128.

Mazumder, U., Sarkar, S., & Khatun, M. (2009). Effect of corticosteroids on perinatal outcomes in preterm premature rupture of membranes. *Journal of Mymensingh Medicine, 18*(Suppl. 1), S45–49.

Melamed, N., Hadar, E., Benn-Haroush, A., Kaplan, B., & Yogev, Y. (2009, June 11). Factors affecting the duration of the latency period in preterm premature rupture of membranes. *Journal of Maternal Fetal Neonatal Medicine*, 1–6.

Noehr, B., Jensen, A., Frederiksen, K., Tabor, A., & Kjaer, S. K. (2009). Loop electrosurgical excision of the cervix and subsequent risk for spontaneous preterm delivery: A population-based study of singleton deliveries during a 9-year period. *American Journal of Obstetrics & Gynecology, 201*(1), 33.e1–33.e6. Retrieved from http://www.sciencedirect.com

Ohlsson, A., & Shah, V. S. (2009). Intrapartum antibiotics for known maternal Group B streptococcal colonization. *Cochrane Database of Systematic Reviews 2009* (3), Art. No.: CD007467. doi: 10.1002/14651858.CD007467.pub2

Pelaez, L. M., Fox, N. S., & Chasen, S. T. (2008). Negative fetal fibronectin: Who is still treating preterm labor and does it help? *Journal of Perinatal Medicine, 36*(3), 202–205.

Ross, M. G., & Eden, R. D. (2009). *Preterm labor*. Retrieved from http://emedicine.com.medscape.com/article/260998-overview

Simpson, K. R., & Creehan, P. A. (2008). *AWHONN perinatal nursing* (3rd ed.). Philadelphia, PA: Lippincott, Williams & Wilkins.

Whitworth, M., & Quenby, S. (2008). Prophylactic oral betamimetics for preventing preterm labour in singleton pregnancies. *Cochrane Database Systematic Reviews, 23*(1), CD006395.

Wilson, B. A., Shannon, M. T., & Shields, K. M. (2010). *Pearson nurse's drug guide 2010*. Upper Saddle River, NJ: Pearson.

Yeganegi, M., Watson, C. S., Martins, A., Kim, S. O., Reid, G., Challis, J. R., & Bocking, A. D. (2009). Effect of lactobacillis rhamnosus GR-1 supernatant and fetal sex on lipopolysaccharide-induced cytokine and prostaglandin-regulating enzymes in human placental trophoblast cells: Implications for treatment of bacterial vaginosis and prevention of preterm labor. *American Journal of Obstetrics & Gynecology, 200*(5), 532.e1–8.

CHAPTER 27

Childbirth at Risk: Labor-Related Complications

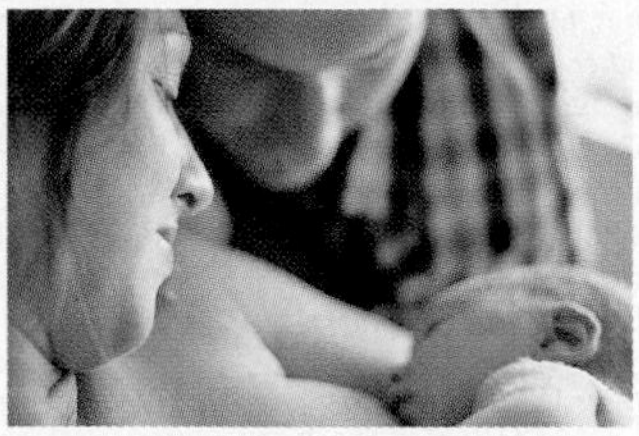

I couldn't wait to begin labor. I wasn't afraid. We had wonderful plans for our labor and birth. My nurse helped me with my breathing as I entered transition. Everything was going so well. Suddenly, the baby began having decelerations. The nurse assisted me onto my side and called for assistance. Time seemed to stand still as the once rapidly beating heart suddenly sounded so slow. It seemed like it took forever to return to its previous rapid pace. For an instant, I was terrified, but after that one episode, there were no further problems.

LEARNING OUTCOMES

1. Describe psychologic disorders that may contribute to difficulty in coping during labor and birth.
2. Discuss dysfunctional labor patterns.
3. Identify the potential maternal risks of precipitous labor and birth.
4. Describe the impact of postterm pregnancy on the childbearing family.
5. Summarize various types of fetal malposition and malpresentation and possible associated problems.
6. Discuss the implications of macrosomia and hydrocephalus on the woman and the fetus.
7. Analyze the implications of abnormal placenta and umbilical cord variations.
8. Discuss the interventions needed in caring for a woman with a prolapsed umbilical cord.
9. Discuss the identification, management, and nursing care of women with amniotic fluid embolus.
10. Identify the signs and symptoms associated with a uterine rupture.
11. Delineate the effects of pelvic contractures on labor and birth.
12. Identify complications related to uterine rupture.
13. Discuss complications of the third and fourth stages of labor.

KEY TERMS

Active management of labor (AMOL) *698*
Amniotic fluid embolism *718*
Anaphylactoid syndrome of pregnancy *718*
Brachial plexus injury *712*
Cephalopelvic disproportion (CPD) *719*
Dystocia *696*
Macrosomia *711*
Persistent occiput posterior (OP) position *702*
Placenta accreta *721*
Placenta increta *721*
Placenta percreta *721*
Postterm pregnancy *700*
Precipitous labor and birth *699*
Prolapsed umbilical cord *717*
Psychologic disorders *693*
Retained placenta *721*
Uterine rupture *719*

The successful completion of the 40-week gestational period requires the harmonious functioning of the five critical factors we discussed in chapter 22 ∞: the birth passage, the fetus, the relationship between the passage and fetus, forces of labor, and psychosocial considerations. Disruptions in any of these components may result in dystocia (at-risk or difficult labor). Some of the most common at-risk conditions during labor are discussed in this chapter.

Care of the Woman at Risk Because of Psychologic Disorders

Anxiety and fear are common emotions in many women in labor. Joy, happiness, excitement, fear of the unknown, and anxiety related to pain sensations may all occur. Even women who are well prepared can experience anxious feelings. Although these reactions are expected in the woman with normal coping mechanisms and adequate social support, women with psychologic disorders may face additional emotional challenges and need additional nursing care and support in the intrapartum period.

The prevalence of psychologic disorders of adults in the United States is 26.2% or roughly 1 in 4 adults (Table 27-1). **Psychologic disorders** are characterized by alterations in thinking, mood, or behavior. Each year, more than half a million women with psychiatric illnesses become pregnant (American College of Obstetricians and Gynecologists (ACOG), 2008). It is further estimated that one third of all pregnant women are exposed to psychotrophic medications at some time during their pregnancies (ACOG, 2008). Although there are many different types of psychologic disorders, only the most common are presented here. Because an in-depth description is beyond the scope of this text, we focus on the impact of these disorders on labor and birth (Table 27-2). Postpartum psychologic disorders are discussed in chapter 39 ∞.

Maternal Implications

Depression affects millions of Americans annually. More women are affected than men (National Institute of Mental Health [NIMH], 2009). Depression is believed to be caused by a central nervous system (CNS) imbalance in serotonin and other neurotransmitters. The hormonal changes associated with pregnancy can directly impact a woman with a previous history of depression. Individuals with depression may have persistent sad mood, anxiety, physical slowing, agitation, energy loss, feelings of worthlessness, difficulty thinking or concentrating, and sleep disturbances (NIMH, 2009).

Depression can affect the labor process in a variety of ways. The woman may be unable to concentrate or process information being provided by healthcare team members. Because depression often causes difficulty sleeping, she may begin labor fatigued or sleep deprived. The labor process may overwhelm her physically and emotionally, because she has no energy "reserves" on which to draw. She may feel unworthy of motherhood or experience hopelessness about the outcome of her labor. However, she may not be able to articulate any of these feelings and may instead appear irritable or withdrawn.

Women with depression are more likely to deliver a low birth weight infant, have decreased fetal growth, and are more likely to have postnatal complications when compared to nondepressed women (ACOG, 2008). It is estimated that 1 in 10 women will experience depression during the pregnancy or postpartum period. Treatment of pregnant women with selective serotonin reuptake inhibitors (SSRIs) should be individualized on a case-by-case basis. Women who take SSRIs are not at greater risk for birth defects and therefore should be managed with pharmacologic agents as needed (ACOG, 2007). Infants commonly have higher cortisol and catecholamine levels, cry more often, and are more frequently admitted to the neonatal intensive care nursery (ACOG, 2008). This is also true of infants of women with bipolar disorder.

TABLE 27-1 Prevalence of Psychologic Disorders

DISORDER	U.S. PREVALENCE	PREVALENCE IN WOMEN/MEN	MATERNAL IMPLICATION
Generalized anxiety disorder (GAD)	6.8 million (3.1%)	Two times higher in women	Anxiety related to the birth process or medical interventions
Bipolar disorder	5.7 million (2.6%)	Women and men equally affected	Depressive or manic symptoms during labor
Depression	18.1 million (8.2%)	Two times higher in women	Withdrawn behavior, physical fatigue due to insomnia, crying spells, sadness, hopelessness, feelings of guilt, lack of interest in baby, thoughts of suicide, headaches during pregnancy
Obsessive-compulsive disorder (OCD)	2.2 million (1.0%)	Equal in men and women	Ritualistic behaviors or thoughts, difficulty focusing on directions
Panic disorder	6 million (2.7%)	Two times higher in women	Intense fear or sense of panic related to birth process
Phobias	19.2 million (8.7%)	Higher in women	May have specific fear related to an individual(s) or a procedure or place
Post-traumatic stress disorder (PTSD)	7.7 million (3.5%)	Higher in women	Repressed memories may be triggered during labor, causing intense anxiety, fear, and emotional distress
Schizophrenia	2.4 million (1.1%)	Affects men and women equally	Typically starts in the late 20s and early 30s. May have hallucinations or delusions, lack of sense of present events, high risk for suicide

Source: Adapted from National Institute of Mental Health (NIMH). (2009). Prevalence of psychologic disorders. *Rockville, MD: Author.*

TABLE 27-2 Psychologic Disorders That Can Affect Labor and Birth

ANXIETY DISORDERS	PERSONALITY DISORDERS
Generalized anxiety disorder (GAD)	Antisocial personality
	Avoidant personality
Social anxiety disorder	Borderline personality
Obsessive-compulsive disorder (OCD)	Dependent personality
	Narcissistic personality
Post-traumatic stress disorder (PTSD)	Obsessive-compulsive personality
	Schizoid personality
Panic disorder	Schizotypal personality
Specific phobias	Paranoid personality
Depression	**Dissociative Identity Disorder**
Major depression	**Schizophrenia**
Dysthymia	**Schizoaffective Disorder**
Bipolar depression	

Individuals with *bipolar disorder* can have depressive symptoms that alternate with episodes of mania. Although a complete discussion of bipolar disorder is beyond the scope of this text, students should refer to a psychiatric nursing text for a more complete discussion. Individuals with bipolar disorder experience the same symptoms as depression (previously discussed) during the depressive phase. Mania is characterized by expansiveness, elation, agitation, hyperactivity, and increased speed of thought and ideas (NIMH, 2009). During manic phases, individuals commonly exhibit poor judgment and hyperexcitability. A pregnant woman experiencing a manic episode may engage in behaviors that are dangerous for herself or her fetus, including alcohol or drug use, fast driving, driving without a seat belt, or engaging in unprotected intercourse with individuals at high risk for sexually transmitted infections (see chapter 6 ∞). There is also a higher risk of suicide in individuals with mood disorders. Women with a previous diagnosis of bipolar depression are at greater risk for developing a mood disorder in the postpartum period (ACOG, 2008). Although postpartum psychosis is a rare disorder (see chapter 39 ∞), it is more common in women with bipolar disorder.

Anxiety disorders include a cluster of diagnoses, such as panic disorder, obsessive-compulsive disorder (OCD), post-traumatic stress disorder (PTSD), generalized anxiety disorder (GAD), social phobia, and other specific phobias. These disorders can cause a wide range of symptoms in laboring women. Following childbirth, 16% of women may have an anxiety disorder (Ford & Ayers, 2009). Specifically, women with panic attacks can experience intense feelings of terror without warning that result in physical symptoms (chest pain, shortness of breath, weakness, faintness, or dizziness) and/or psychologic symptoms (fear, terror, or anxiety) (ACOG, 2008). Other serious medical conditions need to be excluded (e.g., amniotic fluid embolism, cardiac complications, asthma attack). Women with OCD may need to repeat specific rituals as a means of coping in labor. Ritualistic activities that are safe for the mother and the fetus can be used to reduce anxiety. Women who have a history of rape or sexual abuse may suffer from PTSD (ACOG, 2008). Following birth, 2% of women experience PTSD (Ford & Ayers, 2009). The events of labor may trigger flashbacks, avoidance behaviors, or anxiety symptoms. Generalized anxiety disorder, although not acutely disabling, may make the woman very uncomfortable as she enters labor. A woman with social phobia may feel overwhelmed or embarrassed, especially if excessive numbers of staff are needed to care for her or her newborn. These women may also exhibit symptoms that mimic more serious medical conditions (ACOG, 2008). Women with specific phobias may exhibit fears that seem irrational to healthcare providers, such as fear of needles or of their own contractions. Such phobias may be difficult to manage intrapartally and may require pharmacologic intervention.

Schizophrenia is the most disabling psychologic disorder. It is often difficult to treat schizophrenia in pregnant women because many of the medications are contraindicated because they are teratogenic. Women with uncontrolled schizophrenia may have difficulty managing emotions, interacting with the healthcare team, or thinking clearly. The woman's behavior may be dramatically inappropriate or she may simply be withdrawn. Women with schizophrenia are at risk for medication-related congenital malformations. Specifically, antipsychotics can cause cardiovascular defects. These women have an increased incidence of preterm birth, low birth weight, small for gestational age, placental abnormalities, and antenatal hemorrhage (ACOG, 2008). Infants born to schizophrenic mothers have higher postnatal death rates (ACOG, 2008).

> "As a nurse-midwife, all of the women I care for are special, but Karen was one person I will never forget. Karen was diagnosed with bipolar disorder with psychotic episodes that became uncontrolled in pregnancy as a result of discontinuing her medication. In labor, she arrived in a manic state. Her speech was excessively fast-paced, and she rocked in her bed violently throughout the labor. We ensured her physical safety throughout the labor, monitored her contractions and the baby as infrequently as possible, and provided continuous encouragement. At one point, Karen was adamant everyone must "get low" and sit on the floor to facilitate fetal descent. Although it did not seem rational to us, we did sit on the floor. Remarkably, her anxiety dramatically decreased and the sense of control she felt enabled her to focus and 15 minutes later, she pushed her baby out. At her 6-week postpartum visit, Karen was back on medication and enjoying her new role as a mother."

In general, women with psychologic disorders tend to exhibit somewhat exaggerated behaviors during labor. They may need absolute control of everything that happens and refuse to participate until they feel secure (Ford & Ayers, 2009). Although responses vary with different disorders, the woman may not be able to articulate her fears or needs, may not respond to supportive nursing measures, may be unaware of what will happen in labor and birth, may be unable to understand what is happening, or may be suddenly overwhelmed by terrifying memories.

> “One young woman I'll call Cheryl Ann was in preterm labor. I was evaluating her, and she was cooperative but anxious. Then the on-call physician began the vaginal exam. Suddenly, Cheryl Ann's face changed, and she began screaming over and over: "Don't hurt me, I'll do anything you want. No, keep the fire away, please, please, please." She was not with us in the room, she was in another event in her life, and she was terrified! I didn't know what to do. I stayed right beside her and kept talking softly. "It's all right, Cheryl Ann, you are here in the birth center. I'm your nurse. I will stay with you, and I won't let anyone hurt you. There is no fire here. Can you look at me? Hold my hand. You are safe here." She held my hand and in a few moments was able to look at me. She became less anxious and finally was able to be present in her experience.”

Clinical Therapy

The goal of clinical therapy is to provide support that will help decrease the woman's anxiety, keep her oriented to reality, and promote optimal functioning while in labor. The physician or certified nurse-midwife (CNM) may prescribe a sedative, as needed, to help with symptoms and may seek the assistance of the on-call psychiatrist to assess and talk with the woman. The physician or CNM may also provide written orders for analgesic medications because relieving the pain may decrease the psychologic symptoms.

NURSING CARE MANAGEMENT

Nursing Assessment and Diagnosis

Unless birth is imminent or severe complications exist, the nurse begins the assessment by reviewing the woman's background. Factors such as age, parity, family support, culture, past and present experiences, and knowledge of the labor process affect the woman's psychologic response to labor. Past or current history of psychologic disorders should be evaluated. Current and past treatment can also yield helpful information. A careful history should include documentation of all psychotrophic medications used during pregnancy, because some medications can have adverse effects on pregnancy (ACOG, 2008).

As labor progresses, the nurse remains alert for the woman's verbal and nonverbal behavioral responses to the pain and anxiety of labor. The woman who is agitated and seems uncooperative or too quiet and compliant may require further appraisal for psychologic symptoms. Questions such as, "Is everything okay?" or "What's going on?" usually indicate some degree of anxiety and concern. Some women may be irritable, require frequent explanations, or repeat the same questions. The nurse further observes for nonverbal cues, including a tense posture, clenched hands, or pain out of context to the stage of labor. Recognizing the impact of fatigue on pain and anxiety is another important nursing responsibility. Women with sudden physical complaints need extensive evaluation to determine if the etiology is physical or psychologic. The nurse should assess what coping mechanisms have been effective for the woman in the past.

Nursing diagnoses that may apply to the woman with a psychologic disorder include the following:

- ***Ineffective Coping*** related to increased anxiety and stress
- ***Compromised Family Coping*** related to anxiety associated with labor and birth
- ***Fear*** related to invasive medical procedures and unknown outcome of birth process
- ***Anxiety*** related to unfamiliar surroundings and care by unknown medical personnel
- ***Disturbed Visual Sensory Perception*** related to reactivation of traumatic memories

Nursing Plan and Implementation

Primary nursing interventions center on supporting the laboring woman and her family and support persons. If the woman begins to lose her ability to cope or her orientation to reality, the nurse may be able to help her regain control and orientation by:

- Ensuring that the woman's external environment is free from excessive stimuli.
- Maintaining consistency in care providers to the extent possible.
- Encouraging her to identify and to use coping mechanisms that work well for her.
- Identifying and reducing the source of distress if possible.
- Acknowledging the woman's fears, pain, and other symptoms.
- Repeatedly orienting the woman to person, place, and time by statements such as "Janine, I am Tony Martinez and I am your nurse. It is Tuesday and you are in the birthing center because you are in labor now."
- Offering methods to promote relaxation and comfort.
- Providing clear but succinct information about the labor process, medical procedures, the environment, simple breathing exercises, and relaxation techniques.
- Employing a calm, caring, confident, and nonjudgmental approach.
- Providing frequent attention and therapeutic interaction.

Although providing emotional support and comfort measures is imperative, some women with severe uncontrolled psychologic disorders may continue to have excessive symptoms throughout labor and birth. Care for these women should focus on maintaining a safe environment and ensuring maternal and fetal well-being. Pharmacologic interventions may be needed to control excessive symptoms. In addition, some women may warrant referral for focused psychiatric support.

Evaluation

Expected outcomes of nursing care include the following:

- The woman experiences a decrease in physiologic and psychologic stress and an increase in physiologic and psychologic comfort.

- The woman remains oriented to person, place, and time.
- The woman uses effective coping mechanisms to manage her stress and anxiety in labor.
- The woman's and the family's fear is decreased.
- The woman verbalizes feelings about her labor.

Care of the Woman Experiencing Dystocia Related to Dysfunctional Uterine Contractions

Dystocia is an abnormal labor pattern in which abnormalities occur with the power (uterine contractions or maternal expulsion forces), the passenger (fetal size, position, or presentation), or the passage (soft tissues or pelvis). Dystocia encompasses many problems in labor, the most common of which is dysfunctional (or uncoordinated) uterine contractions that result in a prolongation of labor. This form of dystocia is the most common indication for cesarean birth in nulliparous women, accounting for 60% of cesarean births in this group (Gabbe, Niebyl, & Simpson, 2007).

Although there is considerable controversy regarding the definition of a normal labor, there is agreement that women enter the active phase of labor when the cervix is dilated 3 to 4 cm. During this time, contractions occur in a regular pattern and the cervix changes rapidly as plotted against time. As the cervix dilates, the fetal part progressively descends. Alternatively, cervical dilatation may be slower than normal (protraction disorders) or cease altogether (arrest disorders). Figure 27-1 ■ depicts normal and hypotonic uterine contraction patterns.

Tachysystole Labor Patterns

In tachysystole latent labor patterns, ineffectual uterine contractions of poor quality occur in the latent phase of labor, and the resting tone of the myometrium increases. Tachysystole labor patterns are most common in nulliparous women (Gabbe et al., 2007). Contractions usually become more frequent and are more than 5 contractions in a 10 minute period that have occurred over at least 30 minutes (Macones, Hankins, Spong, et al., 2008). Although the contractions are painful, they are ineffective in dilating and effacing the cervix, and a prolonged latent phase may result.

Maternal risks of tachysystole labor include the following:

- Increased discomfort due to uterine muscle cell anoxia.
- Fatigue as the pattern continues and no labor progress results.
- Stress on coping abilities.
- Dehydration and increased incidence of infection if labor is prolonged.

Fetal-neonatal risks include the following:

- Nonreassuring fetal status because contractions and increased resting tone interfere with the uteroplacental exchange.
- Prolonged pressure on the fetal head, which may result in cephalhematoma, caput succedaneum, or excessive molding.

Clinical Therapy

Management of tachysystole labor may include bed rest and sedation to promote relaxation and reduce pain. Typically, the woman will enter active labor, and cervical effacement and dilatation will begin to occur. If the tachysystole pattern continues and develops into a prolonged latent phase, oxytocin infusion or amniotomy may be considered (Strasser, Kwee, & Visser, 2009) (see chapter 28 ∞). These methods are instituted only after cephalopelvic disproportion (CPD) and fetal malrepresentation have been ruled out. CPD is a disparity between the size of the maternal pelvis and the size of the presenting fetal head due to position, presentation, or increased fetal weight that precludes a vaginal birth. When an oxytocin infusion is used to stimulate uterine contractions, the physician or certified nurse-midwife (CNM) needs to assess whether vagi-

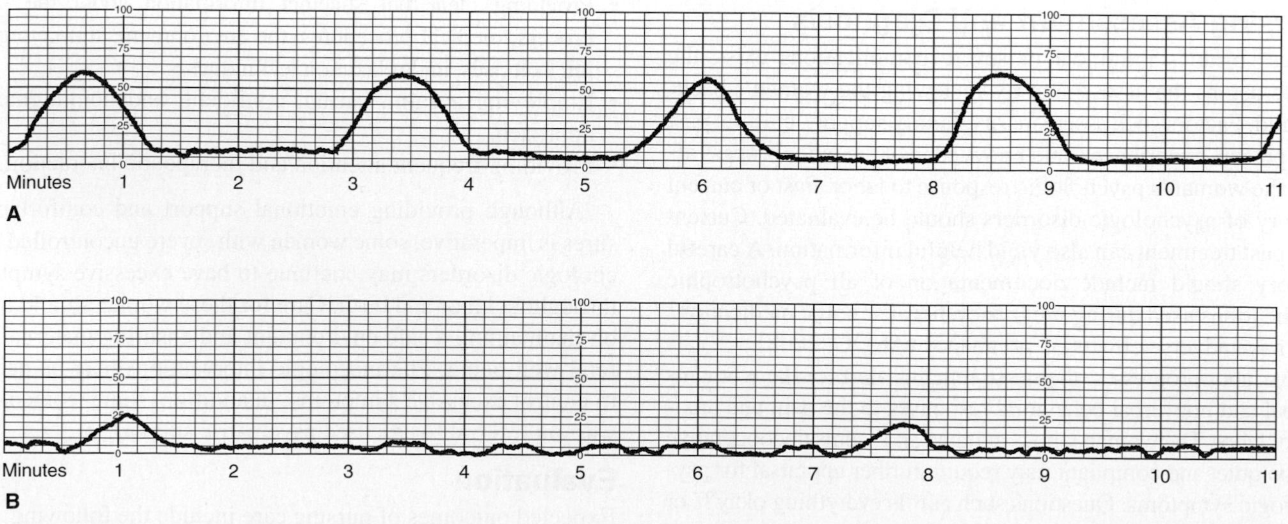

Figure 27-1 ■ Comparison of labor patterns. A. Normal uterine contraction pattern. Note that the contraction frequency is every 3 minutes; duration is 60 seconds. The baseline resting tone is below 10 mm Hg. B. Hypotonic uterine contraction pattern. Note in this example that the contraction frequency is every 7 minutes with some uterine activity between contractions, duration is 50 seconds, and intensity increases approximately 25 mm Hg during contractions.

nal birth is possible (i.e., whether the maternal pelvis is large enough for the fetus to pass through) (Strasser et al., 2009). If the maternal pelvis diameters are less than average, or if the fetus is particularly large or is in a malpresentation or malposition, CPD is said to be present. In the presence of true CPD, labor is not stimulated because vaginal birth is not possible.

NURSING CARE MANAGEMENT

Nursing Assessment and Diagnosis

As part of the labor assessment, the nurse should evaluate the relationship between the intensity of the pain being experienced and the degree to which the cervix is dilating and effacing. The nurse should also note whether anxiety is negatively affecting labor progress. Evidence of increasing frustration and discouragement on the part of the mother and her partner may indicate that the nurse needs to provide some additional information or assurance.

Nursing diagnoses that may apply to the woman in tachysystole labor include the following:

- ***Acute Pain*** related to the woman's inability to relax secondary to tachysystole uterine contractions
- ***Ineffective Coping*** related to ineffectiveness of breathing techniques to relieve discomfort
- ***Anxiety*** related to slow labor progress

Nursing Plan and Implementation

A key nursing responsibility is to provide comfort and support to the laboring woman and her partner. The woman experiencing a tachysystole labor pattern will probably be very uncomfortable because of the increased force of contractions. Her anxiety level and that of her partner may be high. The nurse attempts to reduce the woman's discomfort and promote a more effective labor pattern.

The nurse may suggest supportive measures such as a change of position: left lateral side-lying, high Fowler's, rocking in a rocking chair, sitting up, or walking. Soothing measures include a warm shower, whirlpool, quiet environment, backrub, Therapeutic Touch, and visualization. Mouth care, change of linens, effleurage, and relaxation exercises may provide comfort. If sedation is ordered, the nurse ensures that the environment is conducive to relaxation. The labor partner may also need assistance in helping the woman cope. A calm understanding approach by the nurse offers the woman and her partner further support. Providing information about the cause of the tachysystole labor pattern and assuring the woman that she is not overreacting to the situation are important nursing actions.

Patient education is key for the woman experiencing tachysystole labor. She needs information about the dysfunctional labor pattern and the possible implications for herself and her baby. Information will help relieve anxiety and thereby increase relaxation and comfort. The nurse needs to explain treatment options and offer opportunities to ask questions.

Evaluation

Anticipated outcomes of nursing care include the following:

- The woman has increased comfort and decreased anxiety.
- The woman and her partner are able to cope with the labor.
- The woman experiences a more effective labor pattern.

Hypotonic Labor Patterns

The specific cause of hypotonic contractions is unknown; however, genetic factors may control the normal physiologic processes of labor. Cesarean birth and operative vaginal birth (use of forceps or vacuum extractor), for example, tend to run in families. Some research suggests there is a relationship between uterine dysfunction and advancing maternal age (Beckmann et al., 2008). The familial tendencies for difficult labor give rise to the theory that genetic processes control normal labor. It is hypothesized that there may be an inheritable tendency toward poor uterine contractions and/or soft-tissue relaxation (Beckmann et al., 2008).

CLINICAL TIP

Normal cervical dilatation in a first-time mother—commonly known as a "primip"—is just over 1 cm per hour, and dilatation in a "multip" is about 1.5 cm per hour. If your assessments reveal that this expected pattern is not occurring, consider that a problem may be developing. The most likely causes of the problem are related to either the contractions or to fetal position or size.

Clinical Therapy

When uterine contractions are irregular and of low amplitude and there is commonly less than 1 cm cervical dilatation per hour (called protracted labor) or there has been no change of cervical dilatation for 2 hours (arrest of progress), the physician or CNM evaluates the woman for the presence of any factor that would preclude the use of oxytocin (Pitocin) augmentation. The physician or CNM evaluates the size of the maternal pelvis, the position and presentation of the fetus, and fetal weight. The physician or CNM carefully considers the possibility of CPD. Station is a key component when evaluating for CPD. If the presenting part is not engaged ("out of the pelvis"), especially in a nulliparous woman, it is possible that CPD is present. The physician or CNM may attempt to push the presenting part into the pelvis with fundal pressure to assess if CPD exists. If CPD exists, oxytocin (Pitocin) augmentation should not be used and a cesarean birth is indicated.

When CPD is ruled out, an amniotomy (artificial rupture of membranes [AROM]) can be performed if membranes are intact. Amniotomy is associated with a reduction of labor duration and a decrease in use of oxytocin (Pitocin) (Beckmann et al., 2008). According to a Cochrane Review, amniotomy can reduce duration of labor and cesarean section birth rates (Wei et al., 2009). Amniotomy should not be performed if the presenting part is not well applied to the cervix because this increases the risk of cord prolapse (discussed later in the chapter). However, it is an accepted procedure with the diagnosis of dystocia secondary to uterine hypocontractility. Oxytocin (Pitocin) augmentation can be implemented if adequate contractions do not occur. Oxytocin should be used with caution since it is a drug that appears on the high-alert list due to its ability to cause tachysystole. (See Drug Guide: Oxytocin [Pitocin] in chapter 28 ∞.)

ACOG has outlined two regimens of oxytocin administration: a low-dose regimen and a high-dose regimen (see complete discussion in chapter 28 ∞). Although low-dose regimens are associated with less uterine tachysystole, fetal outcomes have not differed between the two groups. High-dose regimens are said to shorten the mean length of labor, decrease the length of second stage, decrease the incidence of chorioamnionitis and neonatal sepsis, and reduce the incidence of cesarean births related to dystocia (Gabbe et al., 2007). High-dose regimens are mainly used for augmentation of labor and not labor induction (Gabbe et al., 2007). The current data do not support the notion that low-dose regimens are safer or superior to high-dose regimens (Beckmann et al., 2008). Continuous electronic fetal monitoring (EFM) is used to provide ongoing information regarding fetal response to the augmentation. With augmentation of labor, the contraction pattern and progressive cervical dilatation pattern should improve, and fetal descent (measured by station) should occur. If there is no improvement in these areas, cesarean birth may be necessary.

Some practitioners support the use of **active management of labor (AMOL)**. This method of labor management of nulliparous women has four components: (1) standardized criteria for diagnosis of labor, (2) standardized method of labor management, (3) one-to-one nursing care throughout the course of labor, and (4) prenatal education to teach women about the protocol (Chaillet & Dumont, 2007). In this process labor is managed from the beginning with amniotomy, timed cervical examinations, and augmentation of labor with intravenous oxytocin if adequate progress is not made. AMOL begins with careful assessment of the laboring woman, AROM (if the membranes are still intact) within 1 hour of diagnosis of the presence of actual labor, and hourly cervical examinations for the first 3 hours. Thereafter cervical examinations are performed every 2 hours, and at least an additional 1 cm of dilatation is expected at each examination. If cervical dilatation is less than expected, augmentation with an intravenous oxytocin infusion is begun. AMOL also incorporates a strong one-to-one nursing care program, in which the nurse remains with the woman. This permits ongoing assessment and provides the beneficial aspect of constant nursing support. Recent large-scale studies have shown that AMOL does not increase maternal and infant mortality or morbidity. Proponents have voiced support because it does shorten labor in nulliparous women. Interestingly, the rates of caesarean births are not decreased with AMOL (Cunningham et al., 2010).

Those who oppose AMOL contend that labor needs to be considered a normal process and allowed to progress without automatic intervention. Frequent examinations can increase the risk of maternal fever, intrauterine infection, and fetal compromise. Although some women may not strictly adhere to the expected normal time limits of labor, many will go on to give birth without complications if given an opportunity to progress through labor at their own pace. Just as all women do not have the same emotional reactions to labor, all women do not go through labor at the same pace and speed. Frequent examinations and interventions can also lead to maternal anxiety. Only if problems occur should the labor be augmented.

NURSING CARE MANAGEMENT

Nursing Assessment and Diagnosis

Assessing maternal vital signs, contractions, cervical dilatation, fetal descent, and fetal heart rate (FHR) characteristics provides the nurse with data to evaluate maternal-fetal status. The nurse also assesses for signs and symptoms of infection and dehydration. During the vaginal examination, the fetal presenting part (usually vertex) is assessed for the development of a caput. If the fetal vertex presses down on the cervix during contractions without further descent, a *caput succedaneum* may occur. As hypotonic labor continues, the caput increases in size; it seems that the head is descending, but it is not (Figure 27-2 ■).

Because labor progress is slow, the nurse assesses the woman's stress and coping, noting whether anxiety is having a deleterious effect on labor progress. Evidence of increasing frustration and discouragement on the part of the mother and her partner may become apparent as labor continues.

The laboring woman should maintain adequate fluid and nourishment throughout labor. Oral fluid intake or intravenous fluids can be provided. Women can eat light snacks in early labor as well. The nurse should ensure adequate urinary output is occurring.

Nursing diagnoses that may apply to the woman experiencing dysfunctional labor include the following:

- ***Acute Pain*** related to rapid increase in frequency and intensity of uterine contractions
- ***Ineffective Coping*** related to ineffectiveness of breathing techniques to relieve discomfort
- ***Anxiety*** related to slow labor progress

Nursing Plan and Implementation

Nursing measures are aimed at promoting maternal and fetal well-being. The nurse frequently monitors maternal vital signs; notes the frequency, duration, and strength of contractions; and assesses the fetal heart rate (FHR). Once the amniotic membranes are ruptured, the nurse assesses the amount of fluid and the presence of blood or meconium (dark green or black stool present in the large intestine of the fetus). Because meconium can be associated with a compromised fetus, ongoing observation of the amniotic fluid is critical. Maternal hydration status can be monitored by recording intake and output. The nurse assesses the bladder every 2 hours for distention; an in-and-out catheterization can be performed for women unable to void on their own. Alternatively, a Foley catheter may be inserted during the first stage of labor to reduce the need for multiple in-and-out catheterizations, which can increase the risk of urinary

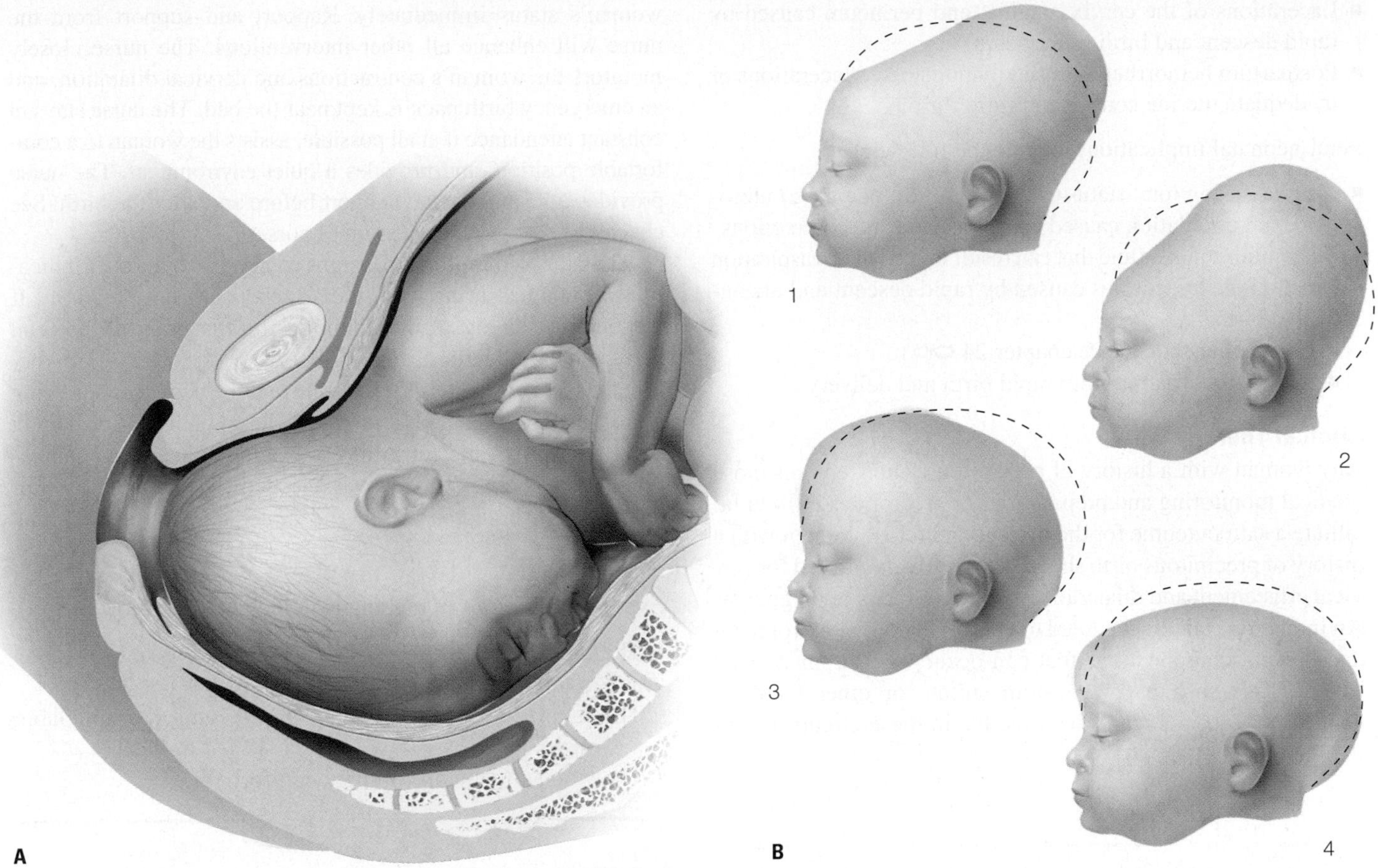

Figure 27-2 ■ Effects of labor on the fetal head. A. Caput succedaneum formation. The presenting portion of the scalp area is encircled by the cervix during labor, causing swelling of the soft tissue. B. Molding of the fetal head in cephalic presentations: (1) occiput anterior, (2) occiput posterior, (3) brow, (4) face.

tract infections. The catheter should be removed before maternal pushing.

Ongoing evaluation for symptoms of infection should be performed, especially for prolonged labors. These symptoms include fever, chills, foul-smelling amniotic fluid, and fetal tachycardia. Vaginal examinations should be kept to a minimum to reduce the incidence of infections.

The laboring woman needs information about the hypotonic labor pattern and the possible implications for herself and her baby. It is particularly important to address the couple's concerns and questions with clear, accurate information. They need to be informed of progress and possible treatment measures. Disadvantages and treatment alternatives also need to be discussed and understood by the woman and her support person.

Evaluation

Expected outcomes of nursing care include the following:

- The woman and her partner understand the labor pattern and its possible implications.
- The woman and her partner are able to cope with the labor.
- The woman's comfort increases and her anxiety decreases.
- The woman experiences a more effective labor pattern.

Care of the Woman and Fetus at Risk for Precipitous Labor and Birth

Precipitous labor and birth occurs when the entire process of labor and birth occurs within 3 hours. The most common causes are abnormally low resistance in maternal soft tissues, which allows for rapid cervical dilatation and fetal descent, and abnormally strong uterine contractions (Cunningham et al., 2010). In precipitous labor, cervical dilatation is 5 cm or more per hour in the primigravida and up to 10 cm per hour for the multigravida.

Precipitous labor and birth and precipitous birth are not the same. A precipitous birth is a sudden, and often unattended, birth. See chapter 24 ∞ for a discussion of precipitous birth and nurse-attended births. The incidence of precipitous birth in the United States is about 2% (Battista & Wing, 2007).

Risks of Precipitous Labor and Birth

Maternal risks of precipitous labor include the following (Cunningham et al., 2010):

- Loss of coping abilities
- Anxiety and fear

- Lacerations of the cervix, vagina, and perineum caused by rapid descent and birth of the fetus
- Postpartum hemorrhage caused by undetected lacerations or inadequate uterine contractions after birth

Fetal-neonatal implications include the following:

- Nonreassuring fetal status or hypoxia from decreased uteroplacental circulation caused by intense uterine contractions
- Meconium stained fluid that can result in meconium aspiration
- Brachial plexus injuries caused by rapid descent and uncontrolled birth
  - Low Apgar scores (see chapter 24 ∞)
  - Intracranial trauma from rapid birth and delivery

Clinical Therapy

Any woman with a history of precipitous labor requires close medical monitoring and preparation for precipitous birth to facilitate a safe outcome for the mother and fetus. Women with a history of precipitous birth should be closely monitored for cervical effacement and dilatation in the final weeks of pregnancy. An induction can be scheduled to control the birth environment and prevent complications that can occur with an unattended birth. Drugs such as magnesium sulfate or other tocolytic agents have not proven to be effective in these circumstances (Cunningham et al., 2010).

NURSING CARE MANAGEMENT

Nursing Assessment and Diagnosis

During the intrapartal nursing assessment, the nurse can identify a woman at increased risk of precipitous labor (for example, a previous history of precipitate or short labor places a woman at risk). During the labor, accelerated cervical dilatation and fetal descent and intense contractions with little uterine relaxation between contractions are indicative of precipitous labor. During labor one or both of the following factors may indicate potential problems:

- Accelerated cervical dilatation (more than 2 cm/hr in multigravidas or more than 1.2 cm/hr in primiparous women) and rapid fetal descent (more than 2 cm/hr in a multiparous and more than 1.2 cm hour in a primiparous woman)
- Intense uterine contractions with less than 60 seconds of relaxation between contractions

Nursing diagnoses that may apply to the woman with precipitous labor include the following:

- ***Risk for Injury*** related to rapid labor and birth
- ***Acute Pain*** related to rapid labor process
- ***Anxiety*** related to rapid labor progress

Nursing Plan and Implementation

If the woman has a history of precipitous labor, it is imperative that the nurse establish rapport quickly because the nurse and woman may be involved in another precipitous labor and birth, and the situation has the potential to be tense. The physician or certified nurse-midwife (CNM) should be notified of the woman's status immediately. Rapport and support from the nurse will enhance all other interventions. The nurse closely monitors the woman's contractions and cervical dilatation, and an emergency birth pack is kept near the bed. The nurse stays in constant attendance if at all possible, assists the woman to a comfortable position, and provides a quiet environment. The nurse provides information and support before and after the birth. See chapter 24 ∞ for a discussion of nurse-managed birth.

The fetus is monitored for signs of hypoxia and other indications of nonreassuring fetal status such as late decelerations. If meconium staining of the amniotic fluid is present, the fetal nares and mouth will be suctioned just after the head is born (before the birth of the shoulders) to prevent the baby from drawing more meconium-stained fluid into the lungs with the first breath. After the birth of the baby, the cords will be visualized and additional suctioning carried out as needed. The neonatologist or nursery staff should be present for immediate care of the infant.

Evaluation

Expected outcomes of nursing care include the following:

- The woman and her baby are closely monitored during labor, and a safe birth occurs.
- The couple feels support and enhanced comfort during labor and birth.
- The woman maintains optimal comfort.

CLINICAL JUDGMENT

Case Study: Kim Hahn

Kim Hahn presents in labor with a fetal heart tracing demonstrating the following: baseline fetal heart rate (BL FHR) of 140 with variability of 6 to 10 beats/min. When you compare the fetal heart rate (FHR) with the uterine contractions, you note there is a slowing of the FHR at the time of the contraction and that the FHR tracing looks like the contraction curve, but it is upside down.

Critical Thinking

Based on the tracing, what would you do?

See www.nursing.pearsonhighered.com for possible responses.

Care of the Woman with Postterm Pregnancy

Postterm pregnancy is one that extends more than 294 days or 42 completed weeks past the first day of the last menstrual period. It is important to understand that 42 completed weeks refers to the completion of 42 weeks, meaning that the 7th day has elapsed. The incidence of postterm pregnancy is approximately 10% of all pregnancies in the United States (Norwitz, Snegovskikh, & Caughey, 2007). Most causes of postterm pregnancies are related to inaccurate pregnancy dating. Postterm pregnancy has been associated with primiparity, previous postterm pregnancy, placenta sulfatase deficiency, fetal anencephaly, male fetus, maternal obesity, and genetic predisposition (Caughey, Snegovskikh, & Norwitz, 2008).

A frequent cause of inaccurate pregnancy dating is error in determining the time of ovulation and conception according to the first day of the last menstrual period. This error can be corrected by performing an ultrasound scan in early pregnancy. A first-trimester scan is the most accurate ultrasonic gestational age assessment. During the first trimester, the crown-rump length (CRL) is used. In second-trimester ultrasound, which is less accurate, the biparietal diameter of the fetal head is measured and then compared with conventional dating tables (Caughey, Nicholson, & Washington, 2008). First trimester dating reduces the number of estimated postterm pregnancies and decreases unnecessary interventions (Caughey et al., 2008).

Maternal Risks

Although postterm pregnancy does not pose any significant risk to the woman during the pregnancy, the labor and birth process may be affected. In many instances, labor is induced. Because postterm pregnancy is associated with an increased incidence of large-for-gestational-age (LGA) or macrosomic (weight in excess of 4000 g) fetuses, vaginal birth is frequently associated with the use of forceps or vacuum extractor. Women who deliver postterm fetuses are more likely to encounter perineal damage because of the increased size of the fetus. Maternal hemorrhage may also occur. Cesarean birth rates are doubled in postterm pregnancies. Cesarean births are associated with endometritis, hemorrhage, and thromboembolitic disease (Cunningham et al., 2010). Many women experience anxiety and are emotionally fatigued as their estimated date of birth (EDB) passes. Normal discomforts associated with late pregnancy persist that can lead to irritability and loss of sleep.

> “When I went over my due date, I felt so anxious and overwhelmed. I was mentally prepared to carry my baby until a certain date, but once that date was reached, I felt unable to deal with all of the discomforts of pregnancy. I couldn't sleep well. I was uncomfortable eating, walking, even putting on my shoes. Well-wishing friends and family would call and say, "Haven't you had that baby yet?" The calls just made it worse. I can't tell you how relieved I was when labor started, and I knew I would soon meet my new baby”

Fetal-Neonatal Risks

True postterm pregnancies are frequently associated with placental changes that cause a decrease in the uterine-placental-fetal circulation. The perinatal mortality rate after 42 weeks is twice that of term infants and increases sixfold during the 43rd gestational week (Beckmann et al., 2008). This decrease reduces the blood supply, oxygen, and nutrition for the fetus. Oligohydramnios (decreased amount of amniotic fluid) is frequently present and may increase the risk of umbilical cord compression (because the cord does not have as much fluid to float in). In such cases, the fetus is more likely to be small-for-gestational-age (SGA) or may lag behind the expected growth curve and experience growth alterations because of decreased nutrition associated with decreased uteroplacental-fetal circulation. If uteroplacental-fetal circulation is not compromised, the fetus continues to gain weight until the 42nd week; therefore, the fetus is often LGA and macrosomic. The LGA or macrosomic fetus has a higher incidence of birth trauma or shoulder dystocia (difficulty or inability to deliver the baby's shoulders). Macrosomia is also associated with prolonged labor, increased risk of cesarean birth, and cephalopelvic disproportion (CPD) (Cunningham et al., 2010). During labor, the postterm fetus may have meconium staining of the amniotic fluid, which can be associated with nonreassuring fetal status and meconium aspiration at birth (Cunningham et al., 2010). Some infants born after the 42nd week of pregnancy may have low umbilical artery pH and lower 5-minute Apgar scores (Norwitz et al., 2007). Many practitioners now favor delivering women once they reach 41 weeks gestation to avoid some of these complications (Norwitz et al., 2007).

Approximately 20% of all postterm infants experience *dysmaturity syndrome,* which is associated with uteroplacental insufficiency (resembling intrauterine growth restriction), meconium aspiration, and short-term neonatal complications (Gabbe et al., 2007). Neonatal complications associated with postterm pregnancies include hypoglycemia seizures and respiratory distress. These fetuses frequently experience nonreassuring fetal heart tracings in the antepartum and intrapartum periods.

Clinical Therapy

When the 40th week of gestation is completed and birth has not occurred, most practitioners begin using the nonstress test (NST), biophysical profile (BPP), or a modified BPP (ultrasound measurement of the amniotic fluid volume plus an NST) as assessment tools. While there is no consensus on the frequency of antenatal surveillance, many practitioners use twice-weekly testing providing the amniotic fluid level is normal. Any time that tests indicate fetal problems or there is decreased amniotic fluid volume, induction of labor is recommended (Cunningham et al., 2010).

NURSING CARE MANAGEMENT

Nursing Assessment and Diagnosis

When the woman is admitted into the birthing area, it is important to establish the EDB and ascertain the type of antenatal testing that has been completed. During labor, ongoing assessments of the fetal heart rate (FHR) by continuous electronic fetal monitoring (EFM) are important to identify reassuring characteristics (lack of decelerations, accelerations with fetal movement) and to determine the presence of variable decelerations or late decelerations so that corrective actions may be taken. When amniotic membranes rupture, the nurse assesses the fluid for the presence of meconium. Ongoing assessments of labor progress (contractions, progressive cervical dilatation and effacement, and fetal descent) may provide clues to the presence of a macrosomic fetus because labor may be lengthened and fetal descent may not occur.

Possible nursing diagnoses for the woman with postterm pregnancy include the following:

- ***Fear*** related to the unknown outcome for the baby
- ***Compromised Family Coping*** related to concern regarding the status of the baby
- ***Risk for Injury (Fetus)*** related to the birth of a macrosomic infant
- ***Risk for Injury (Mother)*** related to perineal trauma
- ***Acute Pain*** related to the birthing process

Nursing Plan and Implementation

Community-Based Nursing Care

If the woman has not been assessing fetal activity every day, the nurse teaches her how to do it so that she can identify inadequate fetal movement and contact her healthcare provider (see chapter 21 for further discussion of techniques to detect fetal movement). The nurse encourages the woman to keep all appointments for BPPs and other testing and provides information regarding the postterm pregnancy and the antenatal testing that will be indicated. In addition, the nurse addresses the implications and associated risks for the baby, as well as possible treatment plans, and provides the woman and her partner opportunities to ask questions and clarify information. Most antenatal testing is performed by the nurse who must be knowledgeable regarding the testing procedures, interpretation of results, and collaboration with the physician or certified nurse-midwife (CNM).

Hospital-Based Nursing Care

In the birth setting, the response of the fetus during labor is assessed carefully. Continuous electronic monitoring of the FHR is important to determine whether reassuring characteristics are present and to detect variable decelerations, especially if oligohydramnios is present. If variable decelerations are present, the laboring woman's position is changed to attempt to take pressure off the umbilical cord, and the FHR is reevaluated. When an amnioinfusion is performed to increase the volume of fluid or to dilute meconium-stained fluid, the nurse assists with the procedure and monitors the infusion and the response of the FHR. (See chapter 28 for further discussion.)

Evaluation

Expected outcomes of nursing care include the following:

- The woman is able to explain the implications of the postterm pregnancy.
- The woman and her partner and family feel supported and able to cope with the labor and birth.
- Fetal problems are identified quickly.

Care of the Woman and Fetus at Risk Because of Fetal Malposition

Persistent occiput posterior (OP) position of the fetus is the most common fetal malposition and occurs when the head remains in the direct OP position throughout labor. In early labor approximately 15% of fetuses are in OP position, although only 5% remain in that position at the time of birth (Cunningham et al., 2010). This position may be normal in some races, particularly those in which women tend to have small pelves or in women with anthropoid pelves. The position is related to transverse narrowing of the midpelvis. For a fetus in an OP position to rotate to an occiput anterior (OA) position, it must rotate 135 degrees (right-occiput-posterior [ROP] to right-occiput-transverse [ROT] to right-occiput-anterior [ROA] to OA) (see Figure 22-8 on page 536), and in most cases this rotation is accomplished. In others, however, it is not. Labor progress may cease or the fetus may be born in a posterior position.

Maternal-Fetal-Neonatal Risks

The woman usually experiences intense pain in the small of her back throughout the labor, unless the baby rotates. At birth, if the fetus remains in a posterior position, the woman may suffer a third- or fourth-degree perineal laceration or extension of a midline episiotomy. There is no increased risk of fetal mortality because of the OP position unless labor is protracted or an operative birth is performed. There is a higher incidence of operative vaginal deliveries in fetuses who fail to rotate from the OP position. Maternal risks of OP malposition include the following (Ridley, 2007):

- Higher rates of cesarean birth
- Prolonged first and second stage of labor
- Oxytocin augmentation
- Anal sphincter injury
- Severe perineal lacerations
- Episiotomy
- Blood loss greater than 500 ml
- Postpartum infection
- Accidental lacerations of the lower uterine segment during cesarean
- Instrument delivery

Clinical Therapy

Medical treatment focuses on close monitoring of both maternal and fetal status and labor progress to determine whether vaginal or cesarean birth is the safer method. Prenatally, use of a hands and knees position twice daily has been helpful in correcting the persistent OP position if it is diagnosed prenatally (Hunter, Hofmeyr, & Kulier, 2007). According to Cunningham et al. (2010), vaginal birth is possible via:

1. Spontaneous birth.
2. Forceps-assisted birth with the occiput directly posterior.
3. Forceps rotation of the occiput to the anterior position and birth (Scanzoni maneuver [Figure 27-3 ■]).
4. Manual rotation to the anterior position followed by spontaneous or forceps-assisted birth (Figure 27-4 ■).

If the pelvis has larger diameters and the perineal muscles are relaxed, as found in grand multiparity (a woman who has had five or more children), the fetus may have no particular problem emerging spontaneously in the OP position. If, however, the perineum is rigid, the second stage of labor may be prolonged. A prolonged second stage is one that lasts over an hour in multiparas and 2 hours or more in nulliparas.

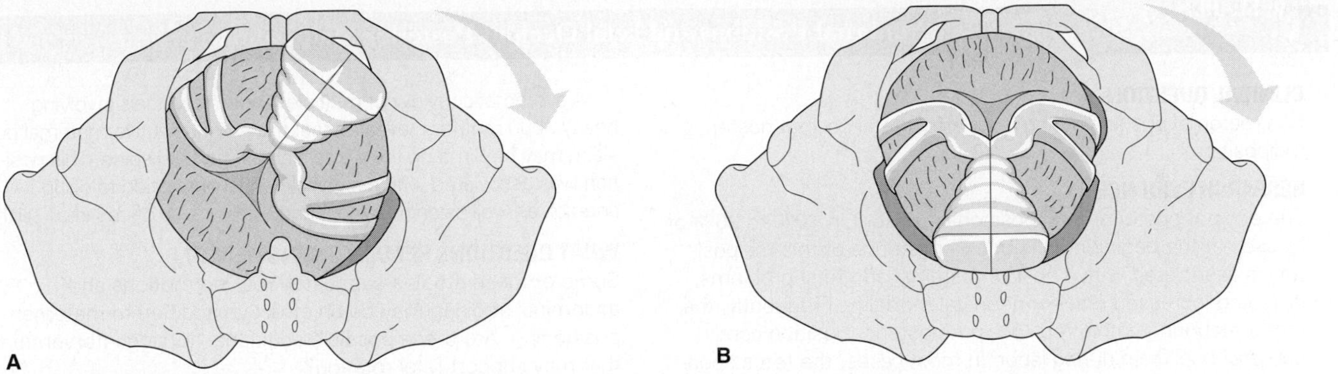

Figure 27-3 ■ Scanzoni maneuver, anterior rotation. A. Forceps are applied to the fetal head, which is in ROP position. Fetal head is then rotated 45 degrees to ROT, then another 45 degrees to ROA, then a final 45 degrees to OA. B. The fetal position has now changed from ROP to OA for a total rotation of 135 degrees. The forceps are now upside down, so they are removed and reapplied to provide the traction necessary for a forceps-assisted birth.

Source: Reprinted with permission from Oxorn, H., and Foote, W. (1986). Human labor and birth *(5th ed., p. 401). Copyright © 1986 The McGraw-Hill Companies, Inc.*

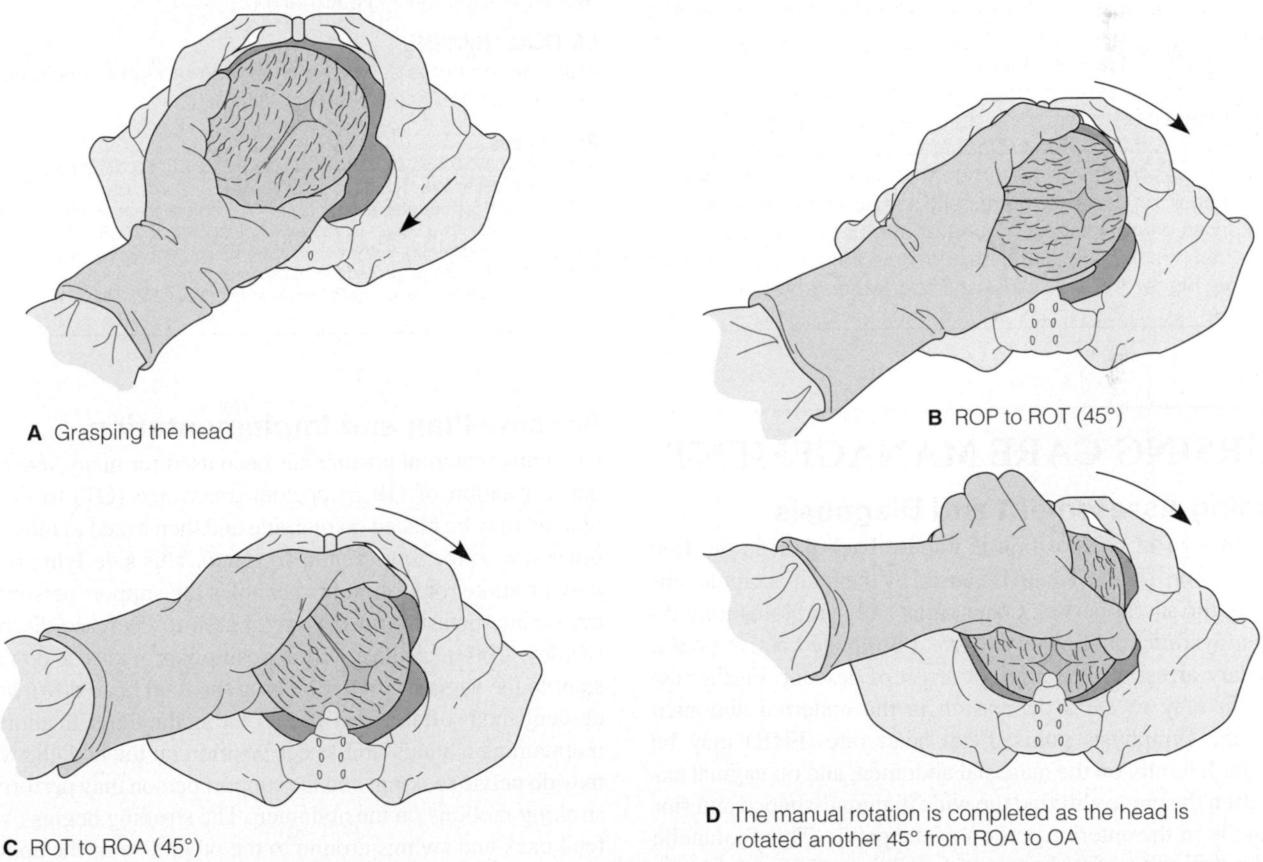

A Grasping the head
B ROP to ROT (45°)
C ROT to ROA (45°)
D The manual rotation is completed as the head is rotated another 45° from ROA to OA

Figure 27-4 ■ Manual rotation of ROP to OA. A. The physician's left hand is inserted into the vagina and the back of the fetal head is grasped. B. The head is flexed and then rotated 45 degrees to ROT. C. The head is rotated another 45 degrees to ROA. D. The manual rotation is completed as the head is rotated another 45 degrees from ROA to OA. During the manual rotation, the physician's other hand is placed on the maternal abdomen, and the body is turned in the same direction as the head by applying pressure to the fetal breech or shoulders.

In the event of a prolonged second stage with arrest of descent due to the OP position, a forceps or manual rotation may be done if no cephalopelvic disproportion (CPD) is present. Forceps rotation has been associated with neonatal high cervical spinal cord injuries in the past. For this reason, obstetricians may choose to perform a cesarean birth (Cunningham et al., 2010). In cases of CPD, cesarean is always the preferred mode of birth. Of women with a persistent OP position, 60% will deliver via cesarean. These account for 12% of all cesarean births performed for dystocia (Cunningham et al., 2010).

RESEARCH EVIDENCE IN PRACTICE Maternal Positions and Fetal Occiput Posterior Malposition

CLINICAL QUESTION

Can maternal position during labor affect fetal occiput posterior malposition?

RESEARCH EVIDENCE

The occiput posterior fetal position is present in 10% to 20% of fetuses at the beginning of labor. Persistence of this malposition is associated with a host of maternal and fetal problems, including increased rates of neonatal mortality. Frequently, the mother laboring with a fetal occiput posterior position complains of back pain during labor. In most cases, the fetus spontaneously rotates into the occiput anterior position during labor. If it does not, risks for both mother and baby can be reduced if interventions are applied to rotate the fetus into a desirable position for birth.

A systematic review of the research literature, combined with information from obstetric textbooks and expert consultation, revealed only weak evidence that the hands-and-knees position was associated with correction of the occiput posterior malposition. However, regardless of whether the fetal position changed, mothers reported this position was comfortable and relieved backache.

One randomized controlled trial studied the effects of the hands-and-knees position on fetal malposition and additional outcomes. Similarly, fetal rotation to the occiput anterior position was greater in the group that used the hands-and-knees position, but only marginally so. However, additional outcomes were achieved in greater numbers with this maternal position, including back pain reduction, less perineal trauma, higher Apgar scores, and shorter length of labor.

A systematic review of multiple randomized trials involving nearly 3000 mothers revealed that the most effective maternal position may be Sims on the same side as the fetal spine. This position was associated with a significant rate of rotation to occiput anterior, as well as shorter labor and a lower rate of cesarean births.

WHAT QUESTIONS REMAIN UNANSWERED?

Some of these studies suggested rocking motions and abdominal stroking may be an effective addition to maternal positioning. Are these possible additional nursing interventions that may support fetal rotation?

WHAT IS BEST PRACTICE?

Most fetuses that present in the occiput posterior position will spontaneously rotate during labor. For those that do not, use of Sims position on the same side as the fetal spine may help the fetus rotate to occiput anterior. The hands-and-knees position may provide some support for fetal rotation, but will likely be most helpful when the baby is appropriately positioned but the mother is experiencing back pain.

CRITICAL THINKING

How can the nurse support the laboring mother in finding a comfortable, yet appropriate, position?

References

Ridley, R. 2007. Diagnosis and intervention for occiput posterior malposition. *JOGNN, 36*(2), 135–143.

Simkin, P. 2010. The fetal occiput posterior position: State of the science and a new perspective. *Birth: Issues in Perinatal Care, 27*(1), 61–72.

Stremler, R., Hodnett, E., Petryshen, P., Stevens, B., Weston, J., & Willan, S. 2005. Randomized controlled trial of hands-and-knees positioning for occipitoposterior position in labor. *Birth: Issues in Perinatal Care, 32*(4), 243–251.

NURSING CARE MANAGEMENT

Nursing Assessment and Diagnosis

The first sign of OP position is intense back pain in the first stage of labor. The back pain is caused by the fetal occiput compressing the sacral nerves. Other signs and symptoms may include a dysfunctional labor pattern, a prolonged active phase, secondary arrest of dilatation, or arrest of descent. Further assessment may reveal a depression in the maternal abdomen above the symphysis pubis. Fetal heart rate (FHR) may be heard far laterally on the maternal abdomen, and on vaginal examination the nurse will find the wide diamond-shaped anterior fontanelle in the anterior portion of the pelvis. This fontanelle may be difficult to feel because of molding of the fetal head. Leopold's maneuvers should also be performed to detect positional changes (see chapter 23 ∞ and Figure 23-7 ∞ on page 571).

Intrapartum ultrasound is another effective tool for detecting fetal malposition (Ridley, 2007). Nursing diagnoses that may apply to women with persistent OP position include the following:

- ***Acute Pain*** related to back discomfort secondary to occiput-posterior position
- ***Ineffective Coping*** related to persistent back pain

Nursing Plan and Implementation

Changing maternal posture has been used for many years to enhance rotation of OP or occiput transverse (OT) to OA. The woman may be placed on one side and then asked to move to the other side as the fetus begins to rotate. This side-lying position may promote rotation; it also enables the support person to apply counterpressure on the sacral area to decrease discomfort (Ridley, 2007). A knee-chest position provides a downward slant to the vaginal canal, directing the fetal head downward on descent and is often effective in rotating the fetus. In addition to maintaining a hands-and-knees position on the bed, the woman may do pelvic rocking, and the support person may perform firm stroking motions on the abdomen. The stroking begins over the fetal back and swings around to the other side of the abdomen. After the fetus has rotated, the woman lies in Sims' position on the side opposite the fetal back. In addition to assuming these positions, the woman may want to sit on the toilet, walk around the room, stand beside the bed and lean forward with her hands on the bed and do the pelvic rock, rest in a whirlpool, or lie on her side in the bed. The use of a birthing ball (see Figure 24-4 ∞ on page 609) has also been helpful in rotating the fetal head.

Evaluation

Expected outcomes of nursing care include the following:

- The woman's discomfort is decreased.

- The woman and her partner apply comfort measures and position changes that assist her.
- The woman's coping abilities are strengthened.
- The woman and her partner state that they feel supported and encouraged.

Care of the Woman and Fetus at Risk Because of Fetal Malpresentation

In a normal cephalic presentation, the occiput is the presenting part and the head is flexed with the chin on the chest (Figure 27-5A ■). Three cephalic malpresentations are possible: military (sinciput), brow, and face (Figure 27-5B–D ■). The fetal body straightens out in these malpresentations from the classic fetal position to an S-shaped position. Of these, the military presentation is probably the least difficult for the woman and fetus. In most cases, as soon as the head reaches the pelvic floor, flexion occurs and a vaginal birth results. Thus, of the cephalic malpresentations, only brow and face are discussed here.

In addition to the cephalic malpresentations, the breech, shoulder (transverse lie), and compound presentations can cause significant difficulty during labor. These malpresentations are also discussed in this chapter.

Brow Presentation

Brow presentations are the least common of all presentations, with an incidence of 1 in 670 births to 1 in 3433 births (Gabbe et al., 2007). In a brow presentation, the forehead of the fetus becomes the presenting part. The fetal head is slightly extended instead of flexed, with the result that the fetal head enters the birth canal with the widest diameter of the head (occipitomental) foremost (Figure 27-5C). Although no specific cause can be identified, proposed causes include high parity, placenta previa, uterine anomaly, hydramnios, fetal anomaly, low birth weight, cephalopelvic disproportion, and large fetus (Bashiri, Burstein, Bar-David, et al., 2008). Primiparity is a protective factor (Bashiri et al., 2008).

In labors in which a brow presentation exists, 33% to 50% will result in a prolonged labor or a secondary arrest of labor (Gabbe et al., 2007). Cesarean birth is preferred in the presence of cephalopelvic disproportion (CPD) or failure of a

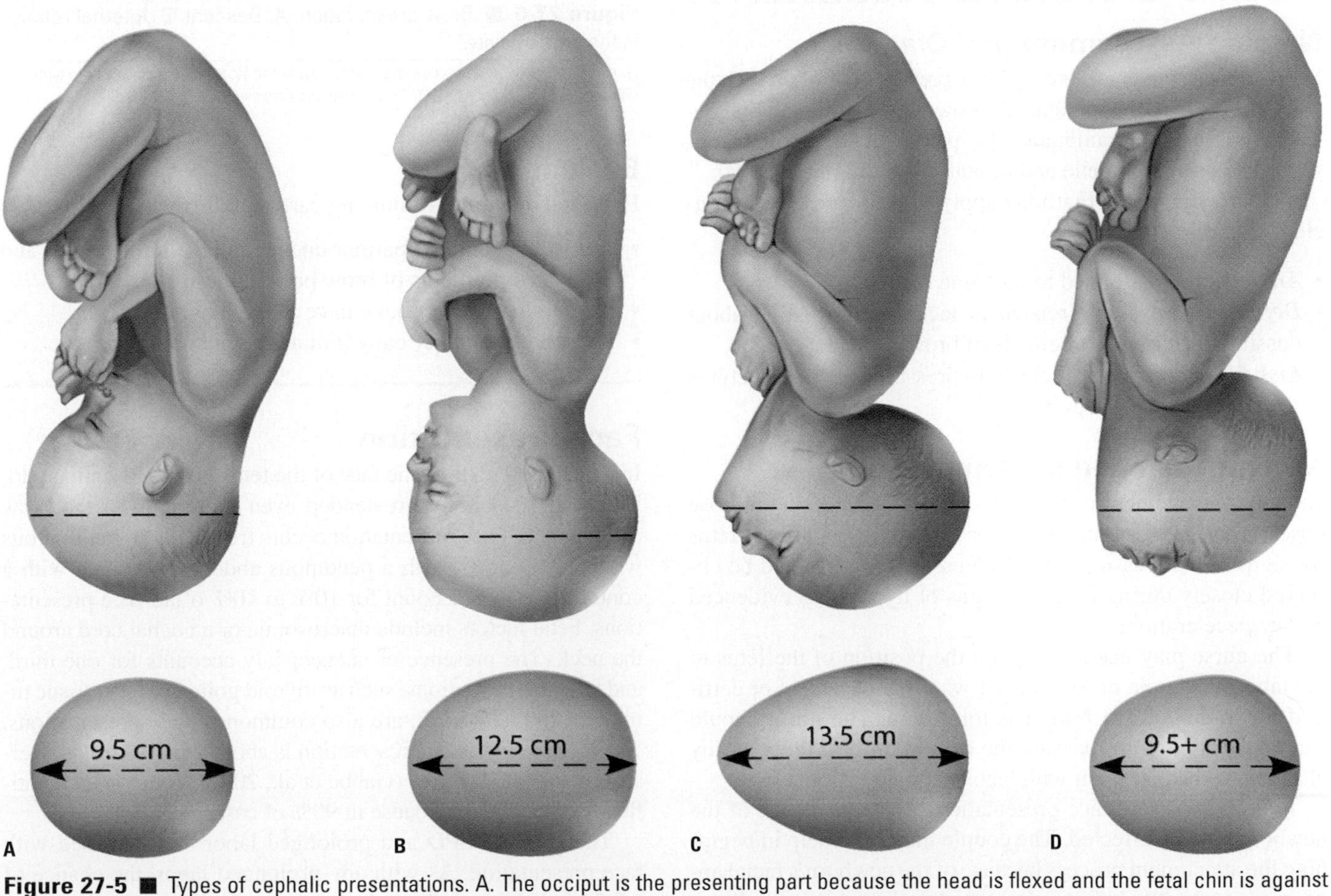

Figure 27-5 ■ Types of cephalic presentations. A. The occiput is the presenting part because the head is flexed and the fetal chin is against the chest. The largest anteroposterior (AP) diameter that presents and passes through the pelvis is approximately 9.5 cm. B. Military (sinciput) presentation. The head is neither flexed nor extended. The presenting AP diameter is approximately 12.5 cm. C. Brow presentation. The largest diameter of the fetal head (approximately 13.5 cm) presents in this situation. D. Face presentation. The AP diameter is 9.5 cm.

Source: From Danforth, D. N., & Scott, J. R. (Eds.). (1990). Obstetrics and gynecology *(5th ed., p. 170, Figure 8–9). Copyright © 1999 Lippincott Williams & Wilkins. Reprinted with permission.*

brow presentation to convert to a normal vertex or face presentation. If a vaginal birth is attempted, the woman will probably have an episiotomy and may require extension of the episiotomy at the moment of birth.

Fetal mortality is increased because of injuries received during the birth. Trauma during the birth process can include cerebral and neck compression and damage to the trachea and larynx.

Clinical Therapy

Active medical intervention is not necessary as long as cervical dilatation and fetal descent are occurring. If labor progress is slow, clinical pelvimetry findings and ultrasound to determine the presence of fetal anomalies are important. Brow presentations should be managed expectedly because a cesarean birth is most frequently warranted (Zayed, Amarin, Obeidat, et al., 2008). Oxytocin may be used with caution to correct an inadequate labor pattern. Use of forceps or manual conversion is contraindicated (Zayed et al., 2008). If problems occur, cesarean birth is indicated.

NURSING CARE MANAGEMENT

Nursing Assessment and Diagnosis

Leopold's maneuvers suggest a brow presentation when both the chin and occiput are palpable. A brow presentation may be detected on vaginal examination by palpation of the diamond-shaped anterior fontanelle and orbital ridges (Figure 27-6 ■).

Nursing diagnoses that may apply to brow presentation include the following:

- ***Anxiety*** or ***Fear*** related to outcome for fetus
- ***Deficient Knowledge*** related to lack of information about possible maternal-fetal effects of brow presentation
- ***Risk for Injury (Fetus)*** related to pressure on fetal structures secondary to brow presentation

Nursing Plan and Implementation

Nursing management of the brow presentation includes close observation of the woman for labor aberrations and of the fetus for signs of nonreassuring fetal status. The fetus should be observed closely during labor for signs of hypoxia as evidenced by late decelerations.

The nurse may need to explain the position of the fetus to the laboring couple or to interpret what the physician or certified nurse-midwife (CNM) has told them. The nurse should stay close at hand to reassure the couple, inform them of any changes, and assist them with labor-coping techniques.

In both brow and face presentations, the appearance of the newborn may be affected. The couple may need help in beginning the attachment process because of the newborn's facial appearance. After the infant is inspected for gross abnormalities, the pediatrician and nurse can assure the couple that the facial edema and excessive molding are only temporary and will subside in a few days.

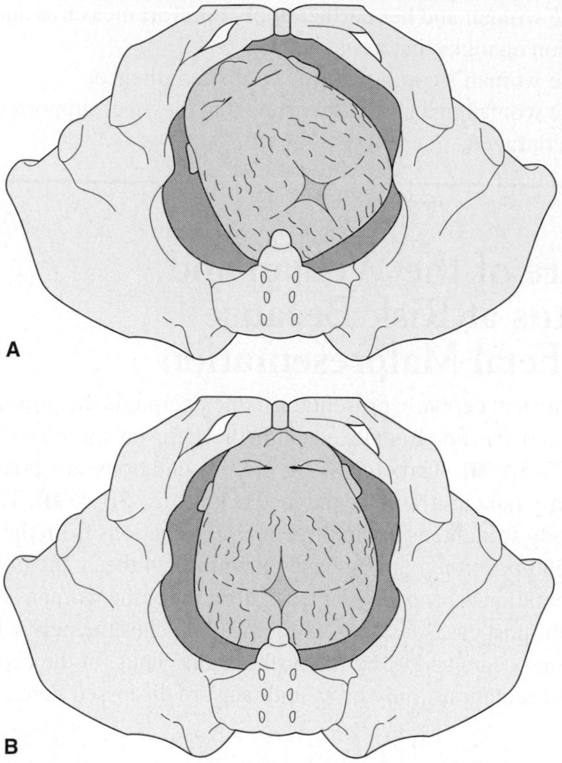

Figure 27-6 ■ Brow presentation. A. Descent. B. Internal rotation in the pelvic cavity.

Source: Reprinted with permission from Oxorn, H., & Foote, W. (1986). Human labor and birth *(5th ed., p. 211). Copyright © 1986 The McGraw-Hill Companies, Inc.*

Evaluation

Expected outcomes of nursing care include the following:

- The woman and her partner understand the implications and associated problems of brow presentation.
- The mother and her baby have a safe labor and birth.
- The woman and her baby initiate the bonding process.

Face Presentation

In a face presentation, the face of the fetus is the presenting part. The fetal head is hyperextended even more than in the brow presentation. Face presentation occurs frequently in multiparous women or women with a pendulous abdomen. Women with a contracted pelvis account for 10% to 40% of all face presentations. Fetal factors include macrosomia or a nuchal cord around the neck. The presence of anencephaly accounts for one third, and fetal malformations, such as thyroid goiter and soft tissue tumors of the fetal neck, are also common in face presentations. The incidence of face presentation is about 1 in 500 births overall or 0.2% of all births (Gabbe et al., 2007). There is an identified fetal or maternal cause in 90% of cases.

The risks of CPD and prolonged labor are increased with face presentation. As with any prolonged labor, the chance of infection is increased.

The fetus may develop edema, making vaginal examination for placement of heart rate electrodes difficult. If a fetal scalp electrode is applied, it should be placed on the mentum. After

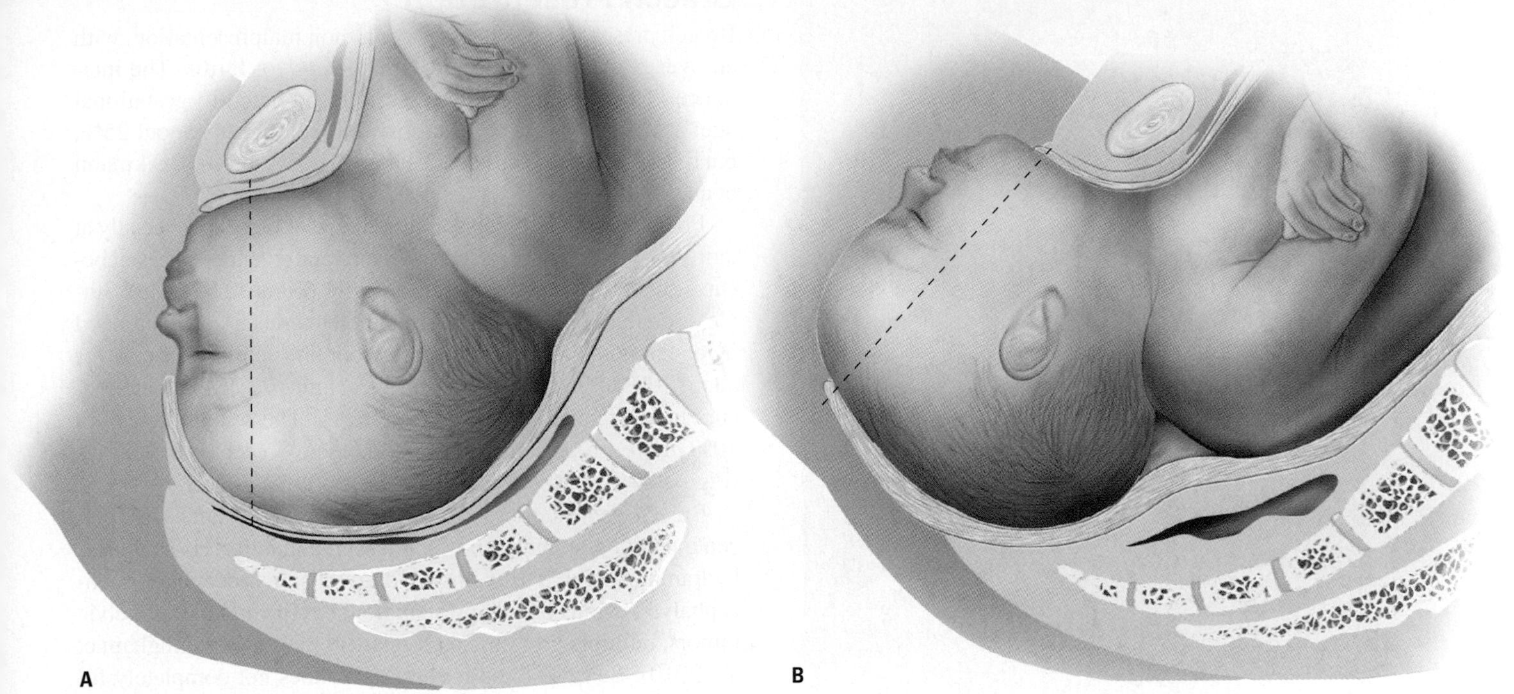

Figure 27-7 ■ Face presentation. Mechanism of birth in mentoanterior position. A. The submentobregmatic diameter at the outlet. B. The fetal head is born by movement of flexion.

birth the edema gives the newborn an unusual appearance. As with the brow presentation, the neck and internal structures may swell as a result of trauma received during descent. Petechiae, swelling, and facial bruising are often seen in the superficial layers of the facial skin because of the birth trauma. The perinatal mortality rate is 2% to 3% not including nonviable malformations and extreme prematurity (Gabbe et al., 2007).

Clinical Therapy

If no CPD is present, the mentum (chin) is anterior, and the labor pattern is effective, the objective of medical treatment is a vaginal birth (Figure 27-7 ■). The success rate of vaginal delivery is 70% to 80%. Oxytocin may be administered as needed for hypotonic labor patterns. Attempts at manual rotation should not be made, because this increases perinatal mortality and maternal morbidity (Creasy, Resnik, Iams, et al., 2009). Mentum posteriors can become wedged on the anterior surface of the sacrum (Figure 27-8 ■). In this case as well as in the presence of CPD, cesarean is the preferred method of birth.

NURSING CARE MANAGEMENT

Nursing Assessment and Diagnosis

When performing Leopold's maneuvers, the nurse finds that the back of the fetus is difficult to outline, and a deep furrow can be palpated between the hard occiput and the fetal back (Figure 27-9 ■). Fetal heart tones can be heard on the side where the fetal feet are palpated. It may be difficult to determine by vaginal examination whether a breech or a face is presenting, especially if facial edema is already present. During the vaginal examination, palpation of the saddle of the nose and the gums should be attempted. When assessing engagement, the nurse needs to remember that the face has to be deep within the pelvis before the biparietal diameter has entered the inlet. The majority

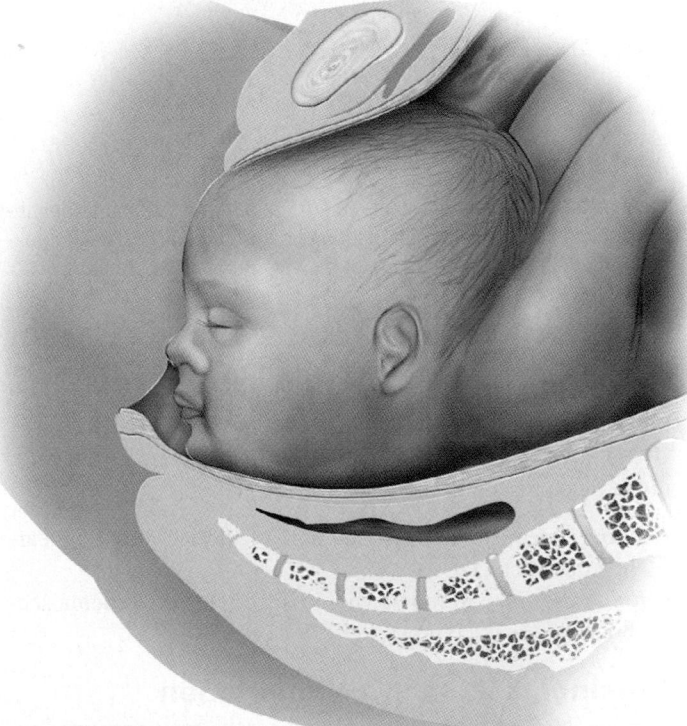

Figure 27-8 ■ Face presentation. Mechanism of birth in mentoposterior position. Fetal head is unable to extend farther. The face becomes impacted.

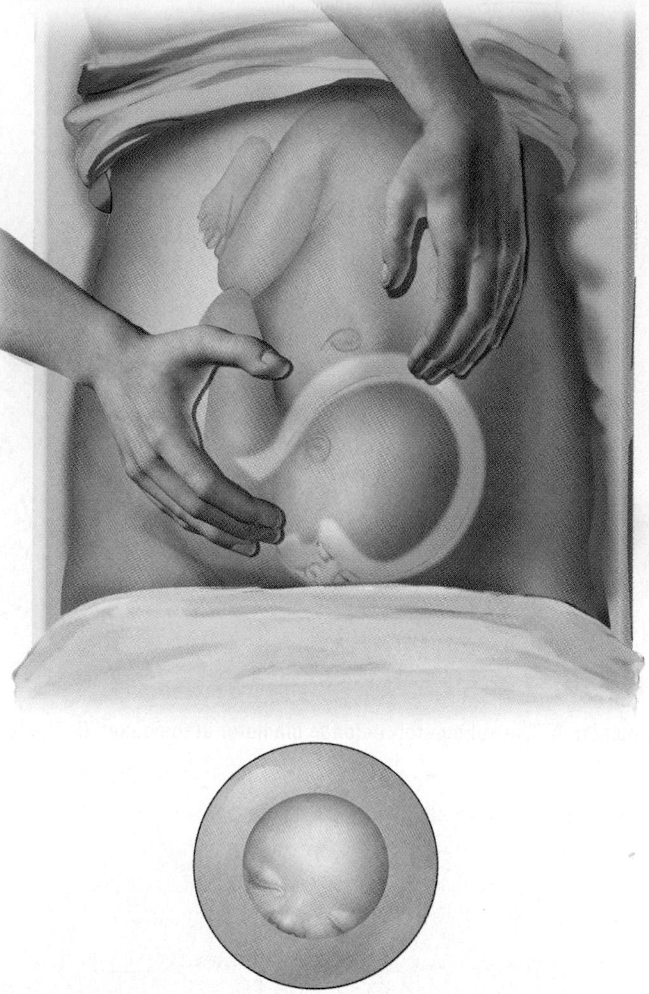

A

B

Figure 27-9 ■ Face presentation. A. Palpation of the maternal abdomen with the fetus in right mentum posterior (RMP). B. Vaginal examination may permit palpation of facial features of the fetus.

of face presentations are diagnosed via vaginal exam later in labor, and some are not diagnosed until the time of birth (Gabbe et al., 2007).

Nursing diagnoses that may apply to the woman with a fetus in face presentation include the following:

- ***Fear*** related to unknown outcome of the labor and appearance of the baby
- ***Risk for Injury*** to the newborn's face related to edema secondary to the birth process

Nursing Plan and Implementation

Nursing interventions are the same as for the brow presentation.

Evaluation

Expected outcomes of nursing care include the following:

- The woman and her partner understand the implications and problems of face presentation.
- The mother and her baby have a safe labor and birth.
- The woman and her baby initiate the bonding process.

Breech Presentation

Breech presentation is the most common malpresentation, with an overall incidence of approximately 4% of births. The incidence of breech presentation is directly related to gestational age: at 25 to 26 weeks' gestation, the incidence is about 25%, but by 32 weeks, the incidence has decreased to 7% (Beckmann et al., 2008).

Frank breech is the most common type of breech (especially at term) and is characterized by flexed hips and extended knees. It occurs in about 50% to 70% of breech births (Figure 27-10A ■). Single or double footling breech (incomplete breech), characterized by one or both hips extended and a foot presenting, accounts for about 10% to 30% of breech births (Figure 27-10B ■) and occurs more frequently in preterm fetuses. The remaining 5% to 10% of breech presentations are complete breech presentations (Figure 27-10C ■) (Beckmann et al., 2008).

Breech presentation is most frequently associated with placenta previa, implantation of the placenta in either cornual area, hydramnios, high parity, oligohydramnios, hydrocephaly, anencephaly, previous breech presentation, uterine anomalies, pelvic tumors, multiple gestation, and fetal anomalies (Cunningham et al., 2010). Because the presenting part does not completely fill the space in the lower uterine segment, once membranes rupture, cord prolapse is more likely. The incidence of cord prolapse is more likely in a breech presentation. Infants born after breech presentation have higher infant mortality and neonatal complications. Factors associated with breech presentation include a decreased muscle tone in the fetus and an abnormal fetal motor ability. Breech fetuses are more likely to have neuromuscular disorders. Children who presented in breech presentation scored lower on motor functioning during the first 5 years of life than children who had presented in cephalic presentation (Creasy et al., 2009). These birth defects can be associated with factors that caused the breech presentation (birth defects or intrauterine growth restriction) or with damage that occurred during birth (Rubio et al., 2009).

Head trauma during vaginal birth is more likely in breech presentation because it does not allow for the slow molding that occurs in a cephalic presentation as the fetal head moves through the birth canal. The head is the largest and least resilient part of the fetal body. It is the last to come through the maternal pelvis in breech presentations; thus molding does not occur. In the case of a preterm breech, a single or double footling and the torso may emerge through a cervix that is not completely dilated, leaving the larger head entrapped by the cervix. Entrapment may also occur with cesarean birth if the incision is inadequate or uterine relaxation is less than optimum. Vaginal breech birth also carries higher risks of meconium aspiration and fetal asphyxia (ACOG, 2006).

Studies have demonstrated that planned cesarean births of breech fetuses had a lower risk of perinatal morbidity and mortality than planned vaginal births (ACOG, 2006). The American College of Obstetricians and Gynecologists now recommends that the mode of birth for a single fetus should be based on the healthcare provider's experience and expertise and notes there is a decrease of expertise in this area of obstetrics. The mother should be informed that there are more com-

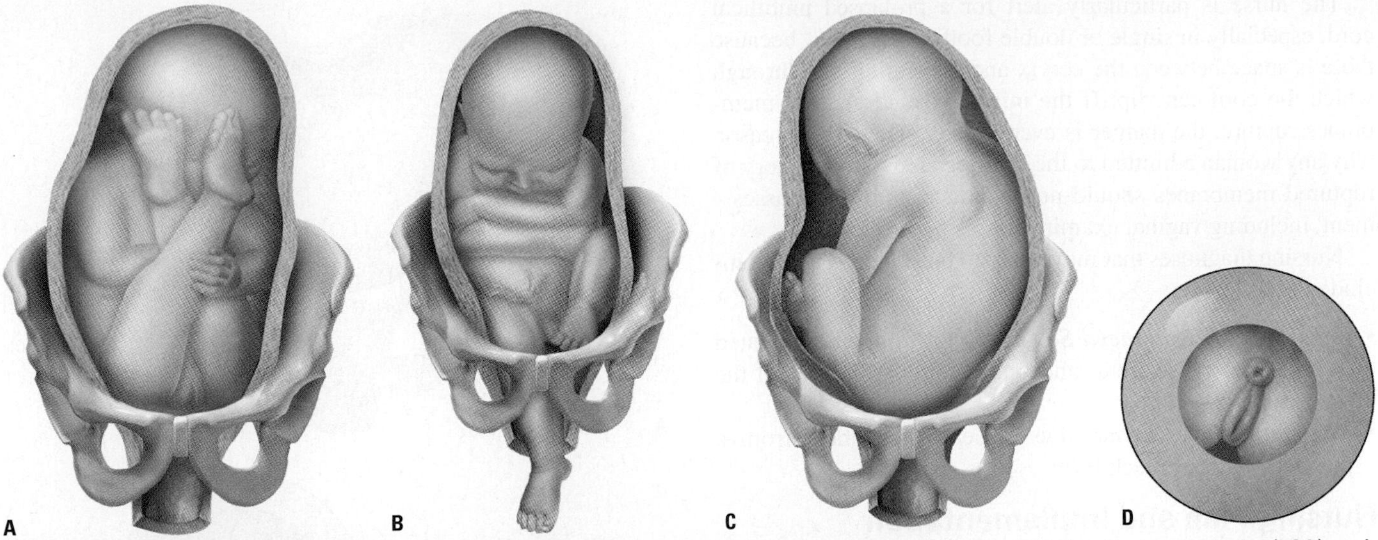

Figure 27-10 ■ Breech presentation. A. Frank breech. B. Incomplete (footling) breech. C. Complete breech in left sacral anterior (LSA) position. D. On vaginal examination, the nurse may feel the anal sphincter. The tissue of the fetal buttocks feels soft.

plications associated with planned vaginal breech delivery than with planned cesarean birth in these fetuses (ACOG, 2006).

Clinical Therapy

An external cephalic version (ECV) is usually attempted at 37 to 38 weeks' gestation. The ECV, which is discussed in detail in chapter 28 ∞, can reduce breech presentation by 50% (Beckmann et al., 2008).

Complementary and alternative therapies have also been used with some success. *Moxibustion* is a traditional Chinese medicine (TCM) technique in which certain herbs are burned close to the skin near a particular acupressure or acupuncture point, thus stimulating the point and allowing energy to flow through it. To promote version in breech presentations, mugwort is burned close to acupoint BL67, located beside the outer corner of the fifth toenail. The heat and pungency of the burning mugwort stimulates the pressure point, much like acupressure or acupuncture does, and energy is released. It is believed that the effect of moxibustion increases fetal activity. Moxibustion has been shown to decrease the need for ECV and reduce the use of oxytocin before and during labor (Gibbs et al., 2008).

Maternal positioning exercises can also be utilized to facilitate the rotation of the fetus. The mother should be advised to assume a position where her hips are higher than her torso, which can give the fetus ample room to move into a cephalic presentation. The mother should be encouraged to perform these exercises 2 or 3 times daily. Once she feels a large movement, however, she should be advised to discontinue the exercises until a care provider has determined if the desirable position has been achieved.

If the version is unsuccessful or the fetus spontaneously turns back into a breech presentation, the physician will evaluate the possibility of a vaginal birth or plan a cesarean birth. Many physicians recommend a cesarean birth when a breech presentation is detected, especially if the woman is nulliparous because breech births have higher mortality and morbidity rates as well as an increased incidence of cord prolapse, birth trauma, and fetal cervical spinal cord injuries due to hyperextension of the head (Beckmann et al., 2008). Contraindications for labor and vaginal birth include the following:

- Fetal weight less than 1500 g or more than 3800 g
- Hyperextension of the fetal neck of more than 90 degrees
- Extension of the fetal arms over the head
- Anomalies, such as hydrocephalus
- Diminished maternal pelvic measurements

If a vaginal birth is being attempted, narcotic agents or an epidural block may be used for pain relief. Epidural anesthesia may be advantageous during the latter portion of labor because it will help prevent the pushing sensation the woman may feel before complete dilatation. If the woman pushes before cervical dilatation is complete, the fetal body may be expelled and the head entrapped. At the time of birth the physician may have an assistant available in case forceps are needed. Once the fetal body is born, an assistant supports the fetal body as the physician applies Piper forceps to assist in birth of the fetal head (called the *aftercoming head*) (Cunningham et al., 2010).

NURSING CARE MANAGEMENT

Nursing Assessment and Diagnosis

At times, the nurse is the first person to recognize a breech presentation. On palpation using Leopold's maneuvers, the nurse feels the hard vertex in the fundus and can perform ballottement of the head independently of the fetal body. The wider sacrum is palpated in the lower part of the abdomen. If the sacrum has not descended, on ballottement the entire fetal body will move. Furthermore, fetal heart tones (FHTs) are usually auscultated above the umbilicus. Passage of meconium from compression of the infant's intestinal tract during descent may occur.

The nurse is particularly alert for a prolapsed umbilical cord, especially in single or double footling breeches, because there is space between the cervix and presenting part through which the cord can slip. If the infant is small and the membranes rupture, the danger is even greater. This is one reason why any woman admitted to the birthing area with a history of ruptured membranes should not ambulate until a full assessment, including vaginal examination, is performed.

Nursing diagnoses that may apply to breech presentation include the following:

- ***Readiness for Enhanced Self-Health Management*** related to an expressed desire to understand the implications of the procedure
- ***Risk for Injury (Fetus)*** due to head entrapment from a planned vaginal breech birth

Nursing Plan and Implementation

During labor, the fetus is at increased risk for prolapse of the cord. Some agency protocols may therefore call for continuous electronic fetal monitoring (EFM) even though there are no current research studies to support the use of EFM. Since women with a breech presentation are at an increased risk for a prolapsed umbilical cord, maternal ambulation is usually not recommended until the presenting part is well engaged. Ongoing assessments of contractions, cervical dilatation, effacement, and fetal descent are also important to monitor labor progress. Emotional support and sharing of information are critical to the childbearing woman and her support person. They need to be kept apprised of the labor's current status as well as the possible treatment plans so they can continue to make informed choices.

During a vaginal birth, the nurse continues to assess the fetal heart rate (FHR) and to provide encouragement and support for the couple. Piper forceps need to be readily available to the physician; the nurse may assist the physician if the forceps are needed for the birth.

Evaluation

Expected outcomes of nursing care include the following:

- The woman and her partner can describe the implications and associated problems with breech presentation.
- The mother and baby have a safe labor and birth.
- Major complications are recognized early, and corrective measures are instituted.

Shoulder Presentation (Transverse Lie) of a Single Fetus

It is not uncommon in multiple gestations for one or more of the fetuses to be in a transverse lie. An incidence of transverse lie of a single fetus is approximately 1 in 300 term births (Cunningham et al., 2010). The infant's long axis lies across the woman's abdomen, and on inspection the contour of the maternal abdomen appears widest from side to side (Figure 27-11 ■).

Maternal conditions associated with a transverse lie are grand multiparity with lax uterine musculature (the most common cause); obstructions such as bony dystocia, placenta previa, neoplasms, and fetal anomalies; hydramnios; and preterm fetus.

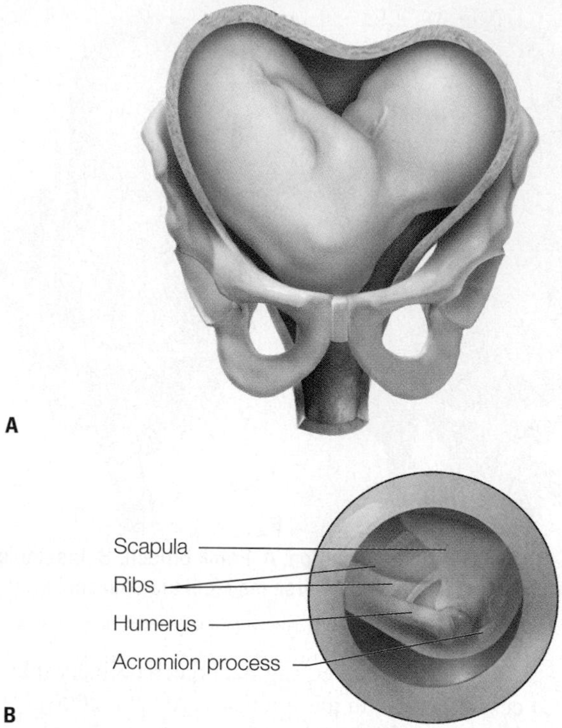

Figure 27-11 ■ Transverse lie. A. Shoulder presentation. B. On vaginal examination, the nurse may feel the acromion process as the fetal presenting part.

Vaginal birth is impossible with a transverse lie. Labor should not be allowed to continue, and a cesarean birth is done quickly. Frequently a vertical incision is made in the uterus because the fetal head and fetal feet lie in the upper portion of the uterus; a low transverse incision may lead to difficulties in extracting the fetus (Cunningham et al., 2010).

If labor is allowed to continue, the fetal shoulder will be forced down into the pelvis and the fetus will become impacted. With no relief, uterine rupture may occur (Cunningham et al., 2010).

Clinical Therapy

Transverse lie may be diagnosed using Leopold's maneuvers and can then be confirmed by ultrasound. At the time of the ultrasound examination, it is important to confirm fetal position, fetal biparietal diameters (to confirm gestational age), and location of the placenta and to carry out an examination for the presence of fetal anomalies and structural abnormalities of the uterus such as leiomyoma (fibroid tumor) or adnexal tumors.

Management varies, depending on the length of gestation, because many transverse lies convert to either cephalic or breech presentation by term (38 weeks). If the fetus is still in a transverse lie at term, an ECV may be done if (1) there is no contraindication to vaginal birth (for example, a fetal anomaly, complete placenta previa, or a structural problem in the uterus), and (2) fetal pulmonary lung maturity is confirmed either by ultrasound measurements or by amniocentesis for assessment of phospholipids (2:1 lecithin/sphingomyelin [L/S] ratio and the presence of phosphatidylglycerol). An ECV is most likely to be successful close to term. Spontaneous version will likely occur if performed before 37 weeks. The use of tocolytics for the procedure may be helpful for nulliparas. The fetus is assessed with a nonstress test (NST) or biophysical profile (BPP) before the procedure. If the version is successful, the woman may be induced if she is at term and her cervix is favorable. However, scientific studies do not support immediate induction as a routine to minimize the chance the fetus will return to the original position (Gabbe et al., 2007).

NURSING CARE MANAGEMENT

Nursing Assessment and Diagnosis

The nurse can identify a transverse lie by inspection and palpation of the abdomen, by auscultation of FHTs in the midline of the abdomen (not conclusive), and by vaginal examination.

On palpation, no fetal part is felt in the fundal portion of the uterus or above the symphysis pubis. The head may be palpated on one side and the breech on the other. FHTs are usually auscultated just below the midline of the umbilicus. On vaginal examination, if a presenting part is palpated, it is the ridged thorax or possibly an arm that is compressed against the chest. Women with a transverse lie may report less shortness of breath, pelvic pressure, and urinary frequency than other women because pressure is not exerted on the diaphragm and the bladder.

Nursing diagnoses that may apply when transverse lie is present include the following:

- ***Risk for Impaired Gas Exchange*** related to decrease in blood flow secondary to cord compression associated with prolapsed cord
- ***Risk for Powerlessness*** related to unknown outcome
- ***Fear*** related to unknown outcome of birth

Nursing Plan and Implementation

The primary nursing actions are to help evaluate the fetal presentation and to provide information and support to the couple. If an ECV has been accomplished and an induction is started, the nurse completes all interventions related to the induction (see the discussion in chapter 28 ∞). If transverse lie is discovered when the woman is admitted to the birthing unit in labor, the nurse provides information regarding the need for either an ECV or a cesarean birth and assists with preparation for the birth. If an ECV is not performed or is unsuccessful, a cesarean birth will be performed. Before the cesarean, the nurse watches for rupture of membranes and the possibility of prolapse of the umbilical cord. (See chapter 28 ∞ for further information regarding teaching with cesarean birth.)

Evaluation

Expected outcomes of nursing care include the following:

- The transverse lie is recognized promptly, and crucial assessments are completed.
- Measures to perform an ECV or a cesarean birth are completed.
- The mother and baby have a safe birth.
- The couple can describe the implications and associated problems of transverse lie.

Compound Presentation

A compound presentation is one in which there are two presenting parts. It can occur when the pelvic inlet is not totally occluded by the primary presenting part. If the prolapsed part is a hand, the birth is generally not difficult. Sometimes the hand slips back, and occasionally it is born alongside the head. This may increase the chance of laceration. Cesarean birth is indicated in the presence of uterine dysfunction or nonreassuring fetal status (Cunningham et al., 2010).

Care of the Woman and Fetus at Risk Because of Macrosomia

Fetal **macrosomia** is defined as weight of more than 4000 g. It is important to remember that the mean birth weight varies throughout the world. For instance, mean birth weight in Sweden is 3490 g, whereas in Pakistan the mean birth weight is 2770 g. In Latino cultures, "fat" babies are more desirable and are viewed as more healthy. Nurses working with Latino women may encounter resistance if counseling is focused on preventing a large baby. Instead, nurses should stress the importance of the baby's health status (Simpson & Creehan, 2007). The definition of macrosomia will thus differ according to the ethnic group being discussed.

A woman who is obese is twice as likely to have a macrosomic fetus (Hillier et al., 2008). Obesity has been defined in a number of ways. For a complete discussion on maternal obesity, see chapter 18 ∞. There is also an association between macrosomia and both pregestational and gestational diabetes. Increased maternal glucose levels have also been shown to increase fetal weight (Hillier et al., 2008). Other risk factors include postterm pregnancy, multiparity, grand multiparity, previous macrosomic infant, previous shoulder dystocia, male sex, and maternal birth weight.

A woman's pelvis that is adequate for an average-sized fetus may be disproportionately small for an oversized fetus. Distention of the uterus causes overstretching of the myometrial fibers, which may lead to dysfunctional labor and an increased incidence of postpartal hemorrhage. If the oversized fetus is not able to descend, the chance of uterine rupture during labor increases. Vaginal birth poses an increased risk of perineal lacerations and extensions of an episiotomy. The mother is also at risk for postpartum hemorrhage and puerperal infection. The incidence of vacuum and forceps birth increases with fetal size.

The most significant complication in macrosomia is *shoulder dystocia,* which is an obstetric emergency. However, shoulder dystocia may occur with fetuses weighing less than 4000 g, and risk factors are not reliable predictors. Following birth of the head, the anterior shoulder of the macrosomic fetus may not emerge either spontaneously or with gentle traction

(Cunningham et al., 2010). If shoulder dystocia is not managed correctly, permanent injury to the baby may result. **Brachial plexus injury** is an injury due to improper or excessive traction applied to the fetal head during birth that results in damage to the network of nerves that send signals from the spine to the shoulder, arm, and hand.

Other injuries that may occur include fractured clavicles, meconium aspiration, asphyxia, hypoglycemia, polycythemia, and hyperbilirubinemia. Other neurologic damage to the fetus can also occur.

In addition, macrosomic infants are more likely to become obese in childhood and adolescence. These children are also at risk to develop diabetes later in life (Landon, Catalano, & Gabbe, 2007).

Clinical Therapy

The occurrence of the maternal and fetal problems associated with macrosomic infants may be somewhat lessened by identifying macrosomia before the onset of labor. The diagnosis is not precise. There is good evidence to show that estimating fetal size with ultrasound is no more accurate than a clinical estimate from Leopold's maneuvers (Heywood, Magann, Rich, et al., 2008; Magliore & Copel, 2007). However, ultrasound is usually employed as an assessment measure in diagnosing macrosomia. If a large fetus is suspected, the maternal pelvis should be evaluated carefully. An estimation of fetal size can be made by palpating the crown-rump length (CRL) of the fetus in utero, but the greatest errors in estimation occur on both ends of the spectrum—the macrosomic fetus and the very small fetus. Whenever the uterus appears excessively large, hydramnios, an oversized fetus, or a multiple pregnancy must be considered.

Labor and vaginal birth for a fetus greater than 4500 g may warrant a cesarean birth to reduce the risks associated with vaginal births. The best method of birth for a fetus weighing 4000 to 4500 g is debated. If a vaginal birth is attempted and difficulty extracting the shoulders occurs during the birth, the obstetrician or certified nurse-midwife (CNM) may direct the woman to sharply flex her thighs up against her abdomen (McRoberts maneuver). This position is thought to change the maternal pelvic angle and therefore reduce the force needed to extract the shoulders, thereby decreasing the incidence of brachial plexus stretching and clavicular fracture (Figure 27-12A–C ■). The maternal head should be lowered and the nurse applies suprapubic pressure directly over the symphysis pubis to aid release of the anterior shoulder. Fundal pressure (pressure exerted at the top of the maternal fundus) should not be performed, because this can further wedge the shoulder against the suprapubic bone.

In addition, the obstetrician or CNM may incorporate other interventions, such as checking the placement of the shoulder, performing an episiotomy, and using the Woods Screw maneuver (which consists of rotating the anterior shoulder 180 degrees to the posterior position). In cases where these interventions fail, the obstetrician or CNM may electively break the clavicle to facilitate extraction of the shoulders.

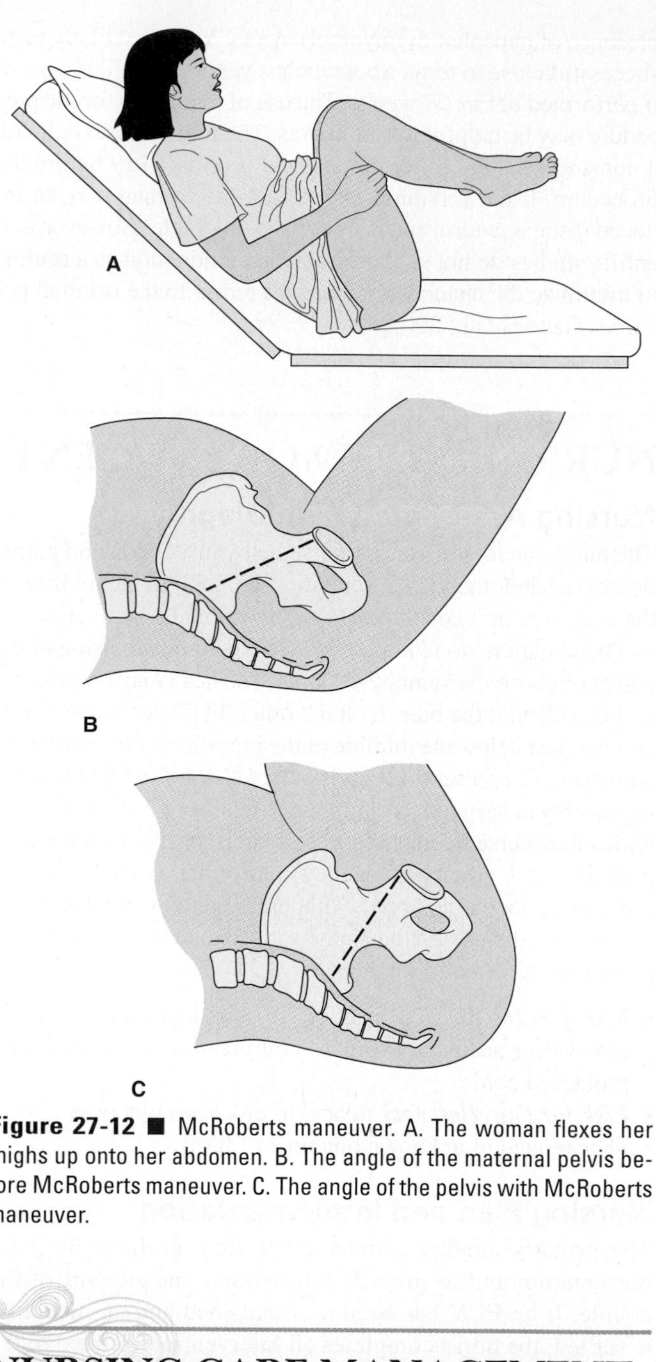

Figure 27-12 ■ McRoberts maneuver. A. The woman flexes her thighs up onto her abdomen. B. The angle of the maternal pelvis before McRoberts maneuver. C. The angle of the pelvis with McRoberts maneuver.

NURSING CARE MANAGEMENT

Nursing Assessment and Diagnosis

The nurse assists in identifying factors associated with macrosomic infants. During the intrapartum period, the risk factors include slow descent of the fetus and prolonged second stage. Because women with these risk factors are prime candidates for dystocia and its complications, the nurse frequently assesses the fetal heart rate (FHR) for nonreassuring heart rate patterns, which may indicate fetal stress; evaluates the rate of cervical dilatation; and assesses fetal descent.

Nursing diagnoses that may apply to the woman with a macrosomic fetus include the following:

- ***Risk for Injury*** to the fetus related to trauma during the birth process

- ***Risk for Infection*** related to traumatized tissue secondary to maternal tissue damage during birth
- ***Risk for Injury*** to the mother related to perineal trauma associated with macrosomic birth

Nursing Plan and Implementation

The nurse monitors labor closely for a dysfunctional pattern, assessing FHR and reporting any sign of labor dysfunction or nonreassuring heart rate patterns to the physician or CNM. The nurse notes any arrest of descent, excessive molding of the fetal head, or the presence of caput succedaneum, which can also indicate a large fetus or cephalopelvic disproportion (CPD).

The nurse provides support for the laboring woman and her partner and information regarding the implications and possible associated problems. The nurse can provide the couple with directions for proper positioning at the time of birth to facilitate extraction of the shoulders. If the nurse anticipates a possible shoulder dystocia, additional staff should be notified and appropriate support personnel for the newborn should be informed. During the birth, the nurse continues to provide support and encouragement to the couple. Informing the woman that possible suprapubic pressure may be needed can help reduce anxiety for the couple.

After the birth, the nurse inspects the newborn for cephalhematoma, Erb palsy (caused by overstretching of the brachial plexus and damage to C_5, C_6, C_7), and fractured clavicles (exhibited by nonmovement of one arm or palpation of the clavicle to detect an irregularity of the bone structure) and informs the admission nursery of any problems. The newborn will need to be observed closely for cerebral and neurologic damage.

Postpartum, the nurse checks the uterus for potential atony and the maternal vital signs for deviations suggesting hypovolemic shock. Frequent fundal checks should be performed to evaluate the woman for postpartum bleeding. If postpartum hemorrhage occurs, intravenous (IV) or intramuscular (IM) Pitocin should be administered to stimulate contraction of the uterus.

Evaluation

Expected outcomes of nursing care include the following:

- The woman and her partner can describe the implications of macrosomia and possible associated problems.
- The mother and baby have a safe labor and birth.

Care of the Woman and Fetus in the Presence of Nonreassuring Fetal Status

When the oxygen supply is insufficient to meet the physiologic demands of the fetus, a nonreassuring fetal status may result. *Nonreassuring fetal status* is the term used to identify data describing the fetal status. Previously, the term fetal distress was used; however, its use implied an ill fetus despite the fact that the condition is often transient, not chronic.

A variety of factors may contribute to a nonreassuring fetal status. The most common are related to cord compression and uteroplacental insufficiency associated with placental abnormalities and preexisting maternal or fetal disease. If the resultant hypoxia persists and metabolic acidosis follows, the situation can be life threatening to the fetus.

The most common initial signs of nonreassuring fetal status are meconium-stained amniotic fluid (in a vertex presentation) and changes in the fetal heart rate (FHR). The presence of ominous FHR patterns, such as late or severe variable decelerations, decrease in or lack of variability, and progressive acceleration in the FHR baseline, are indicative of hypoxia. Fetal scalp blood samples demonstrating a pH value of 7.2 or less provide a more sophisticated indication of fetal problems and are generally obtained when questions about fetal status arise. (See chapter 23 ∞.)

Clinical Therapy

When there is evidence of possible nonreassuring fetal status, treatment centers on relieving the hypoxia and minimizing the effects of anoxia on the fetus. Initial interventions include changing the mother's position, increasing infusion rates of intravenous fluids, and administering oxygen by mask at 6 to 10 L per minute. If electronic fetal monitoring (EFM) has not yet been used, it is usually instituted at this time. If oxytocin is in use, it should be discontinued. Fetal scalp stimulation can be performed. Fetal scalp blood samples can be taken. If EFM is ineffective, the certified nurse-midwife (CNM) or physician may utilize internal monitoring devices to more accurately assess FHR changes. Figure 27-13 ■ depicts intrapartum management of nonreassuring fetal status heart rate patterns.

NURSING CARE MANAGEMENT

Nursing Assessment and Diagnosis

The nurse reviews the woman's prenatal history to anticipate the possibility of nonreassuring fetal status. When the membranes rupture, it is important to assess FHR and to observe for meconium staining. A sterile vaginal examination should be performed to rule out cord prolapse. As labor progresses, the nurse is particularly alert for even subtle changes in the FHR pattern and the fetal scalp pH, if available. Reports by the mother of increased or greatly decreased fetal activity may also be associated with nonreassuring fetal status. For further discussion of FHR patterns and characteristics, see evaluation of fetal status during labor in chapter 23 ∞.

Nursing diagnoses that may apply in the presence of nonreassuring fetal status include the following:

- ***Decreased Cardiac Output (Fetus)*** related to decreased uteroplacental perfusion secondary to maternal hypotension, decreased blood volume, or vasoconstriction with preeclampsia
- ***Anxiety*** related to knowledge of nonreassuring fetal status

Nursing Plan and Implementation

Staff members may become so involved in assessing fetal status and initiating corrective measures that they fail to give explanations and emotional support to the woman, her partner, and other family members. It is imperative that the nurse provide both full

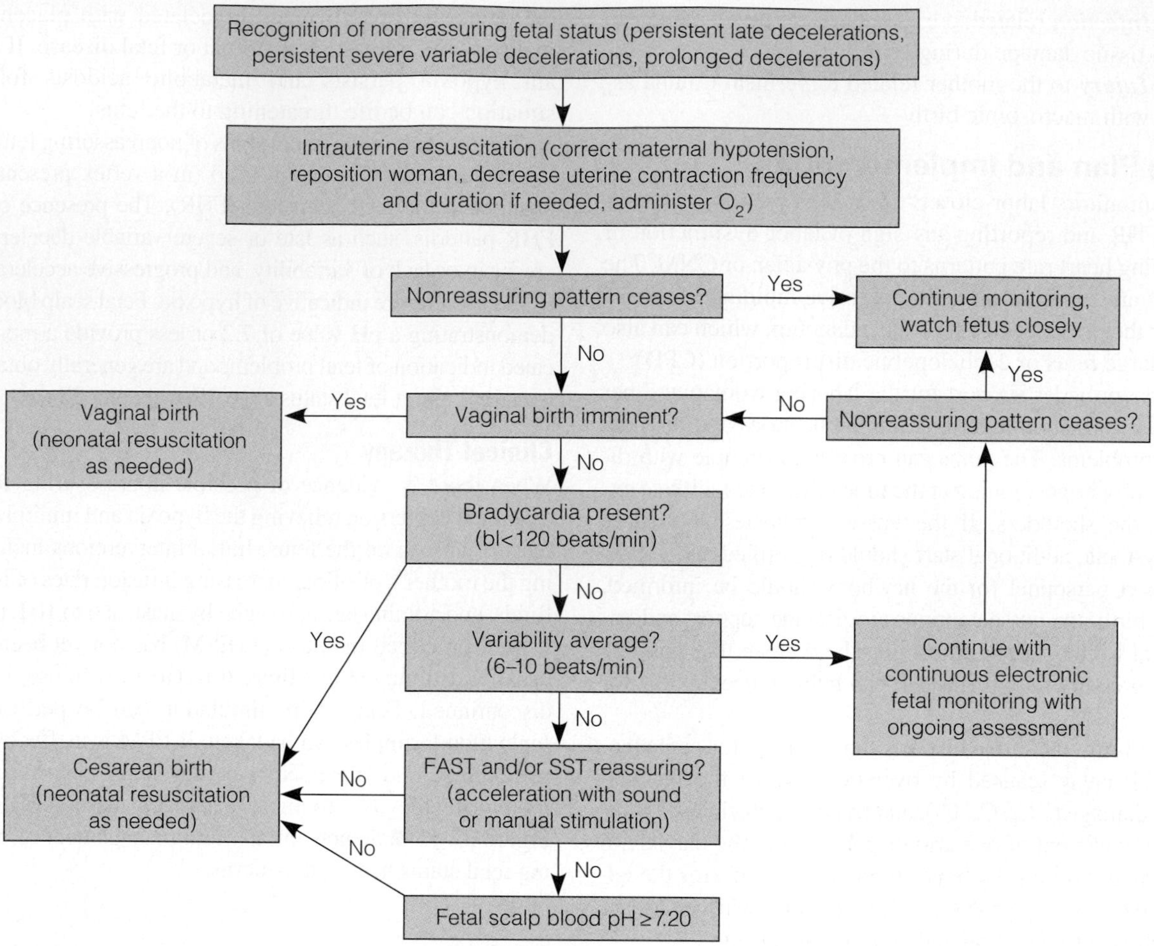

Figure 27-13 ■ Intrapartum management of nonreassuring fetal status.

Note: bl = baseline; FAST = fetal acoustic stimulation test; SST = scalp stimulation test.

Source: From Zuspan, F. P., & Quilligan, E. J. Handbook of obstetrics, gynecology, and primary care. *Copyright 1998, Mosby; reprinted with permission from Elsevier Science.*

explanations of the problem and comfort to the couple. In many instances, if birth is not imminent, the woman must undergo cesarean birth. Anticipation of this surgery may cause fear and frustration for the couple, especially if they were committed to a shared, prepared birth experience.

Evaluation

Expected outcomes of nursing care include the following:

- The woman and her family become less anxious and more able to cope with their situation.
- The FHR remains in normal range, or, alternatively, supportive measures maintain the FHR as normal as possible.

Care of the Woman Experiencing Placental and Umbilical Cord Problems

Placenta Problems

Problems of the placenta can be divided into those that are developmental and those that are degenerative. Developmental problems of the placenta include placental lesions, succenturiate placenta, circumvallate placenta, and battledore placenta (Table 27-3). Degenerative changes include infarcts and placental calcification.

Succenturiate Placenta

In *succenturiate placenta,* one or more accessory lobes of fetal villi have developed on the placenta, with vascular connections of fetal origin (see Table 27-3). Vessels from the major to the minor lobe(s) are supported only by the membranes, thus increasing the risk of the minor lobe's being retained during the third stage of labor.

The gravest maternal danger is postpartal hemorrhage if this minor lobe is severed from the placenta and remains in the uterus. All placentas should be examined closely for intactness. If vessels appear to be severed at the margin of the placenta, the uterus should be explored for retained placental tissue. This condition is not usually diagnosed until after the birth of the placenta.

Fetal/newborn implications can be life threatening if the vascular connections rupture between the placenta lobes because a fatal fetal hemorrhage can result. Examination of the fetal membrane following birth may reveal a small hole with vessels running toward it. This is another indication of a retained lobe (Gibbs et al., 2008). At birth, the infant should be inspected for

TABLE 27-3 Placental and Umbilical Cord Variations

PLACENTAL VARIATION	MATERNAL IMPLICATIONS	FETAL-NEONATAL IMPLICATIONS	
Succenturiate Placenta			
One or more accessory lobes of fetal villi will develop on the placenta.	Postpartal hemorrhage from retained lobe	None, as long as all parts of the placenta remain attached until after birth of the fetus	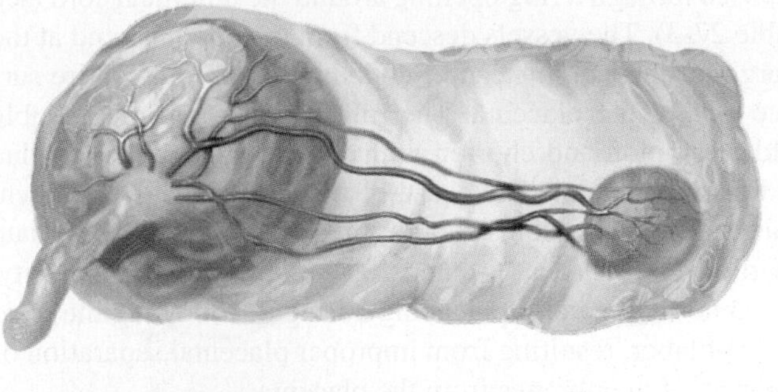
Circumvallate Placenta			
A double fold of chorion and amnion form a ring around the umbilical cord, on the fetal side of the placenta.	Increased incidence of late abortion, antepartal hemorrhage, and preterm labor	Intrauterine growth restriction, prematurity, fetal death	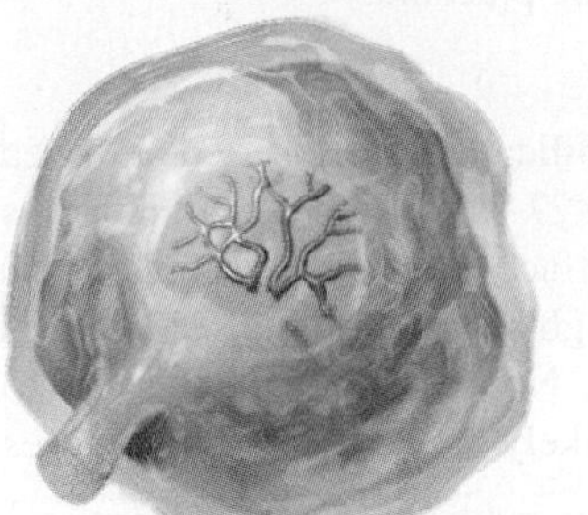
Battledore Placenta			
The umbilical cord is inserted at or near the placental margin.	Increased incidence of preterm labor and bleeding	Prematurity, fetal stress	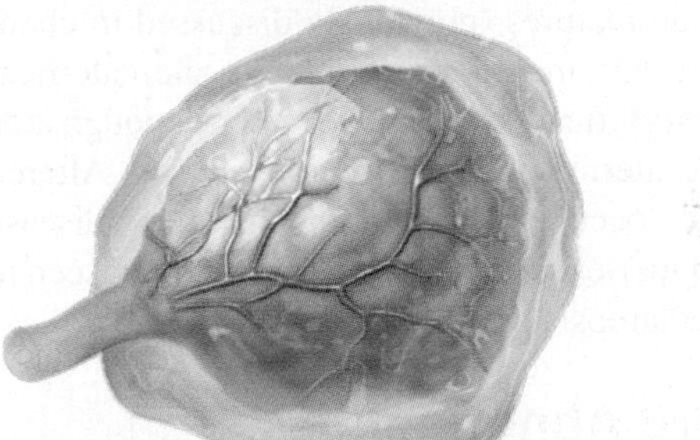
Velamentous Insertion of the Umbilical Cord			
The vessels of the umbilical cord divide some distance from the placenta in the placental membranes.	Hemorrhage if one of the vessels is torn	Fetal stress, hemorrhage	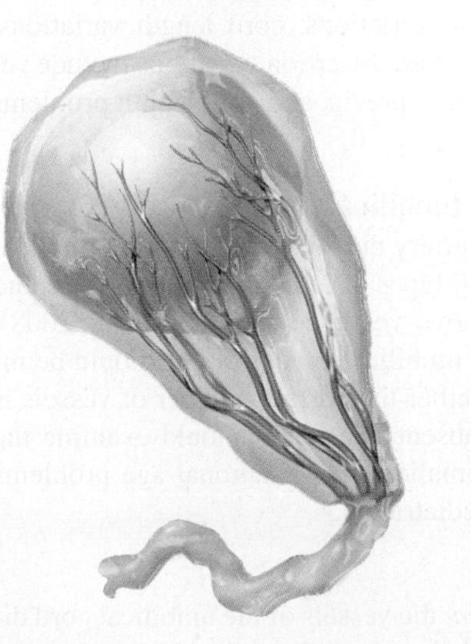

Source: Creasy & Resnik, 2009.

pallor, cyanosis, retractions, tachypnea, tachycardia, and feeble pulse. The infant's cry will be weak and the muscle tone flaccid.

Circumvallate Placenta

In *circumvallate placenta,* the fetal surface of the placenta is exposed through a ring opening around the umbilical cord (see Table 27-3). The vessels descend from the cord and end at the margin of the ring instead of coursing through the entire surface area of the placenta. The ring is composed of a double fold of amnion and chorion with some degenerative decidua and fibrin between. The cause of this condition is unknown. Maternal-fetal problems include an increased incidence of late abortion or fetal death, antepartal hemorrhage, prematurity, and abnormal maternal bleeding during or following the third stage of labor, resulting from improper placental separation or shearing of membranes from the placenta.

Battledore Placenta

In *battledore placenta,* the umbilical cord is inserted at or near the placental margin (see Table 27-3). As a result, all fetal vessels transverse the placental surface in the same direction. The chances of preterm labor are high because of interference with fetal circulation and nutrition. Nonreassuring fetal status or bleeding during labor is also likely because of cord compression or vessel rupture.

Placental Infarcts and Calcifications

As the placenta grade matures (previously discussed in chapter 26 ∞), the placenta may develop infarcts and calcifications. They become significant if they cover a large enough area to interfere with the uterine-placental-fetal exchange. Altered exchange can also occur with certain maternal disease processes, such as hypertension. Infarcts are most often seen in cases of severe preeclampsia and in women who smoke.

Umbilical Cord Abnormalities

Umbilical cord abnormalities include congenital absence of an umbilical artery, insertion variations, cord length variations, and knots and loops of the cord. Insertion variations include velamentous insertion and vasa previa, and cord length problems include long and short cords.

Congenital Absence of Umbilical Artery

Absence of an umbilical artery may have serious fetal implications. The incidence of all types of fetal anomalies is 33% and 74% in infants born with two-vessel cords (Gibbs et al., 2008).

Immediately after the umbilical cord is cut, it should be inspected to determine whether the correct number of vessels is present. If an artery is absent, the nurse should examine the newborn closely for anomalies and gestational age problems and alert the attending pediatrician.

Insertion Variations

In a *velamentous insertion,* the vessels of the umbilical cord divide some distance from the placenta in the placental membranes (see Table 27-3). Velamentous insertions occur more frequently in multiple gestations than in singletons. Other placental anomalies, such as succenturiate placenta, often accompany this condition. The velamentous insertion is more easily compressed or kinked during pregnancy or labor because of the lack of Wharton's jelly to protect it. If the vessels become torn during labor, fetal hemorrhage can occur, and the blood can escape from the vagina. When fetal hemorrhage occurs, it results in fetal heart rate (FHR) abnormalities.

When the vessels of a velamentous insertion transverse the internal os and appear in front of the fetus, a vasa previa has occurred. Fetal hemorrhage with asphyxia is likely to result because as the fetal blood escapes out of the vagina the hemorrhage will probably be diagnosed as maternal.

Cord Length Variations

The average length of the umbilical cord is 55 cm. Although short cords rarely cause complications directly, they have been associated with umbilical hernias in the fetus, abruptio placentae, and cord rupture. Long cords tend to twist and tangle around the fetus, causing transient variable decelerations. A long cord rarely causes fetal death, however, because it is generally not pulled tight until descent at the time of birth. With a long cord and an active fetus, one or more true knots can result. Again, these knots usually are not pulled tight enough to cause fetal stress until the infant has been born, and the cord can then be clamped and cut.

Clinical Therapy

The goals of medical treatment are to prevent serious fetal complications and to examine the newborn for anomalies that coexist with umbilical cord abnormalities.

Any vaginal bleeding during labor warrants continuous monitoring of the fetus, preferably with an external electronic monitor. Any signs of nonreassuring heart rate patterns should be reported immediately. In the presence of bleeding, laboratory tests may be used to differentiate fetal from maternal red blood cells. Fetal hemorrhage is resolved by terminating the pregnancy vaginally or through cesarean birth and by correcting neonatal anemia. Expediting the birth, whether vaginally or surgically, is paramount when a severe nonreassuring heart rate pattern is apparent. Following the birth, the pediatric team identifies and treats any neonatal complications or anomalies.

NURSING CARE MANAGEMENT

Nursing Assessment and Diagnosis

Umbilical abnormalities may not become evident until the birth of the fetus. During labor the nurse should observe for signs of nonreassuring fetal status and excessive bleeding (with velamentous insertion and vasa previa).

Nursing diagnoses that may apply include the following:

- ***Risk for Impaired Gas Exchange (Fetus)*** related to decreased blood flow secondary to placental abnormalities
- ***Deficient Knowledge*** regarding information about placental abnormalities related to an expressed desire to understand the implications of the finding

Nursing Plan and Implementation

The nurse is alert for an unusual amount of bleeding during the labor and birth. Following the birth, the placenta is inspected for abnormalities. Examination of the placenta by a pathologist may be indicated.

Often any mild or moderate variable deceleration can be successfully managed by the nurse. Repositioning of the woman often alleviates pressure on the cord if this is the reason for the deceleration.

Evaluation

Expected outcomes of nursing care include the following:

- The mother and baby have a safe labor and birth.
- The woman's bleeding is assessed quickly, and corrective measures are taken.
- The family is able to cope successfully with fetal or neonatal anomalies, if they exist.

Care of the Woman and Fetus with a Prolapsed Umbilical Cord

An umbilical cord that precedes the fetal presenting part is known as a **prolapsed umbilical cord**. It occurs when the cord falls or is washed down through the cervix into the vagina and becomes trapped between the presenting part and the maternal pelvis. The incidence of cord prolapse is 3% of vertex presentations and 3.7% of all breech presentations. It can also occur in compound presentations. Because of this entrapment, the vessels carrying blood to and from the fetus are compressed. In rare circumstances a prolapsed cord may be visible at the lower edge of the vagina. In other cases, the umbilical cord lies beside or just ahead of the fetal head; this is called *occult cord prolapse.*

Any time that the pelvic inlet is not completely filled by the fetus or the presenting part is not firmly against the cervix, and the membranes rupture, the umbilical cord can be washed down into the birth canal in front of the presenting part (Figure 27-14 ■).

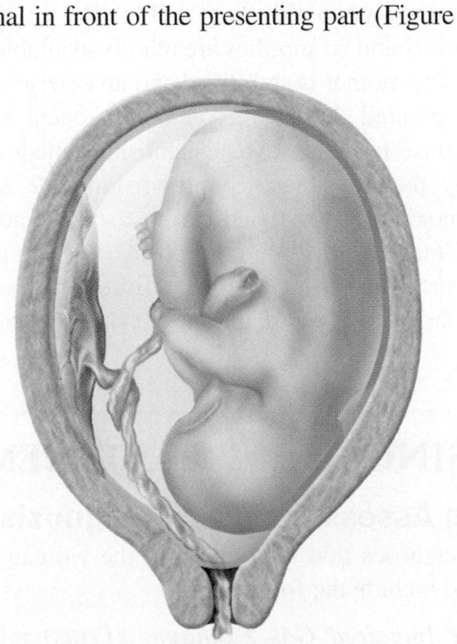

Figure 27-14 ■ Prolapse of the umbilical cord.

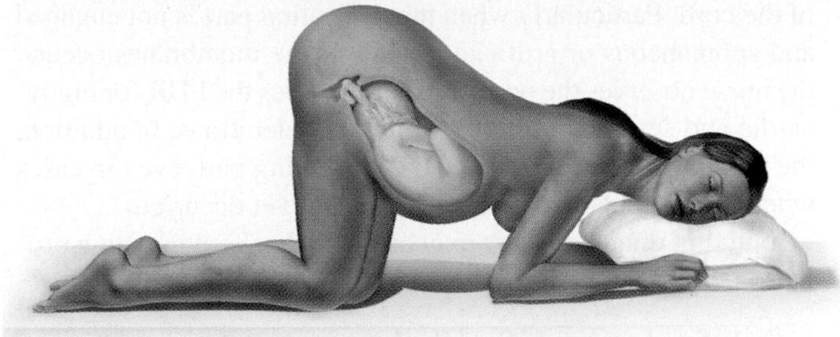

Figure 27-15 ■ Knee-chest position is used to relieve cord compression during cord prolapse emergency.

The incidence of prolapse of the cord is 20 times greater with abnormal axis lie (Cunningham et al., 2010)—especially footling breech and shoulder presentations—low birth weight, a multipara with more than five previous births, multiple gestation, polyhydramnios, unengaged presenting part, obstetric manipulation (amniotomy), and the presence of a long cord (longer than 80 cm). Approximately 50% of cord prolapses occur in the second stage of labor. An additional 47% of cord prolapses occur as a result of some obstetric intervention, such as amniotomy, application of fetal scalp electrode, intrapressure catheter, or external cephalic version (Nasser et al., 2006).

Application: Umbilical Cord Prolapse

Maternal-Fetal-Neonatal Risks

Although a prolapsed cord does not directly precipitate physical alterations in the woman, her immediate concern for the baby creates enormous stress. The woman may need to deal with some unusual interventions, a cesarean birth, and, in some circumstances, death of the fetus.

The fetus is affected because compression of the umbilical cord occludes blood flow through the umbilical vessels. Bradycardia (baseline fetal heart rate [BL FHR]) below 110 beats per minute) and persistent variable decelerations may develop. If labor is occurring, the cord is compressed further with each contraction. If the pressure on the cord is not relieved, the fetus will die.

Care Plan Activity: Prevention of Cord Prolapse

Clinical Therapy

Preventing the occurrence of cord prolapse is the preferred medical approach. For all laboring women with a history of ruptured membranes, bed rest is usually indicated until engagement with no cord prolapse has been documented. When prolapse does occur, it is usually discovered by the nurse, and relieving the compression of the cord by pushing back the presenting part (discussed shortly) is critical for the fetus. It is also effective to place the woman in a knee-to-chest position to relieve pressure on the cord (Figure 27-15 ■). The method of birth will most likely be cesarean unless a vaginal birth is imminent.

NURSING CARE MANAGEMENT

Nursing Assessment and Diagnosis

In the intrapartal area, the nurse reviews the nursing history and ascertains whether the woman is likely to be at risk for prolapse of the cord. Particularly when the presenting part is not engaged and spontaneous or artificial rupture of the membranes occurs, the nurse observes the perineum and assesses the FHR for bradycardia and severe, recurrent, variable decelerations. In addition, the pulsing cord could also be the presenting part, even in cases where dilatation and effacement have not yet occurred.

Nursing diagnoses that may apply to the woman with a prolapsed cord include the following:

- ***Risk for Impaired Gas Exchange (Fetus)*** related to decreased blood flow secondary to compression of the umbilical cord
- ***Fear*** related to unknown outcome

Nursing Plan and Implementation

Because there are few outward signs of cord prolapse, each pregnant woman is advised to call her physician or certified nurse-midwife (CNM) when the membranes rupture and to go immediately to the office, clinic, or birthing facility. A sterile vaginal examination determines whether there is danger of cord prolapse. If the presenting part is well engaged, the risk is minimal and ambulation may be encouraged. If the presenting part is not well engaged, bed rest is recommended to prevent cord prolapse. Maintaining bed rest after rupture of membranes can lead to conflict if the laboring woman and her partner wish to utilize ambulation. The nurse can ease this situation by helping communication between the physician or CNM and the couple.

Amniotic Fluid Problems

If membranes have not yet ruptured when the woman arrives at the facility, at the time of spontaneous rupture or amniotomy the fetal heart rate (FHR) should be monitored by electronic fetal monitoring (EFM) or auscultated for at least a full minute and again at the end of a contraction and after a few contractions. In the presence of cord prolapse, EFM tracings show baseline bradycardia or severe, moderate, or prolonged nonperiodic decelerations. If these patterns are found, the nurse performs a vaginal examination.

If a loop of cord is discovered, the nurse's gloved fingers are left in the vagina, and the presenting part is pushed upward to lift the fetal part off the cord and relieve cord compression until the physician or CNM arrives. This is a lifesaving measure. Oxygen is administered, and FHR is monitored by EFM to see if the cord compression is adequately relieved (baseline will rise above 110 beats per minute, and variable decelerations are lessened or relieved). The nurse may also feel pulsation in the cord; however, in some instances a pulsation cannot be felt, and FHR can be detected only by EFM. A large-gauge intravenous cannula is inserted and intravenous fluids should be initiated. Anesthesia and neonatology services should be notified of impending birth.

In some cases, another nurse may insert an indwelling bladder catheter and, using a sterile asepto syringe or infusion device, fill the bladder with approximately 500 ml of warmed, sterile normal saline. The filled bladder lifts the fetal head upward and relieves pressure on the umbilical cord. Filling her bladder and maintaining the woman in a side-lying position may be all that is needed to relieve the pressure on the cord. If the bladder is not filled, the force of gravity can be incorporated. In this instance, the nurse maintains pressure on the presenting part and instructs the woman to bring her knees to her chest or adjusts the bed to the Trendelenburg position. The nurse maintains pressure on the presenting part while the woman is transported to the birthing or operating room in this position. The nurse maintains this position until the fetus is born via cesarean birth.

Evaluation

Expected outcomes of nursing care include the following:

- The FHR remains in normal range with supportive measures.
- The fetus is born safely.
- The woman and her partner feel supported.
- The woman and her partner understand the problem and the corrective measures that are undertaken.

Care of the Woman and Fetus at Risk Because of Anaphylactoid Syndrome of Pregnancy (Amniotic Fluid Embolism)

Anaphylactoid syndrome of pregnancy or **amniotic fluid embolism** occurs when a bolus of amniotic fluid, fetal cells, hair, or other debris enters the maternal circulation and then the maternal lungs. The cause of this obstetric emergency is unknown but has a 60% to 80% mortality rate (Moore, 2008). It is the second leading cause of maternal deaths, resulting in 5% to 10% of all maternal deaths per year in the United States. It occurs in 1 in 8000 to 1 in 30,000 pregnancies (Moore, 2008). Because amniotic fluid embolism is a rare complication, a national registry was initiated in 1988 to collect retrospective data for analysis.

Clinical Therapy

When an amniotic fluid embolism is suspected, intravenous access is obtained as quickly as possible. The crash cart is accessed and on hand so supplies are readily available if a code is indicated. The mother is stabilized and an emergency cesarean birth is warranted. Symptoms generally occur rapidly so a quick response is imperative. Diagnosis is made by symptomology by the physician. Symptoms include shortness of breath, hypoxia, cyanosis, and cardiovascular and respiratory collapse (Creasy et al., 2009). Supportive nursing measures include preparations for an emergency birth and transfer of the mother to the intensive care unit after surgery is completed.

NURSING CARE MANAGEMENT

Nursing Assessment and Diagnosis

Nursing diagnoses that may apply to the woman with a prolapsed cord include the following:

- ***Risk for Impaired Gas Exchange (Fetus)*** related to decreased blood flow secondary to maternal hypoxia

- ***Risk for Impaired Gas Exchange (Mother)*** related to decreased blood flow secondary to amniotic fluid embolism
- ***Fear*** related to unknown outcome

Nursing Plan and Implementation

In the absence of the physician or certified nurse-midwife (CNM), the nurse administers oxygen under positive pressure until medical help arrives. An intravenous line is quickly established. If respiratory and cardiac arrest occurs, cardiopulmonary resuscitation (CPR) is initiated immediately. The obstetrician and anesthesiologist should be called immediately. If a perinatologist and/or hospital intensivist is on staff, they should also be called.

The nurse readies the equipment necessary for blood transfusion and for the insertion of the central venous pressure (CVP) line. As the blood volume is replaced, using fresh whole blood to provide clotting factors, the CVP is monitored frequently. In the presence of cor pulmonale, fluid overload could easily occur. The fetus is continually monitored. In women who are unresponsive to CPR, an emergent cesarean birth should be performed in an effort to save the fetus. CPR is continued throughout the cesarean procedure.

Evaluation

- The mother is treated with appropriate interventions to achieve stabilization.
- The fetus is delivered safely via cesarean birth.
- The family is informed and supported during emergency procedures.

Care of the Woman with a Uterine Rupture

Uterine rupture is a nonsurgical disruption of the uterine cavity. The incidence of uterine rupture is approximately 1 in 2000 births (Gabbe et al., 2007). A complete rupture is one in which the endometrium, myometrium, and serosa have separated. An *incomplete or partial rupture* is one in which not all layers, but some, have been disrupted. The extent of maternal and fetal distress is proportional to the degree of rupture. Rupture preceding labor is rare. It is most commonly associated with a previous uterine incision that ruptures during the labor process. It can also be caused from uterine manipulation (such as a version), an operative vaginal delivery, abdominal trauma, interval of birth between deliveries less than 18 months, postpartum fever during a previous cesarean birth, or a one-layer closure performed with a previous cesarean birth (Gabbe et al., 2007).

Clinical Therapy

Uterine rupture can only be diagnosed via a surgical incision, but suspected uterine rupture is based on maternal and fetal symptomology. If the rupture is accompanied by vaginal bleeding, the nurse initiates a pad count to keep track of bleeding. Preparations are made for an emergency birth and neonatology services are obtained if available in the practice setting. Neonatal resuscitation should be anticipated.

NURSING CARE MANAGEMENT

Nursing Assessment and Diagnosis

A nonreassuring fetal heart rate is commonly the earliest warning sign of a possible uterine rupture. It is sometimes associated with variable or late decelerations, followed by bradycardia (Gabbe et al., 2007). Upon palpation, there may be loss of a fetal station since the presenting part is no longer being held in place by the uterine wall. Maternal symptoms include constant abdominal pain, uterine tenderness, change in uterine shape, cessation of contractions, hematuria, and signs of shock. Uterine rupture can be suspected clinically but is confirmed surgically.

Nursing Plan and Implementation

When a nonreassuring fetal pattern is identified, the physician or certified nurse-midwife (CNM) is immediately contacted. Risk factors for uterine rupture should be reviewed. Women with a previous history of cesarean birth or uterine surgery are at risk for uterine rupture. Maternal signs and symptoms should be assessed, including pain, bleeding, and hematuria. Leopold's maneuvers and maternal vital signs should be performed. Birth via cesarean is warranted. The nurse prepares the woman for an emergency cesarean birth. The anesthesiologist should be called immediately. Blood should be typed and matched for possible transfusion. An additional intravenous line using an 18 gauge or larger cannula is placed. During the cesarean birth, the degree of rupture is assessed. If the uterus is unable to be repaired or if the mother is hemodynamically unstable, a hysterectomy is performed.

Nursing diagnosis for women experiencing a uterine rupture include the following:

- ***Risk for Impaired Gas Exchange (Fetus)*** related to decreased blood flow secondary to uterine rupture
- ***Risk for Impaired Gas Exchange (Mother)*** related to decreased blood flow secondary to uterine rupture
- ***Fear*** related to unknown outcome
- ***Anxiety*** related to emergency procedures and unknown fetal outcome
- ***Impaired Individual Coping*** due to emergent situation secondary to uterine rupture.

Evaluation

- The mother remains hemodynamically stable throughout emergency cesarean birth.
- The fetus retains optimal oxygenation until a safe birth is achieved.

Care of the Woman with Cephalopelvic Disproportion

The birth passage includes the maternal bony pelvis, beginning at the pelvic inlet and ending at the pelvic outlet, and the maternal soft tissues within these anatomic areas. A contracture (narrowing) in any of the described areas can result in **cephalopelvic disproportion (CPD)**. Abnormal fetal presentations and positions occur in CPD as the fetus moves to accommodate passage through the maternal pelvis.

Cephalopelvic Disproportion

TABLE 27-4 Clues to Contractures of Maternal Pelvis

- Diagonal conjugate less than 11.5 cm (contracture of inlet), outlet less than 8 cm (contracture of outlet)
- Unengaged fetal head in early labor in primigravidas (consider contracture of inlet, malpresentation, or malposition)
- Hypotonic uterine contraction pattern (consider contracted pelvis)
- Deflexion of fetal head (fetal head not flexed on fetal chest; may be associated with occiput posterior)
- Uncontrollable pushing before complete dilatation of cervix (may be associated with occiput posterior)
- Failure of fetal descent (consider contracture of inlet, midpelvis, or outlet)
- Edema of anterior portion (lip) of cervix (consider obstructed labor at the inlet)

The gynecoid and anthropoid pelvic types are usually adequate for vertex birth, but the android and platypelloid types predispose to CPD. Certain combinations of types also can result in pelvic diameters inadequate for vertex birth. (See chapter 10 ∞ for a description of the types of pelves and their implications for childbirth.) Clues that may lead to suspicion of contractures of the maternal pelvis are presented in Table 27-4. Women with a history of pelvic fractures may also be at risk for CPD (Cunningham et al., 2010).

Types of Contractures

There are two types of contractures: contractures of the inlet and contractures of the outlet.

Contractures of the Inlet

The pelvic inlet is contracted if the shortest anterior-posterior diameter is less than 10 cm or the greatest transverse diameter is less than 12 cm. The anterior-posterior diameter may be approximated by measuring the diagonal conjugate, which in the contracted inlet is less than 11.5 cm. Clinical and x-ray pelvimetry are used to determine the smallest anterior-posterior diameter through which the fetal head must pass.

The treatment goal is to allow the natural forces of labor to push the biparietal diameter of the fetal head beyond the potential interspinous obstruction. Although forceps may be used, they cause difficulty because pulling on the head destroys flexion and because they further diminish the available space. A bulging perineum and crowning indicate that the obstruction has been passed.

Contractures of the Outlet

An interischial tuberous diameter of less than 8 cm constitutes an outlet contracture. Outlet and midpelvic contractures frequently occur simultaneously. Whether vaginal birth can occur depends on the woman's interischial tuberous diameters and the fetal posterosagittal diameter.

Implications of Pelvic Contractures

Labor is prolonged and protracted in the presence of CPD, and premature rupture of the membranes (PROM) can result from the force of the unequally distributed contractions being exerted on the fetal membranes. In obstructed labor (the fetus is not able to pass through the birth canal), uterine rupture can also occur. With delayed descent, necrosis of maternal soft tissues can result from pressure exerted by the fetal head. Eventually, necrosis can cause fistulas from the vagina to other nearby structures. Difficult forceps-assisted births can also result in damage to maternal soft tissue.

If the membranes rupture and the fetal head has not entered the inlet, there is a danger of cord prolapse. Extreme molding of the fetal head can result. Traumatic forceps-assisted births can damage the fetal skull and CNS.

Clinical Therapy

Fetopelvic relationships can be assessed by comparing the estimated weight of the fetus as obtained by ultrasound measurements to pelvic measurements obtained by a manual examination before labor and by computed tomography (CT). Occasionally, in high-risk centers magnetic resonance imaging (MRI) is used to identify adequacy of pelvic diameters.

When the pelvic diameters are borderline or questionable, a trial of labor (TOL) may be advised. In this process the woman continues to labor, and careful assessments of uterine contractions, cervical dilatation, and fetal descent are made by the certified nurse-midwife (CNM) or physician and nurse. As long as there is continued progress, the TOL continues. If progress ceases, the decision for a cesarean birth is made.

NURSING CARE MANAGEMENT

Nursing Assessment and Diagnosis

The adequacy of the maternal pelvis for a vaginal birth should be assessed intrapartally as well as antepartally. During the intrapartal assessment, the size of the fetus and its presentation, position, and lie must also be considered. (See chapter 23 ∞ for intrapartal assessment techniques.)

The nurse should suspect CPD when labor is prolonged, cervical dilatation and effacement are slow, and engagement of the presenting part is delayed or lack of fetal descent occurs.

Nursing diagnoses that may apply include the following:

- ***Deficient Knowledge*** related to lack of information about implications of CPD
- ***Fear*** related to unknown outcome of labor

Nursing Plan and Implementation

Nursing actions during the TOL are similar to care during any labor, with the exception that the assessments of cervical dilatation and fetal descent are done more frequently. Contractions should be monitored and the labor progress charted. The fetus should also be monitored frequently. Any signs of fetal stress are reported to the physician or CNM immediately.

The woman may be positioned in a variety of ways to increase the pelvic diameters. Sitting or squatting increases the outer diameters and may be effective in instances where there is failure of or slow fetal descent. Changing from one side to the other or maintaining a hands-and-knees position may assist the fetus in occiput posterior (OP) position to change to an occiput anterior (OA) position. The woman may instinctively want to assume one of these positions. If not, the nurse may encourage a change of position. Women with an epidural may use position changes with adequate support.

A couple may need help in coping with the stresses of complicated labor. The nurse should keep the couple informed of what is happening and explain the procedures that are being used. This should reassure the couple that measures are being taken to resolve the problem.

Evaluation

Expected outcomes of nursing care include the following:

- The woman's fear is lessened.
- The woman has additional knowledge regarding the problems, implications, and treatment plans.

Care of the Woman at Risk Because of Complications of Third and Fourth Stages of Labor

Common complications of the third and fourth stages of labor include retained placenta, lacerations, and placenta accrete (Cunningham et al., 2010).

Retained Placenta

Retention of the placenta beyond 30 minutes after birth is termed **retained placenta**. It occurs in 2% to 3% of all vaginal births. Bleeding as a result of a retained placenta can be excessive. If placenta expulsion does not occur, a manual removal of the placenta by the physician or certified nurse-midwife (CNM) is attempted. In women who do not have an epidural in place, intravenous sedation may be required because of the discomfort caused by the procedure. Retained placenta may be a symptom of an accreta, increta, or percreta (to be discussed shortly). Failure to retrieve the placenta via manual removal usually necessitates surgical removal by curettage. If the woman does not have an epidural in place, the procedure can be performed under general anesthesia.

Lacerations

Lacerations of the cervix or vagina may be present when bright red vaginal bleeding persists in the presence of a well-contracted uterus. The incidence of lacerations is higher among childbearing women who are young, are nulliparous, have an epidural block, undergo forceps-assisted or vacuum-assisted birth, or undergo an episiotomy. Vaginal and perineal lacerations are often categorized in terms of degree:

- First-degree laceration is limited to the fourchette, perineal skin, and vaginal mucous membrane.
- Second-degree laceration involves the perineal skin, vaginal mucous membrane, underlying fascia, and muscles of the perineal body; it may extend upward on one or both sides of the vagina.
- Third-degree laceration extends through the perineal skin, vaginal mucous membranes, and perineal body and involves the anal sphincter; it may extend up the anterior wall of the rectum.
- Fourth-degree laceration is the same as the third degree but extends through the rectal mucosa to the lumen of the rectum; it may be called a third-degree laceration with a rectal wall extension.

Placenta Accreta

In **placenta accreta**, the chorionic villi attach directly to the myometrium of the uterus. Two other types of placental adherence are **placenta increta**, in which the myometrium is invaded, and **placenta percreta**, in which the myometrium is penetrated. These placenta adherent disorders can be life threatening. The adherence itself may be total, partial, or focal, depending on the amount of placental involvement. The incidence of placenta accreta is 1 in 2500 births (Cunningham et al., 2010). Placenta accreta is the most common type of adherent placenta. Previous cesarean births increase the risk of placenta accreta. This is of concern with the rapidly rising cesarean section rate within the United States.

The primary complication of placenta accreta is maternal hemorrhage and failure of the placenta to separate following birth of the infant. An abdominal hysterectomy may be the necessary treatment, depending on the amount and depth of involvement. Chapter 39 ∞ discusses hemorrhage following birth.

The at-risk conditions during labor discussed in this chapter can, in some cases, lead to fetal demise. See chapter 38 ∞ for an in-depth discussion of caring for the family experiencing perinatal loss.

FOCUS YOUR STUDY

- Intense anxiety; fear; loss of orientation to person, place, or time; or other inappropriate behaviors may be associated with an underlying psychologic disorder that results in difficulties with coping.
- Hypotonic labor patterns begin normally and then progress to infrequent, less intense contractions. If there are no contraindications, oxytocin is administered intravenously as treatment.
- Precipitous labor and birth is extremely rapid labor and birth that lasts less than 3 hours. It is associated with an increased risk to the mother and newborn infant.
- Postterm pregnancy is one that extends more than 294 days, or 42 weeks, past the first day of the last menstrual period.
- The occiput-posterior position of the fetus prolongs the labor process, causes severe back discomfort in the laboring woman, and predisposes her to vaginal and perineal trauma and lacerations during birth.
- The types of fetal malpresentations include face, brow, breech, and shoulder.
- A fetus or newborn weighing more than 4000 g is termed *macrosomic.* Macrosomia may lead to problems during labor and birth and in the early neonatal period.
- Prolapsed umbilical cord results when the umbilical cord precedes the fetal presenting part. When this occurs, pressure is placed on the umbilical cord, and blood flow to the fetus is diminished.
- Anaphylactoid syndrome of pregnancy or amniotic fluid embolism occurs when a bolus of amniotic fluid enters the maternal circulation and then enters the maternal lungs. Maternal mortality is very high with this complication.
- Uterine rupture occurs when the layers of the uterine cavity are separated by a nonsurgical event and requires an emergency cesarean birth be performed immediately.
- Cephalopelvic disproportion occurs when there is a narrowed diameter in the maternal pelvis. The narrowed diameter is called a contracture, and it may occur in the pelvic inlet, midpelvis, or outlet. If pelvic measurements are borderline, a trial of labor may be attempted. Failure of cervical dilatation or fetal descent would then necessitate a cesarean birth.
- Third- and fourth-stage complications usually involve a hemorrhage. Causes of hemorrhage include lacerations of the birth canal or cervix, retained placenta, and placenta accreta.
- Nonreassuring fetal status is indicated by persistent late decelerations, persistent severe variable decelerations, and prolonged decelerations. If fetal stress is recognized and treated appropriately, the fetus may be spared any permanent damage.

CRITICAL THINKING IN ACTION

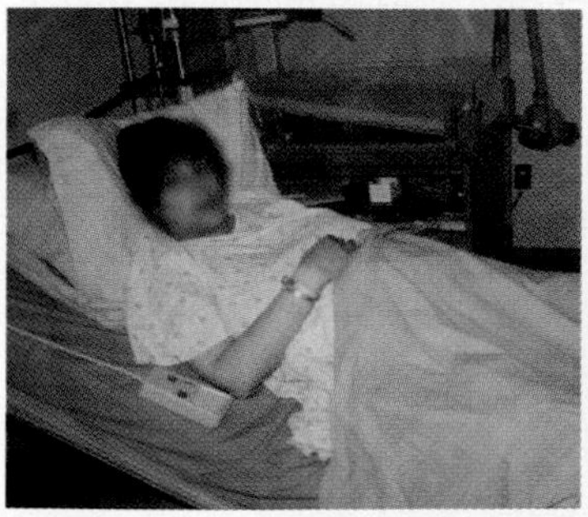

Source: George Dodson/Pearson Education.

June Dice, a 25-year-old G3, P1011, is admitted to labor and delivery at 38 weeks with a moderate amount of dark red vaginal bleeding. June's prenatal history is significant for late prenatal care (20 weeks' gestation by ultrasound) and cocaine abuse. An ultrasound is done upon admission that demonstrates a marginal placenta abruption. You place June on the fetal monitor and observe a fetal heart rate baseline of 146 to 155 with accelerations to 166 with fetal movement. There are occasional mild variable decelerations with a quick return to baseline. Contraction pattern is interpreted as an irritable uterus. An intravenous infusion with Ringer's lactate is started with a #18 intracath. June's vital signs are within normal limits. Her hematocrit is 29%. You assist the physician with a vaginal exam to rupture membranes and insert a fetal scalp electrode and intrauterine pressure catheter. A small amount of light, yellow-green amniotic fluid is observed. The exam shows June is 4 cm dilated, 50% effaced, vertex at –1 station. You follow protocol and start an oxytocin induction/augmentation. June is asking why oxytocin is needed.

1. Explain the goal of labor induction/augmentation in response to June's question.
2. Explain potential risk factors associated with oxytocin induction of labor.
3. You observe a nonreassuring fetal heart rate of 144 to 150 with decreased variability, and persistent late decelerations with each contraction. What interventions would you immediately take?
4. What supportive actions are taken to decrease the risk of hypofibrinogenemia?
5. What complications might be present in the newborn at birth?

See www.nursing.pearsonhighered.com for possible responses.

Pearson Nursing Student Resources
Find additional review materials at
www.nursing.pearsonhighered.com
Prepare for success with additional NCLEX®-style practice questions, interactive assignments and activities, Web links, animations and videos, and more!

REFERENCES

American College of Obstetricians and Gynecologists (ACOG). (2006). *Mode of term singleton breech delivery.* (ACOG Committee Opinion No. 340). Washington, DC: Author.

American College of Obstetricians and Gynecologists (ACOG). (2007). *Treatment with selective serotonin reuptake inhibitors during pregnancy.* ACOG Committee Practice Bulletin No. 354. Washington, DC: ACOG.

American College of Obstetricians and Gynecologists (ACOG). (2008). *Use of psychiatric medications during pregnancy and lactation.* ACOG Practice Bulletin No. 92. Washington, DC: ACOG.

Bashiri, A., Burstein, E., Bar-David, J., Levy, A., & Mazor, M. (2008). Face and brow presentation: Independent risk factors. *Journal of Maternal Fetal Neonatal Medicine, 21*(6), 357–360.

Battista, L. R., & Wing, D. H. (2007). Abnormal labor and induction of labor. In S. G. Gabbe, J. R. Niebyl, & J. L. Simpson (Eds.). *Obstetrics: Normal and problem pregnancies* (5th ed.). Philadelphia, PA: Churchill Livingstone.

Beckmann, C. R. B., Ling, F. W., Barzansky, B. M., Herbert, W. N. P., Laube, D. W., & Smith, R. P. (2008). *Obstetrics & gynecology* (6th ed.). Washington, DC: ACOG.

Caughey, A. B., Nicholson, J. M., & Washington, A. E. (2008). First vs. second trimester ultrasound: The effect on pregnancy dating and perinatal outcomes. *American Journal of Obstetrics & Gynecology, 198*(6), 703.e1–6.

Caughey, A. B., Snegovskikh, V. V., & Norwitz, E. R. (2008). Postterm pregnancy: How can we improve outcomes? *Obstetrical & Gynecological Survey, 63*(11), 715–724.

Chaillet, N., & Dumont, A. (2007). Evidence-based strategies for reducing cesarean section rates: A meta-analysis. *Birth, 12,* 53–64. Published online: February 26, 2007, 12:00 a.m. doi: 10.1111/j.1523-536X.2006.00146.x

Creasy, R. K., Resnik, R., Iams, J. D., Lockwood, C. J., & Moore, T. R. (2009). *Creasy & Resnik's maternal-fetal medicine: Principles and practice* (6th ed.). Philadelphia, PA: Saunders Elsevier.

Cunningham, F. G., Leveno, K. J., Bloom, S. L., Hauth, J. C., Gilstrap, L. C., & Wenstrom, K. D. (2010). *Williams obstetrics* (23rd ed.). New York, NY: McGraw-Hill.

Ford, E., & Ayers, S. (2009). Stressful events and support during birth: The effect on anxiety, mood and perceived control. *Journal of Anxiety Disorders, 23*(2), 260–268. doi:10.1016/j.janxdis.2008.07.009

Gabbe, S. G., Niebyl, J. R., & Simpson, J. L. (2007). *Obstetrics: Normal and problem pregnancies* (5th ed.). Philadelphia, PA: Churchill Livingstone.

Gibbs, R. S., Karlan, B. Y., Haney, A. F., & Nygaard, I. (2008). *Danforth's obstetrics and gynecology.* (10th ed.). Philadelphia, PA: Wolters Kluwer/Lippincott Williams & Wilkins.

Heywood, R. E., Magann, E. F., Rich, D. L., & Chauhan, S. P. (2008). The detection of macrosomia at a teaching hospital. *American Journal of Perinatology, 26*(2), 165–168.

Hillier, T. A., Pedula, K. L., Vesco, K. K., Schmidt, M. M., Mullen, J. A., LeBlanc, E. S., & Pettitt, D. J. (2008). Excess maternal weight gain: Modifying fetal macrosomia risk associated with maternal glucose. *Obstetrics & Gynecology, 112*(5), 1007–1014.

Hunter, S., Hofmeyr, G. J., & Kulier, R. (2007). Hands and knees position posture in late pregnancy and labour for fetal malposition. *Cochrane Database Systematic Review, 17*(4): CD001063.

Landon, M. B., Catalano, P. M., & Gabbe, S. G. 2007. Diabetes mellitus complicating pregnancy. In *Obstetrics: Normal and problem pregnancies* (5th ed.). Philadelphia, PA: Churchill Livingstone.

Macones, G. A., Hankins, G. D., Spong, C. Y., Hauth, J. D., & Moore, T. (2008). The 2008 National Institute of Child Health Human Development workshop report on electronic fetal monitoring: Update on definitions, interpretations, and research guidelines. *Obstetrics & Gynecology, 112,* 661–666; and *Journal of Obstetric, Gynecologic, and Neonatal Nursing, 37,* 510–515.

Magliore, L., & Copel, J. A. How useful a role might US play in full-term laboring patients for estimating fetal weight. *Contemporary OB/GYN,* 01 May 2007, vol./is. 52/5 (81–84), 00903159.

Moore, L. E. (2008). Amniotic fluid embolism. Retrieved from http://emedicine.medscape.com/article/253068

Nasser, N., Roberts, C. L., Barratt, A., Bell, J. C., Olive, E. C., & Peat, B. (2006). Systematic review of adverse outcomes of external cephalic version and persisting breech presentation at term. *Paediatric Perinatal Epidemiology, 20*(2), 163–171.

National Institute of Mental Health (NIMH). (2009). *Prevalence of psychologic disorders,* Rockville, MD: Author.

Norwitz, E. R., Snegovskikh, V. V., & Caughey, A. B. (2007). Prolonged pregnancy: When should we intervene? *Clinical Obstetrics and Gynecology, 50*(2), 547–557.

Ridley, R. T. (2007). Diagnosis and intervention for occiput posterior malposition. *Journal of Obstetric, Gynecologic, and Neonatal Nursing, 36*(2), 135–143.

Rubio, A. S., Griffet, J. R., Caci, H., Bérard, E., El Hayek, T., & Boutté, P. (2009). The moulded baby syndrome: Incidence and risk factors regarding 1,001 neonates. *European Journal of Pediatrics, 168*(5), 605–611. Epub 2008 Sep 16.

Simpson, K. R., & Creehan, P. A. (2007). *AWHONN's perinatal nursing* (3rd ed.). Washington, DC: AWHONN.

Strasser, S. M., Kwee, N., & Visser, G. H. A. (2009). Spontaneous tachysystole as a sign of serious perinatal complications. *Journal of Maternal-Fetal Medicine.* doi: 10.3109/14767050903300951

Wei, S., Wo, B. L., Xu, H., Luo, Z. C., Roy, C., & Fraser, W. D. (2009). Early amniotomy and early oxytocin for prevention of, or therapy for, delay in first stage spontaneous labour compared with routine care. *Cochrane Database of Systematic Reviews* 2009, Issue 2. Art. No.: CD006794. doi: 10.1002/14651858.CD006794.pub2.

Zayed, F., Amarin, Z., Obeidat, B., Alchalabi, H., & Lataifeh, I. (2008). Face and brow presentation in Northern Jordan, over a decade of experience. *Archives of Gynecology & Obstetrics, 278*(5), 427–430.

CHAPTER 28

Birth-Related Procedures

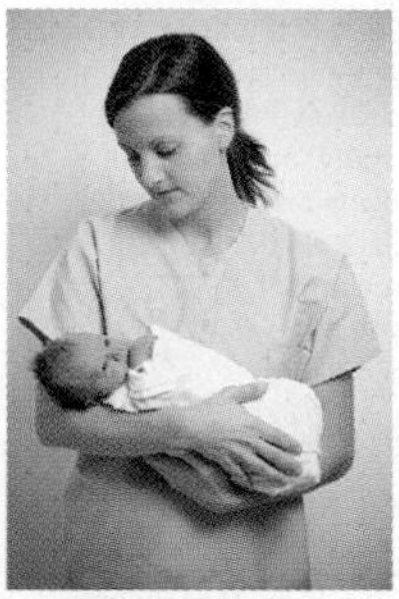

*W*ith our first baby I suddenly had to have a cesarean. Everything happened so fast, but our son was OK, and that's all that mattered. With our second baby, I wanted to try for a vaginal birth but nevertheless I was afraid. I don't know what I would have done without my nurse. She stayed with me the whole time I labored and kept giving me support. She explained everything, so I knew what was happening. I felt safe. I had a beautiful baby girl after 8 hours of labor. Everything went well postpartally, and I am so glad I was able to avoid another cesarean. We don't plan to have another baby, but if we did, I wouldn't be so afraid.

LEARNING OUTCOMES

1. Describe the impact of selected procedures on the childbearing woman and her family or support system.
2. Contrast the methods of external cephalic version and internal version and the related nursing management.
3. Discuss the use of amniotomy in current maternal-newborn care.
4. Compare methods for inducing labor, explaining their advantages and disadvantages.
5. Discuss the use of transcervical intrapartum amnioinfusion.
6. Describe the types of episiotomies performed, the rationale for each, and the associated nursing interventions.
7. Summarize the indications for forceps-assisted birth, types of forceps that may be used, complications, and related interventions.
8. Discuss the use of vacuum extraction, including indications, procedure, complications, and related nursing management.
9. Explain the indications for cesarean birth, impact on the family unit, preparation and teaching needs, and associated nursing management.
10. Discuss vaginal birth following cesarean birth.

KEY TERMS

Amnioinfusion (AI) *740*
Amniotomy *736*
Cervical ripening *728*
Cesarean birth *748*
Episiotomy *741*
External cephalic version (ECV) *725*
Forceps-assisted birth *743*
Labor augmentation *731*
Labor induction *731*
Podalic version *725*
Vacuum extraction *745*
Vaginal birth after cesarean (VBAC) *752*

Most births occur without the need for operative obstetric intervention. In some instances, however, obstetric procedures are necessary to maintain the safety of the woman and the fetus. The most common obstetric procedures are electronic fetal monitoring, version, amniotomy, induction of labor, episiotomy, cesarean birth, and vaginal birth following a previous cesarean birth.

Generally, women are aware of the possible need for an obstetric procedure during their labor and birth, and many women accept whatever procedure is recommended based on the belief that the caregiver knows what is needed and that it is in the baby's best interest. However, some women expect to have a "natural" birth experience and do not desire or anticipate any medical intervention. These women may feel disappointed or even guilty when an unanticipated obstetric procedure is needed. The nurse can provide information regarding any procedure to enhance the understanding of the woman and her partner of what is proposed, the anticipated benefits and possible risks, and any possible alternative treatments.

The nurse must provide emotional support to the woman and her family to assist them in accepting the unanticipated procedure. Although the physical responses to interventions are constantly monitored and documented, it is especially important for nurses to continually assess and document the family's emotional responses to interventions. Many times it is the nurse who plays a key role in emotional support and teaching. The importance of this role is just as imperative to any physical care that the nurse performs for the laboring woman and her family.

Care of the Woman During Version

Version, or turning the fetus, is a procedure used to change the fetal presentation by abdominal or intrauterine manipulation. The most common type of version is **external cephalic version (ECV)** in which the fetus is changed from a breech, transverse, or oblique lie to a cephalic presentation by external manipulation of the maternal abdomen (Figure 28-1 ■). The success rates for version are the highest for transverse presentations. Overall, success rates for version average 60% (Cunningham et al., 2010). Successful ECVs decrease the chances of nonvertex and cesarean births.

The other type of version, called a **podalic version** (also called an *internal version*), is used only with the second twin during a vaginal birth. In an internal version, the obstetrician places a hand inside the uterus, grabs the fetus's feet, and then turns the fetus from a transverse or noncephalic presentation to a breech presentation (Figure 28-2 ■). The fetus is then born in a breech presentation. This maneuver is used only when the second twin is not in a cephalic position. It is considered superior to an external cephalic version because it causes fewer decelerations (Cunningham et al., 2010). Some obstetricians may elect to have the second twin be born by cesarean if the twin is not in a cephalic presentation.

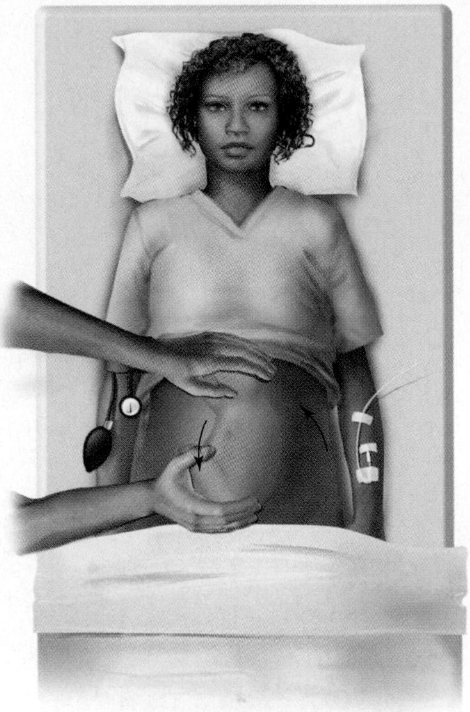

Figure 28-1 ■ External (or cephalic) version of the fetus. A new technique involves applying pressure to the fetal head and buttocks so that the fetus completes a "backward flip" or "forward roll."

External Cephalic Version

If breech or shoulder presentation (transverse lie) is detected in the later weeks of pregnancy, an external cephalic version (ECV) may be attempted. The version is usually done after 36 to 37 weeks' gestation because most fetuses still in breech presentation at this time will not spontaneously change back to a vertex presentation. This provides time for the fetus to assume a vertex position spontaneously. In addition, if complications arise from the procedure, the risk of prematurity is eliminated. Even when ECV is successful, there is some evidence that the stress of the procedure may increase the rate of intrapartum cesarean births. Breech fetuses have been shown to have smaller head circumferences, lower birth weight, and lower fetoplacental ratios. Fetuses that were previously breech tend to have higher rates of nonreassuring fetal status and dystocia. These mothers may also have a smaller pelvis, which may be the cause of the breech presentation in the first place (Creasy, Resnik, Iams, et al., 2008). Factors associated with higher success rates include higher parity, adequate amniotic fluid, lack of fetal engagement, transverse lie, a palpable fetal head, and a relaxed uterus (Cunningham et al., 2010; Kok et al., 2008). Factors associated with higher failure rates include nulliparity, advanced dilatation, fetal weight less than 2500 g, anterior placenta, a low station, maternal obesity, decreased amniotic fluid volume, and anterior or posterior positioning of the fetal spine (Cunningham et al., 2010).

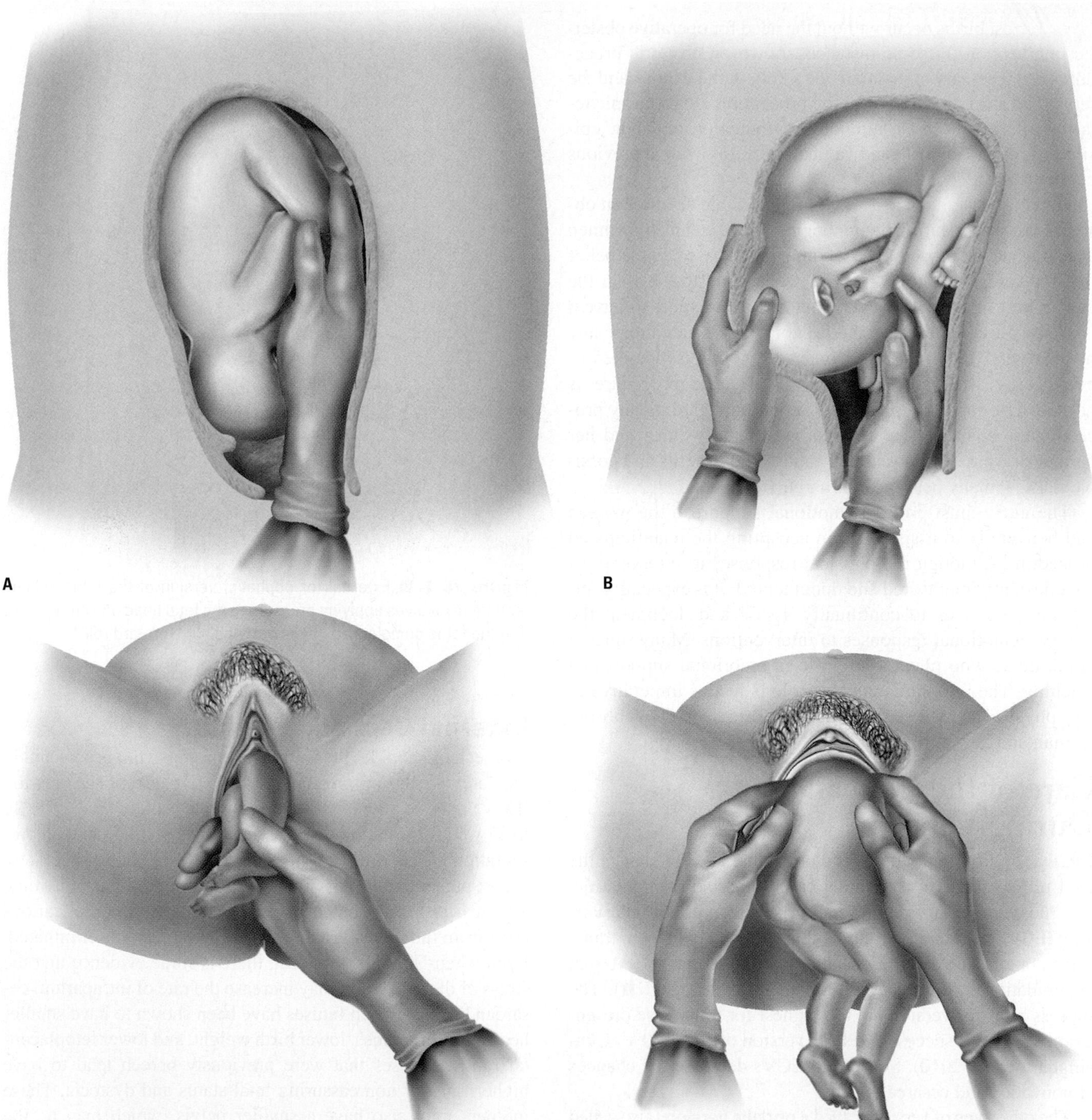

Figure 28-2 ■ Use of podalic version and extraction of the fetus to assist in the vaginal birth of the second twin. A. The physician reaches into the uterus and grasps a foot. Although a vertex birth is always preferred in a singleton birth, in this instance of assisting in the birth of a second twin it is not possible to grasp any other fetal part. The fetal head would be too large to grasp and pull downward, and grasping the fetal arm would result in a transverse lie and make vaginal birth impossible. B. While applying pressure on the outside of the abdomen to push the baby's head up toward the top of the uterus with one hand, the physician pulls the baby's foot down toward the cervix. C. Both feet have been pulled through the cervix and vagina. D. The physician now grasps the baby's trunk and continues to pull downward on the baby to assist the birth.

Criteria for External Version

The following criteria should be met before performing ECV (Creasy et al., 2008):

- A single fetus (also called a singleton) must be present. If a multiple gestation exists, a variety of concerns preclude an external version. For example, a cesarean rather than vaginal birth may need to be considered, and the fetuses might become entangled during a version.
- The fetal breech is not engaged. Once the presenting part is engaged, it is difficult, if not impossible, to do a version.
- An adequate amount of amniotic fluid must exist. The amniotic fluid helps ease movement of the fetus and provides adequate room for the umbilical cord to float without being compressed.
- A reactive nonstress test (NST) should be obtained immediately before performing the version. A reactive NST indicates fetal well-being.
- The fetus must be 36 to 37 or more weeks' gestation. A version may be accompanied by complications that require immediate birth by cesarean. If gestation is less than 37 weeks, a preterm birth would result.

(*Note:* Occasionally, a physician may do an external version while the woman is in early labor before the presenting part has become engaged.)

Contraindications for External Version

Absolute contraindications to ECV include the following (Cunningham et al., 2010):

- ***Suspected intrauterine growth restriction.*** The fetus has been stressed and amniotic fluid may be decreased.
- ***Fetal anomalies.*** This category includes major abnormalities.
- ***Presence of an abnormal fetal heart rate (FHR) tracing.*** A nonreassuring FHR pattern might indicate that the fetus is already stressed and other action needs to be taken.
- ***Rupture of the membranes.*** Rupture of the membranes would result in an inadequate amount of amniotic fluid.
- ***Cesarean birth indicated anyway.*** ECV should not be attempted if there is a contraindication to vaginal delivery.
- ***Maternal problems.*** Maternal problems include gestational diabetes that has required insulin, uncontrolled chronic hypertension, preeclampsia, or maternal cardiac disease.
- ***Amniotic fluid abnormalities.*** Oligohydramnios (amniotic fluid index less than 5 cm) makes the fetus difficult to maneuver and increases risk of umbilical cord compression. Hydramnios (amniotic fluid index greater than 25 cm) stretches the uterine walls, increasing pressure and decreasing the chance the fetus will remain in a cephalic presentation.

Relative contraindications to ECV include the following:

- ***Previous lower uterine segment cesarean birth.*** Prior scarring of the uterus may increase the risk of uterine tearing or uterine rupture.
- ***Nuchal cord.*** A nuchal cord may tighten around the fetal neck and decrease circulation to the fetus.
- ***Multiple gestation.***
- ***Evidence of uteroplacental insufficiency.***
- ***Significant third trimester bleeding.***
- ***Uterine malformation.***

External Version Procedure

The external version is accomplished in a birthing unit, rather than an outpatient setting, in case further intervention (such as emergency cesarean birth) is necessary. There have been no reported fetal deaths from the procedure since 1980. The risk of major complications resulting from an ECV has been reported as 1% to 2%. A systematic review with a total of 2503 women in 11 studies of adverse outcomes of ECV found no increased risk of antepartum fetal death, uterine rupture, placental abruption, prelabor rupture of membranes, or cord prolapse (Nassar et al., 2006).

The woman is instructed to fast for 8 hours preceding the version in case a cesarean birth needs to be performed because of complications. The physician uses ultrasound to confirm the presence of a single fetus, the amount of amniotic fluid, the location of the placenta, the position of the umbilical cord, and that a breech presentation still exists. Maternal vital signs are assessed, and continuous electronic fetal monitoring (EFM) is done to evaluate the fetal heart rate (FHR), to obtain a reactive NST, and to evaluate the presence of uterine activity. Blood work may be drawn, including a complete blood count (CBC) and a blood type and antibody screen (if not already available). The physician explains the procedure and the patient signs a consent form.

An intravenous line is established for medication administration and in case of difficulties. A beta-mimetic agent (a subcutaneous dose of terbutaline) or intravenous infusion of magnesium sulfate (if a beta-mimetic agent is contraindicated because of a medical condition) is administered to achieve uterine relaxation. Occasionally, some physicians do not use a beta-mimetic agent during the version. However, it greatly enhances the comfort of the woman. The use of epidural and spinal analgesia has been found to increase success rates, although further research is needed (Cunningham et al., 2010; Weiniger et al., 2007).

The woman is placed in a supine or slight Trendelenburg position. Once uterine relaxation is achieved, the maternal abdomen is copiously covered with warmed ultrasound gel to decrease excessive manipulation and friction, and the physician grasps the fetal breech between the index finger and the thumb. First the presenting part is gently pushed upward or lifted out of the maternal pelvis by exerting pressure over the skin on the maternal abdomen. If the fetal breech can be lifted out, then the breech and head are rotated or moved out in opposite directions. In most cases, a direction similar to a forward roll is attempted initially. If that is not successful, a roll in the opposite direction is attempted. The procedure should be concluded when any of the following occur: the fetal head is moved to a head-down position; repeated failures have occurred; the woman has indicated that the procedure has become too painful or stressful; or signs of maternal or fetal problems occur, including a nonreassuring FHR pattern (Cunningham et al., 2010). The intravenous tocolytic agent is discontinued, and frequently the fetus is held in the new presentation by either the physician or the nurse until the uterus regains tone. In the event of a failed version, a repeat attempt can be made within a week if the procedure was well tolerated by the woman and her fetus. The risk of maternal-fetal hemorrhage is 2.4% (Boucher, Marquette, Varin, et al., 2008). (See chapter 20 ∞). Ultrasound is performed to confirm the fetal position. A vaginal examination may be performed to evaluate cervical dilatation and fetal descent; however, there is no evidence to support the routine practice of immediate induction of labor to minimize reversion (American College of Obstetricians and Gynecologists (ACOG), 2008). Spontaneous reversion can also occur, but the risk is decreased with term gestations compared with earlier gestations (ACOG, 2008).

External cephalic version has been the subject of several recent systematic evidence reviews. A recent review of interventions (tocolysis, vibroacoustic stimulation of the fetus, epidural or spinal anesthesia, and amnioinfusion) to facilitate ECV in term infants found routine tocolysis was likely to increase the success rates of ECV (Collaris & Tan, 2009).

A recent evidence review of the efficacy of moxibustion to assist in turning a baby from its breech position found positive results. Moxibustion is a type of Chinese medicine that involves burning an herb close to the skin. Evidence was found to support its use in correcting a breech presentation, and it was noted that moxibustion may be beneficial in reducing the need for ECV (Li, Hu, Wang, et al., 2009).

NURSING CARE MANAGEMENT

The nurse begins by ensuring that the expectant woman understands the procedure, knows that the procedure may be uncomfortable or very painful, and realizes that she can tell the physician to stop if the pain is too great.

The possibility of failure of the ECV and the slight risk of a cesarean birth if the fetus exhibits a nonreassuring fetal status should also be discussed. Before the version, the nurse explains the procedure and possible outcomes, then completes initial maternal and fetal assessments, provides ongoing evaluation of FHR, and performs the NST. The nurse obtains blood work and alerts the obstetrical team regarding the procedure in the rare event that a cesarean birth should be necessary. The nurse provides psychologic support through reassurance and continuous explanations throughout the procedure. The nurse continues to monitor maternal blood pressure and pulse about every 2 minutes throughout the period of time the beta-mimetic agent is used and for about 30 minutes after. The FHR is monitored for approximately 1 to 2 hours following the ECV. The nurse also assesses the maternal-fetal response to the tocolytic agent. The nurse continues to provide information by reiterating aftercare instructions, such as monitoring for uterine contractions, being aware of fetal movement (fetal kick counts), and recognizing signs of reversion (excessive movement or a sensation described as the fetus "turning around").

Care of the Woman During Cervical Ripening

Induction of labor may be necessary or beneficial in certain clinical situations. When the cervix is unfavorable, the use of cervical ripening agents increase the likelihood of a successful induction of labor (see Bishop Score and Table 28-3 ∞ on page 732). Misoprostol (Cytotec) and formulations of Prostaglandin E_2 (PGE_2) gel for **cervical ripening** (softening and effacing the cervix) are drugs that may be used for the pregnant woman at or near term when there is a medical or obstetric indication for induction of labor. Mechanical methods designed to ripen the cervix employ the use of balloon catheters to encourage mechanical dilatation.

Use of Misoprostol (Cytotec)

Misoprostol (Cytotec) is a synthetic PGE_1 analogue that can be used to soften and ripen the cervix and to induce labor. It is available as a tablet that is inserted into the vagina, or it can be taken orally or sublingually. The use of Cytotec for cervical ripening has fluctuated. Cytotec was widely used in the 1990s for cervical ripening and induction of labor until several reports showed an increase in the rates of uterine rupture. However, there is now a large body of research that supports its safety and efficacy when used appropriately (ACOG, 2009b). Cytotec is approved by the U.S. Food and Drug Administration (FDA) for prevention of peptic ulcer disease and has had special labeling for indication of cervical ripening and induction of labor since 2002 (ACOG, 2009b).

Research has shown that Cytotec used in ripening the cervix and inducing labor is more effective than oxytocin or prostaglandin agents and is less costly. Women who receive Cytotec to induce labor typically deliver within 24 hours of administration. The use of Cytotec is also associated with lower cesarean birthrates. When compared with women who have been induced using prostaglandin agents or oxytocin, the adverse outcomes do not differ among the three methods (ACOG, 2009b). Most adverse maternal and fetal outcomes associated with misoprostol have been associated with doses beyond the recommended 25 mcg. Misoprostol intravaginally has been found to be as efficacious or superior to dinoprostone gel (Cunningham et al., 2010). Guidelines for misoprostol induction include (ACOG, 2009a):

- The initial dosage should be 25 mcg.
- Recurrent administration should not exceed dosing intervals of more than 3 to 6 hours.
- Pitocin should not be administered less than 4 hours after the last Cytotec dose.
- Cytotec should only be administered where the uterine activity and fetal heart rate (FHR) can be monitored continuously for an initial observation period.

Contraindications for Cytotec include the following (AAP/ACOG, 2007):

- Nonreassuring FHR tracing.
- Frequent uterine contractions of moderate intensity.

DRUG GUIDE Dinoprostone (Cervidil) Vaginal Insert

PREGNANCY RISK CATEGORY: C

OVERVIEW OF MATERNAL-FETAL ACTION

Dinoprostone is a naturally occurring form of prostaglandin E_2. Dinoprostone can be used at term to ripen the cervix and can stimulate the smooth muscle of the uterus to enhance uterine contractions. A single vaginal insert may be used to ripen the cervix and then oxytocin can be administered 30 minutes later (Forest Pharmaceuticals, 2006).

ROUTE, DOSAGE, FREQUENCY

The vaginal insert contains 10 mg of dinoprostone. The insert is placed transversely in the posterior fornix of the vagina, and the patient is kept supine for 2 hours but then may ambulate. The dinoprostone is released at approximately 0.3 mg/hr over a 12-hour period. The vaginal insert should be removed by pulling on the retrieval string upon onset of uterine contractions or after 12 hours (Forest Pharmaceuticals, 2006).

CONTRAINDICATIONS

- Patient with known sensitivity to prostaglandins
- Presence of nonreassuring fetal status
- Unexplained bleeding during pregnancy
- Strong suspicion of cephalopelvic disproportion
- Patient already receiving oxytocin
- Patient with six or more previous term pregnancies
- Patient who is not anticipated to be able to give birth vaginally

Dinoprostone vaginal insert should be used with CAUTION in patients with ruptured membranes, a fetus in breech presentation, presence of glaucoma, or history of asthma (Forest Pharmaceuticals, 2006).

MATERNAL SIDE EFFECTS

Uterine hyperstimulation with or without nonreassuring fetal status has occurred in a very small number (2.8% to 4.7%) of patients. Less than 1% of patients have experienced fever, nausea, vomiting, diarrhea, or abdominal pain (Forest Pharmaceuticals, 2006).

EFFECTS ON FETUS/NEWBORN

Nonreassuring fetal heart rate patterns

NURSING CONSIDERATIONS

- Assess for presence of contraindications.
- Monitor maternal vital signs, cervical dilatation, and effacement carefully.
- Monitor fetal status for presence of reassuring fetal heart rate pattern (baseline 110–160 beats/min, presence of short-term variability, average variability presence of accelerations with fetal movement, absence of late or variable decelerations).
- Remove vaginal insert if uterine hyperstimulation, sustained uterine contractions, nonreassuring fetal status, or any other maternal adverse actions occur.

Source: Forest Pharmaceuticals. (2006). *Cervidil manufacturer's fact sheet.* St. Louis: Forest Pharmaceuticals.

- Prior cesarean section or uterine scar.
- Placenta previa.
- Undiagnosed vaginal bleeding.

Use of Prostaglandin Agents (Cervidil, Prepidil)

The two most commonly used types of prostaglandin gel are Prepidil and Cervidil. Prepidil gel contains 0.5 mg dinoprostone (a form of prostaglandin E_2 for intracervical application) and is placed intracervically. Cervidil is packaged in an intravaginal insert that resembles a 2-cm-square piece of cardboard-like material. It is placed in the posterior vagina and is left in place to provide a slow release of 10 mg dinoprostone at a rate of 0.3 mg/hr over 12 hours (Cunningham et al., 2010). See Drug Guide: Dinoprostone (Cervidil) Vaginal Insert and Drug Guide: Dinoprostone (Prepidil).

Advantages and Disadvantages of Prostaglandin Administration

The advantage of Cervidil is that it can be removed easily if uterine hyperstimulation occurs (Beckmann et al., 2010). Both preparations have been demonstrated to cause cervical ripening, shorter labor, and lower requirements for oxytocin during labor induction. Vaginal birth is achieved within 24 hours for most women. The incidence of cesarean birth is reduced when prostaglandin agents are used before labor induction (Cunningham et al., 2010).

Risks of prostaglandin administration include uterine hyperstimulation, nonreassuring fetal status, higher incidence of postpartum hemorrhage, and uterine rupture that can occur even in the absence of a previous uterine incision (Creasy et al., 2008). Contraindications to labor induction are found in Table 28-1. Women with a previous uterine incision should not receive prostaglandin agents, as the risk of uterine rupture is greatly increased (ACOG, 2009b). Prostaglandin should be used with caution in women with compromised cardiovascular, hepatic, or renal function and in women with asthma or glaucoma (Creasy et al., 2008).

TABLE 28-1 Contraindications to Labor Induction or Augmentation

- Vasa previa or complete placenta previa
- Transverse fetal lie
- Umbilical cord prolapse
- Previous classical cesarean delivery
- Active genital herpes infection
- Previous myomectomy entering the endometrial cavity

Source: From American College of Obstetricians and Gynecologists. Induction of labor. *(Practice Bulletin No. 107). Washington, DC: © ACOG, August, 2009.*

DRUG GUIDE Dinoprostone (Prepidil)

PREGNANCY RISK CATEGORY: C

OVERVIEW OF MATERNAL-FETAL ACTION

Dinoprostone is a synthetically prepared form of prostaglandin E_2. Dinoprostone can be given at term and acts directly on the myometrial fibers to stimulate uterine contractility. Dinoprostone directly softens the cervix, relaxing smooth muscle in the cervix itself, and assists the uterus in producing coordinated contractions with lower doses of pitocin (Wilson, Shannon, & Shields, 2010).

ROUTE, DOSAGE, AND FREQUENCY

Prepidil is packaged as a single-dose syringe that contains 0.5 mg of dinoprostone in a 2.5 ml viscous gel. The package contains two soft plastic catheters that are used for intracervical administration. The plastic catheter is introduced into the external cervical os for placement. The catheters come in two different lengths and have a shield to prevent instillation of the medication into the internal os. The medication can be placed directly during a digital examination, or a speculum can be used to visualize the cervix. The woman is placed in a reclining position and bed rest is maintained to prevent the medication from leaking from the vagina. The woman should be monitored using electronic fetal monitoring for at least 30 minutes and up to 2 hours after placement to assess the contraction pattern and the fetal status. Prepidil may be repeated every 6 hours up to 3 doses. Pitocin should not be administered for at least 6 to 12 hours because the effects of dinoprostone can be heightened when oxytocin is administered (Wilson et al., 2010).

CONTRAINDICATIONS

- Known sensitivity to prostaglandins
- Presence of nonreassuring fetal status
- Unexplained vaginal bleeding during pregnancy
- Current use of oxytocin
- Grandmultiparous women with more than six previous term vaginal births
- Known contraindications for vaginal birth
- Suspected cephalopelvic disproportion
- Previous surgical scar on uterus

Dinoprostone should be used with caution in women with a history of asthma; ruptured membranes; or renal, hepatic, or cardiovascular disease (Wilson et al., 2010).

MATERNAL SIDE EFFECTS

Uterine hyperstimulation can occur, resulting in a nonreassuring fetal heart rate pattern. Rarely, fever, nausea, vomiting, and diarrhea have also been noted to occur. In the past, women who have had a previous cesarean birth and have been given dinoprostone have had a uterine rupture as a result.

EFFECTS ON FETUS/NEWBORN

Nonreassuring fetal heart rate patterns.

NURSING CONSIDERATIONS

- Assess fetal status before administration.
- Assess for contractions.
- Monitor vital signs, cervical changes, and potential side effects.
- Monitor for reassuring fetal status (fetal heart rate of 110–160, presence of variability, accelerations with fetal movement, absence of late or variable decelerations).
- Report uterine hyperstimulation, sustained uterine contractions, nonreassuring fetal status, or adverse maternal reactions to physician or certified nurse-midwife (CNM) immediately.
- Use caution in handling this product to prevent contact with skin. Wash hands thoroughly with soap and water after administration.

Source: Pharmacia & Upjohn. Division of Pfizer, Inc., N.Y., N.Y., 2008.

Prostaglandin Agent Insertion Procedure

It is recommended that prostaglandin gel be used only in a hospital birthing unit and that an obstetrician be readily available in case an emergency cesarean birth is needed. The use of prostaglandin E (PGE) in outpatient settings and birth centers is currently under study. When Prepidil is used, it is introduced by means of a prefilled syringe with a catheter attached to the hub. The catheter is inserted through the vagina and into the endocervix, where the gel is injected. The catheter has a small shield at the top so that the gel cannot be deposited above the internal os. Dinoprostone is available as a gel that may be placed in a diaphragm and applied to the cervix and as a suppository that is placed in the posterior fornix of the vagina.

When Cervidil is used, the vaginal insert is placed in the posterior vagina. The woman should be instructed to call the nurse if it becomes dislodged so it can be reinserted. The woman is then monitored so her contractions and the fetus can be assessed. If hyperstimulation does occur, the insert can be removed. If active labor is established, the insert should also be removed. Women who receive Cytotec typically remain in the acute care setting, and oxytocin is started to facilitate birth.

Mechanical Methods of Cervical Ripening and Labor Induction

Mechanical methods to ripen the cervix or induce labor, such as balloon catheters and extra-amniotic saline infusion (EASI), can be used as an alternative or in conjunction with other agents. Advantages of mechanical agents for cervical ripening are similar efficacy when compared to hormonal agents, less costly, lower incidence of systemic side effects, and less incidence of uterine hyperstimulation (Cunningham et al., 2010).

Balloon catheters have been used for cervical ripening for many years to promote mechanical dilatation. A Foley catheter with a 25-ml to 80-ml balloon is passed through the undilated cervix and then inflated. The weighted balloon applies pressure on the internal os of the cervix and acts to ripen the cervix. This technique can be used alone or in conjunction with other induction methods, such as vaginal misoprostol, intravenous Pitocin, or extra-amniotic saline infusion where additional saline is inserted into the Foley bulb, which is pulled snugly against the cervical os (Cunningham et al., 2010).

One study examined cervical ripening after Foley catheter insertion and found that the mean change in Bishop Score (see the discussion of Bishop Score on p. 732) was 3.56 after placement of a Foley bulb catheter. The average time from Foley bulb expulsion until birth was 8 hours and 27 minutes which indicates that Foley bulb induction is a safe and effective means to induce cervical ripening (Marciniak, Leszczyńska-Gorzelak, Bartosiewicz, et al., 2010). A systematic review of the evidence of mechanical methods of cervical ripening and induction found that in women with an unfavorable cervix, Foley catheter placement prior to induction with oxytocin significantly reduced the duration of labor and reduced the risk of a cesarean section (Gelber & Sciscione, 2006).

NURSING CARE MANAGEMENT

Physicians, certified nurse-midwives (CNMs), and labor and delivery nurses who have had special education and training may administer agents for cervical ripening. Maternal vital signs are assessed for a baseline, and an electronic fetal monitor is applied for at least 30 minutes to obtain an external tracing of uterine activity, fetal heart rate (FHR) pattern, and a reactive nonstress test (NST). If a nonreactive test is obtained, consultation with the physician or CNM is required. After the gel, intravaginal insert, or tablet is inserted, the woman is instructed to remain lying down with a rolled blanket or hip wedge under her right hip to tip the uterus slightly to the left for the first 30 to 60 minutes to maintain the cervical ripening agent in place. Gel may leak from the endocervix. The nurse monitors the woman for uterine tachysystole (hyperstimulation of the uterus) and FHR abnormalities (changes in baseline rate, variability, and presence of decelerations) for 30 minutes to 2 hours if a prostaglandin gel agent is used (ACOG, 2009b). If tachysystole of the uterus greater than five contractions in 10 minutes occurs, the woman is positioned on her left side and oxygen is administered if fetal stress is noted. The administration of a tocolytic agent (such as a subcutaneous injection of 0.25 mg terbutaline) should be considered if the uterine hyperstimulation pattern continues. The gel may be removed if hyperstimulation, severe nausea, vomiting, or tachysystole develops (Wilson et al., 2010). Treatment with antiemetics, antipyretics, and antidiarrheal agents usually is not indicated. Women who receive Cervidil or Cytotec tend to remain in the acute care setting so the contraction pattern and fetal status can be monitored continuously for an initial observation period (ACOG, 2009b).

Women undergoing induction via balloon catheters do not need continuous fetal monitoring. The nurse can perform intermittent monitoring along with the maternal vital signs. The nurse should also assess the location of the catheter to ensure the catheter has not become displaced. This can be achieved by marking the catheter tubing at the introitus and noting whether movement has occurred. After the catheter is inserted, the woman should remain in a recumbent position. Vaginal examinations should not be performed. A bedpan should be used as ambulation should be avoided.

Care of the Woman During Induction or Augmentation of Labor

The American College of Obstetricians and Gynecologists (ACOG) defines **labor induction** as the stimulation of uterine contractions before the spontaneous onset of labor, with or without ruptured fetal membranes, for the purpose of accomplishing birth (ACOG, 2009b). **Labor augmentation** refers to the artificial stimulation of uterine contractions when spontaneous contractions have failed to result in progressive cervical dilation or the descent of the fetus (ACOG, 2009b).

Induction or augmentation may be indicated in the presence of the following (ACOG, 2009b):

- Maternal medical conditions (diabetes mellitus, hypertensive disorders, renal disease, chronic pulmonary disease, antiphospholipid syndrome)
- Preeclampsia, eclampsia
- Premature rupture of membranes (PROM)
- Chorioamnionitis
- Fetal demise
- Postterm pregnancy
- Fetal compromise (severe fetal growth restriction, isoimmunization, oligohydramnios, nonreassuring antepartal testing (poor biophysical profile score)
- Risk of rapid labor or extensive distance from the hospital setting
- Mild abruptio placentae
- Nonreassuring fetal heart rate (FHR)

Contraindications to Labor Induction or Augmentation

All contraindications to spontaneous labor and vaginal birth are contraindications to the induction or augmentation of labor (see Table 28-1).

Before induction is attempted, appropriate assessment must indicate that both the woman and fetus are ready for the onset of labor. Assessment of the individual patient and the clinical situation should be considered. This includes evaluation of fetal maturity and cervical readiness. In order to reduce the likelihood of delivery of a late-preterm infant, confirmation of a gestational age of at least 39 weeks should be ascertained.

The gestational age of the fetus is best evaluated by accurate menstrual dating, ultrasound visualization of the gestational sac between 5 and 6 weeks' gestation, and quickening at 18 to 20 weeks. Serial ultrasounds are helpful in validating gestational age. When needed, amniotic fluid studies for lecithin/sphingomyelin (L/S) ratio and phosphatidylglycerol are also beneficial in assessing fetal lung maturity (see chapter 21 ∞). See Table 28-2 for confirmation of gestational age to ensure a term infant.

TABLE 28-2 Confirmation of Gestational Age

- Ultrasound measurement at less than 20 weeks gestation supports gestational age of 39 weeks or greater.
- Fetal heart tones have been documented as present for at least 30 weeks by Doppler ultrasonography.
- It has been 36 weeks since a positive serum or urine human chorionic gonadotropin pregnancy test result.

Source: ACOG Practice Bulletin 107, Induction of labor, *August, 2009.*

TABLE 28-3 Prelabor Status Evaluation Scoring System

	ASSIGNED VALUE: BISHOP SCORE			
FACTOR	**0**	**1**	**2**	**3**
Cervical dilatation	Closed	1–2 cm	3–4 cm	5 cm or more
Cervical effacement	0% to 30%	40% to 50%	60% to 70%	80% or more
Fetal station	−3	−2	−1, 0	+1, or lower
Cervical consistency	Firm	Moderate	Soft	
Cervical position	Posterior	Midposition	Anterior	

Source: Bishop, E. H. (1964). Pelvic scoring for elective inductions. Obstetrics and Gynecology, *24, 266.*

Bishop Score

The findings on vaginal examination will help determine whether cervical changes favorable for induction have occurred. Bishop (1964) developed a prelabor scoring system that is still helpful in predicting the inducibility of women (Table 28-3). Components evaluated are cervical dilatation, effacement, consistency, and position, as well as the station of the fetal presenting part. A score of 0, 1, 2, or 3 is given to each assessed characteristic. The higher the total score for all the criteria, the more likely that labor will occur. The lower the total score, the higher the failure rate. A favorable cervix is the most important criterion for a successful induction (Cunningham et al., 2010). The presence of a cervix that is anterior, soft, 50% effaced, and dilated at least 2 cm, with the fetal head at +1 station or lower (Bishop score of 9), is favorable for successful induction (Bishop, 1964). Low Bishop scores have been correlated with prolonged labors and a higher incidence of cesarean births (Cunningham et al., 2010).

Fetal fibronectin (fFN) assay has been suggested as a biochemical marker for predicting impending term labor and successful labor induction. The presence of fetal fibronectin in the cervicovaginal secretions has been associated with successful induction of labor; however, in a review of factors that predict labor induction success, fFN was not found to be superior to Bishop score in predicting labor induction success (Droulez, Girard, Dumas, et al., 2008).

Methods of Inducing or Augmenting Labor

When the cervix is favorable, the most frequently used methods of induction or augmentation are stripping the amniotic membranes, amniotomy, intravenous oxytocin (Pitocin) infusion, and complementary methods. Amniotomy is discussed later in this section.

Stripping the Membranes

A nonpharmacologic method of induction or augmentation frequently used by physicians and certified nurse-midwives (CNMs) is called *stripping* (or *sweeping*) *the amniotic membranes.* The CNM or physician inserts a gloved finger as far as possible into the internal cervical os and rotates the finger 360 degrees, twice. This motion separates the amniotic membranes that are lying against the lower uterine segment and internal os from the distal part of the lower uterine segment. The stripping or sweeping is thought to release prostaglandin $F_{2\alpha}$ ($PGF_{2\alpha}$) from the amniotic membranes or prostaglandin E_2 (PGE_2) from the cervix. A systematic review of the membrane sweeping studies found that membrane sweeping tended to promote the onset of labor, reducing the risk for postterm pregnancy and other methods of induction of labor (Hill et al., 2008). Women should be advised that this procedure can cause discomfort. In addition, uterine contractions, cramping, and a bloody discharge can occur after the procedure is performed. Although the procedure is not 100% effective as a labor induction method, if labor is initiated, it typically begins within 24 to 48 hours. As an augmentation method, stripping of the membranes can be performed in the birthing room in an attempt to strengthen contractions without the need for oxytocin administration. If contractions fail to become adequate, however, oxytocin may need to be considered.

Oxytocin Infusion

Intravenous administration of oxytocin is an effective method of initiating uterine contractions. Contraction frequency is only a partial assessment of uterine activity; the duration and intensity of contractions are also important measures of the quality of a contraction. The goal is to achieve an adequate uterine contraction pattern without producing tachysystole. Normal contraction activity is described as five contractions or less in 10 minutes, averaged over a 30-minute window. More than five contractions in 10 minutes (averaged over a 30-minute window) constitutes tachysystole (ACOG, 2009b).

When augmentation is needed because of an arrest of labor or failure of the presenting part to descend, oxytocin is given intravenously to achieve a desirable labor pattern with strong contractions that will result in cervical dilatation and fetal descent. Typically, augmentation is warranted if there are fewer than three contractions in a 10-minute period or if the intensity is less than 25 mm Hg as indicated by an internal uterine pressure catheter during the active phase of labor. An assessment of the maternal pelvis, fetal station, and fetal position is performed before starting the oxytocin infusion. In addition, cephalopelvic disproportion should be ruled out because it is a contraindication. The other contraindications for labor augmentation are the same as for labor induction.

A primary bottle of intravenous fluid is prepared and used to start and maintain the infusion. This avoids the risk of infusing a large dose of oxytocin as the line is begun and provides additional fluids while the oxytocin solution is being kept at a low infusion rate. After the infusion is started, the oxytocin solution is piggybacked into the primary tubing port closest to the catheter insertion. This allows only a small amount of oxytocin to back flow into the tubing and ensures greater dosage accuracy. The oxytocin should be administered with a device that permits precise control of the flow rate. Oxytocin for induction of labor should not be administered intramuscularly or without the aid of an intravenous electric pump. Over the past few years, differences in opinion regarding oxytocin dosage have surfaced.

Ten to 20 units of oxytocin (Pitocin) are added to 1 L of a secondary line of isotonic intravenous fluid (usually 5% dextrose in balanced saline solution—for example, 5% dextrose in lactated Ringer's solution). The resulting mixture will contain 10 or 20 milliunits of oxytocin per milliliter (1 milliunit/min/6 milliunit/hr or 2 milliunit/min/12 milliliters/hr), and the prescribed dose can be calculated easily. Some facilities are now using 30 units of oxytocin (Pitocin) per 500 ml of intravenous fluid to reduce the risk of pulmonary edema in the postpartum period. Other dilutions can also be used. Other dosage concentrations are presented in the following Drug Guide: Oxytocin (Pitocin). It is imperative that the nurse be familiar with the specific dosage used within the institution to avoid medication errors.

DRUG GUIDE Oxytocin (Pitocin)

OVERVIEW OF OBSTETRIC ACTION

Oxytocin (Pitocin) exerts a selective stimulatory effect on the smooth muscle of the uterus and blood vessels. Oxytocin affects the myometrial cells of the uterus by increasing the excitability of the muscle cell, increasing the strength of the muscle contraction, and supporting propagation of the contraction (movement of the contraction from one myometrial cell to the next). Its effect on the uterine contraction depends on the dosage used and on the excitability of the myometrial cells. During the first half of gestation, there is little excitability of the myometrium, and the uterus is fairly resistant to the effects of oxytocin. However, from midgestation on, the uterus responds increasingly to exogenous intravenous oxytocin. Cautious use of diluted oxytocin administered intravenously at term results in a slow rise of uterine activity.

The circulatory half-life of oxytocin is 3 to 5 minutes. It takes approximately 40 minutes for a particular dose of oxytocin to reach a steady-state plasma concentration (Wilson et al., 2010).

The effects of oxytocin on the cardiovascular system can be pronounced. Blood pressure initially may decrease but after prolonged administration increase by 30% above the baseline. Cardiac output and stroke volume increase. With doses of 20 milliunits/min or above, oxytocin exerts an antidiuretic effect decreasing free water exchange in the kidney and markedly decreasing urine output.

Oxytocin is used to induce labor at term and to augment uterine contractions in the first and second stages of labor. Oxytocin may also be used immediately after birth to stimulate uterine contraction and thereby control uterine atony.

ROUTE, DOSAGE, FREQUENCY

For induction of labor: Add 10 units of Pitocin (1 ml) to 1000 ml of intravenous solution. (The resulting concentration is 10 mU oxytocin per 1 ml of intravenous fluid.) Using an infusion pump, administer IV, starting at 0.5–1 milliunit/min and increase by 1–2 milliunits/min every 40–60 minutes. Alternatively, start at 1–2 milliunits/min and increase by 1 milliunit/min every 15 minutes until a good contraction pattern (every 2–3 minutes and lasting 40–60 seconds) is achieved.

MATERNAL CONTRAINDICATIONS

- Severe preeclampsia-eclampsia
- Predisposition to uterine rupture (in nullipara over 35 years of age, multigravida 4 or more, overdistention of the uterus, previous major surgery of the cervix or uterus)
- Cephalopelvic disproportion
- Malpresentation or malposition of the fetus, cord prolapse
- Preterm infant
- Rigid, unripe cervix; total placenta previa
- Presence of nonreassuring fetal status

MATERNAL SIDE EFFECTS

Hyperstimulation of the uterus results in hypercontractility, which in turn may cause the following:

- Abruptio placentae
- Impaired uterine blood flow, leading to fetal hypoxia
- Rapid labor, leading to cervical lacerations
- Rapid labor and birth, leading to lacerations of cervix, vagina, or perineum, uterine atony; fetal trauma
- Uterine rupture
- Water intoxication (nausea, vomiting, hypotension, tachycardia, cardiac arrhythmia) if oxytocin is given in electrolyte-free solution or at a rate exceeding 20 milliunits/min; hypotension with rapid IV bolus administration postpartum

EFFECT ON FETUS-NEWBORN

- Fetal effects are primarily associated with the presence of hypercontractility of the maternal uterus. Hypercontractility decreases the oxygen supply to the fetus, which is reflected by irregularities or decrease in fetal heart rate (FHR).
- Hyperbilirubinemia (Wilson et al., 2010) when administered for augmentation of labor
- Trauma from rapid birth

NURSING CONSIDERATIONS

- Explain induction or augmentation procedure to patient.
- Apply fetal monitor, and obtain 15- to 20-minute tracing and nonstress test (NST) to assess FHR before starting IV oxytocin.
- For induction or augmentation of labor, start with primary IV, and piggyback secondary IV with oxytocin and infusion pump.
- Ensure continuous monitoring of the fetus and uterine contractions.
- The maximum rate is 40 milliunits/min (Blackburn, 2007). Not all protocols recommend a maximum dose. When indicated, the maximum dose is generally between 16 and 40 milliunits/min. Decrease oxytocin by similar increments once labor has

(continued)

DRUG GUIDE Oxytocin (Pitocin) continued

progressed to 5–6 cm dilatation. Protocols may vary from one agency to another.

0.5 milliunit/min = 3 ml/hr

1.0 milliunit/min = 6 ml/hr

1.5 milliunit/min = 9 ml/hr

2 milliunit/min = 12 ml/hr

4 milliunit/min = 24 ml/hr

6 milliunit/min = 36 ml/hr

8 milliunit/min = 48 ml/hr

10 milliunit/min = 60 ml/hr

12 milliunit/min = 72 ml/hr

15 milliunit/min = 90 ml/hr

18 milliunit/min = 108 ml/hr

20 milliunit/min = 120 ml/hr

- Assess FHR, maternal blood pressure, pulse, frequency and duration of uterine contractions, and uterine resting tone before each increase in the oxytocin infusion rate.
- Record all assessments and IV rate on monitor strip and on patient's chart.
- Record oxytocin infusion rate in milliunits/min and ml/hr (e.g., 0.5 milliunits/min [3 ml/hr]).
- Record on monitor strip all patient activities (such as change of position, vomiting), procedures done (amniotomy, sterile vaginal examination), and administration of analgesic agents to allow for interpretation and evaluation of tracing.
- Assess cervical dilatation as needed.
- Apply nursing comfort measures.
- Discontinue IV oxytocin infusion and infuse primary solution when (1) nonreassuring fetal status is noted (bradycardia, late or variable decelerations; (2) uterine contractions are more frequent than every 2 minutes; (3) duration of contractions exceeds more than 60 seconds; or (4) insufficient relaxation of the uterus between contractions or a steady increase in resting tone are noted (Blackburn, 2007). In addition to discontinuing IV oxytocin infusion, turn patient to side, and if nonreassuring fetal status is present, administer oxygen by tight face mask at 7–10 L/min; notify physician.
- Maintain intake and output record.

For Augmentation of Labor

Prepare and administer IV Pitocin as for labor induction. Increase rate until labor contractions are of good quality. The flow rate is gradually increased at no less than every 30 minutes to a maximum of 10 milliunits/min (Blackburn, 2007). In some settings or in a situation when limited fluids may be administered, a more concentrated solution may be used. When 10 units Pitocin are added to 500 ml IV solution, the resulting concentration is 1 milliunit/min = 3 ml/hr. If 10 units Pitocin are added to 250 ml IV solution, the concentration is 1 milliunit/min = 1.5 ml/hr.

For Administration After Expulsion of Placenta

- One dose of 10 units of Pitocin (1 ml) is given intramuscularly or 10 units to 20 units is added to IV fluids for continuous infusion.
- Assess, maternal vital signs.
- Record all assessments and IV rate on patient's chart. Record oxytocin infusion rate in milliunits/min and ml/hr (e.g., 0.5 milliunits/min [3 ml/hr]).
- Apply nursing comfort measures or pharmacologic agents for afterbirth pain associated with pitocin administration.
- Maintain intake and output record.

CLINICAL TIP

Attach the IVPB Pitocin to the medication port closest to the insertion site. If the Pitocin needs to be turned off quickly, there will be little left to infuse through the primary IV line.

ACOG (2009b) cites the use of both a low-dose and a high-dose regimen. The low-dose regimen uses a starting dose of 0.5 to 2 milliunits/min with increases of 1 to 2 milliunits/min every 15 to 40 minutes until an adequate labor pattern is established. The high-dose regimen has a starting dose of up to 6 milliunits/min with incremental increases of 3 to 6 milliunits/min every 20 to 40 minutes. If tachysystole arises with the high-dose regimen, the incremental dose is reduced to 3 milliunits/min; if tachysystole is recurrent, the incremental dose is reduced to 1 milliunit/min. Higher dose regimens have been associated with a shorter labor, less incidence of dystocia, lower cesarean birthrates, and a lower incidence of chorioamnionitis (ACOG, 2009b).

Oxytocin induction is not without some associated risks; however, most side effects are dose-related. The most common side effect of oxytocin administration is tachysystole of the uterus (with or without FHR changes), resulting in uterine contractions that are too frequent (more often than every 2 minutes), uterine contractions that are too intense, or an increased uterine resting tone. Category 2 or 3 FHR tracing changes have been associated with tachysystole (ACOG 2009b).

Other risks include uterine rupture and water intoxication.

Researchers continue to investigate a new method of labor induction with pulsatile oxytocin administration by a computer-controlled pump.

COMPLEMENTARY AND ALTERNATIVE THERAPIES

In addition to the allopathic cervical ripening and induction methods previously discussed, there are a variety of more "natural" and noninvasive methods that CNMs tend to suggest or administer either in the home setting or in tertiary care centers. These methods include the following: sexual intercourse/lovemaking; self or partner stimulation of the woman's nipples and breasts; the use of herbs, such as blue/black cohosh, evening primrose oil, and red raspberry leaves; the use of homeopathic solutions, such as caulophyllum or pulsatilla; castor oil; enemas; and acupressure/acupuncture.

RESEARCH EVIDENCE IN PRACTICE The Relationship Between Labor Induction and Cesarean Birth

CLINICAL QUESTION

Is there an association between labor induction and subsequent cesarean birth?

RESEARCH EVIDENCE

Induction of labor carries with it a cascade of inherent risks. Induction requires an intravenous access line, continuous fetal monitoring, confinement to bed, amniotomy, and the use of pharmacologic agents, each with its own potential for adverse effects. Labor induction is often employed based on medical indications that may preclude a natural labor process. However, some mothers choose elective induction of labor, and currently this is at an all-time high in the United States.

The evidence that links induction of labor and cesarean birth is strong under certain conditions. Induction and cesarean birth appears to be associated most strongly in primiparous mothers. In a retrospective study of more than 62,000 births, the association of labor induction and cesarean birth was evaluated while accounting for demographic variables such as socioeconomic status and location of birth. In this study, cesarean births were associated with labor induction, but only in primiparous women. This relationship is even stronger when the induction is elective. In a retrospective study of more than 1300 women, elective labor induction increased the risk of a cesarean birth by 50% among primiparous women. The association between elective induction and cesarean birth has been demonstrated in multiparous women as well. One large study of more than 11,000 births showed a strong correlation between elective labor induction and cesarean birth.

The association is not apparent when induction is medically indicated. In one study that evaluated only risk-based labor induction in a population of 100 women, cesarean birth was not associated with labor induction. In these mothers, the induction was associated with better birth outcomes.

WHAT QUESTIONS REMAIN UNANSWERED?

Why is this association strongest in primiparous women? Are there factors that could mediate the risk of cesarean birth when labor is induced in primiparous women?

WHAT IS BEST PRACTICE?

When compared with risk-based labor induction, elective labor induction is associated with higher rates of cesarean birth. Risk-based labor induction is not; better outcomes are achieved when induction follows standard medical indications. Primiparous women are at highest risk of cesarean birth, but are particularly so when the induction is not risk-related.

CRITICAL THINKING

What physiologic characteristics of primiparous mothers make them at higher risk of cesarean birth after labor induction? How can the nurse counsel mothers about the risks of elective labor induction?

References

Glantz, J. (2005). Elective induction vs. spontaneous labor: Associations and outcomes. *Journal of Reproductive Medicine, 50*(4), 235–240.

Nicholson, J., Stenson, M., Kellar, L., Caughey, A., & Macones, G. 2009. Active management of risk in nulliparous pregnancy at term: Association between a higher preventive labor induction rate and improved birth outcomes. *American Journal of Obstetrics & Gynecology, 200*(3), 254.e1–254.e13.

Simpson, K. (2010). Reconsideration of the costs of convenience: Quality, operational and fiscal strategies to minimize elective labor induction. *Journal of Perinatal & Neonatal Nursing, 24*(1), 43–52.

Wilson, B. (2007). Assessing the effects of age, gestation, socioeconomic status, and ethnicity on labor inductions. *Journal of Nursing Scholarship, 39*(3), 208–213.

Wilson, B., Effken, J., & Butler, R. (2010). The relationship between cesarean section and labor induction. *Journal of Nursing Scholarship, 42*(2), 130–138.

Although not widely described in nursing and medical textbooks, the use of complementary and alternative medicine (CAM) has risen dramatically. It is estimated that 38% of adults and 12% of children use CAM regularly (National Center for Complementary and Alternative Medicine, 2009). Natural methods are very effective and are frequently the preferred choice of many CNMs and their patients. It is important for nursing students, nurses, and consumers to be aware of all aspects of pregnancy care.

Sexual intercourse is a logical method of stimulating cervical ripening and uterine contractions; female orgasm stimulates uterine contractions, and the male ejaculate contains a rich source of natural prostaglandins (Tan, Andi, Azmi, et al., 2006). Breast and nipple stimulation are also a frequent part of lovemaking, and this stimulates the release of endogenous oxytocin, which in turn stimulates the uterus to contract. Until recently, most literature about sexual intercourse and lovemaking during pregnancy has focused on the possible harmful effects that may arise; however, new research regarding sexual intercourse as a method of labor induction found sexual intercourse will initiate labor and prevent the incidence of postterm gestation (Tan et al., 2006). Sexual intercourse is not used to augment labor.

Nipple stimulation for cervical ripening may be done at term or to augment labor. Nipple stimulation is found to increase endogenous oxytocin and stimulate uterine contractions. It also has been found to initiate spontaneous labor (Cunningham et al., 2010). There are multiple suggested methods, including manual manipulation and use of the electric breast pump. A recent systematic review of clinical trials comparing breast stimulation for third trimester cervical ripening or induction of labor to other or no interventions found that breast stimulation increased the likelihood that women would go into labor. Breast stimulation therefore is not recommended in high-risk women and care should be taken to monitor uterine contractility because hyperstimulation can occur (Creasy et al., 2008).

Herbal preparations such as blue and black cohosh, evening primrose oil, and red raspberry leaf teas are used for both cervical ripening and induction of labor. Although extensive scientific data are not available for many of these preparations, they have been widely used to promote uterine contractions and stimulate and augment labor (Bayles, 2007).

One of the more widely studied herbal preparations is evening primrose oil (*Oenothera biennis*). It has been widely used for centuries by midwives as a means of softening the cervix, vagina, and perineum to facilitate the onset of labor. Evening primrose oil

Case Study: Patient Undergoing Labor Induction

Care Plan Activity: Patient with Pitocin for Labor Augmentation

contains a fatty acid called gamma linolenic acid, which is converted into a prostaglandin compound. Prostaglandins play a key role in ripening the cervix so labor can begin. Women can be advised to begin evening primrose oil supplementation after 38 weeks of pregnancy. The route of delivery is oral or intravaginally. There are a variety of dosing protocols. Side effects are rare but can include headaches, nausea, or skin rashes. Women who experience side effects should be counseled to discontinue the supplement unless advised otherwise by their CNM or physician (Knoche, Selzer, & Smolley, 2008).

Homeopathic solutions, such as caulophyllum, cimicifuga, pulsatilla, and others, are used for cervical ripening and induction of labor. There are no current guidelines for their use in augmenting labor. The midwife or physician needs thorough personal knowledge of homeopathic remedies or ongoing consultation with a homeopathic physician.

Castor oil has been used for many years but has not been studied frequently as a method of labor induction and augmentation. The method by which castor oil stimulates uterine contractions is not understood, but is thought to be a result of the release of prostaglandin E_2 as a consequence of increased peristalsis and diarrhea after ingestion of the drug (Knoche et al., 2008). Although some studies have examined the effectiveness of castor oil, further research is needed to determine the effectiveness of this method (Kavanagh, Kelly, & Thomas, 2009).

Acupressure and acupuncture are not as accepted in the United States as in other countries. However, the rising interest in and use of holistic practices and alternative medicine is prompting a closer look at acupuncture as a method of inducing and augmenting labor and relieving labor pain. In acupuncture, sterile needles are inserted into the body at specific predetermined sites to elicit a desired response, such as initiation of contractions or relief of pain. A systematic review of evidence regarding acupuncture and induction of labor found that women who underwent acupuncture were less likely to require other methods of induction (Moleti, 2009). Although acupuncture requires extensive education and training, some CNMs can work with an acupressurist/acupuncturist to learn manual massage of acupuncture and acupressure points, shiatsu, and other touch techniques.

NURSING CARE MANAGEMENT

No matter which induction or augmentation method is used, close observation and accurate assessments are mandatory to provide safe, optimal care for both woman and fetus. The nurse obtains maternal vital signs (temperature, pulse, respirations, and blood pressure) before beginning an oxytocin infusion. Induction protocols also recommend obtaining a 20- to 30-minute electronic fetal monitor recording demonstrating a reassuring FHR and a reactive nonstress test (NST) and contraction status before the infusion is started. Patient teaching includes the purpose and procedure for the induction, as well as a review of the care that will be provided, including assessments and comfort measures. A Nursing Care Plan for Induction of Labor appears on pp. 737–738.

During the oxytocin infusion, an obstetrician should be readily accessible to manage any complication that occurs (AAP & ACOG, 2007). A fetal monitor is used to provide continuous data. Women may ambulate if a portable or walking monitor is available.

Women who are undergoing alternative methods of induction also need continuous assessment and nursing support. For women who have entered labor after stripping of the amniotic membranes, a normal labor pattern should ensue. Intermittent external fetal monitoring can be used if the fetus is reactive and the maternal vital signs are within normal parameters. Women should be advised that they may continue to have a blood-tinged discharge from the procedure. Women who have their membranes stripped are less likely to go past their due dates. The nurse continues to assess the contraction pattern, including the frequency, intensity, and duration of the contractions.

Women who choose to use nipple stimulation as a means of inducing labor should be continuously monitored with the external fetal monitor while the electric breast pump is in use. Release of oxytocin stimulated by breast pumping can result in surges of oxytocin release, which can lead to nonreassuring fetal status. Some fetuses who are unable to tolerate the release of oxytocin from breast pumping may react without stress to intravenous oxytocin administration, as this results in a small amount of oxytocin being released in a controlled manner.

In cases where homeopathic or herbal remedies have been used to induce labor, normal intermittent monitoring and assessment of maternal vital signs can be performed. If oxytocin is to be administered, the nurse should inform the physician or CNM of what has been given, the dose, the last time administered, and the immediate effects that were achieved. An assessment is performed before administration of pharmacologic substances.

Expected outcomes of nursing care include the following:

- The woman and family are fully informed; understand the induction process; are able to relate the advantages, disadvantages, risks, and possible outcomes; and have had an opportunity to have their questions answered.
- The woman's labor is successfully induced.
- The labor progresses at a normal rate and maternal vital signs remain in normal range.
- The fetal status remains reassuring throughout the labor period.

Care of the Woman During an Amniotomy

Amniotomy is the artificial rupture of the amniotic membranes (AROM). It is probably the most common procedure performed in obstetrics. Because the amniotomy requires that an instrument be inserted through the cervix, at least 2 cm of cervical dilatation must be present. The amniotomy may be performed as a method of induction of labor (to stimulate the beginning of labor), or it

NURSING CARE PLAN For Induction of Labor

INTERVENTION	RATIONALE
1. Nursing diagnosis: Risk for Injury related to hyperstimulation of uterus caused by induction of labor **Goal:** Progression of labor without difficulty or complications	
■ Obtain a baseline for maternal blood pressure, pulse, respirations, temperature, and pain level.	■ Pitocin induction can affect the cardiovascular system. Blood pressure may initially be decreased. If the induction is prolonged the blood pressure may increase by 30%. Respirations can become elevated because of pain sensation, anxiety, or physiologic causes. Temperature is obtained to monitor for infection. The pain level is assessed continuously to determine if pain medication is warranted or changes in vital signs are caused by maternal discomfort.
■ Place patient on external fetal monitor for 20 minutes to obtain a baseline for fetal heart rate (FHR) and variability.	■ Assesses for fetal well-being. Normal FHR ranges from 110 to 160 beats/min. Variability measuring three to five fluctuations in 1 minute is documented as average. Continuous electronic fetal monitoring (EFM) is performed during a Pitocin induction.
■ Perform nonstress test.	■ A nonstress test is performed to assess the fetal heart rate in response to fetal movement. Accelerations of fetal heart rate with fetal movement may indicate the fetus has adequate oxygenation and an intact central nervous system. A reactive nonstress test indicates there were at least two accelerations of 15 beats/min above baseline, lasting 15 seconds in a 20-minute period.
■ Insert IV line and begin primary infusion with 1000 ml of electrolyte solution.	■ An electrolyte solution such as lactated Ringer's is used for the primary solution. A primary IV allows continuous intravenous access and fluid infusion in the event the Pitocin drip needs to be discontinued.
■ Piggyback Pitocin solution into primary IV tubing, via pump, in the port closest to the IV insertion site.	■ Pitocin is mixed in 1000 ml of an electrolyte solution (usually 5% dextrose in lactated Ringer's solution) and piggybacked to main IV line. A pump is used to ensure dosage accuracy.
■ Begin Pitocin infusion per agency protocol.	■ The rate to be used is determined by physician or CNM orders or agency protocol.
■ Monitor infusion pump and connections.	■ This ensures adequate dosing. Early identification of problems with the infusion site, the piggyback connection, or flow rate will minimize effects on uterine contractions and FHR. If a problem is found, correct and restart infusion at the beginning dose.
■ Monitor and evaluate maternal blood pressure and pulse before each increase in the Pitocin infusion rate.	■ Prolonged inductions may increase the blood pressure by 30%. The Pitocin infusion rate should not be advanced if maternal hypertension or hypotension is present or if there are any radical changes in pulse rate.
■ Evaluate urine output.	■ There is an antidiuretic effect with dosages of Pitocin above 20 milliunits/min. This level decreases free water exchange in the kidneys, therefore markedly decreasing urine output.
■ Evaluate and document fetal heart rate before each increase in Pitocin infusion rate.	■ During Pitocin infusion, fetal heart rate should range between 110 and 160 beats/min. Hypercontractility of the maternal uterus may cause nonreassuring fetal status. Fetal bradycardia may occur along with a decrease in variability, leading to fetal hypoxia. Fetal tachycardia may also occur. If persistent fetal bradycardia or fetal tachycardia occurs, the Pitocin is discontinued.
■ Evaluate and document contraction pattern before each increase of the Pitocin infusion rate.	■ Contractions every 2 to 3 minutes, lasting 40 to 60 seconds with moderate intensity, are considered adequate. Cervical dilatation progresses an average of 1.2 cm/hr to 1.5 cm/hr (0.5 in./hr to 0.6 in./hr) during the active phase of labor.
■ Increase Pitocin infusion dosage until adequate contractions are achieved or the maximum dose per agency protocol is reached.	■ Pitocin may be increased every 20 to 40 minutes until an adequate contraction pattern is achieved.

(continued)

NURSING CARE PLAN For Induction of Labor continued

INTERVENTION	RATIONALE
■ Evaluate contraction frequency, duration, and intensity before increasing the infusion rate. Discontinue Pitocin infusion and infuse primary solution if signs of hyperstimulation of the uterus are detected.	■ Signs of hyperstimulation include contraction frequency less than 2 minutes, duration exceeding 60 seconds, and increased resting tone. Hyperstimulation of the uterus puts the patient at risk for abruptio placentae and uterine rupture.
■ Initiate treatment measures to reverse the effects of Pitocin infusion if fetal tachycardia or bradycardia occurs.	■ When the FHR falls outside the normal range (110 to 160 beats/min), treatment measures should be initiated. To reverse the effects of Pitocin, immediately discontinue Pitocin, infuse primary solution, administer oxygen by tight face mask at 7 to 10 L/min, place patient in side-lying position, and notify physician or CNM.

EXPECTED OUTCOME: Contractions will increase in frequency, duration, and intensity. An increase in cervical dilatation, effacement, and intensity will be achieved. The uterus will remain soft between contractions.

may be done to augment labor. A meta-analysis of 12 studies found that if an amniotomy is performed along with early oxytocin administration, the labor will probably be shortened and the incidence of cesarean birth is reduced (Wei et al., 2009). Amniotomy may also be performed during labor to allow access to the fetus in order to apply an internal fetal heart monitoring electrode to the scalp, to insert an intrauterine pressure catheter, or to obtain a fetal scalp blood sample for acid–base determination.

The decision to perform an amniotomy should include the patient. The evidence for advantages and disadvantages should be presented to the patient. Ideally such a discussion would not occur during a vaginal examination (Smyth, Aldred, & Markham, 2007).

Advantages and Disadvantages of Amniotomy

Amniotomy as a method of labor induction has the following advantages:

1. The contractions elicited are similar to those of spontaneous labor.
2. There is usually no risk of hypertonus or rupture of the uterus, as with intravenous oxytocin induction.
3. The woman does not require the same intensive monitoring as with intravenous oxytocin induction.
4. Electronic fetal monitoring (EFM) is facilitated because, once the membranes are ruptured, a fetal scalp electrode may be applied, an intrauterine catheter may be inserted, and scalp blood sampling for pH determinations may be done to assist in evaluating a fetal heart rate (FHR) pattern.
5. The color and composition of amniotic fluid can be evaluated.
6. Amniotomy is a less costly procedure compared to other methods of induction.

The disadvantages of amniotomy are as follows (Smyth, Aldred, & Markham, 2007):

1. Once an amniotomy is done, the risk for infection begins to rise if labor proceeds beyond 24 hours because microorganisms can now invade the intrauterine cavity and cause amnionitis.
2. The danger of a prolapsed cord is increased once the membranes have ruptured, especially if the fetal presenting part is not firmly pressed down against the cervix.
3. Compression and molding of the fetal head are increased because of loss of the cushioning effect of the amniotic fluid for the fetal head during uterine contractions.
4. Fetal injury can occur if the amniohook causes a laceration on the presenting part.
5. Bleeding can occur if an undiagnosed vasa previa is present.
6. Severe variable decelerations can occur, which increases the likelihood of a cesarean birth.
7. The intervention can cause an increase in pain making labor more difficult to manage.

Amniotomy Procedure

Before an amniotomy is performed, the fetus is assessed for presentation, position, station, and FHR. Unless the fetal head is well engaged in the pelvis, some practitioners do not advocate an amniotomy because of the danger of prolapsed cord (refer to chapter 27 for discussion of prolapsed cord). Other risks are abruptio placentae (because of rapid decompression of the uterus with the rapid loss of amniotic fluid), infection (because of the introduction of organisms into the cervix and intrauterine cavity), and amniotic fluid embolus (because of rapid decompression of the uterus and small amounts of fluid entering the maternal vascular system from under the edge of the placenta). These complications may also be associated with spontaneous rupture of membranes (SROM).

While performing a sterile vaginal examination, the physician or certified nurse-midwife (CNM) introduces an amnihook (or other rupturing device) into the vagina, through the cervix, and against the amniotic membrane, which is in front of the fetal presenting part. A small tear is made in the amniotic membrane. Following rupture of the membrane, amniotic fluid is allowed to escape slowly.

Through the Eyes of a Nurse
Labor Induction

Family's Experience

"I can't take it anymore! I can't sleep; I can't bend over; I am exhausted! I have contractions all of the time. We sit and time them, and just when we think it is time to call and come to the hospital, they space out and go away! I am miserable; I just want to get this over. I really want to be induced at this point. I can't take it, I really can't!"

Her husband is concerned as well. "We have been to the hospital twice. She is having contractions on the (electronic fetal) monitor but they keep sending us home. She is crying and miserable. She is up all night and can't rest. What are the dangers of inducing her?"

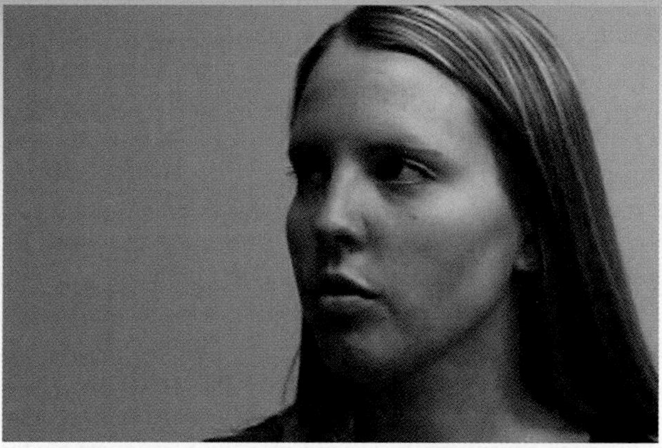

Nurse's Response

"What you are feeling is very typical at this stage of pregnancy. It is often uncomfortable at the end stages of pregnancy. We can certainly let the nurse-midwife know that you would like to consider an induction.

"There are a variety of factors to consider. It is important to determine if there are any contraindications to induction and to review the risks with you. You are overdue, which is one of the indications for induction. The midwife will need to examine your cervix to determine if your cervix is ripe or favorable for induction. You can also explore whether you would like to try complementary methods first or if you would like to schedule a medical induction where oxytocin is administered."

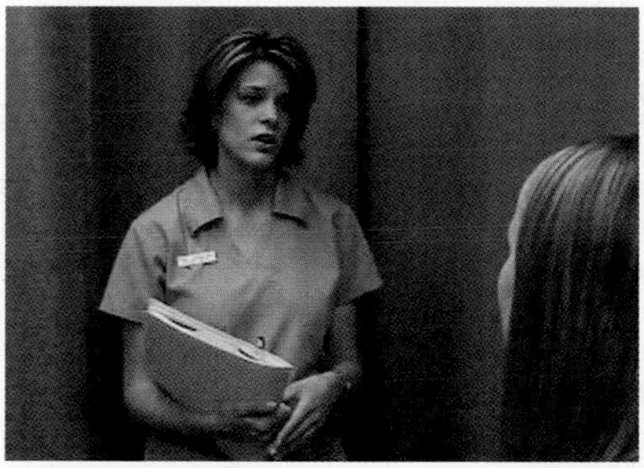

Nurse's Actions and Rationale

The nurse provides reassurance that her feelings and the physical discomforts that she is experiencing are normal at this stage in pregnancy. The nurse explains that there are some contraindications to induction and that these need to be reviewed with the healthcare provider. Table 28-1 lists absolute contraindications to induction. The midwife will perform a vaginal examination to determine if the woman's cervix is favorable for induction. The Bishop score (see Table 28-3) is a measure of prelabor status criteria that is commonly used to determine if induction is likely to be successful. A score of 9 indicates that labor will most likely occur if induction is attempted.

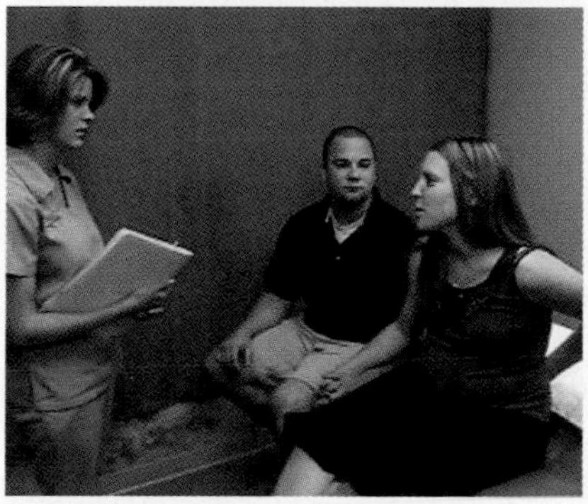

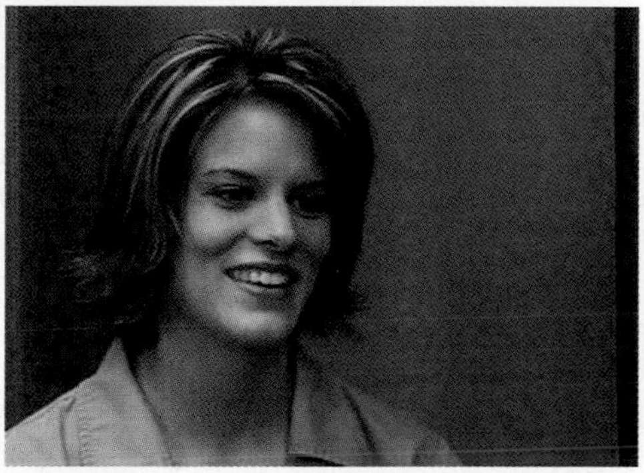

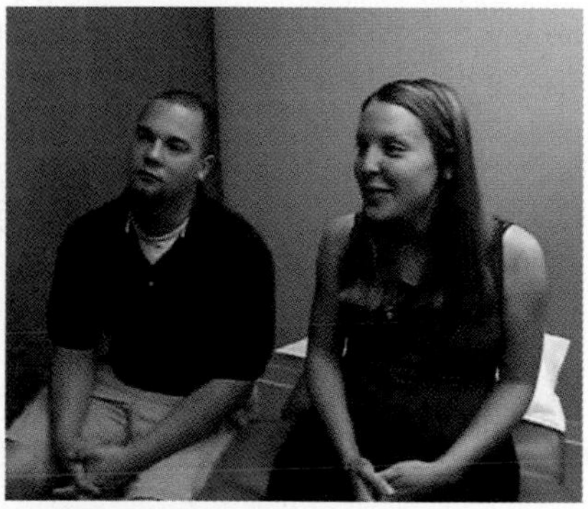

NURSING CARE MANAGEMENT

The nurse explains the procedure to the woman. The fetal presentation, position, and station are assessed because amniotomy is usually delayed until engagement has occurred (to decrease the risk of a prolapsed cord when the fluid is expelled). The woman is positioned in a semireclining position and draped to provide privacy. Disposable underpads and/or towels are placed under the woman's buttocks to absorb the amniotic fluid. The FHR is assessed just before and immediately after the amniotomy, and the two FHR assessments are compared. If there are marked changes, the nurse should check for prolapse of the cord. The amniotic fluid is inspected for amount, color, odor, and the presence of meconium or blood. While wearing disposable gloves, the nurse cleanses and dries the perineal area and changes the disposable underpads. The nurse advises the woman that fluid will continue to be expelled from her vagina. Frequent pericare and pad changes should be done to increase patient comfort. Because there is now an open pathway for organisms to ascend into the uterus, strict sterile technique must be observed during vaginal examinations. In addition, the number of vaginal examinations must be kept to a minimum to reduce the chance of introducing an infection, and the woman's temperature should be monitored every 2 hours. Bed rest is maintained unless the presenting part is engaged and is firmly against the cervix (to decrease the risk of prolapsed cord). The nurse needs to provide information about the amniotomy and the expected effects. Some couples may worry that all the amniotic fluid will be gone and that they will experience a "dry birth." It is important for them to know that amniotic fluid is constantly produced.

Amnioinfusion

Care of the Woman During Amnioinfusion

Amnioinfusion (AI) is a technique by which a volume of warmed, sterile, normal saline or Ringer's lactate solution is introduced into the uterus through the use of an intrauterine pressure catheter (IUPC). AI can be used intrapartally to increase the volume of fluid when oligohydramnios is present and the physician wants either to prevent the possibility of variable decelerations by increasing the volume of amniotic fluid or to treat nonperiodic decelerations that are already occurring. The AI increases the volume of fluid, relieving pressure on the umbilical cord and promoting increased perfusion to the fetus. When AI is used for this indication or for prolonged decelerations in fetal heart rate (FHR) patterns, the abnormal FHR pattern is usually relieved in 20 to 30 minutes (Beckmann et al., 2010).

Amnioinfusion has also been used for meconium dilution in the presence of medium to heavy meconium staining. Debate has ensued regarding the effectiveness of this regimen. A recent systematic review of randomized controlled trials of AI for thick, meconium-stained amniotic fluid found no evidence that AI reduced the incidence of meconium aspiration syndrome (Xu, Hofmeyr, Roy, et al., 2007). The possibility that the meconium had already entered the fetal tracheobronchial tree before the onset of labor or that affected fetuses have been exposed to prolonged periods of nonreassuring fetal status are other factors that may contribute to the review's findings (Xu et al., 2007). Even with these findings, some practitioners continue to administer AIs in the presence of moderate to severe meconium staining. Further research is needed to examine these factors.

Contraindications to AI include patients with a contraindication to vaginal delivery, amnionitis, hydramnios, uterine hypertonus, multiple gestation, known fetal anomaly, uterine anomaly, nonreassuring fetal status requiring immediate birth, nonvertex presentation, scalp pH below 7.2, placenta previa, vasa previa, or abruptio placentae (Cunningham et al., 2010). AI can also be associated with rare serious risk factors, including umbilical cord prolapse, amniotic fluid embolism, and uterine rupture (Beckmann et al., 2010).

There is no one accepted protocol for AI. However, most procedures involve infusing a bolus of from 250 to 500 ml of warmed normal saline through an intrauterine catheter using an infusion pump over 20 to 30 minutes and repeated until the indication resolves. Other protocols include a bolus followed by a constant administration of 180 cc of warmed saline until birth occurs (Queenan, Spong, & Lockwood, 2007).

NURSING CARE MANAGEMENT

The nurse is frequently the first person to detect changes in FHR associated with cord compression or to observe thick, meconium-stained amniotic fluid. When cord compression is suspected, the immediate intervention is to assist the laboring woman to another position in an effort to relieve the compression and to apply O_2 via face mask (see chapter 27 ∞ for further discussion). If this intervention is not successful, an amnioinfusion may be considered. The nurse helps with the AI and monitors the woman's vital signs (blood pressure, pulse, and respiration) and contraction status (frequency, duration, intensity, resting tone, and associated maternal discomfort). Fetal heart rate (FHR) is monitored by continuous electronic fetal monitoring (EFM). The nurse should provide ongoing information to the laboring woman and her partner and answer questions as they arise. Comfort measures and positioning are very important because AI requires the woman to be on bed rest.

The AI should not cause pain or discomfort for the laboring woman other than the need for bed rest. The nurse needs to ensure that the fluid infused is being expelled from the woman's vagina. This is achieved with frequent examination of the woman's sanitary pad or an absorbent pad that is placed beneath her buttocks. The woman should be advised that fluid will leak from her vagina. The nurse should change absorbent pads and provide pericare on a regular basis.

Care of the Woman During an Episiotomy

An **episiotomy** is a surgical incision of the perineal body. Traditionally, some physicians and certified nurse-midwives (CNMs) performed episiotomies to prevent damage to the periurethra, perineum, anal sphincter, and rectum from lacerations during the birth; to prevent damage to the posterior wall of the vagina; to prevent jagged tears from lacerations; to reduce mechanical and metabolic risk to the fetus/newborn; to protect the maternal bladder; and to prevent future perineal relaxation. However, more recent research indicates that routine episiotomy use is driven by local professional norms, experience in training, and individual practitioner preference rather than the needs of the individual woman at the time of delivery (Frankman, Wang, Bunker, et al., 2009).

Although the incidence of episiotomies in the United States has declined, it is still performed in slightly greater than one third of all vaginal births (Frankman et al., 2009). Typically, nurse-midwives tend to perform fewer episiotomies than physicians. Residents and hospital-based physicians tend to perform fewer routine episiotomies than physicians in private practice (Frankman et al., 2009).

Even though the procedure is very common, its routine use has been questioned. The most current research indicates that there are no maternal advantages in performing routine episiotomies (Viswanathan et al., 2009). Research suggests that, rather than protecting the perineum from lacerations, the presence of an episiotomy makes it more likely that the woman will have deep perineal tears. It has also been suggested that perineal lacerations heal more quickly in the absence of episiotomy (Frankman et al., 2009). Major perineal trauma (extension to or through the anal sphincter) is *more* likely to occur if a midline episiotomy is performed. It is estimated that one in five women will experience an anal sphincter injury as a result of a vaginal delivery (Viswanathan et al., 2009). Women who are allowed to tear spontaneously have less sexual dysfunction than women who have undergone episiotomies (Frankman et al., 2009).

Additional complications associated with an episiotomy are blood loss, infection, pain, and perineal discomfort that may continue for days or weeks past birth, including dyspareunia (painful intercourse). Flatal incontinence (uncontrollable passage of gas) has also been reported (Cunningham et al., 2010). There are no scientific data to support the beliefs that episiotomies yield a shorter second stage, improved Apgar scores, or a decrease in perinatal asphyxia (Viswanathan et al., 2009). In light of the debate over the value of episiotomy, it is now suggested that the procedure be used selectively to facilitate birth in the presence of maternal or fetal stress or when a shoulder dystocia is anticipated. There is debate on whether episiotomies should be performed to create more room in the presence of a breech presentation, multiple gestation, or a large-for-gestational-age infant (greater than 4000 g), or for the use of an instrument (forceps or vacuum extractor) to assist birth. Some researchers argue that midline episiotomy and vacuum-assisted birth should be avoided when a large baby is anticipated. Although many practitioners perform episiotomies when an instrument is being used to assist birth, new research suggests this may result in more third- and fourth-degree extensions (Frankman et al., 2009).

Risk Factors That Predispose Women to Episiotomy

Overall factors that place a woman at increased risk for an episiotomy are primigravid status, large or macrosomic fetus, occiput-posterior position, use of forceps or vacuum extractor, shoulder dystocia, and white race (Frankman et al., 2009). Other factors that predispose a woman to episiotomy may be mitigated by nurses and physicians or CNMs. These include the following:

- Use of lithotomy position or other recumbent position (causes excessive perineal stretching)
- Encouraging or requiring sustained breath holding during second-stage pushing (causes excessive perineal stretching, can adversely affect blood flow in the mother and fetus, and encourages the woman to be responsive to caregiver directions rather than to her own urges to push spontaneously)
- Arbitrary time limit placed by the physician or CNM on the length of the second stage

Nursing advocacy is needed to promote selective rather than routine episiotomies. The nurse can begin by encouraging pregnant women to read about prenatal perineal preparation and to talk with the physician or CNM about their personal beliefs and the incidence of episiotomy in their practice. Nurses can share current research with nursing colleagues through staff meetings and explore and strongly encourage nursing care interventions that avoid the lithotomy position. The woman should be encouraged to respond to her body's urges to push during the second stage. Just as patients ask physicians and CNMs about their episiotomy philosophy and incidence, patients may ask labor and birthing nurses to provide information about their actions to help decrease episiotomy rates. It is imperative that each nurse continue to stay current about new information and research in order to maintain current practice standards.

Episiotomy Procedure

The episiotomy is performed with a sharp scissors that has rounded points, just before birth, when approximately 3 to 4 cm of the fetal head is visible during a contraction (Cunningham et al., 2010). There are two types of episiotomy: midline and mediolateral (Figure 28-3 ■). A midline episiotomy is performed along the median raphe of the perineum. It extends down from the vaginal orifice to the fibers of the rectal sphincter. This type of episiotomy avoids muscle fibers and major blood vessels because it divides the insertions of the superficial perineal muscles (Blackburn, 2007). A midline episiotomy is preferred if the perineum is of adequate length and no difficulty is anticipated during the birth, because it entails less blood loss, is easy to repair, and heals with less discomfort for the mother. The major disadvantage is that a tear of the midline incision may extend through the anal sphincter and rectum (Blackburn, 2007).

In the presence of a short perineum, macrosomia, and instrument-assisted birth (use of forceps or vacuum extractor),

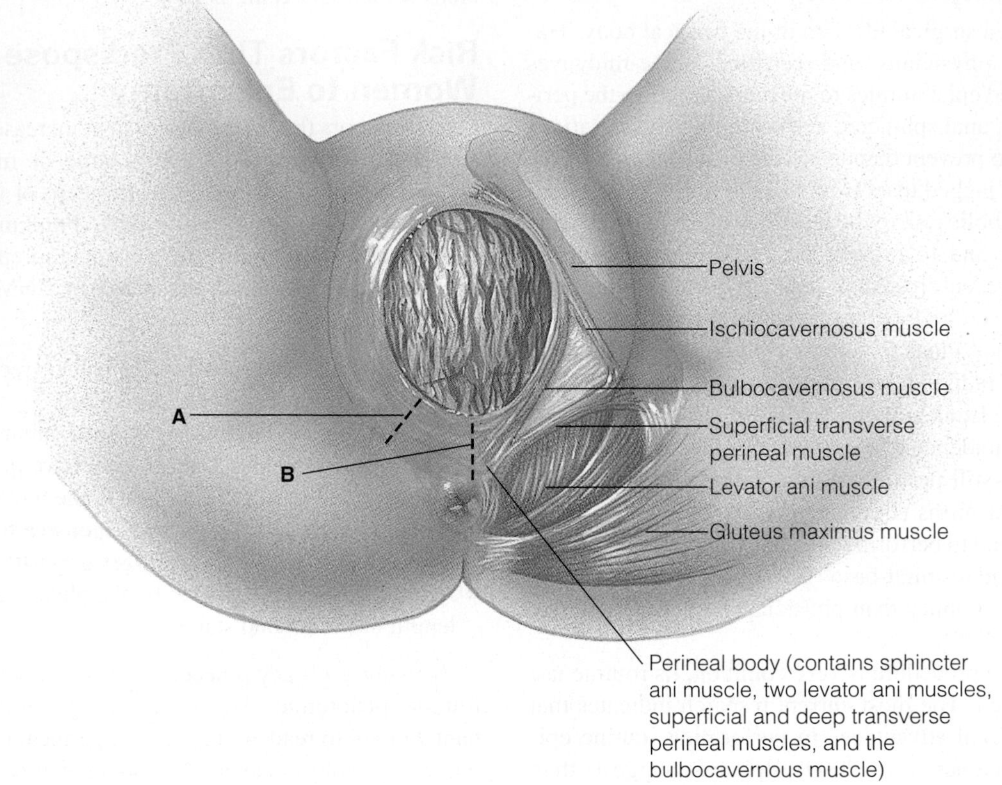

Figure 28-3 ■ The two most common types of episiotomies are midline and mediolateral. A. Right mediolateral. B. Midline.

a mediolateral episiotomy provides more room and decreases the possibility of a traumatic extension into the rectum. The mediolateral episiotomy begins in the midline of the posterior fourchette (to avoid incision into the Bartholin's gland) and extends at a 45-degree angle downward to the right or left (the direction depending on the handedness of the clinician). The mediolateral episiotomy may be complicated by greater blood loss, a longer healing period, and more postpartal discomfort (Frankman et al., 2009).

The episiotomy is usually performed with regional or local anesthesia but may be performed without anesthesia in emergency situations. It is generally suggested that as crowning occurs, the distention of the tissues causes numbing. Adequate anesthesia must be given for the repair.

Repair of the episiotomy (episiorrhaphy) and any lacerations is performed either during the period between birth of the baby and before expulsion of the placenta or after expulsion of the placenta. Many providers wait until after expulsion of the placenta in case a manual removal of the placenta or a uterine exploration is indicated (Blackburn, 2007).

NURSING CARE MANAGEMENT

The woman needs to be supported during the episiotomy and the repair because she may feel some pressure sensations. It is not uncommon for the woman to feel a "pulling" or "tugging" sensation. In the absence of adequate anesthesia, she may feel pain. Placing a hand on her shoulder and talking with her can provide comfort and distraction from the repair process. If the woman is having more discomfort than she can comfortably handle, the nurse needs to act as an advocate in communicating the woman's needs to the physician or CNM. At all times, the woman needs to be the one who decides whether the amount of discomfort is tolerable, and she should never be told, "This doesn't hurt." She is the person experiencing the discomfort, and her evaluation needs to be respected. If there are just a few (three to five) stitches left, she may choose to forgo more local anesthesia, but she should be given the choice. For women with severe pain or anxiety, intravenous medication such as Fentanyl or Nubain can be administered for both pain and anxiety control.

The nurse notes the type of episiotomy on the birth record. This information should also be included in a report to the postpartum nurse so that adequate assessments can be made and relief measures can be instituted if necessary.

Pain relief measures may begin immediately after birth with application of an ice pack to the perineum. For optimal effect, the ice pack should be applied for 20 to 30 minutes and removed for at least 20 minutes before being reapplied. This is advisable because the ice causes vasoconstriction; however, if the ice pack is left in place more than 30 minutes, vasodilation and subsequent edema may occur. The perineal tissues should be assessed frequently to prevent injury from the ice pack. The episiotomy site is inspected every 15 minutes during the first hour after the birth for redness, swelling, tenderness, and hematomas. As a part of postpartal care, the mother will need instruction in perineal hygiene care and comfort measures. (See chapter 36 ∞ for additional discussion of relief measures for the immediate postpartum period.)

It is important for nurses to recognize that perineal pain continues for a period of time. Women who experience prolonged pain tend to have other problems, such as breastfeeding difficulties and depression, and are more reluctant to reestablish sexual activity. Risk factors for subsequent lacerations include use of repeat episiotomy and instrument-assisted births.

DEVELOPING CULTURAL COMPETENCE

Canadian Orthodox Jewish Women

Although many North American women have specific beliefs and expectations for childbirth, other cultural or religious groups may not verbalize specific requests or ideas for their labor experience. Canadian Orthodox Jewish women typically do not express their preferences but instead depend on their healthcare practitioner to make decisions regarding procedures that may be indicated. They typically view healthcare providers as authority figures and participate less in their own healthcare decision making.

Care of the Woman During Forceps-Assisted Birth

Forceps are designed to assist the birth of a fetus by providing traction or by providing the means to rotate the fetal head to an occiput-anterior position. In medical literature and practice, **forceps-assisted birth** is also known as *instrumental delivery, operative delivery,* or *operative vaginal delivery.* There are many different types of forceps, each with special functions. For example, Piper forceps are designed to be used with a breech presentation (buttocks as presenting part); they are applied after the birth of the body, when the fetal head is still in the birth canal and assistance is needed. In conversational language, Piper forceps are said to be applied to the aftercoming head. All other forceps are used in situations when the fetus is in a cephalic (head down) presentation. In such situations, the forceps are applied to the sides of the head. The type of forceps used is determined by the physician assisting with the birth.

Criteria for Forceps Application

ACOG has classified the definitions of forceps applications into three categories: outlet, low, and midforceps. Criteria for *outlet forceps* application are as follows (Cunningham et al., 2010):

1. Forceps are applied when the fetal skull has reached the pelvic floor and is at or on the perineum. (There is bulging of the perineum.)
2. The scalp is visible between contractions without separating the labia. (Earlier in labor, as the woman pushes during the contraction, the fetal scalp may be visible, but when the pushing effort ceases, the scalp recedes and is no longer visible. This criterion indicates that the scalp remains visible even when the woman is not pushing.)
3. The sagittal suture is not more than 45 degrees from the midline. The sagittal suture is the anterior-posterior suture on the top of the fetal head. At this point in a spontaneous birth, extension has almost been completed, external rotation is beginning, and the sagittal suture is between the midline and 45 degrees from the midline. (For example, think of a clock face. If 12:00 is the maternal symphysis pubis and the fetus is in left occiput anterior (LOA), the sagittal suture and the occiput are between 12:00 and 1:30.) (See chapter 22 ∞.) The important aspect of this criterion is that with outlet forceps, the fetal head is moving naturally from extension to external rotation, and the forceps are being used to guide or lift the head out.

The criterion for *low forceps* application is that the leading edge (presenting part) of the fetal skull must be at a station of plus 2 (+2) or below (for example, +3) but not on the pelvic floor. The rotation (internal rotation, which is part of the cardinal movements) of the fetal head is less than 45 degrees (right or left occiput anterior to occiput anterior, or right or left occiput posterior to occiput posterior) (Cunningham et al., 2010).

The criterion for *midforceps* application is that the fetal head must be engaged (largest diameter of the head reaches or passes through the pelvic inlet), but the leading edge (presenting part) of the fetal skull is above a plus 2 (+2) station (for example +1, 0, −1, −2). When midforceps are used, the goal is to apply traction, and, frequently, to rotate the head and facilitate the vaginal birth.

High forceps are not indicated in current obstetric practice. A woman whose fetus is at a station of −3 or is above the pelvic inlet should give birth by cesarean. Types of forceps are depicted in Figure 28-4 ■.

Indications for Use of Forceps

Forceps Delivery

Indications for the use of forceps include the presence of any condition that threatens the mother or fetus and that can be relieved by birth. Conditions that put the woman at risk include heart disease, acute pulmonary edema or pulmonary compromise, certain neurologic conditions, intrapartal infection, prolonged second stage, or exhaustion. Fetal conditions include premature placental separation, prolapsed umbilical cord, and nonreassuring fetal status. Forceps may be used electively to shorten the second stage of labor and spare the woman's pushing effort (when exhaustion or heart disease is present) or when regional anesthesia has affected the woman's motor innervation, and she cannot push effectively. In the past, outlet forceps have been used to protect the head of a preterm infant during birth; however, the advantages of this practice are now being questioned (Cunningham et al., 2010).

Risk factors for a forceps- or vacuum-assisted birth (discussion to follow) are as follows (Cunningham et al., 2010):

- Nulliparity
- Maternal age (35 and over)
- Maternal height of less than 150 cm (4 ft 11 in)
- Pregnancy weight gain of more than 15 kg (33 lb)

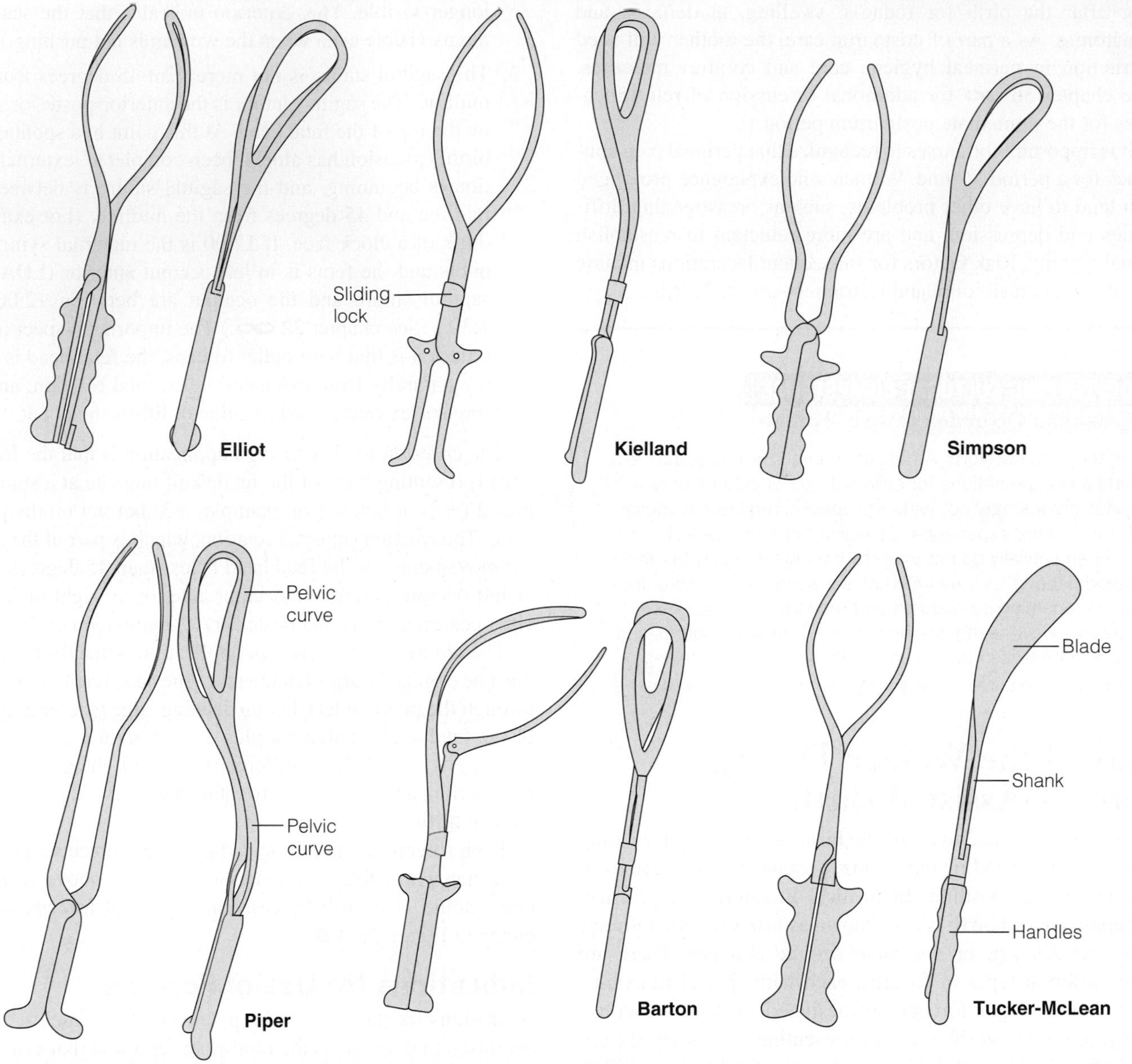

Figure 28-4 ■ Forceps are composed of a blade, shank, and handle and may have a cephalic and pelvic curve. (Note labels on Piper and Tucker-McLean forceps.) The blades may be fenestrated (open) or solid. The front and lateral views of these forceps illustrate differences in blades, open and closed shanks, and cephalic and pelvic curves. Elliot, Simpson, and Tucker-McLean forceps are used as outlet forceps. Kielland and Barton forceps are used for midforceps rotations. Piper forceps are used to provide traction and flexion of the aftercoming head (the head comes after the body) of a fetus in breech presentation.

- Postdate gestation (41 weeks or more)
- Epidural anesthesia
- Infant presentation other than occipitoanterior
- Presence of dystocia
- Presence of a midline episiotomy
- Abnormal fetal heart rate (FHR) tracing

Neonatal and Maternal Risks

Some newborns may develop a small area of ecchymosis or edema, or both, along the sides of the face as a result of forceps application. Caput succedaneum or cephalhematoma (and subsequent hyperbilirubinemia) may occur as well as transient facial paralysis. Other reported complications include low Apgar scores, retinal hemorrhage, corneal abrasions, ocular trauma, other trauma (Erb's palsy, fractured clavicle), elevated neonatal bilirubin levels, and prolonged infant hospital stay (Cunningham et al., 2010).

Maternal risks may include trauma such as lacerations of the birth canal, periurethral lacerations, and extensions of a median episiotomy into the anus, resulting in increased bleeding, bruising, hematomas, and pelvic floor injuries (Beckmann et al., 2010). Women who give birth with the assistance of forceps are more likely to have a third- or fourth-degree laceration and report more perineal pain and sexual problems in the postpartum period (Cunningham et al., 2010). In addition, an increase in postpartum infections, cervical lacerations, and prolonged hospital stays has been reported (Cunningham et al., 2010). Women who have given birth with forceps may also experience urinary and rectal incontinence, anal sphincter injury, and postpartum metritis (Cunningham et al., 2010).

Prerequisites for Forceps Application and Birth

It is very important that all of the prerequisites be met before the forceps procedure is attempted. The prerequisites are as follows (Cunningham et al., 2010):

- The physician must be knowledgeable about the advantages and disadvantages of different types of forceps and their use.
- The cervix must be completely dilated.
- The fetal head must be engaged and the station, presentation, and exact position of the head must be known. The fetus should be in a vertex or a face presentation with the chin anterior.
- Amniotic membranes must be ruptured to allow a firm grasp on the fetal head.
- The type of pelvis should be identified, because certain pelvic types do not permit rotation. In addition, there must be no disproportion between the fetal head and the maternal pelvis.
- Maternal bladder should be empty.
- There must be no obstructions to the birth below the fetal head, such as an incurving coccyx that will not allow the fetus to pass or a disproportion between the size of the head and the outlet or the midpelvis.
- Adequate anesthesia must be given for the type of forceps procedure that is anticipated. For instance, low forceps may be done with a pudendal block; however, midforceps or a rotation of more than 45 degrees requires an epidural, spinal-epidural, or general anesthesia.

Trial or Failed Forceps Procedure

The use of forceps or vacuum may be considered when the clinician believes a successful outcome can occur. In a trial forceps procedure, the physician attempts to use forceps with the knowledge that there could be a degree of cephalopelvic disproportion. A complete setup for immediate cesarean birth needs to be available before the forceps are applied. If a good application cannot be obtained or if no descent occurs with the application, a vacuum technique can be attempted. If this yields no descent, then a cesarean birth is the method of choice.

NURSING CARE MANAGEMENT

The nurse directs nursing care measures toward the variable(s) that may be positively affected by specific nursing interventions. For instance, dystocia may be corrected by changing maternal position, ambulation, rocking, frequent bladder emptying, and so on. FHR abnormalities may be affected by utero-placental-fetal circulation, so the nurse could support ambulation (if not contraindicated), frequent position changes, intake of adequate fluids, and monitoring to detect early FHR changes.

If a forceps-assisted birth is required, the nurse explains the procedure briefly to the woman. With adequate regional anesthesia, the woman should feel some pressure but no pain. The nurse encourages her to avoid pushing during application of the forceps (Figure 28-5 ■ depicts the application). The nurse monitors contractions and advises the physician when one is present because traction is applied only with a contraction. During the contraction, as the forceps are applied, the nurse again advises the woman to avoid pushing. With each contraction, *after the forceps are in place,* the physician provides traction on the forceps as the woman pushes. It is not uncommon to observe mild bradycardia as traction is applied to the forceps. This bradycardia results from head compression and is transient.

Following birth, the newborn is assessed for facial edema, bruising, caput succedaneum, cephalhematoma, corneal abrasion, and any sign of cerebral edema. In the fourth stage, the nurse assesses the woman for perineal swelling, bruising, hematoma, excessive bleeding, and hemorrhage. In the postpartum period it is important to assess for signs of infection if lacerations occurred during the procedure (Beckmann et al., 2010).

The nurse answers questions and reiterates explanations provided, reviews nursing assessments of the woman and her newborn, and provides opportunities for the woman and family to ask further questions. Some women may feel a sense of loss or failure as a result of needing forceps for birth. The nurse provides reassurance to the woman and her family.

Care of the Woman During Vacuum Extraction

Vacuum Extraction

Vacuum extraction is an obstetric procedure used by physicians and certified nurse-midwives (CNMs) to assist the birth of a fetus by applying suction to the fetal head. The vacuum extractor accounts for 68% of all operative vaginal births. Its use has increased by 41% since 1990 and continues to rise (Cunningham et al., 2010). The vacuum extractor is composed of a soft suction cup attached to a suction bottle (pump) by tubing. The suction cup, which comes in various sizes, is placed against the occiput of the fetal head. Care must be taken to ensure that no cervical or vaginal tissue is trapped under the cup. The pump is used to create negative pressure (suction) of approximately 50 to 60 mm Hg in a stepwise sequence or rapid application. An artificial caput ("chignon") is formed as the fetal scalp is pulled into the cup. The physician or CNM then applies traction in coordination with uterine contractions. The fetal head should descend with each contraction until it emerges from the vagina (Figure 28-6 ■).

Research indicates that negative suction applied for more than 10 minutes is associated with a greater incidence of scalp injury. The longer the duration of suction, the more likely the newborn will have scalp injury. Although there are no data on the duration of use, ACOG advises a 30-minute time limit (Simpson & Creehan, 2008). Many practitioners limit the time to 20 minutes. Although there are no specifications on the number of attempts, failure to descend with multiple attempts is an indicator that a cesarean birth may be needed. In addition, if more than three "pop-offs" occur (the suction cup pops off the

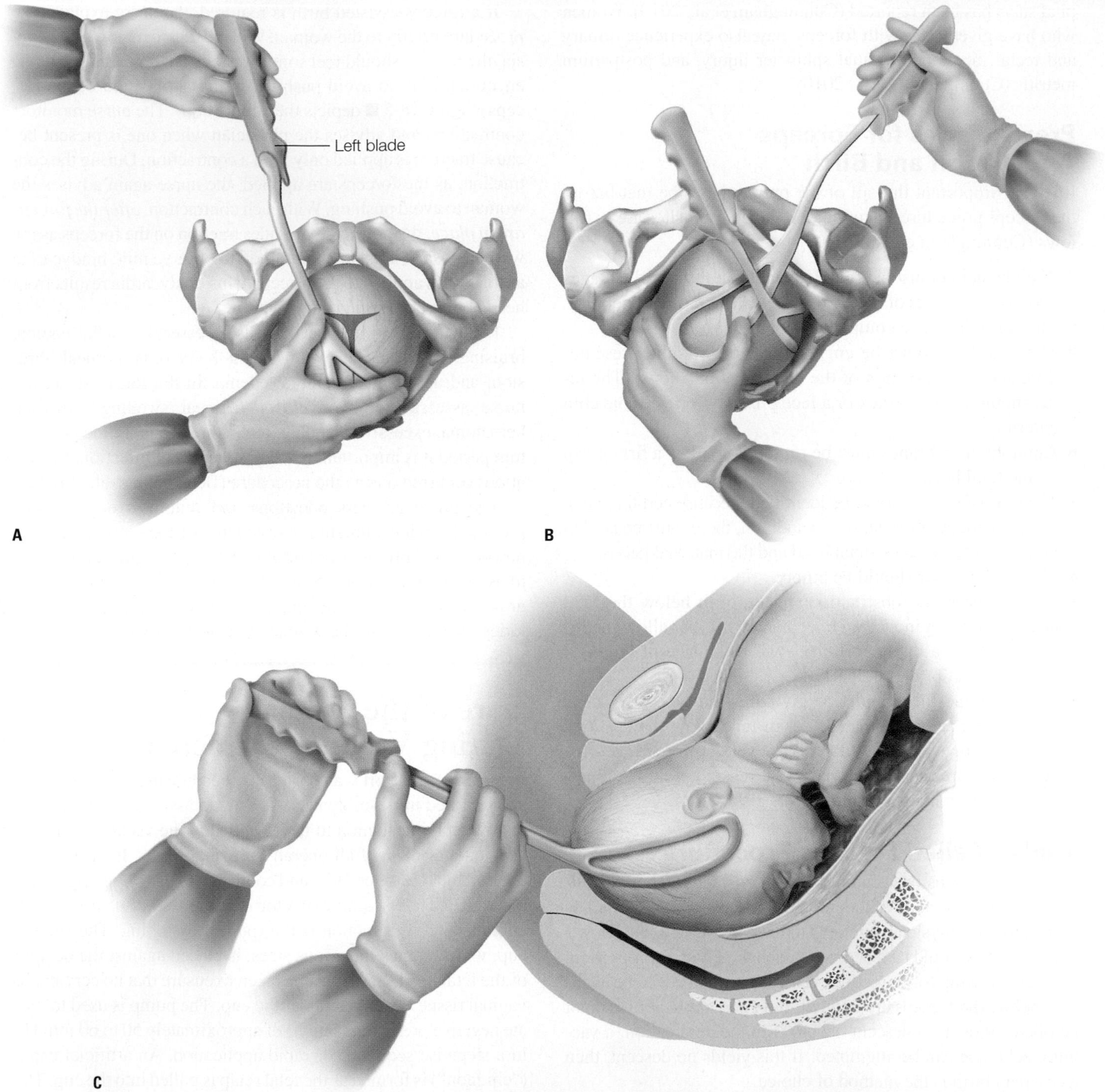

Figure 28-5 ■ Application of forceps in occiput-anterior (OA) position. A. The left blade is inserted along the left side wall of the pelvis over the parietal bone. B. The right blade is inserted along the right side wall of the pelvis over the parietal bone. C. With correct placement of the blades, the handles lock easily. During uterine contractions, traction is applied to the forceps in a downward and outward direction to follow the birth canal.

fetal head), the procedure should be discontinued. The most common indication for the use of the vacuum extractor is a prolonged second stage of labor or nonreassuring heart rate pattern. Vacuum extraction is also used to relieve the woman of pushing effort, or when analgesia or fatigue interferes with her ability to push effectively, or in cases of nonreassuring fetal status when prompt birth is indicated. The vacuum extractor is preferred to forceps in cases of borderline cephalopelvic disproportion (CPD), when successful passage of the fetal head requires all potential space inside the vaginal canal. True CPD is an absolute contraindication to vacuum extraction. Other contraindications include nonvertex presentations, maternal or suspected fetal coagulation defects, known or suspected hydrocephalus, and fetal scalp trauma (Cunningham et al., 2010). Relative contraindications include suspected fetal macrosomia, high fetal station, face or breech presentation, gestation less than 34 weeks, incompletely dilated cervix, and previous fetal scalp blood sampling (Cunningham et al., 2010).

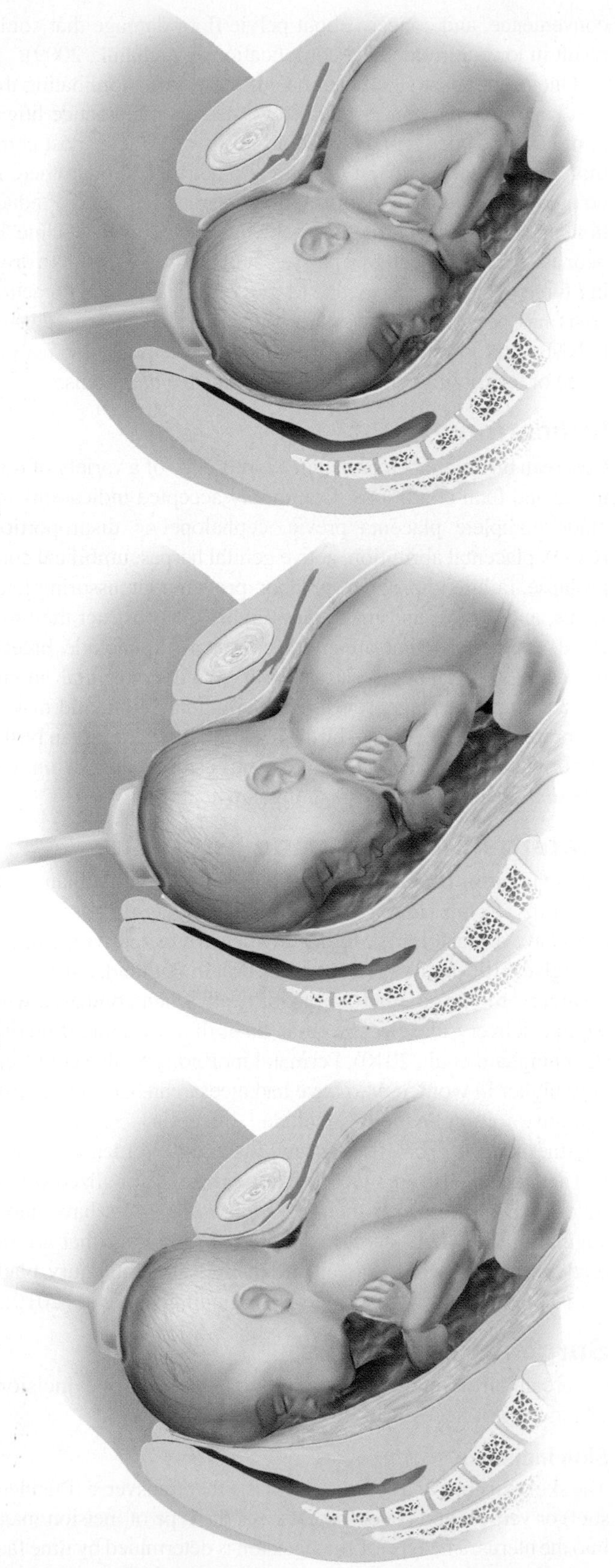

Figure 28-6 ■ Vacuum extractor traction. A. The cup is placed on the fetal occiput, creating suction. Traction is applied in a downward and outward direction. B. Traction continues in a downward direction as the fetal head begins to emerge from the vagina. C. Traction is maintained to lift the fetal head out of the vagina.

Neonatal complications include scalp lacerations, bruising, subgaleal hematomas, cephalhematomas, intracranial hemorrhages, subconjunctival hemorrhages, neonatal jaundice, fractured clavicle, Erb's palsy, damage to the sixth and seventh cranial nerves, retinal hemorrhage, and fetal death. In addition, there is an increased incidence of shoulder dystocia (Cunningham et al., 2010). There appear to be more neonatal complications and injuries with use of a metal suction cup device than with soft cup devices. In the presence of a preterm gestation, risk of periventricular-intraventricular hemorrhage (PV-IVH) has been a concern, and some studies provide conflicting recommendations. Maternal complications include perineal trauma, edema, third- and fourth-degree lacerations, postpartum pain, and infection (Simpson & Creehan, 2008). Women who give birth with the aid of a vacuum extractor report more sexual difficulties in the postpartum period. Maternal genital tract and anal sphincter injuries occur less frequently with the vacuum extractor than with forceps.

In 1998, the U.S. Food and Drug Administration (FDA) released a health advisory statement that vacuum extraction can cause serious or fatal complications. Twelve deaths and nine serious injuries occurred between 1994 and 1998. The FDA recommended caution in using rocking movements when using the device. They also recommended that pediatricians be alerted when a vacuum-assisted birth occurred so the infant can be closely monitored for related injuries. In addition, the following guidelines are recommended when a birth is facilitated by a vacuum extractor (Cunningham et al., 2010):

Application: Vacuum Extraction Delivery

1. The criteria used to evaluate the appropriateness of a forceps birth should also be used to determine the appropriateness of a vacuum birth (station).
2. The same indications and contraindications should be used for both forceps and vacuum births.
3. The presenting part must be vertex and must be at 0 station or below.
4. Vacuum-assisted births should be performed only by an experienced practitioner.
5. The procedure should be terminated immediately if descent does not occur or if the vacuum device pops off more than three times.

NURSING CARE MANAGEMENT

There are different types of vacuum extractors. The nurse must be familiar with the types used within the birthing setting and learn the pressure limits of each type.

The nurse should inform the woman about what is happening during the procedure. If adequate regional anesthesia has been administered, the woman feels only pressure during the procedure. The nurse pumps the vacuum to the appropriate level to provide suction by the physician or CNM. The fetal heart rate (FHR) is auscultated at least every 5 minutes or assessed by continuous electronic fetal monitoring (EFM). The parents need to be informed that the caput (chignon) on the baby's head will disappear within 2 to 3 days.

The nurse continues to assess the newborn for complications such as bruising, newborn jaundice, cephalhematomas, intracranial hemorrhage, and retinal hemorrhages.

Care of the Family During Cesarean Birth

Cesarean birth is the birth of the infant through an abdominal and uterine incision. Cesarean birth is one of the oldest surgical procedures known. Until the 20th century, cesareans were primarily equated with an attempt to save the fetus of a dying woman. As the maternal and perinatal morbidity and mortality rates associated with cesarean birth steadily decreased throughout the 20th century, the rate of cesarean births increased. In 1965, cesarean births constituted 4.5% of all births and progressed to a high of 32.3% in 2008 (Hamilton, Martin, & Ventura, 2010). The cesarean birthrate has risen by 50% since 1996 (Hamilton et al., 2010). In some countries, the incidence has been much lower throughout the 20th century; however, many countries have seen a consistent rise in their cesarean delivery rate. In 2005, the cesarean delivery rate in Australia had risen to 29% (Brennan, Robson, Murphy, et al., 2009). Bolivia has one of the lowest cesarean birthrates in the world, accounting for only 5% of all births. Sweden and the Netherlands have maintained cesarean birthrates of 10% for decades. Many Latin American countries also have low rates, including Peru with a cesarean birthrate below 10%, and Honduras with a rate of 12%. England and Canada have rates below 20%. However, some countries, such as Chile, have rates as high as 40% (Brennan et al., 2009). The rising international cesarean rate is concerning given that the World Health Organization has proposed that a rate greater than 10% to 15% is not justifiable in any region of the world (Brennan et al., 2009).

The rising cesarean birthrate has created marked concern among various practitioner groups. ACOG created a task force in 2000 to address concerns regarding the rise in cesarean birthrates. The committee recommended two benchmarks to be achieved by 2010: a primary cesarean rate of 15.5% for women who were greater than 37 gestational weeks with a cephalic singleton presentation, and a vaginal birthrate of 37% in women who have had one previous cesarean birth after 37 gestational weeks (Cunningham et al., 2010).

Many factors affect the cesarean birthrate, and they need to be considered in discussions about decreasing the current rate in the United States. These factors include a rising number of nulliparous women, who are at an increased risk for cesareans, giving birth; a rise in the maternal age, which is associated with a higher incidence of cesarean birth; changing philosophies regarding the best method of birth with a breech presentation; interpretations of electronic fetal monitoring (EFM) tracings; a decrease in the use of forceps and vacuum extractors to facilitate a vaginal birth; and a dramatic rise in obesity, another risk factor for cesarean birth. Other risks include changing practice related to vaginal birth after cesarean birth, increased use of epidural anesthesia, physician convenience, and type of provider (Cunningham et al., 2010). Interestingly, some women are now requesting a primary cesarean birth because of fear of labor, convenience, and concern about pelvic floor damage that could result in long-term medical complications (Michaluk, 2009).

One of the most significant healthcare factors dominating the 21st century is the concern related to medical malpractice litigation. Failure to perform a cesarean birth is one of the most common malpractice claims in obstetrical practice. Although there is no association between performing a cesarean birth and a reduction in childhood neurologic problems, including a decline in neonatal seizures or cerebral palsy, fear of litigation remains a driving force in obstetrical practice (ACOG, 2009a). The malpractice crisis has become so grave that some certified nurse-midwives (CNMs) and physicians are abandoning obstetrical practice because of fear of litigation and high malpractice premiums.

Indications

Cesarean births are performed in the presence of a variety of maternal and fetal conditions. Commonly accepted indications include complete placenta previa, cephalopelvic disproportion (CPD), placental abruption, active genital herpes, umbilical cord prolapse, failure to progress in labor, proven nonreassuring fetal status, and benign and malignant tumors that obstruct the birth canal. Indications that are more controversial include breech presentation, previous cesarean birth, major congenital anomalies, cervical cerclage, severe Rh isoimmunization, and maternal preference for cesarean birth. The majority of cesarean births performed in the United States are done because of a previous cesarean birth and dystocia (Cunningham et al., 2010).

Maternal Mortality and Morbidity

Cesarean births have a higher maternal mortality rate than vaginal births. In the United States, women undergoing a cesarean birth have a fourfold risk of death when compared with women who give birth vaginally (Lothian, 2006). In England, emergency cesarean birth has a ninefold risk of death when compared with vaginal delivery, and elective cesarean births have a threefold risk (Cunningham et al., 2010). Perinatal morbidity is also considerably higher in women who have had a cesarean. Common postoperative complications include infection, reactions to anesthesia agents, blood clots, and bleeding. Women who have had a cesarean birth are twice as likely to be rehospitalized within 60 days of birth when compared with women who have had a vaginal birth. Other sources of maternal morbidity that are directly associated with cesarean birth include ureteral injury, bladder laceration, and wound infection (Cunningham et al., 2010).

Surgical Techniques

Cesarean birth requires both a skin and a uterine incision, which are not necessarily the same type of incision.

Skin Incisions

The skin incision for a cesarean birth is either transverse (Pfannenstiel) or vertical and is not indicative of the type of incision made into the uterus. The type of skin incision is determined by time factor, patient preference, cosmetic reasons, or physician preference.

The transverse incision is made across the lowest and narrowest part of the abdomen. Because the incision is made just below the pubic hair line, it is almost invisible after healing. Other advantages of this type of incision include less bleeding and better healing. The limitations of this type of skin incision are that it does not allow for extension of the incision if needed. Because it usually requires more time, this incision is used when time is not of the essence (e.g., with failure to progress and no fetal or maternal stress). This type of incision may result in suboptimal visualization, especially in obese women. This type of incision may also develop more scar tissue if subsequent surgeries, such as repeat cesarean, are performed (Creasy et al., 2008).

The vertical (infraumbilical midline) incision is made between the navel and the symphysis pubis. This incision is quicker and is therefore preferred in cases of nonreassuring fetal status when rapid birth is indicated, with preterm or macrosomic infants, or when the woman is obese (Creasy et al., 2008).

Uterine Incisions

The type of uterine incision depends on the need for the cesarean. The choice of incision affects the woman's opportunity for a subsequent vaginal birth and her risks of a ruptured uterine scar with a subsequent pregnancy.

The two major locations of uterine incisions are the lower uterine segment and the upper segment of the uterine corpus (Figure 28-7 ■).

The most common lower uterine segment incision is a transverse incision (Figure 28-7A), which is preferred for the following reasons (Cunningham et al., 2010):

1. The lower segment is the thinnest portion of the uterus and involves less blood loss.
2. It requires only moderate dissection of the bladder from underlying myometrium.
3. It is easier to repair, although repair takes longer.
4. The site is less likely to rupture during subsequent pregnancies.
5. There is a decreased chance of adherence of bowel or omentum to the incision line.

The disadvantages include the following:

1. It takes longer to make a transverse incision.
2. It is limited in size because of the presence of major blood vessels on either side of the uterus.
3. It has a greater tendency to extend laterally into the uterine vessels.

Types of Incisions

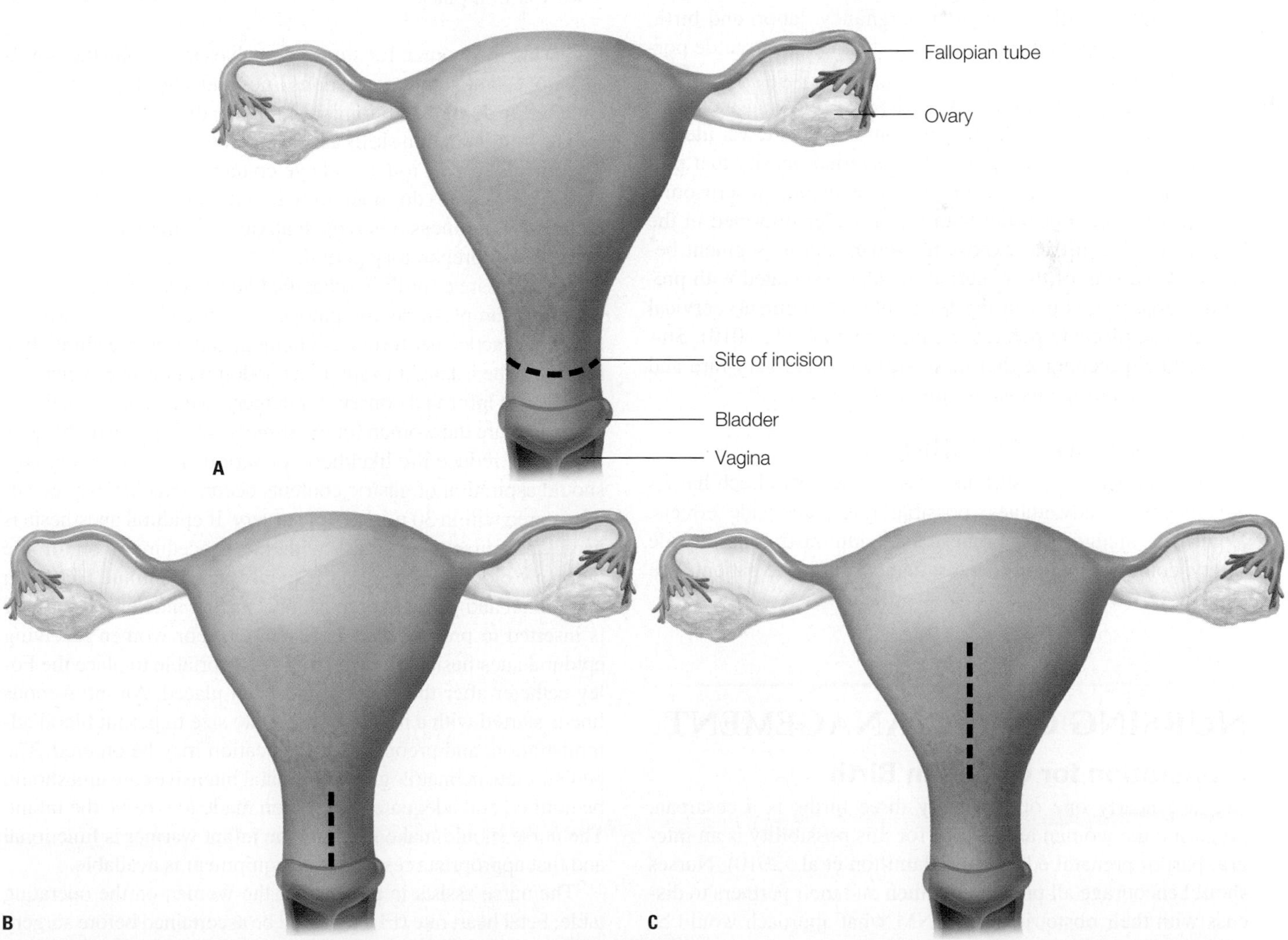

Figure 28-7 ■ Uterine incisions for a cesarean birth. A. This transverse incision in the lower uterine segment is called a Kerr incision. B. The Sellheim incision is a vertical incision in the lower uterine segment. C. This view illustrates the classic uterine incision that is done in the body (corpus) of the uterus. The classic incision was commonly done in the past and is associated with increased risk of uterine rupture in subsequent pregnancies and labor.

4. The incision may stretch and become a thin window, but it usually does not create problems clinically until subsequent labor ensues.

The lower uterine segment vertical incision is preferred for multiple gestation, abnormal presentation, if the woman has had no labor, and for preterm and macrosomic fetuses (Figure 28-7B). Disadvantages of this incision are as follows:

1. The incision may extend downward into the cervix.
2. More extensive dissection of the bladder is needed to keep the incision in the lower uterine segment.
3. If the incision extends upward into the upper segment, hemostasis and closure are more difficult.
4. The vertical incision carries a higher risk of rupture with subsequent labor. Consequently, once a vertical incision is performed, future births need to be via cesarean.

One other incision, the classic incision, was the method of choice for many years but it is used infrequently now (Figure 28-7C). This vertical incision was made into the upper uterine segment. More blood loss resulted, and it was more difficult to repair. Most important, it carried an increased risk of uterine rupture with subsequent pregnancy, labor, and birth, because the upper uterine segment is the most contractile portion of the uterus.

The primary indications for a classical incision include a very small fetus in breech presentation when the lower uterine segment is not thinned out, morbid maternal obesity that precludes safe access to the lower uterine segment, a macrosomic fetus in transverse position with the shoulder impacted in the birth canal, inability to expose the lower uterine segment because of scarring of the maternal bladder associated with previous surgery, myoma in the lower uterine segment, cervical cancer, and placenta percreta (Cunningham et al., 2010). Students should recognize that these situations are very rare and that classical uterine incisions are rarely performed.

Analgesia and Anesthesia

There is no perfect anesthesia for cesarean birth. Each has its advantages, disadvantages, possible risks, and side effects. Goals for analgesia and anesthesia administration include safety, comfort, and emotional satisfaction for the patient. See chapter 25 ∞.

NURSING CARE MANAGEMENT

Preparation for Cesarean Birth

Because nearly one out of every three births is a cesarean, preparing the woman and family for this possibility is an integral part of prenatal education (Hamilton et al., 2010). Nurses should encourage all pregnant women and their partners to discuss with their obstetrician or CNM what approach would be taken in the event of a cesarean. They can also discuss their needs and desires as a couple under those circumstances. Their preferences may include the following:

- Participating in the choice of anesthetic
- Presence of the father (or significant other) during the procedures in the recovery or postpartum room
- Audio or video recording and/or photographing of the birth
- Delayed instillation of eye drops to promote eye contact between parent and infant in the first hour after birth
- Physical contact or holding the newborn while on the operating room table or in the recovery room (If the mother cannot hold the newborn, the father can hold the baby for her.)
- Breastfeeding immediately after the surgery has been completed
- Preparation that may be done, such as abdominal prep, insertion of an indwelling bladder catheter, and starting an intravenous infusion and epidural placement
- Description or viewing of the operating room
- Types of anesthesia for birth and analgesia available postpartum
- Sensations that may be experienced
- Roles of significant others
- Interaction with the newborn
- Immediate recovery phase
- Postpartum phase

Preparing the woman for surgery involves more than the procedures of establishing intravenous lines and a urinary indwelling catheter or doing an abdominal prep. As discussed previously, good communication skills are essential in assisting the couple. Therapeutic use of touch and eye contact (if culturally acceptable and possible) do much to maintain reality orientation and control. These measures reduce anxiety for the woman during the stressful preparatory period.

If the cesarean birth is scheduled and not an emergency, the nurse has ample time for preoperative teaching. The woman needs to practice her turning, coughing, and deep breathing. It is helpful if she is taught to splint her abdominal muscles when she coughs. An informed consent for surgery needs to be signed.

To prepare the woman for the surgery, she is given nothing by mouth. To reduce the likelihood of serious pulmonary damage should aspiration of gastric contents occur, antacids may be administered within 30 minutes of surgery. If epidural anesthesia is used, the nurse may assist with the procedure, monitor the woman's blood pressure and response, and continue EFM. An abdominal and perineal prep is done, and an indwelling catheter is inserted to prevent bladder distention. For women receiving epidural anesthesia, it may be more comfortable to place the Foley catheter after the epidural has been placed. An intravenous line is started with a needle of adequate size to permit blood administration, and preoperative medication may be ordered. The pediatrician, neonatologist, or neonatal intensive care unit should be notified and adequate preparation made to receive the infant. The nurse should make sure that the infant warmer is functional and that appropriate resuscitation equipment is available.

The nurse assists in positioning the woman on the operating table. Fetal heart rate (FHR) should be ascertained before surgery and during preparation because fetal hypoxia can result from aortocaval compression. The operating table may be adjusted so it slants slightly to one side, or a wedge (folded blanket or towels) may be placed under the right hip. The uterus should be displaced about 15 degrees from the midline. This helps relieve the pressure of the heavy uterus on the vena cava and lessens the incidence of vena caval compression and supine maternal hypotension. The woman is strapped onto the table to prevent falls or injuries from occurring during the surgery. If a cauterization device is being used, the grounding source is secured on the woman's leg after the device has been checked to make sure it is in working order. The suction should be in working order, and the urine collection bag should be positioned under the operating table to ensure proper urinary drainage. Auscultation or electronic monitoring of the FHR needs to continue until immediately before the surgery. A last-minute check is done to ensure that the fetal scalp electrode has been removed if the fetus was internally monitored. The nurse should continue to provide reassurance and describe the various procedures being performed, along with a rationale, to ease anxiety and give the woman a sense of control.

Before beginning the procedure, a count of all instruments that will be used during the operative procedure is performed and recorded. Typically, this count is repeated three times throughout the operation to ensure that no instruments are left in the woman's abdomen. The nurse is responsible for ensuring that the instrument count is correct. In the event the count is not correct or if a count was not done initially because of emergency circumstances, a portable x-ray screening is performed to ensure no instruments remain in the maternal abdomen.

Preparation for Repeat Cesarean Birth

When a couple is anticipating a repeat cesarean birth, they have time to reflect on their past experiences, analyze and synthesize the new information they are given, and prepare for the experience. Couples who have had previous negative experiences need an opportunity to describe what they felt contributed to these events. They should be encouraged to identify what they would like to have altered and to list interventions that would make the experience more positive. Those who have had positive experiences need reassurance that their needs and desires will be met in the same manner. In addition, the nurse should provide an opportunity for the couple to discuss any fears or anxieties. Some women undergoing an elective repeat cesarean birth may continue to grieve the loss of the ideal birth experience or continue to exhibit mixed emotions regarding their choices for the birth. These women need reassurance and support throughout the birth process.

Preparation for Emergency Cesarean Birth

The period preceding surgery must be used to its greatest advantage. If possible, the couple needs some time for privacy to assimilate the information given to them and to ask for additional information. It is imperative that caregivers use their most effective communication skills. The nurse must address what the couple may anticipate during the next few hours. Asking the couple, "What questions do you have about the decision?" gives the couple an opportunity for further clarification. The nurse can prepare the woman in stages, giving her information and the rationale for each procedure before commencing. Before carrying out a procedure, it is essential to tell the woman (1) what is going to happen, (2) why it is being done, and (3) what sensations she may experience. This allows the woman to be informed and to consent to the procedure. The woman experiences a sense of control and therefore less helplessness and powerlessness.

Supporting the Father/Partner

Every effort should be made to include the father/partner or support person in the cesarean birth experience. When the father or support person attends the cesarean birth, he or she must wear a surgical gown and mask as do others in the operating suite. The father or support person can sit on a stool placed beside the woman's head to provide physical touch, visual contact, and verbal reassurance to his partner.

Many support persons worry about their own reactions to the operative procedure. A sterile drape is placed between the woman's head and the sterile field. The nurse can advise the support person that this can be used as a partition if he or she does not wish to view the procedure itself. The nurse should encourage support persons to eat if possible before the surgery. Most fathers or support persons who fear "fainting" or "feeling queasy" do not have difficulties in the operating room and frequently forget these fears as they are swept away in the excitement of the birth.

Other measures, such as the following, can be taken to promote the participation of the father or partner who chooses not to be present in the delivery room:

- Allowing the father or partner to be near the operating room, where he can hear the newborn's first cry
- Encouraging the father/partner to carry or accompany the infant to the nursery for the initial assessment
- Involving the father/partner in postpartal care in the recovery room

In the event that a support person cannot be with the woman during the cesarean birth, such as in situations involving emergencies, the nurse may obtain consent from the woman before the surgery and then provide updates to the support person to alleviate undue fear and anxiety.

Immediate Postpartum Recovery Period

After birth, the nurse assesses the Apgar score and completes the initial assessment and identification procedures as after a vaginal birth. Every effort must be made to assist the parents in bonding with the infant. If the mother is awake, one of her arms should be freed to enable her to touch and stroke the infant. The baby can be given to the father to hold until she or he must be taken to the nursery.

The nurse caring for the postpartal woman should check her vital signs every 5 minutes until they are stable, then every 15 minutes for an hour, then every 30 minutes until she is discharged to the postpartal unit. The nurse should remain with the woman until she is stable.

The dressing and perineal pad must be checked every 15 minutes for at least an hour, and the fundus should be gently palpated to determine whether it is remaining firm. The fundus may be palpated by placing a hand to support the incision. Intravenous oxytocin is usually administered to promote the contractility of the uterine musculature. If the woman has had general anesthesia, she should be positioned on her side to facilitate drainage of secretions, turned, and assisted with coughing and deep breathing every 2 hours for at least 24 hours. If she has received a spinal or epidural anesthetic, the level of anesthesia should be checked every 15 minutes. It is important to monitor intake and output and to observe the urine for bloody tinge, which could mean surgical trauma to the bladder. The physician prescribes medication to relieve the mother's pain and nausea, and this should be administered as needed. Some physicians use a single dose of epidural morphine (5 to 7.5 mg) for postsurgical pain relief. Facilitation of parent-infant interaction following birth and postpartum care is discussed in chapter 36 ∞.

Care of the Woman Undergoing Vaginal Birth After Cesarean

In the late 1980s there was an increasing trend to have a trial of labor and **vaginal birth after cesarean (VBAC)** birth in cases of nonrecurring indications for a cesarean (for example, twins, umbilical cord prolapse, placenta previa, nonreassuring fetal status). This trend was influenced by consumer demand and studies that support VBAC as a viable and safe alternative. Recent media reports have reintroduced the debate regarding the safety of VBACs resulting in a decrease in the number of VBACs in the United States.

The American College of Obstetricians and Gynecologists (ACOG) guidelines state that the following aspects should be met when identifying candidates for a trial of labor (Cunningham et al., 2010):

- One previous cesarean birth and a low transverse uterine incision
- An adequate pelvis
- No other uterine scars or previous uterine rupture
- A physician who is able to do a cesarean needs to be available throughout active labor
- In-house anesthesia personnel are available for emergency cesarean births if warranted

Recent debate and research have led to a considerable rise in cesarean births and a significant reduction in women attempting VBACs. In the late 1980s, a movement to increase vaginal births after a previous cesarean birth was advocated because of the increases in morbidity, mortality, and costs associated with cesarean births. This resulted in a decline in the cesarean birthrate and a rise in the VBAC rates. Research in the 1990s, however, changed this trend when reports of rising numbers of uterine ruptures were reported in women attempting VBACs. Although the absolute risks of VBAC are small, there is a 0.1% to 0.7% risk of uterine rupture when women attempt a trial of labor after previously undergoing a cesarean birth (Algert, Morris, Simpson, et al., 2008). The significance is that, in the studies, there were no uterine ruptures in the group of women who had undergone an elective repeat cesarean birth. There is uncertainty about whether a trial of labor after cesarean (TOLAC) increases the risk of perinatal death compared to babies born by elective repeat cesarean section (ERCS). Some studies have found an increased perinatal death rate in babies in the TOLAC groups compared to those in the ERCS group (Richter, Bergmann, & Dudenhausen, 2008). These findings, combined with nonmedical factors (rising malpractice premiums for providers, accessibility to an institution that provides VBAC services, provider attitudes), are primarily responsible in the decline of VBACs in the United States since the 1990s. Other risks associated with VBAC are included in Table 28-4.

Although VBACs remain controversial, success rates for VBAC have been encouraging. Women whose previous cesarean was performed because of nonrecurring indications have been reported to have approximately a 60% to 80% chance of success with VBAC (Harper & Macones, 2008). Women whose previous cesarean was performed for breech presentation had the highest success rates for VBAC (91%). Women who had a previous cesarean birth for nonreassuring fetal status had an 84% success rate, whereas a woman diagnosed with previous dystocia had a 67% success rate. Women who were previously diagnosed with dystocia before 5-cm dilatation had a 67% success rate, whereas women who had previously progressed to 6 to 9 cm had a 73% success rate. Women who had been labeled as having dystocia in the second stage had a 75% success rate (Cunningham et al., 2010).

NURSING CARE MANAGEMENT

The nursing care of a woman undergoing VBAC varies according to institutional protocols. Generally, if the woman is at very low risk (has had one previous cesarean with a lower uterine segment incision), her blood count, type, and screen are obtained on admission; a heparin lock is inserted for intravenous access if needed; continuous electronic fetal monitoring (EFM) is used; and clear fluids may be taken. If the woman is at higher risk, NPO status should be maintained, and, in addition to the care listed, an intrauterine catheter may be inserted to monitor intrauterine pressures during labor.

Supportive and comfort measures are very important. The woman may be excited about this opportunity to experience labor and vaginal birth, or she may be hesitant and frightened about the possibility of complications. The nurse provides information and encouragement for the laboring woman and her partner.

TABLE 28-4 Complications Associated with VBAC

- Uterine rupture
- Uterine dehiscence
- Hysterectomy
- Uterine infection
- Maternal death
- Neonatal death
- Antepartum stillbirth
- Intrapartum stillbirth
- Transfusion
- Hypoxic ischemic encephalopathy

FOCUS YOUR STUDY

- An external (or cephalic) version may be done after 37 weeks' gestation to change a breech presentation to a cephalic presentation, thereby making a lower risk vaginal birth more possible.
- The version is accomplished with the use of tocolytic agents to relax the uterus. An internal (podalic) version is used only when needed during the vaginal birth of a second twin.
- Amniotomy (AROM) is performed to hasten labor. The risks are prolapse of the umbilical cord and infection.
- Prostaglandin E_2 may be used before an induction of labor to soften the cervix (called cervical ripening). These agents are inserted into the vagina to make the cervix more favorable for induction.
- Labor is induced for many reasons. The methods include amniotomy, stripping of the membranes, intravenous oxytocin infusion, and alternative and complementary methods. Nursing responsibilities are heightened during an induced labor.
- Amnioinfusions are used in cases of oligohydramnios or nonperiodic decelerations to increase the volume of amniotic fluid, which relieves cord compression and promotes perfusion to the fetus.
- An episiotomy may be performed just before birth of the fetus. Current evidence shows a limited number of indications for its use.
- Forceps-assisted birth can be accomplished using outlet forceps, low forceps, or midforceps. Outlet forceps are the most common and are associated with few maternal-fetal complications. Midforceps are associated with more complications but, when needed, are an important aid to birth.
- A vacuum extractor is a soft, pliable cup attached to suction that can be applied to the fetal head and used in much the same way as forceps.
- Approximately one in three births is accomplished by cesarean. The nurse has a vital role in providing information, support, and encouragement to the couple participating in a cesarean birth.
- Vaginal birth after cesarean (VBAC) carries a low risk of uterine rupture; however, many physicians perform repeat cesarean births out of fear of malpractice issues. Overcoming the old fears of uterine rupture is a high priority for both the parents and the medical and nursing community.

CRITICAL THINKING IN ACTION

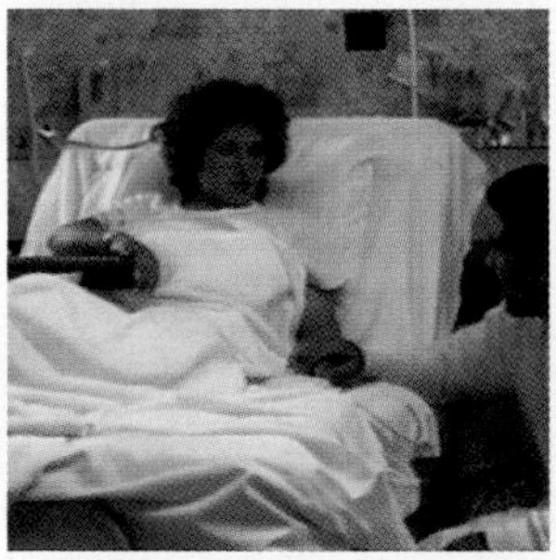
Source: George Dodson/Pearson Education.

Betsy Jones, a 28-year-old G1 PO is at 39 weeks' gestation, and her husband present to you in the labor suite for an external cephalic version procedure by her obstetrician. You introduce yourself and review her prenatal record for any significant risk factors or contraindications to the version procedure. Her prenatal chart is significant in that the fetus has been in a persistent frank breech position. You encourage Betsy and her husband to express their understanding and expectations of the procedure. You discuss certain criteria to be met prior to the procedure and obtain vital signs as follows: T 98.8°F, P 88, R 14, BP 110/80, urine screening negative for sugar, albumin, and ketones. You place Betsy on the external electronic fetal monitor, which demonstrates a fetal heart rate baseline of 140 to 152 with moderate long-term variability. There are no contractions observed by the monitor or Betsy. After explaining how to record fetal movement on the monitor, you proceed with an NST.

1. Explain the contraindications to the version procedure.
2. Discuss the criteria that should be met prior to performing external version.
3. How would you explain to Betsy and her husband what to expect during the version procedure?
4. What support would you give Betsy during the procedure?
5. Explain postversion discharge teaching.

See www.nursing.pearsonhighered.com for possible responses.

REFERENCES

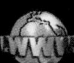

Algert, C. S., Morris, J. M., Simpson, J. M., Ford, J. B., & Roberts, C. L., (2008). Labor before a primary cesarean delivery: Reduced risk of *uterine rupture* in a subsequent trial of labor for vaginal birth after cesarean. *Obstetrics & Gynecology, 112*(5), 1061–1066.

American Academy of Pediatrics (AAP) & American College of Obstetricians and Gynecologists (ACOG). (2007). *Guidelines for perinatal care* (6th ed.). Washington, DC: Author.

American College of Obstetricians and Gynecologists (ACOG). (2008). *External cephalic version* (ACOG Practice Bulletin No.13). Washington, DC: Author.

American College of Obstetricians and Gynecologists (ACOG). (2009a). Catch 22 for New York's obstetricians: Failing state insurance system leaves OBs no options. ACOG News (press release).

American College of Obstetricians and Gynecologists (ACOG). (2009b). *Induction of labor.* (ACOG Practice Bulletin 107). Washington, DC: Author.

Bayles, B. P. (2007). Herbal and other complementary medicine use by Texas midwives. *Journal of Midwifery & Women's Health, 52*(5), 473–478.

Beckmann, C. R., Barzansky, B. M., Herbert, W. N., Douglas, W. N., Laube, W., & Ling, F. W. (2010). *Obstetrics & Gynecology* (6th ed.). Philadelphia, PA: Lippincott Williams & Wilkins.

Bishop, E. H. (1964). Pelvic scoring for elective induction. *Obstetrics and Gynecology, 24,* 266.

Blackburn, S. (2007). *Maternal, fetal, and neonatal physiology: A clinical perspective.* Philadelphia, PA: Saunders.

Boucher, M., Marquette, G. P., Varin, J., Champagne, J., Bujold, E. (2008, July). Fetomaternal hemorrhage during external cephalic version. *Obstetrics & Gynecology 112*(1), 79–84. doi: 10.1097/AOG.0b013e318179978c

Brennan, D. J., Robson, M. S., Murphy, M., & O'Herlihy, C. (2009). Comparative analysis of international cesarean delivery rates using 10-group classification identifies significant variation in spontaneous labor. *American Journal of Obstetrics and Gynecology, 201*(3), 308.e1–8.

Collaris, R. J., & Tan, P. C. (2009). Oral nifepidine versus subcutaneous terbutaline tocolysis for external cephalic version: A double-blind randomized trial. *British Journal of Obstetrics & Gynecology. 116*(1), 74–81.

Creasy, R. K., Resnik, R., Iams, J. D., Lockwood, C. J., & Moore, T. R. (2008). *Creasy and Resnik's maternal fetal medicine* (6th ed.). Philadelphia, PA: Elsevier.

Cunningham, F. G., Leveno, L. J., Bloom, S. L., Hauth, J. C., Gilstrap, L. C., & Wenstrom, K. D. (2010). *Williams obstetrics* (23rd ed.). New York, NY: McGraw-Hill.

Droulez, A., Girard, R., Dumas, A. M., Mathian, B., & Berland, M. (2008). Prediction of successful induction of labor: A comparison between fetal fibronectin assay and the Bishop score. *Journal De Gynécologie, Obstétrique Et Biologie De La Reproduction, 37*(7), 691–696.

Forest Pharmaceuticals. (2006). Cervidil manufacturer's fact sheet. St. Louis, MO: Forrest Pharmaceuticals. FDA Rev date: 11/28/2006.

Frankman, E. A., Wang, L., Bunker, C. H., & Lowder, J. L. (2009). Episiotomy in the United States: Has anything changed? *American Journal of Obstetrics & Gynecology, 200,* 573.e1–573.e8.

Gelber, S. & Sciscione, A. (2006). Mechanical methods of cervical ripening and labor induction. *Clinical Obstetrics & Gynecology, 49*(3), 642–657.

Hamilton, B. E., Martin, J. A., & Ventura, S. J. (2010). Births: Preliminary data for 2008. *National Vital Statistics Reports, 58 (16*), 1–18.

Harper, L. M., & Macones, G. A. (2008). Predicting success and reducing the risks when attempting vaginal birth after cesarean. *Obstetrical & Gynecological Survey, 63*(8), 538–545.

Hill, M. J., McWilliams, G. D., Garcia-Sur, D., Chen, B., Munroe, M., & Hoeldtke, N. J. (2008). The effect of membrane sweeping on prelabor rupture of membranes: A randomized controlled trial. *Obstetrics & Gynecology, 111*(6), 1313–1319.

Kavanagh, J., Kelly, J., & Thomas, J. (2009). Castor oil, bath and/or enema for cervical priming and induction of labor. *Cochrane Database of Systematic Reviews,* 3.

Knoche, A., Selzer, C., & Smolley, K. (2008). Induction of labor. *Practicing Midwife, 11*(9), 38–39.

Kok, M., Cnossen, J., Gravendeel, L., van der Post, J., Opmeer, B., & Willem Mol, B. (2008). Clinical factors to predict the outcomes of external cephalic version: A metaanalysis. *American Journal of Obstetrics & Gynecology, 199,* 630.e1–630.e7.

Li, X., Hu, J., Wang, X., Zhang, H., & Liu, J. (2009). Moxibustion and other acupuncture point stimulation methods to treat breech presentation: A systematic review of clinical trials. *Chinese Medicine, 4,* 4.

Lothian, D. (2006). The cesarean catastrophe. *Journal of Perinatal Education, 15*(1), 42–45.

Marciniak B., Leszczyńska-Gorzelak B., Bartosiewicz J., & Oleszczuk J. (2010). [Effectiveness of intracervical catheter as a labor preinduction method]. *Ginekologia Polska, 81*(1), 31–36.

Michaluk, C. A. (2009). Cesarean delivery by maternal request: What neonatal nurses need to know. Retrieved from http://www.medscape.com/viewarticle/703390

Moleti, C. A. (2009). Trends and controversies in labor induction. *American Journal of Maternal Child Nursing, 34*(1), 40–49.

Nassar, N., Roberts, C., Barratt, A., Bell, J., Olive, E., & Peat, B. (2006). Systematic review of adverse outcomes of external cephalic version and persisting breech presentation at term. *Paediatric and Perinatal Epidemiology, 20,* 163–171.

National Center for Complementary and Alternative Medicine. (2009). The use of complementary and alternative medicine in the United States. Retrieved from http://nccam.nih.gov/news/camstats/2007/camsurvey_fs1.htm

Pharmacia & Upjohn Company. (2008). *Prepidil Gel.* New York, NY: Pfizer Inc.

Queenan, J., Spong, C., & Lockwood, C. (2007). *Management of high-risk pregnancy: An evidence-based approach* (5th ed.) Malden, MA: Blackwell Publishing.

Richter, R., Bergmann, R. L., & Dudenhausen, J. W. (2008). Previous caesarean or vaginal delivery: Which mode is a greater risk of perinatal death at the second delivery? *European Journal of Obstetrics, Gynecology, And Reproductive Biology, 132*(1), 51–57.

Simpson, K. R., & Creehan, P. A. (2008). *AWHONN's perinatal nursing* (3rd ed.). Washington, DC: AWHONN.

Smyth, R., Aldred, S., & Markham, C. (2007). Amniotomy for shortening spontaneous labour. *Cochrane Library,* Issue 4, Chichester, UK: John Wiley & Sons, Ltd.

Tan, P. C., Andi, A., Azmi, N., & Noraihan, M. N. (2006). Effect of coitus at term on length of gestation, induction of labor, and mode of delivery. *Obstetrics & Gynecology, 108*(1), 134–140.

Viswanathan, M., Hartmann, K., Palmieri, R., Lux, L., Swinson, T., Lohr, K. N., . . ., Thorp, J. (2009). *The use of episiotomy in obstetrical care.* Rockville, MD: Agency of Healthcare Research and Quality.

Wei, S., Wo, B. L., Xu, H., Luo, Z. C., Roy, C., & Fraser, W. D. (2009). Early amniotomy and early oxytocin for prevention of, or therapy for, delay in first stage spontaneous labour compared with routine care. *Cochrane Database of Systematic Reviews.* Cochrane AN: CD006794.

Weiniger, C., Ginosar, Y., Elchalal, U., Sharon, E., Nokrian, M., & Ezra, Y. (2007). External cephalic version for breech presentation with or without spinal analgesia in nulliparous women at term. *Obstetrics & Gynecology, 110,* 1343–1350.

Wilson, B. A., Shannon, M. T., & Shields, K. M. (2010). *Pearson nurse's drug guide 2010.* Upper Saddle River, NJ: Pearson.

Xu, H., Hofmeyr, J., Roy, C., & Fraser, W. (2007). Intrapartum amnioinfusion for meconium-stained amniotic fluid: A systematic review of randomised controlled trials. BJOG: An *International Journal of Obstetrics and Gynaecology, 114*(4), 383–390.

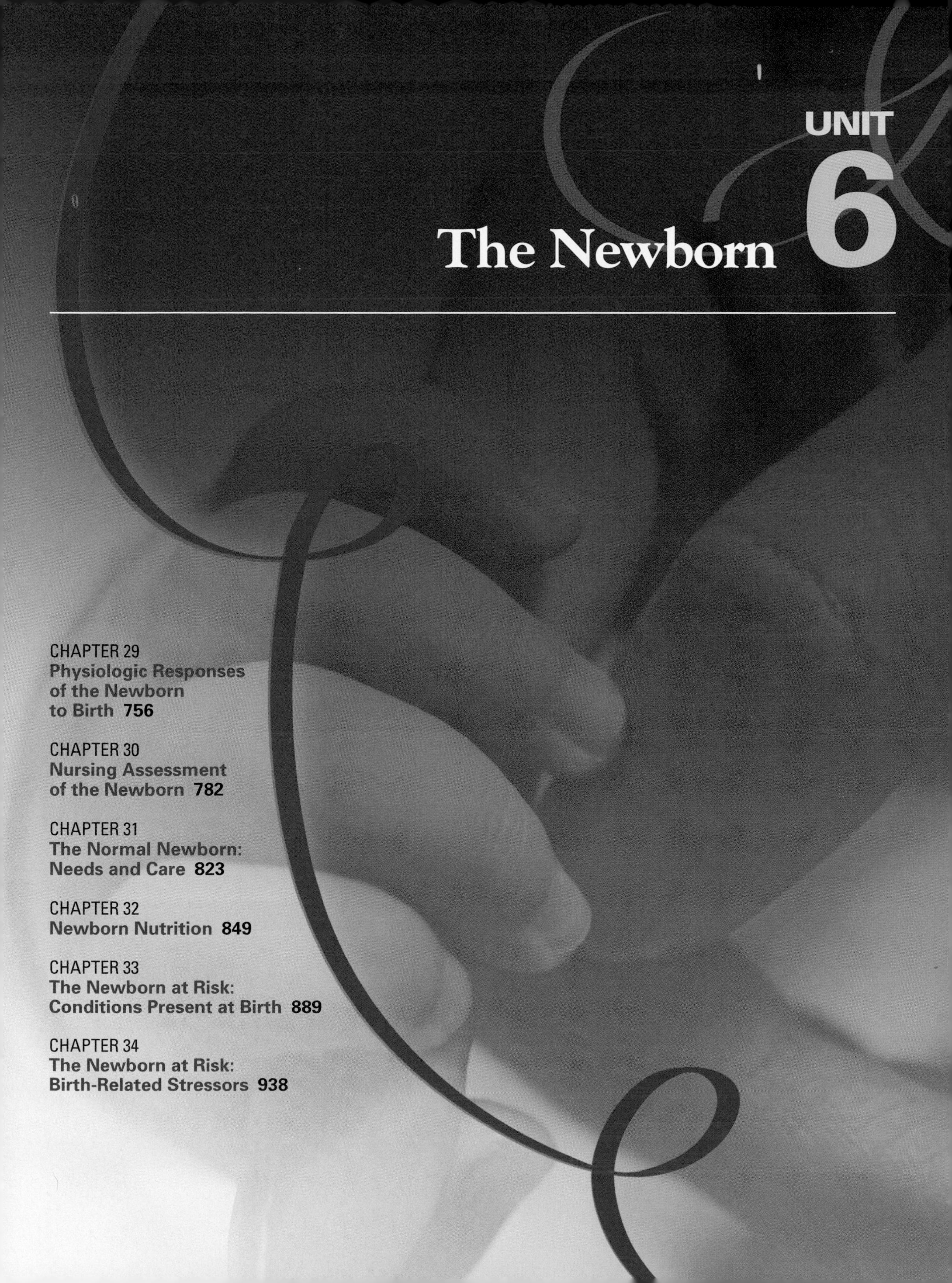

UNIT 6

The Newborn

CHAPTER 29

Physiologic Responses of the Newborn to Birth

The incredible attributes of the newborn have a major purpose. They prepare the baby for interaction with the family and for life in the world.

—Marshall H. Klaus & Phyllis H. Klaus, *The Amazing Newborn*

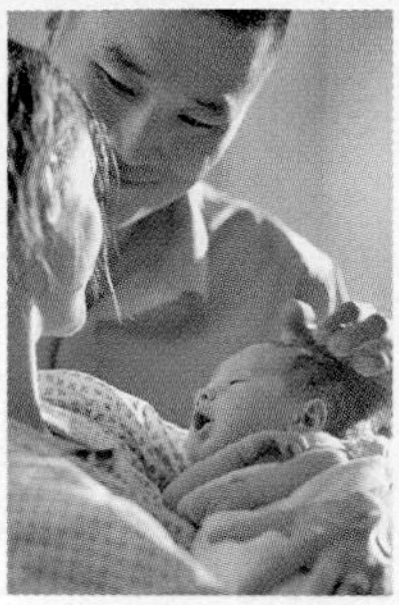

LEARNING OUTCOMES

1. Summarize the respiratory and cardiovascular changes that must occur for the newborn to successfully transition to extrauterine life.
2. Compare the various factors that modify the newborn's blood values to the corresponding results.
3. Relate the process of thermogenesis in the newborn and the major mechanisms of heat loss to the challenge of maintaining newborn thermal stability.
4. Explain the steps involved in the conjugation and excretion of bilirubin in the newborn.
5. Discuss the reasons a newborn may develop hyperbilirubinemia and the nursing interventions that can decrease the probability or the severity of jaundice.
6. Delineate the functional abilities of the newborn's gastrointestinal tract and liver.
7. Relate the development of the newborn kidney to the newborn's ability to maintain adequate fluid and electrolyte balance.
8. Describe basic newborn immunologic responses.
9. Explain the physiologic and behavioral characteristics of newborn neurologic functioning including the patterns of behavior, during periods of reactivity.
10. Describe the normal sensory/perceptual abilities and behavioral states present in the newborn period.

KEY TERMS

Active acquired immunity *775*
Alveolar surface tension *759*
Brown adipose tissue (BAT) *768*
Cardiopulmonary adaptation *760*
Conduction *767*
Convection *767*
Evaporation *767*
Fetal breathing movements (FBM) *757*
Functional residual capacity (FRC) *758*
Habituation *778*
Lung compliance *759*
Meconium *774*
Neonatal transition *757*
Neutral thermal environment (NTE) *766*
Orientation *778*
Passive acquired immunity *775*
Periodic breathing *761*
Periods of reactivity *777*
Physiologic anemia of the newborn *765*
Physiologic jaundice *770*
Radiation *767*
Self-quieting ability *778*
Surfactant *757*
Thermogenesis *768*
Total serum bilirubin *769*

The newborn period is the time from birth through the 28th day of life. During this period, the newborn undergoes physiologic adaptation from intrauterine to extrauterine life. The nurse needs to be knowledgeable about a newborn's normal physiologic and behavioral adaptations and be able to recognize alterations from normal transition.

The first few hours of life, in which the newborn stabilizes respiratory and circulatory functions, are called **neonatal transition**. All other newborn body systems change their level of functioning or become established over a longer period of time during the neonatal period.

Respiratory Adaptations

To begin life as a separate being, the baby must immediately establish respiratory functioning and ventilation. Adequate respiratory gas exchange in conjunction with marked circulatory changes are radical and rapid changes crucial to successful transition to extrauterine life.

Intrauterine Factors Supporting Respiratory Function

Even before the significant respiratory events occur at birth, certain intrauterine factors also enhance the newborn's ability to breathe. Adequate fetal lung development allows the newborn to expand his or her lungs and exchange oxygen and carbon dioxide gases. Even before birth the fetus practices breathing movements that aid in developing lung tissue and strengthening respiratory muscles, allowing him or her to breathe immediately after birth.

Fetal Lung Development

The respiratory system is in a continuous state of development during fetal life, and lung development continues into early childhood. During the first 20 weeks of gestation, lung development is limited to the differentiation of pulmonary, vascular, and lymphatic structures. At 20 to 24 weeks, alveolar ducts begin to appear, followed by primitive alveoli at 24 to 28 weeks. During this time, the alveolar epithelial cells begin to differentiate into type I cells (structures necessary for gas exchange) and type II cells (structures that provide for the synthesis and storage of surfactant). **Surfactant** is composed of surface-active phospholipids (lecithin and sphingomyelin), which are critical for alveolar expansion and stability.

At 28 to 32 weeks of gestation, the number of type II cells increases further, and surfactant is produced by a choline pathway within them. Surfactant production by this pathway peaks at about 35 weeks of gestation and remains high until term, paralleling late fetal lung development. At this time, the lungs are structurally developed enough to maintain good lung expansion and adequate exchange of gases although a fetus born at this gestation may need intensive care to survive.

Clinically, the peak production of lecithin—one component of surfactant—corresponds closely to the marked decrease in incidence of idiopathic respiratory distress syndrome for babies born after 35 weeks' gestation. Production of sphingomyelin—the other component—remains constant during gestation. The newborn born before the lecithin/sphingomyelin (L/S) ratio is 2:1 will have varying degrees of respiratory distress. (See discussion of L/S ratio in chapter 21 ∞ and chapter 34 ∞.)

Fetal Breathing Movements

The newborn's ability to breathe air immediately after birth appears to result from **fetal breathing movements (FBM)**, the intrauterine practice respiratory movements that begin around the 17th to 20th week of gestation. In this respect, breathing can be seen as a continuation of an intrauterine process; the lungs convert from a fluid-filled organ to an air-filled organ capable of gas exchange.

These breathing movements are essential for developing the chest wall muscles and the diaphragm and, to a lesser extent, for regulating lung fluid volume and resultant lung growth.

Initiation of Breathing

To maintain life, two significant changes must take place immediately after birth for the lungs to begin adequate functioning:

1. Pulmonary ventilation must be established through lung expansion.
2. A marked increase in the pulmonary circulation must occur.

The first breath of life—the gasp in response to mechanical, reabsorptive, chemical, thermal, and sensory changes associated with birth—initiates the serial opening of the alveoli. So begins the transition from a fluid-filled environment to extrauterine life as an independent functioning newborn. Figure 29-1 ■ summarizes the initiation of respiration.

Mechanical Events

During the latter half of gestation, the fetal lungs continuously produce fluid. This fluid production expands the lungs almost completely, filling the air spaces. Some of the lung fluid moves up into the trachea and out into the amniotic fluid. The amniotic fluid is then swallowed by the fetus.

In preparation for birth, lung fluid production normally decreases and fetal breathing movement decreases 24 to 36 hours before the onset of true labor (Knuppel, 2007). However, approximately 80 to 100 ml of fluid remains in the respiratory passages of a normal term fetus at the time of birth. Excess fluid must be removed from the alveolar spaces after birth for effective gas exchange to occur (Ramachandrappa & Jain, 2008). As the fetus experiences labor, there is a fetal gasp and active exhalation that initiates the removal of fluid from the lungs (Rosenberg, 2007). During the vaginal birthing process the fetal chest is compressed, increasing intrathoracic pressure and squeezing a small amount of fluid out of the lungs. At delivery, the chest wall recoils, creating negative intrathoracic pressure, which is thought to produce a small, passive inspiration of air that replaces the fluid that was squeezed out. The significance of the "thoracic squeeze" is controversial, and it is now thought that the process of labor is primarily responsible for the initial movement of lung fluid out of the lungs (Rosenberg, 2007).

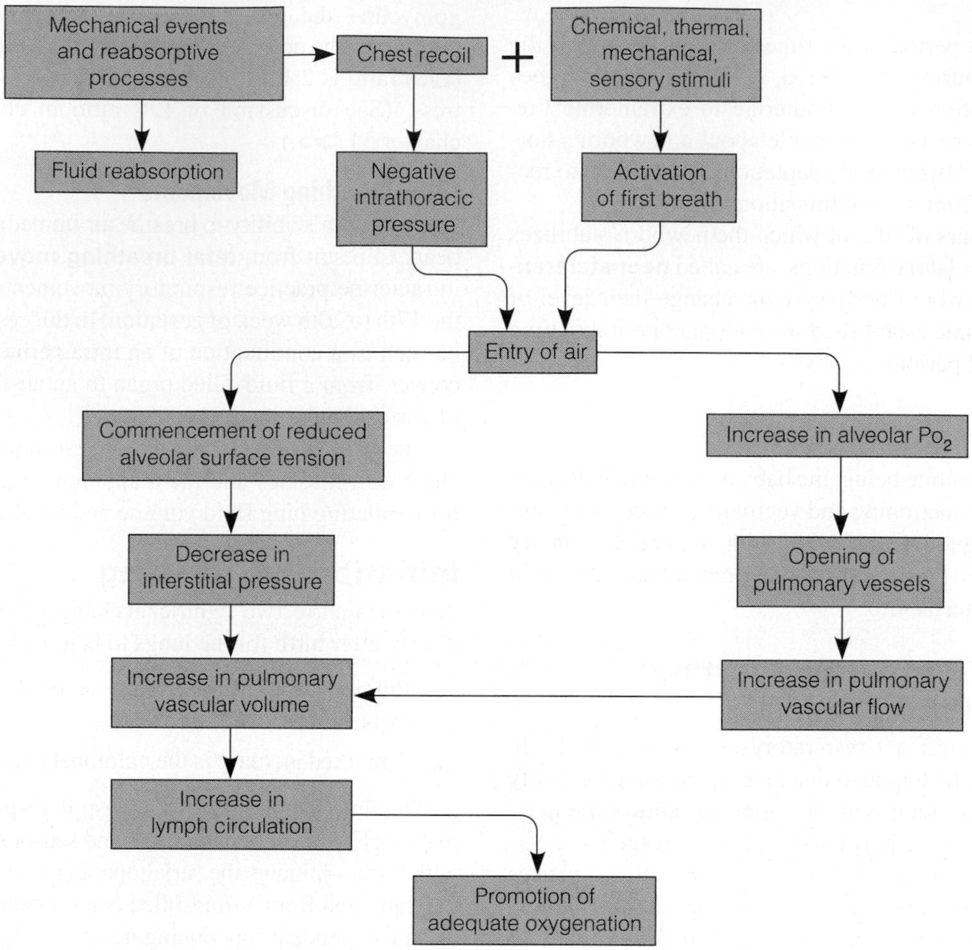

Figure 29-1 ■ Initiation of respiration in the newborn.

After this first inspiration, the newborn exhales and cries against a partially closed glottis, creating a positive intrathoracic pressure. The high positive intrathoracic pressure distributes the inspired air throughout the alveoli and begins the establishment of **functional residual capacity (FRC)**, the amount of air remaining in the lungs at the end of a normal expiration. The higher intrathoracic pressure also increases absorption of lung fluid via the capillaries and lymphatic system. The negative intrathoracic pressure created when the diaphragm moves down with inspiration causes lung fluid to flow from the alveoli across the alveolar membranes into the pulmonary interstitial tissue.

At birth the alveolar epithelium is temporarily more permeable. This, combined with decreased cellular resistance at the onset of breathing, may facilitate passive liquid absorption. With each succeeding breath, the lungs continue to expand, stretching the alveolar walls and increasing the alveolar volume. Protein molecules are too large to pass through capillary walls. The presence of more protein molecules in the pulmonary capillaries than in the interstitial tissue creates oncotic pressure. This pressure draws the interstitial fluid into the capillaries and lymphatic tissue to balance the concentration of protein. Lung expansion helps the remaining lung fluid move into the interstitial tissues. As pulmonary vascular resistance decreases, pulmonary blood flow increases, and more interstitial fluid is absorbed into the bloodstream. In the healthy term newborn, lung fluid moves rapidly into the interstitial tissue but may take several hours to move into the lymph and blood vessels. Figure 29-2 ■ depicts the changes in fetal lung fluid with the first and subsequent breaths. Most of the lung fluid is reabsorbed within 2 hours after birth, and it is completely absorbed within 12 to 24 hours after birth (Rosenberg, 2007).

Although the initial chest compression and recoil should clear the airways of accumulated fluid and permit further inspiration, most clinicians feel it is wise to suction mucus and fluid from the newborn's mouth, nose, and throat. They use a bulb syringe or mucus trap attached to suction as soon as the newborn's head and shoulders are born and again as the newborn adapts to extrauterine life and stabilizes (see Procedure 24-1 ∞ on page 622 and chapter 24 ∞).

Newborns may have problems clearing the fluid in the lungs and beginning respiration for a variety of reasons:

- The lymphatic system may be underdeveloped, thus decreasing the rate at which the fluid is absorbed from the lungs.
- Complications that occur before or during labor and birth can interfere with adequate lung expansion and cause failure to decrease pulmonary vascular resistance, resulting in decreased pulmonary blood flow. Excess fluid must exit the alveoli and pulmonary blood flow must increase to match

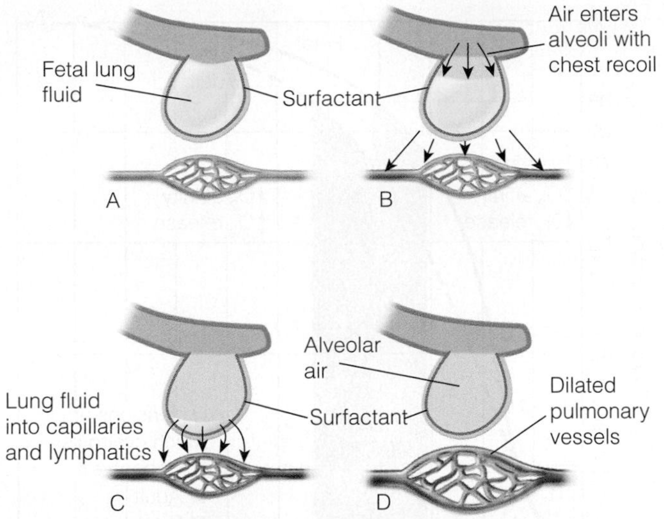

Figure 29-2 ■ Process of absorption of fetal lung fluid during breathing after birth. A. Fetal alveoli filled to functional residual capacity with fetal lung fluid. Fetal lung fluid is produced by the alveoli, fills the airways, and eventually enters the amniotic fluid. B. After fetal chest compression, one third of the fetal lung fluid is squeezed out, allowing air to enter passively as the chest recoils. C. With each subsequent breath, the lungs expand, facilitating the movement of the remaining fetal lung fluid into the capillaries and lymphatic system. Pulmonary blood flow is increasing. D. Normal alveoli after removal of fetal lung fluid and dilatation of pulmonary arteries. Surfactant has lined the inside of the alveoli to prevent collapse.

ventilation with perfusion. These complications include inadequate compression of the chest wall in a very small newborn (small for gestational age [SGA] or very low birth weight [VLBW]) because the immature muscular development causes an overly compliant chest well. Other complications include the absence of the chest wall compression in the newborn delivered by cesarean birth, respiratory depression secondary to maternal analgesia or anesthesia agents, or aspiration of amniotic fluid, blood, or meconium.

Chemical Stimuli

An important chemical stimulator that contributes to the onset of breathing is transitory asphyxia of the fetus and newborn. The first breath is an inspiratory gasp, the result of central nervous system reaction to sudden pressure, temperature change, and other external stimuli (Knuppel, 2007).

This first breath is triggered by normal chest recoil as well as the chemical factors of an elevation in PCO_2 (hypercapnia), decrease in pH (acidosis), and decrease in PO_2 (hypoxia), which are the natural results of normal vaginal labor and birth and cessation of placental gas exchange when the cord is clamped. These stressors, present in all newborns to some degree, stimulate the aortic and carotid chemoreceptors, initiating impulses that trigger the respiratory center in the medulla. Although this brief period of asphyxia is a significant stimulator, prolonged asphyxia is abnormal, depresses respiration, and causes a decrease in pulmonary blood flow. Another chemical factor involves hormonal changes during the labor and delivery process. The levels of prostaglandin, a hormone that suppresses respiration, fall with the clamping of the umbilical cord, thus increasing the infant's respiratory drive (Ramachandrappa & Jain, 2008).

Thermal Stimuli

A significant decrease in ambient temperature after birth—from 37°C to 21–23.9°C (98.6°F to 70–75°F) results in sudden chilling of the moist newborn (Blackburn, 2007). The cold stimulates skin sensory receptors and the newborn responds with rhythmic respirations. Normal temperature changes that occur at birth are apparently within acceptable physiologic limits. Excessive cooling, however, may result in profound respiratory depression and evidence of cold stress (see chapter 34 ∞ for discussion of cold stress).

Sensory Stimuli

During intrauterine life, the fetus is in a dark, sound-dampened, fluid-filled environment and is nearly weightless. After birth the newborn experiences light, sounds, and the effects of gravity for the first time. As the fetus moves from a familiar, comfortable, quiet environment to one of sensory abundance, a number of physical and sensory influences help respiration begin and be sustained after birth. They include the numerous tactile, auditory, visual, and painful stimuli of birth and the normal handling after delivery. Joint movement results in enhanced proprioceptor stimulation to the respiratory center to sustain respirations. Thoroughly drying the newborn and placing him or her in skin-to-skin contact with the mother's chest and abdomen provides stimulation in a far more comforting way and also decreases heat loss.

> **CLINICAL TIP**
> Historically, slapping the buttocks or heels of the newborn was a common way to stimulate breathing, but today the emphasis is on gentle physical contact. Thoroughly drying the newborn and placing the baby in skin-to-skin contact with the mother's chest and abdomen will provide ample external stimulation for the first breaths in a far more comforting way. These actions will also decrease heat loss and promote mother-infant bonding.

Factors Opposing the First Breath

Three major factors may oppose the initiation of respiratory activity: (1) the contracting force between moist surfaces of the alveoli—called **alveolar surface tension**; (2) viscosity of lung fluid within the respiratory tract, which is influenced by surfactant levels; and (3) the ease with which the lung is able to fill with air—called **lung compliance**.

Alveolar surface tension is the contracting force between the moist surfaces of the alveoli. This tension, which is necessary for healthy respiratory function, would cause the small airways and alveoli to collapse after each inspiration if surfactant were not present. Surfactant is important because it reduces surface tension of the fluid lining the alveoli permitting the alveoli to expand. Surfactant stabilizes the alveoli and prevents them from completely collapsing with each expiration and thus promotes lung expansion. Similarly, surfactant promotes lung compliance, the ability of the lung to fill with air easily. When surfactant is decreased, compliance is also decreased, and the pressure needed to expand the alveoli with air increases.

Resistive forces of the fluid-filled lung, combined with the small radii of the airways, necessitates pressures of 30 to 40 cm of water pressure, which are needed to open the lung initially (Niermeyer & Clarke, 2011).

The first breath usually establishes FRC that is 30% to 40% of the fully expanded lung volume. This FRC allows alveolar sacs to remain partially expanded on expiration, decreasing the need for continuous high pressures for each of the following breaths. Subsequent breaths require only 6 to 8 cm H_2O pressure to open alveoli during inspiration. Thus, the first breath of life is usually the most difficult.

Cardiopulmonary Physiology

The onset of respiration stimulates cardiovascular system changes necessary for successful transition to extrauterine life, hence the term **cardiopulmonary adaptation**. As air enters the lungs, PO_2 rises in the alveoli, which stimulates the relaxation of the pulmonary arteries and triggers a decrease in the pulmonary vascular resistance. As pulmonary vascular resistance decreases, the vascular flow in the lung increases very rapidly and achieves 100% normal flow volume at 24 hours of life. This delivery of greater blood volume to the lungs contributes to the conversion from fetal circulation to newborn circulation.

After pulmonary circulation is established, blood is distributed throughout the lungs, although the alveoli may or may not be fully open. For adequate oxygenation to occur, the heart must deliver sufficient blood to functional open alveoli. Shunting of blood is common in the early newborn period. Bidirectional blood flow, or right-to-left shunting through the ductus arteriosus, may divert a significant amount of blood away from the lungs, depending on the pressure changes of respiration, crying, and the cardiac cycle. This shunting of blood away from the lungs in the newborn period is also responsible for the unstable transitional period in cardiopulmonary function.

Oxygen Transport

The transportation of oxygen to the peripheral tissues depends on the type of hemoglobin in the red blood cell (RBC). In the fetus and newborn, a variety of hemoglobin types exist with the most significant being fetal hemoglobin (HbF) and adult hemoglobin (HbA). Approximately 70% to 90% of hemoglobin in the fetus and newborn is HbF. The greatest difference between HbF and HbA relates to the transport of oxygen. The oxygen-carrying capacity of fetal hemoglobin is lower than that of adult hemoglobin. Although each gram of HbF carries less oxygen, it has a greater affinity for the oxygen molecules it carries. At any given arterial oxygen level, HbF has a greater oxygen saturation than HbA. Thus the oxygen-hemoglobin dissociation curve for HbF lies to the left of that for HbA (Figure 29-3 ■). HbF's greater affinity for oxygen benefits the fetus and newborn because it facilitates oxygen transfer across the placenta and into the newborn's tissues. In utero, the fetus has an arterial oxygen tension (PaO_2) between 30 and 40 mm Hg. Because of the nature of the HbF as depicted in the curve, small changes in fetal PaO_2 result in a great amount of oxygen loading in the placenta or unloading to the tissues as compared with the adult. HbF's greater affinity for oxygen also requires that a lower tissue oxygen level exist before oxygen unloading than is required by HbA. Because of this phenomenon, the newborn will have both a lower arterial oxygen level and lower oxygen saturation than the adult before cyanosis becomes clinically apparent.

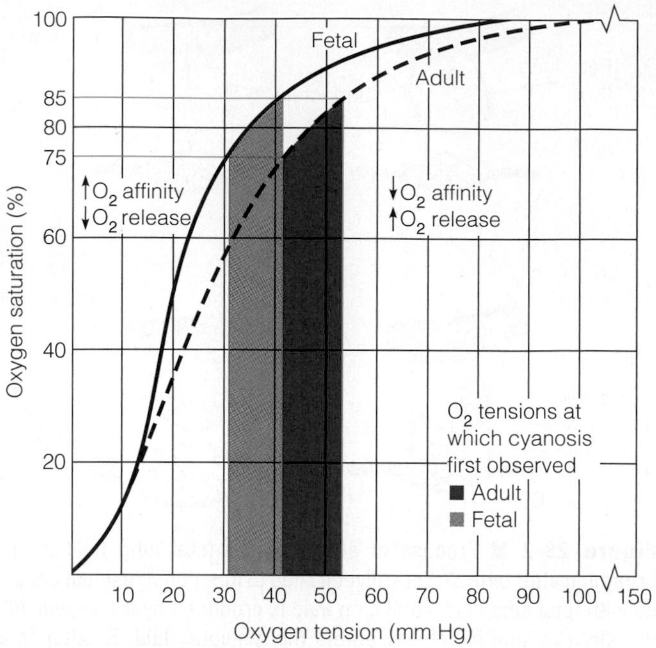

Figure 29-3 ■ Fetal oxygen-hemoglobin dissociation curve.

Source: Reprinted from Care of the High-Risk Infant, *3rd ed., by M. Klaus & A. A. Fanaroff, p. 234. Copyright 1986, with permission from Elsevier Science.*

In addition to the specific characteristics of HbF, other conditions affect the transport of oxygen. Alkalosis (increased pH) and hypothermia can result in less oxygen being available to the body tissues, whereas acidosis, hypercarbia, and hyperthermia can result in less oxygen being bound to hemoglobin and more oxygen being released to the body tissues. Therefore, as blood is perfusing active tissues that are producing acids and carbon dioxide, hemoglobin's affinity for oxygen decreases, allowing oxygen unloading and carbon dioxide and acid uptake. This blood is then transferred to the placenta or the lungs, where its higher carbon dioxide and acid content results in uploading of these waste products from hemoglobin and the uptake of oxygen to be transferred to the tissues.

Other factors that regulate oxygen delivery to the tissues are oxygen-carrying capacity and cardiac output. The oxygen-carrying capacity of blood is defined as the product of the hemoglobin concentration and the maximum amount of oxygen that 1 g of hemoglobin can hold when it is fully saturated. The amount of oxygen bound to hemoglobin divided by the oxygen-carrying capacity yields a percentage that signifies oxygen saturation. Oxygen saturation usually reaches a value between 96% and 98% after several hours of life. Although HbF can hold only 1.26 ml of oxygen per gram of hemoglobin, compared with 1.34 ml of oxygen per gram of HbA, the newborn's hemoglobin level at birth (17 g/dl) is substantially greater than in adults (13 g/dl). Therefore, the absolute oxygen-carrying capacity of fetal blood (21.42 vol %) is greater than in adult blood (17.42 vol %) and allows the fetus to tolerate the relatively hypoxic intrauterine environment.

A significant reduction in the oxygen-carrying capacity results in an increased cardiac output to compensate for hemoglobin's decreased oxygen concentration. Lastly, cardiac output of the fetus and newborn is relatively greater per body weight than in the adult, which contributes to the rapid delivery of oxygenated blood to tissues with high metabolic demands.

Maintaining Respiratory Function

The ability of the lung to maintain oxygenation and ventilation (the exchange of oxygen and carbon dioxide) is influenced by such factors as lung compliance and airway resistance. Lung compliance is influenced by the elastic recoil of the lung tissue and by anatomic differences in the newborn. The newborn has a relatively large heart and mediastinal structures that reduce available lung space. Also, the newborn chest is equipped with weak intercostal muscles, a rigid rib cage with horizontal ribs, and a high diaphragm that restricts the space available for lung expansion. The large abdomen further encroaches on the diaphragm to decrease lung space. Another factor that limits ventilation is airway resistance, which depends on the radii, length, and number of airways. Airway resistance is increased in the newborn when compared with adults.

Characteristics of Newborn Respiration

The normal newborn respiratory rate is 30 to 60 breaths per minute (Tappero & Honeyfield, 2009). Initial respirations may be largely diaphragmatic, shallow, and irregular in depth and rhythm. The abdomen's movements are synchronous with chest movements. Breathing patterns in newborns can be irregular and variable. Periodic breathing is common in preterm infants, but can also be seen in term infants. **Periodic breathing** is defined as "pauses in respiratory movements that last for up to 20 seconds alternating with breathing" (Blackburn, 2007). Periodic breathing is rarely associated with differences in skin color or heart rate changes, and it has no prognostic significance. Tactile or other sensory stimulation stimulates the respiratory center and converts periodic breathing patterns to normal breathing patterns during neonatal transition. With deep sleep, the pattern is reasonably regular. Periodic breathing occurs with rapid eye movement (REM) sleep, and grossly irregular breathing is evident with motor activity, sucking, and crying. Cessation of breathing lasting more than 20 seconds is defined as *apnea* and is abnormal in term newborns. Apnea may or may not be associated with changes in skin color or heart rate (drop below 100 beats per minute [beats/min]). Apnea always needs to be further evaluated.

Newborns tend to be obligatory nose breathers because the nasal route is the primary means of air entry. This is because of the high position of the epiglottis and the position of the soft palate (Blackburn, 2007). Although many term newborns can breathe orally when nasally occluded, nasal obstructions can cause respiratory distress. Any obstruction will cause some degree of respiratory distress, so it is important to keep the throat and nose clear. Immediately after birth and for about the next 2 hours, respiratory rates of 60 to 70 breaths per minute (breaths/min) are normal. Some cyanosis and acrocyanosis are normal for several hours; thereafter the infant's color improves steadily. If respirations drop below 20 or exceed 60 per minute when the baby is at rest, or if dyspnea, central cyanosis, nasal flaring, chest wall retractions, or expiratory grunting occur, the clinician should be notified. Any increased use of the intercostal muscle (retractions) may indicate respiratory distress. (See Respiratory Distress Syndrome in chapter 34 ∞ and Table 34-1 ∞ on page 948 for signs of respiratory distress.)

Cardiovascular Adaptations

As described earlier, the onset of respiration triggers increased pulmonary blood flow after birth. This greater blood volume contributes to the conversion from fetal circulation to neonatal circulation.

Fetal-Newborn Transitional Physiology

During fetal life, blood with the highest oxygen content is directed to the heart and brain. Blood in the descending aorta is less oxygenated and supplies the kidneys and intestinal tract before it is returned to the placenta. Limited amounts of blood, pumped from the right ventricle toward the lungs, enter the pulmonary vessels. In the fetus, increased pulmonary resistance forces most of the blood through the ductus arteriosus into the descending aorta (Table 29-1). See the fetal heart animation on www.nursing.personhighered.com.

TABLE 29-1 Fetal and Neonatal Circulation

SYSTEM	FETAL	NEONATAL
Pulmonary blood vessels	Constricted with very little blood flow (high pulmonary vascular resistance); lungs not expanded and fluid-filled.	Vasodilatation and increased blood flow (decreasing pulmonary vascular resistance); lungs expanded; increased PaO_2 stimulates vasodilation.
Systemic blood vessels	Dilated with low peripheral vascular resistance; blood mostly in placenta.	Arterial pressure rises due to cord clamping with loss of placental reservoir; increased systemic blood volume causes increased peripheral vascular resistance.
Ductus arteriosus	Large with no tone; blood flow from pulmonary artery to aorta (right to left shunting).	Reversal of blood flow. Now from aorta to pulmonary artery (left to right shunting) because of increased left atrial pressure and increased systemic vascular pressures.
		Ductus is sensitive to increased PaO_2 and a decline in circulating prostaglandins and begins to constrict.
Foramen ovale	Patent with large blood flow from right atrium to left atrium.	Increased pressure in left atrium attempts to reverse blood flow and shuts one-way valve.

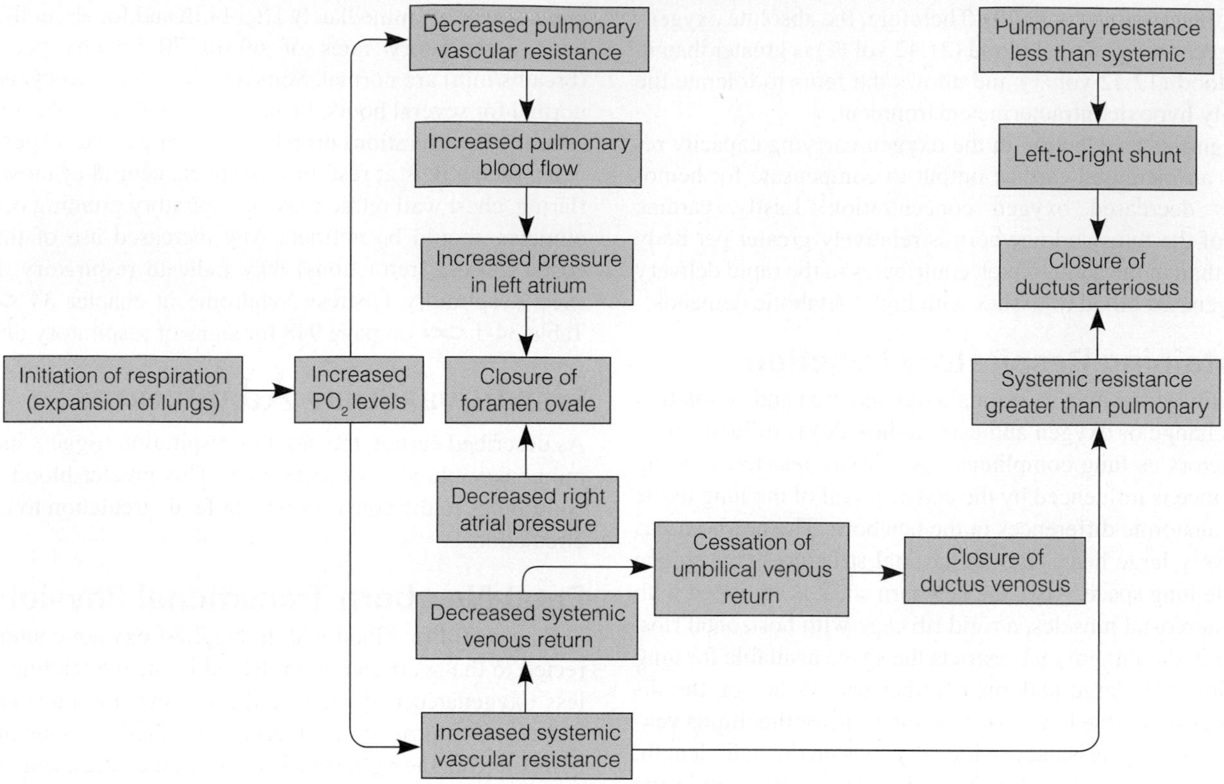

Figure 29-4 ■ Transitional circulation: Conversion from fetal to neonatal circulation.

Marked changes occur in the cardiovascular system at birth. Expansion of the lungs with the first breath decreases the pulmonary vascular resistance and increases pulmonary blood flow. Pressure in the left atrium increases as blood returns from the pulmonary veins. Pressure in the right atrium drops, and systemic vascular resistance increases as umbilical venous flow is halted when the cord is clamped. These physiologic mechanisms mark the beginning of transition from fetal to neonatal circulation and show the interplay of the cardiovascular and respiratory systems (Figure 29-4 ■).

Five major areas of change in cardiopulmonary adaptation (Figure 29-5 ■) are the following:

1. ***Increased aortic pressure and decreased venous pressure.*** Clamping of the umbilical cord eliminates the placental vascular bed and reduces the intravascular space. Consequently, aortic (systemic) blood pressure increases. At the same time, blood return via the inferior vena cava decreases, resulting in decreased right atrial pressure and a small decrease in pressure within the venous circulation.
2. ***Increased systemic pressure and decreased pulmonary artery pressure.*** With the loss of the low-resistance placenta, systemic resistance increases, resulting in greater systemic pressure. At the same time, lung expansion increases pulmonary blood flow, and the increased blood PO_2 associated with initiation of respirations dilates pulmonary blood vessels. The combination of vasodilation and increased pulmonary blood flow decreases pulmonary artery resistance. As the pulmonary vascular beds open, the systemic vascular pressure increases, enhancing perfusion of the other body systems.
3. ***Closure of the foramen ovale.*** Closure of the foramen ovale is a function of changing atrial pressures. In utero, pressure is greater in the right atrium, and the foramen ovale is open after birth, shunting blood from the right atrium to the left. Decreased pulmonary resistance and increased pulmonary blood flow increase pulmonary venous return into the left atrium, thereby increasing left atrial pressure slightly. The decreased pulmonary vascular resistance and the decreased umbilical venous return to the right atrium also cause a decrease in right atrial pressure. The pressure gradients across the atria are now reversed, with left atrial pressure greater, and the foramen ovale is functionally closed 1 to 2 hours after birth. However, a slight right-to-left shunting may occur in the early neonatal period. Any increase in pulmonary resistance or right atrial pressure, such as occurs in crying, acidosis, cold stress, or induced hypoxia, may cause the foramen ovale to reopen, causing a right-to-left shunt. Anatomical closure of the foramen ovale occurs within 30 months (Blackburn, 2007).
4. ***Closure of the ductus arteriosus.*** Initial elevation of the systemic vascular pressure above the pulmonary vascular pressure increases pulmonary blood flow by reversing the flow through the ductus arteriosus. Blood now flows from the aorta into the pulmonary artery. Furthermore, although the presence of oxygen causes the pulmonary arterioles to dilate, an increase in blood PO_2 triggers the opposite response in the ductus arteriosus—it constricts.

In utero the placenta produces prostaglandin E_2 (PGE_2), which causes ductus vasodilation. With the loss of the placenta and increased pulmonary blood flow, PGE_2 levels drop, leaving the active constriction by PO_2 unopposed. If the lungs fail to expand or if PO_2 levels drop, the ductus remains patent. Functional closure in the well newborn starts at 10 to 15 hours after birth, and fibrosis of the ductus occurs within 4 weeks after birth (Blackburn, 2007).

5. ***Closure of the ductus venosus.*** Although the mechanism of initiating closure of the ductus venosus is not known, it appears to be related to mechanical pressure changes that result from severing of the cord, redistribution of blood, and cardiac output. Closure of the ductus venosus forces perfusion of the liver. Fibrosis of the ductus venosus occurs within 2 months, at which time it becomes known as the ligamentum venosum. Figure 29-6 ■ depicts the changes in blood flow and oxygenation as the fetal cardiopulmonary circulation adapts to extrauterine life.

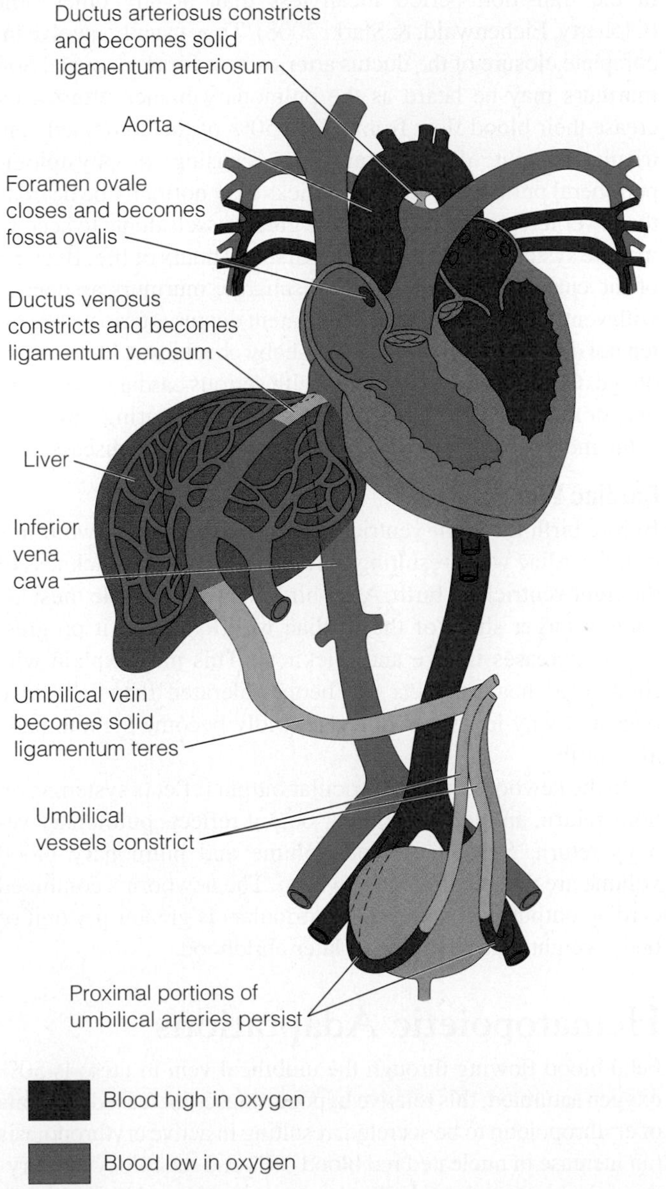
Ductus arteriosus constricts and becomes solid ligamentum arteriosum
Aorta
Foramen ovale closes and becomes fossa ovalis
Ductus venosus constricts and becomes ligamentum venosum
Liver
Inferior vena cava
Umbilical vein becomes solid ligamentum teres
Umbilical vessels constrict
Proximal portions of umbilical arteries persist
Blood high in oxygen
Blood low in oxygen

Figure 29-5 ■ Major changes that occur in the newborn's circulatory system.

Source: Reprinted with permission from Hole, J. W. (1990). Human anatomy and physiology *(5th ed.). Copyright © 1990 The McGraw-Hill Companies, Inc.*

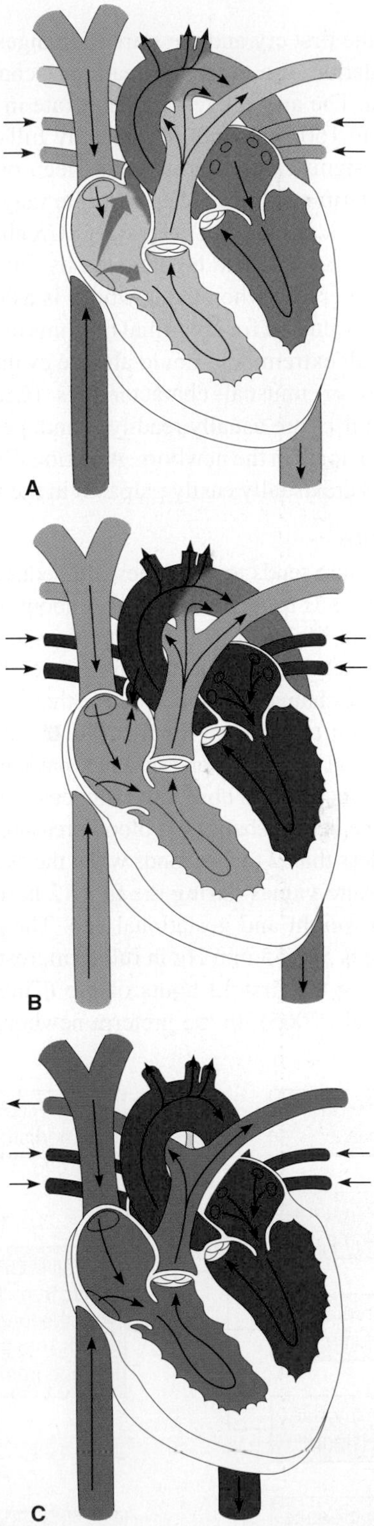
A
B
C

Figure 29-6 ■ Fetal-neonatal circulation. A. Pattern of blood flow and oxygenation in fetal circulation. B. Pattern of blood flow and oxygenation in transitional circulation of the newborn. C. Pattern of blood flow and oxygenation in neonatal circulation.

Characteristics of Cardiac Function

Evaluation of the newborn's heart rate, blood pressure, heart sounds, and cardiac workload provides data for evaluating cardiac function.

Heart Rate

Shortly after the first cry and the start of changes in cardiopulmonary circulation, the newborn heart rate can accelerate to 180 beats/min. The average resting heart rate in the first week of life is 110 to 160 beats/min in a healthy full-term newborn but may vary significantly during deep sleep or active awake states. In full-term newborns, the heart rate may drop to a low of 80 to 100 beats/min during deep sleep (Creehan, 2008).

Apical pulse rates should be obtained by auscultation for a full minute, preferably when the newborn is asleep. The heart rate should be evaluated for abnormal rhythms or beats. Peripheral pulses of all extremities should also be evaluated to detect any inequities or unusual characteristics (Creehan, 2008). While radial pulses are usually readily found, pedal pulses can be difficult to palpate in the newborn. Additionally, brachial and femoral pulses are usually easily palpated in the well newborn.

Case Study: Normal Range of Newborn's Vital Signs

Blood Pressure

The blood pressure tends to be highest immediately after birth, and then it descends to its lowest level at about 3 hours of age. By 4 to 6 days of life, the blood pressure rises and plateaus at a level approximately the same as the initial level. Blood pressure is sensitive to the changes in blood volume that occur in the transition to newborn circulation. Figure 29-7 ■ diagrams this response. Peripheral perfusion pressure is a particularly sensitive indicator of the newborn's ability to compensate for alterations in blood volume before changes in blood pressure. Capillary refill should be less than 2 to 3 seconds when the skin is blanched.

Blood pressure values during the first 12 hours of life vary with the birth weight and gestational age. The average mean blood pressure is 5 to 55 mm Hg in full term, resting newborns over 3 kg during the first 12 hours of life (Thureen, Deacon, Hernandez, et al., 2005). In the preterm newborn, the average mean blood pressure varies according to weight and degree of illness. Crying may cause an elevation of 20 mm Hg in both the systolic and diastolic blood pressure; thus accuracy is more likely in the quiet newborn. The measurement of blood pressure is best accomplished by using the Doppler technique, with a size- and weight-appropriate cuff over the brachial artery.

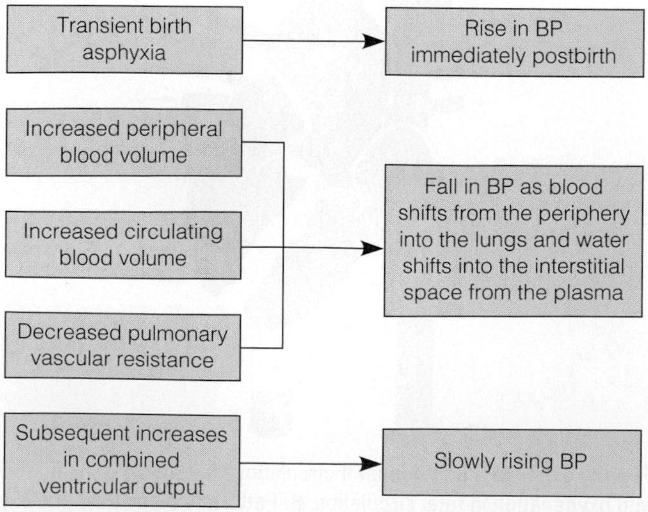

Figure 29-7 ■ Response of blood pressure (BP) to changes in neonatal blood volume.

Heart Murmurs

Murmurs are usually produced by turbulent blood flow through a narrowed opening. Murmurs may be heard when blood flows across an abnormal valve or across a stenosed valve, when there is an atrial or ventricular septal defect, or when there is increased flow across a normal valve. In newborns, 90% of all murmurs are transient and *not associated with anomalies*. Cardiac murmurs are often present in the initial newborn period as transition from fetal to neonatal circulation occurs. These murmurs heard in the transition period mean less than at any other time (Cloherty, Eichenwald, & Stark, 2008). They usually involve incomplete closure of the ductus arteriosus or foramen ovale. Soft murmurs may be heard as the pulmonary branch arteries increase their blood flow from 7% to 50% of the combined ventricular output during transition, causing a physiologic peripheral pulmonary stenosis. Clicks may normally be heard at the lower left sternal border as the great vessels dilate to accommodate systolic blood flow in the first few hours of life. Because of the current practice of early discharge, murmurs associated with ventricular septal defect and patent ductus arteriosus are often not detected until the first well-baby checkup at 4 to 6 weeks of age. Consequently, newborns with serious cardiac anomalies may or may not exhibit murmurs. Oftentimes hearing a murmur is the most common means of recognizing cardiac disease.

Cardiac Workload

Before birth the right ventricle does approximately two thirds of the cardiac work resulting in increased size and thickness of the right ventricle at birth. After birth the left ventricle must assume a larger share of the cardiac workload, and it progressively increases in size and thickness. This may explain why right-sided heart defects are better tolerated than left-sided ones and why left-sided defects rapidly become symptomatic after birth.

In the newborn, right ventricular output reflects systemic venous return, and left ventricular output reflects pulmonary venous return. Systemic blood volume and pulmonary blood volume are not equal in the newborn. The newborn's combined cardiac output (left and right ventricular) is greater per unit of body weight than it will be in later childhood.

Hematopoietic Adaptations

Fetal blood flowing through the umbilical vein in utero is 50% oxygen saturated; this relative hypoxia causes increased amounts of erythropoietin to be secreted, resulting in active erythropoiesis (an increase in nucleated red blood cells and reticulocytes). Erythropoiesis is regulated by the hormone erythropoietin, which is produced postnatally in the kidneys. Levels of erythropoietin rise in response to hypoxia and anemia. After birth, the increases in oxygen saturation and arterial oxygen levels shut off the production of erythropoietin. In the first days of life, hemoglobin (the major iron-containing component of the red blood cell [RBC]) concentration may rise 1 to 2 g/dl above fetal levels as a result of placental transfusion, low oral fluid intake, and diminished extracellular fluid volume. By 1 week postnatally, peripheral hemoglobin is comparable to fetal blood counts. Then the hemoglobin level declines progressively thereafter during the first 2 months after birth. This initial decline in hemoglobin creates a phenomenon known as **physiologic anemia of the newborn** (Blackburn, 2007). The lowest hemoglobin level is reached at about 3 months of age, called the physiologic nadir. The newborn usually tolerates this physiologic state without any clinical difficulties. A factor that influences the degree of physiologic anemia is the nutritional status of the newborn. Supplies of vitamin E, folic acid, and iron may be inadequate given the amount of growth in the later part of the first year of life. Hemoglobin values fall, mainly from a decrease in red cell mass rather than from the dilutional effect of increasing plasma volume. The fact that red cell survival is lower in newborns than in adults, and that red cell production is less, also contributes to this anemia. Neonatal RBCs have a lifespan of 80 to 100 days, approximately two thirds of an adult's RBC lifespan. Erythropoiesis resumes normally when levels of erythropoietin rise in response to low hemoglobin levels and tissue oxygen needs (Blackburn, 2007). Once erythropoiesis resumes, iron stores will be used to produce new RBCs. Most infants require supplemental iron to maintain adequate iron stores.

Leukocytosis is a normal finding because the stress of birth stimulates increased production of neutrophils during the first few days of life. Neutrophils then decrease to 35% of the total leukocyte count by 2 weeks of age. Lymphocytes play a role in antibody formation and eventually become the predominant type of leukocyte, and the total white blood count falls. Blood volume of the term infant is estimated to be 85 ml/kg of body weight (Bagwell, 2007). For example, a 3.6 kg (8 lb) newborn has a blood volume of about 306 ml. Blood volume varies according to the amount of placental transfusion received during the expulsion of the placenta as well as other factors, including the following:

1. ***Delayed cord clamping and the normal shift of plasma to the extravascular spaces.*** Newborn hemoglobin and hematocrit values are higher when a placental transfusion occurs at birth. Placental vessels contain about 75 to 125 ml of blood at term, most of which can be transfused into the newborn through the umbilical vein by holding the newborn below the level of the placenta and by delaying clamping of the cord (Figure 29-8 ■). Blood volume increases by 61% with delayed cord clamping (Bagwell, 2007). The increase is reflected by a rise in hemoglobin level and an increase in the hematocrit. For greatest accuracy, the initial hemoglobin and

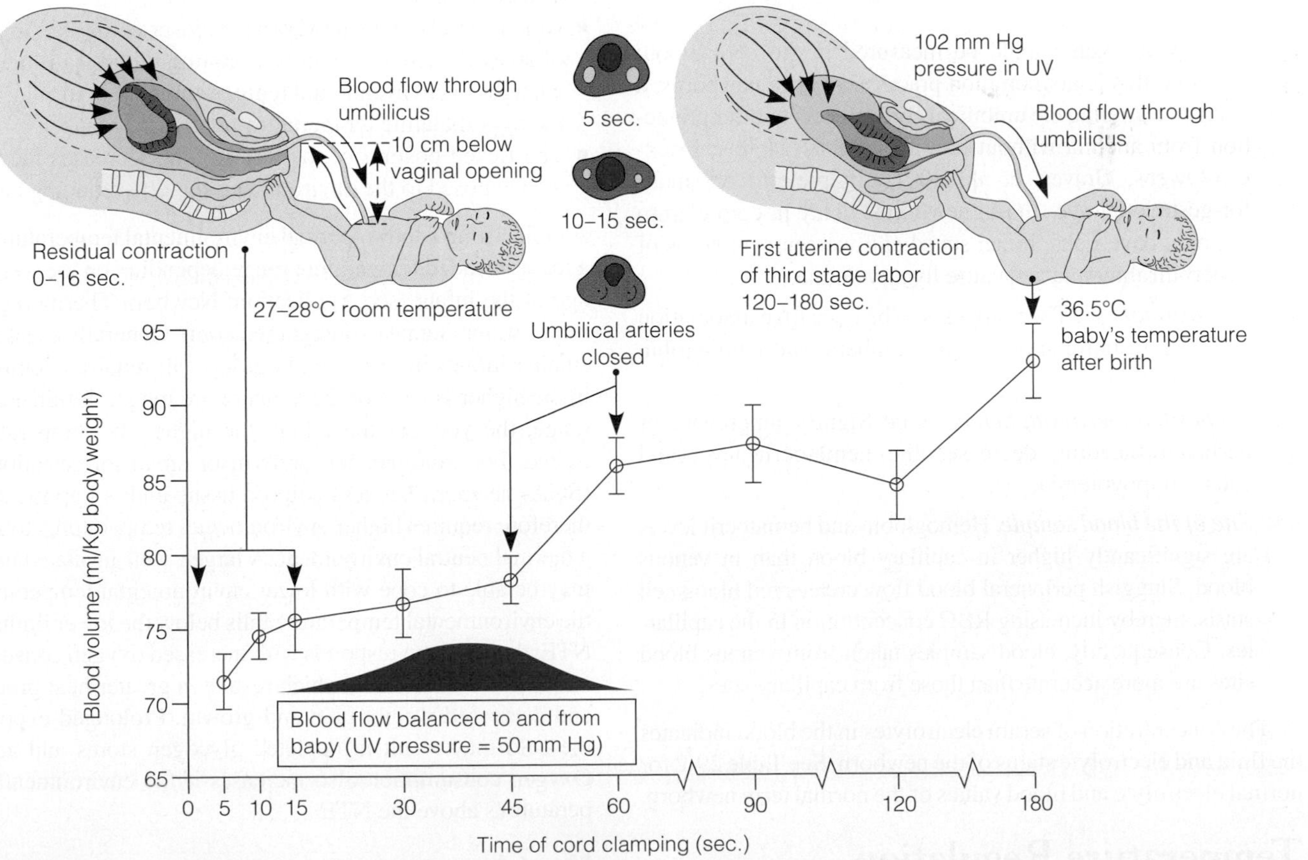

Figure 29-8 ■ Schematic illustration of the mechanisms in placental transfusion (normal term births) through the umbilical vein. The mean neonatal blood volume at 30 minutes is plotted against the time of cord clamping after birth (mean + 1 SE, data from 114 full-term infants). Note episodic, stepwise increments in blood volume at 10, 60, and 180 seconds.

Source: From Yao, A. C., & Lind, J. (1982). Placental transfusion: A clinical and physiological study. *Courtesy of Charles C. Thomas Publisher Ltd., Springfield, Illinois.*

TABLE 29-2 Normal Term Newborn Cord Blood Values

LABORATORY DATA	NORMAL RANGE
Hemoglobin	14–20 g/dl
Hematocrit	43%–63%
WBC	10,000–30,000/mm^3
WBC differential	
Neutrophils	40%–80%
Lymphocytes	20%–40%
Monocytes	3%–10%
Platelets	150,000–350,000/mm^3
Reticulocytes	3%–7%
Blood volume	82.3 ml/kg (third day after early cord clamping), 92.6 ml/kg (third day after delayed cord clamping)
Sodium	129–144 mEq/l
Potassium	3.4–9.9 mEq/l
Chloride	103–111 mEq/l
Bicarbonate	18–23 mEq/l
Carbon dioxide	13–29 mmol/l
Calcium	8.2–111 mg/dl
Glucose	45–96 mg/dl
Total protein	4.8–7.3 g/dl

Source: Adapted from Fanaroff, A. A., & Martin, R. J. (Eds.). (2006). Neonatal-perinatal medicine *(8th ed., pp. 1801, 1810). St. Louis, MO: Mosby.*

hematocrit levels should be measured in the cord blood; however, this is not common practice. In term newborns, a delay in clamping the umbilical cord appears to offer protection from anemia without harmful effects (Mercer, Erickson-Owens, Graves, et al., 2007). In preterm or small-for-gestational-age (SGA) newborns, delay in cord clamping may have risks. It can speed and worsen symptoms of hyperbilirubinemia and cause hypervolemia.

2. ***Gestational age.*** There appears to be a positive association between gestational age, RBC numbers, and hemoglobin concentration.
3. ***Prenatal or perinatal hemorrhage.*** Significant prenatal or perinatal bleeding decreases the hematocrit level and causes hypovolemia.
4. ***Site of the blood sample.*** Hemoglobin and hematocrit levels are significantly higher in capillary blood than in venous blood. Sluggish peripheral blood flow creates red blood cell stasis, thereby increasing RBC concentration in the capillaries. Consequently, blood samples taken from venous blood sites are more accurate than those from capillary sites.

The concentration of serum electrolytes in the blood indicates the fluid and electrolyte status of the newborn. See Table 29-2 for normal electrolyte and blood values of the normal term newborn.

Neonatal Thermoregulation

Temperature Regulation

Temperature regulation is the maintenance of thermal balance by losing heat to the environment at a rate equal to heat production. It is a critical function necessary for survival and optimum health in the infant. Newborns are *homeothermic;* they attempt to stabilize their internal (core) body temperatures within a narrow range in spite of significant temperature variations in their environment. At birth, the fetus moves from a warm, moist intrauterine environment to the relatively colder, drier extrauterine environment. The newborn's temperature may fall 2°C to 3°C after birth mainly because of evaporative losses; this triggers cold-induced metabolic responses and heat production. Term newborns can increase their metabolic rate by 200% to 300% after birth in an attempt to accelerate heat production (Blackburn, 2007).

Thermoregulation in the newborn is closely related to the rate of metabolism and oxygen consumption. Within a specific environmental range called the **neutral thermal environment (NTE)**, the rates of oxygen consumption and metabolism are minimal, and internal body temperature is maintained because of thermal balance (Brand & Boyd, 2010). For an unclothed full-term newborn, the NTE range is an ambient environmental temperature of about 32°C to 34°C (89.6°F to 93.2°F) within 50% relative humidity and adjusted according to the needs of individual infants (Brand & Boyd, 2010). Thus the normal newborn requires higher environmental temperatures to maintain a neutral thermal environment than adults.

Several newborn characteristics affect establishment of thermal stability.

- The newborn has less subcutaneous fat than an adult and a thin epidermis.
- Blood vessels of the newborn are closer to the skin than those of an adult. Therefore, the circulating blood is influenced by changes in environmental temperature and in turn influences the hypothalamic temperature-regulating center.
- The flexed posture of the term infant decreases the surface area exposed to the environment, thereby reducing heat loss.

A table listing neutral thermal environmental temperatures gives a recommended temperature range depending on the weight and age of the infant (see Application: Newborn Thermoregulation on www.nursing.pearsonhighered.com). Generally speaking, the smaller infants in each weight group will require a temperature in the higher portion of the temperature range. Within each time range, the younger the infant, the higher the temperature required. For example, the preterm or small-for-gestational-age (SGA) newborn has less adipose tissue and is hypoflexed, and therefore requires higher environmental temperatures to achieve a thermal neutral environment. A larger, well-insulated newborn may be able to cope with lower environmental temperatures. If the environmental temperature falls below the lower limits of the NTE, the newborn responds with increased oxygen consumption and raised metabolism, which results in greater heat production and decreased weight gain and growth. Prolonged exposure to the cold may result in depleted glycogen stores and acidosis. Oxygen consumption also increases if the environmental temperature is above the NTE.

Heat Loss

A newborn is at a distinct disadvantage in maintaining a normal temperature. With a large body surface in relation to mass and a limited amount of insulating subcutaneous fat, the full-term newborn loses about four times as much heat as an adult does. The newborn's poor thermal stability is due primarily to excessive heat loss rather than to impaired heat production. Because of the risk of hypothermia and possible cold stress, minimizing heat loss in the newborn after birth is essential. (See Provision of Initial Newborn Care in chapter 24 ∞ and chapter 31 ∞ for nursing measures.)

Two major routes of heat loss are from the internal core of the body to the body surface and from the external body surface to the environment. Usually the core temperature is higher than the skin temperature, and the greater the difference in temperatures between core and skin, the more rapidly heat transfer occurs. The transfer is accomplished through an increase in oxygen consumption, depletion of glycogen stores, and metabolizing of brown fat. Heat loss from the body surface to the environment takes place in four ways—convection, radiation, evaporation, and conduction (Figure 29-9 ■).

- **Convection** is the loss of heat from the warm body surface to the cooler air currents. Air-conditioned rooms, air currents with a temperature below the infant's skin temperature, unwarmed oxygen by mask, and removal of the infant from an incubator for procedures increase convective heat loss of the newborn. The amount of heat transferred depends on the velocity of the moving air, the temperature difference between the air and the infant's skin, and the proportion of body surface area exposed.
- **Radiation** losses occur when body heat is transferred to cooler surfaces and objects not in direct contact with the body. The walls of a room or of an incubator are potential causes of heat loss by radiation, even if the ambient temperature of the incubator is within the neutral thermal range for the infant. Placing cold objects (such as ice for blood gases) onto the incubator or near the infant in the radiant warmer will increase radiant heat losses.
- **Evaporation** is the loss of heat incurred when water is converted to a vapor. The newborn is particularly prone to heat loss by evaporation immediately after birth (when the baby is wet with amniotic fluid) and during baths; thus drying the newborn is critical. Evaporation accounts for 25% of heat loss immediately after delivery (Brand & Boyd, 2010). Evaporation also occurs from expired air from the respiratory tract. Babies of lower gestational age have a higher incidence of evaporative heat loss because their skin is immature and they have a large body surface area to weight ratio. Radiant warming beds and bank phototherapy lights also accentuate evaporative loss.
- **Conduction** is the loss of heat to a cooler surface by direct skin contact. Chilled hands, cool scales, cold examination tables, and cold stethoscopes can cause heat loss by conduction. Even if objects are warmed to the incubator temperature, there still may be a significant temperature difference between the infant's core temperature and the ambient temperature. This difference results in heat transfer.

Once the infant has been dried after birth, the highest losses of heat generally result from radiation and convection. The newborn can respond to the cooler environmental temperature

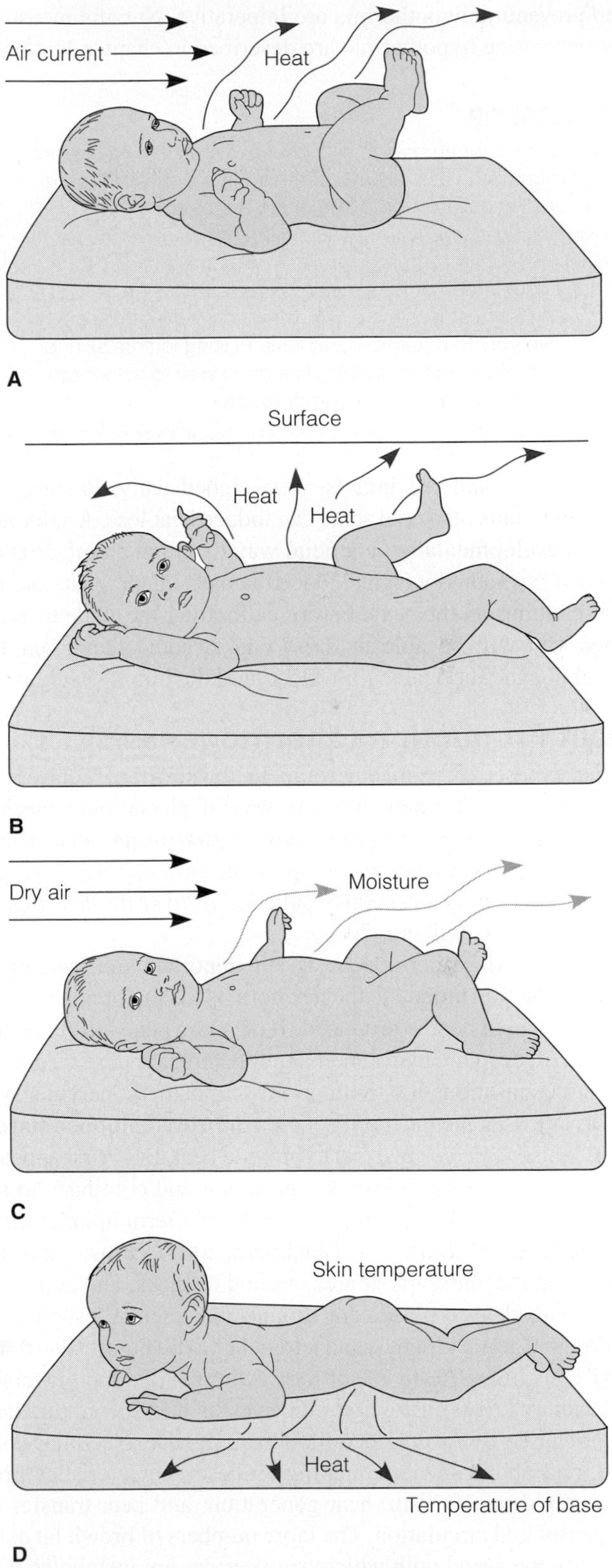

Figure 29-9 ■ Methods of heat loss. A. Convection. B. Radiation. C. Evaporation. D. Conduction.

with adequate peripheral vasoconstriction, but this mechanism is less effective because of the minimal amount of fat insulation present, the large body surface, and ongoing thermal conduction. Because of these factors, minimizing the baby's heat loss and preventing hypothermia are imperative. Nursing measures for preventing hypothermia are described in chapter 31.

CLINICAL TIP

Bath time is when many newborns experience cold stress. To minimize the risk, always bathe infants in a warm room, gather all supplies prior to beginning the bath and prewarming soaps or shampoos. Dry infants with warmed blankets and dress immediately. The infant's head accounts for a large portion of body surface area and has great capacity for heat loss, so placing a hat on the infant is an effective way to minimize heat loss. Placing infants skin to skin with mother after bathing is a good way to help them rewarm and maintain body temperature.

Most hospitalized infants are weighed daily. Placing unclothed infants on a cold scale can induce heat loss. A safer and more developmentally beneficial way to weigh an infant is by doing a "swaddled weight." Place blankets, diaper, hat, and infant clothing on the scale before calibrating the scale to zero. Then you will be able to dress and swaddle the infant for weighing and the scale will reflect only the infant's weight.

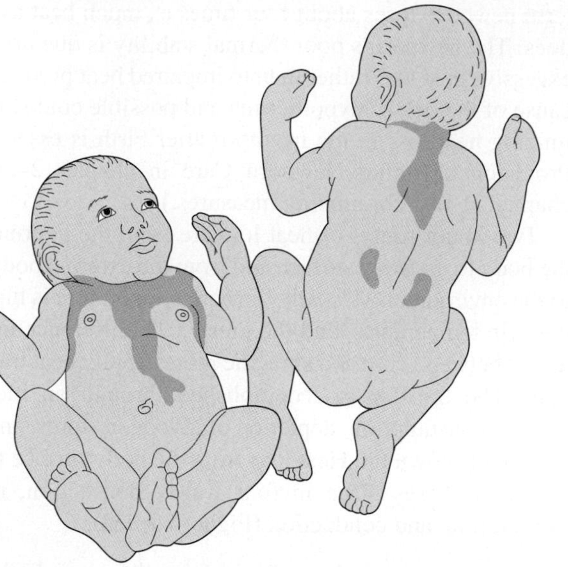

Figure 29-10 ■ The distribution of brown adipose tissue (brown fat) in the newborn.

Source: Adapted with permission from Davis, V. (1980). Structure and function of brown adipose tissue in the neonate. Journal of Obstetric, Gynecologic, & Neonatal Nursing, 9, *364. Copyright © 1980 by the Association of Women's Health, Obstetric and Neonatal Nurses. All rights reserved.*

Heat Production (Thermogenesis)

When exposed to a cool environment, the newborn requires additional heat. The newborn has several physiologic mechanisms that increase heat production, or **thermogenesis**. These include increased basal metabolic rate, muscular activity, and chemical thermogenesis (also called *nonshivering thermogenesis [NST]*) (Rosenberg, 2007).

Nonshivering thermogenesis, an important mechanism of heat production unique to the newborn, is the major mechanism through which heat is produced. It occurs when skin receptors perceive a drop in environmental temperature and, in response, transmit sensations to stimulate the sympathetic nervous system. NST uses the newborn's stores of **brown adipose tissue (BAT)** (also called *brown fat*) to provide heat. BAT first appears in the fetus at 26 to 30 weeks' gestation and continues to increase until 2 to 5 weeks after the birth of a term infant, unless it is depleted by cold stress (Blackburn, 2007). Brown fat is deposited in the midscapular area, around the neck, and in the axillas, with deeper placement around the trachea, esophagus, abdominal aorta, kidneys, and adrenal glands (Figure 29-10 ■). BAT constitutes 2% to 7% of the newborn's total body weight (Blackburn, 2007). Brown fat receives its name from the dark color caused by its enriched blood supply, dense cellular content, and abundant nerve endings. These characteristics promote rapid metabolism, heat generation, and heat transfer to the peripheral circulation. The large numbers of brown fat cells increase the speed with which triglycerides are metabolized to produce heat but cause increased oxygen consumption and caloric output in the already compromised infant.

Shivering, a form of muscular activity common in the cold adult, is rarely seen in the newborn, although it has been observed at ambient temperatures of 15°C (59°F) or less (Polin et al., 2004). If the newborn does shiver, it means the newborn's metabolic rate has already doubled. The increase in muscular activity does little to produce the needed heat to meet the demands of true hypothermia. NST from BAT is the primary source of heat in the hypothermic newborn. Thermographic studies of newborns exposed to cold show an increase in the skin heat over the brown fat deposits in the newborn between 1 and 14 days of age (Polin et al., 2004). If an infant is SGA, intrauterine growth restricted, or premature, his or her brown fat stores will be inadequate to produce sufficient heat. Brown fat stores cannot be replenished once they are used.

An increase in basal metabolism as a result of hypothermia results in an increase in oxygen and glucose consumption. The normal term newborn is usually able to cope with the increase in oxygen requirements, but a decrease in the environmental temperature of 2°C, from 33°C to 31°C, is a drop sufficient to double the oxygen consumption of a term newborn and can cause the newborn to show signs of respiratory distress.

When exposed to cold, the preterm newborn may be unable to increase ventilation to the necessary level of oxygen consumption. (See chapter 34 for a discussion of cold stress.) Because oxidation of fatty acids depends on the availability of oxygen, glucose, and adenosine triphosphate (ATP), the newborn's ability to generate heat can be altered by pathologic events such as hypoxia, acidosis, and hypoglycemia or by medications that block the release of norepinephrine. The effect of certain drugs such as meperidine (Demerol) may also prevent metabolism of brown fat. Neonatal hypothermia prolongs as well as potentiates the effects of many analgesic and anesthetic drugs in the newborn.

Response to Heat

Sweating is the usual initial response of the term newborn to hyperthermia. The newborn sweat glands have limited function until after the fourth week of extrauterine life; heat is lost through peripheral vasodilation and evaporation of insensible water loss. Vasodilatation caused by overheating predisposes the infant to

DEVELOPING CULTURAL COMPETENCE
Newborn Baths in Jordan and Nigeria

In Jordan, the birth of a male infant is a much celebrated event. The newborn is bathed daily during the first week of life. During the final bath, salt is added to the water to help the newborn's skin adjust to the external environment and protect it from changes in the weather.

In Southeastern Nigeria, the *omugwo* is the practice of ritual of cares observed after the birth of a baby. Among the cares is a bathing regime for the newborn that includes physical exercises and routines like flexing the joints, holding the baby upside down, immersing the baby underwater, and even throwing the baby up in the air several times during bathing. These practices are thought to promote general health and physical strength, as well as promoting courage and fearlessness in the baby (Liamputtong, 2007).

hypotension. In term SGA infants, the onset of sweating is delayed; it is virtually nonexistent in preterm infants of less than 30 weeks' gestation because of the underdevelopment of the sweat glands. The term infant will be flaccid and assume a position of extension to facilitate heat loss (Blackburn, 2007). Oxygen consumption and metabolic rate also increase in response to hyperthermia. Severe hyperthermia can lead to death or to gross brain damage if the baby survives.

Hepatic Adaptations

The newborn's liver is frequently palpable 1 to 2 cm below the right costal margin at the midclavicular line (Tappero & Honeyfield, 2009). It is relatively large and occupies about 40% of the abdominal cavity. The newborn's liver plays a significant role in iron storage, carbohydrate metabolism, conjugation of bilirubin, and coagulation.

Iron Storage and Red Blood Cell Production

As red blood cells (RBCs) are destroyed after birth, their iron content is stored in the liver until needed for new RBC production. Newborn iron stores are determined by total body hemoglobin content and length of gestation. The term newborn has about 270 mg of iron at birth, and about 140 to 170 mg of this amount is in the hemoglobin. If the mother's iron intake has been adequate, enough iron will be stored to last until 5 months of age. After about 6 months of age, foods containing iron or iron supplements must be given to prevent anemia.

Carbohydrate Metabolism

At term, the newborn's cord blood glucose level is 15 mg/dl lower than maternal blood glucose level (Rosenberg, 2007). Neonatal carbohydrate reserves are relatively low. One third of this reserve is in the form of liver glycogen and are twice that of the adult. The newborn experiences an energy crunch at the time of birth with the cutting of the umbilical cord and resultant removal of the maternal glucose supply and the increased energy expenditure associated with the birth process and extrauterine life. Fuel sources are consumed at a faster rate because of the work of breathing, loss of heat when exposed to cold, activity, and activation of muscle tone.

Glucose is the main source of energy in the first 4 to 6 hours after birth. During the first 2 hours of life, the serum blood glucose level declines, then rises, and finally reaches a steady state by 3 hours after birth (Rosenberg, 2007).

The nurse may assess the glucose level on admission to the newborn nursery if risk factors or clinical symptoms are present, or per agency protocol. As stores of liver and muscle glycogen and blood glucose decrease, the newborn compensates by changing from a predominantly carbohydrate metabolism to fat metabolism. Energy is derived from fat and protein as well as from carbohydrates. The amount and availability of each of these "fuel substrates" depends on the ability of immature metabolic pathways (i.e., lacking specific enzymes or hormones) to function in the first few days of life.

Conjugation of Bilirubin

In the body, the breakdown of heme-containing proteins causes the production of bilirubin. Conjugation, or the changing of bilirubin into an excretable form, is the conversion of the yellow lipid-soluble pigment (unconjugated, indirect) into water-soluble pigment (excretable, direct). Unconjugated bilirubin is fat soluble, has a propensity for fatty tissues, is not in an excretable form, and is a potential toxin. Fetal unconjugated bilirubin crosses the placenta to be excreted, so the fetus does not need to conjugate bilirubin.

Total serum bilirubin is the sum of conjugated (direct) and unconjugated (indirect) bilirubin. Total bilirubin at birth is less than 3 mg/dl unless an abnormal hemolytic process has occurred in utero. After birth, the newborn's liver must begin to conjugate bilirubin. This produces a rise in serum bilirubin in the first few days of life. The unconjugated bilirubin formed, after RBCs are destroyed, is transported in the blood bound to albumin. The bilirubin is transferred into the hepatocytes and bound to intracellular proteins. These proteins determine the amount of bilirubin that is held in the liver cells for processing and consequently determine the amount of bilirubin uptake into the liver. The activity of uridine diphosphoglucuronosyl transferase (UDPGT) enzyme results in the attachment of unconjugated bilirubin to glucuronic acid (a product of liver glycogen), producing bilirubin glucuronides (conjugated, direct bilirubin). Direct (water soluble) bilirubin is excreted into the tiny bile ducts, then into the common duct and duodenum. The (direct) conjugated bilirubin then progresses down the intestines, where bacteria transform it into urobilinogen (urine bilirubin) and stercobilinogen. Stercobilinogen is not reabsorbed but is excreted as a yellow-brown pigment in the stools.

Even after the bilirubin has been conjugated and bound, it can be changed back to unconjugated bilirubin via the enterohepatic circulation. In the intestines, β-D-glucuronidase enzyme acts to split off (deconjugate) the bilirubin from bilirubin glucuronides if it is not first acted upon by gut bacteria to produce urobilinogen; the free bilirubin is reabsorbed through the intestinal wall and brought back to the liver via portal vein circulation. This recycling of the bilirubin and decreased ability to clear bilirubin from the system are prevalent in babies who have very high β-D-glucuronidase activity levels as well as delayed bacterial colonization of the gut (such as with the use of antibiotics) and further increases the newborn's susceptibility to jaundice. The longer the direct bilirubin remains in the infant's gut, the greater chance it has of becoming deconjugated. Because of this, infants who establish gut motility and active stooling through early and frequent feedings are less likely to develop physiologic jaundice. Conjugation of bilirubin in newborns is depicted in Figure 29-11 ■.

The newborn liver has relatively less metabolic and enzymatic activity at birth and in the first few weeks of life than an adult liver. This reduction in hepatic activity, along with a relatively large bilirubin load, decreases the liver's ability to conjugate bilirubin and increases susceptibility to jaundice.

Physiologic Jaundice

Physiologic jaundice is caused by accelerated destruction of fetal RBCs, impaired conjugation of bilirubin, and increased bilirubin reabsorption from the intestinal tract. This condition does not have a pathologic basis, but rather is a normal biologic response of the newborn.

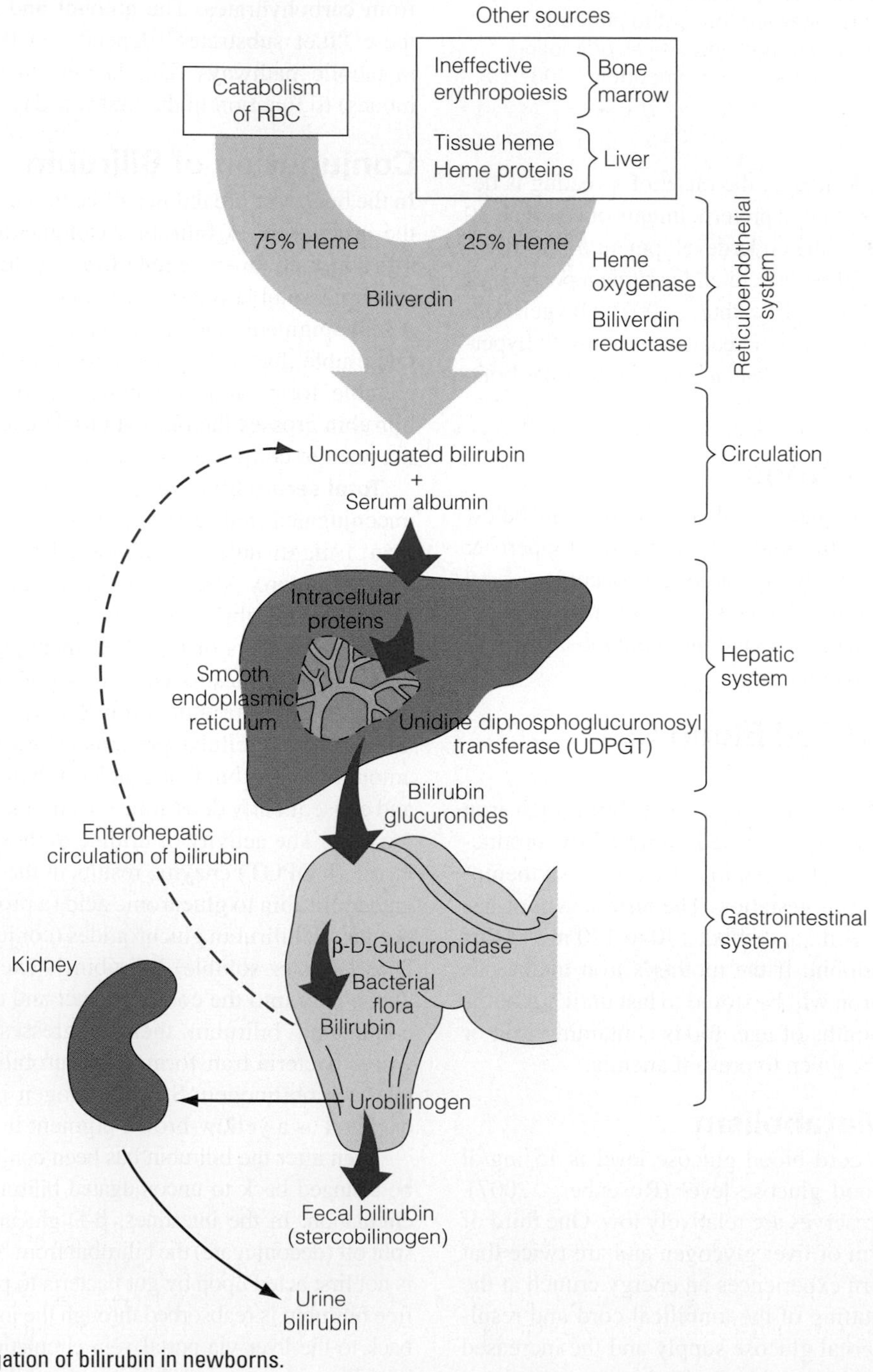

Figure 29-11 ■ Conjugation of bilirubin in newborns.

Source: Adapted from Avery, G. B., Fletcher, M. A., & MacDonald, M. G. Neonatology: Pathophysiology and management of the newborn *(5th ed., p. 767, fig. 38–5). Copyright © 1999 Lippincott, Williams & Wilkins. Reprinted with permission.*

Maisels (2005) describes six factors—several of which can also be related to pathologic events—whose interactions may give rise to physiologic jaundice:

1. ***Increased amounts of bilirubin delivered to the liver.*** The increased blood volume due to delayed cord clamping combined with faster RBC destruction in the newborn leads to an increased bilirubin level in the blood. A proportionately larger amount of nonerythrocyte bilirubin is formed in the newborn. Therefore, newborns have two to three times greater production or breakdown of bilirubin. The use of forceps or vacuum extraction that sometimes causes facial bruising or cephalohematoma (entrapped hemorrhage), or any bruising of the newborn body can increase the amount of bilirubin to be handled by the liver.
2. ***Defective uptake of bilirubin from the plasma.*** If the newborn does not ingest adequate calories, the formation of hepatic intracellular binding proteins diminishes, resulting in higher levels of bilirubin.
3. ***Defective conjugation of the bilirubin.*** Decreased uridine diphosphoglucuronosyl activity, as in hypothyroidism, or inadequate caloric intake causes the intracellular binding proteins to remain saturated and results in greater unconjugated bilirubin levels in the blood. The fatty acids in maternal breast milk compete with bilirubin for albumin binding sites; this process is thought to impede bilirubin processing.
4. ***Defect in bilirubin excretion.*** Delay in introduction of bacterial flora and decreased intestinal motility can also delay excretion and increase enterohepatic circulation of bilirubin.
5. ***Inadequate hepatic circulation.*** Decreased oxygen supplies to the liver associated with neonatal hypoxia or congenital heart disease lead to a rise in the bilirubin level.
6. ***Increased reabsorption of bilirubin from the intestine.*** Reduced bowel motility, intestinal obstruction, or delayed passage of meconium increases the circulation of bilirubin in the enterohepatic pathway, resulting in higher bilirubin values.

About 50% of full-term and 80% of preterm newborns exhibit physiologic jaundice on about the second or third day after birth. The characteristic yellow color results from increased levels of unconjugated bilirubin, which are a normal product of RBC breakdown and reflect a temporary inability of the body to eliminate bilirubin. Serum levels of bilirubin are about 4 to 6 mg/dl before yellow coloration of the skin and sclera appears. The signs of physiologic jaundice appear *after* the first 24 hours postnatally. This differentiates physiologic jaundice from pathologic jaundice (see chapter 34 ∞), which is clinically seen at birth or within the first 24 hours of postnatal life. Major risk factors for developing severe hyperbilirubinemia in late preterm and term infants are total serum bilirubin (TSB) or transcutaneous bilirubin (TcB) level in the high-risk zone on the bilirubin nomogram (Figure 29-12 ■).

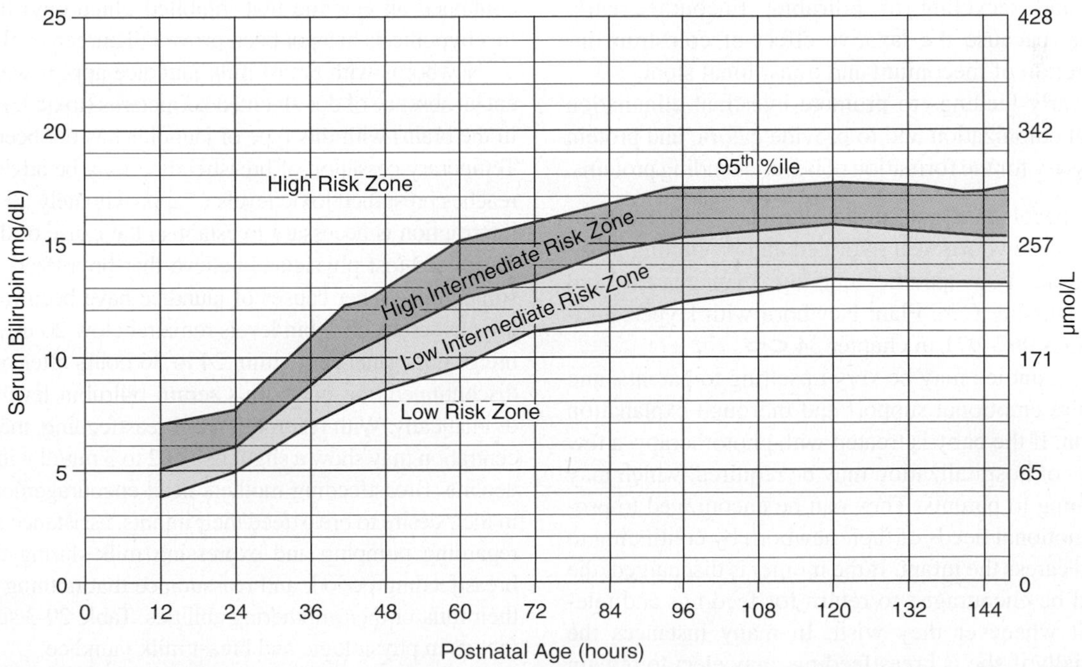

Figure 29-12 ■ Postnatal hour-specific bilirubin nomogram. Note: Nomogram for designation of risk in 2840 well newborns at 36 or more weeks' gestational age with birth weight of 2000 g or more or 35 or more weeks' gestational age and birth weight of 2500 g or more based on the hour-specific serum bilirubin values. The serum level was obtained before discharge, and the zone in which the value fell predicted the likelihood of a subsequent bilirubin level exceeding the 95th percentile (high-risk zone) as shown in Appendix 3, Table 4. Used with permission from Bhutani et al. See Appendix 1 for additional information about this nomogram, which should not be used to represent the natural history of neonatal hyperbilirubinemia.

Source: Reproduced with permission from Pediatrics, *114(1) 297–316 (Fig. 2, p. 301), Management of hyperbilirubinemia in the newborn infant 35 or more weeks of gestation. Copyright © 2004 by the AAP.*

Peak bilirubin levels are reached between days 3 and 5 in the full-term infant and between days 5 and 7 in the preterm infant. But these values are established for European and American Caucasian newborns. Chinese, Japanese, Korean, and Native American newborns have considerably higher bilirubin levels that are not as apparent and that persist for longer periods with no apparent ill effects (Maisels, 2005).

The nursery or postpartum room environment, including lighting, can hinder the early detection of the degree and type of jaundice. Pink walls and artificial lights mask the beginning of jaundice in newborns. Daylight assists the observer in early recognition by eliminating distortions caused by artificial light.

If jaundice is suspected, the nurse can quickly assess the newborn's coloring by pressing the skin, generally on the forehead or nose, with a finger. As blanching occurs, the nurse can observe the icterus (yellow coloring). The newborn develops jaundice in caudal progression, meaning that jaundice is first seen in the face and then travels down the trunk.

Several newborn care procedures will decrease the probability of high bilirubin levels:

- Maintain the newborn's skin temperature at 36.5°C (97.8°F) or above, because cold stress results in acidosis. Acidosis decreases available serum albumin-binding sites, weakens albumin-binding powers, and causes elevated unconjugated bilirubin levels.
- Monitor stool for amount and characteristics. Bilirubin is eliminated in the feces; inadequate stooling may result in reabsorption and recycling of bilirubin. Encourage early breastfeeding because the laxative effect of colostrum increases excretion of meconium and transitional stool.
- Encourage early feedings to promote intestinal elimination and bacterial colonization and to provide caloric and protein intake necessary for the formation of hepatic binding proteins.

If jaundice becomes apparent, nursing care is directed toward keeping the newborn well hydrated and promoting intestinal elimination. For specific nursing management and therapies, see Nursing Care Plan: Newborn with Hyperbilirubinemia on pages 969–971 in chapter 34 ∞.

Physiologic jaundice may be very upsetting to parents, and they will require emotional support and thorough explanation of the condition. If the baby is treated with phototherapy, a few additional days of hospitalization may be required, which may also be disturbing to parents. They can be encouraged to provide for the emotional needs of their newborn by continuing to feed, hold, and caress the infant. If the mother is discharged, the parents should be encouraged to return for feedings and telephone or visit whenever they wish. In many instances the mother, especially if she is breastfeeding, may elect to remain hospitalized with her newborn; the nurse should support this decision. If insurance limitations make this unrealistic, it may be possible to find an empty room for the discharged mother and her family to use while visiting the newborn. As an alternative to continued hospitalization, some newborns are treated with home phototherapy. (See Phototherapy in chapter 34 ∞ for more information.)

Breastfeeding Jaundice and Breast Milk Jaundice

Breastfeeding is implicated in jaundice in some newborns. *Breastfeeding jaundice* occurs in the first days of life in breastfed newborns. It appears to be associated with poor feeding practices and not with any abnormality in milk composition (McGrath & Hardy, 2011). It is related to inadequate fluid intake with some element of dehydration. Prevention of early breastfeeding jaundice includes encouraging frequent (every 2 to 3 hours) breastfeeding, avoiding supplementation, and accessing maternal lactation counseling.

In *breast milk jaundice,* the bilirubin rise is late onset and begins after the first week of life, when physiologic jaundice is waning. This type of jaundice may last from several weeks to several months. The level peaks at 5 to 10 mg/dl at 2 weeks of age and declines over the first several months of life (McGrath & Hardy, 2011).

In contrast to breastfeeding jaundice, breast milk jaundice is related to milk composition promoting increased bilirubin reabsorption from the intestine. Some women's breast milk may contain several times the normal concentration of certain free fatty acids. These free fatty acids may compete with bilirubin for binding sites on albumin and inhibit the conjugation of bilirubin or increase lipase activity, which disrupts the RBC membrane. Increased lipase activity enhances absorption of bile across the gastrointestinal tract membrane, thereby increasing the enterohepatic circulation of bilirubin. In the past it was thought that the breast milk of women whose newborns have breast milk jaundice contained an enzyme that inhibited glucuronyl transferase, but this hypothesis has not been proven (Thureen et al., 2005).

Newborns with breast milk jaundice appear well, and at present an absence of documented kernicterus (toxic levels of bilirubin in the brain) with this type of jaundice has not been documented. Temporary cessation of breastfeeding may be advised if bilirubin reaches presumed toxic levels of approximately 20 mg/dl or if the interruption is necessary to establish the cause of the hyperbilirubinemia. Most physicians believe that breastfeeding may be resumed once other causes of jaundice have been ruled out and as long as serum bilirubin levels remain below 20 mg/dl. In cases of breast milk jaundice, within 24 to 36 hours after breastfeeding is discontinued, the newborn's serum bilirubin levels begin to fall dramatically. With resumption of breastfeeding, the bilirubin concentration may show a slight rise of 2 to 3 mg/dl with a subsequent decline. Breastfeeding mothers need encouragement and support in their desire to breastfeed their infants, assistance and instruction regarding pumping and expressing milk during the interrupted breastfeeding period, and reassurance that nothing is wrong with their milk or their mothering abilities. Table 29-3 summarizes key factors in physiologic and breast milk jaundice.

CLINICAL TIP

Breastfeeding mothers need encouragement and support in their desire to breastfeed their infants, assistance and instruction about pumping and expressing milk during the interrupted breastfeeding period, and reassurance that nothing is wrong with their milk or mothering abilities.

TABLE 29-3 Jaundice

Physiologic Jaundice

- Physiologic jaundice occurs after the first 24 hours of life.
- During the first week of life, bilirubin should not exceed 13 mg/dl. Some pediatricians allow levels up to 15 mg/dl. See Figure 29-12 for the AAP Nomogram for Bilirubin risk for infants > 35 wks gestation.
- Bilirubin levels peak at 3 to 5 days in term infants.

Breast Milk Jaundice

- Bilirubin levels begin to rise about the fourth day after mature breast milk comes in.
- Peak of 5–10 mg/dl is reached at 2 to 3 weeks of age.
- It may be necessary to interrupt breastfeeding for a short period when bilirubin reaches 20 mg/dl.

Coagulation

The liver plays an important part in blood coagulation during fetal life and continues this function following birth. Coagulation factors II, VII, IX, and X (synthesized in the liver) are activated under the influence of vitamin K and therefore are considered vitamin K dependent. The absence of normal intestinal flora needed to synthesize vitamin K in the newborn gut results in low levels of vitamin K and creates a transient blood coagulation alteration between the second and fifth day of life. From a low point at about 2 to 3 days after birth, these coagulation factors rise slowly but do not approach adult levels until 9 months of age or later (Manco-Johnson, Rodden, & Hays, 2011). Other coagulation factors with low umbilical cord blood levels are XI, XII, and XIII. Fibrinogen and factors V and VII are near adult ranges.

Although newborn bleeding problems are rare, an injection of vitamin K (AquaMEPHYTON) is given prophylactically on the day of birth to combat potential clinical bleeding problems. (Hemorrhagic disease of the newborn is discussed in more depth in chapter 34 ∞.)

DEVELOPING CULTURAL COMPETENCE

Interpreting Illness Through Cultural Beliefs

Cultural beliefs lead mothers to interpret illness within their cultural framework, especially when left without clear and understood explanations (D'Avanzo & Geissler, 2008). For example, some Latina women believe that showing strong maternal emotions during pregnancy and during breastfeeding can be detrimental. They may blame jaundice in their newborn on "bili" associated with anger. Such maternal reactions can be lessened by careful explanations to the mothers about the diagnosis, prognosis, duration, and management options for jaundice, and possibility for recurrence.

Platelet counts at birth are in the same range as for older children, but newborns may manifest mild transient difficulty in platelet aggregation functioning. Phototherapy accentuates this platelet problem. Prenatal maternal therapy with phenytoin sodium (Dilantin) or phenobarbital also causes abnormal clotting studies and newborn bleeding in the first 24 hours after birth. Infants born to mothers receiving warfarin (Coumadin) compounds may bleed because these agents cross the placenta and accentuate existing vitamin K-dependent factor deficiencies. Transient neonatal thrombocytopenia may occur in infants born to mothers with severe hypertension or HELLP syndrome (hemolysis, elevated liver enzymes, and low platelet count) (see chapter 20 ∞ for a discussion of HELLP) and in infants born to mothers who have idiopathic isoimmune thrombocytopenic purpura.

Gastrointestinal Adaptations

By 36 to 38 weeks of fetal life, the gastrointestinal tract is adequately mature, with the presence of enzymatic activity and the ability to transport nutrients.

Digestion and Absorption

The full-term newborn has adequate intestinal and pancreatic enzymes to digest most simple carbohydrates, fat, and proteins. The carbohydrates requiring digestion in the newborn are usually disaccharides (lactose, maltose, sucrose), which are split into monosaccharides (galactose, fructose, and glucose) by the enzymes of the intestinal mucosa. Lactose is the primary carbohydrate in the breastfeeding newborn and is generally easily digested and well absorbed. The only enzyme lacking at birth is pancreatic amylase, which remains relatively deficient during the first few months of life. Newborns have trouble digesting starches (changing more complex carbohydrates into maltose), so they should not eat them until after the first few months of life.

Although proteins require more digestion than carbohydrates, they are well digested and absorbed from the newborn intestine. The newborn digests and absorbs fats less efficiently because of the minimal activity of the pancreatic enzyme lipase. The newborn excretes 10% to 20% of the dietary fat intake, compared with 10% for the adult. The fat in breast milk is absorbed more completely by the newborn than is the fat in cow's milk because it consists of more medium-chain triglycerides and contains lipase. (See chapter 32 ∞ for a more detailed discussion of infant nutrition.)

By birth the newborn has experienced swallowing, gastric emptying, and intestinal propulsion. In utero, fetal swallowing is accompanied by gastric emptying and peristalsis of the fetal intestinal tract. By the end of gestation, peristalsis becomes much more active in preparation for extrauterine life. Fetal peristalsis is also stimulated by anoxia, causing the expulsion of meconium into the amniotic fluid in more mature or stressed fetuses.

Air enters the stomach immediately after birth. The small intestine is air filled within 2 to 12 hours, and the large bowel within 24 hours. The salivary glands are immature at birth, and little saliva is manufactured until the infant is about 3 months old. The newborn's stomach has a capacity of 50 to 60 ml. It empties intermittently, starting within a few minutes of the beginning of a feeding and ending between 2 and 4 hours after feeding. Bowel sounds are present within the first 30 to 60 minutes of birth and the newborn can successfully feed during this time. The newborn's gastric pH becomes less acidic about a week after birth and remains less acidic than that of adults for the next 2 to 3 months.

The cardiac sphincter is immature, as is neural control of the stomach, so some regurgitation may be noted in the neonatal period. Regurgitation of the first few feedings during the first day or two of life can usually be lessened by avoiding overfeeding and by burping the newborn well during and after the feeding.

When no other signs and symptoms are evident, vomiting is limited and ceases within the first few days of life. Continuous vomiting or regurgitation should be monitored closely and reported promptly as it may be indicative of a more serious problem. If the newborn has swallowed bloody or purulent amniotic fluid, lavage of the stomach may be indicated in the term newborn to relieve the problem. Bilious vomiting is abnormal and must be evaluated thoroughly because it might represent a condition that warrants prompt surgical intervention.

Adequate digestion and absorption are essential for newborn growth and development. If optimal nutritional support is available, postnatal growth ideally should parallel intrauterine growth. After 30 weeks of gestation the fetus gains 30 g per day and adds 1.2 cm (0.5 in.) to body length daily. To gain weight at the intrauterine rate, the term newborn requires 120 kcal/kg/day. Following birth, caloric intake is often insufficient for weight gain until the newborn is 5 to 10 days old. During this time there may be a weight loss of 5% to 10% in term newborns. A shift of intracellular water to extracellular space and insensible water loss account for the 5% to 10% weight loss. Thus failure to lose weight when caloric intake is inadequate may indicate fluid retention.

CLINICAL JUDGMENT

Case Study: Jonathon Sykes

Jonathon Sykes is a 5-day-old term male infant who has returned to the hospital for a lactation visit. Jonathon's birth weight was 3260 grams (7 pounds, 3 ounces) and his current weight is 2963 grams (6 pounds, 8 1/2 ounces). The lactation nurse is worried about this weight loss and shares her concerns with Jonathon's mother.

Critical Thinking

What would you tell Jonathon's mother about his weight loss since birth?

What are other questions you might ask Jonathon's mother about his daily habits?

Based on his birth weight, what is the appropriate number of kilocalories that Jonathon needs to grow?

See www.nursing.pearsonhighered.com for possible responses.

Elimination

Term newborns normally pass meconium within 8 to 24 hours of life—and almost always within 48 hours. **Meconium** is formed in utero from the amniotic fluid and its constituents, with intestinal secretions and shed mucosal cells. It is recognized by its thick, tarry, black (or dark green) appearance. Transitional (thinner brown to green) stools consisting of part meconium and part fecal material are passed for the next day or two, after which the stools become entirely fecal. Generally, the stools of a breastfed newborn are pale yellow (but may be pasty green); they are more liquid and more frequent than those of formula-fed newborns, whose stools are paler and often the consistency of peanut butter (Figure 29-13 ■). Frequency of bowel movement varies but initially ranges from one every 2 to 3 days to as many as 10 daily. Mothers should be counseled that this is not constipation as long as the bowel movement remains soft. Table 29-4 describes the progression of stools and other physiologic adaptations to extrauterine life.

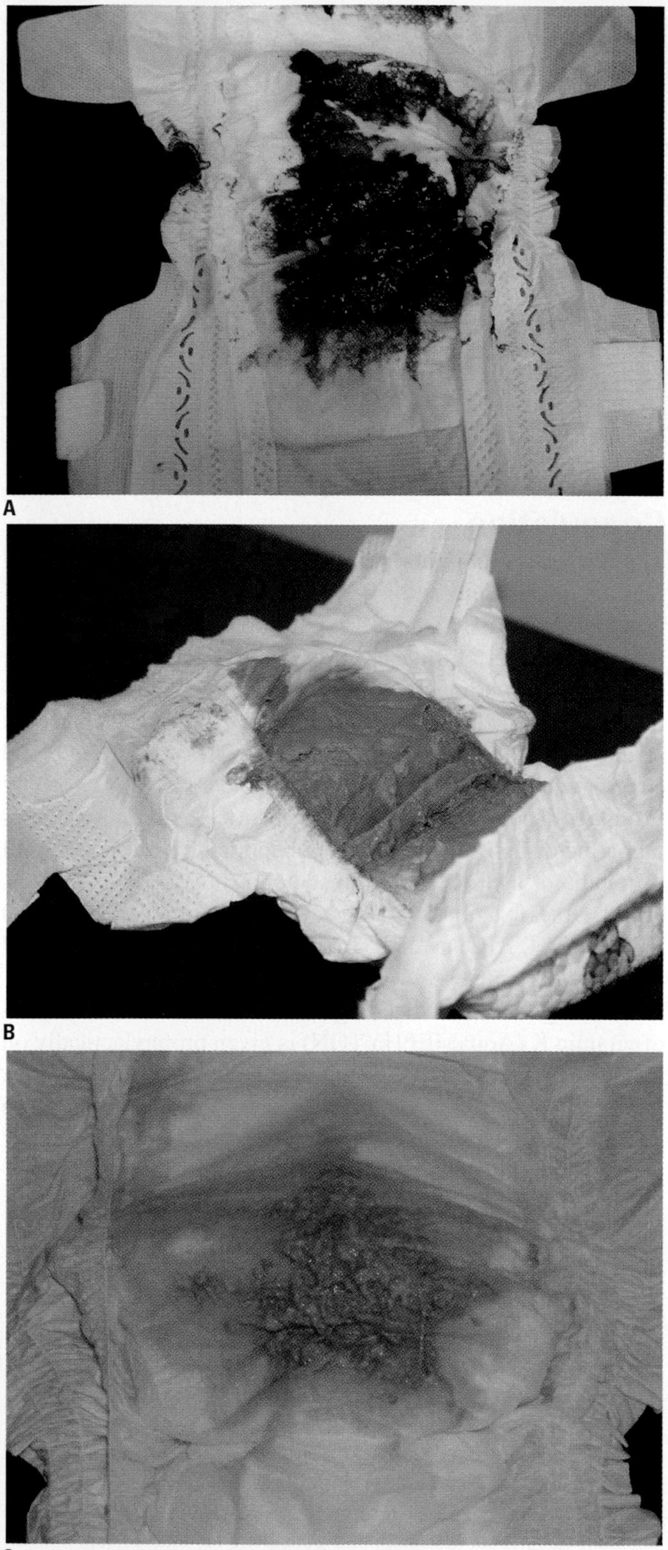

A

B

C

Figure 29-13 ■ Newborn stool samples. A. Meconium stool. B. Transitional stool. C. Breast milk stool.

Source: Courtesy of Brigitte Hall, RNC, MSN, IBCLC.

TABLE 29-4 Physiologic Adaptations to Extrauterine Life

- Periodic breathing may be present.
- Desired skin temperature 36°C–36.5°C (96.8°F–97.7°F), stabilizes 4 to 6 hours after birth.
- Desired blood glucose level reaches 60–70 mg/dl by third postnatal day.
- Stools progress from:
  Meconium (thick, tarry, black; meconium plug may be expelled)
  Transitional stools (thin, brown to green)
  Breastfed infants (yellow gold, soft, or mushy)
  Formula-fed infants (pale yellow, formed, and pasty)

> **“** When the nurse took my first child and put him to my breast his tiny mouth opened and reached for me as if he had known forever what to do. **”**
>
> — *Leslie Kenton, All I Ever Wanted Was a Baby*

Urinary Adaptations

Kidney Development and Function

Certain physiologic features of the newborn's kidneys may affect the newborn's ability to handle body fluids and excrete urine:

1. The term newborn's kidneys have a full complement of functioning nephrons by 34 to 36 weeks of gestation.
2. The glomerular filtration rate of the newborn's kidneys is low in comparison with the adult rate. Because of this physiologic decrease in kidney glomerular filtration, the newborn's kidneys are unable to dispose of water rapidly when necessary.
3. The juxtamedullary portion of the nephron has limited capacity to reabsorb HCO_3 and H and concentrate urine (reabsorb water back into the blood) because the tubules are short and narrow. The limitation of tubular reabsorption can lead to inappropriate loss of substances present in the glomerular filtrate, such as amino acids, bicarbonate, glucose, sodium, potassium, chloride, phosphate, and urea.

The ability to concentrate urine fully is attained by 3 months of age. Feeding practices may affect the osmolarity of the urine but have limited effect on concentration of the urine.

Because the newborn has difficulty concentrating urine, the effect of excessive insensible water loss or restricted fluid intake is unpredictable. The newborn kidney is also limited in its dilutional capabilities. Concentrating and dilutional limitations of renal function are important considerations in monitoring fluid therapy to avoid dehydration and overhydration.

Characteristics of Newborn Urinary Function

Many newborns void immediately after birth, which is usually noticed in the birthing room. Among normal newborns, 93% void by 24 hours after birth, and 100% void by 48 hours after birth (Thureen et al., 2005). A newborn who has not voided by 36 hours should be assessed for adequacy of fluid intake, bladder distention, restlessness, and symptoms of pain. The appropriate clinical personnel should be notified if indicated.

TABLE 29-5 Newborn Urinalysis Values

- Protein less than 5–10 mg/dl
- WBC less than 2–3/hpf
- RBC 0
- Casts 0
- Bacteria 0
- Color pale yellow

The initial bladder volume is 6 to 44 ml of urine. Unless edema is present, normal urinary output is often limited, and the voidings are scanty until fluid intake increases. (The fluid of edema is eliminated by the kidneys, so infants with edema have a much higher urinary output.) The first 2 days postnatally, the newborn may void 2 to 6 times daily, with a urine output of 15 ml/kg/day. The newborn subsequently voids 5 to 25 times every 24 hours, with a volume of 25 ml/kg/day. Observation and documentation of adequate urinary output is necessary given the large number of term infants who have early hospital discharge.

Following the first voiding, the newborn's urine frequently appears cloudy (because of mucus content) and has a high specific gravity, which decreases as fluid intake increases. Occasionally, pink stains ("brick dust spots") appear on the diaper. These are caused by urates and are innocuous. Blood may occasionally be observed on the diapers of female infants. This *pseudomenstruation* is related to the withdrawal of maternal hormones. Males may have bloody spotting from a circumcision. In the absence of apparent causes for bleeding, the clinician should be notified. During early infancy, normal urine is straw colored and almost odorless, although odor occurs when there is a metabolic disorder or when infection is present. Table 29-5 summarizes urinalysis values of the normal newborn.

Immunologic Adaptations

The general purposes of the newborn immune system are those of defense (fighting microorganisms), homeostasis (disposition of worn out cells), and surveillance (recognition and destruction of foreign or aberrant cells). The newborn's immune system is not fully activated until sometime after birth. Because the womb is a relatively sterile environment, the limitations in the newborn's inflammatory response result in failure to recognize, localize, and destroy invasive bacteria. Thus the signs and symptoms of infection are often subtle and nonspecific in the newborn. The newborn also has a poor hypothalamic response to pyrogens; therefore, fever is not a reliable indicator of infection. In the neonatal period, hypothermia is a more reliable sign of infection.

Of the three major types of immunoglobulins primarily involved in immunity—IgG, IgA, and IgM—only IgG crosses the placenta. The pregnant woman forms antibodies in response to illness or immunization. This process is called **active acquired immunity**. When IgG antibodies are transferred to the fetus in utero, **passive acquired immunity** results because the fetus does not produce the antibodies himself or herself. IgG is very active against bacterial toxins.

Because the maternal immunoglobulin is transferred primarily during the third trimester, preterm newborns (especially those born before 34 weeks) may be more susceptible to infection. In addition, postmature infants often have low levels of IgG that suggest decreased transfer with placental damage and aging. In general, newborns have maternally induced immunity to tetanus, diphtheria, smallpox, measles, mumps, poliomyelitis, and a variety of other bacterial and viral diseases. The period of resistance varies: Immunity against common viral infections such as measles may last 4 to 8 months, whereas immunity to certain bacteria may disappear within 4 to 8 weeks.

Although newborn infants are more vulnerable to infection, the normal newborn does produce antibodies in response to an antigen but not as effectively as an older child does. It is customary to begin immunization at 2 months of age so the infant can develop active acquired immunity. Some immunizations for specific viruses (Hepatitis B) are even given in the first day after birth.

IgM immunoglobulins are produced in response to blood group antigens, gram-negative enteric organisms, and some viruses in the expectant mother. Because IgM does not normally cross the placenta, most or all is produced by the fetus beginning at 10 to 15 weeks' gestation. Elevated levels of IgM at birth may indicate placental leaks or, more commonly, fetal antigenic stimulation in utero. Consequently, elevations suggest that the infant was exposed to an intrauterine infection such as syphilis or TORCH syndrome (toxoplasmosis, rubella, cytomegalovirus, or herpes virus hominis type 2 infection). (For in-depth discussion of infection, see chapter 20 ∞ and Table 34-5 ∞ on page 976.) The lack of available maternal IgM in the newborn also accounts for the infant's susceptibility to gram-negative enteric organisms such as *Escherichia coli.*

The functions of IgA immunoglobulins are not fully understood. IgA appears to provide protection mainly on secreting surfaces such as the respiratory tract, gastrointestinal tract, and eyes. Serum IgA does not cross the placenta and is not normally produced by the fetus in utero. Unlike the other immunoglobulins, IgA is not affected by gastric action. Colostrum, the forerunner of breast milk, is very high in the secretory form of IgA. It may provide some passive immunity to the infant of a breastfeeding mother. Newborns begin to produce secretory IgA in their intestinal mucosa at about 4 weeks after birth.

Infant Abilities

Neurologic and Sensory/ Perceptual Functioning

The newborn's brain is about one quarter the size of an adult's, and myelination of nerve fibers is incomplete. Unlike the cardiovascular or respiratory systems, which undergo tremendous changes at birth, the nervous system is minimally influenced by the actual birth process. Because many biochemical and histologic changes have yet to occur in the newborn's brain, the postnatal period is considered a time of risk in regard to the development of the brain and nervous system. For neurologic development—including development of intellect—to proceed, the brain and other nervous system structures must mature in an orderly, unhampered fashion. For discussion of cranial nerves, see chapter 30 ∞.

Intrauterine Factors Influencing Newborn Behavior

Newborns respond to and interact with the environment in a predictable pattern of behavior that is shaped somewhat by their intrauterine experience. This intrauterine experience is affected by intrinsic factors such as maternal nutrition and drug exposure, and external factors such as the mother's physical environment. Depending on the newborn's intrauterine experience and individual temperament, newborn behavioral responses to different stresses vary. Some newborns react quietly to stimulation, others become overreactive and tense, and some may exhibit a combination of the two.

Factors such as exposure to intense auditory stimuli in utero can eventually be manifested in the behavior of the newborn. For example, the fetal heart rate (FHR) initially increases when the pregnant woman is exposed to auditory stimuli, but repetition of the stimuli leads to decreased FHR. Thus the newborn who was exposed to intense noise during fetal life is significantly less reactive to loud sounds postnatally.

Characteristics of Newborn Neurologic Function

Perinatal factors will affect how the infant interacts with the environment. Type of labor and delivery, drugs given to the mother during labor, overall infant health, and of course gestational age of the infant are all matters that affect infant behavior. The environment itself also plays into infant response. A quiet, dim, warm, calming environment will elicit different infant behavior than a noisy, bright, or cold surrounding will.

Normal newborns are usually in a position of partially flexed extremities with the legs near the abdomen. When awake, the newborn may exhibit purposeless, uncoordinated bilateral movements of the extremities. The organization and intensity of the newborn's motor activity are influenced by a number of factors, including the following (Brazelton, 1984):

- Sleep-wake states
- Presence of environmental stimuli, such as heat, light, cold, and noise
- Conditions causing a chemical imbalance, such as hypoglycemia
- Hydration status
- State of health
- Recovery from the stress of labor and birth

Eye movements are observable during the first few days of life. An alert newborn is able to fixate on faces and geometric objects or patterns such as black and white stripes. A bright light shining in the newborn's eyes elicits the optical blink reflex.

The cry of the newborn should be lusty and vigorous. High-pitched cries, weak cries, or no cries are all causes for concern.

The newborn's body grows in a cephalocaudal (head-to-toe), proximal-distal fashion. The newborn is somewhat hypertonic; that is, there is resistance to extending the elbow and knee joints. Muscle tone should be symmetric. Diminished muscle tone and flaccidity may indicate neurologic dysfunction.

Specific symmetric deep tendon reflexes can be elicited in the newborn. The knee jerk is brisk; a normal ankle clonus may involve three or four beats. Plantar flexion is present. Other reflexes, including the Moro, grasping, rooting, Babinski, and sucking reflexes, are characteristics of neurologic integrity. (For further discussion, see chapter 30 ∞.)

Complex behavioral patterns reflect the newborn's neurologic maturation and integration. Newborns who can bring a hand to the mouth are demonstrating motor coordination as well as a self-quieting technique, thus increasing the complexity of the behavioral response. Newborns also possess complex organized defensive motor patterns as exhibited by the ability to remove an obstruction such as a cloth across the face.

Periods of Reactivity

The baby usually shows a predictable pattern of behavior during the first several hours after birth, characterized by two **periods of reactivity** separated by a sleep phase.

First Period of Reactivity

The first period of reactivity lasts from birth to approximately 30 minutes after birth. During this period the newborn is awake and active and may appear hungry and have a strong sucking reflex. This is an optimal period for parent-infant bonding as well as a natural opportunity to initiate breastfeeding if the mother has chosen it (Figure 29-14 ■). Bursts of random, diffuse movements alternating with relative immobility may occur. Respirations are rapid, as high as 80 breaths per minute, and there may be retraction of the chest, transient flaring of the nares, and grunting. The heart rate is rapid, and rhythm may be irregular. Bowel sounds are usually absent.

Period of Inactivity to Sleep Phase

After approximately half an hour, the newborn's activity gradually diminishes. The heart rate and respirations decrease as the newborn enters the sleep phase. The sleep phase may last from a few minutes to 2 to 4 hours. During this period the newborn will be difficult to awaken and will show no interest in sucking. Bowel sounds become audible, and cardiac and respiratory rates return to baseline values.

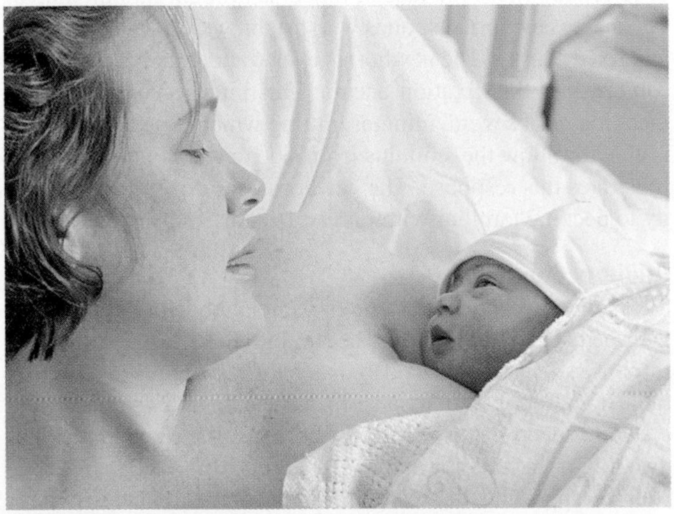

Figure 29-14 ■ Mother and baby gaze at each other. This quiet alert state is the optimal state for interaction.

Source: Superstock Royalty Free.

Second Period of Reactivity

During the second period of reactivity, the newborn is again awake and alert. This period lasts 4 to 6 hours in the normal newborn. Physiologic responses are variable during this stage. The heart and respiratory rates increase; however, the nurse must be alert for apneic periods, which may cause a drop in the heart rate and oxygen level (desaturation). The newborn is stimulated to continue breathing during such times. The newborn may develop rapid color changes and become mildly cyanotic or mottled during these fluctuations. Production of respiratory and gastric mucus increases, and the newborn responds by gagging, choking, and regurgitating.

Care Plan Activity: Physiologic Responses of the Newborn

Continued close observation and intervention may be required to maintain a clear airway during this period of reactivity. The gastrointestinal tract becomes more active. The newborn often passes the first meconium stool and may also have an initial voiding. The newborn shows he or she is ready to be fed by such behaviors as sucking, rooting, and swallowing. If feeding was not initiated in the first period of reactivity, it is done at this time. See Initial Feeding in chapter 32 ∞ for further discussion of the first feeding.

> **CLINICAL TIP**
>
> Because infants are often unable to handle oral secretions effectively enough to protect their airway, parents must be instructed in the proper use of the bulb syringe. The bulb syringe used correctly creates mild suction for removal of oral and nasal secretions. Overuse or vigorous use of the bulb syringe causes unnecessary trauma and inflammation of the small nasal airways resulting in swelling and partial airway obstruction.

Behavioral States of the Newborn

The behavior of the newborn can be divided into two categories: the sleep states and the alert states (Brazelton, 1984; Gardner & Goldson, 2011). These postnatal behavioral states are similar to those that have been identified during pregnancy. Subcategories are identified under each major category.

Sleep States

Newborn Sleep

The sleep states are as follows:

1. ***Deep or quiet sleep.*** The baby has closed eyes with no eye movements, regular even breathing, and jerky motion or startles at regular intervals. Behavioral responses to external stimuli are likely to be delayed. Startles are rapidly suppressed, and changes in state are not likely to occur. Heart rate may range from 100 to 120 beats/min.
2. ***Light sleep (rapid eye movement [REM] or active sleep).*** The baby has irregular respirations, eyes closed with REM, irregular sucking motions, minimal activity, and irregular but smooth movement of the extremities. Environmental and internal stimuli initiate a startle reaction and a change of state.

Newborn sleep cycles have been recognized and defined according to duration. The length of the cycle depends on the age of the newborn. At term, REM active sleep and quiet sleep occur in intervals of 50 to 60 minutes (Gardner & Goldson, 2011).

About 45% to 50% of the total sleep of the newborn is active sleep, 35% to 45% is quiet (deep) sleep, and 10% of sleep is transitional between these two periods. Growth hormone secretion depends on regular sleep patterns. Any disturbance of the sleep-wake cycle can result in irregular spikes of growth hormone. REM sleep stimulates the highest peaks of growth hormone and the growth of the neural system. Over time, the newborn's sleep-wake patterns become diurnal; that is, the newborn sleeps at night and stays awake during the day. (See "Newborn Behavioral Assessment" in chapter 30 ∞ for in-depth discussion of Brazelton's assessment of newborn states.)

Alert States

In the first 30 to 60 minutes after birth, many newborns display a quiet alert state, characteristic of the first period of reactivity. Nurses should use these alert states to encourage bonding and breastfeeding. These periods of alertness tend to be short the first 2 days after birth to allow the baby to recover from the birth process. Subsequent alert states are of choice or of necessity (Gardner & Goldson, 2011). The newborn's increasing choice of wakefulness indicates a maturing capacity to achieve and maintain consciousness. Heat, cold, and hunger are but a few of the stimuli that can cause wakefulness by necessity. Once the disturbing stimuli are removed, the baby tends to fall back asleep.

The following are subcategories of the alert state (Gardner & Goldson, 2011):

1. *Drowsy or semidozing.* The behaviors common to the drowsy state are open or closed eyes; fluttering eyelids; semidozing appearance; and slow, regular movements of the extremities. Mild startles may be noted from time to time. Although the reaction to a sensory stimulus is delayed, it often causes a change of state.
2. *Quiet alert.* In this state, the newborn is alert and follows and fixates on attractive objects, faces, or auditory stimuli. Motor activity is minimal, and the response to external stimuli is delayed.
3. *Active alert.* The eyes are open, and motor activity is quite intense, with thrusting movements of the extremities in the active awake state. Environmental stimuli increase startles or motor activity, but individual reactions are difficult to distinguish because of generalized high activity level.
4. *Crying.* Intense crying is accompanied by jerky motor movements. Crying serves several purposes for the newborn. It may be used as a distraction from disturbing stimuli such as hunger and pain. Fussiness often allows the newborn to discharge energy and reorganize behavior. Most important, crying elicits an appropriate response of help from the parents.

CLINICAL TIP

While the mother/infant couplet is in hospital, the nurse has a perfect opportunity to teach parents techniques to deal with infant crying and fussiness. Most importantly, it is necessary for parents and caregivers to know that for the first several months crying is the only means of communication available to the newborn and usually signifies unmet needs.

Behavioral and Sensory Capacities of the Newborn

Newborns have several behavioral capacities that assist in their adaptation to extrauterine life. For example, **self-quieting ability** is the ability of newborns to use their own resources to quiet and comfort themselves. Their repertoire includes hand-to-mouth movements, sucking on a fist or tongue, and attending to external stimuli.

Neurologically impaired newborns are unable to use self-quieting activities and require more frequent comforting from caregivers when stimulated. For example, drug-positive newborns often exhibit abnormal sleep and feeding patterns and irritability.

Swaddling newborns is a way to provide comfort and security. Swaddling also helps the newborn organize and control his body movements and behaviors. Blanket swaddling should be loose and should allow the infant easy hand to mouth access to promote self-soothing abilities. Tight swaddling, "straitjacket" techniques with arms at sides, is not comforting and may further agitate the infant.

Habituation is the newborn's ability to process and respond to complex stimulation, and to alter his response to a repeated stimulus. For example, when a bright light is flashed into the newborn's eyes, the initial response is blinking, constriction of the pupil, and perhaps a slight startle reaction. However, with repeated stimulation the newborn's response repertoire gradually diminishes and disappears. The capacity to ignore repetitious disturbing stimuli is a neonatal defense mechanism allowing him to shut out overwhelming and disturbing stimuli. Sensory abilities include visual, auditory, olfactory, taste, and tactile capacities.

Visual Capacity

Orientation is the newborn's ability to be alert to, to follow, and to fixate on complex visual stimuli that have a particular appeal and attraction. The newborn prefers the human face and eyes, and high contrast objects and patterns. The newborn is nearsighted and has best vision at a distance of 8 to 15 inches (Kyle & Kyle, 2008). As the face or object is brought into the line of vision, the newborn responds with bright, wide eyes; still limbs; and fixed staring. The newborn's eyes wander and occasionally can cross as this fixation occurs. This intense visual involvement may last several minutes, during which time the newborn is able to follow the stimulus from side to side. Figure 29-15 ■ illustrates this response. The newborn uses this sensory capacity to become familiar with family, friends, and surroundings.

Auditory Capacity

The newborn responds to auditory stimulation with a definite, organized behavior repertoire. The stimulus used to assess auditory response should be selected to match the state of the newborn. A rattle is appropriate for light sleep, a voice for an awake state, and a clap for deep sleep. As the newborn hears the sound, the cardiac rate rises, and a minimal startle reflex may be seen. If the sound is appealing, the newborn will become alert and search for the site of the auditory stimulus. Newborns prefer the sound of the human voice to nonhuman sounds and have very acute hearing immediately after birth (Cheffer & Rannalli, 2011).

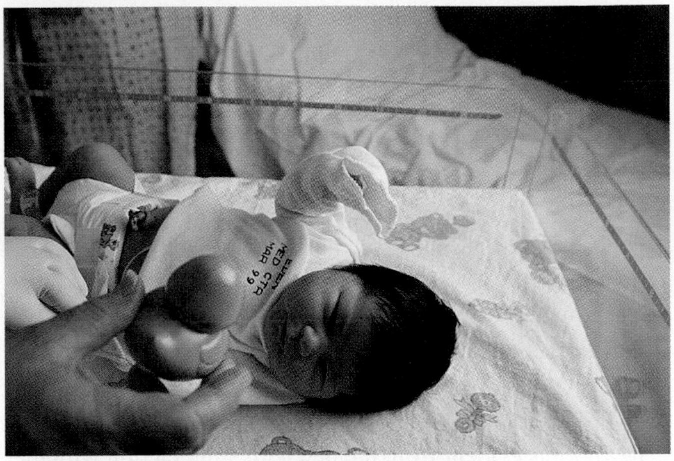

Figure 29-15 ■ Head turning to follow an object.

Source: Photographer, Elena Dorfman.

Olfactory Capacity

Newborns develop the sense of smell rapidly, and can differentiate their mother by smell within the first week of life (Cheffer & Rannalli, 2011). Newborns are able to distinguish their mothers' breast pads from those of other mothers' at just 1 week postnatally, and will turn preferentially toward the mother's smell.

Taste and Sucking

The newborn responds differently to varying tastes. They can distinguish between sweet and sour at 3 days of age (Cheffer & Rannalli, 2011). Sugar, for example, increases sucking, and newborns tend to have a preference for sweet tastes. Newborns fed with a rubber nipple versus the breast also show sucking pattern variations. When breastfeeding, the newborn sucks in bursts with frequent regular pauses. The bottle-fed newborn tends to suck at a regular rate with infrequent pauses.

When awake and hungry, the newborn displays rapid searching motions in response to the rooting reflex. Once feeding begins, the newborn establishes a sucking pattern according to the method of feeding. Finger sucking happens not only postnatally, but also in utero. The newborn frequently uses nonnutritive sucking as a self-quieting activity, which assists in the development of self-regulation. For bottle-fed infants, there is no reason to discourage nonnutritive sucking with a pacifier. Pacifiers should be offered to breastfed infants only after breastfeeding is well established, or during prolonged times away from the mother, or when stressful or painful procedures are required. If the pacifier is offered too soon, a phenomenon called "nipple confusion" may occur in which the breastfed infant has difficulty learning to suck from the breast and may nurse less. (See Supplementary Bottle Feeding in chapter 32 ∞ for a more in-depth discussion.)

Tactile Capacity

The newborn is very sensitive to being touched, cuddled, and held; thus touch may be the most important of all of the senses for the newborn infant. Often a mother's first response to an upset or crying newborn is touching or holding. Swaddling, placing a hand on the abdomen, or holding the arms to prevent a startle reflex are other ways to soothe the newborn. The settled newborn is then able to attend to and interact with the environment. Touch is also used to rouse a drowsy infant making him or her more alert for feeding.

FOCUS YOUR STUDY

- Newborn respiration is initiated primarily by chemical and mechanical events in association with thermal and sensory stimulation.
- The production of surfactant is crucial to keeping the lungs expanded during expiration by reducing alveolar surface tension.
- The newborn is an obligatory nose breather. Respirations move from being primarily shallow, irregular, and diaphragmatic to synchronous abdominal and chest breathing.
- Normal respiratory rate is 30 to 60 breaths per minute.
- Periodic breathing is normal, and newborn sleep states affect breathing patterns.
- The status of the cardiopulmonary system may be measured by evaluating the heart rate, blood pressure, and presence or absence of murmurs. The normal heart rate is 110 to 160 beats/min.
- Oxygen transport in the newborn is significantly affected by the presence of greater amounts of HbF (fetal hemoglobin) than HbA (adult hemoglobin). HbF holds oxygen more efficiently but releases it to the body tissues only at low PO_2 levels.

- Blood values in the newborn are modified by several factors, such as site of the blood sample, gestational age, prenatal or perinatal hemorrhage, and the timing of the clamping of the umbilical cord.
- The newborn is considered to have established thermoregulation when oxygen consumption and metabolic activity are minimal.
- Evaporation is the primary heat loss mechanism in newborns who are wet from amniotic fluid or a bath. In addition, excessive heat loss occurs from radiation and convection because of the newborn's larger surface area compared with weight; and from thermal conduction because of the marked difference between core temperature and skin temperature.
- The primary source for heat production in the cold-stressed newborn is brown adipose tissue.
- Blood glucose levels should reach a steady state by 3 hours of age.
- The newborn's liver plays a crucial role in iron storage, carbohydrate metabolism, conjugation of bilirubin, and coagulation.
- Controversy continues about the relationship of breastfeeding and the development of prolonged jaundice.
- The normal newborn possesses the ability to digest and absorb nutrients necessary for newborn growth and development.
- The newborn's stools change from meconium (thick, tarry, black) to transitional stools (thinner, brown to green) and then to the distinct forms for either breastfed newborns (yellow-gold, soft, or mushy) or formula-fed newborns (pale yellow, formed, and pasty). Most newborns pass their first stool within 48 hours of birth.
- The newborn's kidneys are characterized by a decreased rate of glomerular flow, limited tubular reabsorption, limited excretion of solutes, and limited ability to concentrate urine. Most newborns void within 36 to 48 hours of birth.
- The immune system in the newborn is not fully activated until sometime after birth, but the newborn does possess some immunologic abilities.
- Neurologic and sensory perceptual functioning in the newborn is evident from the newborn's interaction with the environment, presence of synchronized motor activity, and well-developed sensory capacities.
- The first period of reactivity lasts for 30 minutes after birth. The newborn is alert and hungry at this time, making this a natural opportunity to promote attachment.
- The second period of reactivity requires close monitoring by the nurse because apnea, decreased heart rate, gagging, choking, and regurgitation are likely to occur and require nursing intervention.
- Behavioral states in the newborn can be divided into sleep states and alert states.
- Sensory development proceeds in a specific order: tactile/vestibular, olfactory/gustatory, and auditory/visual.

CRITICAL THINKING IN ACTION

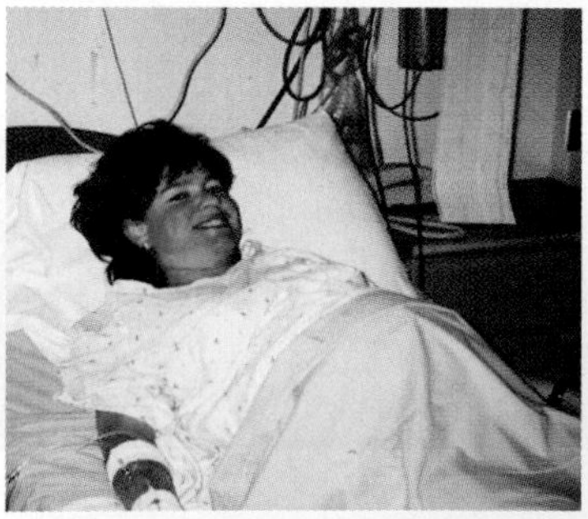

Sandra Dee, a 21-year-old, G1, P0000, at 36 weeks' gestation, has been in labor for the last 12 hours and is fully dilated with caput visible on the perineum. The fetal heart rate is 148 to 152 with early deceleration down to 142 with contraction and pushing. Her contractions are 4 to 5 minutes apart of good quality. Sandra's mother and sister are present for the birth. Her prenatal record shows no significant pregnancy problems or complications, and her vital signs have been stable within normal limits. Sandra has received two doses of Stadol for a total of 2 mg IV for pain relief during her labor. The last dose was given 2 hours ago. You assist with the vaginal birth of a live baby without an episiotomy. You observe the sex and time as the midwife places the infant girl on the mother's abdomen, suctions out the baby's mouth and nose, and proceeds to clamp the cord. You dry and stimulate the infant to breathe, remove the wet blanket and replace it with a dry one, and place the infant skin to skin on the mother's chest. You assess the need for infant resuscitation. The baby has a lusty cry spontaneously less than 30 seconds after birth. You palpate the cord, obtaining a heart rate of 120, and observe that the baby's chest and face are pink, and the legs and arms are flexed with open fist.

1. Explain the changes that must occur in the infant's cardiopulmonary system at birth.
2. What criteria do you look for when you assess the newborn for adequate cardiopulmonary adaptation at birth?
3. What steps do you take to maintain a neutral thermal environment at birth?
4. Sandra plans to breastfeed. When would you initiate the first feeding?
5. Discuss nursing actions that can decrease the probability of high bilirubin levels in the newborn.

See www.nursing.pearsonhighered.com for possible responses.

REFERENCES

Bagwell, G. A. (2007). Hematologic system. In C. Kenner & J. W. Lott (Eds.), *Comprehensive neonatal care: An interdisciplinary approach* (4th ed., pp. 221–253). St. Louis, MO: Saunders.

Blackburn, S. T. (2007). *Maternal, fetal, & neonatal physiology: A clinical perspective* (3rd ed.). St. Louis, MO: Saunders.

Brand, M. C., & Boyd, H. A. (2010). Thermoregulation. In M. T. Verklan & M. Walden (Eds.), *Core curriculum for neonatal intensive care nursing* (4th ed., pp. 110–119). St. Louis, MO: Saunders.

Brazelton, T. B. (1984). *Neonatal behavioral assessment scale* (2nd ed.). London, England: Heineman.

Cheffer, N. D. & Rannalli, D. A. (2011). Transitional care of the newborn. In S. Mattson & J. E. Smith (Eds.), *Core curriculum for maternal-newborn nursing* (4th ed., pp. 345–361). St. Louis. MO: Saunders.

Cloherty, J. R., Eichenwald, E. C., & Stark, A. R. (2008). *Manual of neonatal care.* Philadelphia, PA: Lippincott Williams & Wilkins.

Creehan, P. A. (2008). Newborn physical assessment. In K. R. Simpson & P. A. Creehan, *Perinatal nursing* (3rd ed., pp. 546–574). Philadelphia, PA: Lippincott Williams & Wilkins.

D'Avanzo, C. E., & Geissler, E. M. (2008). *Pocket guide to cultural assessment* (4th ed.). St. Louis, MO: Mosby.

Gardner, S. L., & Goldson, E. (2011). The neonate and the environment: Impact on development. In S. L. Gardner, B. S. Carter, M. Enzman-Hines & J. A. Hernandez (Eds.), *Merenstein & Gardner's handbook of neonatal intensive care* (7th ed., pp. 270–331). St. Louis, MO: Mosby.

Knuppel, R. A. (2007). Maternal-placental-fetal unit: Fetal & early neonatal physiology. In A. H. DeCherney, L. Nathan, T. M. Goodwin, & N. Laufer (Eds.), *Current obstetric & gynecologic diagnosis & treatment* (10th ed., pp. 159–186). New York, NY: Lang Medical Books/McGraw-Hill.

Kyle, T., & Kyle, T. (2008). *Essentials of pediatric nursing.* Philadelphia, PA: Lippincott Williams & Wilkins.

Liamputtong, P. (2007). *Childrearing and infant care issues: A cross-cultural perspective.* (pp. 163–164). New York, NY: Nova Science Publishers.

Manco-Johnson, M., Rodden, D. J., & Hays, T. (2011). Newborn hematology. In S. L. Gardner, B. S. Carter, M. Enzman-Hines, & J. A. Hernandez (Eds.), *Merenstein & Gardner's handbook of neonatal intensive care* (7th ed., pp. 503–530). St. Louis, MO: Mosby.

McGrath, J. M., & Hardy, W. (2011). The infant at risk. In S. Mattson & J. E. Smith (Eds.), *Core curriculum for maternal-newborn nursing* (4th ed., pp. 362–414). St. Louis. MO: Saunders.

Maisels, M. J. (2005). Jaundice. In M. G. MacDonald, M. D. Mullett, & M. Seshia (Eds.), *Avery's neonatology: Pathophysiology & management of the newborn* (6th ed., pp. 768–846). Philadelphia, PA: Lippincott Williams & Wilkins.

Mercer, J. S., Erickson-Owens, D. A., Graves, B., & Haley, M. (2007). Evidence-based practices for the fetal to newborn transition. *Journal of Midwifery and Women's Health, 52*(3), 262–272.

Niermeyer, S., & Clarke, S. (2011). Delivery room care. In S. L. Gardner, B. S. Carter, M. Enzman-Hines, & J. A. Hernandez (Eds.), *Merenstein & Gardner's handbook of neonatal intensive care* (7th ed., pp. 52–77). St. Louis, MO: Mosby.

Polin, R. A., Fox, W. W., & Abman, S. H. (2004). *Fetal and neonatal physiology* (3rd ed.). Philadelphia, PA: Saunders.

Ramachandrappa, A., & Jain, L. (2008). Elective cesarean section: Its impact on neonatal respiratory outcome. *Clinics in Perinatology*, Vol. 35, Issue 2.

Rosenberg, A. A. (2007). The neonate. In S. G. Gabbe, J. R. Niebyl, & J. L. Simpson (Eds.), *Obstetrics: Normal and problem pregnancies* (5th ed., pp. 523–565). Philadelphia, PA: Churchill Livingstone/Elsevier.

Tappero, E., & Honeyfield, M. E. (2009). *Physical assessment of the newborn: A comprehensive approach to the art of physical examination* (4th ed.). Santa Rosa, CA: NICU INK Book Publisher.

Thureen, P. J., Deacon, J., Hernandez, J., & Hall, D. M. (2005). *Assessment and care of the well newborn* (2nd ed.). Philadelphia, PA: Saunders.

CHAPTER 30

Nursing Assessment of the Newborn

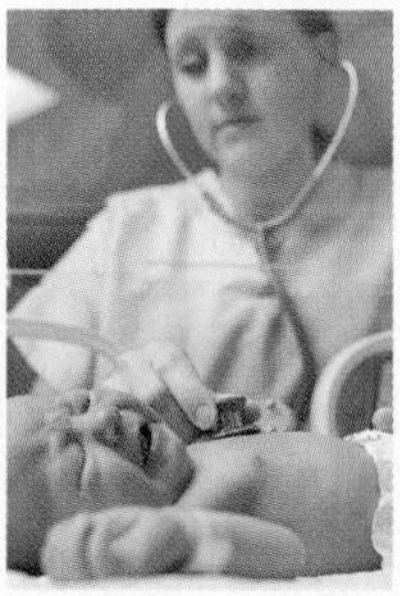

Something very special occurs within the first hour after birth. If the environment is quiet, the birthing without complications, the lights lowered, the handling diminished, newborn infants—aside from all the physiological adaptations they must make—begin in a uniquely human way to adapt to the new experience of being in the world.

—Marshall H. Klaus & Phyllis H. Klaus, *The Amazing Newborn*

LEARNING OUTCOMES

1. Describe the physical and neuromuscular maturity characteristics assessed to determine the gestational age of the newborn.
2. Delineate the normal physical and behavioral characteristics of the newborn.
3. Summarize the components of a systematic physical newborn assessment and the significance of normal variations and abnormal findings.
4. Describe the components of a newborn neurologic assessment.
5. Discuss the neurologic and neuromuscular characteristics of the newborn and the reflexes that may be present at birth.
6. Describe the components of the newborn behavioral assessment.
7. Compare the normal behavioral characteristics of the newborn with the normal variations that may be present.

KEY TERMS

Acrocyanosis *796*
Barlow maneuver *807*
Brazelton's Neonatal Behavioral Assessment Scale *820*
Caput succedaneum *800*
Cephalhematoma *799*
Chemical conjunctivitis *801*
Dubowitz tool *784*
Epstein's pearls *802*
Erb-Duchenne paralysis (Erb's palsy) *806*
Erythema toxicum *796*
Forceps marks *796*
Gestational age assessment tools *784*
Grasping reflex *809*
Harlequin sign *796*
Jaundice *796*
Lanugo *784*
Milia *796*
Molding *799*
Mongolian blue spots *798*
Moro reflex *809*
Mottling *796*
Nevus flammeus (port wine stain) *798*
Nevus vasculosus (strawberry mark) *798*
New Ballard Score (NBS) *784*
Ortolani's maneuver *808*
Pseudomenstruation *806*
Rooting reflex *809*
Skin turgor *796*
Subconjunctival hemorrhage *801*
Sucking reflex *809*
Telangiectatic nevi (stork bites) *798*
Thrush *802*
Tonic neck reflex *809*
Trunk incurvation (Galant reflex) *809*
Vernix caseosa *796*

Unlike adults, newborns communicate their needs primarily by their behavior. Because nurses are the most consistent professional observer of the newborn, they can translate this behavior into information about the newborn's condition and respond with appropriate nursing interventions. This chapter focuses on the assessment of the newborn and interpretation of findings. Assessment of the newborn is a continuous process used to evaluate development and adjustments to extrauterine life. In the birthing area, Apgar scoring and careful observation of the newborn form the basis of the assessment and are correlated with information such as the following:

- Maternal prenatal care history
- Birthing history
- Maternal analgesia and anesthesia
- Complications of labor or birth
- Treatment instituted immediately after birth, in conjunction with determination of clinical gestational age
- Consideration of the newborn's classification by weight and gestational age and by neonatal mortality risk
- Physical examination of the newborn

The nurse incorporates data from these sources with the assessment findings during the first 1 to 4 hours after birth to formulate a plan for nursing intervention.

The various newborn assessments and the data obtained from them are only valuable to the degree to which they are shared with the parents. The parents must be included in the assessment process from the moment of their child's birth. The *Apgar score* and its meaning should be explained immediately to the family (see further discussion in chapter 24 ∞). As soon as possible, the parents should take part in the physical and behavioral assessments as well.

The nurse encourages the parents to identify the unique behavioral characteristics of their newborn and to learn nurturing activities. Attachment is promoted when parents have the opportunity to explore their newborn in private, identifying individual physical and behavioral characteristics. The nurse's supportive responses to the parents' questions and observations are essential throughout the assessment process. The newborn physical examination is the beginning of newborn health surveillance and health education for the newborn's family that continues into the community setting.

Timing of Newborn Assessments

During the first 24 hours of life, the newborn makes the critical transition from intrauterine to extrauterine life. The risk of mortality and morbidity is statistically high during this period. Assessment of the newborn is essential to ensure that the transition is proceeding successfully

There are three major time frames for assessing newborns while they are in the birth facility.

TABLE 30-1 Timing and Types of Newborn Assessments
Assess immediately after birth:
Need for resuscitation
If newborn is stable and can be placed with parents to initiate early attachment/bonding
Assessments within 1 to 4 hours after birth:
Progress of newborn's adaptation to extrauterine life
Determination of gestational age
Ongoing assessment for high-risk problems
Assessment procedures within first 24 hours or before discharge:
Complete physical examination (Depending on agency protocol, the nurse may complete some components independently with the certified nurse-midwife/physician/nurse practitioner completing the exam before discharge.)
Nutritional status and ability to formula-feed or breastfeed satisfactorily
Behavioral state organization abilities

- The first assessment is done in the birthing area immediately after birth to determine the need for resuscitation or other interventions. The stable newborn can stay with the family after birth to initiate early attachment. The newborn with complications is usually taken to the nursery for further evaluation and intervention.
- A second assessment is done by the nursery nurse as part of the routine admission procedure. During this assessment, the nurse carries out a brief physical examination to estimate gestational age and evaluate the newborn's adaptation to extrauterine life. The accuracy of gestational age assessment decreases when performed more than 24 hours after birth. No later than 2 hours after birth, the admitting nursery nurse should evaluate the newborn's status and any problems that place the newborn at risk (American Academy of Pediatrics [AAP] & the American College of Obstetricians and Gynecologists [ACOG], 2007).
- Before discharge a certified nurse-midwife, physician, or nurse practitioner will carry out a behavioral assessment and a complete physical examination to detect any emerging or potential problems.

This chapter presents the procedures for estimating gestational age and performing the complete physical examination and behavioral assessment (Table 30-1). Chapter 24 ∞ discusses the immediate postbirth assessment. Chapter 31 ∞ describes the brief assessment performed during the first 4 hours of life.

Estimation of Gestational Age

It is essential to establish the newborn's gestational age in the first 4 hours after birth so that careful attention can be given to age-related problems. Traditionally, a newborn's gestational age was determined from the date of the pregnant woman's last menstrual period. This method was accurate only 75% to 85%

of the time. Because of the problems that develop with the newborn who is preterm or whose weight is inappropriate for gestational age, a more accurate system was developed to evaluate the newborn. Once learned, the procedure can be done in a few minutes. *It is essential that the nurse wear gloves when assessing the newborn in these early hours after birth and before the first bath until amniotic fluid, vaginal secretions, and blood on the skin are removed.*

Clinical **gestational age assessment tools** have two components: external physical characteristics and neurologic or neuromuscular development evaluations. Physical characteristics generally include sole creases, amount of breast tissue, amount of lanugo, cartilaginous development of the ear, testicular descent, and scrotal rugae or labial development. These objective clinical criteria are not influenced by labor and birth and do not change significantly within the first 12 hours after birth.

Neurologic examination facilitates assessment of functional or physiologic maturation in addition to physical development. However, the newborn's nervous system is unstable during the first 24 hours of life; neurologic evaluation findings based on reflexes or assessments dependent on the higher brain centers may not be reliable. If the neurologic findings drastically deviate from the gestational age derived by evaluation of the external characteristics, a second assessment is done in 24 hours.

The neurologic assessment components (excluding reflexes) are especially helpful in assessing the gestational age of newborns less than 34 weeks' gestation. Between 26 and 34 weeks, neurologic changes are significant, whereas significant physical changes are less evident. One significant neuromuscular change is that muscular tone develops from extension to having the ability to flex the extremity as neurologic maturity develops in a caudocephalad (tail-to-head) progression.

Ballard et al., (1991) developed the *estimation of gestational age by maturity rating*, a simplified version of the well-researched **Dubowitz tool**. The Ballard tool omits some of the neuromuscular tone assessments, such as head lag, ventral suspension (which is difficult to assess in very ill newborns or those on respirators), and leg recoil. In Ballard's tool, each physical and neuromuscular finding is given a point value, and the total score is matched to a gestational age (Figure 30-1 ■). The maximum score on the Ballard tool is 50, which corresponds to a gestational age of 44 weeks.

For example, on completing a gestational assessment of a 1-hour-old newborn, the nurse gives a score of 3 to all the physical characteristics, for a total of 18, and gives a score of 3 to all the neuromuscular assessments, for a total neurologic score of 18. The physical characteristics score of 18 is added to the neurologic score of 18 for a total score of 36, which correlates with 38 or more weeks' gestation. Because all newborns vary slightly in the development of physical characteristics and maturation of neurologic function, scores will usually vary instead of all being 3, as in this example.

Case Study: Newborn Maturity Assessment

Postnatal gestational age assessment tools can overestimate preterm gestational age and underestimate postterm gestational age. The tools have been shown to lose accuracy when newborns of less than 28 weeks' or more than 43 weeks' gestation are assessed. Ballard et al., (1991) in the **New Ballard Score (NBS)** added criteria for more accurate assessment of the gestational age of newborns between 20 and 28 weeks' gestation and less than 1500 g. They suggest that the assessment be made within 12 hours of birth to optimize accuracy, especially in infants of 22 to 28 weeks' gestational age. Also, the Ballard assessment may be overstimulating to infants of less than 27 weeks' gestation (Gardner & Hernandez, 2011).

Some maternal conditions such as preeclampsia, diabetes, and maternal analgesia and anesthesia may affect certain gestational assessment components and warrant further evaluation (see chapter 19 ∞, chapter 21 ∞, and chapter 25 ∞). Maternal diabetes, although it appears to accelerate fetal physical growth, seems to retard maturation. Maternal hypertension states, which retard fetal physical growth, seem to speed maturation.

Newborns of women with preeclampsia have a poor correlation with the criteria involving active muscle tone and edema. Maternal analgesia and anesthesia may cause the baby to have respiratory depression. Babies with respiratory distress syndrome (RDS) tend to be flaccid and edematous and to assume a "froglike" posture (see chapter 34 ∞). These characteristics affect the scoring of the neuromuscular components of the assessment tool used. The NBS gestational age assessment tool is used throughout this chapter to demonstrate the assessment of the physical and neuromuscular criteria associated with gestational age.

Assessment of Physical Maturity Characteristics

The nurse first evaluates observable characteristics without disturbing the baby. Selected physical characteristics common to the Dubowitz and Ballard gestational assessment tools are presented here in the order in which they might be most effectively evaluated:

1. *Resting posture,* although a neuromuscular component, should be assessed as the baby lies undisturbed on a flat surface (Figure 30-2 ■).
2. *Skin* in the preterm newborn appears thin and transparent, with veins prominent over the abdomen early in gestation. As the newborn approaches term, the skin appears opaque because of increased subcutaneous tissue. Disappearance of the protective vernix caseosa promotes skin desquamation, and this is commonly seen in postmature infants (infants greater than 42 weeks' gestational age and those showing signs of placental insufficiency; see chapter 33 ∞).
3. *Lanugo,* a fine hair covering, decreases as gestational age increases. The amount of **lanugo** is greatest at 28 to 30 weeks. It is most abundant over the back (particularly

NEWBORN MATURITY RATING & CLASSIFICATION

ESTIMATION OF GESTATIONAL AGE BY MATURITY RATING

Symbols: X - 1st Exam O - 2nd Exam

NEUROMUSCULAR MATURITY

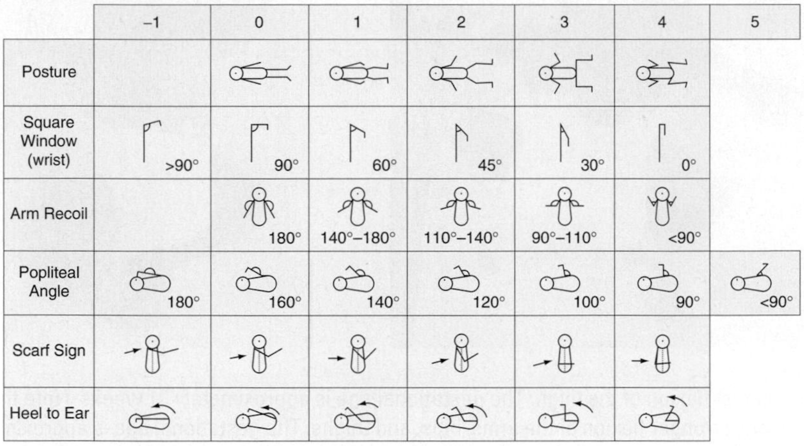

	−1	0	1	2	3	4	5
Posture							
Square Window (wrist)	>90°	90°	60°	45°	30°	0°	
Arm Recoil		180°	140°–180°	110°–140°	90°–110°	<90°	
Popliteal Angle	180°	160°	140°	120°	100°	90°	<90°
Scarf Sign							
Heel to Ear							

Gestation by Dates ______________ wks

Birth Date __________ Hour __________ am pm

APGAR __________ 1 min __________ 5 min

MATURITY RATING

score	weeks
−10	20
−5	22
0	24
5	26
10	28
15	30
20	32
25	34
30	36
35	38
40	40
45	42
50	44

PHYSICAL MATURITY

	−1	0	1	2	3	4	5
Skin	sticky friable transparent	gelatinous red, translucent	smooth pink, visible veins	superficial peeling &/or rash, few veins	cracking pale areas rare veins	parchment deep cracking no vessels	leathery cracked wrinkled
Lanugo	none	sparse	abundant	thinning	bald areas	mostly bald	
Plantar Surface	heel-toe 40–50 mm:–1 <40 mm:–2	>50 mm no crease	faint red marks	anterior transverse crease only	creases ant. 2/3	creases over entire sole	
Breast	imperceptible	barely perceptible	flat areola no bud	stippled areola 1–2 mm bud	raised areola 3–4 mm bud	full areola 5–10 mm bud	
Eye/Ear	lids fused loosely:–1 tightly:–2	lids open pinna flat stays folded	sl. curved pinna; soft; slow recoil	well curved pinna; soft but ready recoil	formed & firm instant recoil	thick cartilage ear stiff	
Genitals male	scrotum flat, smooth	scrotum empty faint rugae	testes in upper canal rare rugae	testes descending few rugae	testes down good rugae	testes pendulous deep rugae	
Genitals female	clitoris prominent labia flat	prominent clitoris small labia minora	prominent clitoris enlarging minora	majora & minora equally prominent	majora large minora small	majora cover clitoris & minora	

SCORING SECTION

	1st Exam = X	2nd Exam = 0
Estimating Gest Age by Maturity Rating	_____Weeks	_____Weeks
Time of Exam	Date _______ Hour_____ am pm	Date _______ Hour_____ am pm
Age at Exam	_____ Hours	_____ Hours
Signature of Examiner	__________ M.D.	__________ M.D.

Figure 30-1 ■ Newborn maturity rating and classification. If a 1-hour-old newborn is given a score of 3 for each of the physical characteristics and neuromuscular assessments, the newborn's total score would be 36. A total score of 36 correlates with 38 or more weeks' gestation.

Source: Reprinted from Journal of Pediatrics, 119, 417, Ballard, J. L., et al. New Ballard score, expanded to include extremely premature infants. Copyright © 1991, with permission from Elsevier.

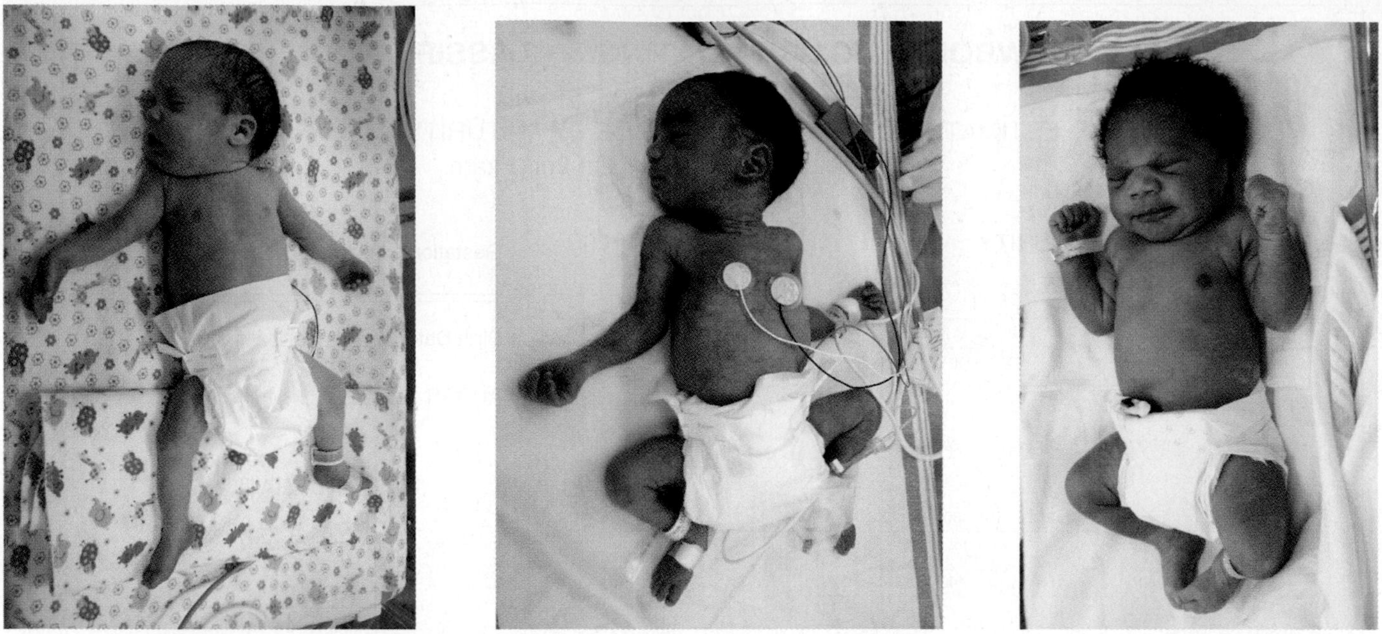

A B C

Figure 30-2 ■ Resting posture. A. Infant exhibits beginning of flexion of the thigh. The gestational age is approximately 31 weeks. Note the extension of the upper extremities. Score 1 or 2. B. Infant exhibits stronger flexion of the arms, hips, and thighs. The gestational age is approximately 35 weeks. Score 3. C. The full-term infant exhibits hypertonic flexion of all extremities. Score 4.

Source: George Dodson/Lightworks Studio/Pearson Education.

between the scapulae), although it will be noted over the face, legs, and arms. Lanugo disappears first from the face, then from the trunk and extremities (Figure 30-3 ■).

4. *Sole (plantar) creases* are reliable indicators of gestational age in the first 12 hours of life. Later, the skin of the foot begins drying, and superficial creases appear. Development of sole creases begins at the top (anterior) portion of the sole and, as gestation progresses, proceeds to the heel (Figure 30-4 ■). Peeling may also occur. Plantar creases vary with race. In newborns of African descent, sole creases may be less developed at term.
5. The nurse inspects the *areola* and gently palpates the breast bud tissue by applying the forefinger and middle finger to the breast area and measuring the tissue between them in centimeters or millimeters (Figure 30-5 ■). At term gestation, the tissue will measure between 0.5 and 1 cm (5 to 10 mm). During the assessment, the nipple should not be grasped firmly because skin and subcutaneous tissue will prevent accurate estimation of size. The nurse must perform this procedure gently to avoid causing trauma to the breast tissue.

   As gestation progresses, the breast tissue mass and areola enlarge. However, a large breast tissue mass can occur as a result of conditions other than advanced gestational age or the effects of maternal hormones on the baby. In the large-for-gestational-age (LGA) infant of a diabetic mother, accelerated development of breast tissue is a reflection of subcutaneous fat deposits. Small-for-gestational-age (SGA) term or postterm newborns may have used subcutaneous fat (which would have been deposited as breast tissue) to survive in utero; as a result their lack of breast tissue may indicate a gestational age of 34 to 35 weeks, even though other factors indicate a term or postterm newborn.
6. *Ear form and cartilage distribution* develop with gestational age. The cartilage gives the ear its shape and substance (Figure 30-6 ■). In a newborn of less than 34 weeks' gestation, the ear is relatively shapeless and flat; it has little cartilage, so the ear folds over on itself and remains folded. By approximately 36 weeks' gestation, some cartilage and slight incurving of the upper pinna are present, and the pinna springs back slowly when folded. (The nurse tests this response by holding the top and bottom of the pinna together with the forefinger and thumb

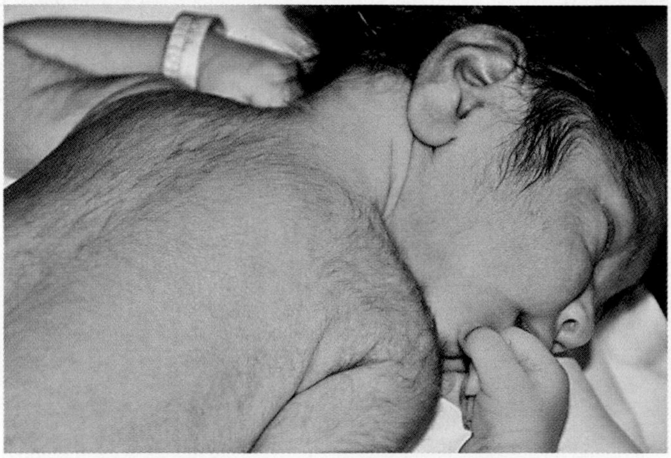

Figure 30-3 ■ Lanugo.

Source: Courtesy of Jo Engle, RN, MSN, NNP-BC and Vanessa Howell, RN, MSN.

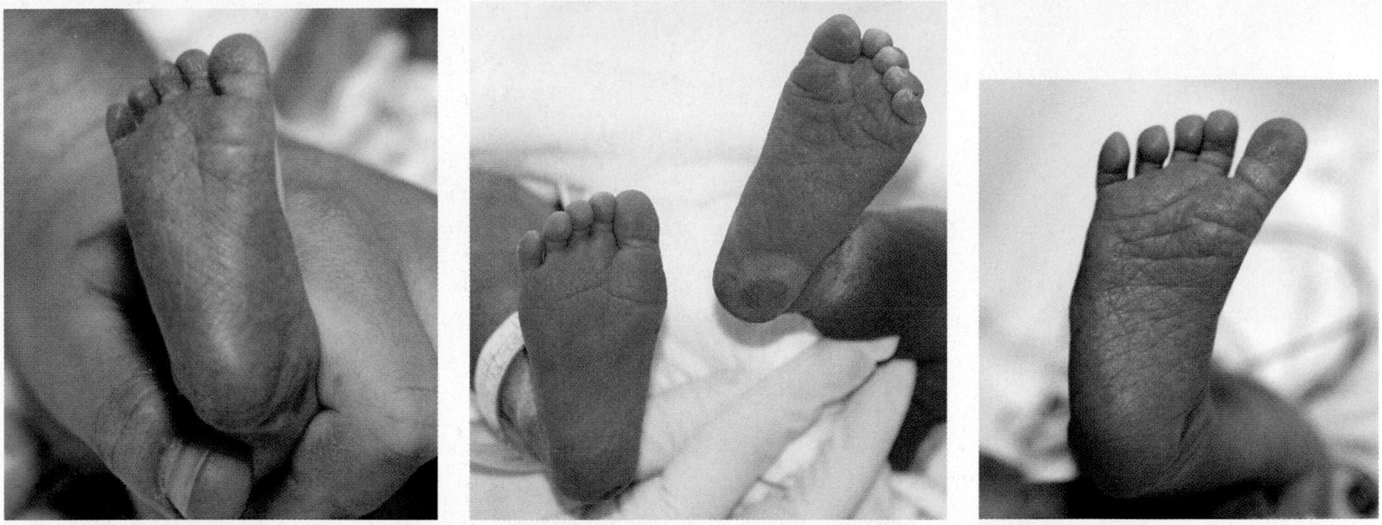

A B C

Figure 30-4 ■ Sole creases. A. Infant has a few sole creases on the anterior portion of the foot. Note the slick heel. Score 2. The gestational age is approximately 35 weeks. B. Infant has a deeper network of sole creases on the anterior two thirds of the sole. Note the slick heel. Score 3. The gestational age is approximately 37 weeks. C. The full-term infant has deep sole creases down to and including the heel as the skin loses fluid and dries after birth. Score 4. Sole (plantar) creases can be seen even in preterm newborns.

Source: George Dodson/Lightworks Studio/Pearson Education.

and then releasing it, or by folding the pinna of the ear forward against the side of the head and releasing it, and observing the response.) By term, the newborn's pinna is firm, stands away from the head, and springs back quickly from the folding.

7. *Male genitals* are evaluated for size of the scrotal sac, the presence of rugae (wrinkles and ridges in the scrotum), and descent of the testes (Figure 30-7 ■). Before 36 weeks, the small scrotum has few rugae, and the testes are palpable in the inguinal canal. By 36 to 38 weeks, the testes are in the upper scrotum, and rugae have developed over the anterior portion of the scrotum. By term, the testes are generally in the lower scrotum, which is pendulous and covered with rugae.
8. The appearance of the *female genitals* depends in part on subcutaneous fat deposition and therefore relates to fetal

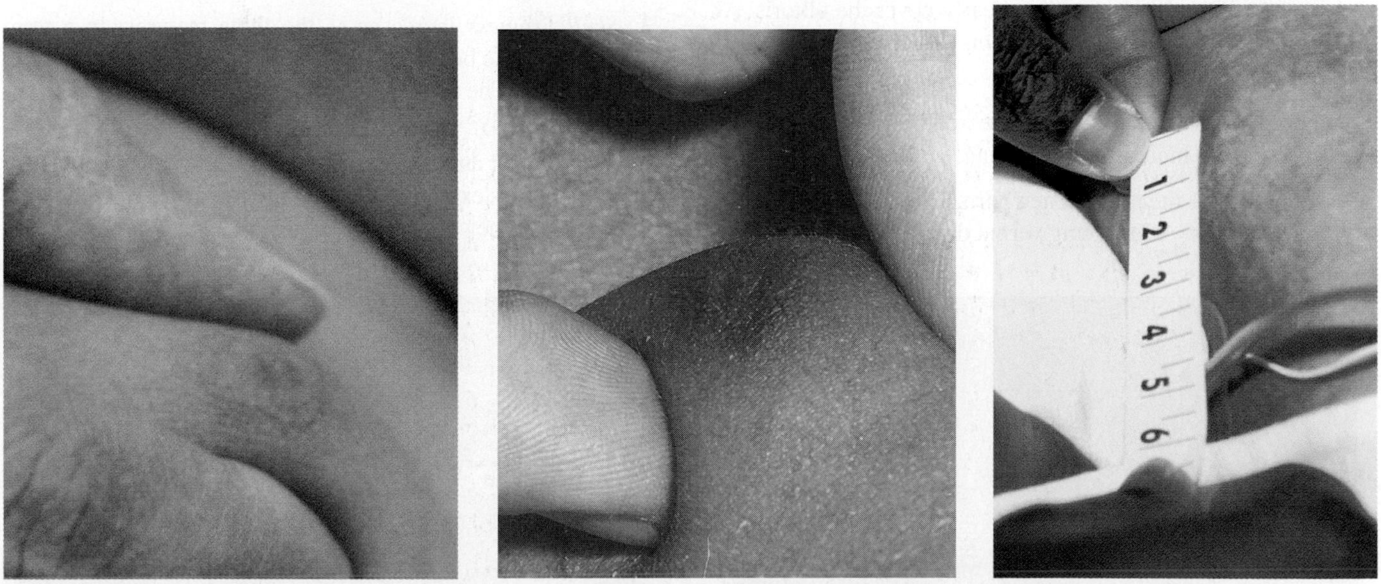

A B C

Figure 30-5 ■ Breast tissue. A. Newborn has a visible raised area greater than 0.75 cm diameter. Score 3. The gestational age is 38 weeks. B. Newborn has a breast tissue area of 10 mm. Score 4. The gestational age is 40 to 44 weeks. C. Gently compress the tissue between the middle and index fingers, and measure the tissue in centimeters or millimeters. Absence of or decreased breast tissue often indicates premature or SGA newborn.

Source: A, C., George Dodson/Lightworks Studio/Pearson Education. B. Dubowitz, L. & Dubowitz, V. (1977). The Gestational Age of the Newborn. Menlo Park, CA: Addison-Wesley. Reprinted by permission of V. Dubowitz, MD, Hammersmith Hospital, London, England.

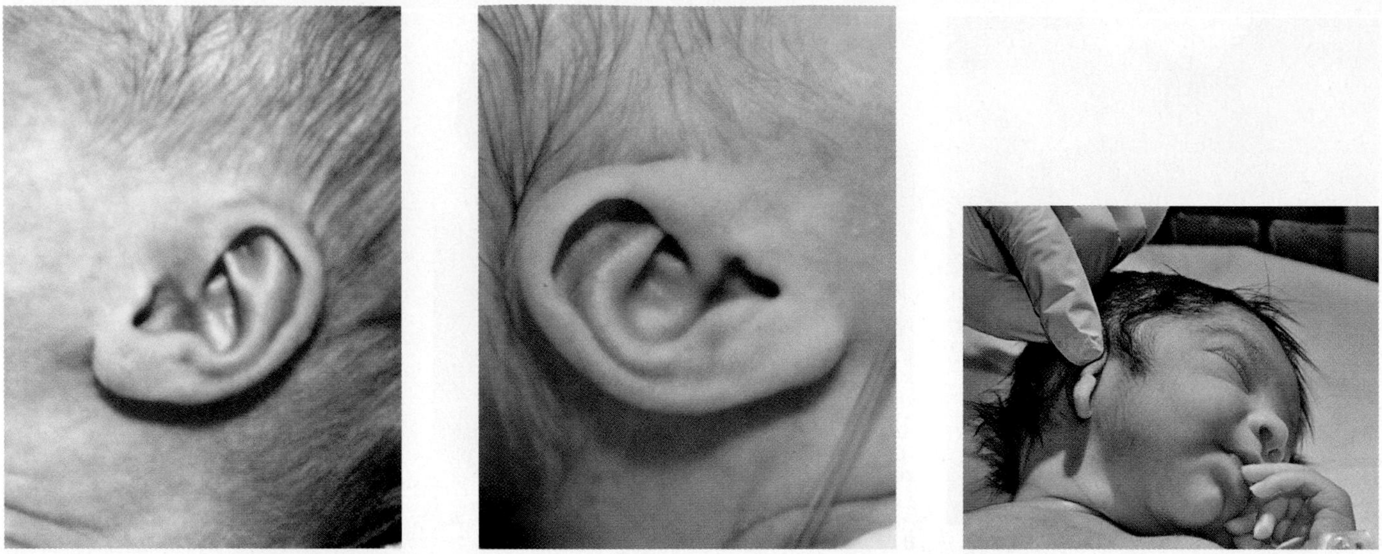

A B C

Figure 30-6 ■ Ear form and cartilage. A. The ear of the infant at approximately 36 weeks' gestation shows incurving of the upper two thirds of the pinna. Score 2. B. Infant at term shows well-defined incurving of the entire pinna. Score 3. C. The pinna is folded toward the face and released. If the auricle stays in the position in which it is pressed or returns slowly to its original position, it usually means that the gestational age is less than 38 weeks.

Source: A–B. George Dodson/Lightworks Studio/Pearson Education. C. Courtesy of Jo Engle, RN, MSN, NNP-BC and Vanessa Howell, RN, MSN.

nutritional status (Figure 30-8 ■). The clitoris varies in size and occasionally is so large that it is difficult to identify the sex of the newborn. This swelling may be caused by adrenogenital syndrome, which causes the adrenals to secrete excessive amounts of androgen and other hormones. At 30 to 32 weeks' gestation, the clitoris is prominent, and the labia majora are small and widely separated. As gestational age increases, the labia majora increase in size. At 36 to 40 weeks, they nearly cover the clitoris. At 40 weeks and beyond, the labia majora cover the labia minora and clitoris.

Other physical characteristics assessed by some gestational age scoring tools include the following:

1. *Vernix* covers the preterm newborn. The postterm newborn has no vernix. After noting vernix distribution, the birthing area nurse (wearing gloves) dries the newborn to prevent evaporative heat loss, thus disturbing the vernix and potentially altering this gestational age criterion. The birthing area nurse must communicate to the neonatal nurse the amount of vernix and the areas of vernix coverage.
2. *Hair* of the preterm newborn has the consistency of matted wool or fur and lies in bunches rather than in the silky, single strands of the term newborn's hair.
3. *Skull firmness* increases as the fetus matures. In a term newborn, the bones are hard, and the sutures are not easily displaced. The nurse should not attempt to displace the sutures forcibly.
4. *Nails* appear and cover the nail bed at about 20 weeks' gestation. Nails extending beyond the fingertips may indicate a postterm newborn.

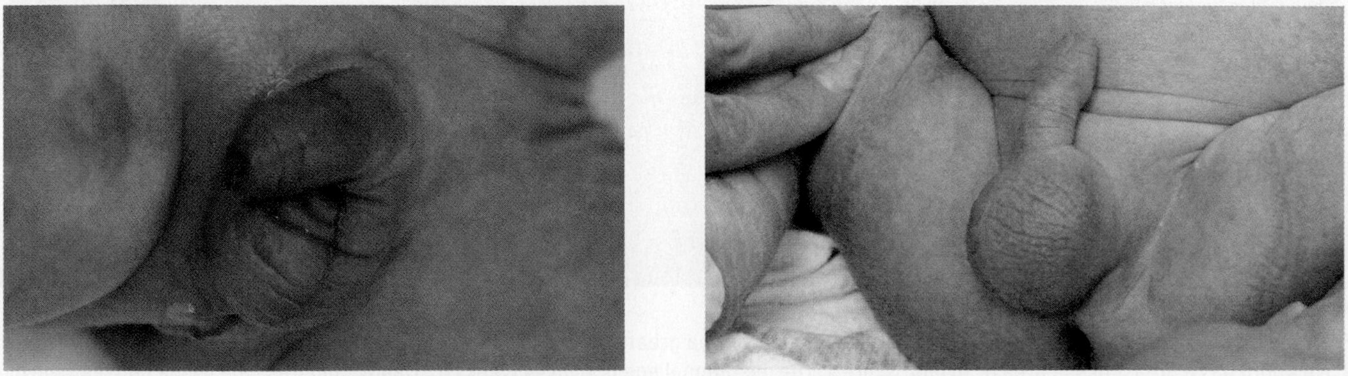

A B

Figure 30-7 ■ Male genitals. A. Preterm infant's testes are not within the scrotum. The scrotal surface has few rugae. Score 2. B. Term infant's testes are generally fully descended. The entire surface of the scrotum is covered by rugae. Score 3.

Source: George Dodson/Lightworks Studio/Pearson Education.

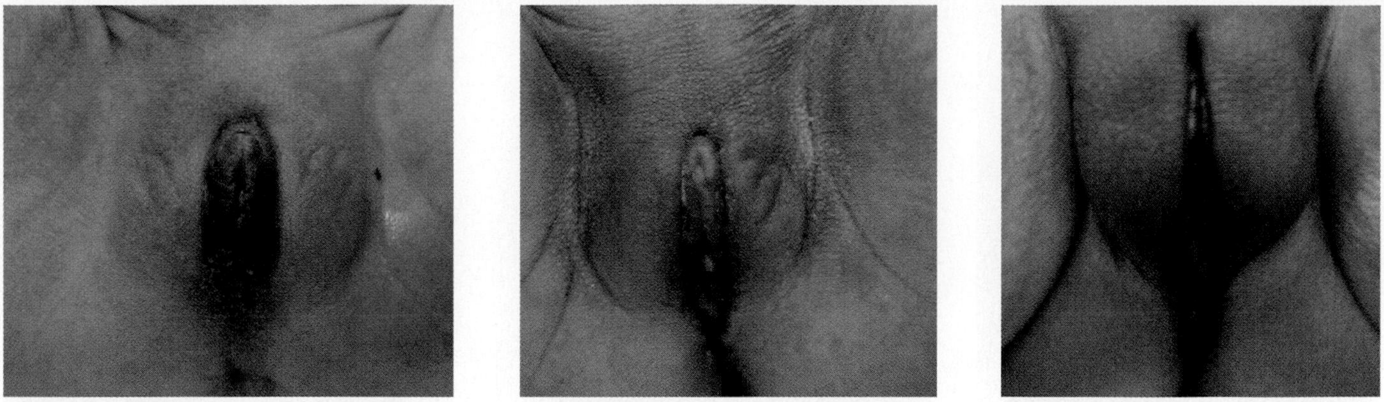

A B C

Figure 30-8 ■ Female genitals. A. Infant has a prominent clitoris. The labia majora are widely separated, and the labia minora, viewed laterally, would protrude beyond the labia majora. Score 1. The gestational age is 30 to 36 weeks. B. The clitoris is still visible. The labia minora are now covered by the larger labia majora. Score 2. The gestational age is 36 to 40 weeks. C. The term infant has well-developed, large labia majora that cover both clitoris and labia minora. Score 3. The labia minora is often dark in some ethnic and racial groups of infants.

Source: George Dodson/Lightworks Studio/Pearson Education.

Assessment of Neuromuscular Maturity Characteristics

The central nervous system of the human fetus matures at a fairly constant rate. Tests have been designed to evaluate neurologic status as manifested by development of neuromuscular tone. As noted earlier, neuromuscular tone in the fetus develops in a caudocephalic direction, from the lower to the upper extremities.

The neuromuscular evaluation requires more manipulation and disturbances than the physical evaluation of the newborn. The neuromuscular evaluation (see Figure 30-1) is best performed when the infant has stabilized. The following characteristics are evaluated:

1. The *square window sign* is elicited by flexing the baby's hand toward the ventral forearm until resistance is felt. The angle formed at the wrist is measured (Figure 30-9 ■).
2. *Recoil* is a test of flexion development. Because flexion first develops in the lower extremities, recoil is first tested in the legs. The nurse places the newborn on his or her back on a flat surface. With a hand on the newborn's knees and while manipulating the hip joint, the nurse places the baby's legs in flexion, and then extends them parallel to each other and flat on the surface. The response to this maneuver is recoil of the newborn's legs. According to gestational age, they may not move, or they may return slowly or quickly to the flexed position. Preterm infants have less muscle tone than term infants so preterm infants have less recoil.

   Arm recoil is tested by flexion at the elbow and extension of the arms at the newborn's side. While the baby is in the supine position, the nurse completely flexes both elbows, holds them in this position for 5 seconds, extends the arms at the baby's side, and releases them. Upon release, the elbows of a full-term newborn form an angle of less than 90 degrees and rapidly recoil back to a flexed position. The elbows of preterm newborns have slower recoil time and form a greater than 90-degree angle. Arm recoil is also slower in healthy but

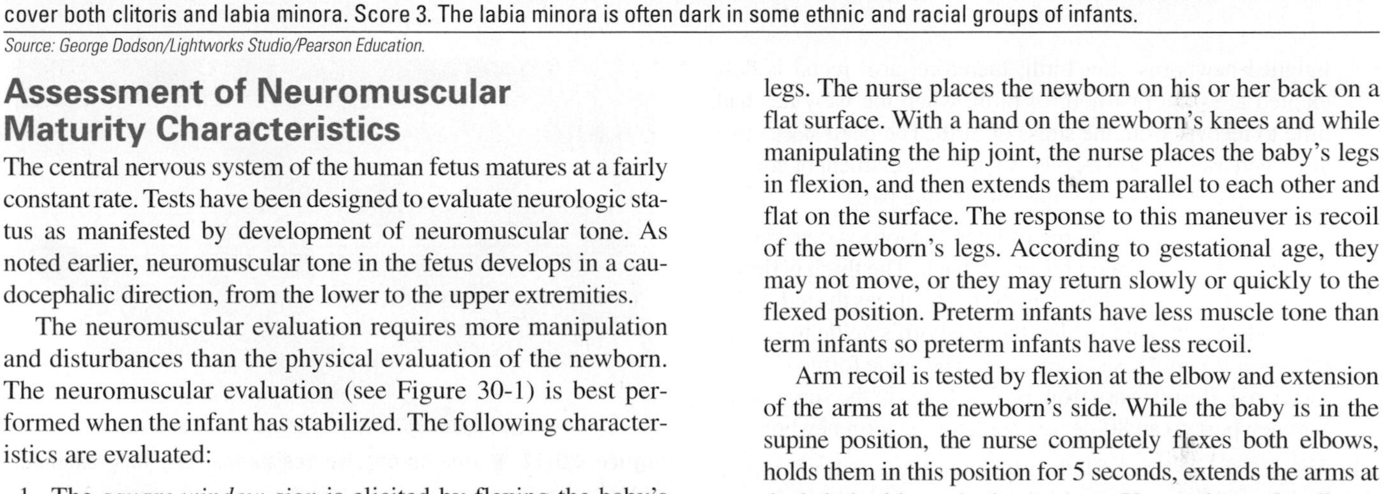

A B C

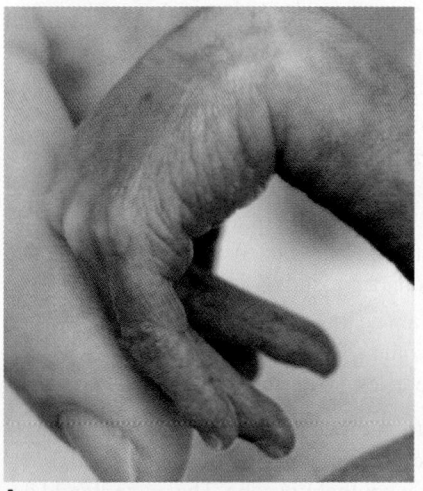

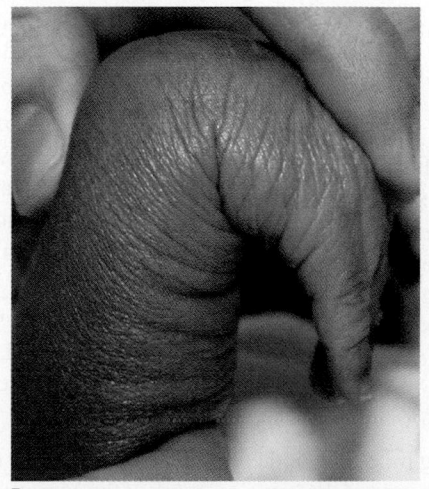

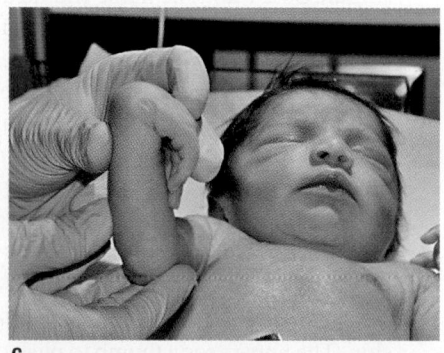

Figure 30-9 ■ Square window sign. A. This angle is 90 degrees and suggests an immature newborn of 28 to 32 weeks' gestation. Score 0. B. A 30–40-degree angle is commonly found in newborns from 38 to 40 weeks' gestation. Score 2–3. C. A 0–15-degree angle occurs in newborns from 40 to 42 weeks' gestation. Score 4

Source: A-B. George Dodson/Lightworks Studio/Pearson Education. C. Courtesy of Jo Engle, RN, MSN, NNP-BC and Vanessa Howell, RN, MSN.

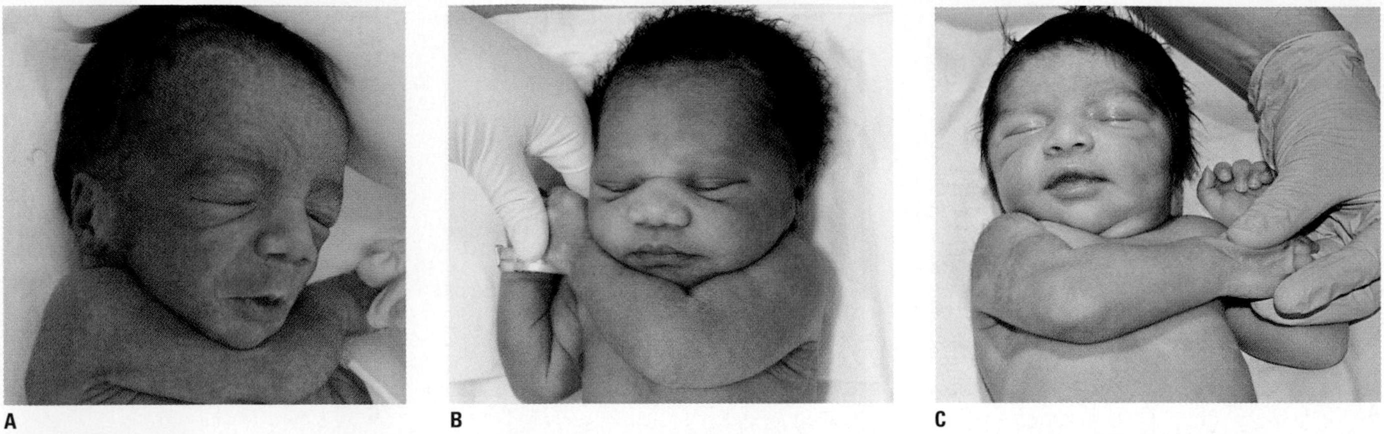

Figure 30-10 ■ Scarf sign. A. No resistance is noted until after 30 weeks' gestation. The elbow can be readily moved past the midline. Score 1. B. The elbow is at midline at 36 to 40 weeks' gestation. Score 2. C. Beyond 40 weeks' gestation, the elbow will not reach the midline. Score 4.

Source: A-B. George Dodson/Lightworks Studio/Pearson Education. C. Courtesy of Jo Engle, RN, MSN, NNP-BC and Vanessa Howell, RN, MSN.

fatigued newborns after birth; therefore, arm recoil is best elicited after the first hour of birth, when the baby has had time to recover from the stress of birth. The deep sleep state also decreases the arm recoil response. Assessment of arm recoil should be bilateral to rule out brachial palsy.

3. The *popliteal angle* (degree of knee flexion) is determined with the newborn flat on his or her back. The thigh is flexed on the abdomen and chest, and the nurse places the index finger of the other hand behind the newborn's ankle to extend the lower leg until resistance is met. The angle formed is then measured. Results vary from no resistance in the very immature newborn to an 80-degree angle in the term newborn.
4. The *scarf sign* is elicited by placing the newborn supine and drawing an arm across the chest toward the newborn's opposite shoulder until resistance is met. The location of the elbow is then noted in relation to the midline of the chest (Figure 30-10 ■). A preterm infant's elbow will cross the midline of the chest, whereas a full term infant's elbow will not cross midline.
5. The *heel-to-ear extension* is performed by placing the newborn in a supine position and then gently drawing the foot toward the ear on the same side until resistance is felt (Figure 30-11 ■). The nurse should allow the knee to bend during the test. It is important to hold the buttocks down to keep from rolling the baby. Both the proximity of foot to ear and degree of knee extension are assessed. The leg of a preterm, immature newborn remains straight and the foot goes to the ear or beyond. With advancing gestational age, the newborn demonstrates increasing resistance to this maneuver. Maneuvers involving the lower extremities of newborns who had frank breech presentation should be delayed to allow for resolution of leg positioning.
6. *Ankle dorsiflexion* is determined by flexing the ankle on the shin. The nurse uses a thumb to push on the sole of the newborn's foot while the fingers support the back of the leg. Then the angle formed by the foot and the interior leg is measured (Figure 30-12 ■). This sign can be influenced by intrauterine position and congenital deformities.

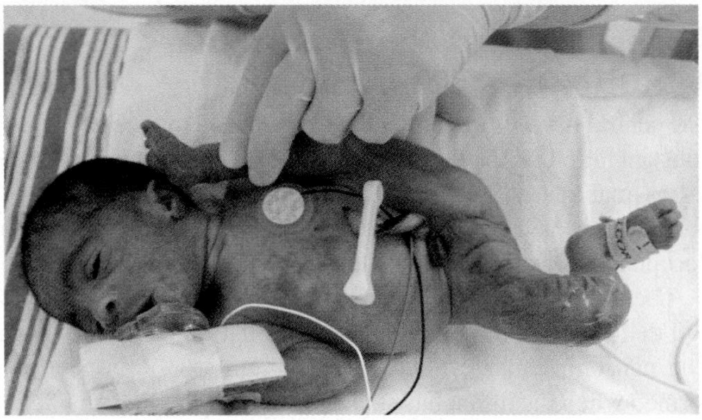

Figure 30-11 ■ Heel-to-ear. No resistance. Leg fully extended. Score 0.

Source: George Dodson/Lightworks Studio/Pearson Education.

7. *Head lag* (neck flexors) is measured by pulling the baby to a sitting position and noting the degree of head lag. Total lag is common in infants up to 34 weeks' gestation, whereas the postmature newborn (42 or more weeks) will hold the head in front of the body line. Full-term newborns are able to support their heads momentarily.
8. *Ventral suspension* (horizontal position) is evaluated by holding the newborn prone on the examiner's hand. The position of head and back and degree of flexion in the arms and legs are then noted. Some flexion of arms and legs indicates 36 to 38 weeks' gestation; fully flexed extremities, with head and back even, are characteristic of a term newborn.
9. Major reflexes such as sucking, rooting, grasping, Moro, tonic neck, Babinski, and others are also evaluated during the newborn exam. These reflexes are discussed later in the chapter.

A supplementary method for estimating gestational age (done by the physician or nurse practitioner) is to view the vascular network of the cornea with an ophthalmoscope. The nurse should delay administration of prophylactic eye ointment until after the eye exam. The amount of vascularity present over the surface of the lens has excellent correlation with infants of 27 through 34 weeks' gestational age. In babies less than 27 weeks' gestation,

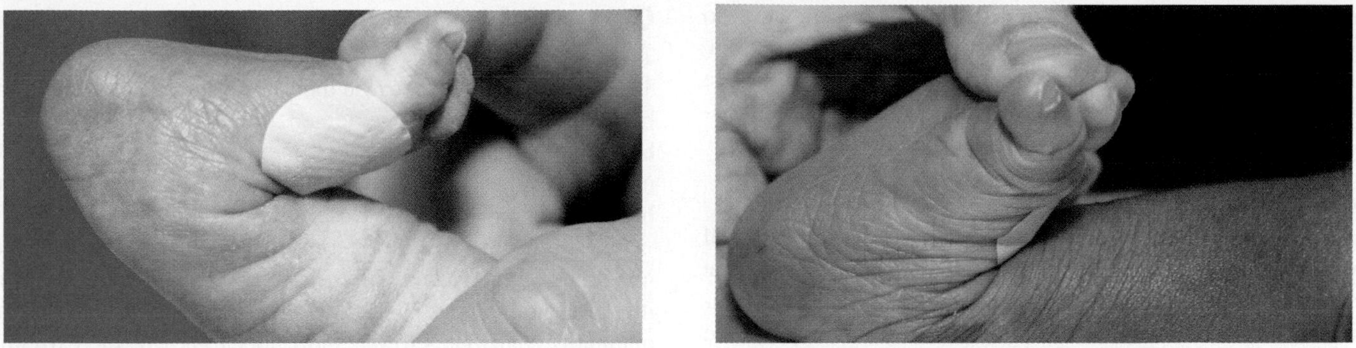

Figure 30-12 ■ Ankle dorsiflexion. A. A 45-degree angle indicates 32 to 36 weeks' gestation. A 20-degree angle indicates 36 to 40 weeks' gestation. Score 2–3. B. A 15- to 0-degree angle is common at 40 weeks' or more gestational age. Score 4.

Source: George Dodson/Lightworks Studio/Pearson Education.

the cornea is cloudy, and the vascular network is not visible; after 34 weeks' gestation the vascular network has generally disappeared completely.

When the gestational age determination and birth weight are considered together, the newborn can be identified as one whose *growth is below the 10th percentile,* or *small for gestational age (SGA); appropriate for gestational age (AGA);* or *above the 90th percentile,* or *large for gestational age (LGA)* (Figure 30-13 ■). This determination enables the nurse to anticipate possible physiologic problems. This information is

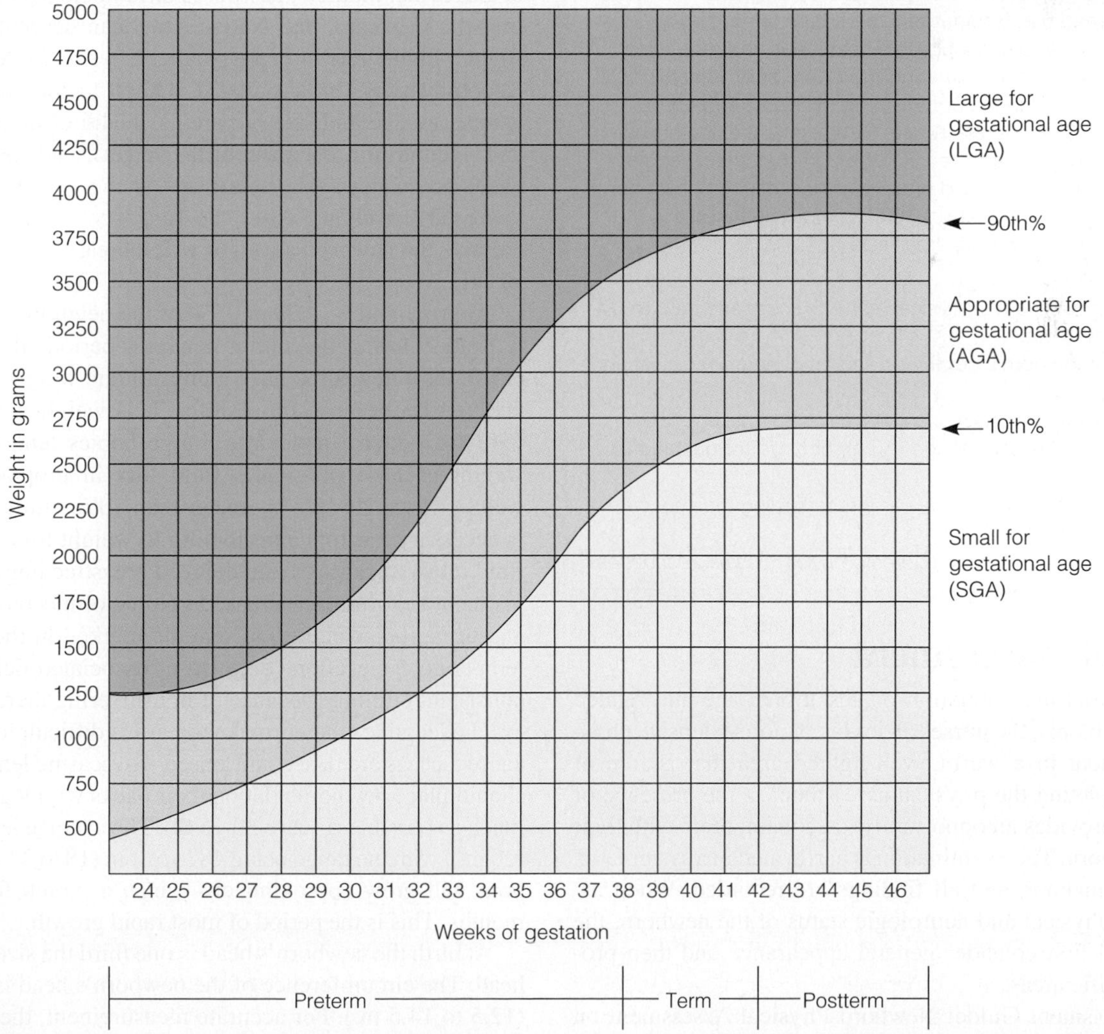

Figure 30-13 ■ Classification of newborns by birth weight and gestational age. The newborn's birth weight and gestational age are placed on the graph. The newborn is then classified as large for gestational age (LGA), appropriate for gestational age (AGA), or small for gestational age (SGA).

Source: Reprinted from Journal of Pediatrics, *71, 161, Battaglia, F. C., & Lubchenco, L. O. A practical classification of newborn infants by weight and gestational age. Copyright © 1967, with permission from Elsevier.*

used in conjunction with a complete physical examination to establish a plan of care appropriate for the individual newborn. For example, an SGA newborn often requires frequent glucose monitoring and early feedings. See chapter 33 ∞ for discussion of these categories and their potential problems.

The nurse also plots the gestational age against the newborn's length, head circumference, and weight on the appropriate growth chart to determine whether these measurements fall within the average range—the 10th to 90th percentile for the corresponding gestational age (Figure 30-14 ■). These correlations further document the level of maturity and appropriate category for the newborn. The comparison of the newborn's ratio of weight to length further facilitates identification of SGA newborns as being symmetrically or asymmetrically growth restricted. See chapter 33 ∞ for more detail.

CLINICAL JUDGMENT

Case Study: Travis Bell

A nurse has completed the gestational assessment on newborn Travis Bell who weighs 3000 g and is 48 cm long with a head circumference of 33 cm. His Apgar scores were 8 at 1 minute and 9 at 5 minutes. Other assessment data include skin dry and cracking with pale areas and rare veins; no lanugo; sole creases covering the entire sole; raised areola 3 mm; well-curved pinna soft with ready recoil; and testes descended with moderate rugae. Reflex data include square window at 0 degree; arm recoil 100 degree; popliteal angle 100 degree; scarf sign yield elbow will not reach midline; heel to ear 90 degree; and posture fully flexed. The parents express concerns over his small size.

Critical Thinking

What are the newborn's physical maturity score and neuromuscular maturity score?

Interpret the newborn's combined scores of neuromuscular and physical maturity.

Determine if the newborn is small for gestational age (SGA), appropriate for gestational age (AGA), or large for gestational age (LGA).

What should the nurse tell the parents regarding their concern over his small size?

See www.nursing.pearsonhighered.com for possible responses.

Physical Assessment

After the initial determination of gestational age and related potential problems, the nurse carries out a more extensive physical assessment in a warm, well-lighted area that is free of drafts. Completing the physical assessment in the presence of the parents provides an opportunity to acquaint them with their unique newborn. The examination is performed in a systematic, head-to-toe manner, and all findings are recorded. When assessing the physical and neurologic status of the newborn, the nurse should first consider general appearance and then proceed to specific areas.

The Assessment Guide: Newborn Physical Assessment on pages 811–819 outlines how to systematically assess the newborn. Normal findings, alterations, and related causes are presented and correlated with suggested nursing responses. The findings are typical for a full-term newborn.

General Appearance

The newborn's head is disproportionately large for the body. The neck looks short because the chin rests on the chest. Newborns have a prominent abdomen, sloping shoulders, narrow hips, and a rounded chest. The center of the baby's body is the umbilicus rather than the symphysis pubis, as in the adult. The body appears long and the extremities short.

Newborns tend to stay in a flexed position similar to the one maintained in utero and will offer resistance when the extremities are straightened. The flexed position that the newborn maintains contributes to the short appearance of the extremities. The hands are tightly clenched. After a breech birth, the feet are usually dorsiflexed, and it may take several weeks for the newborn to assume typical newborn posture.

Weight and Measurements

The normal full-term Caucasian newborn has an average birth weight of 3405 g (7 lb, 8 oz). In the United States, mothers of African descent have smaller newborns at birth at twice the rate of Caucasian mothers; newborns of mothers of Asian, Hispanic (mostly Mexican), and Native American descent have only a slightly higher rate of being smaller at term (Teitler, Reichman, Nepomnyaschy, et al., 2007). Other factors that influence weight are age and size of parents, health of mother (smoking and malnutrition decrease birth weight), and the interval between pregnancies (short intervals, such as every year, result in lower birth weight). After the first week and for the first 6 months, the newborn's weight will increase about 198 g (7 oz) weekly.

Approximately 70% to 75% of the newborn's body weight is water. During the initial newborn period (the first 3 or 4 days), term newborns have a physiologic weight loss of about 5% to 10% because fluid shifts. This weight loss may reach 15% for preterm newborns. Large babies tend to lose more weight because of greater fluid loss in proportion to birth weight. If weight loss is greater than 10%, clinical reappraisal is necessary. Factors contributing to weight loss include small fluid intake resulting from delayed breastfeeding or a slow adjustment to formula, increased volume of meconium excreted, and urination. Weight loss may be marked in the presence of temperature elevation (because of associated dehydration) or consistent chilling (because of nonshivering thermogenesis).

The length of the normal newborn is difficult to measure because the legs are flexed and tensed. To measure length, the nurse should place newborns flat on their backs with legs extended as much as possible (Figure 30-15 ■). The average length is 50 cm (20 in.), with the range being 48 to 52 cm (18 to 22 in.). The newborn will grow approximately 1 inch a month for the next 6 months. This is the period of most rapid growth.

At birth the newborn's head is one third the size of an adult's head. The circumference of the newborn's head is 32 to 37 cm (12.5 to 14.5 in.). For accurate measurement, the nurse places the tape over the most prominent part of the occiput and brings it to just above the eyebrows (Figure 30-16A ■). The circumference of the newborn's head is approximately 2 cm greater than the circumference of the newborn's chest at birth and will

CLASSIFICATION OF NEWBORNS— BASED ON MATURITY AND INTRAUTERINE GROWTH

Symbols: X-1st Exam O-2nd Exam

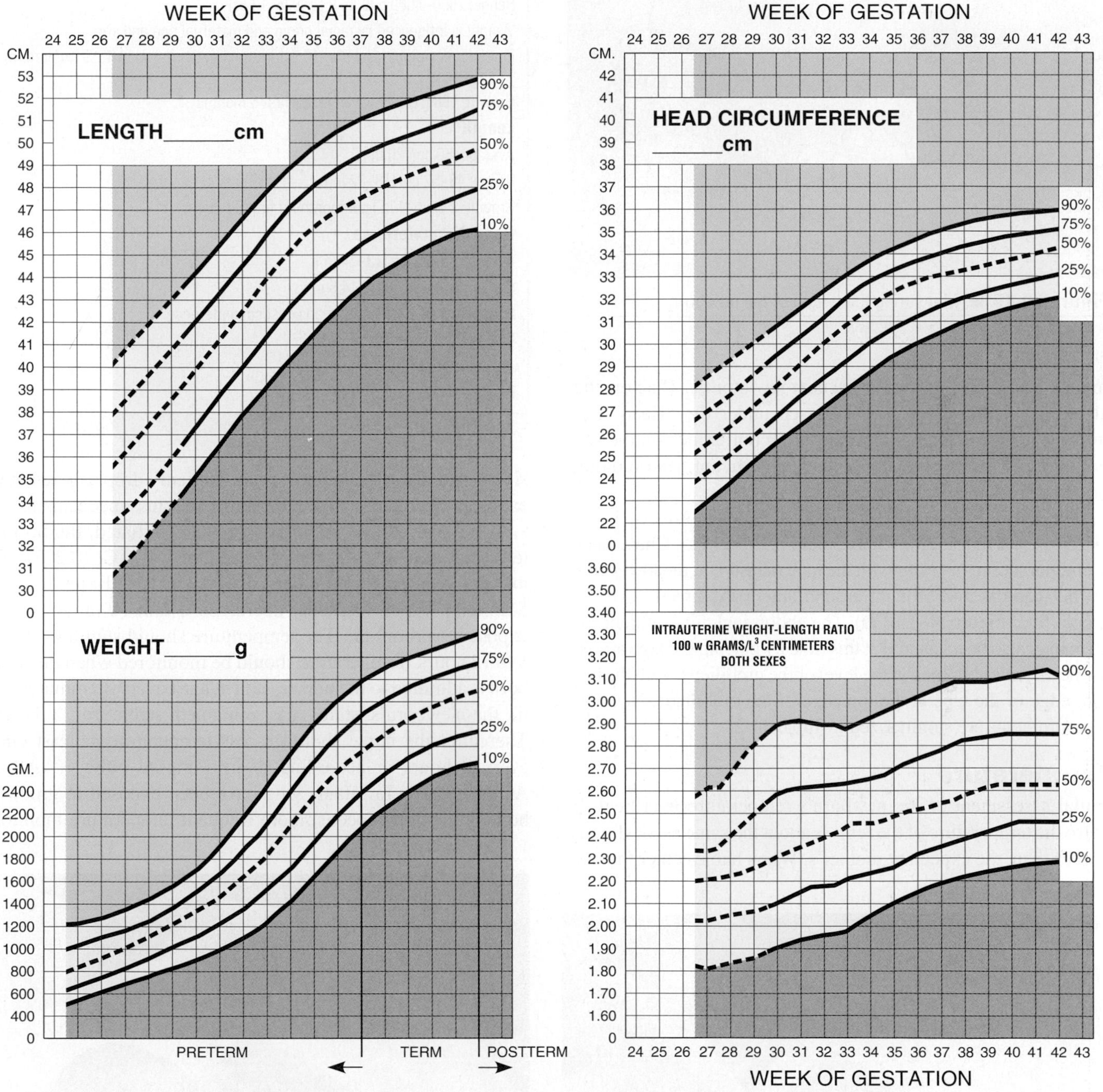

	1st Exam (X)	2nd Exam (O)
LARGE FOR GESTATIONAL AGE (**LGA**)		
APPROPRIATE FOR GESTATIONAL AGE (**AGA**)		
SMALL FOR GESTATIONAL AGE (**SGA**)		
Age at Exam	hrs	hrs
Signature of Examiner	M.D.	M.D.

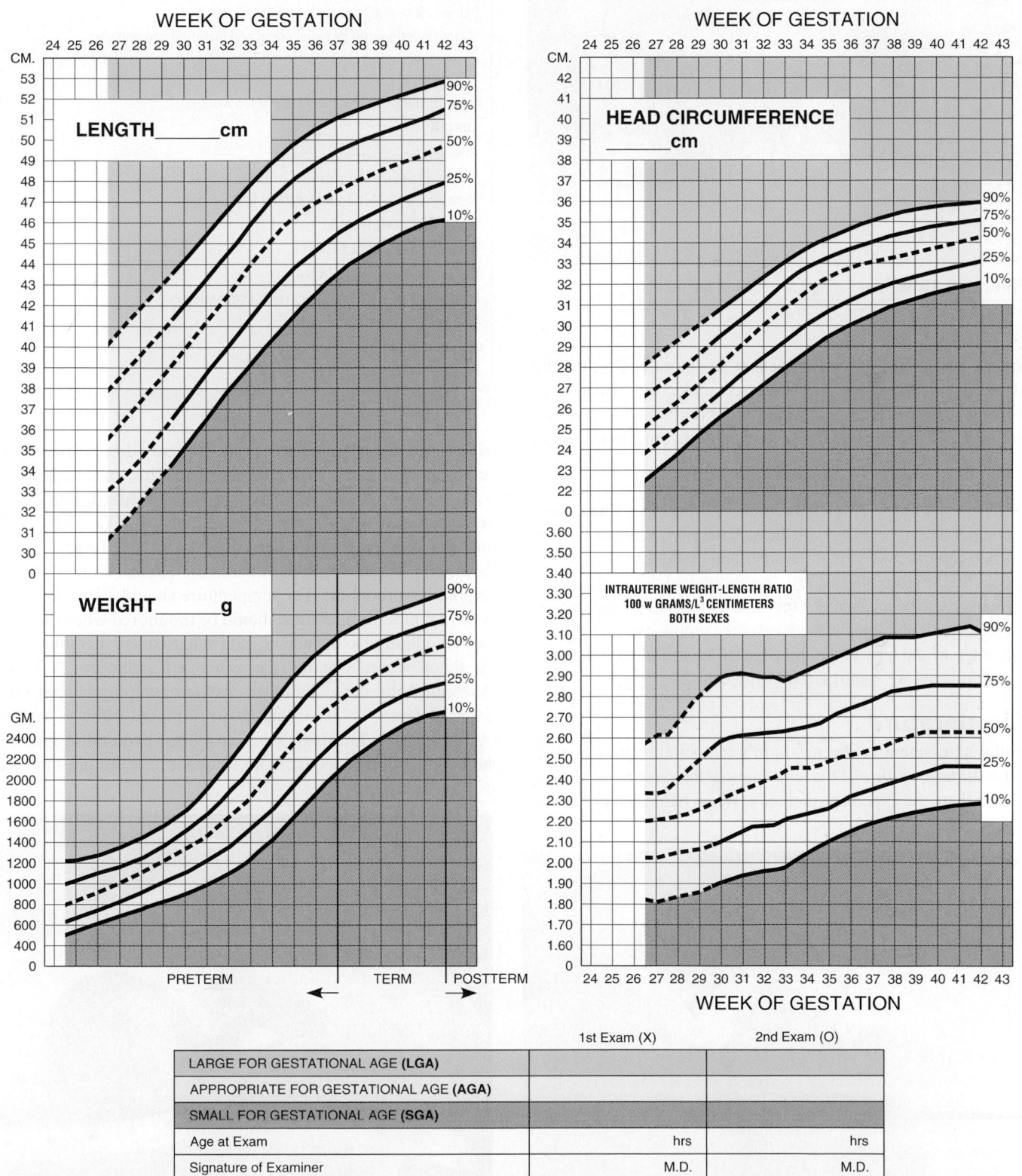

Figure 30-14 ■ Classification of newborns based on maturity and intrauterine growth.

Source: Reprinted from Journal of Pediatrics, *71, 161, Battaglia, F. C., & Lubchenco, L. O., A practical classification of newborn infants by weight and gestational age, copyright © 1967, with permission from Elsevier.*

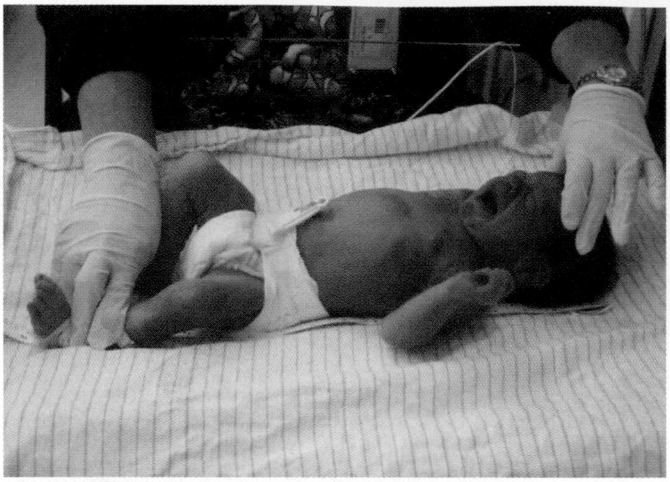

Figure 30-15 ■ Measuring the length of the newborn.

Source: Courtesy of Vanessa Howell, RNC, BSN.

TABLE 30-2 Newborn Measurements

Weight
Average: 3405 g (7 lb, 8 oz)
Range: 2500–4000 g (5 lb, 8 oz–8 lb, 13 oz)
Weight is influenced by racial origin and maternal age and size.
Physiologic weight loss: 5%–10% for term newborns, up to 15% for preterm newborns
Growth: 198 g (7 oz) per week for first 6 months
Length
Average: 50 cm (20 in.)
Range: 48–52 cm (18–22 in.)
Growth: 2.5 cm (1 in.) per month for first 6 months
Head Circumference
Average 33–35 cm (13–14 in.)
Range 32–37 cm (12.5–14.5 in.)
Approximately 2 cm larger than chest circumference
Chest Circumference
Average: 32 cm (12.5 in.)
Range: 30–35 cm (12–14 in.)

remain in this proportion for the next few months. (Factors that alter this measurement are discussed under the "Head" section.) It is best to take another head circumference on the second day if the newborn experienced significant head molding or caput from the birth process.

The average circumference of the chest at birth is 32 cm (12.5 in.) and ranges from 30 to 35 cm (12 to 14 in.). Chest measurements should be taken with the tape measure at the lower edge of the scapulas and brought around anteriorly directly over the nipple line (Figure 30-16B ■). The abdominal circumference or girth may also be measured at this time by placing the tape around the newborn's abdomen at the level of the umbilicus, with the bottom edge of the tape at the top edge of the umbilicus. Newborn measurements are summarized in Table 30-2.

Temperature

Initial assessment of the newborn's temperature is critical. In utero the temperature of the fetus is about the same as, or slightly higher than, the expectant mother's. When babies enter the outside world, their temperatures can suddenly drop as a result of exposure to cold drafts and the skin's heat loss mechanisms.

If no heat conservation measures are initiated, the normal term newborn's core temperature falls 0.1°C (0.2°F) per minute; skin temperature decreases 0.3°C (0.5°F) per minute. Skin temperature markedly decreases within 10 minutes after exposure to room air. The temperature should stabilize within 8 to 12 hours. Temperature should be monitored when the newborn is admitted to the nursery and at least every 30 minutes until the newborn's status has remained stable for 2 hours. Thereafter the nurse should assess temperature at least once every 8 hours or according to institutional policy (AAP & ACOG, 2007). In infants who have been exposed to group B hemolytic streptococcus, more frequent temperature monitor-

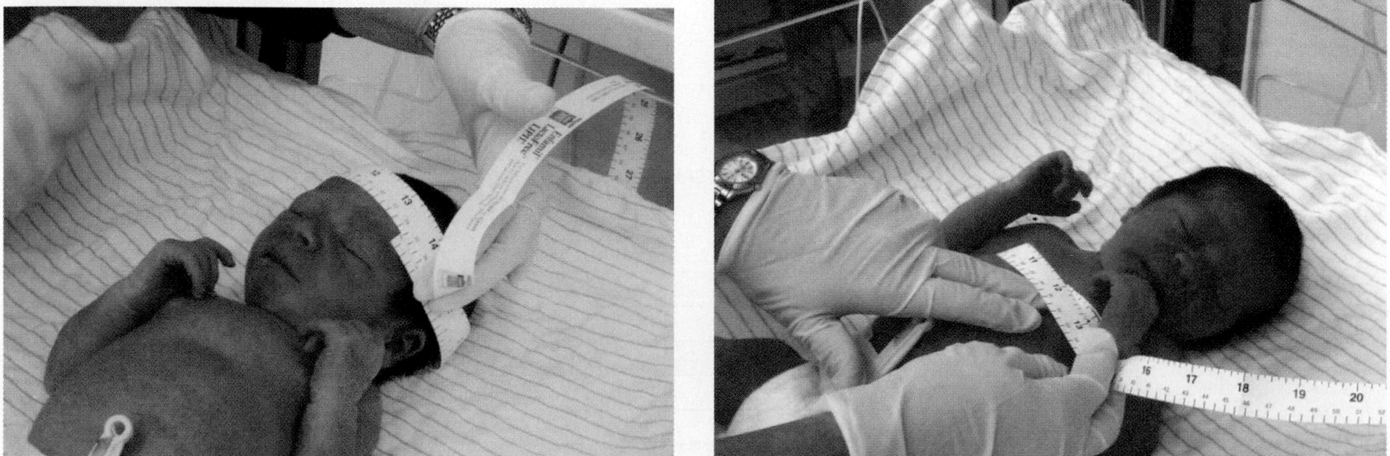

A B

Figure 30-16 ■ A. Measuring the head circumference of the newborn. B. Measuring the chest circumference of the newborn.

Source: Courtesy of Vanessa Howell, RNC, BSN.

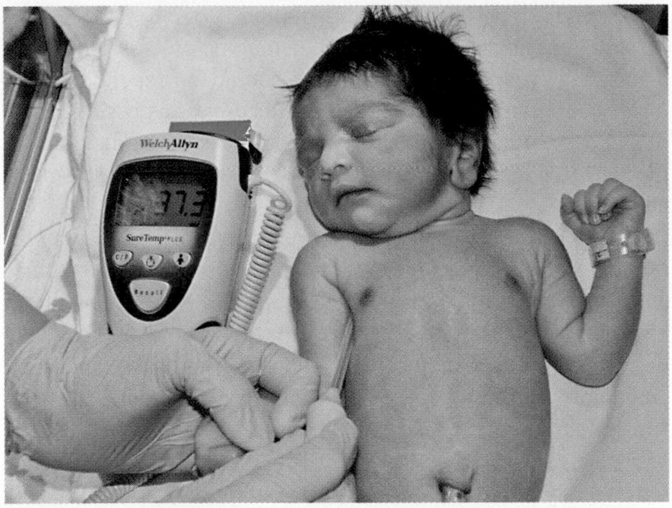

Figure 30-17 ■ Axillary temperature measurement. The axillary temperature should be taken for 3 minutes. The newborn's arm should be tightly but gently pressed against the thermometer and the newborn's side, as illustrated.

Source: Courtesy of Jo Engle, RN, MSN, NNP-BC and Vanessa Howell, RN, MSN.

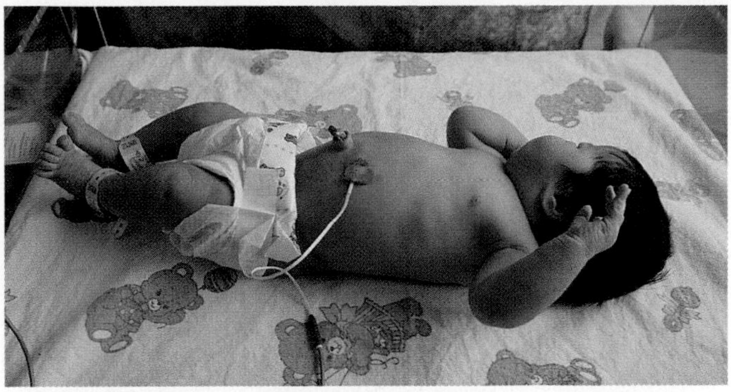

Figure 30-18 ■ Temperature monitoring for the newborn. A skin thermal sensor is placed on the newborn's abdomen, upper thigh, or arm and secured with porous tape or a foil-covered foam pad.

Source: Photographer, Elena Dorfman.

ing may be required. (See chapter 29 ∞ for a discussion of the physiology of temperature regulation.)

Temperature can be assessed by the axillary skin method, a continuous skin probe, or via the rectal route. Axillary temperature reflects body (core) temperature and the body's compensatory response to the thermal environment. Axillary temperatures are the preferred method and are considered to be a close estimation of the rectal temperature. In preterm and term newborns there is less than 0.1°C (0.2°F) difference between the two sites and the axillary method is preferred. If the axillary method is used, the thermometer must remain in place at least 3 minutes, unless an electronic thermometer is used (Figure 30-17 ■). Axillary temperature ranges from 36.4°C to 37.2°C (97.5°F to 99°F). Keep in mind that axillary temperatures can be misleading because the friction caused by apposition of the inner arm skin and upper chest wall and the nearness of brown fat to the probe may elevate the temperature.

Skin temperature is measured most accurately by continuous skin probe, especially for small newborns or newborns maintained in incubators or under radiant warmers. Normal skin temperature is 36°C to 36.5°C (96.8°F to 97.7°F). Assessing skin temperature allows time for interventions to be initiated before a more serious fall in core temperature occurs (Figure 30-18 ■).

Rectal temperature is assumed to be the closest approximation to core temperature, but the accuracy of this method depends on the depth to which the thermometer is inserted. Normal rectal temperature is 36.6°C to 37.2°C (97.8°F to 99°F). The rectal route is **not** recommended as a routine method because it may predispose to rectal mucosal irritation and increase chances of perforation (Blackburn, 2007).

Temperature instability, a deviation of more than 1°C (2°F) from one reading to the next, or a subnormal temperature may indicate an infection. In contrast with an elevated temperature in older children, an increased temperature in a newborn may indicate a reaction to too many coverings, too hot a room, or dehydration. Dehydration, which tends to increase body temperature, occurs in newborns whose feedings have been delayed for any reason. Newborns respond to overheating (temperature greater than 37.5°C or 99.5°F) by increased restlessness and eventually by perspiration. The perspiration is initially seen on the head and face, then on the chest. Many newborns initially cannot perspire, so they increase their respiratory and heart rates, which increases oxygen consumption.

DEVELOPING CULTURAL COMPETENCE
Keeping Newborns Warm

In the Latino culture and others, parents may be overly concerned about keeping their newborn baby warm. Parents should be informed that overdressing babies while they are sleeping is related to a higher risk of Sudden Infant Death Syndrome (SIDS) and that bundling them excessively can be uncomfortable and lead to heat rash.

CLINICAL TIP

Measuring weight and height often aggravate newborns and may alter their vital signs. For better accuracy, take the newborn's vital signs before weighing and measuring.

Skin Characteristics

Although the newborn's skin color varies with genetic background, all healthy newborns have a pink tinge to their skin. The ruddy hue results from increased red blood cell concentration in the blood vessels and from limited subcutaneous fat deposits.

Skin pigmentation is slight in the newborn period, so color changes may be seen even in darker skinned babies. Caucasian newborns have a pinkish-red skin tone a few hours after birth, and African-American newborns can have a pale pink with yellow or red tinge to a reddish-brown skin color. Hispanic and Asian newborns can have a pink or rosy red with yellow tinge to an olive or yellow skin tone (Creehan, 2008). Skin pigmentation deepens over time; therefore, variations in skin color indicating illness are more difficult to evaluate in African-American and Asian newborns (Creehan, 2008). A newborn who is cyanotic at rest and pink only with crying may have choanal atresia (congenital

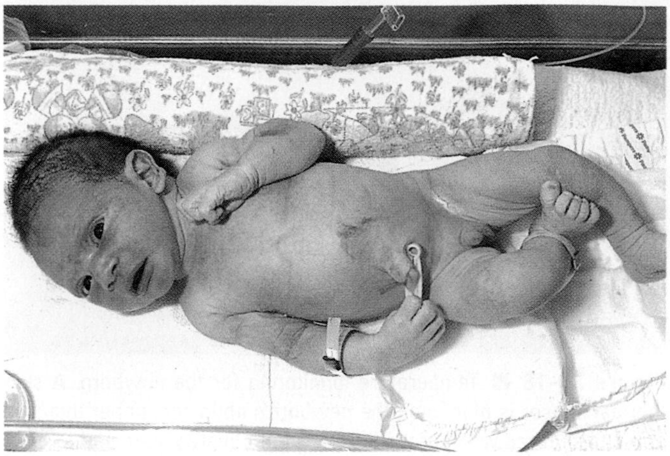

Figure 30-19 ■ Acrocyanosis.

blockage of the passageway between the nose and pharynx). If crying increases the cyanosis, heart or lung problems should be suspected. Very pale newborns may be anemic or have hypovolemia (low blood volume and blood pressure [BP]) and should be evaluated for these problems.

Acrocyanosis (bluish discoloration of the hands and feet) may be present in the first 2 to 6 hours after birth (Figure 30-19 ■). This condition is due to poor peripheral circulation, which results in vasomotor instability and capillary stasis, especially when the baby is exposed to cold. If the central circulation is adequate, the blood supply should return quickly (2 to 3 seconds) to the extremity after the skin is blanched with a finger. Blue hands and nails are a poor indicator of oxygenation in a newborn. The face and mucous membranes should be assessed for pinkness reflecting adequate oxygenation.

Mottling (lacy pattern of dilated blood vessels under the skin) occurs as a result of general circulation fluctuations. It may last several hours to several weeks or may come and go periodically. Mottling may be related to chilling, prolonged apnea, sepsis, or hypothyroidism.

Harlequin sign (clown) color change is occasionally noted. A deep color develops over one side of the newborn's body while the other side remains pale, so that the skin resembles a clown's suit. This color change results from a vasomotor disturbance in which blood vessels on one side dilate while the vessels on the other side constrict. It usually lasts from 1 to 20 minutes. Affected newborns may have single or multiple episodes, but they are transient and clinically insignificant. The nurse should document its occurrence.

Jaundice is first detectable on the face (where skin overlies cartilage) and the mucous membranes of the mouth (Creehan, 2008). Jaundice advances from head to toe and regresses in the opposite direction. It is evaluated by blanching the tip of the nose, the forehead, the sternum, or the gum line. This procedure must be carried out in appropriate lighting. If jaundice is present, the area will appear yellowish immediately after blanching. Another area to assess for jaundice is the sclera. Jaundice must be evaluated and its cause determined immediately to prevent possible serious sequelae. Jaundice may be related to breastfeeding (in some cases), hematomas, immature liver function, or bruises from forceps, or it may be caused by blood incompatibility, oxytocin (Pitocin) augmentation or induction, or a severe hemolytic process. Any jaundice noted before 24 hours of age should be reported to the physician or nurse practitioner. Breastfeeding is a possible cause of late onset jaundice. See Procedure 30-1: Assessing Jaundice in the Newborn. For a detailed discussion of the causes, assessment, and treatment of jaundice, see chapter 34 ∞.

Erythema toxicum is an eruption of lesions in the area surrounding a hair follicle that are firm, vary in size from 1 to 3 mm, and consist of a white or pale yellow papule or pustule with an erythematous base. It is often called "newborn rash" or "flea bite" dermatitis. The rash may appear suddenly, usually over the trunk and diaper area, and is frequently widespread (Figure 30-20 ■). The lesions do not appear on the palms of the hands or the soles of the feet. The peak incidence is at 24 to 48 hours of life. The condition rarely presents at birth or after 5 days of life. The cause is unknown and no treatment is necessary. Some clinicians feel it may be caused by irritation from clothing. The lesions disappear in a few hours or days. If a maculopapular rash (eruption consisting of both macules and papules) appears, a smear of the aspirated papule will show numerous eosinophils on staining; no bacteria will be cultured.

Milia, which are exposed sebaceous glands, appear as raised white spots on the face, especially across the nose (Figure 30-21 ■). No treatment is necessary, because they will clear up spontaneously within the first month. Infants of African heritage have a similar condition called *transient neonatal pustular melanosis*.

Skin turgor is assessed to determine hydration status, the need to initiate early feedings, and the presence of any infectious processes. The usual place to assess skin turgor is over the abdomen, forearm, or thigh. Skin should be elastic and should return rapidly to its original shape.

Vernix caseosa, a whitish cheeselike substance, covers the fetus while in utero and lubricates the skin of the newborn. The skin of the term or postterm newborn has less vernix and is frequently dry; peeling is common, especially on the hands and feet.

Forceps marks may be present after a difficult forceps birth. The newborn may have reddened areas over the cheeks and jaws. It is important to reassure the parents that these will dis-

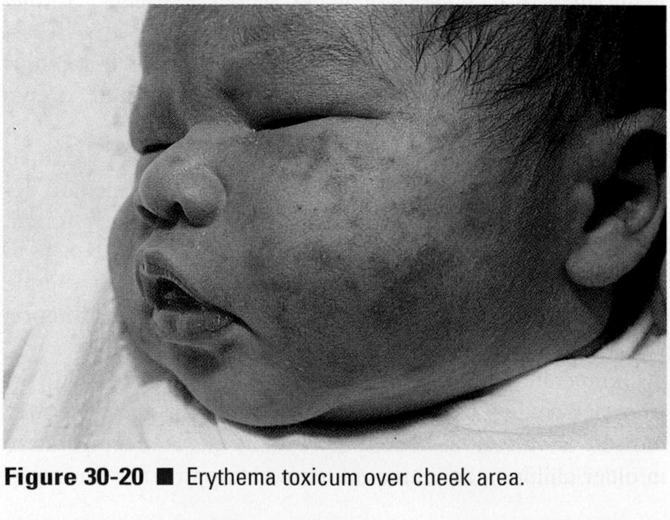

Figure 30-20 ■ Erythema toxicum over cheek area.

PROCEDURE 30-1 Assessing Jaundice in the Newborn

NURSING ACTION

Preparation

- Wash hands
- Assemble equipment

Equipment and Supplies

- Transcutaneous bilimeter

Procedure

1. Observe infant in a well-lit room or near a window during daylight hours. Infant should be specifically checked for jaundice at least twice a shift or with every assessment.
2. Blanch skin on forehead and sternum with digital pressure for 1 second and release. Observe for underlying yellow tinge to skin. If jaundice is observed on the sternum, also check palms, soles, and blanch skin below the knee.

   Rationale: *Progression of jaundice is head to toe (caudal progression). Jaundice is first seen in the face and neck when levels reach 4–8 mg/dl. Jaundice can be seen on palmar and plantar surfaces at levels greater than 15 mg/dl. Visual assessment is often an inaccurate predictor of bilirubin levels.*
3. If infant appears jaundiced, a transcutaneous bilirubin (TcB) level should be checked. TcB levels are monitored with a transcutaneous bilimeter. The device should be used according to manufacturer directions and calibrated as directed. The TcB measurement is obtained from the forehead or sternum and plotted on a nomogram. A total serum bilirubin (TSB) level is still required when treatment with phototherapy or an exchange transfusion is being considered.

   Rationale: *A transcutaneous or total serum bilirubin level should be checked on all infants who appear jaundiced in the first 24 hours of life. A TcB is as reliable as a TSB in most instances and is less invasive. The hour specific nomogram recommended by the AAP provides guidelines for initiating phototherapy in hospitalized infants 35 weeks or greater gestational age. Full term infants receive phototherapy for bilirubin levels > 12 mg/dl. The recommended treatment levels for premature infants are dependent on postnatal age, weight, and contributing factors.*
4. Assessment of jaundice risk requires gathering information about hydration status to include how the infant is being fed, feeding tolerance, amount of urine and stool, and weight. Hemoglobin (Hgb) and hematocrit (Hct) levels are also helpful.

   Rationale: *Infants who are not eating well are more prone to hyperbilirubinemia. Infants born at high altitude develop higher levels of bilirubin than babies born at sea level related to elevated hematocrit and hypoxemia.*
5. The nurse assesses the infant for early signs of bilirubin encephalopathy, which include poor feeding, hypotonia, and lethargy.
6. Document any physical findings and TcB levels, and report jaundice to the primary care practitioner.

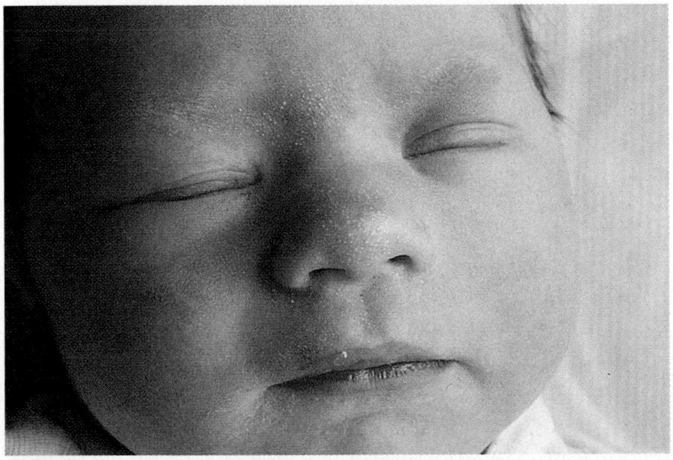

Figure 30-21 ■ Facial milia over bridge of nose.

appear, usually within 1 or 2 days. Transient facial paralysis resulting from the forceps pressure is a rare complication. Vacuum extractor suction marks on the vertex of the scalp are often seen when vacuum extractors are used to assist with the birth. These are benign and do not indicate any underlying brain lesions.

Sucking blisters (vesicles or bullae) may appear on the lips, fingers, or hands of newborns as a result of vigorous sucking, either in utero or after birth. These sucking blisters (Figure 30-22 ■) may be intact or ruptured and require no treatment.

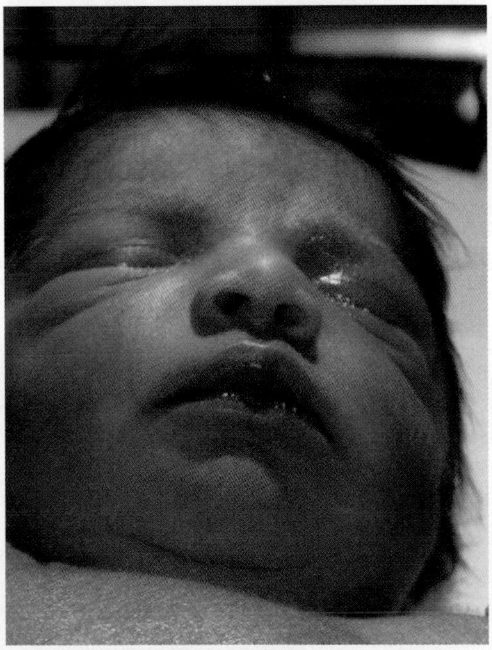

Figure 30-22 ■ Sucking blister in middle of upper lip.

Source: Courtesy of Jo Engle, RN, MSN, NNP-BC and Vanessa Howell, RN, MSN.

Birthmarks

Telangiectatic nevi (stork bites) appear as pale pink or red spots and are frequently found on the eyelids, nose, lower occipital bone, and nape of the neck (Figure 30-23 ■). The lesions are common in light-complexioned newborns and are more noticeable during periods of crying. These areas have no clinical significance and usually fade by the second birthday.

Mongolian blue spots are macular areas of bluish black or gray-blue pigmentation found on the dorsal area and the buttocks (Figure 30-24 ■). They are common in newborns of Asian, Hispanic, and African descent and other dark-skinned races and can be seen in 1% to 9% of Caucasians. They gradually fade during the first or second year of life. They may be mistaken for bruises and should be documented in the newborn's chart.

Nevus flammeus (port wine stain) is a capillary angioma directly below the epidermis. It is a nonelevated, sharply demarcated, red to purple area of dense capillaries (Figure 30-25 ■). In infants of African descent it may appear as a purple-black stain. The size and shape varies, but it commonly appears on the face. It does not grow in size, does not fade with time, and does not blanch as a rule. The birthmark may be concealed by using an opaque cosmetic cream. If convulsions and other neurologic problems accompany the nevus flammeus, the clinical picture is suggestive of *Sturge-Weber syndrome* with involvement of the fifth cranial nerve (the ophthalmic branch of the trigeminal nerve).

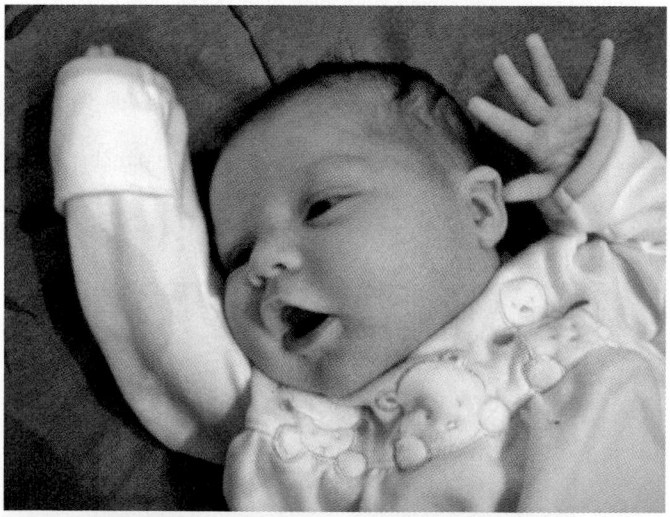

Figure 30-23 ■ Stork bites over left eyelid and near right eyebrow.

Source: Photo courtesy of Anne Garcia.

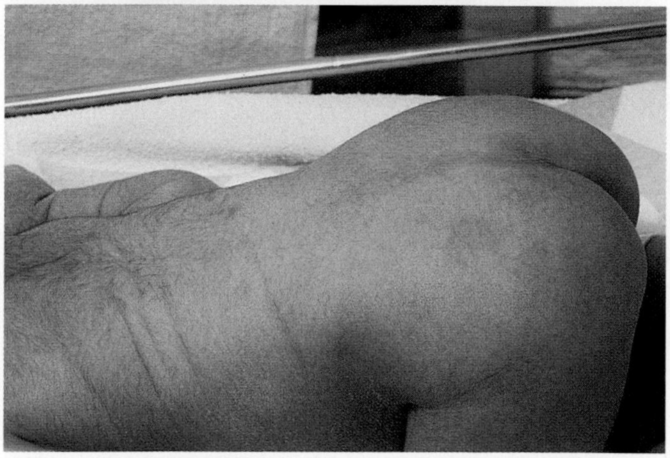

Figure 30-24 ■ Mongolian spots.

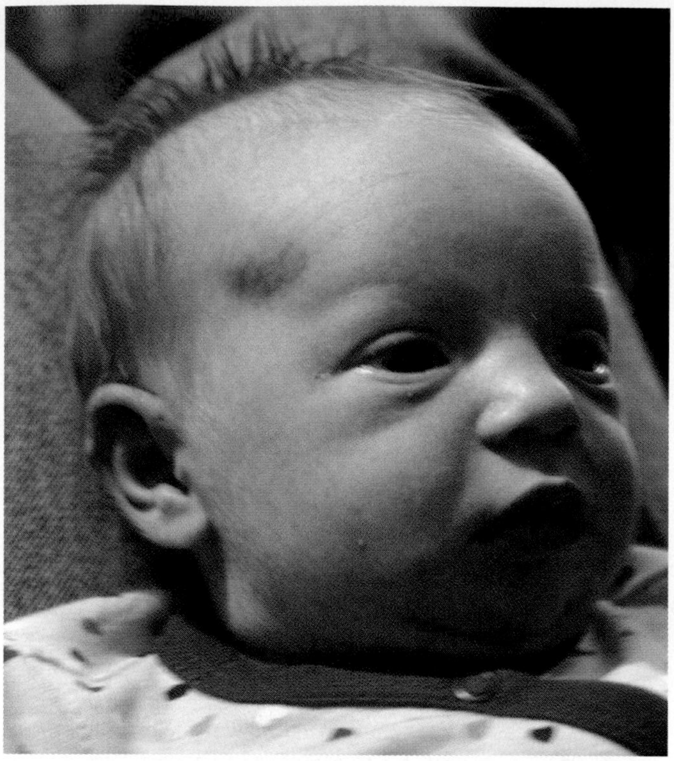

Figure 30-25 ■ Port wine stain over temple area.

Source: Courtesy of Alyssa Torres/Pearson Education.

Nevus vasculosus (strawberry mark) is a capillary hemangioma. It consists of newly formed and enlarged capillaries in the dermal and subdermal layers. It is a raised, clearly delineated, dark red, rough-surfaced birthmark commonly found in the head region. Such marks usually begin to grow (often rapidly) during the second or third week of life and may not reach their full size until about 6 months of age (Tappero & Honeyfield, 2009). They begin to shrink and start to resolve spontaneously several weeks to months after they reach peak growth. A pale purple or gray spot on the surface of the hemangioma signals the start of resolution. The best cosmetic effect is achieved when the lesions are allowed to resolve spontaneously.

Birthmarks are frequently a cause of concern for the parents. The mother may be especially anxious, fearing that she is to blame ("Is my baby marked because of something I did?"). Guilt feelings are common in the presence of misconceptions about the cause. Birthmarks should be identified and explained to the parents. By providing appropriate information about the cause and course of birthmarks, the nurse frequently relieves the fears and anxieties of the family. The nurse should note any bruises, abrasions, or birthmarks seen on the newborn's admission to the nursery.

Head

General Appearance

The newborn's head is large (approximately one fourth of the body size), with soft, pliable skull bones. For most term infants,

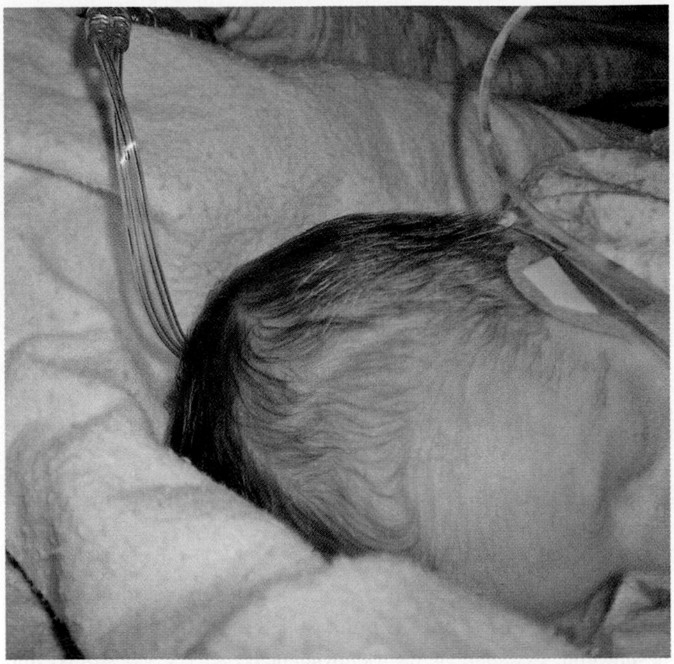

Figure 30-26 ■ Overlapped cranial bones produce a visible ridge in a premature infant. Easily visible overlapping does not occur often in term infants.

Source: Courtesy of Jo Engle, RN, MSN, NNP-BC and Vanessa Howell, RN, MSN.

the occipital-frontal circumference (OFC) is 32 to 37 cm (12.6 to 14.6 in.). The head may appear asymmetric in the newborn of a vertex presentation. This asymmetry, called **molding**, is caused by the overriding of the cranial bones during labor and birth (Figure 30-26 ■). The degree of molding varies with the amount and length of pressure exerted on the head. Within a few days after birth, the overriding usually diminishes, and the suture lines become palpable. Because head measurements are affected by molding, a second measurement is indicated a few days after birth. The heads of breech-born newborns and those born by elective cesarean birth are characteristically round and well shaped because pressure was not exerted on them during birth. Any extreme differences in head size may indicate *microcephaly* (an abnormally small head) or *hydrocephalus* (an abnormal buildup of fluid in the brain). Variations in the shape, size, or appearance of the head may be due to *craniosynostosis* (premature closure of the cranial sutures), which needs to be corrected through surgery to allow brain growth, or *plagiocephaly* (asymmetry resulting in closure of sutures on one side caused by pressure on the fetal head during gestation) (Tappero & Honeyfield, 2009).

Two *fontanelles* ("soft spots") may be palpated on the newborn's head. Fontanelles, which are openings at the juncture of the cranial bones, can be measured with the fingers. Accurate measurement necessitates that the examiner's finger be measured in centimeters. The assessment should be carried out with the newborn in sitting position and not crying. The diamond-shaped *anterior fontanelle* is 3 to 4 cm long by 2 to 3 cm wide. It is located at the juncture of the frontal and parietal bones. The *posterior fontanelle,* smaller and triangular, is formed by the parietal bones and the occipital bone and is 0.5 cm by 1 cm. Because of molding, the fontanelles tend to be smaller immediately after birth than several days later. The anterior fontanelle closes within 18 months, whereas the posterior fontanelle closes within 8 to 12 weeks.

The fontanelles are a useful indicator of the newborn's condition. The anterior fontanelle may swell when the newborn cries or passes a stool or may pulsate with the heartbeat, which is normal. A bulging fontanelle usually signifies increased intracranial pressure, and a depressed fontanelle indicates dehydration (Creehan, 2008). The sutures between the cranial bones should be palpated for amount of overlap. In newborns whose growth has been restricted, the sutures may be wider than normal, and the fontanelle may also be larger because of impaired fetal growth of the cranial bones. In addition to being inspected for degree of molding and size, the head should be evaluated for soft-tissue edema and bruising.

Cephalhematoma

Cephalhematoma is a collection of blood resulting from ruptured blood vessels between the surface of a cranial bone (usually parietal) and the periosteal membrane (Figure 30-27 ■).

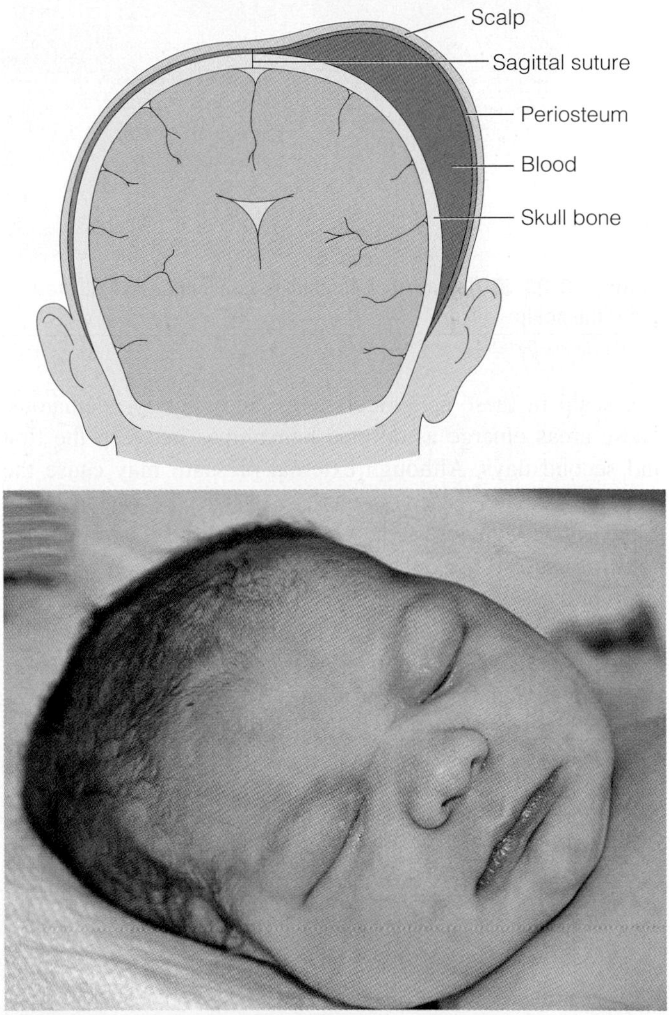

Figure 30-27 ■ Cephalhematoma is a collection of blood between the surface of a cranial bone and the periosteal membrane. This is a cephalhematoma over the right parietal bone.

Source: Courtesy of Jo Engle, RN, MSN, NNP-BC and Vanessa Howell, RN, MSN.

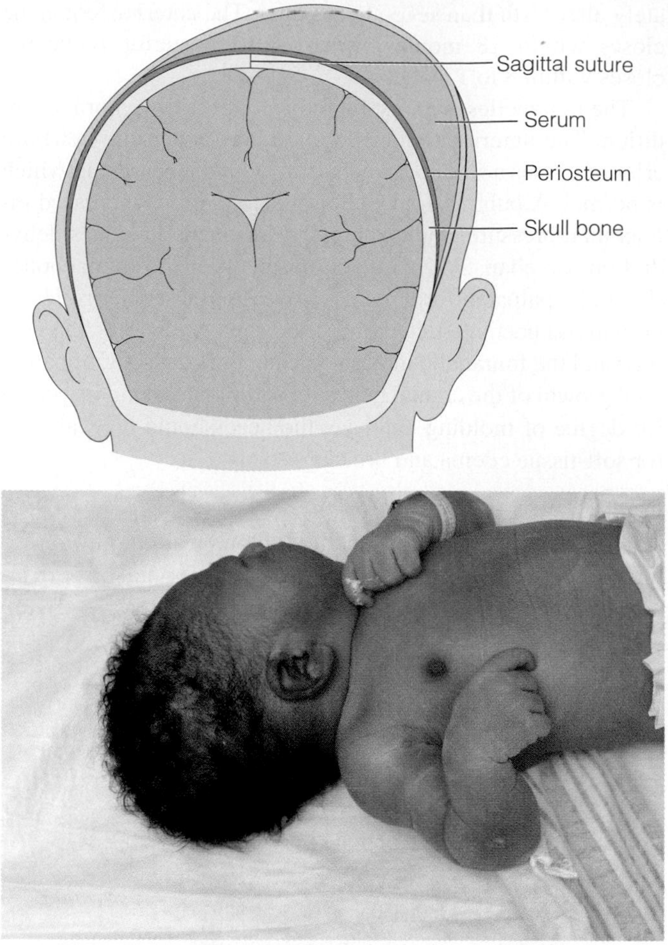

Figure 30-28 ■ Caput succedaneum is a collection of fluid (serum) under the scalp.

Source: B. George Dodson/Lightworks Studio/Pearson Education.

The scalp in these areas feels loose and slightly edematous. These areas emerge as defined hematomas between the first and second days. Although external pressure may cause the mass to fluctuate, it does not increase in size when the newborn cries. Cephalhematomas may be unilateral or bilateral and do not cross suture lines. They are relatively common in vertex births and disappear within 2 weeks to 3 months. They may be associated with physiologic jaundice, because there are extra red blood cells being destroyed within the cephalhematoma. A large cephalhematoma can lead to anemia and hypotension.

Caput Succedaneum

Caput succedaneum is a localized, easily identifiable soft area of the scalp, generally resulting from a long and difficult labor or vacuum extraction. The sustained pressure of the presenting part against the cervix results in compression of local blood vessels, and venous return is slowed. Slowed venous return causes an increase in tissue fluids, an edematous swelling, and occasional bleeding under the periosteum. The caput may vary from a small area to a large area covering a severely elongated head. The fluid in the caput is reabsorbed within 12 hours to a few days after birth. Caputs resulting from vacuum extractors are sharply outlined, circular areas up to 2 cm (0.8 in.) thick. They disappear more slowly than naturally occurring edema. It is possible to distinguish between a cephalhematoma and a caput because the caput overrides suture lines (Figure 30-28 ■), whereas the cephalhematoma, because of its location, never crosses a suture line (Table 30-3). Caput succedaneum is present at birth, whereas cephalhematoma generally is not.

TABLE 30-3 Comparison of Cephalhematoma and Caput Succedaneum

Cephalhematoma
- Collection of blood between cranial (usually parietal) bone and periosteal membrane
- Does not cross suture lines
- Does not increase in size with crying
- Appears on first and second days
- Disappears after 2 to 3 weeks or may take months

Caput Succedaneum
- Collection of fluid, edematous swelling of the scalp
- Crosses suture lines
- Present at birth or shortly thereafter
- Reabsorbed within 12 hours or a few days after birth

Hair

The term newborn's hair is smooth with texture variations depending on ethnic background (Creehan, 2008). Scalp hair is usually high over the eyebrows. Assessment of the newborn's hair characteristics such as color, quantity, hairlines, direction of growth, and hair whorls can identify genetic, metabolic, and neurologic disorders. For example, coarse, brittle, and dry hair may indicate hypothyroidism.

Face

The newborn's face is well designed to help the newborn suckle. Sucking (fat) pads are located in the cheeks. The chin is recessed, and the nose is flattened. The lips are sensitive to touch, and the sucking reflex is easily initiated.

Symmetry of the eyes, nose, and ears is evaluated. See Assessment Guide: Newborn Physical Assessment on pages 811–819 for deviations in symmetry and variations in size, shape, and spacing of facial features.

Facial movement symmetry should be assessed to determine the presence of facial palsy. Facial paralysis appears when the newborn cries; the affected side is immobile, and the palpebral (eyelid) fissure widens (Figure 30-29 ■). Paralysis may result from forceps-assisted birth or pressure on the facial nerve from the maternal pelvis during birth. Facial paralysis usually disappears within a few days to 3 weeks, although in some cases it may be permanent.

Eyes

The eyes of newborns of northern European descent are a blue or slate blue-gray. Dark-skinned newborns tend to have dark eyes at birth. The scleral color tends to be white to bluish white because of its relative thinness. A blue sclera is associated with osteogenesis imperfecta. The infant's eye color is

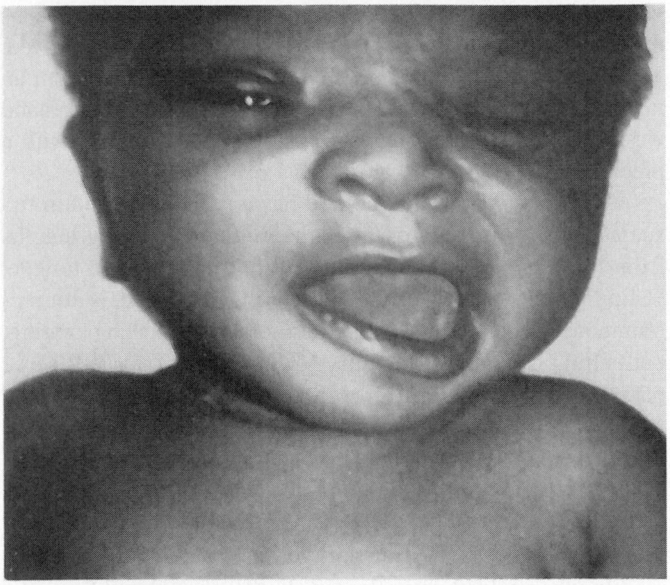

Figure 30-29 ■ Facial paralysis. Paralysis of the right side of the face from an injury to the right facial nerve.

Source: Courtesy of Dr. Ralph Platow. From Potter, E. L., & Craig, J. M. (1975). "Pathology of the fetus and infant" (3rd ed.). Chicago: Year Book Medical Publishers. Reproduced with Permission.

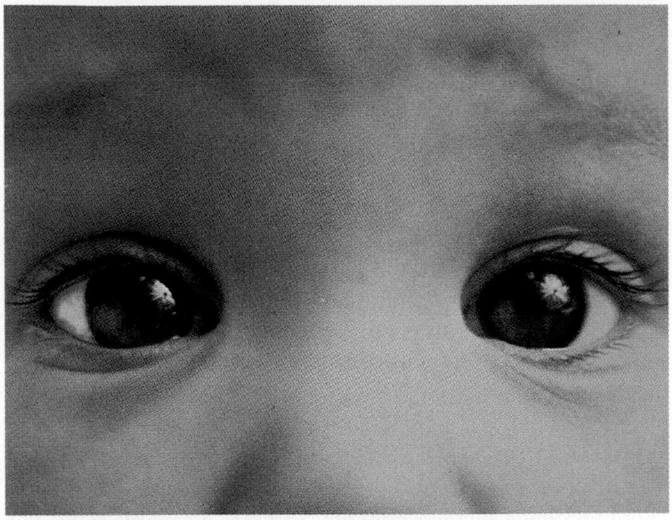

Figure 30-30 ■ Transient strabismus in the newborn may be due to poor neuromuscular control.

Source: Used with permission from Mead Johnson Nutritionals, Evansville, IN.

usually established at approximately 3 months, but it may change any time up to 1 year.

The eyes should be checked for size, equality of pupil size, reaction of pupils to light, blink reflex to light, and edema and inflammation of the eyelids. The eyelids can be edematous during the first few days of life because of the pressure associated with birth.

Erythromycin and tetracycline (in some agencies) are used prophylactically and usually do not cause chemical irritation of the eye (see chapter 31 ∞). The instillation of silver nitrate drops in the newborn's eyes may cause edema and **chemical conjunctivitis**, which may appear a few hours after instillation and disappear in 1 to 2 days (AAP & ACOG, 2007). If infectious conjunctivitis exists, the newborn has the same purulent (greenish yellow) discharge as in chemical conjunctivitis, but it is caused by gonococcus, *Chlamydia,* staphylococci, or a variety of gram-negative bacteria and requires treatment with ophthalmic antibiotics. Onset is usually after the second day. Edema of the orbits or eyelids may persist for several days until the newborn's kidneys can evacuate the fluid.

Small **subconjunctival hemorrhages** appear in about 10% of newborns and are commonly found on the sclera. These hemorrhages are caused by the changes in vascular tension or ocular pressure during birth. They will remain for a few weeks and are of no pathologic significance. Parents need reassurance that the infant is not bleeding from within the eye and that vision will not be impaired.

The newborn may demonstrate transient strabismus (pseudostrabismus) or squinting caused by neuromuscular control of eye muscles (Figure 30-30 ■). It gradually regresses in 3 to 4 months. The "doll's eye" phenomenon is also present for about 10 days after birth. As the newborn's head position is changed to the left and then to the right, the eyes move to the opposite direction. "Doll's eye" results from underdeveloped integration of head-eye coordination.

The nurse should observe the newborn's pupils for opacities or whiteness and for the absence of a normal red retinal reflex. Red retinal reflex is a red-orange flash of color observed when an ophthalmoscope light reflects off the retina. In a newborn with dark skin color, the retina may appear paler or more grayish. The color of the red reflex can also be abnormal with retinoblastoma. Absence of red reflex occurs with cataracts. Congenital cataracts should be suspected in infants of mothers with a prenatal history of rubella, cytomegalic inclusion disease, or syphilis. Brushfield spots (black or white spots on the periphery of the iris) can be associated with Down syndrome (Creehan, 2008).

The cry of the newborn is commonly tearless because the lacrimal structures are immature at birth and are not usually fully functional until the second month of life. However, some babies may produce tears during the newborn period.

Poor oculomotor coordination and absence of accommodation limit visual abilities, but newborns do have peripheral vision and can fixate on near objects (20.3 to 25.4 cm [8 to 10 in.]) in front of their faces for short periods, can accommodate to large objects (7.6 cm [3 in.] tall by 7.6 cm [3 in.] wide), and can seek out high-contrast geometric shapes. Newborns can perceive faces, shapes, and colors and begin to show visual preferences early. Newborns generally blink in response to bright lights, to a tap on the bridge of the nose (glabellar reflex), or to a light touch on the eyelids. Pupillary light reflex is also present. The eye is best examined by rocking the newborn from an upright position to the horizontal a few times or by other methods, such as diminishing overhead lights, which will elicit an opened-eye response.

Nose

The newborn's nose is small and narrow. Infants are characteristically nose breathers for the first few months of life. The newborn generally removes obstructions by sneezing. The nose is patent if the newborn breathes easily with the mouth closed. If respiratory difficulty occurs, the nurse checks for choanal atresia (congenital blockage of the passageway between the nose and pharynx). Historically, choanal atresia can be checked by attempting to gently pass a soft #5 French catheter into both nostrils. Because of possible trauma, a cold, flat metal object may also be held under the nose to observe for fogging (Tappero & Honeyfield, 2009).

The newborn has the ability to smell after the nasal passages are cleared of amniotic fluid and mucus. They will turn their heads toward the milk source, whether bottle or breast. Newborns react to strong odors, such as alcohol, by turning their heads away or blinking.

Mouth

The lips of the newborn should be pink, and a touch on the lips should produce sucking motions. Saliva is normally scant. The taste buds are developed before birth, and the newborn can easily discriminate between sweet and bitter flavors.

The easiest way to examine the mouth completely is to stimulate infants to cry by gently depressing their tongue, thereby causing them to open the mouth fully. It is extremely important to observe the entire mouth to look for a cleft palate, which can be present even in the absence of a cleft lip. The examiner moves a gloved index finger or pinky along the hard and soft palate to feel for any openings (Figure 30-31 ■).

Occasionally, an examination of the gums will reveal precocious teeth over the area where the lower central incisor will erupt. If they appear loose, they should be removed to prevent aspiration. Gray-white lesions (inclusion cysts) on the gums may be confused with teeth. On the hard palate and gum margins, **Epstein's pearls**, small glistening white specks (keratin-containing cysts) that feel hard to the touch, are often present. They usually disappear in a few weeks and are of no significance. **Thrush** may appear as white patches that look like milk curds adhering to the mucous membranes, and bleeding may occur when patches are removed. Thrush is caused by *Candida albicans,* often acquired from an infected vaginal tract during birth, antibiotic use, or poor hand washing when handling the newborn. Thrush is treated with a preparation of nystatin (Mycostatin).

A newborn who is tongue-tied has a ridge of frenulum tissue attached to the underside of the tongue at varying lengths from its base, causing a heart shape at the tip of the tongue. "Clipping the tongue," or cutting the ridge of tissue, is not recommended. This ridge usually does not affect speech or eating, but cutting does create an entry for infection. Transient nerve paralysis resulting from birth trauma may be manifested by asymmetric mouth movements when the newborn cries or by difficulty with sucking and feeding.

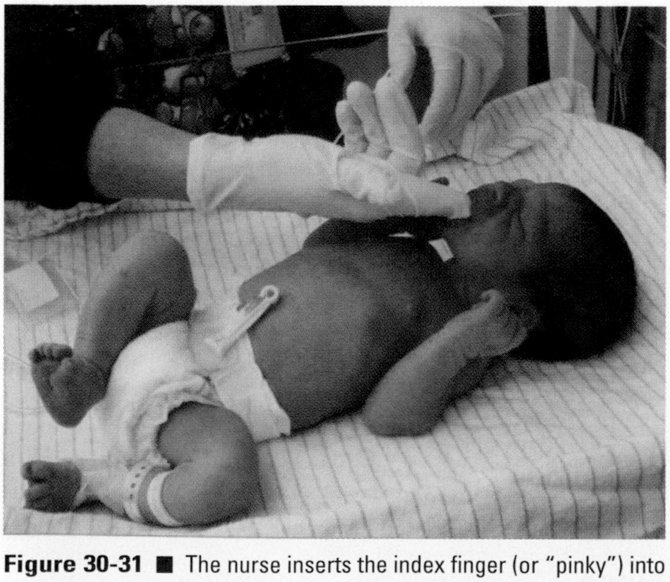

Figure 30-31 ■ The nurse inserts the index finger (or "pinky") into the newborn's mouth and feels for any openings along the hard and soft palates. *Note:* Gloves or a finger cot are always worn to examine the palate.

Source: Courtesy of Vanessa Howell, RNC, BSN.

Ears

The ears of the newborn are soft and pliable and should recoil readily when folded and released. In the normal newborn, the top of the ear (pinna) should be parallel to the outer and inner canthus of the eye. The ears should be inspected for shape, size, position, and firmness of ear cartilage. *Low-set ears* are characteristic of many syndromes and may indicate chromosomal abnormalities (especially trisomies 13 and 18), intellectual disability (mental retardation), or internal organ abnormalities, especially bilateral renal agenesis as a result of embryologic developmental deviations (Figure 30-32 ■). A *preauricular skin tag* may be present just in front of the ear. Visualization of the tympanic membranes is not usually done soon after birth because blood and vernix block the ear canal.

Following the first cry, the newborn's hearing becomes acute as mucus from the middle ear is absorbed, the eustachian tube is aerated, and the tympanic membrane becomes visible. The newborn's hearing initially can be evaluated by response to loud or moderately loud noises unaccompanied by vibrations. The sleeping newborn should stir or awaken in response to the nearby sounds. (This is not a very accurate test, but it may help to alert the examiner to possible problems.) The newborn can discriminate the individual characteristics of the human voice and is especially sensitive to sound levels within the normal conversation range. The newborn in a noisy nursery may be able

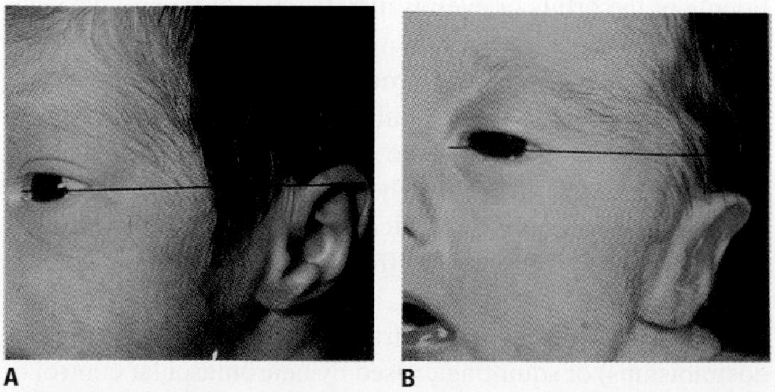

Figure 30-32 ■ The position of the external ear may be assessed by drawing a line across the inner and outer canthus of the eye to the insertion of the ear. A. Normal position. B. True low-set position.

Source: Courtesy of Mead Johnson Nutritionals, Evansville, IN.

to habituate to the sounds and not stir unless the sound is sudden or much louder.

AAP has endorsed universal newborn hearing screening (UNHS) in birthing units as the standard of care (Creehan, 2008) (see chapter 31 ∞ for further discussion). Risk factors (AAP & ACOG, 2007) associated with potential hearing loss include the following:

- The presence of familial hearing loss.
- Serum bilirubin level greater than 20 mg/dl for the full-term newborn or hyperbilirubinemia with a level exceeding indications for exchange transfusion because of toxic drugs.
- Prolonged mechanical ventilation of more than 5 days.
- Congenital infection with rubella, herpes, cytomegalovirus, toxoplasmosis, or syphilis.
- Bacterial meningitis or sepsis.
- Congenital defects of the ear, nose, or throat.
- Small preterm newborns, particularly less than 1500 g at birth.
- Perinatal asphyxia.
- Ototoxic medications.

If congenital hearing loss risk factors exist, two types of tests are commonly used: otoacoustic emissions (OAEs) and auditory brainstem response (ABR).

CLINICAL TIP

Vital sign assessments are most accurate if the newborn is at rest, so measure pulse and respirations first if the baby is quiet. To soothe a crying baby, try placing a pacifier or your moistened gloved finger in the baby's mouth, and then complete your assessment while the baby suckles.

Neck

A short neck, creased with skin folds, is characteristic of the normal newborn. Because muscle tone is not well developed, the neck cannot support the full weight of the head, which rotates freely. The head lags considerably when the newborn is pulled up from a supine to a sitting position, but the prone newborn is able to raise the head slightly. The neck is palpated for masses and presence of lymph nodes and is inspected for webbing. Adequate range of motion and neck muscle function is determined by fully extending the head in all directions. Injury to the sternocleidomastoid muscle (congenital torticollis) must be considered in the presence of neck rigidity.

The clavicles are evaluated for evidence of fractures, which occasionally occur during difficult births or in newborns with broad shoulders. The normal clavicle is straight. If fractured, a lump and a grating sensation (crepitus) during movements may be palpated along the course of the side of the break. The Moro reflex (see pages 809 and 810) is also elicited to evaluate bilateral equal movement of the arms. If the clavicle is fractured, this response will be demonstrated only on the unaffected side.

Chest

The thorax is cylindric and symmetric at birth, and the ribs are flexible. The general appearance of the chest should be assessed. A protrusion at the lower end of the sternum, called the xiphoid cartilage, is frequently seen. It is under the skin and will become less apparent after several weeks as the infant accumulates adipose tissue.

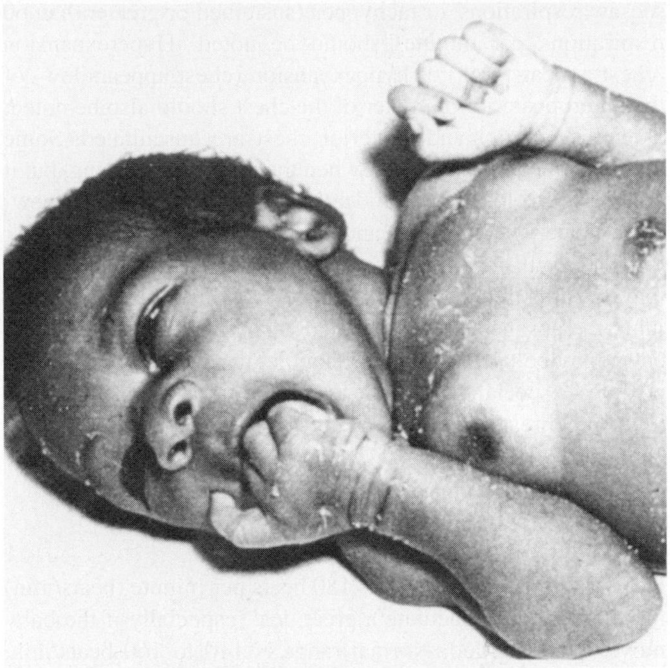

Figure 30-33 ■ Breast hypertrophy.

Source: Reprinted from Korones, S. B. (1986), "High-risk newborn infants", 3rd edition. St. Louis: Mosby-Year-Book Medical Publishers, Inc.

Engorged breasts occur frequently in both male and female newborns. This condition, which appears by the third day, is a result of maternal hormonal influences and may last up to 2 weeks (Figure 30-33 ■). A whitish secretion from the nipples may also be noted. The infant's breast should not be massaged or squeezed because this practice may cause a breast abscess. Extra nipples or supernumerary nipples are occasionally noted below and medial to the true nipples. These harmless pink or brown (in darker skinned newborns) spots vary in size and do not contain glandular tissue. Accessory nipples can be differentiated from a pigmented nevus (mole) by placing the fingertips alongside the accessory nipple and pulling the adjacent tissue laterally. The accessory nipple will appear dimpled.

Cry

The newborn's cry should be strong, lusty, and of medium pitch. A high-pitched, shrill cry is abnormal and may indicate neurologic disorders or hypoglycemia. Periods of crying vary in length after consoling measures are used. A baby's cries are an important method of communication and alert caregivers to changes in the baby's condition and needs (see chapter 29 ∞).

Respiration

Normal breathing for a term newborn is 30 to 60 respirations per minute and predominantly diaphragmatic, with associated rising and falling of the abdomen during inspiration and expiration. Any signs of respiratory distress, nasal flaring, intercostal or xiphoid retractions, expiratory grunting or sighing, seesaw respirations, or tachypnea (sustained or greater than 60 respirations per minute) should be noted. Hyperexpansion (chest appears high) or hypoexpansion (chest appears low) of the anteroposterior diameter of the chest should also be noted. Both the anterior and posterior chest are auscultated. Some breath sounds are heard best when the newborn is crying, but it is difficult to localize and identify breath sounds in the newborn. Upper airway noises and bowel sounds can be heard over the chest wall, making auscultation difficult. Because sounds may be transmitted from the unaffected lung to the affected lung, the absence of breath sounds may not be diagnosed. Air entry may be noisy in the first couple of hours until lung fluid resolves, especially in cesarean births. Brief periods of apnea (episodic breathing) may occur, but no color or heart rate changes occur in healthy, term newborns. Sepsis should be suspected in full-term infants experiencing apneic episodes.

Heart

Heart rates can be as rapid as 180 beats per minute (beats/min) in newborns and fluctuate a great deal, especially if the baby moves or is startled. Normal range is 110 to 160 beats/min. Auscultation provides the nurse with valuable assessment data. The heart is examined for rate and rhythm, position of the apical impulse, and heart sound intensity. Dysrhythmias should be evaluated by a physician.

The pulse rate is variable and is influenced by physical activity, crying, state of wakefulness, and body temperature. Auscultation is performed over the entire heart region (precordium), below the left axilla, and below the scapula. *Apical pulse rates are obtained by auscultation for a full minute,* preferably when the newborn is asleep.

The placement of the heart in the chest should be determined when the newborn is in a quiet state. The heart is relatively large at birth and is located high in the chest, with its apex somewhere between the fourth and fifth intercostal space.

A shift of heart tones in the mediastinal area to either side may indicate pneumothorax, dextrocardia (heart placement on the right side of the chest), or a diaphragmatic hernia. The experienced nurse can diagnose these and many other problems early with a stethoscope. Normally, the heartbeat has a "toc tic" sound. A slur or slushing sound (usually after the first sound) may indicate a murmur. Although 90% of all murmurs are transient and are considered normal, they should be monitored closely by a physician. Many murmurs are secondary to closing of patent ductus arteriosus or patent foramen ovale, which should close 1 to 2 days after birth. Occasionally, aortic or pulmonary stenosis, or small ventricular septal defect murmurs are heard. See chapter 33 ∞ for a discussion of congenital heart defects.

Peripheral pulses (brachial, femoral, pedal) are also evaluated to detect any lags or unusual characteristics. Brachial pulses are palpated bilaterally for equality and compared with the femoral pulses. Femoral pulses are palpated by applying gentle pressure with the middle finger over the femoral canal (Figure 30-34 ■). Decreased or absent femoral pulses may indicate coarctation of the aorta or hypovolemia and require additional investigation. A wide difference in blood pressure between the upper and lower extremities also indicates coarctation.

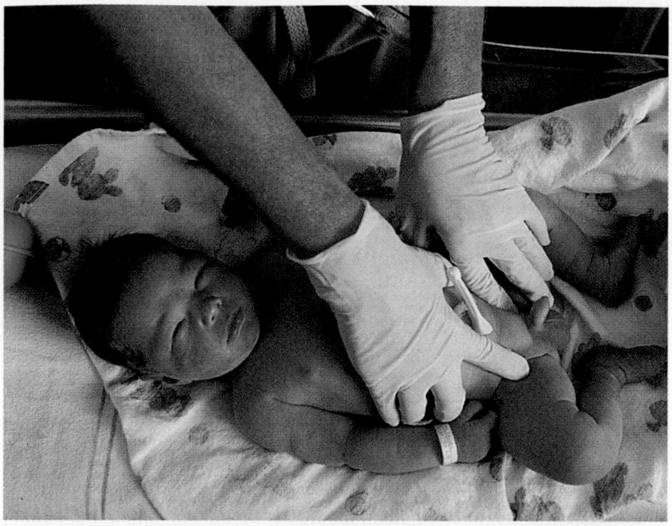

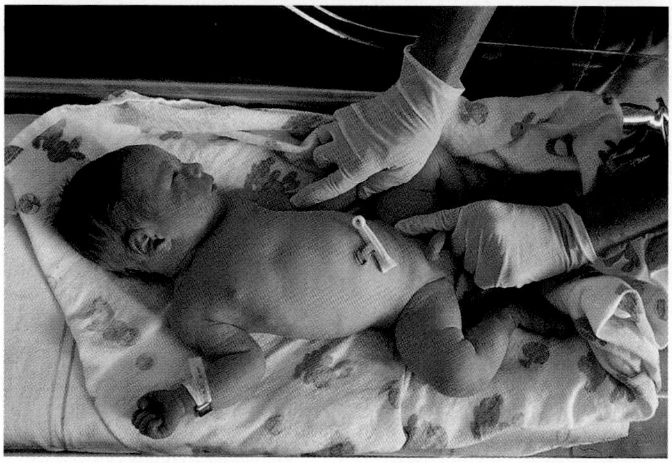

Figure 30-34 ■ A. Bilaterally palpate the femoral arteries for rate and intensity of the pulses. Press fingertip gently at the groin as shown. B. Compare the femoral pulses to the brachial pulses by palpating the pulses simultaneously for comparison of rate and intensity.

Source: Photographer, Elena Dorfman.

The measurement of blood pressure (BP) is best accomplished by using a noninvasive blood pressure device (Figure 30-35 ■). If a blood pressure cuff is used, the newborn's extremities must be immobilized during the assessment, and the cuff should cover two thirds of the upper arm or upper leg. Movement, crying, and inappropriate cuff size can give inaccurate measurements of the blood pressure.

Blood pressure *may not be measured routinely* on healthy newborns but is an essential measurement in newborns who are having distress, are premature, or are suspected of having a cardiac

CLINICAL TIP

If possible, obtain blood pressure (BP) measurement during quiet sleep or sleep state. Place cuff on arm or leg and give infant time to quiet. Obtain average of 2 to 3 measurements when making clinical decisions. Follow mean BP to monitor changes, as it is less likely to be erroneous. Noninvasive BP may overestimate BP in very low-birth-weight infants.

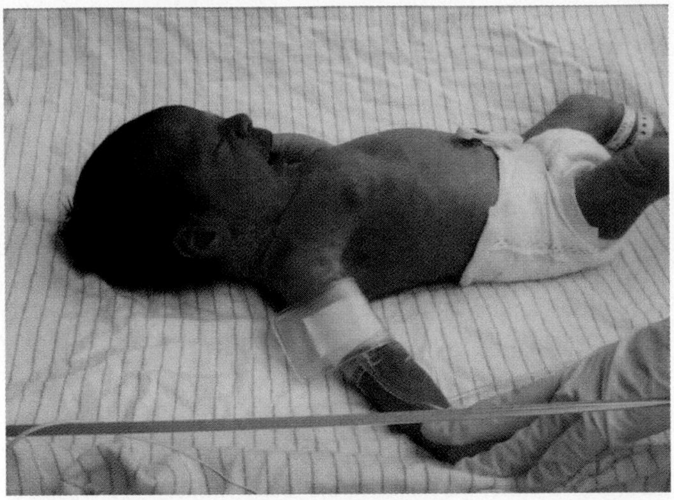

Figure 30-35 ■ Blood pressure measurement using the Dinemapp and Doppler devices. The cuff can be applied to either the newborn's upper arm or the thigh.

Source: Courtesy of Vanessa Howell, RNC, BSN.

anomaly, renal disease, or clinical signs of hypotension (Tappero & Honeyfield, 2009). Infants who have birth asphyxia and are on ventilators have significantly lower systolic and diastolic blood pressures than healthy infants. If a cardiac anomaly is suspected, blood pressure is palpated in all four extremities. At birth, systolic values usually range from 70 to 50 mm Hg and diastolic values from 45 to 30 mm Hg. By the 10th day of life, blood pressure may rise to 90/50 mm Hg. Table 30-4 summarizes newborn vital signs.

Abdomen

The nurse can learn a great deal about the newborn's abdomen without disturbing the infant. The abdomen should be cylindrical, protrude slightly, and move with respiration. A certain amount of laxness of the abdominal muscles is normal. A scaphoid (hollow-shaped) appearance suggests the absence of abdominal contents, seen in diaphragmatic hernia. No cyanosis should be present, and few if any blood vessels should be apparent to the eye. There should be no gross distention or bulging. The more distended the abdomen, the tighter the skin becomes, and engorged vessels appear. Distention is the first sign of many of the gastrointestinal abnormalities.

TABLE 30-4 Newborn Vital Signs

Pulse	**Blood Pressure**
• 110–160 beats/min	• 70–50/45–30 mm Hg at birth
• During deep sleep as low as 70 beats/min; if crying, up to 180 beats/min (Tappero & Honeyfield, 2009)	• 90/60 mm Hg at day 10
• Apical pulse counted for 1 full minute	**Temperature**
	• Normal range: 36.5°C–37.5°C (97.7°F–99.4°F)
Respirations	• Axillary: 36.5°C–37.2°C (97.7°F–99°F)
• 30–60 respirations/minute	• Skin: 36°C–36.5°C (96.8°F–97.7°F)
• Predominantly diaphragmatic but synchronous with abdominal movements	• Rectal: 36.6°C–37.2°C (97.8°F–99°F)
• Respirations are counted for 1 full minute	

Before palpation of the abdomen, the nurse should auscultate the presence or absence of bowel sounds in all four quadrants. Bowel sounds should be present by 1 hour after birth. Palpation can cause a transient decrease in bowel sound intensity.

Abdominal palpation should be carried out systematically. The nurse palpates each of the four abdominal quadrants, moving in a clockwise direction, checking for softness, tenderness, and the presence of masses. The nurse should place one hand under the back for support during palpation. When palpating the abdomen, the nurse may feel for the liver. The newborn's liver is large in proportion to the rest of the body and can usually be felt between 1 and 2 cm below the right costal margin. Depending on institutional protocol, palpation of the kidney may be performed by the staff nurse. Kidneys are more difficult to feel but can be more easily examined within 4 to 6 hours after birth, before the intestines become distended with air and feedings are initiated. The lower pole of the kidney is usually found 1 to 2 cm above the umbilicus. The spleen tip may be palpated in the lateral aspect of the left upper quadrant in the normal newborn (Gardner & Hernandez, 2011).

Umbilical Cord

Initially, the umbilical cord is white and gelatinous in appearance, with the two umbilical arteries and one umbilical vein readily apparent. Because a single umbilical artery is frequently associated with congenital anomalies, the vessels should be counted as part of the newborn assessment. The cord begins drying within 1 or 2 hours after birth and is shriveled and blackened by the second or third day. Within 7 to 10 days it sloughs off, although a granulated area may remain for a few days longer. (Care of the umbilical cord is discussed in chapter 31 ∞.)

Cord bleeding is abnormal and may result because the cord was inadvertently pulled or because the cord clamp was loosened. Foul-smelling drainage is also abnormal and is generally caused by infection, which requires immediate treatment to prevent septicemia. If the newborn has a patent urachus (abnormal connection between the umbilicus and bladder), moistness or draining urine may be apparent at the base of the cord. Another umbilical cord anomaly that can occur is umbilical cord hernia and associated patent omphalomesenteric duct (Figure 30-36 ■). Umbilical hernias are more common in infants of African descent than in Caucasian infants, and seen in low birth weight males (Tappero & Honeyfield, 2009). The umbilical hernias usually close spontaneously by 2 years of age.

Serous or serosanguineous drainage that continues after the cord falls off may indicate a granuloma. It appears as a small, red button deep in the umbilicus (Tappero & Honeyfield, 2009).

DEVELOPING CULTURAL COMPETENCE

Native Americans and Umbilical Cord Care

In the Woodland Indian tribe, upon birth, the umbilical cord is tied and a small piece is saved. This section of the umbilical cord is sewn into a deerskin diamond-shaped pocket. The pocket is hung over the infant's crib to provide protection for the infant.

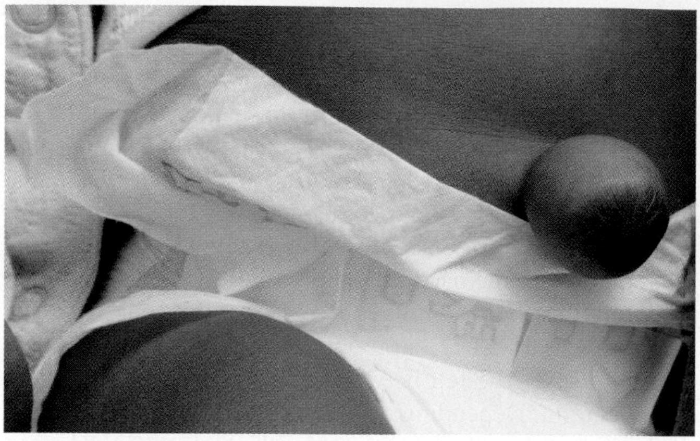

Figure 30-36 ■ Umbilical hernia.

Source: George Dodson/Lightworks Studio/Pearson Education.

Genitals

Female Infants

The nurse examines the labia majora, labia minora, and clitoris, noting the size of each as appropriate for gestational age. A vaginal tag or hymenal tag is often evident and will usually disappear in a few weeks. During the first week of life, the female newborn may have a vaginal discharge composed of thick whitish mucus. This discharge, which can become tinged with blood, is referred to as **pseudomenstruation** and is caused by the withdrawal of maternal hormones. *Smegma,* a white cheeselike substance, is often present between the labia. Removing it may traumatize tender tissue.

Male Infants

The penis is inspected to determine whether the urinary orifice is correctly positioned. *Hypospadias* occurs when the urinary meatus is located on the ventral surface of the penis; *epispadias* occurs when the meatus is located on the dorsal surface of the glans. Hypospadias occurs most commonly among people of Western European descent. *Phimosis* is a condition occurring in newborn males in which the opening of the foreskin (prepuce) is small, and the foreskin cannot be pulled back over the glans at all. This condition may interfere with urination, so the adequacy of the urinary stream should be evaluated.

The scrotum is inspected for size and symmetry. Scrotal color variations are especially prominent in African American, Indian, and Hispanic newborns (Creehan, 2008). The scrotum should be palpated to verify the presence of both testes and to rule out *cryptorchidism* (failure of testes to descend). The testes are palpated separately between the thumb and forefinger, with the thumb and forefinger of the other hand placed together over the inguinal canal. Scrotal edema and discoloration are common in breech births. *Hydrocele* (a collection of fluid surrounding the testes in the scrotum) is common in newborns and should be identified. It usually resolves without intervention. The presence of a discolored or dusky scrotum and solid testis should raise the suspicion of testicular torsion, which should be reported immediately.

Anus

The anal area is inspected to verify that it is patent and has no fissure. Imperforate anus and rectal atresia may be ruled out by observation. A digital examination, if necessary, is done by a physician or nurse practitioner. The passage of the first meconium stool is also noted. Atresia of the gastrointestinal tract or meconium ileus with resultant obstruction must be considered if the newborn does not pass meconium in the first 24 hours of life.

Extremities

Extremities are examined for gross deformities, extra digits or webbing, clubfoot, and range of motion. Normal newborn extremities appear short, are generally flexible, and move symmetrically.

Arms and Hands

Nails extend beyond the fingertips in term newborns. Fingers and toes should be counted. *Polydactyly* is the presence of extra digits on either the hands or the feet. *Syndactyly* refers to fusion (webbing) of fingers or toes. Hands should be inspected for normal palmar creases. A single palmar crease is frequently present in children with Down syndrome.

Brachial palsy, a partial or complete paralysis of portions of the arm, results from trauma to the brachial plexus during a difficult birth. It occurs most commonly when strong traction is exerted on the head of the newborn in an attempt to deliver a shoulder lodged behind the symphysis pubis in the presence of shoulder dystocia. Brachial palsy may also occur during a breech birth if an arm becomes trapped over the head and traction is exerted.

The portion of the arm affected is determined by the nerves damaged. **Erb-Duchenne paralysis (Erb's palsy)** involves damage to the upper arm (fifth and sixth cervical nerves) and is

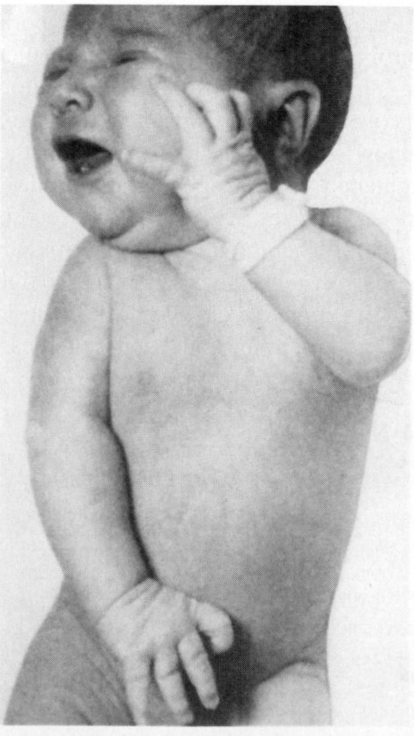

Figure 30-37 ■ Right Erb's palsy resulting from injury to the fifth and sixth cervical roots of brachial plexus.

Source: Photo reprinted from Potter, E. L., & Craig, J. M. Pathology of the fetus and infant (3rd ed.). Copyright © 1975, with permission from Elsevier.

the most common type. Injury to the eighth cervical and first thoracic nerve roots and the lower portion of the plexus produces the relatively rare *lower arm injury.* The *whole arm type* results from damage to the entire plexus.

With Erb-Duchenne paralysis, the newborn's arm lies limply at the side (Figure 30-37 ■). The elbow is held in extension, with the forearm pronated. The newborn is unable to elevate the arm, and therefore the Moro reflex cannot be elicited on the affected side. When a lower arm injury occurs, paralysis of the hand and wrist results; complete paralysis of the limb occurs with the whole arm type.

The nurse carefully instructs the parents in the correct method of performing passive range-of-motion exercises (to prevent muscle contractures and restore function) and arranges supervised practice sessions for the parents and referral to physical therapy follow-up within 2 weeks of discharge. In more severe cases, splinting of the arm is indicated until the edema decreases. The arm is held in a position of abduction and external rotation with the elbow flexed 90 degrees, often called the "Statue of Liberty" position. Prognosis is related to the degree of nerve damage resulting from trauma and hemorrhage within the nerve sheath. Complete recovery occurs within a few months with minimal trauma. Moderate trauma may result in some partial paralysis. Recovery is unlikely with severe trauma, and muscle wasting may develop.

Legs and Feet

The legs of the newborn should be of equal length, with symmetric skin folds. However, they may assume a "fetal posture" secondary to position in utero, and it may take several days for the legs to relax into normal position.

To evaluate for hip dislocation or hip instability, the Barlow and Ortolani maneuvers are performed (Figure 30-38 ■). The nurse (or, more commonly, the physician or nurse practitioner) examiner performs the **Barlow maneuver** to rule out the possibility of developmental dysplasic hip, also called congenital hip dysplasia (hip dislocatability). The examiner grasps and adducts the infant's thigh and applies gentle downward pressure. Dislocation is felt as the femoral head slips out of the acetabulum. The femoral head is then returned to the acetabulum using the Ortolani maneuver, confirming the diagnosis of an unstable or dislocatable hip.

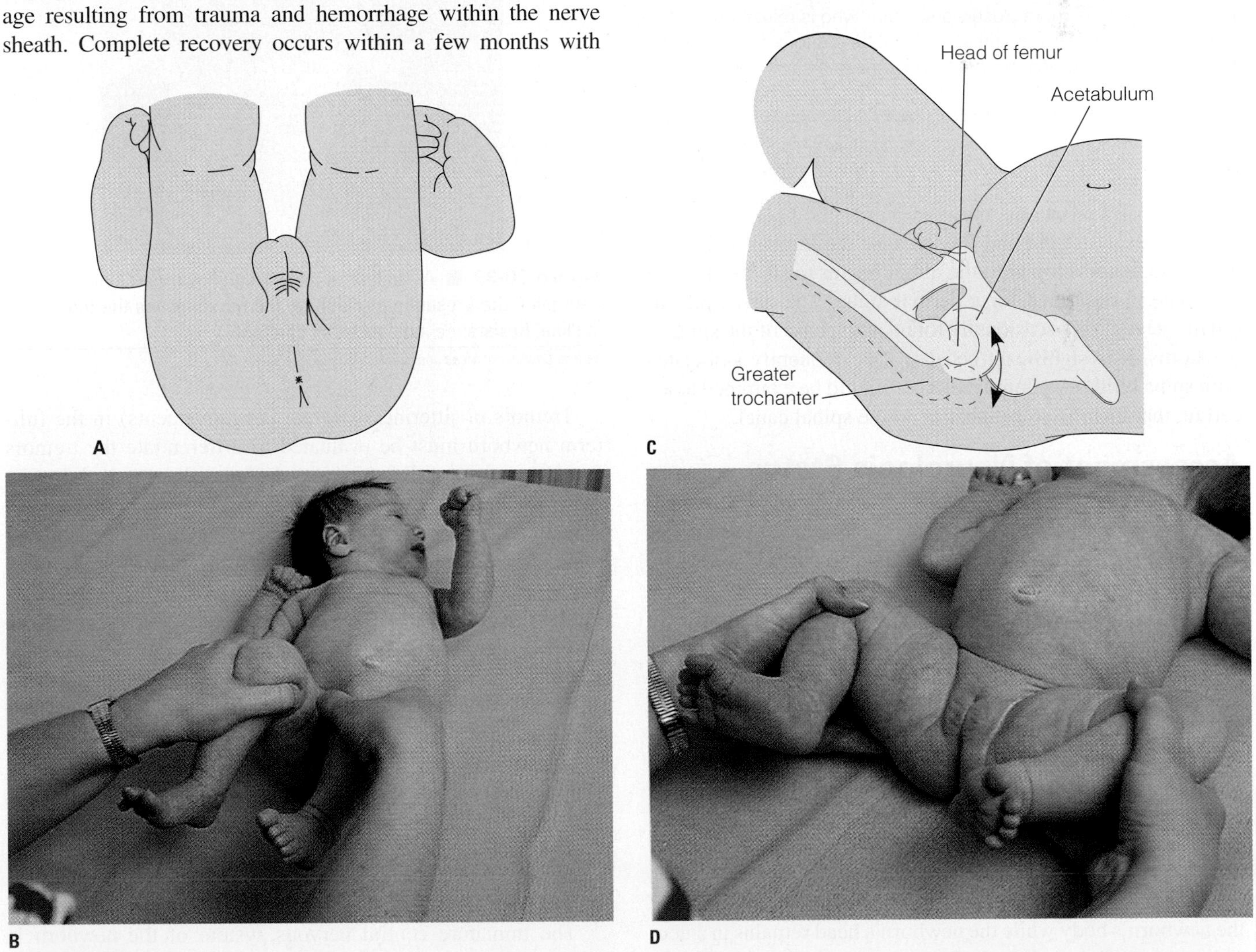

Figure 30-38 ■ A. The asymmetry of gluteal and thigh fat folds seen in infant with left developmental dysplasia of the hip. B. Barlow (dislocation) maneuver. Baby's thigh is grasped and adducted (placed together) with gentle downward pressure. C. Dislocation is palpable as femoral head slips out of acetabulum. D. Ortolani's maneuver puts downward pressure on the hip and then inward rotation. If the hip is dislocated, this maneuver will force the femoral head back into the acetabular rim with a noticeable "clunk."

Ortolani's maneuver should be performed with the newborn relaxed and quiet on a firm surface. With the hips and knees flexed at a 90-degree angle, the examiner grasps the infant's thigh with the middle finger over the greater trochanter and lifts the thigh to bring the femoral head from its posterior position toward the acetabulum. With gentle abduction of the thigh, the femoral head is returned to the acetabulum and the examiner feels a sense of reduction or a "clunk." This reduction is palpable and may be heard.

The feet are then examined for evidence of a talipes deformity (clubfoot). Intrauterine position frequently causes the feet to appear to turn inward (Figure 30-39 ■); this is termed a *"positional" clubfoot.* If the feet can easily be returned to midline by manipulation, no treatment is indicated. Range-of-motion exercises can be taught to the family. Further investigation is indicated when the foot will not turn to the midline position or align readily. This is considered the most severe type of "true clubfoot," or talipes equinovarus.

CLINICAL TIP

Always examine more closely any infant who is reluctant to move an extremity. Fractures are often asymptomatic in the newborn; paralytic injuries are characterized by immobility of an extremity.

Application: Newborn Assessment

Back

With the baby prone, the nurse examines the back. The spine should appear straight and flat because the lumbar and sacral curves do not develop until the infant begins to sit. The base of the spine is examined for a dermal sinus. The nevus pilosus ("hairy nevus") is occasionally found at the base of the spine in newborns. It is significant because it is frequently associated with spina bifida. A pilonidal dimple should be examined to ascertain that there is no connection to the spinal canal.

Assessment of Neurologic Status

The nurse should begin the neurologic examination with a period of observation, noting the general physical characteristics and behavior of the newborn. Important behaviors to assess are the *state of alertness, resting posture, cry,* and *quality of muscle tone* and *motor activity.*

The usual position of the newborn is partially flexed extremities with the legs abducted to the abdomen. When awake, the newborn may exhibit purposeless, uncoordinated bilateral movements of the extremities. If these movements are absent, minimal, or obviously asymmetric, neurologic dysfunction should be suspected. Eye movements are observable during the first few days of life. An alert newborn is able to fixate on faces and brightly colored objects. Shining a bright light in the newborn's eyes elicits the blinking response.

The nurse evaluates muscle tone by moving various parts of the newborn's body while the newborn's head remains in a neutral position. The newborn is somewhat hypertonic; that is, the newborn resists the examiner's attempts to extend the elbow and knee joints. Muscle tone should be symmetric. Diminished muscle tone and flaccidity require further evaluation.

Videos: Newborn Reflexes

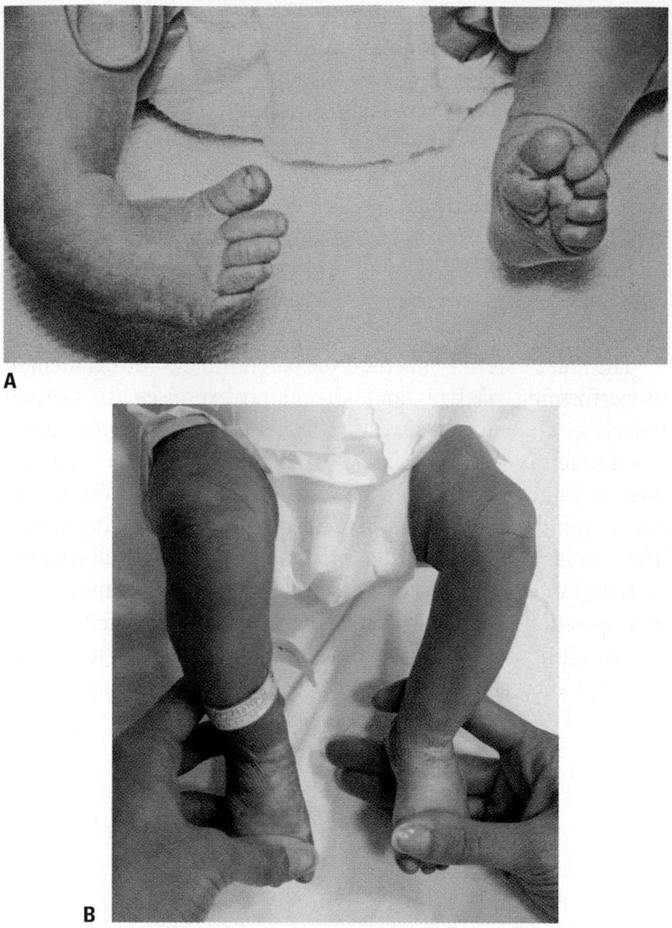

Figure 30-39 ■ A. Unilateral talipes equinovarus (clubfoot). B. To determine the presence of clubfoot, the nurse moves the foot to the midline. Resistance indicates true clubfoot.

Source: Courtesy of Mead Johnson Nutritionals, Evansville, IN.

Tremors or jitteriness (tremorlike movements) in the full-term newborn must be evaluated to differentiate the tremors from convulsions. Tremors may be related to hypoglycemia, hypocalcemia, or substance withdrawal. Environmental stimuli may initiate tremors. Jitteriness may be distinguished from tonic-clonic seizure activity because it usually can be stopped by the infant's sucking on the extremity or by the nurse holding or flexing the involved extremity. A fine jumping of the muscle is likely to be a central nervous system (CNS) disorder and requires further evaluation. Neonatal seizures may consist of no more than chewing or swallowing movements, deviations of the eyes, rigidity, or flaccidity because of central nervous system immaturity. In contrast to tremors, seizures are not usually initiated by stimuli and cannot be stopped by holding.

Specific deep tendon reflexes can be elicited in the newborn but have limited value unless they are obviously asymmetric. The knee jerk is brisk; a normal ankle clonus may involve three or four beats. Plantar flexion is present.

The immature central nervous system of the newborn is characterized by a variety of reflexes. Because the newborn's movements are uncoordinated, methods of communication are limited, and control of body functions is restricted, the reflexes serve a variety of purposes. Some are protective (blink, gag,

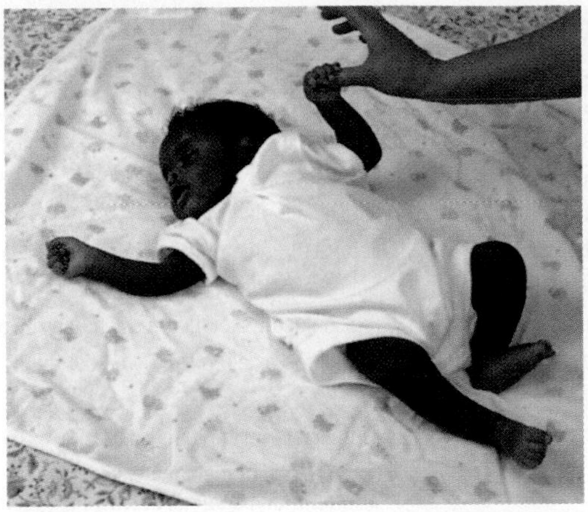

Figure 30-40 ■ Tonic neck reflex.

Source: George Dodson/Pearson Education.

sneeze); some aid in feeding (rooting, sucking) and may not be very active if the infant has eaten recently; and some stimulate human interaction (grasping).

The most common reflexes found in the normal newborn are the following:

- The **tonic neck reflex** (fencer position) is elicited when the newborn is supine and the head is turned to one side. In response, the extremities on the same side straighten, whereas on the opposite side they flex (Figure 30-40 ■). This reflex may not be seen during the early newborn period, but once it appears, it persists until about the third month.
- The **grasping reflex** is elicited by stimulating the newborn's palm with a finger or object. The newborn will grasp and hold the object or finger firmly enough to be lifted momentarily from the crib (Figure 30-41 ■).
- The **Moro reflex** is elicited when the newborn is startled by a loud noise or is lifted slightly above the crib and then suddenly lowered. In response the newborn straightens arms and hands outward while the knees flex. Slowly, the arms return to the chest, as in an embrace. The fingers spread, forming a C, and the newborn may cry (Figure 30-42 ■). This reflex may persist until about 6 months of age.

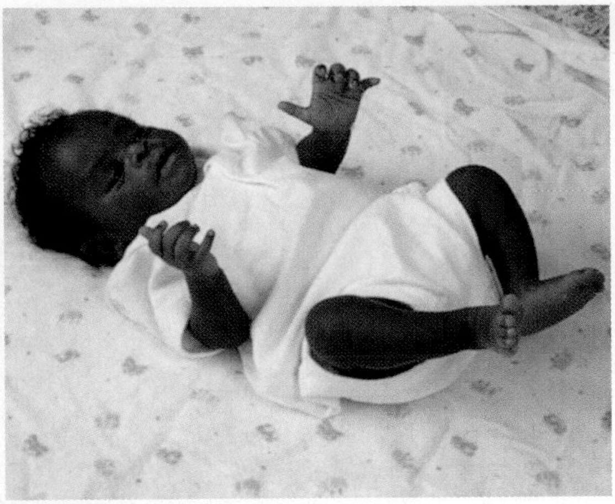

Figure 30-42 ■ Moro reflex.

- The **rooting reflex** is elicited when the side of the newborn's mouth or cheek is touched. In response the newborn turns toward that side and opens the lips to suck (if not fed recently) (Figure 30-43 ■).
- The **sucking reflex** is elicited when an object is placed in the newborn's mouth or anything touches the lips. Newborns suck even while sleeping; this is called nonnutritive sucking, and it can have a quieting effect on the baby.
- **Trunk incurvation (Galant reflex)** is seen when the newborn is prone. Stroking the spine causes the pelvis to turn to the stimulated side.

In addition to these reflexes, newborns can blink, yawn, cough, sneeze, and draw back from pain *(protective reflexes)*. They can even move a little on their own. When placed on their stomachs, they push up and try to crawl *(prone crawl)*. When held upright with one foot touching a flat surface, the newborn puts one foot in front of the other and "walks" *(stepping reflex)* (Figure 30-44 ■). This reflex is more pronounced at birth and is lost in 4 to 8 weeks. Table 30-5 summarizes the stimulus for and response of the common newborn reflexes.

Application: Newborn Reflexes

The nurse uses the following steps to assess CNS integration:

1. Insert a gloved finger into the newborn's mouth to elicit a sucking reflex.

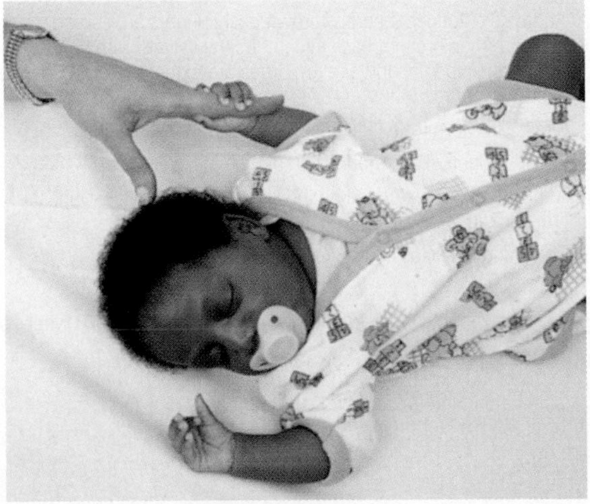

Figure 30-41 ■ Palmar grasping reflex.

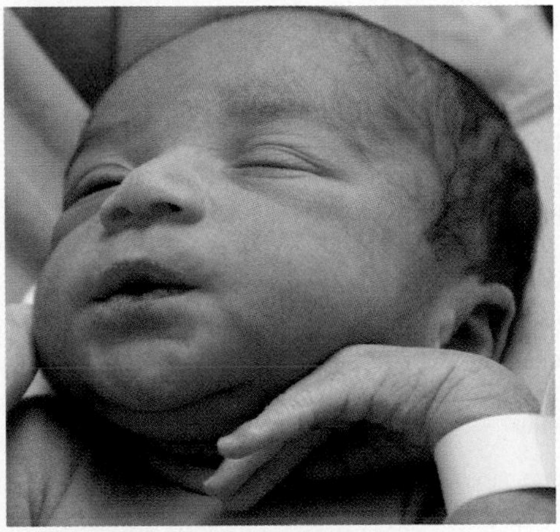

Figure 30-43 ■ Rooting reflex.

Source: George Dodson/Lightworks Studio/Pearson Education.

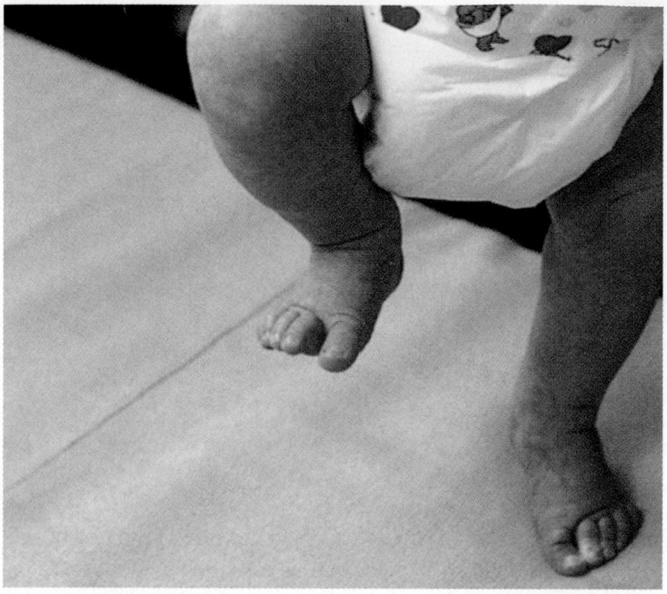

Figure 30-44 ■ The stepping reflex disappears between 4 and 8 weeks of age.

2. As soon as the newborn is sucking vigorously, assess hearing and vision responses by noting sucking changes in the presence of a light, a rattle, and a voice.
3. The newborn should respond with a brief cessation of sucking followed by continuous sucking with repeated stimulation.

This examination demonstrates auditory and visual integrity as well as complex behavioral interactions.

TABLE 30-6 Potential Birth Injuries

CLASSIFICATION	EXAMPLES*
Soft-tissue injuries	Lacerations, abrasions, bruising, fat necrosis
Skull injuries	Cephalhematoma,* fractures
Scalp laceration	Fetal scalp electrode
Scalp abscess	Fetal scalp electrode
Intracranial hemorrhage	Subdural, subarachnoid
Eye injuries	Subconjunctival* and retinal hemorrhages
Fractures	Clavicle,* facial bones, humerus, femur
Dislocations	Hips
Torticollis	Sternocleidomastoid muscle
Nerve injuries	Facial nerve,* brachial plexus,* phrenic nerve, recurrent laryngeal nerve (vocal cord paralysis), Horner syndrome
Spinal cord injuries	Spina bifida
Visceral rupture	Liver, spleen

*Most common birth injuries seen in newborns.

As healthcare providers carry out the newborn physical and neurologic assessment, they are always on the alert to recognize possible alterations and possible injuries related to the birth process that require further investigation and intervention. (See Table 30-6 for potential birth injuries.)

Newborn Physical Assessment Guide

Following is a guide for systematically assessing the newborn (pages 811–819). Normal findings, alterations, and related causes are presented in correlation with suggested nursing responses. The findings are typical for a full-term newborn.

TABLE 30-5 Common Reflexes of the Newborn

REFLEX NAME	EVOKING STIMULUS	RESPONSE
Blinking reflex	Light flash	Eyelids close.
Pupillary reflex	Light flash	Pupil constricts.
Rooting reflex	Light touch of finger on cheek close to mouth	Head rotates toward stimulation; mouth opens and attempts to suck finger. Disappears by about 4 months of age.
Sucking reflex	Finger (or nipple) inserted into mouth	Rhythmic sucking occurs.
Moro reflex	Infant lying on back: slightly raised head suddenly released; infant held horizontally, lowered quickly about 6 in., and stopped abruptly	Arms are extended, head is thrown back, fingers are spread wide; arms are then brought back to center convulsively with hands clenched; spine and lower extremities are extended. Disappears by about 6 months of age.
Startle reflex	Loud noise	Similar to Moro reflex flexion in arms; fists are clenched.
Grasping reflex	Finger placed in palm of hand	Infant's fingers close around and grasp object.
Tonic neck reflex	Head turned to one side while infant lies on back	Arm and leg are extended on the side the infant faces. Opposite arm and leg are flexed.
Abdominal reflex	Tactile stimulation or tickling	Abdominal muscles contract.
Withdrawal reflex	Slight pinprick to the sole of the infant's foot	Leg flexes.
Walking reflex	Infant supported in an upright position with feet lightly touching a flat surface	Rhythmic stepping movement. Disappears at about 4 to 8 weeks of age.
Babinski reflex response	Gentle stroking on the sole of each foot	Fanning and extension of the toes (adults respond to this stimulation with flexion of toes).
Plantar, or toe-grasping, reflex	Pressure applied with the finger against the balls of the infant's feet	A plantar flexion of all toes. Disappears by the end of the first year of life.

Source: Adapted from Mott, S. R., James, S. R., & Sperhac, A. M. (1990). Nursing care of children and families: A holistic approach *(2nd ed.). Menlo Park, CA: Addison-Wesley Nursing.*

ASSESSMENT GUIDE Newborn Physical Assessment

Physical Assessment/Normal Findings	Alterations and Possible Causes*	Nursing Responses to Data[†]
VITAL SIGNS		
Blood pressure (BP): At birth: 70–50/45–30 mm Hg	Low BP (hypovolemia, shock)	Monitor BP in all cases of distress, prematurity, or suspected anomaly.
Day 10: 90–60/50–40 mm Hg (may be unable to measure diastolic pressure with standard sphygmomanometer)		Low BP: Refer to physician immediately so measures to improve circulation are begun.
Pulse: 110–160 beats/min (if in deep sleep, as low as 70 beats/min; if crying, up to 180 beats/min)	Weak pulse (decreased cardiac output) Bradycardia (severe asphyxia, arrhythmia) Tachycardia (over 160 beats/min at rest) (infection, central nervous system (CNS) problems, arrhythmia, stress, hypovolemia)	Assess skin perfusion by blanching (capillary refill test—normal: $<$3 sec). Correlate finding with BP assessments; refer to physician. Carry out neurologic and thermoregulation assessments. Check blood pressure and hematocrit (Hct).
Respirations: 30–60 breaths/min		
Synchronization of chest and abdominal movements Diaphragmatic and abdominal breathing	Tachypnea (pneumonia, respiratory distress syndrome [RDS])	Identify sleep-wake state; correlate with respiratory pattern.
	Rapid, shallow breathing (hypermagnesemia due to large doses given to mothers with preeclampsia)	Evaluate for all signs of respiratory distress; report findings to physician.
	Respirations below 30 breaths/min (maternal anesthesia or analgesia)	
Transient tachypnea	Expiratory grunting; subcostal and substernal retractions; flaring of nares (respiratory distress); apnea (cold stress, respiratory disorder)	Evaluate for cold stress. Report findings to physician or neonatal nurse practitioner.
Crying: Strong and lusty Moderate tone and pitch	High pitched, shrill (neurologic disorder, hypoglycemia)	Discuss newborn's use of cry for communication. Assess and record abnormal cries.
Cries vary in length from 3 to 7 min after consoling measures are used	Weak or absent (CNS disorder, laryngeal problem)	Reduce environmental noises.
Temperature: Axilla 36.4–37.2°C (97.5–99°F)	Elevated temperature (room too warm, too much clothing or covers, dehydration, sepsis, brain damage)	Notify physician of elevation or drop.
	Subnormal temperature (brain stem involvement, cold, sepsis)	Counsel parents on possible causes of elevated or low temperatures, appropriate home care measures, when to call physician.
Heavier newborns tend to have higher body temperatures	Swings of more than 2°F from one reading to next or subnormal temperature (infection)	Teach parents how to take an axillary temperature; assess parents' knowledge regarding use of thermometer; provide teaching as needed.
Weight: 2500–4000 g (5 lb, 8 oz–8 lb, 13 oz)	Less than 2748 g (less than 6 lb) = SGA or preterm infant Greater than 4050 g (greater than 9 lb) = large-for-gestational-age (LGA) or infants of diabetic mothers	Plot weight and gestational age on growth chart to identify high-risk infants. Ascertain body build of parents. Counsel parents regarding appropriate caloric intake.
Within first 3 to 4 days, normal weight loss of 5%–10% Large babies tend to lose more due to greater fluid loss in proportion to birth weight except infants of diabetic mothers	Loss greater than 15% (low fluid intake, loss of meconium and urine, feeding difficulties, diabetes insipidus)	Notify physician of net losses or gains. Calculate fluid intake and losses from all sources (insensible water loss, radiant warmers, phototherapy lights). Daily weights and before discharge.
Length: 48–52 cm (18–22 in.)	Less than 45 cm (congenital dwarf)	Assess for other signs of dwarfism.
Grows 10 cm (3 in.) during first 3 months	Short/long bones proximally (achondroplasia)	Determine other signs of skeletal system adequacy.
	Short/long bones distally (Ellis-van Creveld syndrome)	Plot progress at subsequent well-baby visits.
POSTURE		
Body usually flexed, hands may be tightly clenched, neck appears short because chin rests on chest	Only extension noted, inability to move from midline (trauma, hypoxia, immaturity)	Record spontaneity of motor activity and symmetry of movements.
In breech births, feet are usually dorsiflexed	Constant motion (maternal caffeine intake or drug withdrawal)	If parents express concern about newborn's movement patterns, reassure and further evaluate if appropriate.
SKIN		
Color: Color consistent with ethnic background	Pallor of face conjunctiva (anemia, hypothermia, anoxia)	Discuss with parents common skin color variations to allay fears. Skin color can vary widely within African-American infants.
	*Possible causes of alterations are placed in parentheses.	[†]This column provides guidelines for further assessment and initial nursing interventions.

(continued)

ASSESSMENT GUIDE **Newborn Physical Assessment** continued

Physical Assessment/Normal Findings	Alterations and Possible Causes*	Nursing Responses to Data†
SKIN (continued)		
Newborns of European descent: pink-tinged or ruddy color over face, trunk, extremities Newborns of African or Native American descent: pale pink with yellow or red tinge Newborns of Asian descent: pink or rosy red to yellow tinge	Beefy red (hypoglycemia, immature vasomotor reflexes, polycythemia)	Document extent and time of occurrence of color change.
Common variations: acrocyanosis, circumoral cyanosis, harlequin color change, or mongolian spots	Meconium staining (nonreassuring fetal status) Jaundice (hemolytic reaction from blood incompatibility within first 24 hours, sepsis)	Obtain Hgb and hematocrit values; obtain bilirubin levels. Assess for respiratory difficulty and temperature instability. Differentiate between physiologic and pathologic jaundice.
Mottled when undressed	Cyanosis (choanal atresia, CNS damage or trauma, respiratory or cardiac problem, cold stress)	Assess degree of (central or peripheral) cyanosis and possible causes; refer to physician.
Minor bruising over buttocks in breech presentation and over eyes and forehead in facial presentations		Discuss with parents cause and course of minor bruising related to labor and birth.
Texture: Smooth, soft, flexible; may have dry, peeling hands and feet	Generalized cracked or peeling skin (small-for-gestational-age [SGA] or postterm; blood incompatibility; metabolic, kidney dysfunction) Seborrheic-dermatitis (cradle cap) Absence of vernix (postmature) Yellow vernix (bilirubin staining)	Report to physician. Instruct parents to shampoo the scalp and anterior fontanelle areas daily with mild soap or baby shampoo; rinse well; avoid use of oil.
Turgor: Elastic, returns to normal shape after pinching	Maintains tent shape (dehydration)	Assess for other signs and symptoms of dehydration.
Pigmentation: Clear; milia across bridge of nose, forehead, or chin will disappear within a few weeks		Advise parents not to pinch or prick these pimplelike areas.
Café-au-lait spots (one or two)	Six or more spots (neurologic disorder such as von Recklinghausen disease, cutaneous neurofibromatosis)	If there are six or more café-au-lait spots, refer for genetic and neurologic consult.
Mongolian blue spots common over dorsal area and buttocks in dark-skinned infants		Assure parents of normality of this pigmentation; it will fade in first year or two.
Erythema toxicum	Impetigo (group A β-hemolytic streptococcus or *Staphylococcus aureus* infection)	If impetigo occurs, instruct parents about hand washing and linen precautions during home care.
Telangiectatic nevi	Hemangiomas: Nevus flammeus (port-wine stain) Nevus vasculosus (strawberry hemangioma) Cavernous hemangiomas	Collaborate with physician. Counsel parents about birthmark's progression to allay misconceptions. Record size and shape of hemangiomas. Refer for follow-up at well-baby clinic.
Rashes	Rashes (infection)	Assess location and type of rash (macular, papular, vesicular). Obtain history of onset, prenatal history, and related signs and symptoms.
Petechiae of head or neck (breech presentation, cord around neck)	Generalized petechiae (clotting abnormalities)	Determine cause; advise parents if further health care is needed.
HEAD		
General appearance, size, movement Round, symmetric, and moves easily from left to right and up and down; soft and pliable	Asymmetric, flattened occiput on either side of the head (plagiocephaly) Head held at angle (torticollis) Unable to move head side to side (neurologic trauma)	Instruct parents to change infant's positions frequently when awake. When awake, needs to spend "tummy time." Infants should be placed supine for sleep per "Back to Sleep" guidelines (see chapters 31 and 37). Determine adequacy of all neurologic signs.
Circumference: 32–37 cm (12.5–14.5 in.); 2 cm greater than chest circumference Head one fourth of body size	Extreme differences in size may be due to microencephaly (Cornelia de Lange syndrome, cytomegalic inclusion disease [CID]), rubella, toxoplasmosis, chromosome abnormalities, hydrocephalus (meningomyelocele, achondroplasia), anencephaly (neural tube defect) Head is 3 cm or more larger than chest circumference (preterm, hydrocephalus)	Measure circumference from occiput to frontal area using metal or paper tape. Measure chest circumference using metal or paper tape and compare to head circumference. Record measurements on growth chart. Reevaluate at well-baby visits.
	*Possible causes of alterations are placed in parentheses.	†This column provides guidelines for further assessment and initial nursing interventions.

ASSESSMENT GUIDE Newborn Physical Assessment continued

Physical Assessment/Normal Findings	Alterations and Possible Causes*	Nursing Responses to Data†
HEAD (continued)		
Common variations: Molding	Cephalhematoma (trauma during birth, may persist up to 3 months)	Evaluate neurologic response.
Breech and cesarean newborns' heads are round and well shaped	Caput succedaneum (long labor and birth; disappears in 1 week)	Observe for hyperbilirubinemia. Check Hct. Reassure parents regarding common manifestations due to birth process and when they should disappear.
Fontanelles: Palpation of juncture of cranial bones	Overlapping of anterior fontanelle (malnourished or preterm newborn)	Discuss normal closure times with parents and care of "soft spots" to allay misconceptions.
Anterior fontanelle; 3–4 cm long by 2–3 cm wide, diamond shaped	Premature closure of sutures (craniosynostosis)	Refer to physician. Assess fontanelles and sutures daily.
Posterior fontanelle: 1–2 cm at birth, triangle shaped	Late closure (hydrocephalus)	Observe for signs and symptoms of hydrocephalus.
Slight pulsation	Moderate to severe pulsation (vascular problems)	Refer to physician.
Moderate bulging noted with crying, stooling; pulsations with heartbeat	Bulging (increased intracranial pressure, meningitis) Sunken (dehydration)	Report to physician. Evaluate neurologic status. Evaluate hydration status.
HAIR		
Texture: Smooth with fine texture variations (*Note:* Variations depend on ethnic background.)	Coarse, brittle, dry hair (hypothyroidism) White forelock (Waardenburg syndrome)	Instruct parents regarding routine care of hair and scalp.
Distribution: Scalp hair high over eyebrows (Spanish, Mexican hairline begins midforehead and extends down back of neck)	Low forehead and posterior hairlines may indicate chromosomal disorders	Assess for other signs of chromosomal aberrations. Refer to physician.
FACE		
Symmetric movement of all facial features, normal hairline, eyebrows and eyelashes present		Assess and record symmetry of all parts, shape, regularity of features, sameness or differences in features.
Spacing of features: Eyes-ears at same level, nostrils equal size, cheeks full, and sucking pads present	Eyes wide apart—ocular hypertelorism (Apert syndrome, Cri-du-chat, Turner syndrome)	Observe for other signs and symptoms indicative of disease states or chromosomal aberrations.
Lips equal on both sides of midline	Abnormal face (Down syndrome, cretinism, gargoylism)	
Chin recedes when compared with other bones of face	Atypical small jaw—micrognathia (Pierre Robin syndrome, Treacher Collins syndrome)	Maintain airway; may do best in prone position. Initiate surgical consultation and referral.
Movement: Makes facial grimaces	Inability to suck, grimace, and close eyelids (cranial nerve injury)	Initiate neurologic assessment and consultation.
Symmetric when resting and crying	Asymmetry (paralysis of facial cranial nerve)	Assess and record symmetry of all parts, shape, regularity of features, and sameness or differences in features.
EYES		
General placement and appearance: Bright and clear; even placement; slight nystagmus (involuntary cyclic eye movements)	Gross nystagmus (damage to third, fourth, and sixth cranial nerves)	
Concomitant strabismus	Constant and fixed strabismus	Reassure parents that strabismus is considered normal up to 6 months.
Move in all directions Blue-gray or slate–blue-gray	Lack of pigmentation (albinism) Brushfield spots may indicate Down syndrome (a light or white speckling of the outer two thirds of the iris)	Discuss with parents any necessary eye precautions. Assess for other signs of Down syndrome.
Brown color at birth in dark-skinned infants		Discuss with parents that permanent eye color is usually established by 3 months of age.
Eyelids: Position: above pupils but within iris, no drooping	Elevation or retraction of upper lid (hyperthyroidism). "Sunset sign" lid retraction and downward gaze (hydrocephalus), ptosis (congenital or paralysis of oculomotor muscle)	Assess for signs of hydrocephalus and hyperthyroidism. Evaluate interference with vision in subsequent well-baby visits.
Eyes on parallel plane	Upward slant in non-Asians (Down syndrome)	Assess for other signs of Down syndrome.
Epicanthal folds in Asian and 20% of newborns of northern European descent	Epicanthal folds (Down syndrome, Cri-du-chat syndrome)	
Movement: Blink reflex in response to light stimulus. Eyes open wide in dimly lighted room	Blink absent (CNS injury)	Evaluate neurologic status Refer to physician.
	*Possible causes of alterations are placed in parentheses.	†This column provides guidelines for further assessment and initial nursing interventions.

(continued)

ASSESSMENT GUIDE Newborn Physical Assessment continued

Physical Assessment/Normal Findings	Alterations and Possible Causes*	Nursing Responses to Data[†]
EYES (continued)		
Inspection: Edematous for first few days of life, resulting from birth; no lumps or redness	Purulent drainage (infection); infectious conjunctivitis (gonococcus, chlamydia, staphylococcus, or gram-negative organisms) Marginal blepharitis (lid edges red, crusted, scaly)	Initiate good hand washing. Refer to physician. Evaluate infant for seborrheic dermatitis; scales can be removed easily.
Cornea: Clear	Ulceration (herpes infection); large cornea or corneas of unequal size (congenital glaucoma)	Refer to ophthalmologist.
Corneal reflex present	Clouding, opacity of lens (cataract)	Assess for other manifestations of congenital herpes; institute nursing care measures.
Sclera: May appear bluish in newborn, then white; slightly brownish color frequent in newborns of African descent	True blue sclera (osteogenesis imperfecta)	Refer to physician.
Pupils: Pupils equal in size, round, and react to light by accommodation	Anisocoria—unequal pupils (CNS damage) Dilation or constriction (intracranial damage, retinoblastoma, glaucoma) Pupils nonreactive to light or accommodation (brain injury)	Refer for neurologic examination.
Slight nystagmus in newborn who has not learned to focus	Nystagmus (labyrinthine disturbance, CNS disorder)	
Pupil light reflex demonstrated at birth or by 3 weeks of age		
Conjunctiva: Chemical conjunctivitis Subconjunctival hemorrhage	Pale color (anemia)	Obtain hematocrit and hemoglobin. Reassure parents that chemical conjunctivitis will subside in 1 to 2 days and subconjunctival hemorrhage disappears in a few weeks.
Palpebral conjunctival (red but not hyperemic)	Inflammation or edema (infection, blocked tear duct)	
Vision: 20/200 Tracks moving object to midline Fixed focus on objects at a distance of about 10–20 inches; may be difficult to evaluate in newborn Prefers faces, geometric designs, and black and white to colors	Cataracts (congenital infection)	Record any questions about visual acuity and initiate follow-up evaluation at first well-baby checkup. May suggest toys for parents to purchase—see chapter 34 ∞.
Lashes and lacrimal glands: Presence of lashes (lashes may be absent in preterm newborns)	No lashes on inner two thirds of lid (Treacher Collins syndrome), bushy lashes (Hurler syndrome), long lashes (Cornelia de Lange syndrome)	
Cry commonly tearless	Excessive tearing (plugged lacrimal duct, natal narcotic withdrawal), glaucoma	Demonstrate to parents how to milk blocked tear duct. Refer to ophthalmologist if tearing is excessive before third month of life.
NOSE		
Appearance of external nasal aspects: May appear flattened as a result of birth process	Continued flat or broad bridge of nose (Down syndrome)	Arrange consultation with specialist. May be normal racial variation—Asian or African ancestry.
Small and narrow in midline, even placement in relationship to eyes and mouth	Low bridge of nose, beaklike nose (Apert syndrome, Treacher Collins syndrome) Upturned (Cornelia de Lange syndrome)	Initiate evaluation of chromosomal abnormalities.
Patent nares bilaterally (nose breathers)	Blockage of nares (mucus or secretions), choanal atresia	Inspect for obstruction of nares.
Sneezing common to clear nasal passages	Flaring nares (respiratory distress)	Maintain oral airway until surgical correction is made.
Responds to odors, may smell breast milk	No response to stimulating odors	Inspect for obstruction of nares.
MOUTH		
Function of facial, hypoglossal, glossopharyngeal, and vagus nerves: Symmetry of movement and strength	Mouth draws to one side (transient seventh cranial nerve paralysis due to pressure in utero or trauma during birth, congenital paralysis)	Initiate neurologic consultation.
	Fishlike shape (Treacher Collins syndrome)	Administer artificial tears if eye on affected side of face is unable to close.
Presence of gag, swallowing, coordinated with sucking reflexes	Suppressed or absent reflexes	Evaluate other neurologic functions of these nerves.
Adequate salivation		
	*Possible causes of alterations are placed in parentheses.	[†]This column provides guidelines for further assessment and initial nursing interventions.

ASSESSMENT GUIDE Newborn Physical Assessment continued

Physical Assessment/Normal Findings	Alterations and Possible Causes*	Nursing Responses to Data[†]
MOUTH (continued)		
Palate (soft and hard): Hard palate dome shaped. Uvula midline with symmetric movement of soft palate	High-steepled palate (Treacher Collins syndrome), bifid uvula (congenital anomaly)	Assess for other congenital anomalies.
Palate intact, sucks well when stimulated	Clefts in either hard or soft palate (polygenic disorder)	Initiate a surgical consultation referral. Use special feeding devices.
Epithelial (Epstein's) pearls appear on mucosa		Assure parents that these are normal and will disappear at 2 or 3 months of age.
Esophagus patent, some drooling common in newborn	Excessive drooling or bubbling (esophageal atresia)	Test for patency of esophagus.
Tongue: Free moving in all directions, midline	Lack of movement or asymmetric movement (neurologic damage) Tongue-tied Fasiculations (fine tremors) Spinal muscular atrophy	Further assess neurologic functions. Test reflex elevation of tongue when depressed with tongue blade.
Pink color, smooth to rough texture, noncoated	Deviations from midline (cranial nerve damage) White cheesy coating (thrush) Tongue has deep ridges	Check for signs of weakness or deviation. Differentiate between thrush and milk curds by wiping: if white patches don't come off easily, it is thrush. Reassure parents that tongue pattern may change from day to day.
Tongue proportional to mouth	Large tongue with short frenulum (cretinism, Down syndrome, other syndromes)	Evaluate in well-baby clinic to assess development delays. Initiate referrals.
EARS		
External ear: Without lesions, cysts, or nodules	Nodules, cysts, or sinus tracts in front of ear Adherent earlobes Low set (genetic abnormality or syndrome) Preauricular skin tags	Evaluate characteristics of lesions. Counsel parents to clean external ear with washcloth only; discourage use of cotton-tip applicators. Refer to physician for ligation.
Hearing: Eustachian tubes are cleared with first cry		
Absence of all risk factors	Presence of one or more risk factors	Assess history of risk factors for hearing loss.
Attends to sounds; sudden or loud noise. Elicits Moro reflex	No response to sound stimuli (deafness)	Test for Moro reflex.
NECK		
Appearance: Short, straight, creased with skin folds	Abnormally short neck (Turner syndrome) Arching or inability to flex neck (meningitis, congenital anomaly)	Report findings to physician.
Posterior neck lacks loose extra folds of skin	Webbing of neck (Turner syndrome, Down syndrome, trisomy 18)	Assess for other signs of the syndromes.
Clavicles: Straight and intact	Knot or lump on clavicle (fracture during difficult birth)	Obtain detailed labor and birth history; apply figure-eight bandage. Consider oral analgesic.
Moro reflex elicitable	Unilateral Moro reflex response on unaffected side (fracture of clavicle, brachial palsy, Erb-Duchenne paralysis)	
Symmetric shoulders	Hypoplasia	
CHEST		
Appearance and size: Circumference: 32.5 cm, 1–2 cm less than head		Measure at level of nipples after exhalation.
Wider than it is long		
Normal shape without depressed or prominent sternum	Funnel chest (congenital or associated with Marfan syndrome)	Determine adequacy of other respiratory and circulatory signs.
Lower end of sternum (xiphoid cartilage) may be protruding; less apparent after several weeks	Continued protrusion of xiphoid cartilage (Marfan syndrome, "pigeon chest")	Assess for other signs and symptoms of various syndromes.
Sternum 8 cm long	Barrel chest	
	*Possible causes of alterations are placed in parentheses.	[†]This column provides guidelines for further assessment and initial nursing interventions.

(continued)

ASSESSMENT GUIDE Newborn Physical Assessment continued

Physical Assessment/Normal Findings	Alterations and Possible Causes*	Nursing Responses to Data†
CHEST (continued)		
Expansion and retraction: Bilateral expansion	Unequal chest expansion (pneumonia, pneumothorax, respiratory distress)	Assess respiratory effort regularity, flaring of nares, difficulty on both inspiration and expiration.
No intercostal, subcostal, or supraclavicular retractions	Retractions (respiratory distress) Seesaw respirations (respiratory distress)	
Auscultation: Breath sounds are louder in infants	Decreased breath sounds (decreased respiratory activity, atelectasis, pneumothorax)	Obtain transilluminator. Record findings and consult physician.
Chest and axilla clear on crying	Increased breath sounds (resolving pneumonia or in cesarean births)	Perform assessment and report to physician any positive findings.
Bronchial breath sounds (heard where trachea and bronchi closest to chest wall, above sternum and between scapulae):		
Bronchial sounds bilaterally Air entry clear Rales may indicate normal newborn atelectasis Cough reflex absent at birth, appears in 2 or more days	Adventitious or abnormal sounds (respiratory disease or distress)	Evaluate color for pallor or cyanosis. Monitor every shift or more frequently. Report to physician.
Breasts: Flat with symmetric nipples	Lack of breast tissue (preterm or SGA)	
Breast tissue diameter 5 cm or more at term	Discharge	Evaluate for infection.
Average distance between nipples 8 cm	Breast abscesses	
Breast engorgement occurs on third day of life; liquid discharge may be expressed in term newborns	Enlargement	Reassure parents of normality of breast engorgement.
Nipples	Supernumerary nipples Dark-colored nipples	No intervention is necessary.
HEART		
Auscultation: Location: lies horizontally, with left border extending to left of midclavicle		
Regular rhythm and rate	Arrhythmia (anoxia), tachycardia, bradycardia	Refer all arrhythmia and gallop rhythms. Initiate cardiac evaluation.
Determination of point of maximal impulse (PMI)	Malpositioning (enlargement, abnormal placement, pneumothorax, dextrocardia, diaphragmatic hernia)	
Usually lateral to midclavicular line at third or fourth intercostal space		
Functional murmurs No thrills	Location of murmurs (possible congenital cardiac anomaly)	Evaluate murmur: location, timing, and duration; observe for accompanying cardiac pathology symptoms; ascertain family history.
Horizontal groove at diaphragm shows flaring of rib cage to mild degree	Marked rib flaring (vitamin D deficiency) Inadequacy of respiratory movement	Initiate cardiopulmonary evaluation; assess pulses and blood pressures in all four extremities for equality and quality.
ABDOMEN		
Appearance: Cylindric, with some protrusion; appears large in relation to pelvis; some laxness of abdominal muscles	Distention, shiny abdomen with engorged vessels (gastrointestinal abnormalities, infection, congenital megacolon)	Examine abdomen thoroughly for mass or organomegaly. Measure abdominal girth.
No cyanosis, few vessels seen	Scaphoid abdominal appearance (diaphragmatic hernia)	Report deviations of abdominal size.
Diastasis recti—common in infants of African descent	Increased or decreased peristalsis (duodenal stenosis, small bowel obstruction)	Assess other signs and symptoms of obstruction.
	Localized flank bulging (enlarged kidneys, ascites, absent abdominal muscles)	Refer to physician.
Umbilicus: No protrusion of umbilicus (protrusion of umbilicus common in infants of African descent) Bluish white color	Umbilical hernia Patent urachus (congenital malformation)	Measure umbilical hernia by palpating the opening and record; it should close by 1 year of age; if not, refer to physician. Be aware of cultural practices. Taping or belly bands do not enhance closure.
	Omphalocele (covered defect) Gastroschisis (uncovered defect)	Cover omphalocele and gastroschisis with sterile, moist dressing or plastic sterile bag.
	*Possible causes of alterations are placed in parentheses.	†This column provides guidelines for further assessment and initial nursing interventions.

ASSESSMENT GUIDE **Newborn Physical Assessment** continued

Physical Assessment/Normal Findings	Alterations and Possible Causes*	Nursing Responses to Data[†]
ABDOMEN (continued)		
Cutis navel (umbilical cord projects), granulation tissue present in navel	Redness or exudate around cord (infection) Yellow discoloration (hemolytic disease, meconium staining)	Instruct parents on cord care and hygiene.
Two arteries and one vein apparent	Single umbilical artery (congenital anomalies)	Refer anomalies to physician.
Begins drying 1 to 2 hours after birth	Discharge or oozing of blood from the cord	
No bleeding		
Auscultation and percussion: Soft bowel sounds heard shortly after birth every 10–30 seconds	Bowel sounds in chest (diaphragmatic hernia) Absence of bowel sounds Hyperperistalsis (intestinal obstruction)	Collaborate with physician. Assess for other signs of dehydration or infection.
Femoral pulses: Palpable, equal, bilateral	Absent or diminished femoral pulses (coarctation of aorta)	Monitor blood pressure in upper and lower extremities.
Inguinal area: No bulges along inguinal area	Inguinal hernia	Initiate referral.
No inguinal lymph nodes felt		Continue follow-up in well-baby clinic.
Bladder: Percusses 1–4 cm above symphysis	Failure to void within 24–48 hours after birth	Determine whether baby voided at birth.
Emptied about 3 hours after birth; if not, at time of birth	Exposure of bladder mucosa (exstrophy of bladder)	Consult with clinician. Cover exstrophy with sterile moist gauze.
Urine—inoffensive, mild odor	Foul odor (infection)	Obtain urine specimen if infection is suspected.
GENITALS		
Gender clearly delineated	Ambiguous genitals	Refer for genetic consultation.
MALE		
Penis: Slender in appearance, about 2.5 cm long, 1 cm wide at birth	Micropenis (congenital anomaly) Meatal atresia	Observe and record first voiding.
Normal urinary orifice, urethral meatus at tip of penis	Hypospadias, epispadias	Collaborate with physician in presence of abnormality. Delay circumcision.
Noninflamed urethral opening	Urethritis (infection)	Palpate for enlarged inguinal lymph nodes and record painful urination.
Foreskin adheres to glans	Ulceration of meatal opening (infection, inflammation)	Evaluate whether ulcer is due to diaper rash; counsel regarding care.
Uncircumcised foreskin tight for 2 to 3 months	Phimosis—if still tight after 3 months	Instruct parents on how to care for uncircumcised penis.
Circumcised		Teach parents how to care for circumcision. Check for voiding after procedure and evaluate for excessive bleeding.
Erectile tissue present		
Scrotum: Skin loose and hanging or tight and small; extensive rugae and normal size	Large scrotum containing fluid (hydrocele) Red, shiny scrotal skin (orchitis)	Shine a light through scrotum (transilluminate) to verify diagnosis.
Normal skin color Scrotal discoloration common in breech	Minimal rugae, small scrotum	Assess for prematurity.
Testes: Descended by birth; not consistently found in scrotum	Undescended testes (cryptorchidism)	If testes cannot be felt in scrotum, gently palpate femoral, inguinal, perineal, and abdominal areas for presence.
Testes size 1.5–2 cm (0.6–0.8 in.) at birth	Enlarged testes (tumor) Small testes (Klinefelter syndrome or adrenal hyperplasia)	Refer to and collaborate with physician for further diagnostic studies.
FEMALE		
Mons: Normal skin color, area pigmented in dark-skinned infants		
Labia majora cover labia minora in term and postterm newborns; symmetric size appropriate for gestational age	Hematoma, lesions (trauma) Labia minora prominent	Evaluate for recent trauma. Assess for prematurity.
Clitoris: Normally large in newborn Edema and bruising in breech birth	Hypertrophy (hermaphroditism)	Refer for genetic workup.
Vagina: Urinary meatus and vaginal orifice visible (0.5 cm circumference)	Inflammation; erythema and discharge (urethritis) Congenital absence of vagina	Collect urine specimen for laboratory examination. Refer to physician.
Discharge; smegma under labia	Foul-smelling discharge (infection)	Collect data and further evaluate reason for discharge.
Bloody or mucoid discharge	Excessive vaginal bleeding (blood coagulation defect)	
	*Possible causes of alterations are placed in parentheses.	[†]This column provides guidelines for further assessment and initial nursing interventions.

(continued)

ASSESSMENT GUIDE Newborn Physical Assessment continued

Physical Assessment/Normal Findings	Alterations and Possible Causes*	Nursing Responses to Data†
BUTTOCKS AND ANUS		
Buttocks symmetric	Pilonidal dimple	Examine for possible sinus. Instruct parents about cleansing this area.
Anus patent and passage of meconium within 24–48 hours after birth	Imperforate anus, rectal atresia (congenital gastrointestinal defect)	Evaluate extent of problems. Initiate surgical consultation.
No fissures, tears, or skin tags	Fissures	Perform digital examination to ascertain patency if patency uncertain.
EXTREMITIES AND TRUNK		
Short and generally flexed; extremities move symmetrically through range of motion but lack full extension	Unilateral or absence of movement (spinal cord involvement) Fetal position continued or limp (anoxia, CNS problems, hypoglycemia)	Review birth record to assess possible cause.
All joints move spontaneously; good muscle tone, of flexor type, birth to 2 months	Spasticity when infant begins using extensors (cerebral palsy, lack of muscle tone, "floppy baby" syndrome) Hypotonia (Down syndrome)	Collaborate with physician.
Arms: Equal in length	Brachial palsy (difficult birth)	Report to clinician.
Bilateral movement	Erb-Duchenne paralysis	
Flexed when quiet	Muscle weakness, fractured clavicle Absence of limb or change of size (phocomelia, amelia)	
Hands: Normal number of fingers	Polydactyly (Ellis-van Creveld syndrome) Syndactyly—one limb (developmental anomaly) Syndactyly—both limbs (genetic component)	Report to clinician.
Normal palmar crease	Single line on palm (Down syndrome)	Refer for genetic workup.
Normal-sized hands	Short fingers and broad hand (Hurler syndrome)	Evaluate for history of distress in utero.
Nails present and extend beyond fingertips in term newborn.	Cyanosis and clubbing (cardiac anomalies) Nails long or yellow stained (postterm)	Carry out cardiac and respiratory assessments. Check pulse oximetry.
Spine: C-shaped spine	Spina bifida occulta (nevus pilosus)	Evaluate extent of neurologic damage; initiate care of spinal opening.
Flat and straight when prone	Dermal sinus	
Slight lumbar lordosis	Myelomeningocele	
Easily flexed and intact when palpated	Head lag, limp, floppy trunk (neurologic problems)	
At least half of back devoid of lanugo		
Full-term infant in ventral suspension should hold head at 45-degree angle, back straight		Elicit reflex to assess degree of involvement.
Hips: No sign of instability	Sensation of abnormal movement; jerk, or snap of hip dislocation	Physician or nurse practitioner examines all newborn infants for dislocated hip prior to discharge from birthing center.
Hips abduct to more than 60 degrees		If this is suspected, refer to orthopedist for further evaluation. Reassess at well-baby visits.
Inguinal and buttock skin creases: Symmetric inguinal and buttock creases	Asymmetry (dislocated hips)	Refer to orthopedist for evaluation. Counsel parents regarding symptoms of concern and discuss therapy.
Legs: Legs equal in length	Shortened leg (dislocated hips)	Refer to orthopedist for evaluation.
Legs shorter than arms at birth	Lack of leg movement (fractures, spinal defects)	Counsel parents regarding symptoms of concern and discuss therapy.
Feet: Foot is in straight line	Talipes equinovarus (true clubfoot)	Discuss differences between positional and true clubfoot with parents.
Positional clubfoot—based on position in utero		Teach parents passive manipulation of foot. Refer to orthopedist if not corrected by 3 months of age.
Fat pads and creases on soles of feet	Incomplete sole creases in first 24 hours of life (premature)	
Talipes planus (flat feet) normal under 3 years of age		Reassure parents that flat feet are normal in infants.
	*Possible causes of alterations are placed in parentheses.	†This column provides guidelines for further assessment and initial nursing interventions.

ASSESSMENT GUIDE Newborn Physical Assessment continued

Physical Assessment/Normal Findings	Alterations and Possible Causes*	Nursing Responses to Data[†]
NEUROMUSCULAR		
Motor function: Symmetric movement and strength in all extremities	Limp, flaccid, or hypertonic (CNS disorders, infection, dehydration, fracture)	Appraise newborn's posture and motor functions by observing activities and motor characteristics.
May be jerky or have brief twitchings	Tremors (hypoglycemia, hypocalcemia, infection, neurologic damage)	Evaluate for electrolyte imbalance, hypoglycemia, and neurologic functioning.
Head lag not over 45 degrees	Delayed or abnormal development (preterm, neurologic involvement)	
Neck control adequate to maintain head erect briefly	Asymmetry of tone or strength (neurologic damage)	Refer for genetic evaluation.
REFLEXES		
Blink: Stimulated by flash of light; response is closure of eyelids	Lack of blink response (damage to cranial nerve, CNS injury)	Assess neurologic status.
Pupillary reflex: Stimulated by flash of light; response is constriction of pupil	Lack of reflex (damage to cranial nerve, CNS injury)	
Moro: Response to sudden movement or loud noise should be one of symmetric extension and abduction of arms with fingers extended; then return to normal relaxed flexion.	Asymmetry of body response (fractured clavicle, injury to brachial plexus)	Discuss normality of this reflex in response to loud noises or sudden movements.
Infant lying on back: slightly raised head suddenly released; infant held horizontally, lowered quickly about 6 inches, and stopped abruptly	Consistent absence (brain damage)	Absence of reflex requires neurologic evaluation.
Fingers form a C		
Present at birth; disappears by 6 months of age		
Rooting and sucking: Turns in direction of stimulus to cheek or mouth; opens mouth and begins to suck rhythmically when finger or nipple is inserted into mouth; difficult to elicit after feeding; disappears by 4 to 7 months of age	Poor sucking or easily fatigable (preterm, breastfed infants of drug-addicted mothers, possible cardiac problem) Absence of response (preterm, neurologic involvement, depressed newborns)	Evaluate strength and coordination of sucking. Observe newborn during feeding, and counsel parents about mutuality of feeding experience and newborn's responses.
Sucking is adequate for nutritional intake and meeting oral stimulation needs; disappears by 12 months		
Palmar grasp: Fingers grasp adult finger when palm is stimulated and held momentarily; lessens at 3 to 4 months of age	Asymmetry of response (neurologic problems)	Evaluate other reflexes and general neurologic functioning.
Plantar grasp: Toes curl downward when sole of foot is stimulated; lessens by 8 months	Absent (defects of lower spinal column)	Assess for other lower extremity neurologic problems.
Stepping: When held upright and one foot touching a flat surface, will step alternately; disappears at 4 to 8 weeks of age	Asymmetry of stepping (neurologic abnormality)	Evaluate muscle tone and function on each side of body. Refer to specialist.
Babinski: Fanning and extension of all toes when one side of sole is stroked from heel upward across ball of foot; disappears at about 12 months	Absence of response (low spinal cord defects)	Refer for further neurologic evaluation.
Tonic neck: Fencer position—when head is turned to one side, extremities on same side extend and on opposite side flex; this reflex may not be evident during early neonatal period; disappears at 3 to 4 months of age	Absent after 1 month of age or persistent asymmetry (cerebral lesion)	Assess neurologic functioning.
Response often more dominant in leg than in arm		
Prone crawl: While on abdomen, newborn pushes up and tries to crawl	Absence or variance of response (preterm, weak, or depressed newborns)	Evaluate motor functioning. Refer to specialist.
Trunk Incurvation (Galant): In prone position, stroking of spine causes pelvis to turn to stimulated side	Failure to rotate to stimulated side (neurologic damage)	
	*Possible causes of alterations are placed in parentheses.	[†]This column provides guidelines for further assessment and initial nursing interventions.

CLINICAL JUDGMENT

Case Study: Maria Reyes

Maria Reyes, a 19-year-old G2 (now P2) mother, delivered a 40-week-old female newborn 24 hours ago. The newborn exam was normal. Mrs. Reyes asks about the newborn's exam. She says she has noticed that the baby cries more than her first child did and seems to require holding for longer periods of time after feeding before "quieting down." She is concerned that there is something she is doing wrong and wants to know when her newborn will start to act like her first baby.

Critical Thinking

What should you discuss with her about newborn behavior?
See www.nursing.pearsonhighered.com for possible responses.

Newborn Behavioral Assessment

Two conflicting forces influence parents' perceptions of their newborn. One is the parents' preconceptions, based on hopes and fears, of what their newborn will be like. The other is their initial reaction to their baby's temperament, behaviors, and physical appearance. Nurses can assist parents in identifying their baby's specific behaviors.

> "One of the newborn's first responses is to move into a quiet but alert state of consciousness. The baby is still; his body molds to yours; his hands touch your skin; his eyes open wide and are bright and shiny. He looks directly at you.
>
> This special alert state, this innate ability to communicate, may be the initial preparation for becoming attached to other human beings. One feels awed by the intensity and appealing power of this little bud of humanity meeting the world for the first time."
>
> THE AMAZING NEWBORN

Brazelton's Neonatal Behavioral Assessment Scale The behavioral assessment tool attempts to identify the newborn's repertoire of behavioral responses to the environment and also documents the newborn's neurologic adequacy and capabilities. (For a complete discussion of all test items and maneuvers, see Brazelton & Nugent, 1995.) It provides a way for the healthcare provider, in conjunction with the parents (primary caregivers), to identify and understand the individual newborn's states, temperament, capabilities, and individual behavior patterns. Families learn which responses, interventions, or activities best meet the special needs of their newborn, and this understanding fosters positive attachment experiences.

Because the first few days after birth are a period of behavioral disorganization, the complete assessment should be done on the third day after birth. The nurse should make every effort to elicit the best response. This may be accomplished by repeating tests at different times or by testing during situations that facilitate the best possible response, such as when parents are holding, cuddling, rocking, or singing to their baby.

Care Plan Activity: Assessment of the Uncomplicated Newborn

The behavioral assessment of the newborn should be carried out initially in a quiet, dimly lighted room, if possible. The nurse should first determine the newborn's state of consciousness, because scoring and introduction of the test items correlate with the sleep or awake state. The newborn's state depends on physiologic variables, such as the amount of time from the last feeding, positioning, environmental temperature, and health status; presence of such external stimuli as noises and bright lights; and the sleep-wake cycle of the infant. An important characteristic of the neonatal period is the pattern of states, as well as the transitions from one state to another. The pattern of states is a predictor of the newborn's receptivity and ability to respond to stimuli in a cognitive manner. Babies learn best in a quiet, alert state and in an environment that is supportive and protective and that provides appropriate stimuli.

The nurse should also observe the newborn's sleep-wake patterns (as discussed in chapter 29) and the rapidity with which the newborn moves from one state to another, the newborn's ability to be consoled, and the newborn's ability to diminish the impact of disturbing stimuli. The following questions provide the nurse with a framework for assessment:

- Does the newborn's response style and ability to adapt to stimuli indicate a need for parental interventions that will alert the newborn to the environment so that the baby can grow socially and cognitively?
- Are parental interventions necessary to lessen the outside stimuli, as in the case of the baby who responds to sensory input with intensity?
- Can the baby control the amount of sensory input to be dealt with?

The behaviors and the sleep-wake states in which they are assessed are categorized as follows:

- ***Habituation.*** The newborn's ability to diminish or shut down innate responses to specific repeated stimuli, such as a rattle, bell, light, or pinprick to heel.
- ***Orientation to inanimate and animate visual and auditory assessment stimuli.*** How often and where the newborn attends to auditory and visual stimuli are observed. Orientation to the environment is determined by an ability to respond to cues given by others and by a natural ability to fix on and to follow a visual object horizontally and vertically. This capacity and parental appreciation of it are important for positive communication between infant and parents; the parents' visual (*en face*) and auditory (soft, continuous voice) presence stimulates their infant to orient to them. Inability or lack of response may indicate visual or auditory problems. It is important for parents to know that their newborn can turn to voices usually soon after birth or by 3 days of age and can become alert at different times with a varying degree of intensity in response to sounds.
- ***Motor activity.*** Several components are evaluated. Motor tone of the newborn is assessed in the most characteristic state of responsiveness. This summary assessment includes overall use of tone as the newborn responds to being handled—whether

during spontaneous activity, prone placement, or horizontal holding—and overall assessment of body tone as the newborn reacts to all stimuli.

- *Variations.* Frequency of alert states, state changes, color changes (throughout all states as examination progresses), activity, and peaks of excitement are assessed.
- *Self-quieting activity.* Assessment is based on how often, how quickly, and how effectively newborns can use their resources to quiet and console themselves when upset or distressed. Considered in this assessment are such self-consolatory activities as putting hand to mouth, sucking on a fist or the tongue, and attuning to an object or sound (Figure 30-45 ■). The newborn's need for outside consolation must also be considered—for example, seeing a face; being rocked, held, or dressed; using a pacifier; and being swaddled.
- *Cuddliness or social behaviors.* This area encompasses the infant's need for and response to being held. Also considered is how often the newborn smiles. These behaviors influence the parents' self-esteem and feelings of acceptance or rejection. Cuddling also appears to be an indicator of personality. Cuddlers appear to enjoy, accept, and seek physical contact; are easier to placate; sleep more; and form earlier and more intense attachments. Noncuddlers are active, are restless, have accelerated motor development, and are intolerant of physical restraint. Smiling, even as a grimace reflex, greatly influences parent-infant feedback. Parents identify this response as positive.

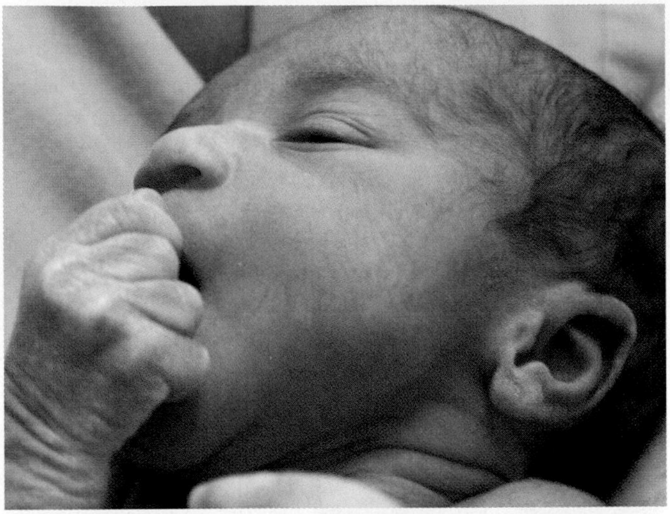

Figure 30-45 ■ The newborn can bring hand to mouth as a self-soothing activity.

Source: George Dodson/Lightworks Studio/Pearson Education.

FOCUS YOUR STUDY

- A perinatal history, determination of gestational age, physical examination, and behavioral assessment form the basis for complete newborn assessment.
- The common physical characteristics included in the gestational age assessment are skin, lanugo, sole (plantar) creases, breast tissue and size, ear form and cartilage, and genitals.
- The neuromuscular components of gestational age scoring tools are usually posture, square window sign, popliteal angle, arm recoil, heel-to-ear extension, and scarf sign.
- By assessing the physical and neuromuscular components specified in a gestational age tool, the nurse can determine the gestational age of the newborn.
- After determining the gestational age of the baby, the nurse can assess how the newborn will make the transition to extrauterine life and can anticipate potential physiologic problems.
- The nurse identifies the newborn as small for gestational age (SGA), appropriate for gestational age (AGA), or large for gestational age (LGA), and prioritizes individual needs.
- Normal ranges for vital signs assessed in newborns are heart rate of 110 to 160 beats per minute; respiratory rate of 30 to 60 respirations per minute; axillary temperature of 36.5°C to 37.2°C (97.7°F to 99°F); skin temperature of 36°C to 36.5°C (96.8°F to 97.7°F); rectal temperature of 36.6°C to 37.2°C (97.8°F to 99°F); and blood pressure of 70/45 to 50/30 mm Hg (at birth).
- Normal newborn measurements include weight from 2500 to 4000 g (5 lb, 8 oz to 8 lb, 13 oz), with weight dependent on maternal size and age; length from 48 to 52 cm (18 to 22 in.); and head circumference from 32 to 37 cm (12.5 to 14.5 in.). Head circumference is approximately 2 cm larger than the chest circumference.

- Commonly elicited newborn reflexes are tonic neck, Moro, grasping, rooting, sucking, and blink.
- Newborn behavioral abilities include habituation, orientation to visual and auditory stimuli, motor activity, cuddliness, and self-quieting activity.
- An important role of the nurse during the physical and behavioral assessments of the newborn is to teach parents about their newborn and involve them in their baby's care. This facilitates the parents' identification of their newborn's uniqueness and allays their concerns.

CRITICAL THINKING IN ACTION

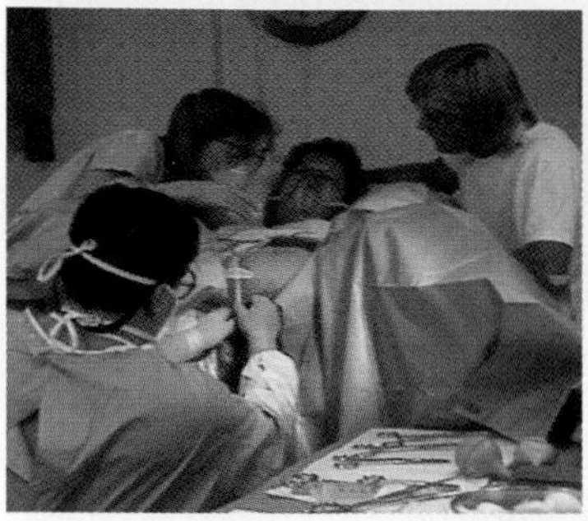

Susan Pine, a 21-year-old G2, now P1011, delivers a 39 2/7-weeks gestation female newborn. The vaginal birth is assisted with a vacuum extractor. The prenatal record is significant for an increase of maternal blood pressure to 140/90 on the day of birth. Susan is treated with magnesium sulfate during her labor and has an epidural analgesia for the pain of labor. The baby's Apgar is 8 and 9 at 1 and 5 minutes, and she has been admitted to the newborn nursery. The newborn's admission exam is normal except for a 2-cm round caput succedaneum.

Now, 8 hours later, the baby's condition is stable and she needs to be bottle-fed. You take her to her mother's room where you observe that Susan does not reach out to take her from you. She seems unsure when handling her baby. Susan asks you about the swelling on her baby's head and wonders if it will ever go away.

1. How would you explain the cause of Susan's baby's caput succedaneum?
2. Compare the difference between a cephalhematoma and caput succedaneum.
3. Explore with Susan her baby's reflexes and state of alertness.
4. Susan asks you how she will know what her baby needs. How would you respond?

See www.nursing.pearsonhighered.com for possible responses.

Pearson Nursing Student Resources

Find additional review materials at
www.nursing.pearsonhighered.com

Prepare for success with additional NCLEX®-style practice questions, interactive assignments and activities, Web links, animations and videos, and more!

REFERENCES

American Academy of Pediatrics (AAP) Committee on Fetus and Newborn & American College of Obstetricians and Gynecologists (ACOG) Committee on Obstetrics. (2007). *Guidelines for perinatal care* (6th ed.). Evanston, IL: Author.

Ballard, J. L., Khoury, J. C., Wedig, K., Wang, L., Eilers-Walsman, B. L., & Lipp, R. (1991). New Ballard score, expanded to include extremely premature infants. *Journal of Pediatrics, 119*(3), 417–423.

Blackburn, S. T. (2007). *Maternal, fetal, neonatal physiology: A clinical perspective* (3rd ed.). London, England: MacKeith.

Brazelton, T. B., & Nugent, J. K. (1995). *The neonatal behavioral assessment scale* (3rd ed.). London, England: MacKeith.

Creehan, P. A. (2008). Newborn physical assessment. In K. R. Simpson & P. A. Creehan, *Perinatal nursing* (3rd ed.) (pp. 546–574). Philadelphia, PA: Lippincott Williams & Wilkins.

Gardner, S. L. & Hernandez, J. A. (2011). Initial nursery care. In S. L. Gardner, B. S. Carter, M. Enzman-Hines, & J. A. Hernandez (Eds.), *Merenstein & Gardner's handbook of neonatal intensive care* (7th ed., pp. 78–112). St. Louis, MO: Mosby.

Tappero, E. & Honeyfield, M. E. (2009). *Physical assessment of the newborn: A comprehensive approach to the art of physical examination* (4th ed.). Santa Rosa, CA: NICU INK Book Publisher.

Tietler, J. O., Reichman, N. E., Nepomnyaschy, L., & Martinson, M. (2007). A cross-national comparison of racial and ethnic disparities in low birth weight in the United States and England. *Pediatrics, 120*(5), e1182–e1189.

CHAPTER 31

The Normal Newborn: Needs and Care

In the sheltered simplicity of the first days after a baby is born, one sees again the magical closed circle, the miraculous sense of two people existing only for each other.

—Anne Morrow Lindbergh

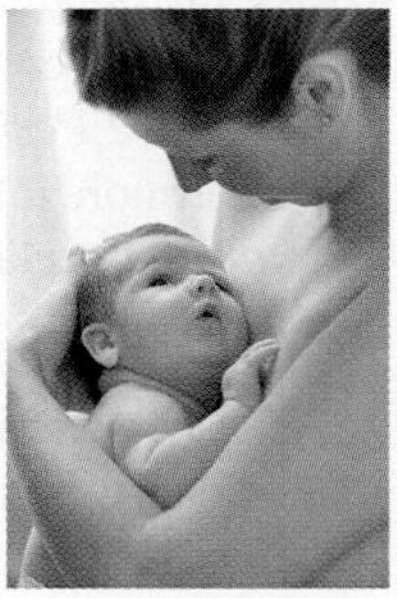

LEARNING OUTCOMES

1. Summarize the essential areas of information to be obtained about a newborn's birth experience and immediate postnatal period.
2. Explain how the physiologic and behavioral responses of a newborn during the first 4 hours after birth (admission and transitional period) determine the newborn's nursing care.
3. Identify activities that should be included in a daily care plan for a normal newborn.
4. Discuss the common concerns of families regarding their newborns.
5. Identify opportunities to individualize parent teaching and enhance each parent's abilities and confidence while providing infant care in the birthing unit.
6. Explain how the common and specific concerns of families can be included in parent teaching during daily newborn and infant care and discharge planning.

KEY TERMS

Circumcision *834*
Newborn screening tests *843*
Parent-newborn attachment *832*

At the moment of birth, numerous physiologic adaptations begin to take place in the newborn's body. Because of these dramatic changes, newborns require close observation to determine how smoothly they are making the transition to extrauterine life. Newborns also require special care that enhances their chances of making the transition successfully.

The two broad goals of nursing care during this period are (1) to promote the physical well-being of the newborn, and (2) to support the establishment of a well-functioning family unit. The nurse meets the first goal by providing comprehensive care to newborns while in the mother-baby unit. The nurse meets the second goal by teaching family members how to care for their new baby and by supporting their efforts so that they feel confident and competent. Thus, the nurse must be knowledgeable about family adjustments that need to be made as well as the healthcare needs of the newborn. It is important that the family return home with the positive feeling that they have the support, information, and skills to care for their newborn. Equally important is the need for each member of the family to begin a unique relationship with the newborn. The cultural and social expectations of individual families and communities affect the way normal newborn care is carried out.

The previous two chapters present an informational database of the physiologic and behavioral changes occurring in the newborn and the pertinent nursing assessments that are needed. This chapter discusses nursing care management while the newborn is in the birthing unit.

Nursing Care During Admission and the First Four Hours of Life

Immediately after birth, the baby is formally admitted to the healthcare facility.

Nursing Assessment and Diagnosis

Before the birth of an infant, the nurse reviews the prenatal record of the mother for information concerning possible risk factors for the infant. These include infectious disease screening results, drug or alcohol use by the mother, gestational diabetes, and any other data determined to be of use in anticipating the needs of the newborn. In addition, the nurse reviews the birth record for prolonged rupture of membranes, instrument or vacuum delivery, use of narcotic analgesia, presence of meconium, and any other data that may impact the infant's ability to successfully transition to the extrauterine environment.

During the first hours after birth, the nurse carries out a preliminary physical examination, including an assessment of the newborn's physiologic adaptations. In many birthing units, the nurse performs and documents the initial head-to-toe physical assessment during the first hour of transition. The nurse is responsible for notifying the physician or nurse practitioner of any deviations from normal. A complete physical examination is also performed later by the physician or nurse practitioner, within the first 24 hours after birth and within 24 hours before discharge. This can be accomplished with one physical examination (American Academy of Pediatrics [AAP] & American College of Obstetricians and Gynecologists [ACOG], 2007). (See chapter 30 ∞.)

Nursing diagnoses are based on an analysis of the assessment findings. Physiologic alterations of the newborn form the basis of many nursing diagnoses, as does the family's incorporation of them in caring for their new baby. Nursing diagnoses that may apply to the newborn include the following:

- ***Ineffective Airway Clearance*** related to presence of mucus and retained lung fluid
- ***Risk for Imbalanced Body Temperature*** related to evaporative, radiant, conductive, and convective heat losses
- ***Ineffective Peripheral Tissue Perfusion*** related to ineffective thermoregulation or poor peripheral circulation
- ***Acute Pain*** related to heel sticks for glucose or hematocrit tests, vitamin K injection, or Hepatitis B immunization

As discussed in chapter 29 ∞, the newborn's physiologic adaptation to extrauterine life occurs rapidly. All body systems are affected. Therefore, many of these nursing diagnoses and associated interventions must be identified and implemented in a very short period (Table 31-1).

Nursing Plan and Implementation

The nurse initiates newborn admission procedures and evaluates the newborn's need to remain under observation. This evaluation may take place in a special transition area or at the mother's bedside. It includes the following:

- Maternal and birth history
- Airway clearance
- Vital signs
- Body temperature
- Neurologic status
- Ability to feed
- Evidence of complications and/or illness

TABLE 31-1 Signs of Newborn Transition

Normal findings for the newborn during the first few days of life include the following:

Pulse: 110–160 beats/minute

- During sleep as low as 100 beats/minute
- If crying, up to 180 beats/minute
- Apical pulse is counted for 1 full minute because rate may fluctuate

Respirations: 30–60 respirations/minute

- Predominantly diaphragmatic but synchronous with abdominal movements
- Brief periods of apnea (less than 15 seconds) with no color or heart rate changes

Temperature:

- Axillary: 36.4°C–37.2°C (97.5°F–99°F)
- Skin: 36°C–36.5°C (96.8°F–97.7°F)

Blood pressure: 70–50/45–30 mm Hg at birth; 90/60 mm Hg at day 10

Blood glucose: greater than or equal to 40 mg%

Hematocrit: less than 65% to 70% central venous sample

If the evaluation is normal, the baby is successfully making the transition to extrauterine life and may need less frequent observations. In some settings, this may also be a time for moving the mother and baby to another care unit.

Initiation of Admission Procedures

After birth the baby is formally admitted to the healthcare facility. The admission procedures include a review of prenatal and birth information for possible risk factors, a gestational age assessment, and an assessment to ensure that the newborn's adaptation to extrauterine life is proceeding normally. This evaluation for risk factors and the status of the newborn must be done no later than 2 hours after birth (AAP & ACOG, 2007).

If the initial assessment indicates that the newborn is not at risk physiologically, the nurse performs many of the routine admission procedures in the presence of the parents and others in the birthing area. Some care measures indicated by the assessment findings may be performed by the nurse or by family members under the guidance of the nurse in an effort to educate and support the family. Other interventions might best be delayed if the newborn must be transferred to an observational nursery.

The nurse responsible for the newborn first checks and confirms the newborn's identification with the mother's identification and then obtains and records all significant information. The essential data to be recorded as part of the newborn's chart include the following:

1. ***Condition of the newborn.*** Pertinent information includes the newborn's Apgar scores at 1 and 5 minutes, resuscitative measures required in the birthing area, physical examination, vital signs, voidings, and passing of meconium. Complications to be noted include excessive mucus, delayed spontaneous respirations or responsiveness, abnormal number of cord vessels, abnormal vital signs, and obvious physical abnormalities.
2. ***Labor and birth record.*** A copy of the labor and birth record should be placed in the newborn's chart or be accessible on computer. The record contains all the significant data about the birth, for example, duration, course, and status of mother and fetus throughout labor and birth and any analgesia or anesthesia administered to the mother. Particular care is taken to note any variation or difficulties such as prolonged rupture of membranes, abnormal fetal position, meconium-stained amniotic fluid, signs of nonreassuring fetal status during labor, nuchal cord (cord around the newborn's neck at birth), precipitous birth, use of forceps or vacuum extraction assisted device, maternal analgesia and anesthesia received within 1 hour of birth, and administration of antibiotics during labor.
3. ***Antepartum history.*** Preexisting maternal conditions or any maternal problems that may have compromised the fetus in utero—such as preeclampsia, spotting, illness, recent infections, rubella status, serology results, hepatitis B screen results, exposure to group B streptococci, or a history of maternal substance abuse—are of immediate concern in newborn assessment. The chart should also include information about maternal age, estimated date of birth (EDB), previous pregnancies, and presence of any congenital anomalies. An HIV test result, if obtained, is also relevant. State statutes vary as to who may have access to this information (AAP & ACOG, 2007).
4. ***Parent-newborn interaction information.*** The nurse notes parents' interactions with their newborn and their desires regarding care, such as rooming-in, circumcision, and type of feeding. Information about other children in the home, available support systems, interactional patterns within each family unit, situations that compromise lactation (breast surgery, previous lactation failure), and any high risk circumstances (adolescent mother, domestic violence, history of child abuse) help in providing comprehensive care (AAP & ACOG, 2007).

As part of the admission procedure, the nurse weighs the newborn in both grams and pounds (Figure 31-1 ■). In the United States, parents understand weights best when stated in pounds and ounces. The nurse cleans and covers the scale each time a newborn is weighed to prevent cross-infection and heat loss from conduction.

The nurse then measures the newborn, recording the measurements in both centimeters and inches. Three routine measurements are length, circumference of the head, and circumference of the chest. In some facilities, abdominal girth may also be measured. The nurse rapidly assesses the baby's color, muscle tone, alertness, and general state. Remember that the first period of reactivity may have concluded, and the baby may be in the sleep-inactive phase, which makes the infant hard to arouse. The nurse does basic assessments for estimating gestational age and completes the physical assessment. (For more discussion of the process of newborn assessment, see chapter 30 ∞.)

In addition to obtaining vital signs, the nurse performs hematocrit and blood glucose evaluations on at-risk newborns or as clinically indicated (such as for small-for-gestational-age [SGA] or large-for-gestational-age [LGA] infants or if the newborn is jittery). These procedures may be done on admission or

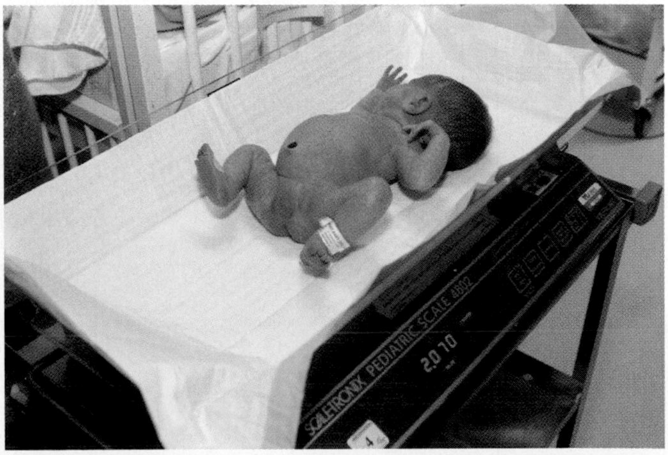

Figure 31-1 ■ Weighing a newborn. The scale is balanced before each weighing, with the protective pad in place.

Source: George Dodson/Lightworks Studio/Pearson Education.

CLINICAL PATHWAY For Newborn Care

Category	First 4 Hours	4–12 Hours Past Birth	8–24 Hours Past Birth
Referral	Review labor/birth record Review transitional nursing record Check ID bands and security alarms if present Consult prn: orthopedics, genetics, infectious disease	Check ID bands and security alarms Transfer to mother-baby care at 4–6 hours of age if stable for at least 2 hours As parents desire, obtain circumcision permit after their discussion with physician Check ID bands and crib cards to ensure they are in the correct crib Lactation consult prn	Check ID bands and security alarm q shift ■ ***Expected Outcomes*** Mother/baby ID bands correlate at time of discharge; security alarms in place at all times; consults completed prn
Assessments	Continue assessments begun first hour after birth Vital signs: TPR, BP prn, q1h × 4 (skin temp 96.8°F–97.7°F (36°C–36.5°C), resp may be irregular but within 30–60 per min) ■ ***Newborn Assessments*** • Respiratory status with resp distress scale × 1 then prn. If resp distress, assess every 5–15 min • Cord: bluish white color, clamp in place and free of skin • Color: skin, mucous membranes, extremities, trunk pink with slight acrocyanosis of hands and feet • Wt (5 lb, 8 oz–8 lb, 13 oz) 2500–4000 g, length (18–22 in.) 46–56 cm, HC (12.5–14.5 in.) 32–37 cm, CC (32.5 cm, 1–2 cm less than head) • Extremity movement—may be jerky or brief twitches • Gestational age classification—term AGA • Anomalies (cong. anomalies can interfere with normal extrauterine adaptation)	Assess newborn's progress through periods of reactivity Vital signs: TPR q8h; and prn or per agency protocol, BP prn ■ ***Newborn Assessments*** • Skin color q4h prn (circulatory system stabilizing, acrocyanosis decreased) • Auscultate lungs q4h (noisy, wet breath sounds clear and equal) • Eyes for drainage, redness, hemorrhage • Umbilical cord base for redness, drainage, foul odor, drying, damp in place • Increased mucus production (normal in 2nd period of reactivity) • Check apical pulse q4h • Temp before and after admission bath • Extremity movements q4h • Check for expected reflexes (suck, rooting, Moro, grasp, blink, yawn, sneeze, tonic neck, Babinski) • Note common normal variations • Assess suck and swallow during feeding • Note behavioral characteristics	VS q8h; normal ranges: T, 97.5°F–99°F (36.4°C–37.2°C) axillary; P, 110–160; R, 30–60; BP, 70–50/45–30 mm Hg ■ ***Continue Newborn Assessments*** • Skin color q4h prn • Signs of drying or infection in cord area • Check that clamp is in place until removed before discharge • Check circ for bleeding after procedure, then q30 min × 2, then q4h and prn • Observe for jaundice, obtain total serum bili (TSB) if infant visibly jaundiced before 24 hours of age. Obtain transcutaneous bili on all infants not previously tested before discharge ■ ***Expected Outcomes*** Vital signs medically acceptable, color pink, assessments WNL, circ site without s/s infection, cord site without s/s of infection and clamp removed; newborn behavior WNL
Teaching/ psychosocial	Admission activities performed at mother's bedside if possible, orient to nursery prn, hand washing, assess teaching needs Teach parents use of bulb syringe, signs of choking, positioning, and when to call for assistance Teach reasons for use of radiant warmer, infant hat, and warmed blankets when out of warmer Discuss/teach infant security, identification	Reinforce teaching about choking, bulb syringe use, positioning, temperature maintenance with clothing and blankets Teach infant positioning to facilitate breathing and digestion Teach new parents holding and feeding skills Teach parents soothing and calming techniques Teach parents about introducing newborn to sibling	Final discharge teaching: diapering, normal void and stool patterns, bathing, nail, and cord care, circumcision/uncircumcised penis/genital care and normal characteristics, rashes, jaundice, sleep-wake cycles, soothing activities, taking temperatures, thermometer reading Explain s/s of illness and when to call healthcare provider Infant safety: car seats, immunizations, metabolic screening ■ ***Expected Outcomes*** Mother/family verbalize comprehension of teaching; demonstrate care capabilities
Nursing care management and reports	Place under radiant warmer Place hat on newborn (decreases convection heat loss) Suction nares/mouth with bulb syringe prn Keep bulb syringe with infant Attach security sensor Obtain lab tests: blood glucose, as needed Obtain blood type, Rh, Coombs on cord blood, HSV culture if parental hx Notify physician's office of infant's birth and any change in status Maintain standard precautions	Wean from radiant warmer (T 98.6°F [37°C] axillary) Glucose testing prn; BP prn Suction nares prn (esp during 2nd period of reactivity) Oxygen saturation prn Bathe infant if temp greater than 97.7°F (36.5°C) axillary Position on back Obtain peripheral Hct per protocol Cord care per protocol Fold diaper below cord (for plastic diapers, turn plastic layer away from skin)	Check for hearing test results Weigh before discharge Cord assessment every shift DC cord clamp before discharge[1] Perform newborn metabolic screening blood tests before discharge Circumcision if indicated; circumcision care: change diaper prn, noting ability to void; follow policy for circumcision clamp or Plastibell care ■ ***Expected Outcomes*** Newborn maintains temp, lab test WNL, cord dry without s/s infection and clamp removed, screening tests accomplished, circ site without s/s infection or bleeding

1. In the case of very early discharge, the cord may still be moist enough that the decision may be made to leave it in place until the follow-up visit with the physician.

CLINICAL PATHWAY For Newborn Care continued

Category	First 4 Hours	4–12 Hours Past Birth	8–24 Hours Past Birth
Activity and comfort	Place under radiant warmer or wrap in prewarmed blankets until stable Soothe baby as needed with voice, touch, cuddling, nesting in warmer	Leave in warmer until stable, then swaddle Position on back after each feeding	Place in open crib Swaddle to allow movement of extremities in blanket, including hands to face ■ ***Expected Outcomes*** Infant maintains temp WNL in open crib; infant attempts self-calming
Nutrition	Assist newborn to breastfeed as soon as mother/baby condition allows Supplement breast only when medically indicated or per agency policy Initiate formula-feeding within first hour Gavage feed if necessary to prevent hypoglycemia	Breastfeed on demand, at least q3–4h Teach positions, observe/assist with feeding, breast/nipple care, establishing milk supply, breaking suction, feeding cues, latching-on techniques, nutritive suck, burping Formula-feed on demand, at least q3–4h Determine readiness to feed and feeding tolerance	Continue breastfeeding or formula-feeding pattern Assess feeding tolerance q4h Discuss normal feeding requirements, signs of hunger and satiation, handling feeding problems, and when to seek help ■ ***Expected Outcomes*** Mother verbalizes knowledge of feeding information; breastfeeds on demand without supplement; bottle: tolerates formula feeding, nipples without problems
Elimination	Note first void and stool if not noted at birth	Note all voids, amount and color of stools q4h	Evaluate all voids and stool color q8h ■ ***Expected Outcomes*** Voids qs; stools qs without difficulty; stool character WNL, diaper area without s/s of skin breakdown or rashes
Medication	Prophylactic ophthalmic ointment both eyes after baby makes eye contact with parents within 1 hr after birth Administer AquaMEPHYTON IM, dosage according to infant weight per MD/NP order	Hepatitis B injection as ordered by physician after consent signed by parents	Hepatitis B vaccine within 2 hr of birth or before discharge ■ ***Expected Outcomes*** Baby has received ophthalmic ointment and vitamin K injection; baby has received first Hep B vaccine if ordered and parental permission received
Discharge planning/ home care	Hepatitis B consent signed Hearing screen consent signed Plan discharge call with parent or guardian in 24 hr to 2 days Assess parents' discharge plans, needs, and support systems	Review/reinforce teaching with mother and significant other Review home preparedness Present birth certificate instructions	Initial newborn screening tests (hearing, blood tests, genetic/metabolic screen) before discharge Bath and feeding classes, videos, or written information given Give written copy of discharge instructions Newborn photographs Set up appointment for follow-up PKU test Have car seat available before discharge. All discharge referrals made, follow-up appt. scheduled ■ ***Expected Outcomes*** Infant discharged home with family; mother verbalizes follow-up appt. time/date
Family involvement	Facilitate early investigation of baby's physical characteristics (maintain temp during unwrapping), hold infant *en face* Dim lights to help infant keep eyes open	Assess parents' knowledge of newborn behaviors, such as alertness, suck and rooting, attention to human voice, response to calming techniques Facilitate parent interaction with infant by performing care in presence of parents and encouraging parents to participate in care	Assess mother-baby bonding/interaction Incorporate father and siblings in care Enhance parent-infant interaction by sharing characteristics and behavioral assessment Support positive parenting behaviors Identify community referral needs and refer to community agencies ■ ***Expected Outcome*** Demonstrates caring and family incorporation of infant
Date			

Abbreviations: AGA, average for gestational age; Appt, appointment; CC, chest circumference; cong, congenital; esp, especially; HC, head circumference; Hct, hematocrit; Hx, history; ID, identification; PKU, phenylketonuria; qs, quantity sufficient; s/s, signs and symptoms; temp, temperature; TPR, temperature, pulse, respirations; VS, vital signs; WNL, within normal limits.

within the first 2 hours after birth (AAP & ACOG, 2007). (See Procedure 34-1 ∞: Performing a Heel Stick on a Newborn on page 961.)

> **CLINICAL JUDGMENT**
>
> **Case Study: Baby Johannson**
>
> You overhear Mr. Johannson speaking to his mother on the phone. He is telling her about the "cute little noises" his 30-minute-old baby makes. The infant is in the room with the mother.
>
> **Critical Thinking**
>
> What is your best course of action?
>
> *See www.nursing.pearsonhighered.com for possible responses.*

Maintenance of a Clear Airway and Stable Vital Signs

Free-flow oxygen should be readily available. The nurse positions the newborn on his or her back (or side, if the infant has copious secretions). If necessary, a bulb syringe or DeLee wall suction (see Procedure 24-1 ∞: Performing Nasal Pharyngeal Suctioning on page 622) is used to remove mucus from the nasal passages and oral cavity. A DeLee catheter attached to suction may be used to remove mucus from the stomach to help prevent possible aspiration. When possible, this procedure should be delayed for 10 to 15 minutes after birth, reducing the potential for severe vasovagal reflex apnea.

In the absence of any newborn distress, the nurse continues with the admission by taking the newborn's vital signs. The initial temperature is taken by the axillary method. A wider range of normal exists for axillary temperature, specifically 36.4°C to 37.2°C (97.5°F to 99°F).

Once the initial temperature is taken, the nurse monitors the core temperature either by obtaining axillary temperatures at intervals or by placing a skin sensor on the newborn for continuous reading. The usual skin sensor placement site is on the newborn's abdomen, but placement on the upper thigh or arm can give a reading closely correlated with the mean body temperature. The vital signs for a healthy term newborn should be monitored at least every 30 minutes until the newborn's condition has remained stable for 2 hours (AAP & ACOG, 2007). The newborn's respirations may be irregular yet still be normal. Brief periods of apnea, lasting only 5 to 10 seconds with no color or heart rate changes, are considered normal. The normal pulse range is 110 to 160 beats per minute (beats/min), and the normal respiratory range is 30 to 60 respirations per minute.

Maintenance of a Neutral Thermal Environment

A neutral thermal environment is essential to minimize the newborn's need for increased oxygen consumption and use of calories to maintain body heat in the optimal range of 36.4°C to 37.2°C (97.5°F to 99°F). If the newborn becomes hypothermic, the body's response can lead to metabolic acidosis, hypoxia, and shock.

The nurse can best achieve a neutral thermal environment by performing the assessment and interventions with a newborn unclothed and under a radiant warmer. The radiant warmer's thermostat is controlled by the thermal skin sensor taped to the newborn's abdomen, upper thigh, or arm (Figure 31-2 ■). The sensor indicates when the newborn's temperature exceeds or falls below the acceptable temperature range. The nurse should be aware that leaning over the newborn may block the radiant heat waves from reaching the newborn. It is common practice in some institutions to cover the newborn's head with a cap made of stockinette or other material to prevent additional heat loss, in addition to placing the newborn under a radiant warmer (Blackburn, 2007).

> **CLINICAL TIP**
>
> A cap can be fashioned from a piece of stockinette to help reduce heat loss from the head.

In light of early discharge practices (12 to 48 hours), healthy term infants can be safely bathed immediately after the admission assessment is completed. The baby is bathed while still under the radiant warmer and should, when possible, take place in the parents' room or with parents present. Bathing the newborn offers an excellent opportunity for teaching and welcoming parent involvement in the care of their baby. If there is any doubt regarding the infant's condition, the baby may be given a sponge bath when the newborn's temperature is normal and vital signs are stable (about 2 to 4 hours after birth), when the newborn's condition dictates, or when the parents wish to give the first bath.

The nurse rechecks the temperature after the bath and, if it is stable, dresses the newborn in a shirt, diaper, and cap; wraps the baby; and places the baby in an open crib at room temperature. If the baby's axillary temperature is below 36.5°C (97.7°F), the nurse returns the baby to the radiant warmer. The rewarming process should be gradual to prevent the possibility of hyperthermia. Once the newborn is rewarmed, the nurse implements measures to prevent further neonatal heat loss, such as keeping the newborn dry, swaddled in one or two blankets with hat on, and away from cool surfaces or instruments. The nurse also protects the newborn from drafts, open windows or doors, and air conditioners. Blankets and clothing are stored in a warm place. See "Temperature" in chapter 30 ∞ and Procedure 31-1. Newborns are often "double-wrapped" in two or more blankets for temperature maintenance.

> **CLINICAL TIP**
>
> Take action to help the newborn maintain a stable temperature:
>
> - Keep the newborn's clothing and bedding dry.
> - Double-wrap the newborn and put a stocking cap on him or her.
> - Use the radiant warmer during procedures.
> - Reduce the newborn's exposure to drafts.
> - Warm objects that will be in contact with the newborn (e.g., stethoscopes).
> - Encourage the mother to snuggle with the newborn under blankets or to breastfeed the newborn with hat and light cover.

Prevention of Vitamin K Deficiency Bleeding

A prophylactic injection of vitamin K_1 (AquaMEPHYTON) is given to prevent hemorrhage, which can occur because of low

PROCEDURE 31-1 Thermoregulation of the Newborn

NURSING ACTION

Preparation

- Pre-warm the incubator or radiant warmer. Make sure warm towels and/or lightweight blankets are available.
- Maintain the temperature of the birthing room at 22°C (71°F), with a relative humidity of 60% to 65%.

Rationale: *The change from a warm, moist intrauterine environment to a cool, dry, drafty environment stresses the newborn's immature thermoregulation system.*

Equipment and Supplies

Pre-warmed towels or blankets

Infant stocking cap

Servocontrol probe

Infant T-shirt and diaper

Open crib

Procedure: Clean Gloves

1. Don gloves.

   Rationale: *Gloves are worn whenever there is the possibility of contact with body fluids—in this case, a newborn wet with amniotic fluid, vernix, and maternal blood.*

2. Place the newborn under the radiant warmer. Wipe the newborn free of blood, fluid, and excess vernix, especially from the head, using pre-warmed towels.

   Rationale: *The radiant warmer creates a heat-gaining environment. Drying is important to prevent the loss of body heat through evaporation.*

3. If the newborn is stable, wrap him or her in a pre-warmed blanket, apply a stocking cap, and carry the newborn to the mother. The mother and her support person can hold and enjoy the newborn together. Alternatively, carry the wrapped newborn to the mother, loosen the blanket, and place the infant skin to skin on the mother's chest under a warmed blanket.

   Rationale: *Use of a pre-warmed blanket reduces convection heat loss and facilitates maternal-newborn contact without compromising the newborn's thermoregulation. Skin-to-skin contact with the mother or father helps maintain the newborn's temperature.*

4. After the newborn has spent time with the parents, return him or her to the radiant warmer and apply a diaper. Leave the newborn uncovered (except for the cap and diaper) under the radiant warmer.

   Rationale: *Radiant heat warms the outer skin surface, so the skin needs to be exposed.*

5. Tape a servocontrol probe on the newborn's anterior abdominal wall, with the metal side next to the skin. Do not place it over the ribs. Secure the probe with porous tape or a foil-covered aluminum heat deflector patch. Figure 31-2 shows a newborn with a skin probe. Note that in this picture the newborn is no longer wearing a stocking cap.

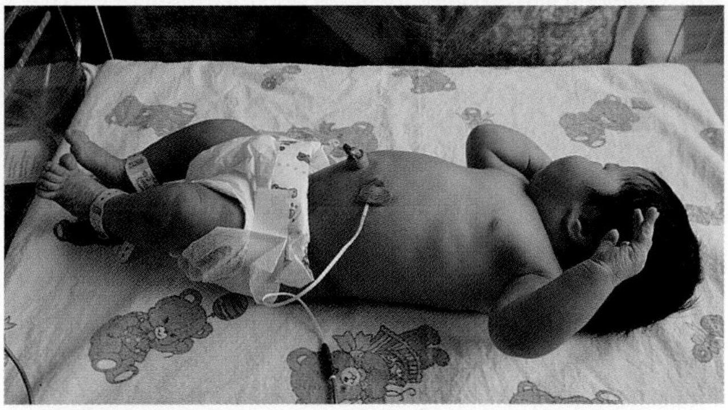

Figure 31-2 ■ Temperature monitoring for the newborn. A skin thermal sensor is placed on the newborn's abdomen, upper thigh, or arm and secured with porous tape or a foil-covered foam pad.

Source: Photographer, Elena Dorfman.

6. Turn the heater to servocontrol mode so that the abdominal skin is maintained at 36.0°C to 36.5°C (96.8°F to 97.7°F).

7. Monitor the newborn's axillary and skin probe temperatures per agency protocol.

   Rationale: *The temperature indicator on the radiant warmer continually displays the newborn's probe temperature. The axillary temperature is checked to ensure that the machine is accurately recording the newborn's temperature.*

8. When the newborn's axillary temperature reaches 37°C (98.6°F), add a T-shirt, double-wrap the infant (two blankets), and place the newborn in an open crib.

9. Recheck the newborn's temperature in 1 hour and regularly thereafter according to agency policy.

   Rationale: *It is important to monitor the newborn's ability to maintain his or her own thermoregulation.*

10. If the newborn's temperature drops below 36.1°C (97°F), rewarm the infant gradually. Place the infant (unclothed except for a diaper) under the radiant warmer with a servocontrol probe on the anterior abdominal wall.

    Rationale: *Rapid heating can lead to hyperthermia, which is associated with apnea, insensible water loss, and increased metabolic rate.*

11. Recheck the newborn's temperature in 30 minutes, then hourly.

12. When the temperature reaches 37°C (98.6°F), dress the newborn, remove him or her from the radiant warmer, double-wrap, and place in an open crib. Check the temperature hourly until stable, then regularly according to agency policy.

Note: *An infant who repeatedly requires rewarming should be observed for other signs and symptoms of illness and a physician notified, because it may warrant screening for infection.*

DRUG GUIDE Vitamin K_1 Phytonadione (AquaMEPHYTON)

OVERVIEW OF NEONATAL ACTION

Phytonadione is used in prophylaxis and treatment of vitamin K deficiency bleeding (VKDB), formerly known as hemorrhagic disease of the newborn. It promotes liver formation of the clotting factors II, VII, IX, and X. At birth, the newborn does not have the bacteria in the colon that are necessary for synthesizing fat-soluble vitamin K_1. Therefore, the newborn may have decreased levels of prothrombin during the first 5 to 8 days of life, reflected by a prolongation of prothrombin time.

PREGNANCY RISK CATEGORY: C

ROUTE, DOSAGE, FREQUENCY

Intramuscular injection is given in the vastus lateralis thigh muscle. A one-time-only prophylactic dose of 0.5 to 1 mg is given intramuscularly in the birthing area or within 1 hour of birth or may be delayed until after first breastfeeding in the birthing area (Wilson et al., 2010).

If the mother received anticoagulants during pregnancy, an additional dose may be ordered by the physician and is given 6 to 8 hours after the first injection. IM concentration: 1 mg/0.5 ml (neonatal strength); can use 10 mg/ml concentration to minimize volume injected.

NEONATAL SIDE EFFECTS

Pain and edema may occur at the injection site. Allergic reactions, such as rash and urticaria, may also occur.

NURSING CONSIDERATIONS

- Protect the drug from light.
- Observe for signs of local inflammation.
- Observe for jaundice and kernicterus, especially in preterm infants.
- Give vitamin K_1 before circumcision procedure.
- Observe for bleeding (usually occurs on second or third day). Bleeding may be seen as generalized ecchymoses or bleeding from the umbilical cord, circumcision site, nose, or gastrointestinal tract. Results of serial prothrombin time (PT) and international normalized ratio (INR) should be assessed.
- Observe for jaundice and kernicterus, especially in preterm infants.

prothrombin levels in the first few days of life (see Drug Guide: Vitamin K_1 Phytonadione [AquaMEPHYTON]). The potential for hemorrhage results from the absence of gut bacterial flora, which influences the production of vitamin K in the newborn. (See chapter 34 ∞ for further discussion.) Current recommendations underscore the need for treatment in infants who are exclusively breastfed (Blackburn, 2007).

Vitamin K injection is given intramuscularly in the vastus lateralis muscle that lies along the midanterior lateral aspect of the thigh (Figure 31-3 ■). Before injecting, the nurse must clean the newborn's skin site for the injection thoroughly with a small alcohol swab. The nurse uses a 25-gauge, 5/8-inch needle for the injection. An alternative site is the rectus femoris muscle in the anterior aspect of the thigh. However, this site is near the sciatic nerve and femoral artery and should be used with caution (Figure 31-4 ■).

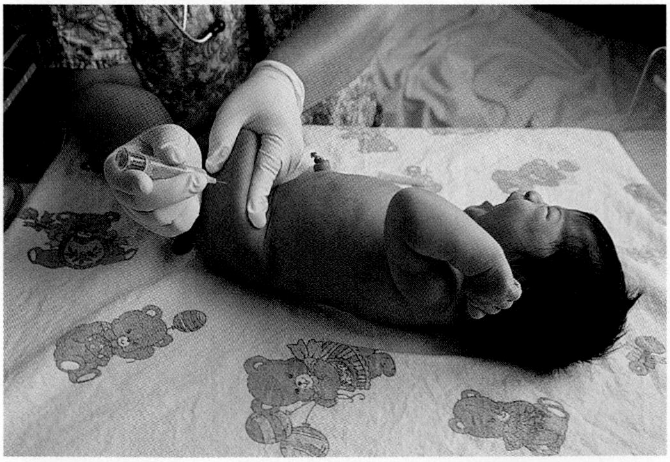

Figure 31-3 ■ Procedure for vitamin K injection. Cleanse area thoroughly with alcohol swab, and allow skin to dry. Bunch the tissue of the midanterior lateral aspect of the thigh (vastus lateralis muscle) and quickly insert a 25-gauge 5/8-inch needle at a 90-degree angle to the thigh. Aspirate, then slowly inject the solution to distribute the medication evenly and minimize the baby's discomfort. Remove the needle and massage the site with an alcohol swab.

Source: Photographer, Elena Dorfman.

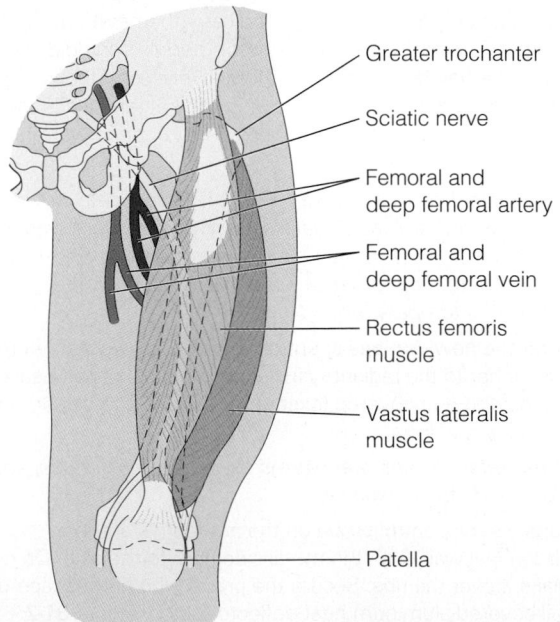

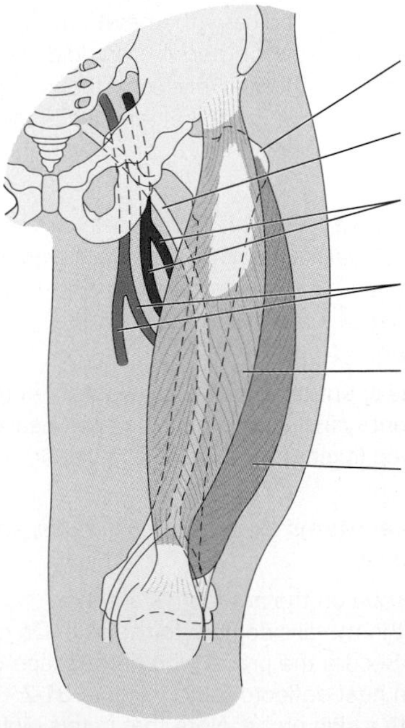

Figure 31-4 ■ Injection sites. The middle third of the vastus lateralis muscle is the preferred site for intramuscular injection in the newborn. The middle third of the rectus femoris is an alternative site, but its proximity to major vessels and the sciatic nerve necessitates caution in using this site for injection.

Prevention of Eye Infection

The nurse is also responsible for giving the legally required prophylactic eye treatment for *Neisseria gonorrhoeae,* which may have infected the newborn of an infected mother during the birth process. A variety of topical agents appear to be equally effective. Ophthalmic ointments that are used include 0.5% erythromycin (Ilotycin Ophthalmic) (see Drug Guide: Erythromycin Ophthalmic Ointment [Ilotycin Ophthalmic]), 1% tetracycline, or per agency protocol. All are also effective against chlamydia, which has a higher incidence rate than gonorrhea.

Successful eye prophylaxis requires that the medication be instilled into the lower conjunctival sac of each eye (Figure 31-5 ■).

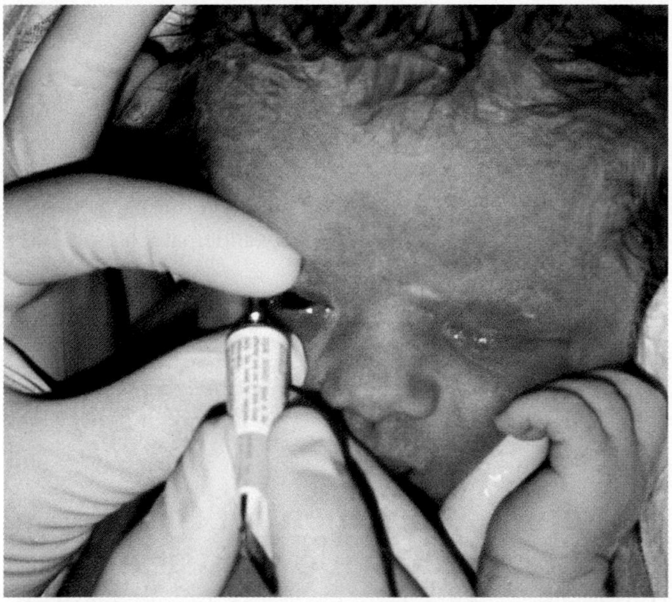

Figure 31-5 ■ Ophthalmic ointment. Retract lower eyelid outward to instill a 1/4-inch strand of ointment from a single-dose ampule along the lower conjunctival surface.

The nurse massages the eyelid gently to distribute the ointment. Instillation may be delayed up to 1 hour after birth to allow eye contact during parent-newborn bonding.

Eye prophylaxis medication can cause chemical conjunctivitis, which gives the newborn some discomfort and may interfere with the baby's ability to focus on the parents' faces. The resulting edema, inflammation, and discharge may cause concern if the parents have not been informed that the side effects will clear in 24 to 48 hours and that this prophylactic eye treatment is necessary for the newborn's well-being.

Early Assessment of Neonatal Distress

During the first 24 hours of life, nurses are constantly alert for signs of distress. If the newborn is with the parents during this period, the nurse must take extra care to teach them how to maintain their newborn's temperature, recognize the hallmarks of newborn distress, and respond immediately to signs of respiratory problems. The parents should learn to observe the newborn for changes in skin color or activity, rapid breathing with chest retractions, nasal flaring, or facial grimacing. Their interventions should include nasal and oral suctioning with bulb syringe, positioning, and vigorous fingertip stroking of the newborn's spine to stimulate respiratory activity if necessary. The nurse must be immediately available to provide appropriate interventions should the newborn develop distress (Table 31-2).

A common cause of neonatal distress is early-onset group B streptococcal (GBS) disease. Infected mothers transmit GBS infection to their infants during labor and birth; thus it is recommended that at-risk mothers receive intrapartum antimicrobial prophylaxis (IAP) for GBS disease. All infants of mothers identified as at risk should be assessed and observed for signs and symptoms of sepsis. It is important to know the policy and procedures that your hospital follows for surveillance of at-risk infants.

DRUG GUIDE Erythromycin Ophthalmic Ointment (Ilotycin Ophthalmic)

OVERVIEW OF NEONATAL ACTION

Erythromycin (Ilotycin Ophthalmic) is used as prophylactic treatment of ophthalmia neonatorum, which is caused by the bacteria *Neisseria gonorrhoeae.* Preventive treatment of gonorrhea in the newborn is required by law. Erythromycin is also effective against ophthalmic chlamydial infections. It is either bacteriostatic or bactericidal, depending on the organisms involved and the concentration of the drug.

PREGNANCY RISK CATEGORY: B

ROUTE, DOSAGE, FREQUENCY

Ophthalmic ointment (0.5%) is instilled as a narrow ribbon or strand, 0.5 to 1 cm long, along the lower conjunctival surface of each eye, starting at the inner canthus. It is instilled only once in each eye. The ointment may be administered in the birthing area or, alternatively, later in the nursery so that eye contact between infant and parent is facilitated and the bonding process immediately after birth is not interrupted. After administration, gently close the eye and manipulate to ensure spread of ointment (Wilson et al., 2010).

NEONATAL SIDE EFFECTS

Sensitivity reaction; may interfere with ability to focus and may cause edema and inflammation. Side effects usually disappear in 24 to 48 hours.

NURSING CONSIDERATIONS

- Wash hands immediately before instillation to prevent introduction of bacteria.
- Do not irrigate the eyes after instillation. Use new tube or single-use container for ophthalmic ointment administration shortly after birth. May wipe away excess after 1 minute.
- Observe for hypersensitivity.
- Teach parents about need for eye prophylaxis. Educate them regarding side effects and signs that need to be reported to the healthcare provider.

TABLE 31-2 Signs of Neonatal Distress

- Increased respiratory rate (more than 60/minute) or difficult respirations
- Sternal, substernal, intercostal retractions
- Nasal flaring
- Grunting
- Excessive mucus
- Facial grimacing
- Cyanosis (central: skin, lips, tongue)
- Abdominal distention or mass
- Vomiting of bile-stained material
- Absence of meconium elimination within 24 hours of birth
- Absence of urine elimination within 24 hours of birth
- Jaundice of the skin within 24 hours of birth or because of hemolytic process
- Temperature instability (hypothermia or hyperthermia)
- Jitteriness or glucose less than 40 mg%

Source: Adapted from Tappero, E. P., & Honeyfield, M. E. (1996). Physical assessment of the newborn *(2nd ed.). Petaluma, CA: NICU Inc.*

Initiation of First Feeding

The timing of the first feeding varies, depending on whether the newborn is to be breastfed or formula-fed and whether there were any complications during pregnancy or birth, such as maternal diabetes or intrauterine growth restriction (IUGR).

Mothers who choose to breastfeed their newborns should be encouraged to put their baby to breast during the first period of reactivity. This practice should be encouraged because successful, long-term breastfeeding during infancy appears to be related to beginning breastfeedings in the first few hours of life. Sleep-wake states affect feeding behavior and need to be considered when evaluating the newborn's sucking ability (Tedder, 2008).

Formula-fed newborns usually begin the first feedings by 5 hours of age, during the second period of reactivity, when they awaken and appear hungry. Signs indicating newborn readiness for the first feeding are licking of the lips, placing a hand in or near the mouth, mouthing the blanket, active bowel sounds, absence of abdominal distention, and a lusty cry that quiets with rooting and sucking behaviors when a stimulus is placed near the lips. Observing the earlier, more subtle cues that baby is ready to nurse provides an opportunity for the nurse to teach the parents to recognize these cues and respond before the baby is frustrated and crying.

Facilitation of Parent-Newborn Attachment

To facilitate **parent-newborn attachment**, eye-to-eye contact between parents and their newborn is extremely important during the early hours after birth, when the newborn is in the first period of reactivity. The newborn is alert during this time, the eyes are wide open, and direct eye contact is made with human faces within optimal range for visual acuity (7 to 8 inches). Eye contact is an important component of the emerging parent-baby bond (Klaus & Klaus, 1985). Consequently, the prophylactic eye medication is often delayed, but no more than 1 hour, to provide an opportunity for this period of eye contact between parents and their newborn, thus facilitating the attachment process (AAP & ACOG, 2007). Parents who cannot be with their newborns in this first period because of maternal or infant distress may need reassurance that the bonding process can proceed normally as soon as both mother and baby are stable.

Another situation that can facilitate attachment is the interactive bath. While bathing their newborn for the first time, parents attend closely to their baby's behavior. In this way the newborn becomes an active participant and parents are drawn into an interaction with their newborn. The nurse can interpret the infant's behavior, model ways to respond to the behavior, and support parental strategies for doing so (Tedder, 2008).

> “Now I believe in love at first sight!”
>
> — A New Mother Holding Her Infant for the First Time

Evaluation

When evaluating the nursing care provided during the period immediately after birth, the nurse may anticipate the following outcomes:

- The newborn baby's adaptation to extrauterine life is supported and complete.
- The baby's physiologic and psychologic integrity is supported.
- Positive interactions between parent and infant will be supported.

Nursing Management of the Newborn Following Transition

Once healthy newborns have demonstrated successful adaptation to extrauterine life, they need appropriate observations for the first 6 to 12 hours after birth and the remainder of their stay in the birthing facility.

Nursing Diagnosis

Examples of nursing diagnoses that may apply during daily care of the newborn include the following:

- *Risk for Ineffective Breathing Pattern* related to periodic breathing
- *Imbalanced Nutrition: Less Than Body Requirements* related to limited nutritional or fluid intake and increased caloric expenditure
- *Impaired Urinary Elimination* related to meatal edema secondary to circumcision
- *Risk for Infection* related to umbilical cord healing, circumcision site, immature immune system, or potential birth trauma (forceps or vacuum extraction birth)
- *Readiness for Enhanced Knowledge* related to lack of information about basic baby care, male circumcision, and breast- and/or formula-feeding
- *Readiness for Enhanced Family Relationship* related to integration of newborn into family unit or demands of newborn care and feeding
- *Risk for Injury* related to hyperbilirubinemia

CLINICAL JUDGMENT

Case Study: Aisha Khan

Aisha Khan gave birth to a healthy girl 2 hours ago. Now she calls you to her room. She sounds frightened and says her baby can't breathe. You find Aisha cradling her newborn in her arms. The baby is mildly cyanotic, is waving her arms, and has mucus coming from her nose and mouth.

Critical Thinking

What would you do?

See www.nursing.pearsonhighered.com for possible responses.

Nursing Plan and Implementation

Maintenance of Cardiopulmonary Function

The nurse assesses vital signs every 6 to 8 hours or more, depending on the newborn's status. The newborn should be placed on his or her back (supine) for sleeping. A bulb syringe is kept within easy reach should the baby need oral-nasal suctioning. If the newborn has respiratory difficulty, the airway is cleared. Vigorous fingertip stroking of the baby's spine will frequently stimulate respiratory activity. A cardiorespiratory monitor can be used on newborns who are not being observed at all times and are at risk for decreased respiratory or cardiac function. Indicators of risk are pallor, cyanosis, ruddy color, apnea, or other signs of instability. Changes in skin color may indicate the need for closer assessment of temperature, cardiopulmonary status, hematocrit, glucose, and bilirubin levels.

Maintenance of a Neutral Thermal Environment

The nurse makes every effort to maintain the newborn's temperature within the normal range. The nurse must make certain the newborn is dried completely after the bath, dressed, and exposed to the air as little as possible. A head covering should be used initially and continued with the small newborn, who has less subcutaneous fat to act as insulation in maintaining body heat. Ambient temperature of the room where the newborn is kept should be monitored to prevent excessive cooling. Parents may be advised to dress the newborn in one more layer of clothing than is necessary for an adult to maintain thermal comfort. The use of clothes layering allows for flexibility as the infant is moved from one area to another.

A newborn whose temperature falls below optimal levels will use calories to maintain body heat rather than for growth. Chilling also decreases the affinity of serum albumin for bilirubin, thereby increasing the likelihood of newborn jaundice. It also increases oxygen use and may cause respiratory distress. An infant who is overheated will have an increased respiratory and heart rate and may also become more active, burning up precious caloric reserves. The increase in respiratory rate also results in insensible fluid loss.

CLINICAL JUDGMENT

Case Study: John Fredericks

John Fredericks, the father of a child less than a day old, has the child lying on its back with only a diaper. When you suggest that the baby may need more covering, he responds: "He doesn't like all that stuff on. After all, he's been naked until now."

Critical Thinking

What actions and teaching are appropriate in this situation?

See www.nursing.pearsonhighered.com for possible responses.

Promotion of Adequate Hydration and Nutrition

The nurse records the newborn's caloric and fluid intake and enhances adequate hydration by maintaining a neutral thermal environment and offering early and frequent feedings. Early feedings promote gastric emptying and increase peristalsis, thereby decreasing the degree of hyperbilirubinemia by limiting the amount of time fecal material is in contact with the enzyme β-glucuronidase in the small intestine. This enzyme acts to free the bilirubin from the stool, allowing bilirubin to be reabsorbed into the vascular system. The nurse records voiding and stooling patterns. The first voiding should occur within 24 hours and passage of stool within 48 hours. When they do not occur, the nurse continues the normal observation routine while assessing for abdominal distention, bowel sounds, hydration, fluid intake, voiding pattern, and temperature stability.

The newborn should be weighed at the same time each day for accurate comparisons and must be kept warm during the weighing. A weight loss of up to 10% for term newborns is considered within normal limits during the first week of life. This weight loss is the result of limited intake, loss of excess extracellular fluid, and passage of meconium. Parents should be told about the expected weight loss, the reason for it, and the expectations for regaining the birth weight. Birth weight should be regained by 2 weeks if feedings are adequate.

Excessive handling can cause an increase in the newborn's metabolic rate and calorie use and cause fatigue. The nurse should be alert to the baby's subtle cues of fatigue, including a decrease in muscle tension and activity in the extremities and neck, as well as loss of eye contact, which may be manifested by fluttering or closing the eyelids. The nurse quickly ceases stimulation when signs of fatigue appear and demonstrates to the parents the need to be aware of newborn cues of fatigue and to wait for periods of alertness for contact and stimulation. The nurse is also responsible for assessing the woman's comfort and latching-on techniques, if breastfeeding, or bottle-feeding techniques. Newborn nutrition is addressed in depth in chapter 32 ∞.

Promotion of Skin Integrity

Newborn skin care, including bathing, is important for the health and appearance of the individual newborn and for infection control within the nursery. Ongoing skin care involves cleansing the buttock and perianal areas with fresh water and cotton, or with a mild soap and water, with diaper changes. If commercial baby wipes are used, those without alcohol should be selected. Wipes that are perfume- and latex-free are also available.

Care Plan Activity: Infant Care During Transition

The umbilical cord is assessed for signs of bleeding or infection. Removal of the cord clamp within 24 to 48 hours of birth reduces the chance of tension injury to the area. Keeping the umbilical stump clean and dry can reduce the chance for infection (Figure 31-6 ■). Many types of routine cord care are practiced, including the use of triple-dye or an antimicrobial agent such as bacitracin or application of 70% alcohol to the cord stump. These practices are largely based on tradition rather than current research findings. The skin absorption and toxicity of triple-dye agents in newborns have not been carefully studied. No single method of umbilical cord care (topical antimicrobials [triple-dye, iodophor ointment, or hexachlorophene powder] or alcohol)

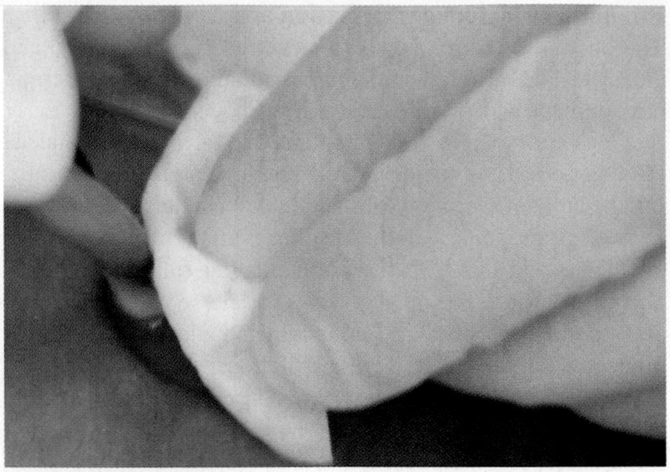

Figure 31-6 ■ The umbilical cord base is carefully cleaned.

Source: George Dodson/Lightworks Studio/Pearson Education.

has been proven to be superior in preventing colonization and disease (AAP & ACOG, 2007). The use of sterile water or air drying results in umbilical cords separating more quickly than those treated with alcohol (Askin, 2008).

Folding the diaper down to prevent coverage of the cord stump can prevent contamination of the area and promote drying. The nurse is responsible for cord care per agency policy. It is also the nurse's responsibility to instruct parents in caring for the cord and observing for signs and symptoms of infection after discharge, such as foul smell, redness and greenish yellow drainage, localized heat and tenderness, or bright red bleeding or if the area remains unhealed 2 to 3 days after the cord has sloughed off.

Promotion of Safety

Safety of the newborn is paramount. It is essential that the nurse and other caregivers verify the identity of the newborn by comparing the numbers and names on the identification bracelets of mother and newborn before giving a baby to a parent (Askin, 2008). Another form of identification band attached to the ankle or umbilical cord has a built-in sensor unit that sounds an alarm if the baby is transported beyond set birthing unit boundaries. Individual birthing units should practice safety measures to prevent infant abduction and provide information to parents regarding their role in this area, as well as in general newborn safety measures (Vincent, 2009). Parental measures to prevent abduction and promote newborn safety include the following:

Security

- Checking that identification bands are in place as they care for their infant and, if missing, asking that they be replaced immediately
- Allowing only people with proper birthing unit identification to remove their baby from their room. If parents do not know the staff person, they should call the nurse for assistance.
- Reporting the presence of any suspicious people on the birthing unit

Safety

- Never leaving their newborn alone in their room. If parents walk in the halls or take a shower, they should have a family member watch the newborn or they should return the newborn to the nursery.
- Never lifting the newborn if a parent feels weak, faint, or unsteady on his or her feet. Instead, the parent should call for assistance.
- Always keeping an eye and hand on the newborn when he or she is out of the crib.
- Protecting from infection, even though newborns do possess some immunity. Parents should ask visitors to leave if they have any of the following: cold, diarrhea, discharge from sores, or contagious disease.

Prevention of Complications

Newborns are at continued risk for the complications of hemorrhage, late-onset cardiac symptoms, jaundice, and infection. Pallor may be an early sign of hemorrhage and must be reported to the physician. The newborn is placed on a cardiorespiratory monitor to permit continuous assessment. Several newborn conditions or procedures such as circumcision put the newborn at risk for bleeding. Cyanosis that is not relieved by oxygen administration requires emergency intervention, may indicate a congenital cardiac condition or shock, and requires immediate and ongoing assessment.

Infection in the nursery is best prevented by requiring that all personnel having direct contact with newborns scrub for 2 to 3 minutes from fingertips to and including elbows at the beginning of each shift. The hands must be washed with soap and rubbed vigorously for 15 seconds before and after contact with every newborn or after touching any soiled surface, such as the floor or one's hair or face. Parents are instructed to practice good hand washing and/or use of an antiseptic hand cleaner before touching the baby. They are also instructed that anyone holding the baby should wash hands as well, even after the family returns home. In some clinical settings family members are requested to wear a gown (preferably disposable) over their street clothes during contact with infants. These are good opportunities for the nurse to reinforce the efficacy of hand washing in preventing the spread of infection.

Jaundice occurs in most newborn infants. Most jaundice is benign, but because of the potential toxicity of bilirubin, newborn infants must be monitored to identify those who might develop severe hyperbilirubinemia and, in rare cases, acute bilirubin encephalopathy or kernicterus (see chapter 34 ∞ for a more detailed discussion) (AAP & ACOG, 2007). Current recommendations include obtaining a total serum bilirubin level in any infant who is visibly jaundiced in the first 24 hours of life, and obtaining either a serum or transcutaneous bilirubin level before discharge. Nomograms for evaluating risk factors based on bilirubin levels and age of infant are available (see chapter 29 ∞ for discussion).

Circumcision

Circumcision is a surgical procedure in which the prepuce, an epithelial layer covering the tip of the penis, is separated from the glans penis and excised. This permits exposure of the glans for easier cleaning.

Circumcision was originally a religious rite practiced by Jews and Muslims. The practice gained widespread cultural acceptance in the United States but is much less common in Europe. Families make the decision about circumcision for their newborn male child. Many parents choose circumcision because they want the male child to have a physical appearance similar to that of the father or the majority of other children, or they may feel that it is expected by society. Another commonly cited reason for circumcising newborn males is to prevent the need for anesthesia, hospitalization, pain, and trauma should the procedure be needed later in life (AAP & ACOG, 2007). To ensure informed consent, parents should be advised during the prenatal period about possible long-term medical effects of circumcision and noncircumcision.

CURRENT RECOMMENDATIONS The 2005 AAP policy statement reaffirmed that it does not recommend *routine* circumcision but acknowledges that medical indications for circumcision still exist (AAP & ACOG, 2007). The policy recommends that analgesia (e.g., dorsal penile nerve block [DPNB] or subcutaneous ring block) be used during circumcision to decrease procedural pain (American Academy of Pediatrics (AAP) & Canadian Paediatric Society (CPS), 2006). The DPNB and subcutaneous ring block are the most effective options. If a circumcision is to be performed it should be done using the least painful method. Recent studies show that using oral sucrose for painful procedures can be effective in managing pain for newborns and it should be used with other nonpharmacologic measures to enhance its effectiveness (AAP & CPS, 2006).

Circumcision *should not be performed* if the newborn is premature or compromised, has a known bleeding problem, or is born with a genitourinary defect, such as hypospadias or epispadias, which may necessitate the use of the foreskin in future surgical repairs.

NURSE'S ROLE A well-informed nurse can allay parents' anxiety by sharing information and allowing them to express their concerns. In order for parents to make a truly informed decision, they must be knowledgeable about the potential risks and outcomes of circumcision. Hemorrhage, infection, difficulty in voiding, separation of the edges of the circumcision, pain, and restlessness are early potential problems. Later there is the risk that the glans and urethral meatus can become irritated and inflamed from contact with ammonia from urine. Ulcerations and progressive stenosis may develop. Adhesions, progressive stenosis, entrapment of the penis, and damage to the urethra are all potential complications that could require surgical correction (AAP & ACOG, 2007).

The parents of an uncircumcised male infant require information from the nurse about good hygiene practices. They should be told that the foreskin and glans are two similar layers of cells that separate from each other. The separation process begins prenatally and is normally completed at between 3 and 5 years of age. In the process of separation, sterile sloughed cells build up between the layers. This buildup looks similar to the smegma secreted after puberty, and it is harmless. Occasionally during the daily bath, the parents can gently test for retraction. If retraction has occurred, daily gentle washing of the glans with soap and water is sufficient to maintain adequate cleanliness. The parents should teach the child to incorporate this practice into his daily self-care activities. Most uncircumcised males have no difficulty doing so.

Circumcision Resources

If circumcision is desired, the procedure should be performed after the newborn is well stabilized and has received his initial physical examination by a healthcare provider. The parents may also choose to have the circumcision done after discharge. However, they need to be advised that if the baby is older than 1 month, the current practice is to hospitalize him for the procedure.

Before a circumcision, the nurse ascertains that the physician has explained the procedure, determines whether the parents have any further questions about the procedure, and verified that the circumcision permit is signed. As with any surgical procedure, the identification band of the infant should be checked to verify his identity before the procedure begins. The nurse gathers the equipment and prepares the newborn by removing the diaper and placing him on a padded circumcision board or some other type of restraint, but restraining only the legs. These restraint measures along with the application of warm blankets to the upper body increase comfort during the procedure. In Jewish circumcision ceremonies, the infant is held by the father or grandfather and given wine before the procedure.

Application: Circumcision

There are a variety of devices (Gomco clamp, Plastibell, Mogen clamp) used for circumcision (Figures 31-7 ■ and 31-8 ■), and all produce minimal bleeding. Therefore the nurse should make special note of infants with a family history of bleeding disorders or with mothers who took anticoagulants, including aspirin, prenatally. During the procedure, the nurse assesses the newborn's response. One important consideration is pain experienced by the newborn. A DPNB or ring block using 1% lidocaine without epinephrine or similar anesthetic significantly minimizes the pain and the shifts in behavioral patterns, such as crying, irritability, and erratic sleep cycles associated with circumcision. Other studies of pain control measures involve the use of topical anesthetic applied 60 to 90 minutes before prepuce removal and the use of sucrose pacifiers before and during the procedure, acetaminophen, and cryoanalgesia. Studies indicate that a combination of methods is most effective in reducing pain during circumcision (AAP & CPS, 2006).

During the procedure, the nurse can provide comfort measures such as lightly stroking the baby's head, providing a pacifier, and talking to him. Following the circumcision, the infant should be held and comforted by a family member or the nurse. The nurse must be alert to any cues that these measures are overstimulating the newborn instead of comforting him. Such cues include turning away of the head, increased generalized body movement, skin color changes, hyperalertness, and hiccuping.

Ideally, the circumcision should be assessed for signs of hemorrhage and infection every 30 minutes for at least 2 hours following the procedure. It is important to observe for the first voiding after a circumcision to evaluate for urinary obstruction related to penile injury and/or edema. Petroleum and gauze are applied to the site immediately following the procedure to help prevent bleeding and can be used to protect the healing tissue afterward.

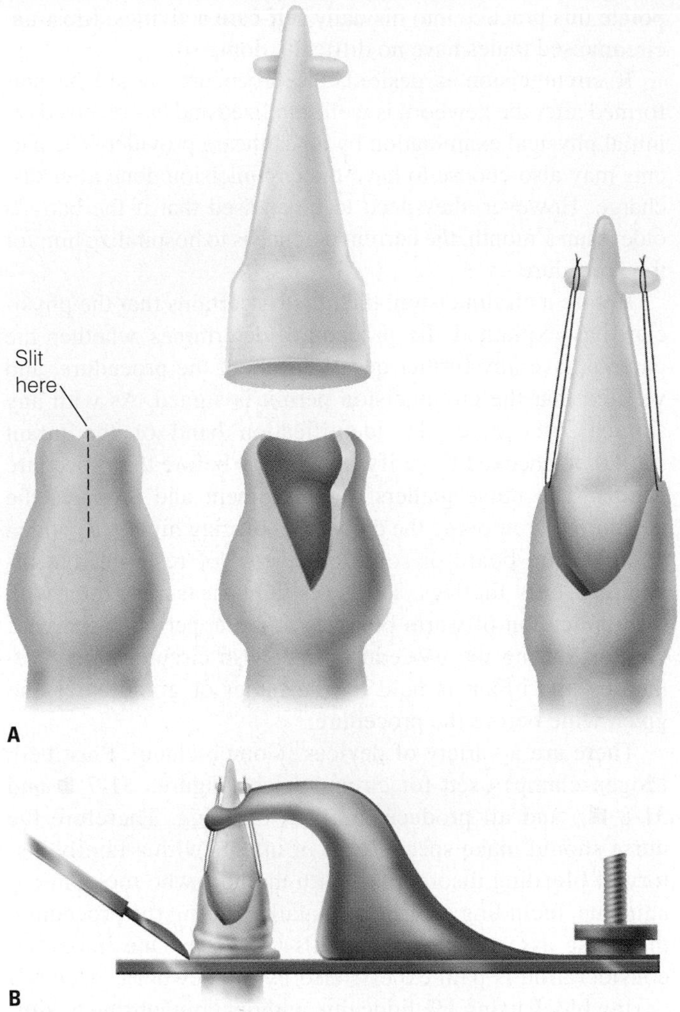

Figure 31-7 ■ Circumcision using the Yellen or Gomco clamp. A. The prepuce is drawn over the cone. B. The clamp is applied. Pressure is maintained for 3 to 4 minutes, and then excess prepuce is cut away.

The nurse must also teach family members how to assess for unusual bleeding, how to respond if it is present, and how to care for the newly circumcised penis. Parents of babies circumcised with a method other than Plastibell should receive the following information:

- Clean with warm water with each diaper change.
- Apply petroleum ointment for the next few diaper changes to help prevent further bleeding (Figure 31-9 ■).
- If bleeding does occur, apply light pressure with a sterile gauze pad to stop the bleeding within a short time. If this is not effective, contact the physician immediately, or take the baby to the healthcare provider's office.
- The glans normally has granulation tissue (a yellowish film) on it during healing. Continued application of a petroleum ointment (or ointment suggested by the healthcare provider) can help protect the granulation tissue that forms as the glans heals.
- Report to the care provider any signs or symptoms of infection, such as increasing swelling, pus drainage, and cessation of urination.
- When diapering, ensure that the diaper is not loose enough to cause rubbing with movement, or tight enough to cause pain.

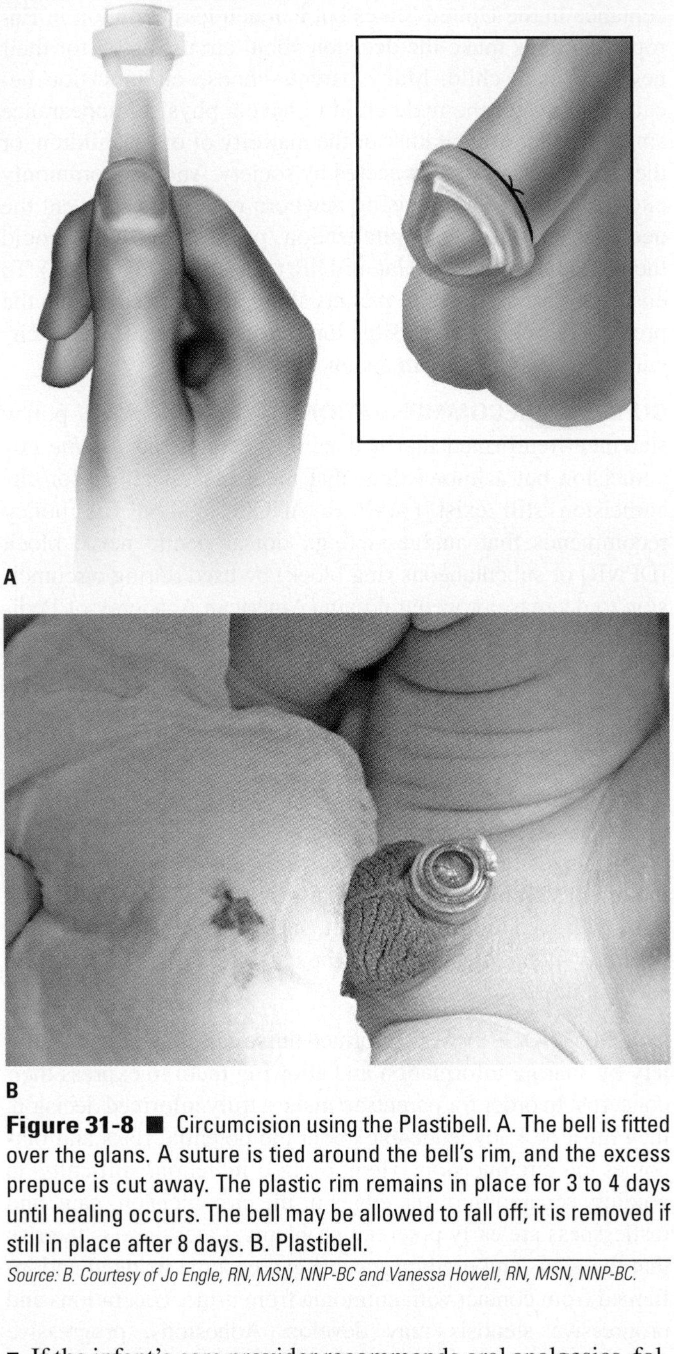

Figure 31-8 ■ Circumcision using the Plastibell. A. The bell is fitted over the glans. A suture is tied around the bell's rim, and the excess prepuce is cut away. The plastic rim remains in place for 3 to 4 days until healing occurs. The bell may be allowed to fall off; it is removed if still in place after 8 days. B. Plastibell.

Source: B. Courtesy of Jo Engle, RN, MSN, NNP-BC and Vanessa Howell, RN, MSN, NNP-BC.

- If the infant's care provider recommends oral analgesics, follow instructions for proper measuring and administration.

If the Plastibell is used, parents should receive information about normal appearance and how to observe for infection. The parents are informed that the Plastibell should fall off within 8 days. If it still remains after 8 days, they should consult with their physician. Though no ointments or creams should be used while the bell remains, use of petroleum ointment to protect granulation tissue may be useful afterward.

Enhancement of Parent-Newborn Attachment

Parent-newborn attachment is promoted by encouraging all family members to be involved with the new member of the family. Some specific interventions are examined in chapters 24 ∞ and 36 ∞ and the accompanying Patient Teaching: Enhancing At-

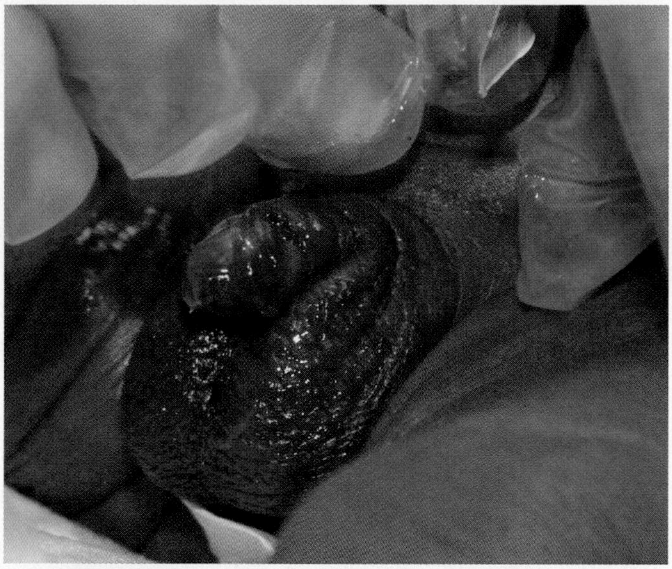

Figure 31-9 ■ Following circumcision, petroleum ointment may be applied to the site for the next few diaper changes.

Source: George Dodson/Lightworks Studio/Pearson Education.

tachment. Infant massage is a common childcare practice in many parts of the world, especially Africa and Asia, and has recently gained attention in the United States. Parents can be taught to use infant massage as a method to facilitate the bonding process and to reduce the stress and pain associated with teething, inoculations, constipation, and colic. Infant massage not only induces relaxation for the infant, but also provides a calming and "feel good" interaction for the parents, which fosters the development of warm, positive relationships.

DEVELOPING CULTURAL COMPETENCE
Infant Naming in Kenya

In Kenya, the naming of the child is an important event. Names are commonly selected to mirror important or current events. For example, an infant who is born while traveling may be given a name that means "wanderer" or "traveler." Other names may be chosen after a relative who is among the "living-dead" (deceased). It is believed that this results in a partial reincarnation of that relative, especially if the child has characteristics in common with that individual. It is also believed there is a connection between newborns and the spirit world. In some parts of the country, the name is chosen when the child is crying. Different names of the living-dead are called, and when the child stops crying when a particular name is called, that becomes the child's given name. In some areas, the name is given on the third day and is marked by a celebration with feasting and rejoicing. On the fourth day, the father of the child commonly hangs an iron necklace on the child's neck. It is at this time that the infant is considered a full human being and the connection with the spirit world is lost.

The nurse can discuss waking activities such as talking with the baby while making eye contact, holding the baby in an upright position (sitting or standing), gently bending the baby back and forth while grasping under the knees and supporting the head and back with the other hand, and gently rubbing the baby's hands and feet. Quieting activities may include swaddling the baby to increase a sense of security; using slow, calming movements; and talking softly, singing, or humming to the baby (Figure 31-10 ■).

A Letter From Your Baby

Dear Parents:

I come to you a small, immature being with my own style and personality. I am yours for only a short time; enjoy me.

1. Please take time to find out who I am, how I differ from you, and how much I can bring you joy.
2. Please feed me when I am hungry. I never knew hunger in the womb, and clocks and time mean little to me.
3. Please hold, cuddle, kiss, touch, stroke, and croon to me. I was always held closely in the womb and was never alone before.
4. Please don't be disappointed when I am not the perfect baby that you expected, nor disappointed with yourselves that you are not the perfect parents.
5. Please don't expect too much from me as your newborn baby, or too much from yourself as a parent. Give us both six weeks as a birthday present—six weeks for me to grow, develop, mature, and become more stable and predictable, and six weeks for you to rest and relax and allow your body to get back to normal.
6. Please forgive me if I cry a lot. Bear with me and in a short time, as I mature, I will spend less and less time crying and more time socializing.
7. Please watch me carefully and I can tell you the things that soothe, console, and please me. I am not a tyrant who was sent to make your life miserable, but the only way I can tell you that I am not happy is with my cry.
8. Please remember that I am resilient and can withstand the many natural mistakes you will make with me. As long as you make them with love, you cannot ruin me.
9. Please take care of yourself and eat a balanced diet, rest, and exercise so that when we are together, you have the health and strength to take care of me.
10. Please take care of your relationship with others. Relationships that are good for you, support both you and me.

Although I may have turned your life upside down, please realize that things will be back to normal before long.

Thank you,

Your Loving Child

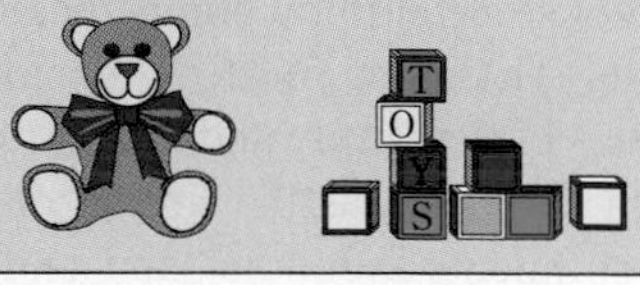

Figure 31-10 ■ A letter from your baby.

PATIENT TEACHING Enhancing Attachment

PATIENT GOALS At the completion of teaching, the parents will be able to:

1. Demonstrate appropriate nurturing behaviors such as touching, bonding, talking to, kissing, and holding their baby.
2. Discuss the normal characteristics and emotional needs of the newborn.
3. List at least three comforting techniques.

TEACHING PLAN

Content	Teaching Method
■ Present information on periods of reactivity and expected newborn responses.	Focus on open discussion.
■ Describe normal physical characteristics of the newborn (see chapter 30 ∞).	Present slides showing newborn characteristics, or in teaching an individual family, point out the normal physical characteristics of their child.
■ Explain the bonding process, its gradual development, and the reciprocal interactive nature of the process.	
■ Discuss the infant's capabilities for interaction, such as nonverbal communication abilities. The nonverbal communications include movement, gaze, touch, facial expressions, and vocalizations—including crying. Emphasize that eye contact is considered one of the cardinal factors in developing infant-parent attachment and will be integrated with touching and vocal behaviors.	Show a video on the interactive capabilities of newborns. In the mother-baby or newborn setting, this teaching is effectively done by nurses who point out the communication that babies are exhibiting throughout the day, enhancing the parents' awareness of the responses of their own infant.
■ Explain that touching, including stroking, patting, massaging, and kissing, will progress to interactive touch between the parents and their infant; discuss their need to assimilate these behaviors into their daily routine with the baby.	Provide handouts, and use a doll to demonstrate behaviors, because repeating even soothing touch, as each family member practices it, can be overstimulating to the infant, thus use of a doll to reinforce teaching can be very helpful.
■ Describe and demonstrate comforting techniques, including the use of sound, swaddling, rocking, massage, and stroking.	Demonstrate the techniques and ask for a return demonstration.
■ Describe the progression of the infant's behaviors as the infant matures, and the importance of the parents' consistent response to their infant's cues and needs.	Allow time for questions and discussion.
■ Provide information about available pamphlets, videos, classes, and support groups in the community.	

Evaluation

Evaluate the learning by providing time for discussion, questions, and return demonstrations in the birthing unit, and during the postpartal return visit or home visit. Continue to observe the parents' positive interaction with their baby during the remainder of their stay in the birthing unit.

Documentation

The nurse should document the information that was given, the type of teaching method used, indicate if the parent performed nurturing behaviors such as touching and comfort techniques, and if verbal or written directions were given. Verbalization of understanding and clarification of any information should be documented. Safety issues and instructions on newborn physical characteristics and normal progression of infant behaviors were given.

Caring for newborns in the birthing setting means that the nurse will have contact with patients from a wide variety of racial, religious, and cultural backgrounds. Though it may not be possible to be conversant with all cultures, the nurse can demonstrate cultural competence with both colleagues and patients. The nurse must be sensitive to the cultural beliefs and values of the family and be aware of cultural variations in newborn care such as the timing of naming the newborn, giving compliments about the baby, and using good luck charms. The nurse plays a vital role in fostering parent-infant attachment. It is important to be sensitive to the cultural beliefs and values of the family.

Several methods may be used to teach parents about newborn care. Daily newborn care videos or classes are a nonthreatening way to convey general information. Individual instruction is helpful to answer specific questions or to clarify an item that may have been confusing in class. Currently many birthing centers have 24-hour educational video channels or videos to be viewed in the mother's room on a variety of postpartum and newborn care issues.

DEVELOPING CULTURAL COMPETENCE

Examples of Cultural Beliefs and Practices Regarding Baby Care*

UMBILICAL CORD

- People of Latin American or Filipino cultural background may use an abdominal binder or bellyband to protect against dirt, injury, and umbilical hernia. They may also apply oils to the stump of the cord or tape metal to the umbilicus to ward off evil spirits (D'Avanzo & Geissler, 2008).
- People of northern European ancestry may expect a sterile cutting of the cord at birth. They may allow the stump to air-dry and discard the cord once it falls off.
- Some Latin American cultures cauterize the stump with a hot flame, hot coal, or the like (World Health Organization [WHO], 1999).
- In Kenya, women may express colostrum to the cord stump (WHO, 1999).
- In Ecuador, the cord is left long in girls to prevent a small uterus and problems with childbirth (WHO, 1999).

PARENT-INFANT CONTACT

- People of Asian ancestry may pick up the baby as soon as he or she cries, or they may carry the baby at all times.
- Some Native Americans, notably the Navajos, may use cradle boards so the infant can be with the family even during work (Andrews, 2008).
- The Muslim father traditionally calls praise to Allah in the newborn's right ear and cleans the infant after birth.

FEEDING

- Some women of Asian heritage may breastfeed their babies for the first 1 to 2 years of life. Many Cambodian refugees practice breastfeeding on demand without restriction, or, if formula-feeding, provide a "comfort bottle" in between feedings (Lipson & Dibble, 2008).
- People of Iranian heritage may breastfeed female babies longer than male babies.
- Some people of African ancestry may wean their babies after they begin to walk.
- Some Asians, Hispanics, Eastern Europeans, and Native Americans may delay breastfeeding because they believe colostrum is "bad" (D'Avanzo & Geissler, 2008).
- Haitian mothers may believe that "strong emotions" spoil breast milk (Lipson & Dibble, 2008).

CIRCUMCISION

- People of Muslim and Jewish ancestry practice circumcision as a religious ritual (Lipson & Dibble, 2008).
- Many natives of Africa and Australia practice circumcision as a puberty rite.
- Native Americans and people of Asian and Latin American cultures rarely perform circumcision (Lipson & Dibble, 2008).
- As of 2006, global estimates are that about 30% of males are circumcised (WHO, 2008).

HEALTH AND ILLNESS

- Some people from Latin American cultural backgrounds may believe that touching the face or head of an infant when admiring it will ward off the "evil eye." They may also neglect to cut the baby's nails to avoid nearsightedness and instead put mittens on the baby's hands to prevent scratching. They also may believe that fat babies are healthier (Andrews, 2008).
- Some people of Asian heritage may not allow anyone to touch the baby's head without asking permission.
- Some Orthodox Jews believe that saying the baby's name before the formal naming ceremony will harm the baby.
- Some Asians and Haitians delay naming their infants (D'Avanzo & Geissler, 2008).
- Some people of Vietnamese ancestry believe that cutting a baby's hair or nails will cause illness.

*Note: The information is meant only to provide examples of some of the behaviors that may be found within certain cultures. Not all members of a culture practice the behaviors described.

Evaluation

When evaluating the nursing care provided during the newborn period, the nurse may anticipate the following outcomes:

- The baby's physiologic and psychologic integrity is supported.
- The newborn feeding pattern will be satisfactorily established.
- The parents express understanding of the bonding process and display attachment behaviors.

Nursing Management in Preparation for Discharge

Although the adjustment to parenting is a normal process, going home presents a critical transition for the family. The parents become the primary caregivers for the newborn and must provide a nurturing environment in which the emotional and physical needs of the newborn can be met. Nursing interventions focus on promoting health and preventing possible problems.

Nursing Assessment and Diagnosis

When preparing for discharge, assess whether parents have realistic expectations of the newborn's behavior and the depth of their knowledge in caring for their newborn.

Nursing diagnoses that may apply to the newborn's family include the following:

- *Readiness for Enhanced Parenting* related to appropriate behavioral expectations for the newborn
- *Readiness for Enhanced Family Processes* related to integration of newborn into family unit or demands of newborn care and feeding

Planning and Implementation

HEALTH PROMOTION EDUCATION

To meet parent needs for information, the nurse who is responsible for the daily care of the mother and newborn should assume the primary responsibility for parent education. Nearly every contact with the parents presents an opportunity for sharing information that can facilitate their sense of competence in newborn care. The nurse also needs to recognize and respect the fact that there are many good ways to provide safe care. Unless their care methods are harmful to the newborn, the parents' methods of giving care should be reinforced rather than contradicted.

The information that follows is provided to increase the nurse's knowledge of newborn care and is used to meet parents' needs for information. Parents may be familiar with handling and caring for infants, or this may be their first time to interact with a newborn. If they are new parents, the sensitive nurse gently teaches them by example and provides instructions geared to their needs and previous knowledge about the various aspects of newborn care.

The nurse observes how parents interact with their infant during feeding and caregiving activities. Even during a short stay, there will be opportunities for the nurse to provide information and evaluate whether the parents are comfortable with changing diapers and wrapping, handling, and feeding their newborn (Figure 31-11 ■). Do both parents get involved in the infant's care? Is the mother depending on someone else to help her at home? Does the mother give excuses ("I am too tired," "My stitches hurt," or "I will learn later") for not wanting to be involved in her baby's care? As the family provides care, the nurse can enhance parental confidence by giving them positive feedback. If the family encounters problems, the nurse can express confidence in the family's abilities to master the new skill or information, suggest alternatives, and serve as a role model. All these considerations need to be taken into account when evaluating the educational needs of the parents. Providing mother-baby-care and home-care instruction on the night shift assists with education needs for early discharge parents.

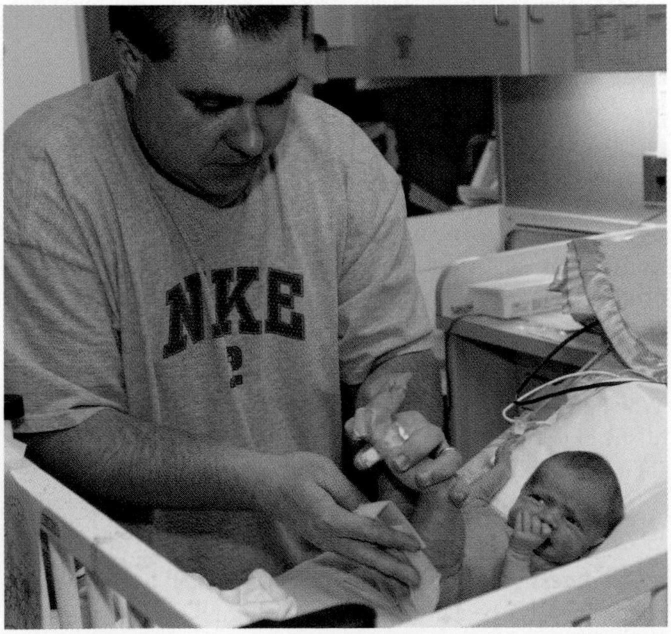

Figure 31-11 ■ A father demonstrates competence and confidence in diapering his newborn daughter.

Source: George Dodson/Lightworks Studio/Pearson Education.

Case Study: Newborn Care

CLINICAL TIP

For patients who are hearing-impaired, videotapes with information in both spoken and signed formats are most helpful. Also, birthing centers should have handouts available for families who do not speak English, as well as either interpreters (not family members) or language interpreter phones.

One-to-one teaching while the nurse is in the mother's room is shown to be the most effective educational model. Both first-time and experienced postpartum mothers rate individual teaching as the most effective method of instruction. Individual instruction is helpful both to answer specific questions and to clarify something that the parents may have found confusing in the educational video. With shorter stays, most teaching unfortunately tends to focus on infant feeding and immediate physical needs of the mothers, with limited anticipatory guidance provided in other areas. (Table 31-3 shows the broad range of information important to share with new parents. These topics are discussed in more detail next.)

> "I felt something impossible for me to explain in words. Then, when they took her away, it hit me. I got scared all over again and began to feel giddy. Then it came to me . . . I was a father."
>
> — *Nat King Cole*

General Instructions for Newborn Care

One of the first concerns of anyone who has not had the experience of picking up a baby is how to do it correctly. The newborn is easily picked up by sliding one hand under the neck and shoulders and the other hand under the buttocks or between the legs, then gently lifting the newborn. This technique provides security and support for the head (which the baby is unable to consistently support until 3 or 4 months of age).

The nurse can be an excellent role model for families in the area of safety. Safety topics include proper positioning of the newborn on the back to sleep and correct use of the bulb syringe (discussed shortly). The baby should never be left alone anywhere but in the crib. The mother is reminded that while she and the newborn are together in the birthing unit, she should never leave the baby alone for security reasons and because newborns spit up frequently the first day or two after birth. Other newborn safety measures are discussed in detail in chapter 37 ∞.

TABLE 31-3 What Parents Need to Know About Newborn Care

Immediate Safety Measures for the Newborn

- Watch for excessive mucus: use bulb syringe to remove mucus.
- Have baby sleep on his or her back in crib or in someone's arms.

Voiding and Stool Characteristics and Patterns

- Urine is straw to amber color without foul smell. Small amounts of uric acid crystals are normal in first days of life (may be mistaken by parents as blood in diaper because of reddish "brick dust" appearance).
- At least 6 to 10 wet diapers a day after the first few days of life.
- Normal progression of stool changes: (1) meconium (thick, tarry, dark green); (2) transitional stools (thin, brown to green); (3a) breastfed infant: yellow gold, soft or mushy stools; (3b) formula-fed infant: pale yellow, formed and pasty stools.
- Only 1 to 2 stools a day for formula-fed baby.
- Six to 10 small, loose yellow stools per day or only one stool every few days after breastfeeding is well established (after about 1 month).

Cord Care

- Wash hands with clean water and soap before and after care. Keep the cord dry and exposed to air or loosely covered with clean clothes. (If cultural custom demands binding of the abdomen, a sanitary method such as the use of a clean piece of gauze can be recommended.)
- Clean cord and skin around base with a cotton swab or cotton ball. Clean 2 to 3 times a day or with each diaper change. Touching the cord, applying unclean substances to it, and applying bandages should be avoided. Do not give tub baths until cord falls off in 7 to 14 days.
- Fold diapers below umbilical cord to air-dry the cord (contact with wet or soiled diapers slows the drying process and increases the possibility of infection).
- Check cord each day for any odor, oozing of greenish yellow material, or reddened areas around the cord. Expect tenderness around the cord and darkening and shriveling of cord. Report to healthcare provider any signs of infection.
- Normal changes in cord: Cord should look dark and dry up before falling off. A small drop of blood may present when cord falls off.
- Never pull the cord or attempt to loosen it.

Care Required for Circumcision and Uncircumcised Infants

Circumcision Care

- Squeeze water over circumcision site once a day.
- Rinse area off with warm water and pat dry.
- Apply small amount of petroleum jelly (unless a Plastibell is in place) with each diaper change.
- Fasten diaper over penis snugly enough so that it does not move and rub the tender glans.
- Because the glans is sensitive, avoid placing baby on his stomach for the first day after the procedure.
- Check for any foul-smelling drainage or bleeding at least once a day.
- Let Plastibell fall off by itself (about 8 days after circumcision).
- Plastibell should not be pulled off.
- Light, sticky, yellow drainage (part of healing process) may form over head of penis.

Uncircumcised Care

- Clean uncircumcised penis with water during diaper changes and with bath.
- Do not force foreskin back over the penis; foreskin will retract normally over time (may take 3 to 5 years).

Techniques for Waking and Quieting Newborns

Techniques for Waking Baby

- Loosen clothing, change diaper.
- Hand-express milk onto baby's lips.
- Talk with baby while making eye contact.
- Hold baby in upright position (sitting or standing).
- Have baby do sit-ups (gently and rhythmically bend baby back and forth while grasping the baby under his or her knees and supporting baby's head and back with your other hand).
- Play patty-cake with baby.
- Stimulate rooting reflex (brush one cheek with hand or nipple).
- Increase skin contact (gently rub hands and feet).

Techniques for Quieting Baby

- Check for soiled diaper.
- Swaddle or bundle baby (bring arms and legs into midline, which increases sense of security).
- Hold swaddled baby upright against mid-chest, supporting bottom and back of head. Baby can hear heartbeat, feel warmth, and hear your softly spoken words or calming sounds.
- Use slow, calming movements with baby.
- Softly talk, sing, or hum to baby.

Signs of Illness and Use of Thermometer

- See Table 31-4: When Parents Should Call Their Healthcare Provider.

CLINICAL JUDGMENT

Case Study: Sarah Feldstein

You are caring for Sarah Feldstein, who had her first child, a daughter, about 4 hours ago. She appears visibly upset when changing her infant's diaper, and says she thinks something is wrong because her daughter has tissue protruding from her vagina and some bleeding in her diaper.

Critical Thinking

What would you do?

See www.nursing.pearsonhighered.com for possible responses.

Demonstrating a bath (see chapter 37 ∞), cord care, and temperature assessment is the best way for the nurse to provide information on these topics to parents. Parents should be told to call their healthcare provider if redness, foul odor, bright red bleeding, or greenish yellow drainage occurs at the cord site or if the area remains unhealed 2 to 3 days after the cord stump has sloughed off. Current evidence does not support the routine application of topical antimicrobials to the drying cord (WHO, 1999). See Table 31-3: What Parents Need to Know About Newborn Care.

The nurse demonstrates and reviews the taking of an axillary or tympanic temperature with the family and discourages the use of mercury thermometers. It is important that families understand the differences and know how to select a thermometer. The newborn's temperature needs to be taken only when signs of illness are present. Parents are advised to call their physician or pediatric nurse practitioner immediately if they observe any signs of illness.

Nasal and Oral Suctioning

Most newborns are obligatory nose breathers for the first months of life. They generally maintain air passage patency by coughing or sneezing. During the first few days of life, however, the newborn has increased mucus, and gentle suctioning with a bulb syringe may be indicated. The nurse can demonstrate the use of the bulb syringe in the nose and mouth and have the parents do a return demonstration. The parents should repeat this demonstration before discharge so they will feel more confident and comfortable with the procedure. Care should be taken to apply only gentle suction to prevent nasal bleeding.

To suction the newborn, the bulb syringe is compressed and the tip is placed in the nostril. The nurse or parent must take care not to occlude the passageway. The bulb is permitted to reexpand slowly by releasing the compression on the bulb (Figure 31-12 ■). The bulb syringe is removed from the nostril, and drainage is then compressed out of the bulb onto a tissue. The bulb syringe may also be used in the mouth if the newborn is spitting up and unable to handle the excess secretions. The bulb is compressed, the tip of the bulb syringe is placed about 1 inch to one side of the newborn's mouth, and compression is released. This draws up the excess secretions. The procedure is repeated on the other side of the mouth. The roof of the mouth and back of the throat are avoided because suction in these areas might stimulate the gag reflex. The bulb syringe should be washed in warm, soapy water and rinsed in warm water daily and as needed after use. Rinsing with a half-strength white vinegar solution followed by clear water may help to extend the useful life of the bulb syringe by inhibiting bacterial growth. A bulb syringe should always be kept near the newborn. New parents and nurses who are inexperienced with babies may fear that the baby will choke and may be relieved if they know how to take action if such an event occurs. They should be advised to turn the newborn's head to the side or hold the newborn with his or her head down as soon as there is any indication of gagging or vomiting and to use the bulb syringe as needed.

SIDS Resources for Parents

Some infants may have transient edema of the nasal mucosa following suctioning of the airway after birth. The nurse can demonstrate the use of normal saline to loosen secretions, and instruct parents in the gentle and moderate use of the bulb syringe to avoid further irritation of the mucous membranes. If parents will be using humidifiers at home, they should be instructed to follow the manufacturer's cleaning instructions carefully so that molds, spores, and bacteria from a dirty humidifier do not enter the baby's environment.

Swaddling the Newborn

Swaddling (wrapping) helps the newborn maintain body temperature, provides a feeling of closeness and security, and may be effective in quieting a crying baby by having the newborn's hands near the mouth to allow for sucking (Iannelli, 2007). If the infant is not resting, placing its hands at its sides then swaddling reduces the amount of stimulation of hand-to-mouth movement and may allow the child to rest. When wrapping the infant, a blanket is placed on the crib (or secure surface) in the shape of a diamond. The top corner of the blanket is folded down slightly, and the newborn's body is placed with the head at the upper edge of the blanket. The right corner of the blanket is wrapped around the infant and tucked under the left side (not too tightly—newborns need a little room to move and to allow for hands to get to the mouth). The bottom corner is then pulled up to the chest, and the left corner is wrapped around the baby's right side (Figure 31-13 ■). The nurse can show this wrapping technique to a new mother so she will feel more skilled in handling her baby.

CLINICAL TIP

You'll find that left-handed people tend to hold the baby over their right shoulder, and right-handed people do the opposite. This keeps the dominant hand free. However, most health personnel wear their name tags on the left side. To avoid scratching the baby's face, wear your name tag on the same side as your dominant hand.

Sleep and Activity

The National Institute of Child Health and Human Development and the American Academy of Pediatrics recommend that healthy term infants be placed on their back to sleep. Parents are taught the importance of following "Back to Sleep Guidelines" to reduce the incidence of sudden infant death syndrome (SIDS) (American Academy of Pediatrics [AAP] Task Force on Sudden

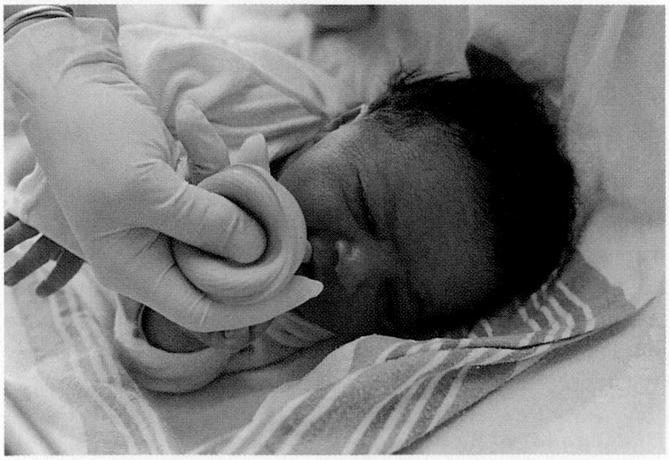

Figure 31-12 ■ Nasal and oral suctioning. The bulb is compressed, the tip is placed in either the mouth or the nose, and the bulb is released.

Source: © Stella Johnson (www.stellajohnson.com).

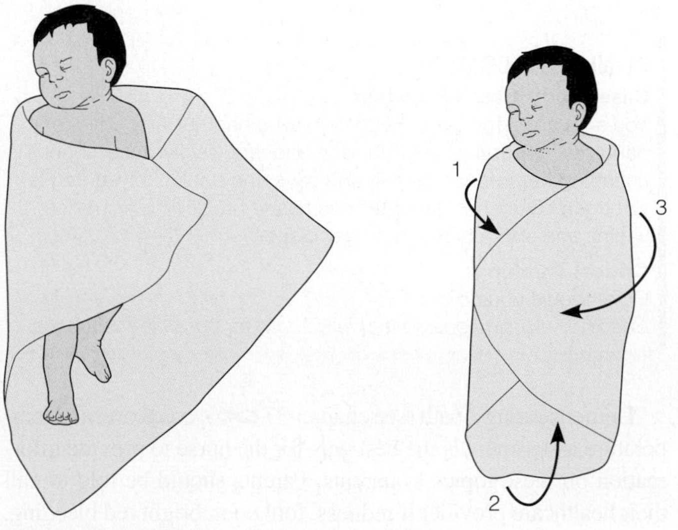

Figure 31-13 ■ Steps in wrapping a baby.

Infant Death Syndrome, 2005). Though infants may need to be placed on their sides initially because of copious or thick secretions, placing them on their backs in the newborn period serves to educate parents regarding infant positioning. Studies indicate that parents position their babies in the same positions they observe in the hospital setting, so nurses must demonstrate this behavior to reduce the risk of SIDS. If exceptions are warranted, these should be explained to families so they do not misinterpret what they observe. The placement of babies in a prone position during wakeful play sessions ("tummy time") should be encouraged as well (AAP & ACOG, 2007). Parents are also encouraged to hold their babies and not allow them to remain in infant carriers for prolonged periods of time.

Perhaps nothing is more individual to each baby than the sleep-activity cycle. It is important for the nurse to recognize the individual variations of each newborn and to assist parents as they develop sensitivity to their infant's communication signals and rhythms of activity and sleep. See chapter 30 ∞ for more detailed discussion of the sleep-activity cycle.

Car Safety Considerations

Half the children killed or injured in automobile accidents could have been protected by the use of a federally approved car seat. Newborns must go home from the birthing unit in a car seat adapted to fit newborns (Figure 31-14 ■). Babies should never be in the front seat of a car equipped with a passenger-side air bag. The safest spot in any car is the middle of the back seat. The car seat should be positioned to face the rear of the car until the baby is a year old or weighs 20 pounds (9.09 kg) (AAP, 2010). Nurses need to ensure that all parents are knowledgeable about the benefits of child safety seat use and proper installation. Nurses can encourage parents to have their infant safety seats checked by local groups trained specifically for that purpose. The Seat Check Initiative provides locations and information about child safety seats.

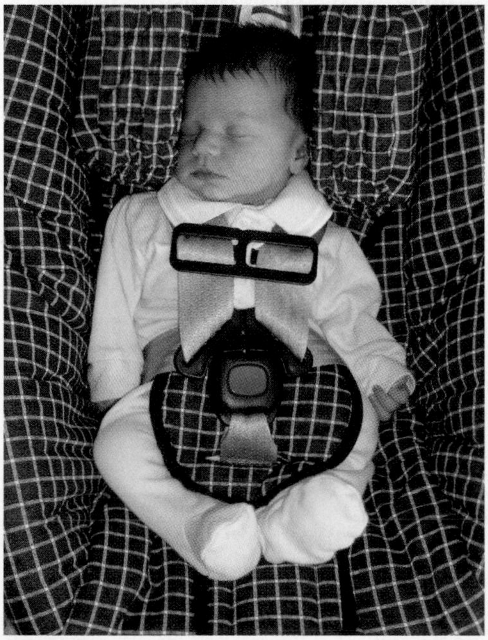

Figure 31-14 ■ Infant car restraint for use from birth to about 12 months of age.

Source: George Dodson/Lightworks Studio/Pearson Education.

Immunization Initiatives

Newborn Screening and Immunization Program

Before the newborn and mother are discharged from the birthing unit, the nurse informs the parents about **newborn screening tests** and tells them when to return to the birthing center or clinic if further tests are needed.

Several of the disorders that can be identified from a few drops of blood obtained by a heel stick are cystic fibrosis, galactosemia, congenital adrenal hyperplasia, hypothyroidism, maple syrup urine disease (MSUD), sickle cell trait, biotinidase deficiency, phenylketonuria (PKU), and hemoglobinopathies. The Expanded Newborn Screening Program allows parents to have their babies screened for more than 20 disorders. Although controversy exists over the need for such comprehensive testing, it is recommended that states test for a core panel of 29 treatable congenital conditions and an additional 25 conditions that may be detected by screening (AAP, Newborn Screening Authoring Committee, 2008).

Phenylketonuria and congenital hypothyroidism are the only tests that are performed in all 50 states and the District of Columbia. Early newborn discharge puts infants at risk for delayed or even missed diagnosis of PKU and congenital hypothyroidism because of decreased sensitivity of screening before 24 hours of age. The likelihood of detecting PKU increases as the infant grows older; the infant must be at least 24 hours old for a valid test. A second test is required in most states, usually between 1 week and 1 month of age, to minimize the chance of a positive child going undetected.

PROFESSIONALISM IN PRACTICE

Evidence-Based Routine Newborn Metabolic Disorders Screening

Best practice for routine screening of newborns for metabolic and other disorders that are initially asymptomatic has been elevated from a Level II (good evidence category) to a Level I (best evidence) based on latest evidence (Institute for Clinical Systems Improvement Guidelines, 2008).

Hearing loss is found in 1 to 3 per 1000 infants in the normal newborn population (Healthy Children, 2010). Hearing screenings before discharge are now conducted in all 50 states. The recommended initial newborn hearing screening should be accomplished before discharge from the birthing unit with appropriate follow-up if the newborn fails to pass the initial screen in all hospitals providing obstetric services (AAP & ACOG, 2007; Creehan, 2008).

According to the National Center for Hearing Assessment & Management, 95.7% of all infants obtained hearing screening in the United States. Sometimes infants fail to pass these tests for reasons other than hearing loss. Amniotic fluid in the ear canals is a frequent cause of suboptimal test results. In these cases, infants are retested in a week or two. The current goal is to screen all infants by 1 month of age, confirm hearing loss with audiologic examination by 3 months of age, and treat with comprehensive early intervention services before 6 months of

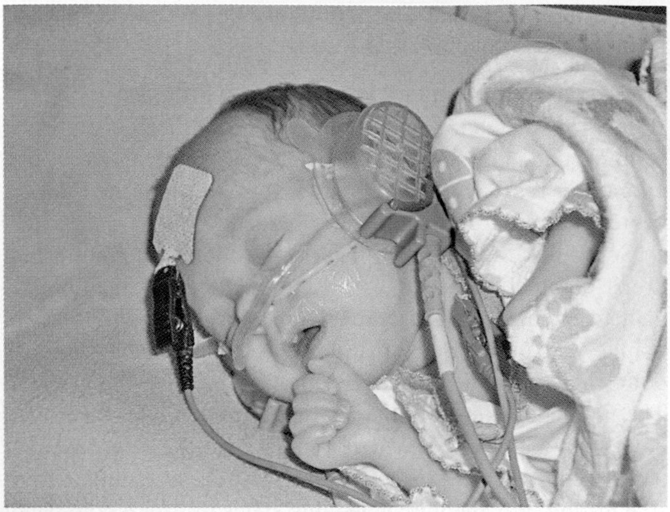

Figure 31-15 ■ Newborn hearing screen.

Source: Courtesy of Jo Engle, RN, MSN, NNP-BC and Vanessa Howell, RN, MSN, NNP-BC.

Application: Newborn Screening Tests

age (AAP & ACOG, 2007). Typically, screening programs use a two-stage screening approach (otoacoustic emissions [OAE] repeated twice, OAE followed by auditory brainstem response [ABR], or automated ABR repeated twice). Families need to be educated about appropriate interpretation of screening test results and appropriate steps for follow-up (Figure 31-15 ■).

Immunization programs against the hepatitis B virus during the newborn period and infancy are in place in many states, at least 20 countries, and high-incidence areas such as American Samoa. Universal vaccination of infants is recommended. See Drug Guide: Hepatitis B Vaccine (Engerix-B, Recombivax HB). Parents need to be advised as to whether their birthing center provides newborn hepatitis vaccination so that an adequate follow-up program can be set in motion (AAP & ACOG, 2007).

The nurse should teach the family all necessary caregiving methods before discharge. A checklist may be helpful to determine whether the teaching has been completed and to verify the parents' knowledge on leaving the birthing unit (Figure 31-16 ■). The nurse needs to review all areas for understanding or any outstanding questions with the mother and father, without rushing and taking time to answer all queries. Any concerns of the parents or nurse are noted.

HEALTH PROMOTION EDUCATION

The nurse discusses with parents ways to meet their newborn's needs, ensure safety, and appreciate the newborn's unique characteristics and behaviors. By assisting parents in establishing links with their community-based healthcare provider, the nurse can get the new family off to a good start. Parents also need to know the signs of illness, how to reach the pediatrician or after-hours clinic, and the importance of follow-up after

RESEARCH EVIDENCE IN PRACTICE: Universal Newborn Hearing Screening

CLINICAL QUESTION

Does universal newborn hearing screening improve early treatment of hearing deficits, enhance language acquisition, and increase childhood communication skills?

RESEARCH EVIDENCE

People who work with children who have hearing loss believe that early identification and intervention are primary factors in a child's subsequent success. Learning language through hearing and the development of speech ultimately help children achieve successful communication skills. Development and testing of automated technologies for screening hearing in newborns led to the implementation of programs for universal hearing screening in hospitals for babies in the first 3 months of life.

Three large retrospective reviews of studies involving more than 1000 babies focused on the effects of universal screening for hearing deficits within the first 3 months of life, with a goal of intervention by 6 months of age. Longitudinal studies of 700 of these children focused on language skills through early school age.

Children who were screened were referred, diagnosed, and treated significantly earlier (6.9 months) than children who were not screened but referred for hearing evaluation later in life (39.5 months). In addition, there was an inverse relationship between degree of loss and age of diagnosis, with children with more severe to profound hearing loss diagnosed very early. There was also a general increase in the identification of children with mild to moderate hearing loss. Children who had early screening had earlier interventions applied, such as hearing aids and cochlear implants.

Longitudinal follow-up indicated that those who had early versus late screening had better receptive language skills and increased communication abilities at school age.

WHAT QUESTIONS REMAIN UNANSWERED?

While improvements in receptive language were found at school age in those who had been screened and treated, expressive language and speech quality had not. What accounts for these differences? Is treatment focusing on auditory aspects of the hearing deficits rather than the acquisition of speech?

WHAT IS BEST PRACTICE?

Universal newborn hearing screening enhances the early identification and treatment of hearing loss in children. This early treatment means that children will have less difficulty acquiring language and communication skills.

CRITICAL THINKING

Usual parental reactions to an initial screen positive for hearing loss include worry, anxiety, and distress. How can the nurse mediate these expected responses?

References

Durieux-Smith, A., Fitzpatrick, E., & Whittingham, J. (2008). Universal newborn hearing screening: A question of evidence. *International Journal of Audiology, 47*, 1–10.

Halpin, K., Smith, K., Widen, J., & Chertoff, M. (2010). Effects of universal newborn hearing screening on an early intervention program for children with hearing loss, birth to 3 years of age. *Journal of the American Academy of Audiology, 21*, 169–175.

Nelson, H., Bougatsos, C., & Nygren, P. (2008). Universal newborn hearing screening: Systematic review to update the 2001 US preventive services task force recommendation. *Pediatrics, 122*(1), e266–e276. doi:10.1542/peds.2007–1422

NURSERY TEACHING CHECKLIST

Please read the *Mother/Baby* information booklet given to you after birth. After reading it, please go through the following list and check whether you understand each topic or need to know more.

		I know this already	Doesn't apply to me	I need to know more	FOR NURSES ONLY: Taught/ reviewed/ demonstrated
Baby Care	What to do if baby is choking or gagging				
	Safety				
	How to do skin care/cord care				
	How to take care of the circumcision or genital area				
	How to know if my baby is sick and what to do				
	What is jaundice and how to detect it				
	Use of thermometer				
	Use of bulb syringe				
	How and when to burp baby				
	Newborn behavior: crying/comforting				
	How to position baby after feeding				
	What does demand scheduling mean?				
Breastfeeding	I attended breastfeeding class/watched breastfeeding video	YES ☐	NO ☐		
	How to position baby for feeding				
	How to get baby to latch on to my nipple properly				
	When and how long to breastfeed				
	Removal of baby from my nipple				
	What is the supply and demand concept?				
	What is the let-down reflex?				
	When does breast milk come in?				
	Supplementing				
	Proper diet for breastfeeding mothers				
	Prevention and comfort measures for sore nipples				
	Prevention and comfort measures for engorgement				
	When and how to use a breast pump				
	How to express milk by hand				
	How to go back to work and continue to breastfeed				
Bottle-Feeding	How to feed my baby a bottle				
	Reasons for NOT propping bottles				
	How to clean nipple/bottle				
	How to prepare formula				
	What formula should my baby drink				
Safety	**Use of infant car seat**				
	Back to Sleep				
	Shaken Baby Syndrome				

Other information: ____________________

Videos viewed/ Literature given: ____________________

Language Spoken by Mother:

☐ English ☐ Spanish ☐ Other ________

Interpreter Used? ☐ Yes ☐ No ☐ Family Interprets

Nurse's Signature(s): ____________________

I have received and understand the instructions given on the above topics.

MOTHER'S SIGNATURE ____________ DATE ____________

Figure 31-16 ■ An infant teaching checklist is completed by the time of discharge.

Source: Adapted from Presbyterian/St. Luke's Medical Center, Denver, CO.

DRUG GUIDE Hepatitis B Vaccine (Engerix-B, Recombivax HB)

OVERVIEW OF NEONATAL ACTION

Recombinant hepatitis B vaccine is used as a prophylactic treatment against all subtypes of the hepatitis B virus. It provides passive immunization for newborns of HBsAg-negative and HBsAg-positive mothers. Hepatitis B can be transmitted across the placenta, but most newborns are infected during birth.

The vaccine is produced from baker's yeast and plasmid containing the HBsAg gene.

Hepatitis B (thimerosal free) vaccine contains more than 95% HBsAg protein and is an inactivated (noninfective) product. Universal immunization is recommended.

Infants of HBsAg-positive mothers should concurrently receive 0.5 ml of hepatitis B immunoglobulin (HBIG) prophylaxis at separate injection sites (Centers for Disease Control and Prevention [CDC], 2010; Wilson, Shannon, & Shields, 2010).

PREGNANCY RISK CATEGORY: C

ROUTE, DOSAGE, FREQUENCY

The first dose of 0.5 ml (10 mcg) is given intramuscularly into the anterolateral thigh within 12 hours of birth for infants born to HBsAg-positive mothers. The second dose of vaccine is given at 1 month of age. The third dose should be administered at least 4 months after the first dose and at least 2 months after the second dose, but not before 6 months of age (CDC, 2010).

Infants born to HBsAg-negative mothers receive their first dose of vaccine at birth, the second dose at 1 to 2 months, and the third dose at 6 to 18 months (AAP & ACOG, 2007).

Infants whose mother's HBsAg status is unknown should receive the same doses of vaccine as infants born to HBsAg-positive mothers.

NEONATAL SIDE EFFECTS

The only common side effect is soreness at the injection site. Occasionally, there is erythema, swelling, warmth, and induration at the injection site; irritability; or a low-grade fever (37.7°C [99.8°F]).

NURSING CONSIDERATIONS

Delay administration during active infection; the vaccine will not prevent infection during its incubation period.

- The vaccine should be used as supplied. Do not dilute. Shake well.
- Do not inject intravenously or intradermally.
- Monitor for adverse reactions. Monitor temperature closely.
- Have epinephrine available to treat possible allergic reactions.
- Responsiveness to the vaccine is age dependent. Preterm infants weighing less than 1000 g have lower seroconversion rates. Consider delaying the first dose until the infant is term postconceptual age (PCA) or use a 4-dose schedule.

TABLE 31-4 When Parents Should Call Their Healthcare Provider

- Temperature above 38°C (100.4°F) axillary or below 36.6°C (97.8°F) axillary
- Continual rise in temperature
- More than one episode of forceful vomiting or frequent vomiting over a 6-hour period
- Refusal of two feedings in a row
- Lethargy (listlessness), difficulty in awakening baby
- Cyanosis (bluish discoloration of skin) with or without a feeding
- Absence of breathing longer than 20 seconds
- Inconsolable infant (quieting techniques are not effective) or continuous high-pitched cry
- Discharge or bleeding from umbilical cord, circumcision, or any opening (except vaginal mucus or pseudomenstruation)
- Two consecutive green watery or black stools or increased frequency of stools
- No wet diapers for 18 to 24 hours or fewer than six to eight wet diapers per day after 4 days of age
- Development of eye drainage

discharge (see Table 31-4). Parents should also check with their clinician for advice about over-the-counter medications to be kept in the medicine cabinet.

The family should have the care provider's phone number, address, and any specific instructions. Having the birthing unit or nursery phone number is also reassuring to a newborn's family. They are encouraged to call with questions. Follow-up calls lend added support by providing another opportunity for parents to have their questions answered.

Some institutions have initiated postpartum and/or newborn follow-up visits 48 hours after birth. The follow-up infant examination should be within 48 hours of discharge if the family is unable to visit their primary care physician within that time period (Creehan, 2008). The home visit focuses on normal newborn care, assessment for hyperbilirubinemia (jaundice), extreme weight loss, feeding problems, and knowledge deficits related to newborn care and feeding within the family unit.

Routine well-baby visits should be scheduled with the clinic, pediatric nurse practitioner, or physician. Regardless of the type of follow-up services available in the community, the nurse contributes to the newborn's health by stressing the importance of routine care and by helping families who have no follow-up plans to connect to local resources for care. (For detailed discussion of home care, see chapter 37 ∞.)

Evaluation

When evaluating the nursing care provided during the newborn period, the nurse may anticipate the following outcomes:

- The parents demonstrate safe techniques for caring for their newborn.
- The parents verbalize developmentally appropriate behavioral expectations of their newborn and knowledge of community-based newborn follow-up care.

FOCUS YOUR STUDY

- The overall goal of newborn nursing care is to provide comprehensive care while promoting the establishment of a well-functioning family unit.
- The period immediately following birth, during which adaptation to extrauterine life occurs, requires close monitoring to identify any deviations from normal.
- Nursing goals during the first hours after birth (admission and transitional period) are to maintain a clear airway, maintain a neutral thermal environment, prevent hemorrhage and infection, initiate oral feedings, and facilitate attachment.
- The newborn is routinely given prophylactic vitamin K to prevent possible hemorrhagic disease of the newborn.
- Prophylactic eye treatment for *Neisseria gonorrhoeae* is legally required on all newborns.
- Nursing goals in daily newborn care include maintaining cardiopulmonary function, maintaining a neutral thermal environment, promoting adequate hydration and nutrition, preventing complications, promoting safety, and enhancing attachment and family knowledge of child care.
- Essential daily care includes assessing vital signs, weight, overall color, intake, output, umbilical cord and circumcision, newborn nutrition, parent education, and attachment.
- Following a circumcision, the newborn must be observed closely for signs of bleeding, inability to void, and signs of infection.
- Signs of illness in newborns include temperature above 38°C (100.4°F) axillary or below 36.6°C (97.8°F) axillary, more than one episode of forceful vomiting, refusal of two feedings in a row, lethargy, cyanosis with or without a feeding, and absence of breathing for longer than 20 seconds.
- Newborn screening for congenital hypothyroidism and phenylketonuria may be done on all newborns in the first 1 to 3 days.

CRITICAL THINKING IN ACTION

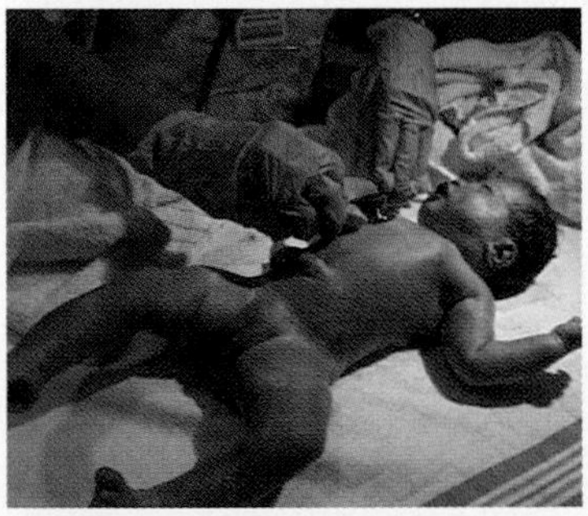
Source: George Dodson/Pearson Education.

Alice Fine, age 32, G1, now P1001, spontaneously delivers a 7.25 pound baby girl over a median episiotomy. The baby's Apgars are 7 and 9 at 1 and 5 minutes. The baby is suctioned, stimulated, and given free flow oxygen at birth. As the nurse on duty, you admit baby Fine to the newborn nursery, place her under a radiant heater, and perform a newborn assessment. You obtain the vital signs of temperature 97°F, heart rate 128, respiration 55. A physical exam demonstrates no abnormalities, and you note that there were no significant problems with the pregnancy, the mother's blood type is A+, and she plans to bottle-feed. You monitor the baby until her vital signs are stable and then take her to the mother's room for her first bottle-feeding at 60 minutes old.

1. How would you explain the technique to suction the newborn with a bulb syringe?
2. How would you review measures to promote the safety of the newborn from abduction?
3. Describe the care of the newborn's cord.
4. How would you review bottle-feeding with the mother?

See www.nursing.pearsonhighered.com site for possible responses.

Pearson Nursing Student Resources

Find additional review materials at
www.nursing.pearsonhighered.com

Prepare for success with additional NCLEX®-style practice questions, interactive assignments and activities, Web links, animations and videos, and more!

REFERENCES

American Academy of Pediatrics (AAP). (2010). Car safety seats: A guide for families 2010. Retrieved from www.aap.org/family/carseatguide

American Academy of Pediatrics (AAP) Committee on Fetus and Newborn & American College of Obstetricians and Gynecologists (ACOG) Committee on Obstetrics. (2007). *Guidelines for perinatal care* (6th ed.). Evanston, IL: Author.

American Academy of Pediatrics (AAP), Newborn Screening Authoring Committee. (2008). Newborn screening expands: Recommendations for pediatricians and medical homes—implications for the system. *Pediatrics, 121*(1), 192–217. doi: 10.1542/peds.2007-3021

American Academy of Pediatrics (AAP) & Canadian Paediatric Society (CPS). (2006). Prevention and management of pain in the neonate: An update. *Pediatrics, 118*(5), 2231–2241. doi: 10.1542/peds.2006-2277

American Academy of Pediatrics (AAP) Task Force on Sudden Infant Death Syndrome 2005). The changing concept of sudden infant death syndrome: Diagnostic coding shifts, controversies regarding the sleeping environment, and new variables to consider in reducing risk. *Pediatrics, 116*(5) 1245–1255. doi: 10.1542/peds.2005-1499

Andrews, M. M. (2008). Transcultural perspectives in the nursing care of children and adolescents. In M. M. Andrews & J. S. Boyle (Eds.), *Transcultural concepts in nursing care* (5th ed., pp. 116–145). Philadelphia, PA: Lippincott.

Askin, D. (2008). Newborn adaptations to extrauterine life. In K. R. Simpson & P. A. Creehan (Eds.), *Perinatal nursing* (3rd ed., pp. 527–545). Philadelphia, PA: Lippincott Williams & Wilkins.

Blackburn, S. T. (2007). *Maternal, fetal, & neonatal physiology: A clinical perspective.* (3rd ed.). St. Louis, MO: Saunders.

Centers for Disease Control and Prevention (CDC) Advisory Committee on Immunization Practices. (2010). *Recommended childhood and adolescent immunization schedule, United States 2010.* Retrieved from www.cdc.gov/vaccines/recs/acip

Creehan, P. A. (2008). Newborn physical assessment. In K. R. Simpson & P. A. Creehan (Eds.), *Perinatal nursing.* (3rd ed., pp. 546–574). Philadelphia, PA: Lippincott Williams & Wilkins.

D'Avanzo, C. E., & Geissler, E. M. (2008). *Pocket guide to cultural assessment* (4th ed.). St. Louis, MO: Mosby.

Healthy Children. (2010). Newborn hearing screening and your baby. Retrieved from www.healthychildren.org/english/ages-stages/baby/pages/purpose-of-newborn-hearing

Iannelli, V. (2007). Swaddling a baby. Retrieved from http://pediatrics.about.com/od/weeklyquestion/a/0607_swaddling.htm

Institute for Clinical Systems Improvement. (2008). Preventive services for children and adolescents, *Institute for Clinical Systems Improvement,* 2008 October. Retrieved from www.guidelines.gov/summary/summary.aspx?doc_id=13314&nbr=006758&string=%22preventive+services+for+children%22+and+adolescents

Klaus, M., & Klaus, P. (1985). *The amazing newborn.* Menlo Park, CA: Addison-Wesley.

Lipson, J. G., & Dibble, S. L. (2008). *Culture & clinical care* (7th ed.). San Francisco, CA: The Regents, University of California.

Tedder, J. L. (2008). Give them *The HUG*: An innovative approach to helping parents understand the language of their newborn. *Journal of Perinatal Education. 17*(2), 14–20. doi: 10.1624/105812408X298345

Vincent, J. L. (2009). Infant hospital abduction: Security measures to aid in prevention. *American Journal of Maternal/Child Nursing, 34*(3), 179–183. doi: 10.1097/01.NMC.0000351706.81502.d0

Wilson, B. A., Shannon, M. T., & Shields, K. M. (2010). *Prentice Hall nurse's drug guide 2010.* Upper Saddle River, NJ: Pearson Education.

World Health Organization (WHO). (1999). Care of the umbilical cord: A review of the evidence. Retrieved from http://www.whoint/en/documents/MSM98-4

World Health Organization (WHO). (2008). Male circumcision information package. [On-line]. Retrieved from www.who.int/hiv/pub/malecircumcision/infopack/en/index.html

CHAPTER 32

Newborn Nutrition

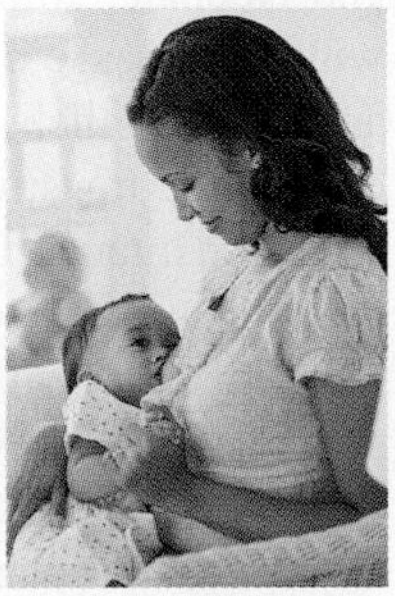

I felt prepared for breastfeeding when my baby was born—I had taken a breastfeeding class and read several books. Breastfeeding started off well. I was a little surprised about the frequent feedings in the beginning, but we got through that just fine. The biggest surprise was that my baby developed allergy symptoms when she was 3 weeks old. It was determined that my daughter is allergic to cow's milk protein. To continue feeding her just breast milk, I had to cut out milk and foods containing milk, which severely limited what I could eat. I did that because I was determined not to let anything stop me from nursing my child for my goal of at least the first year. Fortunately, the allergy is slowly going away as she grows older. At 9 months I can now have a little cheese in my diet again.

—Allyssa, age 25

LEARNING OUTCOMES

1. Compare the nutritional value and composition of human milk and formula preparations in relation to the nutritional needs of the newborn.
2. Explain the advantages and disadvantages of breastfeeding and formula-feeding in determining the nursing care of both mother/family and newborn.
3. Formulate guidelines for helping both breastfeeding and formula-feeding mothers to feed their infants successfully in hospital and community-based settings.
4. Explain the influence of cultural values on infant feeding practices.
5. Describe the nutritional needs and normal growth patterns of infants.
6. Illustrate ways to educate parents about their infant's nutritional needs and normal growth patterns.

KEY TERMS

Colostrum *859*
Foremilk *859*
Hindmilk *859*
La Leche League International (LLLI) *883*
Let-down reflex *859*
Mature milk *859*
Milk/plasma ratio *863*
Oxytocin *859*
Prolactin *858*
Transitional milk *859*

There is nothing so rewarding—and potentially so frustrating—as providing your newborn with nourishment. The very word runs the gamut of meaning from the mundane to the sublime:

Nourish (verb): to provide food/to sustain/to nurture/to cherish

Perhaps this is why something apparently so basic engenders such strong emotions. Feeding your newborn can involve inadequate sleep, loss of freedom, and feeling trapped by unpredictable demands that compromise your ability to get anything else done. On the other hand, it offers the chance to bond at a most basic level, the experience of unconditional love, and the reward of knowing that you are providing the basis for growth and future development.

Early nutrition has a significant impact on the present and future health and well-being of the infant because this is a period of rapid growth and brain development. In addition, infant feeding itself is an important component of newborn socialization that promotes cognitive and emotional development.

It is important that the nurse is well informed about infant nutrition and feeding methods because the parents look to the nurse for this guidance. Parents need accurate and consistent information from the nursing staff. They need to learn the skills to feed their infant successfully. Through each interaction with the parents, there is an opportunity for the nurse to support the parents and promote the family's sense of confidence.

In this chapter we will look at the nutritional needs of the full-term newborn of normal weight in the context of both breast milk and formula composition, discuss feeding methods, explore community-based nursing care, and finally look at a nutritional assessment of the newborn.

Nutritional Needs and Breast Milk/Formula Composition

The newborn's diet must supply all the nutrients required by the body to meet the rapid rate of physical and neurologic growth and development. A neonatal diet should provide adequate hydration and sufficient calories as well as protein, carbohydrates, fat, vitamins, and minerals. Exclusive breast milk and/or iron-fortified 20-calorie/ounce formula are sufficient as sole sources of nutrition to meet the dietary needs of the newborn from birth up to 6 months of age. Complementary solid foods are introduced in the second half of the first year, while the infant continues to receive human milk and/or formula until at least 12 months of age (American Academy of Pediatrics [AAP], 2005). The following several sections discuss the nutritional requirements of the newborn and how these are met by human milk and standard cow's milk–based formula.

Dietary Reference Intakes

The *dietary reference intake (DRI)* encompasses four aspects of nutrient-based reference values: (1) estimated average requirement (EAR), (2) recommended daily allowance (RDA), (3) adequate intake (AI), and (4) tolerable upper intake level (UL). The DRIs represent a framework that links nutrition and health across the lifespan.

Growth

It is physiologically appropriate for both breastfed and formula-fed infants to lose weight in the first 3 to 4 days of life. Formula-fed infants generally lose up to 3.5% of their birth weight; breastfed infants should not exceed a weight loss greater than 7% of their birth weight (Association of Women's Health, Obstetric and Neonatal Nurses (AWHONN), 2007). Infants lose weight with the passage of meconium, with loss of extracellular fluids, and because their fluid intake is normally low in the first few days while transitioning to enteral feedings, especially among breastfed infants. This loss is normal and does not result in dehydration, as infants draw on their extracellular water reserves. Infants should begin gaining weight by day 5 of life or sooner and should be at or above birth weight by 10 to 14 days of age. Weight gain during the first 4 weeks should be about 35 gm (1 oz) per day at 1 month whereas formula-fed infants gain an average of 34.4 gm per day at 1 month. In general, infants gain about 10 g/kg/day or 5 to 7 oz/week (Riordan & Wambach, 2010).

Breastfed and formula-fed babies have different growth rates. This is understandable because the compositions of human milk and formula are different. See Table 32-1 to compare human milk and formula compositions. Most healthcare providers (as well as representatives of formula companies) consider breastfeeding to be the "gold standard" for neonatal nutrition, and the outcomes associated with its use are the norm to which other forms of nutrition should be compared (AAP, 2005; Lawrence & Lawrence, 2005).

Formula-fed infants tend to regain their birth weight earlier than breastfed infants because the formula-fed infant has a greater fluid intake early on. The breastfed infant's fluid intake depends on the mother's milk supply and breastfeeding efficiency. It is noteworthy that breastfed infants born to multiparous mothers who have previously breastfed often do not lose as much weight as infants born to primiparous mothers, because the multiparous mother's milk typically becomes more abundant sooner (Lawrence & Lawrence, 2005). If a healthy full-term infant with normal birth weight has a weight loss exceeding 7%, a feeding evaluation is indicated. If an infant has a weight loss of 10% or greater, an evaluation, an intervention, and a follow-up weight check are indicated to make certain that the infant is receiving sufficient fluid and calories and to determine if the feeding problem is resolved.

Growth rates for breastfed and formula-fed infants are somewhat different once feedings are established. Exclusively breastfed infants have the same or slightly higher weight gain than their formula-fed and mixed-fed peers in the first 3 to 4 months. *Thereafter*, formula-fed and mixed-fed infants have a greater weight gain pattern compared with breastfed infants (Riordan & Wambach, 2010). This characteristic weight gain pattern results in a leaner body build in the breastfed group by the latter half of the first year of life. Measurements of length and head circumference are the same for both groups. An infant typically grows 1 inch per month in the first 6 months, and then

TABLE 32-1 Comparison of Selected Nutrients in Milk

NUTRIENTS PER 30 ML	HUMAN MILK	SIMILAC ADVANCE	ENFAMIL LIPIL	WHOLE MILK
Calories	20	20	20	19
Protein, grams	0.31	0.41	0.42	1.1
% of cal	6%	8%	8%	22%
Source	Human milk	Nonfat milk, Whey protein	Nonfat milk, Whey protein	Cow's milk
Whey: casein	90:10 initially 50:50* eventually	52:48	60:40	20:80
Fat, grams	1.15	1.1	1.1	1.1
% of cal	52%	49%	48%	49%
Source	Human milk (contains DHA, ARA**, etc.)	Safflower, soy, coconut DHA, ARA**	Palm, soy, coconut, sunflower, DHA, ARA**	Butterfat
Carbohydrate, grams	2.1	2.2	2.2	1.5
% of cal	42%	43%	43%	31%
Source	Lactose (human milk)	Lactose (nonfat milk)	Lactose (nonfat milk)	Lactose (whole milk)
Linoleic acid, mg	110	200	172	26
Calcium, mg	8.2	15.6	15.6	39
Phosphorus, mg	4.2	8.4	10.6	30.4
Iron, mcg	8	360	360	16
Copper, mcg	7.4	18	15	4.2
Selenium, mcg	0.4	0.4	0.6	0
Sodium, mg	5.2	4.8	5.4	16
Potassium, mg	15.6	21	21.6	49.8
Chloride, mg	12.4	13	12.6	32.8
Solute load, mOsm	2.9	3.7	3.8	10
Osmolality, mOsm/L	286	300	300	285
Vitamin A, international unit	66	60	60	41
Vitamin D, international unit	0.6	12	12	13.4
Vitamin E, international unit	0.12	0.3	0.4	0.02
Vitamin K, mcg	0.06	1.6	1.6	1.2
Folate, mcg	1.4	3	3.2	1.6

*Whey: casein ratio in human milk changes after birth. In early lactation the ratio is 90:10, later with mature milk the ratio is 60:40, and in late lactation the ratio is 50:5.

**Docosahexaenoic acid (DHA), arachidonic acid (ARA) additives derived from algae, mycotic sources.

Source: Data from Mead-Johnson Nutrition. (2010). Pediatric products handbook. *New York, NY: Bristol-Myers Squibb Company and Abbott Nutrition. (2009).* Pediatric nutritionals product guide. *Columbus, OH: Abbott Laboratories;.*

0.5 inch for the next 6 months. Infants generally double their birth weight by 5 months, triple their birth weight by 1 year of age, and quadruple their birth weight by 2 years (Riordan & Wambach, 2010). Growth charts for tracking an infant's weight, length, and head circumference can be downloaded from the Centers for Disease Control and Prevention (CDC) Web site.

CLINICAL TIP

The following are newborn caloric and fluid needs:

- Caloric intake: 45.5 to 52.5 kcal/lb/day or 100 to 115 kcal/kg/day
- Fluid requirements: 64 to 73 ml/lb/day or 140 to 160 ml/kg/day
- Weight gain in the first few weeks: 1 oz/day (or about a half pound per week)

Fluid

Fluid requirements during the neonatal period are high (140 to 160 ml/kg/day) because of the newborn's decreased ability to concentrate urine and increased overall metabolic rate. Although the infant's total body water content is high (75% to 80%) compared with an adult's (60%), the infant has an increased surface area to mass ratio and decreased renal absorptive capacity that makes the infant more susceptible to dehydration from insufficient fluid intake or increased fluid loss due to diarrhea, vomiting, or other source of fluid loss. Parents and caretakers should be aware of the signs of dehydration. Dry or chapped lips, dry oral cavity, decreased urine output, concentrated urine, general weakness, lethargy, poor skin turgor, sunken eyes, and sunken fontanelle are some of the signs of dehydration. The infant's fluid intake should be increased above the baseline fluid needs when the infant has a fever or is in a warm environment for an extended period of time. The increased fluid requirements should be met with additional breast milk or formula, rather than water because the increased water can cause hyponatremia and may result in seizures if water consumption is excessive.

CLINICAL TIP

A newborn with fever or an infant with persistent diarrhea or vomiting should be evaluated by a physician.

Energy

The basal metabolic rate (BMR) refers to the energy needed for thermoregulation, cardiorespiratory function, cellular activity, and growth. The healthy full-term infant's BMR is about twice that of an adult's, based on body weight (Rolfes, Pinna, & Whitney, 2006). A newborn requires 100 to 115 kcal/kg/day at 1 month and 85 to 95 kcal/kg/day from 6 to 12 months of age. When an infant does not receive sufficient calories, the infant risks losing weight, may experience tissue breakdown, and is at risk for delayed growth and development (Riordan & Wambach, 2010).

Fats

Infants receive approximately 50% of their calories from fat. Fats also help the body absorb the fat-soluble vitamins A, D, E, and K. Fats are a precursor of prostaglandins and other hormones. Essential fatty acids and their derivatives docosahexaenoic acid (DHA) and arachidonic acid (ARA) are associated with improved visual acuity and cognitive ability (Cloherty, Eichenwald, & Stark, 2008; Riordan & Wambach, 2010).

Milk Composition

Approximately 98% of the human milk fat is in the form of triglycerides, and a very small but clinically significant amount is from cholesterol. Cholesterol levels in breast milk may also stimulate the production of enzymes that lead to more efficient metabolism of cholesterol, thereby reducing its harmful long-term effects on the cardiovascular system.

Fatty acids are another key component to brain development. Omega-3 and omega-6 fatty acids are two classes of essential fatty acids found in breast milk, although the level can vary with maternal diet. Docosahexaenoic acid (DHA) and arachidonic acid (ARA) are long-chain polyunsaturated fatty acids (LCPUFAs) derived from linoleic acid and α-linolenic acid. Along with oleic acid, these LCPUFAs are needed for myelination of the spinal cord and other nerves, and impact on visual acuity and cognitive and behavioral functions.

Fat content is the most variable component in human milk, ranging from 30 to 50 grams/liter. Fat content is influenced by maternal parity, duration of pregnancy, the stage of lactation, diurnal regulation, and changes in fat content even during a single feeding. Multiparous mothers produce milk with a lower content of fatty acids. For example, the milk of a mother who delivers a preterm infant has a greater concentration of DHA and ARA than does the milk of a mother who gives birth to a full-term infant during the first few weeks postpartum. Babies born prematurely miss receiving the continuous placental transfer of DHA and ARA while developing during the third trimester. By receiving breast milk, these infants receive the increased concentrations of the preterm mother's DHA and ARA intended for the premature infant (Lawrence & Lawrence, 2005).

Phospholipids and cholesterol levels are higher in colostrum compared with mature milk, although overall fat content is higher in mature breast milk compared with colostrum (see the discussion of colostrum and mature milk in "Stages of Human Milk" on page 859). Fat content is generally higher in the evening and lower in the early morning. Within a single feeding session an infant initially receives the low-fat foremilk before receiving the higher calorie, high-fat hindmilk (see the discussion of foremilk and hindmilk in "Physiologic and Endocrine Control of Lactogenesis" on page 858). Finally, the fat content of breast milk is also affected by maternal diet and maternal fat stores. Mothers on low-fat diets have increased production of medium chain fatty acids (C6–C10), and mothers with high levels of body fat produce breast milk with a higher fat content (Lawrence & Lawrence, 2005).

The fats in the milk-based formulas are modified to parallel the fat profile of human milk by removing the butterfat from cow's milk and adding vegetable oils. There are quite a few differences in the fat sources and amounts used among the major formula brands. Since 2002 infant formulas have been supplemented with DHA and ARA. However, breast milk also contains 167 other fatty acids of uncertain function, and these are absent from formula (Cloherty et al., 2008).

Carbohydrates

Carbohydrates (sugars) serve as the other main source of energy for the infant, providing about 40% of the calories in the infant's diet. By weight, both human milk and formula contain more carbohydrates than fat.

Milk Composition

In breast milk, the primary carbohydrate is lactose. In addition to providing a cellular energy source especially for the brain in the form of glucose, lactose enhances the absorption of calcium, magnesium, and zinc (Lawrence & Lawrence, 2005).

Human milk also contains trace amounts of other carbohydrates such as glucosamines and nitrogen-containing oligosaccharides. Glucosamines are one of the building blocks for connective tissues and help strengthen and hold together ligaments and tendons. Oligosaccharides promote the growth of *Lactobacillus bifidus,* which promotes an intestinal acidic environment creating a hostile environment for bacteria to thrive (Riordan & Wambach, 2010).

In comparing carbohydrates among the standard milk-based formulas, both Enfamil and Similac provide all of their carbohydrate calories from lactose. Nestlé Good Start uses a blend of 70% lactose and 30% corn maltodextrin (a table sugar–like carbohydrate) (Sears, 2009).

Protein

Proteins are the building blocks for muscle and organ structure. They are key to just about every metabolic process in the body, including energy metabolism, cell-signaling, growth, and immune function. The protein requirement for an infant is about 0.8 to 0.9 gram per deciliter (Riordan & Wambach, 2010).

Milk Composition

Milk proteins are often grouped into casein and whey proteins. Whey protein is the predominant dietary protein in human milk. During digestion this type of protein creates soft curds that are easily and quickly broken down. Because of this, breastfeeding babies digest their meals in 90 minutes and need to feed often, about 8 to 12 feedings per day. It is rare for exclusively breastfeeding babies to have constipation. Casein is the major phosphoprotein found in milk. Cow's milk contains a high amount of casein (a low ratio of whey to casein—approximately 20:80) compared with mature human milk (60:40 whey:casein). Because of its tendency to form curds, milk with high amounts of casein is less easily digested.

Cow's milk–based formulas are usually modified to get closer to the whey:casein ratio profile of mature human milk. For example, the whey:casein ratio in Enfamil is 60:40. Although Similac has a ratio of 48:52; the company claims this produces an amino acid profile in the blood that is closer to that found in the breastfeeding infant. Nestlé Good Start (hydrolyzed) and Enfamil Gentlease (partially hydrolyzed formula) reportedly targets fussy, gassy babies and reduces the incidence of spitting up and constipation according to its manufacturer (Sears, 2009). It should also be noted that the whey and casein components in breast milk are not static and change over time to meet the needs of the growing infant. In early lactation, the whey:casein ratio is 90:10. As lactation progresses, the whey:casein ratio in mature breast milk is 60:40. Finally, during late lactation, the whey:casein ratio is 50:50 (Riordan & Wambach, 2010).

Whey protein in human milk is composed of five major components: (1) alpha-lactalbumin, (2) serum albumin, (3) lactoferrin, (4) immunoglobulins, and (5) lysozyme. The latter three components are believed to be non-nutritional proteins and serve immunologic functions in the body. For instance, one of the functions of lactoferrin is to prevent infections in the gastrointestinal tract by binding to free iron and thereby limiting its availability to iron-dependent enteric pathogens. Immunoglobulins (Ig), in particular secretory IgA, is abundant in human milk. Secretory IgA (SIgA) antibodies are made in the breast by the mother in response to exposure to antigens in her environment and passed along in her milk to her infant. Hence, the infant gradually builds up antibodies to the common pathogens in the immediate environment. Lysozymes are enzymes that destroy specific pathogens and also function to enhance the growth of "friendly" intestinal bacteria, namely, lactobacilli. Other kinds of non-nutritional proteins include other enzymes, growth modulators, and hormones (Riordan & Wambach, 2010).

Vitamins, Minerals, and Trace Elements

Vitamins

Most healthy full-term infants receive sufficient vitamin intake in their diets whether receiving human milk or formula, with only a few exceptions. Infants need vitamins for the body's metabolic functions. Vitamins are grouped by how they are absorbed by the body.

Vitamins A, D, E, and K are absorbed in the presence of fat or bile and are stored in fat tissue and the liver for future use. These vitamins are known as the fat-soluble vitamins. Excessive intake of fat-soluble vitamins can result in toxicity, therefore supplementation is not generally recommended, except in the case of Vitamin D (see the following section for further discussion).

Milk Composition

Vitamins in human milk are influenced by the mother's vitamin intake, general nutritional status, and genetic differences, and vary as lactation progresses. Many healthcare providers encourage new mothers to continue their prenatal vitamins after delivery and throughout the lactation period, unless the mother generally eats a well-balanced diet (Riordan & Wambach, 2010).

Vitamin A is needed for general maintenance of healthy skin, hair, nails, gums, glands, bones, and teeth. It helps prevent infections. In developing countries where malnutrition is of great concern, human milk provides a vital source of vitamin A and helps prevent blindness (Lawrence & Lawrence, 2005).

Human milk contains little vitamin D (needed in development of strong teeth and bone mineralization), although historically this was generally sufficient to meet the needs of most infants who are also exposed to an adequate amount of sunlight. However, cases of rickets and other evidence of vitamin D deficiency due to inadequate vitamin D intake and decreased exposure to sunlight are reported in the United States and other Western countries. The American Academy of Pediatrics recommended that all infants and children should receive 400 IU of vitamin D daily, beginning within the first few days after birth. The AAP recommends that breastfed infants (including those receiving some formula supplementation) should stay on vitamin D supplementation from birth. Although not recommended prior to 1 year of age, fortified whole milk contains 400 IU of vitamin D per liter and can provide sufficient vitamin D in later childhood if intake is at least 1 liter per day (AAP Clinical Report, 2008a). Because cow's milk–based formulas are currently supplemented with at least 400 IU of vitamin D per liter, the AAP recommends that formula-fed infants should receive additional supplementation until their intake reaches 1 liter per day (generally about 3 months of age).

Vitamin E (antioxidant and free radical scavenger) is naturally present in human milk, and mothers of preterm infants produce a slightly higher level in their colostrum than mothers of term infants. This is particularly important to premature infants in the NICU who may have damage to their lungs and retina from oxygen toxicity. Iron levels impact the ability of vitamin E to stabilize cell membranes and preserve fatty acids. Iron causes destruction of vitamin E in the gastrointestinal tract, which increases the release of harmful free radicals. Thus vitamin E needs are increased. Vitamin E also serves a role in the formation of red blood cells and prevents hemolytic anemia (especially in the premature infant who may be deficient in vitamin E and whose condition is aggravated by also receiving iron supplementation).

Vitamin K is present in human milk in small quantities. After the infant begins feeding, bacteria will colonize the intestinal tract. These bacteria synthesize additional vitamin K and form the primary source of the vitamin. Within a few days, infants generally will have produced sufficient amounts of vitamin K to prevent excessive bleeding. Vitamin K deficiency resulting in hemorrhage occurs in 0.25% to 1.7% of healthy-appearing newborns during the first week of life. In order to prevent this disorder, it has been the standard of care to give vitamin K prophylaxis after birth until the infant becomes naturally vitamin K sufficient (AAP, 2003 [reaffirmed 2009]).

The eight B vitamins and vitamin C (antioxidant) are water-soluble vitamins that pass readily from serum to breast milk. Breastfeeding mothers can ingest adequate amounts of B vitamins in their natural form from plant and animal food sources with the exception of vitamin B_{12}. Vitamin B_{12} is naturally found only in foods of animal origin. Breastfeeding mothers who follow a strict vegetarian diet or macrobiotic diet may have insufficient vitamin B_{12} in their milk unless they eat plant derived foods with vitamin B_{12} fortification (e.g., cereals) or receive vitamin B_{12} supplementation. Formula is fortified with adequate amounts of the water-soluble vitamins to meet the DRI. Unlike fat-soluble vitamins, any excess water-soluble vitamins ingested are simply excreted and the threat of toxicity is low (Lawrence & Lawrence, 2005).

See Table 32-2 for the vitamin content of human milk during the various stages of lactation (colostrum, transitional, and mature) and cow's milk.

Minerals

Minerals have diverse regulatory functions throughout the body. For example, calcium is important in the clotting mechanisms; phosphorus is a component in adenosine triphosphate (ATP), deoxyribonucleic acid (DNA), ribonucleic acid (RNA), and phospholipids; calcium and phosphorus are necessary for bone formation; sodium is involved in fluid balance; calcium, sodium, and potassium are needed for nerve and muscle function; chlorine is involved in acid–base balance; cobalt works with vitamin B_{12} to form blood cells; copper and iron aid in extracting energy from the citric acid cycle and are also involved in blood production; iodine is needed for thyroid hormone synthesis; and magnesium, manganese, and zinc are needed to help with many enzymatic processes (Thibodeau & Patton, 2009).

MILK COMPOSITION Both human milk and infant formulas contain several major and trace minerals to satisfy the needs of the growing infant. Breast milk provides newborns with minerals in more appropriate doses than do formulas (Blackburn, 2007). The mineral content of human milk does not appear to be influenced by maternal diet. The vitamins and minerals among the formulas being compared are essentially the same, although all generally contain higher levels of minerals than human milk to compensate for their lower bioavailability.

The amount of iron transferred to the fetus during the third trimester of pregnancy is influenced by maternal iron status (Riordan & Wambach, 2010). Iron is an important mineral required by the body to make hemoglobin and is needed for neurologic function. Neurotransmitters require adequate iron levels to function properly; therefore, infants with chronic anemia are at risk for cognitive and developmental delays. Infants deficient in iron may look pale, appear sleepy or tire easily while feeding, and be tachycardic or tachypneic at rest. The infant's iron status is affected by the amount of iron accumulated in utero, the infant's diet after birth, and the general health of the infant.

The AAP recommends against the use of low-iron fortified formulas because of the increased risk for anemia associated with their use (American Academy of Pediatrics (AAP) &

TABLE 32-2 Vitamins and Other Constituents of Human Milk and Cow's Milk*

MILK ELEMENTS	COLOSTRUM	TRANSITIONAL	MATURE	COW'S MILK
Vitamin A (μg)	151.0	88.0	75.0	41.0
Vitamin B_1 (μg)	1.9	5.9	14.0	43.0
Vitamin B_2 (μg)	30.0	37.0	40.0	145.0
Nicotinic acid (μg)	75.0	175.0	160.0	82.0
Vitamin B_6 (μg)	—	—	12.0–15.0	64.0
Pantothenic acid (μg)	183.0	288.0	246.0	340.0
Biotin (μg)	0.06	0.35	0.6	2.8
Folic acid (μg)	0.05	0.02	0.14	0.13
Vitamin B_{12} (μg)	0.05	0.04	0.1	0.6
Vitamin C (mg)	5.9	7.1	5.0	1.1
Vitamin D (μg)	—	—	0.04	0.02
Vitamin E (mg)	1.5	0.9	0.25	0.07
Vitamin K (μg)	—	—	1.5	6.0
Ash (g)	0.3	0.3	0.2	0.7
Calories (kcal)	57.0	63.0	65.0	65.0
Specific gravity	1.050	1.035	1.031	1.032
Milk (pH)	—	—	7.0	6.8

*Per deciliter

Source: Reprinted with permission from Lawrence, R. A., & Lawrence, R. M. (2005). Breastfeeding: A guide for the medical profession *(6th ed.). Copyright Elsevier 2005.*

American College of Obstetricians and Gynecologists (ACOG), 2007). Low-iron formula is fortified with only 2 mg of iron per liter compared with "iron-fortified" formula, which is fortified with 12 mg of iron per liter. It should be noted that the iron concentration in human milk is 0.5 to 1 mg per liter, which is considerably lower than in iron-fortified formulas. However, the iron in human milk is much more completely absorbed—the infant receiving human milk absorbs 50% to 80% of the iron in human milk compared with less than 12% of the iron in formula. Healthy term infants with normal birth weights receiving breast milk or an iron-fortified infant formula during the first 5 to 6 months of life are unlikely to develop iron-deficiency anemia because these infants have sufficient iron stores to sustain them until they start solid feedings in the second half of the first year of life (Riordan & Wambach, 2010).

Some parents have a misconception that infants fed iron-fortified formula are likely to have constipation. Nurses have a responsibility to educate parents and help them understand that the iron added to formula is in an ionic form and does not cause constipation (Levin, Cotton, Patrick-Miller, et al., 2010). The casein in formula (which is different from the casein in human milk) creates firm, rubbery curds that are slow to metabolize and have been associated with constipation in formula-fed infants. In addition, palm olein oil is added to some formulas to provide palmitic acid in an attempt to match the natural palmitic acid profile in human milk. However, the chemical arrangements are different. Palmitic acid derived from olein oil is poorly absorbed. The unabsorbed palmitic acid in formula reacts with calcium to create insoluble soaps during digestion and contribute to constipation.

Trace Elements

Other additives to formulas not yet mentioned include nucleotides (building blocks for DNA and RNA that appear to enhance the immune system, among other things), carnitine (derived from the amino acid lysine and functioning in part to transport fatty acids to the mitochondria for oxidation), and taurine (a conditionally essential nonprotein sulfur amino acid with a number of functions, including a role in growth, and in central nervous system and auditory function development). There are many other components in human milk not yet duplicated in formula and not all components in breast milk have been identified. In general though, formula companies are always striving to improve their products to develop the best "humanized" milk possible. There is no question that formulas today are far superior to formulas in the past.

The Evolution of Formula

Finding an acceptable breast milk substitute following maternal death, infant abandonment, low milk supply, and other situations has been a challenge for centuries. Although there are no written records describing infant feedings from ancient times to the Renaissance period, there is physical evidence of societies using alternative feedings dating back to 2000 BC. Throughout Europe, spouted feeding cups and other feeding receptacles have been found in the graves of infants. Records from written works show that from 1500 to 1700, "wet nurses" (a lactating woman whose purpose of employment was to nurse another woman's infant, sometimes abandoning her own infant to gain employment) were hired at foundling homes (orphanages) and by wealthy European women, because it was customary for noblewomen to delegate all physical work, including infant care (Lawrence & Lawrence, 2005; Stevens, Patrick, & Pickler, 2009).

By the 19th century wet-nursing was falling out of favor, and "dry-nursing" was attempted. Dry-nursing is the practice of feeding an infant milk obtained from another mammal (i.e., goats, cows, mares, donkeys, etc.) (Stevens et al., 2009). Milk from cows was most commonly used because of its availability, not because it was closer in composition to human milk. This practice was used in foundling homes and was associated with very high infant mortality (Lawrence & Lawrence, 2005).

Recognizing the need for an improved breast milk substitute, a few physicians continued attempts to develop a "humanized" animal milk substitute. In the late 1830s, a report of the content of human milk and cow's milk was published. This served as the basis for developing a baby milk substitute by means of modifying milk from a cow to make it more like human milk. Around the 1860s, the first commercially available baby food and infant formula was developed in Europe and became available in the United States by the 1870s. The first formula was comprised of only malt, cow's milk, and wheat flour and required reconstitution with water (Schuman, 2003). It was severely lacking in nutrient composition and quality. Only the most desperate would consider feeding it. Between 1860 and 1920 there were additional scientific discoveries that contributed to the further advancement of the development of an artificial baby milk. These included the discovery of the germ theory and subsequent development of pasteurization of milk, the invention of the bottle and rubber nipple to replace feeding devices that required skill to use and were difficult to clean, and the invention of the "ice box" to refrigerate the baby milk (Stevens et al., 2009).

Two of the biggest commercial advances in milk science were the invention of sweetened condensed milk in the 1830s and evaporated milk in 1883. Condensed milk was made by boiling milk and permitting it to evaporate to one-fourth its original volume, and then adding 6 ounces of sugar per pint to the milk as a preservative (Schuman, 2003). The invention of sweetened condensed milk and evaporated milk meant that for the first time in history, a family did not have to have access to a cow in order to feed their infant milk (if not breastfeeding). From evaporated milk, a homemade evaporated milk formula recipe was created and made available to the public. The evaporated milk formula was a simple mixture of evaporated milk, water, and sugar or corn syrup. The evaporated milk formula gained acceptance because it was affordable, it appeared to support growth equal to that of breastfed infants, and it was widely available. When world events created a need for women to work in factories to fill in for men who went off to fight in the war, this generation of women felt compelled to help out. Bottles and formula made it a viable option for them. Following WWII, formula use was becoming widespread. It is estimated that by 1960 about 80% of bottle-fed infants were being fed with evaporated milk formula and given supplements of vitamins and iron. However, poor infant outcomes were still being observed.

In the 1960s proprietary commercial formulas had improved upon the quality of evaporated milk formulas. Parents were impressed with the advances in science and wanted to raise their children scientifically "by the book." Using formula seemed to be a progressive idea to embrace. By this time more and more women were working outside the home than ever before. "Modern women" saw formula use as more convenient than breastfeeding. Formula companies appealed to these women. In addition to a changing social climate in America, advances in agriculture created a surplus of cow's milk and offered a new marketing opportunity for global commercialization of formula (Schuman, 2003).

Artificial baby milk that was originally intended as a lifesaving product for extreme situations was now being aggressively marketed as a food for all infants. To this end formula companies began an aggressive marketing campaign. One of their marketing tactics was to provide free formula to hospitals, enabling hospitals to phase out their formula preparation rooms. Mothers viewed commercial formula as an acceptable breast milk substitute that appeared to have medical endorsement, was easy to use and affordable, and freed her to do other things such as work outside the home. By 1972, formula use peaked and breastfeeding rates in the United States plummeted (only 25% of women were breastfeeding at hospital discharge) (Schuman, 2003). Again, the public was led to believe that commercial formula was as good as, if not better than, breast milk.

Research efforts beginning in the 1970s showed that human milk was unquestionably superior to evaporated milk and proprietary infant formulas as evidenced by a significant rise in infant morbidity and mortality, especially in developing countries (Schuman, 2003). The revelation of the research findings from the 1970s up to the present has led to resurgence in breastfeeding.

Over the last 50 years or so, considerable time, effort, and money have been allocated to the development of commercial infant formulas in an attempt to better imitate the content and performance of human milk. In 1954, the executive board of the AAP established a Committee on Nutrition to set the standards for nutritional requirements and feeding practices for infants, children, and adolescents. This committee makes recommendations for nutritional requirements in infant formulas to the Food and Drug Administration (FDA). In 1980 Congress passed the Infant Formula Act, which was later amended in 1986. The safety and nutritional quality of formula are now significantly regulated. Despite this, there are several recalls of formula every year. In 1995 the National Alliance for Breastfeeding Advocacy was formed to educate the public, state and federal legislators, policymakers, and healthcare systems about such hazards and to advocate on all matters concerning breastfeeding.

Specialty Formulas

The American Academy of Pediatrics (2005) recommends breastfeeding for all infants, with rare exceptions. When breastfeeding is not an option or is not chosen, then standard cow's milk–based formula is the first choice among the formulas. However, there are situations in which standard cow's milk–based formula is not tolerated, is contraindicated, or is not acceptable to the parents. Before switching to a specialty formula, the parents should first consult with their baby's healthcare provider (Abbott Nutrition, 2009).

Milk-Based Lactose-Free Formulas

Similac Sensitive is a milk-based formula containing milk protein isolate and lactose-free. In place of lactose, the formula manufacturer substitutes a blend of corn syrup solids and sucrose. (Bear in mind that use of non-lactose products should be reserved for those rare infants with clinically proven lactose intolerance.)

Soy-Based Formulas

Soy protein–based formulas include the following products: Enfamil ProSobee with LIPIL, Similac Isomil Advance, Similac Isomil DF (marketed for infants older than 6 months who have diarrhea), and Nestlé Good Start Soy Plus. They all are iron-fortified formulas and meet the nutrient specifications as established by the FDA. They use soy harvested from soybeans and supplemented with methionine (an essential amino acid), carnitine, and taurine. Soy protein–based formulas do not contain any bovine protein (cow protein) or lactose, the formula is usually sweetened with corn syrup, corn maltodextrin, or sucrose. (The latter may cause dental decay after the teeth have erupted.) The fat content varies as well. The formula companies use vegetable oils such as soy, palm, sunflower, olein, safflower, and coconut to meet the fat requirement. Phytates present in soy formulas decrease the absorption of iron, calcium, and zinc, so greater concentrations of minerals and vitamins are added to soy formulas. Also, phytoestrogens (specifically isoflavones), which are estrogen-like compounds found in plants, are consumed in high quantity among infants being fed soy formula. So far, there is no conclusive evidence from studies that phytoestrogens cause harm to infants (AAP Clinical Report, 2008b). Further studies are warranted.

The American Academy of Pediatrics recommends against the use of soy protein–based formula for preterm infants who weigh less than 1800 grams or infants with renal failure because of the high aluminum level in soy formulas. Human milk contains 4 to 65 ng/ml of aluminum; soy protein–based formulas contain 600 to 1300 ng/ml (AAP Clinical Report, 2008b). Soy formula is also not medically indicated for infants having risk factors for allergies, or supplementation for the breastfeeding infant unless specifically indicated (AAP Clinical Report, 2008b).

Although the AAP (2008b) states that the "isolated soy protein-based formulas are safe and effective alternatives to provide appropriate nutrition for normal growth and development," for *term* infants whose nutritional needs are not being met by human milk or cow's milk–based formulas, soy protein–based formula is not intended as a first-choice formula except for infants with primary lactase deficiency or galactosemia, for term infants of formula-feeding vegan parents, and or if the infant develops secondary (transient) lactase deficiency following an acute bout with diarrhea.

Despite the few genuine indications for using soy protein–based formulas, soy formula accounts for almost 25% of the formula market in the United States (AAP Clinical Report, 2008b). The demand for its use appears to be driven by healthcare providers and parents (Vartabedian, 2007). When a newborn is fussy and gassy, many parents mistakenly believe that their infant is "lactose intolerant" because an adult family member is lactose intolerant. On the other hand, cow protein in standard cow's milk–based formula can cause colicky symptoms in sensitive infants. Switching to soy formula will not always solve the cause of the colic symptoms, because infants who are sensitive to the protein in cow's milk–based formula may also be sensitive to the soy protein in soy protein–based formula (Greer, Sicherer, Burks, et al., 2008). Therefore, the AAP recommends using hypoallergenic formulas rather than soy formula for infants with documented cow's milk allergy (AAP Clinical Report, 2008b).

Feeding Intolerances

All too often, fussy breastfeeding or cow's milk–based formula-fed infants are switched to a lactose-free formula because of concerns about lactose intolerance. It is important to distinguish true lactose intolerance from cow's milk protein allergy or other source of feeding intolerance.

Lactose intolerance is defined as a "deficiency of the intestinal enzyme lactase that splits lactose into two smaller sugars, glucose and galactose, and allows lactose to be absorbed from the intestine" (Marks, 2008). This condition causes diarrhea, flatulence, abdominal pain, and, sometimes, abdominal bloating, abdominal distension, and nausea. There are three causes of lactose intolerance: (1) congenital lact*ase* deficiency, (2) secondary lact*ose* intolerance, and (3) developmental or acquired lact*ose* intolerance.

The most common cause of lactose intolerance is developmental or acquired. Many parents will assume that their infant has lactose intolerance because they or the child's older sibling has lactose intolerance. However, this is an age-related condition that develops after 2 to 5 years of age and is therefore not a condition affecting newborns.

Up to 15% of infants have milk protein allergy (mostly because of the beta-lactoglobulin component in cow's milk) or to some other antigen (Brill, 2008). Infants with a *cow's milk protein allergy (CMPA)* who are being fed breast milk or formula may exhibit a variety of symptoms and involves multiple body systems. Gastrointestinal symptoms include copious gas, reflux (spitting up frequently), very loose stools or diarrhea or constipation, mucous and blood (gross or occult) in the stool, may refuse to feed or want to eat small meals frequently due to discomfort and feeling bloated, and may develop failure to thrive. Infants frequently exhibit allergic respiratory symptoms, and cutaneous manifestations include skin rash. Lastly, allergies affect a baby's disposition, hence being labeled a "colicky" baby. They tend to be especially fussy in the first hour after feeding and it impacts their sleep because babies usually go to sleep after feeding. These babies may awaken early due to reflux or gas pain.

Breastfeeding babies may not be allergic to the mother's milk but rather to the cow's milk protein (an antigen) in the mother's milk. By eliminating the culprit (e.g., the bovine protein) from the mother's diet and therefore from the breast milk, the mother can continue to breastfeed, providing optimal nutrition and immune factors to her infant. However, a dietary elimination of cow's milk and milk products (and hidden sources of milk in prepared foods), is a very difficult lifestyle change to make. These mothers need a lot of support and praise for their sacrifice. They also need to know alternate food sources to receive their daily requirement for calcium and vitamin D. Encourage families to read labels and find foods fortified with calcium and vitamin D (e.g., fortified orange juice). Some mothers tolerate rice milk or goat milk on their fortified cereal, although there can be a cross-reaction or sensitivity with goat milk. The silver lining in all of this is that many infants outgrow their cow's milk allergy as early as a year of age. Some sensitive babies take longer to outgrow this problem.

Other Specialized Formulas

For infants who do not have cow's milk–based formula allergy but may have formula intolerance, the formula companies offer hydrolyzed or partially hydrolyzed formula. *(Note: "hydrolyzed" simply means the protein has been broken down into smaller components mimicking digestion.)* These include Nestlé Good Start Gentle Plus and Enfamil Gentlease. Nestlé Good Start Gentle Plus provides 100% hydrolyzed whey protein (no casein protein) for easier digestion, and the carbohydrate requirement is met with a blend of lactose and corn maltodextrin. Fats come from a combination of vegetable oils. Enfamil Gentlease provides hydrolyzed whey and casein proteins with a profile similar to mature human milk, but the lactose amount is reduced to one fifth the amount found in standard milk-based formula (Nestlé Nutrition, 2009). Lactose-free formulas raise concerns about the long-term use of lactose-free formulas when an infant's sole source of food is formula. These specialty formulas are widely available at most food stores and pharmacies that sell infant formula.

For infants with documented cow's milk–based allergies or infants with a metabolic disorder or malabsorption syndrome, the first choice formula is a hypoallergenic formula such as Nutramigen or Alimenum. Both formulas use extensively hydrolyzed casein protein supplemented with a high percentage of free amino acids such as L-cystine, L-tyrosine, and L-tryptophan with the remainder as small peptides. Both are lactose-free. Both use a combination of vegetable fats that are different from each other to meet the fat requirement.

In rare cases, some extremely sensitive infants do not tolerate Nutramigen or Alimentum, and require a "superhypoallergenic" formula. This category of formulas may be prescribed for infants who may have severe food allergies or multiple food allergies, short-bowel syndrome, or other severe GI tract disorder. Both EleCare and Neocate are used in these extreme situations. These formulas provide 100% free amino acids as their protein source, corn syrup solids for their carbohydrate source, and each has a unique fat profile. These expensive specialty formulas are available by prescription only. There are still other specialty formulas developed for infants with other medical conditions such as prematurity, heart disease, kidney disease, and specific metabolic diseases. There are commercial formulas or nutrient supplements designed for their special needs. These formulas are available by prescription only.

HEALTH PROMOTION EDUCATION: CHOICE OF FEEDING

Feeding their newborn is an exciting, satisfying, but often worrisome task for parents. Meeting this essential need of their new child helps parents strengthen their attachment to their child and fosters their self-images as nurturers and providers, yet carries great responsibility. Whether a woman chooses to breastfeed or formula feed, she can be reassured that she can adequately meet her infant's needs. As questions about feeding arise, the nurse works with the woman to help her develop skill in her chosen method. In every interaction, it is the nurse's responsibility to support the parents and promote the family's sense of confidence.

The mother usually decides to breastfeed or formula feed by the sixth month of pregnancy and often even before conception. However, she may not make her final decision until admission to the birth center. The decision is often influenced by relatives, especially the baby's father and the maternal grandmother (AWHONN, 2007), by friends, and by social customs rather than being based on knowledge about the nutritional and psychologic needs of the mother and her newborn.

The *Healthy People 2010* National Health Promotion and Disease Prevention program states that at least 75% of all mothers will initiate breastfeeding, at least 50% will continue to breastfeed until their infants are 6 months old, and at least 25% of mothers continue to breastfeed until their infants are 12 months old. A recent survey of breastfeeding in the United States showed a slow rise to 77% of hospital-born infants receiving some breast milk but the continuation of breastfeeding until 6 months of age still falls short of the desired goal (McDowell, Wang, & Kennedy-Stephenson, 2008). In the last few years, the CDC also began tracking the rate of *exclusive breastfeeding* among infants at 3 months and 6 months of age. The *Healthy People 2010* objective for exclusive breastfeeding at 3 months is 40%; the current rate is 33%. The *Healthy People 2010* objective for exclusive breastfeeding at 6 months is 17%; the current rate is 13.6% (Centers for Disease Control and Prevention [CDC], 2009). It is the healthcare provider's responsibility to provide the parents with accurate information about the distinct advantages of breastfeeding to the mother and infant. In these times of short stays, the Baby-Friendly Hospital Initiative program promotes breastfeeding by designating hospitals as centers for breastfeeding education.

Once the parents have made an informed choice of feeding method, the nurse's primary responsibilities are to support the family's decision and to help the family achieve a positive result. No woman should be made to feel either inadequate or superior because of her choice in feeding. There are advantages and disadvantages to breastfeeding and bottle-feeding, but positive bonds in parent-child relationships can be developed with either method.

Breastfeeding

Breast Milk Production

The female breast is divided into 15 to 20 lobes, separated from one another by fat and connective tissue, and interspersed with blood vessels, lymphatic vessels, and nerves. These lobes are subdivided into lobules composed of small units called alveoli where milk is synthesized by the alveolar secretory epithelium. The lobules have a system of lactiferous ducts that eventually open onto the nipple surface. Mothers are often surprised to see milk coming out of multiple nipple pores when they express their milk. See Figure 32-1 ■ to view the anatomy of the breast.

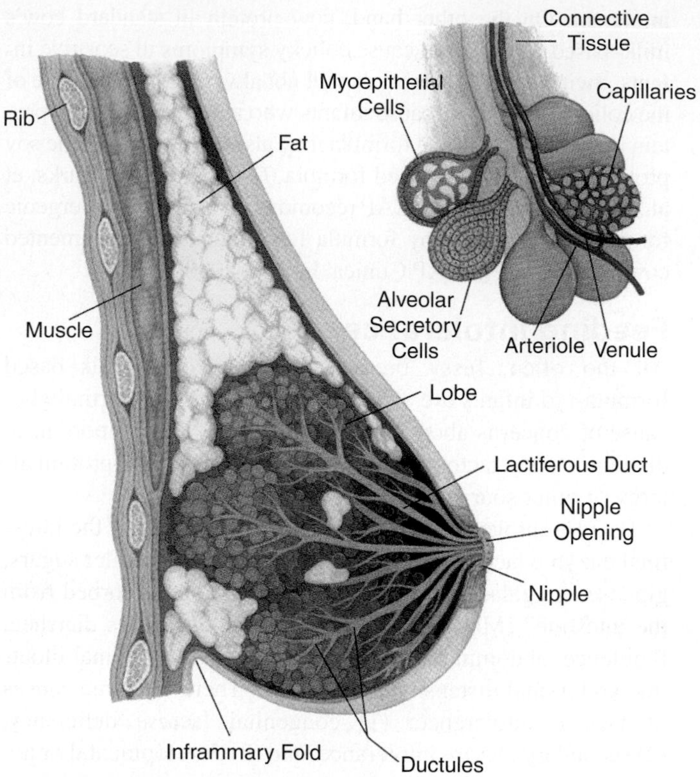

Figure 32-1 ■ Anatomy of the breast.

Source: From Riordan, J. (2005). Breastfeeding and human lactation *(3rd ed., pp. 118–119). Boston: Jones & Bartlett. Copyright © 2005 Jones and Bartlett Publishers, Sudbury, MA. www.jbpub.com. Reprinted with permission.*

Physiologic and Endocrine Control of Lactogenesis

During pregnancy, increased levels of estrogen stimulate breast duct proliferation and development, and elevated progesterone levels promote the development of lobules and alveoli in preparation for lactation. Prolactin levels rise from approximately 10 ng/ml prepregnancy to 200 ng/ml at term. However, lactation is suppressed during pregnancy by elevated progesterone levels secreted by the placenta. Once the placenta is expelled at delivery, progesterone levels fall and the inhibition is removed, triggering milk production. This occurs whether the mother has breast stimulation or not. However, if by the third or fourth day breast stimulation is not occurring, prolactin levels begin to drop.

Initially, lactation is under endocrine control. The hormone **prolactin** is released from the anterior pituitary in response to breast stimulation from suckling or the use of a breast pump. Prolactin stimulates the milk-secreting cells in the alveoli to produce milk, then rapidly drops back to baseline. If more than approximately 3 hours occurs between breast stimulation, prolactin levels begin to drop below baseline. To reverse the overall decline in prolactin levels, the mother can be encouraged to breastfeed/pump more frequently (e.g., every 1.5 to 2 hours during day hours) for a few days to get baseline prolactin raised. This is especially important if the infant is not an effective feeder or if the mother is separated from her infant. Prolactin receptors are established during the first 2 weeks postpartum in response to frequency of breast stimulation (Human Milk Banking Association of North America [HMBANA], 2006). Inadequate development of prolactin receptors during this time is likely to negatively impact the mother's long-term milk volume. By 2 weeks (14 days) postpartum, prolactin levels will be back to prepregnancy levels and milk production will cease if stimulation of the breasts by breastfeeding or pumping does not occur (Lawrence & Lawrence, 2005).

The milk that flows from the breast at the start of a feeding or pumping session is called **foremilk**. The foremilk is watery milk, high in lactose, high in protein, and low in fat (1% to 2%). This is milk that has trickled down from the alveoli between feedings to fill the lactiferous ducts. It is low-fat milk because the fat globules made in the alveoli stick to each other and to the walls of the alveoli and do not trickle down.

In addition to prolactin release, stretching of the nipple and compression of the areola signal the hypothalamus to trigger the posterior pituitary gland to release oxytocin. **Oxytocin** acts on the myoepithelial cells surrounding the alveoli in the breast tissue to contract, ejecting milk, including the fat globules present, into the ducts. This process is called the *milk-ejection reflex*, better known in lay terms as the **let-down reflex** response. The average initial let-down response occurs about 2 minutes after an infant begins to suckle, and there will be 4 to 10 let-down responses during a feeding session. The milk that flows during let-down is called **hindmilk**. As noted, hindmilk is rich in fat (can exceed 10%) and therefore high in calories. In a sample of expressed human milk, the average total fat concentration is about 4% and the total caloric content is about 20 calories/ounce.

By 6 months of breastfeeding, prolactin levels are only 5 to 10 ng/ml, yet milk production continues. A whey protein called feedback inhibitor of lactation (FIL) has been identified as influencing milk production through a negative feedback loop. FIL is present in breast milk and functions to decrease milk production. The more milk that remains in the breast and the longer it remains, the more milk production is decreased. On the other hand, the more often the breasts are emptied, the lower the level of FIL and the faster milk is produced. This mechanism of regulating milk at the local level is called *autocrine control*. This process is key to understanding how a mother maintains or loses her milk supply (Riordan & Wambach, 2010).

There are a number of risk factors that can delay or impair lactogenesis. Maternal factors include cesarean birth, primiparity, long duration of stage I or stage II of labor, postpartum hemorrhage, premature delivery, diabetes type 1, untreated hypothyroidism, obesity, polycystic ovary syndrome or other endocrine disturbances, retained placenta fragments, history of previous breast surgery, insufficient glandular breast tissue, and significant stress (Riordan & Wambach, 2010). Other factors that can interfere with the breast milk supply include smoking and the use of alcohol and some prescription and over-the-counter medications (e.g., antihistamines, combined birth control pills).

Stages of Human Milk

During the establishment of lactation there are three stages of human milk: colostrum, transitional milk, and mature milk.

Colostrum is the initial milk that begins to be secreted during mid-pregnancy and is immediately available to the baby at delivery. Although the volume of colostrum is small, this encourages the newborn to nurse frequently, helping to stimulate milk production. No supplementation with other fluids is necessary unless there is a medical indication. Colostrum is a thick, creamy yellowish fluid with concentrated amounts of protein, fat-soluble vitamins, and minerals, and it has lower amounts of fat and lactose compared with mature milk. It also contains antioxidants and high levels of lactoferrin and secretory immunoglobulin A (IgA). It promotes the establishment of *Lactobacillus bifidus* flora in the digestive tract, which helps to protect the infant from disease and illness. Colostrum also has a laxative effect on the infant, which helps the baby pass meconium stools, which in turn helps decrease hyperbilirubinemia.

The onset of copious milk secretion begins between 32 and 96 hours postpartum. For most women this is observed on day 3. Lay people refer to this as the milk "coming in." The milk produced during this period is called **transitional milk**. Transitional milk has qualities intermediate to colostrum and mature milk but may look indistinguishable from colostrum. It is still yellow in color like colostrum but is more copious and contains more fat, lactose, water-soluble vitamins, and calories. See Figure 32-2 ■ to view a picture of transitional milk. By day 5, most mothers are producing about 16 oz/day (Riordan & Wambach, 2010).

Mature milk is white or can be slightly blue-tinged in color. It is present by 2 weeks postpartum and continues thereafter until lactation ceases. Mature milk contains about 13% solids (carbohydrates, proteins, and fats) and 87% water. Although mature human milk appears similar to skim cow's milk and may

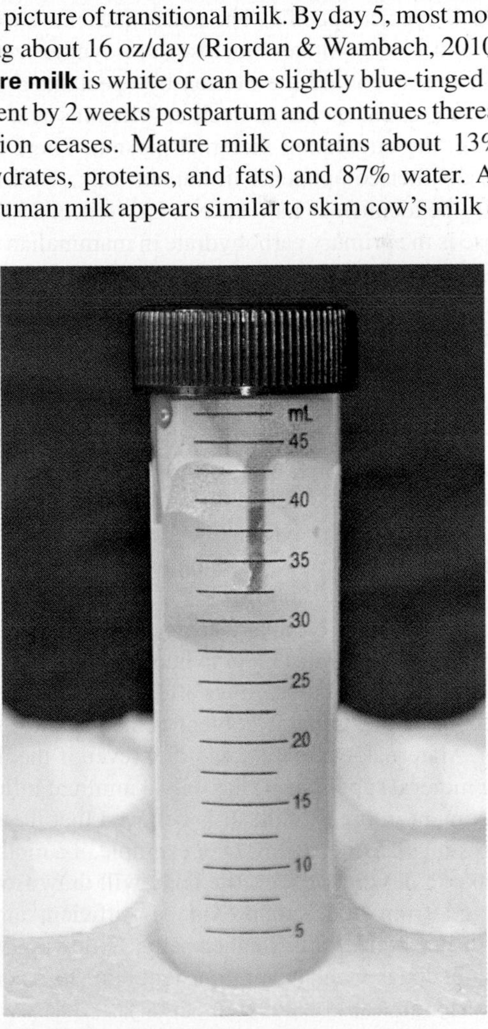

Figure 32-2 ■ Transitional human milk.

Source: Courtesy of Brigitte Hall, RNC, MSN, IBCLC/Pearson Education.

cause mothers to question whether their milk is "rich enough," mothers should be reassured that this is the normal appearance of mature human milk and that it provides the infant with all the necessary nutrients. Although gradual changes in composition do occur continuously over periods of weeks to accommodate the needs of the growing newborn, in general the composition of mature milk is fairly consistent, with the exception of the fat content as noted previously. Milk production continues to increase slowly over the first month. By 6 months postpartum a mother produces about 800 ml/day (Blackburn, 2007).

Advantages of Human Milk

In its breastfeeding policy statement, the AAP recommends exclusive breastfeeding as the preferred feeding for all infants, with a few exceptions, for the first 6 months and continued breastfeeding during the introduction of solids until the infant is 12 months old or older, as desired. There is compelling scientific evidence that indicates that breastfeeding provides infants with specific nutritional, immunologic, and psychosocial advantages over formula-feedings (AAP & ACOG, 2007).

Nutritional Advantages

Human milk provides optimum nutrition for the human infant because it is species specific. The macronutrients such as protein, fat, and carbohydrates (lactose) are synthesized by the mother in the alveoli of the breasts by specialized secretory cells. Micronutrient elements such as vitamins and minerals derive from the circulating maternal plasma. There are more than 200 distinct components in human milk, with more remaining to be identified (Lawrence & Lawrence, 2005).

Lactose is the primary carbohydrate in mammalian milk and plays a crucial role in the nourishment of our offspring. Human milk has a very high lactose content compared with the milk of other mammal species. After lactose is hydrolyzed into galactose and glucose, the galactose is used in the formation of cerebral galactolipids and contributes to brain and central nervous system (CNS) development. Glucose is used by many tissues, but especially by the brain, which consumes 20% of the body's energy requirements and derives this almost exclusively from glucose. In addition to providing a cellular energy source, lactose enhances the absorption of calcium, magnesium, and zinc (Lawrence & Lawrence, 2005).

Fats in breast milk give an advantage to infants who receive human milk. The mineral content in human milk (colostrum) is a little higher for the first few days after birth, and then after a slight decrease, the mineral content remains fairly constant thereafter. Maternal age, parity, and diet (even if the mother is receiving mineral supplement) has only a minimal influence on mineral content in breast milk. It is believed that the maternal body stores regulate the process. For example, if a mother's calcium intake in her diet is poor, the body will draw from its reserves (e.g., from bone) to provide a sufficient amount of calcium in her breast milk for her baby. Following weaning, through a feedback mechanism, transient bone loss normalizes (Bezerra, Mendonca, Lobato, et al., 2004).

As mentioned earlier in this chapter, the iron found in human milk, even though much lower in concentration than that of prepared formulas, is much more readily and fully absorbed facilitated by the high vitamin C and lactose levels in the breast milk and appears sufficient to meet the infant's iron needs for the first 6 months. Excess iron is not desirable because any extra iron that is not absorbed may promote the growth of pathogenic enteric bacteria as well as cause cellular oxidative injury. Lactoferrin, an iron-binding protein found only in breast milk, scavenges iron in the gut and enhances its absorption, eliminating excess iron (Lawrence & Lawrence, 2005).

There is research supporting additional health advantages for the breastfed infant. Breastfed infants have a reduced risk of developing type 1 or type 2 diabetes mellitus, lymphoma, leukemia, Hodgkin's disease, obesity, hypercholesterolemia, and asthma (AAP, 2005).

The mother benefits from breastfeeding as well. When breastfeeding is initiated right after delivery, there is decreased risk for postpartum bleeding. As breastfeeding continues in the early postpartum period, the elevated oxytocin levels stimulate rapid uterine involution.

The benefits of breastfeeding are dose related. However, both mother and baby benefit from even some breastfeeding compared to no breastfeeding at all. In a large study, the authors suggested that breastfeeding has a protective function against premenopausal breast cancer (Riordan & Wambach, 2010). In addition, breastfeeding mothers have a decreased risk of developing ovarian cancer (Lawrence & Lawrence, 2005); and may have a decreased risk of developing postmenopausal osteoporosis (AWHONN, 2007).

The breastfeeding mother also benefits from breastfeeding by burning additional calories making milk (quicker return to prepregnancy weight), thus losing more weight in the postpartum period than the mother who never breastfed. Breastfeeding frequency and total duration also influence weight loss.

Immunologic Advantages

The immunologic advantages of human milk include varying degrees of protection from respiratory tract and gastrointestinal tract infections, necrotizing enterocolitis, urinary tract infections, otitis media, bacterial meningitis, bacteremia, and allergies (AWHONN, 2007). Transplacental passage of maternal immunoglobulin gradually diminishes over the first 6 months of life until the infant can begin to produce his or her own immunoglobulins. Human milk-derived immunologic protection helps supplement this protection.

Secretory IgA, an immunoglobulin present in colostrum and mature breast milk, has antiviral, antibacterial, and antigenic-inhibiting properties, specifically across mucosal surfaces such as the intestinal tract. Secretory IgA plays a role in decreasing the permeability of the small intestine to help prevent large protein molecules from triggering an allergic response. Other constituents of colostrum and mature breast milk that act to inhibit the growth of bacteria or viruses are *Lactobacillus bifidus,* lysozymes, lactoperoxidase, lactoferrin, transferrin, and various immunoglobulins.

Some mothers wonder if there are special considerations for breastfed infants regarding immunizations. Although breastfeeding mothers pass along antibodies and other immune factors in their milk to their infant, breastfeeding is not a substitute for routine immunizations. All infants should receive vaccinations following a schedule as recommended by the Centers for Disease Control and Prevention (CDC, 2010). The current vaccination schedule can be viewed online at the CDC Web site.

Some mothers also wonder if it is safe for them to receive vaccinations while breastfeeding. Mothers should be reassured that most vaccines can safely be taken during the lactation period. According to the CDC, *General Recommendations on Immunization* (2010), "Neither inactivated nor live vaccines administered to a lactating woman affect the safety of breast-feeding for mothers or infants. Breast-feeding does not adversely affect immunization and is not a contraindication for any vaccine."

Psychosocial Benefits of Breastfeeding

The psychosocial advantages of breastfeeding include increased self-esteem, enhanced bonding, and a decrease in stress for the mother and infant.

A mother's self-esteem is increased in knowing that she has provided the perfect food for her baby and provided protection with her antibodies with her own body. For many mothers breastfeeding takes effort, understanding, and an emotional commitment to endure the demands of this lifestyle choice. The mother's sense of accomplishment in being able to satisfy her baby's needs for nourishment and comfort can be a tremendous source of personal satisfaction.

Women who breastfeed, by its nature, have close contact with their infants. Newborns are very responsive to touch, and it is vital for the infant's emotional well-being. The tactile stimulation associated with breastfeeding can communicate warmth, closeness, and comfort. The increased closeness provides both the mother and newborn with the opportunity to learn each other's behavioral cues and needs. From the release of prolactin and oxytocin while breastfeeding, mothers may feel more affectionate toward their newborns, have improved let-down response, and breastfeed more frequently and for longer periods of time (Klaus, 1998; Mohrbacher & Kendall-Tackett, 2005).

Mothers who breastfeed save money and this reduces stress for many families. There are significant cost savings for the family who chooses breastfeeding. The cost of standard formula is approximately $1,300 annually per infant for standard formulas and more for specialty formulas (AWHONN, 2007). There are also healthcare cost savings for families resulting from the decreased incidence of illness in the infant. Because breastfed babies access healthcare resources less often, the family saves money on medical visits and prescription medications and loses less time from work.

Potential societal benefits to breastfeeding include decreased spending on public assistance programs (e.g., Women Infant Children Supplemental Nutrition Program [WIC]), and environmental benefits in terms of use of natural resources and solid waste disposal. Breastfeeding is not dependent on modern technology and can provide the infant with a fresh, clean, naturally warm source of nutrition independent of transportation, supply, electricity, refrigeration, clean water, bottles, nipples, and so on. There are also substantial medical cost savings to society, estimated to be approximately $400 in excess medical costs per never-breastfed infant (AWHONN, 2007). With current breastfeeding initiation rates of approximately 66%, this amounts to an additional $544 million per year in potential healthcare costs that could be saved by breastfeeding. Table 32-3 compares several factors for parents to consider when choosing between breastfeeding and formula-feeding.

Breastfeeding

> "Another challenge I had occurred when I went back to work full-time and had to fight to keep up my milk supply. Because my baby has allergies, it was especially important for her to have only breast milk for the first 6 months. I achieved that goal, but I could not have made it without the help I got from family, friends, the staff at the lactation center, my OB, and my daughter's pediatrician. Also, my boss and co-workers have been very supportive, allowing me breaks to pump my milk 3 times a day at work. Now I know why they say "It takes a village to raise a child." In the end, there is nothing more rewarding than knowing that I'm providing the best nutrition possible and seeing my daughter smile back at me while she nurses. She is healthy and happy and that means the world to me."
>
> — *Alyssa*

Potential Disadvantages and Contraindications to Breastfeeding

Care Plan Activity: Breastfeeding Concerns

Disadvantages

The following is a list of sometimes cited potential disadvantages to breastfeeding:

1. ***Pain with breastfeeding.*** Breastfeeding is a natural process but requires a certain knowledge base that formerly was passed along from generation to generation. With the decline in the extended family structure, this source of knowledge and assistance is often missing for the new mother. Nipple tenderness is the most common source of discomfort and is usually related to improper positioning and/or not obtaining a proper attachment of the infant on the breast. Pain can also be related to engorgement or infection. Breastfeeding with proper technique should not hurt and these mothers should be encouraged to seek assistance from a knowledgeable person skilled in lactation.
2. ***Leaking milk.*** Some women will leak milk when their breasts are full and it is nearly time to breastfeed again or whenever they experience let-down, which can be triggered by hearing, seeing, or even thinking of their baby. If this causes concern to the mother, she can be instructed on how to apply gentle pressure directly over her nipple for a minute or so to stop the leaking momentarily. The mother can wear nursing pads inside her bra (with instructions to change wet pads frequently), or she might want to wear printed tops that camouflage small leaks. Mothers should be given reassurance that this problem diminishes over time.

TABLE 32-3 Comparison of Breastfeeding and Formula-Feeding

BREASTFEEDING	FORMULA (IRON-ENRICHED)-FEEDING
Infant Nutrition	
An ideal balance of nutrients, efficiently absorbed. High bioavailability of iron leaves little excess iron available for bacterial growth, cell injury.	Derived from bovine milk and/or plant sources. Lower bioavailability of nutrients requires higher concentrations in milk. Additives may cause intolerance.
Higher levels of essential fatty acids, lactose, cystine, and cholesterol, necessary for brain and nerve growth.	Still missing numerous ingredients. Formulas do not contain cholesterol. Soy and hydrolysate formulas do not contain lactose. DHA and ARA now added.
Composition varies according to gestational age and stage of lactation, meeting changing nutritional needs.	Nutritional value not varied. Nutritional adequacy depends on proper preparation/dilution.
Long-term decreased incidence of diabetes, cancer, obesity, asthma.	
Contains unsaturated fats.	Contains saturated fats.
Infants determine the volume of milk consumed.	Parents or healthcare provider determine the volume consumed. Overfeeding may occur if caregiver is determined that baby empty bottle.
Frequency of feeding is determined by infant's cues. May feed more frequently as milk digestion is faster.	Frequency of feeding is determined by infant's cues. May feed less frequently as milk digestion is slower.
Immunologic Properties	
Contains immunoglobulins, enzymes, and leukocytes that protect against pathogens. Nutrients promote growth of *Lactobacillus,* protective bacteria. Lower rates of urinary tract infections, otitis media, and other infectious diseases.	No antibodies or anti-infective properties. Formula is linked to an increased incidence of gastrointestinal and respiratory tract infections.
Anti-infective properties present in the milk permit longer storage duration.	Potential for bacterial contamination exists during preparation and storage.
Human milk is hypoallergenic, with minimal risk of protein allergy/intolerance.	Cow's milk protein intolerance relatively common.
Maternal Health	
Faster return to prepregnancy weight.	Provides complete (or supplemental) infant nutrition when human milk not available because of maternal illness, medication/drug use, lactation failure (breast surgery, endocrine disease), or if not chosen as a feeding choice.
Breastfeeding associated with lower risk of breast, ovarian cancer.	
Psychosocial Aspects	
Skin-to-skin contact enhances bonding. Maternal empowerment from satisfaction with providing optimal nourishment and antibody protection for her infant.	Both parents can participate in positive parent-infant interaction during feeding from the start.
Hormones of lactation promote maternal feelings and sense of well-being.	Father can assume feeding responsibilities.
The value system of modern society can create barriers to successful breastfeeding.	Mothers can receive more rest in the beginning because others can help assume feeding responsibilities.
Some mothers may feel ashamed or embarrassed.	
Breastfeeding after returning to work may be difficult.	
Cost	
Healthy diet for mother.	Hypoallergenic formula is more expensive than standard formula.
Savings for infant medical costs: approximately $400 average in first year of life.	Ancillary costs: bottles or bottle liners, nipples, cleaning costs.
Ancillary costs: nursing pads, nursing bras.	Refrigeration is needed if preparing more than one bottle at a time.
A breast pump may be needed.	
Refrigeration is necessary for storing expressed milk.	
Convenience	
Milk is always the perfect temperature. No preparation time is needed.	Formula must be purchased commercially. Preparation is time consuming.
The mother must be available to feed or will need to provide expressed milk to be given in her absence.	Less convenient for traveling or for night feedings.
If she misses a feeding, the mother must express milk to maintain lactation.	Mother need not be present—anyone can feed the infant.
The mother may experience discomfort in the early days of lactation.	

3. ***Embarrassment.*** Some mothers feel uncomfortable about breastfeeding because they are modest, or may feel embarrassed because our society views breasts as sexual objects, and/or an unfriendly social environment makes it difficult to breastfeed in public. This is not an easy issue to overcome. Some mothers will feel more confident after learning how to breastfeed discreetly while in public.

4. ***Stress.*** Many mothers feel a lot of stress juggling work or school and the demands of home life. Some mothers cite this reason for wanting to wean. There are multiple options to suggest for this concern. Mothers can learn about "double pumping" to save time. A double electric breast pump allows the mother to pump both breasts simultaneously, which cuts the pumping time in half. If a mother

struggles to keep up her milk supply, she can try taking an herbal supplement to give her milk supply a boost, unless contraindicated for her. (See Complementary and Alternative Therapies later in the chapter.) Finally, it is still preferable to decrease the frequency of pumping rather than quitting altogether, if that makes things more manageable for the mother. Babies who get some breast milk are still receiving more of the benefits of breast milk than babies who do not receive any breast milk.

5. ***Unequal feeding responsibilities/fathers left out.*** Some parents want feedings to be a shared responsibility. The parents should be informed that it is advisable for the father to wait to bottle feed the baby with expressed breast milk until after the milk supply and breastfeeding are established, generally when their baby is about 3 to 4 weeks old. In the meantime, encourage the father to be supportive of the breastfeeding mother, to have a lot of skin-to-skin contact with his infant, and to share the responsibilities of all other aspects of infant care (bathing, dressing, diapering, burping, rocking, etc.).
6. ***Diet restriction.*** Some mothers think that they have to give up eating certain foods when they breastfeed. This is generally not true. Most mothers can still eat all the foods they are accustomed to eating. Mothers do need to restrict alcohol intake and keep caffeine to a minimum. In the uncommon case where an infant has intolerance or allergy symptoms, as discussed earlier in the chapter, the mother should consult with a lactation consultant or the baby's healthcare provider to help her work through this complication.
7. ***Limited hormonal birth control options.*** Some mothers think that they cannot use a hormonal method of birth control while breastfeeding. Mothers should be informed that using birth control pills containing progesterone and estrogen can cause a decrease in milk volume and may affect the quality of their milk. It is preferred that the mother who wants to use a hormonal birth control method consider using the progestin-only minipill (i.e., Micronor, Nor-QD, Aygestin, or Norlutate); receive Depo-Provera, a progestin-only injection administered every 90 days; or have a progestin-only implant. Although progestin-only hormonal birth control is compatible with lactation, it should not be administered after delivery or at the time of hospital discharge. It is recommended that the mother wait 6 weeks before taking the hormonal medication to ensure a good milk supply (AAP & ACOG, 2007). Mothers can be reassured that barrier methods of birth control and natural family planning do not interfere with lactation at all and are good options to consider as well.
8. ***Vaginal dryness associated with breastfeeding.*** Some mothers experience vaginal dryness related to a low level of estrogen while lactating. Mothers can be given reassurance that this is only a temporary side effect while breastfeeding. A water-based lubricant such as K-Y jelly or Astroglide can be used during intercourse until she weans and estrogen levels increase again.
9. ***Medications and breastfeeding.*** Some mothers are concerned about the safety of breastfeeding while they are taking medications. Mothers can be reassured that most prescription and over-the-counter medications are safe for the breastfeeding infant.

   The mother should be advised to inform her healthcare provider and her infant's healthcare provider that she is breastfeeding when a drug is prescribed for her. In counseling the breastfeeding mother, the healthcare provider should weigh the benefits of the medication against the possible risk to the infant and its possible effects on the breastfeeding process. If the medication is not compatible with breastfeeding but is needed for only a short time, the mother can use a breast pump to maintain lactation and discard the milk. For additional information on medications and their compatibility with breastfeeding, see the list of resources on www.nursing.pearsonhighered.com.

Medications

It has long been recognized that medications taken by the breastfeeding mother may penetrate human milk to some degree. But having a better understanding of the kinetics of drug entry into human milk, as well as factors influencing its bioavailability to the nursing infant is important, because use of medication has been identified as a barrier to breastfeeding and a major reason women cite for discontinuing breastfeeding (Hale, 2010).

It should be noted that (1) most drugs penetrate into human milk, (2) almost all medications appear in only small amounts in human milk (usually less than 1% of the maternal dosage), and (3) very few drugs are contraindicated for breastfeeding women (AAP Committee on Drugs, 2001; Briggs, Freeman, & Yaffe, 2008; Hale, 2010).

Characteristics of a drug that influence its passage into human milk include the following:

- ***Degree of protein binding.*** Unbound drugs are more likely to enter the breast milk.
- ***Degree of ionization.*** Drugs tend to cross into breast milk in un-ionized form.
- ***Molecular weight.*** Drugs with lower molecular weight are more likely to cross into breast milk.
- ***Degree of solubility in fat and water.*** Lipid-soluble drugs pass into breast milk easily because of the high fat content in human milk.
- ***Mechanism of transport.*** Most drugs enter human milk by simple diffusion, but occasionally active transport or carrier-mediated diffusion may be involved.
- ***The pH.*** Human milk, which is acidic, attracts drugs that are weak bases.
- ***Half-life.*** Rates of absorption, metabolism, and excretion determine a drug's half-life, or how fast it leaves the body. The longer the half-life is, the greater the risk of accumulation in breast milk.

The net measurement of these effects determines the **milk/plasma ratio**, which relates the concentration of the drug in the milk to the concentration in the maternal plasma. For drugs that have equivalent dosing levels for the mother *and* equivalent safety profiles in the infant, it is preferable to use the drug with a lower milk/plasma ratio. Also, for any particular drug, it is preferable to use the lowest effective dose in the mother. Finally, the route and timing of the maternal dosing affects the maternal plasma level and therefore also the amount of drug reaching the baby.

Five adjustments should be made when administering drugs to a nursing mother to decrease the effects on the infant (Blackburn, 2007).

1. Avoid long-acting forms of drugs. The infant may have difficulty metabolizing and excreting them, and accumulation may be a problem.
2. Consider absorption rates and peak blood levels in scheduling the administration of the drugs. Less of the drug crosses into the milk if the infant is fed before the mother is given the oral medication.
3. Use preparations that can be given at longer intervals (once versus three to four times per day).
4. When alternatives are available, select the drug that shows the least tendency to pass into breast milk.
5. Use single-symptom drugs versus multisymptom drugs (e.g., a decongestant for allergy rather than a multisymptom drug, especially because liquid forms may contain alcohol).

Potential Contraindications

There are some instances when breastfeeding is or may be contraindicated:

- If mother is HIV positive or has AIDS, she is counseled against breastfeeding except in countries where the risk of neonatal death from diarrhea and other disease (excluding AIDS) is high (AWHONN, 2007).
- Mother has active, untreated tuberculosis, has varicella, or mother is HTLV1-positive (human T-cell leukemia virus type 1).
- Mother has active herpes on her breast—the infant may still feed on the unaffected side only until the lesion has healed.
- Mother has another illness, on a case-by-case basis.
- Mother uses illicit drugs (e.g., cocaine, heroin) or is an alcoholic.
- Maternal smoking poses health risks to the mother and potential second-hand exposure risks to her baby. Research shows that smoking by breastfeeding mothers can significantly alter infants' sleep-wake cycles, causing infants to sleep less and also affects milk flavor (Mennella, Yourshaw, & Morgan, 2007). Maternal smoking can result in breast milk concentrations of nicotine of 1.5 to 3 times the maternal plasma concentration. However, babies who receive breast milk from mothers who smoke are healthier than babies who receive formula and live in a household with smokers. Mothers who smoke cigarettes can breastfeed. To minimize effects on the baby, mothers should time their smoking to immediately *after* breastfeeding and should not smoke in the same room as the infant (American Academy of Family Physicians [AAFP], 2008).
- Specific medications (e.g., radioactive isotopes, antimetabolites, chemotherapy drugs, and a few others). A mother with a diagnosis of breast cancer should not breastfeed so that she can begin treatment immediately.
- Infant has galactosemia.

Potential Problems in Breastfeeding

Because mothers are discharged from the birthing unit before breastfeeding is well established, they are frequently alone when they encounter changes in the breastfeeding process. Many women stop nursing if the situations they encounter seem to pose problems. Nurses can offer anticipatory guidance regarding common breastfeeding phenomena and provide resources for the woman's use after discharge. (See chapter 37 for a detailed discussion of self-care measures the nurse can suggest to a woman with a breastfeeding problem after discharge from the birthing unit.)

COMPLEMENTARY AND ALTERNATIVE THERAPIES

It is estimated that more than a third of Americans use herbal medicine to promote health and treat disease. Nurses working with women of childbearing years should become familiar with common herbal preparations considered for use by lactating women. *Galactogogues* are commonly used to increase a mother's milk production when her supply is decreased, to assist in reestablishing a milk supply after weaning, and to assist in initiating lactation such as when an adoptive mother desires to nurse her infant. They include fenugreek, goat's rue, milk thistle, anise, basil, blessed thistle, fennel seeds, and marshmallow, to name a few (Academy of Breastfeeding Medicine [ABM], 2004). Some of these herbs are not recommended for a nursing mother if she is also pregnant.

Most mothers taking a galactogogue notice an increase in their milk supply within 1 to 3 days. Mothers should be counseled that taking a galactogogue alone will not solve her low milk supply problem. It must be stressed to her that she must also increase the frequency of breastfeeding (or pumping with a good quality breast pump) to have the best results. Ideally, the mother should be stimulating her breasts 8 to12 times a day, especially while lactation is getting reestablished. She also needs to balance the demands in her life and try to get rest when she can and lessen her stress. (Stress has a negative impact on a mother's milk supply.) She must also continue to drink to thirst and eat a healthy diet, which includes receiving a minimum of 1800 calories per day. These behaviors will also help to increase her milk supply.

Herbal galactogogues can be consumed as a tea, or can be taken as capsules or as a tincture added to liquid to drink. The dosage of herbs in tea is not as consistent as it is for herbals in capsules or tinctures due to variable quality of the herbal leaves, differences in steeping time, and the method of tea bag storage. (Tea bags should be stored in a closed container away from light and stored in an environment with low humidity to retain their potency.)

Fenugreek is probably the most well-known herbal galactogogue among lactation consultants in the United States. To avoid potential side effects such as diarrhea in the mother, it is advisable for the mother to build up to the suggested dosing over several days. It is not uncommon for mothers to note that their urine and sweat smells like maple syrup while taking fenugreek due to the plant's fragrant seeds. Mothers should be cautioned that if the *infant's* urine smells like maple syrup, this can be a sign of an inborn error of metabolism not related to the mother's diet, and should be evaluated by their baby's health-care provider. Mothers with diabetes, asthma, allergies to peanuts, soy, chickpeas, or garbanzo beans, or who are taking warfarin sodium (Coumadin) should consult with their healthcare provider before taking this herb (West & Marasco, 2009). Other herbs thought to increase milk supply include alfalfa, dandelion, fennel, horsetail, red raspberry, caraway, and anise. Women with lupus should read labels to avoid preparations that include alfalfa which can exacerbate their disease (West & Marasco, 2009). The following herbs may decrease milk supply, so they should be avoided until a woman is no longer breastfeeding: black walnut, sage, parsley, and yarrow.

There are also anti-galactogogues (e.g., sage, parsley, and peppermint) that may or may not be used in combination with applying cabbage leaves or ice to the breasts to decrease severe engorgement, to diminish an oversupply of milk, and to "dry up" when weaning an infant from the breast (West & Marasco, 2009). See chapter 37 ∞ for further discussion of breast engorgement.

CLINICAL TIP

To treat severe engorgement that typically occurs on day 3 and 4 postpartum, some mothers find relief applying raw chilled, green cabbage leaves topically to their breasts. The mother applies the rinsed and dried cabbage leaves after first "crunching" the "veins" in the leaves using her fist or a rolling pin. The prepared cabbage leaves are applied directly on the bare breasts (avoiding the nipple) and held in place with the mother's bra. The leaves are changed out every couple of hours when they have become wilted or when the mother awakens during the night. This remedy is discontinued as soon as the mother notices the breast swelling has decreased.

The type of herb, the dosage, and the method of administration are variable depending on the problem to resolve and personal preference. Some of these herbal products are commercially available. Women who are pregnant or nursing, or who have chronic health problems and take prescription medications, should be directed to consult with their healthcare provider before taking herbal medication. The healthcare provider will want to obtain a thorough lactation assessment so that the cause of the underlying problem can be determined, guidance and support can be offered for the management of the problem, and contraindications to any galactogogue can be considered.

CLINICAL TIP

Oil of Peppermint, an essential oil, can be added to a cold compress to be placed on the breast to provide some relief to a mother experiencing breast engorgement. Place 4 to 5 drops of peppermint oil in a basin of ice cold water. Dip a piece of clean fabric into the water so that the cloth picks up the essential oil on the surface. Wring out the fabric and place it on the breasts for about 15 to 20 minutes at a time. The breast should be washed completely before feeding. Some babies may find breathing strong fragrances emitted irritating to them. Mothers also need to avoid applying fragrances on or near their breasts because their babies might ingest them.

Timing of Newborn Feedings

The timing of newborn feedings is ideally determined by physiologic and behavioral cues rather than a set schedule. Early signs of hunger in a newborn can include any of the following behaviors: waking up, squirming, bringing hands to mouth, smacking of lips, extending the tongue repeatedly, and rooting. It is ideal to feed the baby before he or she begins to cry. When these symptoms are ignored, the infant will begin to cry (a late feeding cue). Sometimes the crying escalates and the infant becomes frantic. If his or her need for feeding is still not met, then he or she will become exhausted from crying and then fall back to sleep. Breastfed babies should feed 8 to 12 times in a 24-hour period whenever they exhibit hunger cues regardless of when they last fed. Newborns that cry can become disorganized and have difficulty latching onto the breast. The parents should be taught in this case how to calm the baby down before offering the breast. One strategy is to have either parent hold the baby vertically on his or her chest and let the baby suck on a clean finger for a minute or so. Another is to have either parent rock the baby in his or her arms or have a parent hold the infant upright on his or her chest and pat the baby's back. The baby may burp while being rocked and patted, expelling any air he or she swallowed while crying. Once the baby is calm, he or she will be ready to attempt latching on again.

Initial Feeding

If there are no complications at the birth and the mother is not overly sedated, after being dried the infant should be placed on the mother's chest. This skin-to-skin contact after birth helps the baby maintain his or her body temperature, helps with self regulation, increases maternal oxytocin levels, helps the mother to notice subtle feeding cues, and promotes bonding (Figure 32-3 ■).

Throughout the first 2 hours after birth, but especially during the first hour of life, most infants are usually alert and ready to breastfeed. This first feeding should not be forced. Some babies are content just licking the nipple or nuzzling up against the breast initially. Early breastfeeding can enhance maternal-infant bonding and facilitate release of oxytocin, which helps contract the uterus, expelling the placenta and decreasing the

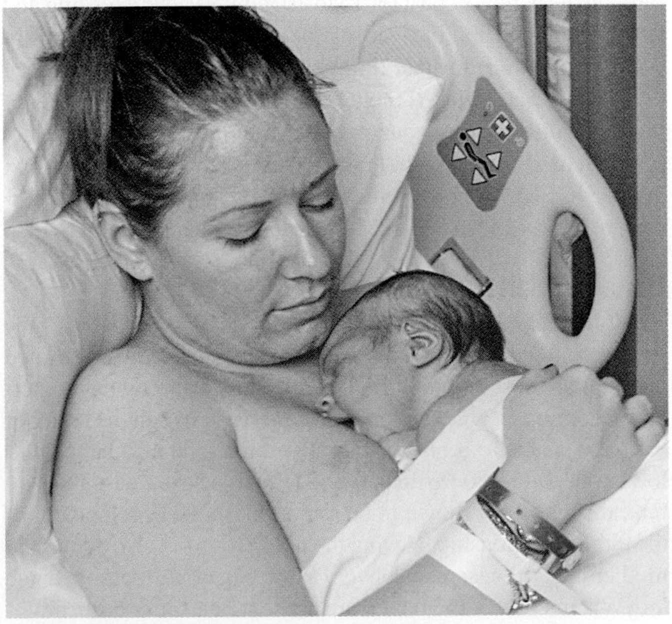

Figure 32-3 ■ Mother and infant skin-to-skin.

Source: Courtesy of Brigitte Hall, RNC, MSN, IBCLC/Pearson Education.

risk of postpartum hemorrhage. Early feedings benefit the newborn because they help prevent hypoglycemia, promote the passage of meconium, provide the newborn with immunologic protection from colostrum, and begin to stimulate further maternal milk production, helping prevent later feeding difficulties.

If the mother plans to bottle-feed, she and her newborn can still enjoy and benefit from skin-to-skin contact initially after birth as well. Formula-feedings are not typically initiated in the birthing room. Formula-feeding newborns are offered formula as soon as they show interest/feeding cues or per agency policy. For both breastfed and formula-fed infants, early feeding stimulates peristalsis which helps the newborn to eliminate the by-products of bilirubin conjugation that have been stored up in the bowel while in utero. Early passage of the meconium stool decreases the newborn's risk of jaundice.

Assessment of the newborn's physiologic status is a primary and ongoing concern to the nurse throughout the first feeding. Extreme fatigue coupled with tachypnea, dusky in color, and diaphoretic while feeding is most likely symptomatic for respiratory and/or cardiac problems or rarely esophageal anomalies (see chapter 33). Findings associated with esophageal anomalies include maternal polyhydramnios and increased oral secretions in the infant. In cases of esophageal atresia, the feeding is taken well initially, but as the esophageal pouch fills, the infant quickly gags and regurgitates. If a fistula is present, the infant gags, chokes, regurgitates mucus, and may become cyanotic as fluid passes through the fistula into the lungs. Although the nurse is always on the alert for any complications, keep in mind that it is not unusual for healthy newborns to regurgitate a small amount of mucus, fluid, or milk shortly after feeding, or to develop hiccups. Most babies have "wet burps" at some point and so virtually all have some degree of reflux. The LES sphincter tone increases to adult pressures for most infants when the infant is 3 to 6 weeks old, though 70% of all 4-month old infants still spit up at least once a day (Vartabedian, 2007). Holding the baby upright on the parent's chest for 15 to 20 minutes after a feeding and not placing the baby in a car seat or swing (which increases abdominal pressure) for that time can help decrease the incidence of reflux. When reflux is ongoing and causes consistent feeding problems due to inflammation of the esophagus, then the reflux problem has become pathologic (called gastroesophageal reflux disease [GERD]). This problem is not evident in the early postpartum period and is managed by the baby's healthcare provider.

Establishing a Feeding Pattern

An "on-demand" feeding program facilitates each baby's own rhythm and helps a new mother establish lactation. Unrestricted feedings are best accomplished by hospitals that provide mother-baby rooming-in practices on a 24-hour basis. When the father of the baby is able to room-in with the mother and new baby, it allows both parents to participate and learn how to care for their infant; this has been shown to be important in the development of the family relationship. Having the father room-in also allows the mother with the cesarean delivery to keep her baby at the bedside too. When mothers and babies are not separated after birth, mothers and fathers are better able to respond to their baby's needs more quickly than the nursery staff may be able to, resulting in less infant crying, natural feeding intervals, and an adequate number of feedings in a 24-hour period.

Case Study: Patient Undecided on Formula Feeding or Breastfeeding

Following the initial alert period (approximately the first 2 hours after birth), the newborn typically falls into a deep sleep for several hours. Mothers should be encouraged to rest during this time too. When the newborn awakens, he or she will likely want to nurse frequently, alternating between relatively short periods of light sleep and quiet wakefulness. As wakefulness and interest in nursing increase, the infant will often cluster 5 to 10 feeding episodes over 2 to 3 hours (Riordan & Wambach, 2010). Mothers may misinterpret "cluster feedings" in the first few days of life to mean that her infant is not satisfied because the mother ought to be producing more milk. The nurse should take this opportunity to reinforce the mother's perception that the infant wants additional milk, but point out that cluster feeding is a normal and necessary pattern to stimulate mother's milk production. Formula supplementation is not indicated and will actually delay milk production.

Some healthy infants are uninterested in nursing and just want to sleep for the first few days after birth. This pattern is noted in babies whose mothers have had a difficult labor, or a prolonged pushing stage during delivery, or have had medication (especially multiple dosing) for labor pain or for a cesarean birth. Late-preterm infants (infants born between 35 weeks but less than 38 weeks gestation) also tend to be very sleepy for the first few days, much more so than full-term infants. In addition, male infants who have undergone a circumcision procedure oftentimes become very sleepy after surgery. These sleepy babies are at risk of losing an excessive amount of weight, becoming dehydrated, and developing exaggerated jaundice in just a few days after birth. In addition, mothers may develop pathologic engorgement if her baby does not wake up to breastfeed frequently and effectively during this time.

To avoid these complications, parents can be taught techniques to wake their sleepy baby whenever the infant shows signs of being in the light state of sleep cycle (see chapter 29). With a little help, this baby may be gently aroused to breastfeed. One method is to remove the baby's blanket and clothing so that the infant is wearing only a diaper and T-shirt. Babies feed better when they are not bundled, and they can actually achieve a better attachment without the bulk of extra clothing and blankets in the way. If the room is too cool for the newborn to feed in just a diaper and T-shirt, have the mother apply a blanket over the top of her baby *after* the baby has attached to the breast. Another technique is to undo and check the baby's diaper. Sitting the baby in a burping position and gently "walking" fingers along the back will usually arouse the baby. Parents should also be encouraged to talk or sing to their baby while trying these techniques to further arouse their baby from sleep.

If the newborn falls asleep after the first few suckles, encourage the mother to use tactile stimulation while the newborn is still attached to the breast. The mother can also be encouraged to use breast compression or breast massage while the infant is breastfeeding to keep milk trickling into the infant's mouth until the infant stimulates the mother to release her milk. If this is not sufficient to keep the baby actively feeding, suggest that the mother remove the baby from the breast momentarily and try to burp the infant. The infant may not actually burp but the burping technique may help wake the infant.

An infant's feeding pattern may change again when the mother's breasts become fuller. Mothers' breasts begin to look and feel noticeably heavier between the second and fourth day postpartum. When milk production has noticeably increased, the "cluster feeding" pattern ceases until the infant has his first growth spurt at about 2 weeks of age. Now an infant generally feeds every 1 1/2 to 3 hours around the clock, about 8 to 12 feedings per day. Feeding intervals are counted from the time of the start of one feeding to the start of the next feeding. During this engorgement phase of lactation some infants may struggle initially with latch-on, especially if the mother allows greater than 3 hours to lapse between feedings. If the newborn is not breastfeeding often or effectively enough to soften the breasts, then the breasts may become quite firm and the mother's nipple may become less pliable and this can lead to a shallow latch attachment and sore nipples. If this occurs, the mother can try to express some milk to soften her areola before latching her infant. When her baby breastfeeds on this fuller than usual breast, it is not uncommon for the infant to only want to feed on just the one side. This feeding pattern usually does not last long either. Within days the infant will be back to breast feeding at both breasts again.

Breastfeeding and formula-feeding infants have the same fluid requirements and receive the same amount of calories per ounce, and both feed around the clock in the beginning, but because they have different diets, their rates of digestion are different. Digestion of formula produces harder to digest casein curds that take about 3 to 4 hours to digest compared with the softer, smaller curds produced from breast milk that are digested in only 90 minutes. For this reason formula-fed newborns generally sleep longer at a stretch and awaken to feed every 3 to 4 hours, typically feeding only 6 to 8 feedings per day. To compensate for sleeping longer between feedings, formula-fed infants feed a larger volume at each feeding. It will be awhile before the baby sleeps through the night.

Regardless of whether a mother is breastfeeding or formula-feeding her infant, many parents are distressed by their infant's erratic feeding pattern. Parents need to be informed about normal infant feeding and sleeping patterns and be aware that these patterns vary among babies and change over days, weeks, and months according to the infant's growth and development. In the beginning, the "average" newborn sleeps a total of 16 hours a day. Infants wake to feed and generally fall back to sleep within an hour. By a month of age, infants are able to sleep one long stretch of sleep, maybe 4 to 5 hours at nighttime, so long as they are not given the opportunity to sleep the long stretch of sleep during the day (Jana & Shu, 2005).

Satiety behaviors are the same for formula-fed babies as for breastfed babies. These behaviors include longer pauses toward the end of the feeding, noticeable total body relaxation (the baby lies limp with hands down at his or her side and unclenched), the infant may release his mother's nipple or the bottle nipple, and many fall asleep. If a baby is satiated and content following feedings, is meeting daily output expectations, and is gaining weight as expected, then feedings are going well. On the other hand, if a breastfeeding baby awakens shortly after feeding and is exhibiting feeding cues, this baby should be offered the breast again regardless as to when he or she was last fed. The newborn may be cluster feeding or may not have fed efficiently at the previous feeding. Also, pacifier use in response to this early waking is especially inappropriate. The pacifier needlessly postpones the feeding, which is indicated based on hunger cues and can have a negative consequence for the mother's milk supply and the infant's weight. The American Academy of Pediatrics recommends waiting to introduce a pacifier in the breastfeeding newborn until breastfeeding is well established, generally when the infant is 3 to 4 weeks old. A formula-feeding infant can be offered a pacifier any time after birth and is thought to help reduce the risk for sudden infant death (AAP, 2010).

CLINICAL TIP

Parents should be instructed never to put honey or corn syrup on their infant's pacifier to encourage an infant to accept it. Honey and possibly corn syrup may be contaminated with *Clostridium botulinum*, a bacterium that causes infantile botulism. Botulism is rare, but when it occurs it causes serious illness.

Both breastfed and formula-fed infants experience growth spurts at certain times and require increased feeding volume. The breastfeeding mother may meet these increased demands by nursing more frequently to increase her milk supply. It takes up to 72 hours for the milk supply to increase adequately to meet the new demand. A slight increase in volume also meets the formula-fed infant's needs. Once the formula feeding infant appears satiated, the infant should not be forced to continue to feed in order to finish the bottle.

Some mothers may find fixed feeding schedules attractive. These mothers should be informed that feeding schedules may work for some formula-fed babies, if they allow some flexibility and increase volume as indicated; however, fixed feeding schedules do not work for breastfeeding babies and can be quite harmful. For breastfeeding babies, fixed feeding schedules do not take into account differences among breastfeeding women (breast storage capacity, as one example) and differences among infants (slow feeders, as an example). A fixed feeding schedule does not incorporate extra breast stimulation, the "cluster feedings" that are needed in order for the breastfeeding mother's milk production to accommodate growth spurts in her continuously growing infant. There are documented cases of infants diagnosed with failure to thrive, poor weight gain, dehydration, breast milk supply failure, and involuntary early weaning associated with fixed feeding schedules for the breastfeeding baby. Nourishing their newborn is a major concern of new parents. Their feelings of success or failure may influence their self-concept as they assume the role of parents. Breastfeeding mothers in particular, as primary caregivers, are especially sensitive about their ability to provide for their infants. With proper instruction, support, and encouragement from professionals, feeding becomes a source of pleasure and satisfaction to both the parents and infant.

Cultural Considerations in Infant Feeding

As healthcare professionals, we can learn about an individual patient's cultural background by engaging in discussions with them and asking questions in a sensitive and respectful way. This provides opportunity to validate healthy practices and to exert a positive influence on other matters (Callister, 2008). An occasion for this kind of dialogue might arise during interactions with a new mother who may have misconceptions about breastfeeding. For example, if a new mother says that she heard that getting upset or angry will spoil her milk, you can point out that this belief likely stems from the correct observation that the breastfeeding infant can sense maternal tension (which also may delay let-down) and may therefore act fussy as well, appearing to behave as if he or she were getting "spoiled milk." Then reassure the mother that there is no evidence that the milk composition itself is changed. This will allow you to focus on the real issues of bonding and relaxation technique. You may also note that simply understanding what is really going on may help the mother to be more relaxed.

Breastfeeding in public is another frequently expressed concern that can create a barrier to achieving *Healthy People 2010* breastfeeding goals. Although people agree that breastfeeding is the most natural and healthy way to feed a baby, mothers feel conflicted because in America breast exposure is often viewed in a sexual context and this may lead to disapproval of attempts to breastfeed in public. As national and state efforts are being made to promote breastfeeding duration to improve the health of mothers and babies, this barrier is slowly being broken down. Public places are incorporating "mother rooms" to provide a comfortable, private area for the nursing mother. There is no state that prohibits breastfeeding in a public place, and there are now 43 states and the District of Columbia and the Virgin Islands that have created laws that specify that a woman is permitted to breastfeed in any location in which she is authorized to be (National Conference of State Legislatures, 2009). Mothers may also be taught how to breastfeed discreetly in public. This is often taught at breastfeeding classes or mother-to-mother support group meetings. See Figure 32-4 ■ to observe a mother discreetly breastfeeding. Some mothers may prefer a baby blanket or shawl to drape over their chests, which will provide more coverage. Finally, mothers who prefer not to breastfeed even discreetly in public can be encouraged to at least pump their breasts and feed the expressed milk in a bottle so they have the option of getting out of the house.

In women of African descent, higher rates of initiation of breastfeeding were associated with increased age, education, and income (McCarter-Spaulding & Gore, 2009). Social support for breastfeeding primarily came from other women, especially maternal grandmothers, but the social support was very limited and early formula and cereal supplementation is common. In many ethnic groups, self efficacy has been shown to predict breastfeeding duration and pattern (exclusive breastfeeding or breastfeeding in combination with formula feeding (McCarter-Spaulding & Gore, 2009).

Another cultural implication related to breastfeeding concerns colostrum. Among some traditional cultures around the world, it is believed that colostrum is "unclean" or even harmful to a newborn. This belief is found among some groups of Hispanics, Navajo Indians, Filipinos, and Vietnamese (D'Avanzo & Geissler, 2008). Because of this ancient belief, mothers living in regions of Central America, sub-Saharan Africa, the Middle East, and parts of Asia even today discard their colostrum or wait until 2 to 4 days to begin breastfeeding when their "true milk" arrives. While waiting for their milk to come in, mothers feed their infant a culturally specific colostrum substitute. These prelacteal feeds include cereal or gruel, animal milk, sugar water, and a variety of herbal teas (Department for International Development, 2009; Geckil, Sahin & Ege, 2009). Not only are these newborns receiving an inferior quality food that is not appropriate for their development and possibly prepared with contaminated water, they are denied vital immunity-building substances, and they

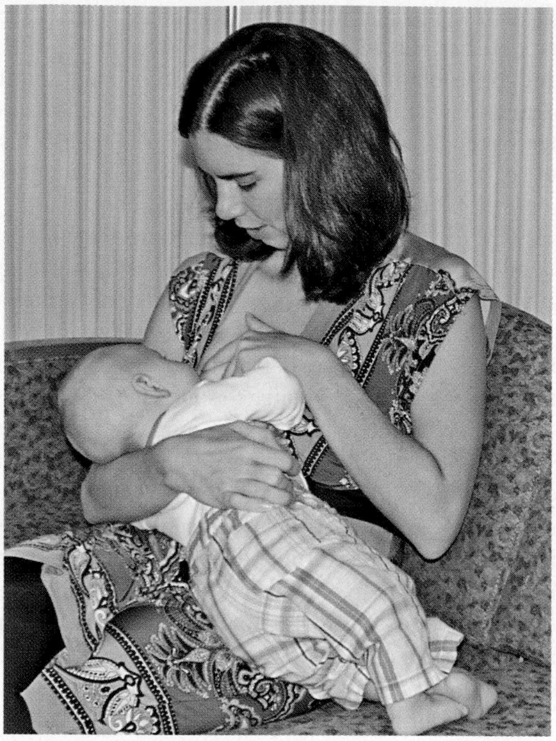

Figure 32-4 ■ Breastfeeding discreetly.

Source: Courtesy of Brigitte Hall, RNC, MSN, IBCLC/Pearson Education.

PROFESSIONALISM IN PRACTICE

Breastfeeding Promotion Legislation

It is important to be a patient advocate and be involved in legislative initiatives on the national and local level. A recently proposed piece of legislation is The Breastfeeding Promotion Act of 2009, H.R. Bill 2819/Senate Bill 1244. If enacted into law, it will protect breastfeeding in the workplace by providing five provisions. These include:

Title I: Amending the Civil Rights Act of 1964 to protect lactating women from being fired or discriminated against in the workplace.

Title II: Giving tax incentives to businesses that establish a private space in the workplace for their employees to breastfeed or express their milk. Employers can also receive tax credits for supplying breastfeeding equipment and providing lactation consultation services for their employees.

Title III: Establishing set standards for breast pumps to ensure that they are safe and effective.

Title IV: Expanding the Internal Revenue Code definition of "medical care" to include breastfeeding equipment and lactation services as tax-deductible for families.

Title V: Requiring employers with 50 or more employees to provide lactating employees break time and a private area to express their milk.

DEVELOPING CULTURAL COMPETENCE
Breastfeeding in Other Cultures

Among traditional societies around the world, weaning from the breast occurs when a child is between 2 and 4 years of age.

In Sweden both parents are entitled to share post-birth parental leave of up to 13 months paid time off. Their national social insurance system pays them 80% of their lost wages. They are also allowed an additional 90 days off without pay (International Labour Organization, 2004).

Many women in Mexico assume that not eating well and not drinking enough fluids result in low milk supply (Sacco, Caulfield, Gittelsohn, et al., 2006).

Chinese women go through a 30-day period of home confinement following delivery, during which she is also not permitted to bathe or wash her hair. This is a century's old tradition to nurture the mother back to her prenatal state and intended to keep her body warm to ward off *fong* (flatulence) and other future health ailments. A *Pui Yuet* (companion) is hired to provide total care for the mother and infant. The Pui Yuet will cook traditional confinement foods daily (provide "heating foods" and avoid "cooling foods"). Most foods must be cooked in sesame oil and old ginger. The mother drinks hot herbal tea with her meals and is not permitted to drink any water because water is thought to cause water retention (Teh, undated).

Muslim women generally breastfeed their children until their children are 2 years of age. This is encouraged in the Koran. Although Muslim women do not breastfeed in public, they will breastfeed in front of family members and relatives as long as the breast is not exposed (Ott, Al-Khadhuri, & Al-Junaibi, 2003).

Haitian mothers may believe that "strong emotions" spoil breast milk; and that thick breast milk causes skin rashes and thin milk results in diarrhea (Callister, 2008; Lipson & Dibble, 2008).

In Malaysia, the ingestion of breast milk represents a great deal more than simple nutrition for newborn infants. It is believed that the mother's milk enters the baby's blood. This is thought to cultivate a long life. Breast milk is thought to bind the mother and baby together, creating a sense of respect and closeness. While milk develops the infant's spirit and body, it also develops faith and character. It is thought that the consumption of breast milk formulates a maternal-infant bond that lasts throughout life. This bond cannot be broken by any means.

miss out on the laxative effect that colostrum provides to rid the body of bilirubin, which reduces the risk of jaundice. Nurses should be aware that some immigrant mothers may have this misconception about their colostrum. In a situation like this, in which a cultural custom is harmful or denies the infant benefit, it is the nurse's responsibility to try to educate the family about the value of colostrum.

Language is a fundamental aspect of a person's culture and can be a source of miscommunication in a healthcare system geared toward serving people who speak English. The most obvious language barrier is when a person does not speak English at all. Whenever possible, it is best to have a female, non-family member translator present to interpret for a mother. For Muslim women, it is culturally unacceptable for them to speak about intimate matters in front of their families. Therefore, it would be inappropriate to ask the new mother's husband or her children to be her interpreter. Even among those who speak English, language barriers and miscommunications still exist due in part to words having different meanings to people of different cultures. It is important to make sure that you give enough explanation to ensure that the mother clearly understands the information provided. These are but a few of the numerous cultural influences related to feeding. (See Developing Cultural Competence: Breastfeeding in Other Cultures.) When nurses are faced with an infant care practice different from the ones to which they are accustomed, nurses need to evaluate the effect of the practice. Different practices are not necessarily inferior. The nurse should intervene only if the practice is actually harmful to the mother or baby.

HEALTH PROMOTION EDUCATION: BREASTFEEDING TECHNIQUE

Breastfeeding Position and Latching On

Breastfeeding is not instinctive, it is learned. It is a natural process, but it takes "know-how." Ideally, each breastfeeding mother should have a breastfeeding evaluation to determine any knowledge deficits, acknowledge any concerns, provide instructions, and assist with breastfeeding.

Application: Breastfeeding

POSITIONING There are multiple breastfeeding positions, but only the four classic breastfeeding positions are discussed here. In addition, there are minor variations of hand placement and body position even among the four classic positions. The four positions discussed here include (1) modified cradle position, (2) cradle position, (3) football (or clutch) hold position, and (4) side-lying position (Figures 32-5 ■ through 32-8 ■). After a mother has fed using one position, encourage her to try a different position when she offers her second breast. Alternating positions facilitates drainage of the breasts and changes the pressure points on the breast. This will provide some relief to the mother with sore nipples.

CLINICAL TIP

When supporting the infant's head in preparation to breastfeed, regardless of the feeding position, it is best not to allow any fingers to be placed on the back of the baby's head. If fingers are placed on the back of the baby's head, it may inadvertently be tilted forward. Whenever the baby's chin is tucked in (chin toward chest), the angle for attachment will not be lined up correctly. This causes the infant to attach with the upper jaw first (rather than the lower jaw first, as preferred), and this will result in a shallow latch attachment and subsequent nipple trauma. Instead, encourage the mother to support her infant's head with her hand at the base of her infant's neck or upper back. This allows for the infant's head to extend slightly back so the infant leads chin first during attachment. If the infant is lined up "nose to nipple" to start with, then the infant will attach to the breast with the lower jaw first. This technique will allow for a deeper latch attachment and a pleasant breastfeeding experience.

Modified cradle position

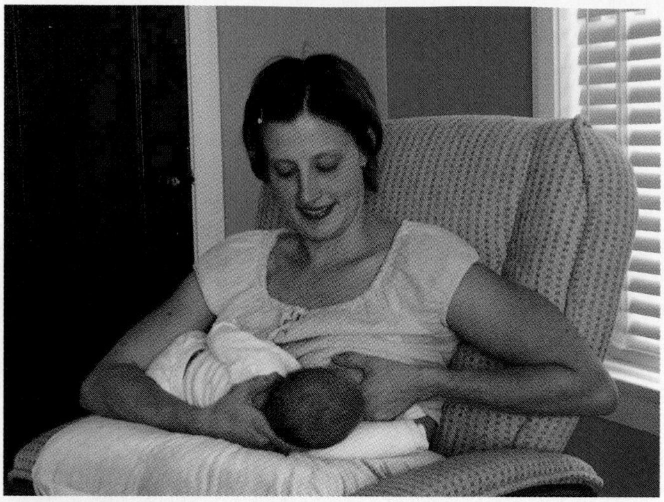

- Have mother sit comfortably in upright position using good body alignment. Use pillows for support (may use Boppy, body pillow, or standard bed pillows). Lap pillow should help bring baby up to breast level so mother does not lean over baby.
- Place baby on mother's lap and turn baby's entire body toward mother (baby is in side-lying position). Position baby's body so that the baby's nose lines up to the nipple. Maintain baby's body in a horizontal alignment.
- To feed at left breast, mother supports baby's head with her right hand at nape of baby's neck (allow head to slightly lag back), mother's right thumb by baby's left ear, and right forefinger near baby's right ear.
- With mother's free left hand, she can offer her left breast.

Figure 32-5 ■ Modified cradle position.

Source: Courtesy of Brigitte Hall, RNC, MSN, IBCLC.

Cradle position

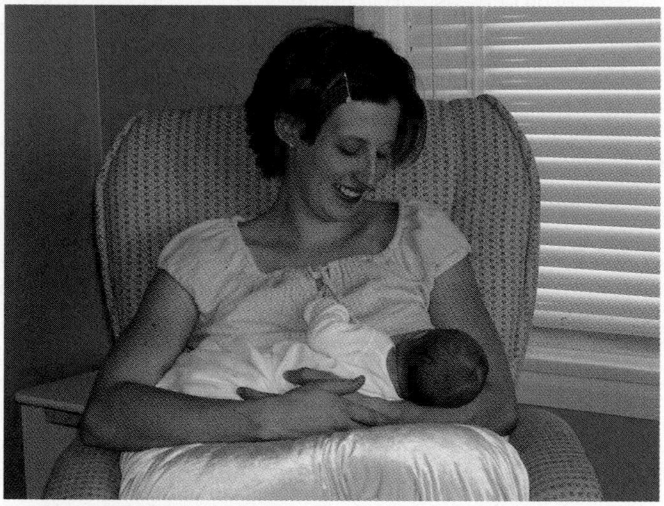

- Have mother sit comfortably in upright position using good body alignment. Use pillows for support (may use Boppy, body pillow, or standard bed pillows). Lap pillow should help bring baby up to breast level so mother does not lean over baby.
- Place baby on mother's lap and turn baby's entire body toward mother (baby is in side-lying position). Position baby's body so that the baby's nose lines up to the nipple. Maintain baby's body in a horizontal alignment.
- If feeding from the left breast, have mother cradle baby's head near the crook of her left arm while supporting her baby's body with her left forearm.
- With mother's free right hand, she can offer her left breast.

Figure 32-6 ■ Cradle position.

Source: Courtesy of Brigitte Hall, RNC, MSN, IBCLC.

Football hold position

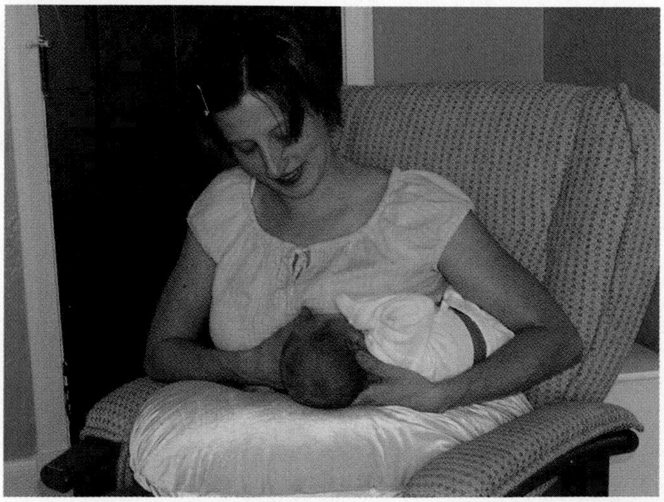

- Have mother sit comfortably and use pillows to raise baby's body to breast level. If using a Boppy and the Boppy is in "normal" position on mother's lap, turn it counterclockwise slightly (if feeding at left breast) to provide extended support for baby's body resting along mother's left side and near the back of mother's chair.
- If feeding at left breast, place baby on the left side of mother's body, heading baby into position feet first. Baby's bottom should rest on the pillow near mother's left elbow.
- Turn baby slightly on her side so that she faces the breast.
- Mother's left arm clutches baby's body close to mother's body. Baby's body should feel securely tucked in under mother's left arm.
- Have mother support baby's head with her left hand. With mother's free right hand, she can offer her breast. (Good position for mother with c-section).

Figure 32-7 ■ Football hold position.

Source: Courtesy of Brigitte Hall, RNC, MSN, IBCLC.

Side-lying position

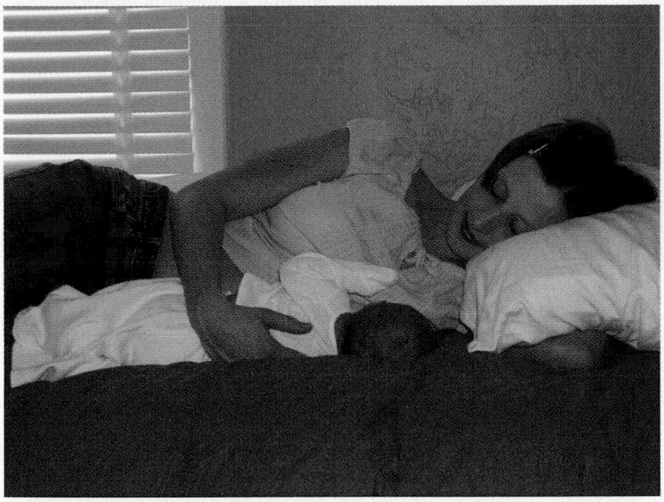

- Have mother rest comfortably lying on her side (left side for this demonstration). Use pillows to support mother's head and back, and provide support for mother's hips by placing a pillow between her bent knees.
- Place baby in side-lying position next to mother's body. Baby's body should face mother's body. Baby's nose should line up to mother's nipple. Place a roll behind baby's back, if desired.
- With mother's free right hand, she can offer her left breast. After baby is securely attached, mom can rest her right hand anywhere that is comfortable for her.

Figure 32-8 ■ Side-lying position.

Source: Courtesy of Brigitte Hall, RNC, MSN, IBCLC.

LATCHING ON It is important to have the mother and baby positioned properly in order to achieve an optimal attachment. If, for example, the infant is lying flat on his or her back (supine position) to feed in the modified cradle position, cradle position, or side-lying position, the infant can obtain only a shallow latch (not attached far back onto the areola). The infant's shoulder becomes an obstacle putting distance between the infant's mouth and the mother's breast. Anything that contributes to a shallow latch is going to cause sore nipples and other complications. Nipple trauma, although relatively common, is not normal. See chapter 37 ∞ for a discussion of breastfeeding with inverted or flat nipples.

The infant needs to attach his or her lips onto the breast, or more accurately, far back onto the areola, not on the actual nipple. If the infant attaches just to the nipple, the mother will have sore nipples, and pain may inhibit the let-down reflex. To obtain a deep latch, the mother needs to be taught how to elicit the infant's rooting reflex, stimulating the infant to open his or her mouth as widely as possible (like a big yawn). Once the infant does this, the mother should quickly but gently draw her baby in toward her. During the first few days of life, the newborn typically only opens his or her mouth widely for a second or so, and then begins to close the mouth again. If the mother misses her chance to get her baby latched on, she simply needs to start over again.

Figures 32-9 ■ through 32-14 ■ demonstrate various positions and techniques used in latching on.

C-hold hand position

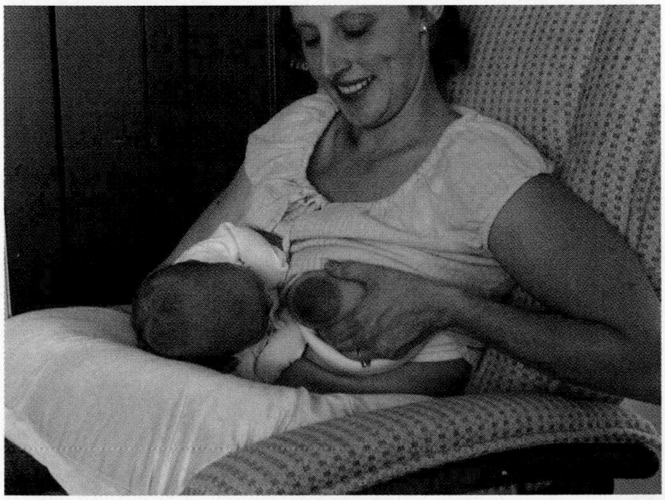

To be ready to draw baby's mouth onto mother's breast, as soon as the baby opens her or his mouth widely enough, the mother needs to have her hand supporting her breast in ready position. She can use various hand holds, but she needs to keep her fingers well behind the areola. One such hand position is called the "C-hold." In this hold, the thumb is placed on top of the breast near 12 o'clock position and the other four fingers are placed on the underside of the breast near the 6 o'clock position (depends on mother's hand size and length of fingers). The key point is in keeping the fingers at least 1 1/2 inches back from the base of the nipple as the fingers support the breast. Mothers are not often aware of where they place their fingers, especially on the underside of the breast. If the fingers are too far forward (too close to the nipple), then the infant cannot grasp a large amount of areola in her or his mouth and this results in a "shallow" latch. A shallow latch is associated with nipple pain and ineffective drainage of the breast.

An alternate hand hold not shown is a "U-hold" hand position. The thumb and forefinger are near the 3 o'clock and 9 o'clock positions on the breast again with fingers at least 1 1/2 inches back from the base of the nipple; the body of the hand rests on the lower portion of the breast. Using this hand hold, the mother's arm position is down at her side rather than sticking outward as it is when supporting the breast using the C-hold position.

Figure 32-9 ■ C-hold hand position.

Source: Courtesy of Brigitte Hall, RNC, MSN, IBCLC.

Scissor hold hand position

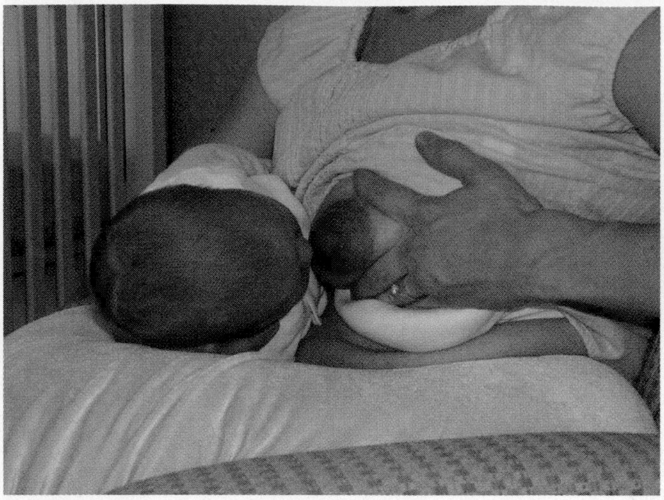

The scissor hold is often discouraged because mothers (especially mothers with small hands) have a difficult time keeping their fingers off the areola or at least $1^1/_2$ inches back from the base of the areola. Here, the mother is able to support her breast well without letting her fingers encroach onto the areola.

The mother should be instructed to gently support the breast and not press too deeply, which can obstruct the flow of milk through the ducts.

Figure 32-10 ■ Scissor hold hand position.

Source: Courtesy of Brigitte Hall, RNC, MSN, IBCLC.

Nose to nipple

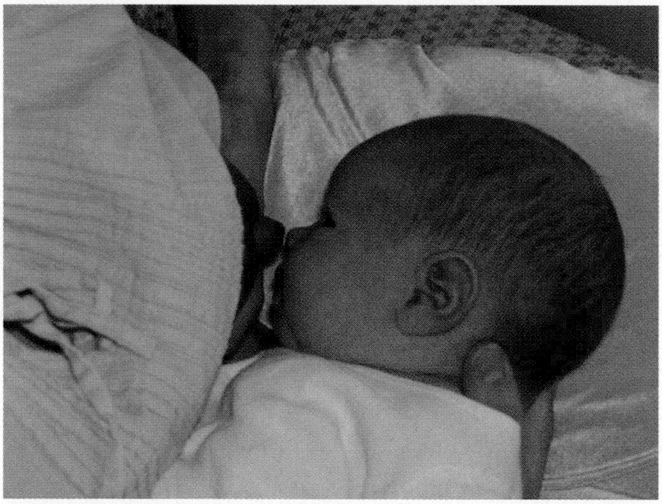

Before eliciting the rooting reflex, it is important to have the baby in good alignment. When the infant opens her or his mouth to latch on, the goal is to achieve a deep, asymmetric latch attachment. The goal is *not* to center the nipple in the baby's mouth. The rationale for this is to optimize oral-motor function. The jaw is a hinge joint. The upper jaw is immobile; the lower jaw compresses the breast. The breast is efficiently drained if more areola is drawn into the baby's mouth from the inferior aspect of the breast and a smaller amount drawn in from the superior aspect of the areola. Aligning the infant to the mother with baby's nose facing mother's nipple permits the jaw to be in a lower position. The next step is to let the infant drop his or her head back (head in "sniff position"), so that the infant leads into the breast with the chin.

Figure 32-11 ■ Nose to nipple.

Source: Courtesy of Brigitte Hall, RNC, MSN, IBCLC.

Initial attempt to elicit the rooting reflex

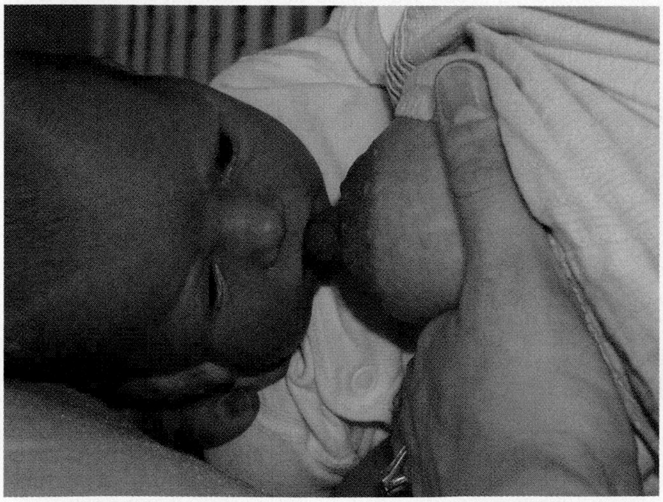

To trigger the rooting reflex, teach the mother to use her nipple to stroke downward in a vertical motion across the middle of baby's lower lip. Initially, the infant may respond by licking or smacking. This is a normal response to the stimulus. Encourage the mother to keep stimulating the infant's lower lip until the infant finally opens her or his mouth widely. If the infant is not responding at all, then the infant is probably too sleepy and may need help waking up. After trying wake up techniques, the infant may be ready to try breastfeeding again.

Figure 32-12 ■ Initial attempt to elicit the rooting reflex.

Source: Courtesy of Brigitte Hall, RNC, MSN, IBCLC.

Continued attempt to elicit rooting reflex

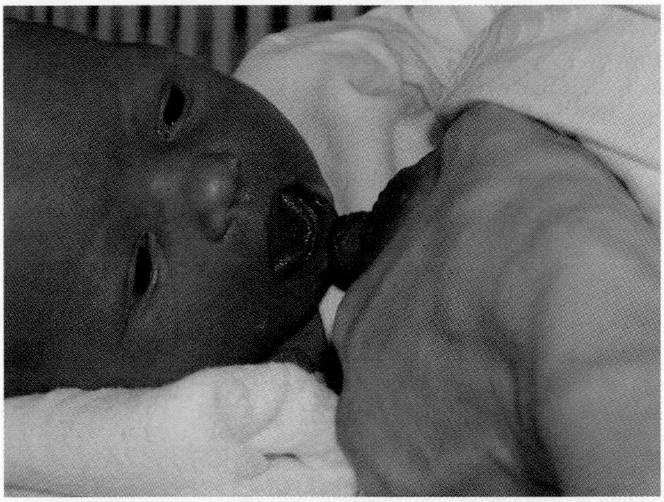

Teach the mother to be patient and wait for the infant's mouth to gape open as widely as possible. Here the infant needs to open the mouth even wider before the mother draws her baby toward the breast. The mother should be encouraged to continue stroking the infant's lip until the infant opens the mouth wider.

Figure 32-13 ■ Continued attempt to elicit the rooting reflex.

Source: Courtesy of Brigitte Hall, RNC, MSN, IBCLC.

Baby is latched-on

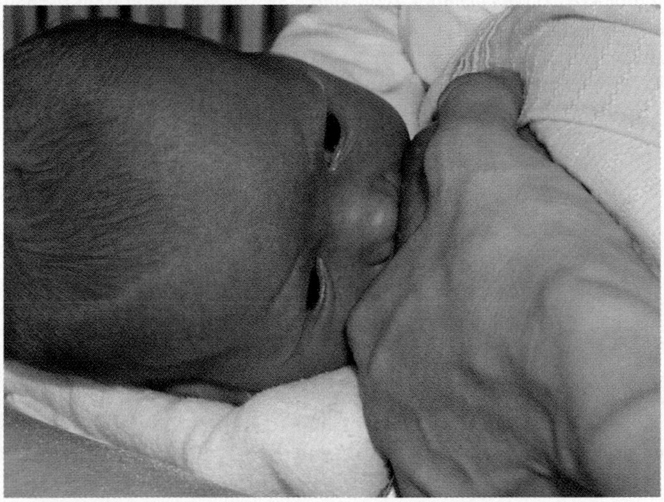

Once baby has latched onto the breast, the mother should check that baby is latched on properly. The infant's chin should be embedded into the mother's breast. The infant's nose should be very close but not actually touching the breast. The nose should be centered. If the mother feels a little pinch on her areola, she can slowly release the hand supporting her breast so she can have a free hand to attempt to move her baby's jaw gently downward. To do this maneuver, the mother needs to place her thumb or forefinger of her free hand (the hand that just released the breast) on baby's lower jaw (there is a horizontal groove to use as leverage—the groove on baby's chin is parallel with the baby's lips). With gentle downward pressure the mother should feel relief of any persistent tenderness. This procedure opens the jaw wider and it also helps to roll out the infant's lower lip that may have been inadvertently drawn into the baby's mouth. As the baby begins to suckle, there should be no dimpling of the infant's cheeks and no smacking or clicking noises.

Figure 32-14 ■ Baby is latched on.

Source: Courtesy of Brigitte Hall, RNC, MSN, IBCLC.

CLINICAL TIP

As you assist new mothers with breastfeeding, it is important to create a relaxed environment and approach to breastfeeding. Encourage the mother to get into a comfortable position, well supported with pillows. Remind her to bring the baby to her breast rather than leaning forward to the baby.

Breastfeeding Assessment

During the birthing unit stay, the nurse must carefully monitor the progress of the breastfeeding pair. A systematic assessment of several breastfeeding episodes provides the opportunity to teach the new mother about lactation and the breastfeeding process, provide anticipatory guidance, and evaluate the need for follow-up care after discharge. Criteria for evaluating a breastfeeding session include maternal response to infant cues, latch-on technique, positioning, signs of active feeding, let-down response, nipple condition, maternal comfort during feeding, infant's weight from previous measurement (usually from the night before), infant's report of intake and output. The literature provides various tools to guide the assessment and documentation of the breastfeeding efforts. The LATCH Scoring Table is one example (Figure 32-15 ■). Table 32-4 identifies signs of successful breastfeeding.

Breastfeeding Efficiency

Parents are often concerned because they have no visual assurance of the amount of breast milk consumed. The mother should be taught other signs of effective, active breastfeeding. The infant should have a rhythmic suckling pattern (the slight pause between jaw compressions on the breast permits the mouth to fill with milk before swallowing) with only

	0	1	2
L Latch	Too sleepy or reluctant No latch achieved	Repeated attempts Hold nipple in mouth Stimulate to suck	Grasps breast Tongue down Lips flanged Rhythmic sucking
A Audible swallowing	None	A few with stimulation	Spontaneous and intermittent > 24 hours old Spontaneous and frequent < 24 hours old
T Type of nipple	Inverted	Flat	Everted (after stimulation)
C Comfort (breast/ nipple)	Engorged Cracked, bleeding, large blisters or bruises Severe discomfort	Filling Reddened/small blisters or bruises Mild/moderate discomfort	Soft Nontender
H Hold (positioning)	Full assist (staff holds infant at breast)	Minimal assist (e.g., elevate head of bed, place pillows for support) Teach one side; mother does other Staff holds and then mother takes over	No assist from staff Mother able to position and hold infant

Figure 32-15 ■ LATCH: A breastfeeding charting and documentation tool. LATCH was created to provide a systematic method for breastfeeding assessment and charting. It can be used to assist the new mother in establishing breastfeeding and to define areas of needed intervention.

Source: Used with permission from AWO. (1994). Jensen, D., Wallace, S. & Kelsay, P. A breastfeeding charting system and documentation tool. Journal of Obstetric, Gynecologic, and Neonatal Nursing, *23(1)27–32. (Table 1 Latch Scoring Table, p. 29.) Washington, DC: Author. © 1994 by the Association of Women's Health, Obstetric and Neonatal Nurses. All rights reserved.*

TABLE 32-4 Successful Breastfeeding Evaluation

A baby is probably getting enough milk if:

- The infant is nursing at least eight times in 24 hours.
- In a quiet room, the mother can hear her infant swallow while nursing, once her milk supply has become abundant.
- The mother's breasts appear to soften after breastfeeding.
- The number of wet diapers increases daily by a minimum of one additional diaper until the fifth day after birth; after day 5, the infant should have six to eight wet diapers daily.
- The infant's stools are beginning to lighten in color by the third day after birth, or have changed to yellow no later than day 5.

Note: Offering a supplemental bottle is not a reliable indicator because most newborns will take a few ounces even if they are getting enough breast milk.

brief pauses lasting seconds between spurts of active feeding. To assess if the jaw compressions are strong enough, the mother can observe or feel if there is movement at the temporomandibular joint located in front of the infant's ears. The mother should visually observe for swallowing and later, as her milk is abundant, she will hear her infant's swallows. The feeding session typically lasts for 10 to 20 minutes on the first breast; the infant may feed only a few minutes on the second breast or not at all. Discourage the mother from watching the clock to determine when the infant needs to switch breast sides but rather encourage her to watch the newborn's feeding pattern to note when active feeding ceases. When satiated, the infant will either pull away from the breast or fall asleep with the mother's nipple still in his or her mouth, though oral muscle tone will be loose. The infant will be extremely relaxed at the end of the feeding and will sleep at least an hour until the next feeding is due (unless cluster feeding). As the infant matures, the feeding intervals will lengthen. Another indicator of breastfeeding efficiency is softening of mother's breasts, although this is not a reliable indicator in the first few days postpartum while breast milk volume is low. Within a week, however, this is a good indicator of milk transfer.

The infant who feeds well will have a characteristic output. Output is a reflection of intake. See Figure 32-16 ■ for breastfeeding intake and output expectations. The infant should also have the characteristic weight loss followed by weight gain pattern discussed earlier in this chapter.

In situations where there is a question regarding milk transfer effectiveness, it can be most reliably measured by obtaining pre- and post-breastfeeding weight checks using an accurate infant scale. The difference in pre-feed and post-feed weights is the amount of milk (each gram increase reflects 1 ml) transferred to the infant and may be useful with assessing breastfeeding efficiency and maternal milk volume.

CLINICAL TIP

With a sleepy baby, unwrap the baby, and place the baby skin-to-skin with his or her mother so the mother can recognize subtle early feeding cues. Encourage the mother to offer her breasts whenever she notices her baby's eyes fluttering under his or her eyelids, or she observes her baby beginning to wriggle around and stretch, or she notices lip smacking and rooting behavior, or observes hand-to-mouth activity.

- Infants should breastfeed 8 to 12 times per day and should appear relaxed after feeding.
- Colostrum is all that a newborn needs in the first few days of life in most cases.
- It is normal for an infant to lose up to 7% of birth weight in the first few days; however, up to 10% weight loss is tolerated if the mother's breasts are full, the infant is observed to breastfeed well, and the infant is not dehydrated.
- Infants should gain 10 grams/kg/day after the mother's milk supply is abundant (about day 4 of life).
- Infants should be back to their birth weight by 2 weeks of age.
- Infant's stool should change in color, consistency, and frequency during the first few days of life. The photo images noted below depict stool color progression. Some babies progress faster to yellow milk stools, as early as day 3.

Day 1

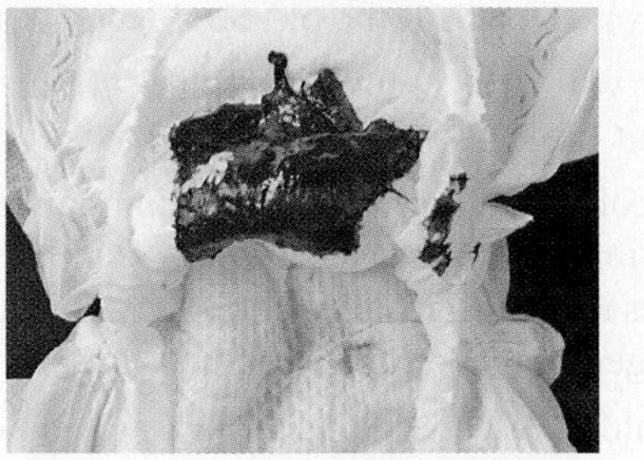

Minimum Output

On day 1, the infant should produce at least one wet diaper and one meconium stool by 24 hours of age.

Note the pinkish-red "brick dust" appearance on the diaper. The uric acid crystals produced by the kidneys is associated with concentrated urine. A red flag is raised if their presence is continued beyond day 2 or 3 of life.

Day 2

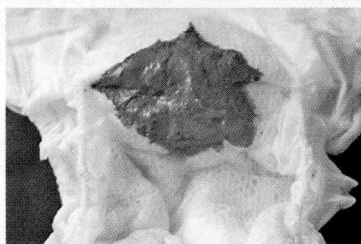

On day 2, the infant should produce at least two wet diapers and two early transitional stools in a 24-hour period by 48 hours of age.

Day 3

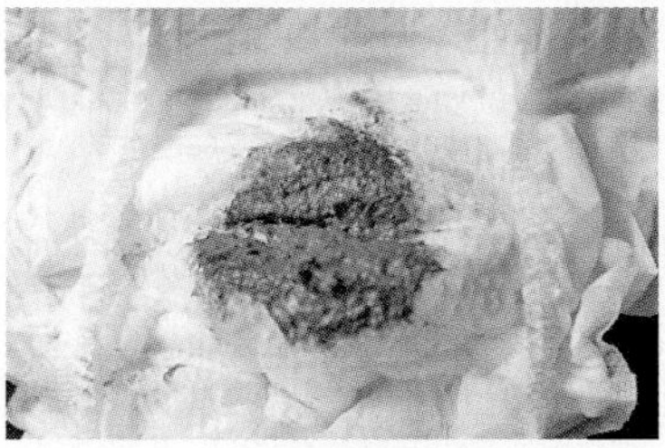

On day 3, the infant should produce at least three wet diapers and three transitional stools in a 24-hour period by 72 hours of age.

When a mother's milk supply is abundant on day 2, some babies will have transitioned to yellow milk stools as early as day 3.

Day 4

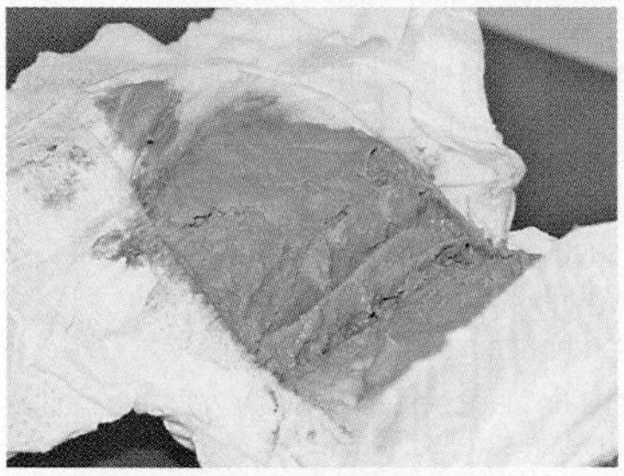

On day 4, the infant should produce at least four wet diapers and three to four yellow-green transitional stools or yellow milk stools in a 24-hour period by 96 hours of age.

Day 5

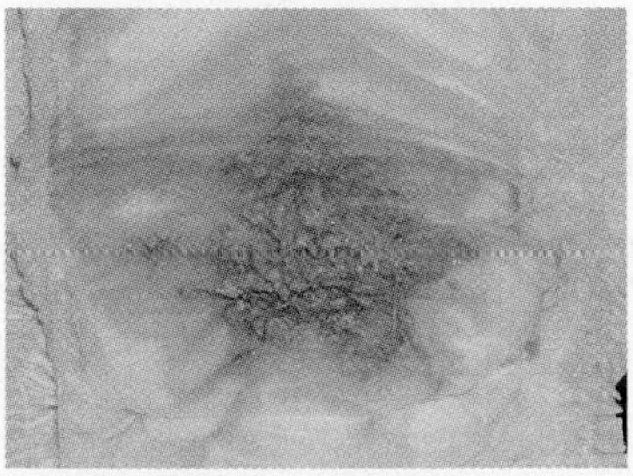

On day 5, the infant should produce at least five wet diapers and three to four yellow milk stools per day; the stools are typically explosive and have a curdy or seedy appearance.

Hereafter, breastfeeding infants will consistently produce at least six well-saturated wet diapers per day. These infants will typically continue to produce at least three to four yellow milk stools daily, but may have up to 10 stools per day until they are about a month old. Infants 4 weeks or older may suddenly decrease their stool frequency, even skipping days.

Figure 32-16 ■ Breastfeeding intake and output expectations.

Source: Days 1–2, 3–4: Courtesy of Brigitte Hall, RNC, MSN, IBCLC/Pearson Education.

Bottle-Feeding Human Milk (Expression, Pumps, Storage)

There are a number of different reasons for bottle-feeding expressed breast milk. The nurse should evaluate the indications in order to recommend the best technique for the mother and her particular need.

Hand Expression

Some mothers prefer to hand express their milk rather than use a breast pump, and many find that in the immediate postpartum period hand expression of milk may be a more effective method of removing drops of colostrum than using an electric breast pump. Nurses should teach all mothers the skill of hand expressing breast milk as it is possible the mother will find herself in a situation without a breast pump and needing to relieve herself from engorgement.

To help the mother hand express breast milk, have the mother follow steps 1 through 4 of the pumping instructions provided in Table 32-5. Then the mother can use the Marmet technique of hand expression described next. It is important that the mother take care to place her hands exactly as directed. The Marmet technique steps are as follows:

1. The mother will position her thumb at the 12 o'clock position on the top edge of the areola (about 1 to 1 1/2 inches back from the tip of her nipple) and her forefinger and middle finger pads at the 6 o'clock position on the bottom edge of the areola (about 1 to 1 1/2 inches from the tip of her nipple). If positioned correctly, an imaginary line between the thumb and fingers will cross through the nipple. See Figure 32-17 ■.
2. Next the mother will stretch her areola back toward her chest wall without lifting her fingers off her breast.
3. Now she should roll her thumb and fingers simultaneously forward. This action compresses the ducts beneath the areola and stimulates the breast to empty the breast both manually and by triggering the let-down reflex.
4. The mother should repeat the sequence multiple times to completely drain her breasts. She should try to maintain a steady rhythm, cycling 45 to 60 times/minute. It is also more effective if the mother repositions her fingers to other positions on the same breast (3 and 9 o'clock, 1 and 7 o'clock, etc.) when the milk flow slows.

The mother should take care not to traumatize her breasts or nipples. Hand expression should not be painful. Most mothers

TABLE 32-5 Pumping Instructions and Storage Guidelines

1. Once a day rinse the breasts with water while bathing or showering. Avoid applying soap directly on the nipples.
2. Wash hands well with soap and water before preparing to pump.
3. Take a few minutes to massage the breasts and relax. Do some slow, deep breathing and think about or look at a picture of your baby. Being relaxed is very important for releasing milk from the breasts. (Stress can inhibit or delay let-down because stress hormones, such as cortisol and adrenalin, can block receptors for let-down.)
4. Sit up straight or lean slightly forward. A pillow placed behind your back may facilitate the slightly tilted forward posture, as gravity aids in the flow of milk from the breasts.
5. For single-sided pumping, pump each breast for 10 to 20 minutes. Some mothers find that they empty their breasts more efficiently if they switch back and forth from one breast to the other as the milk flow diminishes, until they have stimulated each breast for 15 to 20 minutes. The entire pumping session will last 30 to 40 minutes.
6. Pump the expressed milk preferably into glass or plastic bottles. Mothers of healthy infants may also use bottle bags or liners intended for human milk collection and storage; however, note that up to 60% of secretory IgA (SIgA) is lost when milk is stored in these kinds of containers for 48 hours because of the attraction of the antibodies to the polyethylene material used in making the bottle bags/liners (Lawrence & Lawrence, 2005). Because of the loss of antibodies that can occur with bottle bags or liners, mothers of preemies and fragile infants should especially avoid using these kinds of storage containers. Do not fill milk storage containers more than 3/4 full, because milk expands during freezing.
7. Feed *freshly* expressed breast milk whenever there is a need to give a supplement, when possible. Reserve the stored milk for times when fresh milk is not available (e.g., when separated from baby). Fresh breast milk retains more nutrients than refrigerated or frozen milk, although these are still preferred over formula. Expressed human milk may be stored in the refrigerator for up to 8 days, but if intended to be frozen, this should be done within 48 hours of initial refrigeration. Avoid placing human milk in the freezer door or on the bottom of a self-defrosting freezer because the temperature fluctuates more in those areas.
8. Store expressed human milk in volumes the infant is likely to consume at a single feeding or in a volume the infant will consume in a day.
9. Human milk should never be thawed in a microwave oven or placed in a pan and warmed up on the stove. These methods may cause the milk to warm up too hot (and unevenly) and can burn an infant as well as cause heat-sensitive nutrients to be destroyed. Frozen milk can be thawed safely using one of two methods:
   - For a quick thaw, remove the container of frozen milk from the freezer, place the container in a bowl in the sink, and run warm water over it for no longer than 15 minutes. Take care not to immerse the container in water because water may leach into the container of milk possibly contaminating it and diluting it.
   - For a slow thaw overnight, take the frozen container of milk from the freezer the day before or several hours before it is needed and let it defrost in the refrigerator (not on the kitchen counter) over several hours. The time it takes to defrost depends on the volume in the container. Note that breast milk that has been sitting for awhile will normally separate. See Figure 32-18 ■ to view breast milk that has separated. To remix it, simply swirl the bottle (avoid vigorous shaking) until the milk is evenly mixed. Make certain that the fat that clings to the wall of the container has mixed into the milk. If the volume in the bottle is more than can be used in one feeding, pour only the amount needed into a clean bottle, and put the rest of the milk immediately back in the refrigerator. Place the feeding bottle in a bowl in the sink and run warm water over it for no longer than 15 minutes. The bottle should remain fairly upright and the water level in the bowl should remain below the lid of the bottle or milk container to prevent water from inadvertently entering the bottle.
10. Previously frozen thawed breast milk is good in the refrigerator for 24 hours only. It must be used in that time frame or discarded. Thawed milk should never be refrozen.
11. Check the temperature of the milk before feeding it. Babies will drink milk when the milk temperature is between room temperature and body temperature (roughly 65 to 100 degrees).
12. Any milk left over from a feeding should be discarded within an hour of starting the feeding. The reason for this is because saliva "back washes" into the bottle while nipple feeding, and the saliva contains bacteria that can multiply and potentially make a baby sick.

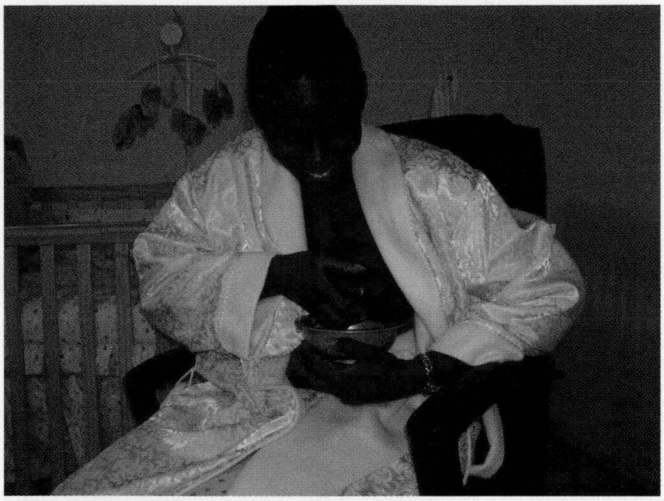

Figure 32-17 ■ Hand Expression.

Source: Courtesy of Brigitte Hall, RNC, MSN, IBCLC.

will need assistance in learning this technique initially. Reassure the mother that it is a skill that is learned, and with practice, she can become an expert at hand expression.

Breast Pumps

Although hand expression can be efficient, many mothers will choose to use a mechanical breast pump to express their milk. Not all breast pumps are of the same quality, even within the same category (see Table 32-6 and Figure 32-19 ■ through Figure 32-21 ■). A desirable breast pump should be able to cycle from low to high suction at a frequency similar to that of a breastfeeding infant (about 45 to 60 cycles per minute). However, differences in the quality of the pump motor or the presence or absence of controls over suction pressure mean that some pumps will generate inadequate pressure or cycle too slowly to be effective, whereas others may exert too high a suction that can cause injury. Breast flange fit and comfort are other variables to consider. Some good quality pumps have multiple flange sizes available to accommodate the various nipple sizes of mothers. Excessive rubbing of the mother's nipple in the flange tunnel can cause discomfort and result in a decreased volume expressed. The nurse should refer the mother to a lactation consultant for a flange fitting if the mother has particularly large nipples.

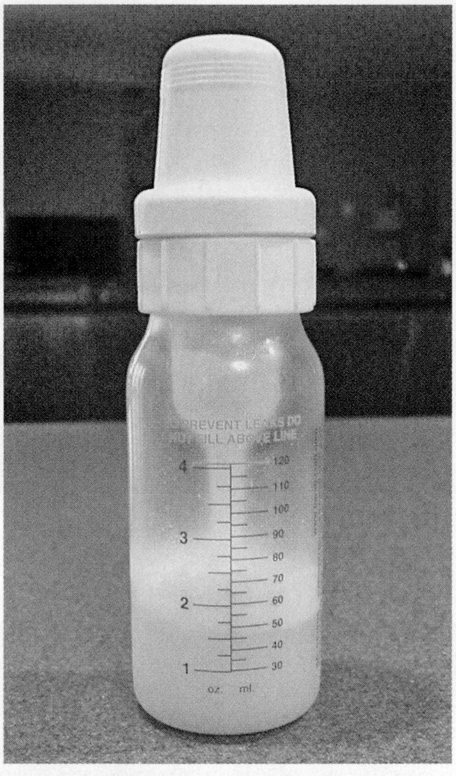

Figure 32-18 ■ Expressed breast milk that has separated.

Source: Courtesy of Brigitte Hall, RNC, MSN, IBCLC/Pearson Education.

Storing Human Breast Milk and Formula

There are different guidelines for storage of expressed breast milk (EBM) depending on whether the infant is a healthy

TABLE 32-6 Types of Breast Pumps and Indications for Use

INDICATION	MANUAL BREAST PUMP (FIGURE 32-19)	SMALL BATTERY/ELECTRIC BREAST PUMP	INDIVIDUAL DOUBLE ELECTRIC BREAST PUMP (FIGURE 32-20)	HOSPITAL-GRADE MULTI-USER DOUBLE ELECTRIC BREAST PUMP (FIGURE 32-21)
A missed feeding	■	▲		
An evening out	■	▲		
Working part-time	■	▲		
Convenience—occasional use	■	▲		
Working full-time			*	*
Premature/hospitalized infant				*
Low milk supply				*
Sore nipples/engorgement			*	*
Latch-on problems/infection			■	*
Drawing out flattish nipples	■	▲	*	*

Source: Modified from the Medela Breastfeeding Information Guide Tips and Products. (2002). Table: Which Breast Pump Is Best for You? *(p. 3). McHenry, IL: Medela, Inc.*

■ Good ▲ Better * Best

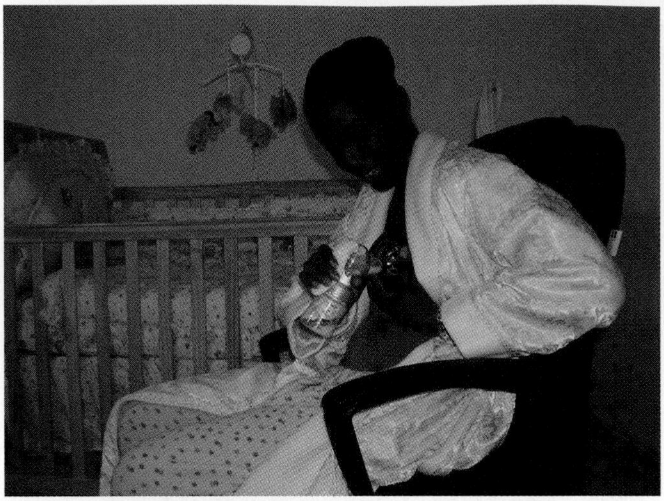

Figure 32-19 ■ Manual breast pump.

Source: Courtesy of Brigitte Hall, RNC, MSN, IBCLC.

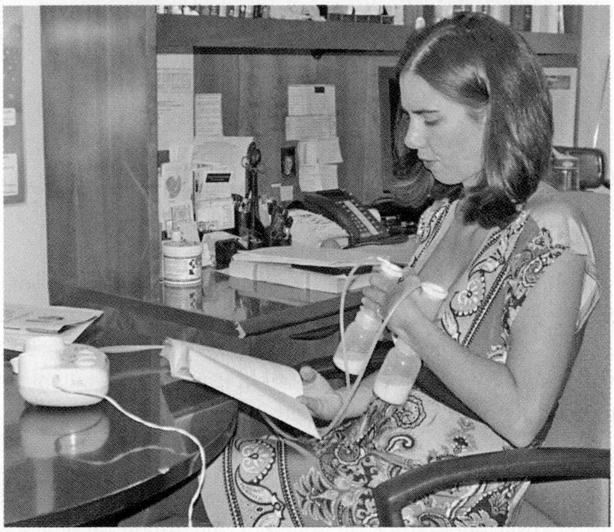

Figure 32-20 ■ Individual double electric breast pump.

Source: Courtesy of Brigitte Hall, RNC, MSN, IBCLC/Pearson Education.

full-term infant or a premature or sick infant in the hospital. The guidelines in Table 32-7 are intended as a resource for the mother of a healthy, full-term infant.

Supplementary Bottle-Feeding

Supplementary bottle-feedings with formula for the breastfeeding infant after birth are not routinely recommended. Supplementation should only be given when medically indicated (ABM, 2009). Routine supplements are not only unnecessary in the early days after birth, but bottle feeding in itself may cause the infant to develop an incorrect sucking pattern, or may cause the infant to refuse the breast altogether (Riordan & Wambach, 2010). Early supplementation with formula may contribute to a delay in early maternal milk production, may result in maternal engorgement after the mother's milk production has increased, and may possibly sensitize an at-risk infant for milk-protein allergy. These types of problems have been implicated in early breastfeeding terminations (Mercer, Teasley, Hopkinson, et al., 2010).

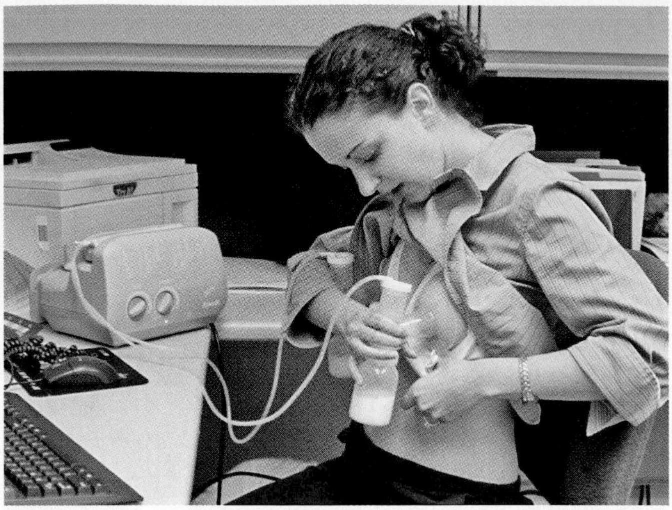

Figure 32-21 ■ Hospital-grade multi-user breast pump.

Source: Courtesy of Brigitte Hall, RNC, MSN, IBCLC/Pearson Education.

TABLE 32-7 Storage Guidelines for Human Milk and Formula

MILK	ENVIRONMENT	TIME UNTIL DISCARD
Human milk or formula, opened/reconstituted	Being fed	Finish feed within 1 hour
Fresh human milk	Room temperature 72–79°F	4 hours
Fresh human milk	Room temperature 66–72°F	6–10 hours
Fresh human milk	Cooler w/ frozen ice packs 59°F	24 hours
Formula, opened/reconstituted	Room temperature	2 hours
Thawed human milk	Refrigerator	24 hours
Formula, opened/reconstituted	Refrigerator	24–48 hours (see label)
Fresh human milk	Refrigerator	8 days
Formula powder, opened can	Room temperature	1 month
Fresh human milk	Freezer	3–4 months
Formula/powder in sealed container	Avoid excessive heat	Printed expiration date
Thawed human milk	Freezer	Do not refreeze
Formula	Freezer	Do not freeze

Sources: Data from Human Milk Banking Association of North America (HMBANA), (2006); Abbott Laboratories (2009); Ameda/Hollister (undated); Mead-Johnson & Company, (2009).

An infant's refusal to breastfeed after receiving bottles in the early post-delivery period may be related to a phenomenon referred to as *nipple confusion* or more accurately termed, *nipple preference*. This potential problem occurs because the techniques for breastfeeding and bottle-feeding are different. In breastfeeding, the infant has to open his or her mouth very wide in order to latch on to the breast. To transfer milk the baby has to extend the tongue forward, cupping the nipple and drawing the mother's nipple deep into the infant's mouth until the teat reaches the "comfort zone" near the junction of the infant's hard and soft palate. After the infant creates suction from the

TABLE 32-8 Factors Requiring Consideration of Supplementation

Risk factors for inadequate intake:

- Maternal/infant separation
- Maternal barriers to breastfeeding (e.g., medications, fatigue, pain, cultural)
- Congenital malformation or illness interfering with ability to breastfeed
- Delayed lactogenesis after day 3 or 4
- Primary lactation failure (usually due to breast pathology or prior breast surgery)
- Low birth weight or infant with illness/disorder requiring nutrient requirements that may exceed that available through breastfeeding

Signs of potential inadequate intake:

- Weight loss > 7% from birth weight
- Delayed bowel movements or continued meconium stools beyond day 2
- Hypoglycemia not responding to frequent breastfeeding attempts
- Hyperbilirubinemia due to breastfeeding jaundice

tongue and cheeks and seals the latch with his or her lips, then the infant rhythmically compresses the breast with his or her jaw while the tongue moves in an undulating motion to move fluid toward the infant's pharynx before swallowing, in coordination with breathing. Also, on average, it takes a couple of minutes before the breastfeeding mother's milk flow increases during let-down. With bottle-feeding, the infant keeps the tongue retracted and uses the tip of the tongue to block the flow of milk, which otherwise drips continuously by gravity even when suction is not applied. The bottle-feeding baby merely needs to create suction with his or her mouth on the bottle nipple and the fluid easily flows.

For the mother who wants her breastfeeding baby to be able to take a bottle from time to time, without risking bottle preference by her baby, it is recommended that the mother wait until her milk supply is well established, and the infant has mastered the skills of breastfeeding. Therefore, the earliest it is recommended to introduce a bottle to a breastfeeding infant is when the infant is 3 to 4 weeks old (AWHONN, 2007).

At times there are valid medical indications for supplementing a breastfeeding infant in the early postpartum period. See Table 32-8 for a list of factors requiring consideration for supplementation. When supplementation is indicated, the first choice is to use the mother's own milk (fresh, previously expressed, or frozen/thawed). If maternal milk is not available, pasteurized donor milk is the next choice, and then formula (HMBANA, 2006). Supplementation can be administered using various methods based on the particular situation, parental preference, and hospital policy. Methods of delivering the feeding supplement include: use of a supplemental nursing device at the breast, cup feeding, spoon or dropper feeding, finger-feeding, or bottle feeding (ABM, 2009).

Formula Feeding

With more attention placed on promoting and assisting breastfeeding mothers, the teaching needs of the mother who is formula-feeding may inadvertently get overlooked. Nurses may assume that families can simply follow the formula preparation instructions on the side of the formula containers. However, research shows that these parents also need teaching, counseling, and support in regard to formula preparation and bottle-feeding technique. In a systematic review of five studies from developed countries looking at how parents prepare formula, all the studies revealed "errors in reconstitution with a tendency to over-concentrate feeds, although under-concentrating also occurred" (Morin, 2005). Parents need to learn about the normal feeding pattern for a formula-feeding infant and recognize symptoms of formula intolerance. They need to know intake and output expectations, the recommended type of formula for their infant, how to prepare and store formula, what equipment they will need, the feeding technique, and safety precautions.

HEALTH PROMOTION EDUCATION: FORMULA-FEEDING GUIDELINES AND TECHNIQUE

Commercial formulas are available in three forms: powder, concentrate, and ready-to-feed. There are situations in which one formula may be better to use than another, but, in general, convenience and cost usually influence the parents' decision.

- *Powdered formula* is the least expensive type of formula. This formula can be made up one bottle at a time, or multiple bottles can be prepared, but they must be used within 24 to 48 hours depending on the manufacturers' instructions. Standard powdered formula is made by adding one level *unpacked* scoop of powdered formula to 60 ml of water (the powder is added to the water). Powdered formulas are not sterile. Preparation of any infant formula, but especially powdered formulas, requires careful handling to avoid contamination with microorganisms. Also it is a little more difficult to mix well to obtain a uniform composition throughout compared to concentrate and ready-to-feed formulas. Vigorous shaking to mix it creates foam, and babies can potentially ingest more gas. It is best to let the bottle sit for a few minutes after being shaken to allow the bubbles to dissipate.
- *Formula concentrate* is more expensive than powder but is not as expensive as ready-to-feed formula. Formula concentrate is commercially sterile. This formula requires being diluted with an equal part of water.
- *Ready-to-feed* formula is the easiest to use because it does not require any mixing; however, this convenience comes at a cost—it is the most expensive formula. It is indicated for use when adequate water is not available, when the infant has a compromised immune system and requires commercially sterile (pasteurized) formula, when an inexperienced babysitter will be feeding the infant, and at other times simply for convenience.

Whatever the type of formula chosen, the nurse should underscore the importance of proper preparation and prompt refrigeration. Parents will need to be briefed on safety precautions during formula preparation. A primary concern is proper mixing to reconstitute formula. Parents need clear instructions to avoid unintentional harm to their infant. Parents should be instructed to follow the directions on the formula package label precisely as written. They should know that adding too much water during preparation dilutes the nutrients and caloric density. This contributes to undernourishment, insufficient weight gain, and possibly water intoxication, which can cause hyponatremia and seizures if the dilution is excessive. Not adding enough water concentrates nutrients and calories and can tax an infant's immature kidneys and digestive system as well as cause dehydration (Morin, 2005). See Table 32-7 for storage guidelines for human milk and formula.

Recommended sanitary precautions and additional safety precautions include:

- Check the expiration date on the formula container.
- Ensure good hand washing before preparing formula; never dip into the can without clean hands.
- Clean bottles, nipples, rings, disks, and bottle caps.
  - Wash in a dishwasher when available (small items and heat-sensitive items on top rack secured in a basket), or
  - Boil briefly (1 to 2 minutes) in a pot of water, or
  - Clean using a microwave sterilization kit, or
  - Clean using very warm soapy water and a nipple and bottle brush
  - Inspect and replace bottle nipples as soon as they show wear—worn nipples can break apart and can become a choking hazard.
- Wash the top of the formula container before piercing the lid. Shake the liquid formulas well before pouring out desired amount.
- Shake prepared formula that has been sitting in the refrigerator before feeding.
- Allow tap water to run for 1 minute before obtaining water to use for mixing—this helps clear any lead standing in the pipes. Also, always use cold tap water because warm tap water tends to contain higher levels of lead as well.
- Use only the scoop supplied in the can of formula when formula preparation instructions call for a "scoop" of powdered formula. A scoop should not be "packed" and should be leveled off (e.g., with the back of a knife).
- Do not add anything else to the bottle, except under direction of baby's healthcare provider.
- Warm up formula in a bottle by placing the bottle in a bowl of warm tap water for no longer than 15 minutes. Do not fill the bowl with water higher than the rim of the bottle.
- Newborns can be fed formula at room temperature but most young infants will prefer it warm. Once a bottle of formula is warmed up, it must be used within an hour or discarded.
- Left over formula remaining in a bottle after feeding should be discarded within an hour of starting the feeding. Allow freshly prepared (unused) formula to sit out at room temperature for no longer than 2 hours; use an insulated pack to transport formula.
- In warm weather, transport reconstituted or formula concentrate from an open can in an insulated pack with frozen gel packs.
- Travel with water and formula separated—carry the premeasured water bottles and carry bottles with premeasured amounts of powdered formula, or carry premeasured commercially prepared formula packets, or have the can of formula available.
- Hold the infant during feedings (even later on when an older infant can hold the bottle for himself or herself) to promote bonding and prevent supine feedings.
- Do not allow the infant to bottle-feed in a supine position because this increases the risk of otitis media and dental caries in the older infant.
- Never prop a bottle—this is a choking hazard.
- Allow infants to take what they want *and* to stop when they want. Overfeeding can lead to obesity.

TABLE 32-9 Water Sources

TYPE	DESCRIPTION
Distilled Water	Minerals and most other impurities have been removed. It will not contain any fluoride. An acceptable water source for reconstituting formula.
Filtered Tap Water	Some minerals and impurities removed during filtration, including fluoride. This is an acceptable water source for reconstituting formula.
Natural Mineral Water	Comes from protected groundwater and by law cannot be treated. Naturally contains high levels of minerals and sodium and so is not suitable for infants or for reconstituting formula.
Spring Water	Comes from a single nonpolluted groundwater, but unlike natural mineral water, it can be further treated. Because there is no regulation requiring the mineral content to be printed on the bottle label, it is best to avoid this water source for reconstituting formula.
Tap Water	Water from the municipal water supply and regulated by drinking water regulations. It is treated and considered safe for use in reconstituting formula.
Well Water	Needs to be tested before use. Higher risk of nitrate poisoning. Untested water is not recommended for use in reconstituting formula.

Parents also need guidance about what kind of water to use to reconstitute formula (see Table 32-9 to review types of water sources) and should discuss with their infant's healthcare provider whether to boil the water before use. If boiling water is used, parents need to be instructed to heat the water until it reaches a rolling boil, continue to let the water boil for 1 to 2 minutes, and, most importantly, allow the water to cool before using it to reconstitute the formula. Parents should also be instructed not to let the water boil down to a low level in the pan because this can cause minerals in the water to become concentrated.

Use of distilled bottled water and filtered tap water raises concerns with regard to fluoride. The AAP recommends that no fluoride supplements should be given to an infant before 6 months of age, but does recommend supplementary fluoride for infants and children aged 6 months to 3 years of age if the water source contains less than 0.3 ppm (AAP & ACOG, 2007). Parents should be encouraged to read the labels on bottled water to see if fluoride has been added and to determine if the water source is suitable for their infant depending on his or her age.

Bottles and Nipples

Parents often have questions about the kind of bottles and nipples to purchase. Plastic, glass, or disposable bottle bags may all be used based on preference. Many newly designed bottles are marketed to lessen air intake while an infant feeds. There is not a particular bottle design that is best for all babies. A key point to emphasize to the families is feeding technique. Parents should try to avoid situations in which an infant is crying for a prolonged time. Crying results in increased ingestion of air even before the infant has started feeding. Infants who are very hungry also gulp more air. For these situations, instruct the parents to burp their infant frequently to prevent the infant from having a large emesis (Figure 32-22 ■ and Figure 32-23 ■). The parent may even want to attempt to pat the baby's back briefly before starting the feeding to calm a crying infant and possibly burp as well. Another tip to avoid excessive ingestion of air is to have the parent hold the infant cradled in his or her arms while

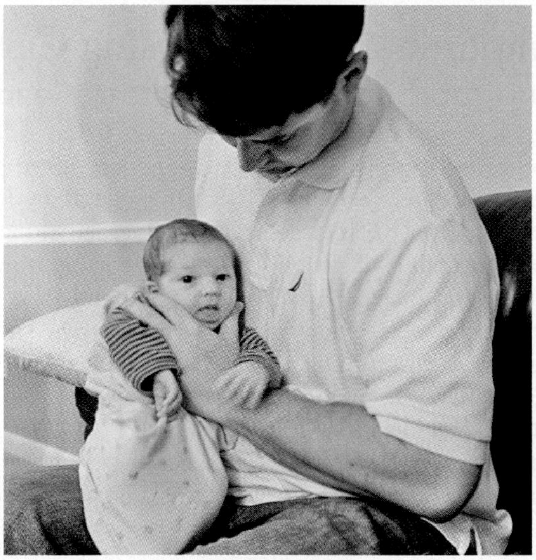

Figure 32-22 ■ Burping baby sitting up on lap.

Source: Courtesy of Brigitte Hall, RNC, MSN, IBCLC/Pearson Education.

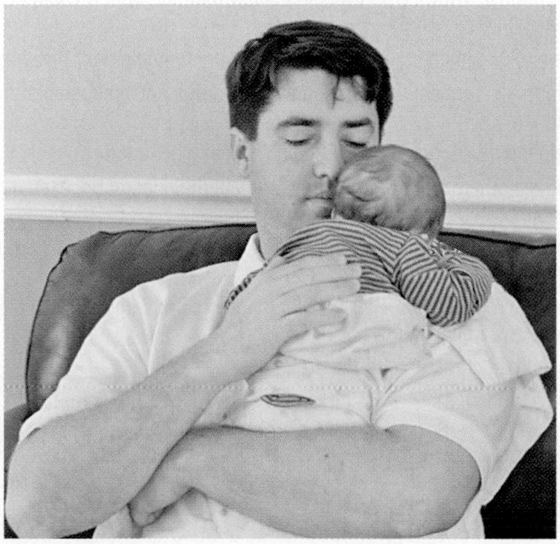

Figure 32-23 ■ Burping baby over the shoulder.

Source: Courtesy of Brigitte Hall, RNC, MSN, IBCLC/Pearson Education.

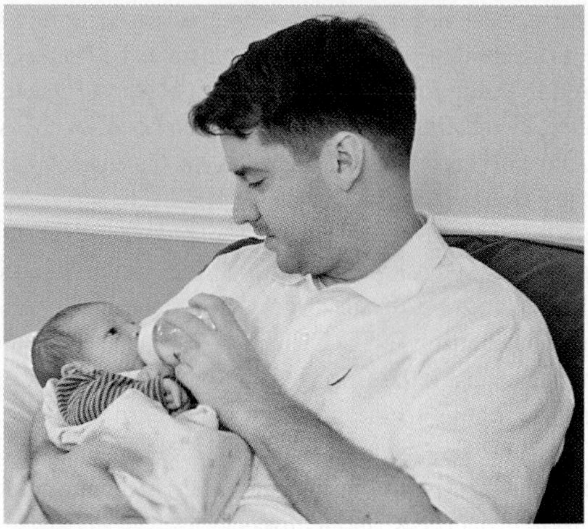

Figure 32-24 ■ Bottle feeding.

Source: Courtesy of Brigitte Hall, RNC, MSN, IBCLC/Pearson Education.

bottle-feeding, and tilting the bottle at a 45-degree angle in order for fluid to cover the nipple. This prevents the infant from sucking in air and swallowing it. The vented bottle design eliminates the negative effects of a vacuum and channels air through an internal vent system above the milk avoiding air bubbles in the milk. See Figure 32-24 ■ to view an infant bottle feeding.

Parents will want to consider a slow-flow nipple for all newborns and for older breastfeeding babies learning to bottle-feed—over time the infant will graduate to medium-flow and high-flow nipples. Generally, nipple shape is of greater importance for breastfeeding babies receiving expressed breast milk or supplemental formula in a bottle. Breastfed babies transition best going from breast to bottle and back to breast again when using a bottle nipple that is not too firm, one that has a relatively wide base (to help maintain a wide-open latch), and one that has a medium nipple length. Nipples are generally made from either rubber or silicone. Families with a history of sensitivity to latex are advised to use the clear silicone nipples. Silicone nipples also have less of an odor, which may be an issue for some infants who are breastfed.

To know if an infant is bottle-feeding well, the nurse needs to observe a bottle-feeding session. Parents should be informed that if the infant is sucking effectively, the parents should observe bubbles rising in the fluid of standard bottles. (If a family is using vented bottles or bottles with liners that retract as fluid is removed, bubbles will not be detected.) No bubbles will be observed if the parent unintentionally places the bottle nipple under the infant's tongue, preventing their infant from sucking effectively. Some infants, especially premature infants, raise their tongue to the roof of their mouth and so it is sometimes a challenge to place the nipple on top of the tongue. Infants who persistently leak milk from the side of the mouth may be getting fluid too quickly. The nurse could suggest using a slower flowing nipple. If symptoms persist, the infant should have an oral evaluation. The infant could have a short lingual frenulum that is restricting tongue mobility (tongue-tied) and may not be able to properly cup his or her tongue under the nipple and channel fluid to the back of the throat, or the infant may have an oral-motor dysfunction and need speech therapy or occupational therapy evaluation.

Recently, there has been a growing concern regarding specific chemicals used in the manufacture of plastic baby bottles, the material used in lining formula cans, and soft plastics. Researchers at the University of Missouri reported that bisphenol-A (BPA) could leach from polycarbonate plastic used in the manufacturing of some baby bottles and may transfer BPA into the baby's milk (Vom Saal et al., 2007). Animal studies show that BPA can cause developmental, neural, and reproductive problems (National Toxicology Program Center for the Evaluation of Risks to Human Reproduction [NTP-CERHR], 2008). There is also concern about bottles made from polyvinyl chloride (PVC), which sometimes contains lead, and there is concern about soft PVC (containing phthalates which are used to soften plastic), which is another hormone-disrupting chemical used in the manufacture of bottle nipples, pacifiers, and teethers.

Although virtually everyone is exposed to these chemicals, infants who are being fed bottles of formula are at greatest risk for exposure. Many leading bottle manufacturing companies and other companies making plastics have changed their products to contain no BPA, PVC, lead, or phthalates. Parents need to be instructed to read product labels to see if the merchandise they are purchasing is free of these potentially harmful chemicals. If product labels do not explicitly state that they are free of these chemicals, then it cannot be assumed that they are BPA-free, PVC-free, lead-free, and phthalates-free.

If parents cannot afford to purchase new BPA-free bottles, then encourage them to limit heating the bottles (avoid using the dishwasher and bottle warmers) and throw out old bottles with scratches. The harmful chemicals are leached most when the plastic is heated or damaged.

Involving Fathers

Our traditional view of the family following the birth of a child places most of the attention on the mother and newborn, oftentimes leaving the father out. Nurses need to recognize this and make every effort to speak to both parents when entering the patient's room. Fathers play a vital role in the family by providing support to the mother and care for their newborn. If a mother has chosen not to breastfeed, then the father can be involved with bottle feedings from the start. However, if the mother is breastfeeding, it is important to ask the father to wait to introduce a bottle until the mother's milk supply and breastfeeding are well established, generally by 3 to 4 weeks post-delivery. The father can be encouraged to assist with breastfeeding in the meantime. He can help the mother get in position and help tweak the baby's latch if the mother complains of any discomfort. The father can also massage the mother's breasts during breastfeeding to help stimulate the sleepy baby to feed better and to relieve any engorgement. The father can help with other aspects too. He can help burp the baby, change diapers, bathe, and comfort the baby. The father can also provide skin-to-skin contact that enhances bonding, provides comfort to the newborn, and calms the baby down before offering the breast. One strategy is to have the father hold the baby vertically on his chest and let the baby suck on a clean finger for a minute or so (see Figure 32-25 ■). These are just a few ways to involve the father after the birth of the baby. These interactions promote father-mother-infant bonding and are important for paternal role development.

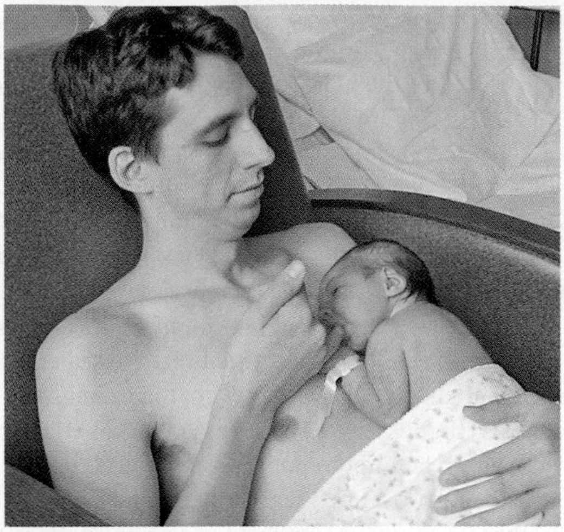

Figure 32-25 ■ Father and infant skin-to-skin.

Source: Courtesy of Brigitte Hall, RNC, MSN, IBCLC/Pearson Education.

Community-Based Nursing Care

Promotion of Successful Infant Feeding

To promote a supportive hospital environment for breastfeeding, the World Health Organization (WHO) and the United Nations Children's Emergency Fund (UNICEF)'s the Baby-Friendly Hospital Initiative (BFHI) recognize hospitals and birthing centers that offer optimal lactation services and comply with the 10 steps outlined in Table 32-10. Baby-friendly status is not easy to achieve. One obstacle, among many, is having to agree not to accept free or low-cost formula (WHO/UNICEF, 2009). There are approximately 91 hospitals in the United States with Baby-Friendly designation as of April 2010 (BFHI USA, 2010).

Seven of the BFHI steps focus on maternity services and newborn care in the hospital, but the third step (antenatal breastfeed-

TABLE 32-10 Baby-Friendly Requirements

Ten Steps to Successful Breastfeeding

1. Maintain a written breastfeeding policy that is routinely communicated to all healthcare staff.
2. Train all healthcare staff in skills necessary to implement this policy.
3. Inform all pregnant women about the benefits and management of breastfeeding.
4. Help mothers initiate breastfeeding within 1 hour of birth.
5. Show mothers how to breastfeed and maintain lactation, even if they should be separated from their infants.
6. Give newborn infants no food or drink other than breast milk, unless medically indicated.
7. Practice rooming in—that is, allow mothers and infants to remain together 24 hours a day.
8. Encourage unrestricted breastfeeding.
9. Give no pacifiers or artificial nipples to breastfeeding infants.
10. Foster the establishment of breastfeeding support groups and refer mothers to them on discharge from the hospital or clinic.

Source: World Health Organization/United Nations Children's Emergency Fund (WHO/UNICEF). (1994). U.S. Committee for UNICEF Interim Program in the United States to Promote the Baby Friendly Ten-Steps to Successful Breastfeeding. Washington, DC: Government Printing Office.

RESEARCH EVIDENCE IN PRACTICE Strategies to Promote Breastfeeding

CLINICAL QUESTION
What interventions are effective in the pre- and postnatal periods to promote breastfeeding as an exclusive source of nutrition for babies?

RESEARCH EVIDENCE
Breastfeeding has health advantages for both babies and their mothers. Babies that are breastfed have fewer infections and allergies, and are less likely to develop asthma, type 2 diabetes, obesity, and childhood leukemia later in life. Mothers who breastfeed are at lower risk for type 2 diabetes, breast cancer, and ovarian cancer than women who have never breastfed. Still, nearly 30% of American children have never been breastfed, and only 35% are breastfed until they are 6 months old. Strategies that can effectively encourage exclusive breastfeeding—or any breastfeeding at all—can have an impact on the health of both babies and mothers.

While a great deal of research has been conducted on strategies to promote breastfeeding, there is little in the way of definitive conclusions because the interventions tested in these studies are not standard. Promotion methods that have been tested include prenatal and postnatal interventions; efforts around the time of delivery; after birth, while breastfeeding is under way; formal education for mothers, fathers, and families; direct support of mothers during breastfeeding observation; peer support; and training of professional staff.

It is clear that interventions to promote breastfeeding can increase the rate, exclusivity, and length of breastfeeding. The characteristics of interventions that seem the most effective are those that are begun before birth and continued into the postnatal period. Programs that involve the father or parental partner are more successful in promoting exclusive breastfeeding. Peer support and education is also effective in promoting breastfeeding.

WHAT QUESTIONS REMAIN UNANSWERED?
Is there a standard approach that can be demonstrated to be effective overall in supporting exclusive breastfeeding?

WHAT IS BEST PRACTICE?
Interventions that begin during the prenatal period, involve the spouse or parental partner, and continue through the postnatal period are most effective in promoting breastfeeding. Providing these support services using a peer or trained breastfeeding coach is an effective way to encourage breastfeeding.

CRITICAL THINKING
What content would be effective in providing breastfeeding education and support? How can the nurse initiate support services in the prenatal period?

References
Chung, M., Raman, G., Trikalinos, T., Lau, J., & Ip, S. 2008. Clinical guidelines. Interventions in primary care to promote breastfeeding: An evidence review for the U.S. Preventive Services Task Force. *Annals of Internal Medicine, 149*(8), 565–582.
Komara, C., Simpson, D., Teasdale, C., Whalen, G., Bells, S., & Giovanetto, L. 2007. Intervening to promote early initiation of breastfeeding in the LDR. *MCN: The American Journal of Maternal Child Nursing, 32*(2), 117–121.
Susin, L., & Giugliani, E. 2008. Inclusion of fathers in an intervention to promote breastfeeding: Impact on breastfeeding rates. *Journal of Human Lactation, 24*(4), 386–392.

ing education) and tenth step (establishment of breastfeeding support groups), connect the mother to community-based breastfeeding promotion and support services.

Research has shown that social and community support is needed for a mother to initiate and sustain breastfeeding (WHO, 2003). Community-based support for breastfeeding mothers often focuses on breastfeeding support groups. **La Leche League International (LLLI)** is the first (not-for-profit international educational and service organization) mother-to-mother breastfeeding support group formally recognized in the United States. It also has expanded to provide educational breastfeeding conferences for professionals, and it is one of the few organizations to have a peer counselor breastfeeding training program, among other things. (See www.nursing.pearsonhighered.com for more information.) Encourage mothers to visit the International Lactation Consultant Association (ILCA) Web site to find lactation consultants in their geographic areas. Another professional organization, The Academy of Breastfeeding Medicine (ABM) provides many research-based breastfeeding protocols that are being implemented in hospitals and agencies around the country that support breastfeeding. To access the protocols, visit the ABM Web site.

Peer counseling is another type of mother-to-mother community support program targeted to low-income women, minorities, and other groups with a low incidence of breastfeeding and counselors are usually hired to work for the Supplemental Nutrition Program for Women, Infants, and Children (WIC). Peer counselors are typically economically disadvantaged mothers themselves in the community who have previously breastfed or are currently breastfeeding and desire helping other disadvantaged women breastfeed successfully. The primary role for peer counselors is providing counseling to pregnant and breastfeeding mothers on a one-to-one basis in the clinic, during home visits, and by telephone follow-up. In a recent systematic review, the use of peer counselors was shown to have a positive impact on infant feeding behavior and is an effective strategy for increasing breastfeeding rates (Chung, Raman, Trikalinos, et al., 2008).

Breastfeeding Resources

WIC

The Supplemental Nutrition Program for Women, Infants, and Children (WIC) functions primarily to provide low-income women and children who are at risk for medical or nutritional problems with nutritious foods to supplement their diets, nutrition education and counseling, and screening and referrals to other health, welfare, and social programs. The WIC program serves 45% of all infants born in the United States. More than half of the formula used in the United States is distributed free of charge to mothers whose babies are enrolled in the WIC program (Kent, 2006). To be eligible for WIC benefits, an applicant's gross income must fall at or below 185% of the U.S. Poverty Income Guidelines. For example, a family of four must not earn more than $40,793 (gross income) per year, effective July 1, 2009 to June 30, 2010. Although WIC provides formula to eligible mothers who are not exclusively breastfeeding, the monthly allotment is not enough to meet the full nutritional needs of a growing infant over time. Mothers need to understand that they will have to purchase additional formula out of pocket as their infant's feeding requirement increases.

Families who are eligible to be enrolled in the WIC program are usually also eligible for other need-based programs. The staff at the WIC office often makes referrals for families to these other programs where indicated. The U.S. Department of Health and Human Services, Administration for Children & Families provides 1000 government benefit and assistance programs for eligible families. Among the numerous programs available, families are likely to want information on enrollment in their state Medicaid program and information about acquiring food stamps from the Supplemental Nutrition Assistance Program (SNAP).

There are many organizations within a community at the local level that provide various kinds of support to families. At the local level hospitals, clinics, and private practice lactation consultants provide some of the following services: parenting classes, breastfeeding classes, breastfeeding consultation visits, breastfeeding support group meetings, postpartum depression support group meetings, boot camp for dads, new parent support group meetings, and infant care classes. Some home health agencies, through physician referral and self-referral, provide home visits for families to check on the newborn and mother after hospital discharge. Food banks, shelters, and churches help low income families when other community resources are not in place yet. Libraries also provide local community service to families. Besides providing books on parenting, feeding, and other related topics, libraries provide families with access to available computers for those needing Internet access.

Communities have an integral role in the promotion and support of successful infant feeding practices by providing programs that meet the emotional, informational, and instructional needs of families. It is very important that nurses discharging mothers from a hospital or birthing center provide the new mother with a list of relevant resources that are available to her in the community. Communities can make a difference in improving quality of life for infants and their families.

Nutritional Assessment

A nutritional assessment is an integral part of a thorough health appraisal and is commonly performed by the infant's primary care provider, a nurse, a lactation consultant, a registered dietitian, or a speech therapist. The nutritional assessment will include all or some of the following parameters to measure wellness:

- Nutritional intake (breast milk, type of formula, other foods)
- Anthropometric measurements (measurements of weight, length, and head circumference)
- Biochemical status (the newborn metabolic screening, iron level, etc.)
- Physical examination (vital signs, total body examination, developmental milestones)
- Sociodemographic data (parity, maternal age, impact of cultural practices on feeding)

Parents will be asked to present a feeding diary for the provider to review, or the parents will need to recall the infant's feeding pattern over the last 24 to 48 hours. The parents will also be asked to describe the infant's urine and stool output, including quantity and quality. The healthcare professional is interested in the infant's behavior pattern, especially during and immediately after feeding. If the newborn is not gaining sufficient weight, the infant's feeding history must be examined more closely. If the infant is breastfeeding, a relevant maternal history is needed to determine if the mother is having breastfeeding difficulties and to help determine the root cause of the problem. If the infant is formula-feeding, the healthcare professional will first want to investigate the family's formula-feeding practices (including formula preparation technique). While gathering these data, the healthcare professional should be sensitive to the family's cultural practices. However, if a cultural practice has harmful effects, then the provider needs to tactfully educate the family to that fact.

The provider should plot the infant's measurements for length, head circumference, and weight on a growth chart, denoting the infant's individual percentile measurement compared with the general population. Because there are variations among infants at the same age, it is important to monitor the infant's individual growth pattern over time. Ideally, the provider wants to see an infant track along the same growth curve. A drop of 20 percentile or more on the growth curve is cause for concern.

As the healthcare provider begins the infant's physical exam, the provider first obtains a subjective impression of the infant's overall appearance. The provider performs a head-to-toe physical examination, carefully noting any deviations from normal. If the infant's primary healthcare provider has any concerns about the infant's nutritional status, the provider may order relevant laboratory studies (i.e., newborn metabolic screening, iron level), may evaluate the infant for malabsorption disorders, and may refer the infant to a pediatric gastroenterologist for further evaluation.

With all the infant data available, it is now possible to determine an infant's nutritional status and potential risks.

The following example shows the effectiveness of these assessments and interventions:

> **Scenario:** *Baby girl Smith was born at 37 weeks' gestation to an 18-year-old, G1P0 via cesarean section. The father of the baby was not present. Baby Smith is now 76 hours postpartum and she and her mother are expected to go home today. While weighing the infant for a discharge weight, the mother mentions that she does not think her daughter is getting much breast milk when she feeds because her infant keeps falling asleep at the breast during the feeding. Baby Smith weighed 3542 grams at birth and her present weight is 3173 grams. (The difference is 369 grams. 369/3542 = 0.104 × 100 = 10.4% weight loss.) An assessment of the mother's breasts reveals symmetric, soft breasts and normal-shaped nipples, with nipples intact. After contacting the infant's healthcare provider to report the significant weight loss, the nurse is now ready to formulate a plan of care.*

The nurse makes the following nursing diagnoses:

Ineffective Breastfeeding related to:

- Mother's lack of knowledge about breastfeeding
- Mother's not responding to infant's feeding cues
- Mother's inability to facilitate effective breastfeeding

As evidenced by a weight loss of 10.4% in baby.

Interrupted Breastfeeding related to:

- Insufficient knowledge regarding newborn's reflexes and breastfeeding techniques
- Lack of support by father of baby or other support persons
- Lack of maternal self-confidence
- Maternal fatigue
- Possible maternal ambivalence
- Poor infant sucking reflex
- Difficulty waking the sleepy baby

Imbalanced Nutrition: Less Than Body Requirements related to:

- Mother's increased caloric and nutrient needs status post-cesarean section
- Infant's inability to correctly latch on and transfer milk

Expected Outcomes of Care

The expected outcomes for the infant include:

- Infant will arouse to feed at least every 3 hours and will stay awake until the end of each feeding.
- The infant will correctly latch on to the breasts and effectively breastfeed 8 to 12 times per day.
- The infant will gain at least 10 g/kg/day and be back to birth weight no later than day 14 of life.
- The infant will have four wet diapers, three to four bowel movements on day 4; five wet diapers, three to four bowel movements on day 5; and six to eight wet diapers, three to four bowel movements every day thereafter during the first month of life.
- Infant's stools will transition from black to yellow by day 5 and will change in consistency from thick and sticky to loose and explosive with small curds or seedy appearance.
- Infant will not have any uric acid crystals in her diaper after day 3 or 4.
- Infant will be satiated after feeding, as evidenced by relaxed muscle tone and sleepiness.

The expected outcomes for the mother include:

- Mother will verbalize/demonstrate an understanding of breastfeeding technique, including positioning and latch on, signs of adequate feeding, self-care.
- Mother will breastfeed pain-free.
- Mother will express satisfaction with the breastfeeding experience.
- Mother will consume a nutritionally balanced diet with appropriate caloric and fluid intake to support breastfeeding.

Plan of Care and Interventions

1. Review the mother's history.
   - Maternal demographics—for example, mother's date of birth, parity, marital status, cultural feeding practices
   - Pregnancy history—for example, complications during pregnancy, gestation at delivery
   - Complications of delivery—for example, cesarean section, excessive blood loss
   - Current medical issues—for example, hypothyroidism? diabetes?
   - History of breast surgery or radiation—for example, breast reduction, radiation to treat previous breast cancer
   - Use of medications, herbs, alcohol, cigarettes
   - Psychosocial history—maternal support system, history of depression, and so on
   - History of previous breastfeeding experience
2. Maternal assessment.
   - Assess the breasts and nipples.
   - Obtain a description of lochia drainage.
3. Infant assessment.
   - Obtain the infant's weight and compare with previous weight measurements.

Note: If this were an older infant, then it would be appropriate to obtain head circumference, length, and weight measurements and track the infant's trend on the growth chart; however, because this infant is only 3 days old, daily tracking of the other growth parameters is not applicable for this situation.

   - Examine the infant, with emphasis on oral anatomy and oral-motor function, infant reflexes, overall behavior, skin color (jaundice).
   - Assess the infant for signs of dehydration.
4. Infant feeding history.
   - Diet
   - Feeding frequency and duration
   - History of supplementation
   - Review elimination pattern: Number of wet diapers, quality of urine, bowel movements, quality of stool.
5. Pre- and post-breastfeeding weight check.
   - Calculate milk transfer during breastfeeding.

Note: Post-feed weight minus pre-feed weight equals net breast milk transfer. The nurse must use a digital electronic scale accurate within 2 grams. The infant does not have to be naked but the clothing and diaper the infant is wearing cannot be changed during this next measurement.

6. Observation of breastfeeding technique.
   - Positioning and latch-on technique, infant responses, suckling pattern, satiated after feeding
7. Review feeding requirement/caloric requirement based on the infant's birth weight (3.542 kg).
   - Fluid requirement: 140 to 160 ml/kg/day
     - Should be up to full volume by day 6 or so; should then receive 496 to 567 ml/day. To convert ml to oz: take 496 ml/day, divide by 30 ml/oz, this equals 16.5 oz/day. For this scenario, the infant should receive 16.5 to 18.9 oz/day.
   - The infant should feed 8 to 12 times per day. If the infant feeds 10 times per day, then the infant should feed 496/10 = 49.6 ml/feeding.
   - On day 3, the infant will *not* be expected to feed approximately 50 ml/feeding (minimum *full* volume);

based on physiologic stomach capacity, the infant may only feed about 30 ml/feeding on day 3 of life but will be increasing volume daily as tolerated until up to full volume in the next couple of days.

- Caloric requirement 100 to 115 kcal/kg/day.
    - Should be up to full caloric requirement by about day 6; should receive 354 to 407 kcal/day. Human milk has 20 kcal/oz; standard infant formula has 20 kcal/oz. To determine how many ounces the infant will require per day, take 354 kcal/day divided by 20 kcal/oz equals 17.7 oz/day. *Note: The infant should be gradually increasing her volume of milk each day and will soon be up to full volume.*

8. Assess teaching needs and provide verbal and written instructions.
    - Review benefits of breastfeeding. *Provide frequent skin-to-skin contact.*
    - Review breastfeeding technique (positioning and latch on).
    - Watch the infant for early feeding cues. *If the infant is too sleepy to exhibit these feeding behaviors, then teach the mother to watch for signs that her infant is in a light state of sleep. When the infant is in a light state of sleep, then the mother can try "wake up techniques" to help her infant wake up at least every 3 hours to feed.*
    - Provide breast pump instructions and review collection and storage.
        - *May start pumping to increase breast stimulation. All expressed breast milk should be fed to the infant. If the mother is not able to express enough milk, then the infant should be supplemented with formula.*
        - Review the process of breastfeeding (principle of supply and demand) and practice proper breastfeeding technique. *Encourage the mother to breastfeed as often as possible and observe for signs of effective breastfeeding.*
    - Review infant intake and output, weight gain expectations. *Maintain a feeding diary to monitor the infant's intake and output; call a lactation consultant or the infant's health-care provider if the infant is not meeting expectations.*
    - Provide information on maternal nutrition and fluid requirements.
        - *Rest as much as possible and be concerned only about self-care needs (i.e., prevention of engorgement, etc.) and caring for the infant right now.*
        - *Eat healthy foods and drink plenty of fluids to quench thirst.*
        - *Plan for a follow-up weight check on infant in 1 to 2 days to assess nutritional status.*

Arrange for a follow-up lactation consultation visit in 2 days to reassess the mother and infant at that time and revise the plan of care.

FOCUS YOUR STUDY

- The American Academy of Pediatrics (AAP) recommends exclusive breastfeeding for the first 6 months and continued breastfeeding until the infant is 1 year old or older.
- During the first few days after birth, the minimum output expectations for an exclusively breastfeeding infant will be: one wet/one stool on day 1; two wets/two stools on day 2; three wets/three to four stools on day 3; four wets/three to four stools on day 4; five wets/three to four stools on day 5. Thereafter, an exclusively breastfeeding infant has a minimum of six to eight wet diapers and three to four yellow milk stools each day, generally during the first month of life.
- Infants' stools start as black and sticky at birth and transition to yellow, curdy, or seedy by day 5, or sooner.
- Formula-feeding infants lose about 3.5% of their birth weight. Breastfeeding infants lose up to 7% of their birth weight. A weight loss of more than 7% is excessive and requires an evaluation and follow-up. A weight loss exceeding 10% requires an intervention that demonstrates sufficient intake for the infant, and adequate breast stimulation for the mother, and requires a plan for follow-up within a couple of days. Infants should be back to their birth weight no later than day 14 of life.
- Growth rate over the lifespan is greatest during infancy. The healthy full-term infant gains approximately 10 g/kg/day for the first month of life. Exclusively breastfed infants have the same or slightly greater weight gain in the first 3 to 4 months of life than mixed-fed and formula-fed infants. Thereafter, formula-fed and mixed-fed infants are heavier than breastfed infants.
- Increases in body length and head circumference between breastfed and formula-fed infants is the same. An infant gains 1 inch per month in the first 6 months, and then 0.5 inch for the following 6 months.

- Generally, infants double their birth weight by 5 months, triple their birth weight by 1 year of age, and quadruple their birth weight by 2 years.
- The dietary reference intake (DRI) for calories for the newborn is 100 to 115 kcal/kg/day.
- The dietary reference intake (DRI) for fluid intake for the newborn is 140 to 160 ml/kg/day.
- Human milk has immunologic and nutritional properties that make it the optimal food for the first year of life.
- Mature human milk and standard commercially prepared formulas provide 20 kcal/oz.
- The breastfed infant's iron stores from in-utero placental transfer is usually depleted by the time the infant is 6 months old. Breastfeeding infants over 6 months of age who are eating complementary foods rich in iron, and infants consuming iron-enriched formula need no other vitamin or mineral supplements with the possible exception of vitamin D.
- There are five types of commercial infant formulas: (1) standard cow's milk–based formulas, such as Enfamil and Similac; (2) soy milk–based formulas, such as ProSobee and Isomil; (3) partially hydrolyzed formulas, such as Nestlé Good Start and Enfamil Gentlease; (4) extensively hydrolyzed hypoallergenic formulas, such as Nutramigen and Alimentum; and (5) essentially nonallergenic amino acid–based formulas, such as Neocate and EleCare.
- Neither cow's milk nor soy milk should be given to infants before 1 year of age. The use of skim milk or low-fat cow's milk is not recommended for children under 2 years old.
- Signs indicating a newborn's readiness to feed include hand-to-mouth movements, rooting, smacking, fussing, and crying (a late-feeding cue).
- By learning about cultural variations, the nurse will gain an understanding of the "context" or unstated assumptions that influence behavior, thus avoiding misunderstanding and improving the ability of the nurse to communicate with patients.
- Infants should not receive water supplements until they start solid foods, generally beginning at 6 months of age.
- Although most maternal medications are transmitted through human milk to some degree, few are actually contraindicated. The bioavailability of transmitted drugs to the infant depends on a variety of factors, including route of administration, protein binding, degree of ionization, molecular weight, timing of the dose with respect to feeding time, and absorption across the infant's intestinal tract. Mothers needing to take medications or herbs should consult with a healthcare provider knowledgeable about medications and lactation.
- Breastfeeding mothers should be taught to use proper positioning and latch-on technique. The mother should be advised to alternate feeding positions periodically to promote efficient drainage of all the ducts in the breast.
- The formula-feeding mother may need help learning about the types of formulas and how to prepare and store formula. Like the breastfeeding mother, she will benefit from understanding feeding cues and proper technique for feeding her infant.
- Nutritional assessment of the infant includes the infant's dietary history, anthropometric measurements, physical examination, and laboratory tests, if indicated.

CRITICAL THINKING IN ACTION

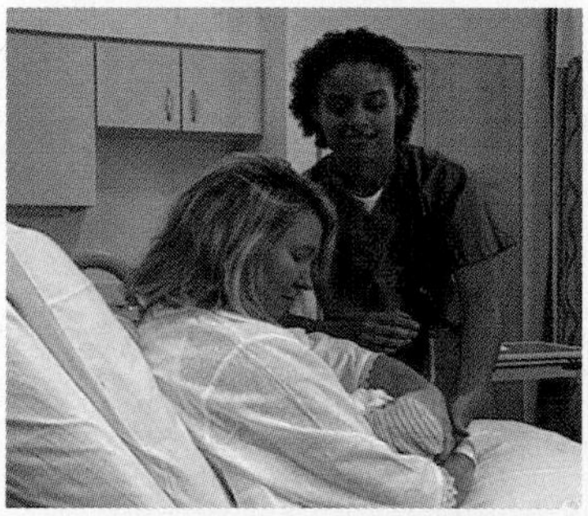

Patty Kline, age 28, G1, now P1, delivers a 7.3 pound baby girl by spontaneous vaginal birth over a median episiotomy. The newborn's Apgar scores are 8 and 9 at 1 and 5 minutes. The infant is suctioned in the nose and mouth and given free-flow oxygen on the mother's abdomen. Patty received an epidural during her labor and birth. Patty initiated breastfeeding within the first hour after the birth, but at that time the newborn did not latch on. The infant was held to the mother's breast, rooted, and licked the nipple. You are the nurse caring for the infant at 2 hours of age. The admission assessment is significant for asymmetric head with a 3-cm caput succedaneum. The infant's temperature is stable. You bring the infant to the mother's room to assist her with breastfeeding.

1. Describe clues that indicate the infant is ready to breastfeed with the mother.
2. How would you explain how to position the infant at the breast?
3. Explain what to observe for the infant's proper latch-on.
4. Explain the basics of milk production.
5. Explore helpful measures the mother can attempt in support of breastfeeding.

See www.nursing.pearsonhighered.com for possible responses.

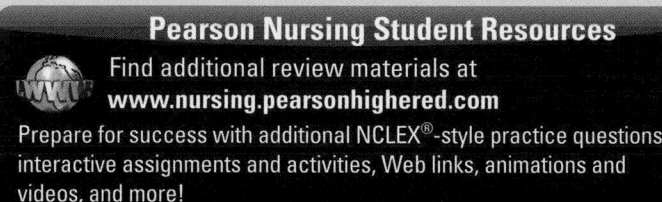

REFERENCES

Abbott Laboratories. (2009). *Formula Prep and Storage*. Retrieved from http://similac.com/baby-formula/bottle-preparation-and-storage

Abbott Nutrition. (2009). Pediatric nutrition product guide. Columbus, OH: Abbott Laboratories.

Academy of Breastfeeding Medicine (ABM). (2004). Protocol #9: Use of galactogogues initiating or augmenting maternal milk supply. *ABM News and Views, 10*(3), 20–22. Retrieved from http://www.bfmed.org/Resources/Protocols.aspx

Academy of Breastfeeding Medicine (ABM). (2009). Protocol #3: Hospital guidelines for the use of supplementary feedings in the healthy term breastfed neonate, revised 2009. *Breastfeeding Medicine, 4*(3), 175–182. doi:10.1089/bfm.2009.9991

Ameda/Hollister. (undated). Milk storage guidelines. Retrieved from http://ameda.com/milkstorage/guidelines.aspx

American Academy of Family Physicians (AAFP). (2008). Breastfeeding, family physicians supporting (position paper). Retrieved from http://www.aaafp.org/online/enhome/policy/policies/b/breastfeedingpositionpaper

American Academy of Pediatrics (AAP) Clinical Report. (2008a). Prevention of rickets and vitamin D deficiency in infants, children, and adolescents. *Pediatrics, 122*(5), 1142–1152. doi:10.1542/peds.2008-1862

American Academy of Pediatrics (AAP) Clinical Report. (2008b). Use of soy protein-based formulas infant feeding. *Pediatrics, 121*(5), 1062–1068. doi:10.1542/peds.2008-0564

American Academy of Pediatrics (AAP) Committee on Drugs. (2001). Transfer of drugs and other chemicals into human milk. *Pediatrics, 108*(3), 776–789. Retrieved from http://www.aap.org/healthtopics/breastfeeding.cfm

American Academy of Pediatrics (AAP) Committee on Fetus and Newborn. (2003, reaffirmed 2009). Policy statement: Controversies concerning vitamin K and the newborn. *Pediatrics, 112*(1), 191–192.

American Academy of Pediatrics (AAP) Healthy Children. (2010). Sleep position: Why back is best. Retrieved from http://www.healthychikldren.org/English/ages-stages/baby/sleep/pages/Sleep-Position

American Academy of Pediatrics (AAP) Section on Breastfeeding. (2005). Policy statement: Breastfeeding and the use of human milk. *Pediatrics, 115*(2), 496–506.

American Academy of Pediatrics (AAP) Committee on Fetus and Newborn & American College of Obstetricians and Gynecologists (ACOG) Committee on Obstetrics. (2007). *Guidelines for perinatal care* (6th ed.). Evanston, IL: Author.

Association of Women's Health, Obstetric, and Neonatal Nurses (AWHONN). (2007). *Breastfeeding support: Prenatal care through the first year. Evidence-based clinical practice guideline.* (2nd ed., pp. 1–89). Washington, DC: AWHONN.

Baby-Friendly Hospital Initiative USA (BFHI USA). (2010). *Implementing the UNICEF/WHO baby-friendly hospital initiative in the U.S.* Retrieved from http://www.babyfriendlyusa.org/eng/index.html

Bezerra, F. F., Mendonca, L., Lobato, E. C., O'Brien, K. O., & Donangelo, C. M. (2004). Bone mass is recovered from lactation to postweaning in adolescent mothers with low calcium intakes. *American Journal Clinical Nutrition, 80*, 1322–1326.

Blackburn, S. T. (2007). *Maternal, fetal, & neonatal physiology: A clinical perspective* (3rd ed.). St. Louis, MO: Saunders.

Briggs, G. G., Freeman, R. K., & Yaffe, S. J. (2008). Drugs in pregnancy and lactation: A reference guide to fetal and neonatal risk (8th ed.). Baltimore, MD: Lippincott Williams & Wilkins.

Brill, H. (2008). Approach to milk protein allergy in infants. *Canadian Family Physician, 54*, 1258–1264.

Callister, L. C. (2008). Integrating cultural beliefs and practices when caring for childbearing women and families. In K. R. Simpson & P. A. Creehan, *Perinatal nursing* (3rd ed., pp. 29–57). Philadelphia, PA: Lippincott Williams & Wilkins.

Centers for Disease Control and Prevention (CDC). (2009). Breastfeeding among U.S. children born 1999–2006, CDC national immunization survey. Retrieved from http://www.cdc.gov/breastfeeding/data/NIS_data/

Centers for Disease Control and Prevention (CDC). (2010). *General Recommendations on Immunization* [PDF version]. Retrieved from http://www.cdc.gov/mmwr/PDF/rr/rr5102.pdf

Chung, M., Raman, G., Trikalinos, T., Lau, J., & Ip, S. (2008). Interventions in primary care to promote breastfeeding: An evidence review for the U.S. preventative task force. *Annals of Internal Medicine, 149*, 565–582.

Cloherty, J. P., Eichenwald, E. C., & Stark, A. R. (2008). *Manual for neonatal care* (6th ed.). Philadelphia, PA: Lippincott Williams & Wilkins.

D'Avanzo, C. E., & Geissler, E. M. (2008). *Pocket guide to cultural assessment* (4th ed.). St. Louis, MO: Mosby.

Department for International Development. (2009). Breast still best for poor babies. Retrieved from http://www.developments.org.uk/articles/breast-still-best-for-poor-babies/

Geckil, E., Sahin, T., & Ege, E. (2009). Traditional postpartum practices of women and infants and the factors influencing such practices in South Eastern Turkey. *Midwifery, 25*, 62–71. doi: 10.1016/j.midw.2006.12.007

Greer, F. R., Sicherer, S. H., Burks, W., & Committee on Nutrition and Section on Allergy and Immunology. (2008). Effects of early nutritional interventions on the development of atropic disease in infants and children: The role of maternal dietary restriction, breastfeeding, timing of introduction of complementary foods, and hydrolyzed formulas. *Pediatrics, 121*(1), 183–191.

Hale, T. W. (2010). *Medications and mothers' milk* (14th ed.). Amarillo, TX: Pharmasoft.

Human Milk Banking Association of North America (HMBANA). (2006). *Best practice for expressing, storing and handling human milk in hospitals, homes and child care settings.* Raleigh, NC: HMBANA. Inc.

International Labour Organization. (2004). Parental leave act—Sweden. Retrieved from http://www.ilo.org/public/english/employment/gems/eeo/law/sweden/l_plas.htm

Jana, L. A., & Shu, J. (2005). *Heading home with your newborn: From birth to reality.* Washington, DC: AAP Association of American Publishers, Inc.

Kent, G. (2006). WIC's promotion of infant formula in the United States. *International Breastfeeding Journal, 1*(8), 1–8. Retrieved from http://www.internationalbreastfeedingjournal.com/content/1/1/8

Klaus, M. (1998). Mother and infant: Early emotional ties. *Pediatrics, 102*(5), 1244–1246.

Lawrence, R. A., & Lawrence, R. M. (2005). *Breastfeeding: A guide for the medical profession* (6th ed.). Philadelphia, PA: Mosby.

Levin, M. B., Cotton, J. M., Patrick-Miller, T. J., Tesoro, L. J., & Rose, H. M. (2010). The pediatric group brochure on formula feeding: Formula feeding information. Retrieved from http://www.pedgroup.com/frmlabrc.htm

Lipson, J. G., & Dibble, S. L. (2008). *Culture & Clinical Care* (7th ed.). San Franciso, CA: The Regents, University of California.

Marks, J. W. (2008). *Lactose intolerance (lactase deficiency)* (D. Lee, Ed.). Retrieved from http://www.medicinenet.com/lactose_intolerance/article.htm

McCarter-Spaulding, D., & Gore, R. (2009). Brestfeeding self-efficacy in women of African descent. *JOGNN, 38*(2), 230–243.

McDowell, M. M., Wang, C. Y., & Kennedy-Stephenson, J. (2008). Breastfeeding in the United States: Findings from the National Health and Nutrition Examination Surveys 1999–2006. NCHS Data Brief, No. 5, April 2008.

Mead-Johnson & Company. (2009). *Preparing your baby's bottle.* Retrieved from http://www.enfamil.com/app/iwp/enfamil/article.do?dm=enf&id=/Consumer_Home2/Enf_Feeding/Enf_Feeding_Guide/preparingbottle&iwpst=B2C&ls=0&csred=1&r=3430830610

Mead-Johnson Nutritionals. (2010). *Pediatric products handbook.* New York, NY: Bristol-Myers Squibb Company.

Mennella, J. A., Yourshaw, L. M., & Morgan, L. K. (2007). Breastfeeding and smoking: Short-term effects on infant feeding and sleep. *Pediatrics, 120*(3), 497–502. doi: 10.1542/peds.2007-488

Mercer, A. M., Teasley, S. L., Hopkinson, J., McPherson, D. M., Simon, S. D., & Hall R. T. (2010). Evaluation of a breastfeeding assessment score in a diverse population. *Journal of Human Lactation, 26*(1), 42–48.

Mohrbacher, N., & Kendall-Tackett, K. (2005). *Breastfeeding made simple: Seven natural laws for nursing mothers.* Oakland, CA: New Harbinger Publications, Inc.

Morin, K. (2005). Information parents need about preparing formula. *American Journal of Maternal/Child Nursing, 30*(5), 334.

National Conference of State Legislatures. (2009). Breastfeeding laws. Retrieved from http://www.ncsl.org/default.aspx?tabid=14389

National Toxicology Program Center for the Evaluation of Risks to Human Reproduction (NTP-CERHR). (2008). *NTP-CERHR Monograph on the potential human reproductive and developmental effects of bisphenol A. NIH Publication No 08-5994.* Research Triangle Park, NJ: National Toxicology Program. Available at: http://cerhr.niehs.nih.gov/chemicals/bisphenol/bisphenol.pdf

Nestlé Nutrition. (2009). How to prepare your baby's bottle. Retrieved from http://www.gerber.com/Articles/How_to_prepare_your_babys_bottle.aspx

Ott, B. B., Al-Khadhuri, J., & Al-Junaibi, S. (2003). Preventing ethical dilemmas: Understanding Islamic health care practices. *Pediatric Nursing, 29*(3), 227–230.

Riordan, J., & Wambach, K. (2010). *Breastfeeding and human lactation* (4th ed.). Boston, MA: Jones & Bartlett.

Rolfes, S. R., Pinna, K., & Whitney, E. (2006). *Understanding normal and clinical nutrition* (7th ed.). Belmont, CA: Thomson Wadsworth.

Sacco, L. M. Caulfield, L. E., Gittelsohn, J., & Martínez, H. (2006). The conception of perceived insufficient milk among Mexican mothers. *Journal of Human Lactation, 22*(3), 277–286. doi:10.1177/08903344062

Schuman, J. (2003). A concise history of infant formula (twists and turns included). *Contemporary Pediatrics*. Retrieved from http://www.contemporarypediatrics.com/contpeds/article/articleDetail.jsp?id=111702

Sears, W. (2009). A word about bottle-feeding. Retrieved from http://www.askdrsears.com/html/0/T000100.asp#T031010

Stevens, E. E., Patrick, T. E., & Pickler, R. (2009). A history of infant feeding. *Journal of Perinatal Education. 18*(2), 32–39. doi:10.1624/105812409X426314

Teh, L. (undated). No bathing, no visiting, and no drinking water: The confinement of Chinese mothers. Retrieved from http://www.geocities.com/Wellesley/3321/win14c.htm

Thibodeau, G., & Patton, K. T. (2009). *The human body in health & disease* (4th ed.). St. Louis, MO: Mosby.

Vartabedian, B. (2007). *Colic solved.* New York, NY: Ballantine Books.

Vom Saal, F. S., Akingbemi, B. T., Belcher, S. M., Birnbaum, L. S., Crain, D. A, Eriksen, M. et al. (2007). Chapel Hill bisphenol A expert panel consensus statement: Integration of mechanisms, effects in animals and potential to impact human health at current levels of exposure. *Reproductive Toxicology, 24*, 131–138.

West, D., & Marasco, L. (2009). *The breastfeeding mother's guide to making more milk.* New York, NY: McGraw-Hill.

World Health Organization (WHO), Department of Child and Adolescent Health and Development (CAH). (2003). *Community-based strategies for breastfeeding promotion and support in developing countries.* Geneva, Switzerland: WHO.

World Health Organization/United Nations Children's Emergency Fund (WHO/UNICEF). (1994). *U.S. committee for UNICEF interim program in the United States to promote the baby friendly ten steps to successful breastfeeding.* Washington, DC: Government Printing Office.

World Health Organization/United Nations Children's Emergency Fund (WHO/UNICEF). (2009). *Acceptable medical reasons for use of breast-milk substitutes.* Retrieved from http://www.who.int/nutrition/publications/infantfeeding/WHO_NMH_NHD_09.01_eng.pdf

CHAPTER 33

The Newborn at Risk: Conditions Present at Birth

When I approach a child,
He inspires me in two sentiments:
Tenderness for what he is,
And respect for what he may become.

—Louis Pasteur

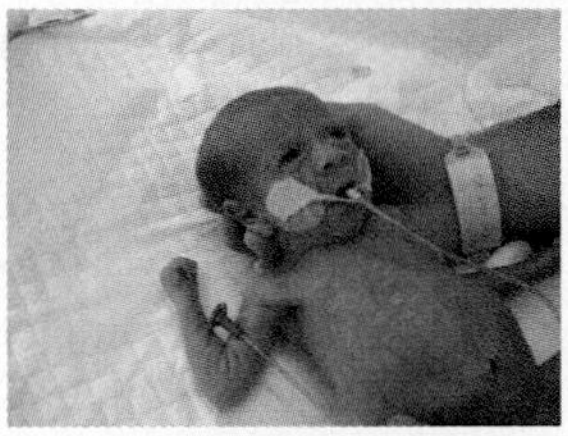

LEARNING OUTCOMES

1. Identify the factors present at birth that indicate an at-risk newborn.
2. Compare the underlying etiologies of the physiologic complications of small-for-gestational-age (SGA) newborns and preterm appropriate-for-gestational-age (Pr AGA) newborns and the nursing care management for each.
3. Describe the impact of maternal diabetes mellitus on the newborn.
4. Compare the characteristics and potential complications that influence nursing management of the postterm newborn and the newborn with postmaturity syndrome.
5. Discuss the physiologic characteristics of the preterm newborn that predispose each body system to various complications and are used in development of a plan of care that includes nutritional management.
6. Summarize the nursing assessments of and initial interventions for a newborn born with selected congenital anomalies.
7. Explain the special care needed by an alcohol or drug-exposed newborn.
8. Relate the consequences of maternal HIV/AIDS to the management of and issues for caregivers of infants at risk for HIV/AIDS in the neonatal period.
9. Identify physical examination findings during the early newborn period that would make the nurse suspect a congenital cardiac defect or congestive heart failure.
10. Explain the special care needed by a newborn with an inborn error of metabolism.

KEY TERMS

Fetal alcohol spectrum disorder (FASD) *921*
Fetal alcohol syndrome (FAS) *921*
Inborn errors of metabolism *931*
Infant of diabetic mother (IDM) *898*
Infant of substance-abusing mother (ISAM) *921*
Intrauterine growth restriction (IUGR) *891*
Large for gestational age (LGA) *897*
Neonatal morbidity *890*
Neonatal mortality risk *890*
Phenylketonuria (PKU) *931*
Postmaturity *900*
Postterm newborn *900*
Preterm infant *901*
Small for gestational age (SGA) *891*

The field of neonatology has expanded greatly. Many levels of nursery care have evolved in response to increasing knowledge about the newborn: special care, intensive care, and convalescent care. Along with the newborn's parents, the nurse is an important caregiver in all these settings. As a professional member of the multidisciplinary healthcare team, the nurse provides the holistic care necessary in the often high-tech perinatal environment.

In addition to the availability of excellent intensive care services, a variety of other factors influences the outcomes of at-risk infants, including the following:

- Birth weight
- Gestational age
- Type and length of newborn illness
- Environmental factors
- Maternal factors
- Maternal-infant separation

Identification of At-Risk Newborns

An at-risk newborn is one who is susceptible to illness (morbidity) or even death (mortality) because of dysmaturity, immaturity, physical disorders, or complications during or after birth. In most cases, the infant is the product of pregnancy involving one or more predictable risk factors, including the following:

- Low socioeconomic level of the mother.
- Limited access to health care or no prenatal care.
- Exposure to environmental dangers, such as toxic chemicals and illicit drugs.
- Preexisting maternal conditions, such as heart disease, diabetes, hypertension, hyperthyroidism, and renal disease.
- Maternal factors such as age or parity.
- Medical conditions related to pregnancy and their associated complications.
- Pregnancy complications such as abruptio placentae, placenta previa, oligohydramnios, preterm labor, premature rupture of membranes, preeclampsia, uterine rupture.

Various risk factors and their specific effects on the pregnancy outcome are identified in Table 15-1 ∞ on page 321. Because these factors and the perinatal risks associated with them are known, the birth of at-risk newborns can often be anticipated. The pregnancy can be closely monitored, treatment can be started as necessary, and arrangements can be made for birth to occur at a facility with appropriate resources to care for both mother and baby.

Whether or not prenatal assessment indicates that the fetus is at risk, the course of labor and birth and the infant's ability to withstand the stress of labor cannot be predicted. The nurse's use of electronic fetal heart monitoring or fetal heart auscultation by Doppler plays a significant role in detecting stress or distress in the fetus. Immediately after birth, the Apgar score is a helpful tool in identifying the at-risk newborn, but it is not the only indicator of possible long-term outcome.

The newborn classification and neonatal mortality risk chart is another useful tool in identifying newborns at risk. Before this classification tool was developed, birth weight of less than 2500 g was the sole criterion for determination of immaturity. Clinicians then recognized that newborns could weigh more than 2500 g but still be immature. Conversely, an infant weighing less than 2500 g might be functionally mature at term or beyond. Birth weight and gestational age together became the criteria used to assess neonatal maturity and mortality risk.

According to the newborn classification and neonatal mortality risk chart, gestation is divided as follows (Gardner & Hernandez, 2011):

- Preterm: less than 37 (completed) weeks
- Late preterm: 34 to 36 6/7 weeks
- Term: 38 to 41 (completed) weeks
- Postterm: greater than 42 weeks

Late preterm is an emerging classification that refers to subgroups of infants between 34 and 37 weeks' gestation; however, it is not yet used consistently for a single age range (Gardner & Hernandez, 2011). (See chapter 37 ∞ for discussion of long-term needs of late preterm infants.)

As shown in Figure 33-1 ■, large-for-gestational-age (LGA) infants are those who plot above the 90th percentile growth curve. Appropriate-for-gestational-age (AGA) infants are those between the 10th percentile and 90th percentile growth curve. Small-for-gestational-age (SGA) infants are those below the 10th percentile growth curve. A newborn is assigned to a category depending on birth weight, length, occipital-frontal circumference, and gestational age. For example, a newborn classified as Pr SGA is preterm and small for gestational age. The full-term newborn whose weight is appropriate for gestational age is classified F AGA. It is important to remember that the intrauterine growth curve charts are influenced by altitude and the ethnicity of the newborn population used to create the chart. Also the assigned newborn classification may vary according to the intrauterine growth curve chart used; therefore, the chart used should correlate with the characteristics of the patient population.

Neonatal mortality risk is the chance of death within the neonatal period, that is, within the first 28 days of life. Seventy-five percent of all neonatal deaths occur within the first week, with the highest rates occurring during the first day of life. As indicated in Figure 33-1, the neonatal mortality risk decreases as both gestational age and birth weight increase. Infants who are Pr SGA have the highest neonatal mortality risk. The previously high mortality rates for LGA infants have decreased at most perinatal centers because of improved management of diabetes in pregnancy and recognition of potential complications of LGA newborns.

Neonatal morbidity can also be anticipated based on birth weight and gestational age. In Figure 33-2 ■, the infant's birth weight is located on the vertical axis, and the gestational age in weeks is found along the horizontal axis. The area where the two meet on the graph identifies common problems. This tool assists in determining the needs of particular infants for special observation and care. For example, an infant of 2000 g at 40

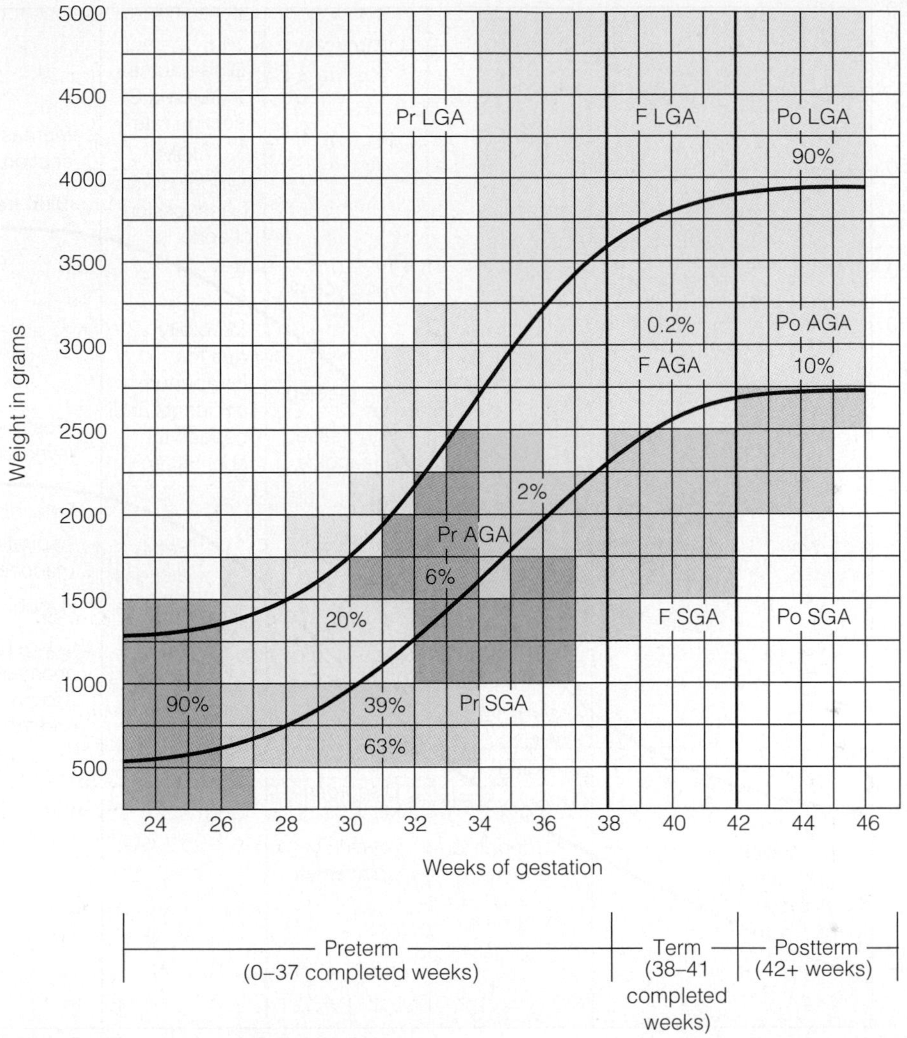

Figure 33-1 ■ Newborn classification and neonatal mortality risk chart. Infants are classified according to weight as small for gestational age (SGA), appropriate for gestational age (AGA), or large for gestational age (LGA) and by weeks of newborn as preterm (Pr), term (F), or postterm (Po). Corresponding neonatal mortality risks are indicated by the percentages in the various colored regions.

Source: Reprinted from Koops, B. L., Morgan, L. P., & Battaglia, F. C., Neonatal mortality risk in relationship to birth weight and gestational age. Journal of Pediatrics, 101*(6), 969. Copyright 1982, with permission from Elsevier.*

weeks' gestation should be carefully assessed for evidence of nonreassuring fetal status, hypoglycemia, congenital anomalies, congenital infection, and polycythemia.

Identifying the nursing care needs of the at-risk newborn depends on minute-to-minute observations of the changes in the newborn's physiologic status. Nursing care management should be directed toward the following:

- Decreasing physiologically stressful situations.
- Constantly observing for subtle signs of change in clinical condition.
- Interpreting laboratory data and coordinating interventions.
- Conserving the infant's energy for healing and growth.
- Providing for developmental stimulation and maintenance of sleep cycles.
- Assisting the family in developing attachment behaviors.
- Involving the family in planning and providing care.

Care of the Small-for-Gestational-Age/Intrauterine Growth Restricted Newborn

Currently infants are considered **small for gestational age (SGA)** when they are less than the 10th percentile for birth weight; very small for gestational age is when they are two standard deviations below the population norm or at less than the third percentile (Cunningham et al., 2010) (see Figure 33-1). When possible, the birth weight charts used to assign the SGA classification to a newborn should be based on the local population into which the newborn is born. A SGA newborn may be preterm, term, or postterm. An undergrown newborn may be also said to have **intrauterine growth restriction (IUGR)**, which describes the pregnancy circumstance of advanced gestation and limited fetal growth. This classification of abnormal growth is

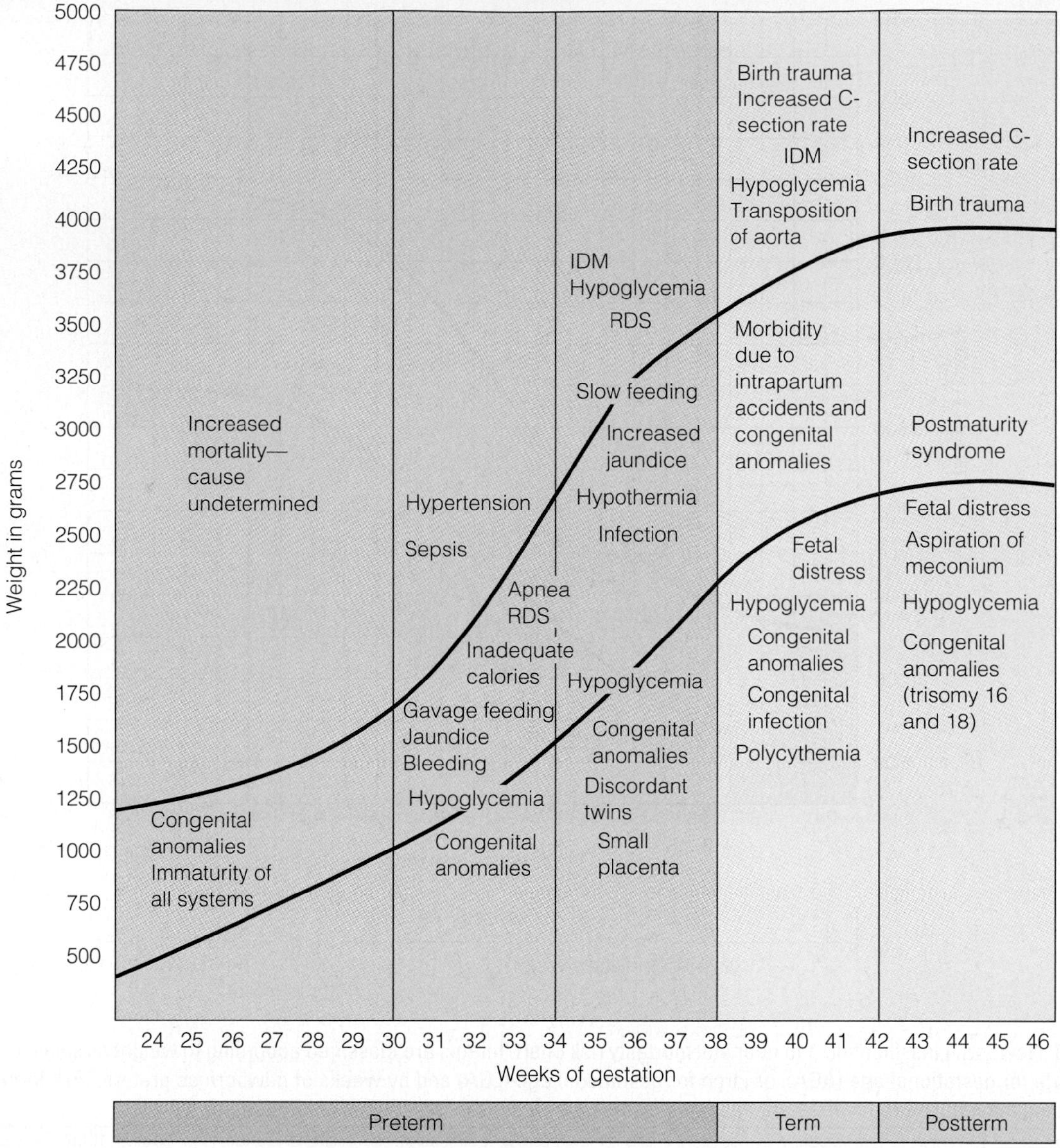

Figure 33-2 ■ Neonatal morbidity by birth weight and gestational age.

Source: Reprinted from Lubchenco, L. O., The high-risk infant, *p. 122. Copyright 1976, with permission from Elsevier.*

also enhanced by looking at growth potential by adjusting birth-weight reference limits for first trimester maternal height, birth order, and fetal neonatal sex. The terms SGA and IUGR are not necessarily interchangeable.

SGA infants are commonly seen with mothers who smoke or have high blood pressure, causing these infants to have an increased incidence of perinatal asphyxia and perinatal mortality when compared with AGA infants (Resnik & Creasy, 2009). The incidence of polycythemia and hypoglycemia are also higher in this group of infants.

Factors Contributing to Intrauterine Growth Restriction

IUGR may be caused by maternal, placental, or fetal factors and may not be apparent antenatally. In the normal pregnancy, intrauterine growth is linear (follows expected growth line) from approximately 28 to 38 weeks' gestation. After 38 weeks, growth is variable, depending on the genetic growth potential of the fetus and placental function. The most common causes of growth restriction are the following:

- ***Maternal factors.*** Primiparity, grand multiparity, multiple-gestation pregnancy (twins and higher order multiples), lack of prenatal care, age extremes (under 16 or over 40), and low socioeconomic status (which can result in inadequate health care, inadequate education, inadequate living conditions, and malnutrition) affect IUGR (Resnik & Creasy, 2009). Before the third trimester, the nutritional supply to the fetus far exceeds his or her needs. Only in the third trimester are maternal malnutrition and drug abuse limiting factors in fetal growth.
- ***Maternal disease.*** Maternal heart disease, substance abuse (drugs, tobacco, alcohol), sickle cell anemia, phenylketonuria (PKU), lupus erythematosus, and asymptomatic pyelonephritis are associated with SGA. Complications asso-

ciated with preeclampsia, chronic hypertensive vascular disease, and advanced diabetes mellitus can diminish blood flow to the uterus, thereby decreasing oxygen delivery to the fetus.

- ***Environmental factors.*** High altitude, exposure to x-rays, excessive exercise, work-related exposure to toxins, hyperthermia, and maternal use of teratogenic drugs, such as nicotine, alcohol, antimetabolics, anticonvulsants, narcotics, and cocaine affect fetal growth (Resnik & Creasy, 2009).
- ***Placental factors.*** Placental conditions such as small placenta, infarcted areas, abnormal cord insertions, placenta previa, reverse end-diastolic blood flow, or thrombosis may affect circulation to the fetus, which becomes more deficient with increasing gestational age.
- ***Fetal factors.*** Congenital infections such as TORCH infections (*t*oxoplasmosis, *o*ther, *r*ubella, *c*ytomegalovirus, *h*erpes simplex virus), syphilis, congenital malformations, discordant twins (see chapter 11 ∞), sex of the fetus (females tend to be smaller), chromosomal abnormalities (trisomies 13, 18, and 21), two-vessel umbilical cord, and inborn errors of metabolism can all predispose a fetus to growth disturbances.

Identifying fetuses with IUGR is the first step in detecting common disorders associated with affected newborns. The perinatal history of maternal conditions, early dating of pregnancy by first trimester ultrasound measurements, antepartal testing (nonstress test, contraction stress test, biophysical profile—see chapter 21 ∞), Doppler velocimetry of the placenta, gestational age assessment, and the physical and neurologic assessment of the newborn are also important (Cloherty et al., 2008).

Patterns of IUGR

Intrauterine growth occurs by an increase in cell number and cell size. If insult occurs early during the critical period of organ development in the fetus, fewer new cells are formed, organs are small, and organ weight is subnormal. In contrast, growth failure that begins later in pregnancy does not affect the total number of cells, only their size. The organs are normal, but their size is diminished. There are two clinical pictures of IUGR newborns.

Symmetric (proportional) IUGR is caused by long-term maternal conditions (such as chronic hypertension, severe malnutrition, chronic intrauterine infection, substance abuse [drugs, alcohol, tobacco], and anemia) or fetal genetic abnormalities (Resnik & Creasy, 2009). Symmetric IUGR can be noted by ultrasound in the first half of the second trimester. In symmetric IUGR there is chronic, prolonged restriction of growth in size of organs, body weight, body length, and, especially, head circumference.

Asymmetric (disproportional) IUGR is associated with an acute compromise of uteroplacental blood flow. Some causes are placental infarcts, preeclampsia, and poor weight gain in pregnancy. The growth restriction may not be evident before the third trimester because although weight is decreased, length and head circumference remain appropriate for that gestational age. In these infants, head growth is usually spared. After 36 weeks' gestation, the abdominal circumference of a normal fetus becomes larger than the head circumference. In asymmetric IUGR, the head circumference remains larger than the abdominal circumference. Thus measuring only the biparietal diameter on ultrasound will not reveal asymmetric IUGR. An early indicator of asymmetric SGA is a decrease in the growth rate of the abdominal circumference, reflecting subnormal liver growth, a reduction in glycogen stores, and a scarcity of subcutaneous fat (Resnik & Creasy, 2009). Birth weight is below the 10th percentile, whereas head circumference, and/or length, may plot between the 10th and 90th percentiles. Asymmetric SGA newborns are particularly at risk for perinatal asphyxia, pulmonary hemorrhage, hypocalcemia, and hypoglycemia in the newborn period.

Despite growth restriction, physiologic maturity develops according to gestational age. Therefore, the term SGA newborn's chances for survival are better than those of the preterm AGA newborn and less predisposed to complications of prematurity such as respiratory distress syndrome and hyperbilirubinemia because of organ maturity. This newborn, however, still faces many other potential difficulties.

Common Complications of the SGA Newborn

The complications occurring most frequently in the SGA newborn include the following:

- ***Fetal hypoxia.*** The SGA infant suffers from chronically lower-than-normal oxygen levels in utero because of placental insufficiency, which leaves little reserve to withstand the demands of labor and birth. Thus intrauterine asphyxia can occur with its potential systemic problems. Cesarean birth may be necessary.
- ***Aspiration syndrome.*** In utero, hypoxia can cause the fetus to gasp during birth, resulting in aspiration of amniotic fluid into the lower airways. It can also lead to relaxation of the anal sphincter and passage of meconium. This may result in aspiration of the meconium in utero or with the first breaths after birth.
- ***Hypothermia.*** Diminished subcutaneous fat (used for survival in utero), depletion of brown fat in utero, and a large surface area decrease the IUGR newborn's ability to conserve heat. The flexed position assumed by the term SGA newborn diminishes the effect of surface area.
- ***Hypoglycemia.*** An increase in metabolic rate in response to heat loss and poor hepatic glycogen stores cause hypoglycemia. In addition, the infant is compromised by inadequate supplies of enzymes to activate gluconeogenesis (conversion of nonglucogen sources, such as fatty acids and proteins, to glucose).
- ***Polycythemia.*** The number of red blood cells is increased in the SGA newborn. This finding is considered a physiologic response to in utero chronic hypoxic stress. Polycythemia may contribute to hypoglycemia.

Newborns with significant IUGR tend to have a poor prognosis, especially when born before 37 weeks' gestation. Factors contributing to poor outcome include:

- ***Congenital malformations.*** Congenital malformations occur in 5% of SGA infants (Cloherty et al., 2008). The more severe the IUGR, the greater the chance for malformation as a result of impaired mitotic activity and cellular hypoplasia.

- ***Intrauterine infection.*** Fetuses exposed to intrauterine infections such as rubella and cytomegalovirus are profoundly affected by direct invasion of the brain and other vital organs by the offending virus, resulting in IUGR.
- ***Continued growth difficulties.*** SGA newborns tend to be shorter than newborns of the same gestational age. Asymmetric IUGR infants can be expected to catch up in weight and approach their inherited growth potential when given an optimal environment.
- ***Cognitive difficulties.*** Often SGA newborns can exhibit subsequent learning disabilities. The disabilities are characterized by hyperactivity, short attention span, and poor fine motor coordination (writing and drawing). Some hearing loss and speech defects also occur (Cunningham et al., 2010).

CLINICAL TIP

In assessing a growth-restricted infant resulting from unexplained maternal etiology (e.g., hypertension, placental insufficiency), an in utero viral infection may be the answer.

Clinical Therapy

The goal of medical therapy for SGA infants is early recognition and implementation of medical management of the potential problems.

NURSING CARE MANAGEMENT

Nursing Assessment and Diagnosis

The nurse is responsible for assessing gestational age and identifying signs of potential complications associated with SGA infants. All body parts of the symmetric IUGR infant are in proportion, but they are below normal size for the baby's gestational age. Therefore, the head does not appear overly large or the length excessive in relation to the other body parts. These newborns are generally vigorous.

The asymmetric IUGR infant appears long, thin, and emaciated, with loss of subcutaneous fat tissue and muscle mass (Figure 33-3 ■). The baby may have loose skin folds; dry, desquamating skin; and a thin and often meconium-stained cord. The head appears relatively large (although it approaches normal size) because the chest size and abdominal girth are decreased. The baby may have a vigorous cry and appear alert and wide eyed.

Nursing diagnoses that may apply to the SGA newborn include the following:

- ***Impaired Gas Exchange*** related to aspiration of amniotic or meconium-stained fluid
- ***Hypothermia*** related to decreased subcutaneous fat
- ***Risk for Injury*** related to decreased glycogen stores and impaired gluconeogenesis
- ***Imbalanced Nutrition: Less Than Body Requirements*** related to SGA's increased metabolic rate
- ***Ineffective Peripheral Tissue Perfusion*** related to polycythemia and increased blood viscosity

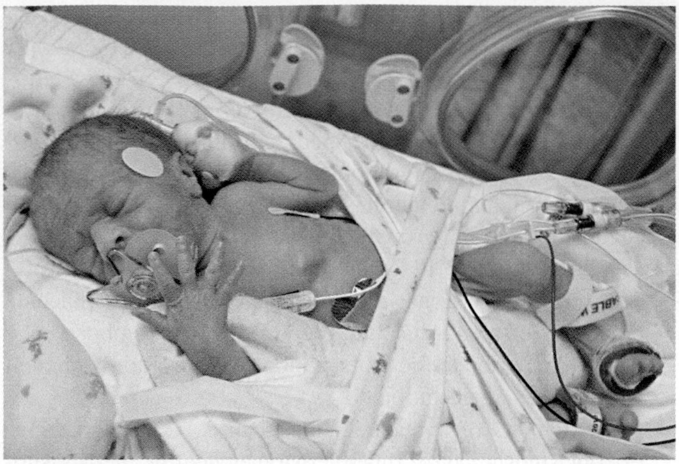

Figure 33-3 ■ Thirty-one-week gestational age, 2-day-old baby girl.

Source: Courtesy of Carol Harrigan, RN, MSN, NNP-BC.

- ***Risk for Impaired Parenting*** related to prolonged separation of newborn from parents secondary to illness

Nursing Plan and Implementation

Hospital-Based Nursing Care

Hypoglycemia, the most common metabolic complication of IUGR, produces such sequelae as central nervous system abnormalities and intellectual disability (mental retardation). Conditions such as asphyxia, hyperviscosity, and cold stress may also affect the baby's outcome. Paying meticulous attention to physiologic parameters is essential for immediate nursing management and reduction of long-term disorders (see the following Nursing Care Plan: For the Small-for-Gestational-Age Newborn on pages 895–897).

Community-Based Nursing Care

The long-term needs of the SGA newborn include careful follow-up evaluation of patterns of growth and possible disabilities that may later interfere with learning or motor functioning. Long-term follow-up care is especially necessary for those infants with congenital malformations, congenital infections, and obvious sequelae from physiologic problems. Parents of the IUGR newborn need support, because a positive atmosphere can enhance the baby's growth potential and the child's ultimate outcome.

Evaluation

Expected outcomes of nursing care include the following:

- The SGA newborn is free from respiratory compromise.
- The SGA newborn maintains a stable temperature.
- The SGA infant is free from hypoglycemic episodes and maintains glucose hemostasis.
- The SGA newborn gains weight and takes breast- or formula-feedings without physiologic distress or fatigue.
- The parents verbalize their concerns surrounding their baby's health problems and understand the rationale behind management of their newborn.

NURSING CARE PLAN For the Small-for-Gestational-Age Newborn

INTERVENTION	RATIONALE
1. Nursing Diagnosis: Impaired Gas Exchange related to amniotic fluid or meconium aspiration **Goal:** The newborn's respirations will be within normal limits, no periods of apnea or evidence of worsening distress.	
■ Obtain maternal prenatal, labor, and birth records.	■ Provides information of fetal stress that may have occurred during the prenatal or intrapartal period. In addition, the birth record will provide information concerning the infant's respiratory status at birth; for example, the Apgar score.
■ Maintain airway patency through judicious suctioning.	■ Respiratory distress in small-for-gestational-age (SGA) newborns is due to in utero hypoxia and aspiration of meconium.
■ Observe for worsening signs of respiratory distress such as generalized cyanosis; worsening retractions, grunting, and nasal flaring, as evidenced by Silverman respiratory index; sustained tachypnea; apnea episodes; inequality of breath sounds; presence of rales and rhonchi, decreased oxygenation saturation (less than 86%).	
■ Monitor and maintain adequate axillary body temperature (36.4°C to 37.2°C [97.5°F to 99°F]) to avoid increased oxygen consumption.	■ Temperature elevation may cause metabolic rate and oxygen needs to increase when associated with meconium aspiration.
■ Administer oxygen or other interventions (e.g., nasal continuous positive airway pressure [CPAP], intubation) per order for relief of respiratory distress signs. (See chapter 34 ∞ for nursing care and treatment of meconium aspiration, infant resuscitation.)	■ Provides healthcare personnel with information on cardiac and pulmonary status.
■ Implement treatment plan for respiratory distress.	
■ Monitor glucose levels.	■ Respiratory distress increases consumption of glucose.
Collaborative: Obtain arterial blood gases (ABGs) and chest x-ray per physician/neonatal nurse practitioner (NNP) orders.	
■ Monitor infant's cardiac status, pulmonary status, pulse oximetry, and ABGs.	■ Oxygen demands increase with meconium aspiration. Obtaining serial ABGs and chest x-ray will provide medical personnel baseline information of infant's respiratory status, and effective medical interventions can be initiated.
EXPECTED OUTCOMES:	The newborn will maintain adequate respiratory gas exchange as evidenced by: respirations of 30–60/min with pulse oximetry and arterial blood gases within normal limits, and show no signs and symptoms of respiratory distress.
2. Nursing Diagnosis: Risk for Ineffective Thermoregulation and Cold Stress secondary to decreased subcutaneous fat **Goal:** The infant's temperature will be stable and maintained within normal limits.	
■ Provide neutral thermal environment (NTE) range for infant based on postnatal weight.	■ Neutral thermal environment charts used for preterm infant are not reliable for weight of SGA infant.
■ Place a skin probe to maintain infant's temperature at 36°C to 36.5°C.	■ A neutral thermal environment requires minimal oxygen consumption to maintain a normal core temperature.
■ Obtain axillary temperatures and compare with registered skin probe temperature. If discrepancy exists, evaluate potential cause.	■ Discrepancies between axillary and skin probe monitor temperatures may be due to mechanical causes or the burning of brown fat.
■ Adjust and monitor incubator or radiant warmer to maintain skin temperature.	
■ Minimize heat losses and prevent cold stress by: 1. Warming and humidifying oxygen without blowing over face to avoid increasing oxygen consumption 2. Keeping skin dry, especially immediately following delivery 3. Keeping incubators, radiant warmers, and cribs away from windows and cold external walls and out of drafts 4. Avoiding placing infant on cold surrounding objects such as metal treatment tables, cold x-ray plates, and scales 5. Padding cold surfaces with diapers and using radiant warmers during procedures 6. Warming blood for exchange transfusions	■ Physical principles of heat loss effects include: 1. Evaporation—loss of heat from infant by water evaporation from the skin 2. Convection—loss of heat from infant to the surrounding air 3. Conduction—loss of heat from infant to the surface in which he or she is in direct contact with 4. Radiation—loss of heat from infant to cooler, surrounding surfaces (not in direct contact)

(continued)

NURSING CARE PLAN For the Small-for-Gestational-Age Newborn continued

INTERVENTION	RATIONALE
■ Observe for signs and symptoms of cold stress: decreased temperature, lethargy, pallor (for further discussion see chapter 34)	■ Hypothermia is a potential problem for an SGA infant because: 1. SGA infant has decreased stores of brown fat available for thermogenesis, because SGA infant has used these stores in utero for survival. 2. SGA infant has poor insulation due to use of subcutaneous tissues in utero for survival.

EXPECTED OUTCOMES: The infant will not exhibit signs and symptoms of hypothermia as evidenced by axillary temperature maintenance of 36.4°C–37.2°C (97.5°F–99°F) and no signs and symptoms of respiratory distress.

3. Nursing Diagnosis: Risk for Injury related to decreased glycogen stores and impaired gluconeogenesis
Goal: Newborn will have a normal blood glucose level.

INTERVENTION	RATIONALE
■ Monitor blood glucose levels per SGA protocol and report values less than 45 mg/dl. (The exact definition of hypoglycemia varies in the literature; it is best to follow your hospital's guidelines.)	■ Combined with depletion of glycogen stores, impaired gluconeogenesis predisposes SGA infants to profound hypoglycemia within first 2 days of life.
■ Observe, record, and report signs of hypoglycemia: cyanosis, lethargy, hypotonia, poor feeding, temperature instability, jitteriness, seizure activity, and apnea.	■ Hypoglycemia in SGA infant is indicated by whole blood sugar less than 20 mg/dl.
■ Initiate feeding schedule for SGA newborns after assessing for low blood glucose levels and signs of respiratory distress per agency protocol.	■ Frequent monitoring of heel stick glucose assists in identifying decreasing glucose levels.
■ Provide glucose intake either through early enteral feeding (before 4 hr) or by intravenous (IV) per physician/NNP order.	■ Provision of glucose through early feedings (begin before 4 hr of age) assists in maintaining glucose levels.

See further discussion of hypoglycemia in chapter 34.

EXPECTED OUTCOMES: The infant will not exhibit signs and symptoms of hypoglycemia as evidenced by a euglycemic state and blood glucose greater than 20 mg/dl.

4. Nursing Diagnosis: Altered Nutrition: Less Than Body Requirements related to increased metabolic needs in the infant
Goal: Newborn will gain weight and tolerate nipple feedings without tiring.

INTERVENTION	RATIONALE
■ Assess suck, swallow, gag, and cough reflexes.	■ Sterile water may be used to test gag & swallow reflex because it causes fewer pulmonary complications in the presence of gastrointestinal tract abnormalities and/or aspiration of feeding. ■ Prevents feeding problems and assists in determining the best method of feeding for infant.
■ Initiate formula-feeding per protocol at 1 hour of age; move early to formula-feeding every 2–3 hr.	■ SGA newborns require more calories/kg for growth than appropriate-for-gestational-age (AGA) newborns because of increased metabolic activity and oxygen consumption secondary to increased percentage of body weight made up by visceral organs.
■ Supplement oral feedings with IV intake per orders. ■ Use concentrated formulas that supply more calories in less volume, such as 22 or 24 cal/oz.	■ Small, frequent feedings of high caloric formula are used because of limited gastric capacity and decreased gastric emptying.
■ Promote growth by providing caloric intake of 120–150 cal/kg/day in small amounts.	■ Growth is evaluated by increase in weight (about 20 g/day), length, and body measurements.
■ Observe, record, and report signs of respiratory distress or fatigue occurring during feedings.	■ Decrease in exhaustion is an important consideration in feeding SGA infant. ■ Adequate nutritional intake promotes growth and prevents such complications as metabolic catabolism and hypoglycemia.
■ Supplement gavage or nipple feedings with IV therapy per physician order until oral intake is sufficient to support growth.	■ Gavage feedings require less energy expenditure on the part of the newborn.
■ Establish a nipple feeding program that is begun slowly and progresses slowly, such as nipple feed once per day, nipple feed once per shift, and then nipple feed every other feeding.	

NURSING CARE PLAN For the Small-for-Gestational-Age Newborn continued

INTERVENTION	RATIONALE
■ Monitor daily weight with anticipation of small amount of weight loss when nipple feedings start.	■ Nipple feeding, an active rather than passive intake of nutrition, requires energy expenditure and burning of calories by infant.

EXPECTED OUTCOMES: The infant will maintain steady weight gain as evidenced by less than 2%/day weight loss, tolerates oral feedings, and urine output is 1–3 ml/kg/hour.

5. Nursing Diagnosis: Risk for Impaired Parenting related to lack of knowledge of infant care and prolonged separation of infant and her or his parents secondary to illness

Goal: Parents will bond with their infant and have realistic expectations about their infant. Parents are comfortable taking infant home. They are able to demonstrate normal infant care and assessments of possible complications, and know when to return for follow-up.

INTERVENTION	RATIONALE
■ Support emotionally the psychologic well-being of family, including positive parent-infant attachment and sensory stimulation of infant.	■ Parent-infant attachment begins in first few hours or days following birth. SGA infants may experience prolonged periods of separation from their parents, which necessitates intervention to ensure parent-infant bonding.
■ Include parents in determining infant's plan of care and encourage their participation. Encourage parents to visit frequently. Provide opportunities for parents to touch, hold, talk to, and care for infant. Determine the type and amount of appropriate sensory stimulation and implement sensory stimulation program.	
■ Prepare for discharge by instructing parents in such areas as feeding techniques, formula preparation, and breastfeeding; bathing, diapering, and hygiene; temperature monitoring; administration of vitamins; care of complications and preventing exposure to infections; normal elimination patterns, normal reflexes and activity, and how to promote normal growth and development without being overprotective; returning for continued medical care; and availability of community resources if indicated.	■ Parents should receive the same postpartum teaching as any parent taking a new infant home. ■ Parents need to understand the changes to expect in color of the infant's stool and number of bowel movements plus odor from formula- or breastfeeding to avoid unnecessary concern. SGA infants usually do not require referral to community agencies such as visiting nurse associations unless there is a specific problem requiring assistance.

EXPECTED OUTCOMES: The parent will demonstrate ability to perform basic infant care tasks as evidenced by exhibiting appropriate attachment behaviors (i.e., talking and holding infant), feeding infant, and bathing infant.

Care of the Large-for-Gestational-Age Newborn

A newborn whose birth weight is at or above the 90th percentile on the intrauterine growth curve (at any week of gestation) is considered **large for gestational age (LGA)**. Some appropriate-for-gestational-age (AGA) newborns have been incorrectly categorized as LGA because of miscalculation of the date of conception due to postconceptional bleeding. Careful gestational age assessment is essential to identify the potential needs and problems of such infants.

The best known condition associated with excessive fetal growth is maternal diabetes (see White's Classification, Table 19-3 ∞ on page 423). Not all LGA newborns are infants of diabetic mothers. The cause of the majority of cases of LGA infants is unclear, but certain factors or situations have been found to correlate with their births (Cloherty et al., 2008):

- It is estimated that 3% to 10% of all pregnancies are complicated by diabetes and 90% of these women are gestational diabetics.
- Genetic predisposition is correlated proportionally to the mother's pre-pregnancy weight and to weight gain during pregnancy. Large parents tend to have large infants.
- Multiparous women have two to three times the number of LGA infants as primigravidas.
- Male infants are typically larger than female infants.
- Infants with erythroblastosis fetalis, Beckwith-Wiedemann syndrome (a genetic condition associated with macroglossia, omphalocele, and newborn hypoglycemia and hyperinsulinemia), or transposition of the great vessels are usually large.

The increase in the LGA infant's body size is characteristically proportional, although head circumference and body length are in the upper limits of intrauterine growth. The exception to this rule is the infant of the diabetic mother, whose body weight is higher but whose length and head circumference may be in the normal range. Macrosomic infants have poor motor skills and have more difficulty in regulating behavioral states. LGA infants tend to be more difficult to arouse and may have problems maintaining a quiet alert state. They may also have feeding difficulties.

Common Complications of the LGA Newborn

Complications of the LGA infant can include the following:

- ***Birth trauma due to cephalopelvic disproportion (CPD) and macrosomia.*** Often LGA newborns have a biparietal diameter greater than 10 cm (4 in.) or are associated with a maternal fundal height measurement greater than 42 cm (16 in.) without the presence of polyhydramnios. Because of their excessive size or macrosomia, there are more breech presentations and shoulder dystocia. These complications may result in asphyxia, fractured clavicles, fractured humerus, brachial plexus palsy, facial paralysis, phrenic nerve palsy, depressed skull fractures, cephalhematoma, and intracranial hemorrhage, all due to birth trauma.
- ***Increased incidence of cesarean births and oxytocin-induced births due to fetal size.*** Mothers and infants have all the risk factors associated with cesarean births.
- ***Hypoglycemia, polycythemia, and hyperviscosity.*** These disorders are most often seen in infants of diabetic mothers and infants with erythroblastosis fetalis or Beckwith-Wiedemann syndrome.

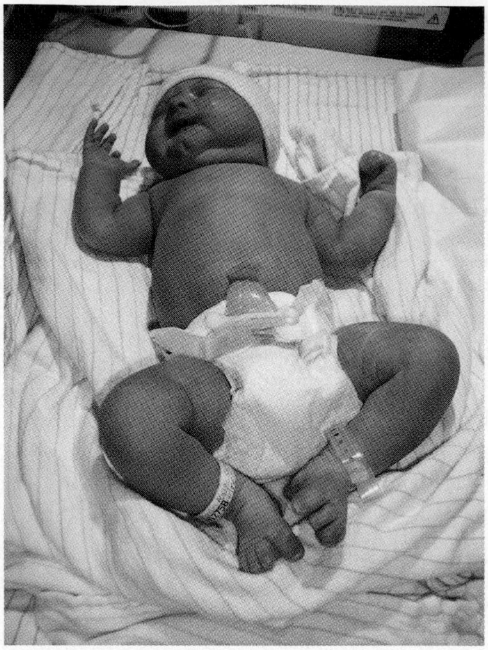

Figure 33-4 ■ Macrosomic infant of a Class B insulin-dependent diabetic mother born at 38 weeks' gestation weighing 3402 grams.

Source: Courtesy of Carol Harrigan, RN, MSN, NNP-BC.

NURSING CARE MANAGEMENT

The perinatal history, in conjunction with ultrasonic measurement of fetal skull (biparietal diameter) and gestational age testing, is important in identifying an at-risk LGA newborn. Nursing care is directed toward early identification and immediate treatment of the common disorders. Essential components of the nursing assessment are monitoring vital signs, screening for hypoglycemia and polycythemia, and observing for signs and symptoms related to birth trauma. The nurse should address parental concerns about the visual signs of birth trauma and the potential for continuation of the overweight pattern. The nurse should help parents learn to arouse and console their newborn and facilitate nutritional intake and attachment behaviors. Mothers of LGA infants with bruising of the face or head may be reluctant to interact with their infants because they fear hurting their infants. The nursing care for complications associated with LGA newborns is similar to the care needed by the infant of a diabetic mother and is discussed in the next section.

Care Plan Activity: Infant of a Diabetic Mother

Care of the Infant of a Diabetic Mother

Infants of diabetic mothers (IDMs) are considered at risk and require close observation the first few hours to the first few days of life. Mothers with severe diabetes or diabetes of long duration associated with renal, retinal, cardiac, or vascular disease may give birth to small-for-gestational-age (SGA) infants. The typical IDM, when the diabetes is poorly controlled or gestational, is large for gestational age (LGA). The infant is macrosomic, ruddy in color, and has excess adipose (fat) tissue (Figure 33-4 ■). The umbilical cord is thick and the placenta is large. There is a higher incidence of macrosomic infants born to certain ethnic groups (Native Americans, Mexican Americans, African Americans, and Pacific Islanders).

IDMs have decreased total body water, particularly in the extracellular spaces, and are therefore not edematous. Their excessive weight is due to increased weight of the visceral organs, cardiomegaly (hypertrophy), and increased body fat. The only organ not affected is the brain.

The excessive fetal growth of the IDM is caused by exposure to high levels of maternal glucose, which readily crosses the placenta. The fetus responds to these high glucose levels with increased insulin production and hyperplasia of the pancreatic beta cells. The main action of insulin is to facilitate the entry of glucose into muscle and fat cells. Once in the cells, glucose is converted to glycogen and stored. Insulin also inhibits the breakdown of fat to free fatty acids, thereby maintaining lipid synthesis; increases the uptake of amino acids; and promotes protein synthesis. Insulin is an important regulator of fetal metabolism and has a "growth hormone" effect that results in increased linear growth. IDMs may be obese as children (Cunningham et al., 2010).

Common Complications of the IDM

Although IDMs are usually large, they are immature in physiologic functions and exhibit many of the problems of the preterm (premature) infant. The complications most often seen in an IDM are as follows:

- ***Hypoglycemia.*** Hypoglycemia is defined as a blood sugar less than 45 mg/dl. Once the fetus is delivered and the maternal glucose supply is severed, the IDM continues to produce high levels of insulin, which deplete the infant's blood glucose within hours after birth. IDMs also have less ability to release glucagon and catecholamines, which normally stimulate glucagon breakdown and glucose release. The incidence of hypoglycemia in IDMs varies according to the degree of success in controlling the maternal diabetes, the maternal blood sugar level at the time of birth, the length of labor, the class of maternal diabetes, and early versus late feedings of the newborn (Moore & Catalano, 2009). Signs and symptoms of hypoglycemia, which usually present within 1 to 2 hours following delivery, include tremors, cyanosis, apnea, temperature instability, poor feeding, and hypotonia. Seizures may occur in severe cases.

CLINICAL TIP

When beginning fluids on an IDM, it is sometimes best to start at a higher concentration of dextrose to avoid hypoglycemic episodes.

- ***Hypocalcemia.*** Hypocalcemia is defined as a serum calcium of less than 7 mg/dl. Tremors are the obvious clinical sign of hypocalcemia. They may be caused by the IDM's increased incidence of prematurity and to the stresses of difficult pregnancy, labor, and birth, which predispose any infant to hypocalcemia. Diabetic women tend to have decreased serum magnesium levels at term secondary to increased urinary calcium excretion, which causes secondary hypoparathyroidism in their infants. Other factors may include vitamin D antagonism, which results from elevated cortisol levels, hypophosphatemia from tissue catabolism, and decreased serum magnesium levels.
- ***Hyperbilirubinemia.*** This condition may be seen at 48 to 72 hours after birth. It may be caused by slightly decreased extracellular fluid volume, which increases the hematocrit level. This elevation facilitates an increase in red blood cell breakdown, thereby increasing bilirubin levels. The presence of hepatic immaturity may impair bilirubin conjugation. Enclosed cranial hemorrhages resulting from a complicated vaginal birth may also contribute to hyperbilirubinemia.
- ***Birth trauma.*** Because most IDMs are macrosomic, trauma may occur during labor and vaginal birth resulting in shoulder dystocia, brachial plexus injuries, subdural hemorrhage, cephalhematoma, and asphyxia.
- ***Polycythemia.*** Fetal hyperglycemia and hyperinsulinism result in increased oxygen consumption, which can lead to fetal hypoxia (Armentrout, 2010). Hemoglobin A_{1c} binds to oxygen, decreasing the oxygen available to the fetal tissues. This tissue hypoxia stimulates increased erythropoietin production, which increases both the hematocrit level and the potential for hyperbilirubinemia. See chapter 19 ∞ for discussion of hemoglobin A_{1c}.
- ***Respiratory distress syndrome (RDS).*** This complication occurs more frequently in newborns of White's classes A through C diabetic mothers who are not well controlled (Cloherty et al., 2008). Insulin antagonizes the cortisol-induced stimulation of lecithin synthesis that is necessary for lung maturation. Thus IDMs may have lungs that are less mature than expected for their gestational age. There is also a decrease in the phospholipid phosphatidylglycerol (PG), which stabilizes surfactant. The insufficiency of PG increases the incidence of RDS. Therefore, it is important to test for fetal lung maturity, or the presence of PG, in the amniotic fluid before birth.

  Transient tachypnea of the newborn, commonly known as "wet lung" syndrome due to retained fetal lung fluid, may also occur in the IDM especially after an elective cesarean delivery. There is a delay in reabsorption of fetal lung fluid from the pulmonary lymphatic system causing a decrease in lung compliance resulting in tachypnea, grunting, and retractions, resolving in 3 to 5 days.

  RDS does not appear to be problematic for infants born to diabetic mothers in White's classes D through F; instead, the stresses of poor uterine blood supply may lead to increased production of steroids, which stimulates lung maturation. IDMs may also have a delay in closure of the ductus arteriosus and an increase in pulmonary vascular resistance (Cloherty et al., 2008; Moore & Catalano, 2009).
- ***Congenital malformations.*** These can include transposition of the great vessels, ventricular septal defect, left or right ventricular wall hypertrophy, small left colon syndrome, intestinal atresia, hydronephrosis, cystic kidneys, and sacral agenesis (caudal regression) (Cloherty et al., 2008). Early careful regulation of maternal glucose before and during pregnancy, especially during the first trimester, decreases the risk of birth defects. See chapter 19 ∞.

Clinical Therapy

Prenatal management is directed toward controlling maternal glucose levels, which minimizes the common complications of IDMs. Because the onset of hypoglycemia occurs within 1 and 2 hours following birth in IDMs (with a spontaneous rise to normal levels by 4 to 6 hours), blood glucose determinations should be performed on capillary or venous blood samples hourly during the first 4 hours after birth and at 4-hour intervals until the risk period (about 48 hours) has passed or per agency protocol.

IDMs whose serum glucose falls below 45 mg/dl should have early feedings with formula or breast milk (colostrum). If normal glucose levels cannot be maintained with oral feeding, an intravenous (IV) infusion of glucose will be necessary. An infusion of D10W at a rate of 6 to 8 mg/kg/min usually maintains normoglycemia in the IDM. If higher glucose concentrations (greater than 12.5%) are needed to maintain normal serum glucose levels, a central line will need to be placed to minimize tissue extravasation. Once the blood glucose has been stable for 24 hours, the infusion rate can be decreased as oral feedings are increased. The newborn's blood glucose levels must be carefully monitored. Repeated dextrose as a bolus infusion is contraindicated because it may lead to severe rebound hypoglycemia following an initial brief increase in glucose level. Newborns with refractory hypoglycemia will need an endocrinology workup and the administration of IV corticosteroids may be indicated.

NURSING CARE MANAGEMENT

Nursing Assessment and Diagnosis

The nurse should not be lulled into thinking that a big baby is a mature baby. In almost every case, because of the infant's large size, the IDM will appear older than gestational age scoring indicates. The nurse must consider both the gestational age and whether the baby is appropriate-for-gestational-age (AGA) or LGA in planning and providing safe care. In caring for the IDM, the nurse assesses for signs of respiratory distress, hyperbilirubinemia, birth trauma, and congenital anomalies.

Nursing diagnoses that may apply to IDMs include the following:

- ***Imbalanced Nutrition: Less Than Body Requirements*** related to increased glucose metabolism secondary to hyperinsulinemia
- ***Impaired Gas Exchange*** related to respiratory distress secondary to delayed production of pulmonary surfactant
- ***Imbalance in Calcium Homeostasis*** related to inappropriate parathyroid response
- ***Ineffective Peripheral Tissue Perfusion*** secondary to polycythemia related to increased synthesis of erythropoietin, chronic intrauterine hypoxia, and increased metabolic rate
- ***Compromised Family Coping*** related to the illness of the baby

Nursing Plan and Implementation

Nursing care of the IDM is directed toward early detection and ongoing monitoring of hypoglycemia (by performing glucose tests) and polycythemia (by obtaining central hematocrits), respiratory distress, and hyperbilirubinemia. (These conditions are presented in chapter 34 ∞.) The nurse also assesses for signs of birth trauma and congenital anomalies.

Parent teaching is directed toward preventing macrosomia and the resulting fetal-newborn problems and instituting early and ongoing diabetic control. Parents are advised that with early identification and care, most IDMs' complications have no significant sequelae.

Evaluation

Expected outcomes of nursing care include the following:

- The IDM's respiratory and metabolic alteration problems are minimized.
- The parents understand the etiology of the baby's health problems and preventive steps they can initiate to decrease the impact of maternal diabetes on subsequent pregnancies.
- The parents verbalize their concerns surrounding their baby's health problems and understand the rationale behind management of their newborn.

Care of the Postterm Newborn

The **postterm newborn** is any newborn born after 42 weeks' gestation. Postterm or prolonged pregnancy occurs in approximately 4% to 14% of all pregnancies (Resnik & Resnik, 2009). The cause of most postterm pregnancies is not completely understood, but several factors are known to be associated with it (see chapter 27 ∞ for a discussion of maternal factors). Many pregnancies classified as prolonged are thought to be a result of inaccurate determination of the estimated date of birth (EDB). Postterm pregnancy is more common in Greek and Italian ethnic groups and the aboriginal people of Australia.

Most babies born as a result of prolonged pregnancy are of normal size and health; some keep on growing and are over 4000 g at birth, which supports the contention that the postterm fetus can remain well nourished. Potential intrapartal problems for these healthy but large fetuses include cephalopelvic disproportion (CPD) and shoulder dystocia. See chapter 27 ∞ for discussion of the necessary assessments and interventions for CPD and shoulder dystocia.

Common Complications of the Newborn with Postmaturity Syndrome

The term **postmaturity** applies only to the infant who is born after 42 completed weeks of gestation and also demonstrates characteristics of *postmaturity syndrome.* Only about 5% of postterm newborns show signs of postmaturity syndrome.

The truly postmature newborn is at high risk for morbidity and has a mortality rate two to three times higher than that of term infants. Although today the percentages are extremely low, the majority of postmature fetal deaths occur during labor, because the fetus has used up necessary body reserves.

Decreased placental function, which impairs nutrition transport and oxygenation, leaves the fetus prone to hypoglycemia and hypoxemia when the stresses of labor begin. The following are common disorders of the postmature newborn:

- Hypoglycemia from nutritional deprivation resulting in depleted glycogen stores.
- Meconium aspiration in response to in utero hypoxia. Oligohydramnios increases the danger of aspirating thick meconium. Severe meconium aspiration syndrome increases the baby's chance of developing persistent pulmonary hypertension, pneumothorax, and pneumonia.
- Polycythemia due to increased production of red blood cells (RBCs) in response to hypoxia.
- Congenital anomalies of unknown cause.
- Seizures due to hypoxic insult.
- Cold stress due to loss or poor development of subcutaneous fat.

The long-term effects of postmaturity syndrome are unclear. At present, studies do not agree on the effect of postmaturity syndrome on weight gain and IQ scores (Resnik & Resnik, 2009).

Prolonged pregnancy by itself is not responsible for the postmaturity syndrome. The characteristics of the postmature newborn are caused primarily by a combination of placental aging and subsequent insufficiency and continued exposure to amniotic fluid.

Clinical Therapy

The aim of antenatal management is to differentiate the fetus that has postmaturity syndrome from the fetus who is large, well nourished, and active and who is tolerating the prolonged (postterm) pregnancy. Antenatal tests that can be done to evaluate fetal status and determine obstetric management are discussed in more depth in chapter 21 and chapter 27. If the amniotic fluid is meconium stained, an amnioinfusion may be done during labor. This procedure dilutes the meconium by directly infusing either normal saline or Ringer's lactate into the uterus, minimizing the risk of meconium aspiration syndrome. (For detailed discussion of clinical management and care of the newborn at risk for meconium aspiration, see chapter 34.)

Hypoglycemia is monitored by serial glucose determinations as per agency hospital protocols. The baby may be placed on glucose infusions or given early feedings if respiratory distress is not present, but these measures must be instituted with caution because of the frequency of asphyxia in the first 24 hours. Postmature newborns are often voracious eaters.

For the small-for-gestational-age (SGA) infant who is postmature, peripheral and central hematocrits are tested to determine the presence of polycythemia. Fluid resuscitation can be initiated. In extreme cases a partial exchange transfusion may be necessary to manage polycythemia and adverse sequelae such as hyperviscosity. Oxygen is provided for respiratory distress. In addition, decreased liver glycogen stores can cause temperature instability and excessive loss of body heat. See chapter 31 for thermoregulation techniques.

NURSING CARE MANAGEMENT

Nursing Assessment and Diagnosis

The newborn with postmaturity syndrome appears alert. This wide-eyed, alert appearance is not necessarily a positive sign because it may indicate chronic intrauterine hypoxia. The infant has dry, cracking, parchmentlike skin without vernix or lanugo (Figure 33-5 ■). Fingernails are long, and scalp hair is profuse. The infant's body appears long and thin. The wasting involves depletion of previously stored subcutaneous tissue, causing the skin to be loose. Fat layers are almost nonexistent.

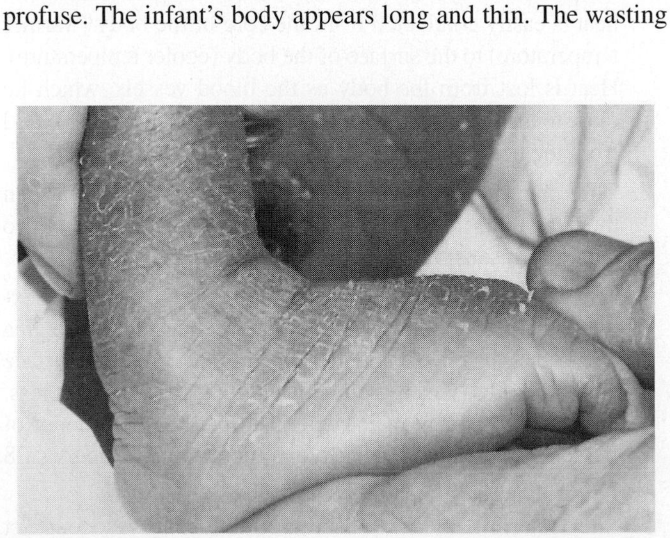

Figure 33-5 ■ The skin of the postterm infant exhibits deep cracking and peeling.

Source: Dubowitz, L., & Dubowitz, V. (1977). The gestational age of the newborn. *Menlo Park, CA: Addison-Wesley. Reprinted by permission of V. Dubowitz, MD, Hammersmith Hospital, London, England.*

Postmature newborns frequently have meconium staining, which colors the nails, skin, and umbilical cord. The varying shades (yellow to green) of meconium staining can give some clue about whether the expulsion of meconium was a recent or a chronic problem; green coloring indicates a more recent event.

Nursing diagnoses that may apply to the postmature newborn include the following:

- ***Hypothermia*** related to decreased liver glycogen and brown fat stores
- ***Imbalanced Nutrition: Less Than Body Requirements*** related to increased use of glucose secondary to stress in utero and decreased placental perfusion
- ***Impaired Gas Exchange*** related to airway obstruction from meconium aspiration
- ***Ineffective Peripheral Tissue Perfusion*** related to polycythemic hyperviscosity

Nursing Plan and Implementation

Hospital-Based Nursing Care

Nursing interventions are primarily supportive measures. They include the following:

- Monitor cardiopulmonary status because the stresses of labor are poorly tolerated and can result in hypoxemia in utero and possible asphyxia at birth.
- Provide warmth via an external heat source to counterbalance the infant's poor response to cold stress and decreased liver glycogen and brown fat stores.
- Frequently monitor blood glucose and initiate early feeding (at 1 or 2 hours of age) or intravenous (IV) glucose per physician/neonatal nurse practitioner (NNP) order.
- Obtain a central hematocrit to determine accurately the presence of polycythemia.

Case Study: Infant with Postmaturity Syndrome

The nurse encourages parents to express their feelings and fears regarding the newborn's condition and potential long-term problems. The nurse also gives careful explanations of procedures, includes the parents in developing care plans for their baby, and encourages follow-up care as needed.

Evaluation

Expected outcomes of nursing care include the following:

- The postterm newborn establishes effective respiratory function.
- The postmature baby is free of metabolic alterations (hypoglycemia) and maintains a stable temperature.

Care of the Preterm (Premature) Newborn

A **preterm infant** is an infant born through 37 completed weeks' gestation (Gardner & Hernandez, 2011) (Figure 33-6 ■). With the help of modern technology, infants are surviving at younger gestational ages but not without significant morbidity. The incidence

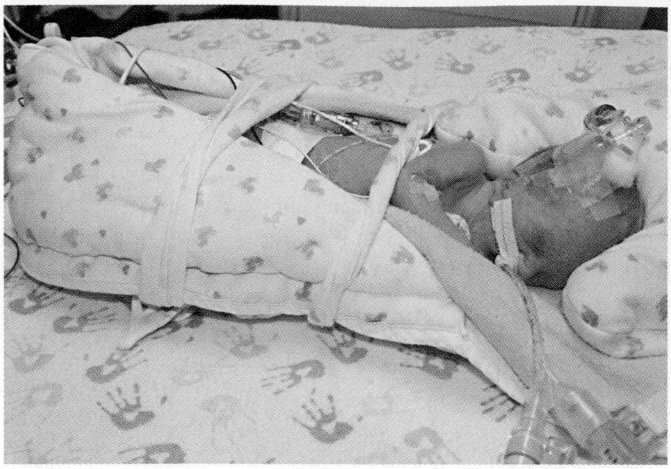

Figure 33-6 ■ A 6-day-old, 28 weeks' gestational age, 960-g preterm infant.

Source: Courtesy of Carol Harrigan, RN, MSN, NNP-BC.

of all preterm births in the United States is approximately 12%. In addition, 18% of African American newborns are preterm (Vargo & Trotter, 2007). The rise in multiple birthrates has markedly influenced overall rates of low-birth-weight (LBW) infants. Prematurity and LBW are common in single women and adolescents. (See chapter 20 ∞ for a discussion of preterm labor.)

The major problem of the preterm newborn is variable immaturity of all systems, the degree of which depends on the length of gestation. The preterm newborn must traverse the same complex, interconnected pathways from intrauterine to extrauterine life as the term newborn. Immaturity means the premature newborn is ill equipped to make this transition smoothly.

Alteration in Respiratory and Cardiovascular Physiology

The preterm newborn is at risk for respiratory problems because the lungs are not fully mature and not fully ready to take over the process of oxygen and carbon dioxide exchange until 37 to 38 weeks' gestation. Critical factors in the development of respiratory distress syndrome (RDS) include the following:

1. The preterm infant is unable to produce adequate amounts of surfactant. (See chapter 29 ∞ for a discussion of respiratory adaptation and development.) Inadequate surfactant lessens compliance (ability of the lungs to fill with air easily), thereby increasing the inspiratory pressure needed to expand each alveoli with air. This progressive atelectasis leads to an inability to develop a functional residual capacity (FRC) causing an ineffective exchange of oxygen and carbon dioxide. As a result, the infant becomes hypoxic, pulmonary blood flow is inefficient, and the preterm newborn's available energy is depleted.
2. The muscular coat of the pulmonary blood vessels is incompletely developed. Consequently the pulmonary arterioles do not constrict as well in response to decreased oxygen levels. This lowered pulmonary vascular resistance leads to increased left-to-right shunting through the ductus arteriosus, which increases the blood flow back into the lungs.
3. Normally the ductus arteriosus responds to increasing oxygen and prostaglandin E levels by vasoconstriction; in the preterm infant, who has higher susceptibility to hypoxia, the ductus may remain open. A patent ductus increases the blood volume to the lungs, causing pulmonary congestion, increased respiratory effort, carbon dioxide retention, and bounding femoral pulses.

The common complications of the cardiopulmonary system in preterm infants are discussed later in the chapter and in chapter 34 ∞.

Alteration in Thermoregulation

Heat loss is a major problem in preterm newborns that the nurse can do much to prevent. Two limiting factors in heat production, however, are the availability of glycogen in the liver and the amount of brown fat available for heat production. Both of these limiting factors appear in the third trimester. In the cold-stressed newborn, norepinephrine is released, which in turn stimulates the metabolism of brown fat for heat production. As a complicating factor, the hypoxic newborn cannot increase oxygen consumption in response to cold stress because of the already limited reserves and thereby becomes progressively colder. Because the muscle mass is small in preterm infants and voluntary muscular activity is diminished (they are unable to shiver), heat production is further limited.

Five physiologic and anatomic factors increase heat loss in the preterm infant:

1. The preterm baby has a high ratio of body surface to body weight. This means that the baby's ability to produce heat (based on body weight) is much less than the potential for losing heat (based on surface area). The loss of heat in a preterm infant weighing 1500 g is five times greater per unit of body weight than in an adult.
2. The preterm baby has very little subcutaneous fat, which is the human body's insulation. Without adequate insulation, heat is easily conducted from the core of the body (warmer temperature) to the surface of the body (cooler temperature). Heat is lost from the body as the blood vessels, which lie close to the skin surface in the preterm infant, transport blood from the body core to the subcutaneous tissues.
3. The preterm baby has thinner, more permeable skin than the term infant. This increased permeability contributes to a greater insensible water loss as well as heat loss.
4. The posture of the preterm baby influences heat loss. Flexion of the extremities decreases the amount of surface area exposed to the environment. Extension increases the surface area exposed to the environment and thus increases heat loss. The gestational age of the infant influences the amount of flexion, from completely hypotonic and extended at 28 weeks to strong flexion displayed by 36 weeks.
5. The preterm baby has a decreased ability to vasoconstrict superficial blood vessels and conserve heat in the body core.

In summary, gestational age is directly proportional to the ability to maintain thermoregulation; thus the more preterm the newborn, the less the infant is able to maintain heat balance.

Preventing heat loss by providing a neutral thermal environment (NTE) using a servo control skin probe is one of the most important considerations in nursing management of the preterm infant. Cold stress, with its accompanying severe complications, can be prevented (see chapter 34 ∞).

Alteration in Gastrointestinal Physiology

The basic structure of the gastrointestinal (GI) tract is formed early in gestation. Maturation of the digestive and absorptive processes is more variable, however, and occurs later in gestation. As a result of GI immaturity, the preterm newborn has the following ingestion, digestion, and absorption problems:

- A marked danger of aspiration and its associated complications due to the infant's poorly developed gag reflex, incompetent esophageal cardiac sphincter, and poor sucking and swallowing reflexes.
- Difficulty in meeting high caloric and fluid needs for growth due to small stomach capacity.
- Limited ability to convert certain essential amino acids to nonessential amino acids. Certain amino acids, such as histidine, taurine, and cysteine, are essential to the preterm infant but not to the term infant.
- Inability to handle the increased osmolarity of formula protein due to kidney immaturity. The preterm infant requires a higher concentration of whey protein than casein.
- Difficulty absorbing saturated fats due to decreased bile salts and pancreatic lipase. Severe illness of the newborn may also prevent intake of adequate nutrients.
- Difficulty with lactose digestion initially because processes may not be fully functional during the first few days of a preterm infant's life. The preterm newborn can digest and absorb most simple sugars.
- Deficiency of calcium and phosphorus may exist because two thirds of these minerals are deposited in the last trimester. Rickets and significant bone demineralization due to deficiency of calcium and phosphorus, which are deposited primarily in the last trimester, are also problems.
- Increased basal metabolic rate and increased oxygen requirements due to fatigue associated with sucking.
- Feeding intolerance and necrotizing enterocolitis (NEC) due to diminished blood flow and tissue perfusion to the intestinal tract due to a combination of contributing factors including prematurity, formula feeding, bacterial colonization, and hypoxemia/ischemic events.

Alteration in Renal Physiology

The kidneys of the preterm infant are immature in comparison with those of the full-term infant, which poses clinical problems in the management of fluid and electrolyte balance. Specific characteristics of the preterm infant include the following:

- The glomerular filtration rate (GFR) is lower because of low renal blood flow. The GFR is directly related to lower gestational age, so the more preterm the newborn, the lower the GFR, which increases steadily after 34 weeks post-conceptional age (PCA). The GFR is also decreased in the presence of diseases or conditions that decrease renal blood flow and perfusion, such as severe respiratory distress, hypotension (low blood pressure [BP]), and asphyxia. Anuria or oliguria may also be observed. A low systolic blood pressure can reflect any disease that decreases cardiac output and affect renal blood flow. Systolic blood pressure varies with gestational age and post-conceptual age. (See Table 33-1 Systolic Blood Pressure Guidelines.)

CLINICAL TIP

A gradual decline in urine output may be associated with a drop in the baby's blood pressure.

TABLE 33-1 Systolic Blood Pressure Guidelines

Day of Life #1			Post-Conceptual Age		
GESTATIONAL AGE	RANGE SYSTOLIC BP	AVERAGE SYSTOLIC BP	WEEKS	RANGE SYSTOLIC BP	AVERAGE SYSTOLIC BP
23	23–55	39	24	35–67	48
24	26–58	42	26	38–70	52
26	29–61	45	28	41–73	56
28	32–65	48	30	45–77	60
30	35–68	51	32	49–81	64
32	38–71	54	34	52–84	68
34	41–75	57	36	56–88	72
36	44–78	60	38	60–91	76
38	47–81	63	40	63–94	80
40	51–85	67	42	66–97	83
42	54–88	71	44	70–100	87
			46	72–103	90

Source: Courtesy of NICU, Cardon Children's Hospital at Banner Desert Medical Center, Mesa, AZ, 2008.

- The preterm infant's kidneys are limited in their ability to concentrate urine or to excrete excess amounts of fluid, due to a blunted response to antidiuretic hormone (ADH). This means that if excess fluid is administered, the infant is at risk for fluid retention and overhydration. If too little is administered, the infant will become dehydrated because of the inability to retain adequate fluid.
- The preterm kidneys begin excreting glucose at a lower serum glucose level than those of the term infant. Therefore, glycosuria with hyperglycemia can lead to osmotic diuresis and polyuria.
- The kidney's buffering capacity is reduced, predisposing the infant to metabolic acidosis. Bicarbonate is excreted at a lower serum level, and acid is excreted more slowly. Therefore, after periods of hypoxia or insult, the preterm infant's kidneys require a longer time to excrete the lactic acid that accumulates. Sodium bicarbonate is frequently required to treat the metabolic acidosis.
- The immaturity of the renal system affects the preterm infant's ability to excrete drugs. Because excretion time is longer, many drugs are given over longer intervals (for example, every 24 hours instead of every 12 hours). Urine output must be carefully monitored when the infant is receiving nephrotoxic drugs, such as gentamicin and vancomycin. In the event of oliguria, drugs can become toxic in the infant much more quickly than in the adult.

Alteration in Hepatic and Hematologic Physiology

Immaturity of the preterm newborn's liver predisposes the infant to several problems. After birth, the glycogen stores in the liver are rapidly used for energy. Glycogen deposits are affected by asphyxia in utero and after birth by both asphyxia and cold stress. The baby born preterm has decreased glycogen stores at birth and frequently experiences stress, which rapidly uses up these limited stores. Therefore, the preterm newborn is at high risk for hypoglycemia and its complications.

Iron is also stored in the liver, especially during the last trimester of pregnancy. Therefore, the preterm newborn is born with low iron stores. If subject to hemorrhage, rapid growth, and excess blood sampling, the preterm infant is likely to become iron depleted more quickly than the term infant. Many preterm babies require transfusions of packed cells to treat symptomatic anemia as a consequence of frequent blood sampling. As the premature infant grows and convalesces, oral iron supplementation may be started, as well as doses of erythropoietin, to enhance red blood cell (RBC) production.

Conjugation of bilirubin in the liver is impaired in the preterm infant. Thus bilirubin levels increase more rapidly and to a higher level than in the full-term infant. Early clinical assessment of jaundice associated with indirect hyperbilirubinemia is more difficult in preterm newborns because they lack subcutaneous fat. (For a further discussion of the newborn with jaundice, see "Pathophysiology of Hyperbilirubinemia" in chapter 34 ∞.)

The normal cord hemoglobin in an infant of 34 weeks' gestation is approximately 16.8 g/dl, and total blood volume ranges from 80 ml/kg to 100 ml/kg (Blackburn, 2007). Because of the small total blood volume, any blood loss is highly significant to the preterm infant. Therefore, periodic assessments of hemoglobin values are performed during the first weeks of life.

Alteration in Immunologic Physiology

Prematurity is the single most significant factor associated with the incidence of sepsis, thus placing the preterm infant at greater risk for infection and bacteria than the term infant. This increased susceptibility may be the result of an infection acquired in utero that may have precipitated preterm labor and birth. Pathogens also may be acquired during the birth process. However, all preterm infants have immature specific and nonspecific immunity.

In utero the fetus receives passive immunity against a variety of infections from maternal IgG immunoglobulins, which cross the placenta (see chapter 29 ∞). Because most of this immunity is acquired in the last trimester of pregnancy, the preterm infant has few antibodies at birth. These provide less protection and become depleted earlier than in a full-term infant. This may be a contributing factor in the higher incidence of recurrent bacterial infection during the first year of life as well as in the immediate neonatal period.

The other immunoglobulin significant for the preterm infant is secretory IgA, which does not cross the placenta but is found in breast milk in significant concentrations. Breast milk's secretory IgA provides immunity to the mucosal surfaces of the GI tract, protecting the newborn from enteric infections such as those caused by *Escherichia coli* and *Shigella.*

Another altered defense against infection in the preterm infant is the skin surface. In very small infants the skin is easily excoriated, and this factor, coupled with many invasive procedures, places the infant at great risk for nosocomial infections. It is vital to use good hand washing techniques in the care of these infants to prevent unnecessary infection.

CLINICAL TIP

The sudden onset of apnea and bradycardia, coupled with metabolic acidosis in an otherwise healthy, growing premature infant, may be suggestive of bacterial sepsis, especially if there is a central line present.

Alteration in Neurologic Physiology

The general shape of the brain is formed during the first 6 weeks of gestation. Between the second and fourth months of gestation the brain's total complement of neurons proliferate; these neurons migrate to specific sites throughout the central nervous system (CNS), and nerve impulse pathways organize. The final step in neurologic development is the covering of these nerves with myelin, which begins in the second trimester of gestation and continues into adult life (Volpe, 2008).

Because the period of most rapid brain growth and development occurs during the third trimester of pregnancy, the closer to term an infant is born, the better the neurologic prognosis. A common interruption of neurologic development in the preterm infant is caused by intraventricular hemorrhage (IVH) and intracranial hemorrhage (ICH). Hydrocephalus may develop as a consequence of an IVH due to the obstruction at the cerebral aqueduct (Volpe, 2008).

Alteration in Reactivity Periods and Behavioral States

The newborn infant's response to extrauterine life is characterized by two periods of reactivity, as discussed in chapter 31. The preterm infant's periods of reactivity are delayed. In the very ill infant, these periods of reactivity may not be observed at all because the infant may be hypotonic and unreactive for several days after birth.

As the preterm newborn grows and the condition stabilizes, identifying behavioral states and traits unique to each infant becomes increasingly possible. In general, stable preterm infants do not demonstrate the same behavioral states as term infants. Preterm infants are more disorganized in their sleep-wake cycles and are unable to attend as well to the human face and objects in the environment. Neurologically, their responses (sucking, muscle tone, states of arousal) are weaker than full-term infants' responses.

By observing each infant's patterns of behavior and responses, especially the sleep-wake states, the parents and nurse can plan nursing care around the times when the infant is alert and best able to attend. The more knowledge parents have about the meaning of their infant's responses and behaviors, the better prepared they will be to meet their newborn's needs and to form a positive attachment with their child. See discussion of developmental care for the preterm newborn later in this section.

CLINICAL TIP

After observing an infant's pattern of behavior and responses, especially the sleep-wake states, use the time when the infant is alert and best able to attend to help parents learn about and provide newborn care and form a positive attachment with their child.

Management of Nutrition and Fluid Requirements

Early feedings are extremely valuable in maintaining normal metabolism and lowering the possibility of such complications as hypoglycemia, hyperbilirubinemia, hyperkalemia, and osteopenia of prematurity. However, the preterm newborn is at risk for complications that may develop because of the immaturity of the digestive system.

Nutritional Requirements

Oral (enteral) caloric intake necessary for growth in an uncompromised healthy preterm infant is 95 to 130 kcal/kg/day (Blackburn, 2007). In addition to these relatively high caloric needs, the preterm infant requires more protein than full-term infants. To meet these needs, many institutions use fortified breast milk or special preterm formulas.

Whether breast milk or formula is used, feeding regimens are established based on the infant's weight and estimated stomach capacity (Table 33-2). Initial formula-feedings are gradually increased as the infant tolerates them. It may be necessary to supplement the oral feedings with parenteral fluids to maintain adequate hydration and caloric intake until the baby is on full oral feedings. Those preterm infants who cannot tolerate any oral (enteral) feedings are given nutrition by total parenteral nutrition (TPN).

In addition to a higher calorie and higher protein formula, preterm infants should receive supplemental multivitamins, which include vitamins A, D, and E, iron, and trace minerals. A diet high in polyunsaturated fats (which preterm infants tolerate best) increases the requirement for vitamin E. Preterm infants fed iron-fortified formulas have higher red cell hemolysis and lower vitamin E concentrations and thus require additional vitamin E. Preterm formulas also need to contain medium-chain triglycerides (MCT) and additional amino acids such as cysteine, as well as calcium, phosphorus, and vitamin D supplements to increase mineralization of bones. Rickets and significant bone

TABLE 33-2 Neonatal Feeding Initiation and Advancement Practice Guidelines

BIRTH WEIGHT	FEEDING TYPE	SCHEDULE	INITIAL FEEDING RATE (ML/KG/DAY)	RATE OF ADVANCEMENT (ML/KG/DAY)	GOAL RATE (ML/KG/DAY)
750 g	EBM/PF24	q3h	10*	20	150–160
750–1000 g	EBM/PF24	q3h	10*	20	150–160
1001–1250 g	EBM/PF24	q3h	10*	20	150–160
1251–1500 g	EBM/PF24	q3h	20	20	150–160
1501–1800 g	EBM/PF24	q3h	30	30	150–160
1801–2500 g	EBM/PD22	q3h	40	40	180
>2500 g	EBM/T20	q3h	50	50	180

Note: Feeding Type key:
EBM: expressed breast milk
PD22: post-discharge formula 22 kcal/oz
PF24: premature formula 24 kcal/oz
T20: term formula 20 kcal/oz

*Continue trophic feedings of 10 ml/kg/day × 3–5 days before advancing

Source: Courtesy of NICU, Cardon Children's Hospital at Banner Desert Medical Center, Mesa, AZ, 2008.

demineralization have been documented in very-low-birth-weight infants and otherwise healthy preterm infants.

Nutritional intake is considered adequate when there is consistent weight gain of 20 to 30 g per day. Initially, no weight gain may be noted for several days, but total weight loss should not exceed 15% of the total birth weight or more than 1% to 2% per day. Some institutions add the criteria of head circumference growth and increase in body length of 1 cm (0.4 in.) per week once the newborn is stable.

Methods of Feeding

The preterm infant is fed by various methods, depending on the infant's gestational age, health and physical condition, and neurologic status. The three most common oral feeding methods are bottle, breast, and gavage.

BOTTLE-FEEDING Preterm infants who have a coordinated as well as rhythmic suck-swallow-breathing pattern are usually between 33 and 34 weeks' postconceptual age and may be fed by bottle. Oral readiness to feed is best described by the following behaviors: remaining engaged in the feeding, able to organize oral-motor functioning, to coordinate the suck-swallow-breath skill, and to maintain physiologic stability (Thomas, 2007). Those premature infants who root when their cheek is stroked and actively search for the nipple are neurodevelopmentally ready to initiate oral feeding. To avoid excessive expenditure of energy, a soft, yellow, single-hole nipple is usually used (milk flow is less rapid). The infant is fed in a semisitting position and burped gently after each half ounce or ounce. The feeding should take no longer than 15 to 20 minutes (nippling requires more energy than other methods). Preterm infants who are progressing from gavage feedings to bottle-feeding should be assessed for feeding readiness and started with one session of bottle-feeding a day. The number of times a day a bottle is offered should be increased slowly until the baby tolerates all feedings from a bottle.

The nurse assesses the infant's ability to suck. Sucking may be affected by postconceptional age, asphyxia, chronic lung disease, intraventricular hemorrhage, or other neurologic insult. Before initiating nipple feeding, the nurse observes the infant for any signs of stress, such as tachypnea (more than 60 respirations per minute), respiratory distress, or hypothermia, which may increase the risk of aspiration. During the feeding, the infant should be observed for signs of difficulty with feeding (tachypnea, a decrease in oxygen saturation levels, bradycardia, lethargy, and uncoordinated suck and swallow). Difficulty in bottle-feeding is often associated with a milk bolus that is too large for the infant's oral cavity, which can lead to aspiration. Demand feeding protocols, based on the infant's hunger cues, should be considered for a growing premature infant only when there is sufficient caloric intake to promote consistent weight gain (Kenner & Lott, 2007).

BREASTFEEDING Mothers who wish to breastfeed their preterm infants should be given the opportunity to put the infant to breast as soon as the infant has demonstrated a coordinated suck and swallow reflex, is showing consistent weight gain, and can control body temperature outside of the incubator, regardless of weight. Preterm infants tolerate breastfeeding with higher transcutaneous oxygen pressures and better maintenance of body temperature than during bottle-feeding. Besides breast milk's many benefits for the infant, it allows the mother to contribute actively to the infant's well-being (Figure 33-7 ■). Mothers should be encouraged to breastfeed if they choose to do so. It is important for the nurse to be aware of the advantages of breastfeeding as well as the possible disadvantages if breast milk is the sole source of food for the preterm infant. See chapter 32 ∞ for a detailed discussion of the advantages and disadvantages of breastfeeding and the contraindications.

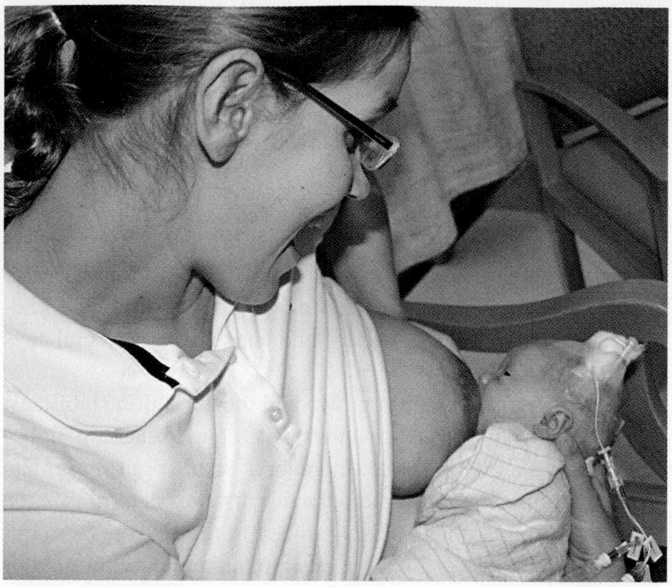

Figure 33-7 ■ Mother breastfeeding her premature infant.

Source: Courtesy of Carol Harrigan, RN, MSN, NNP-BC.

By initiating skin-to-skin holding of LBW infants in the early intensive care phase, mothers can significantly increase milk volume, thereby overcoming lactation problems (Turnage-Carrier, 2010).

Many mothers of preterm infants seem to find that the football hold (see Figure 32-7 ∞ on page 870) is a convenient position for breastfeeding preterm babies. Feeding time may take up to 45 minutes, and babies should be burped as they alternate breasts. Length of feeding time must be monitored so that the preterm infant does not expend too many calories.

The nurse should coordinate a flexible feeding schedule so babies can breastfeed during alert times and be allowed to set their own pace. Feedings should be on demand, but a maximum number of hours between feedings should be set. A similar regimen should be used for the baby who is progressing from gavage feeding to breastfeeding. The mother begins with one feeding at the breast and then gradually increases the number of times during the day that the baby breastfeeds. Even if the infant cannot be put to the breast, mothers can pump their breasts, and the breast milk can be given via gavage. A double-pumping system produces higher levels of prolactin than sequential pumping of the breasts (see Figure 32-20 ∞ on page 878). When breastfeeding is not possible because the infant is too small or too weak to suck at the breast, an option for the mother may be to express her breast milk into a cup. The milk touches the infant's lips and is lapped by the protruding motions of the tongue.

GAVAGE FEEDING The tube or gavage feeding method is used with preterm infants (less than 34 weeks' gestation) who lack or have a poorly coordinated suck-swallow-breathing pattern or are ill and ventilator dependent. Gavage feeding may be used as an adjunct to nipple feeding if the infant tires easily or as an alternative if an infant is losing weight because of the energy expenditure required for nippling, which increases the chance of aspiration. See Procedure 33-1: Performing Gavage Feeding on pages 908–909. Gavage feedings are administered by either the nasogastric or orogastric route and by intermittent bolus or continuous drip method. Currently, there are no conclusive studies supporting one method over the other. In common practice, bolus feedings are usually initiated, but if intolerance occurs, then the feedings are changed to infuse on a pump over a set amount of time (i.e., over an hour) or continuously (Anderson, Wood, Keller, et al., 2011).

Early initiation of minimal enteral nutrition (MEN) via gavage is now advocated in the preterm newborn as a supplement to parenteral nutrition. MEN refers to small-volume feedings of formula or human milk (usually less than 24 ml/kg/day) which are designed to "prime" the intestinal tract, thereby stimulating many of its hormonal and enzymatic functions (American Academy of Pediatrics (AAP) & American College of Obstetricians and Gynecologists (ACOG), 2007). Benefits of early feedings (as early as 24 to 72 hours of life) include the following: no increase in the incidence of necrotizing enterocolitis; fewer days on TPN, thereby decreasing the incidence of cholestatic jaundice; increased weight gain; increased muscle maturation of the gut as well as muscle growth; increase in gut peristalsis; increased gut hormone levels, which can lead to improved feeding tolerance; lower risk of osteopenia; and a possible decrease in the total number of hospital days in the neonatal intensive care unit (NICU).

CLINICAL TIP

Persistent bilious residuals >20% of the feeding and bloody stools may be a cardinal sign of necrotizing enterocolitis (NEC) at which time an x-ray of the abdomen should be obtained.

TOTAL PARENTERAL NUTRITION (TPN) TPN is used in situations when feeding is contraindicated through the GI tract. Contraindications include GI anomalies requiring surgical intervention, NEC, intolerance of feedings, sepsis, and birth depression. TPN may also be used in adjunct with enteral feedings during the early stages of feeding advancement.

The TPN method provides complete nutrition for metabolic requirements and growth to the infant intravenously. TPN includes use of hyperalimentation and intralipids. Hyperalimentation provides vitamins, minerals, protein (in the form of amino acids), and glucose. Appropriate amino acid intake (1 to 4 g/kg/day) is necessary to avoid catabolism and maintain the newborn in a positive-nitrogen balance, and it can be initiated on the first day of life. A percutaneous central venous catheter (PCVC/PICC) is often used with the LBW infant to deliver higher concentrations of glucose (greater than D12.5) as well as to provide an energy substrate. Intralipids (1 to 3 g/kg/day) are also administered to provide essential fatty acids for normal body growth and development.

The nurse needs to monitor serum glucose levels and serum chemistries carefully during the infusion of TPN. The IV rate is monitored hourly to maintain accurate intake. The rate should not be increased to "catch up" if administration lags behind. The IV site should be observed hourly for signs of infiltration—hyperalimentation is extremely caustic and causes severe tissue destruction if it infiltrates. Intake and output are carefully monitored (hyperglycemia causing an osmotic diuresis can lead to dehydration). If hyperglycemia occurs, continuous insulin infusions may be initiated to enhance glucose uptake and utilization. Prolonged administration of TPN combined with little to no enteral intake can result in cholestatic jaundice. Monitoring liver enzymes as well as fractionated bilirubin levels is essential in long-term TPN use. The nurse needs to be aware of the potential complications associated with intralipid infusions, including increased free bilirubin concentrations, impaired pulmonary functions, and interference with platelet function. Therefore, serum triglyceride levels need to be followed. Daily lipid infusion should be spread out over a 24-hour period.

Fluid Requirements

The calculation of fluid requirements takes into account the infant's weight and postnatal age. Recommendations for fluid therapy in the preterm infant are approximately 80 to 100 ml/kg/day for day 1, 100 to 120 ml/kg/day for day 2, and 120 to 150 ml/kg/day by day 3 of life. These amounts may be increased up to 200 ml/kg/day if the infant is extremely premature, receiving phototherapy, or under a radiant warmer facilitating an increase in insensible water losses. If the infant is not hydrated properly, excessive insensible water loss can lead to hypernatremia, hyperkalemia, hypovolemia, hypotension, and oliguria. Fluid losses can be minimized through the use of heat shields and added humidification in the incubator. Daily weights, and sometimes twice-a-day weights, are the best indicator of fluid status in the preterm infant. The expected weight loss during the first 3 to 5 days of life in a preterm infant is 15% to 20% of birth weight.

Common Complications of Preterm Newborns and Their Clinical Management

The goals of medical and nursing care are to meet the growth and development needs of the preterm newborn and to anticipate and manage the complications associated with prematurity. Complications associated with prematurity that require clinical intervention are respiratory distress syndrome (RDS), patent ductus arteriosus (PDA), apnea, pulmonary interstitial emphysema (PIE), intraventricular hemorrhage, and sepsis. Long-term problems include retinopathy of prematurity, bronchopulmonary dysplasia (BPD) leading to chronic lung disease (CLD), and posthemorrhagic hydrocephalus.

PROCEDURE 33-1 Performing Gavage Feeding

NURSING ACTION

Preparation

- When choosing the catheter size, consider the size of the infant, the area of insertion (oral or nasal), and the desired rate of flow.

  Rationale: *The size of the catheter will influence the rate of flow.*
- Explain the procedure to the parents.
- Elevate the head of the bed and position the infant on the back or side to allow easy passage of the tube.
- Measure the distance from the tip of the ear to the nose to the xiphoid process, and mark the point with a small piece of paper tape (Figure 33-8 ■) to ensure enough tubing to enter the stomach.

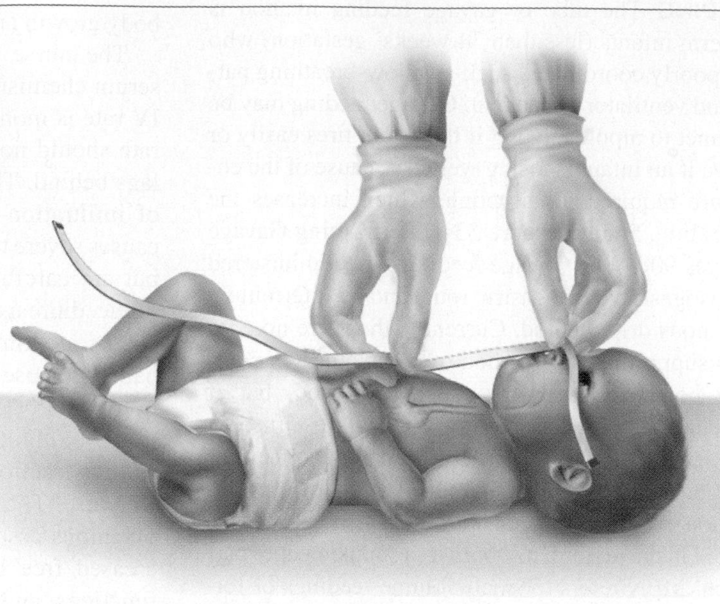

Figure 33-8 ■ Measuring gavage tube length.

Equipment and Supplies

No. 5 or no. 8 Fr. feeding tube. See the Clinical Tip below for guidelines for choosing tube size.

3- to 5-ml syringe, for aspirating stomach contents

1/4-inch paper tape, to mark the tube for insertion depth and to secure the catheter during feeding

Stethoscope, for auscultating the rush of air into the stomach when testing the tube placement

Appropriate formula

Small cup of sterile water to act as lubricant

Clean gloves

> **CLINICAL TIP**
>
> The very small infant (less than 1600 g) requires a 5 Fr. feeding tube; an infant greater than 1600 g may tolerate a larger tube. Long-term indwelling enteral feeding tubes may be used as an alternative to the standard "in and out" gavage tubes, and they come in sizes 5 Fr. and 8 Fr.
>
> Orogastric insertion is preferable to nasogastric because most infants are obligatory nose breathers. If nasogastric is used, a 5 Fr. catheter should be used to minimize airway obstruction.

Procedure: Clean Gloves

Inserting and Checking Placement of Tube

1. If inserting the tube nasally, lubricate the tip in a cup of sterile water. Use water instead of an oil-based lubricant, in case the tube is inadvertently passed into a lung. Shake any excess drops to prevent aspiration.
2. If inserting the tube orally, the oral secretions are enough to lubricate the tube adequately.
3. Stabilize the infant's head with one hand and pass the tube via the mouth (or nose) into the stomach to the point previously marked. If the infant begins coughing or choking or becomes cyanotic or phonic, remove the tube immediately as the tube has probably entered the trachea.
4. If respiratory distress is not apparent, lightly tape the tube in position, draw up 0.5 to 1.0 ml of air in the syringe, and connect the syringe to the tubing. Place the stethoscope over the epigastrium and briskly inject the air (Figure 33-9 ■). You will hear a sudden rush as the air enters the stomach.
5. Aspirate the stomach contents with the syringe, and note the amount, color, and consistency to evaluate the infant's feeding tolerance. Return the residual to the stomach unless you are requested to discard it. It is usually not discarded because of the potential for electrolyte imbalance.

Administering the Feeding

1. Hold the infant for feeding, or position the infant on the right side.

   Rationale: *This position decreases the risk of aspiration in case of emesis during feeding.*
2. Separate the syringe from the tube, remove the plunger from the barrel, reconnect the barrel to the tube, and pour the formula into the syringe.
3. Elevate the syringe 6 to 8 inches over the infant's head, and allow the formula to flow by gravity at a slow, even rate. You may need to initiate the flow of formula by inserting the plunger of the syringe into the barrel just until you see formula enter the feeding tube. Do not use pressure.
4. Regulate the rate to prevent sudden stomach distention leading to vomiting and aspiration. Continue adding formula to the syringe until the infant has absorbed the desired volume.

PROCEDURE 33-1 Performing Gavage Feeding continued

NURSING ACTION

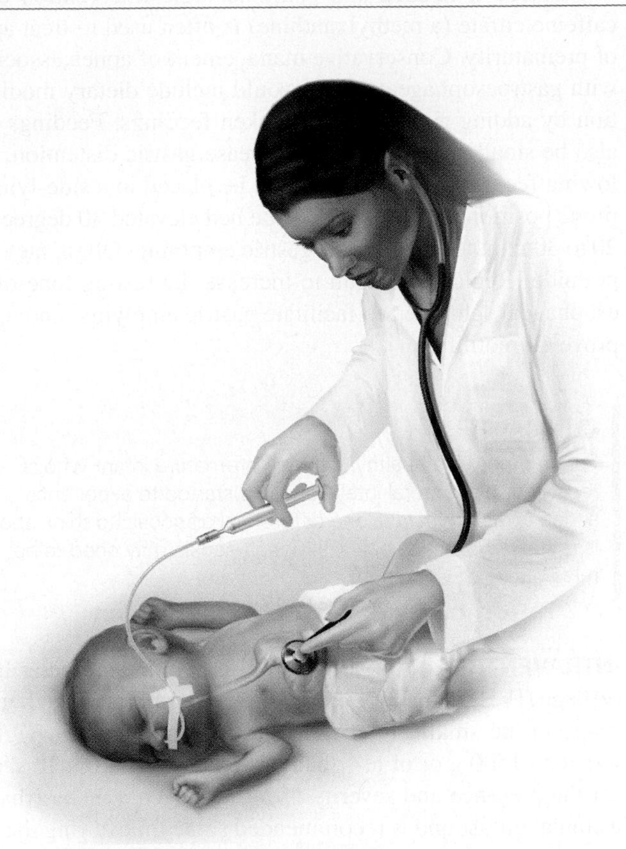

Figure 33-9 ■ Auscultation for placement of gavage tube.

Clearing and Removing the Tube

1. Clear the tubing with 2 to 3 ml of air.

   Rationale: *This ensures that the infant has received all of the formula. If the tube is going to be left in place, clearing it will decrease the risk of occlusion and bacterial growth in the tube.*

2. To remove the tube, loosen the tape, fold the tube over on itself, and quickly withdraw the tube in one smooth motion to minimize the potential for fluid aspiration as the tube passes the epiglottis. If the tube is to be left in, position it so that the infant is unable to remove it. Replace the tube per hospital policy.

Maximize the Feeding Pleasure of the Infant

1. Whenever possible, hold the infant during gavage feeding. If it is too awkward to hold the infant during feeding, be sure to take time for holding after the feeding.

   Rationale: *Feeding time is important to the infant's tactile sensory input.*

2. Offer a pacifier to the infant during the feeding.

   Rationale: *Sucking during feeding comforts and relaxes the infant, making the formula flow more easily. Infants can lose their sucking reflexes when fed by gavage for long periods.*

3. Document procedure, including untoward complications, in the baby's bedside chart or computerized electronic chart.

In-depth discussions of RDS, BPD/CLD, and sepsis, including pathophysiology, clinical management, and nursing care, are contained in chapter 34 ∞. PDA, apnea, intraventricular hemorrhage (IVH), retinopathy of prematurity, and other complications are discussed as follows.

PATENT DUCTUS ARTERIOSUS (PDA) By definition, the ductus arteriosus is the large vessel that is a conduit between the left pulmonary artery and the descending aorta. In the fetus, the ductus arteriosus shunts blood away from the fluid-filled lungs, which are nonfunctional during gestation, toward the placenta for gas exchange. The functional closure of the ductus arteriosus is related to birth weight; the incidence of a symptomatic PDA increases with a decrease in birth weight. For example, in infants 30 weeks and less, functional closure may take several days to weeks to occur.

The incidence of a PDA in an infant weighing less than 1000 g is approximately 80%. Initially, as the pulmonary vascular resistance (PVR) falls and the systemic vascular resistance (SVR) rises, a left-to-right shunt via the PDA results. Blood flows from the aorta into the pulmonary artery, thereby increasing pulmonary blood flow. This leads to left ventricular volume overload, pulmonary edema, and congestive failure. Oxygenation is compromised, and ventilator requirements will increase, leading to the possible difficulty in weaning from the ventilator and long-term pulmonary sequelae. Clinical findings include tachypnea, hyperactive precordium, bounding peripheral pulses, hypotension, widened pulse pressure, tachycardia, and hepatomegaly.

Early identification of symptomatic infants and prompt clinical intervention will minimize long-term complications. There are a multitude of medical management regimens of the PDA. Initial medical management consists of providing adequate respiratory support, restricting fluids, and using diuretics (to decrease pulmonary edema) and perhaps digoxin (to treat congestive heart failure) while waiting for spontaneous closure of the ductus to occur. The administration of prostaglandin synthetase inhibitors, such as indomethacin (Indocin), impairs synthesis of the E series prostaglandins responsible for dilatation of the ductus and can cause ductal closure. Courses of indomethacin therapy vary; the standard, short course consists of three doses of indomethacin, 0.2 mg/kg IV every 12 hours. As an alternative, a long course of indomethacin may be chosen involving dosing over approximately 7 days. A decrease in renal side effects is thought to be the advantage of the longer dosing schedule. Indomethacin is effective, but it is not without side effects and must be used cautiously. Ibuprofen lysine (Neoprofen) is another pharmacologic agent used to close the ductus; the three-dose course consists of one dose of 10 mg/kg IV followed by two subsequent doses of 5 mg/kg IV at 24- and 48-hour intervals after the initial dose. Adverse side effects of both medications include transient renal dysfunction, oliguria, platelet dysfunction, and GI bleeding.

If medical management is unsuccessful or contraindicated, then the ductus may need to be surgically ligated. PDA will often prolong the course of illness in a preterm newborn and may lead to chronic pulmonary dysfunction.

CLINICAL TIP

A growing premature infant showing clinical signs of worsening respiratory status (i.e., increased oxygen needs, increased ventilatory settings), acidosis, and hypotension may be exhibiting signs and symptoms of a patent ductus arteriosus (PDA).

APNEA *Apnea of prematurity* refers to cessation of breathing for 20 seconds or longer or for less than 20 seconds when associated with cyanosis, pallor, and bradycardia. Apnea is the most common problem in the preterm infant $<$ 36 weeks, presenting between day 2 and day 7 of life. The etiology of apnea is multifactorial but is thought to be primarily a result of neuronal immaturity, a factor that contributes to the preterm infant's irregular breathing patterns (central apnea). Obstructive apnea can occur in the premature infant when there is a cessation of airflow associated with blockage of the upper airway (small airway diameter, increased pharyngeal secretions, improper body alignment and positioning).

Differential diagnoses with regard to apnea include sepsis, electrolyte disturbances, hypoglycemia, lung disease (atelectasis, pneumonia, inadequate ventilation), cardiovascular changes (PDA, hypotension, congestive heart failure [CHF]), CNS disturbances (seizures, intraventricular hemorrhage, meningitis, hydrocephalus), medication use (narcotics, opioids, maternal administration of magnesium sulfate), thermoregulation problems (hypo- and hyperthermia), hematologic disturbances (anemia), and GI disturbances (NEC, distention, obstruction, feeding intolerance, gastroesophageal reflux). Gastroesophageal reflux is defined as a movement of gastric contents into the lower esophagus due to poor lower esophageal sphincter tone, activating the laryngeal chemoreflex causing apnea. Apnea of prematurity is then a diagnosis of exclusion.

Apneic onset is often insidious; cardiorespiratory monitoring allows for early recognition and intervention, thus decreasing the need for resuscitative efforts. Apnea may occur during feeding, suctioning, or stooling. However, there may be no observable activity related to apnea. All episodes of apnea are documented. The documentation includes activity at the time of apnea, length of episode (along with any bradycardia, color change, or desaturation on pulse-oximeter associated with the apneic episode), and treatment required to bring the baby out of the apneic spell. These data are useful in determining etiology and the possible course of treatment.

The nurse makes careful observations, quickly assessing the need for intervention or ascertaining that the infant is having periodic breathing. The intervention required depends on the severity of the apneic episode and the baby's response. Gentle stimulation of the infant may be sufficient. Respiratory support is provided if needed and pharmacologic intervention using caffeine citrate (a methylxanthine) is often used to treat apnea of prematurity. Conservative management of apnea associated with gastroesophageal reflux would include dietary modification by adding rice cereal to thicken feedings. Feedings may also be small and frequent to decrease gastric distention. Following feedings, the infant should be placed in a side-lying or prone position with the head of the bed elevated 30 degrees for 20 to 30 minutes to facilitate gastric emptying. Often, metoclopramide (Reglan) is begun to increase the resting tone of the esophageal sphincter, to facilitate gastric emptying, and to improve GI motility.

CLINICAL TIP

For an otherwise healthy, growing premature infant who is receiving total enteral intake and has started to experience apnea and bradycardia, one differential diagnosis to think about is reflux rather than sepsis, although sepsis may need to be ruled out.

INTRAVENTRICULAR HEMORRHAGE Intraventricular hemorrhage (IVH) is the most common type of intracranial hemorrhage in the small preterm infant, especially those weighing less than 1500 g or of less than 34 weeks' gestation. To screen for the presence and severity of intraventricular hemorrhages, a cranial ultrasound is recommended some time during the first week of life and periodically through the infant's hospitalization based upon the initial findings.

The most common site of hemorrhage is the periventricular subependymal germinal matrix in the lateral ventricles of the brain, where there is a rich blood supply and the capillary walls are thin and fragile. The matrix provides little supportive tissue for the fragile blood vessels. Before 32 weeks' gestation, an infant is much more susceptible to hemorrhage of these tiny vessels because they are vulnerable to wide fluctuations in blood pressure and to hypoxic events (such as respiratory distress, birth trauma, birth depression) that damage and rupture vessel walls.

Prenatal interventions include preventing premature birth, administering antenatal steroids, transporting the pregnant mother to a tertiary care center, and cesarean section delivery. Administration of phenobarbital and vitamin K to the mother is being studied for their preventive effect. Postnatal preventive interventions include careful resuscitation efforts, slow correction of acid–base abnormalities, prevention of large fluctuations in blood pressure, and correction of coagulation abnormalities. Potential postnatal preventive pharmacologic interventions include phenobarbital to control seizures and narcotics for sedation (Volpe, 2008).

The outcome for the infant depends on the size of the intraventricular bleed and the gestational age of the infant. The most severe hemorrhages may cause significant motor deficits, lower IQ scores, post-hemorrhagic hydrocephalus, hearing loss, and blindness. Less severe bleeds may have no observable effects. In caring for the infant with an IVH, the nurse provides continuing support for the parents, identifying their level of understanding and facilitating interdisciplinary communication with them.

> **CLINICAL TIP**
> An extremely premature, low-birth-weight infant who presents with a sudden drop in hemoglobin along with the onset of severe metabolic acidosis, a "waxy" color, and hypotension may have experienced an intraventricular hemorrhage.

ANEMIA OF PREMATURITY The preterm infant is at risk for anemia because of the rapid rate of growth required, shorter RBC life, excessive blood sampling, decreased iron stores, and deficiency of vitamin E. The hemoglobin usually reaches its lowest level by 8 to 12 weeks and remains low for 3 to 6 months. Interventions include iron supplementation and administration of recombinant human erythropoietin (r-HuEPO). Iron supplementation ensures adequate stores for RBC production once erythropoiesis starts. The use of r-HuEPO is reported to increase neonatal erythropoiesis, thereby increasing the hematocrit and reticulocyte count. In addition, it has been shown to reduce the need for late blood transfusions (those beyond 2 to 3 weeks of age) in preterm infants (Blackburn, 2007).

Long-Term Complications

The care of the preterm infant and the family does not stop on discharge from the nursery. Follow-up care is extremely important because many developmental problems are not noted until the infant is older and begins to demonstrate motor delays or sensory disability.

Within the first year of life, LBW preterm infants face higher mortality than term infants. Causes of death include sudden infant death syndrome (SIDS)—which occurs about five times more frequently in the preterm infant—respiratory infections, and neurologic defects. Morbidity is also much higher among preterm infants, with those weighing less than 1500 g at highest risk for long-term complications.

The most common long-term problems observed in preterm infants are discussed in the following four sections.

RETINOPATHY OF PREMATURITY Extremely premature newborns are particularly susceptible to injury of the delicate capillaries of the retina causing characteristic retinal changes known as retinopathy of prematurity (ROP). It is this injury to the developing vascular system of the retina that leads to ischemia resulting in hemorrhage, scarring, and, in extreme cases, retinal detachment and impaired vision. The disease is now viewed as multifactorial in origin with hyperoxemia (increased oxygen levels) as one factor. Other risk factors include in vitro fertilization (IVH), CLD, apnea, hypoxia, sepsis, acidosis, anemia, multiple gestation, exposure to bright lights, and blood transfusions. Increased survival of very-low-birth-weight infants may be the most important factor in the increased incidence of ROP.

Judicious use of supplemental oxygen therapy in the premature infant has become the norm in NICUs across the country whereby oxygen saturations are kept $< 93\%$ in an attempt to reduce ROP. Treatment of the acute stages of ROP with laser photocoagulation and cryotherapy is an option. Because most acute cases of ROP regress spontaneously with no long-term visual impairment, the possibility of regression must be weighed against the risk of an unfavorable outcome from treatment. For infants with bilateral traction and retinal detachment, surgical vitrectomy and scleral buckling are performed. Nursing care for the visually impaired infant must concentrate on parental support and education. When the crisis of premature birth is quickly followed by the devastating news of suspected visual impairment (poor visual acuity, myopia, strabismus, amblyopia, and glaucoma) or blindness, the parents will need extensive support by all members of the interdisciplinary health team. The parents again experience overwhelming anxiety and uncertainty about their infant's future abilities. Premature infants with blindness due to ROP may be at increased risk of cognitive and emotional problems. The evidence suggests that this increased risk may be due to environmental factors rather than to inherent intellectual or neurologic factors.

> **CLINICAL TIP**
> According to the AAP & ACOG (2007), all newborns born at 32 weeks or less need to be screened for retinopathy of prematurity (ROP) at 36 weeks corrected gestational age.

NEUROLOGIC DEFECTS The most common neurologic defects include cerebral palsy, hydrocephalus, seizure disorders, lower IQ scores, and learning disabilities. However, the socioeconomic climate and family support systems have been shown to be important factors influencing the child's ultimate school performance in the absence of major neurologic defects. Families can be reminded that risk does not equal injury, injury does not equal damage, and description of damage does not allow a precise prediction about recovery or outcome.

AUDITORY DEFECTS Preterm infants have a 1% to 4% incidence of moderate to profound hearing loss and should have a formal audiologic examination before discharge and at 3 to 6 months (corrected age). One test currently used to measure hearing functions of the newborn is the evoked otoacoustic emissions (EOAE) test. Earphones are used on each ear and independently measure sounds produced in the inner ear in response to acoustic stimuli. Another test, the automated auditory brain response (AABR), measures electroencephalogram (EEG) waves in response to sound waves generated by the test. The AABR provides information about the auditory pathway to the brainstem (Figure 33-10 ■). Any infant with repeated abnormal results should be referred to speech-and-language specialists.

Infants at increased risk include those with congenital viral infections (TORCH), hyperbilirubinemia, severe perinatal asphyxia, meningitis, and birth trauma. Damage from ototoxic drugs such as gentamicin and furosemide (Lasix) is variable and related to multiple factors, including renal function, age, duration of treatment, and concomitant administration of other ototoxic agents.

When evaluating an infant's abilities and disabilities, parents must understand that the developmental progress must be evaluated based on chronologic age from the expected date of

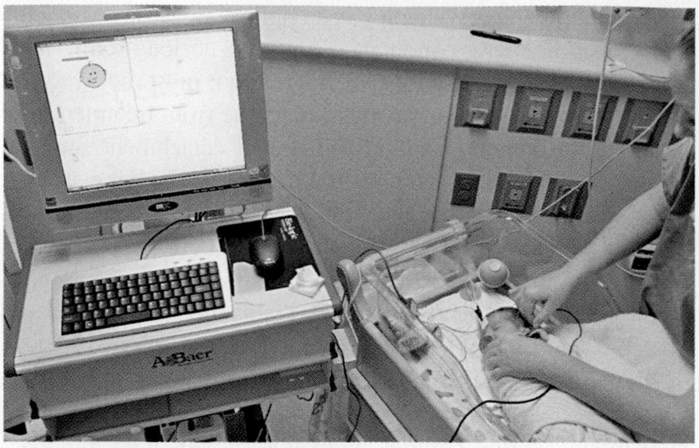

Figure 33-10 ■ Preterm infants should have a formal hearing test prior to discharge.

Source: Courtesy of Carol Harrigan, RN, MSN, NNP-BC.

birth, not from the actual date of birth (corrected age). In addition, the parents need the consistent support of healthcare professionals in the long-term management of their infant. Many new and ongoing concerns arise as the high-risk infant grows and develops; the goal is to promote the highest quality of life possible.

SPEECH DEFECTS The most frequently observed speech defects involve delayed development of receptive and expressive ability that may persist into the school-age years.

NURSING CARE MANAGEMENT

Nursing Assessment and Diagnosis

The nurse needs to assess the physical characteristics and gestational age of the preterm newborn accurately to anticipate the special needs and problems of this baby. Physical characteristics vary greatly, depending on the gestational age, but the following characteristics are frequently present:

- ***Color.*** Usually pink or ruddy but may be acrocyanotic (Cyanosis, jaundice, or pallor are abnormal and should be noted.)
- ***Skin.*** Reddened, translucent, blood vessels readily apparent, lack of subcutaneous fat
- ***Lanugo.*** Plentiful, widely distributed
- ***Head size.*** Appears large in relation to body
- ***Skull.*** Bones pliable, fontanelle smooth and flat, sutures approximated or overriding
- ***Ears.*** Minimal cartilage, pliable, folded over
- ***Nails.*** Soft, short
- ***Genitals.*** Male: nonrugated, small scrotum; testes may or may not be descended. Female: prominent clitoris and labia minora
- ***Posture.*** Flaccid, froglike position
- ***Cry.*** Weak, feeble
- ***Reflexes.*** Poor suck, swallow, and gag
- ***Activity.*** Jerky, generalized movements (Seizure activity is abnormal.)

Determining gestational age in preterm newborns requires knowledge and experience in administering gestational assessment tools. The tool used should be specific, reliable, and valid. For a discussion of gestational age assessment tools, see chapter 30.

Nursing diagnoses that may apply to the preterm newborn include:

- ***Impaired Gas Exchange*** related to immature pulmonary vasculature and inadequate surfactant production
- ***Ineffective Breathing Pattern*** related to immature central nervous system
- ***Risk for Ineffective Cardiac Tissue Perfusion*** related to hypotension secondary to PDA
- ***Ineffective Thermoregulation*** related to hypothermia secondary to decreased glycogen and brown fat stores
- ***Imbalanced Nutrition: Less Than Body Requirements*** related to weak suck and swallow reflexes and decreased ability to absorb nutrients
- ***Ineffective Peripheral Tissue Perfusion*** related to anemia of prematurity
- ***Deficient Fluid Volume*** related to high insensible water losses and inability of kidneys to concentrate urine
- ***Impaired Tisssue Integrity*** related to fragile capillary network in the germinal matrix
- ***Risk for Infection*** related to lack of passive immunity due to preterm birth
- ***Compromised Family Coping*** related to anger or guilt at having given birth to a premature baby

Nursing Plan and Implementation

Maintenance of Respiratory Function

Preterm newborns have increased danger of respiratory obstruction. Their bronchi and trachea are so narrow that mucus can obstruct the airway. The nurse must maintain patency through judicious suctioning, but only on an as-needed basis.

Positioning of the newborn can also affect respiratory function, especially in the preterm newborn. If the baby is in the supine position, the nurse should slightly elevate the infant's head to maintain the airway, being careful not to hyperextend the neck because the trachea will collapse. Also, because the newborn has weak neck muscles and cannot control head movement, the nurse should ensure that this head position is maintained by using a small roll under the shoulders. The prone position splints the chest wall and decreases the amount of respiratory effort used to move the chest wall. The prone position therefore facilitates chest expansion and improves air entry and oxygenation. Weak or absent cough or gag reflexes increase the chance of aspiration in the premature newborn. The nurse should ensure that the infant's position facilitates drainage of mucus or regurgitated formula.

The nurse monitors heart and respiratory rates with cardiorespiratory monitors as well as through physical assessments to identify alterations in the newborn's cardiopulmonary status. Signs of respiratory distress include the following:

- Cyanosis (serious sign when generalized)
- Tachypnea (sustained respiratory rate greater than 60/minute after first 4 hours of life)

- Retractions
- Expiratory grunting
- Nasal flaring
- Apneic episodes
- Presence of crackles or rhonchi on auscultation
- Diminished air entry

If respiratory distress occurs, the nurse administers oxygen per physician or nurse practitioner order to relieve hypoxemia. If hypoxemia is not treated immediately, it may result in PDA or metabolic acidosis. If oxygen is administered to the newborn, the nurse monitors the oxygen concentration with a pulse oximeter. Periodic arterial blood gas sampling to monitor oxygen concentration in the baby's blood is essential because hyperoxemia may lead to ROP.

The nurse also needs to consider respiratory function before initiation of feedings as well as during feeding. To prevent aspiration, increased energy expenditure, and increased oxygen consumption, the nurse needs to assess the infant's gag and suck reflexes before starting oral feedings.

Maintenance of Neutral Thermal Environment

Providing a neutral thermal environment minimizes the oxygen consumption required to maintain a normal core temperature; it also prevents cold stress and facilitates growth by minimizing caloric expenditure to maintain body temperature. The preterm infant's immature CNS, as well as small brown fat stores, provides poor temperature control. A small infant (less than 1200 g) can lose 80 kcal/kg/day through radiation of body heat. The nurse should implement all the usual thermoregulation measures discussed in chapter 31 ∞.

In addition, to minimize heat loss and the effects of temperature instability for preterm and LBW newborns, the nurse should do the following:

1. Allow skin-to-skin contact between mother and newborn to maintain warmth and foster security (see "Kangaroo care" discussion later in this chapter).
2. Warm and humidify oxygen to minimize evaporative heat loss and decrease oxygen consumption.
3. Place the baby in a double-walled incubator, or use a Plexiglas heat shield over small preterm infants in single-walled incubators to avoid radiative heat losses. Some institutions use radiant warmers over the baby and pipe in humidity (swamping). Do not use Plexiglas shields on radiant warmer beds because it blocks the infrared heat.
4. Avoid placing the baby on cold surfaces, such as metal treatment tables and cold x-ray plates (conductive heat loss). Pad cold surfaces with diapers and use radiant warmers during procedures; place the preterm infant on pre-warmed mattresses; and warm hands as well as the stethoscope before examining the baby to prevent heat transfer via conduction.
5. Use warmed ambient humidity. The use of humidity decreases insensible water loss but the optimal level and duration is yet to be determined (Jones, Hayes, Starbuck, et al., 2011). Humidity, however, should only be started once the infant's temperature is within normal limits.
6. Keep the skin dry (evaporative heat loss), and place a cap on the baby's head. The head makes up 25% of the total body size.
7. Keep radiant warmers, incubators, and cribs away from windows and cold external walls (radiative heat loss) and out of drafts (conductive heat loss).
8. Open incubator portholes and doors only when necessary, and use plastic sleeves on portholes to decrease convective heat loss.
9. Use a skin probe to monitor the baby's skin temperature. Correlate ambient temperatures with the skin probe in the incubator on servocontrol. The temperature should be 36°C to 37°C (96.8°F to 98.6°F). Temperature fluctuations indicate hypothermia or hyperthermia. Be careful not to place skin temperature probes over bony prominences; areas of brown fat; poorly vasoreactive areas, such as extremities; or excoriated areas.
10. Warm formula or stored breast milk before feeding.
11. Use reflector patch over the skin temperature probe when using a radiant warmer bed so that the probe does not sense the higher infrared temperature as the baby's skin temperature and therefore decrease the heater output.

Once preterm infants are medically stable, they should be clothed with a double-thickness cap, cotton shirt, and diaper. If possible, they should be swaddled in a blanket. The nurse begins the process of weaning to a crib when the premature infant is medically stable, does not require assisted ventilation, weighs approximately 1500 g, has 5 days of consistent weight gain, and is taking oral feedings, and when apnea and bradycardia episodes have stabilized. The nurse should be familiar with the individual institution's protocol for weaning to crib for preterm infants.

Maintenance of Fluid and Electrolyte Status

Hydration is maintained by providing adequate intake based on the newborn's weight, gestational age, chronologic age, and volume of sensible and insensible water losses. Adequate fluid intake should provide sufficient water to compensate for increased insensible losses and to provide the amount needed for renal excretion of metabolic products. Insensible water losses can be minimized by providing a high-ambient humidity, humidifying oxygen, using heat shields, and placing the infant in a double-walled incubator.

The nurse evaluates the baby's hydration status by assessing and recording signs of dehydration. Signs of dehydration include the following:

- Sunken fontanelles
- Loss of weight
- Poor skin turgor (skin returns to position slowly when squeezed gently)
- Dry oral mucous membranes
- Decreased urine output
- Increased urine specific gravity (greater than 1.013)
- Hypernatremia

The nurse must also identify signs of overhydration by observing the newborn for edema or excessive weight gain and by comparing urine output with fluid intake.

The preterm infant should be weighed at least once daily at the same time each day. *Weight change is the most sensitive indicator of fluid balance.* Weighing diapers is also important for accurate input and output measurement (1 ml equals 1 g). A comparison of intake and output measurements over an 8-hour or 24-hour period provides important information about renal function and fluid balance. Assessment of patterns—in particular, whether they show a net gain or loss over several days—is also essential to fluid management. Monitor blood serum levels and pH to evaluate for electrolyte imbalances.

Accurate hourly intake calculations should be maintained when administering IV fluids. Because the preterm infant is unable to excrete excess fluid, it is important that the nurse maintain the correct amount of IV fluid to prevent fluid overload. This can be accomplished by using neonatal or pediatric infusion pumps. To prevent electrolyte imbalance, overhydration, and dehydration, the nurse must take care to give the correct IV solutions and volumes and concentrations of formulas. Urine specific gravity and pH are obtained periodically. Urine osmolality provides an indication of hydration, although this factor must be correlated with other assessments (e.g., serum sodium). Hydration is considered adequate when the urine output is 1 to 3 ml/kg/hr.

Provision of Adequate Nutrition and Prevention of Fatigue During Feeding

The feeding method depends on the preterm newborn's feeding abilities and health status. Both nipple and gavage methods are initially supplemented with IV therapy until oral intake is sufficient to support growth (110 to 130 kcal/kg/day). Early, small-volume enteral feedings called *minimal enteral nutrition via gavage* have proved to be of benefit to the very-low-birth-weight infant. (See "Methods of Feeding," earlier in this chapter.) Formula or breast milk (with or without fortifiers to increase caloric content) is incorporated into the feedings slowly. This is done to avoid overtaxing the digestive capacity of the preterm newborn.

Before each feeding, the nurse measures abdominal girth and auscultates the abdomen to determine the presence and quality of bowel sounds. Such assessments permit early detection of abdominal distention and decreased peristaltic activity, which may indicate NEC or a paralytic ileus. The nurse also checks for residual formula in the stomach before each feeding. This is done when the newborn is fed by gavage method. This procedure also can be performed when the nipple-fed newborn presents with abdominal distention. The presence of residual formula may indicate intolerance to the type or amount of feeding. Carefully watch for other signs of feeding intolerance including guaiac-positive stools (occult blood in stools), lactose in stools (reducing substance in the stools), vomiting, and diarrhea.

Preterm newborns who are ill or fatigue easily with nipple feedings are usually fed by gavage. The infant is essentially passive with these methods, thus conserving energy and calories. As the baby matures, gavage feedings are replaced with nipple (breast or formula) feedings to assist in strengthening the sucking reflex and meeting oral and emotional needs. Signs that indicate readiness are a strong gag reflex, presence of nonnutritive sucking, and rooting behavior. Both LBW and preterm infants nipple-feed more effectively in a quiet state. The nurse establishes a gradual nipple-feeding program, such as one nipple feeding per day, then one nipple feeding per shift, and then a nipple feeding every other feeding. Daily weights are monitored because often there is a small weight loss when nipple feedings are started. After feedings, the baby is placed on the left side (with support to maintain this position) or on the abdomen to enhance gastric emptying and decrease the chance of aspiration if regurgitation occurs. Gastroesophageal reflux is not uncommon in preterm newborns. Long-term gavage feeding may create nipple aversion that will require developmental occupational therapy interventions.

The nurse involves the parents in feeding their preterm baby (Figure 33-11 ■). This is essential to the development of attachment between parents and infant. In addition, such involvement increases parental knowledge about the care of their infant and helps them cope with the situation.

Prevention of Infection

The nurse is responsible for minimizing the preterm newborn's exposure to pathogenic organisms. The preterm newborn is susceptible to infection because of an immature immune system and thin, permeable skin. Invasive procedures, techniques such as umbilical catheterization, peripheral venipunctures, and mechanical ventilation, and prolonged hospitalization place the infant at greater risk for infection.

Strict hand washing and the use of separate equipment for each infant help minimize exposure of the preterm newborn to infectious agents. Most nurseries have adopted the Standard Precautions recommended by the Centers for Disease Control and Prevention (CDC) of isolating every baby and the Joint Commission on Accreditation of Healthcare Organizations (JCAHO) re-

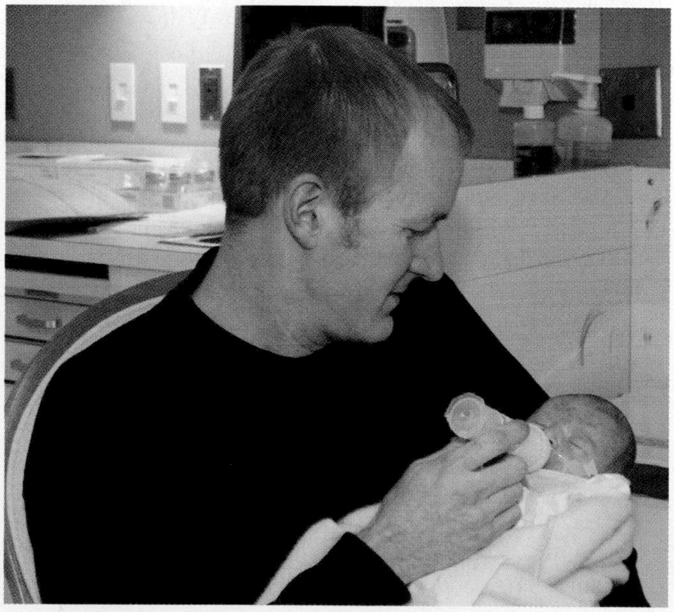

Figure 33-11 ■ Father participating in feeding experience with his premature infant.

Source: George Dodson/Lightworks Studio/Pearson Education.

quirement that staff members have short-trimmed nails and no artificial nails. Staff members are required to scrub 2 to 3 minutes using antibacterial solutions, which inhibit the growth of gram-positive cocci and gram-negative rod organisms. Other nursing interventions include limiting visitors; requiring visitors to wash their hands; and maintaining strict aseptic practices when changing IV tubing and solutions (IV solutions should be changed every 24 hours or per agency protocols), administering parenteral fluids, and assisting with sterile procedures. Incubators and radiant warmers should be changed weekly. Pressure-area breakdown is prevented by changing the baby's position, and using water-bed pillows or a gel mattress. To avoid skin tears, a protective transparent covering can be applied over vulnerable joints, but use it very sparingly (Blackburn, 2007). Chemical skin preps and tape may cause skin trauma and should be avoided as much as possible.

If infection (sepsis) occurs in the preterm newborn, the nurse may be the first to identify the associated subtle clinical signs, such as lethargy and increased episodes of apnea and bradycardia. The nurse informs the clinician of the findings immediately and implements the treatment plan per clinician orders in the presence of infection. For specific nursing care required for the newborn with an infection, see chapter 34 ∞.

Promotion of Parent-Infant Attachment

Preterm newborns can be separated from their parents for prolonged periods after illness or complications that are detected in the first few hours or days following birth. The resultant interruption in parent-newborn bonding necessitates intervention to ensure successful attachment.

Nurses should take measures to promote positive parental feelings toward the newborn. Photographs of the baby are given to parents to have at home or to the mother if she is in a different hospital or too ill to come to the nursery and visit. The infant's first name is placed on the incubator as soon as it is known to help the parents feel that their infant is a unique and special person. A weekly card with the baby's footprint, weight, and length is also sent to promote attachment. The nurse provides the parents with the telephone number of the nursery or intensive care unit and names of staff members so that they have access to information about their baby at any time of the day or night. The nurse encourages visits from siblings and grandparents to foster attachment.

Early involvement in the care and decisions regarding their baby provides parents with realistic expectations for their baby. The unique personality characteristics of the infant and the parents influence bonding and contribute to the interactive process for the family. By observing each infant's patterns of behavior and responses, especially sleep-wake states, the nurse can teach parents optimal times for interacting with their infant. Parents need education to develop caregiving skills and to understand the premature infant's behavioral characteristics. Their daily participation (if possible) is encouraged, as are early and frequent visits. The nurse provides opportunities for the parents to touch, hold, talk to, and care for their baby (change diaper, take an axillary temperature). Skin-to-skin holding *(kangaroo care)* helps parents feel close to their small infants. Kangaroo care has been shown to improve sleep periods and parents' perception of their caregiving ability (DiMenna, 2006; Turnage-Carrier, 2010). See Figure 33-12 ■.

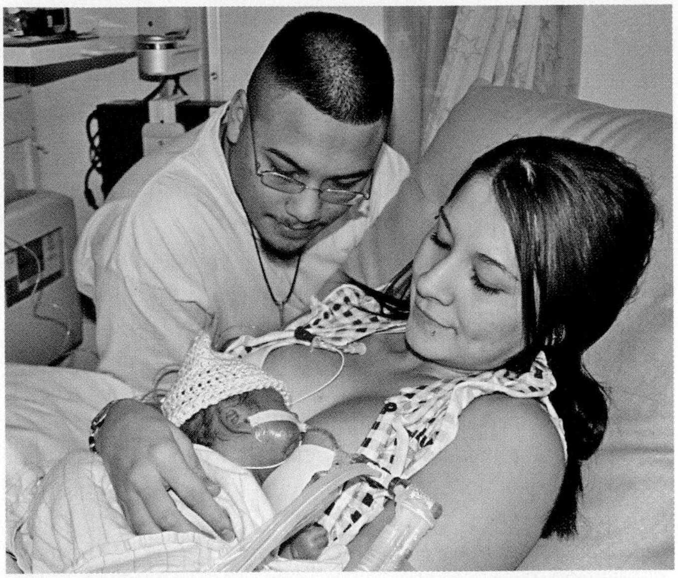

Figure 33-12 ■ Kangaroo (skin-to-skin) care facilitates a closeness and attachment between parents and their premature infant.

Source: Courtesy of Carol Harrigan, RN, MSN, NNP-BC.

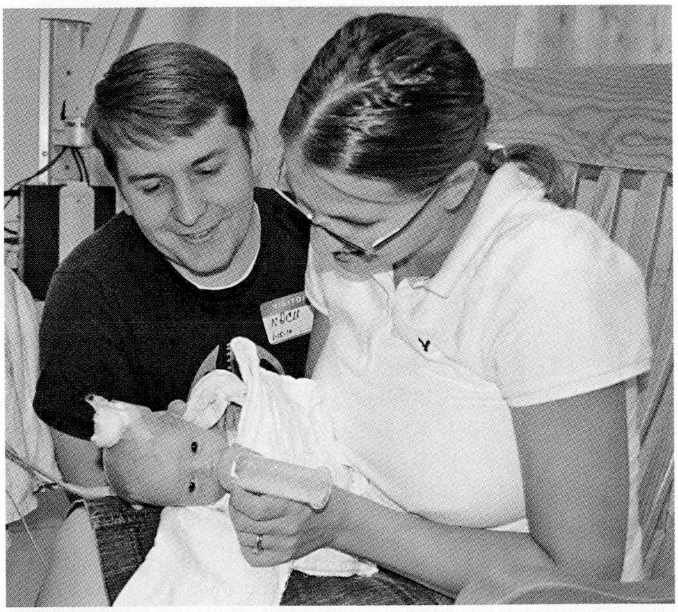

Figure 33-13 ■ Family bonding occurs when parents have opportunities to spend time with their infant.

Source: Courtesy of Carol Harrigan, RN, MSN, NNP-BC.

The parents and nurse can plan nursing care around the times when the infant is alert and best able to attend. The more knowledge parents have about the meaning of their infant's responses, behaviors, and cues for interaction, the better prepared they will be to meet their newborn's needs and form a positive attachment with their child. Parental involvement in difficult care decisions is essential and discussed in greater detail in chapter 34 ∞.

Some parents may progress easily to touching and cuddling their infant; others will not (Figure 33-13 ■). Parents need to know that their apprehension is normal and the progression of acquaintanceship is slow. Rooming-in or "nesting" can provide another opportunity for the stable preterm infant and family to get acquainted. This becomes most beneficial for both the infant and family before discharge, as it offers a quiet, private environment where help is readily available.

Complementary and Alternative Therapies in the NICU

As NICUs are becoming more and more "developmentally" friendly, complementary and alternative medicine (CAM) has now become an adjunct to that nurturing environment. This holistic approach in caring for the LBW infant attempts not only to mimic the intrauterine environment, but also to foster parent-infant bonding by simultaneously caring for the body, spirit, and mind.

Aromatherapy is the use of scent to alter mood or behavior to produce a calming and sedating effect. There is an enhanced bonding process between mothers and newborns associated with the natural body odor emitted from the mother (Turnage-Carrier, 2010). Aromatherapy is utilized in the NICU by placing an article of clothing belonging to the mother next to the infant to produce a soothing and consoling effect on the infant in her absence. Researchers are also investigating other aromatherapies, including peppermint as a respiratory stimulant, chamomile as a method to regulate sleep-wake cycles, Brazilian guava for its analgesic effects, and lavender sitz baths for management of diaper rash.

Skin-to-skin (kangaroo) care has become more prevalent in NICUs across the United States. Skin-to-skin care is defined as the practice of holding infants skin to skin next to their parents. The infant is usually naked, except for a diaper, and placed on his or her parent's bare chest. They are then both covered with a blanket. Benefits of skin-to-skin care as a developmental intervention include the following: improved oxygenation as evidenced by an increase in transcutaneous oxygen levels; enhanced temperature regulation; a decline in the episodes of apnea and bradycardia; increased periods of quiet sleep; stabilization of vital signs; positive interaction between parent and infant, which enhances attachment and bonding; increased growth parameters; and early discharge (Ludington, Morgan, & Abouelfettoh, 2008). Limitations to skin-to-skin care may be due to staff uneasiness when moving the infant while attached to multiple IV lines, monitor leads, and a ventilator, including high-frequency oscillatory ventilation. The restricted confines of the nursery may be another limiting factor as well as the lack of protocols or guidelines to safely maneuver, position, and hold the infant.

Music therapy as a noninvasive auditory stimulus has been shown to be advantageous for the premature infant. The music used in NICUs includes primarily lullabies and soft acoustical pieces which are pleasant, soothing, and calming. Such music has been shown to affect newborn physiologic responses, improving oxygenation, and increasing weight gain. It also has behavioral effects, leading to enhanced parental bonding and increased intervals of nonnutritive sucking periods. Language development is also enhanced if the music is live and sung by the mother or another female, which is preferential to the infant. The overall noise level in the NICU needs to be considered before including any extra auditory stimulation, including music therapy.

Infant massage and gentle human touch (GHT) have been practiced for many centuries. The types of stimulation include massage with stroking, gentle touch without stroking, and Therapeutic Touch or "hands on" containment. When infant massage therapy is applied to preterm infants, physiologic benefits such as stimulating blood and lymphatic flow, promoting weight gain, improving developmental scores, and regulating sleep patterns may be seen. Many emotional and behavioral benefits are also cited by practitioners. Classes are available to teach parents how to perform massage on their infants. Massage demonstrates compassion while increasing the parent's empathy and understanding of the baby. It helps parents learn to interpret their baby's behavioral cues such as facial expression, various crying patterns, and other body language. At the same time it helps infants learn about their various body parts and boundaries and feel how they integrate into the whole. Therapeutic Touch reduces motor activity and energy expenditure by the infant and promotes comfort. Infant massage therapy should be incorporated into the daily developmental care regimen of the stable preterm infant.

Promotion of Developmentally Supportive Care

Prolonged separation and the NICU environment necessitate individualized baby sensory stimulation programs. The nurse plays a key role in determining the appropriate type and amount of visual, tactile, and auditory stimulation.

Some preterm infants are not developmentally able to deal with more than one sensory input at a time. The assessment of preterm infant behavior (APIB) scale identifies the individual preterm newborn behaviors according to five areas of development (Als, Lester, Tronick, et al., 1982). The preterm infant's physiologic and behavioral subsystems are autonomic, motor control, state differentiation, attention maintenance and social interaction, and, finally, overall system regulation or self-regulation. Integration of these subsystems improves with increasing gestational and postconceptual age. If the premature infant's self-regulatory capacity is exceeded and the infant is not able to return to previously integrated subsystem functioning, maladaptive behaviors may result when the infant is confronted with environmental demands. The nurse observes the baby's behavioral reactions to stimulation and then bases developmental interventions on reducing detrimental environmental stimuli to the lowest possible level and providing appropriate opportunities for development (Turnage-Carrier, 2010).

Providing developmentally supportive, as well as family-centered, care has been proven to improve the outcomes of the critically ill neonate. With this in mind, specially designed NICUs with the single-room care concept are becoming more prevalent across the country to minimize lighting and noise exposure as well as to provide privacy for the parents of the convalescing neonate (Gibbins, Hoath, Coughlin, et al., 2008).

The NICU environment contains many detrimental stimuli that the nurse can help reduce. Noise levels can be lowered by replacing alarms with lights or silencing alarms quickly and keeping conversations away from the baby's bedside. Dimmer switches should be used to shield the baby's eyes from bright lights with blankets over the top portion of the incubator. Dimming the lights may encourage infants to open their eyes and be more responsive to their parents. Nursing care should be planned to decrease the number of times the baby is disturbed. Signs (e.g., "Quiet Please") can be placed near the bedside to allow the baby some periods of uninterrupted sleep (Turnage & Carrier, 2010)). Some other suggested developmentally supportive interventions include:

- Facilitate handling by using containment measures when turning or moving the infant or doing procedures such as suctioning. Use the hands to hold the infant's arms and legs, flexed and close to the midline of the body. This helps stabilize the infant's motor and physiologic subsystems during stressful activities.
- Touch the infant gently, and avoid sudden postural changes.
- Promote self-consoling or soothing activities, such as placing blanket rolls or approved manufactured devices next to the infant's sides and against the feet, to provide "nesting." Swaddle the infant to maintain extremities in a flexed position while ensuring that the hands can reach the face. This permits the infant to do hand-to-mouth activities, which can be consoling (Figure 33-14 ■).
- Stimulate the kinesthetic advantages of the intrauterine environment by using soft or fleece-like blankets and Gel beds. Gel bed and pillow use has been reported to improve sleep and decrease motor activity as well as lead to more mature motor behavior, fewer state changes, and a decreased heart rate.
- Provide opportunities for nonnutritive sucking with a pacifier. This improves oxygen saturation; decreases body movement; improves sleep, especially after feedings; and increases weight gain.
- Provide objects for the infant to grasp (e.g., a piece of blanket, oxygen tubing, or a finger) during caregiving. Grasping may comfort the baby.

Teaching the parents to read behavioral cues will help them move at their infant's pace when providing stimulation. Parents are ideally equipped to meet the baby's need for stimulation. Stroking, rocking, cuddling, quiet singing, and talking to the baby can all be an integral part of the baby's care. Visual stimulation in the form of *en face* interaction with the caregivers and the use of mobiles is also important.

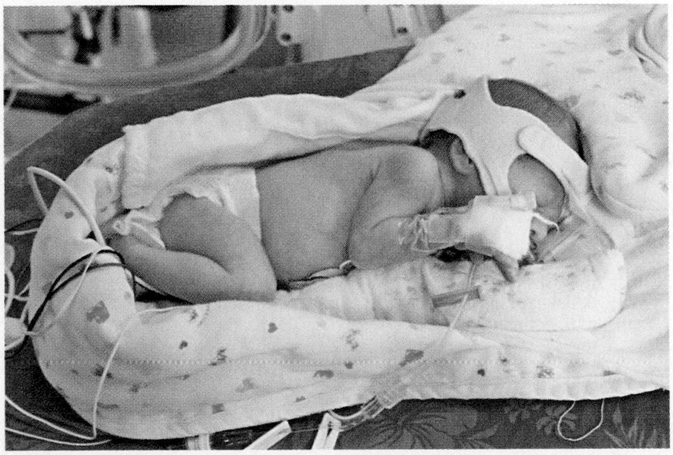

Figure 33-14 ■ A 2-day-old, 31 weeks' gestational age, IUGR infant is "nested." Hand-to-face behavior facilitates self-consoling and soothing activities.

Source: Courtesy of Carol Harrigan, RN, MSN, NNP-BC.

Preparation for Home Care

Parents are often anxious when their premature infant is transferred out of the NICU or is discharged home. Parents of preterm babies should receive the same postpartum teaching as any parent taking a new infant home. In preparing for discharge, the nurse encourages the parents to spend time caring directly for their baby. This familiarizes them with their baby's behavior patterns and helps them establish realistic expectations about the infant. Some hospitals have a special room near the nursery where a mother can spend the night and "nest" with her baby before discharge.

Discharge instruction includes breastfeeding and formula-feeding techniques, formula preparation, and vitamin administration. If the mother wishes to breastfeed, the nurse teaches her to pump her breasts to keep the milk flowing and provide milk even before discharge. The nurse gives information on bathing, diapering, hygiene, and normal elimination patterns and prepares the parents to expect changes in the color of the baby's stool, number of bowel movements, and timing of elimination when the infant is switched from formula-feeding to breastfeeding. This information can prevent unnecessary concern by the parents. The nurse also discusses normal growth and development patterns, reflexes, and activity for preterm infants, especially signs and symptoms of overstimulation. In these discussions, the nurse should emphasize ways to promote bonding behaviors and deal with newborn crying. Care of the preterm infant with complications, preventing infections, recognizing signs of a sick baby, and the need for continued medical follow-up are other key issues. Family-care conferences with all the various disciplines involved in the care of the preterm infant is often helpful just prior to discharge.

Families with preterm infants usually do not need to be referred to community agencies, such as visiting nurse assistance. Referral may be necessary if the infant has severe congenital abnormalities, feeding problems, or complications with infections or respiratory problems or if the parents seem unable to cope with an at-risk baby. Parents of preterm infants can benefit from meeting with others in a similar situation to share common experiences and concerns. Nurses should refer parents to support groups sponsored by the hospital or by others in the community and make connections for parents with early education intervention centers.

Preterm and LBW infants are at greater risk of increased morbidity from vaccine-preventable diseases. Preterm infants who weigh less than 2000 g and are medically stable and thriving do show consistently high rates of seroconversion following the first dose of hepatitis B vaccine even when the first dose is given about 2 months after birth (Domonoske, 2010). The medically stable preterm infant and LBW infant should receive full doses of diphtheria, tetanus, acellular pertussis, *Haemophilus influenzae* type b (Hib), hepatitis B, inactivated poliovirus, rotavirus, and pneumococcal conjugate vaccines (PCV) at a chronologic age consistent with the schedule recommended for full-term infants (Domonoske, 2010). The influenza vaccine should be administered at 6 months of age before the beginning of and during the influenza season. The vaccine for immunoprophylaxis against respiratory syncytial virus (RSV) is given to those high-risk infants prior to discharge from the NICU and monthly thereafter during local RSV season.

Evaluation

Expected outcomes of nursing care include the following:

- The preterm newborn is free of respiratory distress and establishes effective respiratory function.
- The preterm newborn gains weight and shows no signs of fatigue or aspiration during feedings.
- The preterm newborn demonstrates a serial head circumference growth rate of 1 cm per week.
- The preterm infant shows no signs or symptoms of bacteremia.
- The parents are able to verbalize their anger, anxieties, and guilt feelings about the birth of a preterm baby and show attachment behavior such as frequent visits and growing confidence in their participatory care activities.

Care of the Newborn with Congenital Anomalies

The birth of a baby with a congenital defect places both newborn and family at risk. Many congenital anomalies can be life threatening if not corrected within hours after birth; others are very visible and cause the families emotional distress. When one congenital anomaly is found, healthcare providers should look for other ones, particularly in body systems that develop at the same time during gestation. Table 33-3 identifies some of the more common anomalies and their early management and nursing care in the newborn period.

TABLE 33-3 Congenital Anomalies: Identification and Care in Newborn Period

CONGENITAL ANOMALY	NURSING ASSESSMENTS	NURSING GOALS AND INTERVENTIONS
Congenital Hydrocephalus (progressive ventricular enlargement)	Enlarged or full fontanelles Split or widened sutures "Setting sun" eyes Head circumference greater than 90% on growth chart	Assess presence of hydrocephalus: Measure and plot occipital-frontal baseline measurements; then measure head circumference once a day. Check fontanelle for bulging and sutures for widening. Assist with head ultrasound and transillumination. Maintain skin integrity: Change position frequently. Clean skin creases after feeding or vomiting. Use sheepskin pillow under head. Postoperatively, position head off operative site. Watch for signs of infection.
Choanal Atresia (occlusion of posterior nares)	Cyanosis and retractions at rest Noisy respirations Difficulty breathing during feeding Obstruction by thick mucus	Assess patency of nares: Listen for breath sounds while holding baby's mouth closed and alternately compressing each nostril. Assist with passing feeding tube to confirm diagnosis. Maintain respiratory function: Assist with taping airway in mouth to prevent respiratory distress. Position with head elevated to improve air exchange.
Cleft Lip (unilateral or bilateral visible defect)	May involve external nares, nasal cartilage, nasal septum, and alveolar process Flattening or depression of midfacial contour 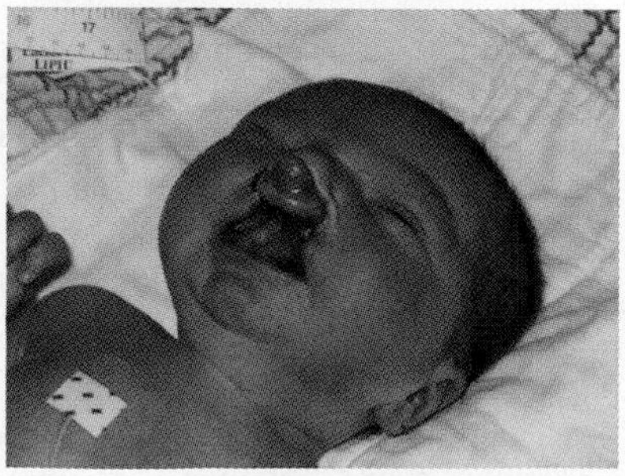	Provide nutrition: Feed with special nipple. Burp frequently (increased tendency to swallow air and reflex vomiting). Clean cleft with sterile water (to prevent crusting on cleft before repair). Support parental coping: Assist parents with grief over loss of idealized baby. Encourage verbalization of their feelings about visible defect. Provide role model in interacting with infant: Parents internalize others' responses to their newborn. (At left) Bilateral cleft lip with cleft abnormality involving both hard and soft palates. *Source: Courtesy of Carol Harrigan, RN, MSN, NNP-BC.*
Cleft Palate (fissure connecting oral and nasal cavity)	May involve uvula and soft palate May extend forward to nostril involving hard palate and maxillary alveolar ridge Difficulty in sucking Expulsion of formula through nose	Prevent aspiration/infection: Place prone or in side-lying position to facilitate drainage. Suction nasopharyngeal cavity (to prevent aspiration or airway obstruction). During newborn period feed in upright position with head and chest tilted slightly backward (to aid swallowing and discourage aspiration). Provide nutrition: Feed with special nipple that fills cleft and allows sucking. Also decreases chance of aspiration through nasal cavity. Clean mouth with water after feedings. Burp after each ounce (tend to swallow large amounts of air).

TABLE 33-3 Congenital Anomalies: Identification and Care in Newborn Period continued

CONGENITAL ANOMALY	NURSING ASSESSMENTS	NURSING GOALS AND INTERVENTIONS
Cleft Palate (continued)		Thicken formula to provide extra calories. Plot weight gain patterns to assess adequacy of diet. Provide parental support: Refer parents to community agencies and support groups. Encourage verbalization of frustrations because feeding process is long and frustrating. Praise all parental efforts. Encourage parents to seek prompt treatment for upper respiratory infection (URI) and teach them ways to decrease URI.
Tracheoesophageal Fistula (type 3) (connection between trachea and lower esophagus; upper segment ends blindly)	History of maternal polyhydramnios Excessive oral secretions Constant drooling Abdominal distention beginning soon after birth Periodic choking and cyanotic episodes Immediate regurgitation of feeding Clinical symptoms of aspiration pneumonia (tachypnea, retractions, rhonchi, decreased breath sounds, cyanotic spells) Inability to pass nasogastric tube	Maintain respiratory status and prevent aspiration. Withhold feeding until esophageal patency is determined. Quickly assess patency before putting to breast in birth area. Place low intermittent suction to control saliva and mucus (to prevent aspiration pneumonia) in pouch. Place in warmed, humidified incubator (liquefies secretions, facilitating removal). Elevate head of bed 20–40 degrees (to prevent reflux of gastric juices). Keep quiet (crying causes air to pass through fistula and to distend intestines, causing respiratory embarrassment). Maintain fluid and electrolyte balance. Give fluids to replace esophageal drainage and maintain hydration. Provide parent education: Explain staged repair—provision of gastrostomy and ligation of fistula, then repair of atresia. Keep parents informed; clarify and reinforce physician's explanations regarding malformation, surgical repair, pre- and postoperative care, and prognosis (knowledge is ego strengthening). Involve parents in care of infant and in planning for future; facilitate touch and eye contact (to dispel feelings of inadequacy, increase self-esteem and self-worth, and promote incorporation of infant into family).

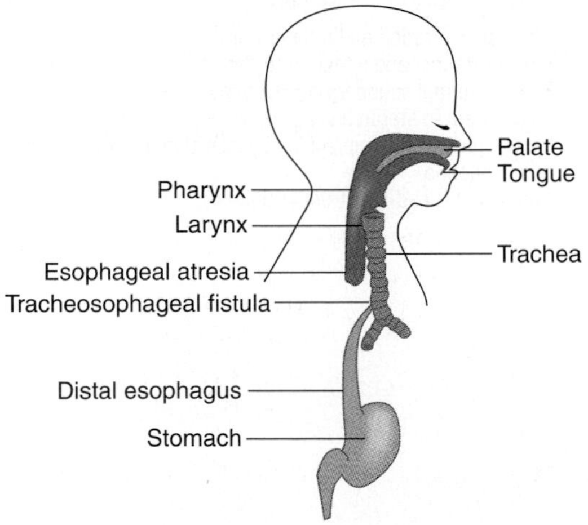

(At left) The most frequently seen type of congenital tracheoesophageal fistula with esophageal atresia.

CONGENITAL ANOMALY	NURSING ASSESSMENTS	NURSING GOALS AND INTERVENTIONS
Diaphragmatic Hernia (portion of intestines in the thoracic cavity through abnormal opening in diaphragm)	Difficulty initiating respirations Gasping respirations with nasal flaring and chest retraction Barrel chest and scaphoid abdomen Asymmetric chest expansion Breath sounds may be absent, usually on left side Heart sounds displaced to right Bowel sounds may be heard in thoracic cavity	Nurse should never ventilate with bag and mask O_2 because the stomach will inflate, further compressing the lungs. Maintain respiratory status: Immediately administer oxygen. Initiate gastric decompression. Place in high semi-Fowler's position (to use gravity to keep abdominal organs' pressure off diaphragm). Turn to affected side to allow unaffected lung expansion. Carry out interventions to alleviate respiratory and metabolic acidosis. Aspirate and irrigate tube with air or sterile water.

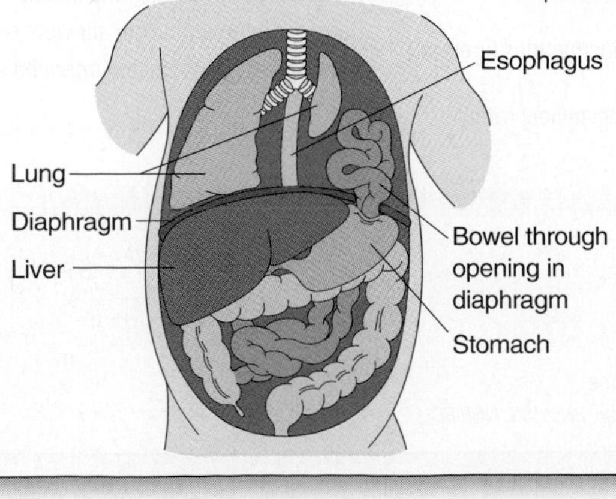

(At left) Diaphragmatic hernia. Note compression of the lung by the intestine on the affected side.
Source: Courtesy of Nancy Houck, RN, BSN, NNP-BC.

(continued)

TABLE 33-3 Congenital Anomalies: Identification and Care in Newborn Period continued

CONGENITAL ANOMALY	NURSING ASSESSMENTS	NURSING GOALS AND INTERVENTIONS
Omphalocele (herniation of abdominal contents into base of umbilical cord) 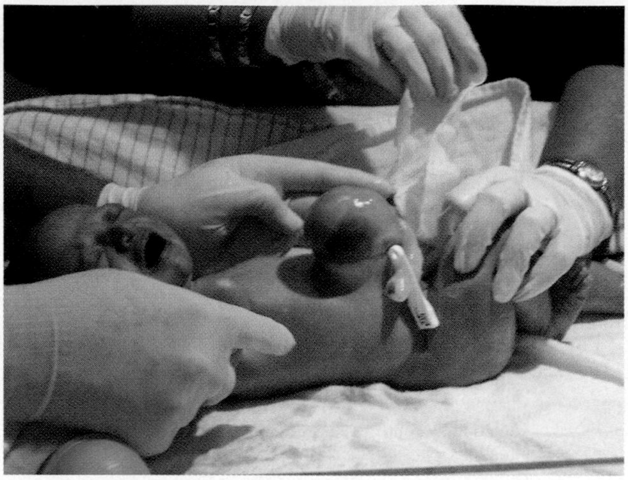	Enclosed transparent sac covering	Maintain hydration and temperature. Provide normal saline for hypovolemia. Place infant in sterile bag up to and covering defect. Initiate gastric decompression by insertion of nasogastric tube attached to low suction (to prevent distention of lower bowel and impairment of blood flow). Prevent infection and trauma to defect. Position to prevent trauma to defect. Administer broad-spectrum antibiotics. (At left) Newborn with omphalocele. *Source: Courtesy of Carol Harrigan, RN, MSN, NNP-BC.*
Gastroschisis (full-thickness defect in abdominal wall allowing viscera outside the body to the right of an intact umbilical cord) 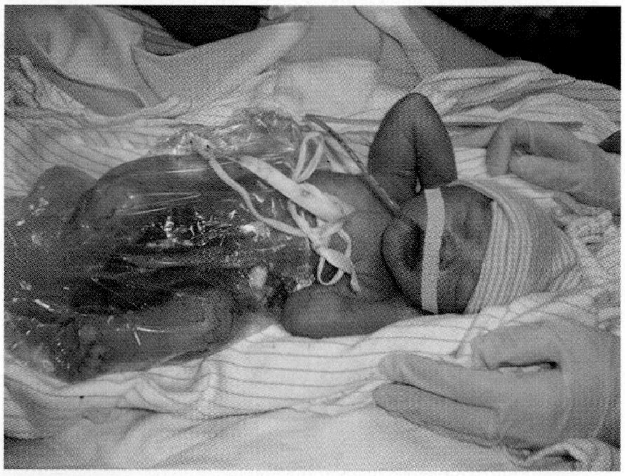	No sac covering. Intestines exposed to the caustic amniotic fluid. Associated with intestinal atresia, malrotation	Maintain hydration and temperature. Prevent trauma and infection to defect. Provide normal saline for hypovolemia Place infant in sterile bag up to axilla. Initiate gastric decompression by insertion of nasogastric tube attached to low suction. Administer broad-spectrum antibiotics. (At left) Term newborn with gastroschisis. Note the externalized loops of bowel visible through the bag. *Source: Courtesy of Carol Harrigan, RN, MSN, NNP-BC.*
Prune Belly Syndrome (congenital absence of one or more layers of abdominal muscles) 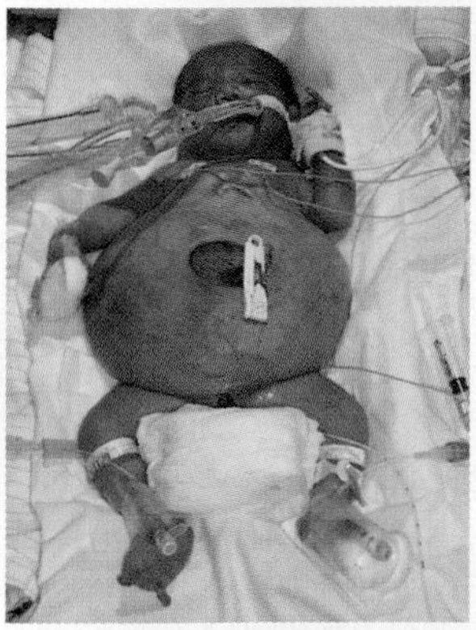	Oligohydramnios leading to pulmonary hypoplasia common Deficiency of the abdominal wall musculature causing the abdomen to be shapeless Skin hangs loosely and is wrinkled in appearance Associated with urinary abnormalities (urethral obstruction) In males, cryptorchidism is common; rarely occurs in females (At left) Prune belly syndrome. *Source: Courtesy of Carol Harrigan, RN, MSN, NNP-BC.*	Maintain respiratory status: May need to be immediately intubated and ventilated. Prevent trauma and infection. Administer broad-spectrum antibiotics. Place a urinary catheter and monitor urinary output. Carry out interventions to alleviate respiratory and metabolic acidosis. Keep parents updated and informed about prognosis.

TABLE 33-3 Congenital Anomalies: Identification and Care in Newborn Period continued

CONGENITAL ANOMALY	NURSING ASSESSMENTS	NURSING GOALS AND INTERVENTIONS
Myelomeningocele (saclike cyst containing meninges, spinal cord, and nerve roots in thoracic and/or lumbar area)	Myelomeningocele directly connects to subarachnoid space so hydrocephalus often associated No response or varying response to sensation below level of defect May have constant dribbling of urine Incontinence or retention of stool Anal wink may or may not be present	Prevent trauma and infection. Position on abdomen or on side and restrain (to prevent pressure and trauma to sac). Meticulously clean buttocks and genitals after each voiding and defecation (to prevent contamination of sac and decrease possibility of infection). May put protective covering over sac (to prevent rupture and drying). Observe sac for oozing of fluid. Credé bladder (apply downward pressure on bladder with thumbs, moving urine toward the urethra) as ordered to prevent urinary stasis. Assess amount of sensation and movement below defect. Observe for complications. Obtain occipital-frontal circumference baseline measurements; then measure head circumference once a day (to detect hydrocephalus). Check fontanelle for fullness and bulging.
	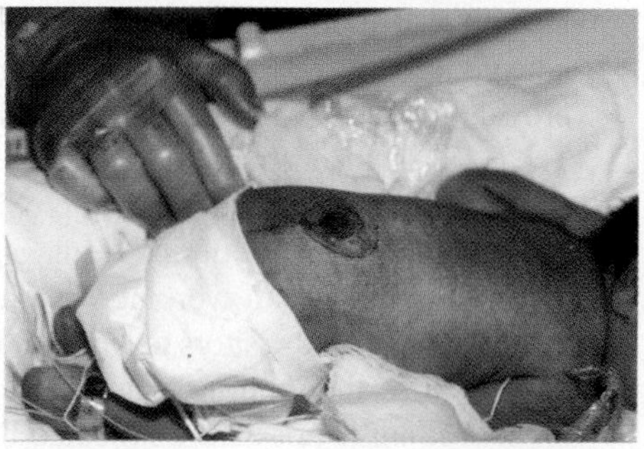	(At left) Newborn with lumbar myelomeningocele. *Source: Courtesy of Carol Harrigan, RN, MSN, NNP-BC.*
Imperforate Anus, Congenital Dislocated Hip, and Clubfoot	See discussion in "Anus and Extremities" in chapter 30 ∞.	Identify defect and initiate appropriate referral early.

Care of the Infant of a Substance-Abusing Mother

An **infant of a substance-abusing mother (ISAM)** may be alcohol or drug (licit or illicit) dependent. After birth, when an infant's connection with the maternal blood supply is severed, the baby may suffer withdrawal. In addition, the drugs the mother ingested may be teratogenic, resulting in congenital anomalies and/or developmental problems.

Alcohol Dependence

Fetal alcohol syndrome (FAS), a leading cause of preventable intellectual disability (mental retardation), includes a group of physical, behavioral, and cognitive malformations frequently found in infants exposed to alcohol in utero. It has been estimated that complete FAS occurs in up to 0.5 to 2 per 1000 live births (Pitts, 2010). FAS rates are increased among Native Americans, Alaska natives, African Americans, and women of low economic status. A new set of guidelines for diagnosis and referral of infants and children with FAS has been developed (Pitts, 2010). The term *fetal alcohol effects (FAE)* was used to describe children who had some, but not all, of the characteristics of FAS; however, it was vague. Recently the term **fetal alcohol spectrum disorder (FASD)** has been used to include all categories of prenatal alcohol exposure, including FAS. FASD, however, is an umbrella term and not meant as a clinical diagnosis. The new diagnostic categories for FAS take into consideration the various clinical manifestations of FAS, the social and family environment, and, if available, the maternal alcohol history. Five diagnostic categories are used to describe effects of alcohol exposure:

1. FAS with a confirmed history of maternal alcohol intake.
2. FAS with phenotypic features but no confirmed history of maternal alcohol intake.
3. Partial FAS with confirmed history of maternal alcohol intake, some facial abnormalities, and one of the following: central nervous system (CNS) abnormalities, growth restriction, or behavioral or cognitive disabilities.
4. *Alcohol-related birth defects (ARBD)* are usually determined only by a positive maternal drinking history. They present with one or more birth defects including malformations and dysplasias of the heart, bone, kidney, vision, or hearing systems and do not exhibit the classic facial dysmorphology of the FAS infant (Pitts, 2010).
5. *Alcohol related neurodevelopmental disorder (ARND).* These children have CNS neurodevelopmental abnormalities and complex behavior and cognitive abnormalities (Pitts, 2010). ARBD and ARND can both occur together.

Although it is known that ethanol freely crosses the placenta to the fetus, it is still not known whether the alcohol alone or the by-products of alcohol breakdown cause the damage. For an in-depth discussion of alcohol abuse in pregnancy, see chapter 19 ∞. The effects of other substances that are often combined with alcohol, such as nicotine, diazepam (Valium), marijuana, and caffeine, as well as poor diet, enhance the likelihood of FAS.

Long-Term Complications for the Infant with FAS

The long-term prognosis for the FAS newborn is less than favorable. Because of the failure-to-thrive appearance, many FAS infants are often evaluated for deficiencies in organic

Fetal Alcohol Syndrome Resources

and inorganic amino acids. These infants have a delay in oral feeding development but have a normal progression of oral motor function. Many FAS infants feed poorly and have persistent vomiting until 6 to 7 months of age. They have difficulty adjusting to solid foods and show little spontaneous interest in food.

CNS dysfunctions are the most common and serious problems associated with FAS. Hypertonicity and increased placidity are seen in these infants. They also have a decreased ability to habituate repetitive stimuli. Children exhibiting FAS can be severely intellectually disabled or have normal intelligence. These children show impulsivity, cognitive impairment, speech and language abnormalities, and learning disabilities indicative of CNS involvement (Pitts, 2010). As they progress through the adolescent years, they change from very thin and underweight children to those who are overweight and often obese. Short stature and microcephaly persist.

NURSING CARE MANAGEMENT

Nursing Assessment and Diagnosis

The nurse assesses the newborn for the following characteristics:

- ***Abnormal structural development and CNS dysfunction.*** These include mental retardation, microcephaly, and hyperactivity.
- ***Growth deficiencies.*** Infants with FAS are often restricted in regard to weight, length, and head circumference being affected. These infants continue to show a persistent postnatal growth deficiency with head circumference and linear growth most affected.
- ***Classic dysmorphic facial features.*** These include short palpebral fissures, epicanthal folds, broad nasal bridge, flattened midface, short upturned or beaklike nose, micrognathia (abnormally small lower jaw), hypoplastic maxilla, thin upper lip or vermilion border, and smooth philtrum (groove on upper lip) (Kenner & Lott, 2007).
- ***Associated anomalies.*** Abnormalities affecting the heart (primarily septal and valvular defects), eyes (optic nerve hypoplasia), ears (conductive and sensorineural hearing loss), kidneys, and skeletal system (especially those involving joints, such as congenital dislocated hips) are often noted.

Alcohol-exposed newborns in the first week of life may show symptoms that include sleeplessness, excessive arousal states, inconsolable crying, abnormal reflexes, hyperactivity with little ability to maintain alertness and attentiveness to environment, jitteriness, abdominal distention, and exaggerated mouthing behaviors such as hyperactive rooting and increased nonnutritive sucking. Seizures may be common. These symptoms commonly persist throughout the first month of life but may continue longer. Alcohol dependence in the infant is physiologic, not psychologic. Signs and symptoms of withdrawal often appear within 6 to 12 hours and at least within the first 3 days of life. Seizures after the neonatal period are rare.

Nursing diagnoses that may apply to the FAS newborn include the following:

- ***Imbalanced Nutrition: Less Than Body Requirements*** related to decreased oral intake and hyperirritability
- ***Risk for Ineffective Cerebral Tissue Perfusion*** related to microcephaly secondary to maternal alcohol use
- ***Ineffective Coping*** related to dysfunctional family dynamics and substance-dependent mother

Nursing Plan and Implementation

Hospital-Based Nursing Care

Nursing care of the FAS newborn is aimed at avoiding heat loss, providing adequate nutrition, and reducing environmental stimuli. The FAS baby is most comfortable in a quiet, dimly lighted environment. Because of their feeding problems, these infants require extra time and patience during feedings. It is important to provide consistency in the staff working with the baby and parents and to keep personnel and visitors to a minimum at any one time.

The nurse should inform the alcohol-dependent mother that breastfeeding is not contraindicated but that excessive alcohol consumption may intoxicate the newborn and inhibit the letdown reflex. The nurse should monitor the newborn's vital signs closely and observe for evidence of seizure activity and respiratory distress.

Community-Based Nursing Care

Infants affected by maternal alcohol abuse are also at risk psychologically. Restlessness, sleeplessness, agitation, resistance to cuddling or holding, and frequent crying can be frustrating to parents as their efforts to relieve the distress are unrewarded. Feeding dysfunction can also result in frustrations for the caregiver and digestive upsets for the infant. Frustration may cause the parents to punish the baby or result in the unconscious desire to stay away from the infant. Either outcome may create an unstable family environment and result in the infant's failure to thrive.

The nurse should focus on providing support for the parents and reinforcing positive parenting activity. Before discharge, parents should be given opportunities to provide baby care so that they can feel confident in their interpretations of their baby's cues and their ability to meet the baby's needs. Referring the family to social services and visiting nurse or public health nurse associations is essential for the well-being of the infant. Follow-up care and teaching can strengthen the parents' skills and coping abilities and help them create a stable, healthy environment for their family. The infant with FAS should be involved in intervention programs that monitor the child's developmental progress, health, and home environment.

Evaluation

Expected outcomes of nursing care include the following:

- The FAS newborn is able to tolerate feedings and gain weight.
- The FAS infant's hyperirritability is controlled, and the baby has suffered no physical injuries.
- The parents are able to identify and meet the special needs of their newborn and accept outside assistance as needed.

Drug Dependence

Drugs of abuse by the pregnant woman can include, but are not limited to, the following singularly or in combination: tobacco, cocaine, phencyclidine (PCP), methamphetamines, inhalants, marijuana, heroin, antidepressants, and methadone. Patterns of abuse of alcohol, marijuana, and heroin in childbearing women have changed very little in the past few years. The incidence of cocaine (especially "crack") use may have stabilized but oxycodone (oxycontin) use has risen dramatically (see "Substances Commonly Abused During Pregnancy" in chapter 19 ∞ for more discussion of maternal substance abuse). Marijuana, alcohol, and nicotine are sometimes used in conjunction with cocaine.

Intrauterine drug-exposed infants are predisposed to a number of problems. Almost all narcotic drugs cross the placenta and enter the fetal circulation, so the fetus can develop problems in utero or soon after birth. The effects of polydrug use on the newborn must always be taken into consideration.

The greatest risks to the fetus of the drug-dependent mother include the following:

- ***Intrauterine asphyxia.*** Asphyxia is often a direct result of fetal withdrawal secondary to maternal withdrawal. Fetal withdrawal is accompanied by hyperactivity with increased oxygen consumption. Insufficiency of oxygen can lead to fetal asphyxia. Moreover, narcotic-addicted women tend to have a higher incidence of hypertension, abruptio placentae, and placenta previa, resulting in placental insufficiency and fetal asphyxia.
- ***Intrauterine infection.*** Sexually transmitted infections, HIV, and hepatitis are often connected with the pregnant addict's lifestyle. Such infections can involve the fetus.
- ***Alterations in birth weight.*** These may depend on the type of drug the mother uses. Women using predominantly heroin or cocaine have infants of lower birth weight who are small for gestational age (SGA). Women maintained on methadone have higher-birth-weight infants, some of whom are large for gestational age (LGA).
- ***Low Apgar scores.*** These may be related to the intrauterine asphyxia or the medication the woman received during labor. The use of a narcotic antagonist (nalorphine or naloxone) to reverse respiratory depression is contraindicated because it may precipitate acute withdrawal in the infant.

Common Complications of the Drug-Exposed Newborn

The newborn of a woman who abused drugs during her pregnancy is predisposed to the following problems:

- ***Respiratory distress.*** The heroin-addicted newborn frequently suffers respiratory stress, mainly meconium-aspiration pneumonia and transient tachypnea. Meconium aspiration is usually secondary to increased oxygen consumption and activity experienced by the fetus during intrauterine withdrawal. In addition, ingestion of heroin will elevate maternal blood pressure causing uterine vasoconstriction, which in turn reduces placental blood flow leading to fetal hypoxia, fetal distress, and meconium aspiration. Transient tachypnea may develop secondary to the inhibitory effects of narcotics on the reflex responsible for clearing the lungs. Respiratory distress syndrome (RDS), however, occurs less often in heroin-addicted newborns, even in those who are premature, because they have tissue-oxygen unloading capabilities comparable to those of a 6-week-old term infant. In addition, heroin stimulates production of glucocorticoids via the anterior pituitary gland.
- ***Jaundice.*** Newborns of methadone-addicted women may develop jaundice due to prematurity. By contrast, infants of mothers addicted to heroin or cocaine have a lower incidence of hyperbilirubinemia because these substances contribute to early maturity of the liver.
- ***Congenital anomalies and growth restriction.*** Infants of cocaine-addicted mothers exhibit congenital malformations involving bony skull defects, such as microencephaly, and symmetric intrauterine growth restriction (IUGR), cardiac defects, and genitourinary defects. Infants exposed to methamphetamines during gestation may show an increased incidence of cardiac anomalies, symmetrical growth restriction, and low birth weight (LBW) (Cunningham et al., 2010). Congenital anomalies, however, are rare.
- ***Behavioral abnormalities.*** Babies exposed to cocaine have poor state organization. They exhibit decreased interactive behaviors when tested with the Brazelton Neonatal Behavioral Assessment Scale. These infants also have difficulty moving through the various sleep and awake states and have problems attending to and actively engaging in auditory and visual stimuli.
- ***Withdrawal.*** The most significant postnatal problem of the drug-exposed newborn is narcotic withdrawal (usually from heroin or methadone). Withdrawal manifestations often begin within the first 24 to 48 hours of life. See Table 33-4 for a discussion of withdrawal symptoms.

Long-Term Effects

During the first 2 years of life, many cocaine-exposed infants demonstrate susceptibility to behavior lability and are unable to express strong feelings such as pleasure, anger, or distress, or even a strong reaction to being separated from their parents. Cocaine-exposed infants may be at higher risk for motor development problems, cognitive impairment, and feeding difficulties due to swallowing problems (Cunningham et al., 2010). Behavior state control is poorly developed in drug-exposed infants, who tend to rapidly progress from sleep to a wakeful state of crying without smooth transition from one state to the next. As a result, these infants have poor social interaction skills; cannot habituate to external stimuli; and become easily overstimulated, having difficulty sleeping.

Infants of drug-addicted mothers often demonstrate a higher incidence of gastrointestinal (GI) and respiratory illnesses. These illnesses can be related not to drug exposure but to the mothers' lack of education regarding proper infant care, feeding, and hygiene. After birth the infant born to a drug-dependent mother may also be subject to neglect or abuse, or both.

Clinical Therapy

For optimal fetal and newborn outcome, the heroin-addicted woman should receive complete prenatal care as early as possible to reduce maternal morbidity and mortality rates and to promote

TABLE 33-4 Clinical Manifestations of Newborn Withdrawal

Central Nervous System Signs	Gastrointestinal Signs	Vasomotor Signs
• Hyperactivity • High-pitched cry • Hyperirritability, difficult to console • Increased muscle tone • Exaggerated reflexes • Tremors, myoclonic jerks, seizures • Sneezing, hiccups, yawning • Short, unquiet sleep • Fever (accompanies the increased neuromuscular activities) **Respiratory Signs** • Tachypnea (greater than 60 breaths per minute when quiet) • Excessive secretions	• Disorganized, vigorous suck • Vomiting • Drooling • Sensitive gag reflex • Hyperphagia • Diarrhea • Poor feeding (less than 15 ml on first day of life; takes longer than 30 minutes per feeding)	• Stuffy nose, yawning, sneezing • Flushing • Sweating • Sudden, circumoral pallor **Cutaneous Signs** • Excoriated buttocks, knees, elbows • Facial scratches • Pressure-point abrasions

fetal stability and growth (Pitts, 2010). Methadone maintenance programs have been the standard to treat the heroin-addicted mother to combat the cravings and to prevent withdrawal. For those women dependent on narcotics, it is not recommended that they be withdrawn completely while pregnant because this induces fetal withdrawal with poor newborn outcomes.

Newborn treatment may include management of complications; serologic tests for syphilis, HIV, and hepatitis B; urine and meconium drug screen; and social service referral. Screening of meconium provides a more comprehensive and accurate indication of exposure over a longer gestational period than does screening of neonatal urine (AAP & ACOG, 2007). Pharmacologic management for opiate withdrawal may include oral morphine sulfate solution, paregoric, tincture of opium, oral methadone, phenobarbital, and diazepam (Pitts, 2010).

Optimal nutritional support to promote adequate weight gain, although a challenge, is important in light of the increase in energy expenditure that withdrawal may entail.

NURSING CARE MANAGEMENT

Nursing Assessment and Diagnosis

Early identification of the newborn needing clinical or pharmacologic interventions decreases the incidence of mortality and morbidity. The identification of substance-exposed newborns is determined primarily by clinical indicators in the prenatal period including maternal presentation, history of substance use or abuse, medical history, or toxicology results. During the newborn period, nursing assessment focuses on the following:

- Discovering the mother's last drug intake and dosage level. Women may be reluctant to disclose this information; therefore, a nonjudgmental interview technique is essential (AAP & ACOG, 2007).
- Assessing for congenital malformations and the complications related to intrauterine withdrawal, such as SGA, asphyxia, meconium aspiration, and prematurity.
- Identifying the signs and symptoms of newborn withdrawal or neonatal abstinence syndrome (see Table 33-5).

Although many of the signs and symptoms of narcotic withdrawal are similar to those seen with hypoglycemia and hypocalcemia, drug-exposed babies have glucose and calcium values within normal limits.

Neonatal abstinence syndrome (NAS) includes both physiologic and behavioral responses. A number of useful systematic scoring systems are available for assessing severity (Pitts, 2010). The severity of withdrawal can be assessed by a scoring system based on observations and measurement of the responses to neonatal abstinence such as the Finnegan scale. It evaluates the infant on potentially life-threatening signs, such as vomiting, diarrhea, weight loss, irritability, tremors, and tachypnea (Table 33-5). NAS scoring helps to guide the need for pharmacologic intervention. For example, pharmacologic treatment is recommended for Finnegan's scores greater than 8 (Pitts, 2010).

Nursing diagnoses that may apply to drug-dependent newborns include the following:

- ***Risk for CNS Injury*** related to perinatal substance abuse
- ***Impaired Breathing Pattern*** related to meconium aspiration syndrome due to fetal stress and hypoxia
- ***Imbalanced Nutrition: Less Than Body Requirements*** related to vomiting and diarrhea, uncoordinated suck and swallow reflex, hypertonia secondary to withdrawal
- ***Impaired Skin Integrity*** related to constant activity, diarrhea
- ***Impaired Parenting*** related to hyperirritable behavior of the infant and lack of knowledge of infant care
- ***Disturbed Sleep Pattern*** related to CNS excitation secondary to drug withdrawal

Nursing Plan and Implementation

Hospital-Based Nursing Care

Care of the drug-exposed newborn is based on reducing withdrawal symptoms and promoting adequate respiration, temperature, and nutrition. See the Nursing Care Plan: The Newborn

TABLE 33-5 Neonatal Abstinence Score Sheet

Neonatal Abstinence Scoring System

SYSTEM	SIGNS AND SYMPTOMS	SCORE	AM	PM	COMMENTS
Central Nervous System Disturbances	Excessive high-pitched (or other) cry	2			Daily weights
	Continuous high-pitched (or other) cry	3			
	Sleeps < 1 hour after feeding	3			
	Sleeps < 2 hours after feeding	2			
	Sleeps < 3 hours after feeding	1			
	Hyperactive Moro reflex	2			
	Markedly hyperactive Moro reflex	3			
	Mild tremors disturbed	1			
	Moderate-severe tremors disturbed	2			
	Mild tremors undisturbed	3			
	Moderate-severe tremors undisturbed	4			
	Increased muscle tone	2			
	Excoriation (specific area)	1			
	Myoclonic jerks	3			
	Generalized convulsions	5			
Metabolic/Vasomotor/ Respiratory Disturbances	Sweating	1			
	Fever < 101°F (99°F–100.8°F/37.2°C–38.2°C)	1			
	Fever > 101°F (38.4°C and higher)	2			
	Frequent yawning (> 3–4 times/interval)	1			
	Mottling	1			
	Nasal stuffiness	1			
	Sneezing (> 3–4 times/interval)	1			
	Nasal flaring	2			
	Respiratory rate > 60/min	1			
	Respiratory rate > 60/min with retractions	2			
Gastrointestinal Disturbances	Excessive sucking	1			
	Poor feeding	2			
	Regurgitation	2			
	Projectile vomiting	3			
	Loose stools	2			
	Watery stools	3			
	Total Score				
	Initials of Scorer				

Source: Reproduced from "Neonatal Abstinence Syndrome," by L. P. Finnegan, in Current Therapy in Neonatal-Perinatal Medicine, *2e, N. Nelson (ed.), 1990, by permission of the publisher, BC Decker.*

of a Substance-Abusing Mother on pages 927 to 928 for specific nursing care measures. Some general nursing care measures include the following (Pitts, 2010):

- Performing neonatal abstinence scoring per hospital protocol.
- Monitoring temperature for hyperthermia.
- Carefully monitoring pulse and respirations every 15 minutes and pulse oximetry until stable.
- Providing small, frequent feedings, especially in the presence of vomiting, regurgitation, and diarrhea.
- Properly positioning on the right side-lying or semi-Fowler's to avoid possible aspirations of vomitus or secretions.
- Administering medications as ordered, such as oral morphine, methadone, and tincture of opium. A sedative, such as phenobarbital, is usually used in combination with an opioid, as it does not control any of the GI symptoms associated with NAS (D'Apolito, 2009).
- Monitoring frequency of diarrhea and vomiting, and weighing infant every 8 hours during withdrawal.
- Swaddling with hands near mouth to minimize injury and achieve more organized behavioral state. (Offer a pacifier for nonnutritive, excessive sucking [Figure 33-15 ■]. Gentle, vertical rocking can be successful in calming an infant who is out of control.)
- Protecting face and extremities from excoriation by using mittens and soft sheets or sheepskin.
- Applying protective skin emollient to the groin area with each diaper change.
- Placing newborn in quiet, dimly lighted area of nursery.

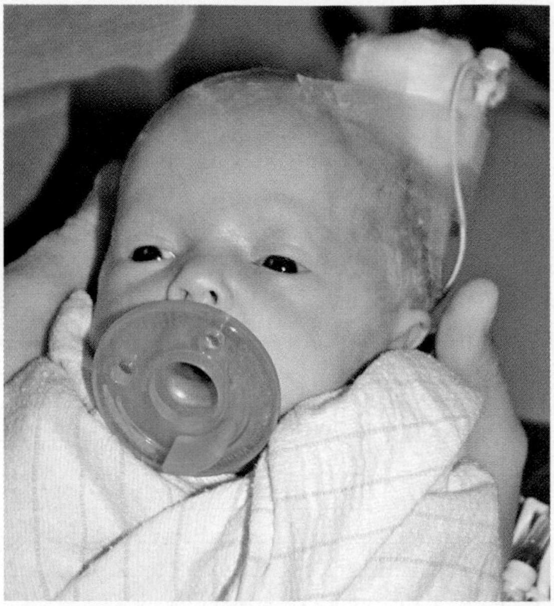

Figure 33-15 ■ Nonnutritive sucking on a pacifier has a calming effect on newborn.

Source: Courtesy of Carol Harrigan, RN, MSN, NNP-BC.

Community-Based Nursing Care

Parents need assistance to prepare for what they can expect for the first few months at home. At the time of discharge, the mother should be instructed to anticipate mild jitteriness and irritability in the newborn, which may persist from 6 days to 8 weeks, depending on the initial severity of the withdrawal (Blackburn, 2007). Infants with neonatal abstinence syndrome are at a significantly higher risk for sudden infant death syndrome (SIDS) when the mother used heroin or cocaine. The infant should sleep in a supine position and home apnea monitoring should be implemented. The nurse should demonstrate and help the mother learn feeding techniques, comforting measures, how to recognize newborn cues, and appropriate parenting responses. Parents are to be counseled regarding available resources, such as support groups, and signs and symptoms that indicate the need for further care. Ongoing evaluation is necessary because of the potential for long-term problems. Follow-up on missed appointments can bring parents back into the healthcare system, thereby improving parent and infant outcomes and promoting a positive, interactive environment after birth (AAP & ACOG, 2007).

Evaluation

Expected outcomes of nursing care include the following:

- The newborn tolerates feedings, gains weight, and has a decreased number of stools.
- The parents learn innovative ways to comfort their newborn.
- The parents are able to cope with their frustrations and begin to use outside resources as needed.

Infants of Mothers Who Are Tobacco Dependent

Despite increased knowledge about the dangers of smoking to the fetus and newborn, 15% to 20% of women continue to smoke during pregnancy (Pitts, 2010). The common consequence of tobacco use is addiction to nicotine. Most smokers report true enjoyment, associated with a sense of relaxation during stress, especially with the first cigarette of the day.

Risks of Tobacco to the Fetus and Newborn

Preconceptual cigarette smoking has been found to increase infertility. Fortunately, the reduction in fertility is reversible if the woman stops smoking. Smoking during pregnancy has been associated with spontaneous abortion, premature birth, placenta previa, and abruptio placentae. See "Tobacco" in chapter 16 ∞ for a discussion of maternal care.

The most studied compound found in cigarette smoke that can adversely affect the intrauterine environment is carbon monoxide. Carbon monoxide binds hemoglobin to form carboxyhemoglobin, which reduces the oxygen-carrying capacity of the blood. Oxygen molecules are then displaced thus lowering fetal oxygen levels and impairing tissue oxygenation. Therefore, the fetus can experience intrauterine hypoxia and ischemia. This chronic hypoxia causes the fetus to produce more red blood cells to increase available oxygen-carrying sites resulting in polycythemia/hyperviscosity, which can further impair placental blood flow. Mothers who smoke during pregnancy are more likely to have low birth weight (LBW) infants and premature infants (Pitts, 2010). These infants typically weigh 150 to 250 g less than infants of nonsmokers (Cloherty et al., 2008). The nicotine in cigarettes acts as a neuroteratogen that interferes with fetal development, specifically the developing nervous system. The greatest risks to the fetus and newborn of the mother who smokes include the following (Barron, 2008):

- *Intrauterine growth restriction and/or prematurity* secondary to cigarette metabolites crossing the placenta, displacing oxygen from hemoglobin, and impairing tissue oxygenation
- *Intrauterine distress* presenting as meconium staining and low Apgar scores
- *Neonatal neurobehavioral abnormalities* such as impaired habituation, orientation, consolability, orientation to sound
- *Hypertonia or hypotonia, tremors, increased Moro reflex*
- *Signs of nicotine toxicity* (tachycardia, irritability, poor feeding, tremors)
- *Sudden infant death syndrome (SIDS)*

Clinical Therapy

Inquiry into tobacco and smoke exposure should be a routine part of the prenatal history. Preconception and prenatal counseling about the effects of cigarette smoking on pregnancy and the fetus should occur. An estimated 5% reduction in perinatal mortality would occur if smoking during pregnancy were eliminated (AAP & ACOG, 2007).

Cotinine, a metabolite of nicotine, has been found in fetal body fluids. There is also a positive correlation between the number of cigarettes smoked per day and concentration of cotinine in maternal urine. Other factors that influence fetal and maternal serum cotinine concentrations are nicotine content of the cigarette and the time elapsed between the last cigarette smoked and the sampling. These findings indicate that cotinine may be used as a marker of maternal-fetal tobacco exposure during pregnancy (Kenner & Lott, 2007).

NURSING CARE PLAN The Newborn of a Substance-Abusing Mother

INTERVENTION	RATIONALE
1. Nursing Diagnosis: Risk for CNS Injury related to perinatal substance abuse **Goal:** The newborn will be free of signs and symptoms of central nervous system (CNS) injury.	
■ Obtain prenatal records and question the mother about history of drug use. Include duration, type of drug or drugs used, time and amount of last dose taken before birth.	■ Noting the mother's last drug ingestion will provide the medical staff with an approximate time frame to expect the infant to exhibit withdrawal symptoms.
■ Assess newborn for signs and symptoms of withdrawal (e.g., high-pitched shrill cry, sneezing, vomiting, diarrhea, hypertonicity, restlessness, and wakefulness) using neonatal abstinence scoring tool every 3 hours.	■ The average symptoms of withdrawal occur 72 hours after birth; however, symptoms may appear as early as 6–24 hours after birth.
■ Provide a quiet, calm, darkened environment. Swaddle infant tightly and place in a side-lying or prone position.	■ Providing a quiet environment decreases stimuli, therefore reducing CNS symptoms.
■ Carefully plan tests and/or treatments to avoid excessive stimuli.	■ Planning care promotes rest and reduces external stimuli.
■ Use soothing techniques such as rocking, cuddling, soft music, and soft tones when speaking.	■ These activities promote comfort, security, and infant bonding.
■ Administer appropriate medications as ordered by physician/neonatal nurse practitioner (NNP). Monitor efficacy and side effects of these medications which may include paregoric and Phenobarbital.	■ These medications aid the infant in alleviating symptoms related to withdrawal.
EXPECTED OUTCOMES:	Infant will have no signs and symptoms of CNS injury as evidenced by reduced hyperactivity, irritability, normal sleep-wake pattern, no jitteriness, and no seizure activity.
2. Nursing Diagnosis: Risk for Ineffective Airway Clearance related to suppression of respiratory system **Goal:** Infant will be free of signs and symptoms of respiratory distress after birth.	
■ Obtain maternal prenatal, labor, and birth records.	■ Provides information about fetal stress that may have occurred during the prenatal or intrapartal period. In addition, the birth record will provide information concerning the infant's respiratory status at birth; for example, the Apgar score.
■ Assess infant's respiratory rate and effort, skin color, heart rate, presence or absence of cough reflex, and symptoms of respiratory distress.	■ Maternal narcotic consumption may depress the cough reflex and respiratory center of the newborn after birth. Symptoms such as cyanosis, tachycardia, grunting, retractions, and nasal flaring may indicate hypoxia.
■ Position infant in a side-lying or semi-Fowler's position.	■ Prevents aspiration.
■ Monitor infant for temperature elevation.	■ Temperature elevation may cause metabolic rate and oxygen needs to increase when associated with CNS stimulation.
Collaborative: Obtain arterial blood gases (ABGs) as ordered by physician.	■ Oxygen demands increase with drug withdrawal. Obtaining ABGs will provide healthcare personnel baseline information on infant's respiratory status, and effective medical interventions can be initiated.
■ Monitor infant's cardiac status and pulmonary status using electrocardiogram (ECG) and pulse oximetry.	■ Provides healthcare personnel with cardiac and pulmonary status.
EXPECTED OUTCOMES:	The newborn will maintain adequate respiratory effort as evidenced by respirations of 30–60/min; no signs of retractions, grunting, or cyanosis; and arterial blood gases are within normal range.
3. Nursing Diagnosis: Imbalanced Nutrition: Less Than Body Requirements related to vomiting and diarrhea, uncoordinated suck and swallow reflex, and hypertonia secondary to withdrawal **Goal:** The infant will gain or maintain weight.	
■ Review gestational age assessment.	
■ Assess infant's sucking and swallowing reflexes.	
■ Monitor regurgitation, vomiting, diarrhea.	■ Gastrointestinal (GI) hypermobility, irritation, and CNS stimulation can increase nutritional needs.
■ Use bulb syringe before feedings if newborn is having problems with nasal stuffiness and congestion.	■ Allows infant to breathe easier by ridding the nasal passages of excessive mucus.

(continued)

NURSING CARE PLAN **The Newborn of a Substance-Abusing Mother** continued

INTERVENTION	RATIONALE
■ Initiate appropriate feedings per physician's orders (e.g., oral, gavage, or IV feedings).	■ Oral feeding may be difficult because of CNS hyperactivity and GI hypermobility.
■ Provide small frequent feedings of a high-calorie formula.	■ Facilitates nutritional intake because small-for-gestational age (SGA) infants require 120–150 kcal/kg/day for adequate nutrition.
■ Position infant on right side after feedings.	■ Prevents regurgitation and promotes gastric emptying.
■ Monitor infant's weight and document on graph.	■ Identifies abnormalities in weight gain/loss and allows for early intervention when necessary.
■ Offer pacifier between feedings for nonnutritive sucking.	■ Nonnutritive sucking allows for sucking practice, management of infant pain, and allows self-consoling behaviors.

EXPECTED OUTCOMES: The infant will tolerate feedings, maintain weight, or gain weight as evidenced by no regurgitation or aspiration of feedings, adequate weight gain according to weight graph.

4. Nursing Diagnosis: Risk for Impaired Parenting related to lack of knowledge of infant care
Goal: The parent will demonstrate ability to independently provide infant care.

INTERVENTION	RATIONALE
■ Assess mother's desire to learn infant care tasks as well as evaluate her present physical and emotional stability.	■ Provides knowledge of mother's ability to care for infant.
■ Instruct mother on coping strategies (e.g., exercise, listening to music, and discussing concerns openly) to manage stressful situations.	■ Gives mother the tools to handle stress, thereby decreasing the chances of exhibiting abusive behavior.
■ Assess mother's insight into her own chemical dependency.	■ Assistance in enrollment into a chemical dependency program may be necessary before mother can independently care for infant.
■ Instruct mother on signs and symptoms of withdrawal and treatment interventions.	■ Assists the mother in understanding infant's behaviors and gives her the tools to intervene without feeling anxious.
■ Offer a night of "nesting in" with infant before discharge.	■ Assists parents to care for infant by themselves, but with nursing support nearby.
■ Encourage mother and family members to perform basic infant care tasks.	■ Facilitates attachment and increases parenting competence.
■ Initiate social service consult as needed.	

EXPECTED OUTCOMES: The parent will demonstrate ability to perform basic infant care tasks as evidenced by exhibiting appropriate attachment behaviors (i.e., talking to and holding infant), feeding infant, and bathing infant.

NURSING CARE MANAGEMENT

Mothers should be counseled that eliminating or reducing smoking even late in pregnancy can improve fetal growth. The use of nicotine patches (instead of smoking) reduces the absorption of nicotine and thereby may result in increased birth weight of the fetus. See "Tobacco" in chapter 16 ∞ for further discussion of prenatal smoking cessation and other intervention programs. Newborns of mothers who are tobacco dependent may be screened with the NICU Network Neurobehavioral Scale (NNNS) to assess their neurologic, behavioral, and stress/abstinence neurobehavioral function (Kenner & Lott, 2007).

The potential for long-term respiratory problems such as asthma, as well as cognitive and receptive language delays that may persist into school age, should be evaluated.

Care of the Newborn Exposed to HIV/AIDS

In the United States, approximately 6000 pregnant women infected with the HIV virus give birth each year. Preventative strategies have reduced the risk of maternal-child transmission of HIV to approximately 1% to 2% (Havens & Mofenson, 2009). Most HIV transmissions during the perinatal and newborn periods can occur across the placenta or through breast milk or contaminated blood (Lott, 2010). The risk of vertical transmission in mothers not receiving antiretroviral (ARV) drug regimen such as oral zidovudine (ZDV) during gestation is 13% to 39% (Venkatesh, Adams, & Weisman, 2011). Pregnant women should be universally tested (with patient notification) for HIV infection as part of the routine battery of prenatal blood tests unless they decline the test (i.e., opt-out approach) as permitted by local and state regulation (Havens & Mofenson,

2009). Refusal of testing should be documented. For further discussion of maternal and fetal HIV/AIDS, see chapter 19 ∞. Some infants infected by maternal-fetal transmission suffer from severe immunodeficiency, with HIV disease progressing more rapidly during the first year of life.

Early identification of babies with or at risk for HIV/AIDS is essential during the newborn period. HIV-1 diagnostic testing for infants and children younger than 18 months differs from older children. Currently available HIV serologic tests (enzyme-linked immunosorbent assay [ELISA] and Western blot test) cannot distinguish between maternal and infant antibodies; therefore, they are inappropriate for infants up to 18 months of age. It may take up to 18 months for infected infants to form their own antibodies to HIV (Havens & Mofenson, 2009). Testing by HIV-1 nucleic acid amplification tests (NAATs) are the preferred tests. Results can be made available within 24 hours (Venkatesh et al., 2011). The first NAAT tests should be performed on the newborn before 12 hours of age (Havens & Mofenson, 2009). Umbilical cord blood should not be used for HIV testing because of the possibility of maternal blood contamination leading to false positive results. A repeat test should be performed at 1 to 2 months of age and again at 4 to 6 months of age (Havens & Mofenson, 2009). Most clinicians confirm the absence of HIV-1 infection with a negative HIV-1 antibody assay result at 12 to 18 months of age (Havens & Mofenson, 2009).

For term infants, AZT (zidovudine [ZDV]) is started prophylactically 2 mg/kg/dose PO every 6 hours beginning at 8 to 12 hours of life and continuing for 6 weeks (Havens & Mofenson, 2009; Venkatesh et al., 2011). If the infant is confirmed to be HIV positive, ZDV is changed to a multidrug antiretroviral regimen. Breastfeeding in developed countries should be avoided with an HIV-positive mother as transmission of the HIV virus to the newborn in breast milk is well documented (Havens & Mofenson, 2009).

NURSING CARE MANAGEMENT

Nursing Assessment and Diagnosis

Many newborns exposed to HIV/AIDS are premature or small for gestational age (SGA), or both, and show failure to thrive during the newborn and infant periods. They can show signs and symptoms of disease within days of birth. Signs that may be seen in the early infancy period include enlarged spleen and liver, swollen glands, recurrent respiratory infections, rhinorrhea, interstitial pneumonia (rarely seen in adults), recurrent gastrointestinal (GI) problems (diarrhea and weight loss), organic failure to thrive, urinary system infections, persistent or recurrent oral and genital candidiasis infections, and loss of developmental milestones (Venkatesh et al., 2011). There is also a high risk of acquiring *Pneumocystis carinii* pneumonia. Opportunistic diseases such as gram-negative sepsis and problems associated with prematurity are the primary causes of mortality in HIV-infected babies.

Nursing diagnoses that may apply to the infant exposed to HIV/AIDS include the following:

- ***Imbalanced Nutrition: Less Than Body Requirements*** related to formula intolerance and inadequate intake
- ***Risk for Impaired Skin Integrity*** related to chronic diarrhea
- ***Risk for Infection*** related to perinatal exposure and immunoregulation suppression secondary to HIV/AIDS
- ***Impaired Physical Mobility*** related to decreased neuromuscular development
- ***Delayed Growth and Development*** related to lack of attachment and stimulation
- ***Impaired Parenting*** related to diagnosis of HIV/AIDS and fear of future outcome

Nursing Plan and Implementation

Hospital-Based Nursing Care

Nursing care of the newborn exposed to HIV/AIDS includes all the normal care required for any newborn in a nursery. In addition, the nurse must include care for a newborn suspected of having a blood-borne infection, as with hepatitis B. Standard Precautions should be used when caring for the newborn immediately after birth until all maternal blood is removed and when obtaining blood samples via vein puncture or heel stick. (The blood of all newborns must be considered potentially infectious because the status of the infant's blood is often not known until after the infant is discharged. Most institutions recommend that their caregivers wear gloves during all diaper changes, especially in the presence of diarrhea because blood may be in the stool, and during examination of the newborn [AAP & ACOG, 2007]. There is a window of time before seroconversion occurs, during which the baby is still considered infectious.)

See Table 33-6 for some general issues for all caregivers of the newborn at risk for HIV/AIDS. In addition, the nurse provides for comfort; keeps the newborn well nourished and protected from opportunistic infections; provides good skin care to prevent skin rashes; and facilitates growth, development, and attachment.

CLINICAL JUDGMENT

Case Study: Jean Corrigan

Mrs. Jean Corrigan, a 23-year-old GIPI positive for HIV, has just given birth to a 7 lb, 1 oz baby girl. As she watches you assessing her daughter in the birthing room, she asks why you are wearing gloves and whether her daughter will have to be in isolation.

Critical Thinking

What will your response be to the new mother?
See www.nursing.pearsonhighered.com for possible responses.

Community-Based Nursing Care

Hand washing is crucial when caring for newborns at risk for AIDS; thus, parents must be taught proper hand washing technique. Nutrition is essential because failure to thrive and weight loss are common. Small, frequent feedings and food supplementation are helpful. The nurse should discuss with the parents sanitary techniques for preparing formula. The nurse should also inform parents that the baby should not be put to bed with juice or formula because of potential bacterial growth. Parents need to be alert to the signs of feeding intolerance, such

TABLE 33-6 Issues for Caregivers of Infants at Risk for HIV/AIDS

Resuscitation	For suctioning use a bulb syringe, mucus extractor, or meconium aspirator with wall suction on low setting. Use masks, goggles, and gloves.
Admission Care	To remove blood from baby's skin, give warm water-mild soap bath using gloves as soon as possible after admission.
Hand Washing	Thorough hand washing is indicated before and after caring for infant. Hands must be washed immediately if contaminated with blood or body fluids. Wash hands after removal of gloves.
Gloves	Gloves are indicated with touching blood or other high-risk fluids. Gloves should also be worn when handling newborns before and during their initial baths, cord care, eye prophylactics, and vitamin K administration.
Mask, Goggle, and Gown	Not routinely needed unless coming in contact with placenta or the blood and amniotic fluid on the skin of the newborn.
Needles and Syringes	Used needles should not be recapped or bent; they should be disposed of in a puncture-resistant plastic container belonging specifically to that baby. After the newborn is discharged the container is discarded.
Specimens	Blood and other specimens should be double bagged and/or sealed in an impervious container and labeled according to agency protocol.
Equipment and Linen	Articles contaminated with blood or body fluids should be discarded or bagged according to isolation or institution protocol.
Body Fluid Spills	Blood and body fluids should be cleaned promptly with a solution of 5.25% sodium hypochlorite (household bleach) diluted 1:10 with water. Apply for at least 30 seconds then wipe after the minimum contact time.
Education and Support	Provide education and psychologic support to family and staff. Caregivers who avoid contact with the baby at risk or who overdress in unnecessary isolation garb subtly exacerbate an already difficult family situation.
	Information resources include the National AIDS Hotline (1-800-342-2437) and the AIDS Clinical Trials Information Service (1-800-TRIALS-A).
Exempted Personnel	Immunologically compromised staff (pregnant women may be included in this group) and possibly infectious staff members should not care for these infants.

Source: Adapted from American Academy of Pediatrics, Committee on Pediatric AIDS and Committee on Infectious Diseases. (1999). Issues related to human immunodeficiency transmission in schools, child care, medical settings, the home, and community. Pediatrics, *104(2), 318–324; Mendez, H., & Jule J. E. 1990. Care of the infant born exposed to AIDS.* Obstetric and Gynecologic Clinics of North America, *17(3), 637; Krist, A. H., & Crawford-Faucher, A. (2002). Management of newborns exposed to maternal HIV infection.* American Family Physician, *65(10), 2049–2056.*

as increasing regurgitation, abdominal distention, and loose stools. The newborn should be weighed three times a week.

The baby should have his or her own skin care items, towels, and washcloths. Most clothing and linens can be washed with other household laundry. Linen that is visibly soiled with blood or body fluids should be kept separate and washed separately in hot, sudsy water with household bleach. Prompt diaper changing and perineal care can prevent or minimize diaper rash and promote comfort. The diaper-changing area in the home should be separate from the food preparation and serving areas. Soiled diapers are to be placed in plastic bags, sealed, and disposed of daily. Diaper-changing areas should be cleaned with a 1:10 dilution of household bleach after each diaper change. Toys should be kept as clean as possible, and they should not be shared with other children. Toys should be checked for sharp edges to prevent scratches.

The nurse should instruct parents in what signs of infection to be alert for and when to call their healthcare provider. The inability to feed without pain may indicate esophageal yeast infection and may require administration of oral nystatin (Mycostatin) for oral thrush. Topical Mycostatin or Desitin ointment is used for diaper rashes. If diarrhea occurs, the baby requires frequent perineal care and fluid replacements. Antidiarrheal medications are often ineffective. Taking rectal temperatures should be avoided, as it may stimulate diarrhea. Fluids, antipyretics, and sponging with tepid water are of use in managing fever. Irritability may be the first sign of fever.

Preventive care for exposed infants includes routine immunizations, except the combined measles-mumps-rubella-varicella (MMRV). HIV-1 exposed and infected infants should receive the rotavirus vaccine at 2, 4, and 6 months of age (Havens & Mofenson, 2009).

Parents and family members need to be reassured that there are no documented cases of people contracting HIV/AIDS from routine care of infected babies. Emotional support for the family is essential because of the stress and social isolation they may face. Because of these stresses, parents may not bond with the baby or may fail to provide the baby with enough sensory and tactile stimulation. The nurse should instruct the parents to hold the baby during feedings because the infant will benefit from frequent, gentle touch. Auditory stimulation may also be provided using music or tapes of parents' voices. The nurse should offer information to families about support groups, available counseling, and information resources.

All infants born to HIV-positive mothers require regular clinical, immunologic, and virologic monitoring. At 1 month of age, the baby's physical examination should include a developmental assessment and a complete blood count, including differential blood count, CD4+ count, and platelet count. Prophylaxis for *Pneumocystis carinii* pneumonia for all infants born to HIV-infected women should be begun after completion of the ZDV prophylaxis regimen (Venkatesh et al., 2011). Pediatric HIV disease raises many healthcare issues for the family. The parents, depending on their health status, may or may not be able to care for their infant, and they must deal with many psychosocial and economic issues.

Evaluation

Expected outcomes of nursing care include the following:

- The parents are able to bond with their infant and have realistic expectations about the baby.
- Potential opportunistic infections are identified early and treated promptly.

- The parents verbalize their concerns surrounding their baby's existing and potential health problems and accept outside assistance as needed.

Care of the Newborn with Congenital Heart Defect

Congenital heart defects (CHD) occur in 3% to 8% of live births (depending on severity of the structural defects). Because accurate diagnosis and surgical treatments are now available, many deaths can be prevented (Cloherty et al., 2008). Corrective cardiac surgery is being done at earlier ages; for example, more than one half of children undergoing surgery are less than 1 year of age, and one fourth are less than 1 month old. It is crucial for the nurse to have comprehensive knowledge of congenital heart disease to detect deviations from normal and to initiate interventions.

Overview of Congenital Heart Defects

In the majority of the cases of congenital heart malformations, the cause is multifactorial with no specific trigger with the diagnosis usually made within the first week of life. Other factors that might influence development of congenital heart malformations can be classified as environmental or genetic. Infections of the pregnant woman, such as rubella, cytomegalovirus, coxsackie B, and influenza, have been implicated. Steroids, alcohol, lithium, and some anticonvulsants have been shown to cause malformations of the heart. Seasonal spraying of pesticides has also been linked to an increase in congenital heart defects. Clinicians are also beginning to see cardiac defects in infants of mothers with phenylketonuria who do not follow their diets. Infants with Down syndrome, Turner's syndrome, Holt-Oram syndrome, trisomy 13, and trisomy 18 frequently have heart lesions. Increased incidence and risk of recurrence of specific defects occur in families.

The common cardiac defects seen in the first 6 days of life are left ventricular outflow obstructions (mitral stenosis, aortic stenosis, or atresia), hypoplastic left heart, coarctation of the aorta, patent ductus arteriosus (PDA) (the most common defect), transposition of the great vessels, tetralogy of Fallot, and large ventricular septal defect or atrial septal defects.

CLINICAL TIP

When cyanosis occurs in an otherwise healthy 12- to 24-hour-old newborn displaying no respiratory distress and is unresolved with oxygen, think about a cardiac, especially a ductal-dependent, lesion.

NURSING CARE MANAGEMENT

The primary goals of the neonatal nurse are early identification of cardiac defects and initiation of referral to the physician. The three most common manifestations of a cardiac defect are cyanosis, detectable heart murmur, and signs of congestive heart failure (tachycardia, tachypnea, diaphoresis, hepatomegaly, and cardiomegaly). Table 33-7 presents the clinical manifestations and medical/surgical management of these cardiac defects.

Initial repair of heart defects in the newborn period is becoming more commonplace. The neonatal intensive care unit (NICU) staff is now more involved in both the preoperative and postoperative care of cardiac newborns. The benefits for the cardiac infant of being cared for by NICU staff include the staff's knowledge of neonatal anatomy and physiology, experience in supporting the family, and an awareness of the developmental needs of the newborn.

After the baby is stabilized, decisions are made about the special ongoing care needs. The parents need careful and complete explanations and the opportunity to take part in decision making. They also require ongoing emotional support. Families of all babies born with congenital abnormalities need genetic counseling regarding future conception. Parents need to verbalize their concern about their baby's health maintenance and to understand the rationale for follow-up care.

Care of the Newborn with Inborn Errors of Metabolism

Inborn errors of metabolism are a group of hereditary disorders that are transmitted by mutant genes. Each causes an enzyme defect that blocks a metabolic pathway and leads to an accumulation of toxic metabolites and in some cases, irreversible brain damage. Most of the disorders are transmitted by an autosomal recessive gene, requiring two heterozygous parents to produce a homozygous infant with the disorder. Heterozygous parents carrying some inborn errors of metabolism disorders can be identified by special tests, and some inborn errors of metabolism can be detected and treated in utero. Some of the inborn errors of metabolism (especially those associated with intellectual disability [mental retardation]) are now detected neonatally through newborn screening programs. With new laboratory technology and the introduction of tandem mass spectrometry (MS/MS), a spot of blood from a newborn can deduct more than 50 inborn errors of metabolism (Matthews & Robin, 2011). For a discussion of other newborn screening tests, such as cystic fibrosis (CF), see chapter 31 ∞.

Types of Inborn Errors of Metabolism

Phenylketonuria (PKU) is the most common of the group of metabolic errors known as amino acid disorders. Newborn screenings have set its incidence at about 1 in 12,000 live births in the United States; however, the incidence varies considerably among ethnic groups (Sterk, 2010). The highest incidence worldwide is noted in white populations from northern Europe and the United States. It is rarely observed in people of African, Hispanic, Chinese, or Japanese descent (Kaye & Committee on Genetics, 2006).

Phenylalanine is an essential amino acid (found in dietary protein) used by the body for growth, and in the normal individual any excess is converted to tyrosine. The newborn with PKU lacks this converting ability, which results in an accumulation of

TABLE 33-7 Cardiac Defects of the Early Newborn Period

CONGENITAL HEART DEFECT	CLINICAL FINDINGS	MEDICAL/SURGICAL MANAGEMENT
Increased Pulmonary Blood Flow		
Patent Ductus Arteriosus (PDA) ↑ in females, maternal rubella, respiratory distress syndrome (RDS), less than 1500 g preterm newborns, high-altitude births	Harsh grade 2–3 machinery murmur upper left sternal border (LSB) just beneath clavicle ↑ difference between systolic and diastolic pulse pressure Can lead to right heart failure and pulmonary congestion ↑ left atrial (LA) and left ventricular (LV) enlargement, dilated ascending aorta ↑ pulmonary vascularity	Indomethacin—0.2 mg/kg IV Q12h × 3 doses Neoprofen—10 mg/kg IV × 1 dose then 5 mg/kg IV @ 24 & 48 hrs from first dose (both prostaglandin inhibitors) Surgical ligation, occlusion coil Use of O_2 therapy and blood transfusion to improve tissue oxygenation and perfusion Fluid restriction, Digoxin, and diuretics

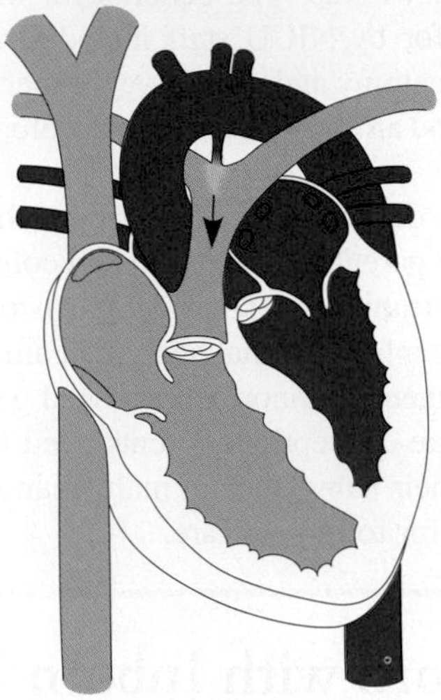

The patent ductus arteriosus is a vascular connection that, during fetal life, short-circuits the pulmonary vascular bed and directs blood from the pulmonary artery to the aorta. Postnatally, blood shunts through the ductus from the aorta to the pulmonary artery.

Source: © 2010 Abbott Laboratories, used with permission.

CONGENITAL HEART DEFECT	CLINICAL FINDINGS	MEDICAL/SURGICAL MANAGEMENT
Atrial Septal Defect (ASD) ↑ in females and Down syndrome	Initially frequently asymptomatic Systolic murmur second left intercostal space (LICS) With large ASD, diastolic rumbling murmur lower left sternal (LLS) border Failure to thrive, upper respiratory infection (URI), poor exercise tolerance	Surgical closure with patch or suture Umbrella occluder
Ventricular Septal Defect (VSD) ↑ in males	Initially asymptomatic until end of first month or large enough to cause pulmonary edema Loud, blowing systolic murmur between the third and fourth intercostal space (ICS) pulmonary blood flow Right ventricular hypertrophy Rapid respirations, growth failure, feeding difficulties Congestive right heart failure at 6 weeks–2 months of age	Follow medically—some spontaneously close Use of Digoxin and diuretics in congestive heart failure (CHF) Surgical closure with Dacron patch or umbrella occluder
Obstruction to Systemic Blood Flow		
Coarctation of Aorta Can be preductal or postductal	Absent or diminished femoral pulses Increased brachial pulses Late systolic murmur left intrascapular area Systolic BP in lower extremities Enlarged left ventricle Can present in CHF at 7–21 days of life	Surgical resection of narrowed portion of aorta Prostaglandin E_1 to maintain patency of PDA to ensure systemic blood flow No afterload reducer drugs

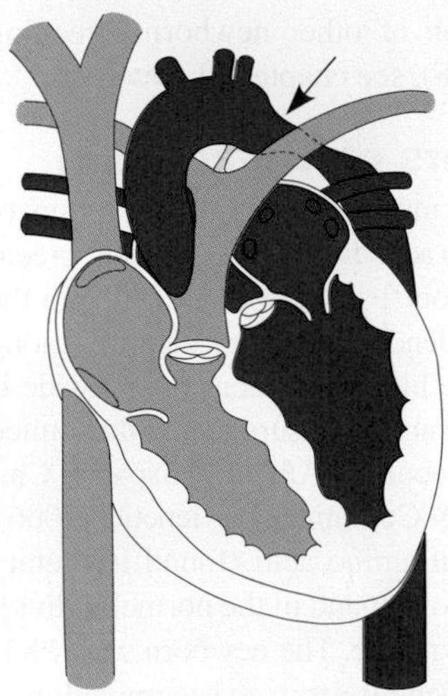

Coarctation of the aorta is characterized by a narrowed aortic lumen. The lesion produces an obstruction to the flow of blood through the aorta, causing an increased left ventricular pressure and workload.

Source: © 2010 Abbott Laboratories, used with permission.

TABLE 33-7 Cardiac Defects of the Early Newborn Period continued

Hypoplastic Left Heart Syndrome	Normal at birth—cyanosis and shocklike congestive heart failure develop within a few hours to days Soft systolic murmur just left of the sternum Diminished pulses Aortic and/or mitral atresia Tiny, thick-walled left ventricle Large, dilated, hypertrophied right ventricle X-ray examination: cardiac enlargement and pulmonary venous congestion	Prostaglandin E_1 (PGE_1) until decision made Norwood procedure Fontan procedure Transplant Compassionate care
Decreased Pulmonary Blood Flow		
Tetralogy of Fallot (TET) Pulmonary stenosis Ventricular septal defect (VSD) Overriding aorta Right ventricular hypertrophy	May be cyanotic at birth or within first few months of life Harsh systolic murmur LSB Crying or feeding increases cyanosis and respiratory distress X-ray: boot-shaped appearance secondary to small pulmonary artery Right ventricular enlargement	Prevention of dehydration, intercurrent infections Alleviation of paroxysmal dyspneic attacks Palliative surgery to increase blood flow to the lungs Corrective surgery—resection of pulmonic stenosis, closure of VSD with Dacron patch
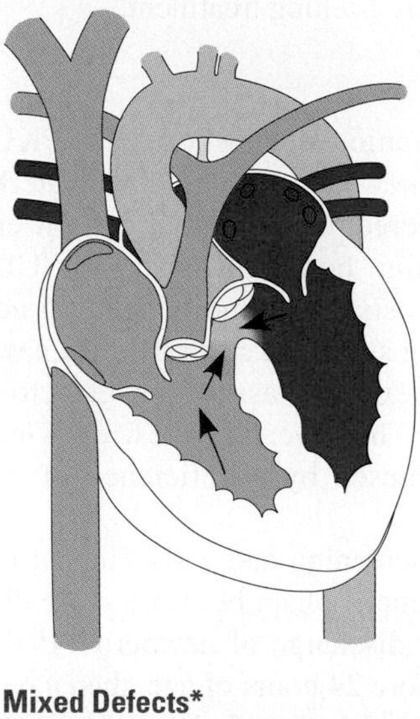	In tetralogy of Fallot, the severity of symptoms depends on the degree of pulmonary stenosis, the size of the ventricular septal defect, and the degree to which the aorta overrides the septal defect. *Source: © 2010 Abbott Laboratories, used with permission.*	
Mixed Defects*		
Transposition of Great Vessels (TGA) (Most common cyanotic heart defect) ↑ females, infants of diabetic mothers (IDMs), LGAs	Cyanosis at birth or within 3 days Possible pulmonic stenosis murmur Right ventricular hypertrophy Polycythemia "Egg on its side" x-ray finding	Prostaglandin E to maintain patency of the PDA Initial surgery to create opening between right and left side of heart if none exists Total surgical repair—usually the arterial switch procedure—done within first few days of life
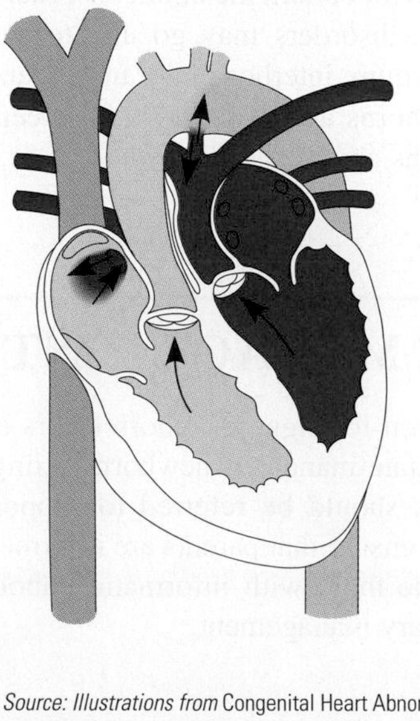	Complete transposition of great vessels is an embryologic defect caused by a straight division of the bulbar trunk without normal spiraling. As a result, the aorta originates from the right ventricle, and the pulmonary artery from the left ventricle. An abnormal communication between the two circulations must be present to sustain life. *Source: © 2010 Abbott Laboratories, used with permission.*	

Source: Illustrations from Congenital Heart Abnormalities. *Clinical Education Aid No. 7, Ross Laboratories, Columbus, OH.*

**Note:* Mixed defects-postnatal survival is dependent upon mixing of systemic and pulmonary blood flow.

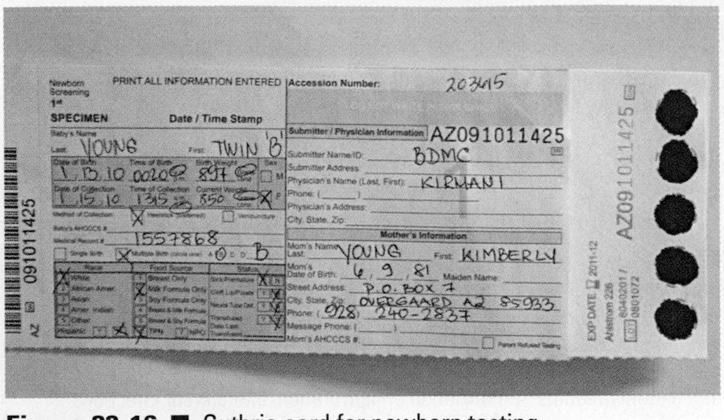

Figure 33-16 ■ Guthrie card for newborn testing.

Source: Courtesy of Carol Harrigan, RN, MSN, NNP-BC.

phenylalanine in the blood. Phenylalanine produces two abnormal metabolites, phenylpyruvic acid and phenylacetic acid, which are eliminated in the urine, producing a musty odor. Excessive accumulation of phenylalanine and its abnormal metabolites in the brain tissue leads to progressive intellectual disability. The Guthrie blood test for PKU is required for all newborns before discharge. The Guthrie test uses a drop of blood collected from a heel stick and placed on filter paper (Figure 33-16 ■). Because phenylalamine metabolites begin to build up in the PKU baby once milk feedings are initiated, the test is done at least 24 hours after the initiation of feedings containing the usual amounts of breast milk or formula. At-risk newborns should be receiving a 60% milk intake, with no more than 40% of their total intake coming from nonprotein IV fluids. The PKU testing of high-risk newborns should be deferred for at least 48 hours after hyperalimentation is initiated. It is vital that the parents understand the need for the screening procedure, and a follow-up check is necessary to confirm that the test was done.

Maple syrup urine disease (MSUD) is an inborn error of metabolism that, when untreated, is a rapidly progressing and often fatal disease caused by an enzymatic defect in the metabolism of the branched chain amino acids leucine, isoleucine, and alloisoleucine. Diagnosis of MSUD is made by analyzing blood levels of leucine, isoleucine, and alloisoleucine. Confirmation of the diagnosis depends on plasma amino acid assay.

Homocystinuria is a disorder caused by a deficiency of the enzyme cystathionine beta-synthase (CBS), which alters the pathway of the conversion of methionine to cysteine. Screening is done by a bacterial inhibition assay (BIA) to detect increased blood methionine (Kaye & Committee on Genetics, 2006). No symptoms are usually seen in the newborn period. Treatment consists of high doses of vitamin B_6.

Galactosemia is an inborn error of carbohydrate metabolism in which the body is unable to use the sugars galactose and lactose. Enzyme pathways in liver cells normally convert galactose and lactose to glucose. In galactosemia, one step in that conversion pathway is absent, either because of the lack of the enzyme galactose 1-phosphate uridyltransferase or because of the lack of the enzyme galactokinase. High levels of unusable galactose circulate in the blood, causing cataracts, brain damage, and liver damage. There appear to be ethnic differences in age of onset of symptoms and in severity of course. Caucasians have more severe symptoms and earlier onset (3 to 14 days) than people of African descent (14 to 28 days).

Another disorder frequently included in mandatory newborn blood screening tests is *congenital hypothyroidism (CH)*. An inborn enzymatic defect, lack of maternal dietary iodine, or maternal ingestion of drugs that depress or destroy thyroid tissue can cause CH. An elevated thyroid-stimulating hormone (TSH) and low T_4 are commonly seen in the premature infant following birth; it may be necessary to repeat levels at 2 to 6 weeks of age. Congenital hypothyroidism occurs more often in Hispanic and Native American/Alaska native people. Infants with Down syndrome are also at increased risk of having CH (Kaye & Committee on Genetics, 2006).

The incidence of metabolic errors is relatively low, but for affected infants and their families these disorders pose a threat to survival and frequently require lifelong treatment.

Clinical Therapy

All states have universal screening of newborns for PKU, CH, and galactosemia (Matthews & Robin, 2011; Sterk, 2010). Mandatory newborn screening for other inborn errors of metabolism, including homocystinuria, MSUD, sickle cell anemia, cystic fibrosis (CF), and congenital adrenal hypoplasia, varies among states. In several states newborn screening includes an enzyme assay for galactose 1-phosphate uridyltransferase; however, this test does not detect galactosemia if it is caused by a deficiency of the enzyme galactokinase.

Identification via newborn screening and early clinical intervention for inborn errors of metabolism becomes more difficult with the advent of early discharge of newborns. If the initial specimen is obtained before 24 hours of age, then a second specimen should be obtained before 5 days of age, although few states currently require the second test (Kaye & Committee on Genetics, 2006). Early collection of specimens may yield false-positive results for certain metabolic disorders. Conversely, certain metabolic disorders may go undetected. Newborns in the NICU who require interhospital transfers and early-discharged healthy newborns are at risk for nonscreening. Newborn screen specimens are always collected before a blood transfusion.

NURSING CARE MANAGEMENT

The nurse assesses the newborn for signs of inborn errors of metabolism and carries out state-mandated newborn testing. Parents of affected newborns should be referred to support groups. The nurse should also ensure that parents are informed about centers that can provide them with information about biochemical genetics and dietary management.

Infant with PKU

The clinical picture of a PKU baby involves a normal appearing newborn, most often with blond hair, blue eyes, and fair complexion. Decreased pigmentation may be related to the competition between phenylalanine and tyrosine for the available enzyme tyrosinase. Tyrosine is needed for the formation of melanin pigment and the hormones epinephrine and thyroxine. Without treatment, the infant fails to thrive and develops vomiting and eczematous rashes. By about 6 months of age, the infant exhibits behavior indicative of intellectual disability and other central nervous system (CNS) involvement, including seizures and abnormal electroencephalogram (EEG) patterns.

The nurse advises parents that once identified, an afflicted PKU infant can be treated by a special diet that limits ingestion of phenylalanine. Special formulas low in phenylalanine, such as Lofenalac, Minafen, and Albumaid XP, are available. Special food lists are helpful for parents of a PKU child (Blackburn, 2007). If treatment is begun before 1 month of age, CNS damage can be minimized. There is an increased risk of producing an intellectually disabled child if the mother with PKU is not on a low-phenylalanine diet during pregnancy. It is recommended that the woman reinstate her low-phenylalanine diet a few months before becoming pregnant (Blackburn, 2007).

Infant with Maple Syrup Urine Disease (MSUD)

Newborns with MSUD have feeding problems and neurologic signs (seizures, spasticity, opisthotonos) during the first week of life. A maple syrup odor of the urine is noted, and when ferric chloride is added to the urine, its color changes to gray-green. An ear swab within 6 to 12 hours after birth has a similar smell. Diagnosis is confirmed with plasma amino analysis.

Newborns with MSUD must be given a formula that is low in the branched-chain amino acids leucine, isoleucine, and valine, which is continued indefinitely. Dietary treatment before 12 days of life has been reported to result in normal intelligence.

Infant with Homocystinuria

Homocystinuria varies in its presentation, but the more common characteristics are skeletal abnormalities, dislocation of ocular lenses, intravascular thromboses, and intellectual disability. Abnormalities occur because of the toxic effects of the accumulation of methionine and the metabolite homocystine in the blood.

Infants with homocystinuria are managed on a diet that is low in methionine but supplemented with cystine and pyridoxine (vitamin B_6). Early diagnosis and careful management may prevent intellectual disability.

Infant with Galactosemia

Clinical manifestations of galactosemia include vomiting soon after ingestion of milk-based formula or breast milk, diarrhea, poor weight gain, hepatosplenomegaly, jaundice, and intellectual disability. The condition is frequently associated with anemia, sepsis, and cataracts in the newborn period (Sterk, 2010). Except for cataracts and intellectual disability, those findings are reversible when galactose is excluded from the diet. Intellectual disability can be prevented by early diagnosis and careful dietary management.

A baby with galactosemia is placed on a galactose-free diet. Galactose-free formulas include Nutramigen (a protein hydrolysate process formula), meat-based formulas, or soybean formulas. As the infant grows, parents must be educated not only to avoid giving their child milk and milk products but also to read all labels carefully and avoid any foods containing dry milk products. Even with early treatment, children may have learning disabilities, speech problems, and female ovarian failure (Kaye & Committee on Genetics, 2006).

Infant with Congenital Hypothyroidism (CH)

Approximately 5% of infants with CH, generally those who are more severely affected, have recognizable features at birth, including a large tongue, umbilical hernia, cool and mottled skin, low hairline, hypotonia, and large fontanelles (especially the posterior fontanelle in term infants) (Kaye & Committee on Genetics, 2006). Early symptoms include prolonged newborn jaundice, poor feeding, constipation, low-pitched cry, poor weight gain, inactivity, and delayed motor development. In addition, premature infants of less than 30 weeks' gestation frequently have lower T_4 and thyroid-stimulating hormone (TSH) values than those of term infants. This difference may reflect the premature infant's inability to bind thyroid hormone and a risk for hypothyroidism.

Babies with CH need frequent laboratory monitoring and adjustment of thyroid medication to accommodate their growth and development. With adequate treatment, children remain free of symptoms, but if the condition is untreated, stunted growth (slowed linear growth) and intellectual disability occur.

Evaluation

Expected outcomes of nursing care include the following:

- The risk of inborn errors of metabolism is promptly identified, and early intervention is initiated.
- The parents verbalize their concerns about their baby's nutritional status, health problems, long-term care needs, and potential outcomes.
- The parents are aware of available community health resources and use them as indicated.

FOCUS YOUR STUDY

- Early identification of potential high-risk fetuses through assessment of preconception, prenatal, and intrapartal factors facilitates strategically timed nursing observations and interventions.
- High-risk newborns, whether they are premature, small for gestational age (SGA), large for gestational age (LGA), postterm, or infants of a diabetic or substance-abusing mother, have many similar problems, although their problems are based on different physiologic processes.
- SGA newborns are associated with perinatal asphyxia and resulting meconium aspiration syndrome, hypothermia, hypoglycemia, hypocalcemia, polycythemia, congenital anomalies, and intrauterine infections. Long-term problems include continued growth and learning difficulties.
- LGA newborns are at risk for birth trauma as a result of cephalopelvic disproportion, meconium aspiration syndrome, hypoglycemia, polycythemia, and hyperviscosity.
- Infants of diabetic mothers are at risk for hypoglycemia, hypocalcemia, hyperbilirubinemia, polycythemia, and respiratory distress due to delayed maturation of their lungs.
- Postterm newborns often encounter intrapartal problems such as cephalopelvic disproportion (CPD), shoulder dystocia, and birth traumas, hypoglycemia, polycythemia, meconium aspiration, cold stress, and possible seizure activity.
- The common problems of the preterm newborn are results of the baby's immature body systems. Potential problem areas include respiratory distress syndrome (RDS), patent ductus arteriosus (PDA), hypothermia and cold stress, feeding difficulties and necrotizing enterocolitis (NEC), marked insensible water loss and loss of buffering agents through the kidneys, infection, anemia of prematurity, apnea and intraventricular hemorrhage (IVH), retinopathy of prematurity, and behavioral state disorganization. Long-term needs and problems include chronic lung disease, speech defects, sensorineural hearing loss, and neurologic sequelae.
- Newborns of alcohol-dependent mothers are at risk for alterations in physical characteristics and the long-term complications of feeding problems; central nervous system (CNS) dysfunction, including lower IQ, hyperactivity, and language abnormalities; and congenital anomalies.
- Newborns of drug-dependent mothers experience drug withdrawal as well as respiratory distress, jaundice, congenital anomalies, and behavioral abnormalities. With early recognition and intervention, the potential long-term physiologic and emotional consequences of these difficulties can be avoided or at least lessened in severity.
- Newborns of mothers with AIDS require early recognition and treatment so that the physiologic and emotional consequences may be lessened in severity and Centers for Disease Control and Prevention (CDC) guidelines implemented.
- Cardiac defects are a significant cause of morbidity and mortality in the newborn period. Early identification and nursing and medical care of newborns with cardiac defects are essential to the improved outcome of these infants. Care is directed toward lessening the workload of the heart and decreasing oxygen and energy consumption.
- Inborn errors of metabolism such as galactosemia, phenylketonuria (PKU), homocystinuria, and maple syrup urine disease (MSUD) are usually included in a newborn screening program designed to prevent intellectual disability through dietary management and medication.
- The nursing care of the newborn with special problems involves understanding normal physiology, the pathophysiology of the disease process, clinical manifestations, and supportive or corrective therapies. Only with this theoretical background can the nurse make appropriate observations concerning responses to therapy and development of complications.
- The nurse facilitates interdisciplinary communication with the parents. Parents of at-risk newborns need support from nurses and healthcare providers to understand the special needs of their baby and feel confident in their ability to care for their baby at home.

CRITICAL THINKING IN ACTION

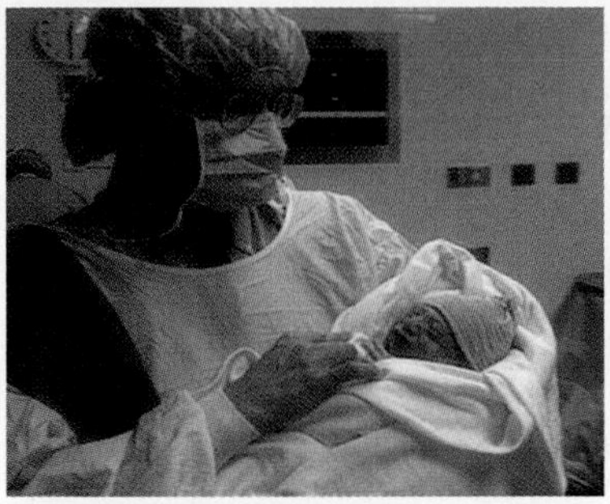

As the nurse on duty, you are caring for baby Erin, a 38-week IDM female born by repeat cesarean birth to a 32-year-old G3 now P3 mother. Erin's Apgar scores are 7 and 9 at 1 and 5 minutes. At 2 hours of age, the baby has an elevated respiratory rate of 100 to 110, heart rate of 165 with Grade II/VI intermittent machinery murmur, and mild cyanosis. She is now receiving 30% oxygen and has a respiratory rate of 70 to 80. The baby's clinical course, chest x-ray, and lab results are all consistent with transient tachypnea of the newborn and patent ductus arteriosus. The mother calls you to ask about how her baby is doing. She tells you that her last child was born at 30 weeks and had to be hospitalized for 6 weeks. She says, "I really tried to do it right this time," and asks you if this baby will have the same respiratory problem.

1. What should you tell the mother?
2. What can you do to facilitate mother-infant attachment?
3. Discuss the emotional response of parents to the birth of an ill or at-risk infant.
4. Discuss the four psychologic tasks essential for coping with the stress of an at-risk newborn and providing a basis for the maternal-infant relationship.
5. Baby Erin is being discharged tomorrow. Review the elements of discharge and home care instructions.

See www.nursing.pearsonhighered.com for possible responses.

Pearson Nursing Student Resources

Find additional review materials at
www.nursing.pearsonhighered.com

Prepare for success with additional NCLEX®-style practice questions, interactive assignments and activities, Web links, animations and videos, and more!

REFERENCES

Als, H., Lester, B. M., Tronick, E., & Brazelton, T. B. (1982). Assessment of preterm infant behavior (APIB). In B. M. Fitzgerald Lester & M. W. Yogman (Eds.), *Theory and research in behavioral pediatrics* (Vol.1). New York, NY: Plenum.

American Academy of Pediatrics (AAP) & American College of Obstetricians and Gynecologists (ACOG). (2007). *Guidelines for perinatal care* (6th ed.). Elk Grove Village, IL: Author.

Anderson, M. S., Wood, L. L., Keller, J. A., & Hay, W.W. (2011). Enteral nutrition. In S. L. Gardner (Ed.), *Merenstein & Gardner's Handbook of neonatal intensive care* (7th ed., pp. 398–433). St. Louis, MO: Mosby.

Armentrout, D. (2010). Glucose management. In M. T. Verklan & M. Walden (Eds.), *Core curriculum for neonatal intensive care nursing* (4th ed., pp. 172–181). St. Louis, MO: Saunders/Elsevier.

Barron, M. L. (2008). Antenatal care. In K. R. Simpson & P. A. Creehan, *AWHONN's perinatal nursing* (3rd ed., pp. 88–124). Philadelphia, PA: Lippincott Williams & Wilkins.

Blackburn, S. (2007). *Maternal-fetal-neonatal physiology: A clinical perspective* (3rd ed.). Philadelphia, PA: Saunders.

Cloherty, J. R., Eichenwald, E. C., & Stark, A. R. (2008). *Manual of neonatal care*. Philadelphia, PA: Lippincott Williams & Wilkins.

Cunningham, F. G., Leveno, K. J., Bloom, S. L., Hauth, J. C., Rouse, D. J., & Spong, C. Y. (2010). *Williams obstetrics* (23rd ed.). New York: McGraw-Hill.

D'Apolito, K. (2009). Neonatal opiate withdrawal: Pharmacologic management. *Newborn & Infant Reviews, 9*, 62–69. doi: 10.1053/j.nainr.2008.12.009

DiMenna, L. (2006). Considerations for implementation of a neonatal kangaroo care protocol. *Neonatal Network, 25*, 405–412.

Domonoske, C. D. (2010). Pharmacology. In M. T. Verklan & M. Walden (Eds.), *Core curriculum for neonatal intensive care nursing* (4th ed., pp. 233–251). St. Louis, MO: Saunders/Elsevier.

Gardner, S. L., & Hernandez, J. A. (2011). Initial nursery care. In S. L. Gardner (Ed.), *Merenstein & Gardner's Handbook of neonatal intensive care* (7th ed., pp. 78–112). St. Louis, MO: Mosby.

Gibbins, S., Hoath, S.B., Coughlin, M., Gibbins, A., & Franck, L. (2008). The universe of developmental care: A new conceptual model for application in the neonatal intensive care unit. *Advances in Neonatal Care, 8*(3), 141–147.

Havens, P., & Mofenson, L. (2009). Committee on pediatrics AIDS: Evaluation and management of the infant exposed to HIV-1 in the United States. *Pediatrics, 123*, 175–187. doi: 10.1542/peds.2008-3076

Jones, J. E., Hayes, R. D., Starbuck, A. L., & Porcelli, P. J. (2011). Fluid and electrolyte management. In S. L. Gardner (Ed.), *Merenstein & Gardner's Handbook of neonatal intensive care* (7th ed., pp. 333–352). St. Louis, MO: Mosby.

Kaye, C. I., & Committee on Genetics. (2006). Newborn screening fact sheets. *Pediatrics, 118*(3), 934–963. doi:10.1542/peds.2006-1782

Kenner, C., & Lott, J. W. (2007). *Comprehensive neonatal care: An interdisciplinary approach* (4th ed.). St. Louis, MO: Saunders/Elsevier.

Lott, J. W. (2010). Immunology and infectious disease. In M. T. Verklan & M. Walden (Eds.), *Core curriculum for neonatal intensive care nursing* (4th ed., pp. 694–723). St. Louis, MO: Saunders/Elsevier.

Ludington, S., Morgan, K., & Abouelfettoh, A. (2008). A clinical guideline for implementation of kangaroo care with premature infants of 30 or more weeks postmenstrual age. *Advances in Neonatal Care, 8*(3S): S3–S23. doi: 10.1097/01.ANC.0000324330.25734.b6

Matthews, A., & Robin, N. H. (2011). Genetic disorders, malformation, and inborn errors of metabolism. In S. L. Gardner (Ed.), *Merenstein & Gardner's Handbook of neonatal intensive care* (7th ed., pp. 78–112). St. Louis, MO: Mosby.

Moore, T. R., & Catalano, P. (2009). Diabetes in pregnancy. In R. K. Creasy & R. Resnik (Eds.), *Maternal-fetal medicine: Principles and practice* (6th ed., pp. 953–993). Philadelphia, PA: Saunders.

Nash, P., & Smith, J. R. (2008). Common neonatal complications. In K. R. Simpson & P. A. Creehan, *AWHONN's perinatal nursing* (3rd ed., pp. 612–646). Philadelphia, PA: Lippincott Williams & Wilkins.

Pitts, K. (2010). Perinatal substance abuse. In M. T. Verklan & M. Walden (Eds.), *Core curriculum for neonatal intensive care nursing* (4th ed., pp. 41–71). St. Louis, MO: Saunders/Elsevier.

Resnik, J. L., & Resnik, R. (2009). Post-term pregnancy. In R. K. Creasy & R. Resnik (Eds.), *Maternal-fetal medicine: Principles and practice* (6th ed., pp. 613–699). Philadelphia, PA: Saunders.

Resnik, R., & Creasy, R. K. (2009). Intrauterine growth restriction. In R. K. Creasy & R. Resnik (Eds.), *Maternal-fetal medicine: Principles and practice* (6th ed., pp. 636–650). Philadelphia, PA: Saunders.

Sterk, L. (2010). Congenital anomalies. In M. T. Verklan & M. Walden (Eds.), *Core curriculum for neonatal intensive care nursing* (4th ed., pp. 782–812). St. Louis, MO: Saunders/Elsevier.

Thomas, J. A. (2007). Guidelines for bottle feeding your premature baby. *Advances in Neonatal Care, 7*(6), 311–318. doi: 10.1097/01.ANC.0000304971.69578.f7

Turnage-Carrier, C. S. (2010). Development support. In M. T. Verklan & M. Walden (Eds.), *Core curriculum for neonatal intensive care nursing* (4th ed., pp. 208–232). St. Louis, MO: Saunders/Elsevier.

Vargo, L. E., & Trotter, C. W. (2007). *The premature infant: Nursing assessment and management* (2nd ed.). White Plains, NY: March of Dimes Foundation.

Venkatesh, M., Adams, K. M., & Weisman, L. E. (2011). Infection in the neonate. In S. L. Gardner (Ed.), *Merenstein & Gardner's Handbook of neonatal intensive care* (7th ed., pp. 553–580). St. Louis, MO: Mosby.

Volpe, J. J. (2008). *Neurology of the newborn* (5th ed.). Philadelphia, PA: Saunders.

CHAPTER 34

The Newborn at Risk: Birth-Related Stressors

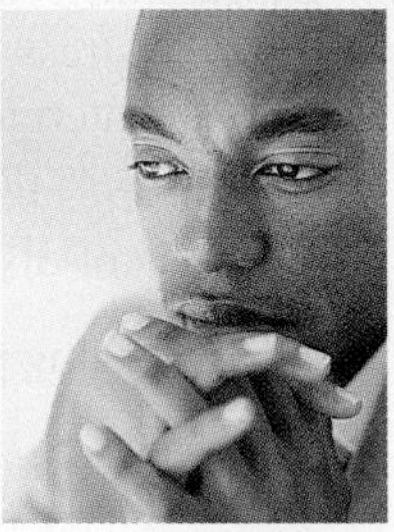

I watched her breathe every precious breath on the respirator. I saw her covered with wires and tubes. I kept watch. She was special to me and I would tell her over and over, "Daddy is here. Daddy loves you." The three days she lived were hell—not knowing if she would make it, uncertain about what plans we should make. Somehow I thought she would live; I was hopeful. When she died, at least I was there with her. The grief was unbearable. But there was also a sense of relief. The uncertainty, the waiting, were finally over.

—Susan Borg, *When Pregnancy Fails*

LEARNING OUTCOMES

1. Explain how to identify newborns in need of resuscitation.
2. Describe the appropriate method of resuscitation of a newborn based on the prenatal/labor record and observable physiologic indicators.
3. Differentiate, based on clinical manifestations, among the various types of respiratory distress (respiratory distress syndrome, transient tachypnea of the newborn, meconium aspiration syndrome, and persistent pulmonary hypertension) in the newborn and their related nursing care.
4. Discuss the types of metabolic abnormalities (cold stress and hypoglycemia), their effects on the newborn, and their nursing implications.
5. Differentiate between physiologic and pathologic jaundice according to timing of onset (in hours), cause, possible sequelae, and specific management.
6. Explain how Rh incompatibility or ABO incompatibility can lead to the development of hyperbilirubinemia.
7. Identify the nursing responsibilities in caring for the newborn receiving phototherapy.
8. Explain the causes and nursing care of infants with anemia and polycythemia.
9. Describe the nursing assessment results that would lead the nurse to suspect newborn sepsis.
10. Discuss the nursing care of the newborn with an infection.
11. Relate the consequences of maternally transmitted infections, such as maternal syphilis, gonorrhea, herpesviridae family (HSV or CMV), and chlamydia, to the management of the infant in the neonatal period.
12. Describe interventions to facilitate parental attachment and meet the special initial and long-term needs of parents of at-risk newborns.

KEY TERMS

Acute bilirubin encephalopathy (ABE) *963*
Bronchopulmonary dysplasia (BPD) *957*
Chronic lung disease (CLD) of prematurity *957*
Cold stress *958*
Erythroblastosis fetalis *963*
Hemolytic disease of the newborn *963*
Hydrops fetalis *964*
Hyperbilirubinemia *963*
Hypoglycemia *959*
Jaundice *963*
Kernicterus *963*
Meconium aspiration syndrome (MAS) *953*
Persistent pulmonary hypertension of the newborn (PPHN) *955*
Phototherapy *966*
Physiologic anemia of infancy *973*
Polycythemia *974*
Respiratory distress syndrome (RDS) *944*
Sepsis neonatorum *975*

Marked homeostatic changes occur during the transition from fetal to newborn life. The most rapid anatomic and physiologic changes of this period occur in the cardiopulmonary system. Thus the major problems of the newborn are usually related to this system. These problems include asphyxia, respiratory distress syndrome (RDS), cold stress, jaundice, hemolytic disease, and anemia. Ideally, problems are anticipated and identified prenatally, some treatment may be initiated in the prenatal/intrapartal period, and appropriate intervention measures are begun prior to, at, or immediately after birth.

Care of the Newborn at Risk Due to Asphyxia

Perinatal asphyxia occurs in 1% to 1.5% of live births, and the incidence increases as the gestational age decreases (Cloherty, Eichenwald, & Stark, 2008). Newborn asphyxia results from circulatory, respiratory, and biochemical factors. Circulatory patterns that accompany asphyxia indicate an inability to make the transition to extrauterine circulation—in effect, a return to fetal circulatory patterns, with the majority of the blood bypassing the lungs. Failure of lung expansion and establishment of respiration rapidly produces serious biochemical changes, including hypoxemia (decreased oxygen in blood), metabolic acidosis (increased acidity of blood reflected by low pH), and hypercapnia (excess levels of carbon dioxide in the blood) (Askin, 2009; Niermeyer & Clarke, 2011).

These biochemical changes produce the following results:

- Pulmonary vasoconstriction and high pulmonary vascular resistance in relation to the lower systemic vascular resistance (following birth the pulmonary vascular resistance should be markedly lower than the systemic vascular resistance)
- Hypoperfusion of the lungs
- A large right-to-left shunt through the ductus arteriosus, bypassing the lungs and impeding oxygenation of the blood

As right atrial pressure exceeds left atrial pressure, the foramen ovale reopens, and blood flows from right to left (Askin, 2009). See chapter 29 ∞ for a review of normal newborn cardiopulmonary adaptation.

However, the most serious biochemical abnormality caused by hypoxia is a change from aerobic to anaerobic metabolism. This change results in the buildup of lactate, combining with hydrogen to form lactic acid, and subsequently developing metabolic acidosis. Lactic acidosis can develop after prolonged tissue hypoxia (oxygen starvation) as active cells rely on anaerobic metabolism.

Simultaneously, respiratory acidosis may also occur in response to a rapid increase in carbon dioxide (PCO_2) during asphyxia. In response to hypoxia and anaerobic metabolism, the amounts of free fatty acids (FFA) and glycerol in the blood increase. Glycogen stores are mobilized to provide a continuous glucose source for the brain. Hepatic and cardiac stores of glycogen may be used up rapidly during an asphyxial incident.

The newborn has several protective mechanisms against hypoxic insults:

- Relatively immature brain
- Resting metabolic rate lower than that observed in the adult
- Ability to mobilize substances within the body for anaerobic metabolism and to use the energy more efficiently
- Intact circulatory system able to redistribute lactate and hydrogen ions in tissues still being perfused

Severe prolonged hypoxia will overcome these protective mechanisms, resulting in brain damage or death of the newborn. The newborn suffering apnea requires immediate resuscitative efforts. The need for resuscitation can be anticipated if specific risk factors are present during the pregnancy or labor and birth period.

Risk Factors Predisposing to Asphyxia

The need for resuscitation may be anticipated if the mother demonstrates the antepartum and intrapartum risk factors described in Table 15-1 ∞ on page 321 and Table 23-1 ∞ on page 559. Fetal/neonatal risk factors are as follows (Gomella et al., 2009; Pappas & Walker, 2010):

- Nonreassuring fetal heart rate (FHR) pattern/sustained bradycardia
- Impairment of maternal oxygenation (maternal asthma/cardiac disease)
- Anything affecting blood flow through the placenta
- Significant intrapartum bleeding
- Difficult birth, prolonged labor
- Fetal scalp/capillary blood sample-acidosis pH less than 7.2
- Narcotic use in labor
- History of meconium in amniotic fluid
- Prematurity
- Male infant
- Small for gestational age (SGA) or macrosomia
- Infant of a diabetic mother (IDM)
- Multiple births
- Structural lung abnormality/oligohydramnios (congenital diaphragmatic hernia, lung hypoplasia)
- Congenital heart disease
- Anemia: isoimmunization, fetal-maternal hemorrhage, parvovirus

Risk factors are not always apparent prenatally. Particular attention must be paid to all at-risk pregnancies during the intrapartal period. Certain aspects of labor and birth challenge the oxygen supply to the fetus, and often the at-risk fetus has less tolerance to the stress of labor (indicated by decelerations, a fixed baseline heart rate, or lack of variability of the FHR) and birth (Ingemarsson, 2009).

Clinical Therapy

The initial goal of clinical management is to identify the fetus at risk for asphyxia so that resuscitative efforts can begin at birth.

Fetal biophysical assessment (see chapter 21 ∞) combined with monitoring of fetal pH, FHRs, and fetal oximetry, if available, during the intrapartum period may help identify the presence of nonreassuring fetal status. If nonreassuring fetal status is present, appropriate measures can be taken to deliver the fetus immediately, before major damage occurs, and to treat the asphyxiated newborn.

The fetal biophysical profile enhances the ability to predict an abnormal perinatal outcome. In addition, fetal scalp blood sampling may indicate asphyxic insult and the degree of fetal acidosis (normal is pH >7.2 with a base deficit <6.0), when considered in relation to the stage of labor, uterine contractions, and nonreassuring FHR patterns (Cloherty et al., 2008). The stress of labor causes an intermittent decrease in exchange of gases in the placental intervillous space, which causes the fall in pH and fetal acidosis. The acidosis is primarily metabolic.

During labor, a fetal pH of 7.25 or higher is considered normal (nonacidemia). A pH value of 7.20 or less is considered an ominous sign of intrauterine asphyxia (acidemia), whereas a pH of less than 7 is considered pathologic acidemia (Cloherty et al., 2008). However, low fetal pH without associated hypoxia can be caused by maternal acidosis secondary to prolonged labor, dehydration, and maternal lactate production.

Assessment of the newborn's need for resuscitation begins at the time of birth by assessing color, heart rate, and respirations of the newborn. The nurse should note the time of the first gasp, first cry, and onset of sustained respirations in order of occurrence. The Apgar score (see chapter 24 ∞) may be helpful in describing the status of the newborn at birth and his or her subsequent adaptation to the extrauterine environment but should not be used to determine whether certain steps need to be taken during resuscitation. If indicated, resuscitation should be started before the 1-minute Apgar score is obtained. The AAP Committee on Fetus and Newborn has recommended the use of an assisted Apgar scoring system that documents the assistance the infant is receiving at the time his or her score is assigned (American Academy of Pediatrics (AAP) & American College of Obstetricians and Gynecologists (ACOG), 2007). The Apgar score at 1 minute tends to relate to intrapartal depression and umbilical cord blood pH and subsequent scores relate to adequacy of resuscitative efforts. Retrospective Apgar scores are likely to be assigned when stabilizing critically ill newborns (Pinheiro, 2009).

Resuscitative efforts are required by 10% of all newborns to begin breathing with 1% of all newborns requiring more extensive resuscitative efforts (Bry, 2008). The AAP and ACOG (2007, pg. 207) recommend identification of newborns *who do not require resuscitation* by carrying out a rapid assessment of these four characteristics:

1. Is the baby full term?
2. Is the amniotic fluid clear of meconium and evidence of infection?
3. Is the baby breathing or crying?
4. Does the baby have good muscle tone?

If the answers to these questions are "yes" then the baby does not need resuscitation and should not be separated from the mother. If the answer to *any* of the previous questions is "no," the infant should receive resuscitative assistance (Pappas & Walker, 2010). The infant should receive one or more of the following categories of action:

- Initial steps in stabilization (warmth, positioning, clearing the airway as necessary, drying, stimulating, and repositioning)
- Oxygen administration
- Positive pressure ventilation
- Chest compressions
- Administration of epinephrine, volume expansion, or both (AAP & ACOG, 2007)

In the birthing room exposure to blood or other body fluids is inevitable. Standard Precautions must be practiced by wearing caps, goggles or glasses, gloves, and impervious gowns until the cord is cut and the newborn is dried and wrapped (Cloherty et al., 2008).

Resuscitation Management

Suctioning (clearing airway) is always performed before resuscitation measures are started so that mucus, blood, or meconium is not aspirated into the lungs. Caregivers should keep the newborn in a head-down position before the first gasp to avoid aspiration of the oropharynx secretions and must suction the oropharynx and nasopharynx immediately. Clearing the nasal and oral passages of obstructive fluids, with a bulb syringe or suction catheter attached to low continuous suction, establishes a patent airway. Vigorous suctioning of the posterior pharynx should be avoided because it can produce significant reflex bradycardia and damage the oral mucosa (Pappas & Walker, 2010). Although clear mucus routinely is suctioned from the mouth in most birthing units, there is no evidence to support the value of this practice (AAP & ACOG, 2007).

After the first few breaths, the nurse places the newborn in a level position under a radiant heat source and dries the baby quickly with warm blankets to maintain abdominal skin temperature at about 36.5°C–37°C (97.7°F–98.6°F) (Angert & Adam, 2009). The stable newborn may be placed on the mother's chest or abdomen "skin to skin" as another heat source. The extremely preterm newborn (<28 weeks estimated gestational age [EGA] or <1000 grams) may be covered with a plastic wrap or placed in a plastic bag up to the neck to attempt to prevent evaporative heat loss under the radiant warmer (Gomella et al., 2009). Drying is also a good stimulus for breathing. Heat loss through evaporation is tremendous during the first few minutes of life. The temperature of a wet 1500-g baby in a cold room (16°C [62°F]) drops 1°C every 3 minutes. Hypothermia increases oxygen consumption. In an asphyxiated infant, it increases the hypoxic insult and may lead to severe acidosis and development of respiratory distress.

Breathing is established by employing the simplest form of resuscitative measures initially, with progression to more complicated methods, as required. For example:

1. Position and clear airway as necessary. Simple stimulation is provided by rubbing the back with a blanket or towel, while simultaneously drying the baby.
2. If respirations have not been initiated or are inadequate (gasping or occasional respirations), the lungs must be inflated with positive pressure. The proper sized mask is positioned securely on the face (over the nose and mouth,

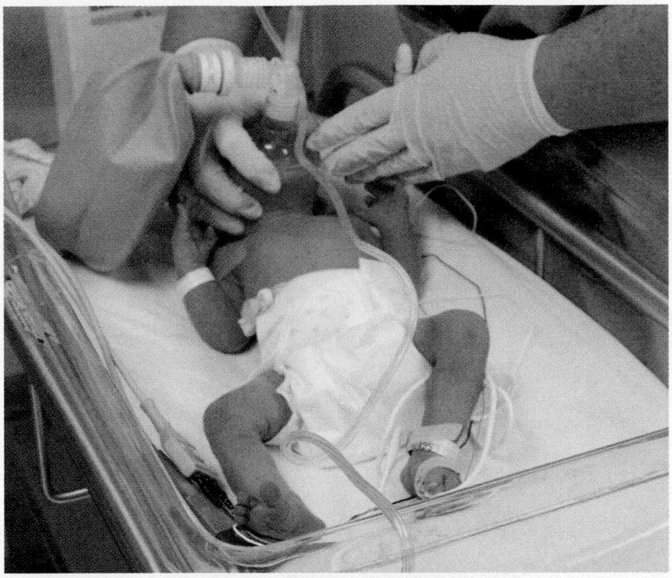

Figure 34-1 ■ Demonstration of resuscitation of an infant with bag and mask. Note that the mask covers the nose and mouth and that the head is in a neutral position. The resuscitation bag is placed to the side of the baby so that chest movement can be seen.

Source: George Dodson/Lightworks Studio/Pearson Education.

avoiding the eyes) with the infant's head in a "sniffing" or neutral position (Figure 34-1 ■). Hyperextension of the infant's neck will obstruct the trachea and must be avoided. An airtight connection is made between the baby's face and the mask (thus allowing the bag to inflate). The lungs are inflated rhythmically by squeezing the bag. Oxygen can be delivered at 100% with an anesthesia bag with an attached manometer or modified self-inflating bag and adequate liter flow of 5–10 L/min (Niermeyer & Clarke, 2011). The self-inflating (Ambu or Hope) bag delivers only 40% oxygen unless it has been adapted with an attached oxygen reservoir (Cloherty et al., 2008). It may not be possible to maintain adequate inspiratory pressure, important in any newborn with surfactant deficiency, with Ambu or Hope bags. In a crisis situation, it is crucial that 100% O_2 be delivered with adequate pressure (Niermeyer & Clarke, 2011).

3. Chest movement is observed for proper ventilation. Air entry and heart rate (HR) are checked by auscultation; HR may be quickly checked by palpating the base of the umbilical cord stump and counting the pulsations for 6 seconds and then multiplying by 10. Manual resuscitation is coordinated with any voluntary efforts. During positive pressure ventilation squeeze the resuscitation bag just enough to improve HR, color, and muscle tone, at a rate of 40–60 breaths per minute. Pressure should be adequate to move the chest wall. The pressure gauge (manometer) must be in place to avoid overdistention of the newborn's lungs and other problems such as pneumothorax or abdominal distention. Increasing the pressure to 30–40 cm H_2O or greater is occasionally necessary if there is no improvement in these parameters (HR, color, muscle tone) (Gomella et al., 2009). If ventilation is adequate, the chest moves symmetrically with each inspiration, bilateral breath sounds are audible, and the lips and mucous membranes become pink. Distention of the stomach is controlled by inserting a nasogastric tube for decompression.
4. Endotracheal intubation (Figure 34-2 ■) may be needed. However, most newborns, except for very-low-birth-weight (VLBW) (less than 1500 g) infants, can be effectively resuscitated by bag-and-mask ventilation. An increasing HR and CO_2 detection are the primary methods for confirming endotracheal tube placement.

Once breathing has been established, the HR should increase to over 100 beats per minute. If the HR is absent or the HR remains less than 60 beats per minute after 30 seconds of effective positive pressure with oxygen concentration of 21% to 100% to elicit an oxygen saturation of 90%, external cardiac massage (chest compression) is begun (Rajani, Chitkara, & Halamek, 2009). Chest compressions are started immediately if there is no detectable heartbeat. The procedure for performing chest compression is as follows:

1. The infant is positioned properly on a firm surface.
2. The resuscitator stands at the foot or head of the infant and the examiner places both thumbs over the lower third of the sternum (just below an imaginary line drawn between the nipples) with the fingers wrapped around and supporting the back (Figure 34-3A ■). Alternatively, the examiner can use two fingers instead of the thumbs (Figure 34-3B ■). The two-thumb method is preferred because it may provide better coronary perfusion pressure; however, it makes access to the umbilical cord for medication administration more difficult (Gomella et al., 2009).
3. The sternum is depressed to sufficient depth to generate a palpable pulse or approximately one third of the anterior-posterior depth of the chest at a rate of 90 beats per minute (Niermeyer & Clarke, 2011). Use a 3:1 ratio of heartbeat to assisted ventilation, 90 chest compressions:30 breaths per minute (Gomella et al., 2009).

Drugs that should be available in the birthing area include those needed in the treatment of shock, cardiac arrest, and narcosis. Oxygen is the drug used most often because of its effectiveness in ventilation. After 30 seconds of ventilation and coordinated cardiac compression, the newborn's cardiopulmonary status is reassessed by palpating the umbilical cord for a pulse. If the newborn has not responded with spontaneous respirations and an HR above 60 beats per minute, resuscitative medications are necessary (Cloherty et al., 2008; Gomella et al., 2009). The most accessible route for administering medications is the umbilical vein (intravenous [IV]). When the HR remains below 60 beats per minute, despite 30 seconds of assisted ventilation followed by another 30 seconds of coordinated chest compression, epinephrine, a cardiac stimulant, is indicated. If persistant bradycardia is present, epinephrine (0.1 to 0.3 ml/kg of a 1:10,000 solution [0.1 mg/ml]) is given through the umbilical vein catheter as rapidly as possible. Endotracheal administration may be considered while IV access is being established. When epinephrine is administered by endotracheal tube, consider a higher dose (0.3 to 1 ml/kg). The

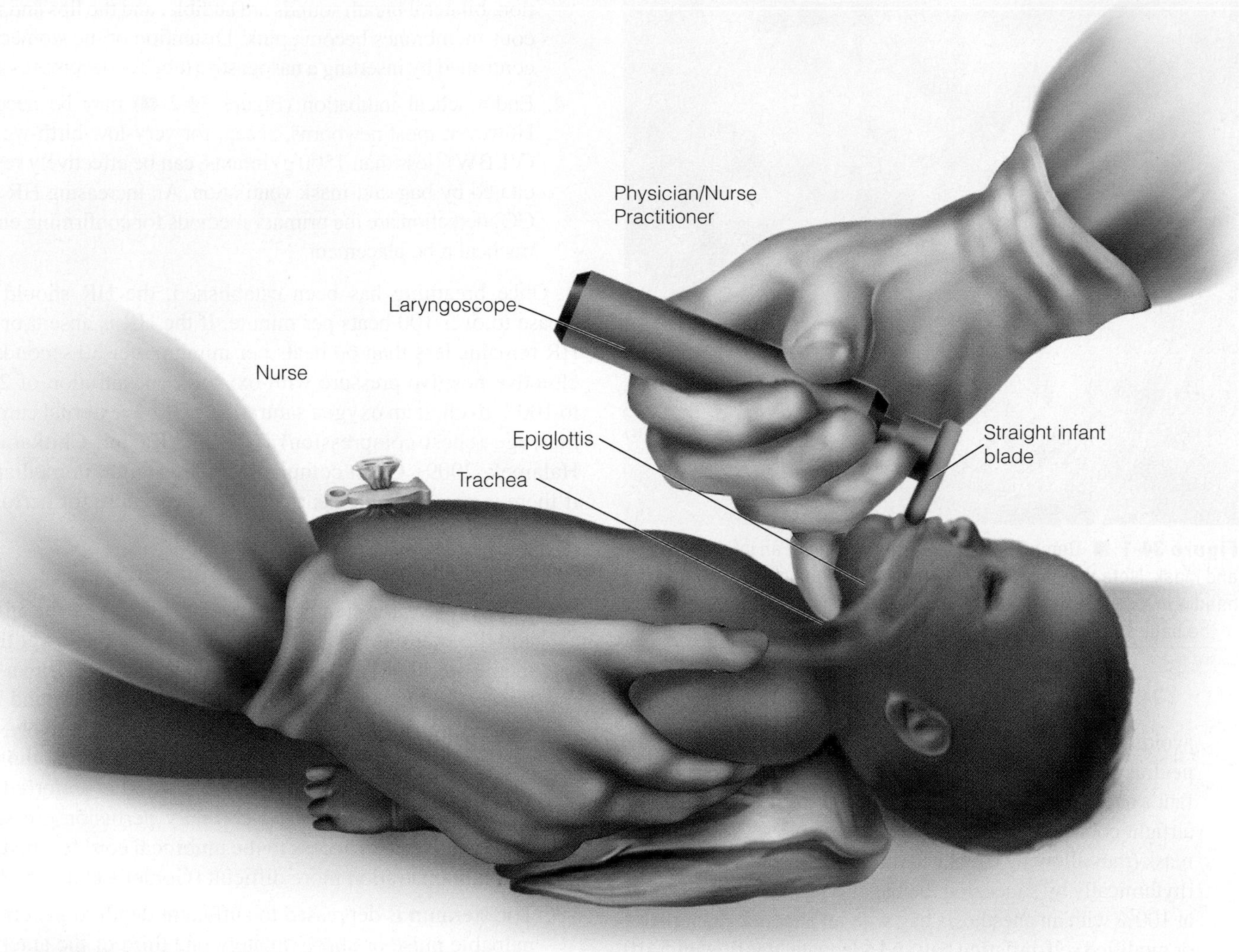

Figure 34-2 ■ Endotracheal intubation is accomplished with the infant's head in the "sniffing" position. The clinician places the fifth finger under the chin to hold the tongue forward and inserts the laryngoscope blade. Once the blade is in position as shown, an endotracheal tube is inserted through the groove in the laryngoscope blade. The endotracheal tube is not seen in this illustration.

endotracheal route is associated with unreliable absorption and may not be effective at the lower dose (Gomella et al., 2009). *Sodium bicarbonate is rarely given in the birthing room.* Sodium bicarbonate is given only to correct metabolic acidosis that results from lactic acid buildup due to insufficient tissue oxygenation and only after effective ventilation is established. Dextrose (2 ml/kg) is given to prevent progression of hypoglycemia. A 10% dextrose in water IV solution ($D_{10}W$) is usually sufficient to prevent or treat hypoglycemia in the birthing area. Naloxone hydrochloride (0.1 mg/kg), a narcotic antagonist, is used to reverse known iatrogenic narcotic depression (Gomella et al., 2009). See Drug Guide: Naloxone Hydrochloride (Narcan).

If shock develops (e.g., low blood pressure [BP], pallor, or poor peripheral perfusion), the baby may be given a volume expander such as normal saline or Ringer's lactate in a dose of 10 ml/kg via umbilical vein route. If there is a known fetal hemorrhage or fetal anemia, whole blood (O Rh-negative crossmatched against the mother's blood) and packed red blood cells (RBCs) given over a 5- to 10-minute period can be used for volume expansion and treatment of hypovolemic shock. In some instances of prolonged resuscitation associated with shock and poor response to resuscitation, dopamine (starting at 5 mcg/kg/min) may be necessary.

NURSING CARE MANAGEMENT

Nursing Assessment and Diagnosis

Communication between the obstetric office or clinic and the birthing area nurse helps in the identification of newborns who may be in need of resuscitation. When the woman arrives in the birthing area, the nurse should have the prenatal/antepartal record and should note any contributory prenatal history factors and assess present fetal status. As labor progresses, nursing assessments include ongoing monitoring of fetal heartbeat and its response to contractions, assisting with fetal scalp blood sampling (if available), and observing for the presence of meconium in the amniotic fluid, when ruptured, to help identify possible fetal asphyxia. In addition, the

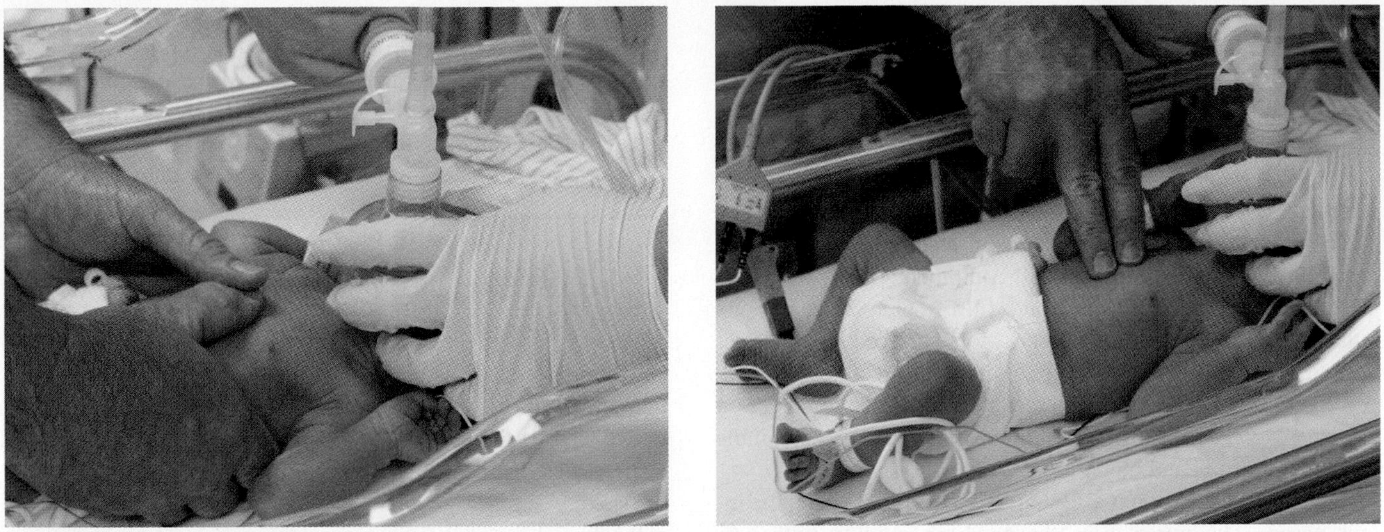

Figure 34-3 ■ External cardiac massage. The lower third of the sternum is compressed with two fingertips or thumbs at a rate of 90 beats per minute. A. In the thumb method, the fingers support the infant's back, and both thumbs compress the sternum. B. In the two-finger method, the tips of two fingers of one hand compress the sternum, and the other hand or a firm surface supports the infant's back.

Source: George Dodson/Lightworks Studio/Pearson Education.

nurse should alert the resuscitation team and the practitioner responsible for the care of the newborn of any potential high-risk laboring women.

Nursing diagnoses that may apply to the newborn with asphyxia and the newborn's parents include the following:

- ***Ineffective Breathing Pattern*** related to lack of spontaneous respirations at birth secondary to in utero asphyxia
- ***Decreased Cardiac Output*** related to impaired oxygenation
- ***Compromised Family Coping*** related to baby's lack of spontaneous respirations at birth and fear of losing their newborn

DRUG GUIDE Naloxone Hydrochloride (Narcan)

OVERVIEW OF NEONATAL ACTION

Naloxone hydrochloride (Narcan) is used to reverse respiratory depression due to acute narcotic toxicity when the mother received a narcotic within 4 hours of delivery. It displaces morphine-like drugs from receptor sites on the neurons; therefore, the narcotics can no longer exert their depressive effects. It is essentially a pure opioid antagonist. Naloxone reverses iatrogenic narcotic-induced respiratory depression, analgesia, sedation, hypotension, and pupillary constriction.

ROUTE, DOSAGE, FREQUENCY

The dose is 0.1 mg/kg (0.25 ml/kg of 0.4 mg/ml preparation) concentration at birth, including premature infants. This drug is usually given through the umbilical vein (IV) or endotracheal tube (ET), although Naloxone can be given intramuscularly (delays onset of action) if adequate perfusion exists. For IV push, infuse over at least 1 minute; for ET administration, dilute in 1 to 2 millimeters of normal saline (NS).

Reversal of drug depression occurs within 1 to 2 minutes after IV administration and within 1 hour of intramuscular (IM) administration. The duration of action is variable (minutes to hours) and depends on the amount of the drug present and the rate of excretion. Duration of narcotic often exceeds that of the Naloxone. Dose may be repeated in 3 to 5 minutes. If initial reversal occurs, repeat dose as needed (Young & Mangum, 2010).

NEONATAL CONTRAINDICATIONS

Naloxone should not be administered to infants of narcotic-addicted mothers or those on methadone maintenance because it may precipitate acute withdrawal syndromes (increased HR and blood pressure (BP), vomiting, seizures, and tremors).

Respiratory depression may result from nonmorphine drugs, such as sedatives, hypnotics, anesthetics, or other nonnarcotic central nervous system (CNS) depressants.

NEONATAL SIDE EFFECTS

Excessive doses may result in irritability, increased crying, and possible prolongation of partial thromboplastin time (PTT).

Tachycardia may occur.

NURSING CONSIDERATIONS

- Monitor respirations—rate and depth—closely for improved respiratory effort.
- Assess for return of respiratory depression when Naloxone effects wear off and effects of longer-acting narcotics reappear.
- Assess continued respiratory depression after positive-pressure ventilation has restored normal HR and color.
- Have resuscitative equipment, O_2, and ventilatory equipment available.
- Note that Naloxone is incompatible with alkaline solutions such as sodium bicarbonate.
- Store at room temperature and protect from light.
- Compatible with heparin.

Nursing Plan and Implementation

Hospital-Based Nursing Care

Following identification of possible high-risk situations, the next step in effective resuscitation is assembling the necessary equipment and ensuring proper functioning.

Check and maintain equipment to ensure its reliability before an emergency arises. The equipment must be cleaned or replaced and restocked immediately after each use and rechecked before every birth. The nurse inspects all equipment—bag and mask, pressure manometer, oxygen and flow meter, laryngoscope bulb/battery, and suction machine—for damaged or nonfunctioning parts before a birth or when setting up an admission bed. A systematic check of the emergency cart and equipment is a routine responsibility of each shift. It is desirable to assemble equipment for pH and blood gas determination as well.

During resuscitation it is essential that the nurse keep the infant warm. The nurse dries the newborn quickly with prewarmed towels or blankets and places a hat to prevent evaporative heat loss, then places the baby under a pre-warmed radiant warmer with servo control set at 36.5°C (97.7°F). The radiant warmer provides an overhead radiant heat source (a thermostatic mechanism that is secured to the infant's abdomen, over a solid organ like the liver, triggers the radiant warmer to turn on or off to maintain a constant temperature). An open bed is necessary for easy access to the newborn. Low-birth-weight (LBW) infants can be placed on a warm chemical mattress to help minimize their heat loss (Reynolds, Pilcher, Ring, et al., 2009).

Training and knowledge about resuscitation are vital to personnel in the birth setting for both normal and high-risk births. Neonatal Resuscitation Program (NRP) certification is renewed every 2 years for personnel working with newborns. Resuscitation is at least a two-person effort, and the nurse should call for additional support as needed. One member must have the skill to perform airway management and ventilation. The resuscitative efforts are recorded on the newborn's chart so that all members of the healthcare team will have access to this information.

Parent Teaching

The new cardiopulmonary resuscitation (CPR) guidelines favor family members being present during resuscitation in the birthing room and in the NICU, but the procedure may be particularly distressing for the parents. If the need for resuscitation is anticipated, the parents should be assured that a team will be present at the birth to care specifically for their newborn. Nurses should advise the parents that a support person will be available for them also. As soon as the infant's condition has been stabilized, a member of the interdisciplinary team needs to discuss the baby's condition with the parents. The parents may have many fears about the reasons for resuscitation and the condition of their baby following the resuscitation.

Evaluation

Expected outcomes of nursing care include the following:

- The newborn requiring resuscitation is promptly identified, and intervention is started early.
- The newborn's metabolic and physiologic processes are stabilized, and recovery proceeds without complications.
- The parents can verbalize the reason for resuscitation and what was done to resuscitate their newborn.
- The parents can verbalize their fears about the resuscitation process and potential implications for their baby's future.

Care of the Newborn with Respiratory Distress

One of the severest conditions to which the newborn may fall victim is respiratory distress—an inappropriate respiratory adaptation to extrauterine life. The nurse caring for a baby with respiratory distress needs to understand the normal pulmonary and circulatory physiology (see "Respiratory Adaptations" in chapter 29 ∞), the pathophysiology of the disease process, clinical manifestations, and supportive and corrective therapies. Only with this knowledge can the nurse make appropriate observations concerning responses to therapy and development of complications. Unlike the verbalizing adult patient, the newborn communicates needs only by exhibiting behaviors or physiologic parameters that must be interpreted by the neonatal intensive care unit (NICU) nurse. The neonatal nurse interprets this behavior as clues about the individual baby's condition. In this section, we discuss respiratory distress syndrome, transient tachypnea of the newborn, meconium aspiration syndrome, and persistent pulmonary hypertension.

Respiratory Distress Syndrome

Respiratory distress syndrome (RDS), also referred to as *hyaline membrane disease (HMD),* is the result of a primary absence, deficiency, or alteration in the production of pulmonary surfactant, a substance produced in the lungs that keeps lungs from collapsing on expiration (Peterson, 2009). Respiratory distress syndrome affects almost 50% of the premature infants born at less than 30 weeks gestation, and the preterm delivery rate in the United States is 12% to 13% (Ramanathan, 2009). The syndrome occurs more frequently in premature Caucasian infants than in infants of African or Hispanic descent and almost twice as often in males as in females.

All the factors precipitating the pathologic changes of RDS have not been determined, but the main factors associated with its development are as follows:

1. ***Prematurity.*** All preterm newborns—whether average for gestational age (AGA), small for gestational age (SGA), or large for gestational age (LGA)—and especially infants of diabetic mothers (IDM) are at risk for RDS. The incidence of RDS increases with the degree of prematurity, with most deaths occurring in newborns weighing less than 1500 g. The maternal and fetal factors resulting in preterm labor and birth, complications of pregnancy, indications for cesarean birth, and familial tendency are all associated with RDS.
2. ***Surfactant deficiency disease.*** Normal pulmonary adaptation requires adequate surfactant, a lipoprotein that coats the inner surface of the alveoli. Surfactant provides alveolar stability by decreasing the alveoli's surface tension and

tendency for collapse. Surfactant is produced by type II alveolar cells starting at about 24 weeks' gestation. In the normal or mature newborn lung, it is continuously synthesized, oxidized during breathing, and replenished. Adequate surfactant levels lead to better lung compliance and permit breathing with less work. RDS is due to alterations in surfactant quantity, composition, function, or production.

CLINICAL TIP

An alveolus can be thought of as a small balloon filled with water and no air. When the balloon is emptied, the water droplets that remain inside the balloon increase the surface tension. As a result, the sides of the balloon stick together. The increased surface tension makes reinflation very difficult and requires an increased amount of energy.

Development of RDS indicates a failure to synthesize adequate surfactant, which is required to maintain alveolar stability (see "Factors Opposing the First Breath" in chapter 29 ∞). Upon expiration, the instability increases atelectasis, which causes hypoxia and acidosis because of the lack of gas exchange (Peterson, 2009). These conditions further inhibit surfactant production and cause pulmonary vasoconstriction. The resulting lung instability causes the biochemical problems of hypoxemia (decreased PO_2), hypercarbia (increased PCO_2), and acidemia (decreased pH), which further increases pulmonary vasoconstriction and hypoperfusion; alveolar endothelial and epithelial damage; and subsequent protein-rich interstitial and alveolar edema (Nash & Smith, 2008). The cycle of events of RDS leading to eventual respiratory failure is diagrammed in Figure 34-4 ■.

Because of these pathophysiologic conditions, the newborn must expend increasing amounts of energy to reopen the collapsed alveoli with every breath, so that each breath becomes more difficult than the last. The progressive expiratory atelectasis upsets the physiologic homeostasis of the pulmonary and cardiovascular systems and prevents adequate gas exchange. Breathing becomes progressively harder as lung compliance decreases, which makes it more difficult for the newborn to inflate the lungs and breathe.

The physiologic alterations of RDS produce the following complications:

1. ***Hypoxia.*** As a result of hypoxia, the pulmonary vasculature constricts, pulmonary vascular resistance increases, and pulmonary blood flow is reduced. Increased pulmonary vascular resistance may precipitate a return to fetal circulation as the ductus arteriosus opens and blood flow is shunted around the lungs in a right-to-left blood flow. This shunting increases the hypoxia and further decreases pulmonary perfusion. Hypoxia also causes impairment or absence of metabolic response to cold; reversion to anaërobic metabolism, resulting in lactate accumulation (acidosis); and impaired cardiac output, which decreases perfusion to vital organs.
2. ***Respiratory acidosis.*** Increased PCO_2 and decreased pH are results of alveolar hypoventilation. A persistent rise in PCO_2 is a poor prognostic sign of pulmonary function and adequacy because increased PCO_2 and decreased pH are results of alveolar hypoventilation.
3. ***Metabolic acidosis.*** Because cells lack oxygen, the newborn begins an anaerobic pathway of metabolism, with an increase

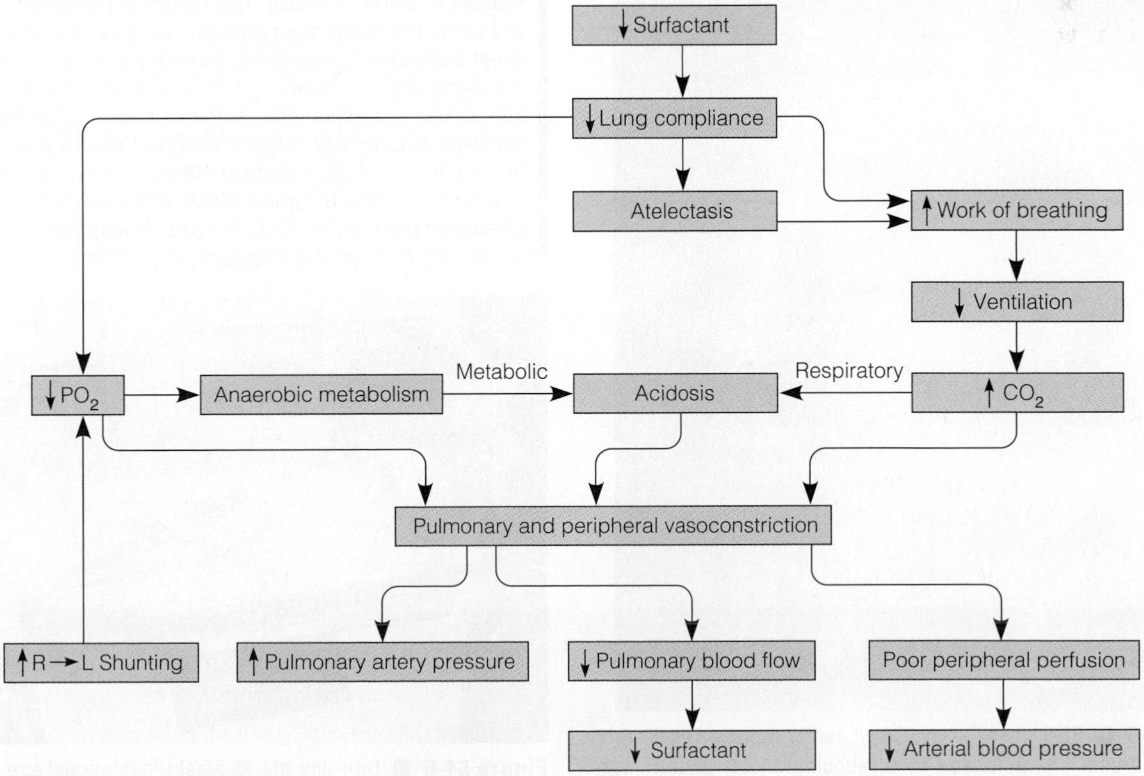

Figure 34-4 ■ Cycle of events of RDS leading to eventual respiratory failure.

Source: Reprinted from Pediatric Clinics of North America, *vol. 20, L. Gluck & M. V. Kulovich,* Fetal lung development *(p. 375). Copyright © 1973, with permission from Elsevier.*

in lactate levels and a resulting base deficit (loss of bicarbonate). As the lactate levels increase, the pH decreases in an attempt to maintain acid–base homeostasis (Askin, 2009).

The classic radiologic picture of RDS is diffuse bilateral reticulogranular (ground glass appearance) density, with portions of the air-filled tracheobronchial tree (air bronchogram) outlined by the opaque ("white-out") lungs with widespread atelectasis, potentially obliterating the heart borders (Figure 34-5 ■). Opacification of the lungs on x-ray image may be due to massive atelectasis, diffuse alveolar infiltrate, or pulmonary edema (Cloherty et al., 2008; Gomella et al., 2009). The progression of x-ray findings parallels the pattern of resolution, which usually occurs in 7 to 10 days, and the time of surfactant reappearance, unless surfactant replacement therapy has been used (Blackburn, 2007). Echocardiography is a valuable tool in diagnosing vascular shunts that shunt blood either away from, right to left reverting to a fetal pattern, or toward the lungs.

Clinical Therapy

The primary goal of prenatal management is to prevent preterm birth through aggressive treatment of preterm labor and administration of steroids to enhance fetal lung development if birth is imminent (see chapter 20 ∞). Antenatal steroids reduce the incidence and severity of RDS and improve survivability of the 24 to 34 weeks' gestation and extremely low-birth-weight newborn (less than 1250 grams) (Cloherty et al., 2008; Gomella et al., 2009).

Postnatal surfactant replacement therapy is available for infants to decrease the severity of RDS in low-birth-weight newborns. Surfactant replacement therapy is delivered through an endotracheal tube and may be given either in the birthing room or the nursery, as indicated by the severity of RDS. Repeat doses are often required. The most frequently reported response to treatment is rapidly improved oxygenation and decreased need for ventilatory support, sometimes occurring quite quickly after the dose is administered.

Supportive medical management consists of ventilatory therapy, blood gas monitoring, pulse oximetry monitoring, correction of acid–base imbalance, environmental temperature regulation, adequate nutrition, and protection from infection. Ventilatory therapy is directed toward preventing hypoventilation and hypoxia. Mild cases of RDS may require only increased humidified oxygen concentrations. Use of continuous positive airway pressure (CPAP) may be required in moderately afflicted infants. Babies with severe cases of RDS require mechanical ventilatory assistance from a respirator (Figure 34-6 ■).

High-frequency ventilation (HFV) can be tried when conventional ventilator therapy is not successful, and it sometimes can be the primary mode of ventilation to minimize lung injury in very small and/or sick infants (Gomella et al., 2009). In some institutions, morphine or fentanyl is used for its analgesic and sedative effects. Sedation may be indicated for infants most likely to have air leak respiratory problems. Use of pancuronium for muscle relaxation or paralysis in infants with RDS is controversial.

CLINICAL TIP

In babies with respiratory distress syndrome (RDS) who are on ventilators, increased urination/diuresis (determined by weighing diapers) may be an early clue that the baby's condition is improving (usually in the second to fourth day). As fluid moves out of the lungs into the bloodstream, alveoli open, and kidney perfusion increases; this results in increased voiding. At this point, the nurse must monitor chest expansion closely. If chest expansion is increasing, pulmonary compliance is improving and ventilator settings may have to be decreased, sometimes quite soon after surfactant dosing. Too high a ventilator setting may "blow the lungs," resulting in pneumothorax. If diuresis does not occur it is a sign that bronchopulmonary dysplasia (BPD), also called *chronic lung disease of prematurity (CLD)* may be developing.

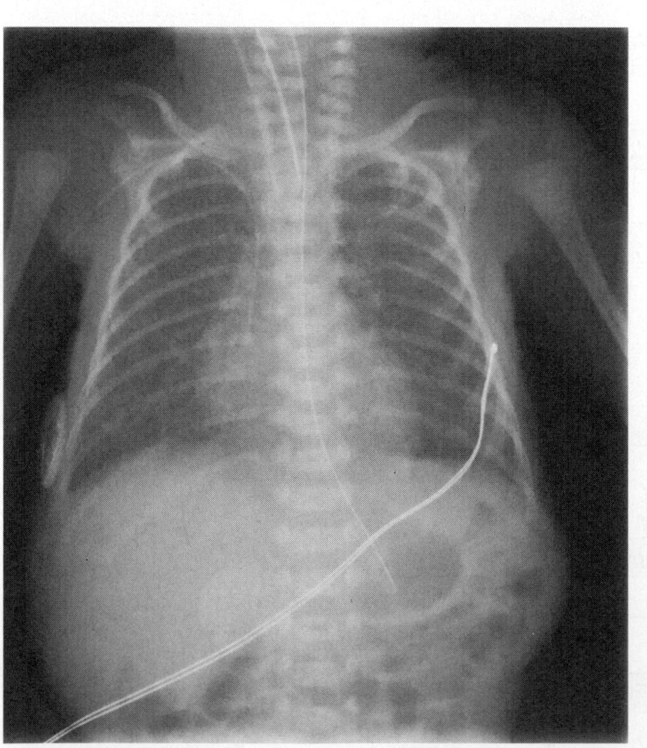

Figure 34-5 ■ RDS chest x-ray. Chest radiograph of respiratory distress syndrome characterized by a reticulogranular pattern with areas of microatelectasis of uniform opacity and air bronchograms.

Source: Courtesy of Carol Harrigan, RN, MSN, NNP-BC.

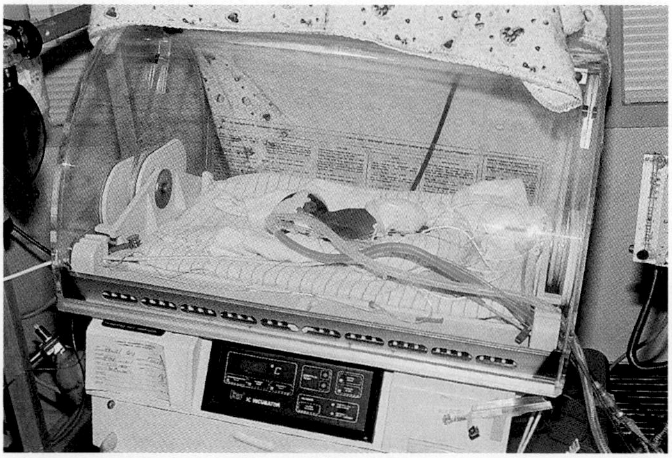

Figure 34-6 ■ One-day-old, 29 weeks' gestational age, 1450-g baby on respirator and in isolette.

Source: Courtesy of Carol Harrigan, RN, MSN, NNP-BC.

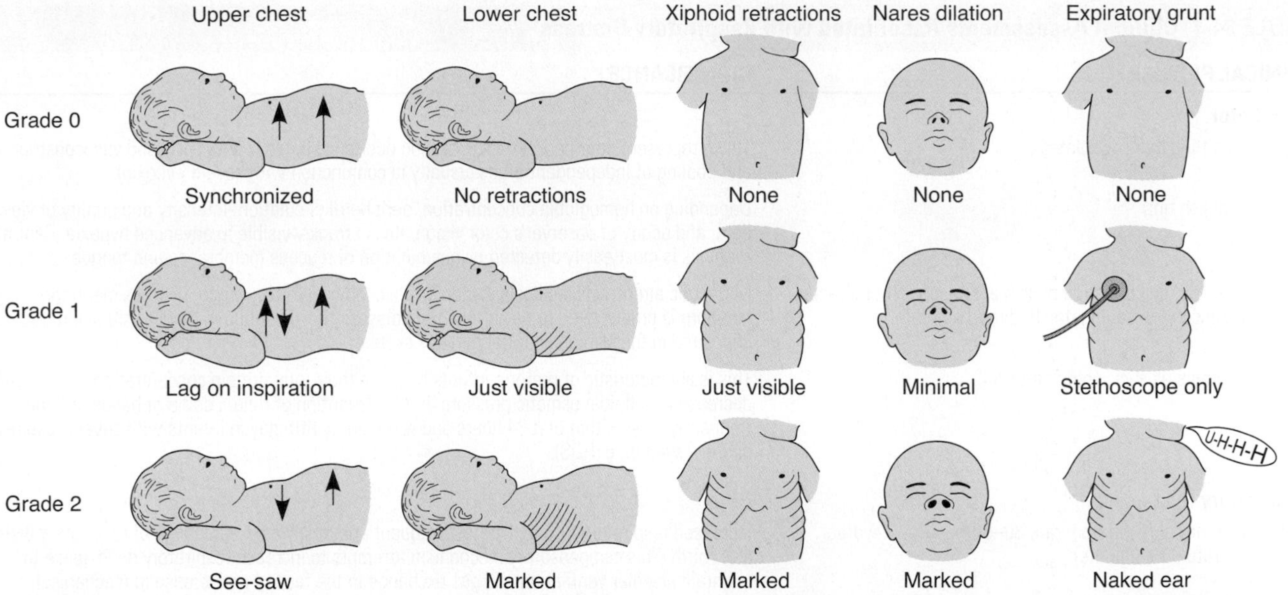

Figure 34-7 ■ Evaluating respiratory status using the Silverman-Andersen index. The baby's respiratory status is assessed. A grade of 0, 1, or 2 is determined for each area, and a total score is charted in the baby's record or on a copy of this tool and placed in the chart.

Source: Used with permission: Clinical Education Series No. 2: Columbus, Ohio: Ross Products Division, Abbott Laboratories. Reproduced with permission from Pediatrics, *17, 1–10, Copyright © 1956 by the AAP.*

NURSING CARE MANAGEMENT

Nursing Assessment and Diagnosis

Characteristics of RDS the nurse should look for are increasing cyanosis, tachypnea (greater than 60 respirations per minute), grunting respirations, nasal flaring, significant retractions, and apnea. Table 34-1 reviews clinical findings associated with respiratory distress in general. The Silverman-Andersen index (Figure 34-7 ■) may be helpful in evaluating the signs of respiratory distress and can be done in the birthing area.

Based on clinical parameters, the neonatal nurse implements therapeutic approaches to maintain physiologic homeostasis and provides supportive care to the newborn with RDS. See Nursing Care Plan: For the Newborn with Respiratory Distress Syndrome on pages 950 to 952.

Nursing interventions and criteria for instituting mechanical ventilatory assistance are done per institutional protocol. Noninvasive oxygen monitoring provides real-time information that is particularly useful in infants showing frequent swings in PaO_2 and oxygen saturation. These methods (pulse oximetry, transcutaneous oxygen monitor) can also reduce the frequency of blood gas sampling. Methods of noninvasive oxygen monitoring and nursing interventions are described in Table 34-2. (The nursing care of infants on ventilators or with umbilical artery catheters is not discussed here. These infants have severe respiratory distress and are cared for in NICUs by nurses with advanced knowledge and training.) Ventilatory assistance with high-frequency ventilators has shown positive results. The parents of a baby born having respiratory distress will need a very supportive environment (Figure 34-8 ■).

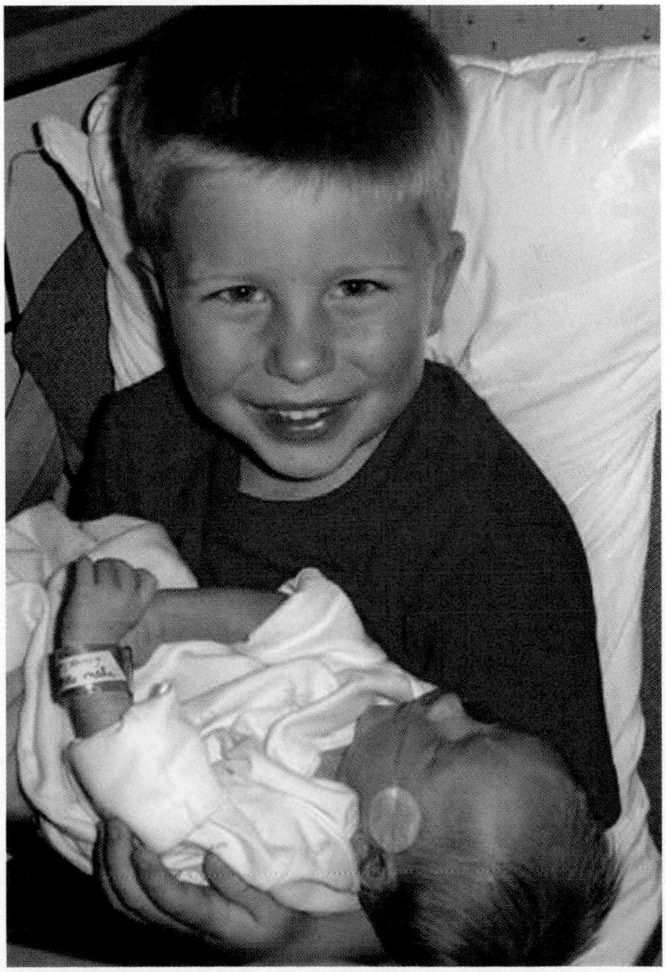

Figure 34-8 ■ This baby born at 36 weeks' gestational age had severe RDS. He has ongoing oxygen needs provided by a nasal cannula but still can be held by his proud big brother.

Source: Courtesy of Lisa Smith-Pedersen, RN, MSN, NNP-BC.

TABLE 34-1 Clinical Assessments Associated with Respiratory Distress

CLINICAL PICTURE	SIGNIFICANCE
Skin Color	
Pallor or mottling (pale or splotchy)	These represent poor peripheral circulation due to systemic hypotension and vasoconstriction and pooling of independent areas (usually in conjunction with severe hypoxia).
Cyanosis (bluish tint)	Depending on hemoglobin concentration, peripheral circulation, intensity and quality of viewing light, and acuity of observer's color vision, this is frankly visible in advanced hypoxia. Central cyanosis is most easily detected by examination of mucous membranes and tongue.
Jaundice (yellow discoloration of skin and mucous membranes due to presence of unconjugated [indirect] bilirubin)	Metabolic alterations (acidosis, hypercarbia, asphyxia) of respiratory distress mean the newborn is predisposed to having bilirubin dissociate from albumin-binding sites and be deposited in the skin and central nervous system.
Edema (presents as slick, shiny taut skin)	This is characteristic of preterm infants because their total protein concentration is low, with a decrease in colloidal osmotic pressure and transudation of fluid. Edema of hands and feet is frequently seen within first 24 hours and resolved by fifth day in infants with severe respiratory distress syndrome (RDS).
Respiratory System	
Tachypnea (normal respiratory rate 30–60/minute, elevated respiratory rate 60+/minute)	Increased respiratory rate is the most frequent and easily detectable sign of respiratory distress after birth. This compensatory mechanism attempts to increase respiratory dead space to maintain alveolar ventilation and gas exchange in the face of an increase in mechanical resistance. As a decompensatory mechanism, it increases workload and energy output by increasing respiratory rate, which causes increased metabolic demand for oxygen and thus increases alveolar ventilation on an already overstressed system. Shallow, rapid respirations increase dead space ventilation, thus decreasing alveolar ventilation.
Apnea (episode of nonbreathing for more than 20 seconds); periodic breathing, a common "normal" occurrence in preterm infants, is defined as apnea of 5–10 seconds alternating with 10–15 seconds of ventilation that is sometimes quite rapid	This poor prognostic sign indicates cardiorespiratory disease, central nervous system (CNS) disease, metabolic alterations, intracranial hemorrhage, sepsis, or immaturity. Physiologic alterations include decreased oxygen saturation, respiratory acidosis, and bradycardia.
Chest	Inspection of the thoracic cage includes shape, size, and symmetry of movement. Respiratory movements should be symmetric and diaphragmatic; asymmetry reflects pathology (pneumothorax, diaphragmatic hernia). Increased anteroposterior diameter indicates air trapping (meconium aspiration syndrome).
Labored respirations (Silverman-Andersen index in Figure 34-7 indicates severity of retractions, grunting, and nasal flaring, which are signs of labored respirations)	Indicates marked increase in the work of breathing.
Retractions (inward pulling of soft parts of the chest cage—suprasternal, substernal, intercostal, subcostal—at inspiration)	These reflect the significant increase in negative intrathoracic pressure necessary to inflate stiff, noncompliant lungs. Infants try to increase lung compliance by using accessory muscles. Lung expansion markedly decreases. Seesaw respirations are seen when the chest flattens with inspiration and the abdomen bulges. Retractions increase the work of breathing and oxygen need so that assisted ventilation may be necessary due to exhaustion.
Flaring nares (inspiratory dilation of nostrils)	This compensatory mechanism attempts to lessen the resistance of the narrow nasal passage.
Expiratory grunt (Valsalva maneuver in which the infant exhales against a closed glottis, thus producing an audible moan)	This increases transpulmonary pressure, which decreases or prevents atelectasis, thus improving oxygenation and alveolar ventilation. Intubation should not be tried unless the infant's condition is rapidly deteriorating, because it prevents this maneuver and allows the alveoli to collapse.
Rhythmic body movement with labored respirations (chin tug, head bobbing, retractions of anal area)	This is a result of using abdominal and other respiratory accessory muscles during prolonged forced respirations.
Auscultation of chest reveals decreased air exchange, with harsh breath sounds or fine inspiratory rales; rhonchi may be present	Decrease in breath sounds and distant quality may indicate interstitial or intrapleural air or fluid.
Cardiovascular System	
Continuous systolic murmur may be audible	Patent ductus arteriosus is common with hypoxia, pulmonary vasoconstriction, right-to-left shunting, and congestive heart failure.
Heart rate usually within normal limits (fixed heart rate may occur with a rate of 110–120/minute)	A fixed heart rate indicates a decrease in vagal control.
Point of maximal impulse usually located at fourth to fifth intercostal space, left sternal border	Displacement may reflect dextrocardia (heart in right side of chest), pneumothorax, or diaphragmatic hernia.
Hypothermia	This is inadequate functioning of metabolic processes that require oxygen to produce necessary body heat.
Muscle Tone	
Flaccid, hypotonic, unresponsive to stimuli	These may indicate deterioration in the newborn's condition and possible CNS damage due to hypoxia, acidemia, or hemorrhage.
Hypertonia and/or seizure activity	

TABLE 34-2 Oxygen Monitors

TYPE	FUNCTION AND RATIONALE	NURSING INTERVENTIONS
Pulse Oximetry—SpO_2		
Estimates beat-to-beat arterial oxygen saturation.	Calibration is automatic.	Understand and use oxyhemoglobin dissociation curve.
Microprocessor measures saturation by the absorption of red and infrared light as it passes through tissue.	Less dependent on perfusion than $TcPO_2$ and $TcPCO_2$; however, functions poorly if peripheral perfusion is decreased due to low cardiac output.	Monitor trends over time and correlate with arterial blood gases.
Changes in absorption related to blood pulsation through vessel determine saturation and pulse rate.	Much more rapid response time than $TcPO_2$–offers real-time readings. Can be located on extremity, digit, or palm of hand, leaving chest free; not affected by skin characteristics. Requires understanding of oxyhemoglobin dissociation curve. Pulse oximeter reading of 88% to 93% reflects a PaO_2 of 50–80 mm Hg (Gomella et al., 2009). Extreme sensitivity to movement; decreases if average of 7th or 14th beat is selected rather than beat to beat. Poor correlation with extreme hyperoxia.	Check disposable sensor at least every 8 hr. Use disposable cuffs (reusable cuffs allow too much ambient light to enter, and readings may be inaccurate).
Transcutaneous Oxygen Monitor–$TcPO_2$		
Measures oxygen diffusion across the skin. Clark electrode is heated to 43°C (preterm) or 44°C (term) to warm the skin beneath the electrode and promote diffusion of oxygen across the skin surface. PO_2 is measured when oxygen diffuses across the capillary membrane, skin, and electrode membrane (Gomella et al., 2009).	When transcutaneous monitors are properly calibrated and electrodes are appropriately positioned, they provide reliable, continuous, noninvasive measurements of PO_2, PCO_2, and oxygen saturation. Readings vary when skin perfusion is decreased. Reliable as trend monitor. Frequent calibration necessary to overcome mechanical drift. Following membrane change, machine must "warm up" 1 hour before initial calibration; otherwise, after turning it on, it must equilibrate for 30 minutes before calibration. When placed on infant, values will be low until skin is heated; approximately 15 minutes required to stabilize. Second-degree burns are rare but possible if electrodes remain in place too long. Decreased correlations noted with older infants (related to skin thickness), with infants with low cardiac output (decreased skin perfusion), and with hyperoxic infants. The adhesive that attaches the electrode may abrade the fragile skin of the preterm infant. May be used for both preductal and postductal monitoring of oxygenation for observations of shunting.	Use $TcPO_2$ to monitor trends of oxygenation with routine nursing care procedures. Clean electrode surface to remove electrolyte deposits; change solution and membrane once a week. Allow machine to stabilize before drawing arterial gases; note reading when gases are drawn and use values to correlate. Ensure airtight seal between skin surface and electrode; place electrodes on clean, dry skin on upper chest, abdomen, or inner aspect of thigh; avoid bony prominences. Change skin site and recalibrate at least every 4 hours; inspect skin for burns; if burns occur, use lowest temperature setting and change position of electrode more frequently. Adhesive disks may be cut to a smaller size, or skin prep may be used under the adhesive circle only; allow membrane to touch skin surface at center.

Transient Tachypnea of the Newborn

Some newborns, primarily LGA, term, and late preterm infants, may develop progressive respiratory distress that can resemble classic RDS. Other risk factors include maternal diabetes and asthma, male sex of the fetus, macrosomia (possibly related to maternal diabetes), and cesarean section delivery, especially elective without spontaneous labor (Guglani, Lakshminrusimha, & Ryan, 2008). Typically, supplemental oxygen of less than 40% will alleviate the hypoxia (Cloherty et al., 2008). They may have had intrauterine or intrapartal asphyxia due to maternal oversedation or poor uterine perfusion, maternal bleeding, prolapsed cord, or breech presentation. The newborn then fails to clear the airway of lung fluid, mucus, and other debris, or an excess of fluid in the lungs due to aspiration of amniotic or tracheal fluid (Gomella et al., 2009; Guglani et al., 2008). Transient tachypnea of the newborn (TTN), which occurs in 11 per 1000 live births (Nash & Smith, 2008), is also more prevalent in cesarean-birth newborns who have not had the thoracic squeeze that occurs during vaginal birth and removes some of the lung fluid (Blackburn, 2007).

Usually the newborn experiences little or no difficulty at the onset of breathing. However, shortly after birth, expiratory grunting, flaring of the nares, subcostal retractions, desaturation, and mild cyanosis may be noted in the newborn breathing room air. Air will become trapped and an increase in the anterior/posterior diameter of the chest will be observed. Tachypnea is usually present by 6 hours of age, with respiratory rates consistently greater than 60 breaths per minute (breaths/min), and reaching 80–100 breaths/min and higher (Guglani et al., 2008). Mild respiratory and metabolic acidosis may be present within the first 6 hours. These clinical signs usually improve within 12 to 24 hours. In mild TTN, the signs

NURSING CARE PLAN For the Newborn with Respiratory Distress Syndrome

INTERVENTION	RATIONALE
1. Nursing Diagnosis: Risk for Ineffective Breathing Pattern related to immature lung development	
Goal: The infant will maintain an effective breathing pattern.	
■ Review maternal birth records, noting medications given to mother before birth and the infant's condition at birth such as Apgar scores and resuscitative measures.	■ Several drugs suppress respiratory function in the newborn.
■ Initiate cardiac and respiratory monitoring and calibrate these monitors every 8 hours or per unit protocol.	■ Close monitoring detects periodic apneic spells and allows for medical intervention if necessary.
■ Monitor infant's respiratory rate and rhythm, pulse, blood pressure, and activity.	■ Increases in respiratory rate and pulse and alteration in rhythm and blood pressure may indicate respiratory distress.
■ Assess skin color; note signs of cyanosis, duskiness, and pallor.	■ Any changes in the normal skin color may indicate a physiologic change occurring.
■ Clear infant's airway by suctioning PRN with bulb syringe.	■ Opens airway by clearing mucus and allows maximum respiratory effort.
■ Administer warmed, humidified oxygen by oxygen hood and monitor the oxygen concentrations every 30 minutes.	■ Prevents mucosal dryness and maintains an even level of oxygen administration.
■ Do not allow oxyhood to touch infant's face; maintain a stable oxygen concentration by increasing and decreasing oxygen by 5% to 10% increments.	■ Allowing oxyhood to touch infant's face may cause apnea by stimulating the facial nerve.
Collaborative: Obtain arterial blood gases (ABGs) per primary care provider/physician orders.	
a. Maintain constant O_2 concentration for 15–30 minutes before sample is obtained. b. Avoid stimulating infant for 15 minutes before obtaining sample. c. Avoid suctioning infant before obtaining sample. d. Obtain sample in heparinized tuberculin syringe and maintain the temperature of the sample. e. Assess the patency of the arterial line to prevent clot formation, then replace blood used to clear line. f. Flush line with 2 ml heparinized solution before restarting flow of IV fluids. g. Monitor transcutaneous pulse oximeter continuously or hourly and record. Rotate sensor site every 3–4 hours.	■ Obtaining ABGs is essential in managing an infant receiving oxygen. Suctioning may cause a discrepancy in ABG readings and should be avoided.
■ Assess infant's need for mechanical ventilation: apnea present, hypoxia (PaO_2 less than 50 mm Hg), hypercapnia ($PaCO_2$ greater than 60 mm Hg), respiratory acidosis (pH less than 7.2).	■ Mechanical ventilation improves oxygenation and ventilation, resulting in rise in PaO_2 and decrease in $PaCO_2$.
■ Administer mechanical ventilation per hospital protocol.	■ Continuous positive airway pressure (CPAP) or positive end-expiratory pressure (PEEP) can be administered by nasal prongs, nasopharyngeal or oral intubation.

EXPECTED OUTCOMES: The infant will maintain an effective breathing pattern as evidenced by respirations of 30–60 breaths/min, arterial blood gases are within normal range, infant is free of signs of retractions or nasal flaring, and blood pH is 7.35–7.45.

INTERVENTION	RATIONALE
2. Nursing Diagnosis: Ineffective Thermoregulation related to increased respiratory effort	
Goal: The infant will exhibit no signs of hypothermia.	
■ Review maternal prenatal and intrapartum records. Note any medications mother received during these times.	■ Medications such as Demerol and magnesium sulfate used by the mother during the prenatal or intrapartum periods significantly interfere with the infant's ability to retain heat.
■ Assess infant's temperature frequently. Place servo probe on infant's skin over a solid organ.	■ Hypothermia leads to pulmonary vasoconstriction because of the increase in oxygen consumption. Cold stress leads to increased oxygen needs; consequently, brown fat is used to maintain body temperature.
■ Observe for signs of increased oxygen consumption and metabolic acidosis.	■ Hypoxia and acidosis further depress surfactant production.

NURSING CARE PLAN For the Newborn with Respiratory Distress Syndrome continued

INTERVENTION	RATIONALE
■ Warm and humidify all inspired gases and record temperature of delivered gases.	■ Cold air/oxygen blown in face of newborn is stimulus for consumption of oxygen and glucose and increased metabolic rate.
■ Use radiant warmers or incubators with servo controls, and open cribs with appropriate clothing.	■ Maintains neutral thermal environment.
■ Note signs and symptoms of respiratory distress, including tachypnea, apnea, cyanosis, acrocyanosis, bradycardia, lethargy, weak cry, and hypotonia.	■ These signs can predispose the infant to metabolic acidosis.

EXPECTED OUTCOMES: The infant will not exhibit signs and symptoms of hypothermia as evidenced by temperature maintenance of 97.7°F–99.1°F and no signs and symptoms of respiratory distress.

3. Nursing Diagnosis: Imbalanced Nutrition: Less Than Body Requirements related to increased metabolic needs in the infant

Goal: Infant will gain weight in a normal curve.

INTERVENTION	RATIONALE
■ Assess suck, swallow, gag, and cough reflexes.	■ Prevents feeding problems and assists in determining the best individualized method of feeding for infant.
■ Assess respiratory status of infant. If any problems are noted, notify physician.	■ In the presence of respiratory distress avoid oral fluids and initiate parenteral nutrition per physician's orders.
■ Monitor IV rates per infusion pump (starting at 80 ml/kg/day) as ordered by physician.	■ Allows for close monitoring of fluid intake.
■ Record hourly intake and output (I&O) and daily weights.	■ IV fluids are administered to replace sensible and insensible water loss, as well as evaporative water loss secondary to respiratory distress. Monitoring I&O will prevent circulatory system overload that can lead to pulmonary edema and cardiac problems.
■ Provide total parenteral nutrition (TPN) when indicated.	■ TPN is used as nutritional alternative if bowel sounds are not present and/or infant remains in acute distress.
■ Advance, based on tolerance, from IV to gastrointestinal (GI) feedings. Gavage or nipple feedings are used, and IV is used as supplement (discontinued when oral intake is sufficient).	■ If IV is discontinued before oral intake is established, baby will not receive adequate calories. ■ Formula or breast milk stimulate GI hormones necessary for a functional absorptive GI tract. ■ Avoid complications associated with nutrition by IV route only.
■ Provide adequate caloric intake: consider amount of intake, type of formula, route of administration, and need for supplementation of intake by other routes.	■ Calories are essential to prevent catabolism of body proteins and metabolic acidosis due to starvation or inadequate caloric intake.
■ Assess infusion site for signs and symptoms of infection including: erythema, edema, and drainage with a foul odor.	■ Appropriate intervention can be initiated when signs and symptoms of infection are detected early. Treatment may avoid infection and sepsis in the infant.

EXPECTED OUTCOMES: The newborn infant will maintain steady weight gain as evidenced by no more than 2%/day weight loss, tolerates oral feedings, and urine output of 1–3 ml/kg/hour.

4. Nursing Diagnosis: Risk for Deficient Fluid Volume related to increased insensible water losses

Goal: The infant will not exhibit signs of dehydration and will display appropriate weight gain.

INTERVENTION	RATIONALE
■ Observe for weight fluctuations by obtaining daily weights.	■ Fluctuations in weight may indicate water imbalance or inadequate caloric intake.
■ Document cumulative balances of intake (IV fluid administration and feedings) and output (urine collection bags, weighing or counting diapers) hourly.	■ Balanced fluid intake and output suggest homeostasis.
■ Obtain urinalysis; monitor closely specific gravity and nitrites.	■ Specific gravity greater than 1.013 and nitrites present in the urine are indicative of not enough fluid intake.
■ Monitor vital signs including blood pressure, pulse, temperature, and mean arterial pressure (MAP).	■ A MAP of less than 20 mm Hg may indicate hypotension.

(continued)

NURSING CARE PLAN For the Newborn with Respiratory Distress Syndrome continued

INTERVENTION	RATIONALE
■ Assess patient for signs of dehydration (i.e., poor skin turgor, pale mucous membranes, and sunken anterior fontanelle).	■ Detecting signs and symptoms of dehydration early in the infant are important because early interventions are vital to prevent further damage.
■ Assess IV site for signs of infection (erythema and edema) and infiltration.	■ If signs and symptoms of infection are noted, intervention is necessary and IV site should be changed.
Collaborative: Obtain labs for hematocrit (Hct), serum calcium, serum magnesium, serum potassium, blood urea nitrogen (BUN), creatinine, and uric acid levels.	■ Determines necessity for TPN administration.
■ Administer fluids, blood products, and electrolytes as ordered by physician.	■ Replaces low nutrient stores and treats anemia if present.

EXPECTED OUTCOMES: The infant will be free of signs and symptoms of dehydration as evidenced by intake equaling output, urine specific gravity in normal range, and a weight gain of at least 20–30 grams/day.

can improve within 24 hours but may continue for 48 to 72 hours when more severe (Cloherty et al., 2008).

Clinical Therapy

Initial x-ray findings may be identical to those showing RDS within the first 3 hours. However, radiographs of infants with transient tachypnea usually reveal a generalized overexpansion of the lungs (hyperaeration of alveoli), which is identifiable principally by flattened contours of the diaphragm. Dense streaks (increased vascularity) radiate from the hilar region and represent engorgement of the lymphatic vessels, which clear alveolar fluid on initiation of air breathing. Within 48 hours the chest x-ray examination is generally normal with the exception of perihilar markings which may remain visible for 3 to 7 days (Gomella et al., 2009; Guglani et al., 2008).

Ambient oxygen concentrations of 30% to 50%, usually under an oxyhood, may be required to correct the hypoxemia (Figure 34-9 ■). Fluid and electrolyte requirements should be met with IV fluids during the acute phase of the disease. Oral feedings are contraindicated because of rapid respiratory rates and the subsequent risk of aspiration, intravenous fluids of $D_{10}W$ at 60–80 ml/kg/day is recommended for a maintenance fluid during the NPO period (Guglani et al., 2008). The duration of the clinical course of transient tachypnea is approximately 72 hours (Gomella et al., 2009).

When hypoxemia is severe and tachypnea continues, persistent pulmonary hypertension must be considered and treatment measures initiated. If pneumonia is suspected initially, antibiotics may be administered prophylactically.

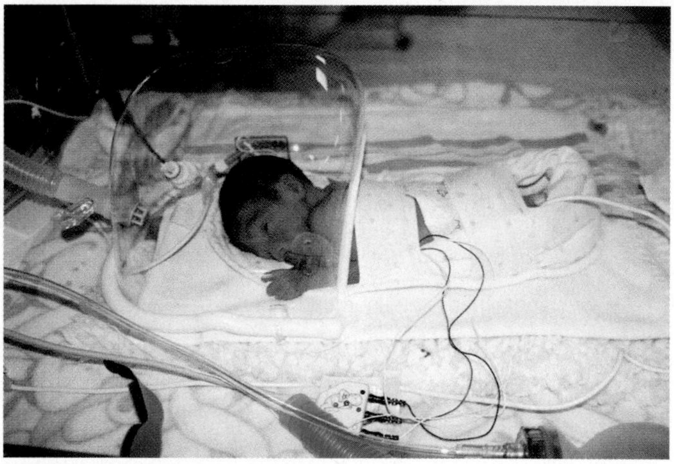

Figure 34-9 ■ Premature infant under oxygen hood. Infant is nested and has a nonnutritive sucking pacifier.

Source: Courtesy of Lisa Smith-Pedersen, RN, MSN, NNP-BC.

CLINICAL JUDGMENT

Case Study: Baby Girl Linn

You are caring for baby girl Linn, who is a 39-week, AGA female born by repeat cesarean birth to a 34-year-old G3, now P3 mother. Baby Linn's Apgar scores were 7 at 1 minute and 9 at 5 minutes. At 2 hours of age, you note an elevated respiratory rate of 70 to 80 and mild cyanosis. The infant is now receiving 30% oxygen and has a respiratory rate of 100 to 120. The baby's clinical course, chest x-ray examination, and lab work are all consistent with transient tachypnea of the newborn. Her mother calls you to ask about her baby. She tells you that her last child was born at 30 weeks' gestation, had respiratory distress syndrome requiring ventilator support, and was hospitalized for 6 weeks. She asks you, "Is this the same respiratory distress?"

Critical Thinking

What will you tell Linn's mother?

See www.nursing.pearsonhighered.com for possible responses.

NURSING CARE MANAGEMENT

For nursing actions, see the Nursing Care Plan: For the Newborn with Respiratory Distress Syndrome on pages 950 to 952.

Care of the Newborn with Meconium Aspiration Syndrome

Because the body's physiologic response to asphyxia/hypoxia is increased intestinal peristalsis and relaxation of the anal sphincter, the presence of meconium in the amniotic fluid indicates that the fetus may be suffering from asphyxia, either in the immediate period during labor or perhaps some time in the recent past. Head or cord compression may illicit a vagal response in the fetus, thus causing passage of meconium in utero (Wiedemann, Saugstad, Barnes-Powell, et al., 2008). However, if the fetus is in a breech position, the presence of meconium in the amniotic fluid does not necessarily indicate asphyxia.

Approximately 8% to 20% of all live-born, late-preterm or term infants are born through meconium-stained amniotic fluid (MSAF). Of the newborns born through MSAF, 5% to 10% develop **meconium aspiration syndrome (MAS)** (Wiedemann et al., 2008). This fluid may be aspirated into the tracheobronchial tree by the fetus in utero or during the first few breaths taken by the newborn. This syndrome primarily affects term, small-for-gestational age (SGA), and postterm newborns and those who have experienced a long labor.

Presence of meconium in the lungs produces (Wiedemann et al., 2008):

- Mechanical obstruction of airways: ball-valve action (air is allowed in but not exhaled), so that alveoli overdistend, with oxygen and carbon dioxide trapping and hyperinflation, air leaks such as pneumothorax are common.
- Chemical pneumonitis leading to the possible development of secondary bacterial pneumonias.
- Inactivation of natural surfactant.
- Vasoconstriction of pulmonary vessels, allowing development of persistent pulmonary hypertension (PPHN).

Clinical Manifestations of MAS

Clinical manifestations of MAS include (1) fetal hypoxia in utero a few days or a few minutes before birth, indicated by a sudden increase in fetal activity followed by diminished activity, slowing of fetal heart rate (FHR) or weak and irregular heartbeat, loss of beat-to-beat variability, and meconium staining of amniotic fluid or particulate meconium; and (2) presence of signs of distress at birth, such as pallor, cyanosis, apnea, slow heartbeat, and low Apgar scores (below 6) at 1 and 5 minutes. Newborns with intrauterine asphyxia, meconium-stained newborns, or newborns who have aspirated particulate meconium often have respiratory depression at birth and require resuscitation to establish adequate respiratory effort.

After the initial resuscitation, the severity of clinical symptoms correlates with the extent of aspiration. Many infants require mechanical ventilation at birth because of immediate signs of distress (generalized cyanosis, tachypnea, and severe retractions). An overdistended, barrel-shaped chest with increased anteroposterior diameter is common. Auscultation reveals diminished air movement with prominent rales and rhonchi. Abdominal palpation may reveal a displaced liver caused by diaphragmatic depression resulting from the overexpansion of the lungs. Yellowish/pale green staining of the skin, nails, and umbilical cord is usually present, especially if the incident occurred some time before birth.

The MAS chest x-ray film reveals asymmetric, coarse, patchy, densities/infiltrates, with possible hyperinflation (9- to 11-rib expansion), atelectasis (collapse of part or all of a lung) which may predispose the newborn to air leak syndromes such as pneumothorax or pneumomediastinum (Wiedemann et al., 2008). Evidence of pulmonary air leak is frequently present. These infants have serious biochemical alterations, which include (1) extreme metabolic acidosis resulting from the cardiopulmonary shunting (bypassing the lungs) and hypoperfusion; (2) extreme respiratory acidosis due to shunting and alveolar hypoventilation; and (3) extreme hypoxia, even in 100% O_2 concentrations and with ventilatory assistance. The extreme hypoxia is also caused by the cardiopulmonary shunting and resultant failure to oxygenate and can lead to persistent pulmonary hypertension of the newborn (PPHN), discussed shortly.

Clinical Therapy

The combined efforts of the maternity and pediatric team are needed to prevent MAS. Previously, the most effective form of preventive management was intrapartum suctioning after the head of the newborn was delivered but the shoulders and chest were still in the birth canal. Current evidence does not support this practice, as routine intrapartum oropharyngeal and nasopharyngeal suctioning does not prevent or alter the course of MAS (AAP & ACOG, 2007; Carbine & Serwint, 2008; Wiedemann et al., 2008).

If the infant is vigorous even if there is meconium-stained amniotic fluid, no subsequent special resuscitation such as tracheal suctioning is indicated. Injury to the vocal cords is also more likely to occur during attempts to intubate a vigorous newborn.

If the infant has absent or depressed respirations, heart rate less than 100 beats per minute, or poor muscle tone, direct tracheal suctioning by specially trained personnel such as a neonatal nurse practitioner, an experienced neonatal intensive care unit (NICU) nurse trained in those skills, a respiratory therapist, or a nurse anesthetist is recommended. The glottis is visualized and the trachea suctioned to remove meconium or other aspirated material from beneath the glottis with use of a DeLee attached to low-pressure wall suction or a meconium aspirator to decrease the possibility of HIV transmission. When using mechanical suction, the suction pressure should be set so that negative pressure does not exceed 100 mm Hg. (This is also done with a cesarean birth.)

Further resuscitative efforts are undertaken as indicated, following the same principles of clinical therapy as for asphyxia (discussed earlier in this chapter). Resuscitated newborns should be immediately transferred to the nursery for closer observation. The infant should be maintained in a neutral thermal environment and tactile stimulation should be minimized. An umbilical arterial line may be used for direct monitoring of arterial blood pressures and blood sampling for pH and blood gases. An umbilical venous catheter may be placed for infusion of intravenous (IV) fluids, blood, or medications.

RESEARCH EVIDENCE IN PRACTICE: Prevention of Meconium Aspiration Syndrome

CLINICAL QUESTION

What is the most effective way to prevent meconium aspiration syndrome after birth?

RESEARCH EVIDENCE

Meconium aspiration syndrome (MAS) is a serious, life-threatening respiratory disorder. Meconium-stained amniotic fluid occurs in approximately 13% of live births and, of these, 5% to 10% subsequently develop MAS. This syndrome remains an important cause of admission for intensive care among term neonates. Traditionally, it was believed that the beginnings of MAS occurred after birth, when the baby took its first breaths and inhaled meconium. Preventive measures included suctioning the baby's upper airway after the head was delivered, and subsequent tracheal intubation and suctioning was standard care for all babies with meconium-stained amniotic fluid. Recent studies have focused on whether these procedures are necessary and result in better outcomes than using these procedures selectively.

Implicit in the traditional treatment is the belief that MAS is a postnatal condition, occurring after the baby takes its first breaths. This belief was tested by the knowledge that babies born via surgical birth also demonstrated MAS under certain conditions. Likewise, randomized trials demonstrated that the majority of babies who were born with meconium-stained amniotic fluid did not develop MAS.

Through randomized trials, systematic reviews, and convening expert panels, it has been determined that some babies are able to protect their airways, even in the presence of meconium-stained amniotic fluid. Other babies, such as the more compromised fetuses with hypoxia and acidosis that gasp in utero, may not protect their airways and, subsequently, develop the complications of meconium aspiration.

Although there is likely no benefit from upper airway suctioning, it is not associated with harm unless it delays handoff of the baby to the neonatal team. Tracheal intubation and suctioning, on the other hand, may carry risks for the baby. A treatment algorithm developed at Baylor University Medical Center provides guidelines for selectively applying upper airway and tracheal suctioning appropriately.

WHAT QUESTIONS REMAIN UNANSWERED?

Is meconium-stained amniotic fluid the cause of fetal distress or a result? Are there symptoms of MAS that are detectable in utero?

WHAT IS BEST PRACTICE?

Upper airway suctioning should be applied after the head—but before the shoulders—is delivered when meconium-stained amniotic fluid is present. Immediate handoff of the baby to the neonatal team should be followed by a second assessment. Vigorous babies need no additional treatment. Tracheal intubation and suctioning should be carried out in depressed newborns, defined as those with a heart rate of <100 beats/min, poor respiratory effort, and poor tone.

CRITICAL THINKING

Develop a checklist that can be used by the neonatal nurse to detect early signs of MAS after a birth with meconium-stained amniotic fluid.

References

Martin, G. I., & Vidyasagar, D. 2008. Proceedings of the first international conference for meconium aspiration syndrome and meconium-induced lung injury. *Journal of Perinatology, 28,* S1–S2, doi:10.1038/jp.2008.176

Singh, B., Clark, R., Powers, R., & Spitzer, A. 2009. Meconium aspiration syndrome remains a significant problem in the NICU: Outcomes and treatment patterns in term neonates admitted for intensive care during a ten-year period. *Journal of Perinatology, 29,* 497–503.

Whitfield, J., Charsha, D., & Ciruvolu, A. 2009. Prevention of meconium aspiration syndrome: An update and the Baylor experience. *Baylor University Medical Center Proceedings, 22*(2), 128–131.

Xu, H., Wei, S., & Fraser, W. 2008. Obstetric approaches to the prevention of meconium aspiration syndrome. *Journal of Perinatology, 28,* S14–S18. doi:10.1038/jp.2008.145

Treatment usually involves delivery of high oxygen concentrations and high-pressure ventilation. Low positive end-expiratory pressures (PEEPs) (4–7 cm H_2O) are preferred to avoid air leaks such as pneumothorax. Unfortunately, high pressures may be needed to cause sufficient expiratory expansion of the obstructed terminal airways or to stabilize airways that are weakened by inflammation so that the most distal atelectatic (collapsed) alveoli are ventilated. Naturally occurring surfactant may be inactivated by the presence of meconium and the subsequent inflammatory response that occurs. Surfactant replacement therapy is most effective when given as a prophylactic measure. Providing exogenous surfactant possibly decreases the incidence of air leaks (Wiedemann et al., 2008). Systemic blood pressure and pulmonary blood flow must be maintained. Dopamine or dobutamine (volume expanders), or both, may be used to maintain systemic blood pressure.

Newborns with respiratory failure who are not responding to conventional ventilator therapy may require treatment with high-frequency ventilation and/or nitric oxide therapy or extracorporeal membrane oxygenation (ECMO) if baby is greater than 1.8 kg and 34 weeks estimated gestational age (EGA) (Gomella et al., 2009). Inhaled nitric oxide has proven successful for newborns with meconium aspiration, pneumonia, and PPHN who are not responding to traditional treatment modalities, and it avoids the need for ECMO.

Treatment also includes chest physiotherapy (chest percussion, vibration, and drainage) to remove the debris. Prophylactic antibiotics are frequently given. Continuous infusion of sodium bicarbonate to correct metabolic acidosis may be necessary for several days for severely ill newborns. Mortality in term and postterm infants is very high because the cycle of hypoxemia and acidemia is difficult to break.

Application: Meconium Aspiration Syndrome

NURSING CARE MANAGEMENT

Nursing Assessment and Diagnosis

During the intrapartum period, the nurse should observe for signs of fetal hypoxia and meconium staining of amniotic fluid. At birth the nurse assesses the newborn for signs of distress. During the ongoing assessment of the newborn, the nurse carefully observes for complications such as pulmonary air leaks; anoxic cerebral injury manifested by seizures/convulsions; myocardial injury evidenced by congestive heart failure or cardiomegaly; disseminated intravascular coagulation (DIC) resulting from hypoxic hepatic damage with depression of liver-dependent clotting factors; anoxic renal damage demonstrated by hematuria, oliguria, or anuria; fluid overload; sepsis secondary to bacterial pneumonia; and any signs of intestinal necrosis from ischemia, including gastrointestinal (GI) obstruction or hemorrhage.

Nursing diagnoses that may apply to the newborn with MAS and the infant's parents include the following:

- ***Impaired Gas Exchange*** related to aspiration of meconium and amniotic fluid during birth
- ***Imbalanced Nutrition: Less Than Body Requirements*** related to respiratory distress and increased energy requirements
- ***Compromised Family Coping*** related to life-threatening illness in a term newborn

Nursing Plan and Implementation

Hospital-Based Nursing Care

Initial interventions are aimed at early identification of meconium aspiration. When significant aspiration occurs, therapy is supportive with the primary goals of maintaining appropriate gas exchange and minimizing complications. Nursing interventions after resuscitation should include maintaining adequate oxygenation and ventilation, regulating temperature, performing glucose testing by glucometer to check for hypoglycemia, observing IV fluids, calculating necessary fluids (which may be restricted in the first 48 to 72 hours because of cerebral edema), providing caloric requirements possibly with total parenteral nutrition (TPN), and monitoring IV antibiotic therapy.

Evaluation

Expected outcomes of nursing care include the following:

- The newborn at risk of MAS is promptly identified, and early intervention is initiated.
- The newborn is free of respiratory distress and metabolic alterations.
- The parents verbalize their concerns about their baby's health problem and survival and understand the rationale behind management of their newborn.

Persistent Pulmonary Hypertension of the Newborn

Persistent pulmonary hypertension of the newborn (PPHN) is a serious disorder that may primarily affect on average 0.2% of live-born term and near-term newborns annually (Konduri & Kim, 2009; Rothstein, Paris, & Quizon, 2009). PPHN has also been called *persistent fetal circulation (PFC)* because the problems that occur are a result of right-to-left (R-L) shunting of blood away from the lungs and through the fetal ductus arteriosus and patent foramen ovale, consequently bypassing the lungs and the ability to be oxygenated, causing worsening hypoxemia and acidosis (Rothstein et al., 2009). The hypoxemia and acidosis are the most potent stimulants of pulmonary vasoconstriction and increased vascular resistance. Once this process has begun, it is self-perpetuating and difficult to interrupt. Clinical deterioration is rapid.

Clinical Therapy

Simultaneous preductal and postductal blood gases or pulse oximetry and/or transcutaneous monitoring can be used to demonstrate ductal shunting. A difference greater than 10% to 15% between preductal and postductal oxygen saturation is indicative of a right-to-left ductal shunt (Gomella et al., 2009). The hyperoxia-hyperventilation test is the most definitive test for PPHN. A positive indication of PPHN is when the PaO_2 increases more than 20 mm Hg or the pulse oximeter exhibits an increase greater than 10% with hyperoxia and hyperventilation (Konduri & Kim, 2009). Oxygen is a potent pulmonary vasodilator. The improved oxygenation can be noted clinically if the infant's mucous membranes turn pink. Echocardiography can show a prolonged ratio of right ventricular ejection period to right ventricular ejection time in infants with PPHN. The goal of therapeutic intervention is to lower the PVR and reverse the process of shunting. This can be accomplished with the use of nitric oxide, which is a selective pulmonary vasodilator, when other methods fail. Oxygenation, ventilation, volume expanders, and drug therapy such as Pavulon, Versed, vasopressors (dopamine or dobutamine) and afterload reducers (nitroprusside) are used until the PaO_2 can be consistently maintained at 60–90 mm Hg (Konduri & Kim 2009).

NURSING CARE MANAGEMENT

The nurse assesses for the onset of symptoms, which usually occur in the first 12 to 24 hours of life. Affected newborns exhibit signs of respiratory distress (grunting, nasal flaring, tachypnea), with increased anteroposterior diameter and cyanosis. They typically fail to respond to conventional methods of oxygenation and ventilation. Significant unexplained hypoxemia exists in the absence of congenital heart disease. The chest radiograph might show no evidence of pulmonary parenchymal disease (depending on the underlying disease). The hypoxemia and cyanosis associated with PPHN are characteristic of extreme changeability. Marked, rapid changes in PaO_2 and color are seen with agitation, stimulation, therapeutic intervention (suctioning), or rapid changes in ambient oxygen.

Infants with PPHN are critically ill and require experienced, highly skilled nurses to provide optimal care with minimal manipulation/stimulation. Any disturbance may cause agitation, which leads to hypoxemia. If a paralyzing agent is used, nursing care includes monitoring the newborn's response to artificial oxygenation and mechanical ventilation. The nurse ensures that the oxygen is delivered in correct amounts and route and records the percentage of oxygen flow. The ventilator settings are checked frequently and recorded per unit policy. The nurse carefully suctions the endotracheal tube only as necessary while assessing the effect of the procedure on the baby's oxygenation and perfusion. The amount and type of secretions are noted. The nurse carefully assesses arterial blood gases and notifies the clinician if the results are out of the acceptable range. Oxygen monitoring is essential for identifying activities that may compromise the infant's status. (Nursing interventions required for noninvasive oxygen monitoring are discussed in Table 34-2.) Continuous monitoring of vital signs and blood pressure is required, and careful inspection of the skin during positioning is necessary to avoid pressure necrosis. Aggressive ventilation poses a potential risk for pneumothorax.

Many infants suffering PPHN are born at or near term at a time when parents least expect problems—especially life-threatening problems—to occur. The magnitude of the infant's illness and the rapid deterioration may be overwhelming to parents. Attachment becomes difficult when the infant responds poorly to touching (as seen by decreased PaO_2). Instead, the nurse can encourage parents to talk very softly to their infant because this will usually not compromise the baby's condition. The nurse should assess their level of understanding and assist them by providing information about their baby's condition and therapies in easily understandable terms. Continuity of nursing care is helpful because it will be less threatening for the parents to relate to a smaller group of nurses.

Care of the Newborn with Complications Due to Respiratory Therapy

Oxygen and mechanical ventilation, although required as therapeutic interventions to reduce hypoxia, hypercarbia, ischemia, and infarction to vital organs, may also have harmful effects. The concentrations of ambient oxygen administered to the newborn must be titrated according to oxygen tension within arterial blood to avoid development of retinopathy of prematurity or bronchopulmonary dysplasia/chronic lung disease.

Pulmonary Interstitial Emphysema

Pulmonary interstitial emphysema (PIE) is the accumulation of air in lung tissues occurring predominantly in very-low-birth-weight (VLBW) neonates who are on mechanical ventilators (Miller & Carlo, 2008). It may be unilateral or bilateral. Air collections outside the lung are a function of lung compliance and use of increased pressures to ventilate. Overdistention of alveoli may progress to PIE when rupture occurs and air escapes and becomes trapped into the interstitial spaces. Air moves along perivascular spaces but not into the pleural space or mediastinum. As the air collections increase, blood vessels are constricted, and blood gas exchange is impaired; thus hypoxia and hypercarbia may develop. The air does not decrease on expiration. This condition is highly associated with subsequent bronchopulmonary dysplasia (BPD). It may also precede pneumothorax or pneumomediastinum (Gomella, et al., 2009; Miller & Carlo, 2008).

Pneumothorax

Pneumothorax, a common complication of respiratory therapy, is an accumulation of air in the thoracic cavity between the parietal and visceral pleura and precedes collapse of the lung (Posner & Needleman, 2008). Asymptomatic pneumothorax occurs in 1% to 2% of newborns. In addition, pulmonary air leaks occur in up to 15% to 30% of mechanically ventilated newborns; however, air leaks can be a consequence of injury due to the disease rather than the mechanical ventilation (Gomella et al., 2009).

Pneumothorax in the newborn causes several physiologic changes: collapse of the lung, compression of the heart and lungs, compromise of venous return to the right heart with mediastinal air, and development of tension in the pleural space. Symptoms of pneumothorax include a sudden, unexplained deterioration in the newborn's condition; decreased breath sounds; apnea; bradycardia; cyanosis; increased oxygen requirements; higher PCO_2; decrease in pH; mottled, asymmetric chest expansion; decreased arterial blood pressure; shock-like appearance; and a shift in the apical cardiac impulses to the side opposite the pneumothorax, often with muffled heart sounds.

Transillumination of the chest is used for rapid evaluation of pneumothorax. However, x-ray examination is the main method of diagnosing this complication (Figure 34-10 ■). Pneumothorax is a potentially life-threatening situation for the newborn

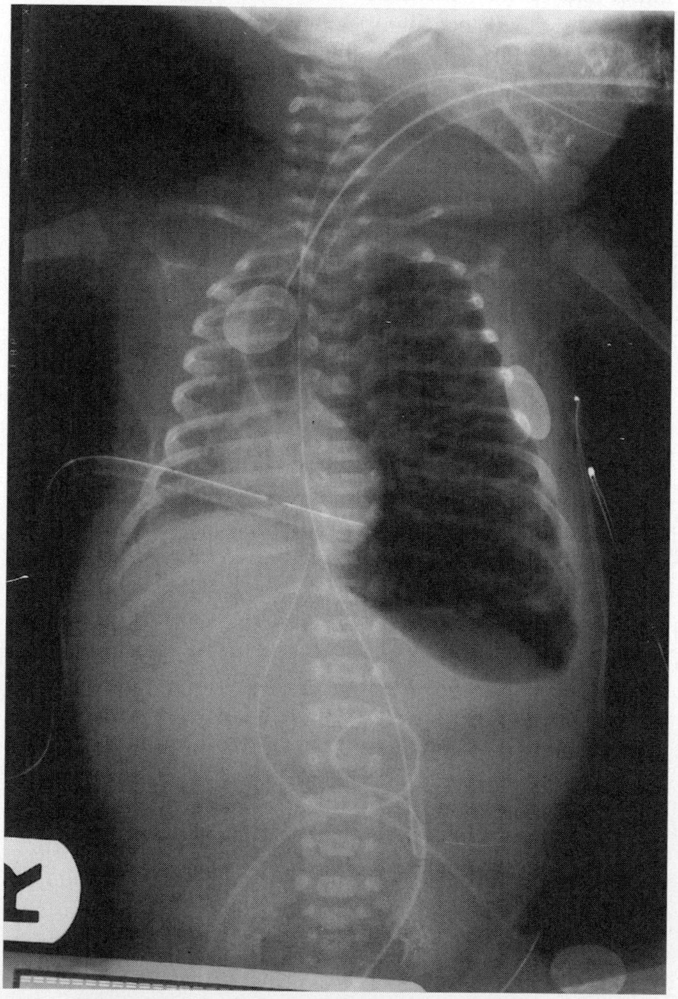

Figure 34-10 ■ Chest x-ray of a left-sided pneumothorax. A rupture of the alveoli sacs allows air to leak through the pleura, forming collections of air outside the lung (air shows on x-ray as dark area over lung).

Source: Courtesy of Carol Harrigan, RN, MSN, NNP-BC.

and may demand immediate removal of the accumulated air. Only skilled and specifically trained personnel should perform a thoracentesis. For complete resolution of the pneumothorax, a chest tube may be inserted (Posner & Needleman, 2008).

Bronchopulmonary Dysplasia/ Chronic Lung Disease

Bronchopulmonary dysplasia (BPD), also known as **chronic lung disease (CLD) of prematurity**, most commonly occurs in very compromised low-birth-weight (LBW) preterm infants who require oxygen therapy, which may cause oxidant injury, and assisted mechanical ventilation, causing volutrauma and barotrauma for the treatment of respiratory distress syndrome (RDS) or other medical condition (Geary, Caskey, Fonseca, et al., 2008). The incidence can reach up to 30% in infants born weighing less than 1 kg at birth (Geary et al., 2009). It has also been associated with neonatal pneumonia, meconium aspiration syndrome (MAS), persistent pulmonary hypertension (PPHN), congenital heart disease (patent ductus arteriosus), other congenital anomalies requiring high levels of oxygen and ventilatory support, and possibly low-grade or asymptomatic pulmonary infection with *Ureaplasma urealyticum* the microorganism frequently located in the amniotic fluid and pulmonary secretions after birth in the preterm newborn (Speer, 2009).

The definition of BPD is dependence on oxygen up to 28 days of age to maintain an oxygen saturation >89%. Mild BPD requires oxygen greater than or equal to 28 days but not at 36 weeks gestational age. Moderate BPD requires the use of oxygen greater than or equal to 28 days at 36 weeks gestational age with less than 30% oxygen required. Severe BPD requires supplemental oxygen greater than or equal to 30% at greater than or equal to 28 days and/or positive pressure support or mechanical ventilation at 36 weeks gestational age (Gomella et al., 2009). The process of BPD is one of continuous lung tissue injury and repair, delaying both lung and body growth.

Clinical Therapy

The goals of therapeutic intervention for the newborn with BPD are to provide adequate oxygenation and ventilation, prevent further lung damage, promote optimal nutrition, and give supportive care to ensure adequate rates of growth and development. Because of the chronic nature of BPD, therapeutic intervention must be individualized to meet the specific needs of the infant. Supplemental oxygen levels are adjusted to consistently keep O_2 saturations between 85% and 93%, depending on associated clinical problems such as poor growth, recurrent bradycardia, and pulmonary hypertension (Gomella et al., 2009). Diuretics and fluid restriction (120 ml/kg/day) are frequently used to control pulmonary fluid retention and to improve lung function; electrolyte supplements are necessary to offset the results of chronic diuretic therapy (Cloherty et al., 2008; Gomella et al., 2009). In addition, bronchodilators are indicated to decrease airway resistance and to control bronchospasm. The infant with chronic lung disease is often on long-term steroids. Serial echocardiography is used to monitor cardiac response to the chronic pulmonary disease.

NURSING CARE MANAGEMENT

Hospital-Based Nursing Care

The nurse observes carefully for any changes in the newborn's oxygenation, giving special attention to maintaining the prescribed oxygen concentration during all activities, especially during periods of stress, such as when the infant is crying; when blood is drawn; while starting an intravenous (IV) infusion; and during a lumbar puncture (LP), suctioning, chest physiotherapy (CPT), and feeding.

The nurse obtains blood gases based on the institution's chronic blood gas protocol—for example, every 3 days, 20 minutes after a permanent change in ambient oxygen concentration (FiO_2), or more frequently if the infant experiences increasing respiratory distress or increasing lethargy. Postural drainage, CPT, and vibration followed by suctioning are carried out with close attention to the baby's tolerance and should be coordinated with rest periods to avoid fatiguing the infant. The nurse maintains the infant's body temperature because hypothermia or hyperthermia will increase oxygen consumption and may increase oxygen requirements. Positioning on the abdomen helps the baby maintain higher transcutaneous oxygen saturation ($TcPO_2$) and improved ventilation.

Bronchodilators such as albuterol, diuretics, steroids, and electrolyte supplements may be used in the clinical management of the BPD infant (Gomella et al., 2009). Many of the side effects of these drugs, such as hypokalemia and mineral losses (fractures), can be avoided by giving the diuretics every other day.

Providing for adequate nutrition enhances formation of new alveoli and enlargement of the airway diameter. The more severely ill the baby, the higher the caloric need to meet the greater expenditure of energy for survival and healing. As soon as tolerated, a 24 kcal/oz formula for preterm infants is started, especially if the baby is on fluid restriction. More oxygen may be required during feeding, and the least energy-consuming feeding method should be used (Figure 34-11 ■). If the feeding schedule

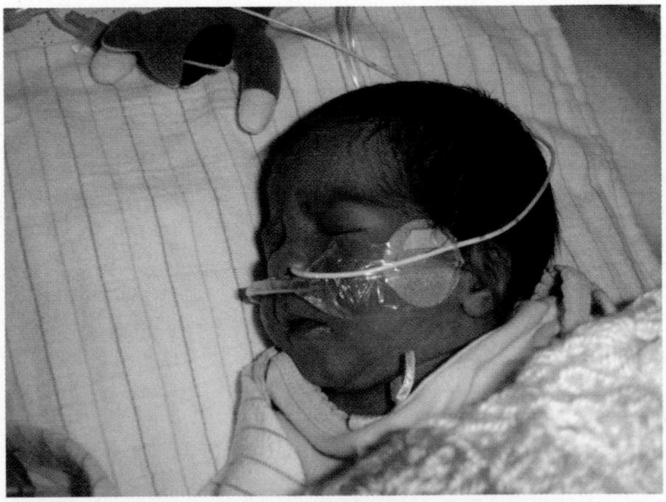

Figure 34-11 ■ A baby with BPD requires oxygen at greater than 36 weeks' gestational age. She still needs to be fed through an NG tube, because she tires with nipple feeds.

Source: Courtesy of Lisa Smith-Pedersen, RN, MSN, NNP-BC.

is too stressful, smaller, more frequent feedings may be initiated (Cloherty et al., 2008; Gomella et al., 2009).

Infants with BPD frequently experience negative oral sensations due to suctioning and intubation. These can adversely affect their transition to nipple or spoon feeding and may require some type of feeding therapy to help them eat successfully. Positioning is often the key to adequate intake and decreasing gastroesophageal reflux (GER). In addition, most infants receive numerous, possibly unpalatable, medications with meals. Attempts must be made to include pleasurable activities such as cuddling at mealtime to develop positive associations with appropriate feeding behaviors.

Infants with BPD are very susceptible to infection, especially if they are on long-term steroids; therefore, it is important to discourage anyone with early signs of infectious disease from having contact with them. The infant's behavior and vital signs should be monitored for changes that might indicate early developing infection. Changes in color, quantity, or quality of pulmonary secretions are noted and reported. The frequency of CPT and suctioning may need to be increased.

Health Promotion Education

When the infant develops BPD and the family becomes aware of the implications of chronic illness and prolonged hospitalization, they may experience despair and find it difficult to cope with this added burden. The nurse can help the family cope by involving them in the plan of care and encouraging them to take an active role in their infant's daily activities. Their involvement will help dispel feelings of inadequacy and prepare them to perform the unique tasks necessary to meet their infant's needs.

Parents need to demonstrate their ability to provide all the care their child will require at home before leaving the hospital. This may include feeding, adjusting O_2 support, O_2 saturation monitoring, suctioning and airway management, CPT, bathing, and giving medications. They also need to know when to call the home health nurse who is providing care. Parents should be taught how to assess the infant's respiratory condition and understand the BPD baseline respiratory pattern (frequency of respiration, rhythm, degree of retractions, and color of skin and mucous membranes). Illness limits the tolerance level for activity, and parents must be taught to evaluate their infant's tolerance of activities and to recognize signs of distress due to poor oxygenation, inadequate ventilation, infection, fluid retention, and bronchospasm. The nurse should give special attention to formulating a program of early stimulation activities because psychomotor delays are frequently seen.

Care of the Newborn with Cold Stress

Cold stress is excessive heat loss resulting in the use of compensatory mechanisms (such as increased respirations and nonshivering thermogenesis/use of brown fat stores) to maintain core body temperature close to 37.0°C/98.6°F (Baumgart, 2008). Heat loss that results in cold stress occurs in the newborn through the mechanisms of evaporation, convection, conduction, and radiation. (See chapter 29 for a detailed discussion of thermoregulation.) Heat loss at birth that leads to cold stress can play a significant role in the severity of respiratory distress syndrome (RDS) and the ultimate outcome for the infant. Both preterm and small-for-gestational-age (SGA) newborns are at increased risk for cold stress because they have decreased adipose tissue, brown fat stores, and glycogen available for metabolism.

As discussed in chapter 29, the newborn's major source of heat production in nonshivering thermogenesis (NST) is brown fat metabolism. The ability of an infant to respond to cold stress by NST is impaired in the presence of several conditions:

- Hypoxemia (PO_2 less than 50 torr)
- Intracranial hemorrhage or any central nervous system (CNS) abnormality
- Hypoglycemia (blood glucose less than 40 mg/dl)

When these conditions occur, the infant's temperature should be monitored more closely and the neutral thermal environment conscientiously maintained. The nurse must recognize these conditions and treat them as soon as possible. The metabolic consequences of cold stress can be devastating and potentially fatal to an infant. Oxygen requirements increase; even before noting a change in temperature, glucose use increases; acids are released into the bloodstream; and surfactant production decreases (Blackburn, 2007). The effects are graphically depicted in Figure 34-12 ■.

NURSING CARE MANAGEMENT

The amount of heat lost by an infant depends to a large extent on the actions of the nurse or caregiver. Following the transfer of a neonatal intensive care unit (NICU) newborn from one bed to another, a transient, although not significant, decrease in temperature for up to 1 hour may be noted. Prevention is especially critical in the very-low-birth-weight (VLBW) infant. Placing the VLBW newborn in a polyethylene wrapping immediately following birth can decrease the postnatal fall in temperature that normally occurs. Using head coverings made of insulated fabrics, wool, polyolefin, or those lined with Gamgee can significantly decrease heat loss after childbirth (Blackburn, 2007). Convective, radiant, and evaporative heat loss can all be reduced. Swaddling and nesting maintain flexion, which reduces exposed surface area and thus convective and radiant losses. Both convective and evaporative heat loss can be reduced.

The nurse observes the baby for signs of cold stress. These include increased movements and respirations, decreased skin temperature and peripheral perfusion, development of hypoglycemia, and, possibly, development of metabolic acidosis.

Vasoconstriction is the initial response to cold stress; because it initially decreases skin temperature, monitor and assess skin temperature instead of rectal temperature. A decrease in rectal temperature means that the infant has long-standing cold stress. By monitoring skin temperature, possible decrease will become apparent before the infant's core temperature is affected.

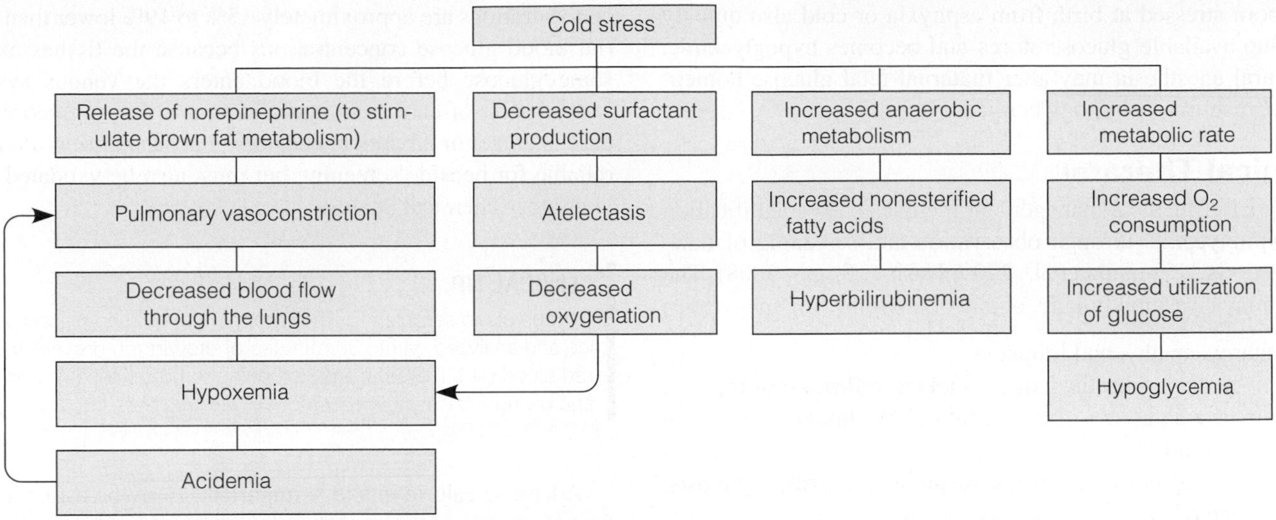

Figure 34-12 ■ Cold stress chain of events. The hypothermic, or cold-stressed, newborn attempts to compensate by conserving heat and increasing heat production. These physiologic compensatory mechanisms initiate a series of metabolic events that result in hypoxemia and altered surfactant production, metabolic acidosis, hypoglycemia, and hyperbilirubinemia.

If a decrease in skin temperature is noted, the nurse determines whether hypoglycemia is present. Hypoglycemia is a result of the metabolic effects of cold stress and is suggested by glucometer values below 40–50 mg/ml, tremors, irritability or lethargy, apnea, or seizure activity.

If hypothermia occurs, the following nursing interventions should be initiated (Gomella et al., 2009):

- Maintain a neutral thermal environment (NTE); adjust based on the gestational age and postnatal age.
- Warm the newborn slowly, because rapid temperature elevation may cause hypotension and apnea.
- Increase the air temperature in hourly increments of 1°C (33.8°F) until the infant's temperature is stable.
- Monitor skin temperature every 15 to 30 minutes to determine whether the newborn's temperature is increasing.
- Remove plastic wrap, caps, and heat shields while rewarming the infant so that cool air as well as warm air is not trapped.
- Warm IV fluids before infusion.
- Initiate efforts to block heat loss by evaporation, radiation, convection, and conduction. Maintain the newborn in NTE.

The nurse assesses the presence of anaerobic metabolism and initiates interventions for the resulting metabolic acidosis. Attempts to burn brown fat increase oxygen consumption, lactic acid levels, and metabolic acidosis. Hypoglycemia may be reversed by adequate glucose intake, as described in the following section.

Care of the Newborn with Hypoglycemia

Hypoglycemia, low blood sugar, can affect 3 to 29 out of 100 babies, both term and preterm (DePuy, Coassolo, Som, et al., 2009). An operational threshold for intervention in newborn hypoglycemia is a plasma glucose concentration of less than 40 mg/dl at any time in any newborn. It requires follow-up glucose measurement to document normal values (Cloherty et al., 2008). Within the first hours of life, normal asymptomatic newborns may have a transient glucose level in the 30s (mg/dl) that will increase either spontaneously or with feedings. Plasma glucose values less than 20 to 25 mg/dl should be treated with parenteral glucose $D_{10}W$, regardless of the age or gestation to raise plasma glucose to greater than 45 mg/dl. There is no absolute threshold that can be applied to all babies. Glucose concentrations must be looked at in conjunction with clinical manifestations.

Hypoglycemia is the most common metabolic disorder occurring in infants of diabetic mothers (IDM), small-for-gestational-age (SGA) infants, the smaller of twins, infants born to mothers with preeclampsia, male infants, and preterm average-for-gestational-age (AGA) infants. The pathophysiology of hypoglycemia differs for each classification (Gomella et al., 2009).

AGA preterm infants have not been in utero a sufficient time to store glycogen and fat. As a result, they have a decreased ability to carry out gluconeogenesis. This situation is further aggravated by increased use of glucose by the tissues (especially the brain and heart) during stress and illness (chilling, asphyxia, sepsis, and respiratory distress syndrome [RDS]).

Infants of White's classes A through C or type 1 diabetic mothers (women with diagnosed or gestational diabetes) have increased stores of glycogen and fat (see chapters 19 ∞ and 33 ∞). Circulating insulin and insulin responsiveness are also higher when compared with other newborns. Because the high glucose loads present in utero stop at birth, and the newborn continues to produce high levels of insulin from their pancreatic beta cells, the newborn experiences rapid and profound hypoglycemia (Gomella et al., 2009). Infants with recurrent episodes of hypoglycemia resulting from congenital hyperinsulinism showed that 50% have long-term neurologic deficits (Nash & Smith, 2008).

The SGA infant has used up glycogen and fat stores because of intrauterine malnutrition and has a blunted hepatic enzymatic response with which to produce and use glucose. Any newborn stressed at birth from asphyxia or cold also quickly uses up available glucose stores and becomes hypoglycemic. Epidural anesthesia may alter maternal-fetal glucose homeostasis, resulting in hypoglycemia.

Clinical Therapy

The goal of medical management includes early identification of hypoglycemia through observation and screening of newborns at risk (Gomella et al., 2009; Nash & Smith, 2008). The baby may be asymptomatic, or any of the following may occur:

- Lethargy, apathy, and limpness
- Poor feeding, poor/inadequate sucking reflex, vomiting
- Hypothermia in low-birth-weight (LBW) infants
- Pallor, cyanosis
- Apnea, irregular respirations, respiratory distress, cyanosis, tachypnea
- Hypotonia, possible loss of swallowing reflex
- Tremors, jerkiness, seizure activity, irritability, eye rolling
- High-pitched cry
- Exaggerated Moro reflex
- Temperature instability

Aggressive treatment is recommended after a single low blood glucose value if the infant shows any of these symptoms. In at-risk infants, routine screening should be done frequently during the first hours of life and then whenever any of the noted clinical manifestations appears or at 1- to 4-hour intervals until the risk period has passed.

Hypoglycemia may also be defined as a *glucose oxidase reagent strip with reflectance meter* below 40 mg/dl, but only when corroborated with laboratory blood glucose (see Procedure 34-1: Performing a Heel Stick on a Newborn). Common bedside methods use whole blood, an enzymatic reagent strip, and a reflectance meter or color chart. Bedside glucose oxidase strip tests can screen for hypoglycemia, but laboratory determinations *must confirm* the results before a diagnosis of hypoglycemia can be made. Glucose reagent strips should not be used by themselves to screen and diagnose hypoglycemia because their results depend on the baby's hematocrit (they react to the glucose in the plasma, not the red blood cells [RBCs]), and there is a wide variance (5 to 15 mg/dl) when compared with laboratory determinations.

CLINICAL TIP

There is no significant evidence to support the use of heel warmers preceding a capillary heelstick of an infant and no evidence of an increased yield of blood with the use of heel warmers (National Association of Neonatal Nurses' Guidelines) (Folk, 2007).

Blood glucose sampling techniques can significantly affect the accuracy of the blood glucose value. It is important to note that whole blood glucose concentrations are 10% to 15% lower than plasma glucose concentration (Cloherty et al., 2008). The higher the hematocrit, the greater the difference is between whole blood and plasma values. Also, venous blood glucose concentrations are approximately 15% to 19% lower than arterial blood glucose concentrations because the tissues extract some glucose before the blood enters the venous system. Newer point-of-care techniques, such as using a glucose oxidase analyzer or an optical bedside glucose analyzer, are more reliable for bedside screening but must also be validated with laboratory chemical analysis.

CLINICAL TIP

Venous blood samples for the laboratory should be placed on ice and analyzed within 30 minutes of drawing to prevent the red blood cells (RBCs) from continuing to metabolize glucose and giving a falsely low reading.

Adequate caloric intake is important. Early breastfeeding or formula-feeding is one of the major preventive approaches. If early feeding or intravenous (IV) glucose is started to meet the recommended fluid and caloric needs, the blood glucose is likely to remain above the hypoglycemic level. During the first hours after birth, asymptomatic newborns may be given oral glucose contained in formula or breast milk (glucose water should not be used because it causes a rapid increase in glucose followed by an abrupt decrease), and then another plasma glucose measurement is obtained within 30 to 60 minutes after feeding.

IV infusions of a dextrose solution D_5W to $D_{10}W$ (5% to 10%) begun immediately after birth should prevent hypoglycemia. Plasma glucose levels are obtained when the parenteral infusion is started. However, in the very small AGA infant, infusions of 10% dextrose solution may cause hyperglycemia to develop, requiring an alteration in the glucose concentration. An IV glucose solution should be calculated based on body weight of the infant and fluid requirements and correlated with blood glucose tests to determine adequacy of the infusion treatment.

In more severe cases of hypoglycemia, corticosteroids may be administered. It is thought that steroids enhance gluconeogenesis from noncarbohydrate protein sources (Gomella et al., 2009).

NURSING CARE MANAGEMENT

Nursing Assessment and Diagnosis

The objective of nursing assessment is to identify newborns at risk and to screen symptomatic infants. For newborns diagnosed with hypoglycemia, assessment is ongoing with careful monitoring of glucose values. Glucose strips, urine dipsticks, and urine volume (monitor only if above 1 to 3 ml/kg/hr) are evaluated frequently for osmotic diuresis and glycosuria.

Nursing diagnoses that may apply to the newborn with hypoglycemia include the following:

- ***Imbalanced Nutrition: Less Than Body Requirements*** related to increased glucose use secondary to physiologic stress
- ***Ineffective Breathing Pattern*** related to tachypnea and apnea
- ***Acute Pain*** related to frequent heel sticks for glucose monitoring

PROCEDURE 34-1 Performing a Heel Stick on a Newborn

NURSING ACTION

Preparation

- Explain to parents what will be done.
- Select a clear, previously unpunctured site.

  Rationale: The selection of a previously unpunctured site minimizes the risk of infection and excessive scar formation.
- The infant's lateral heel is the site of choice because it precludes damaging the posterior tibial nerve and artery, plantar artery, and the important longitudinally oriented fat pad of the heel, which in later years could impede walking (Figure 34-13 ■). This is especially important for infants undergoing multiple heel stick procedures. Toes are acceptable sites if necessary.

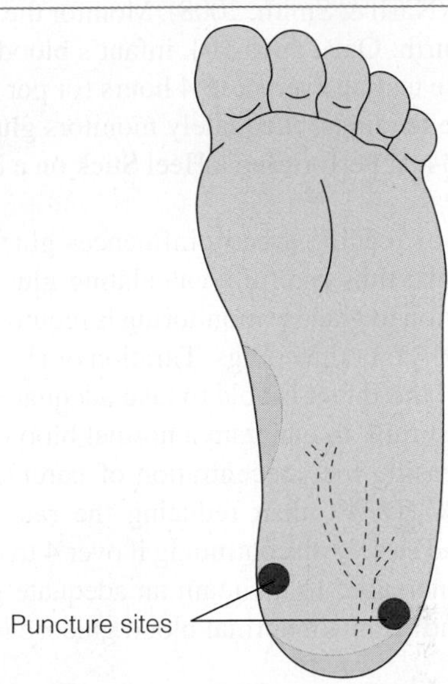

Figure 34-13 ■ Potential sites for heel sticks. Avoid shaded areas to prevent injury to arteries and nerves in the foot and the important longitudinally oriented fat pad of the heel, which in later years could impede walking.

Equipment and Supplies

Microlancet (do not use a needle)

Alcohol swabs

2 × 2 sterile gauze squares

Small bandage (may not use on premature infant with extremely sensitive skin, hold pressure until bleeding ceases)

Transfer pipette or capillary tubes

Glucose reagent strips or reflectance meters

Gloves

Procedure: Clean Gloves

1. Apply gloves.

   Rationale: A needle may nick the periosteum. Gloves are used to implement standard precautions and prevent nosocomial infections.
2. Warming the infant's heel for 5 to 10 seconds to facilitate blood flow is controversial. Check agency policy.

Performing the Heel Stick

1. Grasp the infant's lower leg and foot so as to impede venous return slightly. This will facilitate extraction of the blood sample (Figure 34-14 ■).
2. Clean the site by rubbing vigorously with 70% isopropyl alcohol swab.

   Rationale: Friction produces local heat, which aids vasodilation.
3. Blot the site dry completely with dry gauze square before lancing.

   Rationale: Alcohol is irritating to injured tissue and it may also produce hemolysis, as well as causing a false low reading.
4. With a quick, piercing motion, puncture the lateral heel with a microlancet. Be careful not to puncture too deeply. Optimal penetration is 4 mm.
5. Wipe the first drop of blood away with the gauze.

   Rationale: The first drop may be contaminated by skin contact and the blood cells may have been traumatized during the stick. Blood glucose may be lowered by residual alcohol.

Collecting the Blood Sample

1. Use transfer pipette to place drop of blood on glucose reflectance meter or directly onto the Glucometer test strip.
2. Use capillary tube for hematocrit testing.

Preventing Excessive Bleeding

1. Apply a folded gauze square to the puncture site and secure it firmly with a bandage, or hold pressure until bleeding stops.
2. Check the puncture site frequently for the first hour after sampling.

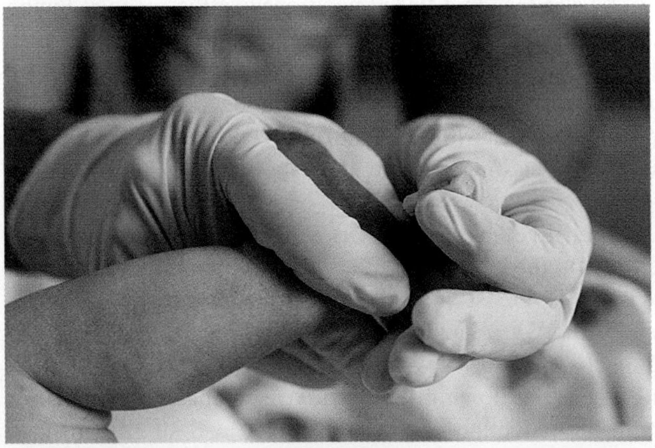

Figure 34-14 ■ Heel stick. With a quick, piercing motion, puncture the lateral heel with a microlancet. Be careful not to puncture too deeply.

Documentation Record the findings on the infant's chart.

Nursing Plan and Implementation

The nurse should monitor all at-risk groups within 30 to 60 minutes after birth and before feedings or whenever there are abnormal signs (Nash & Smith, 2008). Monitor the IDM within 30 minutes of birth. Once an at-risk infant's blood sugar level is stable, glucose testing every 2 to 4 hours (or per agency protocol), or before feedings, adequately monitors glucose levels. See Procedure 34-1: Performing a Heel Stick on a Newborn on page 961.

The method of feeding greatly influences glucose and energy requirements; thus carefully calculating glucose requirements and attention to glucose monitoring is required during the transition from IV to oral feedings. Titration of IV glucose may be required until the infant is able to take adequate amounts of formula or breast milk to maintain a normal blood sugar level. Titrate by decreasing the concentration of parenteral glucose gradually to 5% (D_5W), then reducing the rate of infusion (mg/kg/min), and slowly discontinuing it over 4 to 6 hours. Enteral feeds are increased to maintain an adequate glucose and caloric intake and maintain normal blood glucose levels.

Complementary and Alternative Therapies

The newborn relies on the nurse's observational, assessment, and interventional skills for prompt, safe, and effective pain relief. It is vital that the nurse assist infants to cope with and recover from necessary painful clinical procedures. A variety of nonpharmacologic pain-prevention and relief techniques have been shown to be effective in reducing pain from minor procedures in newborns.

Any unnecessary stimuli (i.e., noise, visual, tactile, and vestibular) of the newborn should be avoided, if possible. Developmental care, which includes limiting environmental stimuli, lateral positioning, the use of supportive bedding, and attention to behavioral cues, assists the newborn to cope with painful procedures (Gardner, Enzman-Hines, & Dickey, 2011).

Containment with swaddling or facilitated tucking (holding the arms and legs in a flexed position) is effective in reducing excessive immature motor responses. Swaddling also may provide comfort through other senses, such as thermal, tactile, and proprioceptive senses. Breastfeeding and skin-to-skin contact with the mother during the painful procedure may help to relieve pain (Weissman, Aranovitch, Blazer, et al., 2009; Gardner et al., 2011).

Nonnutritive sucking (NNS) refers to the provision of a pacifier into the infant's mouth to promote sucking without the provision of breast milk or formula for nutrition. NNS is thought to produce analgesia through stimulation of orotactile and mechanoreceptors when the pacifier is placed into the infant's mouth. Allowing nonnutritive sucking with a pacifier aids in the reduction of procedural pain and stress. Unfortunately a rebound in distress occurs when the NNS pacifier is removed from the infant's mouth (Gardner et al., 2011).

A wide range of oral sucrose doses has been used for procedural pain relief (heel sticks, venipuncture, IM injections), but no optimal dose has been established (Gardner et al., 2011). The sweetness of the sucrose, a disaccharide, elevates the pain threshold through endogenous opioid release in the CNS and produces a calming effect (Gardner et al., 2011). A range of 0.05 to 0.5 ml of 24% sucrose is administered on the anterior part of the tongue via a syringe or nipple approximately 2 minutes before the procedure (Dilli, Kucuk, & Dallar, 2009). Some authors have suggested that multiple doses, such as giving a dose 2 minutes before and 1 to 2 minutes after a procedure, is more effective. It is important to be careful with repeated doses of sucrose, as the concern for hyperglycemia, necrotizing enterocolitis (NEC), and fluid overload may arise. Oral sucrose should be limited to infants greater than 34 weeks gestational age (Gomella et al., 2009). Also, repeated use of sucrose analgesia in preterm infants may affect their neurologic development and behavioral outcomes. Until further research is done, repeated doses of sucrose are not recommended (Gardner et al., 2011). Because oral sucrose reduces but does not eliminate pain, it should be used with other nonpharmacologic measures to enhance effectiveness.

PROFESSIONALISM IN PRACTICE

Litigious Medicolegal Issues in the NICU

Stokowski (2008) cited that the two most litigious medicolegal issues in the neonatal intensive care unit (NICU) are cases involving neonatal resuscitation and hyperbilirubinemia. Neonatal nurses, as do all nurses, have the professional obligation to stay current with all the standards of care in their clinical setting. Cases that involve neonatal resuscitation found some of the following deficiencies:

1. Delay in initiation of resuscitation
2. Miscommunication
3. Equipment unavailable
4. Perception of ineptness
5. Poor documentation—**Need to Chart!**

Some of the deficient areas that were evaluated during cases involving neonatal patients with a diagnosis of jaundice were the following:

1. Not performing baseline bilirubin evaluations (transcutaneous or serum) prior to discharge
2. Charting that is incomplete about jaundice **(if it is not charted, it was not done)**
3. Improper recognition of high-risk conditions predisposing the neonate to jaundice
4. Not following up on clinical assessment of jaundice with serum bilirubin levels
5. Not obtaining a serum bilirubin level if any concerning clinical symptoms are present
6. Incomplete follow-up with any neonate with jaundice

Nurses are considered both independent professionals and institution employees and are increasingly named as individual defendants. In addition, allegations against NICU nurses frequently include, for example: failure to monitor, failure to notify the primary caregiver of clinical changes, treatment delays, not possessing proper competence or knowledge, proper procedure not followed, failure to obtain informed consent, and improper delegation.

The two best recommendations to help prevent legal issues in the NICU environment are:

1. Know the current standards of care/practice and **follow** them.
2. The primary evidence that can be provided is the patient's chart.

Evaluation

Expected outcomes of nursing care include the following:

- The newborn at risk of hypoglycemia is promptly identified, and intervention is started early.
- The newborn's glucose level is stabilized; recovery proceeds without sequelae.

Care of the Newborn with Jaundice

The most common abnormal physical finding in newborns is jaundice (*icterus neonatorum*). Some degree of newborn jaundice, resulting from elevated unconjugated bilirubinemia, occurs in approximately 60% of healthy newborns and 80% of preterm infants (Bhutani and Johnson, 2009; Bradshaw, 2010). **Jaundice** is a yellowish coloration of the skin and sclera of the eyes that develops from the deposit of yellow pigment bilirubin in lipid/fat-containing tissues, as described in chapter 29 ∞. Fetal unconjugated bilirubin is normally cleared by the placenta in utero, so total bilirubin at birth is usually less than 3 mg/L unless an abnormal hemolytic process has been present. Postnatally, the infant must conjugate bilirubin (convert a lipid-soluble pigment into a water-soluble pigment) in the liver.

The rate and amount of conjugation of bilirubin depend on the rate of hemolysis, the bilirubin load, the maturity of the liver, and the presence of albumin-binding sites. See chapter 29 ∞ for discussion of conjugation of bilirubin. A normal, healthy, full-term infant's liver is usually mature enough and produces enough glucuronyl transferase that the total serum bilirubin concentration does not reach a pathologic level. The diagnosis of pathologic jaundice is given to newborns who exhibit jaundice within the first 24 hours of life, have a total serum bilirubin concentration increase of greater than 0.2 mg/dl/hour, surpass the 95th percentile on the nomogram for age in hours, or have persistent visible jaundice after 1 week of age in term infants or after 2 weeks in preterm infants.

Physiologic Jaundice

Physiologic or neonatal jaundice is a normal process that occurs during transition from intrauterine to extrauterine life and appears *after 24 hours of life*. It is typically due to the newborn's increased red cell mass, shorter red cell lifespan (90 days as compared with 120 days in the adult), slower uptake of bilirubin by the liver, lack of intestinal bacteria, and/or poorly established hydration from initial breastfeeding (Gomella et al., 2009). Total bilirubin levels peak around 96 to 120 hours of age, usually after discharge from the hospital (Bhutani & Johnson 2009).

Lab tests reveal a predominance of unconjugated bilirubin. The average level of unconjugated bilirubin in cord blood is approximately 2 mg/dl at birth. This level rises to an average of 5 to 6 mg/dl between the third and fifth days of life. The jaundice is usually not visible after 14 days. The pattern of physiologic jaundice differs between breastfed and formula-fed newborns (for further discussion of physiologic jaundice, see "Physiologic Jaundice" in chapter 29 ∞). Physiologic jaundice remains a common problem for the term newborn and may require treatment with phototherapy.

Pathophysiology of Hyperbilirubinemia

Serum albumin-binding sites are usually able to conjugate enough bilirubin to meet the demands of the normal newborn. However, certain conditions tend to decrease the number or quality of available binding sites. Fetal or neonatal asphyxia and neonatal drugs such as indomethacin decrease the binding affinity of bilirubin to albumin, because acidosis impairs the capacity of albumin to hold bilirubin. Hypothermia and hypoglycemia release free fatty acids (FFAs) that dislocate bilirubin from albumin. Maternal use of sulfa drugs and salicylates interferes with conjugation or with serum albumin-binding sites by competing with bilirubin for these sites. Finally, premature infants have less albumin available for binding with bilirubin. Neurotoxicity is possible because unconjugated bilirubin has a high affinity for extravascular tissue, such as fatty tissue (subcutaneous tissue) and cerebral tissue.

Bilirubin not bound to albumin is free to cross the blood-brain barrier, damage cells of the central nervous system (CNS), and produce **kernicterus** or **acute bilirubin encephalopathy (ABE)** (Moerschel, Cianciaruso, & Tracy, 2008). *Kernicterus* (meaning "yellow nucleus") usually refers to the deposition of unconjugated bilirubin in the basal ganglia of the brain and to permanent neurologic sequelae of untreated **hyperbilirubinemia** (elevation of bilirubin level). The incidence is 0.9 to 1.5 per 100,000 live births (Burke et al., 2009; Manning, Todd, Maxwell, et al., 2007).

The classic bilirubin encephalopathy of kernicterus most commonly found with Rh and ABO blood group incompatibility is less common today because of aggressive treatment with phototherapy and exchange transfusions. Kernicterus cases are reappearing as a result of early discharge and the increased incidence of dehydration (a result of discharge before mother's milk is established when breastfeeding). Unfortunately, current therapy cannot distinguish all infants who are at risk. It is recommended that *all* newborns be screened for their bilirubin level prior to leaving the hospital either using total serum bilirubin (TSB) or transcutaneous bilirubin (TcB) (Maisels et al., 2009).

Causes of Hyperbilirubinemia

A primary cause of pathologic hyperbilirubinemia is **hemolytic disease of the newborn**. All pregnant women who are Rh negative or who have blood type O (possible ABO incompatibility) should be asked about outcomes of any previous pregnancies, including abortions, and history of blood transfusion. Prenatal amniocentesis with spectrophotographic examination may be indicated in some cases. Cord blood from newborns is evaluated for bilirubin level, which normally does not exceed 5 mg/dl. Newborns of Rh-negative and O blood type mothers are carefully assessed for blood type status, appearance of jaundice, and levels of serum bilirubin.

Alloimmune hemolytic disease, also known as **erythroblastosis fetalis**, occurs when an Rh-negative mother is pregnant with an Rh-positive fetus and maternal antibodies cross the placenta. Maternal antibodies enter the fetal circulation, then attach to and destroy the fetal red blood cells (RBCs). The fetal system responds by increasing RBC production. Jaundice, anemia, and compensatory erythropoiesis result. A marked increase in immature RBCs (erythroblasts) also occurs, hence the designation erythroblastosis fetalis. Because of the widespread use of Rh immune globulin (RhoGAM), the incidence of erythroblastosis fetalis has dropped dramatically.

Hydrops fetalis, the most severe form of erythroblastosis fetalis, occurs when maternal antibodies attach to the Rh site on the fetal RBCs, making them susceptible to destruction; severe anemia and multiple organ system failure result. Cardiomegaly with severe cardiac decompensation and hepatosplenomegaly occur. Severe generalized massive edema (anasarca) and generalized fluid effusion into the pleural cavity (hydrothorax), pericardial sac, and peritoneal cavity (ascites) develop. Jaundice is not present until the newborn period because the bilirubin pigments for the fetus are being excreted through the placenta into the maternal circulation. The hydropic hemolytic disease process is also characterized by hyperplasia of the adrenal cortex and pancreatic islets, which predisposes the infant to neonatal hypoglycemia similar to that of infants of diabetic mothers (IDMs). These infants also have increased bleeding tendencies due to associated thrombocytopenia and hypoxic damage to the capillaries. Hydrops is a frequent cause of intrauterine death among infants with Rh disease.

ABO incompatibility (the mother is blood type O and the baby is blood type A or B) may result in jaundice, although it rarely results in hemolytic disease severe enough to be clinically diagnosed and treated. Hepatosplenomegaly may be found occasionally in newborns with ABO incompatibility, but hydrops fetalis and stillbirth are rare.

During pregnancy, predisposing maternal conditions include hereditary spherocytosis, diabetes, intrauterine infections, gram-negative bacilli infections that stimulate production of maternal alloimmune antibodies, drug ingestion (such as sulfas, salicylates, novobiocin, and diazepam), and oxytocin administration. Early prenatal identification of the fetus at risk for Rh or ABO incompatibility allows prompt treatment. (See chapter 20 ∞ for discussion of in utero management of this condition.) Table 34-3 presents risk factors for development of severe hyperbilirubinemia.

DEVELOPING CULTURAL COMPETENCE
Ethnic Variations and Jaundice

Infants of East Asian descent (Japanese, Chinese, and Filipino ethnic groups) have a higher occurrence of hyperbilirubinemia than Caucasian infants. Infants with Asian fathers and Caucasian mothers have a higher incidence of jaundice than if both parents are Caucasian. Other ethnic groups at risk for increased bilirubinemia are Navajo, Eskimo, and Sioux Native American newborns; Greek newborns; Sephardic-Jewish newborns; and some Hispanic newborns.

The prognosis for a newborn with hyperbilirubinemia depends on the extent of the hemolytic process and the underlying cause. Severe hemolytic disease may result in fetal or early neonatal death from the effects of anemia—cardiac decompensation, edema, ascites, and hydrothorax. Hyperbilirubinemia may lead to kernicterus if not aggressively treated. The initial symptoms requiring acute intervention of an exchange transfusion are poor tone, lethargy, and/or feeding/sucking issues. Continuing worsening progression includes neurologic damage, which may cause death, cerebral palsy, cognitive impairment, or hearing loss, or, to a lesser degree, perceptual impairment, delayed speech development, hyperactivity, muscle incoordination, or learning difficulties (Okumura et al., 2009). Intravenous gamma globulin (IVIG) may be used with newborns suffering from isoimmune hemolytic disease, 0.5 to 1 gram per kg over 2 hours and repeat in 12 hours if required (Moerschel et al., 2008).

TABLE 34-3 Risk Factors for Development of Severe Hyperbilirubinemia in Infants of 35 or More Weeks' Gestation (in Approximate Order of Importance)

Major Risk Factors

- Predischarge total serum bilirubin (TSB) or transcutaneous bilirubin (TcB) level in the high-risk or high intermediate zone
- Jaundice observed in the first 24 h after birth
- Blood group incompatibility with positive direct antiglobulin test, other known hemolytic disease (e.g., glucose-6-phosphate dehydrogenase (G6PD) deficiency), elevated $ETCO_2$ (end-tidal carbon dioxide level)
- Gestational age 35–36 weeks (late preterm gestational age)
- Previous sibling received phototherapy
- Cephalhematoma/significant bruising
- Unrecognized hemolysis such as ABO blood type incompatibility or Rh incompatibility
- Infection
- Exclusive breastfeeding, particularly if nursing is not going well and excessive weight loss is experienced
- East Asian or Mediterranean descent*

Minor Risk Factors

- Predischarge TSB or TcB level in the high intermediate risk zone
- Gestational age 37–38 weeks
- Jaundice observed before discharge
- Previous sibling with jaundice
- Macrosomic infant of a diabetic mother
- Maternal age greater than or equal to 25 years
- Male gender

Decreased Risk (these factors are associated with decreased risk of significant jaundice, listed in order of decreasing importance)

- TSB or TcB level in the low-risk zone
- Gestational age greater than or equal to 41 weeks
- Exclusive bottle-feeding
- Black race*
- Discharge from hospital after 72 h

*Descent and race as defined by mother's description.

Source: From American Academy of Pediatrics Subcommittee on Hyperbilirubinemia. (2004). Management of hyperbilirubinemia in the newborn infant 35 or more weeks of gestation. Pediatrics, *114(1), 297–316 (Table 2, p. 301); Maisels, M. J., Bhutani, V. K., Bogen, D., Newman, T. B., Stark, A. R., & Watchko, J. F. (2009). Hyperbilirubinemia in the newborn infant ≥ 35 weeks' gestation: An update with clarifications,* Pediatrics, *124(4), 1193–1198.*

Clinical Therapy

The best treatment for hemolytic disease is prevention. Prenatal identification of the fetus at risk for Rh or ABO incompatibility will allow prompt treatment. See chapter 20 ∞ for discussion of in utero management of this condition.

Laboratory and Diagnostic Assessments

When one or more of the predisposing factors are present, or the appearance of early jaundice, the maternal and neonatal blood types should be tested in the laboratory for Rh or ABO incompatibility (Watchko, 2009). Other necessary laboratory evaluations include Coombs' test, serum bilirubin levels (direct and total), hemoglobin, reticulocyte percentage, white blood cell count, and positive smear for cellular morphology (Table 34-4).

Neonatal hyperbilirubinemia must be considered pathologic if any of the following criteria are met (Bhutani, Johnson, & Keren, 2004; Gomella et al., 2009):

1. Clinically evident jaundice appearing before 24 hours of life or if jaundice seems excessive for the newborn's age in hours
2. Serum bilirubin concentration rising by more than 0.2 mg/dl per hour
3. Total serum bilirubin concentrations exceeding the 95th percentile on the nomogram
4. Conjugated bilirubin concentrations greater than 2 mg/dl or more than 20% of the total serum bilirubin concentration
5. Clinical jaundice persisting for more than 2 weeks in a term newborn

Initial diagnostic procedures are aimed at differentiating jaundice resulting from increased bilirubin production, impaired conjugation or excretion, increased intestinal reabsorption, or a combination of these factors.

Transcutaneous bilirubin (TcB) measurements are a noninvasive method of assessing bilirubin levels and may be used for predischarge risk assessment. A TcB can be performed quickly and painlessly, and repeated measures are easily obtained. TcB can quantify the amount of bilirubin pigment in the infant's skin. Nurses need to measure bilirubin levels to confirm the presence, absence, or suspicion of jaundice. However, it is important to remember that total serum bilirubin levels remain the standard of care for confirmation or diagnosis of hyperbilirubinemia (Gomella et al., 2009).

CLINICAL TIP

Because of exposure to sunlight, sternal transcutaneous bilirubin (TcB) measurements may be more accurate than those taken on the forehead. The sternum, in a dressed infant, is less likely to be affected by the influence of ambient light (such as sunlight) on the skin.

Because of the shorter lifespan of RBCs in the newborn, a significant bilirubin load is produced. When bilirubin breaks down, carbon monoxide (CO) is released. This production of carbon monoxide is being investigated as a marker in the study of bilirubin production. Measuring end-tidal CO (ETCO) has been shown to provide results similar to laboratory measures of bilirubin; however, devices to measure CO are not widely available (Gomella et al., 2009).

TABLE 34-4 Laboratory Evaluation of the Jaundiced Infant of 35 or More Weeks' Gestation

INDICATIONS	ASSESSMENTS
Jaundice in first 24 h	Measure transcutaneous bilirubin (TcB) and/or total serum bilirubin (TSB).
Jaundice appears excessive for infant's age	Measure TcB and/or TSB.
Infant receiving phototherapy or TSB rising rapidly (i.e., crossing percentiles on the nomogram and unexplained by history and physical examination)	Blood type and Coombs' test, if not obtained with cord blood. Complete blood count and smear. Measure direct or conjugated bilirubin. It is an option to perform reticulocyte count, glucose-6-phosphate dehydrogenase (G6PD), and end-tidal carbon dioxide ($ETCO_2$), if available. Repeat TSB in 4–24 h depending on infant's age and TSB level.
TSB concentration approaching exchange levels or not responding to phototherapy	Perform reticulocyte count, G6PD albumin, $ETCO_2$, if available.
Elevated direct (or conjugated) bilirubin level	Do urinalysis and urine culture. Evaluate for sepsis if indicated by history and physical examination.
Jaundice present at or beyond age 3 weeks, or sick infant	Total and direct (or conjugated) bilirubin level. If direct bilirubin elevated, evaluate for causes of cholestasis. Check results of newborn thyroid and galactosemia screen, and evaluate infant for signs or symptoms of hypothyroidism.

Source: From American Academy of Pediatrics Subcommittee on Hyperbilirubinemia. (2004). Management of hyperbilirubinemia in the newborn infant 35 or more weeks of gestation. Pediatrics, 114*(1), 297–316 (Table 1, p. 300).*

Essential laboratory evaluations are Coombs' test, serum bilirubin levels (direct and total), hemoglobin, reticulocyte percentage, white cell count, and positive smear for cellular morphology. The Coombs' test determines whether jaundice is due to Rh or ABO incompatibility. The indirect Coombs' test measures the amount of Rh-positive antibodies in the mother's blood. Rh-positive RBCs are added to the maternal blood sample. If the mother's serum contains antibodies, the Rh-positive RBCs will agglutinate (clump) when rabbit immune antiglobulin is added, which is a positive test result. The direct Coombs' test reveals the presence of antibody-coated (sensitized) Rh-positive RBCs in the newborn. Rabbit immune antiglobulin is added to the specimen of neonatal blood cells. If the neonatal RBCs agglutinate, they have been coated with maternal antibodies, a positive result.

If the hemolytic process is due to Rh sensitization, laboratory findings reveal the following: (1) an Rh-positive newborn with a positive Coombs' test; (2) increased erythropoiesis with many immature circulating RBCs (nucleated blastocysts); (3) anemia, in most cases; (4) elevated levels (5 mg/dl or more)

Infant Receiving Phototherapy

of bilirubin in cord blood; and (5) a reduction in albumin binding capacity. Maternal data may include an elevated anti-Rh titer and spectrophotometric evidence of fetal hemolytic process.

If the hemolytic process is due to ABO incompatibility, laboratory findings reveal an increase in reticulocytes. The resulting anemia is usually not significant during the newborn period and is rare later on. The direct Coombs' test may be negative or mildly positive, whereas the indirect Coombs' test may be strongly positive. Infants with a positive direct Coombs' test have increased incidence of jaundice with bilirubin levels in excess of 10 mg/dl. Increased numbers of spherocytes (spherical, plump, mature erythrocytes) are seen on a peripheral blood smear. Increased numbers of spherocytes are not seen on blood smears from Rh disease infants.

Clinical Therapy

Whatever the cause of hyperbilirubinemia, management of these infants is directed toward alleviating anemia, removing maternal antibodies and sensitized erythrocytes, increasing serum albumin levels, reducing serum bilirubin levels, and minimizing the consequences of hyperbilirubinemia. Early discharge of newborns from birthing centers has significantly influenced the diagnosis and management of neonatal jaundice, increasing the emphasis on outpatient and home care management.

Hemolytic disease may be treated with phototherapy, exchange transfusion, and drug therapy. When determining the appropriate management of hyperbilirubinemia due to hemolytic disease, the three variables that must be taken into account are the newborn's (1) serum bilirubin level, (2) birth weight, and (3) age in hours. If a newborn has hemolysis with an unconjugated bilirubin level of 14 mg/dl, weighs less than 2500 g (birth weight), and is 24 hours old or less, an exchange transfusion may be the best management. However, if that same newborn is over 24 hours old, which is past the time where an increase in bilirubin would result from pathologic causes, phototherapy may be the treatment of choice to prevent the possible complications of kernicterus.

Phototherapy

Phototherapy is the exposure of the newborn to high-intensity light. It may be used alone or in conjunction with exchange transfusion to reduce serum bilirubin levels. Exposure of the newborn to high-intensity light (a bank of fluorescent light bulbs or bulbs in the blue-light spectrum) decreases serum bilirubin levels in the skin by facilitating biliary excretion of unconjugated bilirubin. Phototherapy decreases serum bilirubin levels by changing bilirubin from the non–water-soluble (lipophilic) form to water-soluble by-products that can then be excreted via urine and bile. Photoisomerization occurs when the natural form of bilirubin is exposed to light at a certain wavelength and the bilirubin is converted to a less toxic form. The new isomer, photobilirubin, is created rapidly but is quite unstable. The photobilirubin is bound to albumin, transported to the liver, and incorporated into bile. If it is not quickly eliminated from the bowel, it can convert back to its original form and return to the bloodstream. In addition, the photodegradation products formed when light oxidizes bilirubin can be excreted in the urine.

Case Study: Newborn with Jaundice

Phototherapy is an intervention that is used more for the prevention of hyperbilirubinemia to halt bilirubin levels from climbing dangerously high. The decision to start phototherapy is based on two factors: gestational age and age in hours. Phototherapy is the most effective in the first 24 to 48 hours of usage; frequently the light can be discontinued during or immediately after this time frame. Phototherapy does not alter the underlying cause of jaundice, and hemolysis may continue to produce anemia. Many researchers have recommended initiating phototherapy "prophylactically" in the first 24 hours of life in high-risk, very-low-birth-weight (VLBW), or severely bruised infants. Figure 34-15A ■ shows guidelines for the use of phototherapy. The risk of neonates requiring follow-up/intervention for their hyperbilirubinemia is evaluated by plotting their serum bilirubin level and age in hours on the chart shown in Figure 34-15B ■.

Phototherapy can be provided through halogen spotlights (although these are not widely used because of the risk of thermal burns), conventional banks of phototherapy lights, a fiberoptic blanket attached to a halogen light source around the trunk of the newborn, or a combination of these delivery methods. The bank of bilirubin lights utilize light in the blue spectrum. This is the most effective source available but can mask cyanosis and causes dizziness and nausea in the staff.

With the fiberoptic blanket, the light stays on at all times, and the newborn is accessible for care, feeding, and diaper changes; greater surface area is exposed and there are no thermoregulation issues. The eyes are not covered. Fluid and weight loss are not complications of this system. Furthermore, it makes the infant accessible to the parents and is less alarming to parents than standard phototherapy. Many institutions and pediatricians use fiberoptic blankets for home care. A combination of a fiberoptic light source in the mattress under the baby and a standard light source above may also be used. This is termed *intensive phototherapy.* Intensive phototherapy should reduce the total serum bilirubin (TSB) by 1 to 2 mg/dl within 4 to 8 hours. Levels should continue to decline when phototherapy covers a wider surface area. If a drop in bilirubin levels is not reached then an exchange transfusion should be considered. The nurse uses a photometer to measure and maintain desired irradiance levels. The nurse keeps track of the number of hours each lamp is used so that each can be replaced before its effectiveness is lost (Bradshaw, 2010). Neurotoxicity risk factors such as late prematurity, galactosemia, congenital spherocytosis, asphyxia, sepsis, acidosis, dehydration, albumin <3 mg/dl, G6PD deficiency, Crigler-Najjar syndrome, or isoimmune hemolytic disease are used in making decisions to initiate phototherapy or exchange transfusion (Maisels et al., 2009).

Exchange Transfusion

Exchange transfusion is the withdrawal and replacement of the newborn's blood with donor blood. It is used to treat anemia with RBCs that are not susceptible to maternal antibodies, remove sensitized RBCs that would be lysed soon, remove serum bilirubin, and provide bilirubin-free albumin and increase the binding sites for bilirubin. Concerns over doing an exchange transfusion are related to the use of blood products and associated potential for HIV infection and hepatitis. If the TSB is at or approaching the exchange level, the nurse should send blood

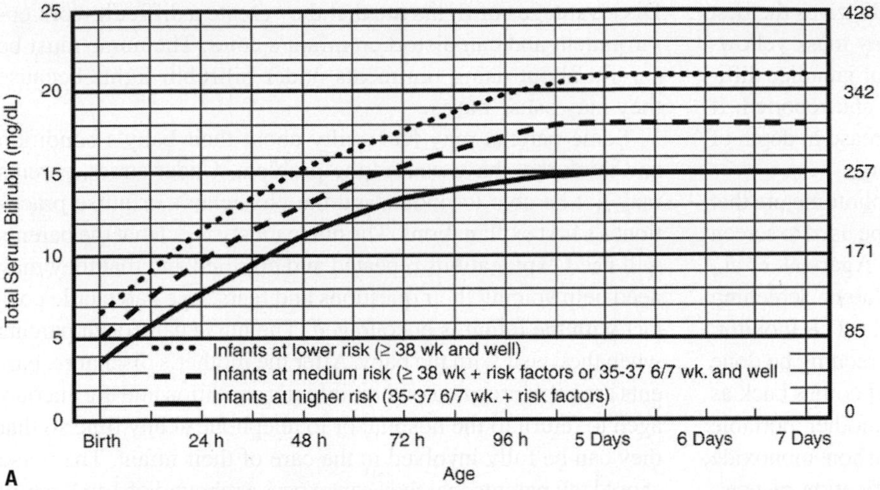

A

- Use total bilirubin. Do not subtract direct reacting or conjugated bilirubin.
- Risk factors = isoimmune hemolytic disease, G6PD deficiency, asphyxia, significant lethargy, temperature instability, sepsis, acidosis, or albumin < 3.0g/dL (if measured)
- For well infants 35–37 6/7 wk can adjust TSB levels for intervention around the medium risk line. It is an option to intervene at lower TSB levels for infants closer to 35 wks and at higher TSB levels for those closer to 37 6/7 wk.
- It is an option to provide conventional phototherapy in hospital or at home at TSB levels 2–3 mg/dL (35–50mmol/L) below those shown but home phototherapy should not be used in any infant with risk factors.

Note: These guidelines are based on limited evidence and the levels shown are approximations. The guidelines refer to the use of intensive phototherapy, which should be used when the TSB (total serum bilirubin) exceeds the line indicated for each category. Infants are designated as "higher risk" because of the potential negative effects of the conditions listed on albumin binding of bilirubin, the blood-brain barrier, and the susceptibility of the brain cells to damage by bilirubin.

Source: American Academy of Pediatrics Subcommittee on Hyperbilirubinemia. (2004). Management of hyperbilirubinemia in the newborn infant 35 or more weeks of gestation. Pediatrics, *114(1), 297–316 (Fig. 3, p. 304).*

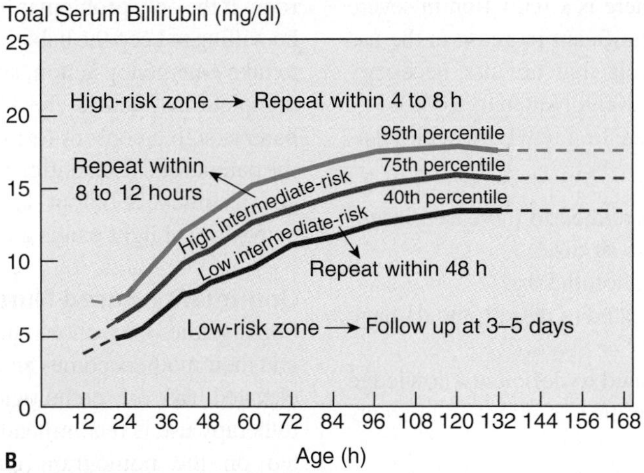

B

Source: Reprinted by permission from Macmillan Publishers Ltd: Journal of Perinatology, *Bhutani, V. K. & Johnson, L. (2009). A proposal to prevent severe neonatal hyperbilirubinemia and kernicterus. 29(Suppl. 1), s61–s67. pg. s64 fig. 3. Copyright © 2009.*

Figure 34-15 ■ A. Guidelines for phototherapy in hospitalized infants of 35 or more weeks' gestation. B. When to follow up a predischarge bilirubin level on an hour-specific bilirubin nomogram.

for immediate type and cross-match. Blood for exchange transfusion is modified whole blood (red cells and plasma) cross-matched against the mother and compatible with the infant.

NURSING CARE MANAGEMENT

Nursing Assessment and Diagnosis

Assessment is aimed at identifying prenatal and perinatal factors that predispose to development of jaundice and identifying jaundice as soon as it is apparent. Significant hyperbilirubinemia in the neonatal population is often due to a multitude of causes including a genetic basis (Watchko et al., 2009). Clinically, ABO incompatibility presents as jaundice and occasionally as hepatosplenomegaly. Fetal hydrops or erythroblastosis fetalis is rare (see chapter 20 ∞). Hemolytic disease of the newborn is suspected if the placenta is enlarged, if the newborn is edematous with pleural and pericardial effusion plus ascites, if pallor or jaundice is noted during the first 24 to 36 hours, if hemolytic anemia is diagnosed, or if the spleen and liver are enlarged. The nurse carefully notes changes in behavior and observes for evidence of bleeding. If laboratory tests indicate elevated bilirubin levels, the nurse checks the newborn for jaundice about every 2 hours and records observations.

To check for jaundice in lighter skinned babies, the nurse should blanch the skin over a bony prominence (forehead, nose, or sternum) by pressing firmly with the thumb. After pressure is released, if jaundice is present, the area appears yellow before normal color returns. The nurse should check oral mucosa and the posterior portion of the hard palate and conjunctival sacs for yellow pigmentation in darker skinned babies. Jaundice progresses in a cephalocaudal direction from the face to the trunk and then to the lower extremities. The overall progression of jaundice should be noted. Assessment in daylight gives the best results, because pink walls and surroundings may mask yellowish tints and yellow light makes differentiation of jaundice difficult. The time at onset of jaundice is recorded and reported. If jaundice appears, careful observation of the increase in depth of color and of the newborn's behavior is mandatory.

In addition to visual inspection, reflectance photometers that measure transcutaneous bilirubin (TcB) should be used to screen and monitor neonatal jaundice (Dalal, Mishra, Agarwal, et al., 2009). Most hospitals have developed a mandatory screening policy for all newborns before discharge using the TcB monitor, and it is recommended that this predischarge screening be done universally (Varvarigou et al., 2009). If the level comes back as high, a follow-up TSB will be performed. Another portable screening tool is the analysis for end-tidal carbon monoxide (ETCO). This analysis allows for rapid identification of newborns with significant hemolytic disease who may be at risk for the sequelae of unconjugated hyperbilirubinemia. Measurements in newborns using the TcB devices are within 2 to 3 mg/dl of the TSB and useful for TSB levels less than 15 mg/dl. When universal screening is performed, there is a reduction in severe hyperbilirubinemia but there is a significant increase in the use of phototherapy, sometimes at levels that are not necessary (Kuzniewicz, Escobar, & Newman, 2009; Newman, 2009).

Nursing diagnoses that may apply to a newborn with jaundice include the following:

- ***Risk for Deficient Fluid Volume*** related to increased insensible water loss and frequent loose stools
- ***Risk for Injury*** related to use of phototherapy
- ***Disturbed Sensory Perception*** related to neurologic damage secondary to kernicterus
- ***Risk for Impaired Parenting*** related to deficient knowledge of infant care and prolonged separation of infant and parents secondary to illness

Nursing Plan and Implementation

Hospital-Based Nursing Care

Hospital-based care is described in Nursing Care Plan: For the Newborn with Hyperbilirubinemia on pages 969–971. Phototherapy success is measured every 12 hours or daily by serum bilirubin levels (more frequently if there is hemolysis or a higher level before initiation of phototherapy). The nurse must turn off the lights while drawing blood for serum bilirubin levels. Because it is not known whether phototherapy injures the delicate eye structures, particularly the retina, the nurse applies eye patches over the newborn's closed eyes during exposure to banks of phototherapy lights (see Figure 34-16 ■ in Procedure 34-2: Infant Receiving Phototherapy on page 971). Conventional phototherapy is discontinued and the eye patches are removed at least once per shift to assess the eyes for the presence of conjunctivitis. Patches are also removed to allow eye contact during feeding (for social stimulation) or when parents are visiting (to promote parental attachment).

Most phototherapy units will provide this level of irradiance 45 to 50 cm below the lamps. The nurse can use a photometer to measure and maintain desired irradiance levels. Disadvantages of lights are that they create a difficult work environment and can distort an infant's color. The nurse must be careful about using ointments under bilirubin lights because they may cause burns.

Some parents may feel guilty about their baby's condition and think they have caused the problem. Under stress, parents may not be able to understand the physician's or nurse practitioner's first explanations. The nurse must expect that the parents will need explanations repeated and clarified and that they may need help voicing their questions and fears. Eye and tactile contact with the infant is encouraged. The nurse can coach parents when they visit with the baby. After the mother's discharge, parents are kept informed of their infant's condition and are encouraged to return to the hospital or to telephone at any time so that they can be fully involved in the care of their infant. The nurse should tell parents that they can expect a rebound of 1 to 2 mg/dl after discontinuation of phototherapy and that a follow-up bilirubin test may be done (Cloherty et al., 2008; Bradshaw, 2010).

While the mother is still hospitalized, some healthcare facilities may allow phototherapy to be carried out in the mother's room if the only problem is hyperbilirubinemia. The mother must be willing to keep the baby in the room for 24 hours a day; be able to take emergency action, such as for choking, if necessary; and complete instruction checklists. Some institutions require that parents sign a consent form. The nurse gives the instructions to the parents but also continues to monitor the infant's temperature, activity, intake & output (I&O), and positioning of eye patches (if conventional light banks are used) at regular intervals.

Community-Based Nursing Care

Some studies have shown that with early discharge of newborns and their mothers comes an increase in hospital readmission and elevated risk of pathologic hyperbilirubinemia. Home phototherapy use is recommended only if the bilirubin level is plotted on the nomogram and found to be in the "optional phototherapy" range. Any newborn with a level in the higher range should be hospitalized for continual phototherapy and serum bilirubin levels closely monitored on a regular schedule.

Jaundice and its phototherapy treatment can be very disturbing to parents and may generate feelings of guilt and fear. The parents' perception of and/or misconceptions about jaundice can affect parent-infant interactions. The nurse should explain the causes of jaundice and emphasize that it is usually a transient problem and one to which all infants must adapt after birth. Reassurance and support are vital especially for the breastfeeding mother, who may question her ability to adequately nourish her newborn.

It is essential that the impact of cultural beliefs be considered. Some Latina women believe that showing strong maternal emotions during pregnancy and breastfeeding can be detrimental. *Bilis* associated with anger may be blamed by some Latina women for jaundice. Cultural beliefs lead mothers to interpret illness within their cultural framework, especially when left without clear and understood explanations. Maternal reactions can be lessened by careful explanations to the mothers about the diagnosis, prognosis, duration, and management options for jaundice and about the possibility of its recurrence.

NURSING CARE PLAN For the Newborn with Hyperbilirubinemia

INTERVENTION	RATIONALE
1. Nursing Diagnosis: Impaired Tissue Integrity related to predisposing factors associated with hyperbilirubinemia **Goal:** Babies at risk for jaundice and early signs of jaundice will be identified.	
■ Evaluate baby's history for predisposing factors for hyperbilirubinemia.	■ Early identification of risk factors enables the nurse to monitor babies for early signs of hyperbilirubinemia. Acidosis, hypoxia, and hypothermia increase the risk of hyperbilirubinemia at lower bilirubin levels.
■ Observe color of amniotic fluid at time of rupture of membranes.	■ Amber-colored amniotic fluid indicates hyperbilirubinemia.
■ Assess baby for developing jaundice in daylight if possible.	■ Early detection is affected by nursery environment. Artificial lights (with pink tint) may mask beginning of jaundice.
1. Observe sclera.	1. Most visible sign of hyperbilirubinemia is jaundice noted in skin, sclera, or oral mucosa. Onset is first seen on face and then progresses down the trunk.
2. Observe skin color and assess by blanching.	2. Blanching the skin leaves a yellow color to the skin immediately after pressure is released.
3. Check oral mucosa, posterior portion of hard palate, and conjunctival sacs for yellow pigmentation in dark-skinned newborns.	3. Underlying pigment of dark-skinned infants may normally appear yellow.
■ Report jaundice occurring within 24 hours of birth.	
EXPECTED OUTCOMES: Baby's jaundice is identified early.	
2. Nursing Diagnosis: Risk for Deficient Fluid Volume related to phototherapy **Goal:** The infant will not exhibit signs of dehydration and will display appropriate weight gain.	
■ Offer feedings every 2 to 3 hr.	■ Adequate hydration increases peristalsis and excretion of bilirubin.
■ Breastfeed on demand with no supplementation unless excessive weight loss or increasing total serum bilirubin (TSB) with adequate feeding.	
■ Provide 25% extra fluid intake.	■ Replace fluid losses due to watery stools, if under phototherapy.
■ Assess for dehydration: 1. Poor skin turgor 2. Depressed fontanelles 3. Sunken eyes 4. Decreased urine output 5. Weight loss 6. Changes in electrolytes	■ Phototherapy treatment may cause liquid stools and increased insensible water loss, which increases risk of dehydration.
■ Monitor intake and output (I&O).	
■ Weigh daily.	
■ Report signs of dehydration.	
■ Administer IV fluids:	
1. Monitor flow rates.	■ Prevents fluid overload.
2. Assess insertion sites for signs of infection.	■ IV fluids may be used if baby is dehydrated or in presence of other complications. IV may be started if exchange transfusion is to be done.
EXPECTED OUTCOMES: Baby will have good skin turgor, clear amber urine output of 1–3 ml/kg/hr, six to eight wet diapers/day, and will maintain weight.	
3. Nursing Diagnosis: Risk for Injury related to use of phototherapy **Goal:** Baby will not have any corneal irritation/drainage, skin breakdown, or major fluctuations in temperature.	
■ Cover baby's eyes with eye patches while under phototherapy lights. Cover testes/penis in male infants.	■ Protects retina from damage due to high intensity light and testes from damage from heat.
■ Make certain that eyelids are closed before applying eye patches.	■ Prevents corneal abrasions.
■ Remove baby from under phototherapy and remove eye patches during feedings.	■ Provides visual stimulation and facilitates attachment behaviors.

(continued)

NURSING CARE PLAN For the Newborn with Hyperbilirubinemia continued

INTERVENTION	RATIONALE
■ Inspect eyes each shift for conjunctivitis, drainage, and corneal abrasions due to irritation from eye patches.	■ Prevents or facilitates prompt treatment of purulent conjunctivitis.
■ Administer thorough perianal cleansing with each stool or change of perianal protective covering.	■ Frequent stooling increases risk of skin breakdown. Prevents infection.
■ Provide minimal coverage—only of diaper area.	■ Provides maximal exposure. Shielded areas become more jaundiced, so maximum exposure is essential.
■ Avoid the use of oily applications on the skin.	■ Prevents superficial burns to skin.
■ Reposition baby every 2 hours.	■ Provides equal exposure of all skin areas and prevents pressure areas.
■ Observe for bronzing of skin.	■ Bronzing is related to use of phototherapy with increased direct bilirubin levels or liver damage; may last for 2 to 4 months.
■ Place Plexiglas shield between baby and light.	■ Hypothermia and hyperthermia are common complications of phototherapy.
■ Monitor baby's skin and core temperature frequently until temperature is stable.	■ Hypothermia results from exposure to lights, subsequent radiation, and convection losses.
■ Check axillary temperature with readings on servo-controlled unit on incubator.	■ Hyperthermia may result from the increased environmental heat.
■ Regulate incubator temperature as needed.	■ Additional heat from phototherapy lights frequently causes a rise in the baby's and incubator's temperatures. ■ Fluctuations in temperature may occur in response to radiation and convection.

EXPECTED OUTCOMES: Baby's eyes are protected, skin is intact, and baby maintains a stable temperature.

4. Nursing Diagnosis: Risk for Impaired Parenting related to deficient knowledge of infant care and prolonged separation of infant and parents secondary to illness

Goals: Parents will bond with infant and have realistic expectations about their infant. Parents are comfortable taking their infant home. They are able to demonstrate normal infant care and assessments of possible complications, and they know when to return for follow-up.

INTERVENTION	RATIONALE
■ Encourage parents to provide tactile stimulation during feeding and diaper changes.	■ Newborn has normal needs for tactile stimulation. ■ Presence of equipment may discourage parents from interacting with newborn.
■ Encourage cuddling and eye contact during feedings.	■ Provides opportunity for parents to bond with their newborn.
■ Offer suggestions to comfort restless infant: ■ Nesting when beneath bili lights ■ Talking softly and singing quietly to infant ■ Taped music or tape recording of evening activities from home ■ Rhythmic patting of buttocks ■ Firm, nonstroking touch, assisting with control of extremities ■ Pacifier for nonnutritive sucking	■ Provides comfort and decreases sensory deprivation.
■ Encourage family/friend support of mother/parents (i.e., meals, rest, child care for siblings, allow expressions of concerns/feelings).	■ Decreases strain on mother/parents by assisting with other responsibilities and allows for additional time with newborn for bonding, care, etc.
■ Evaluate additional psychosocial needs.	■ Parents may not understand what is happening or why.
■ Discuss rationale for treatment and possible side effects of phototherapy with family (stool changes, increased fluid loss, possible temp instability, slight lethargy, rash, altered sleep-wake patterns).	■ Physician preference of treatment modalities may vary. Parents may not understand why their newborn is not receiving a treatment that another with the same condition is receiving.
■ Instruct family on infant's care while undergoing phototherapy: ■ Safety precautions—bili mask (to protect eyes), incubator door closed and latched, covering genitalia per policy. ■ Skin care, cord care, circumcision care as appropriate. ■ Lab draws, rationale I&O.	

NURSING CARE PLAN For the Newborn with Hyperbilirubinemia continued

INTERVENTION	RATIONALE
■ Encourage parent/significant other/sibling involvement in infant care as possible. ■ Give explanation of equipment being used and changes in bilirubin levels. Allow parents an opportunity to ask questions; reinforce or clarify information as needed. ■ Evaluate family's understanding of information.	
■ As necessary, review role of pumping breasts and offering formula for limited time.	■ The etiology of breast milk jaundice remains uncertain. The serum bilirubin levels begin to fall within 48 hr after discontinuation of breastfeeding. Opinion of physicians varies regarding the need for discontinuing breastfeeding.
■ Assist mother to pump her breasts to maintain milk supply.	■ If breastfeeding is temporarily discontinued, assess mother's knowledge of pumping her breasts in regular increments (q 2–3 hours), and provide information and support as needed.

EXPECTED OUTCOMES: The parent will demonstrate ability to perform basic infant care tasks as evidenced by exhibiting appropriate attachment behaviors (i.e., talking and holding infant, feeding infant, and caring for infant under home bili therapy).

Parents verbalize understanding of rationale and possible side effects from phototherapy; parents/family demonstrate safety precautions when caring for infant; parents getting meals, rest, and verbalize support given.

PROCEDURE 34-2 Infant Receiving Phototherapy

NURSING ACTION

Preparation

- Explain the purpose of phototherapy, the procedure itself (including the need to use eye patches), and possible side effects such as dehydration and skin breakdown from more frequent stooling.
- Note evidence of jaundice in the skin, sclera, and mucous membranes (in infants with darkly pigmented skin). Be sure that recent serum bilirubin levels are available.

  Rationale: *The decision to use phototherapy is based on a careful assessment of the newborn's condition over a period of time. The most recent results before starting therapy serve as a baseline to evaluate the effectiveness of therapy.*

Equipment and Supplies

Bank of phototherapy lights

Eye patches

Small scale to weigh diapers

Procedure

1. Obtain vital signs including axillary temperature.

   Rationale: *Provides baseline data.*

2. Remove all of the infant's clothing except the diaper.

   Rationale: *Exposure of the newborn to high-intensity light (a bank of fluorescent light bulbs or bulbs in the blue-white spectrum) decreases serum bilirubin levels in the skin by aiding biliary excretion of unconjugated bilirubin. Because the tissue absorbs the light, best results are obtained when there is maximum skin surface exposure.*

3. Apply eye coverings (eye patches or a bili mask) to the infant according to agency policy. (See Figure 34-16.)

   Rationale: *Eye coverings are used because it is not known if phototherapy injures delicate eye structures, particularly the retina.*

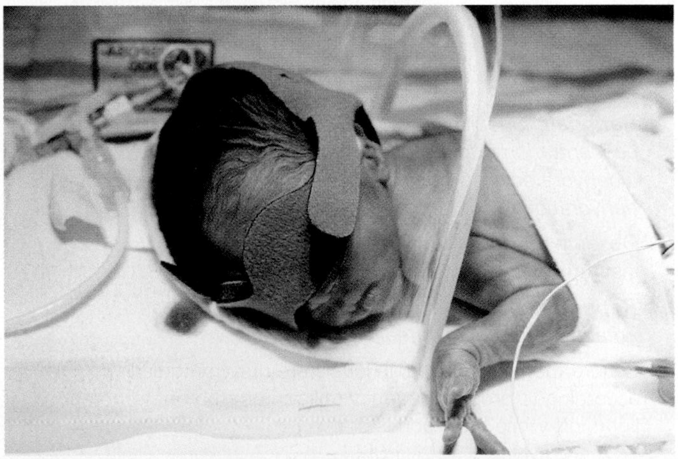

Figure 34-16 ■ Infant receiving phototherapy. The phototherapy light is positioned over the incubator. Bilateral eye patches are always used during photo light therapy to protect the baby's eyes.

Source: Courtesy of Lisa Smith-Pedersen, RN, MSN, NNP-BC/Pearson Education.

(continued)

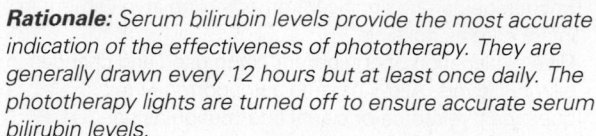

PROCEDURE 34-2 Infant Receiving Phototherapy continued

NURSING ACTION

4. Place the infant in an open crib or isolette (more commonly used in preterm infants and infants who are sicker) about 45 to 50 cm below the bank of phototherapy lights. Reposition every 2 hours.

   Rationale: *The isolette helps the infant maintain his or her temperature while undressed. Repositioning exposes different areas of skin to the lights, prevents the development of pressure areas on the skin, and varies the stimulation the infant receives.*

5. Monitor vital signs every 4 hours with axillary temperatures.

   Rationale: *Temperature assessment is indicated to detect hypothermia or hyperthermia. Deviation in pulse and respirations may indicate developing complications.*

6. Cluster care activities.
7. Discontinue phototherapy and remove eye patches at least every 2 to 3 hours when feeding the infant and when the parents visit.

   Rationale: *Care activities are clustered to help ensure that the newborn has maximum time under the lights. Eye patches are removed to assess for signs of complications such as excessive pressure, discharge, or conjunctivitis. Patches are also removed to provide some social stimulation and to promote parental attachment.*

8. Maintain adequate fluid intake. Evaluate need for IV fluids.
9. Monitor intake and output carefully. Weigh diapers before discarding. Record quantity and characteristics of each stool.

   Rationale: *Infants undergoing phototherapy treatment have increased water loss and loose stools as a result of bilirubin excretion. This increases their risk of dehydration.*

> **CLINICAL TIP**
> If the area of jaundice about the eyes begins to disappear, it is probable that the eye patches are allowing light to enter and better eye protection is needed.

10. Assess specific gravity with each voiding. Weigh newborn daily.

    Rationale: *Specific gravity provides one measure of urine concentration. Highly concentrated urine is associated with a dehydrated state. Weight loss is also a sign of developing dehydration in the newborn.*

11. Observe the infant for signs of perianal excoriation and institute therapy if it develops.

    Rationale: *Perianal excoriation may develop because of the irritating effect of diarrhea stools.*

12. Ensure that serum bilirubin levels are drawn regularly according to orders or agency policy. Turn the phototherapy lights off while the blood is drawn.

    Rationale: *Serum bilirubin levels provide the most accurate indication of the effectiveness of phototherapy. They are generally drawn every 12 hours but at least once daily. The phototherapy lights are turned off to ensure accurate serum bilirubin levels.*

13. Examine the newborn's skin regularly for signs of developing pressure areas, bronzing, maculopapular rash, and changes in degree of jaundice.

    Rationale: *Pressure areas may develop if the infant lies in one position for an extended period. A benign, transient bronze discoloration of the skin may occur with phototherapy when the infant has elevated direct serum bilirubin levels or liver disease. A maculopapular rash is another transient side effect of phototherapy that develops occasionally.*

14. Avoid using lotion or ointment on the exposed skin.

    Rationale: *Lotions and ointments on a newborn receiving phototherapy may cause skin burns.*

15. Provide parents with opportunities to hold the newborn and assist in the infant's care. Answer their questions accurately and keep them informed of developments or changes.

    Rationale: *A sick infant is a source of great anxiety for parents. Information helps them deal with their anxiety. Moreover, they have a right to be kept well informed of their baby's status so that they are able to make informed decisions as needed.*

16. May also provide phototherapy using lightweight, fiberoptic blankets ("bili blankets"). The baby is wrapped in the blanket, which is plugged into an outlet (Figure 34-17 ■).

    Rationale: *With fiberoptic blankets the newborn is readily accessible for care, feedings, and diaper changes. The baby does not get overheated, and fluid and weight loss are not complications of this system. The infant is accessible to the parents and the procedure seems less alarming to parents than standard phototherapy.*

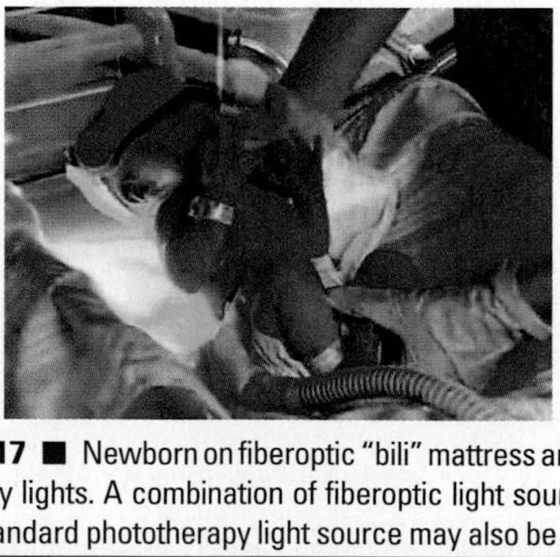

Figure 34-17 ■ Newborn on fiberoptic "bili" mattress and under phototherapy lights. A combination of fiberoptic light source mattress and standard phototherapy light source may also be used.

Note: The color is distorted because of the reflection of the bililight mattress.
Source: George Dodson/Lightworks Studio/Pearson Education.

If the baby is to receive phototherapy at home, parents are taught to record the infant's temperature, weight, fluid I&O, stools, and feedings and to use the phototherapy equipment. In addition, if phototherapy lights are being used, parents must agree that the baby will be exposed to the lights for long periods of time; that they will hold the baby for only short periods for feedings, comforting, and cleansing of the perineal area; and that the room temperature will be regulated to minimize heat loss. Fiberoptic phototherapy blankets eliminate the need for eye patches, decrease heat loss because the baby is clothed, and provide more opportunities for interaction between the baby and parents. The best method of home phototherapy depends on the cause of the hyperbilirubinemia and the rate of progression of the jaundice. Ongoing monitoring of bilirubin levels is essential with home phototherapy and can be carried out in the home, in the follow-up clinic, or in the clinician's office.

CLINICAL JUDGMENT

Case Study: Baby Boy Martin

Baby boy Martin is a term male infant born by vaginal delivery with vacuum assist. His mother has blood type O positive, and Baby Martin has blood type A positive. The baby has a normal complete blood count (CBC) with a hematocrit of 60%. While performing a physical examination on Baby Martin on day 2 of life, the nurse notes that he has a large cephalhematoma, an enlarged liver on palpation (hepatomegaly), and is clinically jaundiced. The nurse suspects that Baby Martin has hyperbilirubinemia and discusses her findings with the neonatal nurse practitioner who orders a total bilirubin level be drawn. When resulted, the level is 16 mg/dl. The decision is made to start this infant on phototherapy treatment.

Critical Thinking

What risk factors and clinical findings does this infant have that predispose him to hyperbilirubinemia?

How would the nurse explain Baby Martin's hyperbilirubinemia and subsequent treatment and nursing care to his mother?

See www.nursing.pearsonhighered.com for possible responses.

Evaluation

Expected outcomes of nursing care include the following:

- The newborns at risk for development of hyperbilirubinemia are identified, and action is taken to minimize the potential impact of hyperbilirubinemia.
- The baby will not have any corneal irritation or drainage, skin breakdown, or major fluctuations in temperature.
- Parents understand the rationale for, goal of, and expected outcome of therapy.
- Parents verbalize their concerns about their baby's condition and identify how they can facilitate their baby's improvement.

Care of the Newborn with Anemia

Neonatal anemia is often difficult to recognize by clinical evaluation alone. The hemoglobin concentration in a full-term newborn is 19.3 ± 2.2 g/dl (Manco-Johnson, Rodden, & Hays, 2011), slightly higher than in premature infants, in whom the mean hemoglobin is 14 to 18 g/dl. Infants with hemoglobin values of less than 11 mg/dl (term) and 7 to 9 g/dl (preterm) are usually considered anemic (Gomella et al., 2009). The most common causes of neonatal anemia are blood loss (preterm babies in the neonatal intensive care unit (NICU) can have 15% to 30% total blood volume loss per week due to lab draws), hemolysis/erythrocyte destruction, and impaired red blood cell (RBC)/erythrocyte production (Widness, 2008).

Blood loss (hypovolemia) occurs in utero from placental bleeding (placenta previa or abruptio placentae). Intrapartal blood loss may be fetomaternal, fetofetal, or the result of umbilical cord bleeding. Birth trauma to abdominal organs (adrenal hemorrhage) or the cranium (subgaleal bleed) may produce significant blood loss, and cerebral bleeding may occur because of hypoxia.

Excessive hemolysis of red cells is usually a result of blood group incompatibilities but may be due to infections. The most common cause of impaired red cell production is a genetically transmitted deficiency in glucose-6-phosphate dehydrogenase (G6PD). Anemia and jaundice are the presenting signs (Gomella et al., 2009).

A condition known as **physiologic anemia of infancy** exists as a result of the normal gradual drop in hemoglobin for the first 8 to 10 weeks of life and corresponds with the decline in fetal hemoglobin (Widness, 2008). Theoretically, the bone marrow stops production of RBCs in response to higher oxygen levels that result from breathing changes after birth. When the amount of hemoglobin decreases, reaching a nadir of 10 to 12 g/dl in the term infant and reaching a nadir at 8 to 10 weeks and 7 to 8 g/dl in preterm infants at about 4 to 8 weeks of age, the bone marrow begins production of RBCs again, and the anemia disappears (Diehl-Jones & Askin, 2010).

Anemia in preterm newborns is seen earlier and is more severe than in term newborns, and increased production of red blood cells does not start until hemoglobin is 7 to 8 g/dl. The preterm baby's hemoglobin reaches a low sooner than does a term newborn's because a preterm infant's red blood cell survival time is shorter than that of a term newborn (Diehl-Jones & Askin, 2010). This difference is a result of several factors: the preterm infant's rapid growth rate, decreased iron stores, and an inadequate production of erythropoietin (EPO). Iatrogenic causes occur more in preterm infants as their condition requires more laboratory assessment (Diehl-Jones & Askin, 2010).

Clinical Therapy

Clinical management depends on the severity of the anemia, whether blood loss is acute or chronic, clinical manifestations, and whether it was anticipated based on the pregnancy history. The age at which anemia is first noted is also of diagnostic value. Clinically, light-skinned anemic infants are very pale when they do not have other symptoms of shock and usually have abnormally low RBC counts. In acute blood loss, symptoms of shock may be present, such as pallor, low arterial blood pressure, and a decreasing hematocrit value.

The initial laboratory workup should include determinations of hemoglobin, hematocrit, bilirubin levels (in hemolytic disease), reticulocyte count, examination of peripheral blood smear, direct Coombs' test of infant's blood, and examination of maternal blood smear for fetal erythrocytes (Kleihauer-Betke test). Mild or chronic anemia in an infant may be treated adequately with iron supplements alone or with iron-fortified formulas. In severe cases of anemia, transfusions with O-negative or typed and cross-matched packed red cells are the preferred method of treatment.

Management of anemia of prematurity includes treating the causative factor (e.g., antibiotics/antivirals used for infection, steroid therapy for disorders of erythrocyte production) and supplemental iron. Blood transfusions (dedicated units of blood ideally from a single donor source) are kept to a minimum. Evidence supports use of recombinant human erythropoietin (rEPO) in only selected cases (Von Kohorn & Ehrenkranz, 2009)—for example, infants in whom it is desirable to maintain a relatively high hematocrit, such as infants with bronchopulmonary dysplasia.

NURSING CARE MANAGEMENT

The nurse assesses the newborn for symptoms of anemia (pallor). If the blood loss is acute, the baby may exhibit signs of shock (a capillary filling time greater than 3 seconds, decreased pulses, tachycardia, and low blood pressure [BP]). Signs of compromise include poor weight gain, tachycardia, tachypnea, and apneic episodes. The baby should be placed on constant cardiac and respiratory monitoring. The nurse promptly reports any symptoms indicating anemia or shock. Continued observations will be necessary to identify physiologic anemia as the preterm newborn grows. The nurse should try to prevent iron deficiency by limiting phlebotomy losses and recording it in tenths of a milliliter. The total blood removed is assessed and replaced by transfusion when necessary or by starting iron therapy at 2 weeks of postnatal age (Aher, Malwatkar, & Kadam, 2008; Diehl-Jones & Askin, 2010).

Care of the Newborn with Polycythemia

Polycythemia, a condition in which blood volume and hematocrit values are increased, is observed more commonly in intrauterine growth restricted (IUGR), late preterm infants; placental transfusion caused by delayed cord clamping or cord stripping; infants receiving maternal-fetal or twin-to-twin transfusions; babies who have been exposed to intrauterine hypoxia; and babies of mothers who smoke, suffer from asphyxia, or take propranolol during pregnancy. Other conditions that may present with polycythemia are chromosomal anomalies such as trisomy 21, 18, and 13 and births at altitudes over 5000 feet (Gomella et al., 2009). The incidence ranges from 1% to 5% in healthy term neonates, and the condition is uncommon in newborns less than 34 weeks' gestation (Diehl-Jones & Askin, 2010).

An infant is considered polycythemic when the central venous hematocrit value is greater than 65%. A potential complication of polycythemia is hyperviscosity, which results in impaired perfusion of the capillary vessels (Diehl-Jones & Askin, 2010).

Clinical Therapy

The goal of therapy is to reduce the central venous hematocrit to a range of 50% to 55% in symptomatic infants (Gomella et al., 2009). To decrease the red cell mass, the symptomatic infant receives a partial exchange transfusion in which blood is removed from the infant and replaced milliliter for milliliter with colloids such as fresh frozen plasma or 5% albumin or crystalloids such as isotonic saline (Diehl-Jones & Askin, 2010). The preference is to use crystalloids because of decreased promotion of infection, incidence of necrotizing enterocolitis (NEC), and their hypoallergenic properties. Supportive treatment of presenting symptoms is required until resolution, which usually occurs spontaneously following the partial exchange transfusion.

NURSING CARE MANAGEMENT

The nurse assesses, records, and reports symptoms of polycythemia. The nurse also does an initial screening of the newborn's hematocrit on admission to the nursery. The peak of term newborn's hematocrit will occur at 2 hours of age and begin to drop slowly by 12 to 18 hours. A capillary hematocrit may be done (see Procedure 34-1: Performing Heel Stick on a Newborn); however, peripheral free-flowing venous hematocrit samples are usually obtained from the antecubital fossa for confirmation.

Many infants are asymptomatic, but as symptoms develop, they are related to the increased blood volume, hyperviscosity (thickness) of the blood, and decreased deformability of red blood cells (RBCs), all of which result in poor perfusion of tissues. The infants have a characteristic plethoric (ruddy) appearance. The most common symptoms observed include the following:

- ***Cardiopulmonary:*** Tachycardia and congestive heart failure due to the increased blood volume.
- ***Respiratory:*** Respiratory distress with grunting, tachypnea, and cyanosis; increased oxygen need; or hemorrhage in respiratory system due to pulmonary venous congestion, edema, and hypoxemia.
- ***Gastrointestinal:*** Feeding intolerance, poor feeding, vomiting, or NEC.
- ***Hematologic:*** Hyperbilirubinemia caused by increased numbers of RBCs breaking down; thrombocytopenia; or elevated reticulocytes and nucleated RBCs.
- ***Renal:*** Renal vein thrombosis with decreased urine output, hematuria, or proteinuria due to thromboembolism; or renal tubular damage.
- ***Central nervous system:*** Jitteriness, irritability, decreased activity and tone, lethargy, stroke (rare), or seizures due to decreased perfusion of the brain, and increased vascular resistance secondary to sluggish blood flow which can result in neurologic or developmental problems.

The nurse observes closely for signs of distress or change in vital signs during the partial exchange. The nurse assesses carefully for potential complications resulting from the exchange such as transfusion overload (which can result in congestive heart failure), irregular cardiac rhythm, bacterial infection, hypovolemia (because of decreased plasma volume), and anemia. Parents need specific explanations about polycythemia and its treatment. The newborn needs to be reunited with the parents as soon after the exchange as the baby's status permits.

Care of the Newborn with Infection

Newborns up to 1 month of age are particularly susceptible to infection, referred to as **sepsis neonatorum**, caused by organisms that do not cause significant disease in older children. Once any infection occurs in the newborn, it can spread rapidly through the bloodstream, regardless of its primary site. The incidence of early onset sepsis (EOS) is 1 to 2 per 1000 live births (0.1% to 0.2%) with a 10 times higher incidence in very-low-birth-weight (VLBW) infants (birth weight <1500 grams) (Puopolo, 2008). The risk of mortality is 5% to 15% in this population. Neonatal sepsis is a blood infection that occurs in an infant younger than 90 days old. Early-onset sepsis is seen in the first week of life. Late-onset sepsis occurs between days 8 and 89.

Nosocomial infections, infections acquired while a baby is in the neonatal intensive care unit (NICU), range from 7% to 24% (Carey, Saiman, & Polin, 2008; Garland & Uhing, 2009). Methicillin-resistant staphylococcus aureus (MRSA) and Candida are two of the most common pathogens causing hospital acquired infections in the NICU population (Venkatesh, Adams, & Weisman, 2011). The general debilitation and underlying illness often associated with prematurity necessitates invasive procedures such as umbilical catheterization, intubation, resuscitation, ventilatory support, monitoring, and parenteral alimentation (especially lipid emulsions), and prior broad-spectrum antibiotic therapy. The incidence of infections caused by umbilical and central line presence in the NICU baby is 3.1 to 9.1 infections for every 1000 days of having the lines in place in the 1001 to 1500 and <1000 gram birth weight babies respectively (Bell, 2008; Curry, Honeycutt, Goins, et al., 2009).

However, even full-term infants are susceptible because their immunologic systems are immature. They lack the complex factors involved in effective phagocytosis and the ability to localize infection or to respond with a well-defined recognizable inflammatory response. In addition, newborns lack IgM immunoglobulin, which is necessary to protect against bacteria, because it does not cross the placenta (refer to chapter 29 ∞ for immunologic adaptations in the newborn period).

Most nosocomial infections in the NICU present as bacteremia/sepsis, urinary tract infections, meningitis, or pneumonia. Maternal antepartal infections such as rubella, toxoplasmosis, cytomegalic inclusion disease, and herpes may cause congenital infections and resulting disorders in the newborn. Intrapartal maternal infections, such as amnionitis and those resulting from premature rupture of membranes (PROM) and precipitous birth, are sources of neonatal infection. (See "Care of the Woman with Perinatal Infection Affecting the Fetus" in chapter 20 ∞ for more detailed information.) Passage through the birth canal and contact with microorganisms in the vaginal flora (β-hemolytic streptococci, herpes, *Listeria,* and gonococci) expose the infant to infection (Table 34-5). With infection anywhere in the fetus or newborn, the adjacent tissues or organs are very easily penetrated, and the blood-brain barrier is ineffective. Septicemia is more common in males, except for those infections caused by group B β-hemolytic streptococcus.

Gram-negative organisms (especially *E. coli, Enterobacter, Proteus, Pseudomonas*, and *Klebsiella*) and the gram-positive organism β-hemolytic streptococcus are the most common causative agents. *Pseudomonas* is a common fomite contaminant of ventilatory support and oxygen therapy equipment. Gram-positive bacteria, especially coagulase-negative staphylococci, are common pathogens in nosocomial bacteremias, pneumonias, and urinary tract infections. Other gram-positive bacteria frequently isolated are *Bacillus, Corynebacterium*, and *Staphylococcus aureus* (Puopolo, 2008).

Protection of the newborn from infections starts prenatally and continues throughout pregnancy and birth. Prenatal prevention should include maternal screening for sexually transmitted infection and monitoring of rubella titers in women who test negative. Intrapartally, sterile technique is essential. Viral cultures are the definitive tests but take time to get results. Visual exam of the lesions is often reported on the labor and birth record to identify a patient with herpes. Placenta and amniotic fluid cultures are obtained if amnionitis is suspected. Local eye treatment with an antibiotic ophthalmic ointment is given to all newborns to prevent damage from gonococcal (occurring 3 days following birth) and possibly chlamydial (occurring 7 to 10 days after birth) infections. Prophylactic antibiotic therapy, for asymptomatic women who test positive for Group B streptococcus (GBS) during the intrapartum period, helps prevent EOS (Venkatesh et al., 2011).

Clinical Therapy

Infants with a history of possible exposure to infection in utero (for example, PROM more than 24 hours before birth or questionable maternal history of infection, maternal fever/chorioamnionitis, or high-risk behavior [such as multiple sexual partners or illicit drug use]) should have cultures taken as soon after birth as possible. Cultures are obtained before antibiotic therapy is begun (Venkatesh et al., 2011).

1. Anaerobic and aerobic blood culture is taken from a peripheral site rather than an umbilical vessel because catheters have yielded false-positive results because of contamination. The skin is prepared by cleaning with a unit-specified antiseptic solution and allowed to dry; the specimen is obtained with a sterile needle/syringe. Correct sterile technique will lessen the likelihood of contamination.
2. Spinal fluid culture is done following a spinal tap/lumbar puncture if there are concerns about central nervous system

TABLE 34-5 Maternally Transmitted Newborn Infections

INFECTION	NURSING ASSESSMENT	NURSING PLAN AND IMPLEMENTATION
Group B Streptococcus 1%–2% colonized, with 1 in 10 developing disease. Early onset—usually within hours of birth or within first week. Late onset—1 week to 3 months (Nash & Smith, 2008).	Severe respiratory distress (grunting and cyanosis). May become apneic or demonstrate symptoms of shock. Meconium-stained amniotic fluid seen at birth.	Early assessment of clinical signs necessary. Assist with x-ray examination—shows aspiration pneumonia or respiratory distress syndrome. Immediately obtain blood, gastric aspirate, external ear canal, and nasopharynx cultures. Administer antibiotics, usually aqueous penicillin or ampicillin combined with gentamicin, as soon as cultures are obtained. Early assessment and intervention are essential to survival.
Congenital Syphilis Spirochetes cross placenta after 16th–18th week of gestation. The more recent the maternal infection the more likelihood of transmission. Most are asymptomatic at birth but develop symptoms within first 3 months of life.	Check perinatal history for positive maternal serology Assess infant for: Elevated cord serum IgM and FTA-ABS (fluorescent treponemal antibody absorbed) IgM Rhinitis (snuffles) Fissures on mouth corners and excoriated upper lip Red rash around mouth and anus Copper-colored rash over face, palms, and soles Irritability, generalized edema, particularly over joints; bone lesions; painful extremities, hepatosplenomegaly, jaundice, congenital cataracts, small for gestational age (SGA), and failure to thrive	Refer to evaluate for blindness, deafness, learning or behavioral problems. Initiate standard precautions until infants have been on antibiotics for at least 24 hours. Administer penicillin. Provide emotional support for parents because of their feelings about mode of transmission and potential long-term sequelae.
Gonorrhea Approximately 30%–35% of newborns born vaginally to infected mothers acquire the infection.	Assess for: Ophthalmia neonatorum (conjunctivitis) Purulent discharge and corneal ulcerations Neonatal sepsis with temperature instability, poor feeding response, and/or hypotonia, jaundice	Administer ophthalmic antibiotic ointment (see Drug Guide: Erythromycin [Ilotycin] Ophthalmic Ointment in chapter 31) or penicillin. If positive maternal test, single dose systemic antibiotic therapy (AAP & ACOG, 2007). Make a follow-up referral to evaluate any loss of vision.
Herpes Type 2 1 in 7500 births. Usually transmitted during vaginal birth; a few cases of in utero transmission have been reported.	Check perinatal history for active herpes genital lesions. Small cluster vesicular skin lesions over all the body about 6 to 9 days of life. Disseminated form—disseminated intravascular coagulation (DIC), pneumonia, hepatitis with jaundice, hepatosplenomegaly, and neurologic abnormalities. Without skin lesions, assess for fever or subnormal temperature, respiratory congestion, tachypnea, and tachycardia	Carry out careful hand washing and contact precautions (gown and glove isolation with linen precautions) (AAP & ACOG, 2007). Obtain throat, conjunctiva, cerebral spinal fluid (CSF), blood, urine, rectal, and lesion cultures to identify herpes virus type 2 antibodies in serum IgM fraction. Cultures positive in 24–48 hours. Administer intravenous acyclovir (Zovirax). Make a follow-up referral to evaluate potential sequelae of microcephaly, spasticity, seizures, deafness, or blindness. Encourage parental rooming-in and touching of their newborn. Show parents appropriate hand washing procedures and precautions to be used at home if mother's lesions are active.
Cytomegalovirus (CMV) Most common cause of congenital infection in the United States—approximately 1% of all newborns (AAP & ACOG, 2007). Transmission occurs in utero, during labor, or may happen postnatally through breast milk.	Congenital CMV disease, including intrauterine growth restriction, jaundice, hepatosplenomegaly, petechiae or purpura (blueberry muffin spots), thrombocytopenia, and pneumonia. Central nervous system (CNS) manifestations are very common and include lethargy and poor feeding, hypertonia or hypotonia, microcephaly, intracranial calcifications, chorioretinitis, and sensorineural deafness.	Diagnosis of congenital CMV infection is established by isolating virus from urine, saliva, or tissue obtained during the first 3 weeks of life. All infants in whom the diagnosis is suspected should have a viral culture performed; a CT scan of the brain is particularly important to document the extent of CNS involvement; eye exam and hearing test; close long-term follow-up evaluating for developmental effects.
Oral Candidal Infection (Thrush) Acquired during passage through birth canal	Assess newborn's buccal mucosa, tongue, gums, and inside the cheeks for white plaques (seen 5 to 7 days of age) Check diaper area for bright-red, well-demarcated eruptions Assess for thrush periodically when newborn is on long-term antibiotic therapy	Differentiate white plaque areas from milk curds by using cotton tip applicator (if it is thrush, removal of white areas causes raw, bleeding areas). Maintain cleanliness of hands, linen, clothing, diapers, and feeding apparatus. Instruct breastfeeding mothers on treating their nipples with nystatin. Administer nystatin swabbed on oral lesions 1 hour after feeding or nystatin instilled in baby's oral cavity and on mucosa. Swab skin lesions with topical nystatin.
Chlamydia Trachomatis Acquired during passage through birth canal.	Assess for perinatal history of preterm birth. Symptomatic newborns present with pneumonia. Chlamydial conjunctivitis presents with inflammation, yellow discharge, and eyelid swelling 5 to 14 days after birth. Assess for chronic follicular conjunctivitis (corneal neovascularization and conjunctival scarring).	Instillation of prophylactic ophthalmic erythromycin is controversial (AAP & ACOG, 2007). Treat chlamydial conjunctivitis or pneumonia with oral erythromycin for 14 days. Monitor for hypertropic pyloric stenosis. Initiate follow-up referral for eye complications and late development of pneumonia at 4 to 11 weeks postnatally.

(CNS) symptoms/pathology. The fluid can be analyzed for culture and gram stain as well as for viral presence (Pacatte, 2008).

3. The specimen for urine culture is best obtained by a suprapubic bladder aspiration or sterile catheterization.
4. Skin cultures are taken of any lesions or drainage from lesions or reddened areas.
5. Tracheal aspirate cultures, if intubated, may be obtained.

Other laboratory investigations include a complete blood count, C-reactive protein (CRP), chest x-ray examination, serology, and Gram stains of cerebrospinal fluid, urine, skin exudate, and umbilicus. White blood cell (WBC) count with differential may indicate the presence or absence of sepsis. A level of 30,000 to 40,000 mm^3 WBC may be normal in the first 24 hours of life, whereas low WBC (less than 5000 to 7500/mm^3) may be indicative of sepsis. A low neutrophil count and high band (immature white cells) count indicate that an infection is present. Stomach aspirate should be sent for culture and smear if a gonococcal infection or amnionitis is suspected. CRP, an acute-phase reactant protein synthesized in response to inflammation, may or may not be elevated initially. Other inflammatory responses may cause an elevation in the CRP, so it should not be used as the only indicator of infection (Hawk, 2008; Lott, 2010; Venkatesh et al., 2011). The CRP may be helpful in watching for improvement once antibiotic therapy is initiated.

Serum IgM levels are elevated (normal level less than 20 mg/dl) in response to transplacental infections. If available, counterimmunoelectrophoresis tests for specific bacterial antigens are performed. In the future, repetitive sequence-based polymerase chain reactions (rep-PCR) will be used to identify specific infectious organisms within hours instead of days (Lott, 2010). Evidence of congenital infections may be seen on skull x-rays or CT scans for cerebral calcifications (cytomegalovirus or toxoplasmosis), on bone x-rays (syphilis or cytomegalovirus), and in serum-specific IgM levels (rubella). Cytomegalovirus infection is best diagnosed by urine culture.

Because neonatal infection causes high mortality, therapy is instituted before results of the sepsis workup are obtained. A combination of two broad-spectrum antibiotics, such as ampicillin and gentamicin, is given in large doses until a culture with sensitivities results is obtained.

After the pathogen and its sensitivities are determined, appropriate specific antibiotic therapy is begun. Combinations of penicillin or ampicillin and kanamycin have been used in the past, but new kanamycin-resistant enterobacteria and penicillin-resistant staphylococcus necessitate increasing use of gentamicin. Rotating aminoglycosides has been suggested to prevent development of resistance. Use of cephalosporins and, in particular, cefotaxime has emerged as an alternative to aminoglycoside therapy in the treatment of neonatal infections. Duration of therapy varies from 7 to 14 days (Table 34-6). However, if cultures are negative and symptoms subside, antibiotics may be discontinued after 2 days/48 hours of negative blood cultures. A normal CRP at 48 hours also supports discontinuing antibiotics if blood cultures are negative. Supportive physiologic care may be required to maintain respiratory, hemodynamic, nutritional, and metabolic homeostasis.

Care Plan Activity: Infection in a Newborn

NURSING CARE MANAGEMENT

Nursing Assessment and Diagnosis

Symptoms of infection are most often noticed by the nurse during daily care of the newborn. The infant may deteriorate rapidly in the first 12 to 24 hours after birth if *B*-hemolytic streptococcal infection is present, with signs and symptoms mimicking respiratory distress syndrome (RDS). In other cases, the onset of sepsis may be gradual, with more subtle signs and symptoms. The most common symptoms include the following:

- Subtle behavioral changes—the infant "isn't doing well" and is often lethargic or irritable (especially after first 24 hours), hypotonic, and hypotensive. Color changes may include pallor, duskiness, cyanosis, or a "shocky" appearance. Skin is cool and clammy.
- Temperature instability, manifested most commonly by hypothermia (recognized by a decrease in skin temperature) or, rarely in newborns, hyperthermia (elevation of skin temperature) necessitates a corresponding increase or decrease in incubator temperature to maintain a neutral thermal environment.
- Feeding intolerance is evidenced by a decrease in total intake, abdominal distention, vomiting, poor sucking, lack of interest in feeding, and diarrhea.
- Hyperbilirubinemia, petechial hemorrhages, hepatosplenomegaly.
- Tachycardia initially, followed by spells of apnea/bradycardia.

Signs and symptoms may suggest CNS disease (jitteriness, tremors, seizure activity). A differential diagnosis is necessary because of the similarity of symptoms to other more specific conditions.

Nursing diagnoses that may apply to the infant with suspected sepsis neonatorum and the family include the following:

- ***Risk for Infection*** related to newborn's immature immunologic system
- ***Deficient Fluid Volume*** related to feeding intolerance
- ***Compromised Family Coping*** related to present illness resulting in prolonged hospital stay for the newborn

Nursing Plan and Implementation

In the nursery, controlling the environment and preventing acquired infection are the responsibilities of the neonatal nurse. An infected newborn can be isolated effectively in an isolette and receive close observation. The nurse must promote strict hand washing technique for all who enter the nursery, including nursing colleagues, physicians, laboratory, x-ray, and respiratory therapists, and parents. Visits to the nursery area by unnecessary personnel should be discouraged. The nurse assists in the aseptic collection of specimens for laboratory tests. Scrupulous care of equipment—changing and cleaning incubators at least every 7 days, removing and sterilizing wet equipment every 24 hours, preventing cross-use of linen and other equipment, cleaning

TABLE 34-6 Neonatal Sepsis Antibiotic/Antiviral Therapy

DRUG	DOSE (MG/KG) TOTAL DAILY DOSE	SCHEDULE FOR DIVIDED DOSES	ROUTE	COMMENTS
Acyclovir (Zovirax)	20 mg/kg	Every 8 hours	IV	Length of treatment is 14 days for skin/eye/mouth (SEM) or 21 days for CNS and disseminated disease: *Herpes.*
Ampicillin	25–50 mg/kg/dose (100 mg/kg/dose if treating meningitis and severe Group B streptococcal sepsis)	Every 12 hours* Every 8 hours† Every 6 hours **	IM or IV	Effective against gram-positive microorganisms, *Listeria,* and most *Escherichia coli* strains. Higher doses indicated for meningitis. Used with aminoglycoside for synergy.
Cefotaxime	50 mg/kg/dose (25 mg/kg/dose Gonococcal infection)	Every 12 hours* Every 8 hours Every 6 hours **	IM or IV	Active against most major pathogens in infants; effective against aminoglycoside-resistant organisms; achieves cerebrospinal fluid (CSF) bactericidal activity; lack of ototoxicity and nephrotoxicity; wide therapeutic index (levels not required); resistant organisms can develop rapidly if used extensively; ineffective against *Pseudomonas, Listeria.*
Gentamicin	4–5 mg/kg/dose	Every 24–48 hours‡ ***	IM or IV	Effective against gram-negative rods and staphylococci; may be used instead of kanamycin against penicillin-resistant staphylococci and *E. coli* strains and *Pseudomonas aeruginosa.* May cause neurotoxicity, ototoxicity, and nephrotoxicity. Need to follow serum levels. Must never be given as IV push. Must be given over at least 30–60 minutes. In presence of oliguria or anuria, dose must be decreased or discontinued. In infants less than 1000 g or 29 weeks, lower dosage 2.5–3 mg/kg/day. Monitor serum levels before administration of second dose.
	4–5 mg/kg/dose (first week of life)	Every 24–48 hours		Peak 5–10 mcg/ml Trough 1–2 mcg/ml
Vancomycin	10–20 mg/kg 30 mg/kg/day	Every 12–24 hours*‡ Every 8 hours†	IV	Effective for methicillin-resistant strains (*Staphylococcus epidermidis*); must be administered by slow intravenous infusion to avoid prolonged cutaneous eruption. For smaller infants, less than 1200 g, less than 29 weeks, smaller dosages and longer intervals between doses. Nephrotoxic, especially in combination with aminoglycosides. Slow IV infusion over at least 60 minutes. Peak 25–40 mcg/ml Trough 5–10 mcg/ml

*Up to 7 days of age.
** ≥45 weeks postmenstrual age.
†Greater than 7 days of age.
‡Dependent on gestational age.
***Dependent on postnatal age.

sink-side equipment such as soap containers periodically, and taking special care with the open radiant warmers (access without prior hand washing is much more likely than with the closed incubator)—will prevent contamination.

Provision of Antibiotic Therapy

The nurse administers antibiotics as ordered by the nurse practitioner or physician. It is the nurse's responsibility to be knowledgeable about the following:

- The proper dose to be administered, based on the weight of the newborn and desired peak and trough levels
- The appropriate route of administration, because some antibiotics cannot be given intravenously
- Admixture incompatibilities. Some antibiotics precipitate in IV solutions when mixed with other antibiotics
- Side effects and toxicity

For term infants being treated for infections, neonatal home infusion of antibiotics should be considered as a viable alternative to continued hospitalization. The infusion of antibiotics at home by skilled registered nurses (RNs) facilitates parent-infant bonding while meeting the ongoing healthcare needs of the infant.

Provision of Supportive Care

In addition to antibiotic therapy, physiologic supportive care is essential in caring for a septic infant. The nurse should carry out the following:

- Observe for resolution of symptoms or development of other symptoms of sepsis.
- Maintain a neutral thermal environment with accurate regulation of humidity and oxygen administration.
- Provide respiratory support: Administer oxygen and observe and monitor respiratory effort.
- Provide cardiovascular support: Observe and monitor pulse and blood pressure; observe for hyperbilirubinemia, anemia, and hemorrhagic symptoms.
- Provide adequate calories, because oral feedings may be discontinued because of increased mucus, abdominal distention, vomiting, or aspiration.
- Provide fluids and electrolytes to maintain homeostasis. Monitor weight changes, urine output, and urine specific gravity.
- Observe for the development of hypoglycemia, hyperglycemia, acidosis, hyponatremia, and hypocalcemia.

Restricting parental visits has not been shown to have any effect on the rate of infection and may be harmful to the newborn's psychologic development. With instruction and guidance from the nurse, both parents should be allowed to handle the baby and participate in daily care. Support of the parents is crucial. They need to be informed of the newborn's prognosis as treatment continues and to be involved in care as much as possible. They also need to understand how infection is transmitted.

Evaluation

Expected outcomes of nursing care include the following:

- The risks for development of sepsis are identified early, and immediate action is taken to minimize the development of the illness.
- Appropriate use of aseptic technique protects the newborn from further exposure to illness.
- The baby's symptoms are relieved, and the infection is treated.
- The parents verbalize their concerns about their baby's illness and understand the rationale behind the management of their newborn.

Care of the Family with Birth of an At-Risk Newborn

The birth of a preterm or ill infant or an infant with a congenital anomaly is a serious crisis situation for a family. Throughout the pregnancy, both parents, together and separately, have felt excitement, experienced thoughts of acceptance, and pictured how their baby would look and act. Both parents have wished for a perfect baby and feared a damaged, unhealthy one. Each parent and family member must accept and adjust when the fantasized fears become reality.

Parental Responses

Family members have acute grief reactions to the loss of the idealized baby they have envisioned. In a preterm birth, the mother is denied the last few weeks of pregnancy that seem to prepare her psychologically for the stress of birth and the attachment process. Attachment at this time is fragile, and interruption of the process by separation can affect the future mother-child relationship. Parents express grief as shock and disbelief, denial of reality, anger toward self and others, guilt, blame, and concern for the future. Self-esteem and feelings of self-worth are jeopardized.

Feelings of guilt and failure often plague mothers of preterm newborns. They may ask themselves, "Why did labor start? What did I do (or not do)?" A woman may have guilt fantasies and wonder what she may have done to cause the early labor: Was it because I had sex with my husband [a week, 3 days, a day] ago?" "Was it because I carried three loads of laundry up from the basement?" "Am I being punished for something I did in the past—even in childhood?"

The period of waiting between suspicion and confirmation of abnormality or dysfunction is a very anxious one for parents because it is difficult, if not impossible, to begin attachment to the infant if the newborn's future is questionable. During the waiting period, parents need support and acknowledgment that this is an anxious time. They must be kept informed about tests and efforts to gather additional data, as well as efforts to improve their baby's outcome. It is helpful to tell both parents about the problem at the same time with the baby present. An honest discussion of the problem and anticipatory management at the earliest possible time by health professionals help the parents (1) maintain trust in the physician and nurse, (2) appreciate the reality of the situation by dispelling fantasy and misconception, (3) begin the grieving process, and (4) mobilize internal and external support.

Nurses need to be aware that anger is a universal response and that it is best directed outward because holding it in check requires great energy, which is diverted away from grieving and physical recovery from pregnancy and giving birth. Anger, aggression, hostility, and irritability may be exhibited and directed unjustifiably at the physician and/or nurse, at the food, at nursing care, or at hospital regulations and routines (Mounts, 2009). Parents rarely show anger with the baby and such responses can precipitate guilt feelings. Perceived maternal stress may be lessened if information is provided regarding preterm behavioral cues. This empowers the mother and allows her to better care for her child. Mothers of preterm babies who have to spend time in a neonatal intensive care unit (NICU) suffer from psychologic distress similar to post-traumatic stress disorder (PTSD). Nurses working with the mothers in the NICU setting have the opportunity to encourage maternal competence and confidence, both during and after hospitalization, by teaching interpretation of their child's behavioral cues, prompting maternal care of the baby while in the NICU, and facilitating expression of their feeling (for more detailed discussion of PTSD see chapter 39 ∞).

Although reactions and steps of attachment are altered by the birth of these infants, a healthy parent-child relationship can occur. Kaplan and Mason (1974) identified four psychologic tasks as essential for coping with the stress of an at-risk newborn and for providing a basis for the maternal-infant relationship:

1. Anticipatory grief as a psychologic preparation for possible loss of the child while still hoping for his or her survival.
2. Acknowledgment of maternal failure to produce a term or perfect newborn expressed as anticipatory grief and depression and lasting until the chances of survival seem secure.
3. Resumption of the process of relating to the infant, which was interrupted by the threat of nonsurvival. This task may be impaired by a continuous threat of death or abnormality, and the mother may be slow in her response of hope for the infant's survival.
4. Understanding of the special needs and growth patterns of the at-risk newborn, which are temporary and yield to normal patterns.

Solnit and Stark (1961) postulated that grief and mourning of the loss of the loved object—the idealized child—mark parental reactions to an infant with abnormalities. *Grief work,* the emotional reaction to significant loss, must occur before adequate attachment to the actual baby is possible. Parental detachment precedes parental attachment. The parents must first grieve the loss of the wished-for perfect child, and then must adopt the imperfect child as the new love object.

Parental responses to an infant with health problems may also be viewed as a five-stage process (Klaus & Kennell, 1982):

1. *Shock* is felt at the reality of the birth of this baby. This stage may be characterized by forgetfulness, amnesia of the situation, and a feeling of desperation.
2. *Denial* is expressed as disbelief of the reality of the situation, characterized by a refusal to believe the child has a problem. This stage is exemplified by assertions such as, "It didn't really happen!" "There has been a mistake; it's someone else's baby."
3. *Depression* over the reality of the situation and a corresponding grief reaction follows acceptance of the situation. This stage is characterized by much crying and sadness. Anger may also occur at this stage. A projection of blame on others or on self and feelings of "why me?" are characteristic of this stage.
4. *Equilibrium and acceptance* are characteristic of a decrease in the emotional reactions of the parents. This stage is variable and may be prolonged because of the continuing threat to the infant's survival. Some parents experience chronic sorrow in relation to their child.
5. *Reorganization* of the family is necessary to deal with the child's problems. Mutual support of the parents facilitates this process, but the crisis of the situation may precipitate alienation between the mother and father.

Postpartum depression occurs in new mothers from 10% to 15% of the time, and rates can be as high as 28% to 70% in mothers with babies in the NICU. Maternal depression can have a negative impact on attachment with the newborn (Mounts, 2009). Fathers also may suffer from depression both before and after the births of their children, adding to the discord in the family unit and compounding the perceived stress experienced by the mothers.

Developmental Consequences

The baby who is born prematurely, is ill, or has a malformation or disorder is at risk for emotional, intellectual, and cognitive development delays. The risk is directly proportional to the seriousness of the problem and the length of treatment. The necessary physical separation of family and infant and the tremendous emotional and financial burdens adversely affect the parent-child relationship. The recent trend to involve the parents with the newborn early, repeatedly, and over protracted periods of time has done much to facilitate positive parent-child relationships.

The parents must have a clear picture of the reality of the disability and the types of developmental hurdles ahead. Unexpected behaviors and responses from the baby because of his or her problem or disorder can be upsetting and frightening. The demands of care for the child and disputes regarding management or behavior stress family relationships. The entire multidisciplinary team may need to pool their resources and expertise to help parents of children born with problems or disorders so that both parents and children can thrive.

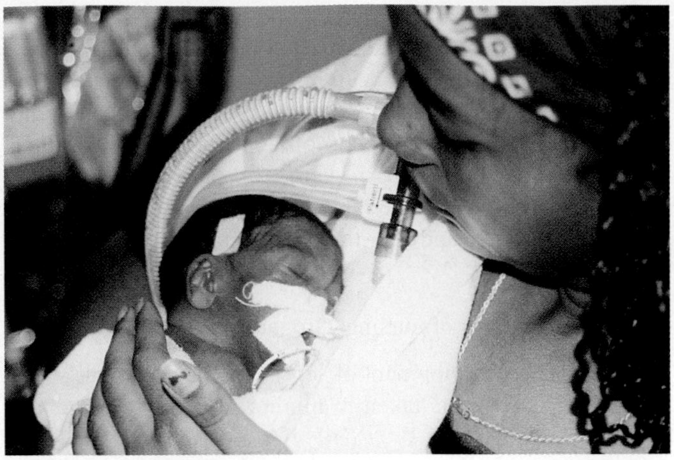

Figure 34-18 ■ Mother of a 26 weeks' gestational age infant with respiratory distress syndrome on a ventilator is getting acquainted with her baby. Physical contact is vital to the bonding process and should be encouraged whenever possible.

Source: Courtesy of Lisa Smith-Pedersen, RN, MSN, NNP-BC.

Early and continued involvement may only mean opportunities to look at or stroke the baby (Figure 34-18 ■). Later, when the mother's and baby's conditions warrant it, the mother should participate in her baby's care (to the extent she is willing) and in planning for the future. This type of involvement facilitates early bonding, attachment, and emotional investment. The parents need a sense of personal success, self-worth, self-esteem, and confidence from the knowledge that they can cope with the situation.

A variety of behavioral patterns may occur. For example, one or more members of the family may make a scapegoat of the child. Another may become the youngster's champion to the exclusion of others. One or the other spouse may feel pushed aside or denied attention and thus may withdraw or leave the family unit. Parents or siblings may feel that their own needs (schooling, material goods, and freedom of movement) are being set aside while all assets (financial and other) go to support the one child's needs. Also there may be an increase in child abuse.

NURSING CARE MANAGEMENT

Nursing Assessment and Diagnosis

A concurrent illness of the mother or other family members or other concurrent stress (lack of health insurance, loss of job, age of parents) may change the family response to the baby. Feelings of apprehension, guilt, failure, and grief that are verbally or nonverbally expressed are important aspects of the nursing history. These observations enable all professionals to be aware of the parental state, coping behaviors, and readiness for attachment, bonding, and caretaking. Appropriate nursing assessments during interviewing and relating to the family include the following:

1. ***Level of understanding.*** Observations concerning the family's ability to assimilate information given and to ask appropriate questions; the need for constant repetition of information.

2. ***Behavioral responses.*** Appropriateness of behavior in relation to information given; lack of response; flat affect.
3. ***Difficulties with communication.*** Deafness (reads lips only); blindness; dysphasia; understanding only a non-English language.
4. ***Paternal and maternal education level.*** Parents who are unable to read or write; parents with eighth-grade–level education; parents with a graduate-level degree or health-care background.

Documentation of such information, gathered through continuing contact and development of a therapeutic family relationship, lets all professionals understand and use the nursing history to provide continuous individualized care.

A record of visits, caretaking procedures, affect (in relating to the newborn), and telephone calls indicates the level or lack of parental attachment. Serial observations, rather than just isolated observations that cause concern, must be obtained. Grant (1978) developed a conceptual framework depicting adaptive and maladaptive responses to parenting of a preterm or less-than-perfect infant (Figure 34-19 ■).

If a pattern of distancing behaviors evolves, the nurse should institute appropriate intervention. Follow-up studies have found that a statistically significant number of preterm, sick, and congenitally defective infants suffer from failure to thrive, battering, or other disorders of parenting. Early detection and intervention may prevent these aberrations in parenting behaviors from leading to irreparable damage or death.

Nursing diagnoses that may apply to the family of a newborn at risk include the following:

- ***Complicated Grieving*** related to loss of idealized newborn
- ***Fear*** related to emotional involvement with an at-risk newborn
- ***Impaired Parenting*** related to impaired bonding secondary to feelings of inadequacy about caretaking activities

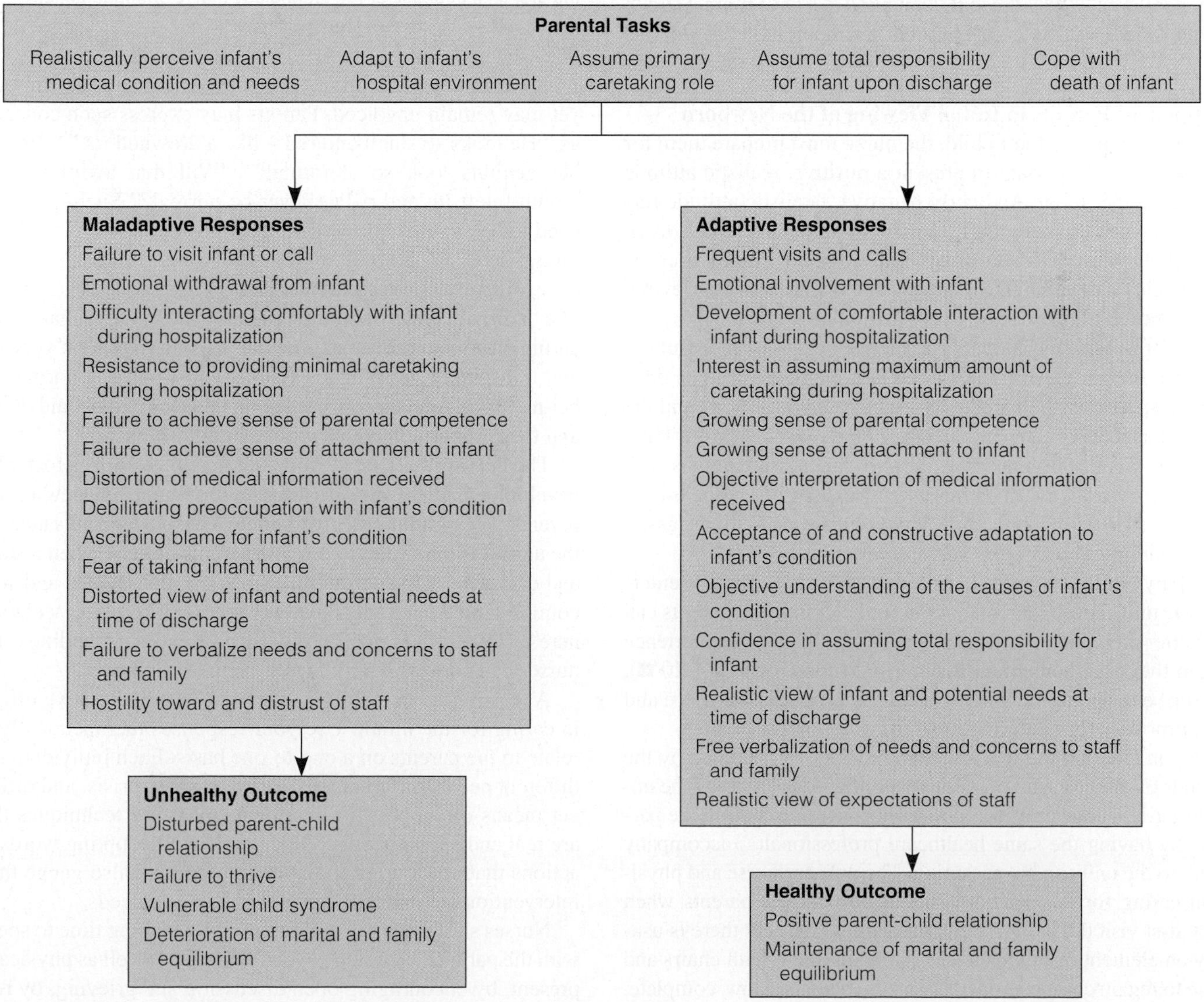

Figure 34-19 ■ Maladaptive and adaptive parental responses during crisis period, showing unhealthy and healthy outcomes.

Source: From P. Grant, Family & community health, *p. 11, fig. 1. Copyright © 1978 Lippincott Williams & Wilkins.*

Nursing Plan and Implementation

Hospital-Based Nursing Care

In their sensitive and vulnerable state, parents are acutely perceptive about others' responses and reactions (particularly nonverbal) to the child. Parents can be expected to identify with the responses of others. Therefore, it is imperative that medical and nursing staff be fully aware of the parents' feelings and come to terms with their own feelings so that they are comfortable and at ease with the baby and the grieving family.

Nurses may feel uncomfortable not knowing what to say to parents or may fear confronting their own feelings as well as those of the parents. Each nurse must work out personal reactions with instructors, peers, clergy, parents, or significant others. It is helpful to have a stockpile of therapeutic questions and statements to initiate meaningful dialog with parents. Opening statements can be as follows: "You must be wondering what could have caused this"; "Are you thinking that you (or someone else) may have done something?"; "How can I help?"; and, "Are you wondering how you are going to manage?" Avoid statements such as, "It could have been worse"; "It's God's will"; "You have other children"; "You are still young and can have more"; and "I understand how you feel." This child is important now.

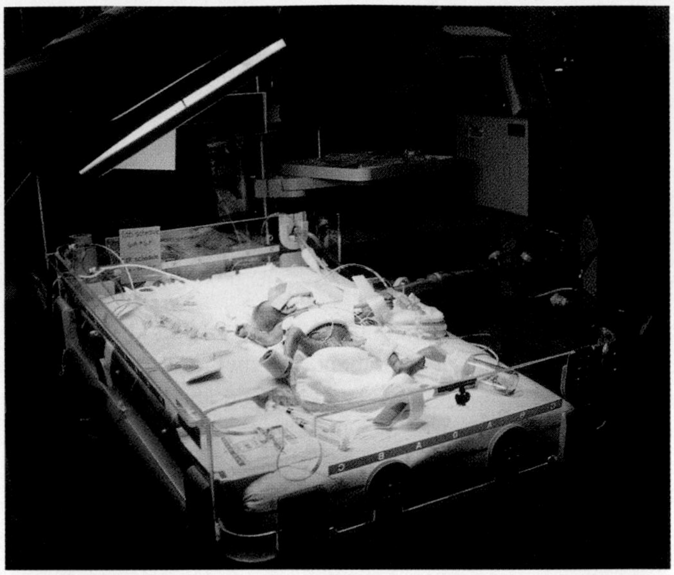

Figure 34-20 ■ This 25 weeks' gestational age infant with respiratory distress syndrome may be frightening for her parents to see for the first time because of the technology that is attached to her.

Source: Courtesy of Lisa Smith-Pedersen, RN, MSN, NNP-BC.

Support of Parents in Initial Viewing of the Newborn

Before parents see their child, the nurse must prepare them for the visit. It is important to present a positive, realistic attitude regarding the infant. An overly negative, fatalistic attitude further alienates the parents from their infant and retards attachment behaviors. Instead of beginning to bond with their child, the parents will anticipate their loss and the process of grieving. Once started, this process is very difficult to reverse.

Before preparing parents for the first view of their infant, observe the baby. All infants exhibit strengths as well as deficiencies; prepare the parents to see both the deviations and the normal aspects of their infant. The nurse may say, "Your baby is small, about the length of my two hands. She weighs 2 lb 3 oz but is very active and cries when we disturb her. She is having some difficulty breathing but is breathing without assistance and in only 35% oxygen and room air is 21%."

Many NICUs have booklets for parents to read before entering the unit. Through explanations and pictures, the parents can be better prepared to deal with the feelings they may experience when they see their infant for the first time (Figure 34-20 ■). Describe the equipment being used for the at-risk newborn and its purpose before entering the unit.

Upon entering the unit, parents may be overwhelmed by the sounds of monitors, alarms, and respirators, as well as by the unfamiliar language and "foreign" atmosphere. Preparing the parents by having the same healthcare professional(s) accompany them to the unit can be reassuring. The primary nurse and physician caring for the newborn should be with the parents when they first visit the baby. Parental reactions vary, but there is usually an element of initial shock. Providing them with chairs and time to regain composure will assist the parents. Slow, complete, and simple explanations—first about the infant and then about the equipment—allay fear and anxiety.

Concern about the infant's physical appearance is common, yet may remain unvoiced. Parents may express such concerns as, "He looks so small and red—like a drowned rat." "Why do her genitals look so abnormal?" "Will that awful looking mouth [cleft lip and palate] ever be normal?" Such questions need to be anticipated by the nurse and addressed. Use of pictures, such as a photo of an infant after cleft lip repair, may be reassuring to doubting parents. Knowledge of the development of a "normal" preterm infant will allow the nurse to make reassuring statements such as "The baby's skin may look very red and transparent with lots of visible veins, but it is normal for her maturity. As she grows, subcutaneous fat will be laid down, and these superficial veins will begin to disappear."

The nursing staff set the tone of the NICU. Nurses foster the development of a safe, trusting environment by viewing the parents as essential caregivers, not as visitors or nuisances in the unit. It is important to provide parents privacy when needed and easy access to staff and facilities. An uncrowded and welcoming atmosphere lets parents know, "You are welcome here." However, even in crowded physical surroundings, the nurses can convey an attitude of openness and trust.

A trusting relationship is essential for collaborative efforts in caring for the infant. Use your responses therapeutically to relate to the parents on a one-to-one basis. Each individual has different needs, different ways of adapting to crisis, and different means of support. Professionals must use techniques that are real and spontaneous to them and avoid adopting words or actions that are foreign to them. Nurses must also gauge their interventions to match the parents' pace and needs.

Nurses show concern and support by planning time to spend with the parents, by being psychologically as well as physically present, by encouraging open discussion and grieving, by repetitious explanations (as necessary), by providing privacy as needed, and by encouraging contact with the newborn. Identifying and clarifying feelings and fears decrease distortions in perception, thinking, and feeling. Nurses invest the baby with value in the eyes of the parents when they provide meticulous care to the newborn, talk and coo (especially in the face-to-face position) while holding or providing care to the newborn, and relate the newborn's activities ("He took a whole ounce of formula"; "She took hold of the blanket and just wouldn't let go"). Nurses should note the "normal" characteristics and capabilities of each newborn as well as the newborn's needs. The nurse should also learn the baby's name and refer to him or her by name. When the baby is physiologically stable and of an appropriate weight, allowing the baby to be dressed in clothes has been determined to aid the mother in perceiving the baby as a "person" or "actual baby" (Bosque & Haverman, 2009).

Facilitation of Attachment If Neonatal Transport Occurs
Transport to a regional referral center some distance from the parents' community may be necessary. It is essential that the mother see and touch her infant before the infant is transported. Bringing the mother to the nursery or taking the infant in a warmed transport incubator to the mother's bedside will allow her to see the infant before transportation to the center. When the infant reaches the referral center, a staff member should call the parents with information about the infant's condition during transport, safe arrival at the center, and present condition.

Support of parents, with explanations from the professional staff, is crucial. Occasionally, the mother may be unable to see the infant before transport, for example, if she is still under general anesthesia or experiencing postpartum complications such as shock, hemorrhage, or seizures. In these cases, take a photograph of the infant to give to the mother, and provide an explanation of the infant's condition and problems and a detailed description of the infant's characteristics. An additional photograph is also helpful for the father to share with siblings or the extended family. With the increased attention to improved fetal outcome, prenatal maternal transports, rather than neonatal transports, are occurring more frequently. This practice gives the mother of an at-risk infant the opportunity to visit and care for her infant during the early postpartal period.

Promotion of Touching and Parental Caretaking
Parents visiting a small or sick infant may need several visits to become comfortable and confident in their abilities to touch the infant without injuring her or him. Barriers such as incubators, incisions, monitor electrodes, and tubes may delay the mother's development of comfort in touching the newborn.

Klaus and Kennell (1982) found a significant difference in the amount of eye contact and touching behaviors of mothers of normal newborns and mothers of preterm infants. Whereas mothers of normal newborns progress within minutes to palm contact of the infant's trunk, the mother of a preterm infant is slower to progress from fingertip to palm contact and from the extremities to the trunk. The progression to palm contact with the infant's trunk may take several visits to the nursery.

Through use of support, reassurance, and encouragement, the nurse can facilitate the mother's positive feelings about her ability and her importance to her infant. Touching facilitates "getting to know" the infant and thus establishes a bond with the infant. Touching as well as seeing the infant helps the mother to realize the "normals" and potentials of her baby (Figure 34-21 ■).

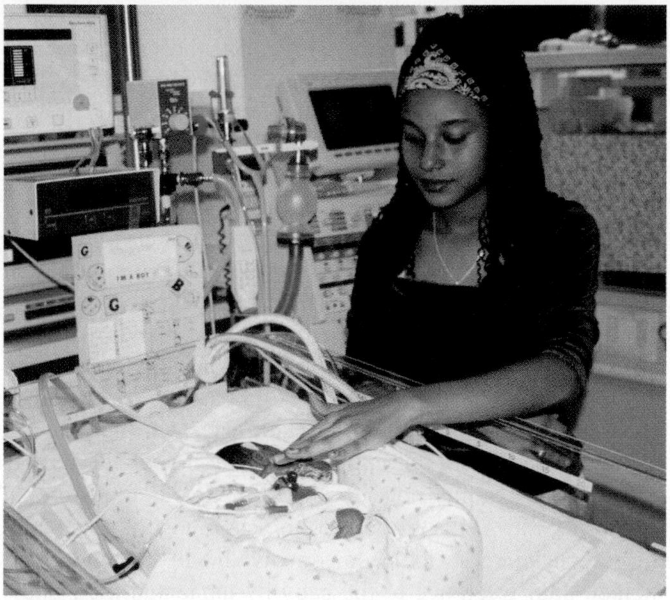

Figure 34-21 ■ Mother of this 26 weeks' gestational age 600-g baby begins attachment through fingertip touch.

Source: Courtesy of Lisa Smith-Pedersen, RN, MSN, NNP-BC.

The nurse can also encourage parents to meet their newborn's need for stimulation. Stroking, rocking, cuddling, singing, and talking should be an integral part of the parents' caretaking responsibilities. Bonding can be facilitated by encouraging parents to visit and become involved in their baby's care (Figure 34-22 ■). When visiting is impossible, the parents should feel free to phone whenever they wish to receive information about their baby. A nurse's warm, receptive attitude provides support. Facilitate parenting by personalizing a baby to the parents, by referring to the infant by name, or relating personal behavioral characteristics. Statements such as, "Jenny loves her pacifier," help make the infant seem individual and unique.

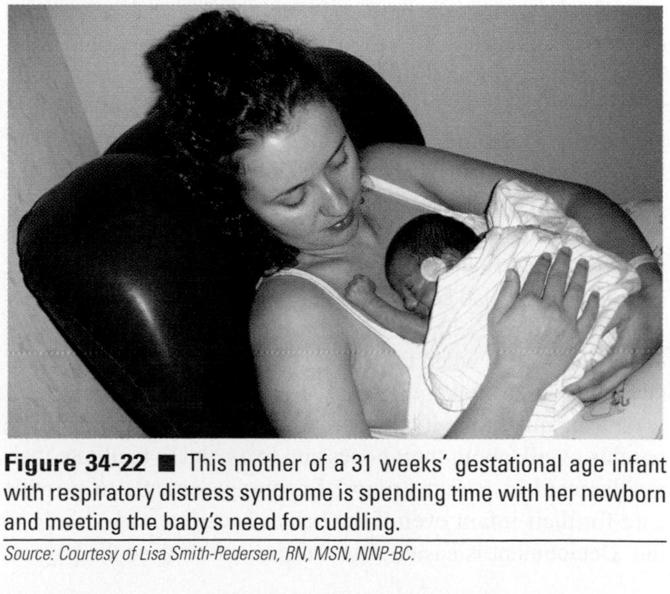

Figure 34-22 ■ This mother of a 31 weeks' gestational age infant with respiratory distress syndrome is spending time with her newborn and meeting the baby's need for cuddling.

Source: Courtesy of Lisa Smith-Pedersen, RN, MSN, NNP-BC.

The variety of equipment needed for life support is hardly conducive to anxiety-free caretaking by the parents. However, even the sickest infant may be cared for, if only in a small way, by the parents. As a facilitator of parental caretaking, the nurse should promote the parents' success. Demonstration and explanation, followed by support of the parents in initial caretaking behaviors, positively reinforce this behavior. Changing the infant's diaper, giving their infant skin care or oral care, or helping the nurse turn the infant may at first be anxiety provoking for the parents, but they will become more comfortable and confident in caretaking and receive satisfaction from the baby's reactions and their ability "to do something." Complimenting the parents' competence in caretaking also increases their self-esteem, which has received recent "blows" of guilt and failure. It is vitally important that the parents never be given a task if there is any possibility they will not be able to accomplish it. Cues that the parents are ready to become involved with the child's care include their reference to the baby by name and their questioning as to amount of feeding taken, sleeping patterns, appearance today, and the like.

Often parents of high-risk infants have ambivalent feelings toward the nurse. These feelings may take the form of criticism of the care of the infant, manipulation of staff, or personal guilt. The nurse should accept this behavior but continue to remind the parents that it is okay and natural to feel disappointment, a sense of failure, helplessness, or anger about the birth. The overprotectiveness and over-optimism are defense mechanisms. To deny the negative feelings only entrenches them further, delays their resolution, and delays realistic planning. Instead of fostering (by silence) these inferiority feelings within mothers, nurses should recognize such feelings and intervene appropriately to enhance mother-infant attachment. The nurse needs to deal with ambivalent feelings that contribute to a competitive atmosphere. For example, the nurse should avoid making unfavorable comparisons between the baby's response to parental and nursing caretaking. Verbalizations that improve parental self-esteem are essential and easily shared. The nurse can point out that, in addition to physiologic use, breast milk is important because of the emotional investment of the mother. Pumping, storing, labeling, and delivering quantities of breast milk is time-consuming and a "labor of love" for mothers. Positive remarks regarding breast milk reinforce the maternal behavior of caretaking and providing for her infant: "Breast milk is something that only you can give your baby" or "You really have brought a lot of milk today" or "Even small amounts of milk are important, and look how rich it is."

If the infant begins to gain weight while being fed breast milk, it is important to point this correlation out to the mother. Parents should also be advised that initial weight loss with beginning nipple feedings is common because of the increased energy expended when the infant begins active rather than passive nutritional intake.

During quiet time it may help for the nurse to encourage the parents to talk about their hopes and fears and to facilitate their involvement in parent groups. Encourage parents to provide care for their infant even if the baby is very sick and likely to die. Detachment is easier after attachment because the parents are comforted by the knowledge that they did all they could for their child while he or she was alive.

Facilitation of Family Adjustment

During crisis, maintaining interpersonal relationships is difficult. Yet in a newborn intensive care area, the parents are expected to relate to many different care providers. It is important that parents have as few professionals as possible relaying information to them. A primary nurse should coordinate and provide continuity for parents. Care providers are individuals and thus will use different terms, inflections, and attitudes. These subtle differences are monumental to parents and only confuse, confound, and produce anxiety. The transfer of the baby from the NICU to a step-down unit or a "regular nursery" or transport back to the home hospital is very anxiety producing for the parents because they must now deal with new healthcare professionals. They may feel that their infant is not being cared for as proficiently because the nurses are not at the bedside as often as they were in the NICU. The nurse not only functions as a liaison between the parents and the wide variety of professionals interacting with the infant and parents, but also offers clarification, explanation, interpretation of information, and support to the parents.

The nurse encourages the parents to deal with the crisis with help from their support system. The support system attempts to meet the emotional needs and provide support for the family members in crisis and stress situations. Biologic kinship is not the only valid criterion for a support system; an emotional kinship is the most important factor. In our mobile society of isolated nuclear families, the support system may be a next-door neighbor, a best friend, or perhaps a schoolmate. The nurse must search out the significant others in the lives of the parents and help them understand the problems so that they can support the parents.

The impact of the crisis on the family is individual and varied. The nurse obtains information about the family's ability to adapt to the situation through the relationship with the family. To institute appropriate interventions, the nurse should view the birth of the infant (normal newborn, preterm infant, or infant with illness or congenital anomaly) as defined by the family. Because the family is a unit composed of individuals who must deal with the situation, it is important to encourage open intrafamily communication. The nurse should discourage the family from keeping secrets from one another, especially between spouses, because secrets undermine the trust of their relationship. Well-meaning rationales such as, "I want to protect her," "I don't want him to worry about it," and so on, can be destructive to open communication and to the basic element of a relationship—trust.

Open communication is especially important when the mother is hospitalized apart from the infant. The first person to visit the infant relays information regarding the infant's care and condition to the mother and family. In this situation, the mother has had minimal contact, if any, with her infant. Because of her anxiety and isolation, she may mistrust all those who provide information (the nurse, physician, father, or extended family) until she can see the infant for herself. This can put tremendous stress on the relationship between the mother and father. The parents (and family) should be given information together. This practice helps overcome misunderstandings and misinterpretations and promotes mutual "working through" of problems.

The needs of siblings should not be overlooked. Siblings have been looking forward to the new baby, and they too suffer a degree of loss. Young children may react with hostility and older ones with shame at the birth of an infant with an anomaly. Both reactions make them feel guilty. Parents, preoccupied with working through their own feelings, often cannot give the other children the attention and support they need. Sometimes another child becomes the focus of family tension. Anxiety thus directed can take the form of finding fault or of overconcern. This is a form of denial; the parents cannot face the real worry—the infant at risk. After assessing the situation, the observant nurse could see to it that another family member or friend step in and give the needed support to the siblings of the affected baby.

The nurse must respect and facilitate the desires and needs of the individuals involved; differences are tolerable and should be able to exist side by side. The nurse can easily elicit the parents' feelings and the meaning of this experience to them by asking, "How are you doing?" The emphasis is on "you," and the interest must be sincere.

Parents from minority cultures must deal with language barriers and cultural differences that can make feelings of isolation and uncertainty more acute. Healthcare providers have the professional responsibility to be aware of cultural needs of all patients and to ensure that their needs are met. Feelings of isolation and uncertainty influence not only the parent's emotional responses to the ill newborn, but also their use of services and their interaction with health professionals. Hospital cultural interpreter programs can assist families with interactions with staff and provide translation during family meetings, multidisciplinary family conferences, and parent support groups (Lipson & Dibble, 2008).

Families with children in the NICU become friends and support one another. To encourage the development of these friendships and to provide support, many units have established parent groups. The core of the groups consists of parents who previously have had an infant in the intensive care unit. Most groups make contact with families within a day or two of the infant's admission to the unit, either through phone calls or visits to the hospital. Early one-on-one parent contacts are more effective than discussion groups in helping families work through their feelings. This personalized method gives the grieving parents an opportunity to share personal feelings about the pregnancy, labor, and birth and their "different from expected" infant with others who have experienced the same feelings and with whom they can identify.

Community-Based Nursing Care

Predischarge planning begins once the infant's condition becomes stable and indications suggest the newborn will survive. Discharge preparation and care conferences should involve a multidisciplinary team approach. The NICU nursing staff is the fulcrum for aiding in the transition of high-risk infants from the intensive care unit to the home. Effective open communication with the families during the entire discharge-planning phase of care empowers the families to assume the role of primary caregiver for their children.

Adequate predischarge teaching helps parents transform any feelings of inadequacy they may have into feelings of self-assurance and attachment. From the beginning the parents should be taught about their infant's special needs and growth patterns. This teaching and involvement are best facilitated by a nurse who is familiar with the infant and his or her family over a period of time and who has developed a comfortable and supportive relationship with them.

Cobedding of twins is often used in the NICU to provide comfort, decrease stress to the twins, and provide a form of developmentally supportive care. Cobedding is also a strategy to maximize the synchronization of sleep-wake cycles (Gardner & Goldson, 2011). Parents of multiples may desire cobedding at home to allow for clustering of care and to facilitate the parents' ability to spend time with both of their children (Figure 34-23 ■). If twins or other multiples experienced cobedding in the NICU, the nurse needs to discuss the advantages and disadvantages of continuing the practice at home. Currently, there is no evidence to establish cobedding of multiples outside the NICU as a safe or unsafe sleep practice (Gardner & Goldson, 2011). The high incidence of prematurity and low birth weight (LBW) in multiple-birth infants and the corresponding risks for sudden infant death syndrome (SIDS) should be considered. As with all families at discharge, parents of multiples should be taught SIDS risk-reduction practices. SIDS reduction practices include supine positioning, babies sleeping in parents' room, firm bedding surface, no loose coverings/items, and no barriers between infants (Bowers et al., 2008).

The nurse's responsibility is to provide home care instructions in an optimal environment for parental learning. Learning should take place over time, to avoid the necessity of bombarding the parents with instructions in the day or hour before discharge. Parents often enjoy doing minimal caretaking tasks with gradual expansion of their role. Many NICUs provide facilities for parents to room in with their infants for a few days before discharge. This

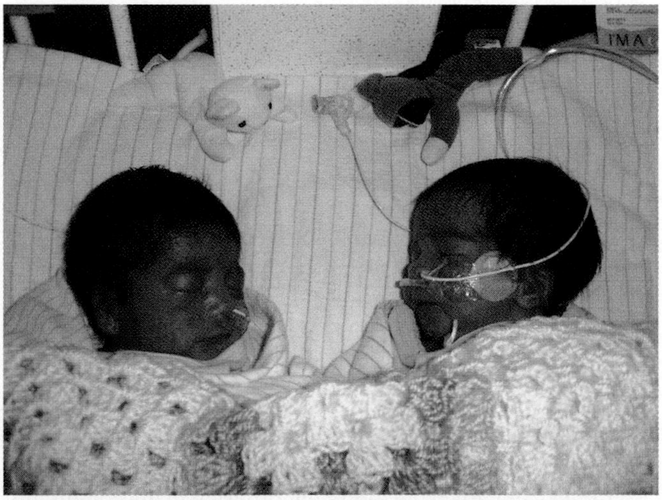

Figure 34-23 ■ Cobedding of twins facilitates delivery of care and parent interaction with healthcare members. These twins were born at 33 weeks' gestation and required oxygen and gavage feeding while in the NICU.

Source: Courtesy of Lisa Smith-Pedersen, RN, MSN, NNP-BC.

allows parents a degree of independence in the care of their infant with the security of nursing help nearby. This practice is particularly helpful for anxious parents, parents who have not had the opportunity to spend extended time with their infant, or parents who will be giving complex physical care at home, such as gastrostomy feeding and care (Collins, Makrides, & McPhee, 2008).

The families are able to interact with the staff while gradually transitioning to sole caretakers of their medically complex high-risk infant. When discharging a medically fragile infant to home, schedule a predischarge home visit by a public health nurse or home health agency. This predischarge visit evaluates the home for any possible issues that may complicate the parents' ability to care for their at-risk infant, especially if there are multiple monitoring equipment needs.

The basic elements of discharge and home care instruction are as follows:

1. Teach parents routine well-baby care, such as bathing, taking a temperature, preparing formula, and/or breastfeeding.
2. Help parents learn to do special procedures as needed by the newborn, such as gavage or gastrostomy feedings, tracheostomy or enterostomy care, medication administration, cardiopulmonary resuscitation (CPR), and operation of an apnea monitor or any required medical equipment. Before discharge, the parents should be as comfortable as possible with these tasks and should demonstrate independence. Written tools and instructions are useful for parents to refer to once they are home with the infant, but they should not replace actual predischarge participation in the infant's care.
3. Make sure that all applicable screening (metabolic, vision, hearing) tests, immunizations, and respiratory syncytial virus (RSV) prophylaxis are done before discharge and that all records are given to the primary care provider and parents.
4. Refer parents to community health and support organizations. The Visiting Nurses Association, public health nurses, or social services can assist the parents in the stressful transition from hospital to home by providing predischarge home visits and then the necessary home teaching and support. Some NICUs have their own parent support groups to help bridge the gap between hospital and home care. Parents can also find support from a variety of community support organizations, such as mothers of twins groups, March of Dimes Birth Defects Foundation, handicapped children services, and teen mother and child programs. Each community has numerous agencies capable of assisting the family in adapting emotionally, physically, and financially to the chronically ill infant. The nurse should be familiar with community resources and help the parents identify which agencies may benefit them.
5. Help parents recognize the growth and development needs of their infant. A developmental care program begun in the hospital can be continued at home, or parents may be referred to an infant development program in the community.
6. Arrange medical follow-up care before discharge. The infant will need to be followed up by a family pediatrician, a well-baby clinic, or a specialty clinic. The first appointment should be made before the infant is discharged from the hospital.

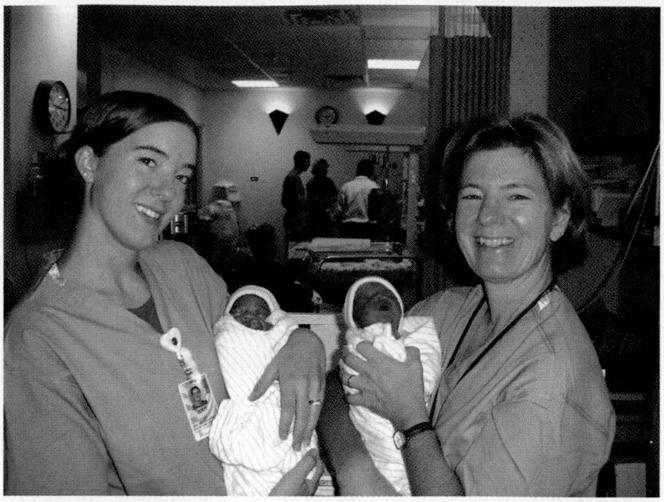

Figure 34-24 ■ Twins on the happy day of discharge, being held by staff in the NICU. This is what is so rewarding about working in the NICU: healthy babies going home to their families.

Source: Courtesy of Lisa Smith-Pedersen, RN, MSN, NNP-BC.

7. Evaluate the need for durable medical equipment for infant care (such as a respirator, oxygen, apnea monitor, feeding pump) in the home. Any extra equipment or supplies should be placed in the home before the infant's discharge.
8. Arrange for neonatal hospice for parents of the medically fragile infant, as needed.

According to a study by Sneath (2009) parents of NICU graduates do not feel adequately prepared for discharge from the NICU with their babies. Teaching that occurs with daily interaction of the NICU staff is not always perceived by the family as adequate, and the stress levels of the family while in the NICU can be a barrier to a learning environment.

Further evaluation after the infant has gone home is useful in determining whether the crisis has been resolved satisfactorily. The parents are usually given the intensive care nursery's telephone number to call for support and advice. The staff can follow up each family with visits or telephone calls at intervals for several weeks to assess and evaluate the infant's (and parents') progress (Figure 34-24 ■).

Evaluation

Expected outcomes of nursing care include the following:

- The parents are able to verbalize their feelings of grief and loss.
- The parents verbalize their concerns about their baby's health problems, care needs, and potential outcome.
- The parents are able to participate in their infant's care and show attachment behaviors.

Considerations for the Nurse Who Works with At-Risk Newborns

The birth of a baby with a problem is a traumatic event with the potential for either disruption or growth of the involved family. The neonatal intensive care unit (NICU) staff nurses may never see the long-term results of the specialized, sensitive care they give to parents and their newborns. Their only immediate evidence of effective care may be the beginning of resolution of parental grief; discharge of a recovered, thriving infant to the care of happy parents; and the beginning of reintegration of family life.

Nurses cannot provide support unless they themselves are supported. Working in an emotional environment of "lots of living and lots of dying" takes its toll on staff. NICUs are among the most stressful areas in health care for patients, families, and nurses. Nurses bear most of the stress and largely determine the atmosphere of the NICU. The nurse's ability to cope with stress is the key to creating an emotionally healthy environment and a positive working atmosphere. The emotional needs and feelings of the staff must be recognized and dealt with to enable them to support the parents. An environment of openness to feelings and support in dealing with their own human needs and emotions is essential for the staff.

As caregivers, nurses may be unaware of their need to grieve for their own losses in the NICU. Working with babies for hours, days, weeks, and sometimes months can foster intimate attachments of the nurses with the baby and family. Nurses must also go through the grief work that parents experience, and they first have to be comfortable with their own feelings about death (Lisle-Porter & Podruchny, 2009). Techniques such as group meetings, individual support, and doing primary care nursing may assist in maintaining staff mental health. Reunions in some nurseries are beneficial for the families and healthcare professionals so they are able to see the children after discharge.

FOCUS YOUR STUDY

- The sick newborn—whether preterm, term, or postterm—must be managed within narrow physiologic parameters.
- These parameters (respiratory, cardiovascular, and thermal regulation) will maintain physiologic homeostasis and prevent introduction of iatrogenic stress to the already stressed infant.
- The nursing care of the newborn with special problems involves understanding normal physiology, the pathophysiology of the disease process, clinical manifestations, and supportive or corrective therapies. Only with this theoretic background can the nurse make appropriate observations concerning responses to therapy and development of complications.
- Asphyxia results in significant circulatory, respiratory, and biochemical changes in the newborn that make the successful transition to extrauterine life difficult. Asphyxia requires early identification and resuscitative management.
- Newborn conditions that commonly present with respiratory distress and require oxygen and ventilatory assistance are respiratory distress syndrome (RDS), transient tachypnea of the newborn, meconium aspiration syndrome (MAS), and persistent pulmonary hypertension of the newborn (PPHN).
- Management of respiratory problems can result in further respiratory compromising conditions such as pulmonary interstitial emphysema, pneumothorax, and bronchopulmonary dysplasia (BPD)/chronic lung disease (CLD).
- Cold stress sets up the chain of physiologic events of hypoglycemia, pulmonary vasoconstriction, hyperbilirubinemia, respiratory distress, and metabolic acidosis.
- Nurses are responsible for early detection and initiation of treatment for hypoglycemia.
- Differentiation between pathologic and physiologic jaundice is key to early and successful intervention.
- Anemia (decreased amount of red blood cell volume) or polycythemia (excess amount) place the newborn at risk for alterations in blood flow and the oxygen-carrying capacity of the blood.
- Nursing assessment of the septic newborn involves identifying very subtle clinical signs that are also seen in other clinical disease states.
- The nurse is the facilitator for interdisciplinary communication with the parents, identifying their understanding of their infant's care and their needs for emotional support.
- Parents of at-risk newborns need support from nurses and healthcare providers to understand the special needs of their baby and to feel comfortable in an overwhelming and often unfamiliar environment.

CRITICAL THINKING IN ACTION

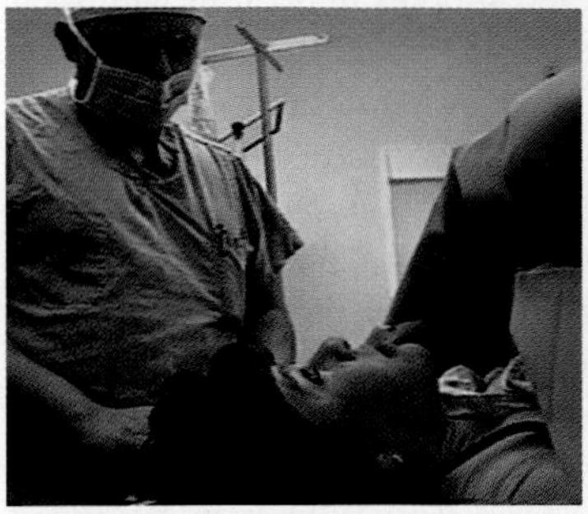

Rebecca Prince, age 21, G2 now P2, gives birth to a 5 pound baby at 38 weeks' gestation by primary cesarean birth for nonreassuring fetal status. The infant's Apgars are 7 and 9 at 1 and 5 minutes. The infant is suctioned and given free-flow oxygen at birth, then is admitted to the newborn nursery for transitional care and does well. You are the nurse caring for baby Prince at 36 hours old. You review the newborn's record and note that the baby's blood type is A+ and his mother is O+. Rebecca wants to breastfeed. You are performing a shift assessment on baby Prince when you observe that the infant has a unilateral cephalhematoma and is lethargic. You blanch the skin over the sternum and observe a yellow discoloration of the skin. Lab tests reveal a serum bilirubin level of 12 mg/dl, hematocrit 55%, a mildly positive direct Coombs' test, and a positive indirect Coombs' test. Baby Prince is diagnosed with hyperbilirubinemia secondary to ABO incompatibility and cephalhematoma. You provide phototherapy by fiberoptic blanket around the trunk of the infant and take the baby to his mother's room.

1. How would you explain the purpose of phototherapy with the mother?
2. Plot the bilirubin on the hour specific nomogram to assess the zone.
3. Explain the follow-up laboratory testing required, and when it will be required.
4. Discuss the advantage of the fiberoptic blanket phototherapy for the newborn.
5. Describe the care the mother can give to the newborn.

See www.nursing.pearsonhighered.com for possible responses.

Pearson Nursing Student Resources

Find additional review materials at
www.nursing.pearsonhighered.com

Prepare for success with additional NCLEX®-style practice questions, interactive assignments and activities, Web links, animations and videos, and more!

REFERENCES

Aher, S., Malwatkar, K., & Kadam, S. (2008). Neonatal anemia. *Seminars in Fetal & Neonatal Medicine 13*(4), 239–247.

American Academy of Pediatrics (AAP), Committee on Fetus and Newborn, & American College of Obstetricians and Gynecologists (ACOG), Committee on Obstetrics. (2007). *Guidelines for perinatal care* (6th ed.). Evanston, IL: Author.

Angert, R., & Adam, H. M. (2009). Care of the very low-birthweight infant. *Pediatrics in Review, 30*(1), 32–35. doi:10.1542/pir.30-1-32

Askin, D. (2009). Fetal-to-neonatal transition—What is normal and what is not? Part 1: The physiology of transition. *Neonatal Network, 28*(3), e33–e36.

Baumgart, S. (2008). Iatrogenic hyperthermia and hypothermia in the neonate. *Clinics in Perinatology, 35*(1), 183–197. doi:10.1016/j.clp.2007.11.002

Bell, S. G. (2008). Vancomycin prophylaxis for late-onset sepsis in very low and extremely low birth weight neonates, *Neonatal Network, 27*(5), 351–354.

Bhutani, V. K., & Johnson, L. (2009). A proposal to prevent severe neonatal hyperbilirubinemia and kernicterus. *Journal of Perinatology, 29*, s61–s67. doi:10.1038/jp.2008.213

Bhutani, V. K., Johnson, L. H., & Keren, R. (2004). Diagnosis and management of hyperbilirubinemia in the term neonate: For a safer first week. *Pediatric Clinics of North America, 51*(4), 843–861.

Blackburn, S. T. (2007). *Maternal, fetal, & neonatal physiology: A clinical perspective* (3rd ed.). St. Louis, MO: Saunders.

Bosque, E. M., & Haverman, C. (2009). Making babies real: Dressing infants in the NICU. *Neonatal Network, 28*(2), 85–92.

Bowers, N. A., Curran, C. A., Freda, M. C., Poole, J. H., Slocum, J., & Sosa, M. E. (2008). High-risk pregnancy. In K. R. Simpson & P. A. Creehan, *AWHONN's perinatal nursing* (3rd ed., pp. 125–299). Philadelphia, PA: Lippincott Williams & Wilkins.

Bradshaw, W. T. (2010). Gastrointestinal disorders. In M. T. Verklan & M. Walden, *Core curriculum for neonatal intensive care nursing* (4th ed., pp. 589–637). St. Louis, MO: Saunders/Elsevier.

Bry, K. (2008). Newborn resuscitation and the lung. *NeoReviews, 9*(11), e506–e512.

Burke, B. L., Robbins, J. M., Bird, T. M., Hobbs, C. A., Nesmith, C., & Tilford, J. M. (2009). Trends in hospitalizations for neonatal jaundice and kernicterus in the United States, 1988–2005. *Pediatrics, 123*(2), 524–532.

Carbine, D. N., & Serwint, J. R. (2008). Meconium aspiration. *Pediatrics in Review, 29*, 212–213. doi:10.1542/pir.29-6-212

Carey, A. J., Saiman, L., & Polin, R. A. (2008). Hospital acquired infections in the NICU: Epidemiology for the new millennium, *Clinics in Perinatology, 35*(1), 223–249.

Cloherty, J. P., Eichenwald, E. C., & Stark, A. R. (2008). *Manual of neonatal care* (6th ed.). Philadelphia, PA: Lippincott Williams & Wilkins.

Collins, C. T., Makrides, M. E., & McPhee, A. J. (2008). Early discharge with home support of gavage feeding for stable preterm infants who have not established full oral feeds. *Cochrane database of systematic reviews, 2*, ID #CD003743.

Curry, S., Honeycutt, M., Goins, G., & Gilliam, C. (2009). Catheter-associated bloodstream infections in the NICU: Getting to zero. *Neonatal Network, 28*(3), 151–155.

Dalal, S. S., Mishra, S., Agarwal, R., Deorari, A. K., & Paul, V. (2009). Does measuring the changes in TcB value offer better prediction of hyperbilirubinemia in healthy neonates? *Pediatrics, 124*(5), e851–e857. doi:10.10542/peds.2008-3623

DePuy, A. M., Coassolo, K. M., Som, D. A., & Smulian, J. C. (2009). Neonatal hypoglycemia in term, nondiabetic pregnancies. *American Journal of Obstetrics and Gynecology, 200*(5), e45–e51. doi:10.1016/j.ajog.2008.10.015

Diehl-Jones, W., & Askin, D. F. (2010). Hematologic disorders. In M. T. Verklan & M. Walden, *Core curriculum for neonatal intensive care nursing* (4th ed., pp. 666–693). St. Louis, MO: Saunders/Elsevier.

Dilli, D., Kucuk, I. G., & Dallar, Y. (2009). Interventions to reduce pain during vaccination in infancy. *Journal of Pediatrics, 154*(3), 385–390. doi:10.1016/jpeds.2008.08.037

Folk, L. A. (2007). Guide to capillary heelstick blood sampling in infants. *Advances in Neonatal Care, 7*(4), 171–178. doi:10.1097/01.ANC.0000286333.67928.04

Gardner, S. L., Enzman-Hines, M., & Dickey, L. A. (2011). Pain and pain relief. In S. L. Gardner, B. S. Carter, M. Enzman-Hines, & J. A. Hernandez, *Merenstein & Gardner's Handbook of neonatal intensive care* (7th ed., pp. 223–269). St. Louis. MO: Mosby/Elsevier.

Gardner, S. L., & Goldson, E. (2011). The neonate and the environment: Impact on development. In S. L. Gardner, B. S. Carter, M. Enzman-Hines, & J. A. Hernandez, *Merenstein & Gardner's Handbook of neonatal intensive care* (7th ed., pp. 270–332). St. Louis. MO: Mosby/Elsevier.

Garland, J. S., & Uhing, M. R. (2009). Strategies to prevent bacterial and fungal infection in the neonatal intensive care unit. *Clinics in Perinatology, 36*(1), 1–13. doi:10.1016/j.clp.2008.09.005

Geary, C., Caskey, M., Fonseca, R., & Malloy, M. (2008). Decreased incidence of bronchopulmonary dysplasia after early management changes, including surfactant and nasal continuous positive airway pressure treatment at delivery, lowered oxygen saturation goals, and early amino acid administration: A historical cohort study. *Pediatrics, 121*(1), 89–96. doi:10.1542/peds.2007-0225

Gomella, T. L., Cunningham, M. D., & Eyal, F. G. (2009). *Neonatology: Management, procedures, on-call problems, diseases, and drugs* (6th ed.). New York, NY: Lange Medical Books/McGraw-Hill.

Grant, P. (1978). Psychological needs of families of high risk infants. *Family and Community Health, 1*(3), 91–102.

Guglani, L., Lakshminrusimha, S., & Ryan, R. M. (2008). Transient tachypnea of the newborn. *Pediatrics in Review, 29*(1), e59–e65. doi:10.1542/pir.29-11-e59

Hawk, M. (2008). C-Reactive protein in neonatal sepsis. *Neonatal Network, 27*(2), 117–120.

Ingemarsson, I. (2009). Fetal monitoring during labor. *Neonatology, 95*, 342–346. doi:10.1159/0000209299

Kaplan, D. M., & Mason, E. A. (1974). Maternal reactions to premature birth viewed as an acute emotional disorder. In H. J. Parad (Ed.), *Crisis intervention*. New York, NY: Family Services Association of America.

Klaus, M. H., & Kennell, J. H. (1982). *Maternal-infant bonding* (2nd ed.). St. Louis, MO: Mosby.

Konduri, G. G., & Kim, U. O. (2009). Advances in the diagnosis and management of persistent pulmonary hypertension of the newborn. *Pediatric Clinics of North America, 56*(3), 579–600. doi:10.1016/j.pcl.2009.04.004

Kuzniewicz, M. W., Escobar, G. J., & Newman, T. B. (2009). Impact of universal bilirubin screening on severe hyperbilirubinemia and phototherapy use. *Pediatrics, 124*(44), 1031–1039. doi:10.1542/peds.2008-2980

Lipson, J. G., & Dibble, S. L. (2008). *Culture & clinical care* (7th ed.). San Francisco, CA: The Regents, University of California.

Lisle-Porter, M. D., & Podruchny, A. M. (2009). The dying neonate: Family-centered end-of-life care. *Neonatal Network, 28*(2), 75–83.

Lott, J. W. (2010). Immunology and infectious disease. In M. T. Verklan & M. Walden (Eds.), *Core curriculum for neonatal intensive care nursing* (4th ed., pp. 694–723). St. Louis, MO: Elsevier/Saunders.

Maisels, M. J., Bhutani, V. K., Bogen, D., Newman, T. B., Stark, A. R., & Watchko, J. F. (2009). Hyperbilirubinemia in the newborn infant ≥35 weeks' gestation: An update with clarifications. *Pediatrics, 124*(4), 1193–1198. doi:10.1542/peds.2009-0329

Manco-Johnson, M., Rodden, D. J., & Hays, T. (2011). Newborn hematology. In S. L. Gardner, B. S. Carter, M. Enzman-Hines, & J. A. Hernandez, *Merenstein & Gardner's Handbook of neonatal intensive care* (7th ed., pp. 503–530). St. Louis. MO: Mosby/Elsevier.

Manning, D., Todd, P., Maxwell, M., & Platt, M. J. (2007). Prospective surveillance study of severe hyperbilirubinemia in the newborn in the UK and Ireland. *Archives of Disease in Childhood. Fetal and Neonatal Edition, 92*(50), f342–f346.

Miller, J. D., & Carlo, W. A. (2008). Pulmonary complications of mechanical ventilation in neonates. *Clinics in Perinatology, 35*(1), 373–381. doi:10.1016/j.clp.2007.11.004

Moerschel, S. K., Cianciaruso, L. B., & Tracy, L. R. (2008). A practical approach to neonatal jaundice. *American Family Physician, 77*(9), 1255–1262.

Mounts, K. O. (2009). Screening for maternal depression in the neonatal ICU. *Clinics in Perinatology, 36*(1), 137–152.

Nash, P., & Smith, J. R. (2008). Common neonatal complications. In K. R. Simpson & P. A. Creehan, *AWHONN's perinatal nursing* (3rd ed., pp. 612–646). Philadelphia, PA: Lippincott Williams & Wilkins.

Newman, T. B. (2009). Universal bilirubin screening, guidelines, and evidence. *Pediatrics, 124*(4), 1199–1202. doi:10.1542/peds.2009-0412

Niermeyer, S., & Clarke, S. B. (2011). Delivery room care. In S. L. Gardner, B. S. Carter, M. Enzman-Hines, & J. A. Hernandez, *Merenstein & Gardner's Handbook of neonatal intensive care* (7th ed., pp. 52–77). St. Louis. MO: Mosby/Elsevier.

Okumura, A., Kidokoro, H., Shoji, H., Nakazawa, T., Mimaki, M., Fujii, K., . . . Shimizu, T. (2009). Kernicterus in preterm infants. *Pediatrics, 123*(6), e1052–e1058. doi:10.1542/peds.2008-2791

Pacatte, K. (2008). Analysis of cerebrospinal fluid in the neonate. *Neonatal Network, 27*(6), 419–422.

Pappas, B. E., & Walker, B. (2010). Neonatal delivery room resuscitation. In M. T. Verklan & M. Walden, *Core curriculum for neonatal intensive care nursing* (4th ed., pp. 91–109). St. Louis, MO: Saunders/Elsevier.

Peterson, S. (2009). Understanding the sequence of pulmonary injury in the extremely low birth weight, surfactant-deficient infant. *Neonatal Network, 28*(4), 221–229.

Pinheiro, J. M. B. (2009). The Apgar cycle: A new view of a familiar scoring system. *Archives of Disease in Childhood. Fetal and Neonatal Edition, 94*, f70–f72. doi:10.1136/adc.2008.145037

Posner, K., & Needleman, J. (2008). Pneumothorax. *Pediatrics in Review, 29*(2), 69–70. doi:10.1542/pir.29-2-69

Puopolo, K. M. (2008). Epidemiology of neonatal early-onset sepsis. *NeoReviews, 9*(12), e571–e579. doi:10.1542/neo.*9-12*-e571 *2008*

Rajani, A. K., Chitkara, R., & Halamek, L. P. (2009). Delivery room management of the newborn. *Pediatric Clinics of North America, 56*(3), 515–535. doi:10.1016/j.pcl.2009.03.003

Ramanathan, R. (2009). Choosing a right surfactant for the respiratory distress syndrome. *Neonatology, 95*, 1–5. doi:10.1159/000151749

Reynolds, R. D., Pilcher, J., Ring, A., Johnson, R., & McKinley, P. (2009). The golden hour: Care of the LBW infant during the first hour of life, one unit's experience. *Neonatal Network, 28*(4), 211–219.

Rothstein, R., Paris, Y., & Quizon, A. (2009). Pulmonary hypertension. *Pediatrics in Review, 30*(2), 39–46. 10.1542/pir.3-2-39

Sneath, N. (2009). Discharge teaching in the NICU: Are parents prepared? An integrative review of parent's perceptions. *Neonatal Network, 28*(5), 237–246.

Solnit, A., & Stark, M. (1961). Mourning and the birth of a defective child. *Psychoanalytic Study of the Child, 16*, 505.

Speer, C. P. (2009). Chorioamnionitis, postnatal factors and proinflammatory response in the pathogenetic sequence of bronchopulmonary dysplasia. *Neonatology, 95*, 353–361. doi:10.1159/000209301

Stokowski, L. A. (2008). The current legal climate in neonatology. Retrieved from http://cme.medscape.com/viewarticle/568009?src=rss

Varvarigou, A., Fouzas, S., Skylogianni, E., Mantagou, L., Bougioukou, D., & Mantagos, S. (2009). Transcutaneous bilirubin nomogram for prediction of significant neonatal hyperbilirubinemia. *Pediatrics, 124*(4), 1052–1059. doi:10.1542/peds.2008-2322

Venkatesh, M. P., Adams, K. M., & Weisman, L. E. (2011). Infection in the newborn. In S. L. Gardner, B. S. Carter, M. Enzman-Hines, & J. A. Hernandez, *Merenstein & Gardner's Handbook of neonatal intensive care* (7th ed., pp. 553–786). St. Louis. MO: Mosby/Elsevier.

Von Kohorn, I., & Ehrenkranz, R. (2009). Anemia in the preterm infant: Erythropoietin versus erythrocyte transfusion—It's not that simple. *Clinics in Perinatology, 36*(1), 111–123. doi:10.1016/j.clp.2008.09.009

Watchko, J. F. (2009). Identification of neonates at risk for hazardous hyperbilirubinemia: Emerging clinical insights. *Pediatric Clinics of North America, 56*(3), 671–687. doi:10.1016/j.pcl.2009.04.005

Watchko, J. F., Lin, Z., Clark, R. H., Kelleher, A. S., Walker, M. W., & Spitzer, A. R. (2009). Complex multifactorial nature of significant hyperbilirubinemia in neonates. *Pediatrics, 124*(5), e868–e877. doi:10.1542/peds.2009-0460

Weissman, A., Aranovitch, M., Blazer, S., & Zimmer, E. Z. (2009). Heel-lancing in newborns: Behavioral and spectral analysis assessment of pain control methods. *Pediatrics, 124*(5), e921–e926. doi:10.1542/peds.2009-0598

Widness, J. A. (2008). Pathophysiology of anemia during the neonatal period, including anemia of prematurity. *NeoReviews, 9*(11), e520–e525. doi:10.1542/neo.*9–11*–e520 *2008*

Wiedemann, J. R., Saugstad, A. M., Barnes-Powell, L., & Duran, K. (2008). Meconium aspiration syndrome. *Neonatal Network, 27*(2), 81–87.

Young, T. E., & Mangum, B. (2010). *Neofax* (23rd ed.). Montvale, NJ: Thomas Reuter.

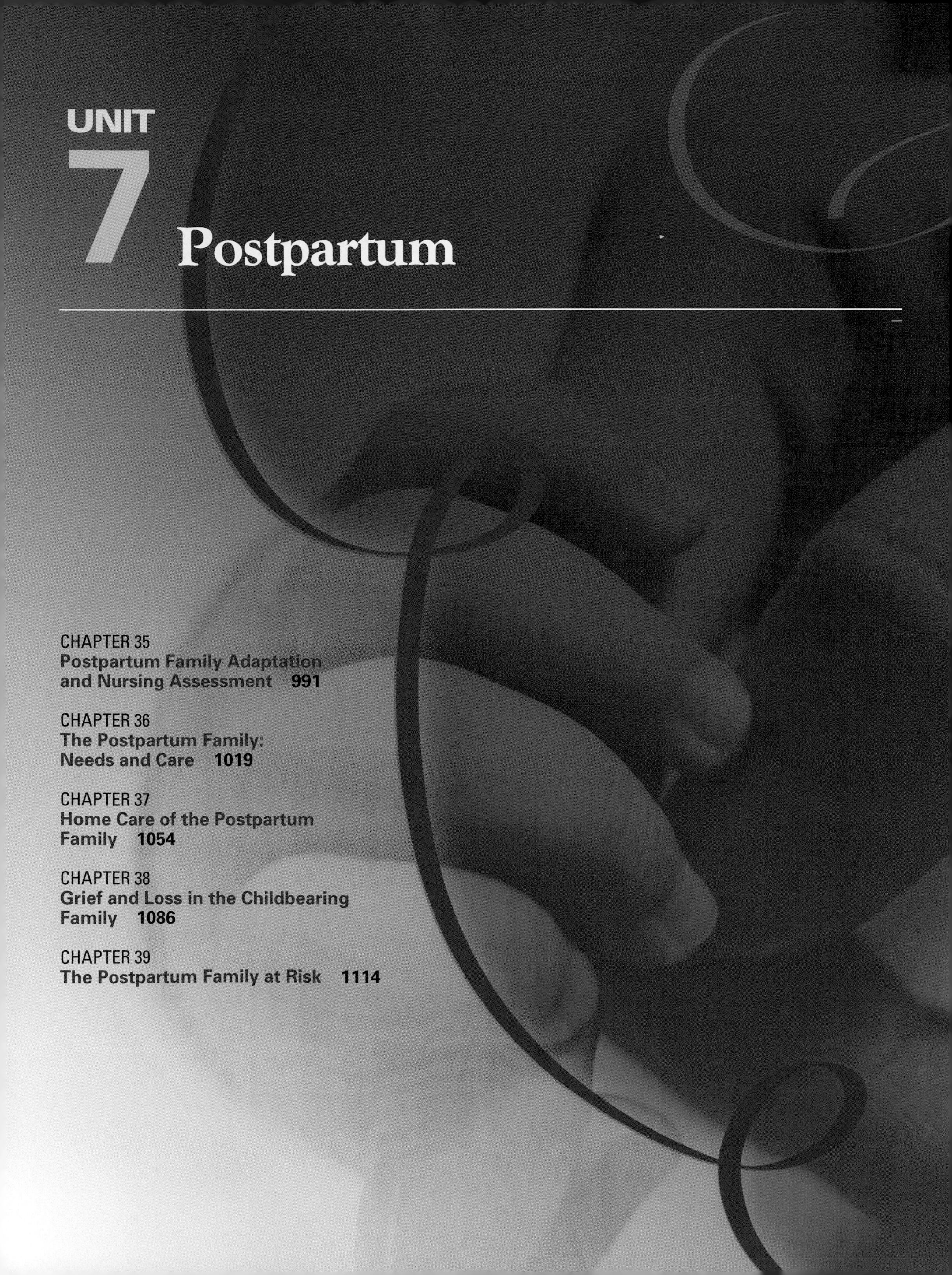

UNIT 7 Postpartum

35 CHAPTER

Postpartum Family Adaptation and Nursing Assessment

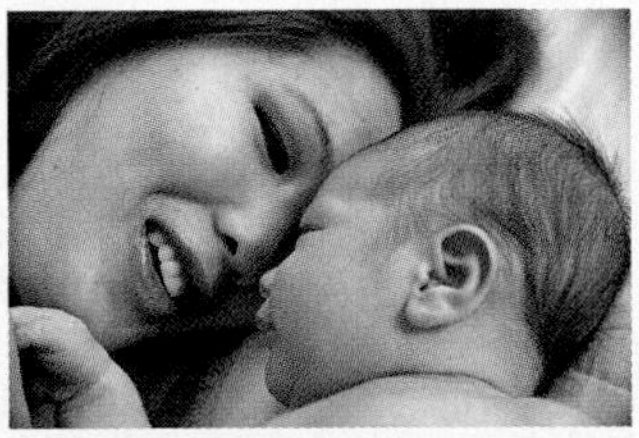

I had heard about the negatives—the fatigue, the loneliness, loss of self. But nobody told me about the wonderful parts: holding my baby close to me, seeing her first smile, watching her grow and become more responsive day by day. How can I describe the way I felt when she stroked my breast while nursing, or looked into my eyes or arched her eyebrows like an opera singer? This was the deepest connection I'd felt to anybody. Sometimes the intensity almost frightened me. For the first time I cared about somebody else more than myself, and I would do anything to nurture and protect her.

—The Boston Women's Health Collective, *The New Our Bodies, Ourselves*

LEARNING OUTCOMES

1. Delineate the basic physiologic changes that occur in the postpartum period as a woman's body returns to its prepregnant state.
2. Describe the psychologic adjustments that normally occur during the postpartum period.
3. Explain the impact of cultural influence upon the postpartum period.
4. Differentiate the physiologic and psychosocial components of a normal postpartum assessment.
5. Describe the normal characteristics and common concerns of the mother that are considered in a postpartum assessment.
6. Examine the physical and developmental tasks that the mother must accomplish during the postpartum period.
7. Identify the factors that influence the development of parent-infant attachment in the nursing assessment of early attachment.

KEY TERMS

Afterpains *998*
Becoming a mother (BAM) *999*
Boggy uterus (uterine atony) *992*
Diastasis recti abdominis *996*
En face *1000*
Engrossment *1001*
Fundus *992*
Involution *992*
Lochia *993*
Lochia alba *993*
Lochia rubra *993*
Lochia serosa *993*
Maternal role attainment (MRA) *999*
Newborns' and Mothers' Health Protection Act (NMHPA) *1016*
Postpartum blues *999*
Puerperium *992*
Reciprocity *1001*

The **puerperium**, or postpartum period, is the period during which the woman readjusts, physically and psychologically, from pregnancy and birth. It begins immediately after birth and continues for approximately 6 weeks or until the body has returned to a near nonpregnant state.

This chapter describes the physiologic and psychologic changes and adaptations that occur postpartally and the basic aspects of a thorough postpartum assessment.

Postpartum Physical Adaptations

Comprehensive nursing assessment is based on a sound understanding of the normal anatomic and physiologic processes of the puerperium. These processes involve the reproductive organs and other major body systems.

Reproductive System

Involution of the Uterus

The term **involution** is used to describe the rapid reduction in size of the uterus and its return to a condition similar to its nonpregnant state, although it remains slightly larger than it was before the first pregnancy. Specifically, the weight of the uterus decreases from 1000 g in the immediate postpartal period to 500 g at the end of the first week. It reaches 300 g by the end of the second week, finally terminating the involution process with a weight of 100 g or less (Cunningham et al., 2010).

Following separation of the placenta, the decidua of the uterus is irregular, jagged, and varied in thickness. The spongy layer of the decidua is cast off as lochia, and the basal layer of the decidua remains in the uterus to become differentiated into two layers within the first 48 to 72 hours after birth. The outermost layer becomes necrotic and is sloughed off in the lochia. The layer closest to the myometrium contains the fundi of the uterine endometrial glands, and these glands lay the foundation for the new endometrium. Except at the placental site, this process is completed in approximately 3 weeks. The placental site can take up to 6 weeks to completely heal (Cunningham et al., 2010). Bleeding from the larger uterine vessels of the placental site is controlled by compression of the retracted uterine muscle fibers. The clotted blood is gradually absorbed by the body. Some of these vessels are eventually obliterated and replaced by new vessels with smaller lumens.

Rather than forming a fibrous scar in the decidua, the placental site heals by a process of exfoliation. The placental site is undermined by the growth of the endometrial tissue, both from the margins of the site and from the fundi of the endometrial glands left in the basal layer of the site. The infarcted superficial tissue then becomes necrotic and is sloughed off (Cunningham et al., 2010). *Exfoliation* is one of the most important aspects of involution. If the healing of the placental site left a fibrous scar, the area available for further implantation would be limited, as would the number of possible pregnancies.

With the dramatic decrease in the levels of circulating estrogen and progesterone following placental separation, the uterine cells atrophy, and the hyperplasia of pregnancy begins to reverse. The process is one in which the *size* of the cells decreases markedly; the *number* of cells does not decrease. Proteolytic enzymes are released, and macrophages migrate to the uterus to promote autolysis (self-digestion). Protein material in the uterine wall is broken down and absorbed. Factors that enhance involution include an uncomplicated labor and birth, complete expulsion of the amniotic membranes and the placenta, breastfeeding, manual removal of the placenta during a cesarean birth, and early ambulation. Factors that slow uterine involution and the rationale for each factor are listed in Table 35-1.

TABLE 35-1 Factors That Retard Uterine Involution

FACTOR	RATIONALE
Prolonged labor	Muscles relax because of prolonged time of contraction during labor.
Anesthesia	Muscles relax.
Difficult birth	The uterus is manipulated excessively.
Grandmultiparity	Repeated distention of uterus during pregnancy and labor leads to muscle stretching, diminished tone, and muscle relaxation.
Full bladder	As the uterus is pushed up and usually to the right, pressure on it interferes with effective uterine contraction.
Incomplete expulsion of placenta or membranes	The presence of even small amounts of tissue interferes with ability of uterus to remain firmly contracted.
Infection	Inflammation interferes with uterine muscle's ability to contract effectively.
Overdistention of uterus	Overstretching of uterine muscles with conditions such as multiple gestation, hydramnios, or a very large baby may set the stage for slower uterine involution.

Changes in Fundal Position

Immediately following the expulsion of the placenta, the uterus contracts firmly to the size of a large grapefruit. The **fundus** (top portion of the uterus) is situated in the midline of the abdomen, one half to two thirds of the way between the symphysis pubis and the umbilicus (Figure 35-1 ■). The walls of the contracted uterus are in close proximity and the uterine blood vessels are firmly compressed by the myometrium. Within 6 to 12 hours after birth, the fundus of the uterus rises to the level of the umbilicus because of blood and clots that remain within the uterus and changes in support of the uterus by the ligaments. A fundus that is above the umbilicus and boggy (feels soft and spongy rather than firm and well contracted) is associated with excessive uterine bleeding. As blood collects and forms clots within the uterus, the fundus rises; firm contractions of the uterine muscle are interrupted, causing a **boggy uterus (uterine atony)**. When the fundus is higher than expected and is not in midline (usually deviated to the right), distention of the bladder should be suspected and the bladder should be emptied immediately and the uterus remeasured (Figure 35-2 ■). If the woman is unable to void, in-and-out catheterization of the bladder may be required. In the immediate postpartal period many women may not be aware of a full bladder. Because the uterine ligaments are still stretched, a full bladder can move the uterus. By the end of

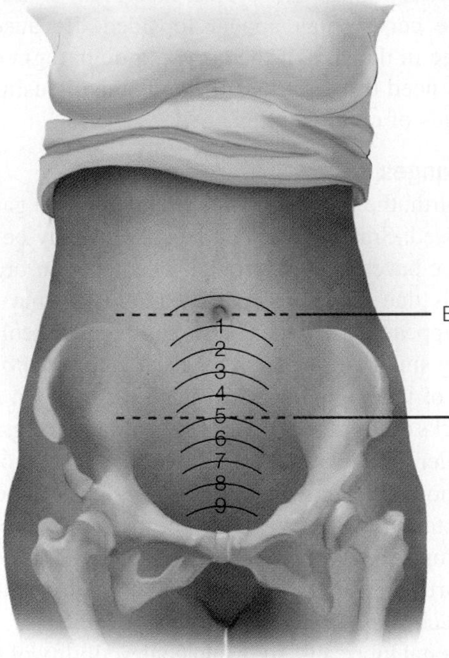

Figure 35-1 ■ Involution of the uterus. (A) Immediately after delivery of the placenta, the top of the fundus is in the midline and approximately two thirds to three fourths of the way between the symphysis pubis and the umbilicus (B). About 6 to 12 hours after birth, the fundus is at the level of (or one fingerbreadth below) the umbilicus. The height of the fundus then decreases about one fingerbreadth (approximately 1 cm) each day.

the puerperium these ligaments have regained their nonpregnant length and tension.

After birth, the top of the fundus remains at the level of the umbilicus for about half a day. On the first postpartum day (first day following birth), the top of the fundus is located about 1 cm below the umbilicus. The top of the fundus descends approximately one fingerbreadth (width of index, second, or third finger), or 1 cm, per day until it descends into the pelvis on the 10th day.

If the mother is breastfeeding, the release of endogenous oxytocin from the posterior pituitary in response to suckling may hasten this process. Barring complications, such as infection or retained placental fragments, the uterus approaches its prepregnant size and location by 5 to 6 weeks. In women who had an oversized uterus during the pregnancy (hydramnios, birth of a large-for-gestational-age [LGA] infant, or multiple gestation), the time frame for immediate uterine involution process is lengthened. If intrauterine infection is present, in addition to the presence of foul-smelling lochia or vaginal discharge, the uterine fundus descends much more slowly. When infection is suspected, other clinical signs such as fever and tachycardia in addition to delay in involution must be assessed. Any slowing of descent is called *subinvolution* (for further discussion of subinvolution, see chapter 39 ∞).

Lochia

The uterus rids itself of the debris remaining after birth through a discharge called **lochia**, which is classified according to its

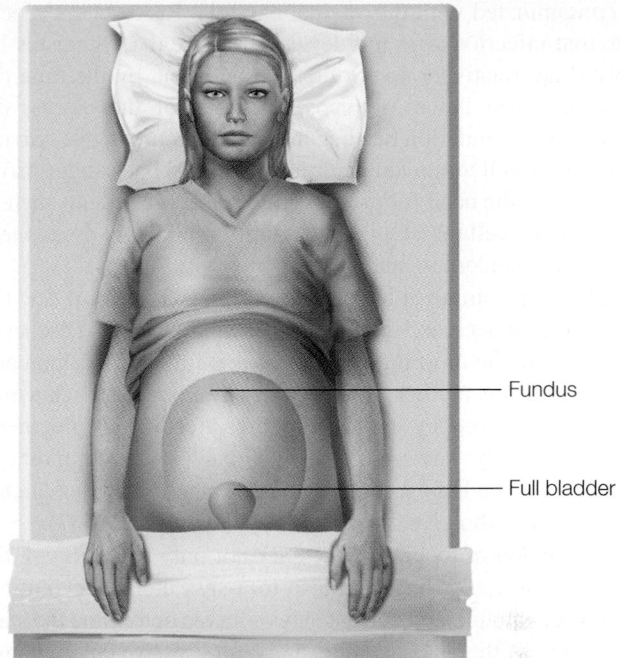

Figure 35-2 ■ The uterus becomes displaced and deviated to the right when the bladder is full.

appearance and contents. **Lochia rubra**, named for the Latin word for *red,* is dark red in color. It is present for the first 2 to 3 days postpartal and contains epithelial cells, erythrocytes, leukocytes, bacteria, shreds of the decidua, and, occasionally, fetal meconium, lanugo, and vernix caseosa. Clotting is often the result of pooling of blood in the upper portion of the vagina. A few small clots (no larger than a nickel) are common, particularly in the first few days after birth. However, lochia should not contain large (plum sized) clots; if it does, the cause should be investigated without delay. **Lochia serosa** is a pinkish color. It follows from about the 3rd to the 10th day. Lochia serosa is composed of serous exudate, shreds of degenerating decidua, erythrocytes, leukocytes, cervical mucus, and numerous microorganisms (Cunningham et al., 2010).

The red blood cell (RBC) component decreases gradually, and a creamy or yellowish discharge persists for an additional week or two. This final discharge, termed **lochia alba** from the Latin word for *white,* is composed primarily of leukocytes, decidual cells, epithelial cells, fat, cervical mucus, cholesterol crystals, and bacteria. Recent studies examining lochia patterns have found that the lochia rubra phase lasts longer than generally assumed and that it varies according to breastfeeding practice and parity (Blackburn, 2007). Variation in the duration of lochia discharge is not uncommon; however, the trend should be toward a lighter amount of flow and a lighter color of discharge. When the lochia stops, the cervix is considered closed, and chances of infection ascending from the vagina to the uterus decrease.

Like menstrual discharge, lochia has a musty, stale odor that is not offensive. Microorganisms are always present in the vaginal lochia, and by the second day following birth the uterus is contaminated with the vaginal bacteria. Researchers speculate that infection does not develop because the organisms involved are relatively nonvirulent. In addition, by the time the bacteria reach the raw, exposed surface of the uterus, the process of granulation has begun, forming a protective barrier. Any foul smell to the lochia or used perineal pads suggests infection and the need for prompt additional assessment, such as white blood cell (WBC) count and differential and assessment for uterine tenderness and fever.

The total volume of lochia is approximately 225 ml, and the daily volume decreases gradually (Blackburn, 2007). Discharge is greater in the morning because of pooling in the vagina and uterus while the mother lies sleeping. The amount of lochia may also be increased by exertion or breastfeeding. Multiparous women usually have more lochia than first-time mothers. Women who undergo a cesarean birth typically have less lochia than women who give birth vaginally (Blackburn, 2007).

Evaluation of lochia is necessary not only to determine the presence of hemorrhage but also to assess uterine involution. The type, amount, and consistency of lochia determine the state of healing of the placental site, and a progressive color change from bright red at birth to dark red to pink to white or clear should be observed. Persistent discharge of lochia rubra or a return to lochia rubra indicates subinvolution or late postpartum hemorrhage (see chapter 39 ∞).

CLINICAL JUDGMENT

Case Study: Patty Clark

You have completed your assessment of Patty Clark, a 24-year-old, G2P2 woman who is 24 hours past childbirth. The fundus is just above the umbilicus and slightly to the right. Lochia rubra is present, and a pad is soaked every 2 hours.

Critical Thinking

What other information do you need in order to determine what to do next?

Why is this finding significant and what outcome would you anticipate?

See www.nursing.pearsonhighered.com for possible responses.

The nurse should exercise caution in evaluating bleeding immediately after birth. The continuous seepage of blood is more consistent with cervical or vaginal lacerations and may be effectively diagnosed when the bleeding is evaluated in conjunction with the consistency of the uterus. Lacerations should be suspected if the uterus is firm and of expected size and if no clots can be expressed.

Cervical Changes

Following birth, the cervix is spongy, flabby, and formless and may appear bruised. The lateral aspects of the external os are frequently lacerated during the birth process (Cunningham et al., 2010). The external os is markedly irregular and closes slowly. It admits two fingers for a few days following birth, but by the end of the first week it will admit only a fingertip.

The shape of the external os is permanently changed by the first childbearing. The characteristic dimplelike os of the nullipara changes to the lateral slit (fish-mouth) os of the multipara. After significant cervical laceration or several lacerations, the cervix may appear lopsided. Because of the slight change in the size of the cervix, a diaphragm or cervical cap will need to be refitted if the woman is using one of these methods of contraception.

Vaginal Changes

Following birth, the vagina appears edematous and gaping and may be bruised. Small superficial lacerations may be evident, and the rugae have been obliterated. The apparent bruising of the vagina is due to pelvic congestion and trauma and will quickly disappear. The hymen, torn and jagged, heals irregularly, leaving small tags called the *carunculae myrtiformes.*

The size of the vagina decreases and rugae begin to return within 3 weeks (Whitmer, 2011). This facilitates the gradual return to smaller, although not to nulliparous, dimensions. By 6 weeks, the nonlactating woman's vagina usually appears normal. The lactating woman is in a hypoestrogenic state because of ovarian suppression, and her vaginal mucosa may be pale and without rugae. This may lead to dyspareunia (painful intercourse), which may be reduced by the addition of a water-soluble personal lubricant. Tone and contractibility of the vaginal opening may be improved by perineal tightening exercises (Kegel exercises are discussed in chapter 16 ∞ and illustrated in Figure 16-13 ∞ on page 365), which may begin soon after birth. The labia majora and labia minora are looser in the woman who has borne a child than in the nullipara.

Perineal Changes

During the early postpartal period, the soft tissue in and around the perineum may appear edematous with some bruising. If an episiotomy or laceration is present, the edges should be approximated. Occasionally, ecchymosis occurs, and this may delay healing. Initial healing of the episiotomy or laceration occurs in 2 to 3 weeks after the birth, although complete healing may take up to 4 to 6 months (Blackburn, 2007). Perineal discomfort may be present during this time.

Recurrence of Ovulation and Menstruation

The return of menstruation and ovulation varies for each postpartal woman. Menstruation generally returns in nonbreastfeeding mothers between 6 and 10 weeks after birth; 50% of the first cycles are anovulatory (Cunningham et al., 2010). The return of ovulation is directly associated with a rise in the serum progesterone level. In nonlactating women the average time to first ovulation can occur within 5 to 11 weeks with a mean time of 7 weeks (Cunningham et al., 2010).

The return of menstruation and ovulation in breastfeeding mothers is usually prolonged and is associated with the length of time the woman breastfeeds and whether formula supplements are used. If a mother breastfeeds for less than 1 month, the return of menstruation and ovulation is similar to the nonbreastfeeding mother. In women who exclusively breastfeed, menstruation is usually delayed for at least 3 months. Sucking by the infant typically results in alterations in the gonadotropin-releasing hormone (GnRH) production, which is thought to be the cause of amenorrhea (Blackburn, 2007). Although exclusive breastfeeding helps to reduce the risk of pregnancy for the first 6 months after

Through the Eyes of a Nurse Postpartum Bleeding and Perineal Changes

Family's Experience

Phone call to the birthing unit from a new mother: "I am still feeling some cramping and having vaginal bleeding at this point although it is easing up some. I am concerned because it had gotten lighter but now it seems to have picked up again. My vaginal area seems to feel better but sometimes it is still sensitive when I wipe after urination. Is this normal?"

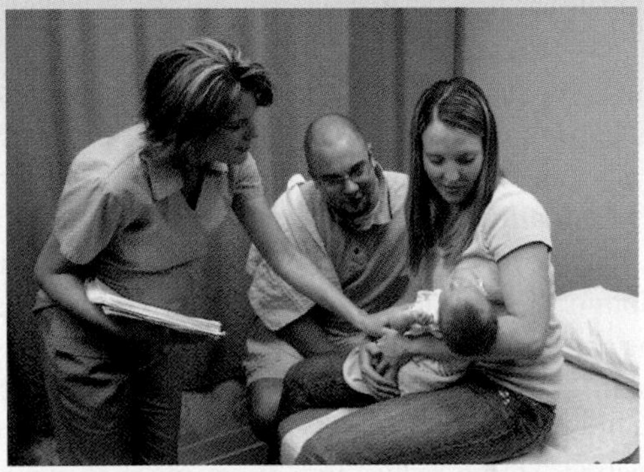

Nurse's Response

"It is normal that the bleeding can increase when your activity level increases. At this point (after 3 to 4 days), the bleeding should be pink in color. You should not be having large clots, although a few small clots may occur. If your bleeding becomes heavy, more than 1 to 2 pads per hour, if there is a foul-smelling odor, if your abdomen becomes tender or painful, or if you have fever or chills, you would need to contact your healthcare provider immediately because those can be warning signs that need further assessing.

"Your uterus will continue to contract in the early postpartum period as a result of *involution*. This helps your uterus return to a prepregnant state and descend behind your pubic bone. You can take an anti-inflammatory medication as directed by your health-care provider. You may notice that the cramping or afterbirth pains occur commonly with breastfeeding. This is also normal.

"The perineal area will continue to heal in the upcoming weeks. It is not unusual for the area to feel tender and to be sensitive. If the area becomes more painful, red, is warm to the touch, or appears to 'come open,' that could be a sign of an infection or a problem with the incision site. You would want to contact your health-care provider if any of those things occur. The sutures that were placed after the birth will continue to heal and will dissolve over time. I would continue to use the topical agents you received in the birth setting and to use the sitz bath."

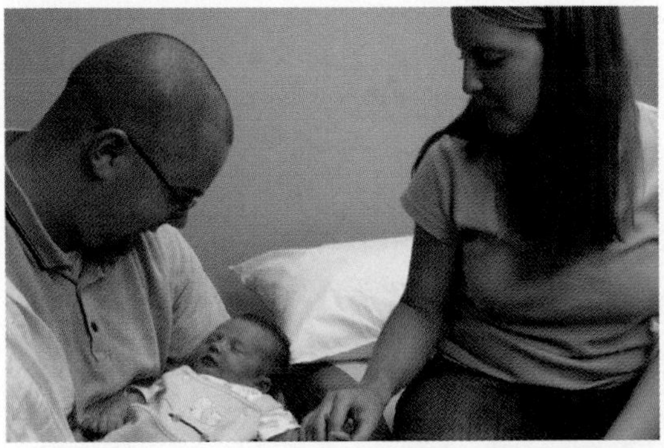

Nurse's Actions and Rationale

The nurse reviews the normal physiologic changes associated with the postpartum period. The signs and symptoms of bleeding and infection should be reviewed. The nurse explains the normal physical changes that occur, including involution of the uterus, cessation of lochia, healing of the laceration or episiotomy site, and breast changes related to lactation. Many women find it helpful if the nurse reviews the various changes that occur as the body returns to a prepregnant state.

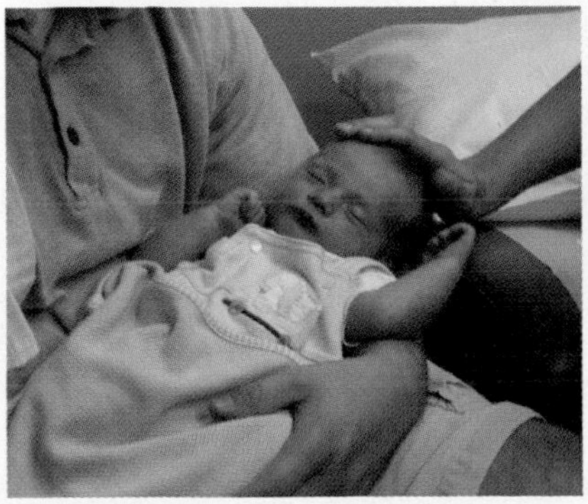

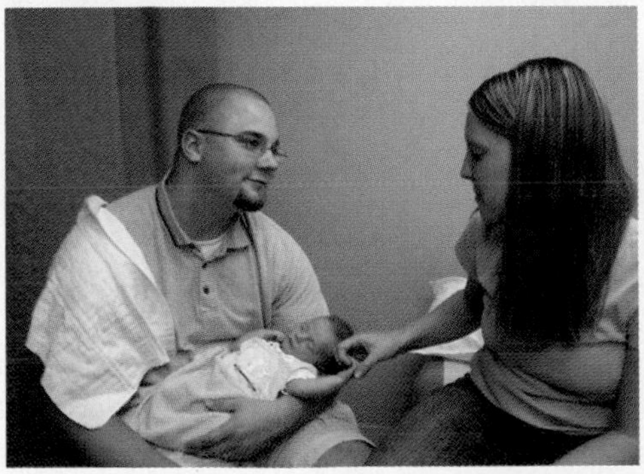

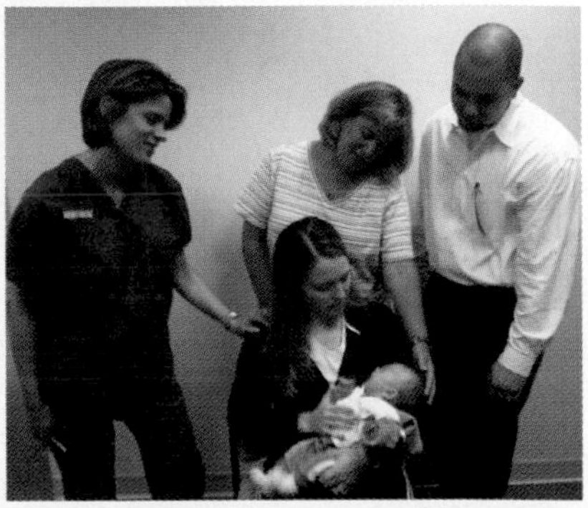

delivery, it should be relied upon only temporarily and if it meets the observed criteria for lactational amenorrhea method (LAM). Furthermore, because ovulation precedes menstruation and women often supplement breastfeeding with bottles and pacifiers, breastfeeding is not considered a reliable means of contraception.

Abdomen

The uterine ligaments (notably the round and broad ligaments) are stretched and require the length of the puerperium to recover. The stretched abdominal wall appears loose and flabby, but it will respond to exercise within 2 to 3 months. In the grandmultipara, in the woman whose abdomen is overdistended, or in the woman whose muscle tone was poor before pregnancy, the abdomen may fail to regain good tone and will remain flabby. **Diastasis recti abdominis**, a separation of the rectus abdominis muscles, may occur with pregnancy, especially in women with poor abdominal muscle tone (Figure 35-3 ■). If diastasis occurs, part of the abdominal wall has no muscular support but is formed only by skin, subcutaneous fat, fascia, and peritoneum. This may be especially pronounced in women who have undergone a cesarean section, as the rectus abdominis muscles are manually separated to access the uterine muscle. Improvement depends on the physical condition of the mother, the total number of pregnancies, pregnancy spacing, and the type and amount of physical exercise. If rectus muscle tone is not regained, support may be inadequate during future pregnancies. This may result in a pendulous abdomen and increased maternal backache. Fortunately, diastasis usually responds well to exercise, and abdominal muscle tone can improve significantly.

The striae (stretch marks), which occurred as a result of stretching and rupture of the elastic fibers of the skin, take on different colors based on the mother's skin color. The striae of Caucasian mothers are red to purple at the time of birth and gradually fade to silver or white. The striae of mothers with darker skin are darker than the surrounding skin and remain darker. These marks gradually fade after a time but remain visible.

Lactation

During pregnancy, the breasts develop in preparation for lactation as a result of the influence of both estrogen and progesterone. After birth, the interplay of maternal hormones leads to the establishment of milk production (see chapter 32 ∞).

Gastrointestinal System

Hunger following birth is common, and the mother may enjoy a light meal. Frequently, she is quite thirsty and will drink large amounts of fluid. Drinking fluids helps replace fluid lost during labor, in the urine, and through perspiration.

The bowels tend to be sluggish after birth because of the lingering effects of progesterone, decreased abdominal muscle tone, and bowel evacuation associated with the labor and birth process. Women who have had an episiotomy, lacerations, or hemorrhoids may tend to delay elimination for fear of increasing their pain or in the belief that their stitches will be torn if they bear down. In resisting or delaying the bowel movement, the woman may cause increased constipation and more pain when elimination finally occurs.

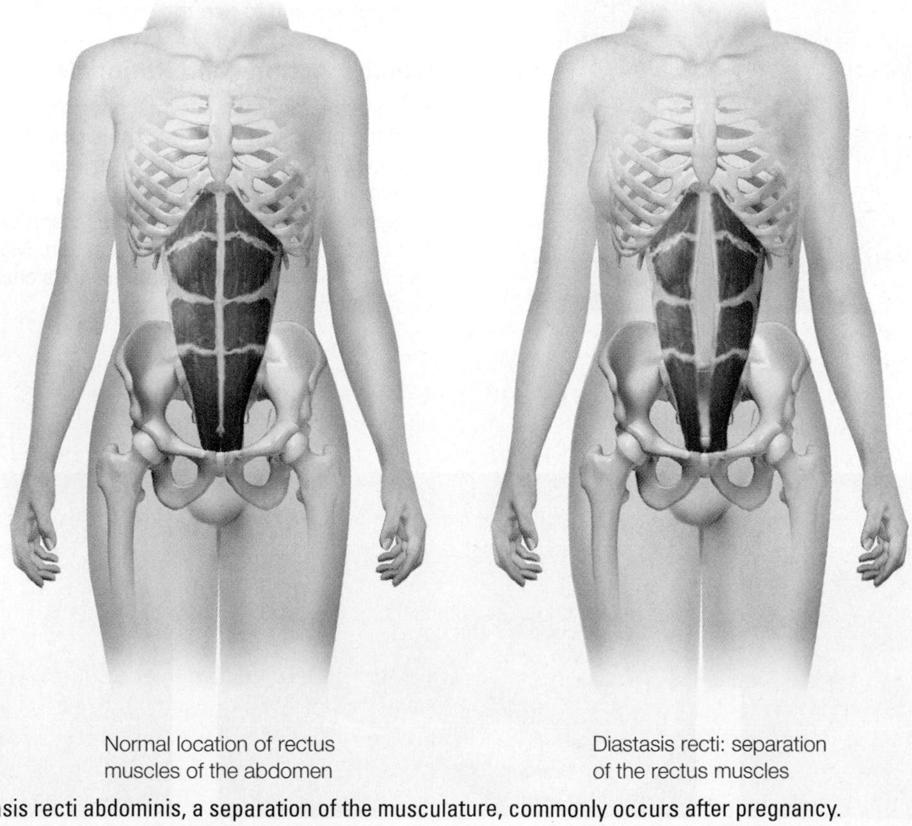

Figure 35-3 ■ Diastasis recti abdominis, a separation of the musculature, commonly occurs after pregnancy.

The woman with a cesarean birth may receive clear liquids shortly after surgery. Once bowel sounds are present, the diet is quickly advanced to solid food. In addition, the woman may experience some initial discomfort from flatulence, which is relieved by early ambulation and use of antiflatulent medications. Chamomile tea and peppermint tea may also be helpful in reducing discomfort from flatulence. It may take a few days for the bowel to regain its tone. The woman who has had a cesarean or a difficult birth may benefit from stool softeners.

Urinary Tract

The postpartal woman has an increased bladder capacity, swelling and bruising of the tissues around the urethra, decreased sensitivity to fluid pressure, and decreased sensation of bladder filling. Consequently, she is at risk for overdistention, incomplete emptying, and buildup of residual urine. Women who have had an anesthetic block have inhibited neural functioning of the bladder and are more susceptible to bladder distention, difficulty voiding, and bladder infections. In addition, immediate postpartal use of oxytocin to facilitate uterine contractions following expulsion of the placenta has an antidiuretic effect. Following cessation of the oxytocin the woman will experience rapid bladder filling (Cunningham et al., 2010).

Urinary output increases during the early postpartal period (first 12 to 24 hours) because of *puerperal diuresis.* The kidneys must eliminate an estimated 2000 to 3000 ml of extracellular fluid with a normal pregnancy, which causes rapid filling of the bladder. Thus adequate bladder elimination is an immediate concern. Women with preeclampsia, chronic hypertension, and diabetes experience even greater fluid retention, and postpartal diuresis is increased accordingly.

If stasis exists, chances increase for urinary tract infection because of bacteriuria and the presence of dilated ureters and renal pelves, which persist for about 6 weeks after birth. A full bladder may also increase the tendency of the uterus to relax by displacing the uterus and interfering with its contractility, leading to hemorrhage. In the absence of infection, the dilated ureters and renal pelves return to prepregnant size by the end of the sixth week.

Hematuria, resulting from bladder or urethral trauma, may occasionally occur after birth, but the presence of lochia may mask this sign. If hematuria occurs in the second or third postpartal week, there may be a bladder infection. Acetone may be present in the urine of women with diabetes or of women with prolonged labor and dehydration. Slight (1+) proteinuria may occur during the first week following birth. However, proteinuria may be associated with an infectious process (cystitis, pyelitis), so it should be evaluated further. A urine specimen contaminated with lochia may falsely indicate proteinuria, so any specimen should be obtained as a midstream or a catheterized specimen.

Vital Signs

During the postpartum period, with the exception of the first 24 hours, the woman should be afebrile. A maternal temperature of up to 38°C (100.4°F) may occur up to 24 hours after birth as a result of the exertion and dehydration of labor. An increase in temperature to between 37.8°C and 39°C may also occur during the first 24 hours after the mother's milk comes in (Cunningham et al., 2010). However, in women not meeting these criteria, infection must be considered in the presence of an increased temperature (see chapter 39 ∞).

Immediately following delivery, many women experience a transient rise in both systolic and diastolic blood pressure, which spontaneously returns to the prepregnancy baseline over the next few days (James, 2008). A decrease may indicate physiologic readjustment to decreased intrapelvic pressure, or it may be related to uterine hemorrhage. Orthostatic hypotension, as indicated by feelings of faintness or dizziness immediately after standing up, can develop in the first 48 hours as a result of abdominal engorgement that may occur after birth. A low or decreasing blood pressure may reflect hypovolemia secondary to hemorrhage, but it is a late sign. Blood pressure elevations may result from excessive use of oxytocin or vasopressor medications. Because preeclampsia can persist into or occur first in the postpartal period, routine evaluation of blood pressure is needed. If a woman complains of headache, hypertension must be ruled out before analgesics are administered.

Puerperal bradycardia with rates of 50 to 70 beats per minute (beats/min) commonly occurs during the first 6 to 10 days of the postpartal period. It may be related to decreased cardiac strain, the decreased blood volume following placental separation, contraction of the uterus, and increased stroke volume. A pulse rate greater than 100 beats/min may be indicative of hypovolemia, infection, fear, or pain and requires further assessment.

Blood Values

Blood values should return to the prepregnant state by the end of the postpartum period. Pregnancy-associated activation of coagulation factors may continue for variable amounts of time after birth. This condition, in conjunction with trauma, immobility, or sepsis, predisposes the woman to development of thromboembolism. The incidence of thromboembolism is reduced by early mobilization. Plasma fibrinogen is maintained at pregnancy levels for a week following childbirth, accounting for the higher sedimentation rate observed in the early postpartal period.

Nonpathologic leukocytosis often occurs during labor and in the immediate postpartal period, with WBC counts up to 25,000 to 30,000/mm^3 (Cunningham et al., 2010). WBC values typically return to normal levels by the end of the first postpartal week. Leukocytosis combined with the normal increase in erythrocyte sedimentation rate may obscure the diagnosis of acute infection at this time (Whitmer, 2011).

Hemoglobin and hematocrit levels may be difficult to interpret in the first 2 days after birth because of the changing blood volume. This loss in blood in the first 24 hours accounts for half of the RBC volume gained during the course of the pregnancy. Blood loss averages 200 to 500 ml with a vaginal birth and 1000 ml or more with a cesarean birth (Rhode, 2011). Lochia constitutes less than 25% of this blood loss (James, 2008). As extracellular fluid is excreted, hemoconcentration occurs, with a concomitant rise in hematocrit. A drop in values indicates an abnormal blood loss. The following is a convenient rule to remember: a 4–3 percentage-point drop in hematocrit equals a blood loss of 500 ml (Whitmer, 2011). After 3 to 4 days, mobilization of interstitial fluid leads to a slight increase in plasma volume. This hemodilution leads to a decrease in hemoglobin, hematocrit, and plasma protein by the end of the first postpartal week. Decreases in plasma volume reach nonpregnant levels by 1 to 2 weeks postpartum (Whitmer, 2011).

Platelet levels typically fall as a result of placental separation. They then begin to increase by the third to fourth postpartum day, gradually returning to normal by the sixth postpartum week. Fibrinolytic activity typically returns to normal during the hours following the birth. The hemostatic system as a whole reaches its normal pregnant status by 3 to 4 weeks postpartal; however, the diameter of deep veins can take up to 6 weeks to return to prepregnant levels (Blackburn, 2007). This is why there is a prolonged risk of thromboembolism in the first 6 weeks following birth.

Cardiovascular Changes

The cardiovascular system undergoes dramatic changes during birth that can result in cardiovascular instability due to an increase in cardiac output. The cardiac output typically stabilizes and returns to pregnancy levels within an hour following birth (Whitmer, 2011). Maternal hypervolemia typically occurs immediately following birth because the maternal circulation has an increase in blood volume that no longer travels through the placenta. Maternal hypervolemia acts to protect the mother from excessive blood loss. Cardiac output declines by 30% in the first 2 weeks and reaches normal levels by 6 to 12 weeks (Blackburn, 2007). Diuresis in the first 2 to 5 days helps to decrease the extracellular fluid and results in a weight loss of 3 kg (James, 2008). Failure to diurese in the immediate postpartal period can lead to pulmonary edema and subsequent cardiac problems. This is seen more commonly in women with a history of preeclampsia or preexisting cardiac problems (Blackburn, 2007; James, 2008).

Neurologic Changes and Conditions

Neurologic problems and disorders can predispose women to higher rates of morbidity and mortality during pregnancy and in the postpartum period. Headaches are the most common neurologic symptoms encountered by postpartal women. Headaches can result from fluid shifts in the first week after birth, leakage of cerebrospinal fluid into the extradural space during spinal anesthesia, pregnancy-induced hypertension, or stress (Aminoff, 2009). It is estimated that up to 40% of postpartum women develop headaches within the first week following birth (James, 2008). There may be an increased incidence in headache if the woman had spinal or epidural anesthesia. Migraine headaches, although less frequent during pregnancy, tend to resume in the postpartal period. Women with epilepsy are nine times more likely to have a seizure during labor or in the first 24 hours after birth than during pregnancy (Samuels & Niebyl, 2007). The postpartum epileptic woman is more likely to be diagnosed with depression, and referral to a therapist or support group should be made (Rousseau, 2008). The physiologic changes of pregnancy that may have required increasing antiepileptic drug (AED) dosage are now removed, and retitration of the AEDs is required to prevent toxicity. Women with multiple sclerosis (MS) and Guillain-Barré syndrome are more likely to have symptoms in the postpartum period than during pregnancy (Samuels & Niebyl, 2007). Myasthenia gravis (autoimmune disease) affects the neuromuscular junctions. The increase in symptoms during pregnancy is variable; however, the first month of pregnancy and the first month of the postpartum period are the most critical (Kalayjian & Goodwin, 2007).

Weight Loss

An initial weight loss of 10 to 12 lb occurs as a result of the birth of infant, placenta, and amniotic fluid. Puerperal diuresis accounts for the loss of an additional 5 lb during the early puerperium. By the sixth to eighth week after birth, many women have returned to approximately prepregnant weight if they gained the average 25 to 30 lb. Women often express concern about the slow pace of their postpartal weight loss. Multiparas tend to have a more positive outlook than primiparas, probably because the multipara's previous experience has prepared her for the fact that the body does not immediately return to a prepregnant state.

Postpartum Chill

Frequently the mother experiences intense tremors that resemble shivering from a chill immediately after birth. Several theories have been offered to explain this shivering: the result of sudden release of pressure on the pelvic nerves after birth, a response to a fetus-to-mother transfusion that occurred during placental separation, a reaction to maternal adrenaline production during labor and birth, or a reaction to epidural anesthesia. If not followed by fever, this chill is of no clinical concern, but it is uncomfortable for the woman. The nurse can increase the woman's comfort by covering her with a warmed blanket and reassuring her that the shivering is a common, self-limiting situation. If she allows herself to go with the shaking, the shivering will last only a short time. Some women may also find a warm drink helpful. Chills and fever later in the puerperium indicate infection and require further evaluation.

Postpartum Diaphoresis

The elimination of excess fluid and waste products via the skin during the puerperium greatly increases perspiration. Diaphoretic (sweating) episodes frequently occur at night, and the woman may awaken drenched with perspiration. This perspiration is not significant clinically, but the mother should be protected from chilling.

Afterpains

Afterpains occur more commonly in multiparas than in primiparas and are caused by intermittent uterine contractions. Although the uterus of the primipara usually remains consistently contracted, the lost tone of the uterus of the multipara results in alternate contraction and relaxation. This phenomenon also occurs if the uterus has been markedly distended, as with multiple-gestation pregnancies or hydramnios, or if clots or placental fragments were retained. These afterpains may cause the mother severe discomfort for 2 to 3 days following birth. The administration of oxytocic agents (intravenous infusion with Pitocin or oral administration of Methergine) stimulates uterine contraction and increases the discomfort of the afterpains. Because endogenous oxytocin is released when the infant suckles, breastfeeding also increases the severity of the afterpains. A warm water bottle placed against the low abdomen may reduce the discomfort of afterpains. In addition, the breastfeeding mother may find it helpful to take a mild analgesic agent approximately 1 hour before feeding her infant. The nurse can assure the mother that the prescribed analgesic agents are not harmful to the newborn and help improve the quality of the breastfeeding experience. An analgesic agent such as ibuprofen is also helpful at bedtime if the afterpains interfere with the mother's rest. See chapter 36 ∞ for a further discussion of analgesics for afterpains.

Postpartum Psychologic Adaptations

The postpartum period is a time of readjustment and adaptation for the entire childbearing family but especially for the mother. The woman experiences a variety of responses as she adjusts to a new family member, postpartal discomforts, changes in her body image, and the reality that she is no longer pregnant. One young mother described her responses well:

> "I feel like it's the day after Christmas. I'm relieved that everything went well and I have a fine baby, but I feel so let down. I had an image of what childbirth would be like, but everything was a little different. I figured that as soon as I gave birth, I would feel fine. Why didn't someone tell me I would still be sore? The pain didn't magically disappear! When I was pregnant, everyone treated me as though I was a little fragile. Now when people call or visit, all they talk about is the baby. I don't think I'm really jealous, but I do miss the attention. During this past day I've started to realize that my life will never, ever be the same again. I've always wanted to be a mother, but I'm not really sure how to do it. Isn't that strange?"

Taking In and Taking Hold Periods

Soon after birth during the *taking-in* period, the woman tends to be passive and somewhat dependent. The new mother follows suggestions, is hesitant about making decisions, and is still rather preoccupied with her needs (Rubin, 1984). She may have a great need to talk about her perceptions of her labor and birth. This helps her work through the process, sort out the reality from her fantasized experience, and clarify anything that she did not understand. Food and sleep are major needs.

After the taking-in period, which may end by the second day, the new mother may be observed to be ready to resume control of her body, her mothering, and her life in general. Rubin (1984) labeled this phase as *taking hold.* If she is breastfeeding, the mother may worry about her technique or the quality of her milk. If her baby spits up following feeding, she may view it as a personal failure. She may also feel demoralized by the fact that the nurse or an older family member handles her baby proficiently while she feels unsure and tentative. She requires assurance that she is doing well as a mother. Today's mothers seem to be more independent and adjust more rapidly, exhibiting behaviors of "taking in" and "taking hold" in shorter time periods than those previously identified.

Becoming a Mother

Maternal role attainment (MRA) is the process by which a woman learns mothering behaviors and becomes comfortable with her identity as a mother. The formation of a maternal identity indicates that the woman has attained the maternal role. This process occurs with each child a woman bears. As the mother grows to know this child and forms a relationship with her or him, the mother's maternal identity gradually and systematically evolves, and she "binds in" to the infant (Rubin, 1984). In most cases, maternal role attainment occurs within 3 to 10 months following birth. Social support, the woman's age and personality traits, the marital or partner relationship, the presence of underlying anxiety or depression, the woman's previous childcare skills, the temperament of her infant, the gestational age and health status of her infant, her birth experience, her own health status, her self-concept, and the family's socioeconomic status all influence the woman's success in attaining the maternal role (Hill & Aldag, 2007).

Mercer proposed replacing the term *maternal role attainment* (MRA) with the term **becoming a mother (BAM)**. She stated that BAM "more accurately encompasses the dynamic transformation and evolution of a woman's persona than does MRA, and the term MRA should be discontinued" (Mercer, 2004, p. 226). BAM more accurately reflects the transition process of becoming a mother that changes throughout the maternal-child relationship (see chapter 36 ∞ for further discussion).

> **PROFESSIONALISM IN PRACTICE**
>
> ***Enhancing Patient-Centered Care***
>
> Mercer (2006) emphasized the importance of individualized dialogue beteen the mother and the nurse, which involves: "a mutual identification by the mother and the nurse of the mother's needs and the available resources among the mother's family and friends, her community, and the larger society. With the mother's input about her preferences for available assistance. . . . Appropriate referrals may be made" (p. 650). Professional nurses who follow Mercer's recommendations enhance the process of a mother and engage in patient-centered care.

Postpartum Blues

The **postpartum blues** consist of a transient period of depression that occurs during the first few days of puerperium. Symptoms may include mood swings, anger, weepiness, anorexia, difficulty sleeping, and a feeling of letdown. This mood change frequently occurs while the woman is still hospitalized, but it may occur at home as well. Changing hormone levels are certainly a factor; an unsupportive environment and insecurity

Postpartum Depression Resources

also have been identified as potential causes. In addition, fatigue, discomfort, and overstimulation may play a part. The postpartum blues usually resolve naturally within 10 to 14 days, but if they persist or if symptoms worsen, the woman may need evaluation for postpartum depression (see chapter 39 ∞). Ideally a depression assessment should be completed each trimester to update a pregnant woman's risk status (Beck, 2008). If not done previously, the nurse assesses the woman for predisposing factors during labor and the postpartum stay. Several depression scales are available for assessing postpartum depression. The routine use of a screening tool, such as the Edinburgh Postnatal Depression Scale or Postpartum Depression Predictors Inventory-Revised, is a matter-of-fact approach that significantly increases the diagnosis (Beck, 2008).

Importance of Social Support

The psychologic outcomes of the postpartum period are far more positive when the parents have access to a support network. Women and their partners may find that family relationships become increasingly important, but the increased family interaction can be a source of stress. The attention that their infant receives from family members is a source of satisfaction to the new parents. In many cases, the ties to the woman's family become especially good. Fathers may report that their relationships with their in-laws become far more positive and supportive. However, the increased family interaction can be a source of stress, especially for the new mother, who often tends to have more contact with both families.

The new parents may also have increasing contact with other parents of small children although contact with coworkers declines. Of great concern are women and their partners who have no family or friends with whom to form a social network. Isolation at a time when the woman feels an increased need for support can result in tremendous stress and is often a contributing factor in situations of postpartum depression, child neglect, or abuse. New mother support groups are helpful for women who lack a social support system.

Postpartum doulas are professionals trained to help the new mother after the birth of the baby. As a "mother's helper," postpartum doula services are tailored to help the new mother feel as rested as possible and well-nourished, and to place her household in good order so that she can focus her energy on her new baby.

Case Study: Mother-Infant Bonding

DEVELOPING CULTURAL COMPETENCE

Middle East Initial Postpartum Experience

In many patriarchal countries in the Middle East, the new mother and her infant stay with the husband's family following the birth of the infant. Frequent visits from the woman's family are discouraged and may even be viewed as burdensome by the husband's family. Typically, only women visit the new mother during the postpartum period. For the birth of the first baby, the wife's parents are expected to purchase all of the supplies and clothing for the baby.

Development of Family Attachment

A mother's first interaction with her infant is influenced by many factors, including her family of origin, her relationships, the stability of her home environment, the communication patterns she has developed, and the degree of nurturing she received as a child. These factors have shaped the person she has become. The following personal characteristics are also important:

- ***Level of trust.*** What level of trust has this mother developed in response to her life experiences? What is her philosophy of childrearing? Will she be able to treat her infant as a unique individual with changing needs that should be met as much as possible?
- ***Level of self-esteem.*** How much does she value herself as a woman and as a mother? Does she feel generally able to cope with the adjustments of life?
- ***Capacity for enjoying herself.*** Is the mother able to find pleasure in everyday activities and human relationships?
- ***Adequacy of knowledge about childbearing and childrearing.*** What beliefs about the course of pregnancy, the capacities of newborns, previous experiences with infants or children, and the nature of her emotions may influence her behavior at first contact with her infant and later?
- ***Prevailing mood or usual feeling tone.*** Is the woman predominantly content, angry, depressed, or anxious? Is she sensitive to her own feelings and those of others? Will she be able to accept her own needs and to obtain support in meeting them?
- ***Reactions to the present pregnancy.*** Was the pregnancy planned? Did it go smoothly? Were there ongoing life events that enhanced her pregnancy or depleted her reserves of energy? How were other life roles changed because of her pregnancy and motherhood?

By the time of birth, each mother has developed an emotional orientation of some kind to the baby based on these factors.

Initial Attachment Behavior

After labor and birth, a new mother demonstrates a fairly regular pattern of maternal behaviors as she continues to familiarize herself with her newborn. In a progression of touching activities, the mother proceeds from fingertip exploration of the newborn's extremities toward palmar contact with larger body areas and finally to enfolding the infant with the whole hand and arms. The time taken to accomplish these steps varies from minutes to days. The mother also increases the proportion of time spent in the **en face** position (Figure 35-4 ■). She arranges herself or the newborn so that she has direct face-to-face and eye-to-eye contact. There is an intense interest in having the infant's eyes open. When the eyes are open, the mother characteristically greets the newborn and talks in high-pitched tones to him or her.

In most instances the mother relies heavily on her senses of sight, touch, and hearing in getting to know what her baby is really like. She also tends to respond verbally to any sounds emitted by the newborn, such as cries, coughs, sneezes, and grunts. The sense of smell may be involved as well.

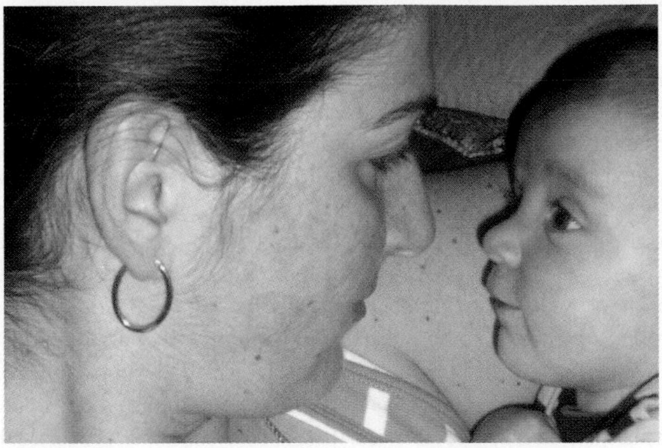

Figure 35-4 ■ The mother has direct face-to-face and eye-to-eye contact in the en face position.

Source: Courtesy of Joanna Allen.

While interacting with her newborn, the mother may be experiencing shock, disbelief, and denial. She may state, "I can't believe she's finally here," or, "I felt he was a stranger." However, the mother may express feelings of connectedness between the newborn and the rest of the family, either in positive or in negative terms: "She's got your cute nose, Daddy," or "Oh, no! He looks just like my first one, and he was an impossible baby." A mother's facial expression or the frequency and content of her questions may demonstrate concerns about the infant's general condition or normality, especially if her pregnancy was complicated or if a previously born baby was not healthy.

During the first few days after her child's birth, the new mother applies herself to the task of getting to know her baby. This is termed the *acquaintance phase.* If the infant gives clear behavioral cues about needs, the infant's responses to mothering will be predictable, which will make the mother feel effective and competent. Other behaviors that make an infant more attractive to caretakers are smiling, grasping a finger, breastfeeding eagerly, cuddling, and being easy to console.

During this time the newborn is also becoming acquainted. Within a few days after birth, infants show signs of recognizing recurrent situations and responding to changes in routine. To the extent that their mother is their world, they are actively acquainting themselves with her.

During the *phase of mutual regulation,* mother and infant seek to deal with the degree of control to be exerted by each in their relationship. In this phase of adjustment, a balance is sought between the needs of the mother and the needs of the infant. The most important consideration is that each should obtain a good measure of enjoyment from the interaction. During the mutual adjustment phase, negative maternal feelings are likely to surface or intensify. Because "everyone knows that mothers love their babies," these negative feelings often go unexpressed and are allowed to build up. If they are expressed, the response of friends, relatives, or healthcare personnel is often to deny the feelings to the mother: "You don't mean that." Some negative feelings are normal in the first few days after birth, and the nurse should be supportive when the mother vocalizes these feelings.

Bonding with the Infant

When mutual regulation arrives at the point where both mother and infant primarily enjoy each other's company, reciprocity has been achieved. **Reciprocity** is an interactional cycle that occurs simultaneously between mother and infant. It involves mutual cuing behaviors, expectancy, rhythmicity, and synchrony. The mother develops a new relationship with an individual who has a unique character and evokes a response entirely different from the fantasy response of pregnancy. When reciprocity is synchronous, the interaction between mother and infant is mutually gratifying and is sought and initiated by both partners (Reyna & Pickler, 2009).

Promoting Attachment in Special Circumstances

Newborns who require immediate care in a special care or intensive care nursery are sometimes taken from their parents immediately after birth. The separation can interfere with the normal attachment process. Consider ways to unite the parents with their newborn as soon as possible. Take into account the health status of the mother, the visitation policy of the nursery, even fear the family may have of the environment in the intensive care nursery. Perhaps the nurse or family can take digital pictures or video clips of the baby and can show them to the mother as soon as possible to reassure her of the baby's status. Education, support, and creativity may be needed to unite the parent(s) with the newborn. If the infant is in an incubator and cannot be held, encourage the parents to stroke the infant's hand, foot, or cheek. Provide reassurances that this will not hurt their infant and is in fact beneficial.

PROFESSIONALISM IN PRACTICE

Promoting Skin-to-Skin Contact

Many hospital units remove infants from their mother following birth to allow convenient assessment and performance of procedures by hospital staff despite a preponderance of evidence that supports immediate skin-to-skin contact (SSC) between mother (or father) and the newborn. Nurses are the professionals most often at the patient's bedside; they have the power and an obligation to serve as leaders and change agents by promoting clinical practices that are supported by research evidence.

Application: Identifying Strategies to Enhance Father-Infant Interactions

Father-Infant Interactions

In Western cultures, commitment to family-centered maternity care has fostered interest in understanding the feelings and experiences of the new father. Evidence suggests that the father has a strong attraction to his newborn and that the feelings he experiences are similar to the mother's feelings of attachment (Figure 35-5 ■). The characteristic sense of absorption, preoccupation, and interest in the infant demonstrated by fathers during early contact has been termed **engrossment**. Differences in involvement still exist among fathers in Western culture and may be influenced by factors other than culture (e.g., previous experience with paternal role or exposure to male/father role models).

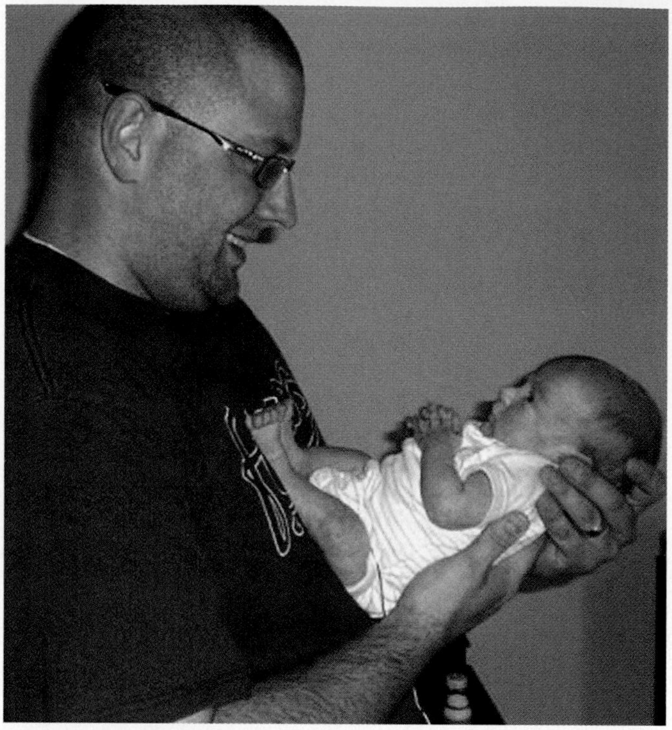

Figure 35-5 ■ The father experiences strong feelings of attraction during engrossment.

Source: Courtesy of Christopher Allen.

DEVELOPING CULTURAL COMPETENCE
Muslim Paternal Attachment

In some cultures there may be little involvement of the father in newborn care. In Muslim culture, for example, emphasis on childrearing and infant care activities is on the mother and female relatives. Nurses need to be aware of cultural differences when evaluating a father's interaction with his newborn.

Siblings and Others

Infants are capable of maintaining a number of strong attachments without loss of quality. These attachments may include siblings, grandparents, aunts, and uncles. The social setting and personality of the individual seem to be significant factors in the development of multiple attachments. Birth centers are especially geared toward the inclusion of the family in the birth process. In the hospital setting, the advent of open visiting hours and rooming-in permits siblings and grandparents to participate in the attachment process.

Cultural Influences in the Postpartum Period

Whereas Western culture places primary emphasis on the events of birth, many other cultures place greater emphasis on the postpartum period. For women not of the dominant American culture, the new mother's primary culture, personal values, and level of acculturation can influence her beliefs about her postpartum care. Her expectations regarding food, fluids, rest, hygiene, medications, relief measures, support, and counsel—as well as other aspects of her life—will be influenced by the beliefs and values of her family and cultural group. Sometimes a new mother's wishes will differ from the expectations of the certified nurse-midwife (CNM) or physician or nurse. (See chapter 2 ∞ for an in-depth discussion.)

All nurses belong to their particular ethnoculture and also share in the culture of health care. As a part of the healthcare cultural group, nurses implement practices that support their general beliefs, such as offering food in the recovery period following birth, providing iced fluids, expecting the woman to ambulate as soon as possible, and assuming the woman will want to shower and perhaps wash her hair soon after birth. It is important for nurses to recognize that they are approaching their patient's care from their own perspective and that, to individualize care for each mother, they need to assess the woman's preferences, her level of acculturation and assimilation to Western culture, her linguistic abilities, and her educational level (Lauderdale, 2008). In addition, the nurse should have the mother exercise her choices when possible, and support those choices, with the help of cultural awareness and a sound knowledge base.

Although describing the practices of different cultural groups always involves some generalization, it is helpful for nurses to understand some of the possible differences in beliefs and practices. Women of European heritage may expect to eat a full meal and have a large amount of iced fluids following the birth, in the belief that the food restores energy and the fluids help replace fluid lost during the labor. She may want to ambulate shortly after the birth, shower, wash her hair, and put on a fresh gown. She may expect a relatively short stay in the hospital and may or may not be interested in educational classes. Women of the Islamic faith may have specific modesty requirements; the woman must be completely covered, with only her feet and hands exposed, and no man, other than the husband or a family member, may be alone with her (Lauderdale, 2008; Reitmanova & Gustafson, 2008).

Some cultures emphasize certain postpartal routines or rituals for mother and baby that are designed to restore the hot-cold balance of the body. Some women of Hispanic, African, and Asian cultures may avoid cold after birth. This prohibition includes cold air, wind, and all water (even if heated). On the other hand, some traditional Mexican women may avoid eating "hot" foods, such as pork, just after the birth of a baby (considered a "hot" experience). It is important to note that each individual or cultural group may define hot and cold conditions as well as hot and cold foods differently. The nurse should ask each woman what she can eat and what foods she thinks would be helpful for healing. The nurse may encourage family members to bring preferred food and drink for the mother. For more detailed discussion of the hot-cold balance concept, see "Cultural Influences Affecting the Family" in chapter 2 ∞.

In many cultures, the extended family plays an essential role during the puerperium. The grandmother is often the primary helper to the mother and newborn. She brings wisdom and experience, allowing the new mother time to rest as well as giving her ready access to someone who can help with problems and concerns as they arise. It is important to ensure access of all family members during the postpartal period. Visiting rules

Application: Exploring Cultural Differences Regarding Postpartum Care may be waived to allow family members or authority figures access to the mother and newborn. These practices show respect and foster a blending of old and new behaviors to meet the goals of all concerned (Purnell & Paulanka, 2008). African American mothers model their mothering skills after their older female relatives. In addition, these same older female relatives usually provide child care as needed (Purnell & Paulanka, 2008). Jewish patients may also request a kosher diet. Some traditional Jewish couples avoid physical contact while the woman is experiencing any vaginal discharge; as a result, unfortunately, the man may be viewed as unsupportive by the staff during the postpartal period (Zauderer, 2009).

DEVELOPING CULTURAL COMPETENCE

Caring for the Orthodox Jewish Couple

The orthodox Jewish couple's beliefs and practices are strictly adhered to in their dress, communication, dietary practices, and activities of daily living in the postpartum time. The nurse should assist the woman in maintaining her modesty in her dress and keeping her hair covered at all times. For the first 7 days after delivery the woman will be given special treatment and will be cared for by family members. Resting after childbirth is considered crucial for the first 6 weeks. The woman will breastfeed her newborn. The baby will not be named nor will the newborn male be circumcised until a later date after discharge from the hospital. Their Sabbath is sacred and begins at sundown on Friday evening and ends after dark on Saturday. During this time neither the man nor the woman will use electricity, travel, or write. They will not tear or cut anything. So if the woman is in the hospital during the Sabbath, the nurse should be sensitive to the fact that any forms that may need to be signed will have to be signed before or after the Sabbath. The woman will need the nurse to adjust an electric bed, turn off/on lights, and tear pieces of toilet paper for her to use. The woman will not leave the hospital and travel home until after the Sabbath (Noble, Rom, Englehardt, et al., 2009).

TABLE 35-2 Postpartum High-Risk Factors

FACTOR	MATERNAL IMPLICATION
Preeclampsia	↑ Blood pressure ↑ CNS irritability → ↑ risk for seizure ↑ Need for bed rest → ↑ risk thrombophlebitis
Diabetes	Need for insulin regulation Episodes of hypoglycemia or hyperglycemia ↓ Healing
Cardiac disease	↑ Maternal exhaustion
Cesarean birth	↑ Healing needs ↑ Pain from incision ↑ Risk of infection ↑ Length of hospitalization
Overdistention of uterus (multiple gestation, hydramnios)	↑ Risk thrombophlebitis (cesarean section [C/S] risk) ↑ Risk of problems breastfeeding (C/S risk) ↑ Risk of hemorrhage ↑ Risk of anemia ↑ Stretching of abdominal muscles ↑ Incidence and severity of afterpains
Abruptio placentae, placenta previa	Hemorrhage → anemia ↓ Uterine contractility after birth→ ↑ infection risk
Precipitous labor (less than 3 hours)	↑ Risk of lacerations to birth canal → hemorrhage
Prolonged labor (greater than 24 hours)	Exhaustion ↑ Risk of hemorrhage Nutritional and fluid depletion ↑ Bladder atony and/or trauma
Difficult birth	Exhaustion ↑ Risk of perineal lacerations ↑ Risk of hematomas ↑ Risk of hemorrhage → anemia
Extended period of time in stirrups at birth	↑ Risk of thrombophlebitis
Retained placenta	↑ Risk of hemorrhage ↑ Risk of infection

Postpartum Nursing Assessment

Comprehensive care is based on a thorough assessment, with identification of individual needs or potential problems. (See Assessment Guide: Postpartum—First 24 Hours After Birth on pages 1005–1006.)

Risk Factors

Ongoing assessment and patient education during the puerperium are designed to meet the needs of the childbearing family and to detect and treat possible complications. Table 35-2 identifies factors that may place the new mother at risk during the postpartum period. The nurse uses this knowledge during the assessment and is particularly alert for possible complications that may occur in an individual because of identified risk factors.

Physical Assessment

There are several principles to remember in preparing for and completing an assessment of the postpartum woman:

- Select the time that will provide the most accurate data. Palpating the fundus when the woman has a full bladder, for example, may give false information about the progress of involution. Ask the woman to void before assessment.
- Consider the patient's need for possible pre-medication before any painful assessments such as fundal massage.
- Provide an explanation of the purposes of regular assessment to the woman.
- Ensure that the woman is relaxed before starting; perform the procedures as gently as possible to avoid unnecessary discomfort.
- Document and report the results according to hospital/unit policy.
- Take appropriate precautions to prevent exposure to body fluids.

The physical assessment is an excellent opportunity for patient teaching. For example, when assessing the breasts of a lactating woman, the nurse can discuss breast care, breast milk production, the let-down reflex, and breast self-examination. A new mother may be very receptive to instruction on postpartum abdominal tightening exercises when the nurse assesses the woman's fundal height and diastasis. The assessment also provides an excellent

TABLE 35-3 Common Postpartum Concerns

Several postpartum occurrences cause special concern for mothers. The nurse will frequently be asked about the following events:

SOURCE OF CONCERN	EXPLANATION
Gush of blood that sometimes occurs when she first arises	Because of normal pooling of blood in vagina when the woman lies down to rest or sleep. Gravity causes blood to flow out when she stands.
Passing clots	Blood pools at top of vagina and forms clots that are passed upon rising or sitting on the toilet.
Night sweats	Normal physiologic occurrence that results as body attempts to eliminate excess fluids that were present during pregnancy. May be aggravated by plastic mattress pad.
Afterpains	More common in multiparas. Caused by contraction and relaxation of uterus. Increased by oxytocin, breastfeeding. Relieved with mild analgesics and time.
"Large stomach" after birth and failure to lose all weight gained during pregnancy	The baby, amniotic fluid, and placenta account for only a portion of the weight gained during pregnancy. The remainder takes approximately 6 weeks to lose. Abdomen also appears large because of decreased muscle tone. Postpartal exercises will help.

time to provide information about the body's postpartum physical and anatomic changes as well as common postpartum concerns (Table 35-3).

Because the time the woman spends in the postpartum unit is limited, nurses should use every available opportunity for patient teaching regarding self-care. To assist nurses in recognizing these opportunities, examples of patient teaching during the assessment have been provided throughout the following discussion.

Vital Signs

The nurse may organize the physical assessment in a variety of ways. Many nurses choose to begin by assessing vital signs because the findings are more accurate when they are obtained with the woman at rest. In addition, establishing whether the vital signs are within the expected normal range will assist the nurse in determining other assessments that might be needed. For instance, if the temperature is elevated, the nurse considers the time since birth and begins to gather information to determine whether the woman is dehydrated or whether an infection is developing.

Temperature elevations (less than 38°C [100.4°F]) due to normal processes should last for only 24 hours. The nurse should evaluate any temperature elevation in light of other signs and symptoms and should carefully review the woman's history to identify other factors, such as premature rupture of membranes (PROM) or prolonged labor that might increase the incidence of infection in the genital tract.

Alterations in vital signs may indicate complications, so they are assessed at regular intervals. After an immediate, transient rise after birth, the blood pressure should remain stable. The pulse often shows a characteristic slowness that is no cause for alarm. Pulse rates return to prepregnant norms very quickly unless complications arise.

CLINICAL TIP

During the first few hours after birth, the woman may have some orthostatic hypotension. This will cause her to have a lower blood pressure reading in a sitting position. For the most accurate reading, measure her blood pressure with the woman in the same position each time, preferably lying on her back with her arm at her side. Because of the propensity for hypotension, the nurse should assist the mother the first few times she attempts to ambulate after delivery.

The nurse informs the woman of the results of the vital signs assessment, providing information regarding the normal changes in blood pressure and pulse. This may also be an opportunity to assess whether the mother knows how to take her own and her infant's temperatures, how to read a thermometer, and how to select a thermometer from the wide variety now available.

Auscultation of Lungs

The breath sounds should be clear. Women who have been treated for preterm labor or preeclampsia are especially at risk for pulmonary edema (see "Care of Woman with a Hypertensive Disorder" in chapter 20 ∞).

Breasts

Before examining the breasts, the nurse dons gloves and then assesses the fit and support of the woman's bra. The nurse provides information about how to select a bra. A properly fitting bra provides support to the breasts and helps maintain breast shape by limiting stretching of supporting ligaments and connective tissue. If the mother is breastfeeding, the straps of the bra should be cloth, not elastic (because cloth has less stretch and provides more support) and easily adjustable. The back should be wide and have at least three rows of hooks to adjust for fit. Traditional nursing bras have a fixed inner cup and a separate half-cup that can be unhooked for breastfeeding while continuing to support the breast. Purchasing a nursing bra one size too large during pregnancy will usually result in a good fit because the breasts increase in size with milk production.

The nurse asks the woman to remove her bra so the breasts can be examined. It is important to note the size and shape of the breasts and any abnormalities, reddened areas, or engorgement. The nurse also palpates the breasts lightly for softness, slight firmness associated with filling, or firmness associated with engorgement, warmth, or tenderness. The nipples are assessed for fissures, cracks, soreness, or inversion. The nurse teaches the woman the characteristics of the breast and explains how to recognize problems such as fissures or cracks in the nipples.

The nurse assesses the nonbreastfeeding mother for evidence of breast discomfort and provides relief measures if necessary. (See discussion of lactation suppression in the nonbreastfeeding mother in chapter 36 ∞.) Breast assessment findings for a nonbreastfeeding woman may be recorded as follows: "Breasts soft, filling, no evidence of nipple tenderness or cracking, nipples everted."

ASSESSMENT GUIDE Postpartum—First 24 Hours After Birth

Physical Assessment/Normal Findings	Alterations and Possible Causes*	Nursing Responses to Data†
VITAL SIGNS		
Blood Pressure (BP): Should remain consistent with baseline BP during pregnancy.	High BP (preeclampsia, essential hypertension, renal disease, anxiety). Drop in BP (may be normal; uterine hemorrhage).	Evaluate history of preexisting disorders and check for other signs of preeclampsia (edema, proteinuria). Assess for other signs of hemorrhage (↑ pulse, cool clammy skin).
Pulse: 50–90 beats/min. May be bradycardia if 50–70 beats/min.	Tachycardia (difficult labor and birth, hemorrhage).	Evaluate for other signs of hemorrhage (↓ BP, cool clammy skin).
Respirations: 16–24/minute.	Marked tachypnea (respiratory disease). Diminished respirations (long-acting epidural narcotics).	Assess for other signs of respiratory disease.
Temperature: 36.2°C to 38°C (97.1°F to 100.4°F)	After first 24 hours, temperature of 38°C (100.4°F) or above suggests infection.	Assess for other signs of infection: notify physician or certified nurse-midwife (CNM).
BREASTS		
General Appearance: Smooth, even pigmentation, changes of pregnancy still apparent: one may appear larger.	Reddened area (mastitis).	Assess further for signs of infection.
Palpation: Depending on postpartal day, may be soft, filling, full, or engorged.	Palpable mass (caked breast, mastitis). Engorgement (venous stasis). Tenderness, heat, edema (engorgement, caked breast, mastitis).	Assess for other signs of infection: If blocked duct, consider heat, massage, position change for breastfeeding. Assess for further signs. Report mastitis to physician or CNM.
Nipples: Supple, pigmented, intact; become erect when stimulated.	Fissures, cracks, soreness (problems with breastfeeding), not erectile with stimulation (inverted nipples).	Reassess technique: recommend appropriate interventions.
LUNGS		
Sounds: clear to bases bilaterally.	Diminished (fluid overload, asthma, pulmonary embolus, pulmonary edema)	Assess for other signs of respiratory distress.
ABDOMEN		
Musculature: Abdomen may be soft, have a "doughy" texture; rectus muscle intact.	Separation in musculature (diastasis recti abdominis).	Evaluate size of diastasis: teach appropriate exercises for decreasing the separation.
Fundus: Firm, midline; following expected process of involution.	Boggy (full bladder, uterine bleeding, deviation from midline).	Massage until firm; assess bladder and have woman void if needed; attempt to express clots when firm. If bogginess remains or recurs, report to physician or CNM.
May be tender when palpated.	Constant tenderness (infection).	Assess for evidence of endometritis.
Cesarean section incision dressing; dry and intact	Moderate to large amount of blood or serosanguineous drainage on dressing.	Assess for hemorrhage. Reinforce dressing and notify healthcare provider.
LOCHIA		
Scant to moderate amount, earthy odor; no clots.	Large amount, clots (hemorrhage). Foul-smelling lochia (infection).	Assess for firmness, express additional clots; begin peripad count. Assess for other signs of infection; report to physician or CNM.
Normal Progression: First 1–3 days: rubra. Following rubra: Days 3–10: serosa (alba seldom seen in hospital).	Failure to progress normally or return to rubra from serosa (subinvolution).	Report to physician or CNM.
PERINEUM		
Slight edema and bruising in intact perineum.	Marked fullness, bruising, pain (vulvar hematoma).	Assess size; apply ice glove or ice pack, analgesic and anesthetic sprays; report to physician or CNM.
Episiotomy: No redness, edema, ecchymosis, or discharge, edges well approximated.	Redness, edema, ecchymosis, discharge, or gaping stitches (infection).	Encourage sitz baths; review perineal care, appropriate wiping techniques.
Hemorrhoids: None present; if present, should be small and nontender.	Full, tender, inflamed hemorrhoids.	Encourage sitz baths, side-lying position; Tucks pads, anesthetic ointments, manual replacement of hemorrhoids, stool softeners, increased fluid intake.
	*Possible causes of alterations are identified in parentheses.	†This column provides guidelines for further assessment and initial nursing action.

(continued)

ASSESSMENT GUIDE Postpartum—First 24 Hours After Birth continued

Physical Assessment/Normal Findings	Alterations and Possible Causes*	Nursing Responses to Data†
COSTOVERTEBRAL ANGLE (CVA) TENDERNESS		
None.	Present (kidney infection).	Assess for other symptoms of urinary tract infection (UTI): obtain clean-catch urine sample; report to physician or CNM.
LOWER EXTREMITIES		
No pain with palpation; negative Homans' sign.	Positive findings (thrombophlebitis).	Report to physician or CNM.
ELIMINATION		
Urinary Output: Voiding in sufficient quantities at least every 4–6 hours; bladder not palpable.	Inability to void (urinary retention). Urgency, frequency, dysuria (UTI).	Employ nursing interventions to promote voiding; if not successful, obtain order for catheterization. Report symptoms of UTI to physician or CNM.
Bowel Elimination: Should have normal bowel movement by second or third day after birth.	Inability to pass feces or hard, small amount of stool (constipation due to fear of pain from episiotomy, hemorrhoids, perineal trauma).	Encourage fluids, ambulation, roughage in diet; sitz baths to promote healing of perineum; obtain order for stool softener.
Cultural Assessment‡	**Variations to Consider**	**Nursing Responses to Data†**
Determine customs and practices regarding postpartum care. Ask the mother whether she would like fluids and ask what temperature she prefers. Ask the mother what foods or fluids she would like. Ask the mother whether she would prefer to be alone during breastfeeding.	Individual preference may include: • Room-temperature or warmed fluids rather than iced drinks. • Special foods or fluids to hasten healing after childbirth. • Some women may be hesitant to have someone with them when their breast is exposed.	Provide for specific request if possible. If woman is unable to provide specific information, the nurse may draw from general information regarding cultural variation. Mexican women may want food and fluids that restore hot-cold balance to the body. Women of European background may ask for iced fluids. Provide privacy as desired by mother.
PSYCHOLOGIC ADAPTATION		
During First 24 Hours: Passive; preoccupied with own needs; may talk about her labor and birth experience; may be talkative, elated, or very quiet.	Very quiet and passive; sleeps frequently (fatigue from long labor; feelings of disappointment about some aspect of the experience; may be following cultural expectation).	Provide opportunities for adequate rest; provide physical comfort measures; provide nutritious meals and snacks that are consistent with what the woman desires to eat and drink; provide opportunities to discuss birth experience in nonjudgmental atmosphere if the woman desires to do so.
Usually by 12 hours; beginning to assume responsibility; some women eager to learn; others easily feel overwhelmed.	Excessive weepiness, mood swings, pronounced irritability (postpartum blues; feelings of inadequacy); culturally prescribed behavior.	Explain postpartum blues; provide supportive atmosphere; determine support available for mother; consider referral for evidence of profound depression.
ATTACHMENT		
En face position; holds baby close; cuddles and soothes; calls by name; identifies characteristics of family members in infant; may be awkward in providing care. Initially may express disappointment over sex or appearance of infant but within 1–2 days demonstrates attachment behaviors.	Continued expressions of disappointment in sex, appearance of infant; refusal to care for infant; derogatory comments; lack of bonding behaviors (difficulty in attachment, following expectations of cultural/ethnic group).	Provide reinforcement and support for infant caretaking behaviors; maintain nonjudgmental approach and gather more information if caretaking behaviors are not evident.
PATIENT EDUCATION		
Demonstrates basic understanding of self-care activities and infant care needs; can identify signs of complications that should be reported.	Unable to demonstrate basic self-care and infant care activities (knowledge deficit; postpartum blues; following prescribed cultural behavior and will be cared for by grandmother or other family member).	Identify predominant learning style. Determine whether woman understands English and provide interpreter if needed; provide reinforcement of information through conversation and through written material (remember that some women and their families may not be able to understand written materials because of language difficulties or inability to read); provide information regarding infant care skills that are culturally consistent; give woman opportunity to express her feelings and demonstrate skills taught; consider social service home referral for women who have no family or other support, are unable to take in information about self-care and infant care, and demonstrate no caretaking activities.
‡These are only a few suggestions. It is not our intent to imply this is a comprehensive cultural assessment.	*Possible causes of alterations are identified in parentheses.	†This column provides guidelines for further assessment and initial nursing action.

> **CLINICAL TIP**
> An easy way to remember the components specific to the postpartum examination is to remember the term BUBBLEHE: B-breast, U-uterus, B-bladder, B-bowel, L-lochia, E-episiotomy/laceration, H-Homans'/hemorrhoids, and E-emotional.

Abdomen and Fundus

The woman should void before her abdomen is examined. This practice ensures that a full bladder is not causing displacement of the uterus or any uterine atony; if atony is present, other causes (such as uterine relaxation associated with a regional block, overstretched uterus, or distended bladder) must be investigated.

The nurse determines the relationship of the fundus to the umbilicus and also assesses the firmness of the fundus. The top of the fundus is measured in fingerbreadths above, below, or at the umbilicus. The nurse notes whether the fundus is in the midline or displaced to either side of the abdomen. If not midline, the uterus position should be located. The most common cause of displacement is a full bladder; thus this finding requires further assessment. If the fundus is in the midline but higher than expected, it is usually associated with clots within the uterus. The results of the assessment should then be recorded. (See Procedure 35-1: Assessing the Status of the Uterine Fundus After Vaginal or Cesarean Birth).

While completing the assessment, the nurse teaches the woman about fundal position and how to determine firmness. The mother can be taught to massage her fundus gently if it is not firm.

> **CLINICAL TIP**
> Assessing the status of the uterine fundus may be uncomfortable. In addition to explaining the importance of the assessment to the mother, you can show her how to perform frequent light massage of the fundus herself to promote uterine involution. She may be delighted to be able to feel the difference between where the fundus is now and where "the top of the uterus" was just prior to delivery. Involving her in her own care encourages her participation. In addition, having her massage her own uterus may lessen bleeding and reduce the need for more thorough massage.

A well-contracted uterus feels as firm as the uterus does during a strong labor contraction. If handled gently, the uterus should not be overly tender. Excessive pain in the uterus during postpartal examination should alert the nurse to possible uterine infection. If the uterus is not firm, the nurse should gently massage the fundus with the fingertips of the examining hand, and then assess the results. If the uterus becomes firm, the chart should read: "Uterus: boggy → firm with light massage." A good habit for the nurse to develop during the postpartal examination is to have the woman lie flat on her back with her head on a pillow and legs flexed. Then the nurse can release the perineal pad to observe the results of uterine massage based on the amount of expelled blood. Occasionally, oxytocic agents, such as an intravenous Pitocin infusion or methylergonovine maleate (Methergine), need to be administered postpartally to maintain uterine contraction and prevent or treat hemorrhage (see Drug Guide: Methylergonovine Maleate [Methergine] in chapter 36 ∞).

> **CLINICAL TIP**
> During postpartum assessment, a firm uterus typically feels like a grapefruit because the muscles are well contracted. If the uterus loses its ability to contract and begins to relax, it is called boggy. A boggy uterus feels softer, like a sponge, or may become so relaxed that you cannot feel it at all. If the uterus is boggy but you can still feel it, massage it until it becomes firm. If you cannot feel it at all, place the side of one hand just above the woman's symphysis pubis to provide stability. Then place the other hand at the level of the umbilicus. (The fundus may have risen to this level because it is relaxed and filling with blood.) Press deeply into the abdomen and massage in a circular motion. You will usually feel the uterus begin to firm up under your hand. If you do not, move your hand slightly lower on the abdomen, and repeat the process.

A boggy uterus that does not contract with light, gentle massage may need more vigorous massage. The nurse assesses the amount and character of any expelled blood obtained while massaging the fundus. When a woman has postpartal uterine atony (the uterus does not remain firm), the nurse should do the following:

1. Reevaluate for full bladder; if the bladder is full, have the woman void.
2. Question the woman on her bleeding history since the birth or last examination. How heavy does her flow seem? Has she passed any clots? How frequently has she changed pads? Were the pads saturated? Look at the discarded pads.
3. For the breastfeeding mother, put the newborn to the mother's breast for feeding to stimulate oxytocin production.
4. Assess maternal blood pressure and pulse to identify hypotension.
5. Reassess the fundus; if the fundus is still boggy, alert the certified nurse-midwife (CNM) or physician immediately, because further interventions, such as intravenous fluids and an oxytocic medication, are needed.

In the woman who has had a cesarean birth, the abdominal incision is exquisitely tender. The nurse should palpate the fundus with extreme care and inspect the abdominal incision for signs of healing, such as approximation (absence of separation between edges of incision), bleeding, and for any signs of infection, including drainage, edema, foul odor, or redness. It is important to document whether internal sutures, steri-strips, or staples are intact. During the assessment, the nurse teaches the woman about her incision. The nurse can also review characteristics of normal healing, incision care, and discuss signs of infection.

Lochia

Lochia is then assessed for character, amount, odor, and the presence of clots. The nurse must wear disposable gloves when assessing the perineum and lochia. Nurses may put on

PROCEDURE 35-1 Assessing the Status of the Uterine Fundus After Vaginal or Cesarean Birth

NURSING ACTION

Preparation

- Consider offering to pre-medicate 30–45 minutes before assessing the fundus, especially if the patient has had a cesarean section.

  Rationale: *The postoperative area will be very tender, and she may be very fearful of the potential pain.*
- Explain the procedure, the information it provides, and what it might feel like.
- Ask the woman to void.

  Rationale: *A full bladder can cause uterine atony.*
- Have the woman lie flat in bed with her head on a pillow. If the procedure is uncomfortable, she may find that it helps to flex her legs. Flexing the legs and providing support under them with folded pillows is especially helpful with post–cesarean section patients.

  Rationale: *The supine position prevents falsely high assessment of fundal height. Flexing the legs relaxes the abdominal muscles.*

Equipment and Supplies

- A clean perineal pad (see Procedure 35-2)

> **CLINICAL TIP**
>
> Gloves may be put on before assessing the abdomen and fundus or when you are ready to assess the perineum and lochia.

Procedure

1. Gently place one hand on the lower segment of the uterus. Using the side of the other hand, palpate the abdomen until you locate the top of the fundus.

   Rationale: *One hand stabilizes the uterus while the other hand locates the top of the fundus. (Support of the uterus prevents stretching of the ligaments that support the uterus.)*
2. Determine whether the fundus is firm. If it is, it will feel like a hard round object (similar to a grapefruit) in the abdomen. If it is not firm, massage the abdomen lightly until the fundus is firm.

   Rationale: *A firm fundus indicates that the uterine muscles are contracted and bleeding will not occur.*
3. Measure the top of the fundus in fingerbreadths above, below, or at the fundus. See Figure 35-6 ■.

   Rationale: *Fundal height gives information about the progress of involution.*
4. Determine the position of the fundus in relation to the midline of the body. If it is not in the midline, locate it and then evaluate the bladder for distention.

   Rationale: *The fundus may deviate from the midline when the bladder is full because the enlarged bladder pushes the uterus aside.*
5. If the bladder is distended, use nursing measures to help the woman void. If she is not able to void after a specified period of time, catheterization may be necessary.
6. Measure urine output for the next few hours until normal elimination is established.

   Rationale: *During the postpartum as diuresis occurs, the bladder may fill far more rapidly than normal, putting the woman at risk for uterine atony and hemorrhage. (Diminished tone of the uterus may cause loss of the urge to void.)*
7. Assess the lochia (see Procedure 35-2).
8. During the first few hours postpartum, if the fundus becomes boggy frequently or is located high above the umbilicus and the woman's bladder is empty, the uterine cavity may be filled with clots of blood. In this case, do the following:
   - Release the front of the perineal pad and lay it back so that you can see the perineum and the pad laying between the woman's legs.
   - *Massage* the uterine fundus until it is firm.
   - Keep one hand in position, stabilizing the lower portion of the uterus. With the hand you used to massage the fundus, put steady pressure on the top of the now-firm fundus and see if you are able to express any clots. (Watch the pad between her legs for clots to pass from the vagina.)

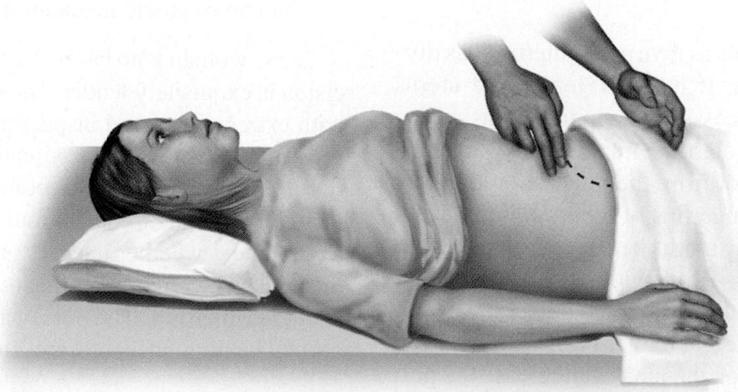

Figure 35-6 ■ Measuring the descent of the fundus for the woman having a vaginal birth. The fundus is located two fingerbreadths below the umbilicus. Always support the bottom of the uterus during any assessment of fundus.

PROCEDURE 35-1 Assessing the Status of the Uterine Fundus After Vaginal or Cesarean Birth continued

NURSING ACTION

Rationale: *If the woman's uterus is filled with blood, it acts as an irritant and the uterus will not remain contracted. When the muscle fibers relax, bleeding results, further aggravating the problem. Pushing on a uterus that is not firm is dangerous because it is possible to cause the uterus to invert, a true emergency.*

9. If measurement of the blood loss is needed, the perineal pads and Chux can be weighed. See Procedure 35-2.

10. Provide the woman with a clean perineal pad.

11. Record findings. Fundal height is recorded in fingerbreadths (e.g., "2 FB ↓ U" or "1 FB ↑ U"). If fundal massage was necessary, note that fact: "Uterus boggy → firm with light massage."

12. Communicate bogginess or heavy flow to primary provider.

13. If the patient is post–cesarean section, inspect the abdominal incision for signs of healing, such as approximation, bleeding, and for any signs of infection, including drainage, edema, foul odor, or redness. Observe whether internal sutures, steri-strips, or staples are intact. If dressing is in place over the incision, observe for the dressing to be clean, dry, and intact.

Rationale: *If drainage is present on the dressing, mark the outline of the drainage and reevaluate 30 minutes later for further bleeding or drainage.*

14. Document findings according to hospital or unit policy.

15. Communicate active bleeding, increasing drainage, redness, foul odor, or incision edges not approximated to primary care provider.

RESEARCH EVIDENCE IN PRACTICE Assessing Risk of Postpartum Hemorrhage

CLINICAL QUESTION

What nursing assessments can identify risk factors and early signs of hemorrhage?

RESEARCH EVIDENCE

Postpartum hemorrhage is the leading cause of pregnancy-related death, causing more than 140,000 maternal deaths a year worldwide. Besides death, postpartum hemorrhage is a significant cause of pregnancy-related morbidity, and is the primary reason for postpartum hysterectomy.

The National Collaborating Center for Primary Care convened a group of obstetric experts to review research literature and develop guidelines for postnatal assessments. While these guidelines do not recommend routine postpartum palpation or measurement of the uterus, assessment of uterine involution and position should be undertaken in women with excessive vaginal blood loss, abdominal tenderness, or fever in the postpartum period. Excessive blood loss is defined as greater than 500 ml for a vaginal birth and more than 1000 ml for a cesarean birth.

Blood loss may be indicated by a mother's complaints of faintness, dizziness, palpitations, or "heart racing." Sudden or profuse blood loss, or blood loss accompanied by signs of shock, should be evaluated as an emergency condition. Diagnostic indications of postpartum hemorrhage include a hematocrit drop of greater than 10%, need for blood transfusion, and hemodynamic instability.

Multiple epidemiological and cross-sectional studies have identified risk factors for postpartum hemorrhage. These factors include labor related causes (induction of labor, precipitous or prolonged labor), uterine overdistention (multiple pregnancies or polyhydramnios), genital tract trauma due to instrument births or cesarean birth, retained placenta or clots, coagulation disorders, and placenta previa. Women who had a third stage of labor longer than 18 minutes had a higher risk of postpartum hemorrhage, and those women with a third stage longer than 30 minutes had a sixfold increase in risk of hemorrhage.

One study focused on risk factors associated with postpartum hysterectomy due to abnormal bleeding. These researchers found that multiparous women with a history of cesarean birth, or women with abnormal placental implantation, were at highest risk for surgical removal of the uterus after birth.

WHAT QUESTIONS REMAIN UNANSWERED?

Many normal vaginal births result in blood loss greater than 500 ml, which has led to questions as to whether this is an appropriate threshold for considering postpartum hemorrhage. What is an appropriate amount of blood loss to expect in a normal vaginal birth?

WHAT IS BEST PRACTICE?

Abdominal palpation of the uterus is not necessary as a routine postpartum assessment after a normal birth. New mothers should be assessed for signs of blood loss, including complaints of faintness, dizziness, or palpitations. Sudden or profuse blood loss, or persistent blood loss after birth, may indicate an emergency situation. Intensive assessment should be focused on women with risk factors for hemorrhage or postpartum hysterectomy.

CRITICAL THINKING

What maternal signs and symptoms should trigger an abdominal assessment for uterine involution and position?

References

Magaan, E., Evans, S., Chauham, S., Lanneau, G., Fisk, A., & Morrison, J. 2005. The length of the third stage of labor and the risk of postpartum hemorrhage. *Obstetrics and Gynecology, 105*(2), 290–293.

National Collaborating Centre for Primary Care. 2006. Postnatal care: Routine postnatal care of women and their babies. *Royal College of General Practitioners,* 392.

Oyelese, Y., & Ananth, C. 2010. Postpartum hemorrhage: Epidemiology, risk factors, and causes. *Clinical Obstetrics and Gynecology, 53*(1), 147–156.

Rossi, A., Lee, R., & Chmait, R. 2010. Emergency postpartum hysterectomy for uncontrolled postpartum bleeding: A systematic review. *Obstetrics and Gynecology, 115*(3), 637–644.

the gloves before beginning the assessment, just before assessing the abdomen and fundus, or when they are ready to assess the perineum and lochia. During the first 1 to 3 days, the lochia should be rubra. A few small clots are normal and occur as a result of blood pooling in the vagina. However, the passage of numerous or large clots is abnormal, and the cause should be investigated immediately. After 2 to 3 days, the lochia becomes serosa.

Lochia should never exceed a moderate amount, such as that needed to partially saturate four to eight peri-pads daily, with an average of six. However, because this number is influenced by an individual woman's pad changing practices, as well as the absorbency of the pad, the nurse must consider the length of time the current pad has been in use, the parity, and the size of the baby and ask whether the amount is normal compared with her typical menstrual period, and whether any clots were passed before the examination, such as during voiding. If heavy bleeding is reported but not seen, the nurse asks the woman to put on a clean perineal pad and reassesses the discharge in 1 hour (see Procedure 35-2 and Figure 35-7 ■).

When a more accurate assessment of blood loss is needed, the perineal pads can be weighed, with 1 g considered equivalent to 1 ml blood.

Clots and heavy bleeding may be caused by uterine relaxation (atony), retained placental fragments, or, rarely, an unknown cervical laceration (seen as heavy bleeding but with firm fundus) that may require further assessment (Table 35-4). Because of the evacuation of the uterine cavity during cesarean birth, women with such surgery usually have less lochia after the first 24 hours than mothers who give birth vaginally. If the woman is at increased risk for bleeding or is actually experiencing heavy flow of lochia rubra, her blood pressure, pulse, and uterus need to be assessed frequently, and the physician may prescribe oxytocin (Pitocin) or methylergonovine maleate (Methergine). See Drug Guide: Methylergonovine Maleate (Methergine) in chapter 36 ∞.

CLINICAL TIP

The parity, length of time since delivery, method of delivery, size of baby/gestation (and other factors that could cause hyperextension of the uterus such as multiple gestation, polyhydramnios, large-for-gestational age, etc.), *must* be considered when deciding whether the amount and color of the lochia is appropriate.

The odor of the lochia is nonoffensive and never foul. If foul odor is present, so is an infection. When using narrative nursing notes, document the amount of lochia first, followed by character. For example:

- Lochia: moderate rubra
- Lochia: small rubra/serosa

Patient teaching that the nurse may address during assessment of the lochia can center on normal changes, effect of position changes on or what can be expected in the amount and color of the flow. Hygienic measures, such as wiping the perineum from front to back and washing her hands after toileting and changing pads, may be reviewed if appropriate. The nurse should approach the timing of teaching hygienic practices delicately, along with the content to be included. By establishing positive goals for the teaching—promoting comfort, enhancing tissue healing, and preventing infection—the nurse can avoid value-laden statements regarding personal beliefs about the need for cleanliness or control of body odor. The nurse should review with the mother the need to notify a healthcare professional if there is regression in the lochia flow pattern (i.e., color or amount).

Perineum

The perineum is inspected with the woman lying in Sims' position. The buttock is lifted to expose the perineum and anus.

If an episiotomy was performed or a laceration required suturing, the nurse assesses the wound. To evaluate the state of healing, the nurse inspects the wound for redness, edema, ecchymosis, discharge, and approximation. After 24 hours, some edema may still be present, but the skin edges should be approximated ("glued" together) so that gentle pressure does not separate them. Gentle palpation should elicit minimal tenderness, and there should be no hardened areas suggesting infection. Ecchymosis interferes with normal healing, as does infection. Foul odors associated with drainage indicate infection. Hematomas sometimes occur, although these are considered abnormal. The nurse next assesses whether hemorrhoids are present around the anus. If present, they are assessed for size, number, and pain or tenderness (see Procedure 35-3 and Figure 35-8 ■).

During the assessment, the nurse talks with the woman to determine the effectiveness of comfort measures that have been used. The nurse provides teaching about the episiotomy or perineal laceration. Some women do not thoroughly understand what an episiotomy is and where it is and may believe that the stitches must be removed, as with other types of surgery. Frequently, when women fear that the stitches must be removed manually, they are afraid to ask about them. While explaining the findings

TABLE 35-4 Changes in Lochia That Cause Concern

CHANGE	POSSIBLE PROBLEM	NURSING ACTION
Presence of clots	Inadequate uterine contractions that allow bleeding from vessels at the placental site.	Assess location and firmness of fundus. Assess voiding pattern. Record and report findings.
Persistent lochia rubra	Inadequate uterine contractions; retained placental fragments; infection; undetected cervical laceration.	Assess location and firmness of fundus. Assess activity pattern. Assess for signs of infection. Record and report findings.

PROCEDURE 35-2 Evaluating Lochia

NURSING ACTION

Preparation

- Explain why lochia occurs, why it is assessed, how it is assessed, and how it changes during the postpartum.
- Ask the woman to void.

  Rationale: *A full bladder can cause uterine atony and increase the amount of lochia.*
- Complete the assessment of uterine fundal height and firmness.

  Rationale: *In almost all cases, fundal height and firmness are evaluated with an assessment of lochia. This practice provides a more thorough assessment.*
- If she has not already done so for the fundal assessment, ask the woman to flex her legs. Then ask her to spread her legs apart. Use the bed sheet as a drape to preserve her modesty.

  Rationale: *This position allows you to see the perineum and the perineal pad more effectively.*

Equipment and Supplies

Note: *Gloves are put on before assessing the perineum and lochia.*

- Gloves
- Clean perineal pad

Procedure: Clean Gloves

1. Don gloves.
2. Lower the perineal pad and observe the amount of lochia on the pad. Because women's pad-changing practices vary, ask her about the length of time the current pad has been in use, whether the amount is normal, and whether any clots were passed before this examination, such as during voiding.

   Rationale: *During the first 1 to 3 days the woman's lochia should be rubra, which is dark red in color. A few small clots are normal and occur as a result of pooling of blood in the vagina when the woman is lying down. The passage of large clots is abnormal and the cause should be investigated immediately.*
3. If the woman reports heavy bleeding or clots, ask her to put on a clean perineal pad and then reassess the pad in 1 hour. Also ask her to call you before flushing any clots she passes into the toilet during voiding.
4. When the uterine fundus is firm and stabilized with the nondominant hand, press down on it with the dominant hand while watching to see if any clots are expelled. (See Procedure 35-1, step 8.)
5. Determine the amount of lochia, using the following guide (see Figure 35-7):
   - Heavy amount—Perineal pad has a stain larger than 6 inches in length within 1 hour; 30 to 80 ml lochia.
   - Moderate amount—Perineal pad has a stain less than 6 inches in length within 1 hour; 25 to 50 ml lochia.
   - Small (light) amount—Perineal pad has a stain less than 4 inches in length after 1 hour; 10 to 25 ml lochia.
   - Scant amount—Perineal pad has a stain less than 1 inch in length after 1 hour or lochia is only on tissue when the woman wipes.

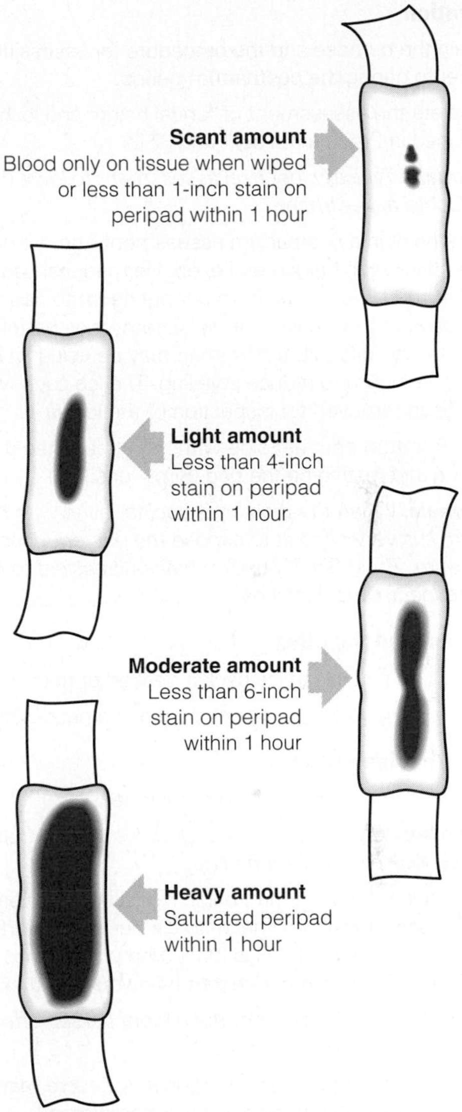

Scant amount
Blood only on tissue when wiped or less than 1-inch stain on peripad within 1 hour
Light amount
Less than 4-inch stain on peripad within 1 hour
Moderate amount
Less than 6-inch stain on peripad within 1 hour
Heavy amount
Saturated peripad within 1 hour

Figure 35-7 ■ Suggested guidelines for assessing lochia volume.

Source: Jacobson, H. A standard for assessing lochia volume. American Journal of Maternal/Child Nursing, 10, *174–175, May–June 1985. Copyright © Lippincott Williams & Wilkins. Reprinted with permission.*

   Rationale: *Lochia should never exceed a moderate amount such as four to eight partially saturated perineal pads daily. Using a consistent standard for measuring lochia improves the accuracy of the information charted and conveyed to others.*

6. In most cases, a woman is discharged while her lochia is still rubra. Provide her with information about lochia serosa and lochia alba.

   Rationale: *Accurate discharge information enables the woman to assess herself more accurately and enables her to judge better when to contact her caregiver.*
7. Document the findings according to hospital/unit policy. For example, "Uterus firm, 1 FB ↓ U, Lochia: moderate rubra, no clots passed."

PROCEDURE 35-3 Postpartum Perineal Assessment

NURSING ACTION

Preparation

- Explain the purpose and the procedure for assessing the perineum during the postpartum period.
- Complete the assessment of fundal height and lochia as described in Procedures 35-1 and 35-2.

  Rationale: *Typically, perineal assessment follows the fundal and lochial assessment.*
- At this point in a postpartum assessment, the woman is lying on her back with her knees flexed. Her perineal pad has already been lifted away from her perineum to permit inspection of the lochia. If an episiotomy was performed or if the birth was difficult, the woman may be using an ice pack on her perineum to reduce swelling. The ice pack would also have been removed for inspection of the lochia.
- Ask her to turn onto her side with her upper knee drawn forward and resting on the bed (Sims' position).

  Rationale: *When the woman is supine, even with her knees flexed, it is very difficult to expose the posterior portion of the perineum. Thus, Sims' position makes it easiest to inspect the perineum and anal area.*

Equipment and Supplies

Clean perineal pad, clean ice pack if desired or needed

Small light source such as a penlight may be necessary

Procedure: Clean Gloves

1. Use a systematic approach to assessment.

   Rationale: *A systematic approach helps ensure that you do not overlook a significant finding.*
2. In evaluating the perineum, begin by asking the woman's perceptions. How does she describe her discomfort? Does it seem excessive to her? Has it become worse since the birth? Does it seem more severe than you would expect?

   Rationale: *Information from the patient herself often helps identify developing problems.*

(**Note:** *Pain that seems disproportionately severe may indicate that the woman is developing a vulvar hematoma.)*

> **CLINICAL TIP**
>
> In evaluating the perineum, use the REEDA scale as a quick reminder of what to assess.
>
> Specifically:
>
> R = redness
> E = edema or swelling
> E = ecchymosis or bruising
> D = drainage
> A = approximation (how well the edges of an incision—the episiotomy—or a repaired laceration seem to be holding together)
>
> Be prepared to respond appropriately to findings.

3. After talking with the woman, assess the condition of the tissue. To allow for full visualization, it may be helpful to ask the woman to lift the knee of her upper leg to expose her perineum more fully. In some cases it may help to use the nondominant gloved hand to lift the buttocks and tissue. Note any swelling (edema) and bruising (ecchymosis).

   Rationale: *The tissue is often traumatized by the birth and mild bruising is not unusual. However, excessive bruising may indicate that a hematoma is developing.*
4. Evaluate the episiotomy, if there is one, or any repaired laceration for its state of healing. Is it reddened? Note the edges of the incision. Are they well approximated? Tell the woman that you are going to palpate the incision gently, then do so. Note any areas of hardness. Note whether the incision is warmer to the touch than the surrounding tissue.

   Rationale: *Gentle palpation should elicit minimal tenderness and there should be no redness, warmth, or areas of hardness, which suggest infection. Both bruising and infection interfere with normal healing. Typically, within 24 hours the edges of the incision should be "glued" together (well approximated).*
5. During the assessment be alert for odors. Typically the lochia has an earthy, but not unpleasant, smell that is easily identifiable.

   Rationale: *A foul odor associated with drainage often indicates infection.*
6. Finally, assess for hemorrhoids. To visualize the anal area, lift the upper buttocks to fully expose the anal area. (See Figure 35-8.) If hemorrhoids are present, note the size, number, and pain or tenderness.

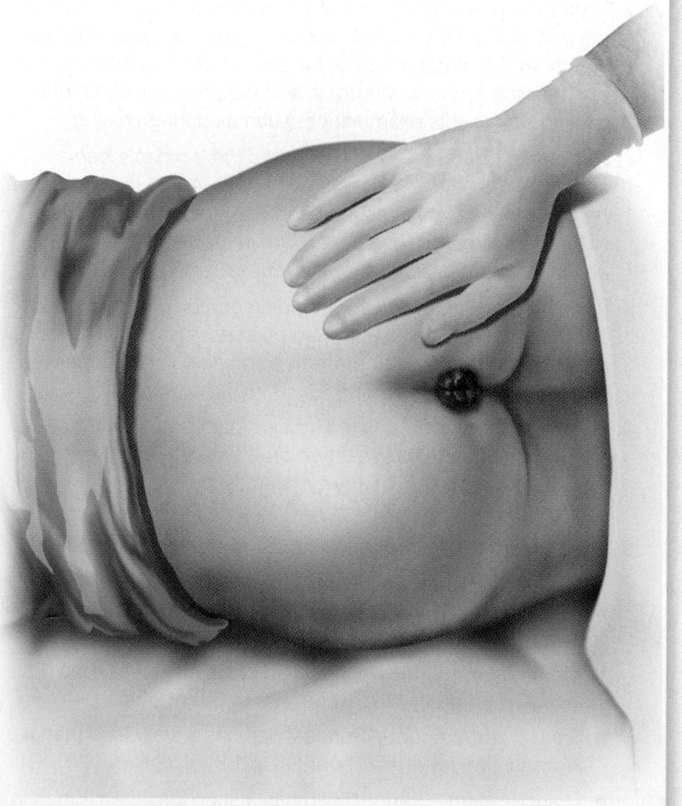

Figure 35-8 ■ Intact perineum with hemorrhoids.

PROCEDURE 35-3 Postpartum Perineal Assessment continued

NURSING ACTION

Rationale: *Hemorrhoids often develop during pregnancy or labor and can cause considerable discomfort. If hemorrhoids are present, the woman may benefit from available comfort measures.*

7. During the assessment, talk to the woman about the effectiveness of comfort measures being used. Provide teaching about care of the episiotomy, hemorrhoids, and the like.

   Rationale: *Health teaching is an important part of nursing care. Many women have concerns about the episiotomy and may not know, for example, that the suture used is dissolvable. This is an excellent time to provide information about good healthcare practices for both the short and long term.*

8. Provide the woman with a clean perineal pad. Replenish the ice pack if necessary.
9. Document findings according to hospital or unit policy. For example: "Midline episiotomy; no edema, ecchymosis, or tenderness. Skin edges well approximated. Woman reports pain relief measures are controlling discomfort"; or "Perineal repair, is approximated, minimal edema, no ecchymosis or tenderness; ice pack to perineum relieves pain."

of the assessment, the nurse can provide information about the episiotomy, its location, and signs that are being assessed. In addition, the nurse can casually add that the sutures are special and will dissolve slowly over the next few weeks as the tissues heal. By the time the sutures are dissolved, the tissues are strong, and the incision edges will not separate. This is also an opportunity to teach comfort measures that may be used and reinforce the need to consult with the healthcare provider before using over-the-counter (OTC) medications or supplements if breastfeeding (see "Relief of Perineal Discomfort" in chapter 36 ∞).

Lysine, an essential amino acid, has been identified as a supplement that decreases the incidence of pain following an episiotomy. Lysine is available as a supplement. The recommended adult dosage is 12 mg/kg of body weight per day. It is present in dietary sources, including meat, cheese, fish, eggs, soybeans, and nuts.

An example of documentation of a perineal assessment might read: "Midline episiotomy; no edema, tenderness, or ecchymosis present. Skin edges are approximated"; or, if a perineal laceration repair, "Skin edges intact, no edema, tenderness or ecchymosis, pain meds helpful. Woman reports sitz bath and Tucks pads or pain relief measures are controlling discomfort."

Lower Extremities

Postpartal women are at increased risk for thrombophlebitis, thrombus formation, and inflammation involving a vein (see "Care of the Woman with Postpartum Thromboembolic Disease" in chapter 39 ∞). If thrombophlebitis occurs, the most likely site will be the woman's legs. Conditions that predispose a patient for thrombophlebitis are hypercoagulability, severe anemia, obesity, and traumatic delivery. To assess for thrombophlebitis, the nurse should have the woman stretch her legs out, with the knees slightly flexed and the legs relaxed. The nurse then grasps the foot and dorsiflexes it sharply. The second leg is assessed in the same way. No discomfort or pain should be present. If pain is elicited, the nurse notifies the CNM or physician that the woman has a positive Homans' sign (see Figure 35-9 ■). The pain is caused by inflammation of a vessel. The nurse also evaluates the legs for edema by comparing both legs, because usually only one leg is involved. Any areas of redness, tenderness, and increased skin temperature are also noted.

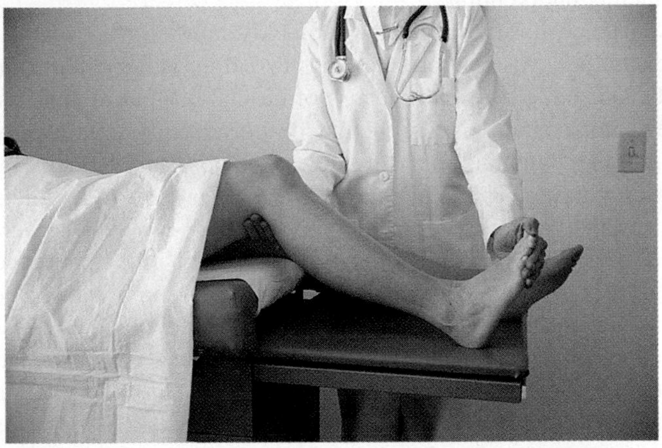

Figure 35-9 ■ Homans' sign: With the woman's knees flexed, the nurse dorsiflexes the foot. Pain in the foot or leg is a positive Homans' sign.

Source: Photographer, Elena Dorfman.

Some facilities have discontinued performing a Homans' sign in the nursing assessment, stating that it is not diagnostic and could lead to an embolus if the clot is dislodged during assessment. Although assessment of Homans' sign is not diagnostic, supporters advocate its use as a screening tool. There are no published reports of an embolus occurring as a result of performing a Homans' sign. In the event of a positive Homans' sign, diagnosis is made by compression or duplex ultrasonography. Low-dose heparin therapy is used in postpartal women who develop a deep vein thrombosis (Cunningham et al., 2010; James, 2008).

Early ambulation is an important aspect of preventing thrombophlebitis. Most women are able to get up shortly after birth or once they have fully recovered from the effects of the regional anesthetic agent, if one has been used. The mother's legs should be assessed for return of sensation following regional anesthesia. The cesarean birth patient requires passive range-of-motion exercises until she is ambulating more freely.

Patient teaching associated with assessment of the lower extremities focuses on the signs and symptoms of thrombophlebitis. In addition, the nurse may review self-care measures to promote circulation and prevent thrombophlebitis, such as leg exercises that may be performed in bed, dorsiflexion on an hourly basis while on bed rest, ambulation, avoiding pressure behind the knees, and avoiding crossing the legs.

Usually, the nurse records the results of the assessment on a flowsheet or a summary nursing note. If tenderness and warmth have been noted, they might be recorded as follows: "Tenderness, warmth, slight edema, and slight redness noted on posterior aspect of left calf—positive Homans'. Woman advised to avoid pressure to this area; lower leg elevated and moist heat applied per agency protocol. Call placed to Dr. Garcia to report findings."

Care Plan Activity: Postpartum Patient Requesting Relief

Elimination

During the hours after birth, the nurse carefully monitors a new mother's bladder status. A boggy uterus, displaced uterus, or a palpable bladder are a sign of bladder distention and requires nursing intervention.

The postpartum woman can quickly show signs of bladder distention, possibly as soon as 1 to 2 hours after childbirth. This distention results because of normal postpartal diuresis. The nurse should assess the bladder for distention frequently until the woman is able to completely empty her bladder with each voiding. The nurse may employ techniques to facilitate voiding, such as helping the woman out of bed to void, pouring warm water on the vulva, running water in the sink, and encouraging the woman to relax and take deep breaths. The physician will order catheterization when the bladder is distended and the woman cannot void, when she is voiding small amounts (less than 100 ml) frequently, or when no voiding has occurred in 8 hours. Although many physicians or CNMs write orders stating that the woman can be catheterized in 8 hours if she has not voided, the nurse needs to assess the bladder and any voiding pattern frequently before the end of the 8-hour period. Some women may require catheterization sooner. The cesarean birth mother may have an indwelling catheter inserted prophylactically. The nurse should perform the same assessments in evaluating bladder emptying once the catheter is removed.

During the physical assessment, the nurse elicits information from the woman regarding the adequacy of her fluid intake, whether she feels she is emptying her bladder completely when she voids, and any signs of UTI she may be experiencing.

In the same way, the nurse obtains information about the new mother's intestinal elimination and any concerns she may have about it. Many mothers fear that the first bowel movement will be painful and possibly even damaging if an episiotomy has been performed. If a woman has a bowel movement during labor or delivery, bowel motility will normally return within 2 to 3 days after a vaginal childbirth. Stool softeners may be ordered to increase bulk and moisture in the fecal material and to allow more comfortable and complete evacuation. Constipation may cause pressure on sutures and increase discomfort and therefore should be prevented. Encouraging ambulation, forcing fluids (up to 2000 ml/day or more), and providing fresh fruits and roughage in the diet enhance bowel elimination and help the woman reestablish her normal bowel pattern.

During the assessment, the nurse may provide information regarding postpartal diuresis, explaining why the woman may be emptying her bladder so frequently. Information about the need for additional fluid intake, with suggestions of specific amounts, may be helpful. The woman should drink at least eight 8-oz glasses of water or juice in addition to other fluids. Breastfeeding mothers will have a higher requirement. The nurse discusses signs of retention and overflow voiding and reviews symptoms of urinary tract infection (UTI) with the mother at this time if it seems an appropriate moment for teaching. The nurse can also review methods of assisting bowel elimination and provide opportunities for the woman to ask questions.

Rest and Sleep Status

Physical fatigue often affects other adjustments and functions of the new mother. The mother requires energy to make the psychologic adjustments to a new infant and to assume new roles. Fatigue is often a highly significant factor in a new mother's apparent disinterest in her newborn. Frequently the woman is so tired from a long labor and birth that everything seems to be an effort.

To avoid inadvertently classifying a very tired mother as one with a potential attachment problem, the nurse should do a psychologic assessment on more than one occasion. After a nap the new mother is often far more receptive to her baby and her surroundings. As part of the postpartum assessment, the nurse evaluates the amount of rest the new mother is getting. If the woman reports difficulty sleeping at night, the nurse should try to determine the cause. If it is simply the strange environment, a warm drink, backrub, or mild sedative may prove helpful. Appropriate nursing measures are indicated if the woman is bothered by normal postpartal discomforts such as afterpains, diaphoresis, or episiotomy or hemorrhoidal pain. The impact of rooming-in on the mother's ability to rest should be assessed. See chapter 36 for more detailed discussion of comfort and pain relief measures.

A daily rest period should be encouraged, and hospital activities should be scheduled to allow time for napping. The nurse can also provide information about the fatigue a new mother experiences and strategies to promote rest and sleep at home, and the impact fatigue can have on a woman's emotions and sense of control.

DEVELOPING CULTURAL COMPETENCE

Rest, Seclusion, and Dietary Restraint in Non-Western Cultures

Rest, seclusion, and dietary restraint practices in many traditional non-Western cultures (African, traditional Mexican, Chinese, Japanese, South Asian groups) are designed to assist the woman and her baby during postpartum vulnerable periods. The period of postpartum vulnerability and seclusion varies between 7 and 40 days. In Ghana, new mothers are relieved from all chores, told to abstain from sex, and not allowed to leave the home (Holtz & Grisdale, 2008; Lauderdale, 2008). Decreased activity and seclusion practices are designed to lessen the influence of spirits or of spreading evil and misfortune. The time of seclusion coincides with the period of lochial flow or postpartum bleeding.

HEALTH PROMOTION EDUCATION: NUTRITION

Postpartum nutritional status is primarily determined based on information provided by the mother and on direct assessment. During pregnancy the daily recommended dietary allowances call for increases in calories, proteins, and most vitamins and minerals. After birth the nonbreastfeeding mother's dietary requirements return to prepregnancy levels, whereas the lactating mother's requirements increase.

Visiting mothers during mealtime provides an opportunity for unobtrusive nutritional assessment and counseling. The nonbreastfeeding mother should be advised about the need to reduce her caloric intake by about 300 kcal and to return to prepregnancy levels for other nutrients. The breastfeeding mother should increase her caloric intake by about 200 kcal over the pregnancy requirements, or a total of 500 kcal over the nonpregnant requirement. Basic discussion will usually prove helpful, followed by referral as needed. In all cases, the nurse should provide literature on nutrition so that the woman will have a source of information following discharge.

The nurse should inform the dietitian of any mother who is a vegetarian, has food allergies or lactose intolerance, or whose cultural or religious beliefs require specific foods. Appropriate meals can then be prepared for her. Many women, especially those who gained more than the recommended number of pounds, are interested in losing weight after birth. The dietitian can design weight reduction diets to meet nutritional needs and food preferences. The nurse may also refer women with unusual eating habits or numerous questions about good nutrition to the dietitian.

New mothers are also advised that it is common practice to prescribe iron supplements for 3 months after birth. Hemoglobin and hematocrit values are then checked at the postpartal visit to detect any anemia.

As a part of the nutritional assessment, the nurse can provide teaching about the nutritional needs of the woman during the postpartum period. See Table 35-5 as well as the discussion in chapter 18 ∞.

Psychologic Assessment

During the first several postpartum weeks, the new mother must accomplish certain physical and developmental tasks:

- Restoring physical condition
- Developing competence in caring for and meeting the needs of her infant
- Establishing a relationship with her new child
- Adapting to altered lifestyles and family structure resulting from the addition of a new member

Adequate assessment of the mother's psychologic adjustment is an integral part of postpartal evaluation. This assessment focuses on the mother's general attitude, feelings of competence, available support systems, and caregiving skills. It also evaluates her fatigue level, sense of satisfaction, and ability to accomplish her developmental tasks.

Some new mothers have little or no experience with newborns and may feel totally overwhelmed. They may show these feelings by asking questions and reading all available material or by becoming passive and quiet because they simply cannot deal with their feelings of inadequacy. Unless a nurse questions the woman about her plans and previous experience in a supportive, nonjudgmental way, the nurse might conclude that the woman is uninterested, withdrawn, or depressed. Clues that may indicate a problem include excessive, continued fatigue; marked depression; excessive preoccupation with physical status or discomfort; evidence of low self-esteem; lack of support systems; marital or relationship problems; inability to care for or nurture the newborn; and current family crises (such as illness or unemployment). These characteristics frequently indicate a potential for maladaptive parenting, which may lead to child abuse or neglect (physical, emotional, intellectual) and cannot be ignored. Referrals to public health nurses or other available community resources may provide greatly needed assistance and alleviate potentially dangerous situations.

TABLE 35-5 Daily Eating to Encourage Healthful Nutrition During the Postpartum Period

- 2–3 servings of milk, yogurt, and cheese group
- 2–3 servings of meat or protein group
- 3–5 servings of vegetable group
- 4 servings of whole grain
- 2–4 servings of fruit group
- 6–11 servings of bread, cereal, rice, and pasta group
- Fats, oils, and sweets sparingly

Assessment of Early Attachment

The nurse in any of the various postpartum settings should periodically observe and note the mother's progress toward attachment. The assessment should include both parents when possible; however, in this section, the behaviors focus primarily on the mother's attachment process. As discussed previously, research shows that fathers experience attachment feelings similar to those experienced by mothers. The following questions can be addressed in the course of nurse-patient interaction:

- Is the mother attracted to her newborn? To what extent does she seek face-to-face contact and eye contact? Has she progressed from fingertip touch to palmar contact to enfolding the infant close to her own body? Is attraction increasing or decreasing? If the mother does not exhibit increasing attraction, why not? Do the reasons lie primarily within her, in the baby, or in the environment?
- Is the mother inclined to nurture her infant? Is she progressing in her interactions with her infant?
- Does the mother act consistently? If not, is the source of unpredictability within her or her infant?
- Is her mothering consistently carried out? Does she seek information and evaluate it objectively? Does she develop solutions based on adequate knowledge of valid data? Does she evaluate the effectiveness of her maternal care and make appropriate adjustments?
- Is she sensitive to the newborn's needs as they arise? How quickly does she interpret her infant's behavior and react to cues? Does she seem happy and satisfied with the infant's

responses to her efforts? Is she pleased with feeding behaviors? How much of this ability and willingness to respond is related to the baby's nature, and how much to her own?

- Does she seem pleased with her baby's appearance and sex? Is she experiencing pleasure in interaction with her infant? What interferes with the enjoyment? Does she speak to the baby frequently and affectionately? Does she call him or her by name? Does she point out family traits or characteristics she sees in the newborn?
- Are there any cultural factors that might modify the mother's response? For instance, is it customary for the grandmother to assume most of the childcare responsibilities while the mother recovers from childbirth?

Once these questions are addressed and the facts are assembled, the nurse can combine the information with personal intuition and knowledge to answer three more unspoken questions: Is there a problem in attachment? What is the problem? What is its source? The nurse can then devise a creative approach to the problem as it presents itself in the context of a unique, developing mother-infant relationship.

Discharge Assessment and Follow-Up

The **Newborns' and Mothers' Health Protection Act (NMHPA)** of 1996 went into effect January 1, 1998. This law states that a woman who has given birth vaginally in a healthcare setting cannot be forcibly discharged within 48 hours of the time of birth for insurance reasons. A woman who had a cesarean birth is covered by her insurance until 96 hours following the time of giving birth. If a mother with an uncomplicated birth and her physician or caregiver mutually decide that discharge before this time frame is required, this can be accomplished. When this occurs it is recommended that the newborn be seen in a follow-up setting within 48 hours (American Academy of Pediatrics [AAP], 2004).

The final discharge assessment should include a physical examination and appropriate discharge teaching that includes both maternal and newborn care guidelines. The mother's laboratory values are examined. If the mother was nonimmune to rubella, a rubella vaccine is administered before discharge. Rh-negative mothers whose infants are Rh positive need RhoGAM before they go home. If either is given, the nurse documents this in the mother's chart. If referrals, such as to social service programs, support groups, a lactation consultant, or a pediatrician, are needed, they should be provided before the family leaves the facility.

Some obstetricians, certified nurse-midwives, and nurse practitioners see all postpartum women 1 to 2 weeks after birth in addition to the routine 6-week checkup. These visits provide opportunities for physical assessment as well as assessment of the mother's psychologic and informational needs and needs of the family. The routine physical assessment, which can be made rapidly, focuses on the woman's general appearance, breasts, reproductive tract, bladder and bowel elimination, and any specific problems or complaints. In addition, the nurse should talk with the mother about her diet, fatigue level, family adjustment, and psychologic status. The nurse explores any problems with child care and refers the mother to a pediatric nurse practitioner or pediatrician if needed. Available community resources, including public health department follow-up visits, are mentioned when appropriate. If not already discussed, teaching about family planning is appropriate at this time, and the nurse provides information regarding birth control methods. The quality of discharge teaching, specifically the relative difference in the amount of information needed and received and the skills of the nurses delivering the teaching, can help the mother feel ready for discharge from the hospital. Likewise, part of the quality of the teaching includes the nurse assessing the *readiness* to be discharged as a general guide for the teaching content, amount of reinforcement of the information, and evaluation of the understanding of the information (Weiss & Lokken, 2009).

Postdischarge care for the postpartum woman may be accomplished by home visits or follow-up phone calls, or both. The optimal time for a home visit or follow-up phone call is between 3 and 4 days after birth; this provides opportunities for further assessment of the mother and her infant and teaching. (See Assessment Guide: Postpartum—First Home Visit and Anticipated Progress at Six Weeks in chapter 37 ∞ on pages 1072–1074.) During this time period, infections, poor infant feeding, excessive weight loss, jaundice, and other problems become apparent (James, 2008). The follow-up phone call is often initiated by a nurse from the postpartum unit of the agency where the mother gave birth. It is made soon after discharge and is designed to provide assessment and, if necessary, care; to reinforce knowledge and provide additional teaching; and to make referrals if indicated. Alternatively, a follow-up phone call from a nurse from the physician or CNM's office can provide new mothers with a source of support and an opportunity to ask questions. Women who appear to be having adjustment problems should be scheduled for an appointment for further evaluation.

In ideal situations, a family approach involving the father, newborn, and other siblings permits a total evaluation and provides an opportunity for all family members to ask questions and express concerns. In addition, a family approach can sometimes enable the nurse to identify disturbed family patterns more readily and suggest, or even institute, therapeutic measures to prevent future problems of neglect or abuse.

FOCUS YOUR STUDY

- The uterus involutes rapidly, primarily through a reduction in cell size.
- Involution is assessed by measuring fundal height. The fundus is at the level of the umbilicus within a few hours after birth and should decrease by approximately one fingerbreadth per day.
- The placental site heals by a process of exfoliation, so no scar formation occurs.
- Lochia progresses from rubra to serosa to alba and is assessed in terms of type, quantity, and characteristics.
- The abdomen may have decreased muscle tone (flabby consistency) initially. The nurse should assess for diastasis recti abdominis, separation of the rectus abdominis muscles.
- Constipation may develop postpartum because of decreased tone in the abdominal muscles, limited diet, and denial of the urge to defecate because of fear of pain.
- Decreased bladder sensitivity, increased capacity, and postpartum diuresis may lead to problems with bladder elimination. Frequent assessment and prompt intervention are indicated. A fundus that is boggy but does not respond to massage, is higher than expected, or deviates to the side usually indicates a full bladder.
- Postpartum, a healthy woman should be normotensive and afebrile. Bradycardia is common.
- The white blood cell (WBC) count is often elevated postpartum. Activation of clotting factors predisposes the woman to thrombus formation.
- Psychologic adaptations of the postpartal woman are traditionally described as "taking-in" and "taking-hold."
- Postpartum "blues" is a common occurrence and ways to prevent and cope with it should be discussed not only with the mother but her significant other(s). Signs of postpartum depression should be discussed as well.
- In consideration of the patient's background, the nurse should recognize and respect cultural variations and individual preferences.
- Postpartum assessment should be completed in a systematic way, usually head to toe, and should include assessment of rest and sleep, nutrition, and attachment. The assessment provides opportunities for informal patient teaching.
- In the weeks following birth, the woman's physical condition returns to a nonpregnant state, and she gains competence in caregiving and confidence in herself as a parent.

CRITICAL THINKING IN ACTION

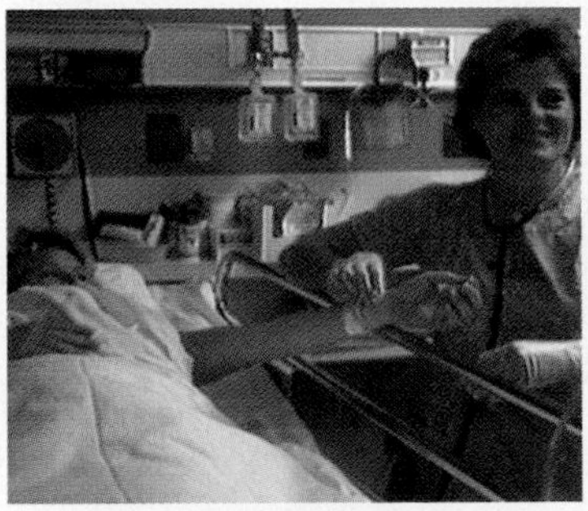

Source: George Dodson/Pearson Education.

Janet Burns, a 25-year-old G3 P3, is 2 hours past a low forceps vaginal birth with a right medial lateral episiotomy of a live 8 pound baby boy. You obtain vital signs of BP 118/70, T 98.8°F, P 76, R 14. You observe the fundus is +1 finger above the umbilicus and slightly to the right. Her episiotomy is slightly ecchymotic and well approximated without edema or discharge. Ice has been applied to the episiotomy for the last 20 minutes. Lochia rubra is present and a pad was saturated in 90 minutes. Janet has an intravenous of Ringer's lactate with 10 units of Pitocin infusing at 100 ml/hr in her lower left arm and is complaining of moderate abdominal cramping. Janet's baby is sleeping peacefully in the bassinet next to her bed. She tells you that she is very tired and requests some pain medication so she can sleep for a while.

1. What nursing assessment is of immediate concern?
2. Discuss care of her episiotomy and perineum.
3. What other self-care measures could you advise?
4. Discuss postpartal occurrences that may cause special concern for the mother.
5. Janet expressed concern about her episiotomy healing. What information can you offer?

See www.nursing.pearsonhighered.com for possible responses.

Pearson Nursing Student Resources
Find additional review materials at
www.nursing.pearsonhighered.com
Prepare for success with additional NCLEX®-style practice questions, interactive assignments and activities, Web links, animations and videos, and more!

REFERENCES

American Academy of Pediatrics. (2004). Hospital stay for healthy term newborns. *Pediatrics, 113*(5), 1434–1436.

Aminoff, M. J. (2009). Neurologic disorders. In R. K. Creasy & R. Resnik (Eds.), *Maternal-fetal medicine: Principles and practice* (6th ed., pp. 613–699). Philadelphia, PA: Saunders.

Beck, C. T. (2008). *Postpartum mood and anxiety disorders: Case studies, research, and nursing care* (2nd ed.). Washington, DC: Association of Women's Health, Obstetric, and Neonatal Nurses.

Blackburn, S. T. (2007). *Maternal, fetal, & neonatal physiology: A clinical perspective* (3rd ed.). St. Louis, MO: Saunders.

Cunningham, F. G., Leveno, K. J., Bloom, S. L., Hauth, J. C., Rouse, D. J., & Spong, C. Y. (2010). *Williams obstetrics* (23rd ed.). New York, NY: McGraw-Hill.

Hill, P. D., & Aldag, J. C. (2007). Maternal perceived quality of life following childbirth. *JOGNN: Journal of Obstetric, Gynecologic, and Neonatal Nursing, 36*(4), 328–334.

Holtz, C., & Grisdale, S. (2008). Global health in reproduction and infants. In C. Holtz, *Global health care: Issues and policies* (1st ed., pp. 437–476). Boston, MA: Jones & Bartlett.

James, D. C. (2008). Postpartum care. In K. R. Simpson & P. A. Creehan, *Perinatal nursing* (3rd ed., pp. 473–526). Philadelphia, PA: Lippincott Williams & Wilkins.

Kalayjian, L., & Goodwin, T. M. (2007). Nervous system & autoimmune disorders in pregnancy. In A. H. Decherney, L. Nathan, T. M. Goodwin, & N. Laufer (Eds.), *Current diagnosis and treatment: Obstetrics & gynecology* (10th ed.). Boston, MA: McGraw-Hill.

Lauderdale, J. (2008). Transcultural perspectives in childbearing. In M. M. Andrews & J. S. Boyle, *Transcultural concepts in nursing care* (5th ed.). Philadelphia, PA: Lippincott Williams & Wilkins.

Mercer, R. T. (2004). Becoming a mother versus maternal role attainment. *Journal of Nursing Scholarship, 36* (3), 226–232.

Mercer, R. T. (2006). Nursing support of the process of becoming a mother. *JOGNN: Journal of Obstetric, Gynecologic, & Neonatal Nursing, 35*(5), 649–651. doi: 10.1111/J.1552-6909.2006.00086.x

Noble, A., Rom, M., Englehardt, K., & Woloski-Wruble, A. (2009). Jewish laws, customs, and practice in labor, delivery, and postpartum care. *Journal of Transcultural Nursing, 20*(3), 323–333.

Purnell, L. D., & Paulanka, B. J. (2008). *Transcultural health care: A culturally competent approach* (3rd ed.). Philadelphia, PA: F. A. Davis.

Reitmanova, S., & Gustafson, D. L. (2008). "They can't understand it": Maternal health and care needs of immigrant Muslim women in St. John's, Newfoundland. *Maternal Child Health Journal, 12*(1), 101–111. doi: 10.1007/s10995-007-0213-4

Reyna, B. A., & Pickler, R. H. (2009). Mother-infant synchrony. *JOGNN: Journal of Obstetric, Gynecologic, and Neonatal Nursing, 38*(4), 470–477. doi: 10.1111/j.1552-6909.2009.01044.x

Rhode, M. A. (2011). Postpartum complications. In S. Mattson & J. E. Smith (Eds.), *Core curriculum for maternal-newborn nursing* (4th ed., pp. 650–666). St. Louis, MO: Saunders/Elsevier.

Rousseau, J. B. (2008). Meeting the needs of the postpartum woman with epilepsy. *MCN: American Journal of Maternal/Child Nursing, 33*(2), 84–89. doi:10.1097/01.NMC.0000313415.77044.10

Rubin, R. (1984). *Maternal identity and the maternal experience.* New York, NY: Springer.

Samuels, P., & Niebyl, J. R. (2007). Neurologic disorders. In S. G. Gabbe, J. R. Niebyl, & J. L. Simpson (Eds.), *Obstetrics: Normal and problem pregnancies* (5th ed., pp. 1132–1152). Philadelphia, PA: Churchill Livingstone/Elsevier.

Weiss, M. E., & Lokken, L. (2009). Predictors and outcomes of postpartum mothers' perceptions of readiness for discharge after birth. *JOGNN: Journal of Obstetric, Gynecologic, and Neonatal Nursing, 38*(4), 406–417. doi: 10.1111/j.1552-6909.2009.01040.x

Whitmer, T. (2011). Physical and psychologic changes. In S. Mattson & J. E. Smith (Eds.), *Core curriculum for maternal-newborn nursing* (4th ed., pp. 301–314). St. Louis, MO: Saunders/Elsevier.

Zauderer, C. (2009). Maternity care for orthodox Jewish couples. *Lifelines, 13*(2), 112–120. doi: 10.1111/j.1751-486X.2009.01402.x

The Postpartum Family: Needs and Care

36 CHAPTER

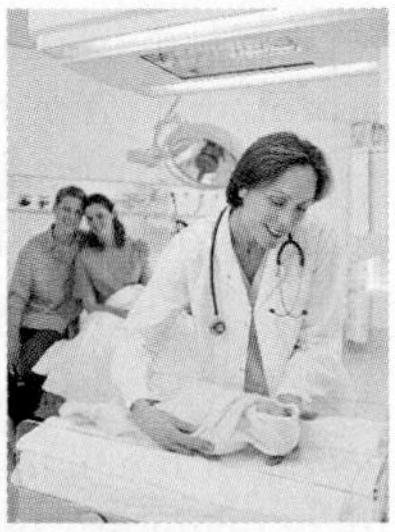

Providing family-centered postpartum care is a challenge that requires creativity, patience, and a sincere desire to help families grow and thrive. Individual families come to the unit with a unique set of values, beliefs, life experiences, challenges, gifts, and expectations. The nurse needs to personalize care to meet their special needs in a manner that helps them to nurture one another and their newborn within the context of their family, their community, and the world. It has been helpful to remember that while it is simply another day of work for me, it is probably one of the most important days in the lives of my patients and their families. The care that I provide shapes their memories of this special time and may affect their health and family processes for many years to come.

LEARNING OUTCOMES

1. Delineate nursing responsibilities for patient teaching during the early postpartum period.
2. Discuss appropriate nursing interventions to promote maternal comfort and well-being.
3. Describe the nurse's role in promoting maternal rest and helping the mother to resume gradually an appropriate level of activity.
4. Identify patient teaching topics for promoting postpartum family wellness.
5. Compare the nursing needs of a woman who experienced a cesarean birth with the needs of a woman who gave birth vaginally.
6. Identify critical physiologic, psychosocial, and safety needs related to the care of obese and morbidly obese postpartum women.
7. Summarize the nursing needs of the childbearing adolescent during the postpartum period.
8. Describe possible approaches to sensitive, holistic nursing care for the woman who relinquishes her newborn.
9. Describe possible approaches to sensitive, holistic nursing care for the postpartum lesbian mother and her partner.
10. Delineate the nurse's responsibilities related to early postpartum discharge.

KEY TERMS

Bogginess *1027*
Couplet care *1039*
Family-centered care *1039*
Mother-baby care *1039*
Patient-controlled analgesia (PCA) *1044*
Relinquishing mother *1048*
Skin-to-skin contact (SSC) *1036*

Certain premises form the basis of effective nursing care during the postpartum period.

- The best postpartum care is family centered and disrupts the family unit as little as possible. This approach uses the family's resources to support an early and smooth adjustment to the newborn by all family members.
- Knowledge of the range of normal physiologic and psychologic adaptations occurring during the postpartum period allows the nurse to recognize alterations and initiate interventions early. Communicating information about postpartum adaptations to the family facilitates their adjustment to their situation.
- Nursing care is aimed at accomplishing specific goals that ultimately meet individual needs. These goals are formulated after careful assessment and consideration of factors that could influence the outcome of care.

Chapter 35 ∞ provides a thorough discussion of postpartum assessment. This chapter describes nursing care during the immediate postpartum period. Specific nursing responses to the mother's physical needs and the family's psychosociocultural needs are described at length and are summarized in the Clinical Pathway for the Postpartum Period on pages 1021–1023.

Nursing Care During the Early Postpartum Period

For most postpartum women, physical recovery proceeds smoothly and is considered a healthy process. Because of this perception, it is all too common for caregivers to think that the woman and her family have no "real" needs and thus no care plan is needed. Nothing can be further from the truth. Every member of the family has needs, although they may not be obvious, especially if they are educational or emotional.

Nursing Diagnosis

The postpartum family's needs, which should be identified during assessment, are the basis for developing nursing diagnoses. Once a nursing diagnosis is made and recorded, systematic action, as delineated in a nursing care plan or clinical pathway, can be used to meet the identified need.

Nursing schools and agencies frequently use NANDA International (Herdman, 2009) approved diagnoses. Examples of diagnoses with defining characteristics and related factors commonly found in postpartum patients include (Herdman, 2009):

- ***Impaired Urinary Elimination.*** Defining characteristics may include (a) dysuria, (b) hesitancy, or (c) retention. Related factors may include (a) anatomic obstruction (urethral swelling), (b) sensory motor impairment (spinal or epidural anesthesia), or (c) multiple causality.
- ***Impaired Skin Integrity.*** Defining characteristics may include (a) destruction of skin layers (abrasions) or (b) disruption of skin surface (lacerations). Related factors may include mechanical factors (tearing/shearing forces during delivery).
- ***Acute Pain.*** Defining characteristics may include (a) guarding behavior, (b) observed evidence of pain, (c) expressive behavior, (d) positioning to avoid pain, (e) protective gestures, or (f) verbal report of pain. Related factors may include (a) physical injuries sustained during labor and delivery (hematomas) or (b) physical changes of postpartum period (uterine contractions).
- ***Risk for Infection.*** Risk factors may include (a) inadequate primary defenses (surgical incision, lacerations, open cervix, etc.), (b) inadequate secondary defenses (decreased hemoglobin), (c) invasive procedures (history of cervical exams or instrumentation during labor and delivery), (d) history of premature rupture of amniotic membranes, or (e) history of prolonged rupture of amniotic membranes.
- ***Risk for Constipation.*** Risk factors may include (a) physiologic (decreased motility of gastrointestinal tract), (b) pharmacologic (opiates), or (c) mechanical (hemorrhoids).

Wellness diagnoses related to family coping, instructional needs, or infant nutrition are also used frequently. Examples of these diagnoses include the following (Herdman, 2009):

- ***Readiness for Enhanced Knowledge.*** Defining characteristics may include (a) expresses an interest in learning (about self- or newborn care), or (b) describes previous experiences pertaining to the topic.
- ***Readiness for Enhanced Coping.*** Defining characteristics may include (a) defines stressors (new family member) as manageable, (b) seeks knowledge of new strategies, or (c) seeks social support.
- ***Effective Breastfeeding.*** Defining characteristics may include but are not limited to (a) effective mother-infant communication patterns, (b) maternal verbalization of satisfaction with the breastfeeding process, (c) mother able to position infant at breast to promote a successful latching-on response, and (d) infant content after feeding. Related factors may include (a) basic breastfeeding knowledge, (b) infant gestational age >34 weeks, (c) maternal confidence, (d) normal breast structure, (e) normal infant oral structure, or (f) support source present.

After completing the assessment and diagnosis steps of the nursing process, the nurse identifies desired outcomes and selects nursing interventions that will promote these outcomes.

Nursing Plan and Implementation

Nursing care management is individualized to meet the needs of each postpartal woman, her newborn, and her family. The plan of care needs to consider the newborn's schedule of activities during the day, such as feeding times, because they frequently determine the mother's schedule. Flexibility is crucial because most breastfeeding infants feed on demand at frequent intervals.

An important component of nursing care is patient teaching, which is designed to help the woman and her family learn how to perform self-care and provide effective newborn care. Sophisticated, detailed forms and guidelines are often available to assist in health teaching. Such tools are a useful adjunct but cannot take the place of the nurse's patient-centered plan. As part of patient teaching, the nurse should discuss cultural beliefs, desired outcomes, and goals with the mother as soon as

CLINICAL PATHWAY For the Postpartum Period

Category	First 4 Hours	4–8 Hours Past Birth	8–24 Hours Past Birth
Referral	Report from labor nurse if not continuing in an LDR room	Lactation consultation as needed	Home nursing, social work, WIC referral if indicated; coordinate universal hearing and state-required newborn metabolic screening ■ ***Expected Outcomes*** Referrals made
Assessments	Postpartum assessments every 15 min × 4, every 30 min × 2, then every 4 h. Includes: • Fundus firm, midline, at or below umbilicus • Lochia rubra less than 2 pad/h; no free flow or passage of clots with massage • Bladder: voids large amounts of urine spontaneously; bladder not palpable following voiding • Incision or dressing clean, dry, and intact if CB • Foley draining if present • Perineum: sutures intact; no bulging or marked swelling; no c/o severe pain. Minimal bruising may be present. If hemorrhoids present, no tenseness or marked engorgement; less than 2 cm diameter • Breasts: soft, colostrum present Vital Signs: • BP WNL; usually between 90/50 and 140/90, consistent with baseline • Temperature: less than 38°C (100.4°F) • Pulse: bradycardia (50 to 70) normal, consistent with baseline • Respirations: 16–24/min; quiet, easy; lungs CTA Comfort level: pain less than 4 on scale of 1–10 Awake, alert, & LOS returning following initial recovery if had anesthesia	Continue postpartum assessment every 4 h Breast: evaluate nipple status; should be no evidence of cracks or bruising Observe feeding technique with newborn Vital signs assessment every 4 h; all WNL; report temperature greater than 38°C (100.4°F) Assess Homans' sign every 8 h Continue assessment of comfort level: pain less than 4 on 1–10 scale	Continue postpartum assessment every 4 h Breasts: nipples should remain free of cracks, fissures, bruising Newborn latches and breastfeeds successfully VS assessment every 4 h; all WNL; Lungs CTA; report temperature greater than 38°C (100.4°F) Continue assessment of comfort level D/C Foley PRN; Pt voids within 4 to 6 h after Foley D/C ■ ***Expected Outcomes*** VS WNL, voids QS, postpartum assessment WNL Incision healthy and intact if CB Comfort level: pain less than 4 on 1–10 scale Involution of uterus in process—fundus may migrate to 1 cm above umbilicus by 12 h; fundal height decreases 1 cm/day thereafter Lochia rubra < 1 pad/h by 24 h Demonstrates and verbalizes appropriate newborn feeding techniques
Teaching/ psychosocial	Explain postpartum assessments Assist with breastfeeding; discuss benefits and AAP recommendations if undecided Teach self-massage of fundus and expected findings; explain rationale for fundal massage Instruct to call for assistance first time OOB and PRN Demonstrate peri care, Surgigator, sitz bath PRN Explain comfort measures Begin newborn teaching: bulb suctioning, positioning, feeding, diaper change, cord care; needs for comfort, warmth, and touch; infant safety and security measures Orient to room if transferred from LDR room Teach TCDB if CB Provide information on early postpartal period Assess mother/infant attachment Encourage SSC between newborn and parent(s) Encourage mother to verbalize her birth story Encourage father to bond and provide newborn care	Discuss psychologic changes of postpartum period; facilitate transition through tasks of taking on maternal role Discuss peri care/hygiene Encourage use of supportive brassiere for all mothers Stress need for frequent rest periods Continue newborn teaching: newborn behavioral states, soothing/comforting techniques, swaddling Return demonstrations indicate woman's understanding Provide opportunities for questions; review and reinforce previous teaching Breastfeeding nipple care: air-drying, proper latch-on technique Formula-feeding breast care: supportive bra, cold compresses, no stimulation, analgesics Assess mother/infant attachment	Reinforce previous teaching, complete teaching evaluation Discuss involution; anticipated physical changes in first 2 weeks postpartum; postpartal exercises; need to limit visitors; baby blues; postpartum fatigue; postpartum depression Discuss postpartal nutrition; balanced diet Breastfeeding: • Increase calories by up to 500 kcal over nonpregnant state (200 kcal over pregnant intake) • Explain milk production, let-down reflex, use of supplements, sore nipples, breast pumping, and milk storage Formula-feeding: • Return to nonpregnant caloric intake • Explain formula preparation and storage Discuss birth control options, sexuality Discuss sibling rivalry and plan for supporting siblings at home Discuss circumcision care PRN Discuss pets; suggestions for improving acceptance of infant by pets Discuss fathering experience Emphasize car seat/vehicle safety, SIDS prevention, "never shake a baby" ■ ***Expected Outcomes*** Mother verbalizes teaching comprehension Positive bonding and emotional behaviors observed (both parents if present) Provides appropriate self- and infant care.

(continued)

CLINICAL PATHWAY For the Postpartum Period continued

Category	First 4 Hours	4–8 Hours Past Birth	8–24 Hours Past Birth
Nursing care management and reports	Ice pack to perineum to decrease swelling and increase comfort Straight catheter PRN × 1 if distended or voiding small amounts Assess LOC, LOS, & lower extremity strength before ambulation If continues unable to void or voiding small amounts, insert Foley catheter and notify CNM or physician	Sitz baths PRN If woman Rh− and infant Rh+, RhoGAM workup; obtain consent; complete teaching Determine rubella status Obtain consent for rubella vaccine if indicated; explain purpose, procedure, implications of vaccine Obtain hematocrit	Continue sitz baths PRN May shower if ambulating without difficulty DC saline lock if present ■ ***Expected Outcomes*** Using sitz bath; voids QS; lab work WNL; performs ADL without sequelae
Activity	Assistance when OOB first time, then PRN SCDs until ambulating if CB Ambulates ad lib Rests comfortably between assessments	Encourage rest periods TCDB & SCDs until ambulating if CB Ambulates ad lib; may leave birthing unit after notifying staff of plan to ambulate off unit	Up ad lib ■ ***Expected Outcomes*** VB: Ambulates ad lib CB: OOB & ambulates by 24 h
Comfort	Institute comfort measures: • Perineal discomfort: peri care; sitz baths, topical analgesics • Hemorrhoids: sitz baths, topical analgesics, Tucks, side-lying or prone position • Afterpains: prone with small pillow under abdomen; warm shower or sitz baths; ambulation • Instruct on use of PCA pump PRN • Administer pain medication PRN	Continue with pain management techniques Offer alternative pain management options: distraction with music, television, visitors; massage; warmed blankets or towels to affected area; using breathing techniques when infant latches on to breast and/or during cramping until medication's action is felt	Continue with pain management techniques ■ ***Expected Outcomes*** Maintains comfort: Pain level less than 4 on 1–10 scale Verbalizes alternative pain management options
Nutrition & Hydration	Regular diet Fluid 2000 ml/day IV fluids if ordered	Continue diet and fluids	Continue diet and fluids ■ ***Expected Outcomes*** Skin turgor WNL Regular diet/fluids tolerated
Elimination	Voiding large amounts straw-colored urine	Voiding large quantities May have bowel movement	Same ■ ***Expected Outcomes*** Voiding QS; passing flatus or bowel movement
Medications	Pain medications as ordered Oxytocin IV infusion and/or Methergine po or IM if ordered Stool softener PRN Tucks pad PRN, perineal analgesic spray PRN, topical hemorrhoid cream PRN	Continue meds Lanolin to nipples PRN; assist with positioning and latch PRN Saline flush to saline lock (if present) every 8 h or as ordered May take own prenatal vitamins and iron—keep secure from siblings	Continue medications RhoGAM and/or rubella vaccine administered PRN ■ ***Expected Outcomes*** Vaccines administered if indicated; pain controlled Saline lock discontinued (site healthy)
Discharge planning/ home care	Evaluate knowledge of normal postpartum and newborn care Evaluate support systems	Discuss typical newborn schedule Plan for periods of rest Birth certificate paperwork completed Evaluate plans for transporting newborn; car seat available	Review discharge instruction sheet/checklist Describe postpartum warning signs and when to call CNM/physician Provide prescriptions Arrangements for baby pictures as per agency protocol Postpartum and newborn visits scheduled ■ ***Expected Outcomes*** Discharged home; mother verbalizes postpartum and newborn warning S/S, follow-up appointment times/dates Hearing and metabolic screens completed with follow-up scheduled if needed

CLINICAL PATHWAY For the Postpartum Period continued

Category	First 4 Hours	4–8 Hours Past Birth	8–24 Hours Past Birth
Family involvement	Identify available support persons Assess family perceptions of birth experience Parenting: demonstrates culturally expected early parenting behaviors	Involve support persons in care, teaching; answer questions Evidence of parental bonding behaviors present	Continue to involve support persons in teaching, involve siblings as appropriate Plans made for providing support to mother following discharge ■ ***Expected Outcomes*** Evidence of parental bonding behavior Support persons verbalize understanding of woman's need for rest, good nutrition, fluids, and emotional support Support persons verbalize understanding of maternal/newborn follow up and S/S of complications requiring additional follow-up

Abbreviations: AAP, American Academy of Pediatrics; ADL, activities of daily living; BP, blood pressure; CB, cesarean birth; CNM, certified nurse-midwife; C/O, complaints of; CTA, clear to auscultation; D/C, discontinue; LDR, labor, delivery, and recovery; LOC, level of consciousness; LOS, level of sensation; OOB, out of bed; PCA, patient-controlled analgesia; PRN, as needed; PP, postpartum; QS, quantity sufficient; SCDs, sequential compression devices; SIDS, sudden infant death syndrome; S/S, signs and symptoms; SSC, skin-to-skin contact; TCDB, turn-cough and deep breathe; VB, vaginal birth; VS, vital signs; WIC, Women, Infants, & Children; WNL, within normal limits

possible after her arrival in the postpartum unit. Examples of these desired patient outcomes include the following:

- Mother and baby remain healthy, safe, and free of injury or complications.
- Mother verbalizes comfort.
- Mother tells birth story and verbalizes feelings and concerns regarding the event.
- Mother reviews educational resources for self- and infant care.
- Mother performs appropriate self- and infant care.
- Parent(s) and newborn demonstrate positive bonding behaviors.
- Parents practice principles of infant safety.
- Mother verbalizes understanding of and demonstrates successful breastfeeding and breast care; or mother describes accurate preparation of infant formula, demonstrates safe bottle-feeding techniques, and verbalizes understanding of lactation suppression care.
- Mother verbalizes sources of support to assist in newborn care and family responsibilities.
- Mother states plan for follow-up health care for self and infant.
- Mother identifies signs and symptoms of maternal or newborn complications and reasons to seek care before routine follow-up visits.

Additional outcomes for the cesarean birth mother include the following:

- Mother states in own words the reason for the cesarean birth and verbalizes feelings related to the event.
- Mother maintains desired comfort level (pain level less than 4 on 1 to 10 scale).
- Mother maintains mobility (up in chair within 12 hours; ambulates within 24).

In summary, all components of nursing care management are designed to achieve the desired outcomes identified for the woman and her family. If the mother is unable to meet these outcomes prior to discharge, the significant other or a family caregiver should verbalize and/or demonstrate understanding of outcomes related to maternal and infant health and safety.

Community-Based Nursing Care

Various services are available to meet the needs of the childbearing family during the immediate postpartum period and beyond. These services range from educational opportunities, such as classes on nutrition, breastfeeding, exercise, infant care and development, and parenting, to specific healthcare programs, such as well-baby checkups, immunization clinics, lactation centers, and family planning agencies. Services may be offered by the birthing unit, private caregivers, volunteer and charitable organizations, or publicly funded agencies. In all cases, the goal is consistent: to meet the health, safety, and psychosocial needs of the mother, the newborn, and the family.

Home health care is one of the most important forms of community-based nursing care offered to postpartum families. Home care visits and phone contacts (telephone follow-up) help ensure that families have the necessary skills and resources to care for an infant and to meet their own health needs. Because of its importance today in caring for childbearing families, home care is discussed in depth in chapter 37 ∞.

Health Promotion Education

Meeting the educational needs of the new mother and her family is one of the primary challenges facing the postpartum nurse. Each woman's educational needs vary according to age, background, culture, experience, and expectations. However, because the mother spends only a brief period of time in the postpartal area, identifying and addressing individual instructional needs can be difficult. Effective education provides the childbearing family with sufficient knowledge to meet many of their own health needs and to seek assistance if necessary.

The nurse assesses the learning needs of the new mother through observation, sensitivity to nonverbal clues, and tactfully phrased questions. For example, "What plans have you made for handling things when you get home?" will elicit a more detailed response than, "Will someone be available to help you at home?" To assess learning needs, some agencies provide a patient handout listing the most frequently identified areas of concern for new mothers. The mother checks those that apply to her or writes in concerns not included. The nurse should plan and implement learning experiences in a logical, nonthreatening way based on knowledge of and respect for the family's cultural values and beliefs.

Timing and Methods of Teaching

Childbearing nursing units must provide education efficiently and effectively in today's healthcare environment, which is characterized by shortened postpartum stays. Assessment of learning needs and patient education should begin when the woman first accesses the healthcare system. Ideally, the woman completes a needs assessment during her pregnancy, which precedes or follows her to the inpatient unit and eventually becomes the discharge teaching tool (James, 2008).

Nursing units may offer a variety of educational options including structured group classes, individualized instruction, printed materials, videotapes, and educational television channels that are available at various times or around the clock to meet the needs of families. Women should have a pencil and paper to write down questions that arise when viewing resources independently. Afterward, nurses need to be available to clarify material or answer any questions about the content. Because more effective learning occurs when there is sensory involvement and active participation, videotapes (sight and hearing) are more helpful than lecture (hearing only). Demonstration, specifically sight, touch, hearing, and, possibly, smell and taste, is even more effective. Opportunities for continued learning through the use of printed materials, access to online educational materials, home visits, postpartum education and support groups, telephone advice lines, and outpatient nurse consultation need to be provided for all patients, especially those who are discharged within 24 to 48 hours following delivery.

Content of Teaching

Maternal learning needs scatter across a variety of topics and vary depending on the mother's age and whether she is a primipara or multipara. Therefore, it is essential that the teaching content be tailored to the individual mother and family. Kanotra et al. (2007) found that postpartum women commonly reported needs for (a) social support; (b) breastfeeding education, support, and assistance; (c) education related to newborn care; (d) education and support related to postpartum depression; (e) adequate length of stay; and (f) maternal insurance coverage following delivery. No list of educational needs is exhaustive, however, and the professional nurse bears the responsibility to assess the specific learning needs of each patient and her family when planning patient-centered care, education, and follow-up.

Teaching should not be limited to "how-to" activities. Anticipatory guidance is essential in assisting the family to cope with role changes, the realities of a new baby, and potential complications such as infant colic, and postpartum health issues. Small-group discussions provide a chance for the new parents to talk about fears and expectations. Questions may arise about sexuality, contraception, childcare, and even the grief associated with giving up the fantasized infant in order to accept the actual one.

Although childbearing is generally considered a natural and healthy experience, the incidence of complications and discomforts in the first year postpartum is common. Runquist (2007) found that both primiparas and multiparas "expressed surprise and distress over the length of the postpartum healing process" (p. 32). Women may experience fatigue, headaches, nausea, backaches, abdominal pain, vaginal pain, dyspareunia, constipation, hemorrhoids, urinary or bowel problems, breast soreness, and emotional disorders. A study that screened 1323 mostly low income, urban women for the problems mentioned above found that 69% experienced problems of minor to major severity within the first year after giving birth, while only 31% reported no problems. The most common problems cited were fatigue, headaches, and nausea, which were experienced by approximately half of the respondents. Backaches were the next most common complaint. Poor emotional health and functional limitations were associated with physical complications (Webb et al., 2008). A national study of 1573 women with a broad range of demographic backgrounds found that 79% of cesarean section patients experienced incisional pain, and approximately half of patients who delivered vaginally experienced perineal pain during the months after childbirth. Many women complained of physical exhaustion as well (Declercq, Cunningham, Johnson, et al., 2008). Therefore, it is important that nurses provide anticipatory guidance to patients regarding potential postpartum health issues and encourage them to seek follow-up care as needed.

Adolescent mothers, patients with cesarean delivery, and parents of newborns with congenital anomalies will have special concerns, as will patients with special needs related to their own physical, mental, or emotional health and abilities. Postpartum nurses need to ensure that special needs families have additional support in place from home care nurses, social workers, chaplains, and other professionals before discharge.

Table 36-1 is a form that identifies important topic areas to be included in postpartum patient teaching. Methods and validation can be checked off as they occur.

Evaluating Learning

Methods for evaluating learning vary according to the objectives and teaching methods. The nurse should validate the knowledge of self- and infant care through patient discussion and return demonstration. Follow-up is indicated if learning needs related to maternal and infant care and safety are not validated as met prior to discharge (James, 2008).

Evaluation of attitudinal or less concrete learning is more difficult. For example, a mother's ability to express her frustrations over an unanticipated cesarean birth or difficulties with breastfeeding as opposed to her desired and expected experience may be the nurse's only clues that learning has occurred. Follow-up phone calls and home visits after discharge may provide additional evaluative information and continue the helping process as the nurse assesses the family's current educational needs and begins planning accordingly.

TABLE 36-1 Areas to Include in Postpartum Teaching

KNOWLEDGE AND SKILLS TO BE TAUGHT	TEACHING METHOD			PATIENT VALIDATION	
	PRINTED MATERIALS	INDICATE VIDEO OR DEMO	VERBAL INSTRUCTION	VERBALIZES UNDERSTANDING	RETURN DEMONSTRATION
Care of the Mother					
Breast care					
Breastfeeding or lactation suppression					
Possible problems and care					
Involutional changes					
Position of fundus					
Afterpains					
Changes in lochia					
Signs of possible problems					
Bladder function					
Fluid needs					
Signs of possible problems					
Bowel function					
Normal patterns					
Dietary assistance					
Perineal care					
Expected healing changes in episiotomy/laceration					
Comfort measures (rinsing with warm water, use of icepacks, use of analgesic/anesthetic spray, sitz bath), home care					
Signs of possible problems					
Rest and activity					
Scheduling rest periods, postpartum fatigue					
Ambulation					
Watching for circulatory problems in legs					
Emotional changes					
Changes in mood, crying, anxiety; "baby blues," postpartum depression, psychosis					
Care of the Father/Partner					
Emotional changes					
Emotional changes and challenges that may occur					
Encouragement to seek support as needed					
Physiologic and psychologic changes that may occur in the mother and newborn					
Infant care concerns					
Possible supportive measures for the new family					
Care of the Baby					
Infant safety and security measures					
Observing the baby					
General appearance					
Five Senses					
Visual					
Hearing					
Touch					
Smell					
Taste					
Vital signs					
Normal parameters					
How to take a temperature					
Skin					
Coloring					
Normal rashes					
Diaper care					
Elimination cycles of stool/urine					
Normal characteristics					
Signs of diarrhea and treatment					
Signs of constipation and treatment					
Emotional and comforting needs					

(continued)

TABLE 36-1 Areas to Include in Postpartum Teaching continued

KNOWLEDGE AND SKILLS TO BE TAUGHT	TEACHING METHOD			PATIENT VALIDATION	
	PRINTED MATERIALS	INDICATE VIDEO OR DEMO	VERBAL INSTRUCTION	VERBALIZES UNDERSTANDING	RETURN DEMONSTRATION
Protective reflexes					
Blinking					
Sneezing					
Swallowing					
Normal reflexes					
Moro					
Fencing					
Head lag					
Stepping					
Feeding the baby					
Schedule					
Breastfeeding					
Positioning, latch, initiating and ending feeding					
Infant cues for feeding					
Identifying problem areas and possible solutions					
Signs of dehydration					
Signs of adequate breastfeeding (output, satiation, weight)					
Formula-feeding					
Positioning					
Preparation of bottles and formula					
Burping or bubbling the baby					
Holding, wrapping, and diapering the baby					
Various holds (cradle, football)					
Securing baby in blanket to provide warmth					
Diapering					
Comparison of reusable (cloth) and single use (paper)					
Methods of diapering and care of soiled diapers					
Perineal skin care					
Circumcision care					
"Back to sleep!"					
Bathing the baby					
Supplies					
Method					
Safety					
Use of bulb syringe and care if choking					
Sudden Infant Death Syndrome (SIDS) prevention (home *and* child care)					
Prevention of battering/shaken baby injuries					
Prevention of falls					
Childproofing the home					
Positioning					
Car seat/vehicle safety					
Health promotion					
When to call healthcare provider					
Temperature					
Diarrhea					
Poor feeding/feeding intolerance					
Malaise/lethargy/"not acting right"					
Protecting baby from infections					
Immunization schedule					
Hearing and metabolic screening					
Aspects of Parenting					
Interaction with newborn					
Newborn behavioral states					
Newborn cues and capacity for interaction					
Parenting needs					
Infant colic					
Acquaintance with individual characteristics of their newborn and possible techniques to use					
Resources available					

Promotion of Maternal Comfort and Well-Being

The nurse promotes and restores maternal physical well-being by assessing the patient on a regular basis and providing the requisite care. Although there is a lack of definitive research data indicating how often maternal status should be assessed, most institutions have assessment protocols for the focused postpartum assessment. At a minimum, blood pressure, pulse, the uterine fundus, the perineum, lochia, and urinary output or need to void are usually assessed at least every 15 minutes for the first hour following delivery of the placenta, every 30 minutes for the second hour, and then every 4 hours for 24 hours. Temperature is assessed at least every four hours (James, 2008).

The nurse performs nursing activities aimed at relieving specific discomforts, such as an edematous perineum or a distended bladder. In addition, medications may be needed to promote comfort, treat anemia, provide immunity to rubella, and prevent development of antibodies in the nonsensitized Rh-negative woman. Finally, the woman may be experiencing alterations in her emotional well-being. Interventions for these conditions are discussed in this section.

Monitoring Uterine Status

The nurse completes an assessment of the uterus as discussed in chapter 35 ∞. The nurse should follow institutional protocol regarding frequency of assessments and use professional judgment to decide when maternal status requires more frequent checks or additional assessments due to issues such as **bogginess** (softening of the uterus due to inadequate contraction of the muscle tissue), positioning out of midline, heavy lochial flow, or the presence of clots (Table 36-2).

The amount, consistency, color, and odor of the lochia are monitored on an ongoing basis. Increased bleeding is most often related to uterine atony and responds to fundal massage, expression of any clots, and emptying the bladder. Nipple stimulation can also be utilized to promote contraction of the uterus. Breastfeeding is an ideal and natural way to stimulate oxytocin release and contract a boggy uterus. Bleeding that does not respond readily requires additional evaluation to rule out complications such as retained placenta, lacerations, coagulation defects, or uterine inversion. Changes in lochia that need to be assessed further, documented, and reported to the physician or certified nurse-midwife (CNM) are presented in Table 35-4 ∞ on page 1010.

Occasionally a medication such as methylergonovine maleate (Methergine) is prescribed to promote uterine contractions. In some cases an intravenous (IV) infusion of oxytocin (Pitocin) may be necessary if the uterus does not remain firm and uterine bleeding is excessive. The nurse will need to ensure patent IV access in this case. See Drug Guide: Methylergonovine Maleate (Methergine) in this chapter and Drug Guide: Oxytocin (Pitocin) in chapter 28 ∞ on page 733. Uterine atony resistant to these drugs can require use of carboprost (Hemabate). See Table 39-1 ∞ on page 1118 regarding the use of uterine stimulants. A Cochrane review noted that research regarding the use of Misoprostyl for postpartum hemorrhage is under way, but additional trials are needed before it can be recommended as a first-line treatment (Mousa & Alfirevic, 2007).

TABLE 36-2 Key Facts to Remember About Monitoring Postpartum Uterine Status

Position of the Uterine Fundus Following Birth

Immediately after delivery of the placenta: The top of the fundus is in the midline about midway between the symphysis pubis and umbilicus.

Six to 12 hours after birth: The top of the fundus is in the midline and at the level of the umbilicus (may migrate to 1 cm above the umbilicus by the 12-hour point and then descend 1 cm/day).

One day after birth: The top of the fundus is in the midline and one fingerbreadth below the umbilicus.

Second day after birth and thereafter: The top of the fundus remains in the midline and descends about one fingerbreadth per day.

Normal Characteristics of Lochia

Lochia rubra is red and is present for the first 2 to 3 days.

Lochia serosa is pinkish red or brown and is present from day 3 to day 10.

Lochia alba is creamy white and is present from day 11 to day 14 (may last 3 to 6 weeks).

PROFESSIONALISM IN PRACTICE

Using Critical Thinking to Anticipate Postpartum Hemorrhage

The nurse uses critical thinking skills to anticipate a postpartum hemorrhage. The nurse needs to be particularly sensitive to a uterus that becomes boggy or to increases in lochial flow. The astute nurse will also be aware of risk factors, such as prolonged second stage, macrosomia, manual removal of placenta, the use of magnesium sulfate, cesarean during second stage, chorioamnionitis, or multiparity. The nurse will monitor closely, maintain intravenous access, have the patient's most recent vital signs in mind, and make certain that oxytocic drugs are readily available when caring for patients at increased risk for postpartum hemorrhage. Optimal communication between the nurse and other members of the healthcare team is essential to the prevention and treatment of this potentially life-threatening complication (Lu, Korst, Fridman, et al., 2009).

HEALTH PROMOTION EDUCATION

The nurse teaches the woman to assess her fundus for firmness and position and to massage the fundus gently to promote uterine contraction. In addition, the nurse instructs her to monitor the amount and color of the lochia. Being aware of normal involutional changes will help the woman identify problems. Discharge instructions should specify that women call their healthcare provider if their bleeding is saturating more than one standard-sized sanitary pad per hour. See Table 35-4 ∞ on page 1010 for changes in lochia that are causes for concern.

DRUG GUIDE Methylergonovine Maleate (Methergine)

OVERVIEW OF ACTION

Methylergonovine maleate (Methergine) is an oxytocic ergot alkaloid that stimulates uterine and vascular smooth muscle. It is used postpartally to stimulate the uterus to contract. Sustained contraction clamps off uterine blood vessels, decreases blood loss, and promotes involution. The drug has a vasoconstrictive effect on all blood vessels, especially the larger arteries. This may result in hypertension, particularly in a woman whose blood pressure is already elevated.

ROUTE, DOSAGE, AND FREQUENCY

Methergine has a rapid onset of action and may be given orally or intramuscularly.

Usual IM dose: 0.2 mg (200 mcg) following expulsion of the placenta. The dose may be repeated every 2–4 hours if necessary (up to 5 doses). Usual onset is 2–5 minutes.

Usual oral dose: 0.2 mg to 0.4 mg (200 mcg to 400 mcg) every 6–12 hours for 2–7 days. Usual onset is 5–10 minutes.

Not for IV use except in emergency—severe hypertension and vasoconstriction may result. Give no more than 0.2 mg (200 mcg)/minute IV. Do not mix with other drugs in syringe or IV line.

MATERNAL CONTRAINDICATIONS

Pregnancy, hypersensitivity. Use caution in hepatic or renal disease, cardiac disease, hypertension, preeclampsia, sepsis, and lactation (may decrease prolactin levels). Administration during the third stage of labor should occur only under immediate supervision of the obstetric provider.

MATERNAL SIDE EFFECTS

Hypertension, nausea, vomiting, headaches, and uterine cramping are common. Dizziness, tinnitus, palpitations, arrhythmias, diaphoresis, dyspnea, chest pain, and allergic reactions may be noted.

Rare and severe side effects include hypertension with seizures, encephalopathy, stroke, myocardial infarction, and pulmonary edema. Hypotension may occur in some women.

EFFECTS ON FETUS OR NEWBORN

Because Methergine has a long duration of action and can thus produce tetanic contractions, it **should never be used during pregnancy or before delivery of the fetus,** when a sustained uterine contraction could cause injury or death to the mother and/or fetus.

NURSING CONSIDERATIONS

- Monitor fundal height and consistency and the amount and character of the lochia.
- Notify provider if uterus remains boggy despite Methergine administration.
- Assess the blood pressure before and routinely throughout drug administration.
- Inform patient that Methergine may cause severe menstrual-like cramps.
- Observe for adverse effects or symptoms of ergot toxicity (ergotism) such as nausea and vomiting, headache, muscle pain, tingling of extremities, cold or numb fingers and toes, chest pain, and general weakness.
- Provide patient and family teaching regarding importance of not smoking during Methergine administration (nicotine from cigarettes constricts vessels and may lead to hypertension), signs of toxicity.
- Refrigeration of ampules is recommended, but it remains stable at room temperature for 60 days.

Sources: Aschenbrenner & Venable, 2009, pp. 1171–1172; Deglin & Valerand, 2009, pp. 806–807; McNulty, 2009, p. 264.

Relief of Perineal Discomfort

Many nursing interventions are available for relieving perineal discomfort. Before selecting a method, the nurse needs to have assessed the perineum to determine the degree of edema and other problems. It is also important to ask the woman whether there are special measures that she feels will be particularly effective and to offer her choices when possible. For instance, some cultures believe that the use of "cold" versus "hot" may alter the recovery or spirit of the new mother (see chapter 35 ∞). These beliefs will affect the choices made by the new mother. The nurse uses disposable gloves while applying all relief measures and washes hands before and after using the gloves. The nurse should be aware that severe perineal discomfort that does not respond to comfort measures may be indicative of a complication such as hematoma and warrants further investigation.

Case Study: Perineal Discomfort

It is important to use good hygienic practices, such as moving from the front (area of the symphysis pubis) to the back (area around the anus) of the perineum. The nurse should follow this principle when placing ice packs and perineal pads and applying topical anesthetic agents or pain relief products. Avoiding contamination between the anal area and the urethral-vaginal area minimizes the risk of infection.

CLINICAL TIP

You may be surprised by how quickly the postpartum woman shows signs of bladder distention, possibly as soon as 1 to 2 hours after childbirth. This is because of normal postpartal diuresis. You can help prevent overdistention by palpating the woman's bladder frequently and encouraging her to void. When urinating the first time after vaginal birth, some mothers may feel the urge to urinate but are unable to begin the flow of urine. Possible interventions include letting her hear running water by turning water on in the sink; running warm water in the sink and having her place one hand in the water; having her place one foot in a basin of warm water; squirting warm water over her perineum using a peri bottle; and placing a few drops of peppermint oil in the urine collection device ("hat"). Be sure to measure the first few voidings. The amount should be at least 150 ml. If she is still unable to void and catheterization becomes necessary, be prepared for difficulty in visualizing the urethra because of localized swelling and discomfort and tenderness in the area. If a patient requires more than one straight catheterization during the postpartum period, the provider may order a Foley for at least 8 to 12 hours to allow the swelling to subside.

PATIENT TEACHING Care of Episiotomy or Laceration

PATIENT GOALS At the completion of the teaching, the woman will be able to:

1. Identify the factors that promote and interfere with wound healing.
2. Summarize self-care activities to promote healing and increase personal comfort.
3. Demonstrate the correct procedure for peri care and taking a sitz bath.
4. Discuss the judicious use of prescribed analgesics or topical anesthetics as needed.

TEACHING PLAN

Content	Teaching Method
■ Describe the process of wound healing. Discuss the risk of contamination of the episiotomy/laceration by bacteria from the anal area.	Discussion helps women understand the importance of good wound care.
■ Explain techniques that are used to keep the episiotomy or laceration clean and promote healing such as: ■ Sitz bath ■ Use of peri bottle following each voiding or defecation ■ Pad change following each elimination and at regular intervals	Focus on open discussion. Demonstrate correct use of the peri bottle or sitz bath if necessary.
■ Describe comfort measures: ■ Ice pack or glove immediately following birth ■ Sitz bath ■ Judicious use of analgesics or topical anesthetics ■ Tightening buttocks before sitting	Focus on discussion and provide an opportunity for questions.
■ Identify signs of episiotomy or laceration infection. Advise the woman to contact her caregiver if infection develops.	Encourage discussion and provide printed handouts. Some of this content may also be covered during a small postpartum class.

Evaluation	Documentation
At the end of the teaching session the woman will be able to verbalize the principles of wound healing and episiotomy or laceration care. She will also be able to demonstrate self-care measures such as peri care, ice packs, taking a sitz bath, and administration of topical anesthetics or analgesics.	Documentation of patient teaching should include the teaching information discussed, the patient's verbalization of understanding, specific interventions or warning signs that were given, along with the patient's understanding of follow-up if needed in the future.

Perineal Care

Perineal care after each elimination (urination or defecation) cleanses the perineum and helps to promote comfort. Many agencies provide "peri bottles" that the woman can use to squirt warm tap water over her perineum following elimination. To cleanse her perineum, the woman may also use a Surgigator (peri bottle), moist antiseptic towelettes, or toilet paper in a blotting (patting) motion. She should be taught to start at the front (area just under the symphysis pubis) and proceed toward the back (area around the anus) to prevent contamination from the anal area. In addition, to prevent contamination, the perineal pad should be applied from front to back, placing the front portion against the perineum first. Perineal pads should be changed regularly to prevent infection.

TEACHING FOR SELF-CARE The nurse demonstrates how to cleanse the perineum and assists the woman as necessary, for example, by offering additional information regarding the use of perineal pads. Many women have never used a perineal pad or belt and will need instruction in using them during the postpartal period. (See Patient Teaching: Care of Episiotomy or Laceration.) Some women may prefer to use the pads designed for urinary incontinence. The pads are also highly absorbent and are usually self-adherent. Postpartum patients with genital piercings should be encouraged to exercise extra vigilance regarding perineal care to prevent infection (Young & Armstrong, 2008).

Ice Pack

If an episiotomy is performed at the time of birth or if a laceration occurs, an ice pack is generally applied to reduce edema and numb the tissues, which promotes comfort. Many agencies offer commercial ice packs or cold gel pads, which should be used according to the manufacturer's instructions. Before applying the ice pack the nurse should ask the woman for permission and consider cultural norms. A Cochrane review (East, Begg, Henshall, et al., 2007) noted that ice packs are commonly applied for 10 to 20 minutes, with no adverse effects. Optimal times and length of application have not been established, however. Use of ice packs may be continued for as long as necessary. Usually, they are needed during the first 24 hours postpartum.

TEACHING FOR SELF-CARE The nurse provides information about the purpose of the ice pack, anticipated effects, benefits, and possible problems.

Case Study: Postpartum Patient

PROCEDURE 36-1 Use of Sitz Baths, Ice Packs, and Perineal Hygiene

NURSING ACTION

Preparation

- Explain the importance and benefits of perineal care. These methods can be used for the woman who has had any type of perineal trauma such as an episiotomy, laceration, extension of the episiotomy, or edema from an extended period of pushing.

  Rationale: *Perineal care promotes healing, prevents infection, and relieves discomfort in the perineal area following a vaginal birth. It may be needed after a cesarean birth if the woman had perineal trauma before having to advance to a cesarean delivery.*

Equipment and Supplies

Peri bottle or squirt bottle

Chemical ice packs *or* exam glove filled with ice chips, tied at top, powder rinsed off and covered with clean cloth

Sitz bath as provided by the facility

Clean towel for drying perineum and one placed on floor around toilet to prevent slipping on wet floor

Rationale: *The woman may need only one of these procedures or she may need to use a combination of two or three. At the very least, the use of peri bottles should be encouraged after each urination or defecation.*

Procedure

Peri Bottle

1. Explain the purpose and use of the peri bottle as well as the benefits and possible problems. Its use can assist with keeping the area clean, provide comfort, prevent infection, and promote healing.
2. Demonstrate and assist the patient as needed to fill a small plastic peri bottle with warm water and reapply the cap. Have patient feel water to assure it is at a comfortably warm temperature. Open the top of the cap and gently squirt the warm water on the entire perineal, urethral, and anal area if able.

   Rationale: *The warm water will aid in increasing blood flow, which promotes healing, and will loosen dried blood that may be present, which aids in cleansing.*
3. Have the woman dry the perineal area with a clean towel, patting dry, beginning at the front (urethral area) and ending at the back (anal area). Apply new peri-pad, ice pack (if using), and underwear.

   Rationale: *Instruct the woman to perform this procedure and apply a new peri-pad after each urination and defecation.*

Ice Packs

1. Explain the purpose and use of the ice packs and expected results, as well as benefits and possible problems.

   Rationale: *Ice packs are generally used to reduce edema due to perineal trauma. Many women find the ice relieves the discomfort by providing temporary numbing of the area.*

   For edema, the ice packs will usually need to be used for 12–24 hours or until the mother no longer feels a need for it.
2. If chemical ice packs are used, activate the pack according to the manufacturer's instructions (written on plastic wrapper), which is usually to squeeze the middle tightly or to bend the ends toward the middle until a "pop" is heard or felt.
3. If chemical ice packs are not available, use an exam glove filled with ice chips and tied off the top of the glove like a balloon. Rinse any powder off the glove and wrap with a clean cloth. Do not apply the glove directly to the skin as it may cause a burn from the extreme cold.
4. The ice pack is to be placed directly on the perineal area, and larger, more absorbent peri-pads can be placed between the ice pack and underwear.
5. The ice pack can remain in place until the next time the woman uses the restroom or until it no longer feels cool to the touch.

   Rationale: *Document use of ice packs per agency guidelines. Report and document any adverse event related to the use of the ice packs.*

Sitz Baths

1. Explain the purpose and use of the sitz bath, anticipated effects, benefits, possible problems, and safety measures to prevent slipping or an injury from hot water. The sitz bath will last approximately 20 minutes.

   Rationale: *The nurse may compare the sitz bath to "sitting in a gentle whirlpool for 20 minutes."*
2. Raise the toilet seat on the toilet.
3. Insert large infusion bag or tube into the back of the sitz-bath basin, anchoring it to the bottom of the basin with the small opening at the end of the tubing facing upward, toward the ceiling.
4. Close the clamp on the tubing.
5. Fill the drainage bag with warm or cool water* up to the top line as indicated on the bag (have bag as full as possible without spilling when carried from the top).

   Rationale: **Warm water (102°F to 105°F or to touch) provides comfort, cleansing, and increases circulation which promotes healing and the prevention of infection. Cool water is effective in reducing edema and decreases pain. Offer both choices and allow the woman to choose which temperature she wants. If using cool water, add ice chips to the water if the woman desires a colder temperature.*
6. Place the basin in the toilet with the side marked "front" facing the front of the toilet.
7. Secure the drainage bag from a hook over the toilet or from the handle used to flush the toilet if it is a few feet higher than the toilet.
8. After placing towels on the floor around the toilet, assist the woman to sit directly on the basin edges as if it were the toilet seat.

   Rationale: *When the woman sits on the basin, excess water may overflow onto the floor around the toilet, thus the need for towels on the floor.*
9. Open the clamp on the tubing. The water will drain from the bag, into the basin, which already has water in it, thus

PROCEDURE 36-1 Use of Sitz Baths, Ice Packs, and Perineal Hygiene continued

NURSING ACTION

producing a gentle swirling movement of the water in the basin and on the perineal area. Water from the basin or bag will flow into the toilet through holes in the sides of the basin.

10. Once the sitz bath is complete, instruct the woman to close the clamp on the tubing, dry perineum with a clean towel, and apply new peri-pad.
11. Rinse the basin and place the tubing and bag inside and set it aside for the next use.
12. Take care to wipe up any spilled water from the floor to avoid slippage and injury.

Documentation

Document the use of the sitz bath as per agency documentation guidelines. Document and report any adverse events related to the use of the sitz bath.

Sitz Bath

The warmth of the water in the sitz bath provides comfort; decreases pain; and increases circulation to the tissues, which promotes healing and reduces the incidence of infection. Sitz baths may be used PRN. The nurse teaches the mother to fill the disposable sitz bath with water at a temperature (warm or cool) that is comfortable for her. The nurse instructs the woman to remain in the sitz bath for 20 minutes. It is important for the woman to have a clean towel to pat dry her perineum after the sitz bath and to have a clean perineal pad ready to apply. The woman should rinse the sitz bath with clean warm water after each use. See Procedure 36-1: Use of Sitz Baths, Ice Packs, and Perineal Hygiene.

Application: Perineal Discomfort

RESEARCH EVIDENCE IN PRACTICE Relieving Postpartum Perineal Pain

CLINICAL QUESTIONS

What are the determinants of postpartum perineal pain? How can it be alleviated?

RESEARCH EVIDENCE

Perineal pain affects nearly three quarters of women in the postnatal period. Pain may be a result of perineal bruising, spontaneous tears, surgical incision (episiotomy), or the use of instruments to assist the birth.

Several epidemiologic and cross-sectional studies have focused on the causes and risk factors associated with perineal pain. Primiparous women experience the highest rate of perineal pain. More significant perineal pain is associated with longer periods of active maternal pushing efforts. Ninety-seven percent of women with episiotomies and 100% of those with more severe tears report pain throughout the first week after birth. As one might expect, women with an intact perineum or first-degree tears had significantly less pain than women with second-, third-, or fourth-degree tears. Women with spontaneous first and even second-degree tears reported less pain than women with episiotomies.

The National Collaborating Center for Primary Care convened a group of obstetric experts to review research literature and provide expert advice on postnatal care. Women in the postnatal period should be asked if they have perineal pain, discomfort, stinging, burning, or offensive odor. If any of these symptoms are reported, the healthcare provider should assess the perineum for signs of inflammation and infection.

Women can be advised to use cold therapy in the form of crushed ice packs or gel pads as an effective method of pain relief for perineal pain. If additional analgesia is required, acetaminophen has been demonstrated to be an effective treatment for pain.

Most perineal pain lessens significantly within the first week after birth. Even women with more severe tears had near complete relief of pain within 6 weeks, and reported no pain at 3 months post-birth.

WHAT QUESTIONS REMAIN UNANSWERED?

Are any topical agents effective in lessening the severity of pain and enhancing healing?

WHAT IS BEST PRACTICE?

Women should be asked if they have postnatal perineal pain, stinging, burning, or offensive odor. The perineum should be assessed if there are concerns about infection or excessive inflammation. Cold therapy and acetaminophen can help reduce the painful symptoms. The mother can be counseled that substantial relief can be expected within a week, and symptoms should subside altogether in the first 2 months.

CRITICAL THINKING

Develop an educational plan for counseling the mother about perineal pain, its treatment, and expected course in the postnatal period.

References

Andrews, V., Thakar, R., Sultan, A., & Jones, P. 2008. Evaluation of postpartum perineal pain and dyspareunia: A prospective study. *European Journal of Obstetrics and Gynecology, 137*(2), 152–156.

Chou, D., Abalos, E., Gyte, G., & Gulmezoglu, A. 2010. Paracetamol/acetaminophen (single administration) for perineal pain in the early postpartum period. *Cochrane Database of Systematic Reviews.* Vol. 3. Issue CD008407.

Leeman, L., Fullilove, A., Borders, N., Manocchio, R., Albers, L., & Rogers, R. 2009. Postpartum perineal pain in a low episiotomy setting: Association with severity of genital trauma, labor care, and birth variables. *Birth, 36*(4), 283–288.

MacArthur, A., & MacArthur, C. 2004. Incidence, severity, and determinants of perineal pain after vaginal delivery. *American Journal of Obstetrics and Gynecology, 191*(4), 1199–1204.

National Collaborating Centre for Primary Care. (2006) Postnatal care. Routine postnatal care of women and their babies. *Royal College of General Practitioners,* 392.

TEACHING FOR SELF-CARE The nurse provides information about the purpose and use of the sitz bath, anticipated effects, benefits, possible problems, and safety measures to prevent injury from possible slipping or extreme water temperature. Home use of sitz baths may be recommended for the woman with an extensive episiotomy or laceration; the woman may use either the disposable sitz bath from the birthing unit or her clean bathtub. When using a bathtub, the woman should draw 4 to 6 inches of water, assess the temperature of the water, and soak in the water for 15 to 20 minutes. If other family members use the bathtub, it should be cleaned prior to her use. The use of a handheld showerhead to irrigate the perineum is another way to cleanse and soothe the traumatized tissue.

Topical Agents

Topical anesthetic agents may be used to relieve perineal discomfort. The woman is advised to apply the anesthetic agent after a sitz bath or perineal care. Anesthetic sprays, foams, ointments, or Tucks pads may be ordered for relief of both perineal and hemorrhoidal pain. It is important for the nurse to emphasize that the woman should wash her hands before and after using the topical treatments.

TEACHING FOR SELF-CARE The nurse provides information about the anesthetic spray or topical agent. The woman needs to understand the purpose, use, anticipated effects, benefits, and possible problems associated with the product. The nurse can combine an explanation with a demonstration of correct application. A return demonstration is a useful method of evaluating the woman's understanding. Directions for self-application should be provided in the woman's primary language and should include instructions to keep the product away from children. Some facilities post instructions with text and photos in postpartum patient restrooms.

> **PROFESSIONALISM IN PRACTICE**
>
> ***Managing Postpartum Perineal Trauma***
>
> The nurse should be aware that approaches to management of postpartum perineal trauma vary between facilities and regions of the country. It is important for baccalaureate-prepared nurses to be familiar with online databases such as the Cochrane Library, to periodically review current literature, and to participate in the development of unit policies and procedures that promote the use of interventions substantiated by research. Nurses who do this are engaged in the Quality and Safety Education in Nursing (QSEN) competency of evidence-based practice.

Relief of Hemorrhoidal Discomfort

Some mothers experience hemorrhoidal pain after giving birth. Relief measures include the use of sitz baths, topical anesthetics, cool packs, or witch hazel pads (Tucks) applied directly to the anal area. Short-term use of topical creams or rectal suppositories containing hydrocortisone is often helpful. Increasing fiber and fluids in the diet, exercising moderately, and using stool softeners as needed prevents straining (Staroselsky, Nava-Ocampo, Vohra, et al., 2008). Women who have had a fourth-degree laceration during birth should not use rectal suppositories.

HEALTH PROMOTION EDUCATION

The woman may find it helpful to maintain a side-lying position when possible or to tighten her buttocks when sitting down to reduce contact of the perineum with the seat and to avoid prolonged sitting. The mother is encouraged to continue a high-fiber diet, maintain adequate fluid intake, and begin moderate exercise such as walking. The nurse can reassure her that hemorrhoids usually disappear a few weeks after birth if the woman did not have them before her pregnancy.

Relief of Afterpains

Afterpains are the pain associated with intermittent uterine contractions that occur when the uterus contracts as it returns to its prepregnant state (see chapter 35). A primipara may not notice afterpains, because her uterus is able to maintain a contracted state. Multiparous women and those who have had an overdistended uterus (due to multiple gestation or hydramnios) frequently experience discomfort from afterpains as the uterus intermittently contracts more vigorously. Breastfeeding women are also more likely to experience afterpains than formula-feeding women because of the release of oxytocin when the infant suckles. The nurse can suggest the woman lie prone with a small pillow under the lower abdomen, explaining that the discomfort may be intensified for about 5 minutes but then will diminish greatly. The prone position applies pressure to the uterus and therefore stimulates contractions. When the uterus maintains a constant contraction, the afterpains cease. Additional nursing interventions include positioning, ambulation, or administration of an analgesic agent, such as ibuprofen or acetaminophen.

Prescription combination drugs such as Lortab or Vicodin (hydrocodone and acetaminophen) and Percocet (oxycodone and acetaminophen) are commonly used for postpartum discomfort, although in June 2009 an FDA advisory panel recommended taking these drugs off the market due to the risk of fatal liver damage when patients take multiple medications, including acetaminophen. While the FDA has not made a final decision, it is likely that narcotics and acetaminophen will be available separately, rather than in combination, in the future. The panel also recommended decreasing the maximum daily dosage of acetaminophen to below 4 grams and recommended that individual dosages of more than 650 mg be available by prescription only (Associated Press [AP], July 1, 2009).

The mother's description of the type and severity of her pain is usually the most reliable method of determining which analgesic agent will best promote the comfort she desires. Many women who are breastfeeding have concerns about the effects of medications on the infant. It is helpful to point out to concerned mothers that mild analgesics such as acetaminophen and ibuprofen pose little risk to their newborns when used judiciously in the short term to allow them the ability to bond and breastfeed in comfort. Short-term use of prescription narcotic agents may be necessary for pain that does not respond to ibuprofen or acetaminophen. Nurses can use references such as *Medications and Mothers Milk* (Hale, 2008) when advising breastfeeding mothers about use of analgesics.

TEACHING FOR SELF-CARE The nurse provides information about the cause of afterpains and methods to decrease discomfort. The nurse also explains any medications that are ordered, expected effect, benefits, possible side effects, and any special considerations such as the possibility of dizziness or sleepiness with particular medications. The nurse must inform patients who take acetaminophen about the risks of accidental overdose. Patients should be instructed to carefully read the labels of any drugs they take concurrently for the presence of acetaminophen.

Relief of Discomfort from Immobility and Muscle Strain

Discomfort may also be caused by immobility and muscle strain. The woman who pushed for a long time during labor may experience muscular aches. It is not unusual for women to experience joint pains and discomfort in both arms and legs, depending on the effort they exerted during the second stage of labor. Early ambulation is encouraged to help reduce the incidence of complications such as constipation and thrombophlebitis. It also helps promote a general feeling of well-being.

The nurse assists the woman the first few times she gets up during the postpartal period. Fatigue, effects of medications, loss of blood, and possibly even lack of food may cause feelings of dizziness or faintness when the woman stands up. Because this may be a problem during the woman's first shower, the nurse should remain in the room, check the woman frequently, and have a chair close by in case the woman becomes faint. Dizziness may be aggravated by standing still and by the warmth of the water, so it is best to wait until the woman has eaten and has shown stability when ambulating. The first shower should be brief. On many postpartum units, ammonia inhalants (referred to as "smelling salts") are available for use in case of fainting. The nurse instructs the woman in the use of the emergency call button in the bathroom prior to the first shower, so the new mother can call for assistance if she becomes faint.

TEACHING FOR SELF-CARE The nurse provides information about ambulation and the importance of monitoring any signs of dizziness or weakness. If she becomes dizzy, the woman should sit down and call for assistance.

Postpartum Diaphoresis

Postpartum diaphoresis (excessive perspiration) may cause discomfort for new mothers. The nurse can offer a fresh dry gown and bed linens to enhance comfort.

Some women may feel refreshed by a shower. It is important to consider cultural practices and realize that some women may prefer not to shower in the first few days following birth. For example, some Hispanic and Asian women prefer to delay showering. Nurses can offer these women a wet washcloth to increase maternal comfort. Because diaphoresis also may lead to increased thirst, the nurse can offer fluids as the woman desires. Again, cultural practices are important to consider. Women of western European background may prefer iced water; Asian women may prefer water at room temperature (see chapter 35 ∞). The nurse should ascertain the woman's wishes rather than operate solely from the nurse's own values or cultural belief system.

TEACHING FOR SELF-CARE The nurse provides information about the normal physiologic changes that cause diaphoresis and methods to increase comfort.

Suppression of Lactation in the Nonbreastfeeding Mother

Many women who do not breastfeed experience some degree of engorgement, accompanied by milk leakage and discomfort. Some women report relief from non-pharmacologic means of suppression such as wearing a support bra continuously for the first week except when showering, avoiding breast stimulation, applying cold packs, or applying cabbage leaves. Although binding the breasts was used in the past, it is no longer recommended. Signs of engorgement usually peak by day 4 and spontaneously resolve by the 10th day postpartum, regardless of treatment. Analgesics such as acetaminophen and ibuprofen can be used until the discomfort subsides. Drugs such as Bromocriptine are no longer used in the United States for lactation suppression due to concerns related to possible rare side effects such as myocardial infarction, cerebral angiopathy, and thromboembolism, although causal relationships between Bromocriptine and these events were not proven. According to a Cochrane review, there is a lack of adequate research regarding side effects of pharmacologic suppression, and "there is currently no evidence to show that nonpharmacologic approaches are more effective than no treatment." Further research is needed (Oladapo & Fawole, 2009, p. 14).

HEALTH PROMOTION EDUCATION

The mother is advised to avoid any stimulation of her breasts and nipples by her baby, herself, breast pumps, or her sexual partner until the sensation of fullness has passed (usually in 7 to 10 days). Such stimulation will increase milk production and delay the suppression process. Heat is avoided for the same reason, and the mother is encouraged to let shower water flow over her back rather than her breasts. The wearing of a 24-hour support bra, the use of analgesics as prescribed, and the use of cabbage leaves and/or cold compresses should be helpful during this period of time (American Academy of Pediatrics [AAP] & The American College of Obstetricians and Gynecologists [ACOG], 2007). Suppression takes only a few days in most cases, but small amounts of milk may be produced up to a month after birth.

Pharmacologic Interventions

Pharmacologic preparations, including pain medications, vaccinations, and Rh immune globulin, are frequently administered in the postpartum period. (See Table 36-3.)

Rubella Vaccine

Women who are not rubella immune as determined by lab studies should receive the rubella vaccine early in the postpartum period. It is administered before discharge, even if she is breastfeeding (AAP & ACOG, 2007; Centers for Disease Control and

TABLE 36-3 Essential Information for Common Postpartum Drugs

TYLENOL NO. 3 (300 mg acetaminophen and 30 mg codeine)

Drug Class: Nonopioid analgesic/opioid analgesic combination.

Dose/Route: Usual adult dose: 1–2 tablets PO every 4 hours PRN.

Indication: For relief of mild to moderate pain.

Adverse Effects: Respiratory depression, apnea, light-headedness, confusion, sedation, dizziness, nausea, vomiting, sweating, dry mouth, constipation, hypotension, facial flushing, suppression of cough reflex, ureteral spasm, urinary retention, pruritus, hepatotoxicity (overdose).

Nursing Implications: Determine whether woman is sensitive to acetaminophen or codeine; has history of impaired hepatic or renal function. Assess pain before and 1 hour after administration. Monitor bowel sounds, respirations, urine output.

Administer with food or milk to minimize gastrointestinal (GI) upset; warn patient that it may cause drowsiness—assistance with newborn care and ambulation may be necessary.

Patient Teaching: Inform patient about name of drug, expected action, and possible side effects; ask if she has any questions.

Nursing Diagnoses Related to Drug Therapy:

Readiness for Enhanced Self-Health Management information regarding drug therapy.

Risk for Injury related to side effects of drugs.

Constipation related to slowed gastrointestinal activity secondary to effects of medications.

PERCOCET 5/325 (325 mg acetaminophen and 5 mg oxycodone)

Drug Class: Nonopioid analgesic/opioid analgesic combination.

Dose/Route: 1–2 tablets PO every 4 hours PRN.

Indication: For moderate to severe pain. Can be used in aspirin-sensitive women.

Adverse Effects: Acetaminophen: Hepatotoxicity, headache, rash, and hypoglycemia.

Oxycodone: Respiratory depression, confusion, sedation, dizziness, blurred vision, apnea, circulatory depression, orthostatic hypotension, euphoria, facial flushing, sweating, constipation, dry mouth, nausea, vomiting, suppression of cough reflex, ureteral spasm, urinary retention.

Nursing Implications: Determine whether woman is sensitive to acetaminophen or codeine; has bronchial asthma; respiratory depression; convulsive disorder; adrenal insufficiency; renal, hepatic, or pulmonary disease.

Assess pain before and 1 hour after administration. Assess blood pressure, pulse, and respirations before and periodically during administration. Increase fluids and fiber, use stool softener to prevent constipation. Warn patient that it may cause sedation—assistance with newborn care and ambulation may be necessary.

Observe woman carefully for respiratory depression if given with barbiturates or sedative/hypnotics or after epidural morphine. Consider that after a cesarean birth, the woman may have depressed cough reflex, so teaching and encouragement to breathe deeply and cough are needed.

Monitor bowel sounds, and urine and bowel elimination.

Patient Teaching: Teaching should include name of drug, expected effect, possible adverse effects, whether the drug is secreted in the breast milk, encouragement to report any signs of adverse effects immediately.

Nursing Diagnoses Related to Drug Therapy:

Ineffective Breathing Pattern related to respiratory depression.

Constipation related to slowed gastrointestinal activity secondary to the effects of medications.

RUBELLA VIRUS VACCINE, LIVE MERUVAX® II (rubella virus vaccine live) or MMR® II (measles, mumps, and rubella virus vaccine live) may be used.

Dose/Route: Single-dose vial of 0.5 ml; inject subcutaneously in outer aspect of the upper arm.

Primary Indication: Stimulate active immunity against rubella virus in the postpartum woman who is susceptible to rubella, in order to protect future pregnancies.

Adverse Effects: Burning, pain, or stinging at the injection site; fever; arthritis/arthralgia; encephalitis; allergic reactions

Nursing Implications: Women who are allergic to neomycin, eggs, or gelatin, or who are immunosuppressed should not receive it. The manufacturer recommends delaying immunization for 3 months following blood transfusions. The immunization is contraindicated during pregnancy, and the patient should avoid pregnancy for 1 month following administration. Patient consent is obtained prior to immunization, and a record of administration is usually filed with the local health department. As with any immunization, epinephrine should be available in case of anaphylactic reaction.

Patient Teaching: Name of drug, expected effect, possible adverse effects, comfort measures to use if adverse effects occur; instruct woman to AVOID PREGNANCY FOR AT LEAST 4 WEEKS following vaccination. Provide information regarding contraceptives and their use.

Nursing Diagnoses Related to Drug Therapy:

Acute Pain Defining characteristics may include guarding, position, or verbal report of pain during or following subcutaneous administration of immunization.

Readiness for Enhanced Immunization Status

Defining characteristics may include expressed desire to receive the immunization, keep a record of the immunization, or learn about possible problems related to the immunization.

Rh_o (D) IMMUNE GLOBULIN (Rh immune globulin specific for D antigen)

Standard intramuscular (IM) formulations include ***RhoGAM®*** or ***HyperRHO S/D Full Dose®***

Microdose intramuscular (IM) formulations include ***HyperRHO S/D Mini-Dose®***, ***MICRhoGAM®***, & ***Mini-Gamulin R®*** (IM formulations are not intended for IV administration).

Dose/Route: Postpartum administration: One vial (300 mcg) IM (deltoid) within 72 hours of birth. Additional vials may be necessary after significant fetal-maternal hemorrhage as indicated by lab results (Kleihauer-Betke test).

Antepartum administration: One standard vial (300 mcg) is given IM at 28 weeks in Rh-negative women. One standard vial (300 mcg) is given IM: (a) after trauma, (b) after amniocentesis, (c) following obstetric manipulation such as version, and (d) following the termination of any pregnancy at 13 weeks or beyond (includes spontaneous or elective abortion, ectopic, etc.).

Antepartum administration prior to 13 weeks gestation: One microdose vial (50 mcg) is given IM following the termination of any pregnancy prior to 13 weeks.

Additional formulations are available. ***WinRho SDF®*** and ***Rhophylac®*** are IV formulations, which may be given IM, but dose may differ from the information above. As always, refer to current manufacturers' recommendations for safe administration.

Indication: Prevention of sensitization in Rh_o (D)-negative women by preventing production of anti-Rh_o (D) antibodies following exposure to Rh_o (D) positive blood. Mother must be Rh negative, not previously sensitized to Rh factor. Infant must be Rh positive, direct antiglobulin negative. Given during pregnancy to prevent erythroblastosis fetalis if fetus is Rh_o (D) positive in current and/or future pregnancies. Given postpartum to protect future pregnancies.

Adverse Effects: Pain at injection site, anemia, fever. May decrease response to live virus vaccines such as rubella.

Nursing Implications: Contraindicated in patients with documented hypersensitivity to human immune globulins. Confirm criteria for administration are present. Review type and crossmatch of mother's and infant's blood and any other labs, as dosage and administration depend on results. Do not confuse IM and IV formulations. If using a pre-filled syringe, allow it to come to room temperature before IM administration. If the mother is Rh (D) negative, and there is any doubt regarding the infant's blood type or lab studies, the medication should be given. **Do not administer to newborn.**

TABLE 36-3 Essential Information for Common Postpartum Drugs continued

Patient Teaching: Name of drug, expected action, possible side effects; report soreness at injection site to nurse; woman should carry information regarding Rh status and dates of RhoGAM injections with her at all times; explain relevance of RhoGAM to subsequent pregnancies.

Nursing Diagnoses Related to Drug Therapy:

Acute Pain: Defining characteristics may include guarding, position, or verbal report of pain during or following intramuscular administration of immunization.

Readiness for Enhanced Immunization Status: Defining characteristics may include expressed desire to receive the immunization, keep a record of the immunization, or learn about possible problems related to the immunization.

MOTRIN, ADVIL (ibuprofen)

Drug Class: nonopioid analgesic; nonsteroidal anti-inflammatory agent.

Dose/Route: 400 to 800 mg orally 3–4 times/day (use as an over-the-counter analgesic not to exceed 1200 mg/day; up to 2400 mg/day may be prescribed for short-term postpartum use)

Indication: Mild to moderate pain.

Adverse Effects: Headache, dizziness, drowsiness, blurred vision, tinnitus, constipation, dyspepsia, nausea, vomiting, hematuria, renal failure, arrythmias, edema, rashes, prolonged bleeding time, blood dyscrasias. Life-threatening adverse effects may include anaphylaxis, GI bleeding, hepatitis, exfoliative dermatitis, Steven-Johnson Syndrome, and toxic epidermal necrolysis.

Nursing Implications: Patients with asthma, aspirin-induced allergy, and nasal polyps are at increased risk for hypersensitivity. Assess pain before and 1 to 2 hours after administration. May cause prolonged bleeding time, which may persist for less than 1 day after discontinuation. Co-administration with opioid analgesics may have additive effects and permit smaller doses. Administer with food, milk, or antacid to decrease GI upset. May cause drowsiness or dizziness—new mothers may require assistance with newborn care and ambulation.

Patient Teaching: Name of drug, expected action, possible side effects. Encourage patient to drink a full glass of water with medication and to remain upright for 15 to 30 minutes. Instruct not to take it on an empty stomach. Inform patient that dosages prescribed for short-term postpartal use are higher than what is recommended for general over-the-counter use of ibuprofen. Ensure that patient knows the trade names (Motrin, Advil, etc.) to avoid accidental overdose. Patient should consult with provider before taking other medications or herbal supplements concurrently.

Nursing Diagnosis Related to Drug Therapy:

Readiness for Enhanced Knowledge: Defining characteristics may include expressing an interest to learn about the medication and how to promote comfort.

Nausea: Defining characteristics may include gagging sensation, report of nausea, and aversion toward food related to ingestion of ibuprofen.

Sources: AAP & ACOG, 2007; Deglin & Vallerand, 2009; Herdman, 2009; Merck, 2008a, pp. 2061–2062; Merck, 2008b, pp. 2054–2056.

Prevention (CDC), 1998, updated 2007). Administering the injection just after childbirth is advantageous because the woman is definitely not pregnant and typically does not want another pregnancy within the near future.

TEACHING FOR SELF-CARE The nurse needs to ensure that the woman understands the purpose of the vaccine and that she must avoid becoming pregnant for at least 1 month. To ensure that the woman understands, an informed consent is usually signed before administration. Because avoiding pregnancy is so important, counseling regarding contraception is necessary.

PROFESSIONALISM IN PRACTICE

How to Address Differing Drug Recommendations

The nurse will find that sources sometimes vary regarding recommendations for various drugs. For example, some sources recommend delaying pregnancy for a minimum of one month following rubella immunization (AAP & ACOG, 2007; Deglin & Vallerand, 2009), but the manufacturer recommends delaying pregnancy for 3 months (Merck, 2008a, 2008b). Both the AAP & ACOG (2007) and Merck (2008a, 2008b) noted that the risk of congenital rubella syndrome from the vaccine is theoretical, and emphasized that cases have not occurred despite accidental administration during pregnancy. The professional nurse should discuss issues such as these with providers, be aware of professional organization recommendations, and read current literature in order to give accurate advice to patients.

Rh Immune Globulin (RhoGam)

All Rh-negative women with Rh-positive babies should receive Rh immune globulin (RhoGAM® or a similar formulation) within 72 hours after childbirth to prevent sensitization from a fetomaternal transfusion of Rh-positive fetal red blood cells (AAP & ACOG, 2007). See discussion of criteria in Procedure 20-2: Intramuscular Administration of Rh Immune Globulin [RhoGAM, HyperRHO, Rhophlac, WinRho-SDF] ∞ on page 482.

TEACHING FOR SELF-CARE The Rh-negative woman needs to understand the implications of her Rh-negative status in future pregnancies. (See chapter 20 ∞ for a detailed discussion.) The nurse provides opportunities for questions during teaching.

Support of Maternal Psychosocial Well-Being

The birth of a child, with the role changes and increased responsibilities it produces, is a time of emotional stress for the new mother. This stress is increased by the tremendous physiologic changes that occur as her body adjusts to a nonpregnant state. Nurses working in maternal-child care should read the works of Rubin (1984) and Mercer (1986, 2004, 2006), two key theorists who have researched and written about the process of developing a maternal identity over the past 40 years. Mercer recommended changing the previous terminology, *maternal role attainment (MRA)*, to *becoming a mother (BAM)* in 2004. Their work also is discussed in chapter 35 ∞.

Mercer (2004) described becoming a mother (BAM) as a life-transforming process through which mothers establish maternal identity, including "(a) commitment, attachment, and preparation (pregnancy); (b) acquaintance, learning, and physical restoration (first 2 to 6 weeks following birth); (c) moving toward a new normal (2 weeks to 4 months); and (d) achievement of the maternal identity (around 4 months)" (p. 231). Mercer (2006) also noted that this process "requires extensive psychological, social, and physical work" and that the second stage, which most women enter after childbirth, might be extended after a complicated pregnancy or birth (p. 649). Postpartum nurses must support the individual woman's process of becoming a mother. An extensive review of the literature by Mercer & Walker (2006) discovered that interactive nurse-patient relationships are necessary to support this transition. Although agencies may use audiovisual approaches to patient education in an era of short stays and cost containment, a portion of patient education and support needs to be offered through individualized patient-nurse interaction.

Immediately following the birth (the taking-in period), the mother may be dependent and inwardly focused on bodily concerns. Although the mother will benefit from rest at some point early in the postpartum period, there is a preponderance of evidence that immediate **skin-to-skin contact (SSC)** between mother and newborn has many positive effects for both (Bystrova et al., 2009; Dabrowski, 2007; Klaus, 2009; Moore, Anderson, & Bergman, 2007). SSC should be encouraged for all mothers and newborns unless complications prevent it. Mother and newborn can rest comfortably together under close nursing supervision, and immediate newborn care such as Apgar scoring and assessment of vital signs can be performed in this position (Romano & Lothian, 2008).

Many women are focused on their own needs during the immediate postpartum period. Once the woman's self-care needs have been met, her focus will shift to the care of her newborn and her ability as a parent (the taking-hold period). During this time the mother is usually receptive to teaching, and tactful instructions and demonstrations assist her in developing mothering skills. The nurse must carefully avoid "taking over" the infant. By functioning as an adviser and allowing the mother to perform the actual care, the nurse demonstrates confidence in the mother's skill and ability, which in turn increases the mother's self-confidence about her effectiveness as a parent. Mercer (2006) emphasized the importance of positive feedback from the nurse regarding the mother's interactions with and provision of care for her newborn. "Mothers need to hear from an expert that it takes time, and trial and error for both mother and infant to know what to expect of the other" (p. 650).

The mother may benefit from the opportunity to tell her birth story during the hours and days following birth. During the postpartal period, the mother must adjust to the loss of her fantasized child and accept the child she has borne. This may be more difficult if the child is not of the desired sex or has birth defects. Parents of newborns requiring special care due to congenital anomalies or prematurity will require extra attention and opportunities to share their concerns, fears, and disappointment.

The incidence of postpartum mood disorders is between 10% and 15% across cultures (AAP & ACOG, 2007). The mother is often discharged before the onset of mood disturbances and disorders associated with the postpartum period. However, an extensive review of the literature, including the research of Beck and Dennis, found that "maternal mood in the immediate postpartum period (or up to 2 weeks postpartum) is a significant predictor of postpartum depression" (McQueen, Montgomery, Lappan-Gracon, et al., 2008, p. 129). Therefore, the nurse needs to individually assess all postpartum patients for mood disorders and coordinate follow-up care for women who exhibit postpartum *blues* prior to discharge (AAP & ACOG, 2007; McQueen et al., 2008). Postpartum blues (also referred to as *baby blues*), postpartum depression, and postpartum psychosis are discussed in detail in chapter 39 ∞. See chapter 35 ∞ for assessment and screening tools for postpartum blues and postpartum depression.

HEALTH PROMOTION EDUCATION

The nurse should advise the mother that physical, psychologic, and hormonal factors all influence an individual's response to childbirth. It is often helpful to discuss normal adaptations in the postpartum period with both the mother and her intimate partner or another family member. This ensures that someone close to her will be aware of the normal patterns of psychologic responses in the early postpartum period. Normal responses include a brief period of irritability, mood swings, crying spells, and other mood-related symptoms associated with postpartum blues. Symptoms are relatively mild and self-limiting, usually resolving within 10 days. Women who experience severe symptoms or symptoms that extend beyond the second postpartum week should be advised to contact their physician or certified nurse-midwife. The nurse should advise families about symptoms of postpartum depression and emphasize the importance of seeking help should they occur.

Promotion of Maternal Nutrition, Rest, and Activity

Promotion of Nutrition

The mother may be hungry and thirsty immediately following delivery, particularly if she had limited oral intake during a prolonged labor. She should be allowed to eat and drink as desired, unless complications prevent it. All postpartum women should be encouraged to eat a healthy, well-balanced diet. A breastfeeding mother will require 500 kcal/day above that which is ordinarily recommended for a woman of her age. Nonbreastfeeding women may return to normal caloric requirements for their age. Many women continue prenatal vitamin and iron supplementation until the postpartum checkup, and breastfeeding mothers may continue supplementation throughout lactation. See chapter 18 ∞ for more information about maternal nutrition, and chapter 35 ∞ for information on nutritional assessment and guidance.

Relief of Fatigue

Following birth, some women feel exhausted and in need of rest. Other women are euphoric and full of psychic energy, ready to retell their experience of birth repeatedly. The nurse evaluates individual needs, always with the goal of providing opportunities for rest (see chapter 35 ∞ for information on assessing rest and sleep status). This may include limiting visitors and providing a comfortable place for the significant other to sleep.

Fatigue is a common occurrence, which should be expected to resolve over the first few postpartal weeks. Additive sleep deprivation related to pregnancy discomforts, labor and delivery, and caring for a newborn, especially if there are other young children in the home, contributes to the problem. Adequate rest is essential to a smooth postpartum transition. The nurse can encourage rest by organizing activities to avoid frequent interruptions for the woman. Ideally, one person close to the mother will be in the room to watch the newborn when the mother sleeps. If this is not possible, the newborn may return to the nursery for a period of time to ensure that the infant remains safe while the mother is sleeping soundly.

Postpartum fatigue can be severe and extended in some women, complicating the recovery process. Runquist (2007) found that "postpartum fatigue emerged as an overwhelmingly negative, distressing, subjective experience that changed every aspect of participants' lives" (p. 30). Severe or prolonged fatigue potentially interferes with the woman's process of becoming a mother, interferes with her ability to care for herself and her baby, slows her return to social and work obligations, and puts her at increased risk for postpartum depression. Conditions such as anemia, infection and inflammation, and thyroid dysfunction predispose to postpartum fatigue, and women diagnosed with or experiencing symptoms of these complications should receive additional assessment and follow-up (Corwin & Arbour, 2007).

Although most mothers feel fatigued, they tend to view themselves as healthy and well if they perceive pregnancy and birth as natural processes. Some cultures have distinct customs regarding rest and activity in the postpartum period. For example, Taiwanese women may follow a traditional recuperation strategy of *doing-the-month* (Ko, Yang, & Chiang, 2008, p. 182), which restricts activity and encourages bedrest for the first month postpartum. Nurses unfamiliar with certain cultural customs may find it stressful if they are expected to perform all maternal-infant care or if women are resistant to Western recommendations for ambulation and exercise following childbirth. Most cultural customs can be accommodated if they are not harmful. The nurse should inform the mother of the health benefits of early ambulation.

HEALTH PROMOTION EDUCATION

Nearly all new mothers experience some degree of fatigue or sleep deprivation during the postpartum period. Women who have had a cesarean birth are coping with both the constant demands of the baby and their own recovery needs. Some women feel self-induced pressure to take care of household chores while the infant is napping. Fatigue and worry about unaccomplished tasks can become continuous and cyclical. Runquist (2007) found that prior experience with newborns, practical support with such things as newborn care, multiple sources of information, and the ability to "let go" of worries about nonessential tasks limited the experience of postpartum fatigue (p. 32). Mothers should be counseled to sleep when the baby sleeps, to utilize family and friends for support, and to delegate or postpone unnecessary chores and activities. Additionally, they should be advised to contact their healthcare provider if they experience signs of infection, anemia, thyroid dysfunction, or unrelenting postpartum fatigue that persists beyond the initial postpartum period.

Resumption of Activity

Ambulation and activity may gradually increase after discharge. The new mother should avoid heavy lifting, excessive stair climbing, and strenuous activity. One or two daily naps are essential and are most easily achieved if the mother sleeps when her baby does.

By the second week at home, the new mother may begin some light housekeeping activities. Although it is customary to delay the return to work outside the home for 6 weeks, most women are physically able to resume practically all activities in 4 to 5 weeks when the lochial flow has stopped. Delaying the return to work until after the final postpartal examination will minimize the possibility of problems.

HEALTH PROMOTION EDUCATION

The nurse can provide the new mother with suggestions for resuming her normal level of activity. Women should be encouraged to limit the number of activities to prevent excessive fatigue, increase in lochia, and negative psychologic reactions, such as feeling overwhelmed. The nurse can encourage the new mother to avoid the temptation to catch up on housework during infant naps, but instead use the time to rest. If excessive fatigue or an increase in lochia occurs, the woman should increase rest periods and decrease extra activities.

Postpartum Exercises

The nurse should encourage the woman to begin simple exercises while in the birthing unit and continue them at home, advising her that increased lochia or pain means she should reevaluate her activity and make necessary reductions. Most agencies provide a booklet describing suggested postpartal activities. (Exercise routines vary for women undergoing tubal ligation following birth and for cesarean birth patients.) See Figure 36-1 ■ for a description of some commonly used exercises. The postpartal woman is more likely to have positive views of her own well-being and less fatigue if she continues to do stretching and/or her own programmed pattern of exercise.

HEALTH PROMOTION EDUCATION

The nurse should advise the woman to begin Kegel exercises immediately after birth. The nurse can explain that these exercises will assist in returning vaginal tone and preventing urinary leakage. If no complications exist, normal exercise can be initiated at 2 weeks after birth. Women should be advised to take short walks outside if the weather is appropriate. Abdominal exercises can be suggested to retone the abdominal muscles. A regular exercise program including vigorous activities such as running, weight lifting, or competitive sports can usually be initiated after her 6-week postpartum examination or when approved by her physician or certified nurse-midwife.

Retention of weight gained during pregnancy contributes to future obesity, placing the woman at increased risk for diabetes, heart disease, and hypertension. Although further research is

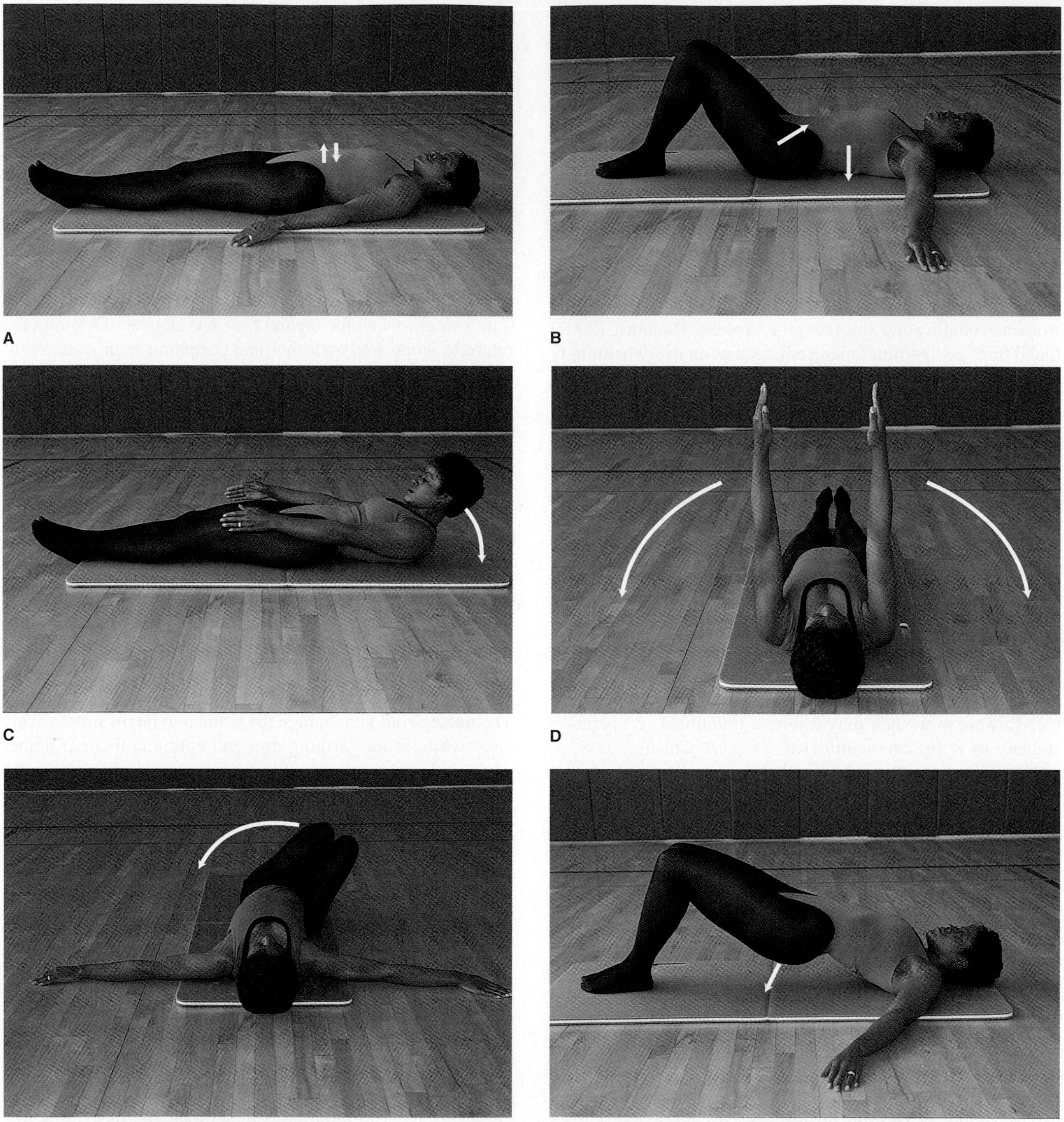

Figure 36-1 ■ Postpartum exercises. Begin with 5 repetitions two or three times daily, and gradually increase to 10 repetitions. First day: A. Abdominal breathing. Lying supine, inhale deeply, using the abdominal muscles. The abdomen should expand. Then exhale slowly through pursed lips, tightening the abdominal muscles. B. Pelvic rocking. Lying supine with arms at sides, knees bent, and feet flat, tighten abdomen and buttocks, and attempt to flatten back on floor. Hold for a count of 10; then arch the back, causing the pelvis to "rock." On the second day, add C. Chin to chest. Lying supine with legs straight, raise head and attempt to touch chin to chest. Slowly lower head. D. Arm raises. Lying supine, arms extended at a 90-degree angle from body, raise arms so that they are perpendicular and hands touch. Lower slowly. On fourth day, add E. Knee rolls. Lying supine with knees bent, feet flat, arms extended to the side, roll knees slowly to one side, keeping shoulders flat. Return to original position, and roll to opposite side. F. Buttocks lift. Lying supine, arms at sides, knees bent, feet flat, slowly raise the buttocks, and arch the back. Return slowly to starting position.

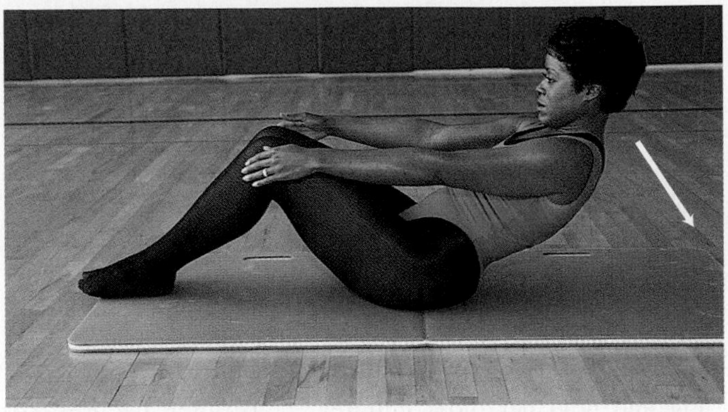
G

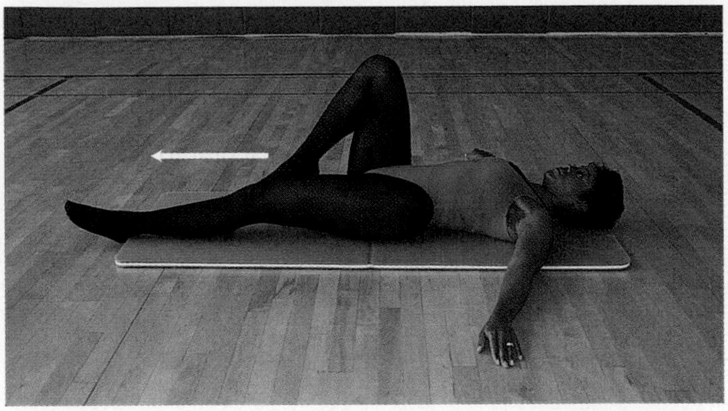
H

Figure 36-1 ■ Continued. On sixth day, add: G. Abdominal tighteners. Lying supine, knees bent, feet flat, slowly raise head toward knees. Arms should extend along either side of legs. Return slowly to original position. H. Knee to abdomen. Lying supine, arms at sides, bend one knee and thigh until foot touches buttocks. Straighten leg and lower it slowly. Repeat with other leg. After 2 to 3 weeks, more strenuous exercises, such as sit-ups and side leg raises, may be added as tolerated. Kegel exercises, begun antepartally, should be done many times daily during postpartum to restore vaginal and perineal tone.

needed, a Cochrane review found that diet alone or a combination of diet and exercise assisted women with weight loss following pregnancy. Although exercise without dietary changes did not contribute to postpartum weight loss in the studies reviewed, it did improve cardiovascular fitness. The authors recommended a combination of diet and exercise to promote heart health and preservation of lean body mass during weight loss (Amorim Adegboye, Linne, & Lourenco, 2007).

PROFESSIONALISM IN PRACTICE

Patient-Centered Care of Anemia

Professional nurses must be sensitive to risk factors for anemia, which contributes to postpartum fatigue. Nurses should pay particular attention to adolescent or low-income patients who may be at high risk for anemia. Education related to diet and iron supplementation is helpful, but the nurse should assess the patient's willingness and ability to comply with recommendations prior to discharge. Some patients stop use of iron supplements due to unpleasant side effects or inability to pay for them. Others lack the financial resources to procure healthy foods that are high in iron. Listening to the mother, providing individualized education, exploring options, and coordinating necessary resources and follow-up are professional nursing responsibilities that fulfill the Quality and Safety Education in Nursing (QSEN) competency of patient-centered care.

Promotion of Family Wellness and Shared Parenting

A satisfactory maternity experience may have a positive impact on the entire family. The new or expanding family who receives appropriate information and has adequate time to interact with its newest member in a supportive environment will feel more comfortable and secure at home.

In the past, newborns were typically separated from their parents immediately after birth. Today most facilities support **family-centered care**, which is focused on keeping the mother and baby together as much as the mother desires. **Mother-baby care**, or **couplet care** (care of both the mother and her baby), is an important part of the family-centered care approach, in which the infant remains at the mother's bedside and both are cared for by the same nurse. Couplet care allows the nurse to teach and role model and to integrate the entire family into the care of the woman and her infant. It also enables the mother to have time to bond with her baby and learn to care for him or her in a supportive environment.

A Cochrane review of 30 research studies involving 1925 mother-infant dyads found that skin-to-skin contact (SSC) immediately following birth helped to stabilize newborn temperature and cardiorespiratory status, promoted breastfeeding and maternal-infant attachment, and was associated with decreased infant crying (Moore et al., 2007). A study of 29 father-infant dyads found that the 15 infants offered SSC with their fathers following cesarean birth cried less and became drowsy sooner than those in the control group (Erlandsson, Dsilna, Fagerberg, et al., 2007). Therefore, the nurse should encourage immediate SSC following delivery of healthy term and late pre-term infants if stable. A warm blanket and hat should be placed over the infant, and these linens should be replaced if they become wet.

In a mother-baby unit, the newborn's crib is placed near the mother's bed, where she can see her baby easily. The crib should be a self-contained unit stocked with items the parents might require in providing care. A bulb syringe for suctioning the mouth or nares should always be accessible, and the mother and father or partner should be familiar with its use. The mother-baby unit is conducive to an on-demand feeding schedule for both breastfeeding and formula-feeding infants. It is essential that parents be oriented to the facility's infant security procedures and protocols to prevent infant abduction. This can be discussed in prenatal courses and upon admission to the birthing unit, and it will need to be reinforced when the infant begins rooming in.

Mothers are frequently very tired after birth, so the responsibility for providing total infant care could be overwhelming. The mother-baby policy must be flexible enough to permit the mother to return the baby to the nursery if she finds it necessary because of fatigue or physical discomfort. Many agencies have unlimited visiting hours for the father or significant others of the mother's choice. These opportunities to hold and care for the child promote paternal self-confidence and foster paternal attachment. Encouraging fathers or significant others to spend the night allows parents to share initial newborn care responsibilities while they still have the support of nursing staff if questions arise.

Although our culture idealistically and theoretically supports involved fathers, new fathers often lack role models, support, and resources. It is imperative that all teaching in the family-centered care unit be directed to both parents at times that are convenient for both and that fathers be encouraged to share their feelings and be actively involved in the childbearing experience. It is also helpful to provide anticipatory guidance for fathers regarding the feelings and situations they may experience, particularly if their baby is breastfed. Encouraging fathers to be involved in infant bathing, the bedtime routine, holding, cuddling, and playing will allow them to develop a relationship and reap the rewards they desire.

Reactions of Siblings

Sibling visitation helps meet the needs of both the siblings and their mother. A visit to the hospital reassures children that their mother is well and still loves them. It also provides an opportunity for the children to become familiar with the new baby. For the mother, the pangs of separation are lessened as she interacts with her children and introduces them to the newest family member.

Most agencies now recognize the importance of providing siblings with opportunities to see their mother and meet the infant during the early postpartal period (Figure 36-2 ■). Approaches to this issue vary from specified visiting hours for siblings to unlimited visiting privileges.

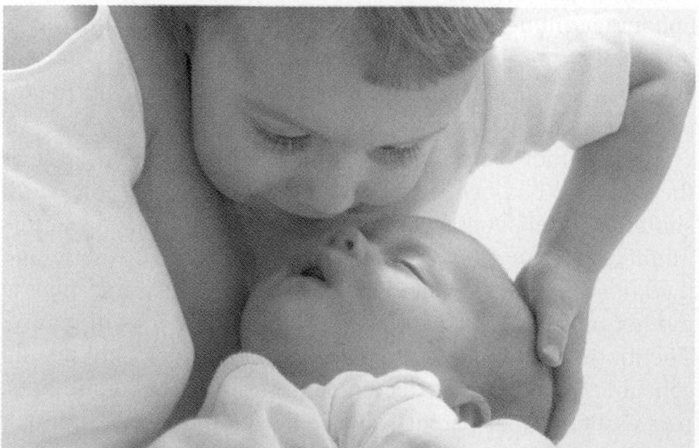

Figure 36-2 ■ The sister of this newborn becomes acquainted with the new family member.

Source: niderlander/shutterstock.

HEALTH PROMOTION EDUCATION

Although the parents have prepared the child(ren) for the presence of a new brother or sister, the actual arrival of the infant requires some adjustments. Some children may be present for the birth and have an opportunity to spend time with their new sibling and their parents immediately following the birth. They may even remain throughout the woman's hospitalization, especially if it is brief, and all go home as a family.

For the mother who is returning home to small children, it is often helpful to have the father carry the new baby inside. This practice keeps the mother's arms free to immediately hug and hold her older children, reaffirming her love for them. Many mothers have found that bringing a doll home with them for an older child is helpful. The child cares for the doll alongside his or her parents, thereby identifying with the parent. This identification helps decrease anger and the need to regress to get attention.

Often older children enjoy working with the parents to care for the newborn. Involvement in care helps the older child develop a sense of closeness to the baby. It also helps the child learn acceptable behavior toward the newborn, feel a sense of accomplishment, and develop tenderness and caring. With constant supervision and assistance as necessary, even very young children can hold the baby or a bottle during feeding.

Regression is a common occurrence even when siblings have been well prepared. The nurse can provide anticipatory guidance so that parents are not surprised or upset if their previously toilet-trained child begins to have accidents or if an older sibling requests a bottle or the breast.

Regardless of age, an older sibling needs reassurance that he or she is still special to the parents, a truly loved and valued family member. Words of love and praise coupled with hugs and kisses are very important. So, too, is special parent-child time. Both parents should spend quality one-on-one time with each of their older children. This may require some careful planning, but its worth cannot be overestimated. It confirms the parents' love for the child and often helps the child accept the new baby.

The child, especially one of the opposite sex from the newborn, may raise queries about the appearance of the genitals as compared to his or her own. A simple explanation, such as, "That's what little girls (boys) look like," is often sufficient.

Resumption of Sexual Activity

Nursing interventions in the postpartal period acknowledge that each parent is also a sexual being. Couples were formerly discouraged from engaging in sexual intercourse until 6 weeks postpartum. Although the earliest time at which the couple can safely resume intercourse has not been demonstrated by research, the risks of hemorrhage and infection are minimal after 2 weeks postpartum (AAP & ACOG, 2007). Currently, the couple is advised to abstain from intercourse until the episiotomy is healed and the lochial flow has stopped (usually by the third to sixth week postpartum). During this period, couples can be encouraged to express their affection and love through kissing,

PATIENT TEACHING Resuming Sexual Activity After Childbirth

PATIENT GOALS At the completion of the teaching, the couple will be able to:

1. Discuss the changes in the woman's body that affect sexual activity.
2. Formulate alternative approaches to sexual activity based on an understanding of these changes.
3. Identify the length of time it is advisable to wait before resuming sexual activity.
4. Discuss information needed to make contraceptive choices.

TEACHING PLAN

Content	Teaching Method
■ Present information about changes that may affect sexual activity, including the following: ■ Tenderness of the vagina and perineum ■ Presence of lochia and the healing process ■ Dryness of the vagina ■ Breast tenderness/escape of milk during sex ■ Fatigue	Discussion is a logical approach. It may be useful to make a universal statement and link it with a question to determine a couple's initial level of knowledge. For example, "Many women experience vaginal dryness when they resume intercourse for the first several weeks after childbirth. Are you familiar with this change and the cause for it?" Use the information gained during this discussion to determine the depth to which to cover the material.
■ Discuss healing at the placental site and stress that the presence of lochia indicates that healing is not yet complete. Explain that vaginal dryness may pose a problem because of postpartal hormonal changes. Dryness may be prolonged if woman is breastfeeding, because of low estrogen levels. This can be managed by using a water-soluble lubricant. In most cases, coitus can resume at some point after 2 weeks, depending on the woman's comfort and desire (AAP & ACOG, 2007). Explain that escape of milk during sexual activity can be minimized by breastfeeding the baby immediately beforehand.	Provide printed information to clarify content and serve as a resource for the couple following discharge.
■ Discuss the importance of contraception during the early postpartal period. Provide information on the advantages and disadvantages of different methods, including special considerations for breastfeeding mothers. The woman's body needs adequate time to heal and recover from the stress of pregnancy and childbirth. Couples who are opposed to contraception may choose abstinence at this time.	Provide samples of different types of contraceptives. Provide literature on specific contraceptive methods.
■ Discuss the impact of fatigue and the new baby's schedule on the woman's feelings of desire. Refer the couple to a physician or certified nurse-midwife for additional information if needed.	Many couples are unprepared for the impact of fatigue and the baby's schedule on lovemaking. Information enables the couple to anticipate this impact.

Evaluation

Determine the couple's learning by providing time for discussion and questions. If the couple indicates that they plan to use a particular contraceptive method, you may ask them about aspects of the method to ascertain that they have correct and complete information.

Documentation

Documentation of patient teaching should include the teaching information discussed, the patient's verbalization of understanding, specific interventions or warning signs that were given, along with the patient's understanding of follow-up if needed in the future.

holding, and talking. Since postpartum women often experience vaginal dryness due to hormonal changes, some form of lubrication, such as K-Y jelly, may initially be necessary during intercourse. This may continue throughout the period of lactation in breastfeeding mothers because of lower estrogen levels. The female-superior or side-by-side positions for coitus may be preferable because they enable the woman to control the depth of penile penetration.

Breastfeeding couples should be forewarned that during orgasm, milk may spurt from the nipples because of the release of oxytocin. Some couples find this pleasurable or amusing; other couples choose to have the woman wear a bra during sexual activity. Breastfeeding the baby before lovemaking may reduce the chance of milk release.

Other factors may inhibit satisfactory sexual experience. The baby's crying may "spoil the mood," the woman's changed body may be unattractive to her or to her partner, and maternal sleep deprivation may interfere with a mutually satisfying experience. Couples may also be frustrated if there is decreased libido or other changes in the woman's physiologic response to sexual stimulation. These changes are due to hormonal changes and may persist for several months.

Maternal fatigue is often a significant factor limiting the resumption of sexual intercourse. Consequently, couples should be encouraged to find a time for lovemaking when both are interested and awake. While interest and desire vary, most couples resume sexual activity within 3 months.

Anticipatory guidance during the prenatal and postnatal periods can forewarn the couple of these eventualities and of their temporary nature. See Patient Teaching: Resuming Sexual Activity After Childbirth on page 1041.

HEALTH PROMOTION EDUCATION

The nurse should discuss normal sexual changes that frequently occur in the postpartum period. A discussion that includes both partners can facilitate an open dialog between them and can provide an opportunity for questions and answers.

Contraception

Because many couples resume sexual activity before the postpartal examination, family-planning information should be made available before discharge. A couple's decision to use a contraceptive is often motivated by a desire to gain control over the number of children they will conceive or to determine the spacing of future children. In choosing a specific method, consistency of use outweighs the absolute reliability of a given method. The nurse must identify risk factors and contraindications of the various methods to help the couple select a contraceptive method that has practical application and is compatible with the couple's health and physical needs.

Often different methods of contraception are appropriate at different times in the couple's life. Thus they should have a clear understanding of all of the methods available to them so that they can make an appropriate choice. The currently available contraceptive methods are discussed in detail in chapter 5 ∞.

HEALTH PROMOTION EDUCATION

The nurse should discuss available contraceptive methods with both partners before discharge. Written information should also be provided for the couple to refer to at a later time. The nurse should stress the fact that pregnancy can occur before the first menstrual period returns and that contraception before that time is necessary to avoid pregnancy. The nurse should be frank and open with the couple, answering questions as needed.

Parent-Infant Attachment

Nursing interventions to enhance the quality of parent-infant attachment should be designed to promote feelings of well-being, comfort, and satisfaction. Table 36-4 describes parental attachment behaviors and those that require further assessment (see chapter 35 ∞ for ways to assess maternal-infant attachment). Following are some suggestions for ways of achieving this.

- Determine the childbearing and childrearing goals of the infant's mother and father, and incorporate them when planning nursing care for the family. This includes considering cultural preferences, and giving the parents choices about their labor and birth experience and their initial time with their new infant.
- Postpone eye prophylaxis for 1 hour after birth to facilitate eye contact between parents and their newborn (eye ointment further clouds the newborn's vision and makes eye contact difficult for the baby).
- Provide private time in the first hour after birth for the new family to become acquainted. Encourage SSC between mother (or father) and baby to promote breastfeeding and bonding.
- Arrange the healthcare setting so that the individual nurse-patient relationship can be developed and maintained. A primary nurse can develop rapport and assess the mother's strengths and needs.
- Encourage the mother to tell her birth story. Clarify information for the mother as necessary.
- Encourage the parents to involve the siblings in integrating the infant into the family by bringing them to the birthing center for sibling visits.
- Use anticipatory guidance from conception through the postpartal period to prepare the parents for expected problems of adjustment.

TABLE 36-4 Parent Attachment Behaviors

ASSESSMENT AREA	ATTACHMENT	BEHAVIOR REQUIRING ASSESSMENT AND INFORMATION
Caretaking	Talks with baby. Demonstrates and seeks eye-to-eye contact. Touches and holds baby "en face." Changes diapers when needed. Baby is clean. Clothing is appropriate for room temperature. Feeds baby as needed, and baby is gaining weight. Positions baby comfortably and checks on baby.	Does not refer or speak to baby. Completes activities without addressing the baby or looking at the baby. Lack of interaction. Does not recognize need for or demonstrate concern for baby's comfort or needs. Feeding occurs intermittently. Baby does not gain weight. Waits for baby to cry and then hesitates to respond.
Perception of the baby	Has knowledge of expected child development. Understands that the baby is dependent and cannot meet parent's needs. Accepts sex of child and characteristics.	Has unrealistic expectations of the baby's abilities and behaviors. Expects love and interaction from the baby. Believes that the baby will fulfill parent's needs. Is strongly distressed over sex of baby or feels that some aspect of the baby is unacceptable.
Support	Has friends who are available for support. Seems to be comfortable with being a parent. Has a realistic belief of parenting role.	Is alone or isolated. Is on edge, tense, anxious, and hesitant with the baby. Demonstrates difficulty incorporating parenting with own wants and needs.

Please note: These are a few of the behaviors that may be associated with attachment. It is vitally important for the nurse to observe the parents on more than one occasion and to take into consideration individual characteristics, values, beliefs, and customs.

- Include parents in any nursing intervention, planning, and evaluation. Give choices whenever possible.
- Initiate and support measures to alleviate fatigue in the parents.
- Help parents identify, understand, and accept both positive and negative feelings related to the birth, the newborn, and the overall parenting experience.
- Support and assist parents in determining the personality and unique needs of their infant.

Whenever possible and culturally acceptable, the mother and father should be allowed to care for their baby. This practice gives them a chance to learn their newborn's normal patterns and develop confidence in caring for him or her. It also allows them to spend more uninterrupted time with their infant in the first days of life. Early discharge may be advantageous if mother and baby are doing well, help is available for the mother at home, and the family and certified nurse-midwife or physician agree.

The nurse may observe beginnings of parent-newborn attachment in the first few hours after birth, and when continuing assessments during home visits after discharge. As the nurse assesses attachment, it is important to remember that cultural values, beliefs, and practices will direct child care activities and self-care practices. For example, traditionally religious-observant Jewish families may not name their newborns until the eighth day following birth at the circumcision ceremony known as the *brit* or *bris milah* (Noble, Rom, Newsome-Wicks, et al., 2009). Nurses should respect cultural norms and incorporate them into the care of the newborn whenever possible. Chapter 35 ∞ discusses this and other cultural practices in the postpartum period.

HEALTH PROMOTION EDUCATION

Some parents, especially first-time parents, may feel awkward in their new role. It is helpful for the nurse to advise parents that they may experience feelings of uncertainty as they grow into the parental role and alter their family processes to accommodate the new family member. The nurse should also provide reassurance and advise new parents of normal infant behavior and activity. The nurse assesses attachment before discharge. If the nurse identifies a possible alteration in attachment, the parents can be referred to a new parent support group, parenting classes, or counseling to assist them with their transition into their new roles. The nurse can explain that new attachments are being formed, and like all new relationships, both the infant and the parents are discovering each other. The nurse should discuss possible risk factors of altered attachment such as inability or lack of desire to care for the infant.

Nursing Care Following Cesarean Birth

Approximately 31.1% of women delivered by cesarean section in the United States in 2006; this represented a 50% increase since 1996 (Menacker & Martin, 2009). Nurses need to be adept at addressing the special needs of this growing population of patients. After a cesarean birth, the new mother has postpartal needs similar to those of women who gave birth vaginally. Because she has undergone major abdominal surgery, however, the woman also has nursing care needs similar to those of other surgical patients.

Care Plan Activity: Postpartum Care Following Cesarean Birth

Promotion of Maternal Physical Well-Being After Cesarean Birth

Care of the patient following cesarean delivery is similar to the care of patients who deliver vaginally, but also includes consideration of the postoperative condition. Nursing interventions will focus on promotion of maternal comfort, promotion of maternal and newborn safety, and prevention of postoperative complications. The nurse will monitor neurologic and neuromuscular status closely until effects of anesthesia have worn off. Routine postpartum assessments will include inspection of the dressing or incision for intactness and signs of complications or infection, as well as increased attention to lung sounds, gastrointestinal status, and genitourinary status.

Immobility after the use of narcotic and sedative agents and alterations in the immune response of postoperative patients increase the chances of pulmonary infection. For this reason, the woman is encouraged to cough and breathe deeply and to use incentive spirometry every 2 to 4 hours while awake for the first few days following cesarean birth.

Immobility increases the risk of abdominal distention and discomfort, deep vein thrombosis, and pulmonary embolism. The patient may wear sequential compression devices (SCDs) until she is ambulating. Within the first 12 hours postoperatively, unless medically contraindicated, the woman should be assisted to dangle her legs on the side of the bed. Once she is awake, alert, and has complete sensation and strength in her lower extremities, the woman should be assisted out of bed. Ambulation should begin no later than 24 hours postoperatively and should be encouraged at least two to three times a day.

The nurse continues to assess the woman's pain level and provide relief measures as needed. Sources of pain include incisional pain, gas pain, referred shoulder pain, periodic uterine contractions (afterpains), and pain associated with voiding, defecation, or constipation.

Nursing interventions are oriented toward preventing or alleviating pain or helping the woman cope with pain. The nurse should undertake the following measures:

- Administer analgesic medications as needed and ordered, especially during the first 24 to 72 hours. Their use will relieve the woman's pain and enable her to be more mobile and active.
- Promote comfort through proper positioning, backrubs, oral care, and the reduction of noxious stimuli, such as noise and unpleasant odors.
- Encourage the presence of the significant other and the newborn. This may provide distraction from the painful sensations and help reduce the woman's fear and anxiety. The presence of a significant other provides a watchful presence over the newborn, allowing the baby to stay in the room with the mother while she may not be alert or comfortable enough to be responsible for the newborn if left alone.
- Encourage the use of breathing, relaxation, and distraction techniques (for example, stimulation of cutaneous tissue) taught in childbirth preparation class.

- Instruct the woman to splint her incision with a pillow when changing positions, coughing, deep breathing, or sneezing.
- Encourage adequate rest periods. This may include limiting excessive visitors and phone calls.
- Encourage early ambulation to prevent abdominal distention that can occur with excess accumulation of gas in the intestines.
- Allow the woman to begin judiciously consuming food and fluids as desired when awake and alert. Although many institutions still withhold oral intake until bowel sounds return, a Cochrane review found no evidence to support this practice. Women experience fewer gastrointestinal complications and discomforts following cesarean when allowed to advance their own diet (Mangesi & Hofmeyr, 2005).

Neuraxial analgesia administered just after the cesarean birth is an effective method of pain relief for most women in the first 24 hours following birth (see Drug Guide: Postpartum Neuraxial Morphine).

The physician may prescribe **patient-controlled analgesia (PCA)**. With this approach, the woman is given a bolus of analgesia, often morphine, at the beginning of therapy. Using a special intravenous (IV) pump system, the woman presses a button to self-administer small doses of the medication as needed. For safety, the pump is preset with a time lockout so that the pump cannot deliver another dose until a specified time has elapsed. Women using PCA feel less anxious and have a greater sense of control with less dependence on the nursing staff. The frequent smaller doses help the woman experience rapid pain relief without grogginess and also eliminate the discomfort of injections. As with any drug therapy, the nurse will monitor the patient for side effects and intervene as necessary.

If general anesthesia was used, abdominal distention from the accumulation of gas in the intestines may produce discomfort for the woman during the first postpartum days. Additional measures to prevent or minimize gas pains include leg exercises, abdominal tightening, avoiding carbonated or very hot or cold beverages, and avoiding the use of straws. The woman may find it helpful to lie prone or on her left side. Lying on the left side allows gas to rise from the descending colon to the sigmoid colon so that it can be expelled more readily. Other women report that a rocking chair helps them obtain relief. Medical interventions for gas pain include the use of antiflatulents (such as Mylicon), suppositories, and enemas.

The nurse can minimize discomfort and promote satisfaction as the mother assumes the activities of her new role. Instruction and assistance in assuming comfortable positions when holding or breastfeeding the infant will do much to increase the mother's sense of competence and comfort. Sitting in a chair or tailor fashion in bed, leaning slightly forward with the infant propped on a pillow in her lap, will prevent irritation to the incision. Use of the football hold and side-lying positions may be most comfortable for breastfeeding during the initial postoperative course.

By the first or second day after the cesarean birth, the mother is usually receptive to learning how to care for herself and her infant. Demonstration of proper body mechanics in getting out of bed without the use of a side rail and ways of caring for the infant that prevent strain and torsion on the incision are also indicated. The nurse needs to place special emphasis on home management, encouraging the woman to let others assume responsibility for housekeeping and cooking. Fatigue not only prolongs recovery but also interferes with breastfeeding and mother-infant interaction.

The woman usually does extremely well postoperatively. If neuraxial anesthesia was used, the side effects of general anesthesia are absent. Even after general anesthesia, however, most women are ambulating by the day after the surgery. Usually the woman can shower by the first or second postpartal day, which seems to provide a mental as well as physical lift. The incision can be covered with plastic if the dressing is still in place. If staples have been used, the incision is sometimes left open to the air, and showering is permitted without covering it. Most women are discharged on the second or third postoperative day.

Women with cesarean births have several special needs following discharge: increased need for rest and sleep; incisional care; assistance with household chores, infant care, and self-care; and relief of pain and discomfort. Nurses need to address these areas during hospitalization and discharge planning. Perhaps one of the most important considerations for cesarean birth mothers is the need to plan for additional assistance at home to enable the new mother to rest and heal.

HEALTH PROMOTION EDUCATION

The nurse can assist the woman in identifying interventions to relieve discomfort or pain. The woman should be encouraged to take pain medication regularly, engage in frequent rest periods, avoid prolonged activity, and observe for signs of "overdoing it" (such as discomfort and fatigue). The nurse should advise the woman that recovery after a surgical procedure involves healing time and that fatigue and soreness are common symptoms of too much activity too quickly. The nurse can assist the family in identifying resources for assisting the new mother at home, such as assistance from friends and family, cleaning services, or food delivery services.

Promotion of Parent-Infant Interaction After Cesarean Birth

Many factors associated with cesarean birth may hinder successful and frequent maternal-infant interaction. These include the physical condition of the mother and newborn and maternal reactions to stress, anesthesia, and medications. The mother and her infant may be separated after birth because of hospital routines, prematurity, or neonatal complications. A healthy infant born by an uncomplicated cesarean birth is no more fragile than an infant born vaginally. Many agencies are beginning to provide time for the family together in the operating room if the mother's and infant's conditions permit. As noted earlier in the chapter, if skin-to-skin contact (SSC) with the mother is not possible immediately following cesarean delivery of a healthy newborn, the nurses should offer SSC with the father.

Signs of depression, anger, or withdrawal in the mother following cesarean birth may indicate a grief response to the loss

DRUG GUIDE Postpartum Neuraxial Morphine

OVERVIEW OF OBSTETRIC ACTION

Neuraxial administration (epidural or intrathecal) of morphine is used to provide relief of pain associated with cesarean births, extensive episiotomies, or third- and fourth-degree lacerations. Morphine binds to opiate receptors in the central nervous system, thereby altering both the perception of and emotional response to pain. Women experience little or no discomfort or pain during recovery and for up to 24 hours following epidural or intrathecal administration of morphine. This may be extended to 48 hours with the use of EREM (Depodur™), a sustained-release formulation. There is no motor or sympathetic block. Onset of analgesia is slower than with fentanyl, but duration is longer.

ROUTE, DOSAGE, AND FREQUENCY

Morphine (preservative-free formulation) is administered intrathecally or epidurally by the anesthesia provider. Dosages up to 200 μg intrathecal morphine, 5 mg epidural morphine, or 10 mg epidural EREM may be given. Larger doses increase the side effects without extending the length of analgesia. According to Carvalho (2008), "intrathecal doses of morphine >100 μg to 200 μg and epidural doses > 2 to 4 mg are unnecessary" for cesarean delivery (p. 958). If a subsequent dose is required, the anesthesia provider, not the nurse, administers it.

MATERNAL CONTRAINDICATIONS

Allergy/hypersensitivity to morphine.

MATERNAL SIDE EFFECTS

Most common: confusion, sedation, constipation, hypotension, pruritus, urinary retention, nausea, and vomiting.

Early-onset respiratory depression (30 to 90 minutes after administration) and late-onset respiratory depression (6 to 18 hours after administration) are rare in young, healthy obstetric patients, but can result in irreversible neurologic injury or death. Women who are obese, concurrently receiving magnesium sulfate, or who have obstructive sleep apnea are at increased risk for respiratory depression. Respiratory depression is managed by administration of Naloxone (Narcan), mask ventilation, and endotracheal intubation with mechanical ventilation if necessary.

NURSING CONSIDERATIONS

- Obtain history: sensitivity (allergy) to morphine.
- Assess vital signs, orientation, level of consciousness, motor function, sensation, reflexes, skin color, breath sounds, depth and rate of respirations, catheter insertion site, and ability to void (unless Foley in place). Notify anesthesia provider of abnormal assessments or complications.
- Monitor and evaluate analgesic effect. Ask patient about comfort level and notify anesthesia provider of inadequate pain relief.
- Check catheter (if still present) to ensure it is intact and not leaking.
- Assess for pruritus (scratching and rubbing, especially around face and neck).
- Administer comfort measures for narcotic-induced pruritus, such as lotion, backrubs, cool or warm packs, or diversional activities. Administer prescribed medications prn.
- If allergic reaction (urticaria, edema, or respiratory difficulties) occurs, administer naloxone or diphenhydramine per provider standing order. Have drugs immediately available.
- Provide comfort measures for nausea or vomiting, such as frequent oral hygiene or gradual increase of activity; administer prescribed prn medications as needed.
- Assess level of consciousness, lower extremity sensation and strength, postural blood pressure, and heart rate before ambulation.
- Assist patient with her first ambulation and then prn.
- Provide assistance and supervision with newborn care.
- According to guidelines approved by the American Society of Anesthesiologists in 2007, respiratory status should be assessed at least hourly for the first 12 hours and at least every other hour for the second 12 hours (12 to 24 hours) following a single administration of neuraxial morphine. Respiratory status should be assessed for 48 hours following administration of EREM. Patients receiving continuous morphine should be assessed for the duration of administration. Pulse oximetry and apnea monitors are sometimes employed as adjuncts to assessment, but they cannot take the place of a thorough nursing assessment. Pulse oximetry is not sensitive to hypercarbia, and neither tool is sensitive to hypoventilation (Carvalho, 2008).
- Assess bladder for distention if unable to void. Assist patient to void. Catheterization may be necessary if unresolved.
- Inform patient that headaches related to epidurals are uncommon, but occasionally occur 2 to 5 days after administration. Bed rest in a quiet dark room, caffeine, and hydration may help. Call anesthesia provider as needed. Blood patch can be administered by anesthesia if unresolved.

Sources: Carvalho, 2008; Deglin & Vallerand, 2009.

of the fantasized vaginal birth experience. Fathers as well as mothers may experience feelings of "missing out," guilt that the surgery was the result of something they did "wrong," and even jealousy toward another couple who had a vaginal birth. The couple may also feel guilty that they are considering their personal needs and not simply the welfare of the infant.

Newborn Safety Following Cesarean Birth

One of the primary concerns regarding the nursing care of the couplet is the promotion of safety. Mothers who have experienced cesareans, particularly unanticipated ones that follow lengthy labors, may be fatigued, sleep deprived, and under the influence of medications that alter their level of consciousness. Vigilant attention must be paid to the mother's level of consciousness and ability to stay awake when holding her infant, providing care, and breastfeeding. Some mothers will require constant support and observation to complete these activities safely, particularly if the father is sleep deprived as well. Nursing units should have risk management guidelines in place to assist nurses in their assessment and support of these vulnerable patients.

CLINICAL TIP

A thorough nursing assessment of respiratory status includes rate, depth, and regularity of respirations; lung sounds; level of consciousness; and color of skin and mucous membranes. The nurse should be sensitive to subtle changes in level of consciousness, including mild anxiety or agitation, which may be early signs of hypoxia. Changes in the mental status of postpartum patients, however, require astute assessment and critical thinking skills on the part of the nurse in order to differentiate physiologic etiologies from possible postpartum psychosis.

The nurse can support the parents in a variety of ways. Initially, nurses must work through their own feelings about cesarean birth. The nurse who considers a vaginal birth "normal" and refers to it as such implies that a cesarean birth is "abnormal," rather than simply an alternative method. Thus language and terminology, though seemingly insignificant, can convey to the couple negative messages about their cesarean birth experience.

The nurse should offer positive support to the couple. They may need the opportunity to tell their story repeatedly to work through their feelings. The nurse can provide factual information about their situation and support the couple's effective coping behaviors. The nurse should provide the parents with choices by allowing them to participate in decision making about the options available to them.

The presence of the father or significant other during the birth process positively influences the woman's perception of the birth event. His or her presence not only reduces the woman's fears but also enhances her sense of control and enables the couple to share feelings and respond to one another with touch and eye contact. Later they have the opportunity to relive the experience and fill in any gaps or missing pieces. This is especially valuable if the mother has had general anesthesia. The father or significant other can take pictures, hold the baby, and foster the discovery process by directing the mother's attention to details about her newborn.

The perception of and reactions to a cesarean birth experience depend on how the woman defines that experience. Her reality is what she perceives it to be. If the woman's attitude is more positive than negative, successful resolution of subsequent stressful events is more likely. Because the definition of events is transitory in nature, the possibility of change and growth is present. Often the mothering role is perceived as an extension of the childbearing role, and inability to fulfill expected childbearing behavior (vaginal birth) might lead to parental feelings of failure and frustration. The nurse can help families alter their negative definitions of cesarean birth and encourage positive perceptions.

HEALTH PROMOTION EDUCATION

The nurse should advise the mother that she is able to hold, cuddle, lift, and feed her infant despite her surgical incision. The nurse can assist the woman in finding positions that are comfortable for holding and feeding the baby. Upon discharge, the woman should be encouraged to care for the infant and to allow family members or friends to assist with other household duties.

Nursing Care of the Obese Postpartum Patient

Obesity is increasing in the United States, and the postpartum nurse will care for a growing number of obese and morbidly obese patients. The obese patient has needs similar to all postpartum patients, but she needs special attention to prevent injury, respiratory complications, thromboembolic disease, and infection, for which she is at high risk.

The nurse should carefully assess the woman for airway obstruction and hypoxia, particularly if she received opioids. Ambulation should be encouraged as soon as possible to prevent pneumonia. The use of sequential compression devices (SCDs) and early ambulation are essential to the prevention of deep vein thrombosis, especially if the patient had a cesarean birth. If mechanical vacuum devices are used to facilitate drainage from her incision following a cesarean birth, the patient should be educated about them. The mother should demonstrate how to visualize, clean, and completely dry her incision prior to discharge. The use of a mirror may be helpful. She needs to recognize and report signs of infection or dehiscence of her surgical incision or episiotomy repair promptly.

The obese patient has special safety concerns. The nurse needs to utilize adequate personnel and appropriate assistive devices to maintain safety for both the patient and staff members during position changes, transport, and ambulation. Additionally, the new mother may need extra supervision and assistance when breastfeeding her baby to ensure newborn safety.

In addition to the health and safety risks, obese women sometimes experience prejudice and humiliation when in the healthcare setting. The nurse needs to be sensitive to special needs in order to promote the woman's dignity. Advance communication and coordination that ensures the woman will have the correct-sized bed, blood pressure cuff, transport equipment, gown, and assistive equipment for ambulation is essential to efficient, compassionate, and respectful patient-centered nursing care (Mahlmeister, 2007).

TEACHING FOR SELF-CARE The nurse should advise the mother to ambulate as early as possible to avoid medical complications. The mother is taught symptoms of infection and should report these symptoms immediately to her healthcare provider.

Nursing Care of the Postpartum Adolescent

The postpartum nurse will provide care for adolescent mothers, some of whom are very young. Following a 14-year decline, the birthrate for teenage women increased in 2006 to 41.9 births per 1000 females ages 15 to 19, resulting in a total of 435,436 births to women in this age group; in 2008 the rate for this age group was 41.5 births per 1000. The birthrate in females ages 10 to 14 continued to decline to a rate of 0.6 births per 1000 women (Martin et al., 2009). The transition to motherhood can be stressful for adult women. Teen mothers have fewer life experiences, and fewer social, educational, and financial resources to help with the transition than do older mothers. Their newborns are also more likely to suffer from low birth weight, preterm birth, and death in infancy than those born to adult women (Martin et al., 2009). Additional teaching, support, referrals, and follow-up may be required, particularly if the young woman has delivered a baby with special concerns due to prematurity or low birth weight.

Adolescent mothers have the same basic physical care needs as older mothers. They usually recover without difficulty, as they are young and healthy. Some adolescents, however, may not have a working knowledge of their own anatomy and physiology or the related terminology, and they may require special assistance with postpartum hygiene and care. Some may never have had a gynecologic exam prior to pregnancy, and they may feel embarrassed by the experience of being examined by a variety of healthcare professionals. A hospital filled with healthcare workers may be intimidating to them as well. The nurse should be sensitive to the patient's needs and ensure that she understands the reason for assessments, demonstrates appropriate self- and newborn care, and feels comfortable to ask questions. The nurse should offer detailed teaching on contraception, as the young woman may have no prior experience with it and may not feel comfortable requesting this information.

The nurse-patient relationship is extremely important when working with an adolescent mother. The nurse should maintain a respectful, nonjudgmental attitude and listen to the patient to learn of individual needs. The nurse must also assess the development and cognitive level of the adolescent in order to communicate effectively and to provide patient-centered care for the young woman (King-Jones, 2008). Peterson, Sword, Charles, et al. (2007) discovered that adolescent mothers valued nursing care that was "friendly, patient, respectful, and understanding of the mothers' individual needs" (p. 204). The young women appreciated nurses who anticipated their needs, respected them as mothers, and talked to them in the same manner used when working with older mothers. They perceived encounters during which the nurse appeared rushed, too serious, judgmental, or not to understand their needs as unsatisfactory. Nurse-patient relationships that made them feel "at ease" (p. 210) and encouraged their participation were highly valued.

Working with the adolescent mother and her family requires sensitivity on the nurse's part. Adolescent mothers still trying to meet their own educational goals rely on the support of their husband or boyfriend, their own parents, teachers, childcare providers, and school nurses. They need support people to talk to, ask questions of, assist with childcare, provide financial support, and offer unconditional support to them and their children. Although each situation is different, adolescent mothers most often rely on their husbands or boyfriends and their own mothers to help with raising their children (Brosh, Weigel, & Evans, 2007). The nurse should work with the family whenever possible to promote healthy and positive interactions during the postpartal period.

The nurse has many opportunities for teaching adolescent parents about their newborn in the postpartum unit, and serves as a role model for new parents when responding to and caring for the newborn. The father, if he is involved, should be included as much as possible. Although the grandmother or another family member may plan to assist with or provide much of the newborn care in some cases, the nurse should always ensure that the adolescent mother has the knowledge and demonstrates the skills to provide care for her newborn before discharge. The young mother appreciates positive feedback about her newborn and her developing maternal responses. This praise and encouragement will increase her confidence and self-esteem.

A newborn physical examination performed at the bedside gives the parent(s) immediate feedback about the newborn's health and demonstrates methods of handling an infant. The nurse can teach as the examination progresses, giving the new mother information about the fontanelles, cradle cap, shampooing the newborn's hair, and so on. The nurse might also use this time to teach the young parent(s) about infant stimulation techniques. Because adolescents tend to concentrate their interactions in the physical domain, they need to comprehend the importance of verbal, visual, and auditory stimulation for newborns as well.

Performing an examination at the bedside also gives the adolescent permission to explore her baby, which she may have been hesitant to do. A Brazelton neonatal assessment (see chapter 30 ∞) will help the mother understand the newborn's response to stimuli, a key factor in the adolescent's response to the individuality of her newborn once she goes home. Parents who have some idea of what to expect from their infants will be less frustrated with the newborn's behavior.

Group classes for adolescent mothers should include infant care skills, information about growth and development, infant feeding, well-baby care, and danger signals in the ill newborn. If classes are offered in the hospital during the postpartum stay, the adolescent mother and father should be strongly encouraged to attend and participate. The nurse can correct misconceptions and unrealistic expectations about growth and development.

During the postpartum period, the adolescent may have special needs, depending on her level of maturity, support systems, and cultural background. Brosh, Weigel, & Evans (2007) found that adolescent mothers reported difficulty accessing services to which they were entitled from some public and community agencies. The nurse should inform teenage mothers of available options and assist them to begin navigating service agencies prior to discharge whenever possible.

Ideally, teenage mothers should visit adolescent clinics where mother and baby are assessed for several years after birth. School systems' classes for young mothers help adolescents finish school and learn how to parent at the same time. Support groups and programs should address the issues discussed above and meet at a time and place that is welcoming and allows the mother and father to attend together. Although the teen mother may already attend or have a plan to attend a local program accessed during the prenatal period, the postpartum nurse should be aware of local programs and support groups offered through schools and healthcare organizations and make referrals as needed.

In the event that a woman decides to keep an unwanted child, the nurse should be aware of the potential for parenting problems. Families with unwanted children are more prone to crisis than others, although in many cases parents grow to love their child after attachment occurs. The nurse should be ready to initiate crisis management strategies or make appropriate referrals as the need arises. Assessment and follow-up by social workers should be coordinated before discharge.

Nursing Care of the Woman Who Relinquishes Her Infant

A **relinquishing mother** is one who chooses an adoption plan for her newborn. It is difficult to determine how many mothers pursue this option each year, as information regarding the characteristics of children adopted independently or through private agencies is not always available (National Center for State Courts, 2009). It was estimated that more than 52,000 women in the United States pursued an adoption plan at the beginning of the 21st century (Kobokovich, as cited in Smith, 2008).

The reasons for relinquishment vary. Although relinquishing mothers were traditionally young and single, 38.5% of births in 2006 were to unmarried women (Martin et al., 2009). Single parenthood is no longer stigmatized to the extent it was in the past, although some single mothers still pursue adoption for their newborns. Some relinquishing mothers are living in poverty or simply unable to care for another child, whereas others do not have the desire or emotional maturity to be mothers. The decision not to parent the newborn may also involve complicated psychosocial issues such as rape, incest, conception outside the woman's current intimate relationship, domestic violence, or the threat of abandonment by her intimate partner or family if the mother keeps the child. The reasons are personal and complex, and the mother may or may not choose to share her decision process with the nurse. The nurse can support the mother by encouraging her to share her feelings, by listening actively, and by simply being there for her.

There are multiple avenues through which adoption occurs, including private independent agreements, private agencies, and public agencies. Adoptions may be considered open, semi-open, or closed. In an identified adoption, the birthparents select the adoptive parents (Smith, 2008). If a relationship already exists, both sets of parents may be present for the delivery and throughout the immediate postpartum period. The nurse may work with the birthmother, the birthfather, the parents planning to adopt the child, social workers, adoption agency personnel, or attorneys when caring for the relinquishing mother and her newborn. This is a potential source of anxiety for the nurse, particularly if controversies occur between the parties or if situations with which the nurse is unfamiliar arise. Birthing units should have policies and resources available to guide the care of relinquishing mothers, and nurses should consult with social workers or other support personnel if they are uncertain how to proceed in given situations.

The nurse's primary responsibility is to provide compassionate patient-centered care that supports the birthmother's adoption plan and promotes a positive experience for her (Smith, 2008). The nurse should make certain that the plan is understood and communicated to other staff members. If no support person is present, the nurse acts as the primary support person and ensures that the woman has a clear understanding of all that occurs. Following delivery, the woman should be given the choice to remain on a childbearing unit or to move to a different inpatient unit. The amount of contact she chooses to have with her newborn should be respected. When the birthfather and/or prospective adoptive parents are present, the nurse will need to take cues from the birthmother as to how to best provide support for all. Nurses should have a familiarity with the rights of birthfathers within their state and provide support to the father whenever possible as well.

Respectful communication that involves choosing words thoughtfully and accurately is important when caring for women who choose adoption for their newborns. The National Council for Adoption (2008) recommended use of the phrases "choosing an adoption plan" or "finding a family to parent your child" rather than terms such as "giving away," "giving up your child," or "putting your child up for adoption."

Finally, the nurse needs to acknowledge the significance of the birthmother's experience. Aloi (2009) noted, "The birthmother experience has been unheard and unacknowledged by the healthcare delivery system and by society, as well, even though the effects are lifelong and profound" (p. 27). It is essential that the nurse acknowledges the woman's loss and supports her decision. Although a thorough discussion of grief and loss is beyond the scope of this section, perinatal nurses should be aware that relinquishing mothers are at risk for *disenfranchised grief*, in which they are unable to proceed through the grieving process and come to resolution with the loss (Robinson, as cited in Aloi, 2009, p. 28). The nurse can support the relinquishing mother by acknowledging her relationship with the newborn, validating her loss, offering her the opportunity to hold and spend time with the baby to create memories, and giving her time to say goodbye (Aloi, 2009).

The woman should be referred to a support group following discharge, as participation is helpful for many women. Charitable and religious organizations that assist birthmothers with the experience of adoption often provide support to these mothers throughout the prenatal and postpartum experience. If she is not already connected in this way, the mother may benefit from a referral to an organization, a therapist, or clergy member if she desires additional support beyond what she expects to receive from family and friends. For additional information, see chapter 38 ∞ regarding nursing care of parents experiencing grief and loss.

PROFESSIONALISM IN PRACTICE

Patient-Centered Care of the Relinquishing Mother

A relinquishing mother who receives only physical care, while providers fail to acknowledge or address her emotional needs, is denied her right to quality, patient-centered nursing care. It is essential for nurses to use active listening, provide nonjudgmental support, show concern and compassion, and personalize care for the relinquishing mother. When the mother is admitted to the birthing unit, the staff should be informed about her decision to relinquish the infant. Any special requests regarding the birth should be respected, and the woman should be encouraged to express her emotions. Birthfathers are often forgotten in this process, and they should be included and supported whenever possible and acceptable to the birthmother. This demonstrates the Quality and Safety Education in Nursing (QSEN) competency of patient-centered care.

Nursing Care of the Lesbian Mother

Although the literature regarding gay and lesbian families is growing, much of it is focused on options for conception, challenges experienced by gay parents, and legal issues. There has been little published about the labor, delivery, and postpartum experiences of lesbian mothers. A qualitative study of lesbian couples in Norway discovered that they were generally happy with the perinatal care they received. They felt somewhat vulnerable in their visibility as lesbian parents, and they took responsibility to be open about their sexuality without being overly assertive when first meeting their healthcare provider(s). The women noted that most providers became more confident while interacting with them over time. When faced with rude or uncaring behaviors, the women sometimes thought it may be related to their sexuality, but acknowledged that perhaps the provider behaved in that way to everyone. The women appreciated healthcare professionals who were warm, respectful, and accepting (Spidsberg, 2007). The women's desire to be treated as any other mothers, with acknowledgment of their intimate relationships, echoed the findings of Wilton and Kaufmann (2001) in the United Kingdom. A review of the literature did not find similar recent studies in the United States, and further research is needed to meet the needs of these mothers.

The nurse should maintain an attitude that is respectful, caring, and open to sexual diversity when working with all patients. Providing quality patient-centered care for any postpartum woman involves acknowledging, welcoming, and involving her intimate partner in care and decision-making. If the nurse has not cared for a postpartum lesbian mother before, it may be helpful to admit this to the patient and to ask her for guidance regarding any special needs or requests that she or her partner may have. The nurse should be aware that standardized postpartum instructions, particularly those related to intercourse and contraception, might need to be individualized and amended.

Nursing Care of the Developmentally Disabled Postpartum Mother

The postpartum time period is one of great growth in the maternal mothering role. New mothers are faced with various challenges and different learning opportunities. Women with developmental or intellectual disabilities are at particular risk during this time period. Material should be presented to them in an easy-to-understand format. Peer mentors are often helpful role models for these women. Teaching should be performed at a level that is achievable for the individual woman. A needs assessment should be performed to determine what needs the mother and new family may have. Community and private resources should be available to make the transition to the postpartum period as flawless as possible.

> **PROFESSIONALISM IN PRACTICE**
>
> ***Caring for a Complex Patient Population***
>
> Nursing students will work with a variety of patients in the postpartum setting, including women at the far ends of the childbearing age spectrum; women across the socioeconomic spectrum; women who abuse substances; women who have experienced a variety of assistive reproductive techniques; women who will return to prison after childbirth; women with a history of trauma, domestic violence, or abuse; and women who are homeless or otherwise disenfranchised. This responsibility may initially be overwhelming to students, particularly as they worry about the future of the woman and/or her newborn. It may also be difficult for students to imagine a professional lifetime of caring for such a complex patient population. Post-conference conversations with faculty members, peers, and staff nurses, if possible, are the appropriate time to discuss such concerns. There are no easy answers, but it is helpful to view problematic issues within the context of guiding principles such as the American Nurses Association (ANA) (2005) Code of Ethics for Nurses, the Association of Women's Health, Obstetric, and Neonatal Nurses (AWHONN) (2009) Standards for Professional Nursing Practice in the Care of Women and Newborns, and the mission of the university, hospital, or nursing school.

Nursing Care of the Mother with a History of Sexual Abuse

Women who have been previously sexually abused tend to have more anxiety and stress related to hospital procedures, interactions with unfamiliar staff, and being touched in general. The postpartum woman who has a history of sexual abuse may have difficulty establishing trust and may feel uncomfortable when private information or demonstrations are being performed. The nurse should treat the woman with respect by providing draping whenever possible. Speaking to the woman in private protects her fragile emotions from being observed by others. Support groups may offer the mother with a history of sexual abuse a safe haven to share her experiences and the impact it has on her mothering.

Discharge Information

Healthy postpartum women and newborns are frequently discharged within 24 to 48 hours of delivery, before many of their important healthcare and educational needs have been addressed. These include establishing breastfeeding, ruling out infections, supporting infant-family bonding, and patient teaching. Home health services are increasingly being recognized as a cost-effective means of meeting the postbirth needs of mothers and newborns. Home care of the postpartum family is the subject of chapter 37 ∞.

CLINICAL JUDGMENT

Case Study: Dana Sullivan

You walk into her room and find Dana Sullivan, a 29-year-old G2P2, crying 48 hours after a repeat cesarean birth. She states "I'm not ready to go home. With my first baby they made me go home after 2 days. Can they make me go home so early again?"

Critical Thinking

What therapeutic nursing questions would you ask Dana to assess her reluctance to go home?

See www.nursing.pearsonhighered.com for possible responses.

Ideally, preparation for discharge begins the moment a woman initially enters the healthcare system for prenatal care. Nursing efforts should be directed toward assessing the couple's knowledge, expectations, and beliefs, and then providing anticipatory guidance and teaching accordingly (see Table 36-1). Because teaching is one of the primary responsibilities of the postpartum nurse, many agencies have elaborate teaching programs and classes. Before the actual discharge, however, the nurse should spend private time with the woman (or couple) to determine whether they have any last-minute questions (Figure 36-3 ■). In general, discharge teaching should include at least the following:

1. The woman should contact her caregiver if she develops any of the signs of possible complications:
   a. Sudden, persistent, or spiking fever (greater than 100.4°F) or chills
   b. Change in the character of the lochia—foul smell, return to bright red bleeding, excessive amount (more than one pad per hour after 24 hours)
   c. Evidence of mastitis, such as breast tenderness, reddened areas, malaise, fever, chills
   d. Evidence of thrombophlebitis, such as calf pain, tenderness, redness, or pain with walking
   e. Evidence of urinary tract infection, such as urgency, frequency, burning on urination
   f. Evidence of infection in an incision (either episiotomy or cesarean), such as redness, edema, pain or discomfort, discharge, or lack of approximation
   g. Continued mood changes or signs of postpartum depression, inability to care for self or baby, feelings of self-harm, or anxiety
   h. Severe pelvic pain or abdominal tenderness
2. The woman should review the literature she has received that explains recommended postpartum exercises, the need for adequate rest, the need to avoid overexertion initially, and the recommendation to abstain from sexual intercourse until lochia has ceased. The woman may take a shower and may continue sitz baths at home if she desires.
3. The woman should be given the phone numbers of the postpartum unit, lactation consultant, and nursery, and should be encouraged to call if she has any questions.
4. The woman should receive information on local agencies or support groups, such as La Leche League and Mothers of Twins, which might be of particular assistance to her.
5. Both breastfeeding and formula-feeding mothers should receive information geared to their specific nutritional needs. They should also be told to continue their vitamin and iron supplements until their postpartal examination.
6. The woman should have a scheduled appointment for her postpartal examination and for her infant's first well-baby examination before they are discharged.
7. The mother should clearly understand the correct procedure for obtaining copies of her infant's birth certificate.
8. The new parents should be able to provide home care for their infant and should know when to anticipate that the cord will fall off, when the infant will need his or her immunizations, and so on. They should also be comfortable feeding and handling the baby and should be aware of basic safety considerations, including the need to use a car seat whenever the infant is in a car, sudden infant death syndrome (SIDS) prevention, and prevention of shaken baby injuries. These topics are covered in chapter 37 ∞.
9. The parents should be aware of signs and symptoms in the infant that indicate possible problems and whom they should contact about them.

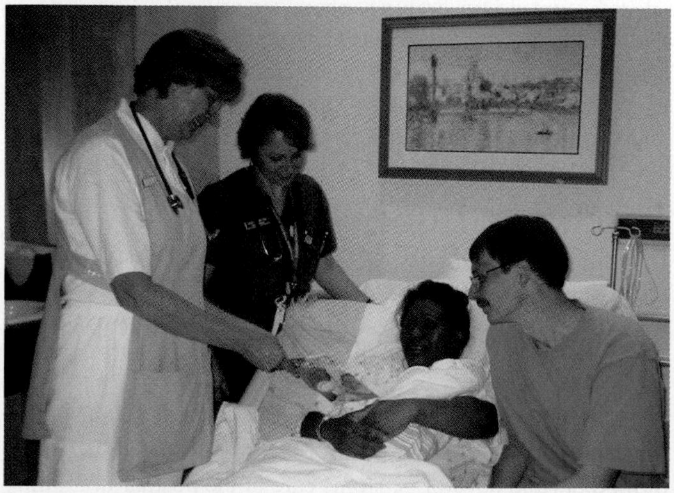

Figure 36-3 ■ The nurse provides discharge instructions to the mother and father before discharge.

The nurse can use this final period to reassure the couple of their ability to be successful parents, stressing the infant's need to feel loved and secure. The nurse can also urge parents to talk to each other and work together to solve any problems that may arise.

The nurse addresses follow-up visits when appropriate. If not already discussed, teaching about family planning is appropriate at this time, and the nurse can provide information regarding contraception.

In ideal situations, a family approach involving the father or significant other, infant, and possibly other siblings would permit a total evaluation and provide an opportunity for all family members to ask questions and express concerns. In addition, a family approach can enable the nurse to identify disturbed family patterns more readily and initiate interventions to prevent future problems of neglect or abuse.

Evaluation of the Postpartum Family

Anticipated outcomes of comprehensive nursing care of the postpartum family include the following:

- The mother and infant remain healthy, safe, and free of injury or complications.
- The mother verbalizes comfort and uses self-comfort measures as appropriate.
- The mother verbalizes feelings and concerns related to the birth event and her newborn.
- The mother performs appropriate self-care measures.
- The new parents demonstrate safe and effective care of their baby.
- The parents and newborn display positive bonding behaviors.
- The mother-infant dyad demonstrates successful breastfeeding (or parents describe safe formula preparation and demonstrate safe bottle-feeding). Mothers describe breast care as appropriate.
- The mother is rested and verbalizes understanding of the importance of gradual return to activities.
- The mother identifies sources of support to assist with newborn care and family responsibilities.
- The mother states plan for follow-up health care for herself and her infant.
- The mother identifies signs and symptoms of maternal-newborn complications and reasons to seek care before routine follow-up visits.
- The cesarean birth mother states in her own words the reason for the cesarean birth and verbalizes feelings.
- The cesarean birth mother verbalizes comfort and maintains mobility.
- The obese patient remains free of injury or complications.
- The adolescent mother has been supported physically and emotionally.
- The woman relinquishing her newborn verbalizes the rationale for her decision and demonstrates acceptance of her decision.
- All women and their significant others have been supported with regards to their cultures (may include special considerations related to age, sexual preference, ethnic background), their abilities, and their histories.
- In summary, all components of nursing care are designed to achieve the desired outcomes identified for the woman and her family.

[redacted]

FOCUS YOUR STUDY

- Effective parent learning requires precise timing of teaching, as well as choice of a teaching method that is effective for the family, such as videotapes, return-demonstration, and so on. Content on self-care, infant care, and anticipatory guidance is important.
- Postpartum discomfort may be due to a variety of factors, including an edematous perineum, an episiotomy or extension, engorged hemorrhoids, hematoma formation, afterpains, immobility, diaphoresis, sore nipples, or engorged breasts. Various self-care approaches are helpful in promoting comfort. Cultural values are incorporated in providing care to the new family.
- Lactation occurs in response to breast stimulation. Nursing support is essential to effective breastfeeding.
- A variety of techniques may be helpful to relieve discomfort during suppression of lactation if breastfeeding is not planned.
- The first day or two following birth are marked by maternal behaviors that are more dependent and oriented to the woman's comfort. Thereafter the woman becomes more independent and ready to assume responsibility.
- The new mother requires opportunities to discuss her childbirth experience with an empathetic listener.
- Maternal rest is promoted by advising the woman to take frequent rest periods, nap when the baby is napping, avoid unnecessary activities, and use her social support system. Ambulation and activity should be resumed gradually.

- Rooming-in provides the childbearing family with opportunities to interact with their newborn during the first hours and days of life. This enables the family to develop some confidence and skill in a "safe" environment.
- Sexual intercourse may resume once the episiotomy has healed and lochia has stopped. Couples should be forewarned of possible changes; for example, the vagina may be "dry," fatigue may inhibit the level of desire, or the woman's breasts may leak milk during orgasm.
- Following cesarean birth, a woman has the nursing care needs of a surgical patient in addition to her needs as a postpartum patient. She may also require assistance in working through her feelings if the cesarean birth was unexpected.
- Following vaginal or cesarean birth, obese and morbidly obese women are at high risk for injury and complications. These new mothers have special physiologic, safety, and psychosocial needs.
- Postpartum, the nurse evaluates the adolescent mother in terms of her level of maturity, available support systems, cultural background, and existing knowledge and then plans care accordingly.
- The mother who decides to relinquish her baby needs emotional support and validation of her loss. She should be able to decide whether to see and hold her baby and should have any special requests regarding the birth honored.
- The lesbian mother and her intimate partner value the same treatment as other couples. Nurses should acknowledge, accept, and involve the partner in care and decision-making.
- Before discharge, the nurse should give the couple any information necessary for the woman to provide appropriate self-care. They should have a beginning skill in caring for their newborn and should be familiar with warning signs of possible complications for mother or baby. Printed information is valuable for reference, as couples will have questions after they return home.
- Because of the trend toward early discharge, follow-up care is more important than ever. Many approaches are used, especially home visits.

CRITICAL THINKING IN ACTION

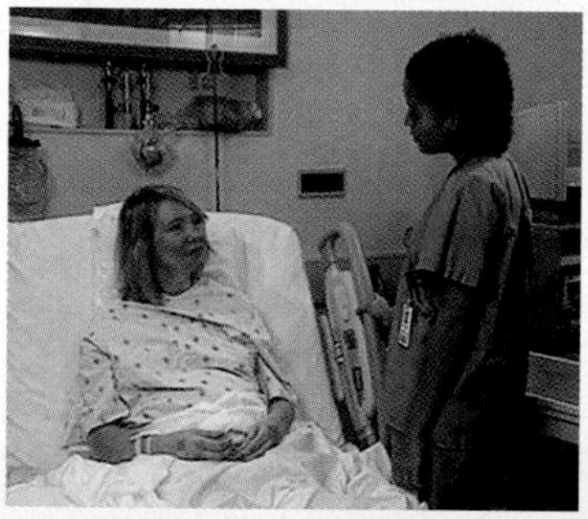

Wendy Calahan, a 31-year-old G3, P2, gave birth to an 8.5 pound baby boy by primary cesarean birth for failure to progress. The baby's Apgar scores were 9 and 9 at 1 and 5 minutes. The baby was admitted to the newborn nursery for transitional observation. Wendy was transferred to the postpartum unit, where you assume her care. You introduce yourself and orient her to the room, call bell, and safety measures. You perform an initial assessment, with all findings within normal limits. Wendy tells you she is very tired and would like to rest while her baby is in the nursery. Her husband and family have left the hospital after spending time with her in the recovery room but will return later. She admits she is disappointed that she could not give birth vaginally even though she pushed for 2 hours. She says, "This baby was just too big."

1. How would you discuss with Wendy the need for frequent assessments after birth?
2. Explain "maternity or baby blues."
3. Explore activities to minimize maternity blues.
4. Discuss concerns of a woman experiencing her second pregnancy.
5. Discuss behaviors that inhibit paternal attachment.

See www.nursing.pearsonhighered.com for possible responses.

Pearson Nursing Student Resources

Find additional review materials at
www.nursing.pearsonhighered.com

Prepare for success with additional NCLEX®-style practice questions, interactive assignments and activities, Web links, animations and videos, and more!

REFERENCES

Aloi, J. A. (2009). Nursing the disenfranchised: Women who have relinquished an infant for adoption. *Journal of Psychiatric and Mental Health Nursing, 16*(1), 27–31. doi:10.1111/j.1365-2850.2008.01324.x

American Academy of Pediatrics (AAP) & The American College of Obstetricians and Gynecologists (ACOG). (2007). *Guidelines for perinatal care* (6th ed.). Elk Grove Village, IL: Author.

American Nurses Association (ANA). (2005). *Code of ethics for nurses with interpretive statements.* Retrieved from http://nursingworld.org/ethics/code/protected_nwcoe813.htm

Amorim Adegboye, A. R., Linne, Y. M., & Lourenco, P. M. C. (2007). Diet or exercise, or both, for weight reduction in women after childbirth. *Cochrane Database of Systematic Reviews* 2007, Issue 3. Art. No.: CD005627. doi:10.1002/14651858.CD005627.pub2

Aschenbrenner, D. S., & Venable, S. J. (2009). *Drug therapy in nursing* (3rd ed.). Philadelphia, PA: Wolters Kluwer Health/Lippincott Williams & Wilkins.

Associated Press (AP). (2009, July 1). FDA panel votes to eliminate Vicodin, Percocet. Retrieved from http://www.msnbc.msn.com/id/31664450/ns/health-more_health_news/

Association of Women's Health, Obstetric, and Neonatal Nurses (AWHONN). (2009). *Standards for professional nursing practice in the care of women and newborns* (7th ed.). Washington, DC: Author.

Brosh, J., Weigel, D., & Evans, W. (2007). Pregnant and parenting adolescents' perception of sources and supports in relation to educational goals. *Child & Adolescent Social Work Journal, 24*(6), 565–578. doi:10.1007/s10560-007-0107-8

Bystrova, K., Ivanova, V., Edhborg, M., Matthiesen, A.-S., Ransjö-Arvidson, A.-B., Mukhamedrakhimov, R., et al. (2009). Early contact versus separation: Effects on mother–infant interaction one year later. *Birth, 36*(2), 97–109. doi:10.1111/j.1523-536X.2009.00307.x

Carvalho, B. (2008). Respiratory depression after neuraxial opioids in the obstetric setting. *Anesthesia & Analgesia, 107*(3), 956–961. doi:10.1213/ane.0b013e318168b443

Centers for Disease Control and Prevention (CDC). (1998; updated 2007). *CDC guidelines for vaccinating pregnant women.* Retrieved from http://www.cdc.gov/vaccines/pubs/downloads/b_preg_guide.pdf

Corwin, E., & Arbour, M. (2007). Postpartum fatigue and evidence-based interventions. *MCN: American Journal of Maternal/Child Nursing, 32*(4), 215–219.

Dabrowski, G. (2007). Skin-to-skin contact: Giving birth back to mothers and babies. *Nursing and Women's Health, 11*(1), 64–71. doi:10.1111/j.1751-486X.2007.00119.x

Declercq, E., Cunningham, D. K., Johnson, C., & Sakala, C. (2008). Mothers' reports of postpartum pain associated with vaginal and cesarean deliveries: Results of a national survey. *Birth, 35*(1), 16–24. doi:10.1111/j.1523-536X.2007.00207.x

Deglin, J. H., & Vallerand, A. H. (2009). *Davis's drug guide for nurses* (11th ed.). Philadelphia, PA: F. A. Davis.

East, C. E., Begg, L., Henshall, N. E., Marchant, P., Wallace, K. (2007). Local cooling for relieving pain from perineal trauma sustained during childbirth. *Cochrane Database of Systematic Reviews, 4.* Art. No.: CD006304. doi:10.1002/14651858.CD006304.pub2

Erlandsson, K., Dsilna, A., Fagerberg, I., & Christensson, K. (2007). Skin-to-skin care with the father after cesarean birth and its effect on newborn crying and prefeeding behavior. *Birth, 34*(2), 105–114. doi:10.1111/j.1523-536X.2007.00162.x

Hale, T. W. (2008). *Medications and mothers' milk* (13th ed.). Amarillo, TX: Hale Publishing.

Herdman, T. H. (2009). *NANDA International nursing diagnoses: Definitions and classification 2009–2011.* Ames, IA: Wiley-Blackwell.

James, D. (2008). Postpartum care. In K. R. Simpson & P. A. Creehan (Eds.), *AWHONN's perinatal nursing* (3rd ed., pp. 473–526). Philadelphia, PA: Wolters Kluwer Health/Lippincott Williams & Wilkins.

Kanotra, S., D'Angelo, D., Phares, T. M., Morrow, B., Barfield, W. D., & Lansky, A. (2007). Challenges faced by new mothers in the early postpartum period: An analysis of comment data from the 2000 Pregnancy Risk Assessment Monitoring System (PRAMS) survey. *Maternal and Child Health Journal, 11*(6), 549–558. doi:10.1007/s10995-007-0206-3

King-Jones, T. C. (2008). Caring for pregnant adolescents: Perils and pearls of communication. *Nursing for Women's Health, 12*(2), 114–119. doi:10.1111/j.1751-486X.2008.00297.x

Klaus, M. (2009). Commentary: An Early, Short, and Useful Sensitive Period in the Human Infant. *Birth, 36*(2), 110–112. doi:10.1111/j.1523-536X.2009.00315.x

Ko, Y., Yang, C., & Chiang, L. (2008). Effects of postpartum exercise program on fatigue and depression during "doing-the-month" period. *Journal of Nursing Research, 16*(3), 177–186. Retrieved from http://www.lww.com/product/?1682_3141 or OVID Database

Lu, M. C., Korst, L. M., Fridman, M., Muthengi, E., & Gregory, K. D. (2009). Identifying women most likely to benefit from prevention strategies for postpartum hemorrhage. *Journal of Perinatology, 29*(6), 422–427. doi:10.1038/jp.2009.2

Mahlmeister, L. R. (2007). Best practices in perinatal nursing: Improving outcomes for obese and morbidly obese women during the intrapartum and postpartum periods. *The Journal of Perinatal & Neonatal Nursing, 21*(2), 86–88. doi:10.1097/01.JPN.0000270621.79831.02

Mangesi, L., & Hofmeyr, G. J. (2005). Early compared with delayed oral fluids and food after caesarean section. *The Cochrane Database of Systematic Reviews, 3.*

Martin, J. A., Hamilton, B. E., Sutton, P. D., Ventura, S. J., Menacker, F., Kirmeyer, S., et al. (2009). Births: Final data for 2006. *National vital statistics reports; Volume 57, Number 7.* Hyattsville, MD: National Center for Health Statistics. Retrieved from http://usgovinfo.about.com/gi/dynamic/offsite.htm?zi=1/XJ&sdn=usgovinfo&cdn=newsissues&tm=49&gps=128_413_1020_507&f=00&tt=2&bt=1&bts=1&zu=http%3A//www.cdc.gov/

McNulty, J. (2009). Postpartum obstetric hemorrhage. In G. G. Briggs & M. Nageotte (Eds.), *Diseases, complications, and drug therapy in obstetrics: A guide for clinicians.* Bethesda, MD: American Society of Health-System Pharmacists.

McQueen, K., Montgomery, P., Lappan-Gracon, S., Evans, M., & Hunter, J. (2008). Evidence-based recommendations for depressive symptoms in postpartum women. *JOGNN: Journal of Obstetric, Gynecologic, & Neonatal Nursing, 37*(2), 127–136. doi:10.1111/j.1552-6909.2008.00215.x

Menacker, F., & Martin, J. A. (2009). BirthStats: Rates of cesarean delivery, and unassisted and assisted vaginal delivery, United States, 1996, 2000, and 2006. *Birth, 36*(2), 167. doi:10.1111/j.1523-536X.2009.00317.x

Mercer, R. T. (1986). *First-time motherhood: Experiences from teens to forties.* New York, NY: Springer.

Mercer, R. T. (2004). Becoming a mother versus maternal role attainment. *Journal of Nursing Scholarship, 36*(3), 226–232. doi:10.1111/j.1547-5069.2004.04042.x

Mercer, R. T. (2006). Nursing support of the process of becoming a mother. *JOGNN: Journal of Obstetric, Gynecologic, & Neonatal Nursing, 35*(5), 649–651. doi:10.1111/J.1552-6909.2006.00086.x

Mercer, R. T., & Walker, L. O. (2006). A review of nursing interventions to foster becoming a mother. *JOGNN: Journal of Obstetric, Gynecologic, & Neonatal Nursing, 35*(5), 568–582. doi:10.1111/J.1552-6909.2006.00080.x

Merck. (2008a). MERUVAX® II. *2009 Physicians' Desk Reference* (63rd ed.). Montvale, NJ: Physicians' Desk Reference, Inc.

Merck. (2008b). M-M-R® II. *2009 Physicians' Desk Reference* (63rd ed.). Montvale, NJ: Physicians' Desk Reference, Inc.

Moore, E. R., Anderson, G. C., & Bergman, N. (2007). Early skin-to-skin contact for mothers and their healthy newborn infants. *Cochrane Database of Systematic Reviews* 2007, Issue 3. Art.No.: CD003519. doi:10.1002/14651858.CD003519.pub2

Mousa, H. A., & Alfirevic, Z. (2007). Treatment for primary postpartum haemorrhage. *Cochrane Database of Systematic Reviews* 2007, Issue 1. Art. No.: CD003249. doi:10.1002/14651858.CD003249.pub2

National Center for State Courts (2009). Family adoption FAQs. Retrieved from http://www.ncsconline.org/wc/CourTopics/FAQs.asp?topic=Adopt#FAQ44

National Council for Adoption. (2008). Correct adoption terminology. Retrieved from http://www.adoptioncouncil.org/resources/adoption_terms.html

Noble, A., Rom, M., Newsome-Wicks, M., & Woloski-Wruble, A. (2009). Jewish laws, customs, and practice in labor, delivery, and postpartum care. *Journal of Transcultural Nursing, 20*(3), 323–333. doi:10.1177/1043659609334930

Oladapo, O. T., & Fawole, B. (2009). Treatments for suppression of lactation. *Cochrane Database of Systematic Reviews* 2009, Issue 1. Art. No.: CD005937. doi:10.1002/14651858.CD005937.pub2

Peterson, W. E., Sword, W., Charles, C., & DiCenso, A. (2007). Adolescents' perceptions of inpatient postpartum nursing care. *Qualitative Health Research, 17*(2), 201–212. doi:10.1177/1049732306297414

Romano, A. M., & Lothian, J. A. (2008). Promoting, protecting, and supporting normal birth: A look at the evidence. *JOGNN: Journal of Obstetric, Gynecologic, & Neonatal Nursing, 37*(1), 95–104. doi:10.1111/J.1552-6909.2007.00210.x

Rubin, R. (1984). *Maternal identity and the maternal experience.* New York: Springer.

Runquist, J. (2007). Persevering through postpartum fatigue. *JOGNN: Journal of Obstetric, Gynecologic, and Neonatal Nursing, 36*(1), 28–37. doi:10.1111/J.1552-6909.2006.00116.x

Smith, K. J. (2008). The hospital-based adoption process: A primer for perinatal nurses. *MCN: The American Journal of Maternal/Child Nursing, 33*(6), 382–388. doi:10.1097/01.NMC.0000341260.10922.4e

Spidsberg, B. D. (2007). Vulnerable and strong—lesbian women encountering maternity care. *Journal of Advanced Nursing, 60*(5), 478–486. doi:10.1111/j.1365-2648.2007.04439.x

Staroselsky, A., Nava-Ocampo, A. A., Vohra, S., & Koren, G. (2008). Hemorrhoids in pregnancy. *Canadian Family Physician, 54*(2), 189–190. Retrieved from www.pubmed.gov

Webb, D. A., Bloch, J. R., Coyne, J. C., Chung, E. K., Bennett, I. M., & Culhane, J. F. (2008). Postpartum physical symptoms in new mothers: Their relationship to functional limitations and emotional well-being. *Birth, 35*(3), 179–187. doi:10.1111/j.1523-536X.2008.00238.x

Wilton, T., & Kaufmann, T. (2001). Lesbian mothers' experiences of maternity care in the UK. *Midwifery, 17*(3), 203–211. doi:10.1054/midw.2001.0261

Young, C., & Armstrong, M. L. (2008). What nurses need to know when caring for women with genital piercings. *Nursing and Women's Health, 12*(2), 128–138. doi:10.1111/j.1751-486X.2008.00299.x

CHAPTER 37

Home Care of the Postpartum Family

Working as a home-care nurse with an early discharge program is the most fulfilling job I have ever had. It is an honor and a privilege to be allowed into the home to share this special time with childbearing families. When I offer breastfeeding support, help new parents to access the resources they need, or recognize a problem and ensure timely follow-up, I know that I am making a difference in their lives. The appreciation expressed by the families and the healthcare providers I serve is a gift that I receive.

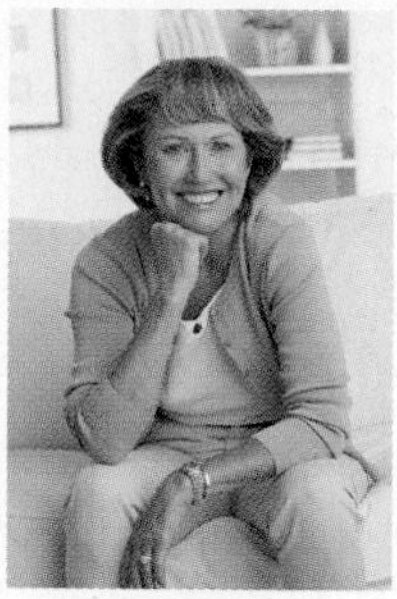

LEARNING OUTCOMES

1. Explain the history of the controversy surrounding length of stay (LOS).
2. Discuss the components of postpartum home care.
3. Identify the main purposes of home visits during the postpartum period.
4. Summarize actions the nurse should take to ensure personal safety during a home visit.
5. Delineate aspects of fostering a caring relationship in the home.
6. Describe assessment, care of the newborn, and reinforcement of parent teaching in the home.
7. Discuss maternal and family assessment and anticipated progress after birth.
8. Describe appropriate nursing interventions for women who are experiencing breastfeeding difficulties.
9. Identify postpartum resources that are available to new families.

KEY TERMS

Active alert state *1068*
Bed sharing *1066*
Cosleeping *1066*
Crying state *1068*
Deep sleep *1068*
Drowsy awake state *1068*
Late preterm infant *1059*
Light sleep *1068*
Postpartum home care *1055*
Quiet alert state *1068*
Room sharing *1065*
Shaken baby syndrome (SBS) *1069*
Sudden infant death syndrome (SIDS) *1065*
Weaning *1080*

Home care is an essential component of perinatal nursing care, particularly as caregivers struggle to find an appropriate balance between providing quality patient care and managing escalating healthcare costs. The hospital length of stay (LOS) following childbirth proved controversial during the last years of the 20th century. Consumers often requested early discharge as an alternative to home delivery in the 1980s. The average LOS decreased further during the early 1990s in an effort to contain healthcare costs, with third-party payers reimbursing only a 24-hour stay following an uncomplicated vaginal delivery. Professional organizations questioned the safety of this trend during the mid-1990s, and Congress responded with the Newborns' and Mothers' Health Protection Act (NMHPA) of 1996 (Bernstein et al., 2007).

Role of Length of Stay and Professional Guidelines and Recommendations in Postpartum Home Care

The Newborns' and Mothers' Health Protection Act (NMHPA) was signed into law in 1997 and took effect in January 1998. Although the bill does not prohibit earlier discharge, it provides for a guaranteed minimum stay of up to 48 hours following an uncomplicated vaginal birth and 96 hours following an uncomplicated cesarean birth at the discretion of the new mother and her healthcare provider (American Academy of Pediatrics [AAP] & the American College of Obstetricians and Gynecologists [ACOG], 2007; Bernstein et al., 2007; Evans, Garthwaite, & Wei, 2008). Despite numerous studies, findings are inconclusive as to whether a shortened length of stay (LOS) is harmful or beneficial to childbearing families.

An analysis of maternal and infant data from approximately 3 million births in California suggested that early discharge was not hazardous following routine pregnancy, but that newborns at highest risk of readmission benefited from laws that guaranteed a minimum LOS (Evans et al., 2008). Another large California study found that after the AAP Subcommittee on Hyperbilirubinemia mandated increased surveillance and follow-up regarding hyperbilirubinemia in 1994, readmissions increased and peaked in 1998. Readmissions decreased following the 1998 legislation regarding length of stay, suggesting again that increased LOS benefited high-risk infants. The authors noted, however, that demonstrating cause and effect is difficult, as many complex issues affect newborn readmission rates (Burgos, Schmitt, Stevenson, et al., 2008).

Optimal timing of discharge needs to be determined by considering the medical, social, and financial factors in each case. Bernstein et al. (2007) found that mothers and physicians do not always agree on readiness for discharge, and they emphasized that the decision regarding LOS needs to be made jointly. The AAP and ACOG (2007) developed guidelines for LOS and follow-up care for mothers and newborns. Newborns discharged prior to 48 hours of age should be examined by a healthcare professional "competent in newborn assessment," (p. 230) within 48 hours of discharge. A qualified nurse can accomplish the visit in a clinical setting or in the home, provided that the results are reported to the physician that day. Suggested discharge criteria and recommendations for follow-up after early discharge are found in Table 37-1.

The American Academy of Pediatrics (AAP) & The American College of Obstetricians and Gynecologists (ACOG) (2007) also recommended provision of adequate screening and follow-up for hyperbilirubinemia, depending on the infant's risk status. Therefore, infants who are discharged at 48 hours or older may require follow-up as well. The assessment is ideally accomplished between 72 and 96 hours, during the time of highest risk for hyperbilirubinemia. The visit(s) should include assessment of the weight and percent change since birth, adequacy of intake, voiding and stooling patterns, and the presence or absence of jaundice. The health professional uses clinical judgment to determine the need for a bilirubin test.

Considerations for the Home Visit

In planning a home visit, the nurse should clearly understand the purpose of the visit and identify the maximum amount of content to be addressed. Other important considerations include ways of creating and fostering relationships with families, techniques for preplanning and executing the visit while maintaining safety, documenting the visit, and ensuring telephone follow-up.

The postpartum home visit differs from community health visits in that only one or two visits are typically planned, and long-term follow-up by the nurse is not anticipated. Although the postpartum home visit is comprehensive, it is specifically focused on a postpartum family's needs and care.

Because of the established guidelines for discharge of the mother and baby (refer to Table 37-1), the nurse can logically expect to find certain levels of health and wellness. However, because the status of the mother and newborn can change, the nurse should stay alert for deviations from the norm.

Purpose and Timing of the Home Visit

Home care for the postpartum family focuses on assessment, teaching, and counseling. The visit frequently occurs on the third to sixth day postpartum, depending on when the couplet was discharged. This time frame encompasses the potential peak times for newborn jaundice and maximal weight loss, and it meets the recommendations set forth by the AAP Subcommittee on Hyperbilirubinemia (2004). Additionally, by this time the milk should be coming in, and breastfeeding is either going well or problems are becoming apparent. Parents frequently have new and different questions, having spent a couple of days and nights caring independently for their newborn since discharge.

Postpartum home care provides opportunities for expanding information and reinforcing self- and infant-care techniques initially presented in the birth setting. The home setting provides an opportunity for the nurse and family to interact in a more relaxed environment, one in which the family has control of the setting. It also provides an invaluable opportunity for the nurse to assess home safety in the setting where the family will grow together. In some instances, a

Postpartum Home Visits

TABLE 37-1 Minimal Criteria for Discharge of Newborns Prior to 48 Hours of Age

1. Antepartum, intrapartum, and postpartum course for both the mother and the newborn is uncomplicated
2. Vaginal delivery
3. Singleton birth at 38 to 42 weeks' gestation, with birth weight appropriate for gestational age according to appropriate intrauterine growth curves
4. Newborn's vital signs are normal and stable for 12 hours before discharge
   - Respiratory rate less than 60/min
   - Heart rate 100 to 160/min
   - Axillary temperature of 36.5°C to 37.4°C (97.7°F to 99.3°F) in an open crib with appropriate clothing
5. Newborn has urinated and passed at least one spontaneous stool
6. Newborn has completed at least two successful feedings
   - Documentation has been made regarding the newborn's ability to coordinate sucking, swallowing, and breathing while feeding
   - If breastfeeding, a knowledgeable caregiver has observed and documented latch, swallowing, and infant satiety
7. Physical exam reveals no abnormalities requiring continued hospital stay
8. No evidence of excessive bleeding from the circumcision site for the previous 2 hours
9. Clinical significance of any jaundice has been determined and appropriate management and follow-up is in place
10. Mother's knowledge, ability, and confidence to care for the newborn are documented to include teaching of the following:
    - Condition of the newborn
    - Appropriate newborn output (urine and stools)
    - Care of the cord, skin, and genitals as well as temperature assessment and measurement
    - Maternal knowledge of signs of illness and common problems, particularly jaundice
    - Instruction in newborn safety to include car seat use and positioning for sleep
11. Family or other support persons and healthcare providers are available to the couplet during the first few days following discharge
12. Instructions given to follow in the event of a complication or emergency
13. Lab data have been reviewed to include maternal syphilis, hepatitis B virus surface antigen, and HIV; umbilical cord or newborn blood type and direct Coombs' if indicated
14. Required screening tests have been accomplished; if a test was performed before 24 hours of milk feeding, a plan for repeat must be in place in accordance with local or state policy
15. Initial hepatitis B vaccine has been administered or an appointment made for its administration
16. Hearing screening has been completed per hospital protocol
17. A physician-directed source of continuing medical care for both mother and baby has been identified; appropriate follow-up within 48 hours by a person qualified to assess the newborn is scheduled
18. Family, environmental, and social risk factors have been assessed. If risk factors are present, the discharge should be delayed until resolved or a plan is in place to safeguard the infant. Factors may include but not be limited to untreated parental substance use, positive maternal or infant toxicology results, history of child abuse or neglect, mental illness in a parent who is in the home, lack of social support, no fixed home, history of domestic violence, adolescent mother—especially with other risk factors, and barriers to follow-up (lack of access to telephone, transportation issues, non–English speaking parents).

Recommended follow-up for infants with a shortened hospital stay of less than 48 hours should include the following within 48 hours of discharge:

- Weigh the infant
- Assess the newborn's general health, hydration, and degree of jaundice; identify any new problems
- Review feeding pattern and technique; observe breastfeeding for adequate position, latch on, and swallowing
- Assess historical evidence of stool and urine patterns for adequacy
- Assess quality of mother-newborn interaction and details of newborn behavior
- Reinforce maternal or family education in neonatal care, particularly feeding and sleep position
- Review results of laboratory tests performed at discharge
- Perform screening tests as required by the state and others as clinically indicated
- Identify a plan for healthcare maintenance, including a method for obtaining emergency services, preventive care and immunizations, periodic evaluations and physical examinations, and necessary screening

Source: Used with permission from American Academy of Pediatrics (AAP) & the American College of Obstetricians and Gynecologists (ACOG). (2007). Guidelines for perinatal care *(6th ed.). Copyright © AAP.*

home provides unique challenges in assessing and enhancing the woman's self-care and infant care, and the nurse has many opportunities to exercise critical thinking and develop creative options with the family.

Fostering a Caring Relationship with the Family

Although the nurse in the birthing center strives to enhance family autonomy and control, the inherent atmosphere of the institutional environment may cause the new mother and family to feel disempowered. It is important for the professional nurse to recognize that the parameters of the home visit are different in many ways from those of the hospital or birthing center environment. In the home, the family has control of their environment and the nurse is an invited visitor. The nurse can rely on the same characteristics of a caring relationship that have been integral to hospital-based practice—regard for patients, genuineness, empathy, and establishment of trust and rapport—but the relationship may take on new elements as the nurse moves into the home setting for the first time (Table 37-2).

Planning the Home Visit

Before the home visit, the nurse prepares by identifying the purpose of the visit and gathering anticipated materials and equipment. Communication with the primary healthcare provider(s) and a thorough review of inpatient records gives the nurse an understanding of current needs and any special concerns for each individual mother-baby couplet. A personal contact while the woman is still in the birth setting or a previsit telephone call is used to arrange the appointment with the woman and her family. During the previsit contact it is important for the nurse to identify clearly the purpose and goals of the visit, to let the patient know approximately how long the visit will take, and to begin establishing a rapport.

Maintaining Safety

In the past, nurses were viewed as a mainstay of communities and could move in most settings without fear or concern for safety. However, in current times some communities are not safe for visiting nurses. Risks noted by home-care nurses include isolated locations, illegal drugs, threatening animals,

TABLE 37-2 Fostering a Caring Relationship

DEMONSTRATED GOAL	APPROACHES TO ACHIEVE GOAL
Regard	Introduce yourself to the family. Call the family members by their surnames until you have been invited to use the given or a less formal name. Ask to be introduced to other members of the family who are present. Allow the mother or spokesperson to assume this role. Use active listening. Maintain objectiveness. Ask permission before sitting.
Genuineness	Mean what you say. Make sure that your verbal and nonverbal messages are congruent. Be nonjudgmental. Don't make assumptions about individuals or settings. Always strive to demonstrate caring behaviors. Be prepared for the visit, honestly answer questions and provide information, and be truthful. If you don't know the answer to a question, tell the patient you will find the information and report back.
Empathy	Listen to the mother and family without judgment, trying to view events and circumstances from their point of view. Be attentive to what the birthing experience means to them so that you will understand their concerns from their perspective. Remember, empathy denotes understanding, not sympathy.
Trust and Rapport	Do what you say you will do. Be prepared for the visit and be on time. Notify the family if you are running late because of patient care. Follow up on any areas that are needed.

gangs, vandalism, inadequate lighting, guns, verbal abuse, robberies, inappropriate sexual comments, adverse weather and road conditions, dilapidated or pest-infested buildings, unsanitary conditions, and violent lifestyles (Anderson, 2008). Thus it is important for the nurse to follow some basic safety rules when conducting a home visit. Specifically, the nurse should:

- Confirm the address, and ask for directions during the previsit contact.
- Trace out the route to the patient's home on a map or the Internet before leaving for the visit, and take the map along; use a GPS device if available.
- Provide a daily schedule of visits, including patient addresses and phone numbers, to supervisors.
- Notify an instructor or supervisor when leaving for a visit and check in as soon as the visit is completed.
- Carry a cellular phone with the battery charged at all times.
- Carry a hard copy of agency and emergency phone numbers that are also programmed into the cellular phone.
- Carry a phone card or enough change to make a call from a pay phone in case of poor cellular transmission in some locations.
- Ensure that the vehicle used for visits is well maintained and has sufficient fuel.
- Pay close attention to traffic conditions and exercise care and caution while driving.
- Exercise caution when using a cellular phone while driving (first pull over to a safe place and stop, use a hands-free device, etc.).
- Wear a name tag and carry identification.
- Carry a flashlight, particularly for night visits.
- Carry food and water for personal use.
- Avoid wearing expensive jewelry.
- Before starting out (or before arriving at the home) lock personal belongings in the trunk of the car, out of sight.
- Call patients when on the way to confirm that they are home and that they are expecting the nurse.
- Identify other individuals present in the home at the start of the visit.
- Pay attention to the body language of all present during the visit.
- Request that threatening or sexually inappropriate behavior stop immediately.
- Be aware of personal body language and how it might be interpreted (for example, avoid crossing arms or shoving hands in pockets; remain calm and convey a sense of respect at all times).
- Leave the home immediately if a weapon is visible and the patient or a family member refuses requests to put it away.
- Ask patients to keep threatening pets secured in a different area of the home during the visit.
- Request that patients and family members avoid the use of illegal substances during the visit.
- If a situation arises that feels unsafe or if the previous requests are not honored, terminate the visit.
- Always have car keys in hand before returning to the vehicle.
- Lock the doors and drive away upon return to the vehicle at the completion of visits—do not sit in the vehicle to chart.
- Inform the supervisor immediately of any threatening situation, assault, or injury.
- Notify authorities if a crime has been committed.

It may be helpful to drive around neighborhoods known to be unsafe before making an initial visit to identify potential cues to violence and to determine whether extra security is necessary. If the visit is in an area that seems very unsafe, it may be wise for two nurses to go together or for the nurse to be accompanied by a security officer. Nurses should avoid entering areas where violence is in progress. In such cases, they should return to the car and contact the appropriate authorities by calling 911. If violence erupts while in the home and the nurse is unable to safely exit, the nurse should stay in a secure room with the door locked, if possible, and call 911.

Home care agencies are required to have violence protection programs as mandated by the Occupational Safety and Health Administration (OSHA) in 1996. This includes having policies in place and providing safety education for new employees and at least annually for all. Agencies in high-risk areas often contract with security and escort services to protect personnel in the community. Agencies should also have code phrases to use and a set plan for all to follow if a nurse calls to report being in an unsafe situation. Incidents should be tracked and reported to authorities. Patients should be informed that they are required to provide a safe environment and may face termination of services otherwise. Agencies may face ethical dilemmas involving the refusal or termination of services to patients in homes deemed to be too risky for nurses. In that case, the physician should be notified and other options considered for the patient (Anderson, 2008).

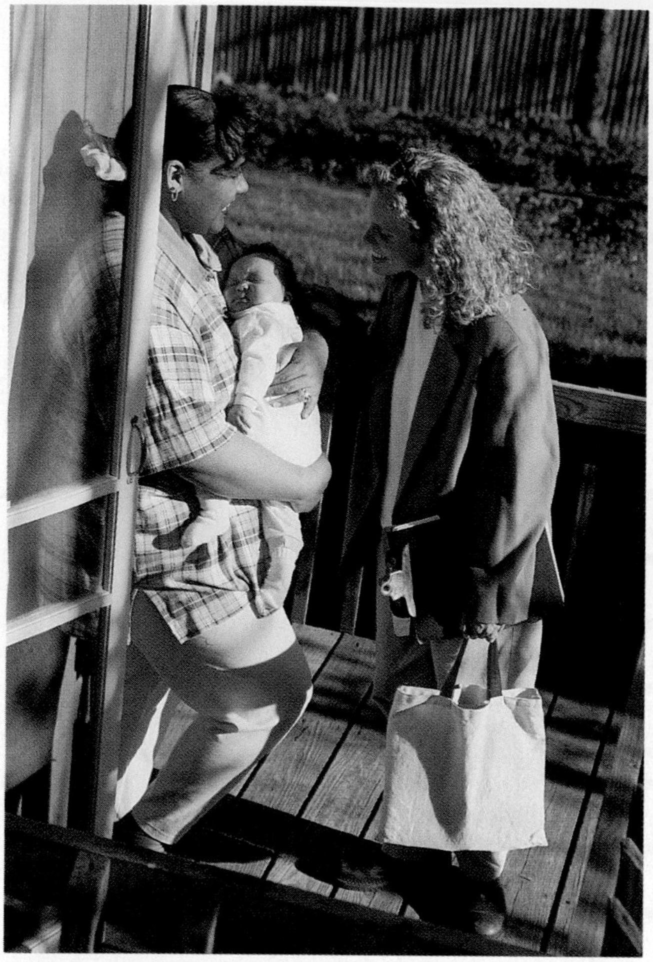

Figure 37-1 ■ Nurse arriving for a home visit.
Source: George Dodson/Pearson Education.

Nurses will want to ask questions about and review the violence protection plan of a home care agency to ensure that their safety will be protected to the extent possible before accepting employment. Nurses may also wish to enroll in further personal safety training independently. Anderson (2008) provides additional recommendations and resources that will be helpful to prospective home-care nurses.

Because postpartum home care frequently involves only one visit, it may be helpful to discuss safety expectations during the previsit telephone contact. Home-care nurses should be familiar with their agency policies and notify supervisors if safety issues requiring agency support are present.

Most people are more comfortable in familiar settings and have some hesitation when entering other residential areas. It is important for nurses to be aware of their surroundings and the people who are nearby. First home visits may feel uncomfortable because they are unfamiliar, but comfort increases with experience (Figure 37-1 ■).

Carrying Out the Home Visit

When the door is answered, the nurse should introduce herself or himself and confirm that the location is correct. The nurse may tactfully request to be introduced to others present if this information is not offered. If a place to sit is not indicated, the nurse may inquire, "Where is the best place to sit so that we can talk for a while?" In some homes, the mother or family may offer refreshments, and this may be an important aspect of welcoming a visitor. In this case, it is beneficial to the relationship to accept the refreshment graciously. Other culturally appropriate customs should be respected in the home setting whenever possible.

Many agencies have developed a uniform assessment tool to be used during postpartum home visits. This ensures that the nurse completes a physical assessment of both the mother and the newborn; assesses infant feeding and weight; evaluates maternal psychosocial adjustment, parental bonding, parenting behaviors, family adaptation, and coping skills; and determines environmental strengths and risk factors. Based on these assessments the nurse may do any of the following:

- Provide direct physical care.
- Carry out patient and family teaching.
- Consult with the physician, midwife, or a specialist, such as a lactation consultant.
- Refer the woman or family to appropriate community agencies.
- Schedule additional home visits or telephone follow-up.

Because home-care nursing is practiced geographically independent of the healthcare facility, the nurse needs to have excellent assessment skills and be adept at noticing variations from the norm. Critical thinking and problem-solving skills are necessary. Effective communication with the families and the appropriate healthcare providers is essential in the coordination of required treatment and follow-up.

The remainder of the chapter focuses on specific aspects of newborn and maternal care that are assessed, addressed, and evaluated during the home visit.

Home Care: The Newborn

When the family provides care for their newborn, the nurse can instill confidence by giving them positive feedback. If the family encounters problems, the nurse can suggest alternatives and serve as a role model. Each newborn has variations in normal physiologic responses and in growth and development patterns. Parents need to learn to interpret these changes in their child. To help parents care for their newborn at home, some physicians encourage prenatal pediatric visits to establish contact before the birth. Public health nurses have long been involved as guides in newborn care and parent education. Some birthing units are now expanding their primary care functions to the new family to include one home visit by a nurse who cared for the family in the birthing unit. The birthing unit nursery staff may also make themselves available as a 24-hour telephone resource for the new family who needs additional support and consultation during the first few days at home with their newborn. Routine well-baby visits should be scheduled with the clinic, pediatric nurse practitioner, or physician.

The family should have been taught all necessary caregiving methods before discharge. However, the home-care nurse may use a checklist to determine that the family clearly understands the material. If not, the nurse should complete pertinent teaching. Parents are frequently overwhelmed, sensory overloaded, and exhausted during their short hospital stay and will require a review of initial teaching.

Parents often have questions regarding infant care, feeding, and signs of illness. Therefore, the home-care nurse will want to address those issues. The nurse also needs to review with the couple all areas for understanding and to answer any questions they may have, making sure that they have the phone number and address of, and any specific instructions from, their healthcare providers. Having the nursery phone number is also reassuring to a new family. The nurse encourages them to call with questions.

Physical Assessment of the Newborn at Home

In the home, a newborn physical exam is performed to assess general appearance and vital signs as well as the skin and the respiratory, cardiovascular, gastrointestinal, genitourinary, musculoskeletal, and neurologic body systems. The infant's behavioral state and the parent-infant interaction should be assessed as well. An exam of the infant's fontanelles, eyes, ears, mouth, nose, neck, color, evidence of jaundice, umbilical cord, circumcision if done, reflexes, hydration, nutritional status and feeding history, elimination of urine and stool, activity, sleep-wake cycles, weight, and percentage of change from birth weight should be documented under the appropriate body systems. See chapter 30 ∞ for a complete, step-by-step newborn assessment.

The home visit is the time to ensure that the appropriate screening exams as required by the state have been accomplished and to obtain the blood for screening if still needed. If the newborn did not pass a universal hearing screen before discharge, the nurse should ensure that the parents have a plan to accomplish the required screening or audiology follow-up. The nurse will also assess and reinforce knowledge related to infant care as detailed in the following sections.

Assessment of Late Preterm Infants

Late preterm infants are those infants born between 34 and 36 6/7 gestational weeks. Late preterm infants typically weigh 4 1/2 to 6 pounds and are at greater risk for a variety of complications due to immaturity of their compensatory mechanisms (March of Dimes, 2010). Because of a greater risk for complications, these infants should receive a home health visit within 24 to 48 hours of discharge (Engle, Tomashek, Wallman, et al., 2007). Late preterm births account for 70% of all premature births (Engle et al., 2007). Late preterm infants have higher infant morbidity and mortality rates than term infants. These infants have more respiratory complications and may have more feeding issues. Some may require a feeding tube before regular feedings can be established. The home health nurse needs to assess the frequency and duration of breast feedings. If the infant is formula fed, the amount of formula being ingested and the frequency of feedings should be recorded because dehydration is often a cause of rehospitalization of these infants. Infants who are breastfed and those that are firstborn are at greatest risk for readmission in the neonatal period (Engle et al., 2007).

Assessment of output, adequate weight gain, and hydration status is imperative. Follow-up visits are indicated to assess ongoing weight-gain patterns. Parent education should include the signs of dehydration, adequate feeding parameters, and expected urinary/stool output, and the symptoms of jaundice should be reviewed at the home visit.

These infants are also more likely to develop hyperbilirubinemia. Some infants may be undergoing home phototherapy. In these cases, the nurse assesses the infant's color, collects a blood sample if indicated, and ensures that phototherapy equipment is being properly used. Some late preterm infants are placed on iron supplements due to anemia, and the nurse should ask the family if the supplement is being given as ordered. The nurse should provide education on the need and use of such supplements. Since late preterm infants are also more likely to acquire infections, the nurse instructs the care provider to use good hand washing techniques and to avoid exposure of the infant to individuals with infections or illnesses. Taking the baby out in large crowded places should also be avoided. Sepsis occurs more commonly in late preterm infants.

Although later preterm infants may be similar in size and appearance to term infants, they require ongoing assessment and care from the family and the health care team. Close observation and intervention can help prevent readmission to the hospital and long-term complications. Since these infants are more prone to behavioral and developmental problems than term infants, healthcare providers should be advised of their premature status at birth (March of Dimes, 2010).

Positioning and Handling of the Newborn

The nurse demonstrates methods of positioning and handling the newborn as needed. When the newborn is out of the crib, one of the following holds can be used (Figure 37-2 ■). The cradle hold is frequently used during feeding. It provides a sense of warmth and closeness, permits eye contact, frees one of the adult's hands, and provides security because the cradling protects the newborn's body. Extra security is provided by gripping the thigh with the hand while the arm supports the newborn's body. The upright position provides security and a sense of closeness and is ideal for burping. One hand should support the neck and shoulders while the other hand holds the buttocks or is placed between the newborn's legs. The newborn may also be held upright in a cloth sling carrier that gently holds the baby against the mother's or father's chest and frees the hands for other tasks. The football hold frees one of the caregiver's hands and permits eye contact. This hold is ideal for shampooing, carrying, or breastfeeding. It frees the caregiver to talk on the telephone, answer the door, or do the myriad tasks that await attention at this busy time.

Skin-to-skin contact (SSC) immediately following delivery has been found to be beneficial to breastfeeding and to have positive effects on the mother-infant relationship over the first year of life (Bystrova et al., 2009; Dabrowski, 2007; Moore, Anderson, & Bergman, 2007; Romano & Lothian, 2008). Klaus (2009) noted that the benefits of skin-to-skin contact and carrying the infant against the chest continue during the first weeks of the newborn's life. Therefore, the nurse can encourage both parents to continue this practice at home, particularly if they had limited opportunities to do so while in the hospital.

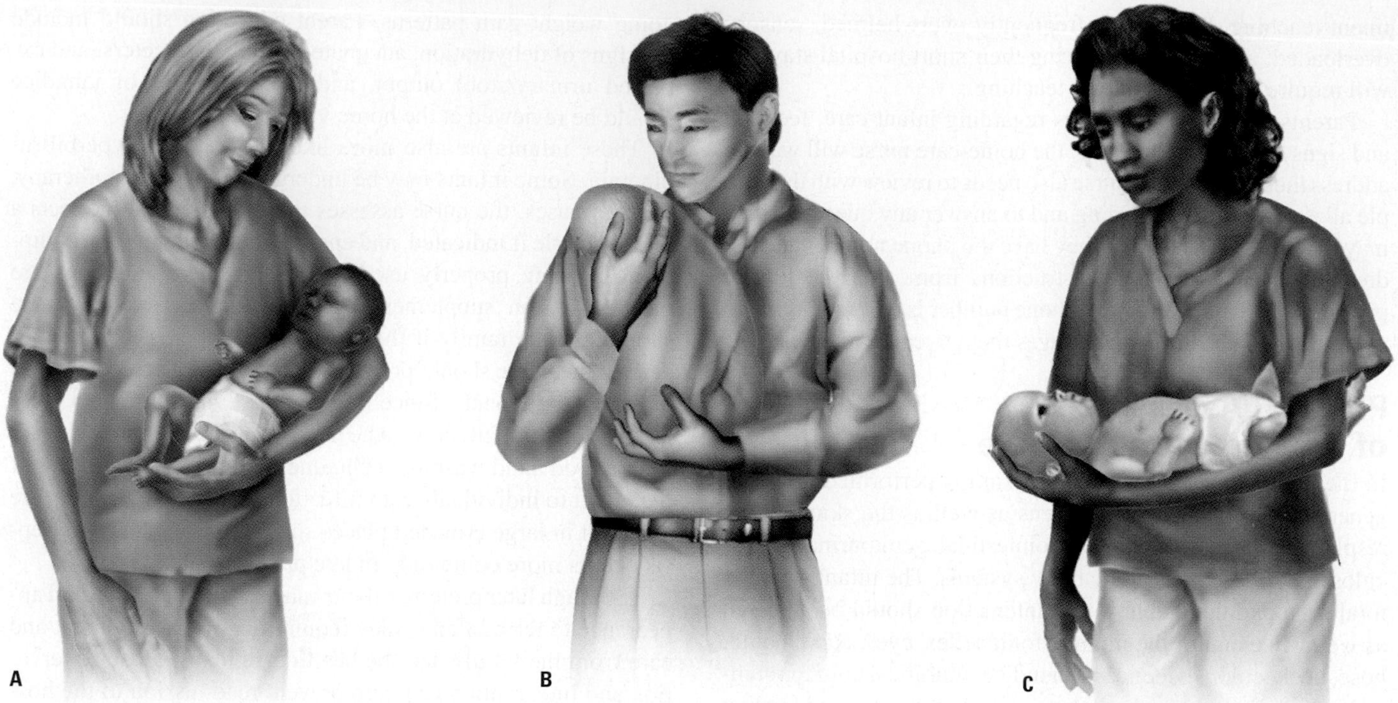

Figure 37-2 ■ Various positions for holding an infant. A. Cradle hold. B. Upright position. C. Football hold.

Skin Care and Bathing

The skin maintains temperature and serves as a barrier between the newborn and the environment. It is also a potential portal of entry for environmental toxins and infectious agents. Keeping the skin healthy and intact is essential to the newborn's health. The requirements of infant skin care include frequent assessment, effective cleansing, effective moisturizing, and maintenance of an effective barrier against external irritants. The following section provides information from the Association of Women's Health, Obstetric, and Newborn Nurses (AWHONN) Neonatal Skin Care Evidence-Based Clinical Practice Guideline (AWHONN, 2007a).

An actual bath demonstration is the best way for the nurse to provide information to parents. Because excess bathing and use of soap removes natural skin oils and dries out the newborn's sensitive skin, bathing should be done only two to three times per week. A mild, nonmedicated skin cleanser may be used as needed. Cleansing agents with a neutral pH (5.5 to 7.0) that are preservative-free are recommended. Because cleansers can be drying to the skin, they need not be used at every bath or in excess. Antimicrobial soaps should be avoided, as they may disturb the infant's normal skin colonization (AWHONN, 2007a).

Sponge baths have traditionally been recommended for the first 2 weeks or until the umbilical cord completely falls off and the umbilicus has healed. However, immersion bathing, in which the parents place the newborn's entire body except for the head and neck into a tub, is better tolerated by some infants, is more pleasurable for some newborns and parents, and results in less heat loss. This practice has been found to be safe prior to cord separation and has not been demonstrated to be associated with more cord infections (AWHONN, 2007a). Therefore, the nurse can reassure parents that either method is safe and that they can choose the method most comfortable for them and their newborn. The parents should take care to keep the room warm and free of drafts while using either method.

Many birthing units and agencies provide videos for parents to watch before bathing their baby for the first time, as a home visit does not usually allow time for a nurse demonstration and a parent return demonstration of a bath. See Patient Teaching: Newborn Bathing.

Supplies can be kept in a plastic bag or container for convenience (Table 37-3). At home, the family may want to use a small plastic dishpan, a clean kitchen or bathroom sink, or a large bowl as the baby's tub. Commercial plastic baby tubs are not necessary, but some parents prefer to purchase them.

Before starting, if no one else is at home, the parent may want to silence phones and place a sign on the door to avoid being disturbed. Having someone home during the first few baths is helpful, because that person can retrieve forgotten items, attend to interruptions, and provide moral support. It is important to have supplies gathered before beginning, as the caregiver will not be able to turn away or break hand contact with the newborn once he or she is positioned for the bath.

Sponge Bath

After the supplies are gathered, the tub (or any of the containers mentioned) is filled with approximately 5 inches of water

TABLE 37-3 Bath Supplies

Washcloths (2)	Shampoo
Towels (2)	Petrolatum product if indicated
Blankets (2)	Diapers
Unperfumed mild skin cleanser	Clean clothes

PATIENT TEACHING Newborn Bathing

Patient Goals

At the completion of the teaching, the family will be able to:

1. Identify safety concerns related to sponge and tub baths for newborns.
2. List appropriate supplies for bathing.
3. Demonstrate proper bathing procedures for both sponge and tub baths.
4. Discuss the use of appropriate skin care agents for newborn use.

TEACHING PLAN

Teaching Method	Content
Clarify information related to sponge bathing and tub bathing for safe newborn bathing. Explain that the proper environment is needed for newborn safety and comfort.	Describe the proper environment (including safety factors) for sponge and tub bathing for newborns.
Encourage the mother to assemble supplies before beginning the newborn bath to avoid cold exposure, and ensure that proper supplies are being used.	Identify proper bathing supplies that are needed for both sponge and tub baths.
Demonstrate proper technique and encourage the family to ask questions as they arise. Help instill confidence in new parents.	Demonstrate sponge bathing. Discuss and demonstrate tub bathing using an infant model.
Clarify the need for appropriate cleansing agents for newborns.	Explain the need for neutral pH, fragrance-free, and dye-free cleansing products for newborn use.

Evaluation

At the end of the teaching session the woman and family will be able to verbalize the principles of proper bathing for the newborn. They will be able to demonstrate the proper techniques to ensure safety during both sponge and tub baths.

Documentation

Document the information that was given, the type of teaching method used, indicate if the patient performed a bath, if it was demonstrated, or if verbal or written directions were given. Verbalization of understanding and clarification of any information should be documented. Safety issues and instructions should also be documented.

that is warm to the touch. Some parents carefully test the water temperature against their forearm. Others may also choose to purchase a thermometer to help them determine when the bath water is comfortable and safe to use. Water should be 38°C to <40°C (100°F to <104°F) (AWHONN, 2007a). Soap should not be added to the water.

The newborn is placed on a flat protected surface, such as a counter or in a bassinet adjacent to the container of water for a sponge bath. The newborn should be wrapped in a blanket, with a T-shirt and diaper on, to keep him or her warm and secure. Parents should be reminded never to leave an infant unattended on an elevated surface or near any amount of water. Parents should be encouraged to keep one hand on their infant at all times and to keep their eyes on their infant at all times while positioned for a bath.

To start the sponge bath, the adult wraps the dampened washcloth around the index finger once. Each eye is gently wiped from inner to outer canthus. This direction prevents the potential for clogging the tear duct at the inner canthus, where the eye naturally drains. A different portion of the washcloth is used for each eye to prevent cross-contamination. Some eye swelling and drainage may be present the first few days after birth as a result of the eye prophylaxis.

The bath giver washes the ears next by wrapping the washcloth once around an index finger and gently cleaning the external ear and behind the ear. Cotton swabs (Q-tips®) are never used in the ear canal, because it is possible to put a swab too far into the ear and damage the eardrum. In addition, a swab may push any discharge farther down into the ear canal.

The caregiver rinses out the washcloth and then wipes the remainder of the baby's face with the warm, dampened soap-free washcloth. Many babies start to cry at this point. The face should be washed every day, and the mouth and chin should be wiped off after each feeding.

The neck is washed carefully but thoroughly with the washcloth. A mild soap may now be used. Formula or breast milk and lint collect in the skin folds of the neck, so it may be helpful to sit the newborn up, supporting the neck and shoulders with one hand while washing the neck with the other hand.

When sponge-bathing, the bath giver will want to bathe the upper and lower body separately to minimize heat loss. Once the face and neck are clean and dry, the bath giver unwraps the blanket, removes the T-shirt, and wets the chest, back, and arms with the washcloth. The bath giver may then lather his or her hands with a mild infant skin cleanser and wash the baby's chest, back, and arms. Soap is rinsed off with the wet washcloth, and the upper part of the body is dried with a towel or blanket. The newborn's upper body is then wrapped with a clean, dry blanket to prevent heat loss.

Next the bath giver unwraps the newborn's legs, wets them with the washcloth, and lathers, rinses, and dries them well. If the newborn has dry skin, a small amount of an emollient such as petrolatum may be used. Products without preservatives, perfumes, or dyes are recommended. Baby oil is not recommended because it clogs skin pores. Families need to be aware that baby powder should be avoided, as it can cause serious respiratory problems if the baby inhales it. The genital area is cleansed after each wet or dirty diaper. Females are washed from the front of the genital area toward the rectum to avoid fecal contamination of the urethra and the bladder. Newborn females often have a thick, white mucous discharge or a slight bloody discharge from the vaginal area. This discharge is normal for the first 1 to 2 weeks after birth. The mucus may come off if wiped gently after diaper changes but should not be intentionally scrubbed off.

Parents of uncircumcised males should cleanse the penis daily. Even minimal retraction of the foreskin is not advised (see in-depth discussion of care of uncircumcised male babies in chapter 31 ∞). Males who have been circumcised also need their penises cleansed daily. A very wet washcloth is squeezed above the baby's penis, allowing clear water to run over the circumcision site. The area is gently patted or fanned dry. Soap is not used around the penis for the first 3 to 4 days following circumcision, as it can be irritating to the tissues. A small amount of an emollient such as petrolatum, or petrolatum-impregnated gauze strips may be applied during each diaper change for the first 24 to 48 hours. Emollients promote comfort and healing and prevent adherence of the diaper to the site. It is important to avoid using ointments if a Plastibell is in place, because ointments may cause the Plastibell ring to slip off the penis too early. The Plastibell usually falls off within 5 to 8 days. If it does not, the family needs to call the healthcare provider.

The newborn should be wrapped in a terry cloth bath towel or bath blanket and gently patted dry at the end of the bath to promote skin integrity and prevent heat loss. It is particularly important that the cord be thoroughly dried if it has become wet during the bath.

The last step in bathing is washing the hair (although some prefer to do this step first). The newborn is swaddled in a dry blanket, leaving only the head exposed, and held in the football hold with the head tilted slightly downward. A cup or cupped hand may be used to pour warm water over the newborn's head, taking care to avoid the eyes and ear canals. Parents should avoid placing the infant's head directly under running water, as changes in water temperature could cause burns or discomfort. The hair is moistened and lathered with a small amount of shampoo. A very soft brush may be used to massage the shampoo over the entire head, including the fontanelles, which families often call the "soft spots." The hair is then rinsed and toweled dry. Oils or lotions are not used on the newborn's head unless prescribed by a healthcare provider.

Tub Baths

When tub-bathing, the bath can be completed efficiently with the newborn's trunk and lower extremities underwater. The newborn's face, eyes, ears, and neck can be washed and dried as described above before undressing him or her for the tub bath. A large, clean kitchen or bathroom sink, plastic container, or commercial infant tub that allows the baby to be immersed to the neck may be used as the infant's tub. A washcloth can be placed in the bottom of the container to prevent slippage. The infant should be held securely at all times (Figure 37-3 ■). Commercial infant tubs often support the infant's head and neck. If desired by the parents and if time allows, the nurse can demonstrate how to securely support the infant while giving an immersion bath.

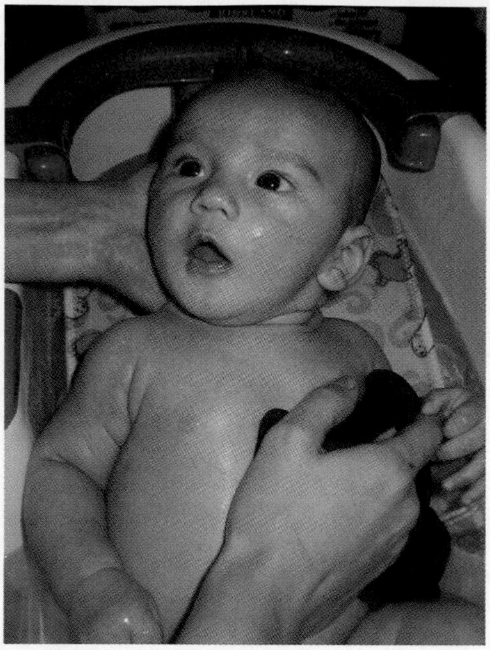

Figure 37-3 ■ When bathing the newborn, the caregiver must support the head. Wet babies are very slippery.

Because wet newborns are slippery, some parents pull a cotton sock (with holes cut out for the fingers) over the supporting arm to provide a "nonskid" surface. The newborn's body is washed with a soapy washcloth or hand. To wash the back, the bath giver places the noncradling hand on the newborn's chest with the thumb under the newborn's arm closest to the adult. Gently tipping the newborn forward onto the supporting hand frees the cradling arm to wash the back. After the bath, the newborn is lifted out of the tub in the cradle position, dried well, and wrapped in a dry blanket. If the cord has not fallen off, it should be thoroughly dried before re-covering with clothing. The hair is then washed in the same way as for a sponge bath.

Once the bath is complete, the parents can double-blanket the newborn in clean dry blankets and a hat for approximately 10 minutes. Once the infant is totally dry, they may dress the baby and apply a clean, dry hat and blanket. The nurse must educate parents that infants and young children can drown even in small amounts of water. It is paramount that adults not allow the infant to be immersed above the neck and that they keep the infant safe by maintaining hand, arm, and eye contact with the infant at all times during the tub bath.

Cord Care

The parents should be instructed to allow the cord to dry naturally. They should be taught to:

- Wash their hands before and after handling the cord.
- Keep the cord clean and dry.

- Keep the cord exposed to air or covered only loosely by clean clothes.
- Keep the diaper folded below the cord to prevent contamination.
- Clean the cord if it becomes soiled with urine or stool.
- Dry the cord thoroughly after each cleansing.

Although some healthcare facilities still apply topical agents such as alcohol or triple dye to the cord, these have not been found to speed separation or to decrease infection. The use of such agents is potentially injurious and is not supported by research or recommended for routine use in developed countries (AWHONN, 2007a). Research continues on best practices related to umbilical cord care, however, and home-care nurses should review the literature frequently.

The nurse should teach the parents to inspect the cord during each diaper change and bath. Parents can be reassured that the stump may smell earthy as it necroses and that it might have a small amount of "cloudy mucoid material" (AWHONN, 2007a) at the stump. The parents should consult their healthcare provider immediately if they notice drainage from the stump or at the point of attachment, if the cord or drainage smells foul, or if they notice redness, swelling, or other discoloration of the surrounding skin. This could indicate omphalitis (infection of the umbilical cord stump) or necrotizing fasciitis (soft tissue infection), potentially fatal complications. Signs of systemic infection such as fever, inability to maintain temperature, poor feeding, or lethargy should always be reported. Parents should also notify the provider if the cord doesn't fall off within 2 weeks, or if the area fails to heal within 2 or 3 days of separation (AWHONN, 2007a).

Nail Care

During the first days of life, the nails may adhere to the skin of the fingers, and cutting is contraindicated. Within a week the nails separate from the skin and frequently break off. If the nails are long or if the newborn is scratching his or her face, the nails may be gently filed using a newborn file. This is most easily done while the infant is asleep. Newborn socks or mittens may be used to cover the newborn's hands and prevent facial scratching.

Dressing the Newborn

Newborns need to wear a T-shirt, diaper (diaper cover if using cloth diapers), and a sleeper. At home, the temperature determines the amount of clothing the newborn wears. Families who maintain their home at 60°F to 65°F should dress the infant more warmly than those who maintain a temperature of 70°F or higher.

Newborns should wear a head covering outdoors to protect their sensitive ears from drafts and to prevent heat loss. Parents can wrap a blanket around the baby, leaving one corner free to place over the head for added protection while outdoors or in crowds. The nurse must advise families about the ease with which a newborn's skin can burn when exposed to the sun. To prevent sunburn, the newborn should remain shaded, wear a light layer of clothing, or be protected with sunscreen specifically formulated for infants. Many healthcare professionals, however, recommend avoiding sunscreen until the infant is at least 6 months old.

Diaper shapes vary and are subject to personal preference. Prefolded and disposable diapers are usually rectangular. Cloth diapers may also be triangular or kite-folded. Extra material is placed in front for males and toward the back for females to increase absorbency.

Baby clothing should be laundered separately with a mild soap or detergent. Diapers are generally presoaked before washing. All clothing should be rinsed twice to remove soap and residue and to decrease the possibility of rash. Some newborns may not tolerate clothing treated with fabric softeners added to the washer or dryer.

Temperature Assessment, Fever, and Illness

As the nurse prepares to teach parents about taking their baby's temperature, it is important to provide opportunities for discussion and demonstration. Families often need a review of how to take their infant's temperature and when to call their primary healthcare provider.

CLINICAL TIP

Dressing a newborn baby with a T-shirt may be quite a challenge. The T-shirt is first pulled over the baby's head. The next challenge is getting the arms in the sleeves, because the newborn grasps at the fabric of the T-shirt as you try to pull it over the hands and arms. It helps to put your hand through the right sleeve of the T-shirt and hold the baby's right hand. Then pull the sleeve over your hand. Repeat the same movements for the left sleeve.

Parents need to take the newborn's temperature only when signs of illness are present. Axillary temperatures are used to determine temperature stability and readiness for discharge in healthy newborns, and a newborn axillary temperature of 36.5°C to 37.4°C (97.7°F to 99.3°F) is considered normal (AAP & ACOG, 2007). Although the axillary temperature doesn't correlate closely with the rectal temperature, this method is convenient, easy for parents to employ, and poses low risk to the newborn.

The rectal method is considered the gold standard for measuring temperatures of febrile infants, as rectal temperature is closer to the true core temperature found in the pulmonary artery and the bladder, but it carries the risk of rectal trauma, which can result in rare but life-threatening perforation, hemorrhage, or necrotizing fasciitis (Christensen, Pysher, & Christensen, 2007; De Curtis, Calzolari, Marciano, et al., 2008; Hutton et al., 2009). Some parents are comfortable taking rectal temperatures, whereas others prefer using the axillary method.

Parents may ask the home-care nurse for information about how to measure their baby's temperature if he or she seems sick. Tympanic thermometer measurements have not been found to be accurate in young infants, so they are not recommended. Although the infrared skin thermometer used on the forehead shows promise, further research is needed (De Curtis et al., 2008; Hutton et al., 2009). Some parents use skin palpation to determine temperature. This is not a reliable way to measure fevers in young infants, yet a study demonstrated that parents were usually able to determine the absence of a fever by using palpation (Katz-Sidlow, Rowberry, & Ho, 2009).

In the absence of one best answer, the nurse can recommend that parents purchase a new thermometer that is designed to measure infant temperature. It is helpful for nurses to periodically check thermometer availability at local retailers and review current academic and manufacturers' literature. The parents may also want to discuss their choice of temperature measurement location and type of thermometer with their primary healthcare provider.

The nurse should ensure that parents do not plan to use a mercury thermometer. Breakage of mercury thermometers has caused symptomatic mercury poisoning in children and adults, and improper disposal contributes to environmental contamination (Agency for Toxic Substances and Disease Registry [ATSDR], 2009; U.S. Environmental Protection Agency [EPA], 2009). Mercury thermometers should not be used or kept in homes and should be disposed of at a hazardous waste collection site. Digital thermometers provide a safe alternative. The nurse should ask parents if they are aware of the hazards of mercury thermometers during the safety assessment and inform parents of local programs or hazardous waste facilities where the thermometers may be turned in. Parents can contact their local health department or review Web sites for the EPA or Centers for Disease Control (CDC) if they need additional information.

Parents should use the same thermometer and measurement site during the course of one illness in order to more accurately monitor trends in the infant's temperature. The parents should inform the pediatric healthcare provider of the temperature, the site, and the type of thermometer used. Most healthcare providers will verify an axillary temperature with a rectal measurement when evaluating an infant for fever.

Traditionally, a rectal temperature of 38°C (100.4°F) has been considered a fever. Because newborns under 90 days of age, and particularly those under 30 days of age, are at high risk for serious bacterial infections, the nurse should tell parents to see their healthcare provider if their newborn has a rectal temperature of 100.4°F or greater or an axillary temperature of 99.4°F or greater. It will be important for the parents to document the measured temperature, time of measurement, and the method used. Parents can expect that their baby will receive a febrile workup if less than 3 months of age and will be admitted for a workup and observation if less than 1 month of age (Berkowitz, 2007).

Parents need to be informed that newborns with systemic infection may not be febrile but may exhibit more subtle manifestations such as temperature instability, poor feeding, abdominal distention, inability to tolerate feedings, apnea, or alterations in behavior such as irritability or lethargy. A baby who is feeding poorly or just not acting right, even in the absence of a fever, may be exhibiting signs of potentially serious infection. Therefore, parents of young infants should call their primary care provider immediately for any signs of illness and/or fever, rather than treating the infant at home.

Parents of older babies will want to discuss the management of colds, flu, teething, constipation, diarrhea, and other common ailments with their clinician before they occur. Although fevers in otherwise healthy older babies do not necessarily require treatment with antipyretics, their healthcare providers can make recommendations regarding over-the-counter analgesics and antipyretic medications, such as acetaminophen or ibuprofen, to increase comfort as necessary.

Aspirin is not recommended, as it was noted to be associated with Reye's syndrome in children with varicella or influenza. The use of ibuprofen or acetaminophen is not contraindicated in infants, but the nurse should instruct parents not to give any medications to a child under 2 years of age without first discussing it with their healthcare provider (Turkoski, 2007). As noted previously, infants under 3 months of age should see a provider for any measured fever or other signs of illness.

The home-care nurse should caution the parents not to administer any over-the-counter (OTC) cough or cold medications to their baby. Use of such OTC antihistamine and decongestant preparations has not been adequately researched in young children, package instructions have been misinterpreted by parents, and administration has been associated with adverse reactions and death in some cases. Therefore, the parents should talk with their healthcare provider regarding the management of coughs and colds. Additionally, parents should never give young children any medication designed for adult use, and parents should not give more than one medication concurrently to their child unless prescribed by their provider (Lokker et al., 2009; Ryan, Brewer, & Small, 2008; U.S. Food and Drug Administration [FDA], 2008a, 2008b).

Stools and Urine

The appearance and frequency of a newborn's stools can cause concern for parents. The nurse prepares them by discussing and showing pictures of meconium stools and transitional stools and by describing the difference between breast milk and formula stools. Although each baby develops his or her own stooling patterns, parents can get an idea of what to expect (see Figure 29-13 ∞ on page 774).

- Babies can be expected to have at least one meconium stool on the first day of life and at least two during the second 24 hours. Three to four stools can be expected each day by 3 to 5 days of age, and three to six stools per day on days 5 through 7 and thereafter (AAP & ACOG, 2007). Stools progress from meconium on the first 2 days to transitional (greenish-brown) stools, to mushy yellow and seedy. Once breastfeeding is well established, usually by 1 month of age, individual babies vary in their stooling patterns. Constipation is unlikely to occur in newborns receiving only breast milk. Infrequent stooling in the first few weeks may indicate inadequate milk intake.
- Formula-fed babies may have only 1 or 2 stools a day; their stools are more formed and may be darker yellow or brown in color

The nurse can show parents pictures of a constipated stool (small, pelletlike) and diarrhea (watery, loose, green). Families should understand that a green color is common in transitional stools so that they do not mistake transitional stools for diarrhea during the first week of a newborn's life.

Babies normally void (urinate) at least once in the first 24 hours and at least twice in the second 24 hours. At least three to five daily voids can be expected on days 3 through 5 and four to six daily voids on days 5 through 7 (AAP & ACOG, 2007).

By the fifth day of life and thereafter, the newborn can be expected to have five or more wet diapers per day. Fewer may indicate that the newborn needs more fluids. Frequency of voiding is easy to assess with cloth diapers. Parents who use superabsorbent single-use disposable diapers may have difficulty determining voiding patterns because the surface of the diaper feels dry. The liquid pools inside the filling of the diaper. Parents can pull the top layer off to check whether the filling is saturated. Although pink or orange uric acid crystals may be found in the diaper during the first few days of life, the presence of crystals beyond the third or fourth day may indicate inadequate hydration.

Diaper Area Care

The diaper area should be cleansed and well dried with each diaper change. Frequent diaper changes minimize contact between the skin and urine or stool, and decrease the risk of diaper dermatitis (DD)—often referred to by parents as diaper rash. It is also helpful to allow the infant to spend short periods of time air-drying with the diaper off in order to prevent maceration and irritation. Minimal soap is required when cleaning the diaper area, and scrubbing should be avoided. If the parents use commercial diaper wipes, they should be alcohol-free. If an emollient with petrolatum is routinely used as a barrier to protect the skin in the diaper area, the parents do not need to scrub all of it off with each diaper change. The urine and feces should be removed from the barrier, and an additional layer of the barrier can be applied once the area is clean and dry (Friedlander, Eichenfield, Leyden, et al., 2009).

Even with proper care many babies experience some type of diaper rash. This can take the form of a contact dermatitis, otherwise known as irritant diaper dermatitis (IDD), a localized, nonimmunologic reaction to the friction, occlusion, moisture, urine, feces, and chemicals in the diaper environment. Moisturizers such as petrolatum provide protection from wetness and promote healing of mildly irritated skin. If diaper rash occurs, the parents should also apply a protective skin barrier containing zinc oxide to prevent further injury. A thin layer of petrolatum can be placed on top of the zinc oxide layer to prevent the diaper from sticking. Fecal material and urine should be removed with each diaper change, but the skin barrier should be maintained if possible and reapplied as necessary.

A variety of commercial newborn care barrier products are available, which contain either petrolatum or zinc oxide. Some products also contain lanolin, which protects the skin but may be allergenic to some infants. The nurse can recommend a commercial product or tell the parents to choose one with petrolatum and another with zinc oxide. Parents should read labels and avoid over-the-counter ointments containing corticosteroids, as their use can be hazardous to newborns (AWHONN, 2007a; Friedlander et al., 2009).

Commercial disposable diapers have improved greatly over the years to keep newborns dry. This generally decreases the incidence of DD, but some newborns may develop an allergic response to fragrances, dyes, or rubber in diapers (Friedlander et al., 2009). Therefore, parents may want to try switching brands of diapers if the DD persists. If the family uses cloth diapers, a different mild detergent, more thorough rinsing, and hanging them in the sun to dry may alleviate the problem.

When the rash is severe or persists beyond 2 to 3 days despite the treatment above, the parents should contact their healthcare provider. DD is frequently complicated by *Candida albicans,* particularly in infants who have recently had diarrhea, oral thrush, or antibiotic exposure. If this is the case, the provider can prescribe Vusion, a topical agent including miconazole, zinc oxide, and petrolatum, which was approved by the FDA for the treatment of DD complicated by *C. albicans* in 2006 (Aschenbrenner & Venable, 2009; Friedlander et al., 2009). Persistent DD should receive further evaluation to rule out rare metabolic, nutritional, or cutaneous disorders; or malignancies (Friedlander et al., 2009).

Sleeping

When, where, and for how long their baby sleeps are common concerns of parents. The following sections address SIDS prevention, crib safety, cosleeping, and the proper positioning of a baby for sleep. The newborn's sleep-wake states are then described.

Sudden Infant Death Syndrome (SIDS) Prevention

Sudden infant death syndrome (SIDS) is defined as "the sudden unexpected death of an infant less than 1 year of age, with onset of the fatal episode apparently occurring during sleep, that remains unexplained after a thorough investigation, including performance of a complete autopsy and review of the circumstances of death and the clinical history" (Krous et al., as cited by Mitchell, 2009, p. 215).

The causes of SIDS are multifactorial and not fully understood. An extensive review of the literature from the past several decades noted that "thermal stress, rebreathing of expired gases, and infection seem the most viable hypotheses for the mechanisms of SIDS" at this point in time (Mitchell, 2009, p. 216). SIDS occurring during prone positioning appears to have a thermal component. As discussed later in this chapter, babies should sleep on their backs as recommended by the AAP and should not be overheated by the use of heavy clothing or blankets during sleep (Omojokun & Moon, 2008).

The AAP published a number of additional recommendations to prevent SIDS in 2005, which will be discussed in the following paragraphs. The AAP recommended a standard sleep surface such as a firm crib mattress that is covered only with a sheet. The infant should sleep in a separate crib or a bassinet next to the parent's bed, a practice which is known as *room sharing* without *bed sharing* (Fu, Colson, Corwin, et al., 2008, p. 503). **Room sharing** is when the infant sleeps in the same room in close proximity to the parents. Soft crib materials and makeshift bedding composed of pillows, comforters, sheepskin, quilts, or similar items should not be used. Infant toys, stuffed animals, and loose blankets and sheets should be removed from the crib as well. If a lightweight blanket is used, it should be secured by tucking it under the mattress. The blanket should not come higher than chest level on a sleeping infant to ensure it does not cover the infant's face. Parents may be advised to instead use sleep clothing or sleep sacks to reduce the danger from unsecured blankets. Nurses should educate parents about the need to maintain proper temperature for the infant, because overheating is also a risk factor for SIDS (Mitchell, 2009; National Institute of Child Health and Human Development [NICHD], 2008; Omojokun & Moon, 2008).

Although a number of positioning devices have been marketed to decrease the risk of SIDS, their efficacy and safety has not been demonstrated, and they are not recommended. Some children require home monitoring for health reasons, but monitors are not recommended for the purpose of SIDS reduction (Omojokun & Moon, 2008).

"After prone sleeping position, maternal smoking is the next major modifiable risk factor for SIDS" (Mitchell, 2009, p. 217). Numerous studies have shown that women who smoke while pregnant have a much greater incidence of having a baby die of SIDS than do nonsmokers. Smoking should be avoided in the home and around children to minimize SIDS risk as well as the numerous additional risks of secondhand smoke. Adequate ventilation in and around the crib should be provided.

The AAP also recommends giving infants a pacifier when napping or sleeping, because the use of pacifiers has decreased the incidence of SIDS. Parents should be advised that the pacifier does not need to be reinserted once it falls out after the infant has fallen asleep. The pacifier should not be coated with sweet substances or sugar, and it should be cleaned and replaced frequently. Infants who do not wish to use a pacifier should not be forced to do so. The incidence of SIDS is very low in the first month of life, so introduction of the pacifier can be delayed until 1 month of age in breastfeeding infants to prevent issues with lactation (Damato, 2007).

These recommendations are for healthy infants, and parents should follow them unless otherwise directed by their health-care provider in response to a particular medical condition. Nurses have the opportunity to assess for risk factors in the home environment and to educate families, particularly patients in groups at high risk for SIDS. Parents can be encouraged to attend infant cardiopulmonary resuscitation (CPR) classes, especially if there is a family history of SIDS, prematurity, or another health problem.

Families often ask nurses additional questions about SIDS, such as whether immunizations are a risk factor. The nurse can reassure the parents that the incidence of SIDS is less in fully immunized infants, and that they can follow current immunization recommendations with confidence (Vennemann, Hoffgen, Bajanowski, et al., 2007). Parents can find additional information at the National Institute of Child Health and Human Development (NICHD) and National Institutes of Health (NIH) Web sites.

The SIDS rate in African Americans continues to remain higher than that in other races. African American mothers have higher rates of bed sharing and are less likely to place their infants on the back to sleep than are other mothers. Cultural values and socioeconomic status may play a role in compliance. Nurses need to reinforce recommendations for placing babies on their backs to sleep, room sharing without bed sharing, and avoidance of smoking. Home-care nurses should inform parents of free crib distribution programs if available, and nurses should work with local agencies and charitable organizations to make approved cribs accessible to low-income families as needed (Bruckner, 2008; Fu, et al., 2008). Research regarding possible genetic links for SIDS in the African American population is ongoing (Cummings, et al., 2009). The NICHD provides a SIDS prevention pamphlet targeted for African American families, which can be downloaded from their Web site.

Crib Safety

During the home visit, the nurse discusses with the family their newborn's sleeping arrangements, and observes the crib, bassinet, cradle, mat, or other devices. If possible, the nurse should observe the infant while sleeping to ensure all safety precautions are being followed.

Parents will want to make certain that their infant's crib meets all federal safety standards as set by the Consumer Product Safety Commission and ASTM (formerly the American Society for Testing and Materials). The crib headboard and footboard should be solid, with no large designs cut out of the wood, as the infant's head could become entrapped in them. Crib slats should be no more than 2 inches apart. If the crib is older and painted, ensure that the paint is not lead-based. If there is any doubt, the crib should not be used unless it is stripped and painted with new lead-free enamel. It is important for parents to be aware that safety regulations today are different from those in years past and that there are safety issues associated with the use of an old crib.

Mattresses should fit snugly to prevent entrapment and suffocation and should always be lowered to a level at which the infant cannot fall out (Forsythe, Maher, Kirchick et al., 2007). Parents should always leave the side rails up when the baby is in the crib, even if they are in the room. Although the Consumer Product Safety Commission issues guidelines for crib safety, safety standards have not been changed since 1982, although changes are expected to be made in late 2010 (Michon, 2010). Parents should inspect the crib regularly to determine whether it is in safe working order, with no splinters, sharp edges, or loose parts. Parents can go to the Consumer Product Safety Commission Web site to check for information about infant products and to sign up for e-mail notifications of updates and recalls.

Cosleeping

The nurse should be aware that the topic of maternal infant cosleeping, which has been the norm in many cultures for centuries, has become a source of debate in the United States and Canada in recent years. The term has a variety of meanings and is sometimes used interchangeably with bed sharing. According to McKenna, Thoman, & Anders (as cited by the Academy of Breastfeeding Medicine Protocol Committee [ABM], 2008), **cosleeping** refers to an infant sleeping "in close social and/or physical contact with a caregiver (usually the mother)" (p. 38). Cosleeping may include sharing any surface, such as a bed, mat, futon, or floor. Bed sharing has been implicated in cases of SIDS and is not recommended by the AAP. **Bed sharing** (mother and infant sharing the same bed) is just one form of cosleeping, however, as cosleeping may also include the infant sleeping on a separate piece of furniture in close proximity to the parent (ABM, 2008).

RESEARCH EVIDENCE IN PRACTICE Bedsharing with an Infant

CLINICAL QUESTION

What are the risks associated with sharing a bed with an infant?

RESEARCH EVIDENCE

Bed sharing with an infant remains a controversial topic. Yet, in one longitudinal study, more than a third of mothers reported frequent bed sharing with their infants, and two thirds reported sometimes sharing their beds with their babies. Mothers who breastfeed are twice as likely to bring their babies to bed with them.

Concerns have been raised about the association of bed sharing, sudden infant death syndrome (SIDS), and infant suffocation. Indeed, in one study, 13% of parents reported that they rolled onto or partly onto their infants while bed sharing. Still, these proposed associations with serious infant outcomes have not been confirmed by carefully controlled studies. Nine large-scale case-control studies focused on the relationship between bed sharing and SIDS. Three found no increased risk for SIDS. Six of the studies reported an increased incidence of SIDS in bed sharing with smoking mothers, but it was not possible to discriminate the effects of smoking from those of bed sharing. The risk of infant suffocation was increased for infants less than 11 weeks of age, but there was no statistical association between suffocation and bed sharing with infants older than 3 months.

In some cultures, bed sharing is commonplace and accepted. Hispanics, African Americans, and Asian/Pacific Islanders all bed share at higher rates than Caucasian women. Some women bed share due to economic limitations. Single mothers and mothers with an annual income of less than $30,000 were nearly twice as likely to bed share as their more economically advantaged counterparts.

One key issue is the finding that maternal sleep is hampered when bed sharing with an infant. Mothers report sleeping more lightly and feeling less rested when their infants share their beds.

WHAT QUESTIONS REMAIN UNANSWERED?

Are there long-term psychologic or physical effects from extensive bed sharing during infancy?

WHAT IS BEST PRACTICE?

Smoking mothers should be counseled to avoid sleeping with their infants at any age. Nonsmoking mothers, however, should not be pressured to abstain from bed sharing with their older infants (3 months or older). Mothers should be counseled that their own sleep will be enhanced if the infant sleeps in a separate bed, but that the risk of SIDS and suffocation are not increased with bed sharing of older infants.

CRITICAL THINKING

Under what conditions should a mother be counseled not to bed share at all?

References

Ateah, A., & Hamelin, K. 2008. Maternal bedsharing practices, experiences, and awareness of risks. *JOGNN: Journal of Obstetric, Gynecologic, and Neonatal Nursing, 37*(3), 274–281.

Lahr, M., Rosenberg, K., & Lapidus, J. 2005. Bedsharing and maternal smoking in a population-based survey of new mothers. *Pediatrics, 116*(4), e530–e542.

Lahr, M., Rosenberg, K., & Lapidus, J. 2007. Maternal infant bedsharing: Risk factors for bedsharing in a population-based survey of new mothers and implications for SIDS risk reduction. *Maternal and Child Health Journal, 11*(3), 277–286.

The ABM (2008) has urged continued research, rather than an across-the-board policy against bed sharing, because sleeping in close proximity increases the frequency and duration of breastfeeding throughout the night. The organization noted that many of the cases of SIDS that occurred during bed sharing involved parents who smoked, were overtired, or under the influence of substances; involved the infant sleeping prone; or involved unsafe surfaces such as couches or waterbeds. The ABM suggested that cosleeping on a firm mattress on the floor might decrease risks related to entrapment and suffocation. Infant beds that attach to the side of the adult bed are available, but have not been researched for safety and efficacy.

Ateah and Hamelin (2008) surveyed 293 mothers of young infants. Despite the fact that 89% of them knew of the risks associated with bed sharing, 72% of the women reported sleeping with their infants at one point or another, in many cases during and/or following a nighttime breastfeeding. Thirteen percent of these women reported a close call, in which they or the father rolled onto their infant or the infant became covered by linens, particularly when the parents were very tired. The researchers published the following clinical implications of bed sharing based on their findings: (a) nurses should promote the practice of infant supine sleep in an approved crib in the parent's room, (b) cosleeping in a crib next to the parent's bed offers convenience to breastfeeding mothers without the risks of bed sharing, (c) recommendations for safe bed sharing cannot be provided, as issues such as maternal exhaustion and infant overheating are not within the parent's control, (d) parents should be informed about the risks of bed sharing as well as the recommendations of the AAP and the Canadian Pediatric Society, and (e) increased public education is needed regarding the benefits of cosleeping by room sharing without bed sharing (p. 280).

As the research continues, the AAP recommendations and those offered by Ateah and Hamelin (2008), which were published in *JOGNN: The Journal of Obstetric, Gynecologic, and Neonatal Nursing,* provide excellent guidance for home-care nurses when educating parents on SIDS prevention and safe infant sleep practices.

PROFESSIONALISM IN PRACTICE

Educating Parents About Bed Sharing

Parents will sometimes inform nurses that they intend to sleep with their infants in the bed for ease of breastfeeding or for personal reasons despite recommendations. It is important for nurses to realize that parents will make their own decisions regarding parenting, yet parent education remains a nursing responsibility. Nurses must make parents aware of AAP recommendations for supine sleep and room sharing without bed sharing, so the parents can make informed decisions regarding their newborn's safety within the context of current research, their culture, and personal beliefs.

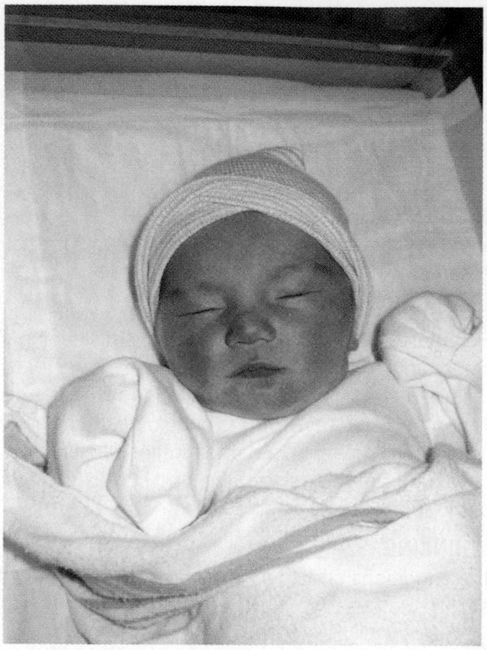

Figure 37-4 ■ Infants should be placed on their backs when sleeping.

Proper Positioning

Newborns and infants should always be placed in the supine position to sleep, as recommended by the AAP since 1992 (Figure 37-4 ∞). Deaths related to SIDS have dramatically decreased since the initiation of "Back to Sleep" campaigns around the globe. However, an increase in the number of children with cranial asymmetry, particularly unilateral flattening of the occiput, has been noted since the campaign began. Some parents resist supine positioning due to concerns about flattening their baby's head (Hutchison, Stewart, & Mitchell, 2007).

Parents should therefore be counseled within the newborn's first 2 to 4 weeks of life to place their infant in the prone position to allow "tummy time" while the infant is awake and under their direct observation (Omojokun & Moon, 2008). This position will promote upper shoulder girdle strength and will help to prevent the development of flat areas on the occiput.

Parents can also be taught to alternate their infant's head position from right to left each night when placing the newborn supine for sleep. Periodically changing the infant's orientation to outside activity such as the bedroom door will encourage the infant to use more than one head position to sleep and rest. This can be accomplished by placing the infant at alternate ends of the crib or bassinet. The home-care nurse can demonstrate these positions for the parents, reinforce the importance of supine sleep in relation to SIDS prevention, and give parents other ideas for carrying and positioning, such as the use of front packs, backpacks, and slings. Parents should read and follow all product information provided by the manufacturer.

Some parents may resist supine positioning due to fears about aspiration. The nurse can encourage parents to hold their infants upright for 10 to 15 minutes following feedings. Additionally, the parents can be reassured that infant deaths related to aspiration have decreased since "Back to Sleep" was initiated (Hutchison, Stewart, & Mitchell, 2007).

Many mothers return to the workforce during the first year of their newborn's life, so the nurse should remind parents to educate caregivers and family members who will care for the newborn in their absence about the importance of supine sleep positioning and insist that it is practiced with their child.

Sleep-Wake States

The newborn demonstrates several different sleep-wake states after the initial periods of reactivity. It is not uncommon for a newborn to sleep almost continuously for the first 2 to 3 days following birth, awakening only for feedings every 3 to 4 hours. Some newborns bypass this stage of deep sleep and require only 12 to 16 hours of sleep. The parents need to know that this is normal.

Sleep states include deep sleep and light sleep. During **deep sleep** the infant will be nearly still except for occasional startles, twitches, and sucking. The infant will arouse to intense stimuli, and care and feeding at this time will be frustrating. **Light sleep** makes up the highest proportion of newborn sleep and usually precedes awakening. It is characterized by some body movements, rapid eye movements (REM), and brief fussing or crying. The infant may arouse, remain in light sleep, or return to deep sleep in response to stimuli. Infants are not usually ready to feed in this state.

Awake states include drowsy awake, quiet alert, active alert, and crying states. During the **drowsy awake state**, infants open and close their eyes, but the eyes appear glazed and the face is often still. They may return to sleep or awaken further in response to stimuli. The **quiet alert state** (also called *wide awake state*) is characterized by a brightening of the eyes and face. Infants are most attentive to their environment in this state and provide positive feedback to caregivers. This is an optimal state during which to initiate breast feeds (Koehn & Riordan, 2010). The **active alert state** (also called *active awake state*) brings about an increase in facial and body movement, with periods of fussiness occurring. The infant in this state has increased sensitivity to disturbing stimuli, and intervention to console the infant at this point is beneficial. The **crying state** is evidenced by increased motor activity, grimaces, eyes tightly closed or open, and extreme responsiveness to stimuli. Infants may be able to console themselves, or they may require consoling from a caregiver.

For newborns, crying is a spontaneous response to unpleasant stimuli, and their only means of expressing their needs vocally. After 2 or 3 days, newborns settle into individual patterns and families learn to distinguish different tones and qualities of their newborn's cry. The amount of crying is also highly individual. Some newborns cry as little as 15 to 30 minutes in 24 hours, or as long as 2 or more hours. When crying continues after causes such as discomfort and hunger are eliminated, the newborn may be comforted by swaddling, rocking, or other reassuring activities. There is some indication that newborns who are held more tend to be calmer and cry less when not being held. Some parents may be afraid that holding will "spoil" the newborn, and need reassurance that this is not the case. On the contrary, picking babies up when they cry teaches them that adults are responsive to them. This helps build a sense of trust in humankind. Of course, the nurse documents and assesses any crying, and provides teaching and referrals as necessary. See Table 37-4 for the characteristics and caregiving implication of each state.

> “It was so exciting to go home with our new baby. That first day went quite well, and Joe and I felt that we were on our way as new parents. Our son had been fed and diapered a number of times, and it was now time for bed. When we snuggled him in his bassinet, he lay quietly and didn't cry. Then we looked at each other and at the same time said, "What if we don't hear him in the middle of the night?" We went on to bed but with much trepidation. Our baby's first cry in the night woke us immediately. We both sat up and simultaneously said, "There he is!"
>
> After a few weeks, we could laugh at the anxiety we had during those first few days. I'm sure all new parents must have had similar experiences.”

Injury Prevention

Accidental injuries were the fifth leading cause of death in infants under 1 year of age in the United States in 2004 and the sixth leading cause of death in this age group in 2005 (Mathews & MacDorman, 2008). The top five most common fatal injuries in infants under 1 year of age in 2005 included unintentional suffocation, motor vehicle accidents, unspecified homicide, classifiable homicide, and drowning. The top five most common nonfatal accidental injuries in infants under 1 year of age who were treated in U.S. emergency departments in 2006 were falls, strikes, bites or stings, foreign bodies, and fires/burns (National Center for Injury Prevention and Control, Centers for Disease Control & Prevention, n.d. [page updated 15 July 09]). It is helpful to keep these causes of injury in mind when counseling new parents regarding safety in the home.

During the home visit, the nurse can share information regarding common injuries and accidents that occur in infants as well as how to prevent them from occurring. The parents should have been instructed on car seat safety before leaving the birthing unit, and the nurse can confirm this. It is essential that the parents understand never to leave a baby unattended on any elevated surface, near water, or near pets or other children who may unintentionally harm them.

If time allows, the nurse observes the environment and identifies future changes that need to be made to childproof the home. Safety related to electrical outlets, appliances, and sources of danger in kitchens and bathrooms will need to be addressed as the infant becomes mobile. Poisonous substances and medications should be secured. It is important for nurses to be aware of the impact they can have on the safety of families through home visits.

Shaken Baby Syndrome

Shaken baby syndrome (SBS) is a traumatic brain injury that results from violent shaking, with or without contact between the infant's head and an exterior surface. Swelling and bleeding are the result, and the infant may sustain permanent neurologic damage. SBS results in death in approximately 20% of cases (Lewin, 2008; Mraz, 2009). The AAP has made a number of recommendations to address and prevent shaken baby injuries, including home visitation programs and any other child abuse prevention efforts that prove efficacious. The Shaken Baby Syndrome Prevention Act of 2007 was introduced in the U.S. 110th legislative session, but did not pass. However, a number of states have passed legislative preventive programs (Govtrack, n.d.; National Conference of State Legislatures, 2009). A variety of educational preventive programs have been introduced by nurses to educate parents and communities regarding the risks of SBS (Goulet, et al., 2009; Smith & deGuehery, 2008).

Risks for SBS include infants who are inconsolable, fragile, premature, special needs, and/or male. Parental risk factors include male caregiver; less educated, young, substance-abusing, poorly supported, or single parent; history of domestic violence; depression; unrealistic expectations; or the belief that the infant is intentionally manipulative (Carbaugh, as cited by Lewin, 2008). Home visits provide an excellent opportunity to educate parents regarding safety and injury prevention, shaken baby injuries, and the hazards of abuse and neglect. Nurses need to directly inform parents to never shake a baby. Home visits are also the ideal time to provide appropriate resources and referrals to local preventive educational and support programs. Home-care nurses can access parent information from sources such as the Web site of the National Center on Shaken Baby Syndrome.

Infant Colic as a Parental Stressor

Infant colic is manifested by persistent, unexplained, inconsolable crying, that can continue for several hours each day, often occurring in the evening. It is a source of great distress and anxiety to new parents, as the colicky infant does not respond to usual methods of soothing. Colic can emerge by 2 to 3 weeks of age, and it can continue until the infant is 4 to 6 months of age. The etiology is unknown, but is believed by many to be gastrointestinal in nature (Cohen-Silver & Ratnapalan, 2009; Jarvis, 2008). Research investigating the differences in the microorganisms found in the gastrointestinal tracts of colicky versus non-colicky infants is ongoing and shows promise (Mentula, Tuure, Koskenala, et al., 2008; Savino et al., 2008).

Interventions including dietary modifications in the infant and/or the breastfeeding mother; administration of pharmacologic agents such as simethicone and anticholinergics; administration of herbal preparations, sucrose, and probiotics; infant massage; vibration of the infant; carrying; changes in the amount and type of infant stimulation; and parental support have been used and researched. Definitive treatment guidelines have not been developed, however (Arikan, Alp, Gözüm, et al., 2008; Cohen-Silver & Ratnapalan, 2009).

Catherine, Ko, and Barr (2008) found 51 articles in 11 parenting magazines popular in Canada and the United States that addressed crying, colic, soothing, or SBS over a 5-year period. The articles presented contradictory advice regarding the etiology and treatment of colic, perhaps reflecting the current state of

TABLE 37-4 Infant Sleep and Awake States*

INFANT STATES	PHYSICAL CHARACTERISTICS	BODY ACTIVITY	EYE MOVEMENTS	FACIAL MOVEMENTS	BREATHING PATTERN	RESPONSES	CAREGIVER IMPLICATIONS
Sleep States							
Quiet sleep (also known as deep sleep)	Anabolic, restorative sleep, increased cell mitosis and replication, lowered oxygen consumption, release of growth hormone.	Typically still, may occasionally startle or twitch.	None.	None or may have occasional sucking movements.	Slow and regular.	Only intense or disturbing stimuli will arouse infant, threshold to stimuli is high.	Difficult to arouse for feedings. Teach parents to time feedings when infant is in a more responsive state. Infant may arouse slightly if an attempt is made to awaken but typically returns to the quiet sleep state.
Active sleep (also light sleep or known as rapid eye movement [REM] state)	Processing and recording information. Often linked to learning. Is the highest proportion of sleep and precedes awakening.	Some body movements.	REM, eyelids flutter beneath closed eyelids.	May smile or make fussing or crying noises.	Irregular.	More responsive to internal stimuli (hunger) and external stimuli (such as being picked up by caregiver). When stimulated may arouse, return to quiet sleep, or remain in active sleep.	Inexperienced care providers may attempt to feed when infant makes normal crying sounds.
Awake States							
Drowsy awake	May return to sleep or awaken further.	Smooth movements with variable activity level. May experience mild startles intermittently.	Eyes may open and close. May appear heavy-lidded, or eyes may appear like slits.	May have no facial movements and appear still, or may have some facial movements.	Irregular.	Usually reacts to stimuli but may be slowed. May change to other states such as quiet alert, active alert, or crying.	To stimulate infant, provide verbal, sight, or oral stimulation. If left alone, infant may return to a sleep state.
Quiet alert (also called *wide awake*)	Attentive to environment, focuses attention on stimuli.	Minimal.	Eyes bright and wide.	Attentive appearance.	Regular.	Most attentive, focuses attention on stimuli.	In the first hours after birth, may experience intense alertness before going into a long sleeping period. This state increases in intensity as the infant becomes older. Providing stimuli will help maintain an active alert state or a drowsy awake or quiet alert state. Infant provides pleasure and positive feedback to care providers. Good time to feed infant.
Active alert (also called *active awake*)	Infant's eyes are open, not as bright as in quiet alert. More body activity than in a quiet alert state.	Smooth movements may be interspersed with mild startles from time to time.	Eyes open with a glazed, dull appearance.	May be still with or without facial movements.	Irregular.	Reacts to stimuli with delayed responses to stimuli, or may change to quiet alert or crying state.	Infant may be fussy and become sensitive to stimuli, may become more and more active and start crying. If fatigue or caregiver interventions disturb this state, infant may return to a drowsy awake or sleep state.
Crying	Communication tool, response to unpleasant stimuli from environment or internal stimuli. Characterized by intense crying for more than 15 seconds.	Increased motor activity, skin color changes to darkened appearance, red, or ruddy.	Eyes may be tightly closed or open.	Grimaces.	More irregular than in other states.	Very responsive to internal or external unpleasant stimuli.	Indicates that the infant's limits have been reached. May be able to console himself or herself and return to an alert or sleep state, or may need intervention from caregiver.

* A *state* is a group of characteristic behaviors and physiologic changes that occur together in a regular pattern.

Source: From Understanding the behavior of term infants. *Copyright © 2003 March of Dimes. Reprinted with permission.*

knowledge about colic. Conflicting information leads to uncertainty and frustration among parents. The authors also expressed concern that very few of the articles mentioned the increased risks of child abuse and SBS related to incessant crying.

It is important for nurses to provide new parents with anticipatory guidance regarding the symptoms of infant colic and the strain that it can cause in family relationships. Parents will want to see their infant's healthcare provider to rule out other causes for prolonged crying, such as urinary tract infection (Freedman, Al-Harthy, & Thull-Freedman, 2009). If no physiologic etiology is found, the parents should be supported and educated regarding the risks of child abuse. Nurses must remind parents to simply lay the baby down safely in his or her crib and take a break if they become frustrated with the crying. Parents should be encouraged to seek support from healthcare providers as well as support from family and friends if colic occurs. It is also important to reassure parents that the condition does resolve in time and that newborns go on to develop normally. Home-care nurses should be aware of local support groups and/or hotlines for colic and share these resources with all new parents.

Newborn Screening and Immunization Program

Before the newborn and mother are discharged from the hospital, the nurse informs parents about the normal screening tests for newborns and tells them when to return for further tests if needed. The home-care nurse ensures that the blood specimens have been obtained and may obtain a specimen as necessary.

Newborn screening tests detect disorders that cause intellectual disability (mental retardation), physical handicaps, or death if left undiscovered. Disorders that can usually be detected from a drop of blood obtained by a heel stick on the second or third day of life include galactosemia, congenital adrenal hyperplasia, congenital hypothyroidism, phenylketonuria (PKU), and sickle cell anemia. Parents should be instructed that a second blood specimen will often be required from the newborn after 7 to 14 days. Nurses should clarify that an abnormal test result is not diagnostic. More definitive tests must be performed to verify the results. It is important to follow protocols that incorporate state laws about newborn testing, as the required screening and protocols vary between states. See chapter 33 ∞ for more information regarding newborn screening.

The nurse should ensure that the family has information regarding the current childhood immunization schedule and has plans to begin or continue immunizations. The nurse should be familiar with current recommendations and should share information about immunizations with the family as necessary.

Home Care: The Mother and Family

Home care of the mother and family involves performing an assessment of the mother and family as well as discussing breastfeeding concerns.

Assessment of the Mother and Family at Home

During the home visit, the nurse will continue the ongoing postpartum assessment that started prior to discharge. The initial goal is to assess the woman's perceptions of her current circumstances, her recovery from childbirth, her adjustment and that of her partner to parenthood, the newborn's condition, family-newborn bonding, and any problems or concerns the woman may have. The nurse asks specifically about the following areas:

- Progression of lochia (color, amount of flow, presence of foul odor or clots)
- Fever or malaise
- Dysuria or difficulty voiding
- Pain in the pelvis or perineum
- Painful, reddened hot spots or shooting pains in the breasts during or between feedings
- Areas of redness, edema, tenderness, or warmth in the legs

The nurse also talks with the mother about her diet, fatigue level, ability to rest and sleep, pain management, signs of postpartal complications, activity level, sexuality issues, self-care ability, social support system, and any pertinent cultural or religious practices related to postpartum or newborn care. Before performing the physical assessment, the nurse ensures privacy. The physical assessment focuses on maternal physical adaptation, which is assessed by evaluating vital signs, heart and lungs, breasts, abdominal musculature, bowel and bladder elimination patterns, fundal height and location, the perineum, lochia, edema, extremities, and laboratory values.

The psychologic assessment focuses on attachment, adjustment to the parental role, maternal emotions, sibling adjustment, and educational needs. When appropriate, the nurse mentions available community resources, including the public health department, which can be used for follow-up visits. In ideal situations, a family approach involving the presence of the father and any siblings provides an opportunity to observe family interactions and opportunities for all family members to ask questions and express concerns. In addition, this approach may bring to the surface any questionable family interaction pattern, such as one suggestive of abuse or neglect; the nurse can consider further referral if needed. See Assessment Guide: Postpartum—First Home Visit and Anticipated Progress at Six Weeks.

During the home visit, the nurse continues to provide teaching to the mother and her family and describes self-care measures as needed. The nurse also reviews the signs of developing illness with the woman and her partner. If signs of potential complications are present, the nurse completes a more in-depth evaluation and determines whether it is necessary for the woman to see her primary care provider. If information about family-planning options has not been addressed previously, the nurse provides it at this time and answers any questions the woman or her partner may have about methods of birth control and their sexual relationship.

Postpartum Fatigue

Postpartum fatigue is a major concern that may trouble new mothers for as long as 19 months postpartum. It is characterized

ASSESSMENT GUIDE Postpartum—First Home Visit and Anticipated Progress at Six Weeks

Physical Assessment/Normal Findings	Alterations and Possible Causes*	Nursing Responses to Data†
VITAL SIGNS		
Blood Pressure: Return to normal prepregnant level.	Elevated blood pressure (anxiety, essential hypertension, renal disease), preeclampsia (can occur postpartum).	Review history, evaluate normal baseline; refer to physician/certified nurse midwife (CNM) if necessary.
Pulse: 60–90 beats/min (or prepregnant normal rate).	Increased pulse rate, tachycardia, chest pain (excitement, anxiety, blood loss, cardiac disorders).	Count pulse for full minute, note irregularities; marked tachycardia or beat irregularities require additional assessment and possible physician/CNM referral.
Respirations: 12–24/min.	Marked tachypnea or abnormal patterns (respiratory or cardiac disorders).	Evaluate for respiratory disease or cardiac complications; refer to physician/CNM if necessary.
Temperature: 36.6°C–37.6°C (98°F–99.6°F).	Increased temperature (infection or engorgement).	Assess for signs and symptoms of infection or disease state.
WEIGHT		
2 days: Possible weight loss of 12–20+ lb.	Minimal weight loss (fluid retention, preeclampsia).	Evaluate for fluid retention, edema, deep tendon reflexes, and blood pressure elevation.
6 weeks: Returning to normal prepregnant weight.	Retained weight (excessive caloric intake).	Determine amount of daily exercise. Provide dietary teaching. Refer to dietitian if necessary for additional dietary counseling.
	Extreme weight loss (excessive dieting, inadequate caloric intake).	Discuss appropriate diets, refer to dietitian for additional counseling if necessary; reinforce need for up to 500 additional kcal/day when breastfeeding.
BREASTS		
Nonbreastfeeding: 2 days: May have mild tenderness; small amount of milk may be expressed.	Some engorgement (incomplete suppression of lactation).	Engorgement may be seen in nonbreastfeeding mothers. Advise patient to wear a supportive, well-fitted bra, avoid very warm showers, avoid pumping or any stimulation of breasts, use ice packs for comfort, evaluate for signs and symptoms of mastitis.
6 weeks: Soft, with no tenderness; return to prepregnant size.	Redness; hardened area, marked tenderness (mastitis). Palpable mass (tumor).	Counsel about nipple care. Observe infant feeding. Evaluate patient condition, evidence of fever; refer to physician/CNM for initiation of antibiotic therapy, if indicated. A breastfeeding mother should examine her breasts monthly, after feeding, when breasts are empty; if palpable mass is felt, refer to physician for further evaluation.
Breastfeeding: Full, with prominent nipples; lactation established.	Cracked, fissured nipples (improper latch). Redness, marked tenderness, hardened area (mastitis or abscess). Palpable mass (plugged milk duct, tumor).	For breast engorgement accompanied by erythema, instruct the mother to: 1. Keep breast empty by frequent feeding. 2. Rest when possible with breasts elevated. 3. Take prescribed pain relief med. 4. Drink adequate fluids. If symptoms persist for more than 24 hours, or if accompanied by fever greater than 100.4°F, or flu-like symptoms, redness, instruct her to call her physician/CNM.
ABDOMINAL MUSCULATURE		
2 days: Improved firmness, although "bread dough" consistency is not unusual, especially in multipara.	Marked relaxation of muscles.	Evaluate exercise level; provide information on appropriate exercise program.
Striae pink and obvious.		
Cesarean incision healing.	Drainage, redness, tenderness, pain, edema (infection).	Evaluate for infection; refer to physician/CNM if necessary.
6 weeks: Muscle tone continues to improve; striae may be beginning to fade, may not achieve a silvery appearance for several more weeks; linea nigra fading.		
ELIMINATION PATTERN		
Urinary Tract: Return to prepregnant urinary elimination routine.	Urinary incontinence, especially when lifting, coughing, laughing, and so on (urethral/perineal trauma, hormonal influences, cystocele).	Assess for cystocele; instruct in appropriate muscle tightening exercises; refer to physician/CNM.
	Pain or burning when voiding, urgency and/or frequency, pus or white blood cells (WBC) in urine, pathogenic organisms in culture (stinging may be due to lacerations or episiotomy; urinary tract infection).	Evaluate for urinary tract infection; obtain clean-catch urine; refer to physician/CNM for treatment if indicated.
	*Possible causes of alterations are placed in parentheses.	†This column provides guidelines for further assessment and initial nursing intervention.

ASSESSMENT GUIDE Postpartum—First Home Visit and Anticipated Progress at Six Weeks continued

Physical Assessment/Normal Findings	Alterations and Possible Causes*	Nursing Responses to Data†
ELIMINATION PATTERN (continued)		
Routine urinalysis within normal limits (proteinuria disappeared).	Sugar or ketone in urine—may be some lactose present in urine of breastfeeding mothers (diabetes).	Evaluate diet; assess for signs and symptoms of diabetes; refer to physician/CNM.
Bowel Habits: 2 days: May be some discomfort with defecation, especially if patient had severe hemorrhoids or third- or fourth-degree extension.	Severe constipation or pain when defecating (trauma or hemorrhoids).	Discuss dietary patterns; encourage fluid, adequate roughage. Continue use of stool softener if necessary to prevent pain associated with straining; continue sitz baths, periods of rest for severe hemorrhoids; assess healing of episiotomy and/or lacerations; severe constipation may require administration of laxatives, stool softeners, and an enema if not contraindicated (check with physician/CNM).
6 weeks: Return to normal prepregnancy bowel elimination.	Marked constipation (inadequate fluid and/or fiber intake).	See previously discussed interventions.
	Fecal incontinence or constipation (rectocele).	Assess for evidence of rectocele; instruct in muscle tightening exercises; refer to physician/CNM.
REPRODUCTIVE TRACT		
Lochia: 2 days: Lochia rubra or lochia serosa, scant amounts, fleshy odor.	Excessive amounts and/or large clots (nonfirm uterus), foul odor (infection), passing tissue (possible retained placenta).	Assess for evidence of infection and/or failure of the uterus to descend and decrease in size; refer to physician/CNM.
6 weeks: No lochia, or return to normal menstruation pattern.	See above.	See above.
Fundus and Perineum: 2 days: Fundus is at least two fingerbreadths below the umbilicus; uterine muscles still somewhat lax; introitus of vagina lacks tone—gapes when intra-abdominal pressure is increased by coughing or straining.	Uterus not decreasing in size appropriately or extremely tender (infection).	Assess fundus for firmness and/or signs of infection; refer to physician/CNM if indicated.
Episiotomy and/or lacerations healing; no signs of infection; may have some bruising and tenderness.	Evidence of redness, severe pain, poor tissue approximation in episiotomy and/or laceration (wound infection).	Continue perineal hygiene care; refer to physician or CNM as necessary.
6 weeks: Uterus almost returned to prepregnant size with almost completely restored muscle tone.	Continued flow of lochia, failure to decrease appropriately in size (subinvolution).	Assess for evidence of subinvolution and/or infection; refer to physician or CNM for further evaluation and treatment if necessary.
HEMOGLOBIN AND HEMATOCRIT LEVELS		
6 weeks: Hemoglobin (Hb) 12 g/dl; Hematocrit (Hct) 37% ± 5%	Hb less than 12 g/dl; Hct less than 32% (anemia).	Assess nutritional status, assess for signs or symptoms of anemia, begin (or continue) supplemental iron; for marked anemia (Hb less than or equal to 9 g/dl) additional assessment and/or physician/CNM referral may be necessary.
ATTACHMENT		
Bonding process demonstrated by soothing, cuddling, and talking to infant; appropriate feeding techniques; eye-to-eye contact; touching; calling infant by name.	Failure to bond demonstrated by lack of behaviors associated with bonding process; calling infant by nickname that promotes ridicule; inadequate infant weight gain; infant is dirty; hygienic measures are not being maintained; severe diaper rash; failure to obtain adequate supplies to provide infant care (malattachment).	Provide counseling; talk with the woman about her feelings regarding the infant; provide support for the caretaking activities that are being performed; refer to public health nurse or social worker for continued home visits; refer if abuse or neglect is suspected.
Parent interacts with infant and provides activities soothing, caretaking activities.	Parent is unable to respond to infant needs (inability to recognize needs, inadequate education and support, fear, family stress).	Provide support for caretaking activities observed; provide information regarding caretaking activities, such as responding to infant cry; methods of wrapping infant; methods of soothing the infant such as swaddling, rocking, increasing stimuli by singing to the infant or decreasing stimuli by putting infant to rest in quiet room; methods of holding the infant; differences in the cry. Identify support system such as friends, neighbors; provide information regarding community resources and support groups; reinforce "Never shake a baby."
	*Possible causes of alterations are placed in parentheses.	†This column provides guidelines for further assessment and initial nursing intervention.

(continued)

ASSESSMENT GUIDE Postpartum—First Home Visit and Anticipated Progress at Six Weeks continued

Physical Assessment/Normal Findings	Alterations and Possible Causes*	Nursing Responses to Data[†]
ATTACHMENT (continued)		
Parents express feelings of comfort and success with the parent role.	Evidence of stress and anxiety (difficulty moving into or dealing with the parent role).	Provide support and encouragement; provide information regarding progression into parent role and assist parents in talking through their feelings; refer to community resources and support groups.
Woman is in the informal or personal stage of maternal role attainment.	Woman is still greatly influenced by others, has not developed an image or style of her own (woman remains in the anticipatory stage).	Provide role modeling for the woman in working through problem solving with the infant; provide encouragement as she thinks through decisions and develops her sense of problem solving; encourage her to make decisions regarding infant care; provide positive reinforcement.
ADJUSTMENT TO PARENTAL ROLE		
Parents are coping with new roles in terms of division of labor, financial status, communication, readjustment of sexual relations, and adjusting to new daily tasks.	Inability to adjust to new roles (immaturity, extremes of maternal age, inadequate education and preparation, ineffective communication patterns, inadequate support, current family crisis).	Provide counseling, provide anticipatory guidance, refer to parent groups.
EDUCATION		
Mother understands self-care measures.	Inadequate knowledge of self-care (inadequate education).	Provide education and counseling.
Parents are knowledgeable regarding infant care.	Inadequate knowledge of infant care (inadequate education).	
Siblings are adjusting to new baby.	Excessive sibling rivalry.	
Parents have a method of contraception.	Birth control method not chosen.	
	*Possible causes of alterations are placed in parentheses.	[†]This column provides guidelines for further assessment and initial nursing intervention.

by feelings of exhaustion and decreased capacity for physical and mental work. Chapter 36 includes an extensive discussion on postpartum fatigue, including risk factors, complications, and management.

Breastfeeding Issues

The home-care nurse should inform mothers that fatigue may be a significant problem, which can increase the risk of postpartum depression. The nurse can emphasize the benefits of good nutrition and periods of uninterrupted sleep. The mother should be encouraged to ask family and friends for assistance with responsibilities, limit visitors, and use an answering machine or voicemail to allow for more rest. The nurse can also reinforce the need for continued use of prescribed prenatal vitamins and iron, particularly if the patient is breastfeeding.

PROFESSIONALISM IN PRACTICE

Privacy During Postpartum Home-Care Visit

Childbearing women should be asked and informed about postpartum depression at every health care encounter, and the home visit is no exception. It is helpful for the nurse to include other family members in this discussion, so everyone is aware of the symptoms. However, the patient may share things with the nurse in private that she would not share in front of others, so it is important that the nurse request at least a few minutes alone with her. Asking others to leave briefly during the perineal exam is one option for the nurse. The private interaction also allows the nurse to screen the patient regarding domestic violence, which often escalates during the childbearing period.

Breastfeeding Concerns Following Discharge

AWHONN supported the *Healthy People 2010* goals related to breastfeeding and encouraged the national goals to be expanded even further. AWHONN (2007b) "supports an exclusive breastfeeding initiation rate of 90%, a 75% 6-month breastfeeding rate and a 50% 1-year breastfeeding goal by 2025" (para 3). The recommendations are based on benefits to mothers and babies, which have been demonstrated by research.

Breastfed infants have decreased risks of infections. Breastfeeding as an infant is also associated with lower rates of SIDS, insulin dependent diabetes, allergies, asthma, lymphoma, ulcerative colitis, and adult-onset hypertension. Breastfeeding benefits maternal-infant attachment, maternal self esteem, and uterine involution. Finally, mothers who breastfeed have decreased risk for subsequent osteoporosis, ovarian cancer, premenopausal breast cancer, and rheumatoid arthritis (AWHONN, 2007b).

The benefits of breastfeeding result in cost savings for parents, insurers, and employers. Therefore, it has a high economic as well as health value for society. However, most mothers are discharged before breastfeeding is well established, and many require anticipatory guidance and support in order to continue once they go home. The U.S. Breastfeeding Committee (2009) proposed that breastfeeding support is important to health care reform, as it has the potential to save $14 billion per year in the United States.

Avery, Zimmerman, Underwood, et al. (2009) found that women who accept breastfeeding as a learned skill and demonstrate a confident commitment to the process, continue to breastfeed. Because many mothers discontinue breastfeeding as a result of problems and concerns early on, the home visit is the ideal time to promote continuation of breastfeeding. The home-care nurse has the opportunity and privilege to not only reinforce initial breastfeeding teaching and answer questions, but also to observe an episode of breastfeeding in the home environment where it will continue until weaning. Guidance and support can be individualized according to the mother's specific needs and living situation. There are numerous books and references available to assist nurses in the care of breastfeeding couplets.

The AAP recommends that all breastfeeding newborns be seen by a pediatrician or other knowledgeable healthcare professional at 3 to 5 days of age to assess weight and to have a physical exam to include assessment of jaundice and hydration, maternal breastfeeding status, infant elimination, and formal observation of a breastfeeding session (AAP & ACOG, 2007). A home visit a few days after discharge meets these requirements and can identify at-risk infants before they lose excessive weight and at a time when intervention can correct most breastfeeding problems before they become complicated by insufficient milk. The home health nurse can assess the infant and the breastfeeding process, provide appropriate education to promote breastfeeding, and initiate referrals to a lactation consultant or primary healthcare provider as needed. Additionally, the nurse can provide individualized support and encouragement as desired by the patient.

Breastfeeding Assessment

The nurse should observe a feeding episode, if possible, to assess for correct position, maternal and infant feeding cues, latch on, position, let-down, sucking pattern, nipple condition, infant response, and maternal response. The nurse can assess the parents' ability to identify infant feeding cues such as rooting, hand-to-mouth movements, sucking, opening of mouth in response to stimulation, and infant transition from sleep to drowsy awake to quiet alert states. Various tools are available to assess the breastfeeding session, including the LATCH Scoring Table (Figure 32-15 ∞ on page 874). Assessment of the mother's ability to perceive infant satiety cues such as a gradual decrease in sucking, pulling away and releasing the nipple, relaxation, sleep, contentment, and a small amount of milk visible in the mouth can be accomplished at this time as well (AWHONN, 2007c).

Concerns Related to the Breastfeeding Infant

According to AAP criteria, the infant's weight should remain within 10% of his or her birth weight, and the infant should feed at least 8 to 10 times per day by the fourth day of life. The infant should have at least three voids and at least three stools per 24 hours by the third day of life. Infants with a weight loss of more than 7% that continues beyond 72 hours of life or inadequate output require more extensive evaluation of breastfeeding to correct potential problems. In this case the nurse should notify the primary healthcare provider (AAP & ACOG, 2007; AWHONN, 2007c).

The nurse can assist the couplet experiencing a 7% to 9% infant weight loss with techniques to increase milk production and promote better milk transfer. The nurse will provide assistance with breastfeeding techniques as needed, encourage breastfeeding every 2 hours for the next 24 hours, and then recheck the newborn's weight the next day. If breastfeeding technique is correct and the milk is just starting to come in, the newborn generally begins gaining weight back within hours. The newborn's primary healthcare provider should be notified regarding a weight loss of more than 9% regardless of when it occurs. Lactation problems beyond the expertise of the nurse always require a lactation consultant and/or provider referral.

Newborns frequently require assistance in awakening to feed at least 8 times a day during the first week of life. The quiet alert state is ideal for latch on, and parents should be taught to recognize this state as well as the presence of early feeding cues. The quiet alert baby has bright eyes and is responsive to stimuli. Early feeding cues include sucking motions, bringing the hands to the mouth, rooting, extending the tongue, turning the head to the side, and whimpering (Koehn & Riordan, 2010). Techniques that are helpful in arousing a sleepy baby to the quiet alert state include undressing the baby, changing the diaper, lightly touching, speaking, turning on lights, placing the baby skin-to-skin on the mother's chest, and gently rocking the baby. Overaroused newborns who are crying or who exhibit closed down behaviors such as tightly closed eyes and uncoordinated movements of extremities require calming techniques to bring them to a quiet alert state. Changing the diaper, comforting, holding, swaddling, gently rocking, and talking softly will assist the newborn to return to the quiet alert state so the breast can be offered (Koehn & Riordan, 2010; Riordan & Hoover, 2010).

Many mothers have concerns related to their breast milk supply. The nurse can educate and reassure the mother regarding the signs of adequate transfer. The baby should feed at least 8 to 12 times in 24 hours for a total of at least 140 minutes of active suckling per day during the first 2 weeks. Audible swallowing should be heard. The mother's nipple should be moist, and mother and baby should be satisfied at the end of feedings. The baby's lips and mucous membranes should look moist. The baby should pass at least three to five loose yellow stools per day by day 4 or 5, and five or more per day by 1 week of age. The baby should have at least six diapers that are saturated with clear urine each day by 1 week of age. Additionally, the baby should return to birth weight by the 2-week well-baby visit (Riordan & Hoover, 2010; Smith & Riordan, 2010). The satiated baby will be content at the end of feedings with arms extended and relaxed. A small amount of milk may be visible at the side of the mouth. If all of the previous criteria are met, the nurse can feel confident in telling the mom that the baby is "getting enough" and that exclusive breastfeeding is the ideal diet for the baby until 6 months of age.

Recommendations at this point would be to continue nursing on demand, at least every 3 hours, and to expect the baby to demand more frequent feedings during growth spurts. The mother can allow the baby who is actively sucking and swallowing to nurse for as long as desired on the first side and then for as long as the baby desires on the second side to encourage consumption of the high-fat hind milk. The mother will need to take the newborn in for periodic weight checks, well-baby exams, and immunizations as directed by the infant's provider. As recommended by the AAP, the parents will want to talk with their provider about vitamin D supplementation within the first 2 months, fluoride supplementation at six months, and adding additional foods that contain iron or an iron supplement at 6 months (AAP & ACOG. 2007).

The home-care nurse will occasionally discover a breastfed baby with a weight loss of up to 7% in a normal newborn. Infants experiencing breastfeeding difficulties whose weight loss is greater than 7% may need supplementation. A call to the pediatrician from the patient's home is warranted to discuss the issue. An infant with a weight loss of more than 9% will almost always need supplementation. Because it is important to begin rehydrating the newborn as soon as possible, the home-care nurse may need to help a patient who has planned only to feed from the breast to formulate an interim contingency plan. The nurse can assist her with pumping or hand expressing.

Some mothers may prefer to feed their breast milk to the baby using a syringe, finger, or cup, rather than a bottle. Additional research needs to be done to make recommendations regarding these approaches, however (AWHONN, 2007c). Therefore, only nurses who are experienced with breastfeeding support and lactation consultants should assist mothers with these alternatives.

Expressed breast milk is the ideal intervention. However, if the mother does not have enough breast milk, the nurse will find it necessary to assist the mother with preparation of formula until her supply is adequate and the baby is rehydrated. Therefore, it is important that the home-care nurse be familiar with infant formulas and preparation. The use of infant formula is discussed later in this chapter.

Concerns Related to Maternal Breastfeeding Difficulties and Formula-Feeding

In addition to problems with milk transfer and concerns about milk supply, many new mothers have breastfeeding difficulties, including leaking, nipple soreness, cracked nipples, breast engorgement, and plugged ducts. The nurse can assess for these complications at the home visit and provide interventions to decrease maternal discomfort.

NIPPLE SORENESS Mothers should be counseled to expect sensations of massaging and stretching as the infant elongates the nipple during nursing. This may be uncomfortable when the infant initially latches for feedings, but the discomfort should decrease after the first few seconds of nursing. Nipple soreness is a common complaint and frequent reason for early discontinuation of breastfeeding. The nipples may exhibit erythema, edema, abrasions, fissures, cracks, bruises, blisters, and bleeding. This early transient discomfort is usually due to mechanical trauma, and it peaks between the third and sixth days. Poor latch and/or suck are the primary causes of mechanical trauma, and a change in nipple shape at the end of a feeding is a common indicator. Therefore, observation of feeding, assistance with proper positioning and latching technique, and observation of the shape of the nipple at the end of the feeding are essential to the prevention and treatment of soreness (AWHONN, 2007c; Dennis, Allen, McCormick, et al., 2008; Smith & Riordan, 2010).

Care Plan Activity: Breastfeeding Pain

The baby's position at the breast is a critical factor in nipple soreness. The mother's hand should be off the areola, and the baby should be tummy to tummy and facing the mother's chest, with ear, shoulder, and hip aligned. The nose is near or just touching the breast, and the lips should be flanged out. The gums are on the areola, and the tongue is over the bottom gum and cupping the nipple. (See Figures 32-11 through 32-14 on pages 872–873.) Because the area of greatest stress to the nipple is in line with the newborn's chin and nose, encouraging the mother to rotate positions when feeding the infant may decrease nipple soreness. Changing positions alters the focus of greatest stress and promotes more complete breast emptying. Although some mothers are initially hesitant to try the side-lying position, this is frequently a helpful position to use when difficulty in latching is encountered. Nipple soreness due to mechanical trauma is frequently related to the infant's sucking pattern or to anatomical variations of the newborn's oral cavity or the mother's nipples. Nipple characteristics such as their size, shape, and ability to elongate may affect comfort during sucking. The size and shape of the infant's oral cavity may also affect the sucking pattern and comfort. A short or tight newborn lingual frenulum (ankyloglossia or tongue-tie) can cause discomfort as well (AWHONN, 2007c; Smith & Riordan, 2010).

An observation of the feeding should assess the baby's oral cavity for anatomical concerns as well as the ability to open the mouth wide enough to attain a deep latch. When latched, the lips should be flanged out, and the newborn should cover as much of the areola as possible. Turning the lips under can cause pain and inadequate transfer of milk. The mother can be taught to observe this and to apply gentle upward pressure on the newborn's upper lip and gentle downward pressure on the infant's chin to correct the position as needed. To prevent trauma, the mother should also be taught to gently insert her finger between the infant's gums to break the latch before removing the baby from the breast.

While nursing, the baby can be expected to suck rapidly at the beginning and more slowly toward the end of a feeding. Sucking should be quiet, with swallowing heard every two to three sucks. The baby's cheeks should be full and rounded. Movement should be seen at the jawline. Dimpling at the cheek may be indicative of a poor or shallow latch or an unusual movement of the tongue. The presence of clicking, smacking, or slurping may indicate an improper seal or suck, and the infant should be re-latched. Persistent clicking may be heard if the infant has ankyloglossia (tongue-tie) (Smith & Riordan, 2010).

Finally, the mother's nipple will be elongated at the end of a feeding, but it should be the same shape as at the beginning. Nipples that are angled, creased, or distorted at the end of feedings indicate anatomical variations or latch problems. Intervention is required if distorted nipples are painful (Smith & Riordan, 2010).

The nurse can instruct the mother in a number of measures to promote comfort and healing and to prevent skin breakdown. Washing the breasts with warm water and avoiding drying soaps is recommended. Simply keeping the nipples clean and dry is adequate for many mothers. Alternatively, warm water compresses can be applied followed by air-drying (Figure 37-5 ■). Gently massaging or pumping the breast before feedings stimulates let-down and flow and may be helpful in decreasing initial latch-on pain related to vigorous nursing. The mother can also apply an ice compress to the nipples just before feeding to decrease sensation (Smith & Riordan, 2010).

Lanolin is sold over the counter and offered to mothers by many healthcare providers for the treatment of sore nipples. However, the practice guidelines developed by AWHONN (2007c) noted that additional research is needed before hydrogel dressing, paraf-

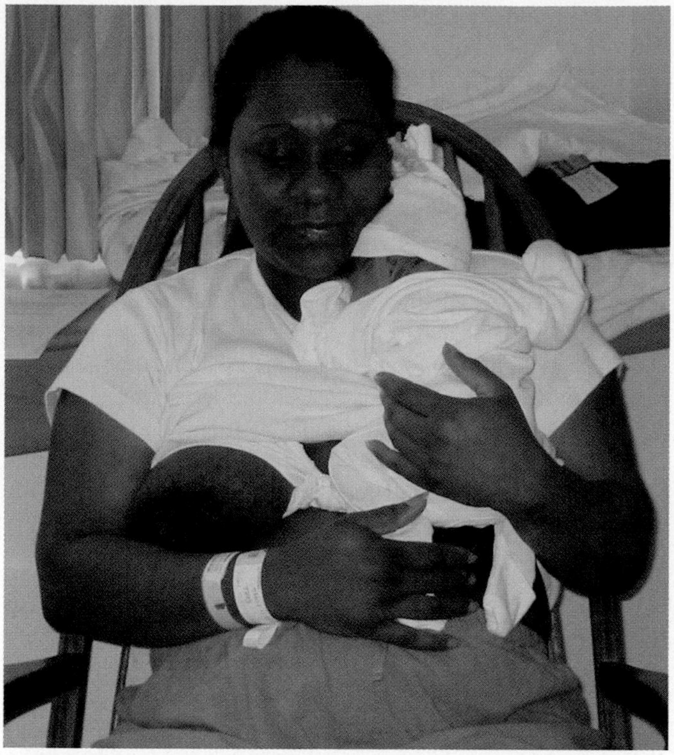

Figure 37-5 ■ Air-drying the nipples can help prevent cracking and fissures.

fin, lanolin, sprays, or antibiotic creams can be recommended. Smith & Riordan (2010) emphasized that ointments should not be applied to infected nipples, with the exception of currently prescribed antifungal or antibiotic preparations. Although application of expressed breast milk was recommended in the past, this may actually spread organisms into wounded nipples (Smith and Riordan, 2010). Dennis et al. (2008) noted that it is unclear which intervention(s) are best, and developed a protocol to conduct a Cochrane review regarding interventions for nipple pain.

If a woman finds that her bra or clothing rubs against her nipples and adds to her discomfort, she may find it helpful to use breast shells between feedings. It is not helpful to limit nursing time at the breast. This may actually increase discomfort related to engorgement and have a negative effect on milk production and infant nutrition. For severe cases, in which the mother is unable to tolerate breastfeeding, the mother will need to pump or hand-express the breast milk until the nipple condition improves (Smith & Riordan, 2010).

The most important factor in decreasing pain is educating the mother about proper latch-on techniques. Anticipatory guidance and informing patients that many mothers experience nipple discomfort on days 3 through 6 and that the discomfort usually improves markedly by the end of the first week should be helpful in encouraging new mothers to continue breastfeeding, knowing that an end to the discomfort is in sight (AWHONN, 2007c).

The home-care nurse can make recommendations for interventions for patients with sore nipples. It is essential that the nurse read the product literature and current research on products recommended by the providers and lactation consultants in the local area. Additionally, the nurse should remind the mother that small amounts of any product applied to her nipples will be ingested by her newborn. Therefore, she will want to consult her primary care provider or a lactation consultant before applying commercial products.

The nurse should talk with a lactation consultant or provider if the patient's discomfort is severe enough to require temporary use of a thin silicone nipple shield and/or pumping rather than nursing. Nipple shields should be used only under close monitoring, as they can potentially affect milk transfer and have a negative impact on the infant. Nipple pain that does not resolve after a few days may indicate infection or other problems and should be referred to a provider so the appropriate therapy can be prescribed.

FLAT OR INVERTED NIPPLES Many women with flat or inverted nipples have the fear that they will be unable to breastfeed. This is not usually the case. Pregnancy and previous breastfeeding often lessen the inversion to the point that it is not an issue with subsequent babies. Breastfeeding mothers with flat or inverted nipples may experience difficulties after discharge if breastfeeding was not successfully established before leaving the hospital. Frequently, positioning the infant well back on the areola will be enough to promote the suckling that stretches and elongates the nipple during feedings. Exercising the nipple before latching loosens the tissue and helps to separate adhesions that cause retraction or inversion. The nurse can teach the mother to stimulate and shape the nipple just before feeding. A cold pack will evert a flat nipple. Inverted nipples that can be everted can be shaped by the mother by placing her thumb 1 1/2 to 2 inches behind the nipple and pulling back into her chest. As noted previously, use of the side-lying position is helpful (Smith & Riordan, 2010; Riordan & Wambach, 2010).

The nurse can also recommend use of a pump to evert the nipple just before latch on. Experienced nurses may feel comfortable assisting mothers to use a thin silicone nipple shield during the initial latch. The shield can be removed once the baby has suckled enough to elongate the nipple. Inverted nipples that are not easily everted by the measures above should be referred to a lactation consultant.

BREAST ENGORGEMENT A distinction exists between breast fullness and engorgement. All lactating women experience a transitional fullness at first, initially because of venous congestion and later because of accumulating milk. However, this fullness generally lasts only 24 hours, the breasts remain soft enough for the newborn to suckle, and there is no pain. Severely engorged breasts are hard, painful, and warm, and may appear taut and shiny. Engorgement can be accompanied by a fever up to 101°F. Engorgement may occur as a result of infrequent feedings, delayed initiation of feedings, use of supplements, time-limited feedings, and too quickly removing the baby from the first side to ensure feeding from both breasts at each feeding (Riordan & Hoover, 2010).

Treatments employed for engorgement may include warm compresses or showers for a short time just before nursing, cold compresses or frozen bags of vegetables applied to breasts after feedings, cabbage compresses, breast massage and milk expression, ultrasound, anti-inflammatory medications, and pumping.

Many women anecdotally express increased comfort with the use of cold compresses, frozen vegetable bags, and the judicious use of cabbage leaves, but anti-inflammatory medications are the only treatments demonstrated by research to be effective (Riordan & Hoover, 2010). A Cochrane review is planned to determine which interventions are most effective for treating engorgement (Mangesi & Muzonzini, 2008).

Although unrelieved engorgement and stasis are not necessarily associated with mastitis, they do lead to involution and decreased milk synthesis. Frequent feedings for a minimum of approximately 160 minutes of nursing every 24 hours are essential to the treatment of engorgement. Although pumping is sometimes discouraged in this situation for fear that it will increase milk production, it is necessary to pump if the infant is unable to nurse to empty the breasts (Riordan & Hoover, 2010; Smith & Riordan, 2010). A technique described as *areolar compression* by Riordan and Hoover and *reverse pressure softening* by Cotterman (2004) is recommended before pumping or attempting to latch if severe breast and alveolar edema is present. It will be helpful for homecare nurses working with breastfeeding mothers to review these references and to work with a lactation consultant to learn this technique as well as to learn more about the use of commercial breast pumps and manual expression of breast milk. See Nursing Care Plan: For the Woman with Engorgement on page 1079.

PLUGGED DUCTS Some mothers experience plugging of one or more ducts. Manifested as an area of tenderness, redness, and heat, or a palpable lump in an otherwise well woman, plugging may be relieved by the use of massage and frequent feedings. The nurse can encourage the mother to massage her breasts from her chest wall forward to the nipple while standing in a warm shower or following the application of moist heat to the breast. The mother should then breastfeed her infant, starting on the affected breast to promote drainage. Frequent breastfeeding and the use of a variety of positions to ensure complete emptying help to prevent and to resolve the problem. The nurse should also encourage the patient to wear a comfortable bra and loose, nonrestrictive clothing (Riordan & Wambach, 2010).

CLINICAL JUDGMENT

Case Study: Ann Nyembe

Ann Nyembe calls you from home in tears on her third postpartum day. She states breastfeeding was going well in the hospital but now her breasts are swollen, hard, and very painful, and her baby is refusing to suckle. Ann expresses some disappointment that "the breastfeeding didn't work" because she truly believes that breastfeeding is best for babies, and she enjoyed her breastfeeding experience in the hospital, especially breastfeeding the baby immediately after birth. But she also states she has been crying all day and can no longer tolerate her painful breasts. In addition, she says the baby "seems happier" with the bottle.

Critical Thinking

What actions can the nurse recommend to Ann to increase the likelihood she will continue breastfeeding and to decrease her discomfort?

See www.nursing.pearsonhighered.com for possible responses.

MASTITIS Plugged ducts and milk stasis increase the risk for *mastitis*, an inflammatory condition of the breast. Stress and fatigue, cracked nipples, and an abundant milk supply are associated with mastitis as well. Symptoms of mastitis include fever (greater than 100.4°F); a hot, red, tender area on the breast; and flulike symptoms. Treatment of mastitis includes continued breastfeeding, application of moist heat, increased fluids, rest, analgesics, and antibiotics as prescribed if necessary (Riordan & Wambach, 2010). For more information about mastitis see chapter 39 ∞ and Figure 39-2 ∞ on page 1132.

A Cochrane review found a lack of research regarding antibiotic treatment for mastitis and urged further studies (Jahanfar, Ng, & Teng, 2009). As with nipple pain and engorgement, a Cochrane review is planned to determine the risks and benefits of the various interventions currently used to prevent mastitis (Crepinsek, Crowe, Michener, et al., 2008).

EFFECT OF MEDICATIONS AND ALCOHOL Analgesics are appropriate as directed by a primary healthcare provider. Avoidance of breastfeeding while the drug levels are peaking in maternal plasma minimizes the amount received by the infant. The peak concentration varies from drug to drug, and it may be difficult to time this during the first week of breastfeeding. Nursing ideally occurs frequently, and the mother may require analgesics to nurse comfortably. Non-narcotic analgesics can be administered approximately 30 minutes prior to nursing if the mother suffers afterpains when nursing (AWHONN, 2007c).

Hale (2010) pointed out that the nonsteroidal anti-inflammatory drug (NSAID) ibuprofen is cleared for infant use and that its levels in milk are generally subclinical. Because most drugs do pass into the breast milk, the mother will want to check with her provider before taking medications. The nurse can use the references listed in Table 37-5 to check recommendations regarding use of specific drugs during lactation.

Alcohol passes into the breast milk. Therefore, it is not recommended for breastfeeding women. Mothers who do occasionally drink while lactating should be advised to consume the alcohol with a meal and after breastfeeding rather than shortly before a breastfeeding in order to minimize the amount the infant receives (Bronner, 2010).

TABLE 37-5 References for Nurses Who Work with Breastfeeding Patients

- Briggs, G. G., Freeman, R. K., & Yaffe, S. J. (2008). *Drugs in pregnancy and lactation* (8th ed.). Baltimore, MD: Lippincott Williams & Wilkins.
- Hale, T. D. (2008). *Medications and mothers' milk* (13th ed.). Amarillo, TX: Hale Publishing.
- Huggins, K., & Ziedrich, L. (2007). *The nursing mother's guide to weaning: How to bring breastfeeding to a gentle close and how to decide when the time is right.* Boston, MA: Harvard Common Press. (written for breastfeeding mothers)
- Lawrence, R. A., & Lawrence, R. M. (2005). *Breastfeeding—a guide for the medical profession* (6th ed.). Philadelphia, PA: Elsevier Mosby.
- Riordan, J., & Wambach, K. (2010). *Breastfeeding and human lactation* (4th ed). Sudbury, MA: Jones & Bartlett.

NURSING CARE PLAN For the Woman with Engorgement

INTERVENTION	RATIONALE
1. Nursing diagnosis: Acute Pain related to increased breast fullness secondary to increased blood supply to breast tissue causing swelling of tissue around milk ducts **Goal:** Patient will remain free of breast fullness and pain.	
■ Instruct patient to nurse frequently.	■ Engorgement may be a result of infrequent or missed feedings. Frequent feedings will prevent the breast from becoming increasingly full which in turn decreases pain caused by engorgement. The newborn should be offered the breast at least eight to ten times in a 24-hour period.
■ Instruct patient to nurse at least 10 to 15 minutes on each breast per feeding.	■ Hind milk may be brought forward when the newborn is able to suckle for 10 to 15 minutes per breast. This will allow the breast ducts to empty with each feeding.
■ Assist patient to pre-express milk onto nipple or baby's lips.	■ Engorgement may be the result of newborns who are too sleepy to suck at each feeding or not eager to nurse vigorously. Expressing some milk onto the nipple may entice the newborn to nurse more aggressively.
■ Initiate pumping or manually express milk at the beginning of the feeding.	■ Engorgement may be the result of the breast not emptying at each feeding. Pumping or manually expressing the breast will allow the breast to empty. Pumping or hand expressing the milk at the beginning of each feeding will help soften the breast so the newborn can latch on to the nipple and facilitate letdown.
■ Instruct patient to pump, hand express, or massage to empty breast when feedings are missed.	■ If patient develops a feeling of fullness in the breast, or the newborn has missed a feeding, then pumping or hand expressing the milk will help keep the milk ducts empty. When the milk ducts become backed up, milk production can be inhibited, eventually decreasing the milk supply. Pumping during engorgement should not affect the milk supply.
■ Administer analgesics before nursing.	■ Acetaminophen and ibuprofen alone or in combination with codeine may be administered just before nursing to relieve pain and discomfort. The medication will reach the milk within 30 minutes.
■ Apply warm and/or cold compresses before nursing.	■ Warm compresses may be applied before nursing to stimulate letdown or soften the breast. This will allow the newborn to grasp the areola. A proper latch on will help prevent plugged ducts and assist in emptying the breast to reduce breast fullness and pain associated with engorgement. Relaxing in the shower with warm water running over the breast may have the same effect. Cold compresses may also be used to help reduce pain.
■ Apply fresh cabbage leaves to the breast between feedings.	■ Placing fresh cabbage leaves inside the bra is a home remedy that may relieve edema associated with engorgement, thereby reducing pain. Relief may be experienced within 30 minutes. Prolonged application of cabbage leaves may reduce the milk supply.

EXPECTED OUTCOMES: There will be no evidence of swelling found in breast tissue. The woman's pain will have decreased, and her breast tissue will be soft and without tenderness.

BREASTFEEDING AND THE WORKING MOTHER Many mothers return to work while still breastfeeding. The home-care nurse can help the woman to explore options and solve problems related to breastfeeding in the workplace to promote continuation. The earlier the breastfeeding mother returns to work, the more often she will need to pump her breasts to express the breast milk. Recommendations for mothers who are using a breast pump can be found in Table 32-5 ∞ on page 876. Because milk production follows the principle of supply and demand, if breasts are not pumped, the milk supply will decrease. The nurse can review pumping and storage of breast milk with the mother, as the mother will want to begin pumping at least a week or two before returning to work. The mother will also want to introduce her baby to expressed milk from a bottle or cup prior to her return. An electric pump and double collection system is optimal for the working mother (see Figure 32-20 on page 878). Working mothers can obtain printed materials on pumping, storage, working while breastfeeding, and related issues from lactation consultants and breastfeeding support groups, such as La Leche League (Lawrence & Lawrence, 2008; Rojjanasrirat & Wambach, 2010).

The nurse can suggest methods of maintaining breast milk supply such as relaxation, stress reduction, proper nutrition, adequate fluid intake, and frequent nursing during the evenings, in the mornings, and on days off. The nurse and patient can explore options such as pumping at work, visiting the infant or having the infant brought to work during the mother's lunch, and having the child care provider give expressed breast milk or formula (Rojjanasrirat & Wambach, 2010).

Use of the side-lying position is less fatiguing and may allow the mother to relax when she does have the opportunity to breastfeed her baby before and after work. Night breastfeeding presents a dilemma. It may help a working mother maintain her milk supply, but it may also contribute to fatigue. Depending on the rigidity and demands of the mother's work schedule, the nurse can explore options with the mother to promote the continuation of breastfeeding as much as possible during the first year of life.

> **PROFESSIONALISM IN PRACTICE**
>
> ***Workplace Issues Related to Breastfeeding***
>
> Mills (2009) and Stewart-Glenn (2008) found that maternal employment continues to be a barrier to long-term breastfeeding. Many employers are uninformed regarding the benefits of breastfeeding and do not view breastfeeding as a workplace issue. Many working mothers, particularly lower-income employees, are not aware of their options to continue breastfeeding after they return to work. Little research has been done on workplace issues related to breastfeeding. The professional nurse can advocate for patients by informing and encouraging them to discuss breastfeeding with their employers. Nurses can engage in public education campaigns related to the benefits of breastfeeding in the workplace, such as less absenteeism related to infant illness. Nurses also need to conduct research that investigates the effects of corporate lactation support programs and work cultures that are supportive of breastfeeding. Finally, as recommended by Thulier and Mercer (2009), nurses should contact their legislators and work to promote legislation that protects and supports breastfeeding mother-infant dyads.

WEANING **Weaning** is a process that begins with the introduction of sources of nutrition other than breast milk and ends when the child no longer breastfeeds and receives all nutrition from other sources. Ideally, the decision to wean is based on the child's nutritional needs, psychologic needs, and developmental milestones (Lawrence & Lawrence, 2008). However, the decision to *wean* the baby from the breast may be made for a variety of reasons, including family or cultural pressures, changes in the home situation, work schedules, pressure from the woman's partner, or a personal opinion about when weaning should occur.

Although the Centers for Disease Control and Prevention (CDC) reported that 77% of infants born in 2005 and 2006 were initially breastfed, many women wean their infants prior to 6 months of age. The home-care nurse will likely visit the mother early in the postpartum period, and it is important to provide anticipatory guidance and support to the mother in order to extend breastfeeding for as long as possible to benefit mother and baby. Many women wean their infants earlier than originally planned, because they don't believe they are adequately nourishing and satisfying their baby with the breast (Gatti, 2008; Li, Fien, Chen, et al., 2008; Thulier & Mercer, 2009). Therefore, education regarding how to establish and maintain sufficient milk supply and how to respond to infant growth spurts is essential. The woman should also receive contact information for support groups and lactation consultants in her local area.

Although some women need to wean abruptly due to medical or logistical reasons, a gradual approach is physically and emotionally comfortable for many mothers and their babies. The mother may wish to start by substituting one or two breast feedings with other sources of nutrition and cup feedings each day. Eventually, the mother may want to breastfeed only once or twice a day prior to stopping entirely.

If a baby initiates weaning during the first year of life and the mother wishes to continue breastfeeding, she can often work through this with the help of a lactation consultant. The infant who is weaned before 12 months should receive iron-fortified newborn formula rather than cow's milk (AAP & ACOG, 2007).

Nurses should inform mothers that lactation consultants will help them with weaning issues in addition to providing support for establishing and continuing lactation. The nurse can also share resources with breastfeeding mothers (see Table 37-5).

CULTURAL CONSIDERATIONS RELATED TO BREASTFEEDING Cultures vary tremendously in their initiation of breastfeeding, support persons important to the continuation of breastfeeding, and weaning practices. Despite increases in breastfeeding in the United States, minority women still breastfeed at lower rates than white women. Many immigrants breastfeed less than family members from their native countries after moving to the United States. African American women, in particular, breastfeed at low rates (Thulier & Mercer, 2009; Wambach & Riordan, 2010). Lack of family support decreases the likelihood that the woman will continue breastfeeding once she goes home, so it is important to find out the important support persons for breastfeeding in each cultural context.

Although cultural considerations related to each group are beyond the scope of this chapter, it is important for the home-care nurse to individualize care for all women by incorporating their cultural beliefs and practices related to breastfeeding. Thulier and Mercer (2009) recommended the use of peer counselor programs to support women who are breastfeeding. The authors also noted the need for research that explores ethnic influences on breastfeeding and investigates interventions designed to promote breastfeeding in minority populations.

For further discussion regarding cultural influences on infant feeding practices, see chapter 2 of this text. Another excellent reference is the chapter, "The Cultural Context of Breastfeeding," in *Breastfeeding and Human Lactation* by Riordan & Wambach (2010).

BREASTFEEDING REFERRALS AND SOCIAL SUPPORT Support from the woman's family and social contacts is very important with regard to the initiation and continuation of breastfeeding, as is support from healthcare professionals. Providers of care need to be educated about breastfeeding physiology and resources in order to educate and support patients. Family members require information and education from professionals in order to support breastfeeding women as well (Clifford & McIntyre, 2008; Thulier & Mercer, 2009). Women who participate in local support groups can learn over time and observe role models to enhance their breastfeeding experience. The home-care nurse should be familiar with local lay support groups and encourage breastfeeding mothers to contact them.

FORMULA-FEEDING The AAP recommends that parents use a commercially prepared, iron-fortified infant formula until 1 year of age if the baby is not breastfed (AAP & ACOG, 2007). Some mothers need or choose to feed their infants formula because of their own health status or personal preference. If the mother does not have a health history that precludes her from breastfeeding, it may be helpful to explore the reasons for her decision. Some mothers have chosen formula because of lack of education about the benefits of breastfeeding, misconceptions about breastfeeding, or lack of support. If that is the case and the mother desires help with breastfeeding, lactation can still be established at this time with proper support. If the mother needs or chooses to use formula, it is important for the nurse to support her choice and provide information related to safe formula feeding.

Most human milk substitutes in this country are available in ready-to-feed, liquid concentrate, and powder forms. Many parents reconstitute the powder, as it is the most economical formulation. Chronic overconcentration can result in hypernatremic dehydration, whereas underconcentration can result in water intoxication and undernourishment. Therefore, it is important to emphasize the importance of mixing the formula exactly as the package directs. Product storage recommendations should be followed, expiration dates should be honored, and parents should date and time the bottles when prepared. Families must use uncontaminated water and employ safe-handling practices during preparation of formula as well.

According to the EPA, between 15% and 20% of U.S. households rely on private wells for the water they use and consume. Private wells are not publicly inspected and regulated, as are municipal water supplies, so the individual family is responsible for testing its water and maintaining its well. Water can be contaminated with microorganisms and with chemicals such as nitrates and pesticides, which are not necessarily removed by filtering or boiling. Infants and children are highly susceptible to waterborne illness. Therefore, the nurse should make certain that families who use private wells are aware that they need to purchase bottled water to reconstitute infant formula until their well water has been tested for safety. Information on safe use of well water can be obtained from sources such as the CDC, the U.S. Environmental Protection Agency (EPA), the U.S. Food and Drug Administration (FDA), the Department of Agriculture, and local public health departments (Rogan, Brady, and the Committee on Environmental Health, and the Committee on Infectious Diseases, 2009). Descriptions of the various types of bottled water and the Web sites and telephone contact numbers for well water resources in every state are found in Rogan et al. (2009).

The World Health Organization (WHO) published new guidelines regarding the preparation of powdered formula in 2007, due to concerns regarding *Enterobacter sakazakii* and *Salmonella enterica*. Guidelines include sterilizing bottles and nipples between uses and boiling the water used to reconstitute the powder. The water should be mixed with the powder when it is still 70°C (158°F) or warmer. Ideally, the formula will be consumed within 2 hours of preparation, but individually prepared bottles that have not been touched can be stored in a refrigerator at 5°C (41°F) or less for a maximum of 24 hours (WHO, 2007).

A large study of women in the United States evaluated mothers' use of four important safe handling practices for infant formula: (a) hand washing before preparation, (b) washing bottles and nipples thoroughly between uses, (c) discarding formula left at room temperature for >2 hours, and (d) never heating formula in microwave ovens. More than half of the women reported that they did not always wash their hands prior to preparation, and a significant number reported not following one or more of the other practices as well. More than 70% of women reported not receiving any information regarding formula preparation from a healthcare provider by the time they were 5 months postpartum (Labiner-Wolfe, Fein, & Shealy, 2008).

Home-care nurses should be aware that there are significant education gaps regarding the safe preparation and storage of infant formula. The home visit is an excellent time to assess the parents' understanding and to inspect the area where the formula will be prepared and stored. The WHO (2007) developed pamphlets describing safe formula preparation, which offer explicit instructions for healthcare workers and for infant caregivers in multiple languages. The pamphlets can be downloaded from the WHO Web site.

CLINICAL JUDGMENT

Case Study: Carla Humphrey

During a home visit, you notice that the new mother, Carla Humphrey, has many bottles and nipples laying at the bottom of the dish drainer. You ask her how she has cleaned them, and she says she usually rinses them at the end of each evening.

You note that the family is in a rural area, and confirm with Mrs. Humphrey that they use well water. You decide to research the current recommendation further, and find that the WHO (2007) recommends sterilizing bottles and nipples between uses, and the FDA (2007, updated 2009) advocates sterilizing bottles and nipples prior to the first use only and then washing with hot water or in the dishwasher between uses if a clean source of tap water is available.

Critical Thinking

What is your best recommendation for sterilizing the bottles and nipples?

See www.nursing.pearsonhighered.com for possible responses.

Other Types of Follow-Up Care

Other types of follow-up care may include return home visits, telephone follow-up, and postpartum classes or support groups.

Return Visits

If the mother and family and physician or certified nurse-midwife have chosen discharge earlier than 48 hours after vaginal birth, the mother may, in some states, request a total of three visits. In such cases, the nurse would schedule the first visit about 24 hours after discharge and then space out the other two visits over the next week. In other instances, the nurse may schedule additional home visits based on the findings of the first home visit and the follow-up phone call.

Telephone Follow-Up

Case Study: Follow-Up with the Patient at Home

The postpartum home-care nurse usually makes a follow-up phone call a few days after the home visit. During the call, the nurse may provide additional information, address questions or areas of confusion, and make referrals.

Some families may be offered or may request a telephone follow-up at the time of discharge. A mutually agreeable time is set for the call, typically within 3 days of discharge, or earlier if desired. Calls typically last about 20 minutes and are preplanned and goal directed.

To perform an effective telephone assessment, the nurse must be able to listen skillfully, use open-ended questions, and wait for answers. The nurse projects a warm, caring attitude so that the mother feels comfortable talking to a faceless caller. When assessment reveals signs of an initial or recurring postpartum complication, the nurse refers the woman to her primary care provider for further evaluation.

The plan of care developed and implemented during a telephone conversation is limited to supportive counseling, teaching, and referral. The new mother may have many questions, especially about newborn care, and is generally at a high level of learning readiness. The nurse can answer the woman's questions and use the questions as a "stepping stone" for further teaching. Many communities have established 24-hour advice lines for new parents to call when they have questions or need support. In areas where help lines are not available, parents may be directed to call the birthing center. If birthing center nurses field parent phone calls, they should follow established protocols regarding the advice to be given and the documentation required. In either case, the home-care nurse provides the number so that it is readily accessible for the family.

Postpartum Classes and Support Groups

Postpartum classes are becoming more common as caregivers recognize the continuing needs of the childbearing family. In many instances, classes are prepared to meet the specific needs of a variety of families so that, for example, single mothers and adolescent mothers can attend class with peers. A series of structured classes may focus on topics such as parenting, postpartal exercise, or nutrition, or there may be loosely structured group sessions that address mothers' concerns as they arise. Such classes offer chances for the new mother to socialize, share her concerns, and receive encouragement. Because babysitting arrangements may be difficult or expensive, it is desirable to provide child care for siblings.

Some cities offer breastfeeding or new-parent support groups through birthing centers or hospitals or as a community effort. Once again, the support group provides an opportunity for parents to interact with one another and to share information and experiences.

Many parents look to Internet resources for additional information on parenting and newborn care. Internet sites can be devised by anyone, so the quality, currency, usefulness, and accuracy of the information may vary. Nurses have an opportunity to assist parents in evaluating the reliability of the information they find. Parents can be encouraged to view Web sites affiliated with government organizations, universities, or healthcare organizations, as such sites are usually credible.

PROFESSIONALISM IN PRACTICE

Reporting Unsanitary Conditions in the Home

As healthcare professionals, nurses are required to report infant neglect or abuse. When practicing in private homes, the nurse will be exposed to a wide range of home management practices with regards to aesthetics and sanitation. For example, the nurse will need to distinguish a home that is simply messy from a home that is unsanitary. It is important to develop rapport with the parents and to provide education as needed when sanitation issues are present. In certain cases, a follow-up visit is warranted. In cases of extreme filth or severe pest infestations, the nurse will need to use critical thinking skills to determine whether the most vulnerable patient—the infant—is at risk for injury. If that is the case, the nurse should notify the appropriate authorities and follow the home care agency plan for such contingencies. If in doubt, the nurse should call upon resource persons and supervisors for assistance.

FOCUS YOUR STUDY

- The Newborns' and Mothers' Health Protection Act took effect in January 1998, and provides for a guaranteed minimum stay of up to 48 hours following an uncomplicated vaginal birth and 96 hours following an uncomplicated cesarean birth. The AAP recommends that all infants discharged before 48 hours be examined within 48 hours after discharge, and, ideally, that all newborns be seen at the 3- to 5-day point for weight, hydration, intake and output, and jaundice screening. Home care nursing meets this requirement.
- The overall goal of postpartum home visits is to enhance opportunities for smooth transition of the new family. The home visit provides opportunities for assessment, teaching, breastfeeding support, and fostering a caring relationship with new families.
- In planning the home visit, the nurse needs to take precautions to maintain safety, such as carrying a cellular phone, notifying supervisors of location of visit, keeping personal belongings out of sight, assessing the neighborhood and home for signs of danger, and, if present, terminating the visit.
- Physical assessment of the newborn during a home visit includes assessments of vital signs, weight, overall color including jaundice, assessment of body systems, intake/output, hydration, umbilical cord and circumcision, newborn nutrition, newborn safety, parent education, and attachment.
- Teaching goals during home visits include reinforcing daily newborn care, including demonstrations of positioning and handling, sponge and tub bathing, nail care, and dressing; discussing temperature assessment and signs of illness; assisting with newborn feeding; discussing expected newborn output; discussing newborn behavioral states; promoting safe and appropriate newborn sleeping, including SIDS prevention; promoting crib safety; encouraging childproofing of the home environment; discussing prevention of unintentional injuries and abuse; and encouraging newborn screening and immunization.
- The physician or pediatric nurse practitioner should be notified if there is evidence of redness around the newborn's umbilicus, if there is bright red bleeding or puslike drainage near the cord stump, or if the umbilical site remains unhealed.
- A primary risk factor for sudden infant death syndrome (SIDS) is sleeping in the prone position. Guidelines that came out in 2005 discourage cosleeping, smoking in pregnancy, and smoking after birth. Further recommendations include placement of the infant crib in close proximity to the parents' bed and the use of pacifiers as measures to further prevent SIDS.
- State-mandated screening is performed on all newborns in the first 1 to 3 days. States vary regarding the conditions for which they screen.
- Universal hearing screening is performed on all newborns. Newborns who do not pass the screening should receive diagnostic testing by age 3 months and interventions by age 6 months as necessary.
- Signs of illness in mothers include pain or burning with urination, passage of clots or placental tissue, excessive pelvic or perineal pain, chest pain, difficulty breathing, excessive or foul-smelling lochia, failure of fundus to descend at the anticipated rate, temperature of 100.4°F or above, elevation of blood pressure, tenderness, redness, or pain in the legs or breasts, and feelings consistent with postpartum depression.
- Difficulties with breastfeeding include sore, cracked, flat, or inverted nipples; breast engorgement; plugged ducts; and mastitis.
- Breastfeeding mothers require information on effects of alcohol and various medications on breast milk; pumping; weaning; and breastfeeding referrals and social support.
- Return visits, telephone follow-up, classes, and support groups can provide valuable information and support to new mothers and their families.

CRITICAL THINKING IN ACTION

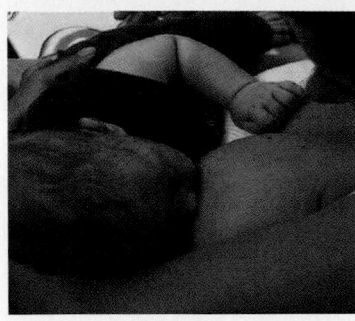

Jane Benne, age 23, G1 gave birth by cesarean for cephalopelvic disproportion to a healthy 7 pound 1 ounce baby boy 5 days ago. You are making a home visit 2 days after Jane was discharged from the hospital to her two-story home. When you arrive the baby is sleeping in a bassinet in Jane's bedroom on the second level. Jane has been trying to breastfeed and complains to you of sore nipples and swollen breasts. She is also having problems getting the baby to latch on and says that she has been supplementing her baby's feedings with a bottle because she is afraid her baby is not getting enough milk from her breasts alone. She also mentions that the baby seems more satisfied after she gives the bottle and seems to sleep longer. You ask her how she has been feeling, and she tells you that she is very tired and upset about her body not making enough milk to feed her child. You assess Jane's breasts and find them to be full and firm, but the nipples are cracked and blistered.

1. What is your focus in the home postpartum visit?
2. What counseling can you give Jane regarding her sore nipples?
3. What suggestion do you give Jane regarding supplemental bottle-feedings?
4. Explain your assessment of Jane's abdominal incision and provide suggestions for healing.
5. How would you discuss the baby's voiding patterns to ensure adequate hydration?

See www.nursing.pearsonhighered.com for possible responses.

Pearson Nursing Student Resources

Find additional review materials at
www.nursing.pearsonhighered.com

Prepare for success with additional NCLEX®-style practice questions, interactive assignments and activities, Web links, animations and videos, and more!

REFERENCES

Academy of Breastfeeding Medicine (ABM) Protocol Committee. (2008). ABM clinical protocol #6: Guideline on cosleeping and breastfeeding. *Breastfeeding Medicine, 3*(1), 38–43. doi:10.1089/bfm.2007.9979

Agency for Toxic Substances and Disease Registry (ATSDR). (2009). *National alert: A warning about continuing patterns of metallic mercury exposure.* Retrieved from http://www.atsdr.cdc.gov/alerts/970626.html

American Academy of Pediatrics (AAP) Subcommittee on Hyperbilirubinemia. (2004). Management of hyperbilirubinemia in the newborn infant 35 or more weeks of gestation. *Pediatrics, 114*(1), 297–316. Retrieved from http://pediatrics.aappublications.org/

American Academy of Pediatrics (AAP) & The American College of Obstetricians and Gynecologists (ACOG). (2007). *Guidelines for perinatal care* (6th ed.). Elk Grove Village, IL: Author.

Anderson, N. R. (2008). Safe in the city. *Home Healthcare Nurse, 26*(9), 534–542. doi:10.1097/01.NHH.0000338512.00571.1b

Arikan, D., Alp, H., Gözüm, S., Orbak, Z., & Cifci, E. K. (2008). Effectiveness of massage, sucrose solution, herbal tea or hydrolysed formula in the treatment of infantile colic. *Journal of Clinical Nursing, 17*(13), 1754–1761. doi:10.1111/j.1365-2702.2007.02093.x

Aschenbrenner, D. S., & Venable, S. J. (2009). *Drug therapy in nursing* (3rd ed.). Philadelphia, PA: Wolters Kluwer Health/Lippincott Williams & Wilkins.

Association of Women's Health, Obstetric, and Neonatal Nurses (AWHONN). (2007a). *Neonatal skin care evidence-based clinical practice guideline* (2nd ed.). Washington, DC: Author.

Association of Women's Health, Obstetric, and Neonatal Nurses (AWHONN). (2007b). *AWHONN position statement: Breastfeeding.* Retrieved from http://www.awhonn.org/awhonn/content.do?name=05_HealthPolicyLegislation/5H_PositionStatements.htm

Association of Women's Health, Obstetric, and Neonatal Nurses (AWHONN). (2007c). *Breastfeeding support: Prenatal care through the first year evidence-based clinical practice guideline* (2nd ed.). Washington, DC: Author.

Ateah, C. A., & Hamelin, K. J. (2008). Maternal bedsharing practices, experiences, and awareness of risks. *JOGNN: The Journal of Obstetric, Gynecologic, and Neonatal Nursing, 37*(3), 274–281. doi:10.1111/j.1552-6909.2008.00242.x

Avery, A., Zimmerman, K., Underwood, P. W., and Magnus, J. H. (2009). Confident commitment is a key factor for sustained breastfeeding. *Birth, 36*(2), 141–148. doi:10.1111/j.1523-536X.2009.00312.x

Berkowitz, C. (2007). Approach to the febrile infant: A changing paradigm. *Family Practice Recertification, 29*(3), 41–47. Retrieved from http://www.acquirecontent.com/titles/family-practice-recertification.

Bernstein, H. H., Spino, C., Finch, S., Wasserman, R., Slora, E., Lalama, C., . . . McCormick, M. C. (2007). Decision-making for postpartum discharge of 4300 mothers and their healthy infants: The life around newborn discharge study. *Pediatrics, 120*(2), e391–e400. doi:10.1542/peds.2006-3389

Briggs, G. G., Freeman, R. K., & Yaffe, S. J. (2008). *Drugs in pregnancy and lactation* (8th ed.). Baltimore, MD: Lippincott Williams & Wilkins.

Bronner, Y. L. (2010). Maternal nutrition during lactation. In Riordan & Wambach (Eds.), *Breastfeeding and human lactation* (4th ed., pp. 497–518). Sudbury, MA: Jones & Bartlett.

Bruckner, T. A. (2008). Economic antecedents of prone infant sleep placement among black mothers. *Annals of Epidemiology, 18*(9), 678–681. doi:10.1016/j.annepidem.2008.07.001

Burgos, A. E., Schmitt, S. K., Stevenson, D. K., & Phibbs, C. S. (2008). Readmission for neonatal jaundice in California, 1991–2000: Trends and implications. *Pediatrics, 121*(4), e864–e869. doi:10.1542/peds.2007-1214

Bystrova, K., Ivanova, V., Edhborg, M., Matthiesen, A.-S., Ransjö-Arvidson, A.-B., Mukhamedrakhimov, R., et al., (2009). Early contact versus separation: Effects on mother–infant interaction one year later. *Birth, 36*(2), 97–109. doi:10.1111/j.1523-536X.2009.00307.x

Catherine, N. L. A., Ko, J. J., & Barr, R. G. (2008). Getting the word out: Advice on crying and colic in popular parenting magazines. *Journal of Developmental and Behavioral Pediatrics, 29*(6), 508–511. doi:10.1097/DBP.0b013e31818d0c0c

Christensen, R. D., Pysher, T. J., & Christensen, S. S. (2007). Case report: Perianal necrotizing fasciitis in a near-term neonate. *Journal of Perinatology, 27,* 390–391. doi:10.1038/sj.jp.7211733

Clifford, J., & McIntyre, E. (2008). Who supports breastfeeding? *Breastfeeding Review 16*(2), 9–19. Retrieved from CINAHL Plus with Full Text.

Cohen-Silver, J., & Ratnapalan, S. (2009). Management of infantile colic: A review. *Clinical Pediatrics, 48*(1), 14–17. doi:10.1177/0009922808323116

Cotterman, K. J. (2004). Reverse pressure softening: A simple tool for easier latching during engorgement. *Journal of Human Lactation, 20*(2), 227–237. doi:10.1177/0890334404264224

Crepinsek, M. A., Crowe, L., Michener, K., & Smart, N. A. (2008). Interventions for preventing mastitis after childbirth. *Cochrane Database of Systematic Reviews* 2008, Issue 3. Art. No.: CD007239. doi:10.1002/14651858.CD007239

Cummings, K. J., Klotz, C., Liu, W.-Q., Weese-Mayers, D. E., Marazita, M. L., Cooper, M. E., . . . Wilson, R. J. A. (2009). Sudden infant death syndrome (SIDS) in African Americans: Polymorphisms in the gene encoding the stress peptide pituitary adenylate cyclase-activating polypeptide (PACAP). *Acta Pædiatrica, 98*(3), 482–489. doi:10.1111/j.1651-2227.2008.01131.x

Dabrowski, G. (2007). Skin-to-skin contact: Giving birth back to mothers and babies. *Nursing and Women's Health, 11*(1), 64–71. doi:10.1111/j.1751-486X.2007.00119

Damato, E. G. (2007). Safe sleep: Can pacifiers reduce SIDS risk? *Nursing for Women's Health, 11*(1), 72–76. doi:10.1111/j.1751-486X.2007.00120.x

De Curtis, M., Calzolari, F., Marciano, A., Cardilli, V., & Gianvincenzo, B. (2008). Comparison between rectal and infrared skin temperature in the newborn. *Archives of Disease in Childhood—Fetal and Neonatal Edition, 93*(1), F55–F57. doi:10.1136/adc.2006.114314

Dennis, C. L., Allen, K., McCormick, F. M., & Renfrew, M. J. (2008). Interventions for treating painful nipples among breastfeeding women. *Cochrane Database of Systematic Reviews* 2008, Issue 4. Art. No.: CD007366. doi:10.1002/14651858.CD007366.

Engle, W. A., Tomashek, K. M., Wallman, C., and the Committee on the Fetus and Newborn. (2007). Late preterm infants: A population at risk. *Pediatrics, 120,* 1390–1401. doi:10.1542/peds.2007.2952

Evans, W. N., Garthwaite, C., & Wei, H. (2008). The impact of early discharge laws on the health of newborns. *Journal of Health Economics, 27*(4), 843–870. doi:10.1016/j.jhealeco.2007.12.003

Forsythe, P. L., Maher, R., Kirchick, C., & Bieda, A. (2007). Family teaching toolbox: Infant safety at home. *Advances in Neonatal Care, 7*(2), 78–79. doi:10.1097/01.ANC.0000267912.58726.ba

Freedman, S. B., Al-Harthy, N., & Thull-Freedman, J. (2009). The crying infant: Diagnostic testing and frequency of serious underlying disease. *Pediatrics, 123*(3), 841–848. doi:10.1542/peds.2008-0113

Friedlander, S. F., Eichenfield, L. F., Leyden, J., Shu, J., & Spellman, M. C. (2009). Diaper dermatitis: Appropriate evaluation & optimal management strategies. *Contemporary Pediatrics, Apr:* Supplement: 2–14. Retrieved from CINAHL Plus with Full Text.

Fu, L. Y., Colson, E. R., Corwin, M. J., & Moon, R. Y. (2008). Infant sleep location: Associated maternal and infant characteristics with sudden infant death syndrome prevention recommendations. *The Journal of Pediatrics, 153*(4), 503–508. doi:10.1016/j.jpeds.2008.05.004

Gatti, L. (2008). Maternal perceptions of insufficient milk supply in breastfeeding. *Journal of Nursing Scholarship, 40*(4), 355–363. doi:10.1111/j.1547-5069.2008.00234.x

Goulet, C., Frappier, J-Y., Fortin, S., Déziel, L., Lampron, A., & Boulanger, M. (2009). Development and evaluation of a shaken baby syndrome prevention program. *JOGNN: Journal of Obstetric, Gynecologic, and Neonatal Nursing, 38*(1), 7–21. doi:10.1111/j.1552-6909.2008.00301.x

Govtrack (n.d.). H. R. 2052: Shaken Baby Syndrome Prevention Act of 2007. Retrieved from www.govtrack.us/congress/bill.xpd?bill=h110-2052

Hale, T. (2008). *Medications and mothers' milk* (13th ed.). Amarillo, TX: Hale Publishing.

Hale, T. (2010). Drug therapy and breastfeeding. In Riordan & Wambach (Eds.), *Breastfeeding and human lactation* (4th ed., pp. 163–196). Sudbury, MA: Jones & Bartlett.

Huggins, K., & Ziedrich, L. (2007). *The nursing mother's guide to weaning: How to bring breastfeeding to a gentle close and how to decide when the time is right.* Boston, MA: Harvard Common Press.

Hutchison, L., Stewart, A., & Mitchell, E. (2007). Infant sleep position, head shape concerns, and sleep positioning devices. *Journal of Paediatrics & Child Health, 43*(4), 243–248. doi:10.1111/j.1440-1754.2007.01054.x

Hutton, S., Probst, E., Kenyon, C., Morse, D., Friedman, B., Arnold, K., & Helsley, L. (2009). Accuracy of different temperature devices in the postpartum population. *JOGNN: Journal of Obstetric, Gynecologic, and Neonatal Nursing, 38*(1), 42–49. doi:10.1111/j.1552-6909.2008.00302.x

Jahanfar, S., Ng, C. J., & Teng, C. L. (2009). Antibiotics for mastitis in breastfeeding women. *Cochrane Database of Systematic Reviews* 2009, Issue 1. Art. No.: CD005458. doi:10.1002/14651858.CD005458.pub2.

Jarvis, S. (2008). The management of infant colic. *GP: General Practitioner, 4/11/2008,* p. 9.

Katz-Sidlow, R. J., Rowberry, J. P., & Ho, M. (2009). Fever determination in young infants: Prevalence and accuracy of parental palpation. *Pediatric Emergency Care, 25*(1), 12–14. doi:10.1097/PEC.0b013e31819dac6

Klaus, M. (2009). Commentary: An early, short, and useful sensitive period in the human infant. *Birth, 36*(2), 110–112. doi:10.1111/j.1523-536X.2009.00315.x

Koehn, M., & Riordan, J. (2010). Infant assessment. In Riordan & Wambach (Eds.), *Breastfeeding and human lactation* (4th ed., pp. 669–703). Sudbury, MA: Jones & Bartlett.

Labiner-Wolfe, J., Fein, S. B., & Shealy, K. R. (2008). Infant formula-handling education and safety. *Pediatrics, 122*(2), S85–S90. doi:10.1542/peds.2008-1315k

Lawrence, R. A., & Lawrence, R. M. (2005). *Breastfeeding—a guide for the medical profession* (6th ed.). Philadelphia, PA: Elsevier Mosby.

Lawrence, R., & Lawrence, R. M. (2008). Approach to breastfeeding. In Duggan, Watkins, & Walker (Eds.), *Nutrition in Pediatrics: Basic Science & Clinical Applications* (4th ed., pp. 363–375). Hamilton, Ontario; Lewiston, NY: B.C. Decker.

Lewin, L. (2008). Shaken baby syndrome: Facts, education, and advocacy. *Nursing for Women's Health, 12*(3), 235–239. doi:10.1111/j.1751-486X.2008.00328.x

Li, R., Fien, S. B., Chen, J., & Grummer-Strawn, L. M. (2008). Why mothers stop breastfeeding: Mothers' self-reported reasons for stopping during the first year. *Pediatrics, 122*(Supplement 2), s69–s76. doi:101542/peds.2008-1315i

Lokker, N., Sanders, L., Perrin, E. M., Kumar, D., Finkle, J., Franco, V., . . . Rothman, R. L. (2009). Parental misinterpretations of over-the-counter pediatric cough and cold medication labels. *Pediatrics, 123*(6), 1464–1471. doi:10.1542/peds.2008-0854

Mangesi, L., & Muzonzini, G. (2008). Treatments for breast engorgement during lactation. *Cochrane Database of Systematic Reviews* 2008, Issue 1. Art. No.: CD006946. doi:10.1002/14651858.CD006946

March of Dimes. (2010). Premature birth. Retrieved from http://www.marchofdimes.com/professionals/685.asp

Mathews, T. J., & MacDorman, M. F. (2008). Mortality statistics from the 2005 period linked birth/infant death data set. *National Vital Statistics Reports, 57*(2). Retrieved from http://www.cdc.gov/nchs/data/nvsr/nvsr57/nvsr57_02.pdf

Mentula, S., Tuure, T., Koskenala, R., Korpela, R., & Könönen, E. (2008). Microbial composition and fecal fermentation end products from colicky infants—a probiotic supplementation pilot. *Microbial Ecology in Health and Disease, 20*(1), 37–47. doi:10.1080/08910600801933846

Michon, K. (2010). Crib recalls, safety, and litigation. Retrieved from http://www.nolo.com/legal-encyclopedia/article-32403.html

Mills, S. P. (2009). Workplace lactation programs: A critical element for breastfeeding mothers' success. *AAOHN Journal, 57*(6), 227–231. doi:10.3928/08910162-20090518-02

Mitchell, E. A. (2009). What is the mechanism of SIDS? Clues from epidemiology. *Developmental Psychobiology, 51*(3), 215–222. doi:10.1002/dev.20369

Moore, E. R., Anderson, G. C., & Bergman, N. (2007). Early skin-to-skin contact for mothers and their healthy newborn infants. *Cochrane Database of Systematic Reviews* 2007, Issue 3. Art.No.: CD003519. doi:10.1002/14651858.CD003519.pub2

Mraz, M. A. (2009). The physical manifestations of shaken baby syndrome. *Journal of Forensic Nursing, 5*(1), 26–30. doi:10.1111/j.1939-3938.2009.01027.x

National Center for Injury Prevention and Control, Centers for Disease Control and Prevention (n.d.; last updated July 15, 2009). *Injury data and statistics: Downloadable leading causes charts.* Retrieved from http://www.cdc.gov/injury/wisqars/LeadingCauses.html

National Conference of State Legislatures. (2009). Shaken baby syndrome prevention legislation. Retrieved from www.ncsl.org/?TabId=17669

National Institute of Child Health and Human Development (NICHD). (2008). *Sudden infant death syndrome (SIDS).* Retrieved from http://www.nichd.nih.gov/health/topics/Sudden_Infant_Death_Syndrome.cfm

Omojokun, O. O., & Moon, R. Y. (2008). Sudden infant death syndrome: A review of the literature. *Current Pediatric Reviews, 4*(1), 31–39. doi:10.2174/157339608783565824

Riordan, J., & Hoover, K. (2010). Perinatal and intrapartum care. In Riordan & Wambach (Eds.), *Breastfeeding and human lactation* (4th ed., pp. 215–251). Sudbury, MA: Jones & Bartlett.

Riordan, J., & Wambach, K. (2010). Breast-related problems. In Riordan & Wambach (Eds.), *Breastfeeding and human lactation* (4th ed., pp. 291–324). Sudbury, MA: Jones & Bartlett.

Rogan, W. J., Brady, M. T., and the Committee on Environmental Health, and the Committee on Infectious Diseases. (2009). Drinking water from private wells and risks to children. *Pediatrics, 123*(6), e1123–e1137. doi:10.1542/peds.2009-0752

Rojjanasrirat, W., & Wambach, K. (2010). Maternal employment and breastfeeding. In Riordan & Wambach (Eds.), *Breastfeeding and human lactation* (4th ed., pp. 551–577). Sudbury, MA: Jones & Bartlett.

Romano, A. M., & Lothian, J. A. (2008). Promoting, protecting, and supporting normal birth: A look at the evidence. *JOGNN: Journal of Obstetric, Gynecologic, & Neonatal Nursing, 37*(1), 95–104. doi:10.1111/J.1552-6909.2007.00210.x

Ryan, T., Brewer, M., & Small, L. (2008). Over-the-counter cough and cold medication use in young children. *Pediatric Nursing, 34*(2), 174–184. Retrieved from http://www.pediatricnursing.net/issues/08marapr/

Savino, F., Cordisco, L., Tarasco, V., Locatelli, E., Petrucci, E., & Matteuzzi, D. (2008). Molecular identification of gas-forming coliforms in breast-fed colicky and healthy infants. *Digestive and Liver Disease, 40*(10), A115–A116. doi:10.1016/j.dld.2008.07.306

Smith, K. M., & deGuehery, K. A. (2008). Shaken baby syndrome education program: Nurses making a difference. *MCN: The American Journal of Maternal Child Nursing, 33*(6), 371–375. doi:10.1097/01.NMC.0000341258.26169.d4

Smith, L. J., & Riordan, J. (2010). Postpartum care. In Riordan & Wambach (Eds.), *Breastfeeding and human lactation* (4th ed., pp. 253–290). Sudbury, MA: Jones & Bartlett.

Stewart-Glenn, J. (2008). Knowledge, perceptions, and attitudes of managers, coworkers, and employed breastfeeding mothers. *AAOHN Journal, 56*(10), 423–429. doi:10.3928/08910162-20081001-02

Thulier, D., & Mercer, J. (2009). Variables associated with breastfeeding duration. *JOGNN: Journal of Obstetric, Gynecologic, and Neonatal Nursing, 38*(3), 259–268. doi:10.1111/j.1552-6909.2009.01021.x

Turkoski, B. B. (2007). Medicating young or very young patients. *Orthopaedic Nursing, 26*(3), 194–201. doi:10.1097/01.NOR.0000276973.32679.a0

U.S. Breastfeeding Committee (2009). *Health care reform: Improving breastfeeding support will save billions.* Retrieved from http://www.usbreastfeeding.org/LinkClick.aspx?link=Publications%2fHealth-Care-Reform-One-Page-USBC.pdf&tabid=36&mid=378

U.S. Environmental Protection Agency (EPA). (2009). *Mercury: Basic facts.* Retrieved from http://www.epa.gov/mercury/about.htm

U.S. Food and Drug Administration (FDA). (2008a). *FDA releases recommendations regarding use of over-the-counter cough and cold products: Products should not be used in children under 2 years of age; evaluation continues in older populations.* Retrieved from http://www.fda.gov/NewsEvents/Newsroom/PressAnnouncements/2008/ucm116839.htm

U.S. Food and Drug Administration (FDA). (2008b). *FDA statement following CHPA's announcement on nonprescription over-the-counter cough and cold medicines in children.* Retrieved from http://www.fda.gov/NewsEvents/Newsroom/PressAnnouncements/2008/ucm116964.htm

U.S. Food and Drug Administration (FDA). (2007; updated 2009). *FDA 101: Infant formula.* Retrieved from http://www.fda.gov/ForConsumers/ConsumerUpdates/ucm048694.htm

Vennemann, M. M. T., Hoffgen, M., Bajanowski, T., Hense, H.-W., & Mitchell, E. A. (2007). Do immunizations reduce the risk for SIDS? A meta-analysis. *Vaccine, 25*(26), 4875–4879. doi:10.1016/j.vaccine.2007.02.077

Wambach, K., & Riordan, J. (2010). The cultural context of breastfeeding. In Riordan & Wambach (Eds.), *Breastfeeding and human lactation* (4th ed., pp. 799–816). Sudbury, MA: Jones & Bartlett.

World Health Organization (WHO). (2007). *Safe preparation, storage, and handling of powdered infant formula guidelines.* Retrieved from http://www.who.int/foodsafety/publications/micro/pif_guidelines.pdf

CHAPTER 38

Grief and Loss in the Childbearing Family

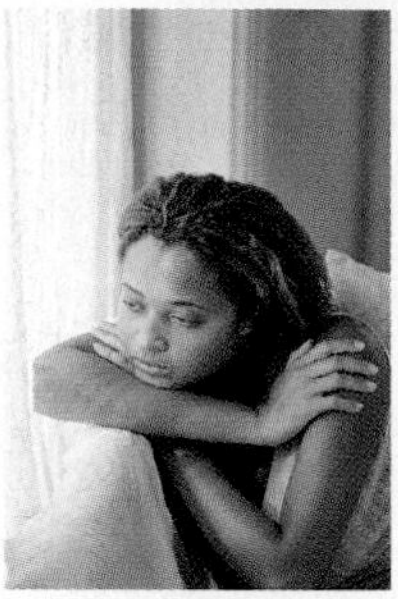

"You have a beautiful baby," the ultrasound technician said quietly. She was studying the flickering images on her screen, staring intently at the shadows of the tiny heart. I think she had already seen that our baby was going to die.

—Amy Kuebelbeck

(Excerpt from *Waiting with Gabriel: A Story of Cherishing a Baby's Brief Life* by Amy Kuebelbeck (Loyola Press, 2003). Reprinted with permission of Loyola Press. To order copies call 1-800-621-1008 or go to www.loyolapress.com.)

LEARNING OUTCOMES

1. Discuss perinatal loss including etiology, diagnosis, and the nurse's role in facilitating the family's mourning process.
2. Describe the physical, cognitive, emotional, behavioral, and spiritual responses experienced by parents during grieving associated with perinatal loss.
3. Delineate the personal, societal, and cultural issues that may complicate responses to perinatal loss.
4. Identify nursing diagnoses and interventions to meet the special needs of parents and their families related to perinatal loss and grief.
5. Differentiate between helpful and nonhelpful responses in caring for families experiencing perinatal loss.

KEY TERMS

Attachment theory *1090*
Bereavement *1089*
Caring theory *1100*
Disenfranchised grief *1090*
Dual process model *1090*
Euphemism *1106*
Grief *1089*
Hospital disposition *1106*
Instrumental styles of coping *1093*
Intuitive styles of coping *1093*
Maceration *1104*
Meaning reconstruction *1091*
Mourning *1090*
Perinatal hospice *1108*
Perinatal loss *1087*
Religion *1093*
Responding model *1100*
Spirituality *1093*

Perinatal loss is the death of a fetus or infant from the time of conception through the end of the newborn period 28 days after birth. This chapter discusses grief and loss in the childbearing family and the nurse's role in facilitating the family's mourning process. Although the primary focus is stillbirth, care of the family experiencing the death of an infant in the newborn period is inclusive. Causes and clinical aspects of spontaneous abortion (miscarriage) in the antepartum period are discussed in chapter 15 ∞, and chapter 27 ∞ discusses labor-related complications that can lead to fetal demise; this section discusses causes and clinical aspects of intrauterine fetal death (IUFD) after 20 weeks' gestation, often referred to as *stillbirth* or *fetal demise.*

Perinatal loss is a tragic event for the couple experiencing it and the family who loves them. Compounding the tragedy are many misconceptions surrounding perinatal loss, a lack of grief education afforded healthcare personnel, and clinical interventions that are out of step with current research. One of the biggest misconceptions about perinatal loss is that it is not as relevant as other losses because of the lack of interaction with the infant. In reality, this could not be further from the truth. Studies have shown that about 90% of couples believe that the loss of their infant was the worst thing that ever happened to them, and more than 80% believe that the death caused a significant decrease in their ability to function for a time (Swanson, Connor, Jolley, et al., 2007). Additionally, the grief for parents is lifelong and nonlinear, often described as the grief that never goes away (Arnold & Gemma, 2008, Cacciatore & Bushfield, 2007).

With regard to education, studies assessing the comfort level of nurses assisting families experiencing perinatal loss clearly demonstrate that many nurses are uncomfortable with death and dying and that more education is needed and, indeed, greatly desired (Chan et al., 2008; Kain, 2007; Kendall & Guo, 2008; Roehrs, Masterson, Alles, et al., 2008; Rogers, Babgi, & Gomez, 2008). The level of comfort, or lack thereof, observed in the study was mostly dependent upon the nature of thinking on a more hopeful level, length of experience in nursing, and palliative care education, with palliative care education making the most significant difference (Feudtner et al., 2007).

Lastly, concerning research and practice, in recent years there has been a paradigm shift in the field of grief and bereavement regarding the components of a "normal" mourning process as well as when, where, and how much intervention is warranted. Much of what has become the traditional standard of care for bereaved individuals has come into question as new research sheds light on the inefficacy of predetermined early and intense intervention. This chapter focuses on providing frameworks for understanding grief and loss, guidelines for effectively responding to a grieving family, and specific nursing interventions for the family experiencing perinatal loss in the clinical setting.

Common Causes of Perinatal Loss

The National Center for Health Statistics' most recent compilation of fetal mortality statistics occurred in 2005, and for the first time in decades, there was a slight reverse to the trend of declining fetal mortality rates from 2003 to 2005. In the United States, the incidence of fetal death after 20 weeks stands at 6.2 per 1000 total births, accounting for 60% of all perinatal deaths (fetal and neonatal) (MacDorman & Kirmeyer, 2009). Stillbirth currently occurs in 1 in 160 deliveries in the United States, (American College of Obstetricians and Gynecologists [ACOG], 2009) and more than 80% of stillbirths occur before term, with approximately half occurring before 28 weeks' gestation (MacDorman & Kirmeyer, 2009).

Antepartal fetal deaths, although infrequent, account for about half of all perinatal mortality in the United States (Druzin, Smith.,Gabbe, et al., 2007). Approximately 25,000 fetal deaths occur annually (ACOG, 2009). The *perinatal mortality rate (PMR)* is defined by the National Center for Health Statistics as late fetal deaths (over 28 gestational weeks) plus the first 6 days of life. It is estimated that 70% to 90% of stillbirths occur before the onset of labor, with more than 50% occurring between 20 and 28 weeks' gestation (Druzin et al., 2007). The cause may be unknown, or it may result from any of a number of physiologic maladaptations including asphyxia; congenital malformations; superimposed pregnancy complications including preeclampsia or eclampsia, diabetes, systemic lupus erythematosus, renal disease, thyroid disorders, cholestasis of pregnancy, abruptio placentae, placenta previa, diabetes, renal disease, cord accidents, fetal growth restriction, and alloimmunization (ACOG, 2009).

Perinatal loss can also occur due to infections such as human parvovirus B19, syphilis, streptococcal infection, and *Listeria* (ACOG, 2009). Perinatal loss is increased in women with multiple gestations and among women who smoke, have lower education attainment levels, advanced maternal age, and those who are obese (ACOG, 2009). Women who have had other pregnancies affected by stillbirth or growth restriction are at greater risk for having a stillborn infant (ACOG, 2009). Perinatal loss associated with birth defects can occur as a result of congenital anomalies or may occur if the fetus is exposed to teratogens late in the pregnancy.

Although the cause is often unknown, several risk factors elevate the chances of stillbirth, including maternal race or ethnicity, age, multiple gestation, and number of previous pregnancies (with nulliparas at highest risk). Most disturbing is the continuing disparity in race and ethnicity. African American women have fetal mortality rates 2.3 times higher than that of Caucasian American women, with Native Americans at 29% and Hispanic Americans at 14% higher respectively (MacDorman & Kirmeyer, 2009). In the United States, black women have higher rates of stillbirth, nearly double that of either white or Hispanic women (ACOG, 2009). Some recent studies have been undertaken to try to determine the cause of the unacceptably higher number of African American women experiencing infant mortality, but further studies are needed (Barnes, 2008).

Twin pregnancies demonstrated a mortality rate 2.7 times higher than singleton pregnancies, and triplets or higher were at 4.6 times the singleton rate. Fetal mortality rates were highest with decreasing maternal age; women under the age of 15 had 2.2 times the rate of stillbirth than that of women from 25 to 29 years of age. Additionally, women of advanced maternal age (greater than 35 years of age) also showed increased risk; in fact, advanced maternal age appeared to be an independent risk factor even when concurrent medical conditions were factored out (MacDorman & Kirmeyer, 2009). Obesity is one of the most common modifiable risk factors, in which the risk appears to increase with gestational age and is a major cause of stillbirth related to placental dysfunction (ACOG, 2009).

Perinatal loss in industrialized countries has declined in recent years as early diagnosis of congenital anomalies and advances in genetic testing techniques have increased the use of elective termination. Surprisingly, other reproductive advances have increased the incidence of fetal death. Pregnancies conceived by in vitro fertilization had higher rates of pregnancy loss, pregnancy complications (placenta abruption, fetal loss after 24 weeks' gestation, gestational hypertension, placenta previa, and cesarean births) (Gibbs, Karlan, Haney, et al., 2008). Conversely, fetal death occurs more frequently in monochorionic twins, which generally are conceived naturally. Most twins conceived via assisted reproductive technology are dichorionic placentation (Fletcher, Zach, Pramanik, et al., 2009). In addition, certain genetic testing procedures such as amniocentesis and chorionic villus sampling (CVS) can actually cause fetal loss.

In industrialized countries, infection plays a significant role in fetal deaths, accounting for 10% to 20% of all fetal demises; however, rates are believed to be much higher in developing countries (Reddy et al., 2009). Infection can be a causal factor in stillbirth by various means:

1. Causing severe maternal illness
2. Infecting the placenta and preventing oxygen and nutrients from crossing to the fetus
3. Infecting the fetus and causing a congenital deformity that is incompatible with life
4. Infecting the fetus and damaging a vital organ such as the brain or heart
5. Precipitating preterm labor, with the fetus dying in labor.

Ascending bacterial organisms include *Escherichia coli,* group B streptococci, and *Ureaplasma urealyticum.* These infections can occur before or after the membranes have ruptured, resulting in fetal demise. Prevalent viral causes of fetal demise include parvovirus and coxsackievirus. *Toxoplasma gondii, Listeria monocytogenes,* and the organisms that cause leptospirosis, Q fever, and Lyme disease have also been identified as causative factors for stillbirth, but the prevalence is unknown. Untreated syphilis is associated with a high stillbirth rate, as is malaria infection when contracted for the first time by the mother during the pregnancy (Reddy et al., 2009). These infections carry a much higher morbidity and mortality rate in developing countries.

Certain maternal conditions can also be associated with higher rates of fetal death. Past maternal exposure to some bacterial and viral antigens can produce an autoimmune response that can result in fetal death. Women with acquired and immune thrombophilia have higher rates of miscarriage and fetal demise than those without hematologic alterations (ACOG, 2009).

Maternal medical conditions contributing to the incidence of stillbirth include (Reddy et al., 2009):

- Hypertensive disorders
- Diabetes mellitus
- Thyroid, renal, or liver disease
- Connective tissue disease (such as systemic lupus erythematosus [SLE])
- Cholestasis

Other maladaptations that can cause stillbirth are:

- Antiphospholipid syndrome
- Heritable thrombophilias
- Red cell and/or platelet alloimmunization
- Congenital anomaly and malformations
- Chromosomal abnormalities including confined placental mosaicism
- Fetomaternal hemorrhage
- Fetal growth restriction
- Placental abnormalities including vasa previa and placental abruption
- Umbilical cord pathology including velamentous insertion, prolapse, occlusion, and entanglement
- Multifetal gestation including twin–twin transfusion syndrome/twin reverses arterial perfusion
- Amniotic band sequence
- Central nervous system lesions

Maternal Physiologic Implications

Prolonged retention of the dead fetus may lead to the development of disseminated intravascular coagulation (DIC), also called consumption coagulopathy, in the mother. After the release of thromboplastin from the degenerating fetal tissues into the maternal bloodstream, the extrinsic clotting system is activated, triggering the formation of multiple tiny blood clots. Fibrinogen and factors V and VII are subsequently depleted, and the woman begins to display symptoms of DIC. Fibrinogen levels begin a linear descent 3 to 4 weeks after the death of the fetus and continue to decrease in the absence of appropriate medical intervention.

Besides DIC, other adverse outcomes can also occur if the onset of labor and subsequent birth are delayed. Women with prolonged retention of a dead fetus are more prone to infection. A resulting infection can cause endometritis or sepsis. The longer the pregnancy continues, the higher the incidence of maternal infection.

Although immediate induction is routinely performed, there may be situations in which induction is delayed, such as maternal refusal or the presence of a multiple gestation.

In cases of multiple gestations, fibrinogen, prothrombin time (PT), partial thromboplastin time (PTT), and platelet count are obtained. If these values are normal, no further monitoring is required. DIC rarely occurs in cases of multiple gestations where the remaining fetus(es) are allowed to grow and mature; however, there is a risk of multicystic encephalomalacia in monochorionic twins.

Clinical Therapy

Many women first report an absence of fetal activity, although some women may fail to recognize this change in fetal activity. Diagnosis of intrauterine fetal death (IUFD) is confirmed by visualization of the fetal heart with absence of heart action on ultrasound. Some practitioners routinely have a second ultrasound performed or have a second practitioner verify the absence of cardiac activity before making the diagnosis. When a fetal demise occurs, maternal estriol levels fall. Without medical intervention, most women have spontaneous labor within 2 weeks of fetal death. The once common practice of waiting for the onset of labor has largely been abandoned in recent years because the risks of complications increase with delaying the birth. It is estimated that 60% of fetal deaths have no known cause. In 25% to 60% of all fetal deaths, the cause remains unknown even after an autopsy (Lindsey, 2010). The specific cause is more difficult to identify if the time since the death is prolonged. Prompt birth increases the ability to identify the cause of death.

In modern practice, most women with a diagnosed fetal demise are given the option of waiting a few days or scheduling an induction procedure immediately. Most women will elect for an induction within a day or two of the final diagnosis. One study determined that women who waited more than 24 hours experienced more prolonged anxiety compared with women who underwent induction within 6 hours of diagnosis (Lindsey, 2010).

The mode of induction is dependent upon the gestational age of the fetus and the readiness of the cervix. Women with an unfavorable cervix may be given vaginal prostaglandin agents, misoprostol, or laminaria tents. Women whose gestations are less than 16 gestational weeks may have a laminaria tent inserted into the cervix before a dilatation and extraction procedure. *Laminaria tents* are made from the stems of brown seaweed which are cut, shaped, dried, sterilized, and packaged in specific sizes. Laminaria tents work by drawing water out of the cervical tissue, allowing the cervix to soften and dilate. They are commonly used to dilate the cervix in preterm gestations when induction is warranted. They may be placed before surgical procedures or inductions of labor.

Women less than 28 weeks' gestation are typically given misoprostol 200 to 400 mg vaginally every 4 to 12 hours until spontaneous labor occurs (ACOG, 2009). Women who are term and have not had a previous cesarean birth or other uterine scar may undergo an induction of labor. Women with an unfavorable cervix may be given cervical ripening agents, such as vaginal prostaglandin agents or misoprostol. Induction with high-dose Pitocin regimen can be performed following the same protocol as any other term induction of labor (ACOG, 2009).

In women who have had a previous low transverse incision cesarean birth over 28 gestational weeks, cervical ripening and transcervical Foley catheter are recommended. Misoprostol 400 micrograms every 6 hours has been given to women between 24 to 28 weeks with a previous uterine incision (ACOG, 2009). Management of women with a previous classical incision or uterine surgery is limited and the method of birth should be individualized.

Postbirth Evaluation

Identifying the causative factor of fetal loss assists many families in progressing through the mourning process. Information obtained from a postmortem examination or postmortem studies can provide vital information related to the cause of the fetal death, the possibility for reoccurrence, and closure for the couple. The types of studies and tests performed depend on the parents' past history, medical history, and the couple's preferences for the depth of testing desired. Chromosome studies should be considered if the couple has a history of other second- or third-trimester losses or if either parent has a suspected balanced translocation or mosaic chromosomal pattern (ACOG, 2009).

If an intra-amniotic infection is the suspected cause, cultures of both the placenta and the fetus should be obtained. If specific infections are being considered, both IgM and IgG antibodies should be drawn to determine if an acute infectious process has occurred.

All stillborn infants should have a careful visual inspection at the time of birth for obvious defects or abnormalities. The placenta and membranes should also be closely examined and the placenta should be sent to pathology for further testing. The umbilical cord should be inspected for true knots, a velamentous insertion, lack of Wharton's jelly, or a short cord to determine if a cord accident was the cause. If a specific cause is suspected, blood tests and x-rays can be performed (Lindsey, 2010). An autopsy is the best mechanism to determine the cause of death; however, in the event that the parents decline an autopsy, magnetic resonance imaging (MRI) can also provide detailed information (Lindsey, 2010).

Most practitioners perform a complete blood count (CBC) and antibody screen upon admission. Because diabetes is a causative factor, a random or postpartum glucose level can be obtained to rule out this cause. Additional maternal factors can also be evaluated. Additional tests that may be performed are listed in Table 38-1.

The Experience of Loss

Application: Grief

The term **bereavement** comes from a root term meaning to be "deprived of something" or to be left "desolate or alone." To be bereaved simply means to have suffered the *event of loss* (Corr, Nabe, & Corr, 2009). **Grief** is an individual's *reaction to the loss,* including physical symptoms, thoughts, feelings, functional limitations, and spiritual responses. Grief reactions may

TABLE 38-1 Tests to Determine Cause of Fetal Loss

FETAL TESTING	MATERNAL TESTING
• Fetal blood tests and x-rays	• Diabetes testing
• Autopsy or magnetic resonance imaging (MRI)	• Complete blood count (CBC) with platelet count
• Placental studies	• Kleihauer-Betke test
• Chromosomal studies (if indicated)	• Abnormal antibody testing (lupus anticoagulant, anticardiolipin antibodies)
	• Thyroid stimulating hormone (TSH) levels
	• Infectious disease testing (rubella, syphilis, malaria, toxoplasmosis, cytomegalovirus)
	• Hereditary thrombophilia testing
	• Toxicology testing

be immediate or delayed, heightened or stunted, and highly variable. Though often used interchangeably, **mourning** is the *process* by which individuals incorporate the experience into their lives. Mourning is influenced by many factors, including personality, gender, family dynamics, and social, religious, and cultural norms (DeSpelder & Strickland, 2005). Mourning may be manifested by certain behaviors and rituals, such as weeping or visiting a gravesite, which help the person experience, accept, and adjust to the loss. The unanticipated loss of an expected child can be devastating and traumatic for parents. Though most people eventually regain a sense of purpose and adjust well, some suffer long-lasting and destructive consequences. "Studies suggest that 15% to 25% of women who experience perinatal loss have enduring adjustment problems and many seek professional help to guide them through this difficult time" (Bennett, Litz, Lee, et al., 2005, p. 180). Bennett et al. suggest that there is nothing in a person's background to prepare him or her for the abrupt transition from a joyous event to the sorrow of perinatal loss. Perinatal loss is also unique in that the parents have not had experiences with the child that was to be, and attachment is based mostly upon hopes and dreams for the future relationship (Callister, 2006).

Society typically does not offer the kind of support for perinatal loss that is offered for other, more recognized losses. This places perinatal loss in the category of disenfranchised grief. **Disenfranchised grief**, as defined by Kenneth Doka (2002), is grief that is not supported by the usual societal customs. Perinatal loss is sometimes referred to as a "silent loss" because of this phenomenon of disenfranchising grief. People are uncomfortable discussing the loss with the parents and often pull away when their support is most needed. "The loss of a child and all the child has to offer, compounded with the societal attitude discounting the loss and the potential withdrawal of social support, may leave the bereaved parents feeling distraught and alone at a time that was supposed to be full of happiness" (Bennett, et al., 2005, p. 181). Parents struggle to come to terms with the devastation of the loss and are often confused and bewildered as to how to make that happen. The nurse caring for a family experiencing perinatal loss can take positive steps to help facilitate the family's mourning process and help them begin their journey to recovery.

Frameworks for Understanding Perinatal Loss

There have been a plethora of models and theories postulated over the years attempting to explain patterns of grief and loss, and there is no consensus for which models should serve as the cornerstones of theory and teaching. There has been some very enlightening research in the last decade, however, that is presenting a vastly different perspective of bereavement than previously offered. Surprisingly, research into the grieving process in the past decade has not successfully replicated data supporting the stage model of grieving made famous by Elisabeth Kubler-Ross (Maciejewski, Zhang, & Block, 2007). For instance, in natural deaths, whether expected or unexpected, acceptance and sense making were the predominant emotions throughout the first 24 months, rather than the previous stage model where the acceptance stage followed the depression stage close to the end of the first year (Neimeyer, 2009). Current evidence-based research supports the belief that the grieving process is entirely variable, and dependent upon many factors, such as the type of death, age of the deceased, and age of the griever. It is nonlinear and more easily understood when simply thought of as a process that encompasses the need of the griever to remain connected to the deceased, while simultaneously finding a way to exist in a changed world without the deceased (Currier, Holland, & Neimeyer, 2006; Neimeyer, 2009). For a mother who loses a baby, this might be phrased as "Am I still a mother? Who am I now?" The *intensity* to which the grief will be experienced is best understood from the aspect of the level of attachment the grieving person had to the deceased and usually entails finding personal meaning in the loss for successful integration into the grieving person's life. Several models explain these concepts.

Worth noting is the **dual process model**, a view of grief encompassing two competing spheres: loss and restoration. The loss orientation is concerned with the individual's need to confront the reality of the loss, and the restoration orientation seeks to regain balance and temper the pain of grief. Both spheres of orientation are important; some people may gravitate more toward the loss side and some more toward the restoration side. The dual process model can be helpful as the griever comes to understand that they have the choice to consciously shift between spheres, allowing grief in the safer moments, while recognizing the necessity of change (Neimeyer, 2009).

With respect to perinatal loss specifically, there are two theories that may provide the best framework for the nurse seeking to understand and assess the grieving family in his or her care. **Attachment theory**, first developed by John Bowlby (1969) and revisited by Brier (2009) and Shaver and Tancredy (2001), begins with the basic premise that human beings are biologically predisposed to bond with emotionally significant persons in their lives. The grief response as seen through the lens of attachment theory is a state of separation anxiety brought on by the disruption in the attachment bond. The intensity of the grief response displayed by parents experiencing perinatal loss can be assessed to some extent by determining the level of attachment to the anticipated infant. For mothers, nine events are important to the formation of attachment to her baby (Bennett, et al., 2005; Klaus & Kennell, 1976):

1. Planning the pregnancy
2. Confirming the pregnancy
3. Accepting the pregnancy
4. Feeling fetal movement
5. Accepting the fetus as an individual
6. Giving birth
7. Seeing the baby
8. Touching the baby
9. Giving care to the baby

Helpful questions to assess the first five levels of attachment could include topics such as naming of the baby, future plans,

TABLE 38-2 Psychologic Process of Becoming a Parent

- Feelings of procreativity or generativity
- A sense of continuity through the generations
- Responses to quickening and bodily changes
- Fears and expectations about the coming baby
- The impact of this exciting process on expectant parents' relationship at home
- Changes that the baby will bring to their careers and to their lives in general
- Attachment to real and idealized aspects of the infant
- Self-esteem building

Source: Reprinted from Loss during pregnancy or in the newborn period: Principles of care with clinical cases and analyses, *1997, p. 7. Reprinted with permission of the publisher, Jannetti Publications, Inc., East Holly Avenue, Box 56, Pitman, NJ 08071-0056. Phone (856) 256-2300; FAX (856) 589-7463. (For more information, visit the Web site at www.ajj.com).*

nursery preparations, and personal stories of the pregnancy. Additionally, there are psychologic processes related to becoming a parent that can help to identify those parents who have a strong level of attachment. These are noted in Table 38-2.

Several researchers and theorists have demonstrated the need for continuing bonds as a means to remain connected to the deceased infant (Arnold & Gemma, 2008; Boelen, Stroebe, Schut, et al., 2006; Boerner & Heckhausen, 2003; Talbot, 2002). Therefore, the goal of recovery, as related to attachment theory, is for the grieving parent to find a way to maintain the bond with the deceased infant while at the same time acknowledging that the infant is not physically present for future interactions.

The second theory centers on a search for meaning and is probably the most prevalent theme for bereaved parents. Robert Neimeyer (2005, 2009) proposes that meaning reconstruction is one of the most important aspects of the grieving process for bereaved individuals. Simply put, **meaning reconstruction** focuses on redefining ourselves and our interactions with the world after a significant loss. There is no question that the unexpected loss of a baby can precipitate a crisis of meaning for the parents. Are they still parents? How do they readapt to the world without their child in it? A large percentage of parents (61%) are troubled by the question, "Why me?" and 70% to 85% find themselves searching for meaning early in the loss. Evidence supporting the conceptualization of parental bereavement as a crisis of meaning is plentiful (Attig, 2004; Cacciatore & Bushfield, 2007; Neimeyer, 2009; Wheeler, 2001). However, it has also been suggested that some individuals do not seek meaning; that of those who do, less than half are able to find it; and that even when they do, the tendency is to continue searching (Currier, Holland, & Neimeyer, 2006). Other studies showed that a significant factor of influence is the particular meaning construct the person places on the loss. People who tend to find positive constructs within the loss fare better than those who tend toward negative constructs (Gamino & Sewell, 2004). Neimeyer concluded, partly in response to the Davis study, that when parents are struggling with meaning making, it is important to facilitate the process; but if they are not, the caregiver should not initiate the process. The goal of recovery, as related to meaning reconstruction, is a positive change in self-identity by assigning the loss a meaning, thereby allowing the individual to assimilate the loss into her or his world.

Once there is an understanding of the frameworks for the mourning process, or the rationale behind the grief, common manifestations of grief can be explored. It is important to note that for purposes of this discussion, only the possible early responses are identified, as these are the ones the nurse is most likely to encounter in the clinical care setting. Initial grief reactions can include shock, numbness, denial, protest, disorientation, guilt, and confusion. In the initial grief reaction, there is a protective brain mechanism at work that activates to prevent us from taking in too much damaging information at one time and going into "meltdown." For a couple experiencing perinatal loss, this might manifest itself in *denial* of the impending or actual death of the fetus or infant. Even when the initial healthcare provider suspects fetal demise, the couple is hoping that a second opinion may be different. Some couples may not be convinced of the death until they see and hold the dead infant after birth. The couple may move rapidly from shock, confusion, and denial into very intense emotions. *Anger,* resulting from feelings of loss, loneliness, and, perhaps, guilt, is a common reaction, as is despair and an intense longing for the event not to have occurred. Anger may be projected at significant others and/or healthcare team members. The mother may attempt to identify a specific event that caused the death and may blame herself for the death. As the couple and their families begin to confront the pain of their loss, many normal manifestations of grief may be present. The nurse should be familiar with these normal reactions, so that abnormal or complicated reactions can be identified when present. See Table 38-3.

Special Issues for Consideration

Many factors will influence a couple's response to perinatal loss, including individual factors such as age, gender, and personality type. A teenage couple is going to react very differently than a couple in their 30s, men and women tend to respond differently, and emotional personalities will display differently than stoic personalities. Family dynamics will greatly factor into the grief response. Is the family chaotic in nature? Is there a family leader? Do they have open communication or closed and guarded interactions? Do they deny the reality of the event and pretend it isn't happening? Answers to these questions can greatly assist the nurse who is caring for the family. Culture and religious beliefs also influence the couple's reaction in a negative or positive manner. Socioeconomic status will play a role, in that for some people, grief is a luxury. If the grieving parent(s) are more concerned with children at home, or putting food on the table, their grief will most likely be delayed to a time when they have the resources to deal with it. Finally, there are special circumstances that will influence the grief response. Early pregnancy loss has a special form of grief attached, fetal reduction and multifetal pregnancy loss entail separate and distinct issues, and grief from infertility is a largely ignored segment of the grieving population. Each of these components bears further discussion.

TABLE 38-3 Normal Physical, Cognitive, Emotional, Behavioral, and Spiritual Early Responses to Loss

PHYSICAL	COGNITIVE	EMOTIONAL	BEHAVIORAL	SPIRITUAL
Physical signs and symptoms of shock Palpitations Shortness of breath Difficulty sleeping Nausea/vomiting Loss of appetite Dry mouth Feeling of emptiness in the pit of the stomach Weakness/lethargy Tightness in throat Sighing Fatigue Oversensitivity to light and sound "Aching" arms	Denial, disbelief Confusion Sense of unreality Disorientation Time confusion Vigilance or obliviousness Focused or detached Poor concentration Preoccupation Sense of presence Hallucinations of the deceased infant	Sadness Anger/rage Guilt/self-reproach Anxiety Numbness Flat affect Indifference Withdrawn or explosive Repetitive storytelling Loneliness Yearning/nostalgia	Withdrawal Dependence Fear of being alone Memorializing the loss Disorientation Sleep and appetite disturbances Absent-minded behavior Dreams of the deceased Crying/sighing Restlessness Avoidant behaviors Treasuring of mementos	Blaming God Hostility toward God Lack of meaning or direction Wishing to join the deceased Isolation Feelings of betrayal Hopelessness Destruction or strengthening of beliefs Feelings of being punished Acceptance as "Divine Will" Assigning of deceased infant as "angel" in heaven

Sources: Data from DeSpelder, L. A., & Strickland, A. L. (2005). The last dance: Encountering death and dying *(7th ed.). New York, NY: McGraw Hill; Eutsey, D. E., et al., (Eds.). (2001).* Palliative care: Patient and family counseling manual. *Gaithersburg, MD: Aspen Publishers, Inc.; Schneider, J. M. (1994). Colfax, WI: Seasons Press; Worden, J. W. (2009).* Grief counseling and grief therapy: A handbook for the mental health practitioner *(4th ed.). New York, NY: Springer Publishing Company, Inc.*

Individual and Family Issues

Age

Age plays a major role in grief reactions. Couples in their 30s may feel that they are running out of time for childbearing; however, they are most likely to have living children at the time of the loss, which may eventually soften the blow somewhat. Couples in their 20s may be experiencing their first significant death, yet often have the sense that they still have time to have another child. With regard to age, however, adolescent parents probably pose the greatest challenge to nursing interventions.

The birthrate for females aged 15 to 19 rose 3% to 41.9 births per 1000 in 2006, the first increase since 1991 (Martin et al., 2009). When adolescents become pregnant, 70% have mixed feelings or do not want to be pregnant and only 41% view themselves as pregnant with a "baby" (Wheeler, 1997). The adolescent who attaches meaning to her pregnancy has the highest rate of grief reaction and life impact. Wheeler's landmark study (1997) showed that grief responses of adolescents were also affected by age of the adolescent, the gestational age at the time of the loss, and the length of time since the loss. Those who were 16 years and younger reported more physical and emotional responses to the loss than did the older adolescents, and those whose losses occurred after 14 weeks' gestation reported more sensitivity to the lack of social support afforded them following the loss.

Though adolescents have a mature concept of death, it is often clouded by their sense of invulnerability, an "It can't happen to me" mentality (Corr et al., 2009). Adolescents rely heavily on peer support and have a natural mistrust of authority figures, which can make assisting them more difficult. It is important to remember that adolescents are already experiencing major life changes, and the death of an infant can have a profound impact on their development. For many adolescents, a pregnancy loss may be the first time they are experiencing the psychologic impact of grief, and normal adolescent growth and development must be taken into consideration when assessing the impact of grief responses (Wheeler & Austin, 2000). Nursing care of the adolescent parent experiencing perinatal loss requires patience and understanding on the part of the nurse. Adolescent parents should be treated with respect and offered the same consideration as adult grievers. They should not be forced into any particular mode of response, but allowed to dictate their own needs within the experience. Gentle and honest guidance are often all that are needed to ensure a healthy nurse-patient interaction.

Family Dynamic

Family dynamics and the presence or lack of cohesion will greatly factor into a couple's grief response. Families who are chaotic and have poor interfamily communication skills are often fractured and of little support to the couple experiencing the loss. Families who demonstrate strong familial ties and open group interaction tend to fare better in the long run. The most difficult family dynamic to assess and assist is the "lie and deny" family. This family deals with bad news and loss events as though they have not occurred. If they do not talk about it, it did not happen. Because a necessary component for the beginning of a healthy mourning process is to accept the reality of the death, the nurse is placed in the tenuous position of mediator between medical personnel and the family members, who do not want to hear anything negative. It is important to discern the possible causes for denial before proceeding. Denial is a normal and necessary process in the beginning of the mourning process, and the family may just need more time to assimilate the difficult information. Persistent denial, however, can be addressed by a gentle review of the facts of the situation with an emphasis on past tense verbiage when discussing the infant.

Gender Issues

Historically, most of the research regarding grief and bereavement has been done on women. As a result, many stereotypes developed regarding how men and women cope with loss. Hallmark research by Martin and Doka (2000) identified a new model for the two major coping styles and reveals a more effective means of supporting the griever. The model identified the two dominant styles of coping as "intuitive" and "instrumental." People with **intuitive styles of coping** generally feel their way through loss and prefer care with an emphasis on emotional and psychosocial support. People with **instrumental styles of coping** generally use more cognitive skills to navigate loss and value care that includes an emphasis on problem solving (Corr et al., 2009). It is important for the nurse to be aware that although gender *influences* mourning, it does not *determine* the experience for the bereaved.

For intuitive grievers, the nurse may initiate discussion of thoughts and feelings concerning the loss. Mobilization of support from nonjudgmental family and friends is generally appreciated, and providing resource materials that include support groups and the opportunity for networking is usually welcome. The nurse should share with intuitive grievers that enlisting the support of others with whom they can talk rather than relying solely on their spouses is favorable for both partners. The nurse should also share that spouses are commonly unable to be emotionally available to each other following loss. The nurse should normalize the lack of emotional accessibility and provide reassurance that the relationship is not doomed to fail because of the death of an infant.

For the instrumental griever, the nurse should specifically address that a parent who seems detached and unaffected by the loss is not uncaring. It is more common for men to fall into this category, as they frequently experience pregnancy through the mother and, when traditionally trained, believe they are not supposed to be emotional but be strong for their partners (Worden, 2009). The parent who is an instrumental griever may not mention the infant, talk about the loss, or view pictures. He or she may resist when the partner shows emotion or attempts to engage him or her in conversation regarding the loss. Instrumental grievers tend to be more active as well as more vocal in assigning blame and commonly use explosive emotion to obtain desired results. Contrary to traditional thought, instrumental grievers' response to loss is not unhealthy, yet they are often criticized for their behavior. Because of their perceived strength, they rarely receive validation and support from others. In supporting instrumental mourners, the nurse should keep in mind that they value acceptance, acknowledgment of their pain, information regarding the loss, what to expect in the aftermath, and tasks that are connected to the loss.

The nurse should inform bereaved couples that both styles of grieving are acceptable and should be honored. Intuitive grievers (most often women) should understand that instrumental grievers may not show emotion or wish to talk about the loss, but are mourning in their own way. Instrumental grievers (most often men) should understand that intuitive grievers will need to talk about the event and help to provide avenues for that outlet. The nurse can instill a measure of hope by reassuring parents that although they may feel as if they cannot bear the pain of the loss, it will not always remain so intense.

Other Features of Bereaved Individuals

In addition to age, family traits, and gender issues, Parkes and Weiss (1983) identified overall features of bereaved individuals that place them at increased risk for pathologic or complicated grief reactions. These features include insecurity, anxiety, or low self-esteem; previous psychiatric history; excessive anger and guilt; a physical disability or illness; previous unresolved losses; inability to express emotion; and concurrent problems of living. Parkes and Weiss also identified features of bereaved individuals' circumstances that will put them at risk; these include an unsupportive or unavailable family, lack of social/religious or other supports, and low socioeconomic status.

Societal Issues

Spirituality

In times of crisis, spirituality brings comfort and strength to some people, and for some it is the single most important factor in quality of life. For others, a life crisis may precipitate a spiritual crisis and catalyze a complete redefining of the belief system, though the new belief system is often stronger than the one previously ascribed to (Frantz, Farrell, & Trolley, 2005).

Religion and spirituality are not one in the same. **Spirituality** is defined as the human search for meaning and connectedness to life, others, God, the universe, and transcendence. **Religion** is defined as structured efforts conducted in a systematic approach to attain holiness (Balk, 2004). Religious practices are based upon the level of a person's assimilation into the particular religion and are too varied and numerous to define for standards of care. With regard to specific religious practices, it is prudent for the nurse simply to ask the family how they can best be assisted in meeting their religious needs.

One study identified six themes affecting the spiritual needs of bereaved parents: honest exchange of information, empathy and presence, continuing bonds, spiritual rites, attachment with others, and grief support (Meert, Thurston, & Briller, 2005). The nurse can facilitate the spiritual needs of the couple by providing an atmosphere of acceptance regarding spiritual rites and encouraging the couple's use of spiritual writings, prayers, and observances. Questions that solicit the spiritual viewpoint of the couple regarding the loss can allow release of parental distress concerning spiritual matters. It is important for the nurse not to answer rhetorical questions, but allow the parents to process their own thoughts and feelings concerning meaning, purpose, and significance of the life and death of their infant. It is also important for the nurse to distinguish between his or her own personal beliefs and those of the parents. Some healthcare professionals get defensive and critical when the spiritual needs of the parents conflict with their own spiritual viewpoint. Recognition of personal limitations is healthy and providing care is not exclusive to direct delivery. The nurse acts as a family advocate by offering to contact the couple's clergyperson, spiritual advisor, or the hospital chaplain. Research

CLINICAL TIP

It is vitally important to respect the family's religious beliefs and not interject our own preferences into the situation. Baptizing an infant whose parents have not requested such is a violation of their rights and disrespecting of their wishes. Allow the parents to dictate all spiritual aspects of their infant's care.

DEVELOPING CULTURAL COMPETENCE

Cultural Responses to Perinatal Loss

There is much information a nurse can learn about a particular culture's response to perinatal loss and grieving. While knowledge of specific beliefs and rituals is helpful when caring for a family from an unfamiliar culture, it is *most* important that the nurse simply remains open, curious, nonjudgmental, and unassuming. There are underlying threads that weave together the relevant factors affecting grief response, yet no two people will grieve alike and even knowledge of a person's cultural and religious background does not offer the nurse a guaranteed blueprint to follow. This is particularly true where culture is concerned. Not only are there many country of origin and regional differences, but the extent of assimilation into American culture will factor in as well. Therefore, to say that all Hispanic Americans will respond to the death of an infant alike because they are all Hispanic Americans would be akin to saying that all Protestants will worship alike because they are Protestant. One only has to consider the vast number of Protestant denominations with varying and often conflicting viewpoints to realize that such a generalization is useless to the nurse assisting grieving parents and families. Perinatal loss is unique in cultural awareness because one can never be sure to what extent culture, religious beliefs, or other factors will dominate the response to such an unexpected and unnatural event as the death of a baby. Even people who have assimilated into American culture will often revert in times of crisis and death.

confirms that providing effective spiritual care to a parent during loss and bereavement is valuable in facilitating healthy parental mourning (Meert et al., 2005).

Remembering that while the family is the most reliable source of information about its own beliefs and how to best assist it, there *are* some commonalities within culture groups that the nurse should be aware of in anticipation of meeting the parents' and family's needs (Table 38-4). The way many cultures experience grieving and death rituals is often heavily influenced by their religious beliefs, and therefore addressed in the table as well.

CLINICAL TIP

A basic rule of thumb for cultural issues is to remember that curiosity is okay; avoidance is not. If you are not sure what the family needs, simply ask them how you can help to accommodate their wishes. Families appreciate an honest and caring attitude.

PROFESSIONALISM IN PRACTICE

Instituting Culturally Competent Care

There are ways that a nurse can provide culturally competent care in such a challenging situation. A good place to start is with a formal or informal cultural awareness questionnaire similar to ones used for general nursing care. Questions pertaining to death, dying, and perinatal losses should provide answers for the following:

- What the families beliefs are about what happens after death
- How the family views the death of an infant, in particular
- How the dying infant should be cared for as he or she approaches death, including who should be present and any ceremonies that should be performed at the moments before and after death
- How the body should be handled after death, including how the body should be cleansed and dressed, who should handle the body, and whether the body should be buried or cremated
- Whether grief should be expressed quietly and privately, or loudly and publicly, such as with public crying, keening, or wailing
- Whether there are different expectations on how a man should grieve versus a woman, or for children versus adults; what the family considers the role for each member in coping with the death
- What ceremonies and rituals should be performed and who should participate, such as children, community members, and friends

(Adapted from Cancer.Net. (2009). Understanding grief within a cultural context. From http://www.cancer.net/patient/Coping/Grief+and+Bereavement/Grief+Among+Cultures; Clements, P. T., Vigil, G. J., Manno, M. S., Henry, G. C. Wilks, J., Das, S., et al. (2003). Cultural perspectives of death, grief, and bereavement. *Journal of Psychosocial Nursing, 41*, 18–26.)

Specific Circumstance

Infertility

Infertility is not an episode, but an ongoing struggle for those who are caught in its grasp. The focus of treatment for infertility is a correct diagnosis, appropriate treatment, and successful live birth, yet infertility brings with it grief and loss issues that affect all realms of the couple's life. Not only are the medical and physical components extremely challenging, but the loss issues of infertility go largely unrecognized by the usual support systems, placing it within the disenfranchised grief category. In the early phase, the patients are trying to assimilate the diagnosis of infertility and what the diagnosis actually means for them. Then they are faced with a gamut of decisions and difficulties such as:

- Treatment available (method that is best for them; when to begin; repercussion of choices; risk involved)
- Waiting (menstrual cycles; pregnancy; failed pregnancy; surgery; hormone treatments; in vitro fertilization)
- Psychologic roller coaster (spiritual impact; the strain on finances and primary, secondary, familial, and workplace relationships)
- When to discontinue treatment.

TABLE 38-4 Common Cultural Practices: Grief, Bereavement, and Perinatal Loss

CULTURE	FAMILY HIERARCHY & REACTION TO MEDICAL COMMUNITY	COMMON BELIEFS AND EXPRESSIONS OF GRIEF	CARE AND HANDLING OF THE BODY: RELIGIOUS & CULTURAL RITUALS
		Before & After Death	***Before & After Death***
African American	Matriarchal; family decision making. Family, religion, and community play a large role in grief recovery; considered collectivists. May distrust majority healthcare system; common to rely on internal resources. Healthcare providers should work to build trust and respect family dynamics.	Vary widely because of diversity in religious beliefs, countries of origin, and geographical regions. Some will cry or wail while others will appear stoic, especially if mistrustful of healthcare providers. Many hold strong religious beliefs; will turn to clergy for assistance. Prayer for healing or comfort around the bedside is a common occurrence for Christians. May be averse to withdrawal of life support.	Will generally want pictures and mementos; naming of the infant is important for family heritage. Death is often called "home going" or "passing on," especially by Christians. May desire pre- or post-death baptism. Common to wait for extended family to arrive for funeral services. Most likely to prefer burial to cremation. May have elaborate caskets and/or services as a way of showing respect and giving the infant a final tribute. Tend to view life as a continuous circle, and therefore many have a steadfast belief of being reunited with their infant.
Old Order Amish	Patriarchal; strong family and community ties. Decisions dictated by religious beliefs; made by both parents, but father will usually relay. Will accept life-supporting medical technology. Most have eighth-grade education, so information should be provided appropriately. Will consent to legal dictates.	Children are a gift from God. Many losses occur due to advanced maternal age and consanguinity. The loss is profound, but viewed as God's will. Very private in grief; will keep to themselves for comfort. Rare for them to share with outsiders, known as the "English."	Do not believe in infant baptism. Family and friends will usually want to wash the body for burial in a white gown. Photos are not permitted (for the living or dead). May not accept mementos as community prepares casket and burial clothes, but offer should be made as less conservative families may accept. Bracelet may be accepted as legal identification. May want to transport body home and burial will be at a designated facility or on the family farm as laws permit.
Asian American	Generally patriarchal, but strong community influence. In the more traditional families, older members are highly respected and should be included. Generally avoid confrontation and more traditional may avoid eye contact. Touching is impolite. Saying "no" directly may be considered rude, so healthcare provider should ask open-ended questions.	Community oriented. May believe that bad *karma* causes illness and death. May believe the number "4" is associated with death. Death of an infant is intensely mourned. Initial grief is acceptable and there may be crying and/or wailing at times. Death is not a usual topic for discussion and overt expressions of prolonged grief may be viewed as mental illness and therefore may alternately be expressed as somatic complaints (safer to be body related than mind related).	Usually a blend of Western and Eastern grieving and death ritual practices. The body should be handled with much care and always with respect. Family members may wear white clothing or headbands to mark mourning. Common to have an elaborate funeral ritual for the soul's passing.
European American	Family hierarchy is dependent upon faith values; Christian families tend toward patriarchy, while secular families tend toward companion marriage with equal decision making. Comfortable with technology and generally utilize to fullest extent possible. More likely to question authority and expect answers from healthcare providers.	Expressions of grief span the spectrum of responses; most often dictated by religious beliefs, geographical regions within the United States, and country of origin. Crying is acceptable; intense grief reactions are dependent upon previous factors noted. Usually no set mourning period and most likely to mourn longer than support is offered.	May or may not wish to bathe infant personally. May or may not wish to view and/or hold the infant. May or may not desire pictures. The nurse should inquire about all, but not place pressure for any. Naming of the baby and use of the name by healthcare providers is important. Burial or cremation preference may be determined by faith practices, financial status, or personal preference. May desire funeral services; infant areas in cemeteries are acceptable, especially to Catholics, who view infants as sinless. Baptism may or may not be desired and should not be done unless the parents request such. Pictures and mementos are usually appreciated.
Hinduism (addressed separately, although Indian Americans are included in the Asian American minority group)	Patriarchal, though family oriented; needs of all over individual emphasized. Husband or eldest male will usually communicate decisions.	Combination of culture, philosophy, and religion. Believe in *karma* and reincarnation; seek to transcend birth and death by good deeds (karma), which ultimately frees the soul.	The body should be bathed, oils applied, and dressed in new clothes. Cremation should take place before the next sunrise in order to release the soul from the body. Eldest male member begins the cremation by physically pushing the button or flipping the switch (or, in older traditions, lighting the funeral pyre).

(continued)

TABLE 38-4 Common Cultural Practices: Grief, Bereavement, and Perinatal Loss continued

CULTURE	FAMILY HIERARCHY & REACTION TO MEDICAL COMMUNITY	COMMON BELIEFS AND EXPRESSIONS OF GRIEF	CARE AND HANDLING OF THE BODY: RELIGIOUS & CULTURAL RITUALS
		Before & After Death	***Before & After Death***
Hispanic & Latino American	Patriarchal; family decision making. Male to female, older to younger concept of *respeto* (respect) in social order. Applies to healthcare providers and mutual respect is expected. More trusting of individual practitioners than system; expect warmth, caring and attention. More traditional will expect handshake and formal use of last name upon introduction (Senor y Senora). Generally view human touch as respect from healthcare professionals.	View loss as God's will. Tend to rely on faith and prayer as tools for coping. Outward expression is encouraged, especially crying among women. Men tend toward stoicism for the family. Both may experience depressive symptoms. Support comes from family and friends. Extended family will usually travel for services. Support is found in family, friends, church, and community. Tend not to look toward medical community for support.	Baptism and naming are usually desired. Generally prefer burial to cremation. Pictures and other mementos are important, as they tend to utilize them for honoring the infant in the home. Country of origin will determine particular rituals involved in grief and death. Catholicism predominates. Prefer open casket ceremonies. May wear traditional dark funeral clothing for an undefined mourning period. Continuing bonds with the deceased are important (hence, the "Day of the Dead" in Mexico). Belief of a fine line between the living and dead. Rituals include the lighting of candles, prayers for the dead, and shrines for honoring them.
Jewish	Traditionally patriarchal; modern Jews tend toward companion marriage with equal decision making.	For observant Jews, having children is commanded by God and considered a great blessing. Loss of an infant is profound and support may be sought from the family's rabbi. Some will tend toward stoicism while others will openly grieve. Believe the soul begins the journey from the body immediately; this is why it is important to bury the body as soon as possible. The parents may not want to view the body as they tend to want to remember the deceased as alive rather than dead.	Perinatal loss is a somewhat controversial topic in Judaism today. Traditionally, neonates (infants under 30 days of age) were not named or provided traditional bereavement practices such as sitting shiva. In recent times, the customs have changed and many will observe full mourning and burial rituals for a perinatal loss. Adherence to traditional Jewish tradition will entail body washing by a special group of people who ritually wash and dress the body in linen shrouds. Naming the infant will depend upon whether the family adheres to the old traditions, as will sitting shiva. The infant may be named at the burial and given a name associated with comfort. Pictures of the dead are not permitted and autopsy not acceptable unless there is benefit to the living. Burial should take place within 24 hours and cremation is forbidden. Bodies should be whole if possible. Burial is sometimes in an infant section, but always in a Jewish cemetery and usually in a wood coffin with no metal to delay decomposition. Prefer monetary donations to charities in lieu of flowers as the withering and dying of the flowers is considered a painful reminder of the loss.
Muslim	Patriarchal, but decision making is shared. Information should be provided to both parents, even though the father may relay all decisions. Autopsy is usually forbidden unless for major concerns or demanded by law.	Death is considered a part of life. Children are a gift from Allah and are returned to Allah if they die, as they are considered sinless. The death of a fetus or infant is not minimized, but regarded as just as significant as that of an adult. Crying and solemn expressions of grief are permitted as long as control is maintained. Excessive grieving is considered not accepting of the will of Allah. The funeral is followed by three formal days of mourning (and 40 days of unofficial mourning), but for infants less than 4 months gestation, the fetus may only be wrapped and buried.	If the child is born alive, but death is imminent, the father may whisper the phrase "There is no God but Allah" in the infant's ear, securing the infant's call to worship. Naming is essential as the mother and infant will be bound together in paradise. Parents may desire to perform a ritual washing of the body, usually by the same sex parent. Conversely, they may not wish to see or hold the baby, as the viewing of bodies unnecessarily is discouraged. The legs should be straightened and sometimes the parents may request that the body face the right and face Mecca. Pictures are not usually desired, but should be offered. Locks of hair should not be removed; the body should be left intact and wrapped in a plain white shroud. Cremation is forbidden.
Native American	Patriarchal, though parents will make decisions together.	Navajo, the second largest Native American population, have traditional customs followed upon death. Tend to be stoic, and grieve privately. Death is viewed as a transitional step on the journey to the next world and the mourners must follow strict burial and bereavement rituals to ensure a successful journey.	Rituals must be completed within 4 days of death. The body is washed and painted for the journey. They do not speak of the dead after the fourth day because it is believed that it will impair the journey of the deceased. After a time, any discussion of the deceased is believed to bring ill health to the surviving family, and therefore support following the loss can be a challenge.

Sources: Adapted from Callister, L. C. (2006). Perinatal loss: A family perspective. Journal of Perinatal and Neonatal Nursing, 20*(3), 227–234; Chichester, M. (2005). Multicultural issues in perinatal loss.* AWHONN Lifelines, *9, 312–320; Chichester, M. (2007). Requesting perinatal autopsy: Multicultural considerations.* MCN, The American Journal of Maternal Child Nursing, 32*(2), 81–86; Clements, P. T., Vigil, G. J., Manno, M. S., Henry, G. C., Wilks, J., Das, S., et al. (2003). Cultural perspectives of death, grief, and bereavement.* Journal of Psychosocial Nursing, 41, *18–26; Hebert, M. P. (1998). Perinatal bereavement in its cultural context.* Death Studies, 22, *61–78; Lobar, S. L., Youngblut, J. M., & Brooten, D. (2006).* Pediatric Nursing, 31*(1), 44–50; Schott, J., & Henley, A. (2007). Pregnancy loss and death of a baby: The new Sands guidelines 2007,* British Journal of Midwifery, 15*(4), 195–198).*

In supporting the patient dealing with infertility, the nurse should assess where the woman is in the process and respond accordingly. The nurse should be compassionate, give accurate and honest information, validate the many losses incurred, and support whatever decisions the couple makes regarding the continuation of treatment or decision to stop treatment. The nurse should not avoid the couple, offer pat answers or reasons for the infertility or the outcome, or relay unsolicited stories of others' successes or failures. For couples finally experiencing a pregnancy following infertility treatment, there may be heightened anxiety for which additional reassurances will need to be offered.

Early Pregnancy Loss

Early pregnancy loss, whether by ectopic or molar pregnancy, blighted ovum, or spontaneous abortion, is devastating for many couples. As attachment is based on the level of emotional bonding, it is necessary for the nurse to assess the situation in order to respond to actual patient needs and validate the loss for those who view the event as the death of their baby. Compounding early pregnancy loss is the extraordinary guilt the couple typically harbors, especially the mother. Mothers will often blame themselves, whether by commission or omission, particularly in cultures where a woman's status is dominated by themes of motherhood and childrearing. The nurse should reassure the couple that they did not do anything to precipitate the loss, and provide support materials specific to the type of loss incurred and what to expect in the immediate aftermath.

Assessment of future pregnancies will need to be dealt with gently, as some couples have no desire to try again. Healthcare professionals sometimes find it easier and more comfortable to refocus on something other than the loss; however, that tends to minimize the loss event and isolate the griever. Even if the parents are expressing an interest in trying again, it is important not to focus exclusively on the future pregnancy, but to provide opportunities to address the current loss. The nurse should prepare the couple for the fact that family members and friends will often underestimate the impact of the loss and may offer well-meaning, though often harmful, remarks or platitudes in an attempt to ease emotional pain. This is a common reaction in early pregnancy loss, as they may have not known about the pregnancy or feel as if the couple "didn't know the baby." The nurse should reassure the parents that they have a right to their feelings, thoughts, emotions, and reactions to the loss. An early pregnancy remembrance box (a remembrance journal, sachet pillow, and a baby ring) provides a sensitive and caring way to give parents something to take with them that contains memories of their baby (Figure 38-1 ■).

Multifetal Pregnancy Loss

In 2006, the U.S. live twin birth rate was 32.1 per 1000, and the high-order multiple-birth rate was 153.3 per 100,000 births, a decline since the 2002 statistics. One of every eight twins, and one of every three triplets are born very premature (less than 32 weeks gestation) and thus death during infancy is much more common in twins and multiples at 29.8 per 1000 and 59.6 per 1000 births, respectively (Martin et al., 2009). Multifetal pregnancy loss (MPL) may occur by spontaneous abortion, elective termination for unwanted pregnancy, selective reduction for fetal malformation, or selective reduction in high-risk multiple pregnancy to provide a greater chance of survival for remaining embryos. The loss of an infant in a multiple pregnancy may also occur by intrauterine demise, twin-to-twin transfusion syndrome, complications of monoamniotic twinning, placental problems, adverse intrapartum events, delayed interval delivery, postoperative complications, and the effects of prematurity. Parents whose multiples die have an increased risk of prolonged or delayed grief (Pector, 2004).

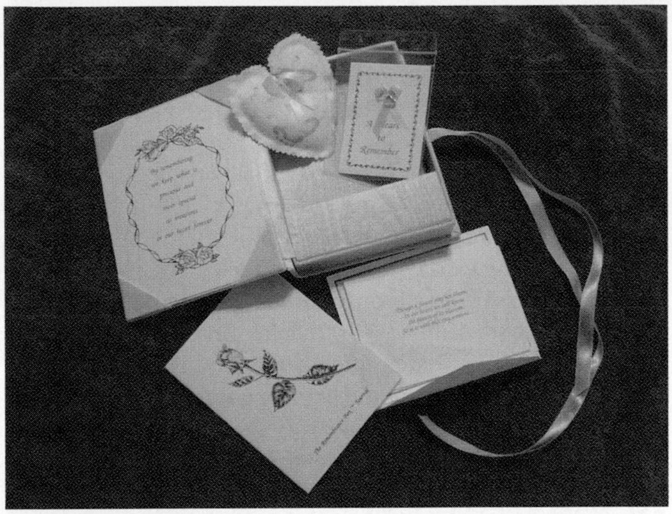

Figure 38-1 ■ Early pregnancy remembrance box.

Source: © Share Pregnancy & Infant Loss Support, Inc. www.nationalshare.org

Many aspects of multifetal pregnancy loss have historically been overlooked by healthcare professionals (Keefe-Cooperman, 2004–2005; Kersting et al., 2005; Pector, 2004). Some of the predominant issues affecting parents are the following:

- Traumatic impact of diagnoses of malformation or birth defects
- Options and impact of difficult decisions
- Sudden death of an infant, fear and anxiety for surviving infants
- Prospect of infertility because of previous abortions
- Last attempt at in vitro fertilization (IVF) or such fertility intervention, guilt
- Cohabitation of mourning and joy, and resurgence of the body's remembering on special days and holidays

In supporting bereaved parents caring for surviving infant(s) in the loss of a multiple, the nurse should resist the urge to suggest the parents refocus on the positive aspect of having surviving siblings. Statements inferring that the death was meant to be, the death allowed the other infant(s) to live, or the child who died would have had a compromised quality of life should never be made. The nurse should understand that the couple might have difficulty mourning their loss as they attempt to balance emotions of joy and sadness while caring for the surviving infant(s). Parents will often imagine what the deceased infant might have looked like, what kind of personality the infant might have developed, and what the relationship with siblings might have been. They may harbor feelings of guilt if they feel relief for not having to care for numerous infants. The nurse should support parents by addressing these distinctive concerns and prepare them for the unique issues related to multifetal loss before they leave the hospital.

When creating visual memories for bereaved parents, an effort should be made to take pictures of the multiples together. The nurse should ask parents how they prefer to address surviving infants, for example, twins, triplets, quadruplets, and so forth. Additionally, the nurse should ask the couple whether they wish to delay funeral services until the mother is able to attend the ceremony. If the couple desires a delay, the nurse should contact appropriate disciplines to arrange for the delay in disposition of fetal remains (Pector, 2004). The nurse should prepare the mother for the likelihood of her body missing and remembering the baby immediately after delivery, while caring for surviving infant(s), and surrounding special days, milestones, and holidays. Finally, the nurse should be aware of the risk for complicated bereavement and refer the couple for appropriate support via resource materials (Keefe-Cooperman, 2004–2005).

Maternal Death

Maternal death is defined by the World Health Organization as "the death of a woman while pregnant or within 42 days of termination of pregnancy, irrespective of the duration and the site of the pregnancy, from any cause related to or aggravated by the pregnancy or its management, but not from accidental or incidental causes (2007)." The most common causes of maternal death are hemorrhage, hypertensive disorders, embolism, infection, and pre-existing chronic conditions, such as diabetes and cardiovascular disease. Obesity is also becoming a significant factor in maternal deaths because of the medical conditions that result (The Joint Commission, 2010). In 2006, the national maternal mortality rate was 13.2 deaths per 100,000 live births (Heron, et al., 2009). A recent number of reports indicate that maternal mortality may be rising in the United States, although there has been a change in the classification system that may have resulted in the identification of more deaths as pregnancy-related (Hoyert, 2007). The numbers of maternal deaths are certainly not decreasing, however, and the death of even one mother on a perinatal unit can be a devastating experience for all involved.

For the husband or father of the child, the death of his partner is shocking (even if she had previous medical problems) and traumatic, somewhat akin to the proverbial knock on the door when there has been an unexpected accident. There is an even deeper shock presenting here, in that the death is surrounding an expectedly joyous event, a birth. The initial shock of maternal death experienced by the husband or father is traumatic and powerful. The grieving process is complicated by a number of factors (such as possibly caring for the newborn infant while grieving his partner) and too comprehensive a topic for this venue. What is important for nurses caring for the father and/or other family members is to recognize that initial grief reactions may be extremely intense. As long as no one is violating the fundamental principles of grief reaction (not hurting themselves, others, or personal property), the father and family should be fully supported through this initial time with all support available to them and the facility in which the nurse is practicing. Interactions should be brief and direct, such as offering tissues, and straightforward condolences (e.g., "I'm so sorry this is happening to you"). As with all losses, it is important to resist offering explanations or platitudes. There are no adequate explanations, and platitudes are not helpful and in most cases prove harmful.

For the staff, a maternal death on the perinatal unit can be traumatic as well. When a death occurs on any unit, there are individual as well as group reactions to the event. The individual nurses involved may experience feelings of shock, sadness, anger, guilt, and other grief-associated reactions. The unit as a whole may experience feelings of inadequacy, anger, guilt, confusion, and depression. For the nurses directly involved, the father and family must still be cared for, and for everyone on the unit, nursing care continues. It is important for management in these situations to step in and provide an opportunity for the staff to express their feelings in a safe environment. Intervention for the staff could include professional debriefing or, where professional assistance is not available, simply calling a staff meeting to allow the nurses to work through some of the emotions while supporting one another (Dietz, 2009). The most important thing for the nurse to remember is to take care of his or her own grief reactions and allow time for personal healing. Focusing on the positive aspects of the situation where they exist (such as personal kindness shown to the mother before the death, or to the family in the aftermath) is an important step in the healing process as well as reflecting objectively on those things out of one's personal control (the mother's underlying medical issues or unforeseen complications). The idea, as with the loss of an infant, is to eventually memorialize the event with a balanced perspective, recognizing where personal effectiveness as well as limitations exist and learning to live with them, both personally and professionally.

NURSING CARE MANAGEMENT

Nursing Assessment and Diagnosis

The Clinical Setting

Cessation of fetal movement reported by the mother to the nurse is frequently the first indication of fetal death. It is followed by a gradual decrease in the signs and symptoms of pregnancy. Fetal heart tones are absent, and fetal movement is no longer palpable. Once fetal demise is established, the nurse assesses the family members' ability to adapt to their loss. Open communication among the mother, her partner, and the healthcare team members contributes to a realistic understanding of the medical condition and its associated treatments. The nurse may discuss prior experiences the family has had with loss and what they feel were their perceived coping abilities at that time. Identifying the family's social supports and resources is also important.

Perinatal loss may also occur in the intrapartum period as a result of an intrapartum complication, such as an unresolved shoulder dystocia, prolapsed umbilical cord, abruptio placentae, or other complication. In such emergent situations, healthcare team members often focus on the physical needs of the mother and an attempt to save the fetus's life. Commonly, it is not until the infant is delivered that the family is advised a perinatal death has occurred. Thus, the parents are faced with the sudden and completely unanticipated death of their infant. The most common response is protest or disbelief.

Although the physician or certified nurse-midwife (CNM) informs the family of the death, the nurse continues one-on-one care with the family, providing both physical and emotional support throughout this crucial period. The nurse assists the family in the mourning process and explores their immediate wishes for viewing and holding their deceased

Nursing diagnoses that may apply include the following:

- ***Grieving*** related to the imminent loss of a child
- ***Powerlessness*** related to lack of control in current situational crisis
- ***Compromised Family Coping*** related to death of a child/unresolved feelings regarding perinatal loss
- ***Interrupted Family Processes*** related to fetal demise
- ***Hopelessness*** related to sudden, unexpected fetal loss
- ***Risk for Spiritual Distress*** related to intense suffering secondary to unexpected fetal loss

Nursing Plan and Implementation

Most facilities have an established protocol to follow in the event of perinatal death. It typically provides a holistic focus for family-centered nursing care. It is important that the entire healthcare team be notified so multidisciplinary care can be initiated. When fetal death has been confirmed before admission, the entire staff on the unit is informed so they can avoid making inappropriate remarks. Many facilities have a symbol, such as a card with a leaf or a cluster of flowers, which is placed on the mother's door so that all of the staff is aware of the loss (Figure 38-2 ■). This is something that should be discussed with the family before placement, as some may view the symbol as an identification of them as "damaged." As is stated throughout the chapter, it is important to allow the family to dictate their own experience.

Figure 38-2 ■ Door card.

Source: © Share Pregnancy & Infant Loss Support, Inc. www.nationalshare.org

Avoiding the Use of Clichés

> **“** There were the inevitable platitudes about God "needing another angel" or God "taking" Gabriel from us for a reason. I can't imagine those concepts being a comfort to anybody. What kind of sadistic God would breathe life into a baby only to snuff it out? After millennia of infant deaths, you'd think God would have plenty. If God needed more babies in heaven, God could simply will some into existence . . . I would be bitter for the rest of my life—and probably beyond—if I thought a higher power had targeted my baby to die. **”**
>
> —*Amy Kuebelbeck**

Inappropriate remarks are a hallmark of uninformed interactions, even though the intent behind them is honorable. The nurse should become familiar with statements that are helpful in facilitating the family's mourning process. Although grieving people often say that it is easier to forgive less-than-helpful remarks than to forgive those who do not reach out to them at all, the use of clichés can be harmful. The nurse can facilitate a healthy mourning process for the family by using active listening techniques and avoiding the use of clichés. Sitting in silence with a family is often the most helpful form of intervention available. For a list of helpful versus unhelpful statements with rationales, see Table 38-5.

Application: Grief

Facilitating the Family's Mourning Process

As mentioned at the opening of this chapter, there has been a recent paradigm shift in the field of grief and bereavement with regard to what constitutes a "normal" mourning process, as well as when and where early intervention is warranted. The standard of care has been centered on the notion that early and intense grief responses should be encouraged and even elicited for healing to begin. The relevant research, however, determined that many people are naturally resilient and will recover in their own time, without the benefit of assistance (Balk, 2004; Bonnano, 2008; Lang, Goulet, & Amsel, 2003; Miller, 2003). For instance, stoic responses, when exhibited because of familial or cultural traits, are not always counterproductive and may not need intervention in order for the person to begin the path to recovery. Furthermore, not only is early intervention not always necessary, it can even be harmful in some instances (Bonnano, 2008; Brier, 2009; Murray, Terry, Vance, et al., 2000). Although the research confirms that traumatic grief is usually best assisted by early intervention, perinatal loss does not *always* fall into this category, which leads to the current quandary: When is early intervention warranted and effective? The debate continues, but for the nurse caring for a family experiencing perinatal loss, avoiding the trap of "cookie cutter" responses is not difficult if simple, caring guidelines are followed rather than rigid rules. The nurse should keep two goals

---

*Excerpt from *Waiting with Gabriel: A Story of Cherishing a Baby's Brief Life* by Amy Kuebelbeck (Loyola Press, 2003). Reprinted with permission of Loyola Press. To order copies call 1-800-621-1008 or go to www.loyolapress.com.

TABLE 38-5 Unhelpful Versus Helpful Interactions with Grieving Families

UNHELPFUL	HELPFUL	RATIONALE
You're young; you can try again. At least you have your other children.	I am sure you'll miss [Sara] and no one will ever take her place in your heart.	Saying that they can try again diminishes their current pain. Saying that no one can ever take the deceased infant's place validates the loss as real and the infant as unique.
At least you didn't know him or her yet.	I'm sure you had many hopes and dreams for the future.	Never start a sentence with the words "at least." It diminishes whatever follows. Speaking of future plans validates the loss of the hoped-for child and the dreams that will never be.
It's a blessing in disguise.	I don't know why this terrible thing has happened to you. I just want you to know that I care and want to help you through it.	Statements like, "It's a blessing in disguise" are often said when there are deformities involved. There is no adequate explanation for the family as to why this tragedy has befallen them and none should be offered. Instead, reassurance that they will not be alone should be given.
God needed another angel in heaven.	I'm so sorry this is happening to you. You are a good person and this is a terrible thing to have to go through. I'm here to listen if you would like to talk about it.	The family may make this statement as an indication of their belief system, and that is perfectly acceptable. It is not acceptable, however, for the nurse to impose her or his own belief system upon the family. It is much more effective to address the issue at hand (they are in pain) and reassure them of your caring presence.

in mind when assisting grieving parents and families. The first is to help the family navigate the medical/hospital system and the second is to facilitate the family's mourning process by allowing them to dictate their own experience.

CLINICAL TIP

Allowing families to meet their own needs in grief offers them the best path to learning to live with their loss; trying to force them into doing things the way that you think is best for them serves your own needs, not theirs, and can prove harmful.

The Caring Theory

The classic caring model developed by Swanson (1991), has sustained the test of time; it is as relevant today as when it was originally developed. Perhaps because of its lack of rigidity and concentration wholly on the overall *attitude* of the caregiver, it can best serve as a solid foundation for good nursing practice related to bereavement care. The **caring theory** consists of five attributes of the caregiver: (1) knowing, (2) being with, (3) doing for, (4) enabling, and (5) maintaining belief.

Knowing is defined as attempting to understand the event as it has meaning in the life of the parents. A thorough nursing assessment will facilitate the nurses' understanding of the significance of the loss to the parents. Nurses who operate from a level of knowing are perceived as sensitive, knowledgeable, and appropriate. Nurses who do not are often perceived as distant, cold, and uncaring. *Being with,* or being emotionally present, is the nurse's ability to reach beyond professionalism and give of herself or himself as a human being. *Doing for* is a restating of the golden rule. It means that the nurse does for the parents as she or he would have things done for her or him in the same situation. This does not mean detail by detail, as every family is unique in their needs; rather, this is an overall, treat-them-as-you-would-your-own-family type of behavior. *Enabling* means facilitation of the parents' passage through life transitions and unfamiliar events. Enabling encompasses all of the interventions listed throughout the text regarding perinatal loss and places the caregiver in the role of facilitator. Finally, *maintaining belief* is defined as believing in the parents' capacity to get through the event and face a future with meaning. The nurse who ascribes to this model of care well serves the needs of bereaved parents by compassionately helping them in the midst of their pain and imprinting positive memories to sustain them.

The Art of Responding

Employing the caring theory of behavior, the nurse can then look to the responding model as a set of guidelines for successful interactions with grieving families. Keeping in mind the uniqueness of each situation, the **responding model** is offered to give the nurse an overall set of guidelines for effectively interacting with families experiencing perinatal loss (see Table 38-6). The specific elements of the model are addressed throughout the rest of the chapter and within the nursing care plan.

Preparing the Family for the Birth and Death

Upon arrival to the facility, the couple with a known or suspected fetal demise should immediately be placed in a private room. When possible, the woman should be in a room that is farthest away from other laboring women. Care should be taken not to

TABLE 38-6 The Essential Elements of Responding Effectively to the Needs of Grieving Families

Recognition and Validation of the Loss
Emotional Availability
Spiritual and Cultural Accommodation
Physical Presence
Open Communication
Normalization of Grief Reactions
Decision-Making Assistance
Interdisciplinary Involvement
Nonjudgmental Attitude
Genuine Caring

Source: Shields, K. (2005). Preparing the family for the birth and death. *Healing Through Hope. Used with permission.*

leave the couple in the waiting room with other expectant parents or visitors waiting for news from other women in labor. The nurse should sit down for a moment, offer an introduction, and acknowledge the loss in the event of a known demise or impending death. A simple statement such as "My name is Brenda and I'll be your nurse today; I'm so sorry; this must be so hard for you. I'd like to help you through it," will go a long way toward establishing a relationship of trust between the nurse and the parents.

The couple should be allowed to remain together as much as they wish. The nurse provides privacy as needed and maintains a supportive environment. The couple should be given complete information about what to expect and what will happen. Questions should be encouraged and answered (Figure 38-3 ■). The nurse stays with the couple so they do not feel alone and isolated; however, cues that the couple wants to be alone should be assessed continuously. Some couples may want outside support, such as family members or friends, to be present during the labor. The nurse facilitates the couple's wishes.

When possible, the same nurse should provide care for the couple so that a therapeutic relationship can be established. As the relationship develops, the nurse provides solace by listening to the couple without offering explanations. The nurse also provides ongoing opportunities for the couple to ask questions. It is not uncommon for the family to ask the same questions repeatedly. This is part of the initial process. Clear explanations and straightforward answers should be provided and the parents treated equally in giving of information. The nurse also arranges for other members of the multidisciplinary team to interact with the family. The team should take great care to avoid inflicting further trauma on the couple by

PERINATAL COMFORT CARE PROGRAM
PLANNING FOR OUR BABY'S BIRTH A PARENT'S REVIEW LIST

- ♥ Let your doctor and Labor/Delivery staff know the name of your baby.
- ♥ Your baby's condition may be different at time of birth than expected right now. Your doctor may need to make immediate medical decisions at the time of your baby's birth in order to give your baby the best chance for a quality life. Some of your plans may not be possible in this situation. Please talk about this with your doctor before your baby's birth.

Mother's Name ______ Father's Name ______ Baby's Name ______

Obstetrician ______ Pediatrician ______ EDC ______ Diagnosis ______

Completed by: ______ (Name/Title) ______ (Date)

Section A

♥ **These are our wishes for the *personal care* of our baby at time of birth.**

		Comments/Date	Revisions/Date
	1. Hold our baby as soon as possible and as much as possible		
	2. Establish a plan for family and friends to celebrate our baby's birth/ visitation on the floor. Designate ______ to give updates to family and friends.		
	3. Designate ______ as adult chaperone for siblings.		
	4. After delivery and when I am stable to celebrate, stay in the same room for labor, delivery, and recovery if possible		
	5. Have a family member cut the umbilical cord		
	6. After delivery, give my baby to me after being quickly wiped, suctioned and wrapped.		
	7. Perform religious ceremonies		
	8. Videotape our baby		
	9. Take pictures of our baby		
	10. Make footprints & handprints of our baby		
	11. Take family photos and handprints		
	12. Have private time with our baby with minimal interruptions		
	13. Bathe our baby		
	14. Hold our baby while dying and after death		
	15. Obtain keepsakes such as : lock of hair, ID band, tape measure, crib card, hat, blanket and clothes		

St. Joseph Hospital
ST. JOSEPH HEALTH SYSTEM

PATIENT ID

PERINATAL COMFORT CARE PROGRAM
PLANNING FOR OUR BABY'S BIRTH
A PARENT'S REVIEW LIST

7401-0053 (6/22/07) Page 1 of 2

Figure 38-3 ■ St. Joseph perinatal comfort care program: planning for our baby's birth, a parent's review list.

Source: Courtesy of St. Joseph Hospital, St. Joseph Health Systems, Orange, CA. www.sjo.org

(continued)

	16. Allow teaching services (Medical residents and/or nursing students) present ☐ YES ☐ NO		
	17. Organ Donation Wishes		
	18. Autopsy -		
	19.		

Section B

	♥ **These are our wishes for the *comfort care* of our baby at time of birth**	**Comments/Date**	**Revisions/Date**
	1. Let me know if our baby has a heartbeat		
	2. Perform oral/nasal suctioning and blow by oxygen for comfort only		
	3. Do not perform advanced life support without explaining why it is necessary		
	4. Delay taking vital signs, weighing our baby, giving medications and obtaining lab work if not medically necessary		
	5. Allow our baby to feed: ___ breastfeed or ___ drops of expressed milk or formula		
	6. Provide our baby with medications if needed for comfort care		
	7.		

Section C

	♥ **Discuss your *medical options* with your doctor prior to birth:**	**Comments/Date**	**Revisions/Date**
	1. Medications to be used during labor		
	2. Management of milk suppression		
	3. Physical comfort measure after birth		
	4. Review your wishes for extended stay		
	5. Discuss plans for taking your baby home if this is an option		
	6.		

Plan of Care reviewed by: ________________________ ____________

(Signed by Hospital Staff) ________________________ ____________

________________________ ____________

The following changes have been made by the parent(s) upon admission to the hospital

____

____

____

St. Joseph Hospital

ST. JOSEPH HEALTH SYSTEM

PERINATAL COMFORT CARE PROGRAM
PLANNING FOR OUR BABY'S BIRTH
A PARENT'S REVIEW LIST

PATIENT ID

7401-0053 (6/22/07)

Page 2 of 2

Figure 38-3 ■ Continued. St. Joseph perinatal comfort care program: planning for our baby's birth, a parent's review list.

Source: Courtesy of St. Joseph Hospital, St. Joseph Health Systems, Orange, CA. www.sjo.org

displaying conflicting words and behavior, such as using a falsely cheerful tone of voice while their body language clearly indicates sorrow (Trulsson & Radestad, 2004). The nurse offers to contact the hospital chaplain or another cleric for them, and a social worker should be involved. The nurse typically coordinates members of the multidisciplinary team so that a comprehensive plan of care can be initiated.

The nurse explains details of the plan of care (Figure 38-4 ■) and allows the family to ask questions and make decisions for their labor and birth preferences. The availability of anesthesia and analgesia should be reviewed. The woman typically can have pain medication whenever she desires. The nurse facilitates the participation of the woman and her partner in the labor and birth process.

It is important to remember that, in contrast to a typical birth experience, the birth of a terminal or stillborn infant marks both the beginning and the end. For this reason, it is imperative that the couple and family have all wishes and preferences respected. The family may be overwhelmed and may have difficulty making decisions in this period. The nurse can strengthen the couples' ability to cope by providing a warm atmosphere of acceptance. The nurse must assist the couple in exploring their feelings and help them to make decisions about who will be present and what rituals will occur during and following the birth. Examples of birth preferences include the following:

- Use of music, dimmed lighting, or other environmental preferences
- Laboring or birthing in a specific position
- Having the infant placed on the mother's chest immediately after birth

A THERAPEUTICALLY EQUIVALENT PRODUCT MAY BE DISPENSED AND ADMINISTERED UNLESS CHECKED IN THE LEFT COLUMN.

✓	DATE	TIME	⬅ DATE AND TIME MUST BE ENTERED	NEONATAL COMFORT CARE ORDERS	ROOM NO.

ALLERGIES: **Weight:** ______ **kg**

Check (✓) all that apply and fill in the blank if applicable

1. **Medical Diagnosis:** ____________
2. **Code Status:** ☐ **Full Code** ☐ **See DNAR Form**
3. **Vital Signs:** every 4 hours and Prn
4. **Diet:** Breast milk or Formula ________ as tolerated by breast, bottle, gavage, or syringe
   ☐ If needed place a Corpak for home care size _____ unweighted
5. **Offer Non-pharmacologic Comfort Measures Prn:** Swaddling, Holding, and Pacifier
6. **Offer Oral Sucrose per policy for mild to moderate pain Neonatal Infant Pain Scale (NIPS) less than 4**
7. **Pain Control:**
   A. **Short-acting or Breakthrough Pain Medications**
   Opioids need not be held for respiratory depression in actively dying patients.
   ☐ Morphine ____mg (0.2 – 0.5 mg/kg/dose) Po q ____ HRS Prn severe pain NIPS score greater than 4
   ☐ Acetaminophen ____mg (10 –15 mg/kg/dose) Po or PR q ____HRS Prn mild pain
   Note: Max dose = 90 mg/kg/day if greater than 36 weeks; 60 mg/kg/day if 32 – 36 weeks
   B. **Long-acting Pain Medications**
   Opioids need not be held for respiratory depression in actively dying patients.
   ☐ Methadone ____mg (0.05 – 0.1 mg/kg/dose) Po q ____HRS
   C. **Gastric Pain**
   ☐ Famotidine suspension (8 mg/mL) ______mg (0.5 mg/kg/dose) Po q 12 hours, **or**
   ☐ Other: ____________
8. **Dyspnea: Order opioids here if patient not already receiving opioids for pain.**
   ☐ Morphine _____mg (0.2 – 0.5 mg /kg/dose) Po q ___HRS Prn dyspnea
   or
   ☐ Lorazepam _____mg (0.1 mg /kg/dose) Po q ___HRS Prn dyspnea
   ☐ _____ % Oxygen _____ liters/min. by nasal cannula (indicated for hypoxemia; may be helpful in other cases)
9. **Anxiety/Agitation**
   ☐ Lorazepam ____mg (0.1 mg /kg/dose) Po q ____HRS Prn agitation.
   or
   ☐ Diphenhydramine ____mg (1 mg /kg/dose) Po q ____HRS Prn agitation
10. **Secretions**
   Control with medications is preferred as suctioning can be uncomfortable for the patient.
   Note: Minimizing fluids will help decrease symptoms
   ☐ Reposition q 2-4 HRS as tolerated
   ☐ Glycopyrrolate ____mCg (40 – 100 mCg /kg/dose) Po q ___HRS Prn secretions
11. **Fever**
   May consider additional non-pharmacologic measures such as bathing.
   ☐ Acetaminophen ____mg (10 –15 mg /kg/dose) Po or PR q ____HRS Prn Temp greater than ____°C
   Note: Max dose = 90 mg/kg/day if greater than 36 weeks; 60 mg/kg/day if 32 – 36 weeks
12. **Diarrhea**
   ☐ Loperamide ____ mg (0.08 – 0.24 mg /kg/DAY in divided doses) Po q ___ HRS Prn diarrhea (Do not exceed 2 mg/dose), **or**
   ☐ Other: ____________

12-hour Chart Check____________ **RN** **DATE:** ____ / ____ / ____ **TIME:**______

T.O. ____________ **Taken by:** ____________ **Title:** ______

TRANSCRIBED BY: ______ ___/___/___, **TIME:**______ **NOTED BY:**______ ___/___/___, **TIME:**______

PHYSICIAN SIGNATURE: ____________ **DATE:**______ **TIME:** ______

PRINTED NAME/ID:. (FOR MEDICATION/BIOLOGICALS T.O. ORDERS ONLY, COUNTER-SIGN ABOVE WITHIN 48 HOURS, AND INCLUDE THE DATE/TIME AUTHENTICATED)

St. Joseph Hospital
ST JOSEPH HEALTH SYSTEM

NEONATAL COMFORT CARE ORDERS

PATIENT ID

6381-2065 (5/07/07)

PHYSICIAN'S ORDERS

Figure 38-4 ■ St. Joseph Hospital Neonatal Comfort Care Orders.

Source: Courtesy of St. Joseph Hospital, St. Joseph Health Systems, Orange, CA. www.sjo.org

- Allowing the father to cut the umbilical cord
- Including other family members or friends present at the birth

Sometimes couples worry that others may view their preferences as "strange" or "wrong." Reassure the family that it is their experience and that there are no right or wrong feelings or wishes.

The couple may have waves of overwhelming grief, disbelief, or sadness. Encourage them to experience the grief that they feel, but do not force the issue. It is not uncommon for one partner to attempt to put on a "brave front," feeling that, by showing grief, he or she will make the other partner feel worse. It is also not uncommon for partners to have intense feelings that they feel unable to share. Encourage partners to express their emotions freely to the extent they are able. Help them understand that they may each experience different feelings.

> ❝ At last, we are holding our beautiful baby. Swaddled in his hospital blanket decorated with pastel teddy bears and hot-air balloons, he is crying with some effort, his eyes squeezed tightly closed. He has the plump newborn cheeks his sisters had and a hint of downy dark hair. He is a little pale, and his fingernails are faintly blue. He is beautiful. We are overwhelmed with pride and love—and concern—for the newest member of our family. ❞
>
> —*Amy Kuebelbeck**

*Excerpt from *Waiting with Gabriel: A Story of Cherishing a Baby's Brief Life* by Amy Kuebelbeck (Loyola Press, 2003). Reprinted with permission of Loyola Press. To order copies call 1-800-621-1008 or go to www.loyolapress.com.

Supporting the Family in Decision Making

It is important to remember that the family will need guidance *throughout* the process. The couple should be offered simple choices all along the way to help them retain as much control over their situation as possible. If the infant is born alive, but suffering from a complication that is incompatible with life, the nurse should make every effort to allow the parents as much time as possible with the infant. In addition, the extended family should be allowed as much access as is comfortable for the parents.

> "I kiss Gabriel's forehead. It is cool . . . I kiss him again and whisper to him, "Don't leave yet." I tell him (Mark) that the nurse seemed concerned about Gabriel's heart rate. She comes back and listens with her stethoscope again. "Six," she said. Six? We don't understand. Her face close to mine, she says gently, "Your baby is dying." No! Not yet! The words scream through my mind, but nothing comes out except a sob."
>
> —Amy Kuebelbeck*

Advocates of seeing the stillborn infant believe that viewing assists in dispelling denial and enables the couple to progress to the next step in the mourning process. In recent years, this has become a topic of controversy in the field of death and dying. A study by Hughes and colleagues in 2002 concluded that adverse outcomes such as higher anxiety levels were reported in higher numbers in mothers who held the infant than in mothers who only saw the infant or did not see or hold the infant (Turton, 2008). One potential explanation for this aberrant finding is the possibility that if nurses who are uncomfortable with death and dying are rigidly following standard bereavement checklists rather than recognizing the uniqueness of each situation, the mother and father may be forced into uncomfortable situations they are not properly prepared for. Another proposed explanation is that when the parents view and hold the infant, further bonding occurs, which leads to a more intense grief reaction. Even more recently, Turton (2008) found an increase in posttraumatic stress disorder among women who held their dead infant. Ironically, though the women wanted to hold and see the infant, the trauma appears to be related to the vivid imagery that is implanted during holding and see the dead infant. It should be noted, however, that numerous other studies did not find an increase in anxiety and instead found that most women who held their infant did not regret it, while many who did not had subsequent feelings of regret (Cacciatore, Radestad, & Froen, 2008; Flenady & Wilson, 2008; Radestad & Christofferson, 2008; Radestad, Saflund, Wredling, et al., 2009). Until more conclusive studies are reported, the nurse should offer the couple the opportunity to see and hold the infant, assess possible motivations behind negative responses (such as a fear of the unknown), and reassure the couple that *any decision they make for themselves is the right one.* Careful listening on the part of the nurse should allow the parent(s) to make clear their wishes. Additionally, the nurse should not allow pressure from others to be put upon the couple to either see and hold or not see and hold their stillborn infant. If they choose to see their stillborn infant, prepare the couple for what they will see by saying "she is going to feel cold," "he is going to be blue," or other appropriate statements. If the parents have shared with you the name they had chosen for their baby, use that name in discussing the baby; for example, "Jessie's face is bruised." If the couple is hesitant to view the infant out of a fear of what the infant will look like, offering a Polaroid picture will sometimes help to allay their fears. With the development of digital bereavement photography, it is becoming easier for nurses to offer the family quality photos of their infant. Most facilities have a digital camera and printer for such use. There are also Web sites where parents can obtain digital photography or have photographs enhanced, edited, or have effects added, such as selective coloring (McCartney, 2007).

> **CLINICAL TIP**
>
> A picture that appears distressing in color may be comforting in black-and-white. A close-up of the infant's hand or foot lying in the parent's hand may provide a loving memory. Use your creativity in taking bereavement pictures.

Postmortem Care

Properly preparing the infant for viewing and holding is an essential step in the process. Stillborn infants are often misshapen, and the skin can be discolored or in a state of maceration. **Maceration** is the process of tissue breakdown, which begins from the moment an undelivered infant dies. It is characterized by sloughing of the skin, which can help determine the interval between death and delivery of the infant; that is, the more sloughing, the greater length of time between the demise and delivery (Pauli, 2005). When bathing the infant for viewing, care should be taken to cause as little additional disruption to the skin as possible. A gloved hand is preferable to a washcloth for these infants. After bathing, the infant should be placed in a suitable-sized gown and then wrapped in a blanket. A hat can be applied to cover birth defects. This allows the parents an opportunity to view the infant before seeing the birth defect. Many parents will eventually remove the covering to inspect the infant; however, applying a covering allows them time to adjust to the appearance at their own pace. In cases of extreme maceration, the parents should be fully informed of the condition of the skin, so that they can decide for themselves if they want to see, hold, and/or fully uncover the infant. Couples will often look to assisting medical and nursing personnel for the "correct" attitude toward their stillborn infant. The nurse should carefully monitor personal reactions and display acceptance of the choices the parents make. For step-by-step postmortem care instructions, see Table 38-7.

In a compromised or dying infant, bathing should be done quickly, so that the infant can be returned to the parents as soon as possible. Some parents may wish to participate in the bath

Rights of Parents When a Baby Dies—Choices or Mandates?

*Excerpt from *Waiting with Gabriel: A Story of Cherishing a Baby's Brief Life* by Amy Kuebelbeck (Loyola Press, 2003). Reprinted with permission of Loyola Press. To order copies call 1-800-621-1008 or go to www.loyolapress.com.

TABLE 38-7 Postmortem Care

Document Time of Death per Physician

Gather Supplies per Hospital Protocol

Appropriate forms.

Bathing—2 basins, absorbent pads, diapers, clothing, washcloths, hat.

Memory kit—memory card with foot or handprint area, memory box.

Morgue kit—identification tags, pads for wrapping, paperwork.

Remove Tubes and Wires When Applicable

Cap and leave all indwelling tubes and catheters if autopsy is to be performed. Plug endotracheal tube (E.T.) with cotton ball and tape over opening to hold in place and prevent seepage.

Bathe and Dress Fetus/Infant

Offer parents opportunity to assist with bathing and dressing infant as appropriate (if infant is stillborn, skin maceration may be traumatic for parents).

With gloved hands, place infant in lukewarm basin of water.

Rinse if skin breakdown is present; if skin integrity is intact, rub gently with washcloth. Soap is optional; based also on integrity of skin.

Place fetus/infant in second basin of lukewarm water to rinse.

Gently pat dry. Do not use scented (especially baby products) lotions or powders.

If seepage present from nasal cavity, place petroleum jelly in nostrils.

Diaper and dress fetus/infant in outfit provided either by parents, hospital, or volunteer organization. Consider the use of a hat, particularly where deformity is present.

Take Pictures

Cover imperfections and deformities when applicable.

Use mementos in pictures when available.

Use soft, yet vibrant, colors in background or consider black and white photos.

Place fetus/infant in a flattering and comforting position (different for every infant).

Offer parents opportunity to participate in picture taking, but do not force the issue.

If Desired by Parents, Wrap in Warm Blanket and Present Infant for Holding

Prepare parents before holding fetus/infant by telling them what they will see, feel, and smell.

Offer a picture before holding.

Model normal nurturing behavior for parents.

Offer time alone with infant and check back frequently within previously specified time frame.

After Holding, Remove Clothing for Weight and Measurements, Footprints, Handprints, Memory Card, and Lock of Hair (When Applicable)

Prepare Fetus/Infant for Pathology/Morgue/Family Transport According to Hospital Protocol

For morgue care:

Complete all hospital paperwork.

Place infant in supine position on top of folded diapers and pad to maintain body position and prevent disfigurement.

Use neck and body rolls to help with alignment.

Wrap infant according to hospital protocol.

Take Memory Box and Bereavement Information to Parents

Memory box should include pictures, ID bracelet, memory card, other personal items, and bereavement clothes.

Bereavement information should include pamphlets on grief and loss as well as local and national resources for support and information.

Document the Events Leading Up to and Following the Death Including

Time and pronouncement of death with physician's name.

Placement of tubes and catheters.

Postmortem care.

Comfort measures and bereavement care provided to family.

Preparation and transport to morgue.

process or complete it themselves. Some parents will hold their infant for a short time before returning him or her to the nurse, whereas others will wish to spend a great deal of time with their infant. The nurse allows the infant to remain with the parents for as long as they desire.

CLINICAL JUDGMENT

Case Study: Lu Chen

Lu Chen, a 23-year-old G1 female of Asian heritage was admitted to the hospital 1 week ago for premature rupture of membranes and preterm labor. By dates, the fetus is 21 weeks gestation and nonviable at this point in time. Lu has been on strict bedrest and a medication regimen to halt her labor, but has developed a fever and nonreassuring fetal heart tones (FHT) and has been brought over to the labor and delivery unit for monitoring with the likelihood of imminent delivery. You have been assigned as Lu's nurse for your shift. In report, you are told that Lu is quiet and withdrawn. She answers questions with "yes" or "no," and does not elaborate. Her mother is in the room with her, but does not speak English. Lu is listed as married, but the father is not present. You are aware that the obstetrician has spoken with Lu regarding the impending delivery and the baby's incompatibility with life at the current gestational age. You do not know how much Lu understands of what she has been told and you are unsure what role, if any, her culture will play in her reaction to the loss of her baby.

The decision is made to stop the medications and let the labor progress. When you ask Lu if she would like you to call her husband to be with her, she says that he is overseas on business and cannot make it back in time. She says that her mother will be with her and that she will be fine.

The delivery takes place and you clean and pat dry the infant, and prepare for holding. You ask Lu if she would like to hold her baby, and she shakes her head no, not making eye contact. You are concerned that she may regret not holding her baby or taking pictures.

Critical Thinking

What might you say to Lu in order to assist her in emotionally preparing for the delivery of her infant?

What questions could you ask Lu that a culturally sensitive plan of care may have answered?

See www.nursing.pearsonhighered.com for possible responses.

Supporting Siblings and Extended Family Members

Some couples may want other family members, friends, or their other children to be with them in their experience, and possibly view and hold the infant. The nurse acts as an advocate to ensure that the family's wishes are respected. Siblings will respond according to their age and maturity level. Children younger than seven may not recognize that the death is permanent, whereas older children may respond with concern for the parents' well-being. It is normal for them to slightly regress in social and cognitive behaviors when under stress. Children should be included as much as desired by the parents and told the truth in a simple, honest, and age-appropriate manner, avoiding the use of euphemisms when describing death and the aftermath. A **euphemism** is a substituted word or expression with a more pleasant association than the one that, although more direct, is considered to be harsher (Corr et al., 2009). Children will need reassurance of two things: that they are still going to be taken care of and that nothing they did caused the event to happen. In facilities in which child life specialists are present, their help can be elicited to assist the family in preparing the children for the death and provide an outlet for the children during the event.

Extended family members, especially grandparents, are "doubly" grieving as they suffer through the pain their children are experiencing and the loss of their grandchild. They will have varied reactions, from the extreme of attempting to completely control the process for their child to a display of total passivity. Most reactions fall somewhere in the middle of the continuum. The nurse can help to validate the grandparents' grief by acknowledging the difficulty of their position and extending her support to them as well as to the parents. Even grandparents who are blaming, questioning, or demanding can be made a part of the team when approached in a nondefensive, nonjudgmental, and aid-enlisting manner.

Family support has been shown to be a major comfort to couples in families in which there is open communication and honest interaction. Less intense grief over time has been reported in families who are able to express their emotions with one another as compared with more stoic families. The nurse should provide every opportunity for family cohesion throughout the process, encouraging as much participation and interaction as desired by the couple.

Actualizing the Loss: Providing Memories

In a fetal demise, the nurse should remember that mementos are some of the few memories the parents have to provide them comfort after the death of their baby. Every effort should be made to offer as many quality mementos as possible, such as pictures and hand- or footprint molds and cards (Figure 38-5 ■). Most facilities prepare a remembrance box or package for the family to take home (Figure 38-6 ■). This typically consists of a photograph taken of the infant or the family, a card with the baby's footprints, a crib card, identification band, a lock of hair, and, possibly, a blanket or clothing worn by the infant. In the event that the couple decline the package, it is common for the hospital to retain these items for a specific period of time in case they change their minds.

> "Our night nurse, Cindy, encouraged us to take Gabriel's footprints before we went to sleep. She tenderly made several prints of his feet and his hands, and she helped us mix the plaster of Paris that we had brought along for a permanent imprint of his feet. While Mark held him, she carefully snipped a tiny lock of almost-black hair from the back of Gabriel's head.
> ... So in the dim fluorescent light, I rearranged the pillows on my bed to make a place for him ... My arm draped over his chest, my cheek touching his cool forehead, I fell asleep with my son for one last time."
>
> —*Amy Kuebelbeck**

Providing Discharge Care

The family usually has three options open to them for disposition of the fetus or infant's body. The first is a traditional burial. Many funeral homes offer reduced fees for infant burial services. The family should contact the funeral home directly to make arrangements. Some families may wish to bury their infant on private land. This is state, county, and locally dictated and it is up to the family to ascertain any restrictive ordinances as to transportation and burial. Hospitals with comprehensive bereavement programs in place usually have access to this information. The second option is cremation at a funeral home. Families will need to decide what to do with the cremains. The third option, and not one generally recommended, is hospital disposition. **Hospital disposition** at most facilities is incineration at regular intervals, usually with other body parts, and the family does not have the option to obtain the ashes. Some institutions, especially private and/or religiously affiliated facilities, offer mass burial options for hospital disposition, but not many.

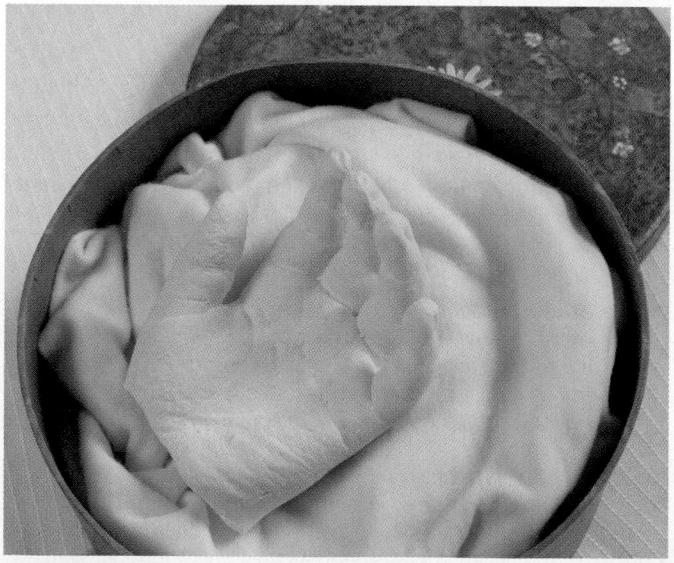

Figure 38-5 ■ Foot and handprint molds.

Source: George Dodson/Pearson Education.

*Excerpt from *Waiting with Gabriel: A Story of Cherishing a Baby's Brief Life* by Amy Kuebelbeck (Loyola Press, 2003). Reprinted with permission of Loyola Press. To order copies call 1-800-621-1008 or go to www.loyolapress.com.

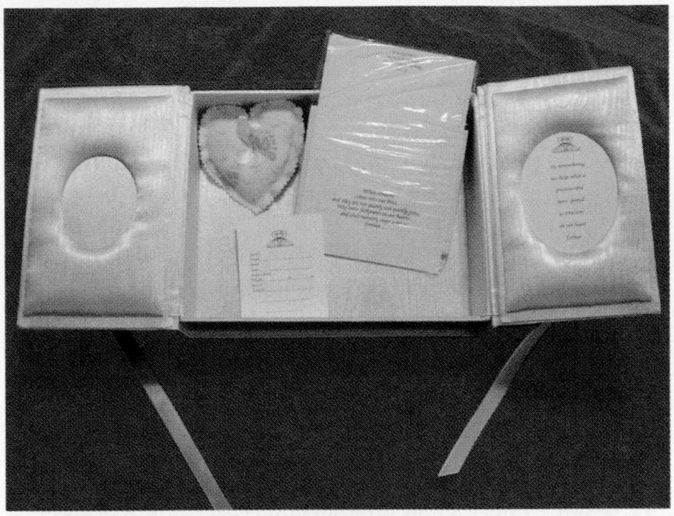

Figure 38-6 ■ Personal Memory Box.

Source: © Share Pregnancy & Infant Loss Support, Inc. www.nationalshare.org

In the last decade or so, a few programs have been initiated that offer more individualized burial options for infants designated for hospital disposition. These programs are usually a coordinated effort between facilities within a specific area and one of the local funeral homes and cemeteries that serve their community. The program is usually offered at little or no charge to the family. Whatever option the family decides upon, the nurse should support their decision and assist them in any way possible to achieve their goal for disposition and/or funeral services.

After the birth, the couple can be given the option of an early discharge (as early as 6 to 8 hours after the birth). Facility protocol will dictate where mothers are transferred after a perinatal loss. Some hospitals have the woman remain on the labor and delivery unit, whereas others will give the mother the option of choosing a postpartum room or one on a medical unit. If the mother is transferred to a postpartum unit, care is given to put her in a room far away from other rooms and the newborn nursery. Again, it is imperative that all staff members, as well as student nurses, housekeeping, dietary, and the like be notified of the mother's status (refer to Figure 38-2).

Discharge focuses on the physical considerations and adaptation of the mother and emotional considerations of the couple. Postpartum directions for follow-up care should be provided. Written materials should be provided and a phone number for questions can be given. The woman should also be given information on her milk coming in and interventions to follow to decrease the discomfort associated with engorgement.

Additional information should be given on the mourning process (Figure 38-7 ■). The nurse can prepare the couple to return home by stressing that others may not know what to say, and that even loved ones may make inappropriate comments because they do not know how to respond to grief and loss. This can prepare the couple for the reactions of others. If there are siblings, each will usually progress through age-appropriate grieving. Provide the parents with information about normal grief reactions, both psychologic and physiologic. The couple should be given information regarding depression as a normal part of grieving. Couples may feel empty and lost and may experience physical symptoms such as sleep disturbances, weight loss or gain, listlessness, fatigue, hyperactivity, inability to concentrate, and a lack of motivation. The onset of the symptoms of depression often coincides with the time when other people have moved on and withdrawn support for the couple, making it harder for them to cope. The couple should be informed that depression following perinatal loss is normal and unless debilitating or prolonged need not be medicated or treated and will subside in time. If depression is prolonged, outside help should be sought. Additionally, as the mourning process ensues, families should be encouraged to implement cultural, religious, or social customs that will assist them in their grief. The nurse should advise the family that certain upcoming milestones, such as holidays, future birthdays, baby showers, Mother's Day, Father's Day, and other social events may trigger their grief. The family can better cope with these events if they are adequately prepared. Finally, the couple should be advised not to make any major life change decisions in the first year following the death, whenever possible. Making major life changes compounds grief reactions by adding other losses (such as moving away from the familiar) on top of the loss of infant, often resulting in complicated mourning.

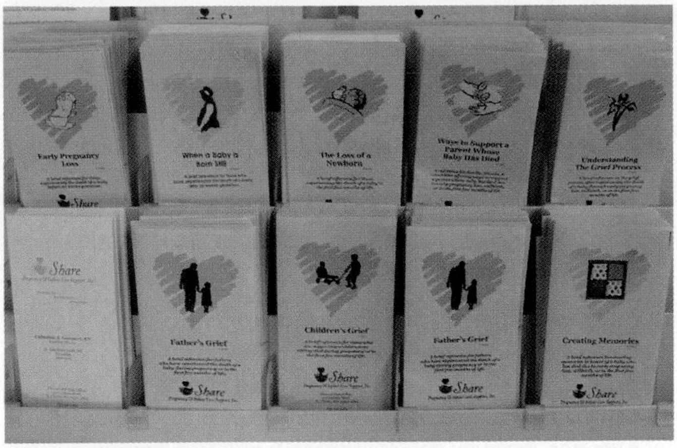

Figure 38-7 ■ Bereavement literature.

Source: © Share Pregnancy & Infant Loss Support, Inc. www.nationalshare.org

When caring for a family suffering from a perinatal loss, it is important to remember that the nurse experiences many of the same grief reactions as the parents of a stillborn infant. It is important to have colleagues and family members available for counseling and support.

Following discharge, some families may need closure of the intrapartum event to continue their mourning process. A consultation can be scheduled with the practitioner who cared for them during the pregnancy and birth. Families may also wish to read the results of tests performed during the intrapartum period and the autopsy report. The couple should be provided with a copy of the medical record and encouraged to ask questions, express their feelings, and ask for clarification.

Families are routinely referred for counseling services after a perinatal loss has occurred. A counselor who specializes in perinatal issues can provide expertise and assist the couple in their grieving. Partners should be allowed to verbalize fears and concerns about future pregnancies. When appropriate, referrals to genetic counselors, religious support persons, and social service agencies also should be provided.

Besides referral information, the parents should receive scheduled follow-up phone calls to assess the family's functioning and their progress with grief work, *if* they indicated the desire for follow-up contact. During these follow-up phone calls, pertinent information can be given and additional resources can be identified.

Referring the Family to Community Services

Perinatal Loss Resources

Although most facilities have an established protocol for families experiencing perinatal loss, programs that are more comprehensive are being established in communities to provide a systematic intervention program to assist these families. Community support groups that focus on perinatal loss can provide an important support network and resources. Specialized groups, such as those focused on early pregnancy loss, stillbirth, and perinatal loss associated with specific congenital anomalies, allow families the opportunity to interact with peers who have lost infants under similar circumstances. The nurse provides the group name, contact person (if possible), and phone number. Bereavement resources can be offered that provide a list of relevant articles and books on death, dying, and grieving the loss of an infant. Information should be provided on supportive organizations such as Share Pregnancy and Infant Loss Support, RTS Bereavement Services, Centering Corporation, and Compassionate Friends.

Internet technology has allowed large numbers of individuals to share resources and information and participate in online support groups. Internet resources can be effective for all families and may be the only resources available for families in rural underserved areas. A study by Capitulo (2004) found that online perinatal loss support groups were "cultures," in that they had distinct beliefs, behaviors, norms, and attitudes that set a pattern of behavior for members of the online community. They were very helpful in allowing mothers to interact with other mothers in similar circumstances.

Perinatal Hospice

Specialized hospice programs are another community resource that assists grieving families. **Perinatal hospice** offers a compassionate, structured program providing a context in which parents can find meaning in the intimate experience of the life and death of their child. In perinatal hospice programs, parents whose fetus has a known lethal congenital anomaly, are given the opportunity to explore options, such as elective termination or waiting for the onset of spontaneous labor or a medically indicated induced labor. For families wishing to continue their pregnancies, the program typically assigns a multidisciplinary team that provides compassionate care, ongoing counseling, referral to support groups, and spiritual guidance (Munson & Leuthner, 2007). Perinatal hospice programs have sprung up in over 40 hospitals in the country, sometimes by request of genetic clinicians who, having given parents devastating news, found themselves with nowhere to refer the parents for assistance (Roush, Sullivan, Cooper, et al., 2007). These programs offer parents much needed support and guidance through the entire process of the pregnancy, birth, discharge, and/or death of the fetus or infant.

Application: Pregnancy After Miscarriage

According to Suzanne Engelder, of the St. Joseph Perinatal Comfort Care program in Orange, California:

> "Regarding the future of perinatal hospice. . . . There has been tremendous growth over the past 4 years. More and more hospitals are looking at providing this special care. I think what is unique about our program (and a few others across the country) is that we are a collaborative program between hospice (outpatient) and hospital (inpatient). Most perinatal hospice care is being provided in the NICU setting and it really is more palliative care in the NICU versus hospice care which focuses on care and support before the birth/death to prepare and educate parents/families. What I would like to see is more hospitals collaborating with hospices to provide care before and after. Another issue is reimbursement. Currently this is a non-reimbursable service. When adult hospice first came to the U.S. in the 1970s, it was run by volunteers and there was no reimbursement for it. In 1983, Medicare made it a benefit. My hope is that perinatal hospice will follow the same path—that insurance companies will see the benefit for the patient and family and be willing to pay for the care. The care provided on the front end saves resources at the time of birth/death and the back end (bereavement)."

The strength and success of these programs are a testament to the progress that has been made in bereavement care in the last decade. The challenge ahead is to move these programs into more awareness and ensure that healthcare providers are offered education to assist them in recognition of the need for these services.

Care of the Couple Who Has Experienced Loss in a Previous Pregnancy

A couple who has had a previous perinatal loss typically enters a subsequent pregnancy with conflicting feelings and may experience ambivalence, fear, and anxiety (Callister, 2006; Côté-Arsenault & Donato, 2007; DeBackere, Hill, & Kavanaugh, 2008). Many times, their experience is relived when another pregnancy occurs. Some couples conceive soon after a loss, whereas others wait years. Some couples enter a subsequent pregnancy with grief work largely completed, whereas others are still experiencing unresolved grief.

The nurse caring for a couple who has had a previous loss needs to be kind, compassionate, and patient. Couples need specific information and clear explanations of all prenatal information. Referrals to a genetic counselor should be made when appropriate (Barr, 2006). Some couples may wish to have a consultation with a perinatologist. If unresolved grief issues are present or the family experiences extreme anxiety, counseling may be beneficial.

Interventions to decrease anxiety can help the couple tremendously. At the first visit, an early ultrasound can be performed to verify the presence of the fetal heartbeat. In early pregnancy, women may be fearful when first-trimester pregnancy symptoms begin to resolve. It may be helpful for these women to come in for weekly visits for a period of time sim-

RESEARCH EVIDENCE IN PRACTICE Pregnancy After a Perinatal Loss

CLINICAL QUESTION

How can families be supported through a subsequent pregnancy after a perinatal loss?

RESEARCH EVIDENCE

One of the most difficult situations in obstetric nursing is helping a family deal with the death of a fetus or baby. The grief process can be severe and enduring. Although one might believe a subsequent pregnancy would alleviate feelings of loss, research shows that these feelings do not disappear when the family becomes pregnant again. Indeed, some research shows that the grief from the previous perinatal loss may extend and impact the subsequent pregnancy. Parents may question whether they will be capable of having a normal pregnancy and carrying a baby to term.

Several studies have focused on the impact of a perinatal loss on subsequent pregnancies. One integrative review summarized the findings from multiple quantitative and qualitative studies. Responses to a subsequent pregnancy included anxiety that was present for both parents, but was higher for women than their partners. The timing of the most severe anxiety was linked to the timing of the fetal loss. In one study, anxiety decreased as the pregnancy advanced.

Depressive symptoms were commonly reported in women who were pregnant but had experienced a previous perinatal loss. These symptoms were higher for women than for men. As a contrast with anxiety, depressive symptoms worsened as the pregnancy progressed and appear to be greater for women who conceive less than a year after their perinatal loss.

Studies did not reveal a clear relationship between perinatal loss and attachment to the subsequent fetus. Findings were conflicting in that some showed decreased prenatal attachments, while other, more controlled, studies reported that prenatal attachment may be delayed to the third trimester but not absent by the time of birth.

The themes from these studies show parents who are trying to balance being hopeful while worried about a subsequent perinatal loss. These are complex emotions that parents may not be willing to share openly with a healthcare provider. Nursing interventions that were found to be helpful were conducting an evaluation of emotional health, encouraging parents to talk and voice their concerns, tailoring childbirth education for expectant parents who have had a previous loss, and encouraging early attachment behaviors.

WHAT QUESTIONS REMAIN UNANSWERED?

More study is needed to determine the effect of perinatal loss on subsequent fetal and infant attachment. How can the nurse encourage fetal and infant attachment when a previous perinatal loss has occurred?

WHAT IS BEST PRACTICE?

Parents with a history of perinatal loss should be encouraged to talk about their losses and voice their concerns. Prenatal education should be modified for these parents to address grief, manage anxiety, and facilitate communication with healthcare providers. Mothers in particular should be assessed for signs of anxiety and depression throughout the pregnancy.

CRITICAL THINKING

How can traditional prenatal education be adapted for parents with a previous perinatal loss?

References

Armstrong, D., Hutti, M., & Myers, J. 2009. The influence of prior perinatal loss on parents' psychological distress after the birth of a subsequent healthy infant. *JOGNN: Journal of Obstetric, Gynecological, and Neonatal Nursing, 38*(6), 656–666.

DeBackere, K., Hilll, P., & Kavanaugh, K. 2008. The parental experience of pregnancy after perinatal loss. *JOGNN: Journal of Obstetric, Gynecological, and Neonatal Nursing, 37*(5), 525–537.

O'Leary, J. 2009. Never a simple journal: Pregnancy following perinatal loss. *Bereavement Care, 29*(2), 12–17.

Wright, P. 2005. Childbirth education for parents experiencing pregnancy after perinatal loss. *Journal of Perinatal Education, 14*(4), 9–15.

ply to hear the fetal heartbeat. This intervention may continue to be helpful until the woman begins to feel fetal movement. Throughout the pregnancy, the office or clinic nurse can play a key role by providing reassurance and answering questions that the woman may have.

Women with a previous loss typically receive additional antepartum testing throughout the pregnancy. Ultrasounds can be used to provide reassurance and assess fetal growth and development, placental functioning, and cord variations. Nonstress testing and biophysical profiles can be performed weekly after 32 weeks to ensure fetal well-being. Fetal kick counts should be initiated at 28 weeks and continue until the birth occurs. Women with a previous loss should be delivered at their expected date of birth or when the pregnancy is at term and should not go over their due date, because placental functioning can decline in postdate pregnancies.

Evaluation

Caring for a family experiencing perinatal loss is a challenging, yet rewarding, opportunity for the nurse who offers his or her humanity, concern, and acceptance. There is nothing quite like helping a family through one of the most difficult events of their lives. The reward is often greater for the giver than for those who are receiving, because the important life lessons learned and the sense of accomplishment achieved when reaching out to others in need is rarely rivaled. Nurses should remember to process their own grief reactions so that they remain healthy responders for the next family in need.

Expected outcomes of nursing care for the family experiencing perinatal loss include the following:

- Family members feel free to express their feelings about the death of their baby if they desire to do so.
- Family members participate in decision making regarding preferences for the labor, birth, and the immediate postpartum period.
- Family members participate in the decision of whether to see their baby and other decisions about the baby.
- The family has resources available for continued support.
- Family members know the community resources available and have names and phone numbers to use if they choose.

Nursing care of a family experiencing perinatal loss is further described in the following Nursing Care Plan.

Case Study: Family with Perinatal Loss

NURSING CARE PLAN For a Family Experiencing Perinatal Loss

INTERVENTION	RATIONALE
1. Nursing Diagnosis: Compromised Family Coping related to perinatal loss as evidenced by crying/sadness, irritability/anger, guilt responses, and/or fear **Goal:** The patient will verbalize thoughts and feelings associated with the loss, and understand the factual events surrounding the loss. The patient begins to form a trust relationship with the nurse and freely asks for and accepts support provided by nursing staff.	
■ Normalize the experience by assuring parents that there is no right or wrong way to express grief.	■ Grief reactions encompass a broad spectrum of thoughts and emotions. Providing a nonjudgmental, supportive environment validates the grief response, thereby establishing a trust relationship, which helps to facilitate a healthy mourning process.
■ Crying. Offer tissues while allowing free expression of emotion.	■ Crying is a normal reaction to the loss event and offering tissues is a tangible form of acceptance.
■ Anger. Avoid defensiveness, state the obvious, and enlist the parent's assistance in exploring possible sources of, and solutions to, their anger.	■ Anger as a part of the grief response usually stems from frustration at the circumstances and should not be taken personally. Allowing for the free expression of anger, as well as remaining neutral in responses, will help to defuse the situation. Utilizing a team approach will assist the patient in viewing hospital personnel as partners in care, rather than adversaries.
■ Guilt responses. Reframe the event in a reality-based forum, reassuring the parents that they did nothing to precipitate the loss.	■ Guilt is a predominant feature of grief following loss, especially in parents experiencing the death of an infant. Reality testing, a companion of factual information versus the parents' perceptions of culpability, assists them in coming to the conclusion that they did the best they could in the circumstance.
■ Fear. Provide honest, simple explanations of what to expect before, during, and after the loss event.	■ Families can cope with extreme situations when they are properly informed in an honest and forthright manner. Maintaining a close presence while providing factual information will help alleviate feelings of fear and isolation. Offering simple choices allows patients to maintain a semblance of control over their circumstances.
EXPECTED OUTCOMES:	The patient and family acknowledge the loss as evidenced by verbalizing an understanding of the factual events surrounding the loss and openly expressing thoughts and feelings regarding the loss in a safe and constructive manner. The patient and family begin to form a trust relationship as evidenced by freely asking for and accepting support provided by nursing staff, and relating to the nurse in an environment of acceptance.
2. Nursing Diagnosis: Interrupted Family Processes related to sudden, unexpected crisis of perinatal loss **Goal:** The patient and family are able to maintain family cohesion necessary for returning to homeostasis.	
■ Gather information regarding the family and the surrounding loss event before initial interaction.	■ Effective intervention requires an extensive knowledge of the situation at hand. Failure to gather essential facts can precipitate a negative interaction with the family, leading to a breakdown in communication.
■ Determine the extent of the family's knowledge regarding the situation before initial interaction.	■ Effective crisis intervention always begins with the point of the family's knowledge and bridges from what they know to what you need them to know. Presenting the facts in an orderly fashion with increasing detail will help the family process difficult information.
■ Assess the family's internal resources necessary for maintaining family cohesion by active listening and asking open-ended questions regarding normal coping styles.	■ Asking open-ended questions will help to identify the family's resources for coping. Identifying the family's internal resources allows the nurse to utilize the family's unique strengths and normal coping mechanisms in dealing with crisis and loss. This will help them regain equilibrium as a family unit.

NURSING CARE PLAN For a Family Experiencing Perinatal Loss continued

INTERVENTION	RATIONALE
■ Mobilize family and hospital support systems.	■ The family support system is preferable because of the comfort factor associated with familiarity and the consistency of long-term support. The hospital support system is supplementary to the family support system and can provide additional resources and support for individual family members, thereby strengthening the family unit.

EXPECTED OUTCOMES: The patient and family maintain the cohesion necessary for returning to homeostasis as evidenced by openly interacting, supporting, and communicating needs within the family and using family, hospital, and community support systems as needed.

[redacted]

FOCUS YOUR STUDY

- Perinatal loss poses a major nursing challenge to provide support and care for the parents.
- Perinatal loss is a tragic and often traumatic event in the life of most families experiencing it.
- Fetal death after 20 weeks accounts for 60% of all fetal deaths per year, with 50% of those deaths occurring before 28 weeks' gestation.
- Bereavement is the *event* of the loss, grief is the *reaction* to that loss, and mourning is the *process* by which we incorporate the loss into our lives with individual, cultural, religious, and social norms.
- Up to 25% of women will need professional help to facilitate their mourning process following the death of their infant.
- Attachment theory with regard to perinatal loss is based upon the premise that human beings are biologically predisposed to bond with emotionally significant persons in their lives and the grief response is a state of separation anxiety brought on by the disruption in the attachment bond.
- For mothers, there are nine events that are important to the formation of attachment to her infant. They are (1) planning the pregnancy, (2) confirming the pregnancy, (3) accepting the pregnancy, (4) feeling fetal movement, (5) accepting the fetus as an individual, (6) giving birth, (7) seeing the baby, (8) touching the baby, and (9) giving care to the baby.
- Meaning reconstruction focuses on redefining ourselves and how we interact with the world after a significant loss. The goal of recovery, as related to meaning reconstruction, is a positive change in self-identity by assigning the loss a meaning, thereby allowing the individual to assimilate the loss into her or his world.
- There are many normal physical, cognitive, emotional, behavioral, and spiritual early responses to loss. The recognition of normal responses helps to identify the presence of abnormal or exaggerated responses.
- Many factors will influence a couple's response to perinatal loss, including individual and family personality traits, as well as social, cultural, and religious customs.
- Cessation of fetal movement reported by the mother to the nurse is frequently the first indication of fetal death. The nurse continues one-on-one care with the family, providing both physical and emotional support throughout this crucial period.
- The nurse can facilitate a healthy mourning process for the family by using active listening techniques and avoiding the use of clichés. Sitting in silence with a family is often the most helpful form of intervention available.
- Traditionally, it was believed that early and intense grieving was necessary for healing, but recent studies show that many people are naturally resilient and will not necessarily grieve initially or intensely.
- The caring theory places the emphasis of care on the attitude adopted by the nurse toward the grieving family as paramount to successful intervention and includes knowing, doing for, enabling, and maintaining belief.

- The responding model describes 10 behaviors and actions necessary for effective interaction with the grieving family and includes recognition of the loss, emotional availability, spiritual and cultural accommodation, physical presence, open communication, normalization of grief reactions, decision-making assistance, interdisciplinary involvement, nonjudgmental attitude, and genuine caring.
- Upon arrival to the facility, the nurse should make introductions, acknowledge the loss, and establish the beginnings of a trust relationship with the family.
- The nurse functions as advocate for the family in organizing interdisciplinary involvement, maintaining continuity of care, offering the opportunity for open communication, and ensuring that the family's wishes regarding their loss experience are honored.
- Couples experiencing perinatal loss should be offered the opportunity to participate in postmortem care and to view, hold, and name their baby. In the event a couple declines the opportunity, the nurse should assess for fear of the unknown as a motivating factor and take steps to alleviate that fear. The couple should never be coerced into viewing and holding their infant if they choose not to, and the nurse should display a nonjudgmental, accepting attitude regardless of the decision made by the couple.
- Siblings and extended family members should be included in the plan of care to whatever extent the couple wishes. Children should be given information in an honest and age-appropriate manner, and grandparents should be recognized for the "double" grief they are experiencing through the pain of their child and death of their grandchild.
- Mementos are important links for the family to their deceased infant. A memory box should be offered with as many personal items of the infant as possible. Hand- and/or footprint cards are especially desired items.
- Follow-up care should include bereavement materials and community support information as well as a telephone call to assess the family's well-being and provide any further desired information.
- Couples experiencing pregnancy following a loss can be expected to have higher levels of fear and anxiety and will need to be treated with care and concern. Information may need to be repeated and details of time lines provided to raise the comfort level of the couple.

CRITICAL THINKING IN ACTION

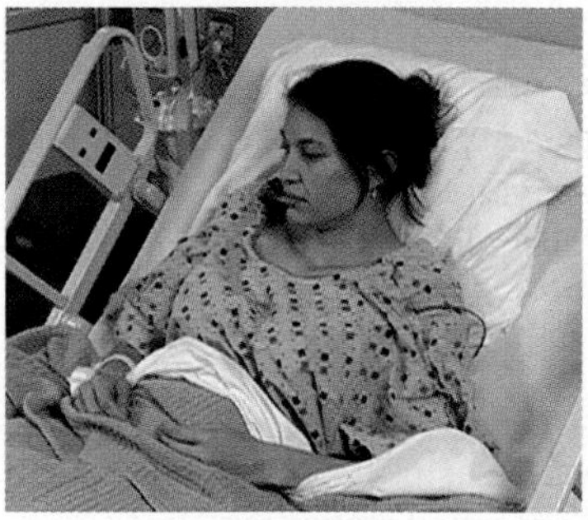

Marguerite, a 25-year-old married woman, is admitted for delivery of a stillborn baby girl. Through tears, Marguerite shares that she has named the baby, Alicia, after her grandmother. She has already decorated the nursery with the many gifts she received at her baby shower. Marguerite apologizes for "crying so much" and frequently expresses a fear that her husband, John, may blame her for Alicia's death because she worked until the time of the final ultrasound. She wonders aloud if he would be right. She communicates a desire to see and hold Alicia, but is very fearful of how the baby will look and whether people will think that she is morbid for wanting to hold a dead baby. Marguerite apologizes again for crying and shares that she does not know who else to talk to because no one seems to understand what she is going through.

1. What should the nurse helping families through the crisis of perinatal loss know about grief in general?
2. What should the nurse know about the unique nature of perinatal loss?
3. What types of nursing behaviors will facilitate the family's mourning process?

See www.nursing.pearsonhighered.com for possible responses.

Pearson Nursing Student Resources

Find additional review materials at **www.nursing.pearsonhighered.com**

Prepare for success with additional NCLEX®-style practice questions, interactive assignments and activities, Web links, animations and videos, and more!

REFERENCES

American College of Obstetricians and Gynecologists (ACOG). (2009). Management of stillbirth. ACOG Practice Bulletin, Number 102, *Obstetrics and Gynecology, 113*(3), 748–761. doi:10.1097/AOG.0b013e31819e9ee2

Arnold, J., & Gemma, P. B. (2008). The continuing process of parental grief. *Death Studies, 32*(7), 658–673. doi:10.1080/07481180802215718

Attig, T. (2004). Meanings of death seen through the lens of grieving. *Death Studies, 28*(4), 341–360. doi:10.1080/07481180490432333

Balk, D. E. (2004). Recovery following bereavement: An examination of the concept. *Death Studies, 28*(4), 361–374. doi:10.1080/07481180490432351.

Barnes, G. L. (2008). Perspectives of African-American women on infant mortality. *Social Work in Health Care, 47*(3), 293–305.

Barr, P. (2006). Relation between grief and subsequent pregnancy status 13 months after perinatal bereavement. *Journal of Perinatal Medicine, 34*(3), 207–211. doi:10.1515/JPM.2006.036

Bennett, S. M., Litz, B. T., Lee, B. S., & Maguen, S. (2005). The scope and impact of perinatal loss: Current status and future directions. *Professional Psychology: Research and Practice, 36*(2), 180–187. doi:10.1037/0735-7028.36.2.180

Boelen, P. A., Stroebe, M. S., Schut, H. A. W., & Zijerveld, A. M. (2006). Continuing bonds and grief: A prospective analysis. *Death Studies, 30*(8), 767–776. doi:10.1080/07481180600852936

Boerner, K., & Heckhausen, J. (2003). To have and have not: Adaptive bereavement by transforming mental ties to the deceased. *Death Studies, 27*(3), 199–226. doi:10.1080/07481180302888

Bonnano, G. A. (2008). Loss, trauma, and human resilience: Have we underestimated the human capacity to thrive after extremely aversive events? *Psychological trauma: Theory, research, practice, and policy,* Vol. S, No. 1, 101–113. doi:10.1037/1942-9681.S.1.101

Bowlby, J. (1969). *Attachment and loss: Attachment* (Vol. 1). New York, NY: Basic Books.

Brier, N. (2009). Grief following miscarriage: A comprehensive review of the literature. *Journal of Women's Health, 17*(3), 451–454. doi:10.1089/jwh.2007.0505

Cacciatore, J., & Bushfield, S. (2007). Stillbirth: The mother's experience and implications for improving care. *Journal of Social Work in End-of-Life Palliative Care, 3*(3), 59–79. doi:10.1300/J457v03n03_06

Cacciatore, J., Radestad, I., & Froen, J. F. (2008). Effects of contact with stillborn babies on maternal anxiety and depression. *Birth, 35*(4), 313–320.

Callister, L. C. (2006). Perinatal loss: A family perspective. *Journal of Perinatal and Neonatal Nursing, 20*(3), 227–234.

Capitulo, K. L. (2004). Perinatal grief online. *American Journal of Maternal/Child Nursing, 29*(5), 305–311.

Chan, M. F., Lou, F. L., Arthur, D. G., Cao, F. L., Wu, L. H., Li, P., et al. (2008). Investigating factors associate to nurses' attitudes toward perinatal bereavement care. *Journal of Clinical Nursing, 17*(4), 509–18. doi:10.1111/j.1365-2702.2007.02007

Corr, C. A., Nabe, C. M., & Corr, D. M. (2009). *Death and dying: Life and living* (6th ed.). Belmont, CA: Wadsworth/Cengage Learning, Inc.

Côté-Arsenault, D., & Donato, K. L. (2007). Restrained expectations in late pregnancy following loss. *JOGNN: Journal of Obstetric, Gynecologic, and Neonatal Nursing, 36*(6), 550–557. doi:10.1111.j.1552-6909.2007.00185.x

Currier, J. M., Holland, J. M., & Neimeyer, R. A. (2006). Sense-making, grief, and the experience of violent loss: Toward a mediational model. *Death Studies, 30*(5), 403–428. doi:10.1080/07481180600614351

DeBackere, K. J., Hill, P. D., & Kavanaugh, K. L. (2008). The parental experience of pregnancy after perinatal loss. *JOGNN: Journal of Obstetric, Gynecological, and Neonatal Nursing, 37,* 525–537. doi:10.1111/j.1552-6909.2008.00275.x

DeSpelder, L. A., & Strickland, A. L. (2005). *The last dance: Encountering death and dying* (7th ed.). New York, NY: McGraw Hill.

Dietz, D. (2009). Debriefing to help perinatal nurses cope with a maternal loss. *Maternal Child Health, 34*(4), 243–248. doi:10.1097/01.NMC.0000357917.41100.c5

Doka, K. J. (Ed.). (2002). *Disenfranchised grief: New directions, challenges, and strategies for practice.* Champaign, IL: Research Press.

Druzin, M. L., Smith, J. F. Jr., Gabbe, S. G., & Reed, K. L. (2007). Antepartum fetal evaluation. In S. G. Gabbe, J. R. Niebyl, & J. L.Simpson (2007). *Obstetrics: Normal and problem pregnancies.* (5th ed.). Philadelphia, PA: Churchill Livingstone.

Feudtner, C., Santucci, G., Feinstein, J. A., Snyder, C. R., Rourke, M. T., & Kang, T. I. (2007). Hopeful thinking and level of comfort regarding providing pediatric palliative care: A survey of hospital nurses. *Pediatrics, 119,* 186–192. doi:10.1542/peds.2006-1048

Flenady, V., & Wilson, T. (2008). Support for mothers, fathers, and families after perinatal death. *Cochrane Database of Systematic Reviews, 23*(1), CD000452.

Fletcher, G. E., Zach, T., Pramanik, A. K., & Ford, S. P. (2009). Multiple births. Retreived from http://emedicine.medscape.com/article/977234.

Frantz, T. T., Farrell, M. M., & Trolley, B. C. (2005). Positive outcomes of losing a loved one. In R. A. Neimeyer (Ed.), *Meaning reconstruction & the experience of loss* (pp. 193–194). Washington, DC: American Psychological Association.

Gamino, L. A., & Sewell, K. W. (2004). Meaning constructs as predictors of bereavement adjustment: A report from the Scott & White Grief Study. *Death Studies, 28*(5), 397–421. doi:10.1080/07481180490437536

Gibbs, R. S., Karlan, B. Y., Haney, A. F., & Nygaard, I. (2008). *Danforth's obstetrics and gynecology.* (10th ed.). Philadelphia, PA: Wolters Kluwer/Lippincott, Williams & Wilkins.

Heron, M. P., Hoyert, D. L., Murphy, S. L., Xu, J., Kochanek, K. D., & Tejada-Vera, B. (2009). Deaths: Final data for 2006. National Center for Health Statistics, *National Vital Statistics Report, 57*(14). Retrieved from www.cdc.gov/nchs/data/nvsr//nvsr57/nvsr57_14.pdf.

Hoyert, D. (2007). Maternal mortality and related concepts. National Center for Health Statistics. *Vital health STAT, 3*(33).

The Joint Commission. (2010). Preventing maternal death. *Sentinel Event Alert,* (44). Retrieved from www.jointcommission.org/SentinelEvents/SentinelEventAlert/sea_44.htm.

Kain, V. J. (2007). Moral distress and providing care to dying babies in neonatal nursing. *International Journal of Palliative Nursing, 13*(5), 243–248.

Keefe-Cooperman, K. (2004–2005). A comparison of grief as related to miscarriage and termination for fetal abnormality. *OMEGA, 50*(4), 281–300.

Kendall, A., & Guo, W. (2008). Evidence-Based neonatal bereavement care. *Newborn and Infant Nursing Reviews, 8*(3), 131–135. doi:10.1053/j.nainr.2008.06.011

Kersting, A., Dorsch, M., Kreulich, C., Reutemann, M., Ohrmann P., Baez, E., et al. (2005). Trauma and grief 2–7 years after termination of pregnancy because of fetal anomalies—A pilot study. *Journal of Psychosomatic Obstetrics & Gynecology, 26*(1), 9–14. doi:10.1080/01443610400022967

Klaus, M. H., & Kennell, J. H. (1976). *Maternal-infant bonding.* St. Louis, MO: Mosby.

Kuebelbeck, A. (2003). *Waiting with Gabriel: A story of cherishing a baby's brief life.* Chicago, IL: Loyola Press.

Lang, A., Goulet, C., & Amsel, R. (2003). Lang and Goulet Hardiness Scale: Development and testing on bereaved parents following the death of their fetus/infant. *Death Studies, 27*(10), 851–880. doi:10.1080/0716100345

Lindsey, J. L. (2010). *Evaluation of fetal death.* Retrieved from http://www.emedicine.com/medscape/article/259165-overview

Lobar, S. L., Youngblut, J. M., & Brooten, D. (2006). Death and dying in multicultural perspective. *Pediatric Nursing, 31*(1), 44–50.

MacDorman M. F., & Kirmeyer S. (2009) Fetal and perinatal mortality, United States, National Vital Statistics Report. *National Center for Health Statistics, 57*(8), 1–102.

Maciejewski, P. K., Zhang, B., & Block, S. D. (2007). An empirical examination of the stage theory. *JAMA, 297*(7), 716–723.

Martin, J. A., Hamilton, B. E., Sutton, P. D., Ventura, S. J., Menacker, F., Kirmeyer, S., & Mathews, T. J. (2009). Births: Final data for 2006. National Vital Statistics Report. *National Center for Health Statistics, 57*(7), 1–102.

Martin, T. L., & Doka, K. J. (2000). *Men don't cry . . . Women do.* Philadelphia, PA: Brunner/Mazel.

McCartney, P. R. (2007). Digital Bereavement Photography. *MCN: The American Journal of Maternal Child Nursing, 32*(5), 322. doi:10.1097/01.NMC.0000288005.18124.b8

Meert, K. L., Thurston, C. S., & Briller, S. H. (2005). The spiritual needs of parents at the time of their child's death in the pediatric intensive care unit and during bereavement: A qualitative study. *Pediatric Critical Care Medicine, 6*(4), 420–427.

Miller, E. D. (2003). Reconceptualizing the role of resiliency in coping and therapy. *Journal of Loss and Trauma, 8,* 239–246. doi:10.1080/15325020305881

Munson, D., & Leuthner, S. R. (2007). Palliative care for the family carrying a fetus with a life-limiting diagnosis. *Pediatric Clinics of North America, 54,* 787–798. doi:10.1016/j.pcl.2007.06.006

Murray, J. A., Terry, D. J., Vance, J. C., Battistutta, D., & Connolly, Y. (2000). Effects of a program of intervention on parental distress following infant death. *Death Studies, 24*(4), 275–305. doi:10.1080/074811800200469

Neimeyer, R. A. (2005). *Meaning reconstruction & the experience of loss.* Washington, DC: American Psychological Association.

Neimeyer, R. A. (2009). *New theories of grief: Going beyond Kubler-Ross.* Association for Death Education and Counseling, Webinar Lecture. Retrieved from www.adec.org.

Parkes, C. M., & Weiss, R. S. (1983). *Recovery from bereavement.* New York, NY: Basic Books.

Pauli, R. M. (2005). *Maceration and the timing of intrauterine death.* Retrieved from http://www.wisc.edu/wissp/wisspers/jan95001.htm

Pector, E. A. (2004). Views of bereaved multiple-birth parents on life support decisions, the dying process, and discussions surrounding death. *Journal of Perinatology, 24,* 4–10. doi:10.1038/sj.jp.7211001

Radestad, I., & Christofferson, L. (2008). Helping a woman meet her stillborn baby while it is soft and warm. *British Journal of Midwifery, 16*(9), 588–591.

Radestad, I., Saflund, K., Wredling, R., Onelov, E., & Steineck, G. (2009). Holding a stillborn baby: Mothers' feelings of tenderness and grief. *British Journal of Midwifery, 17*(3), 178–180.

Reddy, U. M., Goldenberg, R., Silver, R., Smith, G. C. S., Pauli, R., et al. (2009). Stillbirth classification—Developing an international consensus for research: Executive summary of a national institute of child health and human development workshop. [Editorial] *Obstetrics & Gynecology, 114*(4), 901–914. doi:10.1097/AOG.0b013e3181b8f6e4

Roehrs, C., Masterson, A., Alles, R., Witt, C., & Rutt, P. (2008). Caring for families coping with perinatal loss. *JOGNN: Journal of Obstetric, Gynecologic, and Neonatal Nursing. 37*(6), 631–639. doi:10.1111/j.1552-6909.2008.00290.x

Rogers, S., Babgi, A., & Gomez, C. (2008). Educational interventions in end-of-life care: Part I, An educational intervention responding to the moral distress of NICU nurses provided by an ethics consultation team. *Advances in Neonatal Care, 8*(1), 56–65. doi:10.1097/01.ANC.0000311017.02005.20

Roush, A., Sullivan, P., Cooper, R., & McBride, J. W. (2007). Perinatal hospice. *Newborn and Infant Nursing Reviews, 7*(4), 216–221. doi:10.1097/01.ANC.0000311017.02005.20

Shaver, P., & Tancredy, C. (2001). Emotion, attachment, and bereavement: A conceptual commentary. In M. S. Stroebe, R. O. Hansson, W. Stroebe, & H. Schut (Eds.), *Handbook of bereavement research: Consequences, coping and care* (pp. 63–88). Washington, DC: American Psychological Association.

Shields, K. (2005). *Preparing the family for the birth and death.* Lakewood Ranch, FL: Healing Through Hope.

Swanson, K. M. (1991). Empirical development of a middle range theory of caring. *Nursing Research, 40*(3), 161–166.

Swanson, K. M., Connor, S., Jolley, S. N., Pettinato, M., & Wang, T. (2007). Contexts and evolution of women's responses to miscarriage during the first year after loss. *Research in Nursing and Health, 30*(1), 2–16.

Talbot, K. (2002). *What forever means after the death of a child.* London, UK: Brunner-Routledge.

Trulsson, O., & Radestad, I. (2004). The silent child—Mothers' experiences before, during, and after stillbirth. *Birth, 31*(3), 189–195.

Turton, P. (2008). To see or not to see: Should parents hold their stillborn? *RCM Midwives,* April/May 2008 (n. p.).

Wheeler, I. (2001). Parental bereavement: The crisis of meaning. *Death Studies, 25*(1), 51–66. doi: 10.1080/07481180126147

Wheeler, S. R. (1997). Adolescent pregnancy loss. In J. R. Woods & J. L. Esposito (Eds.), *Loss during pregnancy or in the newborn period: Principles of care with clinical cases and analyses* (pp. 387–410). Pittman, NJ: Jannetti.

Wheeler, S. R., & Austin, J. (2000). The loss response list: A tool for measuring adolescent grief responses. *Death Studies, 24*(1), 21–34. doi:10.1080/074811800200676

Worden, J. W. (2009). *Grief counseling and grief therapy: A handbook for the mental health practitioner* (4th ed.). New York, NY: Springer.

World Health Organization. (2007). Maternal mortality in 2005: Estimates developed by WHO, UNICEF, UNFPA, and the World Bank. Retrieved from http://whqlibdoc.who.int/publications/2007/9789241596213_eng.pdf

CHAPTER 39

The Postpartum Family at Risk

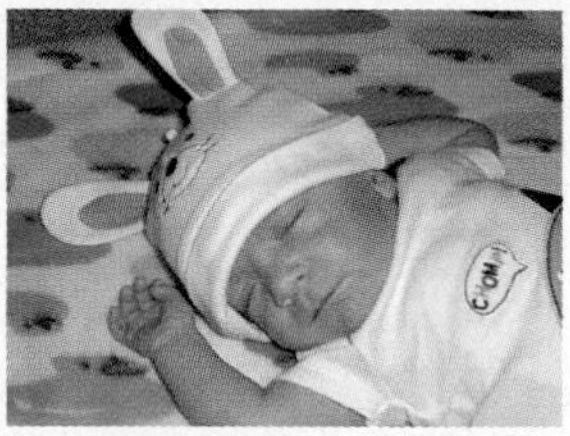

We are surviving. Just. Why don't they give the Croix de Guerre to people who can go without more than 2 hours total daily sleep for 5 weeks? I thought babies ate at 6–10–2–6–10–2—mine does. He also eats at 5–7–9–11 and 4–8–12. I am getting rather used to going around with my breasts hanging out. They are either drying from the last feed or getting ready for the next one. But the love—I never knew, never imagined that I would love him like this. This incredible feeling of boundless, endless love—a wish to protect his innocence from ever being hurt or wounded or scratched. And that awful, horrible, mad feeling in the first week that you'll never be able to keep anything so precious and so vulnerable alive.

—The Boston Women's Health Collective, *The New Our Bodies, Ourselves*

LEARNING OUTCOMES

1. Identify the causes of and appropriate nursing interventions for early and late hemorrhage during the postpartum period.
2. Develop a nursing care plan that reflects knowledge of etiology, pathophysiology, current clinical therapy, nursing and preventive management for the woman experiencing postpartum hemorrhage, reproductive tract infection, urinary tract infection, lactation mastitis, thromboembolic disease, or a postpartum psychiatric disorder.
3. Explain how to evaluate the mother's knowledge of health promotion measures.
4. Delineate signs of complications to be reported to the primary care provider and measures that can be taken to prevent recurrence of complications.
5. Identify ways to provide continuity of nursing care for women with postpartum complications in the community setting.

KEY TERMS

Adjustment reaction with depressed mood *1141*
Early (primary) postpartum hemorrhage *1115*
Late (secondary) postpartum hemorrhage *1115*
Mastitis *1131*
Pelvic cellulitis (parametritis) *1126*
Peritonitis *1124*
Postpartum blues *1141*
Postpartum depression (PPD) *1141*
Postpartum endometritis (metritis) *1125*
Postpartum major mood disorder *1141*
Postpartum psychosis *1143*
Post-traumatic stress disorder (PTSD) *1142*
Puerperal infection *1124*
Puerperal morbidity *1124*
Subinvolution *1120*
Thrombophlebitis *1134*
Uterine atony *1116*

The postpartum period is typically envisioned as a smooth, uneventful time, somewhat anticlimactic, that follows the anticipation of pregnancy and the excitement and work of labor and birth. Often it is, despite the challenges of new parenthood and integration of a new person into the family. Short maternity hospitalization—1.5 days after vaginal childbirth and 2.5 days following cesarean childbirth—may wrongly reinforce the notion that the postpartum recovery is speedy and uncomplicated. Early postpartum discharge challenges the nurse to impart anticipatory information about normal postpartum recovery and self-care for the new mother and care of the newborn. Other issues that make identification difficult include at risk families, limited resources (including transportation), attitudes toward the pregnancy and adolescent pregnancies, and overall access to care. It is equally important for the nurse to be aware of physical or emotional complications that may develop during the postpartum period, and to teach the family the signs of such complications; findings to report to the physician or certified nurse-midwife (CNM); and preventive measures, if available.

Written instructions to supplement any discussion will be of great value to the family in the early weeks at home with a newborn, when life can be chaotic and verbal instructions may be forgotten. The family should have telephone numbers for postpartum follow-up services and other resources for getting answers to questions. By communicating an attitude of willingness to answer questions and to listen to concerns, the nurse enhances the family's comfort in making calls later for what they might otherwise perceive as "too trivial to bother someone about."

When a telephone follow-up or an examination at the home visit, where available, provides evidence of a developing complication, the nurse shares these findings or impressions with the woman, and they mutually plan an appropriate next step. In the case of telephone follow-up, the nurse usually counsels the woman to notify her physician or CNM, and is prepared to schedule an appointment immediately if risk assessment indicates. The nurse who identifies a complication at the home visit will need to communicate the clinical findings to the physician or CNM and document them and any interventions for the permanent record. See chapter 37 ∞ for a more detailed discussion of home care for the postpartum family.

Complications, by their very nature, suggest the need for immediate collaborative management and are inherently stressful. Postpartum complications sometimes necessitate readmission of the woman to the hospital, thereby disrupting the family and adding concerns not only about her health but the way in which infant care will be managed. The most common complications of the postpartum period are hemorrhage, infection, thromboembolic disease, and postpartum psychiatric disorders. These are the major focus of this chapter.

Care of the Woman with Postpartum Hemorrhage

Hemorrhage in the postpartum period is described as either early (immediate or primary) or late (delayed or secondary) postpartum hemorrhage. **Early (primary) postpartum hemorrhage** occurs in the first 24 hours after childbirth and is the more common of the two. **Late (secondary) postpartum hemorrhage** occurs from 24 hours to 6 weeks after birth. Classifying hemorrhage as early or late can be helpful in considering the cause; issues of uterine tone and reproductive tract trauma are more common causes of early hemorrhage while retained placental tissue is more likely associated with later problems. Postpartum hemorrhage (PPH) continues to be a cause of significant maternal mortality and morbidity and accounts for approximately one sixth of maternal deaths attributable to pregnancy in the United States (Poggi, 2007). Worldwide, it is estimated that 140,000 women die from postpartum hemorrhage, about one every four minutes (Oyelese & Ananth, 2010).

The traditional definition of postpartum hemorrhage has been a blood loss of greater than 500 ml following childbirth. This definition is being questioned, because careful quantification indicates that the average blood loss in a normal vaginal birth is actually greater than 500 ml, the average blood loss after cesarean childbirth exceeds 1000 ml, and the average blood loss is more than 1500 ml during repeat cesarean birth (Oyelese & Ananth, 2010). Clinical estimates tend to underestimate actual blood loss by up to 50%. Regardless of clinical experience, healthcare providers tended to overestimate low volumes of loss and significantly underestimate excessive blood loss.

Clinical estimation of blood loss at childbirth may be difficult because blood mixes with amniotic fluid and is obscured as it oozes onto sterile drapes or is sponged away. As the amount of blood loss increases, as in the case of hemorrhage, estimates are likely to be even less accurate than those associated with normal childbirth. Moreover, postpartum hemorrhage may occur intra-abdominally, into the broad ligament, or into hematomas arising from genital tract trauma, wherein the blood loss is concealed. Given the increased blood volume of pregnancy, the clinical signs of hemorrhage—such as decreased blood pressure (BP), increasing pulse, widening pulse pressure, thirst, restlessness, and decreasing urinary output—do not appear until as much as 1800 ml to 2100 ml of blood has been lost, shortly before the woman becomes hemodynamically unstable (Gilstrap & Yeomans, 2008).

To meet the standard of care in cases of postpartum hemorrhage, systems are needed in every obstetrical setting that enable nurses to respond quickly to implement certain actions independently based on evidence-based protocols (Simpson, 2010). In some settings with significant numbers of childbirths, rapid response teams have been initiated for obstetric (OB) emergencies such as postpartum hemorrhage, similar to a call for coding someone experiencing a cardiac arrest. To minimize the "cry wolf" phenomenon, such measures require training and an attitude that these are "our" (the hospital's) patients (Catanzarite, Almyrde, & Bombard, 2007).

Early (Primary) Postpartum Hemorrhage

At term, blood volume and cardiac output have increased so that 20% of cardiac output, or 600–800 ml per minute, perfuses the pregnant uterus, supporting the developing fetus. When the placenta separates from the uterine wall, the many uterine vessels that have carried blood to and from the placenta are severed abruptly. The normal mechanism for hemostasis after expulsion of the placenta is contraction of the interlacing uterine muscles to occlude the open sinuses that previously brought blood into the placenta. Absence of prompt and sustained uterine contraction (uterine atony) can cause significant blood loss. Other causes of hemorrhage include laceration of the genital tract; episiotomy; retained placental fragments; vulvar, vaginal, or subperitoneal hematomas; uterine inversion; uterine rupture; problems of placental implantation; and coagulation disorders.

Uterine Atony

Uterine atony (relaxation of the uterus) is a common cause of early postpartum hemorrhage. As many as 1 in every 20 new mothers will experience some degree of uterine atony. Although uterine atony can occur after any childbirth, its contributing factors include the following (Cunningham et al., 2010):

- Overdistention of the uterus due to multiple gestation, polyhydramnios, or a large infant (macrosomia)
- Dysfunctional or prolonged labor, which indicates that the uterus is contracting abnormally
- Oxytocin augmentation or induction of labor
- Grandmultiparity, because stretched uterine musculature contracts less vigorously
- Use of anesthesia (especially halothane) or other drugs such as magnesium sulfate, calcium channel blockers such as nifedipine, or tocolytics like terbutaline (Brethine), any of which cause the uterus to relax
- Prolonged third stage of labor—more than 30 minutes
- Preeclampsia
- Asian or Hispanic heritage
- Operative birth (includes vacuum extraction or forceps-assisted births)
- Retained placental fragments
- Placenta previa

Hemorrhage from uterine atony may be slow and steady or sudden and massive. The blood may escape vaginally or collect in the uterus, evident as large clots. The uterine cavity may distend with up to 1000 ml or more of blood, while the perineal pad and linen protectors remain suspiciously dry. A treacherous feature of postpartum hemorrhage is that maternal vital signs may not change until significant blood loss has occurred because of the increased blood volume associated with pregnancy. Women with preeclampsia are an exception to this finding because they do not have the normal hypervolemia of pregnancy and cannot tolerate even normal postchildbirth blood loss (Gilstrap & Yeomans, 2008). Any anemia should be treated prior to labor. The nurse will assess the woman's beliefs about blood transfusion and document those findings in the record that follows her throughout her childbirth stay. Knowing whether or not the woman will willingly accept transfusions, if needed, is important to decision making about managing hemorrhage, although the woman will be questioned again about transfusion if such treatment seems warranted.

Ideally, postpartum hemorrhage is prevented, beginning with adequate prenatal care, good nutrition, avoidance of traumatic procedures, risk assessment, early recognition, and management of complications as they arise. Review of maternal records for risk factors will help nurses to plan assessment timelines to maximize early identification and management of excessive bleeding. *It is critical to remember that a woman with no identifiable risk factors may hemorrhage after childbirth as well.* The woman and her partner, sometimes other family members, are excited about the birth and wish to celebrate or to have some private time engaging with the newborn when he or she is appropriately warm and ready for an early visit. But postpartum women must be assessed at frequent intervals, especially in the initial hours after delivery of the placenta when most deaths from hemorrhage occur.

There is some evidence that active management of the third stage of labor through administration of an oxytocic after delivery, controlled traction on the umbilical cord, and uterine massage after birth could prevent half of the cases of postpartum hemorrhage (Oyelese & Ananth, 2010). Any woman at risk should be typed and cross-matched for blood transfusion. After expulsion of the placenta, the fundus is palpated to ensure that it is firmly contracted. If it is not firm, fundal massage is performed until the uterus contracts. Fundal massage is uncomfortable for the woman who has not received regional anesthesia; she will need an explanation for why this uncomfortable procedure is necessary and support as massage is initiated. A reminder to use the same breathing patterns for control of discomfort as she used in labor can serve in this situation as well. Clinical guidelines schedule vital signs and assessment of fundal contractility and lochia at regular intervals (see chapter 35 ∞ and chapter 36 ∞).

Clinical Therapy

If bleeding is excessive, venous access with large bore catheters (18 gauge), sometimes using two concurrent access sites, will be established and crystalloid solutions such as normal saline or Lactated Ringer's are begun to replace blood volume. When excessive bleeding continues despite external uterine massage, the obstetrician may elect to do a bimanual massage (Figure 39-1A ■). Bimanual massage compresses the body of the uterus from below while the abdominal hand massages the fundus from above.

If uterine massage is not effective, uterine stimulants (uterotonic agents) will be administered at a rapid infusion rate to contract the atonic musculature. Oxytocin, ergotamine, and prostaglandin are most often used. Misoprostol, best known for its use in labor induction and medical abortion, is being used to prevent and treat uterine atony after attempts to control bleeding with oxytocics. Table 39-1 summarizes critical nursing information about the use of uterine stimulants to control bleeding.

MANAGEMENT BY SELECTIVE ARTERIAL EMBOLIZATION

For the woman who had a vaginal delivery and unsuccessful tamponade effort to control postpartum bleeding, the next step is arterial embolization.The woman must be hemodynamically stable as the procedure itself takes approximately 30 minutes.

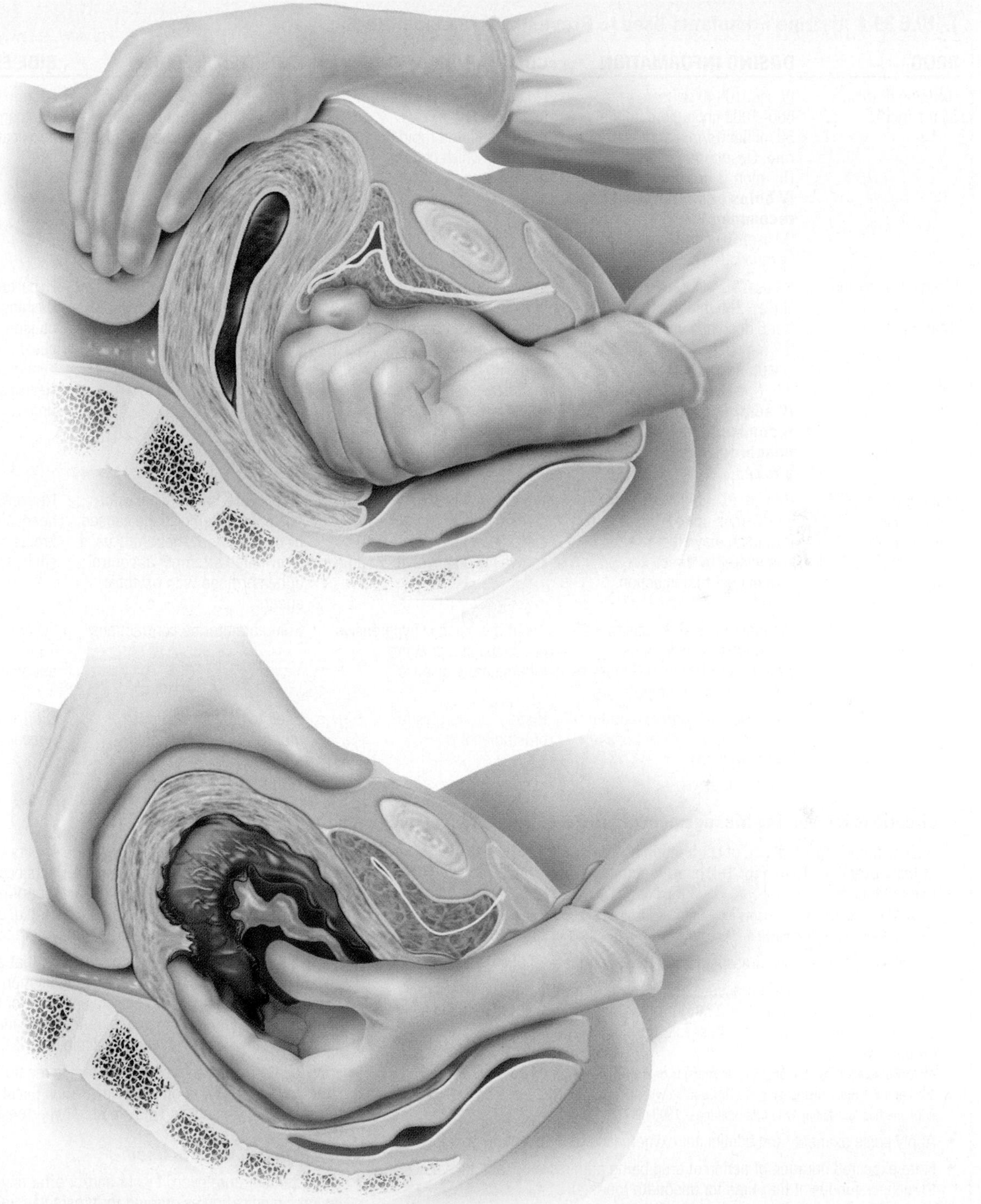
A

B

Figure 39-1 ■ A. Manual compression of the uterus and massage with the abdominal hand usually will effectively control hemorrhage from uterine atony. B. Manual removal of placenta. The fingers are alternately abducted, adducted, and advanced until the placenta is completely detached. Both procedures are performed only by the medical clinician.

Source: Adapted from Cunningham, F. G., MacDonald, P. C., & Gant, N. F. (Eds.). (1989). Williams obstetrics *(18th ed., pp. 417–418). Norwalk, CT: Appleton & Lange.*

A percutaneous catheter is inserted to embolize bleeding vessels using Gelfoam, glue, coils, or polyvinyl alcohol. Arterial embolization also can be used for bleeding that continues after hysterectomy or as an alternative to hysterectomy when the woman wishes to preserve fertility. Regular menstrual cycles follow and women have had successful subsequent pregnancies (Fiori et al., 2009).

SURGICAL MANAGEMENT OF POSTPARTUM HEMORRHAGE Surgical management depends on the clinical situation, institution, available personnel, and available equipment. Packing the uterine cavity tightly with 4-inch-wide sterile gauze provides time for blood and fluid replacement prior to laparotomy and time to provide prophylactic antibiotics. In some settings, the gauze is presoaked with 5000 units of thrombin diluted in 5 ml

TABLE 39-1 Uterine Stimulants Used to Prevent and Manage Uterine Atony

DRUG	DOSING INFORMATION	CONTRAINDICATIONS	EXPECTED EFFECTS	SIDE EFFECTS
Oxytocin (Pitocin, Syntocinon)	IV use: 10–40 units in 500–1000 crystalloid fluid at 50 milliunits/min administration rate. Onset: immediate. Duration: 1 hr. **IV bolus administration not recommended.** IM use: 10 units. Onset: 3–5 min. Duration: 2–3 hr.	None for use in postpartum hemorrhage. Avoid undiluted rapid IV infusion, which causes hypotension.	Rhythmic uterine contractions that help to prevent or reverse postpartum hemorrhage caused by uterine atony.	Uterine hyperstimulation, mild transient hypertension, water intoxication rare in postpartum use.
Methylergonovine maleate (Methergine)	IM use: 0.2 mg every 2–4 hr. Onset: 2–5 min. Duration: 3 hr (for 5 dose maximum). PO use: 0.2 mg every 4 hr (for 6 doses). Onset: 7 to 15 min. Duration: 3 hr (for 1 week). **IV administration not recommended—can cause dangerous hypertension and stroke.**	Women with labile or high blood pressure or known sensitivity to drug, cardiac disease, and Raynaud's disease. Use with caution during lactation.	Sustained uterine contractions that help to prevent or reverse postpartum hemorrhage caused by uterine atony; management of postpartal subinvolution.	Hypertension, dizziness, headache, flushing/hot flashes, tinnitus, nausea and vomiting, palpitations, chest pain. Overdose or hypersensitivity is recognized by seizures; tingling and numbness of fingers and toes.
Prostaglandin ($PGF_{2\alpha}$, Carboprost tromethamine [Hemabate], Prostin/15M)	IM use: 0.25 mg repeated every 15–90 min, up to 8 doses max. Physician may elect to administer by direct intramyometrial injection.	Women with active cardiovascular, renal, liver disease, or asthma or with known hypersensitivity to drug.	Control of refractory cases of postpartum hemorrhage caused by uterine atony; generally used after failed attempts at control of hemorrhage with oxytocic agents.	Nausea, vomiting, diarrhea, headache, flushing, bradycardia, bronchospasm, wheezing, cough, chills, fever.
Dinoprostone Prostin E_2	Vaginal or rectal suppository 20 microgram every 2 hours. Stored in frozen form—must be thawed to room temperature.	Avoid if woman is hypotensive, or has asthma or acute inflammatory disease.	Stimulate uterine contractions	Fever is common and occurs within 15 to 45 min of insertion; bleeding, abdominal cramps, N/V.
Misoprostol (Cytotec)	800–1000 microgram rectally. Rapid effects, contractions within minutes.	History of allergies to prostaglandins.	Used to prevent and treat uterine atony after failed attempts to control bleeding with oxytocics.	Diarrhea, abdominal pain, headache

Implications for Nursing Management of the Postpartum Woman Receiving Uterine Stimulants

- Assess fundus for evidence of contraction and amount of uterine bleeding at least every 10–15 min for 1–2 hr after administration, then every 30–60 min until stable.
  Note: More frequent assessments are determined by the woman's condition or by orders of the physician or certified nurse-midwife (CNM).
- Weigh peripads or Chux dressing for objective estimate of blood loss.
- Monitor pulse and blood pressure every 15 min for at least 1 hr after administration, then every 30–60 min until stable. Often the early sign is a slightly increased heart rate. Assess blood loss by hematocrit and hemoglobin levels.
  Note: Remember that the physiologic changes of pregnancy increased the blood volume by 40% and the RBC volume by 30%. The woman will not show signs of severe hypovolemia until she has lost about 1/3 of her volume—1800 ml.
- Apply pulse oximeter and administer oxygen according to agency protocol.
- Note expected duration of action of drug being administered, and take care to recheck fundus at that time for adequate tone.
- When the drug is ineffective, the fundus remains atonic (boggy or uncontracted), and bleeding continues, massage the fundus. If massage fails to cause sustained contraction, consider the status of the urinary bladder. If uterine tone is not restored after the bladder is empty and fundal massage has been performed, notify the physician or CNM immediately.
- Monitor woman for signs of known side effects of the drug; report to physician or certified nurse-midwife if side effects occur.
  - Continuous electrocardiogram (EKG) monitoring may be indicated for hypotension, continuous bleeding, tachycardia, or shock.
  - Elevate the legs to a 20- to 30-degree angle to increase venous return.
- Remind the woman and her support person that uterine cramping is an expected result of these drugs and that medication is available for discomfort. Administer analgesic medications as needed for pain relief. Provide nonpharmacologic comfort measures. If analgesic medication ordered is insufficient for pain relief, notify the physician or CNM.
- Provide information to woman and family regarding importance of not smoking during Methergine administration (nicotine from cigarettes leads to constricted vessels and may lead to hypertension) and signs of toxicity.

When Prostaglandin Is Used

- Check temperature every 1–2 hr and/or after any chill. Administer antipyretic medication as ordered for prostaglandin-induced fever.
- Auscultate breath sounds frequently for signs of adverse respiratory effects.
- Assess for nausea, vomiting, and diarrhea. Administer antiemetic and antidiarrheal medications as ordered. (In some settings, women are premedicated with these drugs.)

Sources: American College of Obstetrics & Gynecology (2006). ACOG Practice Bulletin: Clinical management guidelines for obstetrician-gynecologists #76. Obstetrics & Gynecology, 108*(4), 1039–1046; Anderson, J. M., & Etches, D. (2007). Prevention and management of postpartum hemorrhage.* American Family Physician, 75*(6), 875–882; Catanzarite, V., Almyrde, K., & Bombard, A. (2007, September). Grand Rounds: OB Team Stat: Developing a better L&D rapid response team.* Contemporary Obstetrics & Gynecology, 52*(9), 52–54, 56, 57. Francois, K. (2006). Critical care in OB Part 1: Managing uterine atony and hemorrhagic shock.* Contemporary OB/GYN, *February, 52–59.*

of normal saline (Gilstrap & Yeomans, 2008). As uterine packing is no longer a favored way for providing uterine tamponade, some clinicians now use one or two Foley catheters or Sengstaken-Blakemore tubes with isotonic saline to provide pressure against the uterine walls. The tubes have open tips, which permit any continuous drainage from the uterus to be visualized even as pressure tamponade is controlling the bleeding. In addition, an SOS Bakri Balloon Tamponade made of silicone, which limits clot adhesion, can be inserted transvaginally past the cervical os with ultrasound guidance and can detect ongoing bleeding..

For non–life-threatening levels of hemorrhage, the uterine artery or internal iliac (hypogastric) artery may be surgically ligated to control bleeding, especially when excessive bleeding occurs during cesarean childbirth. In most cases regular menstrual cycles resume and successful pregnancy can be expected in the future. Several kinds of uterine compression suturing procedures are being investigated such as the B-Lynch compression (brace suture) procedure. When tied, the suture creates uterine compression to control bleeding associated with uterine atony and averting hysterectomy (Cunningham, 2010).

Peripartum hysterectomy provides definitive surgical treatment of uterine bleeding related to uterine atony and placenta accreta (Gilstrap & Yeoman, 2008). Because it ends childbearing for the woman, it is often considered a procedure of last resort. The new mother may experience emotional distress related to loss of fertility and need opportunities to discuss those feelings candidly with a caring professional.

Lacerations of the Genital Tract

Early postpartum hemorrhage also may be associated with lacerations of the perineum, vagina, or cervix. Several factors predispose women to higher risk of reproductive tract lacerations:

- Nulliparity
- Epidural anesthesia
- Precipitous childbirth (less than 3 hours)
- Macrosomia
- Forceps- or vacuum-assisted birth
- Use of oxytocin

Genital tract lacerations should be suspected when bright red vaginal bleeding persists in the presence of a firmly contracted uterus. The nurse who suspects a laceration should notify the clinician so that the laceration can be immediately sutured to control hemorrhage and repair the integrity of the reproductive tract (American Academy of Pediatrics [AAP] & American College of Obstetricians and Gynecologists [ACOG], 2007). The woman is moved to a delivery or surgical area for access to special lighting to facilitate treatment.

Episiotomies can be an underappreciated source of postpartal blood loss because of slow, steady bleeding, especially if it was done early in the birth process. The risk for bleeding is increased with mediolateral episiotomies. To fully assess the episiotomy site, the nurse must position the woman on her side.

Retained Placental Fragments

Retained placental fragments can be a cause of early postpartum hemorrhage; however, they generally are the most common cause of late hemorrhage. Retention of fragments is usually attributable to partial separation of the placenta during massage of the fundus before spontaneous placental separation, so this practice should be avoided.

Following birth, the placenta should always be inspected for intactness and evidence of missing fragments or cotyledons on the maternal side and for vessels that traverse to the edge of the placenta outward along the membranes of the fetal side. The latter finding may indicate succenturiate placenta and a retained lobe. Uterine exploration by the physician may be required at that time to remove missing fragments (see Figure 39-1B ■). This cause should be immediately suspected if bleeding persists and no lacerations are noted. Sonography may be used to diagnose retained placental fragments. Curettage, formerly a standard treatment, is now thought by some to traumatize the implantation site, thereby increasing bleeding and the potential for uterine adhesions. It may be necessitated by the degree of hemorrhage, however (Cunningham et al., 2010).

Vulvar, Vaginal, and Pelvic Hematomas

Hematomas occur as a result of injury to a blood vessel from birth trauma, often without noticeable trauma to the superficial tissue, or from inadequate hemostasis at the site of repair of an incision or laceration. The soft tissue in the area offers little resistance, and hematomas containing 250 to 500 ml of blood may develop rapidly. Hematomas may be vulvar (involving branches of the pudendal artery), vaginal (especially in the area of the ischial spines), vulvovaginal, or subperitoneal. The latter are rare but most dangerous because of the large amount of blood loss that can occur without clinical symptoms until the woman becomes hemodynamically unstable. Subperitoneal hematomas involve the uterine artery branches or vessels in the broad ligaments and require laparotomy for surgical correction.

Risk factors for hematomas include the following: preeclampsia, use of pudendal anesthesia, first full-term birth, precipitous labor, prolonged second stage of labor, macrosomia, forceps- or vacuum-assisted births, and history of vulvar varicosities. Hematomas less than 3 cm in size and nonexpanding are managed expectantly with ice packs and analgesia. Heat may be used after 24 hours to facilitate absorption of the blood within the hematoma. Small hematomas usually resolve over several days. For larger hematomas and those that expand, surgical management is usually required: The hematoma is evacuated using incision and drainage (I&D) (Gilstrap & Yeomans, 2008). The bleeding vessel is ligated, and the wound closed, with or without vaginal packing. A temporary indwelling urinary catheter may be necessary because voiding may be impossible with packing in place. Frequent assessment of the perineum of the woman under the effects of regional anesthesia is important since her pain sensation is disrupted. Once the effects of anesthesia have subsided, vaginal and vulvar hematomas are generally associated with perineal pain, often intense and sometimes disproportionate to the objective findings observed. The hematoma site is an ideal medium for proliferation of flora normally present in the genital tract. Consequently, broad-spectrum antibiotics are usually ordered prophylactically to prevent infection or abscess.

Uterine Inversion

Uterine inversion, a prolapse of the uterine fundus to or through the cervix so that the uterus is, in effect, turned inside out after birth, is a rare (the incidence is 1 in 2000 or more) but life-threatening cause of associated postpartal hemorrhage (Gilstrap & Yeomans, 2008). Although not always preventable, uterine inversion is often associated with these factors: fundal implantation or abnormal adherence of the placenta, weakness of the uterine musculature or other uterine abnormalities, protracted labor, uterine relaxation secondary to anesthesia or drugs such as magnesium sulfate, and excess traction on the umbilical cord or vigorous manual removal of the placenta. Most cases of uterine inversion are managed by immediate repositioning of the uterus within the pelvis by the physician.

Uterine Rupture

Spontaneous rupture of the uterus is rare in the United States but continues to be seen in developing countries where emergency surgery for obstructed labors may be less immediately accessible. The woman with a ruptured uterus will have acute, severe abdominal pain, with minimal to diffuse external bleeding. Concealed hemorrhage may occur in the abdominal cavity or broad ligaments, undetected until the woman becomes symptomatic from hypovolemic shock. Risk factors for uterine rupture include prior uterine surgery, including cesarean birth; fetal malpresentation; grandmultiparity; operative vaginal birth; and oxytocic induction of labor. With uterine rupture, immediate surgery is required with fluid and blood replacement as needed.

Coagulation Disorders (Coagulopathies)

Coagulopathies should be suspected when postpartal bleeding persists with no identifiable cause. A consumptive coagulopathy such as disseminated intravascular coagulation (DIC) may occur during pregnancy as a result of preeclampsia, amniotic fluid embolism, sepsis, abruptio placentae, or prolonged intrauterine fetal demise syndrome (Roberts & Funai, 2009). (See chapter 20 ∞.)

Late (Secondary) Postpartum Hemorrhage

Although early postpartum hemorrhage most often occurs within hours of birth, delayed hemorrhage occurs most often within 1 to 2 weeks after childbirth, most frequently as a result of **subinvolution** (failure to return to normal size) of the placental site or retention of placental tissue. Blood loss at this time may be excessive but rarely poses the same risk as that from immediate postpartum hemorrhage. Late postpartum hemorrhage is much less common but can be extremely stressful for the woman and her family who are at home by this time.

The site of placental implantation is always the last area of the uterus to regenerate after childbirth. In the case of subinvolution, adjacent endometrium and the decidua basalis fail to regenerate to cover the placental site. Deficiency of immunologic factors has been implicated as a cause. Faulty implantation in the less vascular lower uterine segment, retention of placental tissue, or infection may contribute to subinvolution.

Care Plan Activity: Postpartum Perineal Pain

With subinvolution, the postpartum fundal height is greater than expected. In addition, lochia often fails to progress from rubra to serosa to alba normally. Lochia rubra that persists longer than 2 weeks postpartum is highly suggestive of subinvolution (Poggi, 2007). Some women report scant brown lochia or irregular heavy bleeding. Leukorrhea, backache, and foul-smelling lochia may occur if infection is a cause. There may be a history of heavy early postpartal bleeding or difficulty in expulsion of the placenta during the third stage of labor. When portions of the placenta have been retained in the uterus, bleeding continues because normal uterine contraction that constricts the bleeding site is prohibited. Presence of placental tissue within the uterus can be confirmed by pelvic ultrasonography.

Subinvolution is most commonly diagnosed during the routine postpartum examination at 4 to 6 weeks after childbirth. The woman may relate a history of irregular or excessive bleeding or describe the symptoms listed previously. An enlarged, softer-than-normal uterus, palpated bimanually, is an objective indication of subinvolution. Treatment includes oral administration of methylergonovine maleate (Methergine) 0.2 mg every 3 to 4 hours for 24 to 48 hours (see Table 39-1). When uterine infection is present, antibiotics also are administered. The woman is reevaluated in 2 weeks. If retained placenta is suspected or other treatment is ineffective, curettage may be indicated (Poggi, 2007).

NURSING CARE MANAGEMENT

Nursing Assessment and Diagnosis

Careful and ongoing assessment of the woman during labor and birth and evaluation of her prenatal history will help identify factors that put her at risk for postpartum hemorrhage. However, it is critical to remember that postpartum hemorrhage may occur without any risk factors, so that all women must be monitored. Regular and frequent assessment of fundal height and evidence of uterine tone or contractility will alert the nurse to the possible development or recurrence of hemorrhage. Monitoring the bladder for evidence of increasing distention, with immediate intervention can sometimes help to prevent excessive bleeding that occurs when a full bladder displaces the uterus and interferes with contractility. Assessment for bleeding can be done visually, by pad counts, or by weighing the perineal pads or other items that have absorbed blood.

For all complaints of perineal pain, the nurse should examine the perineal area for signs of hematomas: ecchymosis, edema, tenseness of tissue overlying the hematoma, a fluctuant mass bulging at the introitus, and extreme tenderness to palpation. Estimating the size on first assessment of the perineum enables the nurse to better identify increases in size and the potential blood loss. The nurse notifies the physician or certified nurse-midwife (CNM) if a hematoma is suspected. The nurse can decrease the risk of vulvar or vaginal hematoma by applying an ice pack to the woman's perineum during the first hour after birth and intermittently thereafter for the next 8 to12 hours. If a small hematoma develops despite preventive measures, a sitz bath after the first 12 hours will aid fluid absorption once bleeding has stopped and will promote comfort, as will the judicious use of analgesic agents (see chapter 36 ∞). Close monitoring of the woman who has had excessive bleeding is important during sitz baths to ensure safety.

In cases of excess bleeding, nurses should be alert for signs of impending hypovolemic shock. Frequent noninvasive monitoring should continue: heart rate, blood pressure, auscultation of heart sounds and breath sounds, oxygen saturation, skin turgor, color, temperature, color and moisture of mucous membranes, capillary refill, level of consciousness, and urinary output, possible with Foley catheter/urometer and electrocardiogram (ECG) readings. Throughout the bleeding episode, assessment of color and amount of blood loss will be ongoing with pad counts or weighing to estimate loss. The nurse will note the odor of the drainage to enable early diagnosis of infection. The nurse will anticipate the addition of invasive monitoring for a more objective evaluation of status: central venous pressure (CVP) monitoring via a peripheral line and/or Swan-Ganz central line insertion for pulmonary artery wedge pressure monitoring, and arterial blood gases to ascertain acidosis and hypoxia. In some settings, the woman needing invasive hemodynamic monitoring may be transported to an intensive care unit.

Nursing diagnoses that may apply when a woman experiences postpartum hemorrhage include the following:

- ***Deficient Fluid Volume*** related to blood loss secondary to uterine atony, lacerations, hematomas, retained placental fragments, or coagulopathies
- ***Risk for Ineffective Peripheral Tissue Perfusion*** related to hypovolemia
- ***Risk for bleeding*** related to lack of information about signs of delayed postpartum hemorrhage
- ***Risk for Impaired Parenting*** related to separation from newborn, urgency of personal health status, and fatigue
- ***Risk for Infection*** related to surgical procedures, invasive procedures, anemia, and blood transfusions

Nursing Plan and Implementation

If the nurse detects a soft, boggy uterus, it is massaged until firm. If the uterus is not contracting well and appears larger than anticipated, the nurse may express clots during fundal massage. Once clots are removed, the uterus tends to contract more effectively. Overly aggressive massage should be avoided so as not to injure the vessels in the broad ligaments or cause reactive relaxation of the musculature.

If the woman seems to have a slow, steady, free flow of blood, the nurse begins weighing the perineal pads (1 ml = 1 g) and monitors the woman's vital signs at least every 15 minutes, more frequently if indicated (James, 2008). If the fundus is displaced upward or to one side because of a full bladder, the nurse encourages the woman to empty her bladder—or catheterizes her if she is unable to void—to allow for efficient uterine contractions.

CLINICAL TIP

A boggy uterus indicates that the uterus is not well contracted. This results in increased uterine bleeding which may remain in the uterus and form clots or may result in increased flow. To assess the amount of blood loss, you must first massage the uterus until it is firm and then express clots. Even though the woman may have a firm uterus, significant bleeding can occur from causes other than uterine atony. To accurately determine the amount of blood loss, it is not sufficient to assess only the peri-pad. You should also ask the woman to turn on her side so you can assess underneath her for pooling of blood.

When there are risk factors for postpartum hemorrhage or frequent fundal massage has been necessary to sustain uterine contractions, the nurse should maintain the vascular access (the IV line) initiated during labor in case additional fluid or blood becomes necessary. Sometimes physicians and CNMs write orders that specify "discontinue IV after present bottle." The astute postpartum nurse will assess the consistency of the fundus and the presence of normal versus excessive lochia before discontinuing the infusion. If the assessments are not reassuring, the nurse continues the IV and notifies the physician or CNM.

The nurse reviews these findings when available, compares them to the admission baseline, and notifies the physician or CNM if the hematocrit has decreased by 10 percentage points or more. In cases where there is risk of postpartum hemorrhage and blood has been cross-matched earlier, the nurse checks that blood is available in the blood bank. During bleeding episodes, it is important to appreciate that hemoglobin and hematocrit levels will not reflect the volume lost until after equilibration in 6–24 hours (Smith, 2008).

As the woman's blood volume becomes depleted, positioning her with her legs elevated to 30 degrees facilitates venous return and promotes oxygenation. Unlike the Trendelenberg position used in the past for those in shock, this position does not impede breathing or cardiac function and promotes cerebral circulation. Supplemental oxygen may be necessary to keep peripheral tissues oxygenated when blood is shunted to protect vital organs like the brain and kidneys.

Keeping the woman as comfortable as possible with perineal care and frequent changes of disposable pads is important. Frequent position changes will aid in comfort but cannot be allowed to compromise venous return or oxygenation. She will be kept NPO in case surgery is needed, so oral care is important for comfort. There are many interruptions when the patient is experiencing a complication, so the nurse will need to seek opportunities to promote rest whenever possible. Any intervention to help with maternal infant bonding in the interval of separation is of great value to the woman—photographs or videotapes of the newborn, direct reports from the nursery staff, and brief visits to the room if her condition allows. The father also can be encouraged to visit the newborn and bring information to the mother.

If assessment reveals that the woman's condition is deteriorating, the nurse anticipates that more intensive monitoring will be necessary. At times, this will translate to preparing the woman and her family for a transfer to an intensive care setting, helping them to understand the justification for this change, and

Application: Postpartum Hemorrhage

reassuring them about the continued level of quality care, despite leaving a now familiar environment. If the woman will remain on the obstetrical unit, the nurse will anticipate and request necessary resources and personnel to ensure the patient's safety and well-being. In urgent situations, such as escalating postpartum bleeding, it is easy for the woman and her family to feel as if they are the center of attention but not to understand what is happening—only that something is going "badly wrong." The need to provide them with ongoing information about her status and each procedure and its rationale in understandable terms is a critical dimension of quality nursing care. A calm competent approach by the nurse goes a long way to calming the woman and her family, as does offering them opportunities to verbalize their feelings and ask questions or seek clarification.

Clearly, the care of the woman experiencing postpartum hemorrhage depends on good nursing assessment and prompt reporting of nonreassuring findings to the physician. Direct treatment methods, however, require the collaboration of a physician and in some cases, radiography or surgical staff. The nurse becomes an important liaison between these departments, keeping the necessary individuals apprised of the woman's status. For example, if additional transfusions of whole blood or blood products are anticipated, it may be the nurse who keeps the hospital laboratory informed to facilitate timely response. Care may well include the preprocedural preparation of the woman for surgery or for procedures such as arterial embolization performed by a radiologist.

The nurse may assume a prominent role in preparing the woman for insertion of CVP or Swan Ganz catheters and in the administration of crystalloid fluids (normal saline and Lactated Ringer's solution) or of blood and blood products. With rapid attempts to replace depleted blood volume, the nurse must carefully monitor the woman for evidence of fluid overload. When blood products are transfused, watching for transfusion reactions and responding promptly according to hospital procedures becomes a nursing role. Typically, volume is replaced initially with rapid administration of crystalloid solutions, in a 3 ml solution per 1 ml of estimated blood lost ratio (Diepenbrock, 2008). Normal saline must be hung prior to administration of blood since dextrose causes hemolysis and Lactated Ringer's causes agglutination of cells. Once it is evident that fluid replacement alone is not adquate, red blood cells (RBCs) are often transfused to replace depleted oxygen-carrying red cells. If platelets decrease significantly, fresh frozen plasma may be added. Frequent laboratory testing of hemoglobin, hematocrit, platelets, and a coagulation panel are monitored. Table 39-2 provides basic information about blood products used with women experiencing PPH.

When blood loss is significant and vital signs become unstable, crystalloid and colloid fluid replacement can no longer compensate for the loss and transfusion of blood products becomes necessary (see Table 39-2). Initially, colloid and crystalloid solutions are administered to replace lost intravascular volume. Second, RBCs are given to restore oxygen carrying capacity, and then clotting factors and platelets are given to restore physiologic hemostasis (Burtelow et al., 2007). Whole blood is not used routinely; rather the specific components being depleted are replaced without the addition of unnecessary volume of whole blood (Diepenbrock, 2008). Women who require blood products may be concerned about the associated risks. They should receive assurance that follow-up care will monitor for untoward consequences of blood replacement. Adherence to strict clinical protocols while accessing blood products from the lab and administering blood products is imperative to maximize patient safety. More immediately evident transfusion reactions range from a nonhemolytic and self-limited febrile response to life-threatening hemolytic reactions with blood group incompatibility, often because of error. Nurses assess for any type of transfusion reaction and notify the physician immediately. In the case of the hemolytic reaction, the uninfused blood will be returned to the lab for reevaluation (Diepenbrock, 2008).

The nurse evaluates the woman for signs of anemia, such as fatigue, pallor, headache, thirst, and orthostatic changes in pulse or BP, and reviews the results of all hematocrit determinations. All medical interventions, IV infusions, blood transfusions, oxygen therapy, and medications such as uterine stimulants are monitored as necessary and evaluated for effectiveness. Urinary output should be monitored to determine adequacy of fluid replacement and renal perfusion, with amounts less than 30 ml per hour reported to the physician (James, 2008). Good hand washing using Standard Precautions throughout the hospitalization and emphasizing proper hand washing for home care, is important to minimize risk of postpartum infection.

TABLE 39-2 Blood Products for Managing Postpartum Hemorrhage (PPH)

BLOOD PRODUCT	USE IN PPH	VOLUME/UNIT	INFUSION INFORMATION
Cryoprecipitate	Corrects deficiencies of factor VIII, XIII, von Willebrand factor + fibrinogen.	40 ml	Increases fibrinogen levels 10 mg/dl/ per unit transfused.
Fresh Frozen Plasma	Contains increased Factor V, VIII, and fibrinogen, and antithrombin III	200–250 ml	Thawed for use. Must use within 24 hours of thaw. Infuse with blood filter or component filter. May give at 200 ml/hour unless flluid overload.
Packed Red Blood Cells	Contains RBCs, WBCs, and plasma Increases oxygen carrying capacity of blood without adding volume—used for acute blood loss.	250 ml	Filter required for administration. Infusion rate <4 hours/unit. Expected to increase hemoglobin by 1 gram/dl and hematrocit by 3% per unit transfused.
Platelets	Controls or prevents blood loss associated with deficiency in platelets and for prophylactic use for those with platelet counts <10,000.	50–70 ml (taken from 1 unit of blood)	Give within 4 hours of preparation. Use component filter for administration. Increases platelets by 5000–10,000^3 per unit transfused.

Source: Data from Diepenbrock, N. H. (2008). Quick reference to critical care. *Philadelphia, PA: Lippincott Williams & Wilkins.*

The nurse also helps the woman plan activities so that adequate rest is possible.The woman who is experiencing anemia and fatigue may need assistance with self-care and progressive ambulation for several days. When she is able to be out of bed to shower, use of a shower chair permits independence while providing a measure of safety should the woman experience weakness or dizziness. The emergency call light should be easily accessible whenever nurses have left the bedside, even temporarily.

Once her condition has stabilized somewhat, the mother may find it difficult to care for her baby because of the fatigue associated with blood loss. The mother may require additional assistance in caring for her infant. If she has IV lines in place, even carrying the newborn may be awkward. For the mother who feels compelled to do as much as possible, the nurse may also need to "give permission" to the mother to return her infant to the nursery so she can have adequate periods of uninterrupted rest.

If the father of the child is involved in the birth experience, he can support the mother's recovery by helping to meet her physical needs while encouraging her to rest. The mother is likely to feel less concern over her limited opportunities for newborn care if she can witness the father's interactions with and care for the newborn. The couple may wish for arrangements to be made for the father to stay in the hospital room, sleeping on a cot and eating with the mother so that limited rooming-in with the newborn is still an option. In that way, even if the mother is too fatigued to care for the infant, she can enjoy the infant's presence and initiate bonding. The extent to which the father becomes involved with the care of the mother and baby must be carefully balanced with his need to be rested for the extra responsibilities he will assume when his partner and newborn child are discharged from the hospital.

CLINICAL JUDGMENT

Case Study: Betsy Lambert

Betsy Lambert is a primigravida who had a spontaneous vaginal delivery at 0941 today. An overview of her history reveals the following:

23 years old, married, G 1 P0 on admission to Labor Unit. Pregnancy normal. Rh positive. No drug allergies. Labs on admission to L&D normal with exception of Hemoglobin 11 grams and Hematocrit 33%. Labor: 13 hours. Estimated Blood Loss: 450 ml. Delivered female (7 lb 7 oz) spontaneously after epidural anesthesia. APGAR 9/10. Newborn exam was within normal limits and routine newborn orders were implemented. Day shift reports firm fundus, voided 210 ml around 1100, vital signs stable. Baby visited and breastfed briefly with help from lactation nurse. Ate lunch and had Tylenol #3 at 1300 for perineal pain. Has been sleeping for long intervals.

You find Mrs. Lambert still dozing but awaken her for exam and note the following: B/P 112/20, HR 116, R 16, T 100. Breasts—soft, nontender, wearing support bra. Uterus—fundus firm and 2 cm below umbilicus slightly left of midline. Bladder—possibly slightly distended but she feels no urge to void. Lochia—the two perineal pads and blue absorbent underpads are covered with bright red blood. Perineum—covered with blood, as are thighs. Some of the blood has dried on the skin. Slight edema noted—midline episiotomy intact. Ice pack in place but ice melted. Homans' sign—negative. Emotional status—reports her husband went home to rest and will be back at dinnertime. Talks with excitement about first attempt to nurse baby. Asks for something cold to drink. The patient cannot remember when she was last checked for bleeding. You don gloves and wash her perineum gently and her thighs and change all her pads so you can better assess her degree of bleeding. An IV is in place with 10 units of Pitocin (100 ml is left in the IV bag).

You return, as promised, in 15 minutes to reevaluate her lochia and find that her perineal pads are again covered in blood.

Critical Thinking

Based on your assessments and Mrs. Lambert's lab findings, what actions will you take first?

If one of your anticipated actions is to inform the obstetrician, what specific information will you report and what management should you anticipate initially?

What follow-up care will you anticipate performing during the remainder of your shift?

See www.nursing.pearsonhighered.com for possible responses.

Health Promotion Education

The woman and her family or other support persons should receive clear, preferably written, explanations of the normal postpartum course, including progressive changes in the lochia and fundus and signs of abnormal bleeding. Instructions for the prevention of bleeding should include fundal massage, ways to assess the fundal height and consistency, and inspection of the episiotomy and lacerations, if present. The woman should receive instruction in perineal care (see chapter 36 ∞). The woman and her family are advised to contact their caregiver if any of the signs of postpartum hemorrhage occur (Table 39-3). If iron supplementation is ordered, instructions for proper dosage should be provided to enhance absorption and avoid constipation and nausea.

Community-Based Nursing Care

For most postpartum women, routine discharge instructions include advice such as:

> "You take care of the baby, and let someone else care for you, the family, and the household."

TABLE 39-3 Signs of Postpartum Hemorrhage

Excessive or bright red bleeding (saturation of more than one pad per hour)
A boggy fundus that does not respond to massage
Abnormal clots
High temperature
Any unusual pelvic discomfort or backache
Persistent bleeding in the presence of a firmly contracted uterus
Rise in the level of the fundus of the uterus
Increased pulse or decreased BP
Hematoma formation or bulging/shiny skin in the perineal area
Decreased level of consciousness

Because of her fatigue and weakened condition, the woman who experienced postpartum hemorrhage may be unable even to care for her newborn unassisted. The caregivers at home need clear, concise explanations of her condition and needs for recovery. For example, all should understand the woman's need to rest and to be given extra time to rest after any necessary activity. They should also be told that anemia is associated with postpartum depression so that they can be vigilant for and promtly report any change in the woman's affect. To ensure her safety, the woman should be advised to rise slowly to minimize the likelihood of orthostatic hypotension. Until she regains strength, the mother should be seated when holding the newborn.

The person who assumes responsibility for grocery shopping and meal preparation will need advice about the importance of including foods high in iron in the daily menus. Having the woman indicate her preferences from a list of such foods will promote cooperation with the diet. The nurse also explains the rationale for continuing medications containing iron and reminds the woman that vitamin C–containing fluids maximize absorption of iron, and tea or milk products prevent absorption.

The woman should continue to count perineal pads for several days so she can recognize any recurring problem with excessive blood loss (hypovolemia). Invasive procedures, her debilitated condition, and anemia associated with hemorrhage increase the woman's risk of puerperal infection. She and her caregivers should use good hand washing technique and minimize exposure to infection in the home. They should be given a list of signs of infection and should understand the importance of alerting her healthcare provider immediately should signs occur.

In addition to meeting the woman's physical needs, the nurse will assess the couple's coping strategies and resources for dealing with the impending crisis. Providing realistic information, offering to call those in their support network, and exploring effective coping strategies can be of immeasurable value as they try to maintain a sense of balance in this difficult situation. A sense of emergency often exists in the event of late postpartum hemorrhage. Because it commonly occurs 1 to 2 weeks after birth, the couple is generally at home, involved in the day-to-day activities demanded by their new roles, when the unexpected, excessive bleeding begins. Quick decisions about child care arrangements must often be made so that the mother can return to the hospital. Both mother and father are likely to be alarmed by the excessive bleeding and concerned about her prognosis. There will be additional worries about separation from the newborn, especially when the mother is breastfeeding. The father may find himself torn between the needs of the mother and those of the newborn and any other children. Ideally, arrangements can be made to minimize separation of the family members.

Evaluation

Expected outcomes of nursing care include:

- Signs of postpartum hemorrhage are detected quickly and managed effectively.
- Maternal-infant attachment is maintained successfully.
- The woman is able to identify abnormal changes that might occur following discharge and understands the importance of notifying her caregiver if they develop.

Care of the Woman with a Reproductive Tract Infection or Wound Infection

Puerperal infection is an infection of the reproductive tract associated with childbirth that occurs at any time up to 6 weeks postpartum. The most common postpartum infection is endometritis (metritis), which is infection limited to the uterine lining. The cause of postpartum fever is presumed to be endometritis until proven otherwise. However, infection can spread by way of the lymphatic and circulatory systems to become a progressive disease resulting in parametrial cellulitis and **peritonitis** (infection involving the peritoneal cavity). Other causes of postpartum fever should be considered: respiratory complications such as atelectasis or pneumonia, acute pyelonephritis, thrombophlebitis, or breast engorgement, which rarely lasts more than 24 hours (Duff, Sweet, & Edwards, 2009). Careful assessment of all postpartum women with elevated temperatures is clearly essential to ensure early and accurate diagnosis and treatment. Moreover, preventive measures to prevent respiratory infection, urinary tract infection (UTI), and thrombophlebitis are crucial components of postpartum nursing care. The woman's prognosis is directly related to the stage of the disease at the time of diagnosis, the causative organism, the appropriateness of treatment, and the state of her health and immune system. The death rate from postpartum infection is low in the United States, but "infection continues to account for 7% of maternal deaths after live birth in the United States and is the fourth leading cause of death following delivery" (Duff et al., 2009, p. 749).

The standard definition of **puerperal morbidity** established by the Joint Committee on Maternal Welfare is "a temperature of 38°C (100.4°F) or higher, with the temperature occurring on any 2 of the first 10 days postpartum, exclusive of the first 24 hours, and when taken by mouth by a standard technique at least four times a day." During today's short obstetric hospital stays, the temperature is measured every 6 hours in most settings, consistent with the definition for puerperal morbidity. However, serious infections can occur in the first 24 hours or may cause only persistent low-grade temperatures.

The vagina and cervix of approximately 70% of all healthy pregnant women contain pathogenic bacteria that, alone or in combination, are sufficiently virulent to cause extensive infections. Although the uterus is considered a sterile cavity before rupture of the fetal membranes, bacterial contamination of amniotic fluid with the membranes still intact at term is more common than previously believed and may contribute to premature labor. Following rupture of the membranes and during labor, contamination of the uterine cavity by vaginal or cervical bacteria can easily occur. Other factors also must be present for infection to occur, such as the change to an alkaline pH postpartally that favors growth of aerobes. Uterine infections are relatively uncommon following uncomplicated vaginal births but they continue to be a major source of morbidity for women who give birth by cesarean.

Routine antibiotic prophylaxis for cesarean childbirth in conjunction with aseptic technique, fewer traumatic operative births, a better understanding of labor dystocia, improved surgical intervention, and a population that is generally at less risk from malnutrition and chronic debilitative disease have contributed to a reduction in overal postpartal morbidity and mortality.

Because shortened inpatient stays are the norm in maternity care, women will likely be discharged following childbirth before clinical signs of puerperal infection are evident. According to Gorgas (2008), 94% of postpartal infections manifest after hospital discharge and many of the women present to the emergency room. Consequently, birthing center nurses are challenged to analyze the woman's history and clinical course for risk assessment and to recognize the sometimes early subtle signs of infection so that discharge may be delayed as needed. Before discharge, the nurse advises the woman about preventive measures, including scrupulous hand washing, and signs of infection. Nurses should educate the patient and her family about the risk of infection and how to recognize and respond appropriately, should it occur. Community and home care nurses, where available, review the prenatal and birth record for continuity of risk assessment, conduct physical assessment for objective findings of infection, collect specimens as ordered for diagnosing infection, and collaborate with the primary caregiver in managing infection.

Postpartum Uterine Infection

Postpartum uterine infection is known as *metritis* and *endometritis*. Because the infection involves the decidual lining of the uterus, the myometrium, and parametrial tissue, some authorities are proposing the terminology *metritis with parametrial cellulitis* (Cunningham et al., 2010).

Risk factors for postpartum uterine infection include the following:

- Cesarean birth is the single most significant risk (10 times greater than in vaginal births) (James, 2008). If a cesarean occurs after an extended labor with ruptured membranes, the incidence of infection can be as high as 35% without antibiotic prophylaxis and 15% with prophylactic coverage (Duff et al., 2009).
- Prolonged premature rupture of the amniotic membranes (PPROM)
- Prolonged labor preceding cesarean birth
- Multiple vaginal examinations during labor
- Compromised health status (low socioeconomic status, anemia, obesity, smoking, use of illicit drugs or alcohol, poor nutritional state)
- Use of fetal scalp electrode or intrauterine pressure catheter for internal monitoring during labor
- Obstetric trauma—episiotomy, laceration of perineum, vagina, or cervix
- Chorioamnionitis—infection of placenta, chorion, and amnion
- Pre-existing bacterial vaginosis or *Chlamydia trachomatis* infection
- Instrument-assisted childbirth—vacuum or forceps
- Manual removal of the placenta or uterine exploration after delivery
- Retained placental fragments
- Urinary catheters and intravenous lines in place (Smith, 2008)
- Lapses in aseptic technique by surgical staff
- Diabetes mellitus (four times more common than in non–diabetic mothers) (Davies & Gibbs, 2008)
- Immunocompromised status

Postpartum Endometritis

Postpartum endometritis (metritis), an inflammation of the endometrium portion of the uterine lining, may occur postpartally in 1% to 3% of women who give birth vaginally and ranges from 5% to 15% of those who give birth by cesarean (Duff et al., 2009).

Postpartum infection from vaginal delivery primarily affects the placental implantation site, the decidua, and adjacent myometrium. Bacteria that colonize the cervix and vagina gain access to the amniotic fluid during labor and postpartum and begin to invade devitalized tissue (the lower uterine segment, lacerations, and incisions). The same pathogenesis, polymicrobial proliferation and tissue invasion, is associated with cesarean delivery, but surgical trauma, additional devitalization of tissue, blood and serum accumulation, and foreign bodies (sutures, staples) provide additional favorable anerobic bacterial conditions. For highly indigent populations, the risk remains high (Duff et al., 2009). Both aerobic and anaerobic organisms cause endometritis, which is often polymicrobial. See Table 39-4 for a list of common causative organisms.

Clinical findings of metritis in the initial 24 to 36 hours postpartum tend to be related to group B streptococcus (GBS). Late-onset postpartum endometritis/metritis is most commonly associated with genital mycoplasmas and *Chlamydia trachomatis.* These microbes have a longer replication time and latency period than other bacteria and are not consistently eradicated by antibiotics used for early postpartal infections.

In mild cases of metritis, the woman generally has vaginal discharge that is bloody, foul smelling, and either scant or profuse. In more severe cases, she also has uterine tenderness;

TABLE 39-4 Common Causative Organisms in Endometritis

AEROBES	ANAEROBES
• Group A, B, D streptococcus	• *Peptostreptococcus*
• Enterococcus	• *Clostridium* species
• *Staphylococcus* species	• *Bacteroides* species
• *Escherichia coli*	• *Chlamydia trachomatis*
• *Klebsiella pneumoniae*	• Genital mycoplasma
• *Proteus mirabilis*	

Sources: Data from: Duff, W. P., Sweet, R. L., & Edwards, R. K. (2009). Maternal and fetal infectious disorders. In R. K. Creasy & R. Resnik (Eds.), Maternal-fetal medicine: Principles and practice *(6th ed., pp. 739–796). Philadelphia: Saunders; James, D. C. (2008). Postpartum care. In K. R. Simpson & P. A. Creehan,* AWHONN's perinatal nursing *(3rd ed., pp. 473–526). Philadelphia: Lippincott Williams & Wilkins.*

sawtooth temperature spikes, usually between 38.3°C (101°F) and 40°C (104°F) on two separate assessments at least 6 hours apart; tachycardia that parallels temperature increase; and chills. Purulent and foul-smelling lochia is cited as a classic sign of endometritis (Smith, 2008).

Broad spectrum antibiotics are used for treatment. Ampicillin is often added for the nonallergic woman when high fevers begin within the first 24 to 48 hours after delivery, since early spikes are generally associated with enteroccocal infection. Women generally improve within 2 days of initiating antibiotics. If fever continues at 48 hours after antibiotic therapy, an additional workup is necessary to check for refractory pelvic infection (Cunningham et al., 2010). Antibiotics are continued until the woman has been afebrile for a minimum of 24 hours and the clinical exam is benign; then antibiotics may be discontinued.

Pelvic Cellulitis (Parametritis)

Pelvic cellulitis (parametritis) is infection that has ascended to involve the connective tissue of the broad ligament or, in more severe forms, the connective tissue of all the pelvic structures. The infection generally ascends upward in the pelvis by way of the lymphatic vessels in the uterine wall but may also occur if pathogenic organisms invade a cervical laceration that extends upward into the connective tissue of the broad ligament—a direct pathway into the pelvis. This level of infection should be suspected in those whose fever persists when another source cannot be identified.

A pelvic abscess may form and is most commonly found in the uterine ligaments, the cul-de-sac of Douglas, and the subdiaphragmatic space. Parametritis may be a secondary result of pelvic thrombophlebitis. This condition occurs when a clot, usually in the right ovarian vein, becomes infected, and the wall of the vein breaks down from necrosis, spilling the infection into the connective tissues of the pelvis (Cunningham et al., 2010).

A woman suffering from parametritis may demonstrate a variety of symptoms, including marked high temperature (38.9°C to 40°C or 102°F to 104°F), chills, malaise, lethargy, abdominal pain, subinvolution of the uterus, tachycardia, and local and referred rebound tenderness. If peritonitis develops, the woman will be acutely ill with severe pain; marked anxiety; high fever; rapid, shallow respirations; pronounced tachycardia; excessive thirst; abdominal distention; nausea; and vomiting.

Postpartum Wound Infections

Given the degree of bacterial contamination that occurs with normal vaginal birth, it is surprising that more women do not have infections of the episiotomy or repaired lacerations of the perineum, vagina, or vulva. Good aseptic technique is the likely rationale. When perineal wound infection does occur, it is recognized by the classic signs: redness, warmth, edema, purulent drainage, and, later, gaping of the previously approximated wound. Local pain may be severe.

After cesarean delivery, wound infection is most often associated with concurrent endometritis. The wound is typically red, indurated, tender at the margins, and draining purulent exudate. Some women have cellulitis without actual purulent drainage. Clinical exam is usually sufficient for diagnosis but culture of the exudate should be routinely done since methicillin-resistant *Staphylococcus aureus* (MRSA) infections are possible (Duff et al., 2009).

Clinical Therapy

The infection site and causative organism(s) are diagnosed by careful history and complete physical examination, blood tests, aerobic and anaerobic endometrial cultures (although this may be of limited value, because multiple organisms are usually present), and urinalysis to rule out urinary tract infection (UTI). Blood cultures are positive in up to 25% of febrile women but do not reflect accurately the severity of the infection (Smith, 2008).

Localized wound infection is treated with broad-spectrum antibiotics, sitz baths, and analgesics as necessary for pain relief (chapter 36 ∞). Wounds with evidence of pus or serosanguineous effusion or an infected stitch site are opened and drained completely. Once the incision and drainage (I&D) of the wound is complete, it may be packed with saline dampened gauze and repacked 2 to 3 times daily, and covered with clean gauze using aseptic technique. This allows removal of necrotic debris when packing is removed. When the infection is resolved and there is evidence of healthy granulation tissue, secondary closure is considered. Antibiotics with coverage against *Staphyloccus aureus* should be given. Nafcillin, 2 grams IV every 6 hours is a common choice. For allergy to β-lactam antibiotics, an appropriate alternative is vancomycin 1 gram IV every 12 hours. Antibiotics are typically continued until the wound base is clean and any signs of cellulitis have resolved.

The incidence of metritis has been reduced by prophylactic administration of antibiotics to women undergoing cesarean childbirth. Metritis, once diagnosed, is treated by the administration of parenteral broad spectrum antibiotics (Duff et al., 2009; James, 2008). Common standard treatment regimens consist of clindamycin for gram-positive and anaerobic coverage in combination with an aminoglycoside, typically gentamicin, and for gram negative coverage or ampicillin and sulbactan every 6 hours (Cunningham et al., 2010). The route and dosage are determined by the severity of the infection. Careful monitoring is also necessary to prevent the development of a more serious infection. Parametritis and peritonitis are treated with aggressive IV therapy. Broad-spectrum antibiotics effective against the most common causative organisms are chosen initially until the results of culture and sensitivity reports are available. If multiple organisms are present, the approach to antibiotic therapy is continued unless no improvement is observed; then the antibiotic is changed. With appropriate antibiotic coverage, improvement should occur within a few days. Antibiotics are generally continued until the woman is afebrile for 24 to 48 hours (James, 2008). Follow-up with oral antibiotics is not necessary (Cunningham et al., 2010).

An abscess is frequently manifested by the development of a palpable mass and may be confirmed with ultrasound. An abscess usually requires incision and drainage to avoid rupture into the peritoneal cavity and the possible development of peritonitis. After drainage of the abscess, the area may be packed with iodoform gauze to promote drainage and facilitate healing (Duff et al., 2009). Approximately 90% of women with postpartum infection respond quickly to antibiotic therapy or drainage of abscesses and are associated with complete recovery and no long-term sequelae (Smith, 2008).

NURSING CARE MANAGEMENT

Nursing Assessment and Diagnosis

The nurse should inspect the woman's perineum or abdominal wound site every 8 to 12 hours for signs of early infection. The REEDA scale helps the nurse remember to consider *r*edness, *e*dema, *e*cchymosis, *d*ischarge, and *a*pproximation of either the perineal or surgical wound. Any degree of induration (hardening) should be immediately reported to the clinician.

Fever, malaise, abdominal pain, foul-smelling lochia, larger than expected uterus, tachycardia, and other signs of infection should be noted and reported immediately so that treatment can begin. The white blood cell (WBC) count, a usual objective measure of infection, cannot be used reliably because of the normal increase in WBCs during the postpartum period; a postpartum WBC count of 14,000 to 16,000/mm^3 is not an unusual finding. An increase in WBC level of more than 30% in a 6-hour period, however, is indicative of infection.

Nursing diagnoses that may apply to the woman with a puerperal infection include the following:

- ***Risk for Injury*** related to the spread of infection
- ***Acute Pain*** related to the presence of infection
- ***Deficient Knowledge*** related to lack of information about condition and its treatment
- ***Risk for Impaired Parenting*** related to delayed parent-infant attachment secondary to woman's pain and other symptoms of infection as well as possible separation of the newborn from the mother

Nursing Plan and Implementation

Hospital-Based Nursing Care

Careful attention to Standard Precautions, aseptic technique, and good hand washing during labor, birth, and postpartum is essential to minimze the risk of puerperal infection.

The nurse caring for a woman during the postpartum period is responsible for teaching the woman self-care measures that are helpful in preventing infection. The woman should understand the importance of good perineal care, hygiene practices to prevent contamination of the perineum (such as wiping from front to back, changing perineal pads after voiding), and thorough hand washing. Once edema and perineal pain are under control, the nurse can also encourage sitz baths, which are cleansing and promote healing (see chapter 36 ∞). Adequate fluid intake coupled with a diet high in protein and vitamin C, which are necessary to promote wound healing, also helps prevent infection (James, 2008). If the woman has a draining wound or purulent lochia, it is especially important that those in contact with soiled items and linens practice good hand washing. Clear, concise instructions about wound care and how to discard soiled dressings appropriately must be provided to safeguard the woman and her caregivers. Assuming a semi-Fowler's position will facilitate drainage of purulent discharge.

If the woman is seriously ill, ongoing assessment of urine specific gravity and intake and output is necessary. The nurse also carefully administers antibiotics as ordered and regulates the IV fluids rate. Ongoing assessment of the woman's condition is vital to detect subtle changes in her health status. The nurse also recognizes the woman's comfort needs related to hygiene, positioning, oral care, and pain relief.

Promoting maternal-infant attachment can be difficult with the acutely ill woman. The nurse may provide pictures of the infant and keep the mother informed of the infant's well-being. Mementos, such as a footprint, a note written by the father "from the baby," or a videotape of the baby can be comforting to the mother during their separation. If she feels up to it, the new mother will also benefit from brief visits with her newborn.

The woman who wishes to breastfeed when her condition allows can maintain lactation by assistance with pumping her breasts regularly. Understanding that the opportunity to breastfeed is simply delayed, not eliminated by the infectious process may serve as helpful reassurance. The partner of a seriously ill woman will be concerned about her condition and torn about spending time with her or with their newborn. Because maternal-infant bonding may be compromised, father-newborn bonding can be especially important. See Nursing Care Plan: For the Woman with a Puerperal Infection on pages 1128–1129 for specific nursing care measures.

Community-Based Nursing Care

The woman with a puerperal infection needs assistance when she is discharged from the hospital. If the family cannot provide this home assistance, a referral to home care services is needed. Home care services should be contacted as soon as puerperal infection is diagnosed so that the nurse can meet with the woman for a family and home assessment and development of a home care plan.

The family needs instruction in the care of a newborn, including feeding, bathing, cord care, immunizations, and significant observations that should be reported. A well-baby appointment should be scheduled. The woman who has maintained lactation by pumping and discarding her milk may need assistance with early breastfeeding. Breastfeeding mothers receiving antibiotics should be instructed to inspect the infant's mouth for signs of thrush and to report the finding to their physician.

The mother should be instructed regarding activity, rest, medications, diet, and signs and symptoms of complications, and she should be scheduled for a return medical visit. She needs to know the importance of taking the entire course of prescribed antibiotics even though she may begin to feel better before the bottle is empty. She also needs to be informed about the importance of pelvic rest; that is, she should not use tampons or douches nor have intercourse until she has been examined by the physician and told it is safe to resume those activities.

Evaluation

Expected outcomes of nursing care include the following:

- The infection is quickly assessed, and treatment is instituted successfully without further complications.

NURSING CARE PLAN For the Woman with a Puerperal Infection

INTERVENTION	RATIONALE
1. Nursing Diagnosis: Risk for Infection related to traumatized tissues **Goal:** The woman will be free of complications associated with infection.	
■ Encourage the woman, staff, and family members to adhere to a strict hand washing policy.	■ Hand washing kills bacteria and prevents cross-contamination.
■ Review the woman's prenatal, intrapartal, and postpartal records for underlying problems that could contribute to poor wound healing or increased risk for spread of infection.	■ Identifying underlying problems gives the caregiver an opportunity to initiate preventive measures that will promote healthy wound healing and stop the spread of infection.
■ Monitor blood pressure, pulse, respiration, and temperature.	■ Obtain baseline data; signs and symptoms of septic shock produce a decrease in blood pressure and an increase in respirations. Temperature increase of 38°C/100.4°F or greater on any 2 days after the first 24 hours indicates infection.
■ Instruct the woman on proper perineal care including wiping perineum from front to back after voiding, washing the perineum after voiding and defecating, and changing peri-pads frequently, always followed by hand washing.	■ Proper perineal care techniques enhance good hygiene and assist in removing urine and fecal contaminants from perineum. Changing peri-pads frequently decreases skin contact with a moist medium that favors bacteria growth.
■ Encourage a well-balanced diet with adequate protein, calories, and vitamin C. ■ Continue prenatal vitamins and iron as ordered	■ Protein and vitamin C are essential nutrients for tissue healing and repair.
■ Encourage the woman to consume 2000 ml of fluid a day.	■ Maintains hydration and increases circulating volume. Dilutes organisms which are eliminated with voiding.
■ Encourage use of the sitz bath, Surgigator, or the perineal light two to four times a day for at least 10–15 minutes.	■ Moist or dry heat to the perineum increases localized blood flow, promotes healing, and provides comfort.
■ Encourage early ambulation.	■ Enhances circulation and drainage of lochia.
■ Assess and report signs and symptoms of infection in perineum including: redness, erythema, edema, discharge, approximation of wound edges (REEDA), and pain.	■ Identifying signs and symptoms of infection early allows for prompt treatment and healing.
Collaborative: Obtain lab work as ordered by the physician including culture and sensitivity, complete blood count (CBC) with differential, and white blood cell (WBC) count.	■ Identifies abnormal lab values for early intervention. In addition, identifies infection and its causative organism for appropriate antibiotic treatment.
■ Administer antibiotic therapy as ordered by the physician.	■ Fights infection and helps prevent ascension of organisms into further tissue.
■ Encourage semi-Fowler's position at intervals.	■ Uses gravity to assist drainage of infected material.
■ Promote wound drainage by assisting physician in opening the wound if necessary. Also, if the wound is greater than 2–3 cm, pack with iodoform gauze.	■ Iodoform gauze is used to maintain patency of wound opening. This promotes drainage and prevents abscesses from developing.
■ Report signs and symptoms of severe infections: foul-smelling lochia, uterine subinvolution, uterine tenderness, severe lower abdominal pain, elevated temperature, elevated WBC count, general malaise, chills, lethargy, tachycardia, nausea and vomiting, and abdominal rigidity.	■ Reporting signs and symptoms of severe infections early allows for initiation of appropriate therapy by the physician and prevents further spread of the invading pathogen.
EXPECTED OUTCOME: The woman will be free of complications associated with infection as evidenced by practicing behaviors that prevent the spread of infection and promote timely wound healing.	
2. Nursing Diagnosis: Acute Pain related to the infection process **Goal:** The woman will be free of pain or have a level of relief that is acceptable.	
■ Assess pain location and intensity; have the woman describe on a scale from 1 (mild) to 10 (severe). Assess nonverbal signs of pain, including facial grimacing and agitation.	■ Assesses the need for pain management and evaluates interventions already implemented.
■ Teach the woman to request or take analgesic before pain is severe.	■ Allows timing of medication for effective relief. The effects of IV analgesia are almost immediate; the effects of intramuscular (IM) analgesics occur in 20–30 min, while those of oral medications are 30–45 min.

NURSING CARE PLAN For the Woman with a Puerperal Infection continued

INTERVENTION	RATIONALE
■ Encourage the woman to discuss anxiety and fears.	■ Reduces anxiety/fear and may decrease the woman's perception of pain.
■ Encourage frequent rest periods and decrease disturbing environmental stimuli.	■ Frequent rest periods will conserve woman's energy. Excessive environmental stimuli may increase woman's pain perception.
■ Promote relaxation by encouraging diversional activities and the use of exercises including radio/television, reading, guided imagery, deep breathing techniques, massage, visualization, and meditation.	■ Promotes relaxation and refocuses woman's attention away from the intensity of pain.
Collaborative: Administer analgesics as ordered by the physician, evaluating the response to the analgesic and any adverse effects in a timely manner.	■ Relieves pain and interrupts the pain, fear, tension cycle to facilitate relaxation.

EXPECTED OUTCOME: Woman is free of pain or has an acceptable level of pain as evidenced by verbalization of pain relief and the exhibition of a relaxed demeanor.

3. Nursing Diagnosis: Risk For Impaired Parenting/Attachment related to pain secondary to maternal infection and/or separation from infant to minimize exposure

Goal: Mother will have no problems bonding with infant and assuming responsibility for the care of the infant with assistance and later independently

INTERVENTION	RATIONALE
■ Provide quality time for mother and infant contact.	■ Aids in the bonding process.
■ Encourage the partner or family members to give the woman videos and pictures of the infant if the mother's condition requires separation from the infant.	■ Promotes bonding and gives the mother reassurance that the infant is being cared for.
■ Encourage the partner and family members to become involved with the care of the infant and verbalize interaction to the mother.	■ Allows the mother to feel as though she is involved in the care of the infant.
■ Encourage the mother to feed (breast or bottle) infant if her condition is stable. If the mother is unable to breastfeed, encourage and assist her in pumping her breasts to maintain milk production.	■ Hands-on participation in the infant's care gives mother a positive outlook.
■ Assess maternal support systems.	■ As the mother is recovering, she will need assistance in household organization and personal care.
Collaborative: Offer referrals to home health services, doula services, lactation services, and/or support groups.	■ Ensures the woman's well-being, and identifies problems that may require intervention

EXPECTED OUTCOME: Mother will bond with the infant as evidenced by exhibiting appropriate attachment behaviors when interacting with infant, providing care to self and infant, and verbalization of understanding of the parenting role.

- The woman understands the nature of the infection and the purpose of therapy; she carries out any ongoing antibiotic therapy necessary after discharge.
- Maternal-infant attachment is maintained.

Care of the Woman with a Urinary Tract Infection

The postpartum woman is at increased risk of developing urinary tract problems because of the normal postpartum diuresis, increased bladder capacity, decreased bladder sensitivity from stretching or trauma, bacterial shedding with urinary stasis, and possible inhibited neural control of the bladder following the use of general or regional anesthesia and contamination from catheterization. It is important that the mother empty her bladder completely with each voiding.

Overdistention of the Bladder

Overdistention occurs postpartally when the woman is unable to empty her bladder, usually because of trauma or the effects of anesthesia. Women who have not sufficiently recovered from the effects of anesthesia cannot void spontaneously, and catheterization is necessary. After the effects of anesthesia have worn off, if the woman cannot void, postpartal urinary retention is highly indicative of a urinary tract infection (UTI). Other risk factors for urinary retention after childbirth include nulliparity, instrumental delivery, and prolonged first and second stages of labor, episiotomy, lacerations, and nulliparity (Cunningham et al., 2010).

> **CLINICAL TIP**
> Postpartum urinary retention is often defined as "the absence of spontaneous urination within 6 hours of a vaginal delivery or within 6 hours after removal of an indwelling catheter post-Cesarean delivery." The astute nurse will watch the woman's bladder for signs of retention—not the clock! As urinary retention promotes uterine atony and a subsequent increase in bleeding and also contributes to the possibility of UTI, timely intervention is crucial.

Clinical Therapy

Overdistention in the early postpartum period is often managed by draining the bladder with a straight catheter as a one-time measure. If the overdistention recurs or is diagnosed later in the postpartum period, an indwelling catheter may be ordered for 24 hours. An alternate urinary retention protocol involves bladder ultrasound scans with intervention based on the amount of urine volume. For example, if the volume is greater than 200 ml, the bladder is drained and the catheter is left in for another day, whereas if the volume is 200 ml or less, the catheter is removed and the bladder rechecked after 4 hours (Cunningham et al., 2010).

NURSING CARE MANAGEMENT

Nursing Assessment and Diagnosis

The overdistended bladder appears as a large mass, reaching sometimes to the umbilicus and displacing the uterine fundus upward and to one side. There is increased vaginal bleeding, the fundus is boggy, and the woman may complain of cramping as the uterus attempts to contract. Some women also experience backache and restlessness. Nursing diagnoses that may apply when a woman has difficulties due to overdistention include the following:

- ***Risk for Infection*** related to urinary stasis secondary to overdistention of the bladder
- ***Urinary Retention*** related to decreased bladder sensitivity and normal postpartum diuresis

Nursing Plan and Implementation

Diligent monitoring of the bladder during the recovery period and preventive health measures greatly reduce the chance for overdistention of the bladder. Encouraging the mother to void spontaneously and helping her use the toilet, if possible, or the bedpan if she has received conductive anesthesia, prevents overdistention in most cases. The nurse assists the woman to a normal position for voiding (i.e., sitting with the legs and feet lower than the trunk) and provides privacy to encourage voiding. The woman should be medicated for whatever pain she may be having before attempting to void because pain may cause a reflex spasm of the urethra. Perineal ice packs applied after birth will minimize any edema, which may interfere with voiding. Pouring warm water over the perineum or having the woman void in a sitz bath may also be effective. Some women note that hearing running water nearby, blowing bubbles through a straw into a glass of water, or voiding onto a bedpan into which a few drops of tincture of peppermint have been added helps stimulate voiding.

If catheterization becomes necessary, careful, meticulous, aseptic technique should be employed during catheter insertion. The vagina and vulva are traumatized to some degree by vaginal birth, and edema is common. This edema may obscure the urinary meatus; therefore, the nurse needs to be extremely careful in cleansing the vulva and inserting the catheter. It is imperative to discard a catheter that has inadvertently been introduced into the vagina and thus contaminated. Because catheterization is an uncomfortable procedure as a result of the postpartal trauma and edema of the tissue, the nurse should be careful and gentle not only in inserting the catheter but also in handling and cleaning the perineal area.

If the amount of urine drained from the bladder reaches 900 to 1000 ml, the catheter should be clamped and taped firmly to the woman's leg. The nurse should carefully document the procedure, including taking the woman's vital signs before and after the procedure and noting her responses. After an hour, the catheter may be unclamped and placed on gravity drainage. This technique protects the bladder and avoids rapid intra-abdominal decompression. When the indwelling catheter is removed, a urine specimen is often sent to the laboratory. The tip of the catheter may also be removed and sent for culture.

Evaluation

Expected outcomes of nursing care include the following:

- The woman voids adequately to meet the demands of the increased fluid shifts during the postpartum period.
- The woman does not develop infection due to stasis of urine.
- The woman actively incorporates self-care measures to decrease bladder overdistention.

Cystitis (Lower Urinary Tract Infection)

Retention of residual urine, bacteria introduced at the time of catheterization, and a bladder traumatized by childbirth combine to provide an excellent environment for the development of cystitis (lower urinary tract infection). *Escherichia coli* has been demonstrated to be the causative agent in most cases of postpartum cystitis and pyelonephritis (upper urinary tract infection). *Klebsiella pneumoniae* and *Proteus* species are significant pathogens, especially in women with a history of recurrent UTIs (Duff et al., 2009). In most cases, the infection ascends the urinary tract from the urethra to the bladder. If cystitis is not treated, the infection can spread to the kidneys (pyelonephritis) because vesiculoureteral reflux (backward flow of urine) forces contaminated urine into the renal pelvis.

Clinical Therapy

When cystitis is suspected, a clean-catch, midstream urine sample is obtained for microscopic examination, culture, and sensitivity tests. The specimen may require collection by the nurse with the woman on a bedpan because few postpartal women can collect a true midstream, clean-catch specimen without contaminating the specimen with lochia. A catheterized specimen is avoided when possible because of the increased risk of infection. When the bacterial concentration is greater than 100,000 colonies of the same organism per milliliter of fresh urine, infection is generally present. Counts between 10,000 and 100,000 may also suggest infection, particularly if clinical symptoms are noted.

In the clinical setting, antibiotic therapy is often begun before culture and sensitivity reports are available. Frequently used antibiotics include a preparation of trimethoprim-sulfamethoxazole–double strength (Bactrim DS, Septra DS), one of the short-acting sulfonamides, nitrofurantoin (Macrodantin), or, in the case of sulfa allergy, ampicillin or amoxicillin-clavulanic acid. The antibiotic is changed later if indicated by the results of the sensitivity report. Antispasmodic or urinary analgesic agents, such as phenazopyridine hydrochloride (Pyridium), may be given to relieve discomfort.

NURSING CARE MANAGEMENT

Nursing Assessment and Diagnosis

Assessment for urinary distention and developing UTI is a component of postpartum assessment, performed at least daily during hospitalization and more often with risk factors. Intake and output of urine is commonly measured for 24 hours after vaginal delivery and an additional 24 hours after the indwelling catheter is removed from women with cesarean deliveries. Women should be encouraged to void every 2 to 4 hours to prevent urinary stasis and to report any sensations of incomplete emptying of the bladder or dysuria.

Acute cystitis usually causes symptoms of frequency, dysuria, urgency, hesitancy and dribbling, nocturia, and suprapubic pain. Gross hematuria may be noted but high fever and systemic symptoms are not expected.

When a UTI progresses to pyelonephritis, systemic symptons usually occur, and the woman becomes acutely ill. Symptoms include high fever, chills, flank pain (unilateral or bilateral), nausea, and vomiting, in addition to the signs of lower UTI. Costovertebral angle (CVA) tenderness may be noted on exam but is not required for diagnosis. Clean-catch urine specimens show large numbers of white blood cells and are positive for infection (Smith, 2008).

Nursing diagnoses that may apply if a woman develops a UTI postpartally include the following:

- ***Acute Pain*** with voiding related to dysuria secondary to infection
- ***Ineffective Self Health Management*** related to need for information about self-care measures to prevent UTI

Nursing Plan and Implementation

Screening for asymptomatic bacteriuria in pregnancy should be routine. Frequent emptying of the bladder during labor and postpartum should be encouraged to prevent overdistention and trauma to the bladder. Catheterization technique and nursing actions to prevent overdistention (previously discussed) also apply. If symptoms of UTI occur, they should be reported to the physician or certified nurse-midwife (CNM). A clean-catch-midstream specimen for culture and sensitivity may be ordered. A 10- to 14-day course of antibiotics to treat UTI is typically started while culture results are pending. Changes in the regimen can be made once culture results are consulted, if necessary. The woman with pyelonephritis must understand the importance of follow-up care after discharge to prevent recurrence or further complications.

Health Promotion Education

All postpartum women should be taught the signs and symptoms of cystitis and pyelonephritis as symptoms are more likely to be noted later in the postpartum interval.

The nurse should advise the postpartum woman to continue good perineal hygiene following discharge, to maintain a good fluid intake (at least 8 to 10 8-oz glasses daily) especially of water, and to empty her bladder whenever she feels the urge to void, but at least every 2 to 4 hours while awake. Once sexual intercourse is resumed, the new mother should void before (to prevent bladder trauma) and following intercourse (to wash contaminants from the vicinity of the urinary meatus). Wearing cotton-crotch underwear to facilitate air circulation also reduces the risk of UTI. Acidification of the urine is thought to aid in preventing and managing UTI. The nurse thus advises the woman to avoid carbonated beverages, coffee, citrus fruits, tomatoes, and chocolate, which increase alkalinity of urine, and to drink cranberry, plum, apricot, and prune juices and take vitamin C, which increase the acidity of urine (Mengel & Schwiebert, 2009).

Evaluation

Expected outcomes of nursing care include:

- The woman identifies the signs of UTI and her condition is treated successfully.
- The woman uses self-care measures to prevent the recurrence of UTI as part of her personal hygiene routine.
- The woman continues with any long-term therapy or follow-up as appropriate for the diagnosis.
- Maternal-infant attachment is maintained; the woman is able to care for her newborn effectively.

Care of the Woman with Postpartum Mastitis

Mastitis is a unilateral inflammation of the interlobular connective tissue in the breast that occurs primarily in lactating women. (Chapter 37 discusses the breastfeeding difficulties of the woman with mastitis.) Inflammation can occur at any time during breastfeeding but onset is usually between 2 to 8 weeks postpartum or any other time that nursing frequency decreases. It ranges in severity from local inflammation to abscess and septicemia. The incidence of sporadic mastitis is 5%

to 10% of breastfeeding mothers and less than 1% in nonlactating mothers (Duff et al., 2009).

The usual causative organisms are *Staphylococcus aureus, Haemophilus parainfluenzae, H. influenzae, E. coli,* and *Streptococcus* species. Clinical features include fever; chills; headache; flulike muscle aches and malaise because of myalgia; and a warm, reddened, painful area of the breast, often wedge-shaped because of septal distribution of connective tissue (Figure 39-2 ■). The infection usually begins when bacteria invade the breast tissue after it has been traumatized in some way (see the factors commonly associated with mastitis in Table 39-5). Milk serves as a favorable medium for the invasive bacteria to multiply; thus, milk stasis is another risk factor. The most common source of the causative organism is the infant's nose and throat, although other sources include the hands of the mother or hospital staff and the woman's circulating blood. Infants of women with mastitis generally remain well unless the causative organism is *Candida albicans.*

When *Candida albicans* is the causative organism of mastitis, entering the breast through a small fissure or abrasion on the nipple, the baby will often have thrush, a candidal infection of the mouth. There may be a history of a recent course of antibiotics in the woman. Signs include late-onset nipple pain, followed by shooting pain between feedings, often radiating to the chest wall (Lawrence & Lawrence, 2009). Eventually, the skin of the affected breast may become pink, flaking, and pruritic. Women may notice a yeasty odor to their milk. Unless the mother and her newborn are treated for *Candida,* recolonization will occur when breastfeeding is resumed.

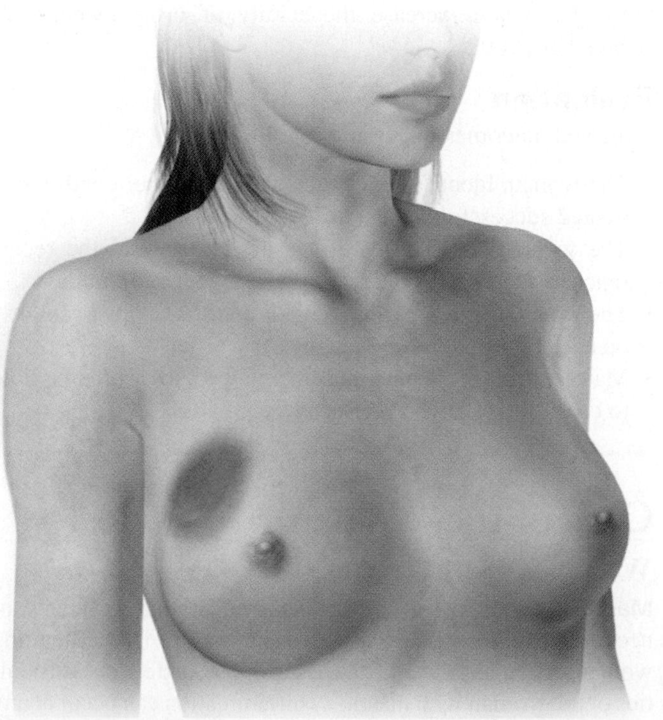

Figure 39-2 ■ Mastitis. Erythema and swelling are present in the upper outer quadrant of the breast. Axillary lymph nodes are often enlarged and tender. The segmental anatomy of the breast accounts for the demarcated, often V-shaped wedge of inflammation.

TABLE 39-5 Factors Affecting Development of Postpartum Mastitis

Milk Stasis
- Failure to change infant position to allow emptying of all lobes
- Failure to alternate breasts at feedings
- Poor suck
- Poor let-down

Actions That Promote Access/Multiplication of Bacteria
- Poor hand washing technique
- Improper breast hygiene
- Failure to air-dry breasts after breastfeeding
- Use of plastic-lined breast pads that trap moisture against nipple

Breast/Nipple Trauma
- Incorrect positioning for breastfeeding
- Poor latch on
- Failure to rotate position on nipple
- Incorrect or aggressive pumping technique
- Cracked nipples

Obstruction of Ducts
- Restrictive clothing
- Constricting bra
- Underwire bra

Change in Number of Feedings/Failure to Empty Breasts
- Attempted weaning
- Missed feeding
- Prolonged sleeping of infant, including sleeping through the night
- Favoring side of nipple soreness

Lowered Maternal Defenses
- Fatigue
- Stress
- Poor diet

Clinical Therapy

Clinical diagnosis is possible in most cases, although culture and sensitivity testing of breast milk may be done. If a culture of the breast milk is ordered either for initial diagnosis or with recurrence or failed treatment of mastitis, it is more reliable with a midstream-type collection process. The nipple is washed first; then the first 3 ml of breast milk are manually expressed and discarded, after which the actual specimen is collected. A leukocyte count greater than 1 million/ml and a bacterial count greater than 10,000 colonies/ml are diagnostic (Newton, 2007).

Treatment of mastitis involves bed rest for at least 24 hours; increased fluid intake (at least 2 to 2.5 L/day); a supportive bra; frequent breastfeeding; local application of warm, moist heat or ice packs; and analgesics that are compatible with breastfeeding (James, 2008). Nonsteroidal anti-inflammatory agents are recommended to treat both fever and inflammation. Some clinicians question the worth of milk culture because it is not ductal tissue that is infected, and recommend antibiotic coverage empirically based on the most common etiologic organisms, for example, a course of 7- to 10-day antibiotics, depending on response, usually a penicillinase-resistant penicillin, such as dicloxacillin

500 mg every 6 hours or a cephalosporin, such as cephalexin 500 mg every 6 hours (Duff et al., 2009). Both drugs have similar safety profiles and are relatively inexpensive. The woman should continue to breastfeed; in fact, regular drainage of both breasts actually helps by preventing milk stasis and abscess formation, and there is virtually no risk to the newborn. If there has been no change in symptomatology in 48 hours, modification of the antibiotic therapy will be considered—perhaps changing to ampicillin/clavulanate (Augmentin) in the nonallergic patient. There have been reported cases of methicillin-resistant *staph aureus* (Academy of Breastfeeding Medicine (ABM), 2008).

Candidal infections can be especially stubborn. Initial treatment generally involves antifungal creams or ointments once or twice daily. Oral Diflucan is excreted in breast milk but is not considered toxic to the infant and can be used if other agents fail. Women should be instructed to cleanse their nipples with warm water and allow air-drying before application of the antifungal medication. For the woman who prefers to avoid medication, an alternative treatment is cleansing of the nipples with a solution of 1 tablespoon of vinegar in 1 cup of water or 1 teaspoon of baking soda in 1 cup of water, followed by air-drying.

Ten percent of cases will progress to abscess formation if mastitis remains untreated, treatment fails, or the infant is abruptly weaned (Cunningham et al., 2010). Abscess is more common when there is a lag of 24 hours or more between onset of symptoms and care seeking. Abscesses are associated with exquisite tenderness of the breast and an undurated area with possible fluctuation. Breast abscess may require incision and drainage, and intravenous (IV) antibiotics; analgesics and antipyretics are commonly ordered. Community-acquired methicillin-resistant *Staphylococcus aureus* (MRSA) is likely to cause abscess formation (Cunningham et al., 2010).

Improved outcome, a decreased duration of symptoms, and decreased incidence of a breast abscess result if the breasts continue to be emptied by either breastfeeding or pumping. Thus, continued breastfeeding is recommended in the process of mastitis. The plan of care should include contacting the woman within 24 hours of initiation of treatment to ensure that symptoms are subsiding.

PROBIOTICS AND OTHER COMPLEMENTARY THERAPIES FOR MASTITIS

Probiotics are a category of dietary supplements consisting of beneficial microorganisms (*pro* means "for" and *biotic* means "life" versus *antibiotic,* which literally means "against life"). Probiotics compete with disease-causing microorganisms in the gastrointestinal tract. When antibiotics are taken, they kill many of the beneficial bacteria that exist naturally in the digestive tract. Supplementing with probiotics after a course of antibiotics is frequently prescribed by nutritionists and complementary practitioners. Commonly used probiotics include *Lactobacillus acidophilus* and *Bifidobacterium bifidum;* there are other species of *Lactobacillus* and *Bifidobacterium* that have been shown to be effective in such conditions as diarrhea and vaginal infections. *Bifidobacterium* also competes against *Candida albicans.* Probiotics can be taken in the form of powder, capsules, and suppositories, or in fermented milk products such as yogurt or *kefir.*

Other complementary therapies used for mastitis include belladonna, acupuncture, oxytocin nasal spray to improve milk ejection, a traditional Chinese herb known as extracts of *Fructus gleditsiae,* and application of cabbage leaves over the affected area to relieve engorgement. (See chapter 37 ∞ for more details.)

NURSING CARE MANAGEMENT

Nursing Assessment and Diagnosis

Daily assessment of breast consistency, skin color, surface temperature, nipple condition, and presence of pain is essential to detect early signs of problems that may predispose to mastitis. The mother should be observed breastfeeding her baby to ensure use of proper technique for positioning, latch on, and disengagement of the infant from the nipple. Consultation with a lactation specialist can be of great value, especially for first-time mothers. During the breast assessment while the breastfeeding woman is still hospitalized, the nurse is advised to teach her about the potential for mastitis, risk factors, preventive measures, recognition of symptoms, and the need to notify the physician promptly if symptoms occur.

If an infection has developed, the nurse should assess for contributing factors such as cracked nipples, poor hygiene, engorgement, supplemental feedings, change in routine or infant feeding pattern, abrupt weaning, or lack of proper breast support so that these factors may be corrected as part of the treatment plan. Nursing diagnoses that may apply to the woman with mastitis include the following:

- ***Risk for trauma*** related to lack of information about appropriate breastfeeding practices
- ***Ineffective Breastfeeding*** related to pain secondary to development of mastitis

Nursing Plan and Implementation

Preventing mastitis is far simpler than treating it. Ideally, mothers should be instructed in proper breastfeeding technique prenatally. The nurse should help the mother breastfeed soon after birth and should review correct technique. Comanagement of breastfeeding between the nurse and a certified lactation specialist is often possible. All women, even those not breastfeeding, are encouraged to wear a good supportive bra at all times to avoid milk stasis, especially in the lower lobes.

Meticulous hand washing by the breastfeeding mother and all personnel is the primary measure for preventing epidemic nursery infections and subsequent maternal mastitis. Prompt attention to mothers who have blocked milk ducts eliminates stagnant milk as a growth medium for bacteria or the development of cracks and fissures, a common portal for bacterial entry. If the mother finds that one area of her breast feels distended, she can rotate the position of her infant for breastfeeding, manually express milk remaining in the breast after feeding (usually only necessary if the infant is not sucking well), or massage the caked area toward the nipple as the infant nurses. Mothers who have developed mastitis can apply warm, moist compresses to the affected area before breastfeeding. The nurse encourages the mother to breastfeed frequently, starting with the unaffected breast until let-down occurs in the affected breast, then encourages feeding from the affected breast until it is emptied completely (James, 2008). After nursing, the mother can leave a small amount of milk on each nipple to prevent cracking and allow nipples to air dry and apply cold packs to reduce pain and edema (ABM, 2008). Early identification of and intervention for sore nipples are also essential, as is prompt assessment of the breastfeeding mother's breasts when thrush is discovered in her newborn's mouth. For a detailed discussion of breastfeeding, see "Breastfeeding Concerns Following Discharge" in chapter 37 ∞.

Health Promotion Education

The woman should be aware of the importance of regular, complete emptying of the breasts to prevent engorgement and stasis. She should also understand the role of let-down in successful breastfeeding, correct positioning of the infant on the nipple, proper latch on, and the principles of supply and demand. If the mother is taking antibiotics, she needs to understand the importance of completing the full course of antibiotics, even if the infection seems to clear quickly. Infants tolerate the small amount of antibiotics in breast milk without difficulty. Postpartum women need to be advised that mastitis may recur. Breastfeeding mothers who will be returning to work outside the home need information on how to do so successfully. Because mastitis tends to develop following discharge, it is important to include information about signs and symptoms in the discharge teaching and printed materials (Table 39-6). All flulike symptoms should be considered a sign of mastitis until proven otherwise. If symptoms develop, the woman should contact her caregiver immediately, because prompt treatment helps to avoid abscess formation.

Community-Based Nursing Care

Because symptoms seldom occur before the second to fourth week postpartum, birthing unit nurses often are not fully aware of how uncomfortable and acutely ill the woman can be. The home care nurse who suspects mastitis on the basis of assessment findings refers the woman to the physician. The nurse may be asked to obtain a sample of breast milk to be cultured for the causative organism.

If the mother feels too ill to breastfeed or develops an abscess that prevents breastfeeding, the home care nurse can help the mother obtain an appropriate breast pump to help her maintain lactation and can provide opportunities for demonstration and return demonstration of pumping. The nurse can assist the mother to deal with her feelings about temporarily being unable to breastfeed. Referral to a lactation consultant or to La Leche League can be invaluable to the woman's physical and emotional adjustment to mastitis.

Evaluation

Expected outcomes of nursing care include the following:

- The woman is aware of the signs and symptoms of mastitis.
- The woman reports her signs and symptoms of mastitis early, and it is treated successfully.
- The woman can continue breastfeeding if she chooses.
- The woman understands self-care measures she can use to prevent recurrence of mastitis.

Care of the Woman with Postpartum Thromboembolic Disease

Thromboembolic disease may occur during pregnancy, but it is generally considered a postpartum complication. *Venous thrombosis* refers to formation of a blood clot (thrombus formation) at an area of impeded blood flow in a superficial or deep vein. When the thrombus is formed in response to inflammation in the vein wall, it is termed **thrombophlebitis**. Pulmonary embolism, a rare but life-threatening condition, occurs when thrombi formed in the deep leg veins are carried to the pulmonary artery, obstructing pulmonary blood flow to one or both lungs. These vascular occlusive processes—venous thrombosis, thrombophlebitis, septic pelvic thrombophlebitis, and pulmonary embolism—are known as thromboembolic diseases (Mengel & Schwiebert, 2009).

Three major causes of thromboembolic disease, often referred to as *Virchow's Triad*, are hypercoagulability of blood, venous stasis, and injury to the epithelium of the blood vessel. Changes in the woman's coagulation system in pregnancy contribute to hypercoagulability, and compression of the common iliac vein by the gravid uterus leads to venous stasis. These factors increase the risk of this phenomenon appropriately 2 to 6 times in pregnant and postpartum women (Poggi, 2007). Super-

TABLE 39-6 Comparison of Findings of Engorgement, Plugged Duct, and Mastitis

CHARACTERISTICS	ENGORGEMENT	PLUGGED DUCT	MASTITIS
Onset	Gradual, immediately postpartum	Gradual, after feedings	Sudden, after 10 days
Site	Bilateral	Unilateral	Usually unilateral
Swelling and heat	Generalized	May shift, little or no heat	Localized, red, hot, and swollen
Pain	Generalized	Mild but localized	Intense but localized
Body temperature	Less than 38.4°C (101.1°F)	Less than 38.4°C (101.1°F)	Greater than 38.4°C (101.1°F)
Systemic symptoms	Feels well	Feels well	Flulike symptoms

Source: Reprinted from Breastfeeding: A guide for the medical profession *by R. A. Lawrence, & R. M. Lawrence (1999). (5th ed., p. 276). Copyright 1999, with permission from Elsevier.*

ficial vein thrombophlebitis complicates the general childbearing period for 1 in 500 to 750 women. Deep vein thrombosis (DVT), which is more serious, occurs most commonly in postpartum women between postpartum days 10 to 20.

Risk factors associated with increased risk of thromboembolic disease include the following:

- Cesarean birth
- Immobility (prolonged)
- Obesity
- Cigarette smoking
- Previous thromboembolic disease or strong family history
- Trauma to extremity (can include injury from incorrect positioning or prolonged interval in stirrups during labor)
- Varicose veins
- Diabetes mellitus
- Advanced maternal age
- Multiparity
- Anemia
- Malignancy
- Inherited coagulation pathway deficiency
- Protein C & S deficiency

Factors contributing directly to the development of postpartum thromboembolic disease include (1) increased amounts of certain blood clotting factors; (2) postpartum thrombocytosis (increased quantity of circulating platelets and their increased adhesiveness); (3) release of thromboplastin substances from the tissue of the decidua, placenta, and fetal membranes; and (4) increased amounts of fibrinolysis inhibitors. These same factors protect childbearing women from exsanguinating from blood loss at delivery. Because women are at risk for thromboembolic disease during the childbearing period, attention should be given to measures that might prevent this complication (Table 39-7).

Women with inherited thrombophilias are at significantly greater risk of thromboembolism than women without these conditions. In these conditions, several regulatory proteins that act as inhibitors in the coagulation cascade are deficient, exacerbating hypercoagulability and contributing to recurrent venous thromboembolism. Most are transmitted by autosomal-dominant inheritance and affect predominantly Caucasian European populations, rarely those with Asian or African ethnic backgrounds. A personal or family history of thrombosis at any age is not uncommon, nor is a history of adverse pregnancy outcomes, such as severe pregnancy-induced hypertension, placental abruption, intrauterine growth retardation, or fetal loss after 20 weeks (Cunningham et al., 2010). Women with thrombophilias may require therapeutic levels of low-molecular-weight or unfractionated heparin throughout pregnancy and continued heparin therapy, followed by warfarin sodium (Coumadin) for at least 6 weeks postpartum.

Superficial Vein Disease

Superficial thrombophlebitis is far more common in postpartum women than during pregnancy. Often the clot involves the saphenous veins. This disorder is more common in women with pre-existing varices (enlarged veins), although it is not limited to that group. Superficial vein disease (SVD) may also occur as a sequelae to IV catheterization. Symptoms—tenderness in a portion of the vein, local heat and redness, normal temperature or low-grade fever, and, occasionally, slight elevation of the pulse—usually become apparent about the third or fourth postpartum day. A tender palpable cord may be noted along a portion of the vein. Treatment involves application of local heat, elevation of the affected limb, bed rest and analgesic agents, and the use of elastic compression support hose. Anticoagulants are usually not necessary unless complications develop. Pulmonary embolism is extremely rare. If improvement is not evident or deep vein involvement is suspected, appropriate diagnostic measures are taken and serve as a basis for treatment decisions (Mengel & Schwiebert, 2009).

Deep Vein Thrombosis

Deep vein thrombosis (DVT) or thrombophlebitis is more frequently seen in women with a history of thrombosis. Obstetric complications such as polyhydramnios, preeclampsia, and operative birth are associated with an increased incidence. After a clinical diagnosis of DVT, a woman's risk in a subsequent pregnancy increases.

TABLE 39-7 Measures to Decrease Risk of Thromboembolic Disease in Childbearing Women

ANTEPARTUM MEASURES	INTRAPARTUM MEASURES	POSTPARTUM MEASURES
Advise woman to avoid sedentary lifestyle and to exercise as much as possible (walking is ideal).	Encourage ambulation unless contraindicated in early labor.	Encourage early ambulation.
Recommend plenty of fluids to avoid dehydration.	Later, encourage leg exercises.	For women on bed rest, advise or assist with turning and leg exercises every 2 hours (woman may be encouraged to rotate ankles and to "write baby's name in air with toes").
Advise to quit smoking.	Do not gatch bed or use pillows under knees.	Encourage fluids to avoid dehydration.
Teach to avoid prolonged standing or sitting in one position or sitting with legs crossed.	Pad stirrups.	Advise no smoking.
Encourage elevation of legs when sitting.	Ensure correct positioning in stirrups that minimizes pressure on the popliteal area.	Use antiembolism stockings with those at risk. Pneumatic compression stockings may be ordered after cesarean birth until ambulation occurs.
Teach to avoid tight knee-high hose or other constrictive garments.	Limit time in stirrups as much as possible. After cesarean birth, initiate leg and foot exercises as soon as possible (in recovery).	Advise against prolonged sitting and crossing legs. Avoid knee gatch in hospital bed.
Encourage to take frequent breaks during long car trips to walk around, thereby preventing prolonged venous stasis.	Use antiembolism stockings for women at risk of deep vein thrombosis (DVT).	Encourage elevation of legs while sitting.

Clinical manifestations may include edema of the ankle and leg and an initial low-grade fever often followed by high temperature and chills. Other findings include tenderness or pain, a palpable cord, changes in limb color, and difference in limb circumference of more than 2 cm (0.8 in.). Depending on the vein involved, the woman may complain of pain in the popliteal and lateral tibial areas (popliteal vein), entire lower leg and foot (anterior and posterior tibial veins), inguinal tenderness (femoral vein), or pain in the lower abdomen (iliofemoral vein). Homans' sign (refer to chapter 35 and Figure 35-9) may or may not be positive. A positive Homans' sign is a specific finding but has a low sensitivity for helping diagnose DVT (Smith, 2008). Most DVTs occur in the left leg. Because of reflex arterial spasm, sometimes the limb is pale and cool to the touch—the so-called *milk leg* or *phlegmasia alba dolens*—and the dorsalis pedis pulse may be diminished or difficult to palpate.

CLINICAL JUDGMENT

Case Study: Wanda Sugiyama

Wanda Sugiyama, G1P1, had a cesarean birth after a prolonged labor and failure to progress. As she is walking in the hallway with her husband, you notice that Wanda is limping slightly, and you comment on that observation. Wanda responds that she is having pain in her right lower leg. She says, "Maybe I pulled a muscle during labor."

Critical Thinking

What would you do?

See www.nursing.pearsonhighered.com for possible responses.

Pulmonary Embolism

Pulmonary embolism (PE) occurs when a thrombus from a lower extremity or the pelvis lodges in the pulmonary vascular bed and restricts circulation to the corresponding area of the lung vasculature. The embolus may be microscopic in size or may be massive enough to occlude the branches of the pulmonary artery (McCaffery & Blum, 2009). Pulmonary embolism is a particularly catastrophic event with a high mortality rate; most fatalities occur within 30 to 60 minutes; however, early recognition and prompt action can decrease the mortality rate significantly and treatment of DVT can often prevent this complication. Although the incidence of DVT in pregnancy is now believed to be almost comparable with that of postpartum DVT, PE develops most commonly in postpartum women. The most common risk factors are proximal DVT and recurrent thromboembolic disease. Diagnosis may be difficult because the most common clinical findings include nonspecific signs and symptoms such as dyspnea, pleuritic chest pain, cough with or without hemoptysis, cyanosis, tachypnea and tachycardia, panic, syncope, or sudden hypotension. Physical assessment will also reveal diaphoresis, friction rub, changes in the heart sounds, and electrocardiogram (ECG) may document a right axis shift (Turrentine, 2008). The nurse who recognizes the clinical findings of this clinical emergency, especially in a woman at risk, should alert the woman's physician immediately, as time can be critical. Elevating the head of the woman's bed may facilitate ease of breathing; oxygen by facemask at 8 to10 L per minute is initiated. Narcotics may be ordered for pain and to decrease anxiety, thereby decreasing the respiratory effort. Several imaging tests are available to assist in diagnosing pulmonary embolism; the choices depend on availability, the woman's condition, and the element of time (McCaffery & Blum, 2009). The woman with pulmonary embolism will be transferred to an intensive care setting where cardiovascular and respiratory status are monitored closely.

Clinical Therapy

Treatment involves the immediate IV administration of either standard unfractionated heparin or low molecular weight heparin (LMWH) using an infusion pump to permit continuous, accurate infusion to stabilize the clot. An example of a possible regimen is a subcutaneous injection of Enoxaparin 1 mg/kg twice daily. Heparin therapy is continued until the international normalized ratio (INR) with oral warfarin is achieved at 2.0–3.0. An advantage of LMWH is a safe profile and dosing not reliant on monitoring the activated partial thromboplastin time (aPTT) at a laboratory. In some cases thrombolytics (streptokinase or urokinase) or an embolectomy may be used. Maintenance with warfarin sodium (Coumadin) is started at 1 to 5 days. An initial dose of 5 to 10 mg/daily PO is titrated based on the prothrombin time (PT) with the INR target rate cited above (Cunningham et al., 2010). Strict bed rest and elevation of the affected leg are required, and analgesics are given as necessary to relieve discomfort. If fever is present, the woman may also be given an antibiotic (Smith, 2008). In most cases thrombectomy (surgical removal of the clot) is not necessary.

Once the symptoms have subsided (usually in several days), the woman may begin walking while wearing elastic support stockings. The woman will continue on warfarin sodium (Coumadin) for 3 to 6 months and for 12 months after recurrence (McCaffery & Blum, 2009). While taking warfarin sodium (Coumadin), prothrombin times are assessed periodically to maintain correct dosage levels. Periodic assessment for signs of bleeding is essential, including those for hematuria and fecal occult blood. In those who cannot be given anticoagulants, a vena cava filtering device may be considered (Smith, 2008). To prevent recurrence in subsequent pregnancies, prophylactic treatment will be considered.

NURSING CARE MANAGEMENT

Nursing Assessment and Diagnosis

The nurse carefully assesses the woman's history for factors predisposing to development of thrombosis or thrombophlebitis. In addition, as part of regular postpartum assessment, the nurse is alert to any patient complaints of pain in the leg, inguinal area, or lower abdomen, because such pain may indicate DVT. The nurse also assesses the woman's legs for evidence of edema, temperature change, or pain with palpation.

Nursing diagnoses that may apply to a postpartal woman with thromboembolic disease include the following:

- ***Ineffective Peripheral Tissue Perfusion*** related to obstructed venous return

- ***Acute Pain*** related to tissue hypoxia and edema secondary to vascular obstruction
- ***Risk for Impaired Parenting*** related to decreased maternal-infant interaction secondary to bed rest and intravenous lines
- ***Interrupted Family Processes*** related to illness of family member
- ***Deficient Knowledge*** related to self-care after discharge on anticoagulant therapy

Nursing Plan and Implementation

Women with varicosities should be evaluated for the need for support hose during labor and postpartum. Adequate fluid intake is necessary during labor to avoid dehydration. Because trauma is often a factor in the development of thrombophlebitis, the nurse avoids keeping the woman's legs elevated in stirrups for prolonged periods. If stirrups are used, they should be comfortably padded and adjusted to provide correct support and prevent pressure on popliteal vessels. Early ambulation is encouraged following birth, and the use of the knee gatch on the bed should be avoided. Women confined to bed following a cesarean birth are encouraged to perform regular leg exercises to promote venous return.

Once the diagnosis of DVT is made, the nurse maintains the heparin therapy, provides for appropriate comfort measures, and monitors the woman closely for signs of PE. The nurse also assesses for evidence of bleeding related to heparin and keeps the antagonist for heparin, protamine sulfate, readily available.

The nurse instructs the woman to avoid prolonged standing or sitting, because these positions contribute to venous stasis. She is also instructed to avoid crossing her legs because of the pressure it causes. The nurse also advises her to take frequent breaks, such as when taking car trips and while working if she sits most of the day. Walking is acceptable because it promotes venous return. The woman is reminded to identify her history of thrombosis or thrombophlebitis to her physician during subsequent pregnancies so that preventive measures may be instituted early. Recurrence is not uncommon (Turrentine, 2008).

Health Promotion Education

Women discharged on warfarin sodium (Coumadin) should be taught about the drug and safety factors associated with its use. Women need to be educated about foods high in vitamin K (a nutrient that lessens warfarin's effectiveness) and the need to strive for consistent daily intake so that accurate dosage of the drug can be achieved. When the dietary intake of these foods, such as cauliflower, soybean and canola oil, mayonnaise, broccoli, green and black tea, peppers, spinach, collard greens, and others increases significantly, the drug's anticoagulant effect can be lessened; when intake decreases significantly, there is a risk of bleeding. Thus consistency of intake is important. Favorites from these foods can be consumed in moderation and others avoided daily. Cranberry juice increases the effects of the drug and, if desired, should be consumed in moderation and with consistency. Binge alcohol use inhibits warfarin metabolism; an occasional alcoholic beverage does not affect coagulation adversely. Several herbals affect the efficacy of warfarin sodium; for example, garlic, ginger, and ginkgo prolong PT and should be avoided. Many multivitamins contain vitamin K; women on warfarin sodium (Coumadin) may take them but, again, should do so consistently. Vitamin C doses up to 500 mg per day and vitamin E doses up to 400 international units per day are considered safe; higher doses can affect coagulation.

While taking anticoagulants, the woman will be asked to undergo frequent coagulant tests to guide dosing. Point-of-care testing is now available to decrease the inconvenience of going into a laboratory environment for testing. Home self-testing involves a single capillary finger stick (Coaguchek, ProTime, Avocet) to test thromboplastin-mediated clotting expressed as prothrombin time (PT) or international normalized ratio (INR). The risk of bleeding increases significantly when the INR is 3 or greater (Lockwood, 2009). Bleeding should be reported if it fails to stop within 10 minutes. The nurse encourages the woman to carry a MedicAlert card or to wear a bracelet in case of emergency, to inform all healthcare providers (including dentists) that she is taking anticoagulants, and to have vitamin K available in case of bleeding.

While on anticoagulants, women should be cautious about using sharp objects such as knives or razor blades to avoid injury. Risky behaviors that could contribute to falls should be avoided. Wearing protective gloves during gardening or heavy housework and always wearing shoes can keep hands and feet safe from injury. For any severe bleeding episode, the woman should seek emergency care where IV vitamin K may be administered and fresh frozen plasma may be used to return her to an appropriate INR level.

Women who are discharged on warfarin must understand the purpose of the medication and be alert to signs of hemorrhage, such as bleeding gums, epistaxis, petechiae or ecchymosis, or evidence of blood in the urine or stool. Because careful monitoring is important, the woman should clearly understand the need to keep scheduled appointments for PT assessment. Certain medications, such as aspirin and other nonsteroidal anti-inflammatory drugs, increase anticoagulant activity, so they should be avoided. In fact, while she is taking warfarin sodium (Coumadin) the woman should check for possible medication interaction before taking *any* other medication. See the Nursing Care Plan: The Woman with Thromboembolic Disease for specific nursing care measures.

Community-Based Nursing Care

Because the mother with postpartum thromboembolic disease will depend on others for much of her initial home care, it is helpful for the father to be involved in preparations for discharge. The nurse should provide ample opportunities to answer questions and clarify instructions, verbally and in writing. The nurse will evaluate the extent to which both mother and father have understood instructions regarding the plan of care. It is especially important before discharge to assess the couple's plans to ensure bed rest for the mother if ordered. They might explore ways for her to maintain bed rest and still spend quality time with her newborn and any other children. For example, young children can sit on the bed for storytelling or play quiet games, and the newborn's crib can be placed adjacent to the mother's bed.

Case Study: Postpartum Thromboembolic Disease

NURSING CARE PLAN The Woman with Thromboembolic Disease

INTERVENTION	RATIONALE
1. Nursing diagnosis: Ineffective Peripheral Tissue Perfusion related to interruption of venous blood flow secondary to complications of labor and birth **Goal:** The woman's presenting signs and symptoms are relieved.	
■ Assess, record, and report signs of thrombophlebitis.	■ Early detection of developing thrombophlebitis permits prompt treatment. As the thrombus increases in size, signs of obstruction also increase. Assessment provides baseline data that may be used to monitor success of treatment.
■ Assess leg for edema, peripheral pulse, temperature, color, and tenderness every 8 hours. Initially note presence of palpable cord.	■ Edema/swelling, diminished or absent peripheral pulse, pallor, cool skin temperature, and tenderness are symptoms of deep vein thrombosis (DVT) and indicate dysfunction of peripheral circulation in the lower extremities. Measure circumference of lower leg to monitor for swelling. Peripheral pulses in both legs should be palpated for pulse rate and pulse strength to allow for comparison. A lower extremity cool to the touch may be due to reflex arterial spasm.
■ Assess Homans' sign every 8 hours (see Figure 35-9 ∞ on page 1013).	■ Normally there is no pain or discomfort associated with this procedure. Pain is caused by inflammation of the vessel. If pain is elicited the nurse documents the response as a positive Homans' sign and reports findings to the physician. Some women with thrombophlebitis never have a positive Homans' sign.
■ Maintain bed rest during the acute phase.	■ Bed rest is ordered to decrease the possibility that a portion of the clot will dislodge and result in pulmonary embolism.
■ Provide warm, moist soaks as ordered.	■ Warmth promotes blood flow to affected area.
■ Maintain limb in elevated position.	■ Elevation of affected limb promotes venous return and helps decrease edema.
■ Add a footboard to the bed and encourage use.	■ Flexion and extension of legs against a footboard activates the calf muscle pump and promotes venous reurn.
■ Initiate progressive ambulation following the acute phase and provide properly fitting compression stockings before ambulation. These should be properly measured.	■ Elastic compression stockings or "TEDs" help prevent pooling of venous blood in lower extremities. Stockings should be carefully measured according to guidelines to ensure proper pressure gradient and avoid "garter-like" roll at top. ■ Woman may begin to ambulate within a few days when symptoms subside.
Collaborative: Administer unfractionated heparin as ordered, by continuous intravenous drip, heparin lock, or subcutaneously, or administer low molecular weight heparin (LMWH) subcutaneously as ordered including: 1. Monitor IV or heparin lock site (if in use) for patency, signs of infiltration, or signs of infection. 2. Obtain international normalized ratio (INR) and partial thromboplastin time (PTT) per physician order and review before administering heparin. 3. Observe for signs of anticoagulant overdose with resultant bleeding including: a. Hematuria b. Epistaxis c. Ecchymosis or petechiae d. Bleeding gums e. Nose bleeds f. Bruising disproportionate to injury g. Cuts, scratches, injection, or venipuncture sites that bleed excessively	■ Heparin does not dissolve blood clot but is administered to prevent further clotting and improve tissue perfusion. It is safe for breastfeeding mothers because heparin is not excreted in breast milk.
4. Provide protamine sulfate, per physician order, to combat bleeding problems related to heparin overdose.	■ Protamine sulfate is a heparin antagonist, given intravenously, which is almost immediately effective in counteracting bleeding complications caused by heparin overdose.

NURSING CARE PLAN The Woman with Thromboembolic Disease continued

INTERVENTION	RATIONALE
5. Monitor and report any signs of pulmonary embolism.	■ Pulmonary embolism is a major complication of DVT/thrombophlebitis.
6. Initiate or support any emergency treatment.	■ Signs and symptoms may occur suddenly and require immediate emergency treatment; prognosis is related to size and location of embolism.
7. Obtain prothrombin time (PT) and review before beginning warfarin. Repeat periodically per physician order.	■ PT is the test most commonly used to monitor the blood of women receiving warfarin.

EXPECTED OUTCOME: Woman will have increased venous return from lower leg as evidenced by decreased edema in lower leg, negative Homans' sign, and no pain or tenderness in lower leg.

2. Nursing Diagnosis: Acute Pain related to tissue hypoxia and edema secondary to vascular obstruction
Goal: Woman will obtain relief of pain or experience level of pain that is acceptable.

INTERVENTION	RATIONALE
■ Administer analgesics per physician order. Notify physician if pain is not relieved.	■ Analgesics act to relieve pain and enable the woman to rest. Aspirin or ibuprofen products are contraindicated because they inhibit platelet adhesiveness. Acetaminophen may be ordered by the physician.
■ Observe or report disruptive effects of pain on emotions and behavior.	■ Once pain decreases, woman is more likely to ambulate, which will help increase venous return and decrease edema.
■ Provide supportive nursing comfort measures such as backrubs, provision of quiet time for sleep, diversional activities, or imagery.	

EXPECTED OUTCOME: Woman will have reduction in pain as evidenced by a pain level less than 5 at all times.

3. Nursing Diagnosis: Risk for Impaired Parenting related to decreased maternal-infant interaction secondary to bed rest and IVs
Goal: Woman will demonstrate evidence of positive physical and social interaction with newborn.

INTERVENTION	RATIONALE
■ Maintain mother-infant attachment when mother is on bed rest: 1. Provide frequent contacts for mother and infant; modified rooming-in if possible by having the crib placed close to the mother's bed and nurse checks often to help mother lift or move infant. 2. Encourage mother to continue feeding infant.	■ Maternal-infant attachment is enhanced by frequent contact and opportunities to interact.

EXPECTED OUTCOME: Woman will develop attachment bonds as evidenced by physical interactions: good eye contact, touching the baby, holding baby close, attempting to comfort baby, and kissing baby and social interactions: calling baby by name, making positive comments about baby, asking questions about baby, asking questions about baby care, and talking to baby.

4. Nursing Diagnosis: Interrupted Family Processes related to illness of family member
Goal: Woman and her family will cope effectively with her illness.

INTERVENTION	RATIONALE
■ Encourage woman to express her concerns to her partner. Assist couple in planning ways to manage while woman is hospitalized and after her discharge.	■ Illness of any family member impacts the entire family. This is especially true when the family situation is such that the mother is the primary nurturer and she is absent. Family members attempt to continue their own roles while also assuming the tasks of the missing mother. This can result in crisis.
■ Encourage partner or support person to bring other children to the hospital to visit mother and meet new sibling.	
■ Encourage partner or support person to bring in family pictures and notes from other children. Encourage phone calls.	
■ Contact social services if indicated to obtain additional assistance for family if needed.	

EXPECTED OUTCOMES: Woman expresses assurance that her family misses her but is coping effectively as evidenced by:

- Family visits woman frequently.
- Woman and family verbalize plan for division of family tasks while the woman is hospitalized, and understanding of potential needs of woman once released from hospital.

(continued)

NURSING CARE PLAN The Woman with Thromboembolic Disease continued

INTERVENTION	RATIONALE
5. Nursing Diagnosis: Risk for Bleeding related to lack of information about DVT/thrombophlebitis, its treatment, preventive measures, and the medication, warfarin sodium (Coumadin). **Goal:** Woman will understand her condition, its treatment, safety during treatment, and long-term implications.	
■ Provide information (both verbal and written supplements) about the woman's condition, its treatment regimen, the importance of compliance, and safety factors. Provide contact information that the woman can access 24/7.	■ Such discussion is essential to help the woman understand the condition, her medication, and its implications. She must have a clear understanding to be able to provide effective self-care.
■ Discuss ways of avoiding circulatory stasis such as avoiding prolonged standing, sitting, crossing legs, and wearing restrictive clothing.	■ Prolonged sitting, standing, and crossing legs should be avoided, as these activities decrease venous return.
■ Discuss safety precautions necessary while taking LMWH and warfarin sodium (Coumadin) (extra care with knives, razors, and other sharp objects; care around animals in the home that may scratch or bite; wear MedicAlert bracelet identifying that she is on anticoagulant therapy, avoiding being barefoot).	■ Anticoagulation places woman at risk of excessive bleeding and requires increased attention to safety issues that typically do not pose a significant risk. During warfarin sodium therapy, the international normalized ratio (INR) levels are monitored regularly to minimize risks.
■ Advise use of soft toothbruth and to avoid aggressive brushing.	
■ Advise to routinely inspect her body for evidence of bleeding.	
■ Advise to wear seatbelt in car.	
■ Advise to monitor menstrual flow, as it may be increased.	
■ Teach importance of compliance with warfarin sodium therapy and interactions of vitamin K with warfarin sodium, and check for interactions when starting new medications.	■ Warfarin sodium interacts with numerous medications that either increase or decrease its effectiveness.
■ Teach woman and partner to advise all healthcare providers, including dentists, that she is taking anticoagulants.	
■ If LMWH is being used at home, teach proper sterile technique for self-injection and safe disposal of syringes.	■ INR levels are monitored initially to facilitate dosage decisions. Once consistent effects are obtained, LMWH may be used without laboratory monitoring. With warfarin therapy, INR results will be monitored and dosage managed on the basis of lab results.
■ Teach importance of consistent level of vitamin K intake while on warfarin sodium and foods high in vitamin K to facilitate planning.	■ Vitamin K interacts with warfarin sodium. A consistent (balanced) intake of foods with vitamin K minimizes the problem of interaction.
■ Explain necessary follow-up testing ordered to maintain target INR.	■ Knowing details of anticipated follow-up care facilitates planning for home and child management issues.

EXPECTED OUTCOMES: Woman has health promotion knowledge as evidenced by:

- Woman verbalizes understanding of ways to avoid circulatory stasis, need to wear supportive stockings, medications dosage and side effects, and the importance of a balanced diet.
- Woman verbalizes understanding of signs and symptoms of bleeding that need to be reported to healthcare provider.

The father may be assuming multiple roles in the circumstances—household manager, parent, worker, and caregiver. Fatigue is inevitable. There may be financial concerns as a result of prolonged health care or his extended time away from work to care for the family. Many concerns will not surface until the couple returns home and fully comprehends the reality of their situation. For that reason it is valuable to provide them with an accessible resource and to plan telephone or home visit follow-up care. Signs of postpartum thrombophlebitis may not occur until after discharge from the birthing unit. Consequently, all couples must be taught about the signs and symptoms and to appreciate the importance of reporting them immediately and of not massaging the affected leg. If signs and symptoms occur after discharge, a short readmission might be required. Every effort is made in that case to allow mother, father, and newborn to remain together.

After DVT, some women continue to have leg pain, edema, and dermatitis of the affected extremity for prolonged periods caused by a residual venous abnormality and can significantly affect one's quality of life. Continuing use of compression stockings for a minimum of 1 year after diagnosis will help to prevent the complication of DVT (McCaffery & Blum, 2009).

Evaluation

Expected outcomes of nursing care include:

- The woman seeks treatment for her thrombophlebitis early and is managed successfully without further complications.
- At discharge, the woman is able to explain the purpose, dosage regimen, and necessary precautions associated with any prescribed medications, such as anticoagulants.
- The woman can discuss self-care measures and ongoing therapies (such as the use of compression stockings) that are indicated.
- The woman has bonded successfully with her newborn and is able to care for the baby effectively.

Care of the Woman with a Postpartum Psychiatric Disorder

The relationship of affective disorders to childbirth is reflected in the fact that the rate of admission to a psychiatric hospital is greater during the year after childbirth than at any other time in a woman's life.

Types of Postpartum Psychiatric Disorders

Many types of psychiatric problems may occur in the postpartum. The *Diagnostic and Statistical Manual of Mental Disorders* (American Psychiatric Association, 2000) has added a postpartum-onset specifier to the mood disorder diagnostic category of psychiatric disorders. It is proposed that postpartum psychiatric disorders be considered one diagnosable syndrome with three subclasses: (1) adjustment reaction with depressed mood, (2) postpartum major mood disorder, and (3) postpartum psychosis. The incidence, etiology, symptoms, treatment, and prognosis vary with each subclass, but the subclasses appear on a continuum from mild to severe.

Adjustment Reaction with Depressed Mood

Adjustment reaction with depressed mood is commonly known as **postpartum blues**, or as *maternal* or *baby blues.* It occurs in as many as 50% to 75% of mothers and is characterized by mild depression interspersed with happier feelings (Beck, 2008b). This adjustment reaction does not consistently affect the woman's ablity to function. Postpartum blues typically begin within 3 to 5 days after the baby's birth and are self-limiting, lasting from a few hours to 1 to 14 days. The depression is more severe in primiparas than in multiparas and seems related to the rapid alteration of estrogen, progesterone, and prolactin levels after birth, challenges of new motherhood, fatigue, and life-style adjustments. New mothers experiencing postpartum blues commonly report feeling overwhelmed, unable to cope, fatigued, anxious, irritable, and oversensitive. A key feature is episodic tearfulness and rapid mood shifts often without an identifiable reason. Not uncommonly, when asked why she is crying, this woman responds that she does not know. Cunningham et al. (2010) identifies several factors that contribute to the "blues":

- Emotional letdown that follows labor and childbirth
- Physical discomfort typical in the early postpartum
- Fatigue
- Anxiety about caring for the newborn after discharge
- Depression during pregnancy or previous depression unrelated to pregnancy
- Severe PMS (premenstrual syndrome)

Validating the existence of this phenomenon, labeling it as a real but normal adjustment reaction, and providing reassurance can offer a measure of relief. Assistance with self and infant care, rest, good nutrition, information, and family support aids recovery. Helping the new mother anticipate a transient emotional letdown after discharge is important guidance from the nurse, as is talking with her about her view of "the perfect mother." Trying to achieve that image can contribute to fatigue and exacerbate the letdown feeling. The partner should be encouraged to watch for and report signs that the new mother is not returning to a more normal mood but is instead slipping into a deeper depression or that happier times are no longer interspersed with the blues.

Postpartum Major Mood Disorder

Postpartum major mood disorder, also known as **postpartum depression (PPD)** has an overall prevalence rate of about 4.5% to 28% of postpartum women across multiple studies (Doucet, Dennis, Letourneau, et al., 2009).

Many of the symptoms of this major depression are indistinguishable from serious depression at other times in life: sadness, frequent crying, insomnia or excessive sleeping, appetite change, difficulty concentrating and making decisions, feelings of worthlessness, obsessive thoughts of inadequacy as a person and parent, lack of interest in activities that are usually associated with pleasure (including sexual relations), and lack of concern about personal appearance. Persistent anxiety further contributes to the woman's feeling of being out of control. Irritability and hostility toward others, including the newborn, may be evident. Women participating in Beck's qualitative research on postpartum depression described a sense of living their daily life in a sort of fog, from which they believed they would never emerge. Once they improved, they often grieved over the time lost with their newborns while in this "fog." The duration of symptoms varies but as many as half continue to be symptomatic at 6 months or longer. Delayed treatment of major depression is associated with a longer duration.

Risk factors for postpartum depression include the following:

- Primiparity
- Ambivalence about maintaining the pregnancy
- Occurrence of postpartum blues
- History of postpartum depression or bipolar illness (recurrence rates are ≥20%)
- Lack of social support
- Lack of a stable and supportive relationship with parents (especially her father, as a child) or partner

- The woman's dissatisfaction with herself, including body image problems and eating disorders
- Poverty
- Depression during pregnancy
- Complications of delivery
- Loss of newborn
- Age (adolescence increases risk)
- Domestic violence

Although it may occur at any time during the first year postpartum, the greatest risk occurs within the first 4 weeks after childbirth. Surprisingly, it is not always associated with depression during pregnancy. Postpartum depression is considered to have a multifactorial cause. When depressive symptoms occur, physical causes, such as thyroid disease, anemia, or drug abuse, are ruled out through clinical and laboratory exams.

Because postpartum depression is complicated to detect when providers wait for the woman to self report or the family to become concerned enough to seek help, routine screening by those providers in contact with this population is imperative. For women considered to be at high risk, telephone follow-up after delivery or an earlier clinic appointment than 6 weeks may be helpful. Nurses in the pediatrician's office assisting with well-child visits have an excellent opportunity to screen women for PPD (Sheeder, Kabin, & Stafford, 2009). Community health nurses who are seeing other members of the family or parish nurses who know new mothers in their congregation can observe for evidence of depression. The Beck Depression Inventory or the Edinburg Postnatal Depression Scale (EPDS) are useful and validated for screening for postpartum depression. For the EPDS, a score of greater than 12 is indicative of depression.

The woman's safety, and that of her child(ren), is a priority. Inquiring about suicidal ideas and assessment for thoughts and feelings toward the infant, hallucinations and delusions, and impulsiveness that might put the infant and siblings at risk is critical. Women with postpartum depression are at risk for suicide, most prominently as they enter or exit the deeply depressed state. In a deep depression, the woman is unlikely to be able to plan and carry out suicide. For that reason, signs of improvement in depression should be celebrated with some caution, and continued observation is necessary. Whereas the woman with postpartum psychosis may attempt suicide because of illogical thought processes, delusions, and hallucinations, the woman with major depression attempts suicide because her suffering is so great that dying seems a more favorable option than continuing to live in such pain. She may also attempt suicide to save her newborn from some perceived or real threat—including the threat that she herself might cause harm. The risk of suicide is greater in those who have attempted suicide previously, have a specific plan, and can access the means or weapon identified within the plan. The more specific the plan, the greater is the probability of an attempt.

The woman and her family need information about the illness and its expected course, including the risk of recurrence, as well as comprehensive information about the treatment plan. They need opprtunities to clarify misconceptions about mental illness and to have answers to questions. Referral to local or online support groups may be helpful.

The expected outcomes for mild to moderate depression treated with antidepressants and psychotherapy are good; recurrence rates are increased after each episode of depression. The serotonin reuptake inhibitors (SSRIs) are used most often. Their most frequently occurring side effects include headache, nausea, diarrhea, sleep disruption, anxiety, and sexual dysfunction (Gjerdingen, Katon, & Rich, 2008). The second-line antidepressant drugs are the tricyclics. They cause dry mouth, constipation, orthostatic hypotension, and weight gain. Monoamine oxidase inhibitors (MAOIs) are rarely used in the treatment of PPD because these drugs have a high profile of interacting with other medications. Women typically continue antidepressants for 1 year after symptoms abate.

All current antidepressant agents are excreted into breast milk. Zoloft, Lustral, Paxil, Seroxat, and Deroxat are considered first-line agents. Because of its prolonged half-life, fluoxetine (Prozac) is not recommended for nursing mothers. Physicians will wish to educate their breastfeeding postpartum patients who need antidepressants about the different alternatives and help them to balance the risks and benefits with the safety profiles. The final decision about continuing to breastfeed and to take antidepressants is the informed woman's. To help in making the decision, she and her significant other need to be helped to consider how she will respond without pharmacologic therapy and how unmedicated depression will affect the maternal-infant relationship and the infant's well-being and development. An invaluable online resource for prescribers with current information on drug safety and toxic effects during pregnancy and lactation is the LacMed Database.

Electroconvulsive therapy (ECT) is used for quicker treatment of those who have severe depression or mania, are unresponsive to other treatment, or are at high risk of suicide. Antidepressants may take 2 to 3 weeks to become effective. ECT results often become noticeable within 1 week (Townsend, 2009).

Post-Traumatic Stress Disorder

Many women envision their own labor and delivery unfolding in a particular way and may experience angst if their labor reality fails to match their expectations. Labor and birth that go awry, including those associated with complications, may cause **post-traumatic stress disorder (PTSD)** (also called *post-traumatic stress syndrome (PTSS),* which the APA's *Diagnostic and Statistical Manual of Mental Disorders*—DSM-IV (2000, p. 463) describes as "exposure to an extreme traumatic event involving direct personal experience of an event that involves actual or threatened death or serious injury . . . a person's response to the event must involve intense fear, helplessness, or horror." These extreme traumatic situations are typically ones outside the realm of usual human experience—situations that would be distressing for anyone.

At particular risk for PTSD are women who are especially anxious or fearful about childbirth, have low coping capacity, and/or prior psychiatric histories (Tham, Christensson, & Ryding, 2007). For the woman, the facts of the labor and birth have become distorted, perhaps because of pain or change in consciousness related to medications she received. Perhaps she underwent an emergency cesarean delivery or her baby had a serious physical anomaly. Perhaps her labor coach could not make the trip to the hospital in time for the birth or she experienced a postpartum hemorrhage. Her perceptions of what occurred and the actions of those involved frequently are far different from the reality, perhaps even seeming delusional.

Clinical features of PTSD include feeling numb, seeming dazed and unaware of her environment, intrusive thoughts and flashbacks to the threatening event, difficulty thinking, difficulty sleeping, irritability, and avoidance of others and reminders of the traumatic event. Tachycardia, hyperventilation, and nausea may occur (Stone, 2009). These signs and symptoms may not be evident until after the woman has left the birth setting. Distress associated with the original traumatic event can recur at anniversaries, and some women are hesitant to consider future pregnancies because of this birth trauma (Beck, 2008a).

Based on her qualitative research and the work of others related to traumatic birth experiences, Beck (2008a, p. 8) suggests the following implications for nursing care: (1) Whenever possible, intervene to prevent traumatic birth experiences; (2) provide technically competent, concerned care for the woman and family; (3) assess for anxiety and fears on admission to labor and provide information to dispel myths; (4) debrief the woman and family after a stressful traumatic childbirth experience ; and (5) visit the woman during her hospitalization to assess for evidence of signs of early trauma. Women should be asked to tell their birth story, to compare and contrast the actual experience with their birth plan or prior visions of the special day, and to tell what went well for them and what part, if any, of the experience was unexpected, troublesome, disappointing, or distressing.

Nurses who work in childbirth settings should appreciate that a woman they are admitting at any point in time may have previously had a traumatic birth. That woman will need sensitive caregivers who provide additional support and information and follow the birth plan to the extent possible. Support for new parents and helpful information is available online from the Trauma and Birth Stress (TABS) charitable trust located in New Zealand.

Postpartum Psychosis

Postpartum psychosis, which has an incidence of 1 to 2/1000, usually becomes evident within the first 1 to 4 weeks after childbirth (Sit, Rothschild, & Wisner, 2006). Although relatively rare, this disorder gains considerable national attention in the media and is considered an emergency, given the risk of infanticide or suicide, especially in teens. Symptoms include agitation, hyperactivity, insomnia, mood lability, confusion, irrational thinking and behaviors, difficulty remembering or concentrating, and poor judgment, as well as delusions and hallucinations, which tend to be related to the infant. Clinical features progress rapidly and include the following (Parry, 2007):

- Sleep disturbances—the woman is unable to sleep, even when her infant is sleeping
- Depersonalization—seeming unaware of or distant from the immediate environment and individuals within it
- Confusion; irrational or disorganized thinking; bizarre behaviors; delusions; hallucinations
- Psychomotor disturbances—stupor or agitated state sometimes with rapid and incoherent speech

Risk factors include (1) previous puerperal psychosis; (2) history of bipolar (manic-depressive) disorder; (3) prenatal stressors, such as lack of social support, lack of a partner, and low socioeconomic status; (4) obsessive personality; and (5) a family history of a mood disorder. There is some question among experts that postpartum psychosis represents a variant of bipolar disorder timed to coincide with the hormonal changes after childbirth, since the majority meet the criteria for a mood disorder and about half of women experience manic behavior (Sit et al., 2006).

The psychotic woman experiences delusions and/or visual, auditory, or tactile hallucinations. In some women, these symptoms support her perceptions that the infant should not be allowed to live or that she should commit suicide. For example, she may believe that her newborn is evil, some form of "changeling," and will harm her or others, or she may believe that her newborn would be "better off dead" than living in such an evil world. She may contemplate suicide because she believes that her child would be better off without a mother than with her as such a "terrible, crazy mother." Illogical thinking or evidence of bonding difficulties may serve as cues to infanticide and suicide risk; however, this assessment is often challenging because of periods of lucidity seen in some psychotic women. Nurses in various clinical settings who come in contact with this woman may note that the child has been neglected or the woman is practicing unsafe behaviors because of the woman's cognitive impairment. For example, a pediatric nurse noticed that one of her women placed the newborn across the room at the edge of the narrow exam table while she paced back and forth across the room, muttering to herself, appearing not to notice the baby. This same woman came to her appointment during heavy snow with both her infant and herself underdressed for warmth.

Provisions for safety of the woman and infant are paramount. This woman needs immediate referral to psychiatric care, usually requiring admission to an inpatient psychiatic hospital. Continued assessment of her symptomatology, safety, and functional capacity is a major nursing role in the setting. An initial history, physical examination, and lab work will help to rule out an organic cause of acute psychosis. If the woman has a fever, a urine culture should be performed, and if drug use is suspected, a urinary drug screen is ordered. A CT or MRI may be ordered if the neurologic exam increases concern about a stroke (Sit et al., 2006).

Treatment for postpartum psychosis is directed at the specific type of psychotic symptoms displayed, and may include antidepressants and a mood stabilizer such as lithium, valproic acid, or carbamazepine, combined with antipsychotics. Electroconvulsive therapy (ECT) is another treatment option if rapid stabilization is required. Psychotherapy and social support are part of the management plan as well.

A dilemma exists for breastfeeding women for whom lithium or psychotropic medication is being considered. Since infants have immature hepatic and renal systems and a more permeable blood-brain barrier, they may be vulnerable to side effects, especially when younger than 2 months of age, premature, or exposed to these medications in utero. With the exception of lithium (which is contraindicated with breastfeeding), the amount of psychotropic drugs excreted into breast milk appears to be modest and not to compromise growth and development (Eberhard-Gran, Eskild, & Opjordsmoen, 2006). Parents of an infant need to be educated to consider these factors in making a decision about the use of psychotropic medications: (1) severity of symptoms and their effect on the infant if medications are not used; (2) benefits of breastfeeding to the baby; (3) potential risks to the baby if psychotropics are used; and (4) preferences of the woman. If psychotropics are prescribed, the lowest dose possible of monotherapy should be used and the infant should be monitored carefully by a pediatrician for difficulty being aroused from sleep, rigidity, tremors, irritability, poor hydration, and poor feeding with failure to gain weight (Sit et al., 2006).

Clinical Therapy

Women with a history of postpartum psychosis or depression or other risk factors should be referred to a mental health professional for counseling and biweekly visits between the second and sixth week postpartum for evaluation. Treatment for postpartum depression includes the following:

- Antidepression medications, usually the selective serotonin reuptake inhibitors. The woman and her partner should be reminded that antidepressants may take several weeks to have an effect.
- Individual or group psychotherapy and cognitive behavioral therapy. These are common treatment measures for both disorders; however, specific therapies used may vary. Cognitive behavioral therapy (CBT)—time limited, problem-focused therapy intended to reduce emotional distress by modifying maladaptive beliefs, assumptions, attitudes, and behaviors. With help, depressed women examine the factors that contribute to depression and attempt to better understand them in an effort to change what is dysfunctional. Interpersonal psychotherapy (IPT)—Depression generally has an interpersonal component, in that it affects one's roles and relationships. Role transitions, conflicts, disputes, loss, and grief are often explored. The first few sessions involve assessment of interpersonal issues that will be the therapy's focus. Maintenance therapy with a psychiatrist, psychologist, or social worker once monthly often follows the short-term phase.
- Psychoeducation (family therapy)—educating the woman and her family about her mental illness and the treatment regime and helpful ways of coping—will be part of the treatment plan.
- Practical assistance with child care and other demands of daily life.

Outpatient treatment may continue after discharge from the hospital. With a support group of postpartum women and their partners, a couple may feel consolation that they are not alone in their experience. Moreover, the support group provides a forum for gaining information about postpartum depression, learning stress-reduction measures, and experiencing renewed self-esteem and support. The most effective support groups provide for safe child care to facilitate attendance. If a support group is not available locally, the woman and her family may be encouraged to contact Depression After Delivery (DAD), or Postpartum Support International, a national Web-based support network. The Mills Depression and Anxiety Symptom-Feeling Checklist focuses on symptoms and feelings the postpartum woman has experienced over the previous 2-week interval. The woman is advised to contact her healthcare provider immediately if she marks the symptoms and feelings highlighted in red—those that relate to harm to herself or the infant. The checklist is not intended to be used for diagnosis but to help the woman put her feelings into context.

NURSING CARE MANAGEMENT

Nursing Assessment and Diagnosis

Assessment for factors predisposing a woman to postpartum depression or psychosis should begin prenatally. Questions designed to detect problems can be included as part of the routine prenatal history interview or questionnaire. Women with a personal or family history of psychiatric disease, particularly postpartum depression or psychosis, need prenatal instructions on the signs and symptoms of depression and may need additional emotional support. Ideally the assessment should be completed each trimester to update a pregnant woman's risk status (Beck, 2002). If the assessment has not been done previously, the nurse assesses the woman for predisposing factors during her labor and postpartum stay. Answers to open-ended questions can be telling: What has been your greatest surprise about motherhood? Your greatest disappointment? Biggest concern? Biggest challenge? Or how does being a mother compare to what you had envisioned?

New mothers and their families expect a challenging adjustment period after bringing home a new baby; they may not realize that their experiences are outside the norm. There is general anticipation that motherhood will be a happy occasion; a woman may not be able to admit her unhappiness out of shame or embarassment that she is somehow different as a mother. The woman might be concerned that telling someone, even a professional, about her symptoms makes her sound "crazy" and that her baby might be taken away (Doucet et al., 2009). One woman reported that she wanted help and sensed she needed it, but did not know which doctor to call. "I had only been home for 3 weeks and my postpartum clinic visit was 3 weeks away when I started feeling so desperate. Should I call my OB? The pediatrician had seen the baby in the hospital nursery but we hadn't visited him yet and, besides, I'm not his patient—I'm an adult. My family doctor doesn't see pregnancy-related problems, so who do I call?"

Several depression scales are available for assessing postpartum depression. The routine use of a screening tool in a matter-of-fact approach significantly increases the diagnosis because the woman does not feel singled out. The Edinburgh Postnatal Depression Scale (Table 39-8) is likely the most widely used screening tool for postpartum depression in large populations of women. Mothers who score above 12 on the Edinburgh Postnatal Depression Scale are likely to be suffering from postpartum depression. Beck's (2002) revised Postpartum Depression Predictors Inventory (PDPI-Revised) tool is a practical and simple screening checklist for use during routine care with all postpartal women to identify those who might be experiencing postpar-

TABLE 39-8 Edinburgh Postnatal Depression Scale

In the past 7 days:

1. I have been able to laugh and see the funny side of things.
As much as I always could
Not quite so much now
Definitely not so much now
Not at all

2. I have looked forward with enjoyment of things.
As much as I ever did
Rather less than I used to
Definitely less than I used to
Hardly at all

***3. I have blamed myself unnecessarily when things went wrong.**
Yes, most of the time
Yes, some of the time
Not very often
No, never

4. I have been anxious or worried for no good reason.
No, not at all
Hardly ever
Yes, sometimes
Yes, very often

***5. I have felt scared or panicky for no very good reason.**
Yes, quite a lot
Yes, sometimes
No, not much
No, not at all

***6. Things have been getting on top of me.**
Yes, most of the time I haven't been able to cope at all
Yes, sometimes I haven't been coping as well as usual
No, I have been coping quite well
No, I have been coping as well as ever

***7. I have been so unhappy that I have had difficulty sleeping.**
Yes, most of the time
Yes, sometimes
Not very often
No, not at all

***8. I have felt sad or miserable.**
Yes, most of the time
Yes, quite often
Not very often
No, not at all

***9. I have been so unhappy that I have been crying.**
Yes, most of the time
Yes, quite often
Only occasionally
No, never

***10. The thought of harming myself has occurred to me.**
Yes, quite often
Sometimes
Hardly ever
Never

Note: Response categories are scored 0, 1, 2, and 3 according to increased severity of the symptoms. Items marked with an asterisk* are reverse scored (3, 2, 1, 0). The total score is calculated by adding together the scores for each of the 10 items. A score above the threshold of 12–13 out of 30 indicates with 86% sensitivity that the woman is suffering from postpartum depression.
Source: Cox, J. L., Holden, J. M., & Sagovsky, R. (1987). Detection of postnatal depression: Development of the 10-item Edinburgh Postnatal Depression Scale. British Journal of Psychiatry, 150, *782–786. Users may reproduce the scale without further permission provided they respect copyright by quoting the names of the authors, the title, and the source of the paper in all reproduced copies.*

tum depression so that early management might be initiated (Table 39-9). No matter what approach the nurse uses to assess for postpartum depression, enabling the woman's voice to be heard about her feelings of maternal role transition and how she is adjusting in this vulnerable time is of inestimable value. Listening to her story provides a critical emic (insider's) view of her circumstances as opposed to an etic (outsider's) view.

In providing daily care, the nurse observes the woman for objective signs of depression—anxiety, irritability, poor concentration, forgetfulness, sleeping difficulties, appetite change, fatigue, and tearfulness—and listens for statements indicating feelings of failure and self-accusation. Severity and duration of symptoms should be noted. Behavior and verbalization that are bizarre or seem to indicate a potential for violence against herself or others, including the infant, are reported as soon as possible for further evaluation. The nurse needs to be aware that many normal physiologic changes of the puerperium are similar to symptoms of depression (lack of sexual interest, indecisiveness, appetite change, sleep disturbance, and fatigue). It is essential that observations be as specific and as objective as possible and that they be carefully documented.

Beck and Indman (2005) found that anxiety was a prominent feature of illness for some women and suggested that women be assessed for their level of anxiety, particularly regarding infant care. Because of the strong association of interrupted sleep and postpartum depression and the finding that severe fatigue was an excellent predictor of postpartum depression (Corwin, Brownstead, Barton, et al., 2005), assessing fatigue level at 2 weeks postpartum by telephone may be helpful in predicting depression risk early. Restorative sleep improves one's ability to cope and make decisions, thereby producing a sense of better self-control.

A central challenge for nursing is identifying women at risk of suicide. Like others with psychologic disorders, the postpartum woman is likely ambivalent about suicide, and may be "rescuable" if suicide ideation is assessed and timely action follows. Assessment of suicide risk reflects the standard of care; contrary to myth, asking a depressed woman about suicidal thoughts does not increase her risk, but it may save her life. Introducing the issue of suicide can be as simple as saying something like, "I'm concerned about the amount of emotional pain you're feeling, and I'm wondering whether you've ever thought of hurting yourself." Ambivalence about suicide is likely to make the woman answer candidly. A suicide prevention contract may be established with the woman to exact an agreement that she will seek help immediately if she begins to consider self-harm. For example, the nurse might say, "Promise me that should you begin to feel as if you are going to hurt yourself, you will telephone me or the hotline immediately—that you will not act without talking to someone." Because of the hope this offers, the woman is likely to respond by seeking help; she does not want to renege on a promise she made to a nurse who has shown such caring for her.

If a woman admits that she has thought of hurting herself, assessment of the risk that she will follow through is imperative. The mnemonic **SAL** is useful for risk assessment: Is there a **S**pecific plan with a designated time? Is there an **A**ccessible weapon or other means? How **L**ethal is the method identified

TABLE 39-9 Postpartum Depression Predictors Inventory (PDPI)—Revised and Guide Questions for Its Use

During Pregnancy	**Check One**	**Yes**	**No**
Marital Status			
1. Single	0		
2. Married/cohabitating	0		
3. Separated	0		
4. Divorced	0		
5. Widowed	0		
6. Partnered	0		
Socioeconomic Status			
Low	0		
Middle	0		
High	0		
Self-Esteem			
Do you feel good about yourself as a person?		0	0
Do you feel worthwhile?		0	0
Do you feel you have a number of good qualities as a person?		0	0
Prenatal Depression			
1. Have you felt depressed during your pregnancy?		0	0
If yes, when and how long have you been feeling this way?			
If yes, how mild or severe would you consider your depression?			
Prenatal Anxiety			
Have you been feeling anxious during your pregnancy?		0	0
If yes, how long have you been feeling this way?			
Unplanned/Unwanted Pregnancy			
Was the pregnancy planned?		0	0
Is the pregnancy unwanted?		0	0
History of Previous Depression			
1. Before this pregnancy, have you ever been depressed?		0	0
If yes, when did you experience this depression?			
If yes, have you been under a physician's care for this past depression?		0	0
If yes, did the physician prescribe any medication for your depression?		0	0
Social Support			
1. Do you feel you receive adequate emotional support from your partner?		0	0
2. Do you feel you receive adequate instrumental support from your partner (e.g., help with household chores or babysitting)?		0	0
3. Do you feel you can rely on your partner when you need help?		0	0
4. Do you feel you can confide in your partner? (repeat same questions for family and again for friends)		0	0
Marital Satisfaction			
1. Are you satisfied with your marriage (or living arrangement)?		0	0
2. Are you currently experiencing any marital problems?		0	0
3. Are things going well between you and your partner?		0	0
Life Stress			
1. Are you currently experiencing any stressful events in your life such as:			
Financial problems		0	0
Marital problems		0	0
Death in the family		0	0
Serious illness in the family		0	0
Moving		0	0
Unemployment		0	0
Job change		0	0
After Delivery, Add the Following Items			
Child Care Stress			
1. Is your infant experiencing any health problems?		0	0
2. Are you having problems with your baby feeding?		0	0
3. Are you having problems with your baby sleeping?		0	0
Infant Temperament			
1. Would you consider your baby irritable or fussy?		0	0
2. Does your baby cry a lot?		0	0
3. Is your baby difficult to console or soothe?		0	0
Maternity Blues			
1. Did you experience a brief period of tearfulness and mood swings during the 1st week after delivery?		0	0
Comments:			

Source: Used with permission from AWHONN. Beck, C. T. (2002). Revision of the postpartum predictors inventory. JOGNN: Journal of Obstetric, Gynecologic, & Neonatal Nursing, 31(4), 394–402. (Table 2 on PDPI, pp. 399–400). Washington, DC: Author.

RESEARCH EVIDENCE IN PRACTICE — Screening for Postpartum Depression

CLINICAL QUESTION

What is the most appropriate method to screen for postpartum depression?

RESEARCH EVIDENCE

Postpartum depression (PPD) occurs in approximately 10% to 20% of mothers and is the most common serious postpartum disorder. PPD can occur at any time in the first year after birth, but usually starts within the first 4 weeks. It can be a debilitating disease that affects the whole family, and may have long-term effects on the child. Despite the potential for negative consequences, rates of diagnosis and treatment are low because of lack of recognition by healthcare providers or an underestimation of its impact.

Symptoms of PPD are severe and may be long-lasting, requiring treatment. However, these symptoms may be subtle and are often confused with other medical or psychologic conditions. Use of a sensitive, valid screening tool can help identify mothers who are exhibiting a range of symptoms that represent PPD.

The most thoroughly researched and recognized screening tool for PPD is the Edinburgh Postnatal Depression Scale (EPDS). This screening tool is a self-report that is quick, easy, and takes only 5 minutes or less. It consists of 10 questions with 4 possible responses, and yields a summary score that can be interpreted to determine the presence of PPD. An equally valid tool is the Postpartum Depression Screening Scale (PDSS) that is more sensitive than the EPDS but requires responses to 35 items. Both screening tools have been administered via the Internet, which was found to be an effective way to solicit participation. The relative anonymity of the Internet screening process actually resulted in a higher level of participation than in-person administration, with larger numbers of ethnic minority women responding via the Internet.

There are no antenatal or prenatal tools that adequately predict postpartum depression. Therefore, all women should be screened before they are discharged from the hospital and screening should continue throughout the first year after birth.

WHAT QUESTIONS REMAIN UNANSWERED?

Is Internet administration of PPD screening tools comparable to in-person completion in terms of accurate diagnosis of postpartum depression?

WHAT IS BEST PRACTICE?

Screening for postpartum depression should be done in the first postpartum follow-up after birth. Of the screening tools available, the EPDS is the quickest and easiest to use, and the PDSS is the most sensitive. Administering the screening tool in person or via the Internet are both effective in identifying women who have PPD.

CRITICAL THINKING

What are ways that the nurse can encourage mothers to complete screening tools for depression during the postpartum period?

References

Le, H., Perry, D., & Sheng, X. 2009. Using the internet to screen for postpartum depression. *Maternal and Child Health Journal, 13*(2), 213–221.

Neiman, S., Carter, S., VanSell, S., & Kindred, C. 2010. Best practice guidelines for the nurse practitioner regarding screening, prevention, and management of postpartum depression. *Critical Care Nurse Quarterly, 33*(3), 212–218.

Schumacher, M., & Zubaran, C. 2008. Screening tools for postpartum depression: Validity and cultural dimensions. *International Journal of Psychiatric Nursing Research, 14*(1), 1752–1765.

in the plan? A specific plan that identifies a highly lethal method that is immediately accessible is evidence of very high risk of suicide. Immediate intervention is critical; emergency psychiatric hospitalization is likely necessary. Those considered a threat to themselves or others may be admitted to involuntary hospitalization for a minimum of 48 hours until further evaluation is complete.

Family members of the depressed woman should also be alert to signals that she may be intent on self-harm; they must be advised that threats should always be taken seriously. Clues to suicide that might be noted by family are comments such as "I don't deserve to live," "Life is no longer worth living," or "You won't have to worry about me for long." Someone who is considering suicide may also telephone or write family or friends to say good-bye or give away prized possessions. Family members should be told to be especially vigilant for suicide when the woman seems to be feeling better.

Possible nursing diagnoses that may apply to a woman with a postpartum psychiatric disorder include the following:

- ***Ineffective Coping*** related to postpartum depression
- ***Risk for Impaired Parenting*** related to postpartum mental illness
- ***Self-Directed Violence*** against self (suicide), newborn, and other children related to depression.

Nursing Plan and Implementation

Nurses working in antepartum settings or teaching childbirth classes play indispensable roles in helping prospective parents appreciate the lifestyle changes and role demands associated with parenthood. Offering realistic information and anticipatory guidance and debunking myths about the perfect mother or perfect newborn may help prevent postpartum depression. Social support teaching guides are available for nurses to help postpartum women explore their needs for postpartum support.

The nurse should alert the mother, partner, and other family members to the possibility of postpartum blues in the early days after birth and reassure them of the short-term nature of the condition. Symptoms of postpartum depression should be described and the mother encouraged to call her healthcare provider if symptoms become severe, if they fail to subside quickly, or if at any time she feels she is unable to function. Encouraging the mother to plan how she will manage at home and providing concrete suggestions on how to cope will aid in her adjustment to motherhood. Table 39-10 provides suggestions for the mother that serve as primary prevention for postpartum depression.

Information, emotional support, and assistance in providing or obtaining care for the infant may be needed. The nurse can

TABLE 39-10 Primary Prevention Strategies for Postpartum Depression

1. Celebrate childbirth but appreciate that it is a life-changing transition that can be stressful—at times it can seem overwhelming. Share your feelings with each other and/or others.
2. Consider keeping a journal where you write down feelings. Not only is it emotionally cathartic, it provides a great memory book.
3. Appreciate that you do not have to know everything to be a good parent—it is okay to seek advice during this transition.
4. Connect to others who are parents—use them as a support and information network.
5. Set a daily schedule and follow it even if you do not feel like it. Structuring activity helps counteract inertia that comes with feeling sad or unsettled.
6. Prioritize daily tasks. Decide what must be done and what can wait. Try to get one major thing done every day. Remember, you do not always have to look like a magazine fashion model.
7. Remember that you do not have to entertain or care for everyone who drops by. Doing something for someone else, however, often tends to make you feel better.
8. If someone volunteers to help you with tasks or baby care, take them up on it. While your volunteer is in action, do something pleasurable or get some rest.
9. Maintain outside interests. Plan some time every day—even if it's just 15 minutes—to do something exclusively for "you" that is pleasurable.
10. Eat a healthful diet. Limit alcohol. Quit smoking. Get some exercise. (All of these can positively affect the immune system.)
11. Get as much sleep as possible. Rest whenever you can, such as when the baby is napping. If you have other young children, bring them onto your bed to read or play quietly while you lie down.
12. Limit major changes (moves, job changes, etc.) the first year insofar as possible.
13. Spend time with others.
14. If things get overwhelming, and you feel yourself slipping into depression, reach out to someone for help.
15. Attend a postpartum support group if one is available. Consider also an international program.

Source: Data from Postpartum Support International (PSI).

assist family members by identifying community resources and making referrals to public health nursing services and social services. Postpartum follow-up is especially important, as well as visits from a psychiatric home-health nurse.

Postpartum Support

Community-Based Nursing Care

Home visits, especially for early discharge families, are invaluable in fostering positive adjustments for the new family constellation. Telephone follow-up at 2 to 3 weeks postpartum to ask whether the mother is experiencing difficulties is also helpful. Monitoring for signs of depression or performing brief screening at well-child follow-ups also can be valuable for early identification and timely intervention.

In all women, the presence of three symptoms on 1 day or one symptom for 3 days may signal serious postpartum depression and requires immediate referral to a mental health professional. Immediate referral should also be made if rejection of the infant or threatened or actual aggression against the infant has occurred. In such cases, the newborn is never left unattended with the mother. Depression does appear to interfere with optimal mothering; there is less interaction between mother and child, more mood and cognitive development problems, and more visits to the doctor in these children (Beck, 2002). A diagnosis of postpartum depression or other psychiatric disorder will pose major problems for the family, especially the father. The symptoms of these disorders are difficult to witness and may be harder to understand than physical problems such as hemorrhage or infection. The father may feel hurt by his partner's hostility and may worry that she is becoming insane, or be baffled by her mood swings and lack of concern about herself, the newborn, or household responsibilities. He may be troubled by their lack of intimacy or deteriorating communication. Certainly, he has cause for concern about how the newborn and any other children are being affected. There may be very real practical matters to handle—running the household; managing the children, including the totally dependent newborn; and caring for the mother—added to his usual routines and work responsibilities. It is not surprising that even in the most supportive families, relationships may suffer in response to these circumstances. It is often a family member who in desperation makes contact with the healthcare agency. This is especially difficult when the mother is reluctant to admit she is suffering emotional difficulty or is too ill to recognize her own needs. The integration of the newborn into the family and care of the newborn and other children can be further compromised by co-occurrent postpartum depression in fathers. With both parents having depressive symptomatology, the infant and other children are further at risk.

Evaluation

Expected outcomes of nursing care include the following:

- The woman's signs of depression are identified and she receives therapy quickly.
- The newborn is cared for effectively by the father or another support person until the mother is able to provide care.
- The mother and newborn will remain safe.
- The newborn is integrated into the family.

FOCUS YOUR STUDY

- Nursing assessment and intervention play a large role in preventing postpartum complications.
- The main causes of early postpartum hemorrhage are uterine atony, lacerations of the vagina and cervix, and retained placental fragments. Late postpartum hemorrhage most often originates from retained placental fragments and, though not usually as catastrophic as early hemorrhage, may require readmission.
- The most common postpartum infection is metritis, which is limited to the uterine cavity.
- A postpartum woman is at increased risk for developing urinary tract problems because of normal postpartum diuresis, increased bladder capacity, decreased bladder sensitivity from stretching or trauma, and possibly inhibited neural control of the bladder following the use of anesthetic agents.
- Mastitis is an inflammation of the breast often caused by *Staphylococcus aureus, Escherichia coli,* and *Streptococcus* species. Mastitis is seen primarily in breastfeeding women. Symptoms seldom occur before the second to fourth postpartal week. Continuation of breastfeeding is recommended as part of the treatment plan.
- Thromboembolic disease originating in the veins of the leg, thigh, or pelvis may occur antepartally or postpartally and carries with it the potential for creating a life-threatening pulmonary embolus.
- Although many different types of psychiatric problems may be encountered in the postpartum period, postpartum blues is the most common. Postpartum blues episodes occur frequently in the week after birth, are associated with hormonal fluctuations, and are typically transient.
- Risk factors for postpartum depression should be screened for during each trimester of pregnancy and during the immediate postpartum period. Nurses should be alert to the risk of suicide and infanticide in cases of severe postpartum depression or psychosis.
- Telephone calls and home visits are effective measures for extending comprehensive care into the home setting of the postpartum family at risk. Support groups in which child care is available also can be an invaluable community service by professional nurses.

CRITICAL THINKING IN ACTION

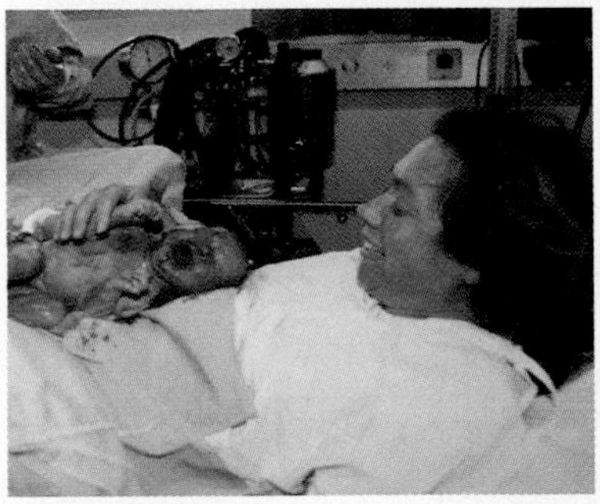

Betty Jones, a 32-year-old G4 P2012, is admitted to the postpartum unit after a precipitous birth of a preterm (35 weeks' gestation) 4-pound baby girl followed by a postpartum tubal ligation. Betty's vital signs and postpartum assessment are within normal limits. She has an abdominal dressing that is dry and intact and she is able to void. Her IV with 10 units of Pitocin is infusing well in her lower left arm. She admits to 3 on a pain scale of 10. Betty admits to active use of crack cocaine throughout her pregnancy, and smoked it most recently 5 hours before she gave birth. She is HIV positive with a CD_4 count of 726 cells/mm^3 and was treated with zidovudine during the pregnancy, labor, and birth. She also has a history of genital herpes and had been treated for chlamydia during the pregnancy. Her infant has been admitted to the special care nursery because of her preterm status. Betty anticipates her baby will be taken into foster care when discharged from the nursery. Wishing to establish as much of a relationship with her infant as possible before that happens, she asks if she can breastfeed the baby while she is in the hospital.

1. What is your response to Betty's request to breastfeed her infant?
2. Over the course of the first postpartum day, Betty appears lethargic and spends most of her time sleeping. After her evening visitors leave, you observe that she is highly energetic and excitable. Would urine testing be useful to help determine if Betty has used cocaine this evening?
3. Discuss supportive nursing care for infants born of HIV-positive mothers.
4. Betty wishes for an early discharge from the hospital. What physical criteria must be met before leaving the hospital?
5. Discuss when she should contact her physician/CNM after her discharge.

See www.nursing.pearsonhighered.com for possible responses.

REFERENCES

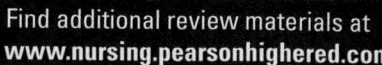

Academy of Breastfeeding Medicine (ABM). (2008). Protocol #4: ABM Clinical Protocol #4 Mastitis, Revision, May 2008. *Breastfeeding Medicine, 3*(3), 177–180. doi:10.1089/bfm.2008.9993

American Academy of Pediatrics (AAP) Committee on Fetus and Newborn & American College of Obstetricians and Gynecologists (ACOG) Committee on Obstetrics. (2007). *Guidelines for perinatal care* (6th ed.). Evanston, IL: Author.

American College of Obstetrics & Gynecology. (2006). *Postpartum hemorrhage* Practice Bulletin No. 76. *Obstetrics & Gynecology, 108*(4), 1039–1046.

American Psychiatric Association (APA). (2000). *Diagnostic and statistical manual of mental disorders: DSM-IV-TR* (4th ed.). Washington, DC: Author.

Anderson, J. M., & Etches, D. (2007). Prevention and management of postpartum hemorrhage. *American Family Physician, 75*(6), 875–882.

Beck, C. T. (2002). Revision of the postpartum depression predictors inventory. *JOGNN: Journal of Obstetric, Gynecologic, & Neonatal Nursing, 31*(4), 394–402.

Beck, C. T. (2008a). *Postpartum mood and anxiety disorders: Case studies, research, and nursing care* (2nd ed.). Washington, DC: AWHONN.

Beck, C. T. (2008b). State of the science on postpartum depression: What nurse researchers have contributed. *MCN: American Journal of Maternal Child Nursing, 33*(3), 151–156. doi:10.1097/01.NMC.0000313421.97236.cf

Beck, C. T., & Indman, P. (2005). The many faces of postpartum depression. *JOGNN: Journal of Obstetric, Gynecologic, & Neonatal Nursing, 34*(5), 569–576.

Burtelow, M., Riley, E., Druzin, M., Fontaine, M., Ville, M., & Goodnough, L. T. (2007). How we treat: Management and life-threatening postpartum hemorrhage with standardized massive transfusion protocol. *Transfusion, 47,* 1564–1572. doi:10.1111/j.1537-2995.2007.01404.x

Catanzarite, V., Almyrde, K., & Bombard, A. (2007, September). Grand Rounds: OB Team Stat: Developing a better L&D rapid response team. *Contemporary Obstetrics & Gynecology, 52*(9), 52–54, 56, 57.

Corwin, E. J., Brownstead, J., Barton, N., Heckard, S., & Merin, K. (2005). The impact of fatigue on the development of postpartum depression. *JOGNN: Journal of Obstetric, Gynecologic, & Neonatal Nursing, 34*(5), 577–586.

Cunningham, F. G., Leveno, K. J., Bloom, S. L., Hauth, J. C., Rouse, D. J., & Spong, C. Y. (2010). *Williams obstetrics* (23rd ed.). New York, NY: McGraw-Hill.

Davies, J. K., & Gibbs, R. (2008). Obstetric and perinatal infections. In R. S. Gibbs, B. Y. Karlan, A. F. Haney, & I. Nygaard, *Danforth's Obstetrics & Gynecology* (10th ed. pp. 340–364). Philadelphia, PA: Lippincott Williams & Wilkins.

Diepenbrock, N. H. (2008). *Quick reference to critical care.* Philadelphia, PA: Lippincott Williams & Wilkins.

Doucet, S., Dennis, C. L., Letourneau, N., & Blackmore, E. R. (2009). Differentiation and clinical implications of postpartum depression and postpartum psychosis. *JOGNN: Journal of Obstetrics, Gynecologic, & Neonatal Nursing, 38*(3), 269–279. doi:10.1111/j.1552-6909.2009.01019.x

Duff, P., Sweet, R. L., & Edwards, R. K. (2009). Maternal and fetal infectious disorders. In R. K. Creasy & R. Resnik (Eds.), *Maternal-fetal medicine: Principles and practice* (6th ed., pp. 739–795). Philadelphia, PA: Saunders.

Eberhard-Gran, M., Eskild, A., & Opjordsmoen, S. (2006). Use of psychotropic medications in treating mood disorders during lactation. *CNS Drugs, 20*(3), 187–198.

Fiori, O., Deux, J., Kambale, J., Uzan, S., Bougdhere, F., & Berkane, N. (2009). Impact of pelvic embolization for intractable postpartum hemorrhage on fertility. *American Journal of Obstetrics & Gynecology, 200*(4), 384E1–384E4. doi:10.1016/j.ajog.2008.11.029

Gilstrap, L. C., & Yeomans, E. R. (2008). Complications of delivery. In R. S. Gibbs, B. Y. Karlan, A. F. Haney, & I. Nygaard. *Danforth's Obstetrics & Gynecology* (10th ed, pp. 452–461). Philadelphia, PA: Lippincott Williams & Wilkins.

Gjerdingen, D. K., Katon, W., & Rich, D. E. (2008). Stepped care treatment of postpartum depression: A primary care-based management model. *Women's Health Issues, 18*(1), 44–52. doi:10.1016/j.whi.2007.09.001

Gorgas, D. L. (2008). Infection related to pregnancy. *Emergency Medical Clinics of North America, 26*(2), 345–366.

James, D. C. (2008). Postpartum care. In K. R. Simpson & P. A. Creehan, *AWHONN's perinatal nursing* (3rd ed., pp. 473–526). Philadelphia, PA: Lippincott Williams & Wilkins.

Lawrence, R. M., & Lawrence, R. A. (2009). The breast and the physiology of lactation. In R. K. Creasy & R. Resnik (Eds.), *Maternal-fetal medicine: Principles and practice* (6th ed., pp. 125–142). Philadelphia, PA: Saunders.

Lockwood, C. J. (2009). Thromboembolic disease in pregnancy. In R. K. Creasy & R. Resnik (Eds.), *Maternal-fetal medicine: Principles and practice* (6th ed., pp. 853–867). Philadelphia, PA: Saunders.

McCaffery, R., & Blum, C. (2009). Venothrombic events: Evidence-based risk assessment, prophylaxis, diagnosis, and treatment. *The Journal for Nurse Practitioners, 5*(5), 326–333. doi:10.1016/j.nurpra.2008.07.009

Mengel, M. B., & Schwiebert, L. P. (2009). *Family medicine: Ambulatory care and prevention* (5th ed.). New York, NY : McGraw-Hill.

Newton, E. R. (2007). Breastfeeding. In S. G. Gabbe, J. R. Niebyl, & J. L. Simpson (Eds.), *Obstetrics: Normal and problem pregnancies* (5th ed., pp. 586–615). Philadelphia, PA: Churchill Livingstone/Elsevier.

Oyelese, Y., & Ananth, C. V. (2010). Postpartum hemorrhage: Epidemiology, risk factors, and causes. *Clinical Obstetrics and Gynecology, 53*(1), 147–156.

Parry, B. L. (2007). Management of depression and psychoses during pregnancy and the puerperium. In S. G. Gabbe, J. R Nielyl, & J. L.Simpson, *Obstetrics: Normal and problem pregnancies* (5th ed., pp. 1261–1265). Philadelphia, PA: Churchill Livingstone Elsevier.

Poggi, S. B. H. (2007). Postpartum hemorrhage & the abnormal puerperium. In A. H. DeCherney, L. Nathan, T. M. Goodwin, & N. Laufer (Eds.), *Current obstetric & gynecologic: Diagnosis & treatment* (10th ed., pp. 477–497). New York, NY: Lange Medical Books/McGraw-Hill.

Roberts, J. M., & Funai, E. F. (2009). Pregnancy-related hypertension. In R. K. Creasy & R. Resnik (Eds.), *Maternal-fetal medicine: Principles and practice* (6th ed., pp. 651–688). Philadelphia, PA: Saunders.

Sheeder, J., Kabin, K., & Stafford, B. (2009). Screening for postpartum depression at well-child visits: Is once enough during the first 6 months of life? *Pediatrics, 123*(66), 992–998.

Simpson, K. R. (2010). Perinatal patient safety: Postpartum hemorrhage. *The American Journal of Maternal/Child Nursing, 35*(2), 124.

Sit, D., Rothschild, A. J., & Wisner, K. L. (2006). A review of postpartum psychosis. *Journal of Women's Health, 15*(4), 352–368.

Smith, R. P. (2008). *Netter's obstetrics and gynecology* (2nd ed.). Philadelphia, PA: Saunders.

Stone, H. L. (2009). Post-traumatic stress disorder in postpartum patients: What nurses can do. *Nursing for Women's Health, 13*(4), 286–291. doi:10.1111/j.1751-486X.2009.01438.x

Tham, V., Christensson, K., & Ryding E. L. (2007). Sense of coherence and symptoms of post-traumatic stress after emergency caesarean section. *Acta Obstetricia et Gynecologica Scandinavica, 86*(9), 1090–1096. doi:10.1080/00016340701507693

Townsend, M. (2009). *Psychiatric mental health nursing: Concepts of care in evidence-based practice* (6th ed.). Philadelphia, PA: F. A. Davis.

Turrentine, J. E. (2008). *Clinical protocols in obstetrics and gynecology.* London, England: Informa Healthcare.

APPENDIX A: Common Abbreviations in Maternal-Newborn and Women's Health Nursing

ABE	Acute bilirubin encephalopathy
AC	Abdominal circumference
accel	Acceleration of fetal heart rate
AFAFP	Amniotic fluid alpha-fetoprotein
AFI	Amniotic fluid index
AFP	Alpha-fetoprotein
AFV	Amniotic fluid volume
AGA	Average for gestational age
AI	Amnioinfusion
AMOL	Active management of labor
AOP	Apnea of prematurity *or* Anemia of prematurity
ARBD	Alcohol-related birth defects
ARBOW	Artificial rupture of bag of waters
ARND	Alcohol related neurodevelopmental disorder
AROM	Artificial rupture of membranes
ART	Artificial reproductive technology
BAM	Becoming a mother
BAT	Brown adipose tissue (brown fat)
BBOW	Bulging bag of water
BBT	Basal body temperature
β-hCG	Beta-human chorionic gonadotropin
BL	Baseline (fetal heart rate baseline)
BOW	Bag of waters
BPD	Biparietal diameter *or* Bronchopulmonary dysplasia
BPP	Biophysical profile
BRB	Bright red bleeding *or* Breakthrough bleeding
BR CA	Breast cancer
BSE	Breast self-examination
BSST	Breast self-stimulation test
BV	Bacterial vaginosis
CC	Chest circumference or Cord compression
CD	Cycle day
CEI	Continuous epidural infusion
C–H	Crown-to-heel length
CID	Cytomegalic inclusion disease
CLD	Chronic lung disease
CMV	Cytomegalovirus
CNM	Certified nurse-midwife
CNS	Clinical nurse specialist
COCs	Combined oral contraceptives
CPAP	Continuous positive airway pressure
CPD	Cephalopelvic disproportion *or* Citrate-phosphate-dextrose
CRL	Crown-rump length
CRNP	Certified registered nurse practitioner
C/S	Cesarean section (or C-section)
CST	Contraction stress test
CVS	Chorionic villus sampling
D&C	Dilatation and curettage
D&E	Dilatation and evacuation
decels	Deceleration of fetal heart rate
DFMR	Daily fetal movement response
dil	Dilatation
DPNB	Dorsal penile nerve block
DRI	Dietary reference intake
DTR	Deep tendon reflexes
DUB	Dysfunctional uterine bleeding
EAB	Elective abortion
EASI	Extra-amniotic saline infusion
ECMO	Extracorporeal membrane oxygenator
ECV	External cephalic version
EDB	Estimated date of birth
EDC	Estimated date of confinement
EDD	Estimated date of delivery
EFM	Electronic fetal monitoring
EFW	Estimated fetal weight
EIA	Enzyme immunoassay
ELF	Elective low forceps
ELISA	Enzyme-linked immunosorbent assay
EOS	Early onset sepsis
EP	Ectopic pregnancy
epis	Episiotomy
EPT	Expedited partner therapy
ERCS	Elective repeat cesarean section
FAB	Fertility awareness-based methods
FAD	Fetal activity diary
FAS	Fetal alcohol syndrome
FASD	Fetal alcohol spectrum disorder
FBM	Fetal breathing movements
FBS	Fetal blood sample *or* Fasting blood sugar test
FCC	Family-centered care
FECG	Fetal electrocardiogram
fFN	Fetal fibronectin
FGM	Female genital mutilation
FHR	Fetal heart rate

FHT	Fetal heart tones
Fhx	Family history
FISH	Fluorescence in situ hybridization
FL	Femur length
FMC	Fetal movement count
FMH	Fetal-maternal hemorrhage
FMR	Fetal movement record
FPG	Fasting plasma glucose test
FSE	Fetal scalp electrode
FSH	Follicle-stimulating hormone
FSHRH	Follicle-stimulating hormone-releasing hormone
$FSPO_2$	Fetal arterial oxygen saturation
G or grav	Gravida
GDM	Gestational diabetes mellitus
GIFT	Gamete intrafallopian transfer
GnRF	Gonadotropin-releasing factor
GnRH	Gonadotropin-releasing hormone
GTD	Gestational trophoblastic disease
GTPAL	Gravida, term, preterm, abortion, living children; a system of recording maternity history
HA	Head-abdominal ratio or headache
HAI	Hemagglutination-inhibition test
HC	Head compression
hCG	Human chorionic gonadotropin
hCS	Human chorionic somatomammotropin (same as hPL)
hMG	Human menopausal gonadotropin
hPL	Human placental lactogen
HPTs	Home pregnancy tests
HPV	Human papilloma virus
HT	Hormone therapy
HRT	Hormone replacement therapy
HSV	Herpes simplex virus
IAP	Intrapartum antimicrobial prophylaxis
ICSI	Intracytoplasmic sperm injection
IDM	Infant of a diabetic mother
IPV	Intimate partner violence
ISAM	Infant of a substance-abusing mother
IUD	Intrauterine device
IUFD	Intrauterine fetal death
IUGR	Intrauterine growth restriction
IUI	Intrauterine insemination
IUPC	Intrauterine pressure catheter
IUS	Intrauterine system
IVF	In vitro fertilization
LADA	Left-acromion-dorsal-anterior
LADP	Left-acromion-dorsal-posterior
LBC	Lamellar body count
LBW	Low birth weight
LDRP	Labor, delivery, recovery, and postpartum
LGA	Large for gestational age
LH	Luteinizing hormone
LHRH	Luteinizing hormone-releasing hormone
LMA	Left-mentum-anterior
LML	Left mediolateral (episiotomy)
LMP	Last menstrual period *or* Left-mentum-posterior
LMT	Left-mentum-transverse
LOA	Left-occiput-anterior
LOF	Low outlet forceps
LOP	Left-occiput-posterior
LOS	Length of stay
LOT	Left-occiput-transverse
L/S	Lecithin/sphingomyelin ratio
LSA	Left-sacrum-anterior
LSP	Left-sacrum-posterior
LST	Left-sacrum-transverse
MAS	Meconium aspiration syndrome
mec	Meconium
MEN	Minimal enteral nutrition
MLE	Midline episiotomy
MSAF	Meconium-stained amniotic fluid
MSAFP	Maternal serum alpha-fetoprotein
multip	Multipara
NAS	Neonatal abstinence syndrome
NEC	Necrotizing enterocolitis
NFP	Natural family planning
NNS	Nonnutritive sucking
NP	Nurse practitioner
NSCST	Nipple stimulation contraction stress test
NST	Nonstress test or Nonshivering thermogenesis
NSVD	Normal sterile vaginal delivery
NT	Nuchal translucency
NTD	Neural tube defects
NTE	Neutral thermal environment
NVP	Nausea and vomiting of pregnancy
OA	Occiput anterior
OCPs	Oral contraceptive pills
OCT	Oxytocin challenge test
OF	Occipitofrontal diameter of fetal head
OFC	Occipitofrontal circumference
OGTT	Oral glucose tolerance test
OM	Occipitomental (diameter)
OP	Occiput posterior

p	Para
PABC	Pregnancy-associated breast cancer
Pap smear	Papanicolaou smear
PAPP-A	Pregnancy-associated plasma protein A
PCEA	Patient-controlled epidural analgesia
PCOS	Polycystic ovarian syndrome
PDA	Patent ductus arteriosus
PG	Phosphatidylglycerol *or* Prostaglandin
PGS	Preimplantation genetic screening
PID	Pelvic inflammatory disease
Pit	Pitocin
PKU	Phenylketonuria
PMR	Perinatal mortality rate
PMS	Premenstrual syndrome
PNV	Prenatal vitamins
PPHN	Persistent pulmonary hypertension
primip	Primipara
PROM	Premature rupture of membranes
PSI	Prostaglandin synthesis inhibitor
PTB	Preterm birth
PTL	Preterm labor
PUBS	Percutaneous umbilical blood sampling
RADA	Right-acromion-dorsal-anterior
RADP	Right-acromion-dorsal-posterior
RDS	Respiratory distress syndrome
REM	Rapid eye movements
RIA	Radioimmunoassay
RLF	Retrolental fibroplasia
RMA	Right-mentum-anterior
RMP	Right-mentum-posterior
RMT	Right-mentum-transverse
ROA	Right-occiput-anterior
ROM	Rupture of membranes
ROP	Right-occiput-posterior *or* Retinopathy of prematurity
ROT	Right-occiput-transverse
RPL	Recurrent pregnancy loss
RRA	Radioreceptor assay
RSA	Right-sacrum-anterior
RSP	Right-sacrum-posterior
RST	Right-sacrum-transverse
SAB	Spontaneous abortion
SBS	Shaken baby syndrome
SET	Surrogate embryo transfer
SGA	Small for gestational age
SIDS	Sudden infant death syndrome
SMB	Submentobregmatic diameter
SOB	Suboccipitobregmatic diameter *or* Shortness of breath
SPA	Sperm penetration assay
SRBOW	Spontaneous rupture of bag of waters
SRMC	Single-room maternity care
SROM	Spontaneous rupture of membranes
STI	Sexually transmitted infection
STS	Serologic test for syphilis
SVE	Sterile vaginal exam
TAB	Therapeutic abortion
TcB	Transcutaneous bilirubin
TCM	Transcutaneous monitoring
TDI or THI	Therapeutic donor insemination (*H* designates mate is donor)
TET	Tubal embryo transfer
TOL	Trial of labor
TOLAC	Trial of labor after cesarean
TORCH	Toxoplasmosis, rubella, cytomegalovirus, herpesvirus hominis type 2
TSS	Toxic shock syndrome
ū	Umbilicus
UA	Uterine activity
UAC	Umbilical artery catheter
UAU	Uterine activity units
UC	Uterine contraction
UNHS	Universal newborn hearing screening
UPI	Uteroplacental insufficiency
US	Ultrasound
VBAC	Vaginal birth after cesarean
VDRL	Venereal Disease Research Laboratories
VIP	Voluntary interruption of pregnancy
VLBW	Very low birth weight
VVC	Vulvovaginal *candidiasis*
WIC	Supplemental food program for women, infants, and children
ZIFT	Zygote intrafallopian transfer

APPENDIX B: Conversions and Equivalents

TEMPERATURE CONVERSION
(Fahrenheit temperature − 32) × 5/9 = Centigrade temperature
(Centigrade temperature × 9/5) + 32 = Fahrenheit temperature

SELECTED CONVERSION TO METRIC MEASURES

Known Value	Multiply by	To Find
inches	2.54	centimeters
ounces	28	grams
pounds	454	grams
pounds	0.45	kilograms

SELECTED CONVERSION FROM METRIC MEASURES

Known Value	Multiply by	To Find
centimeters	0.4	inches
grams	0.035	ounces
grams	0.0022	pounds
kilograms	2.2	pounds

CONVERSION OF POUNDS AND OUNCES TO GRAMS

	Ounces															
Pounds	0	1	2	3	4	5	6	7	8	9	10	11	12	13	14	15
0	—	28	57	85	113	142	170	198	227	255	283	312	340	369	397	425
1	454	482	510	539	567	595	624	652	680	709	737	765	794	822	850	879
2	907	936	964	992	1021	1049	1077	1106	1134	1162	1191	1219	1247	1276	1304	1332
3	1361	1389	1417	1446	1474	1503	1531	1559	1588	1616	1644	1673	1701	1729	1758	1786
4	1814	1843	1871	1899	1928	1956	1984	2013	2041	2070	2098	2126	2155	2183	2211	2240
5	2268	2296	2325	2353	2381	2410	2438	2466	2495	2523	2551	2580	2608	2637	2665	2693
6	2722	2750	2778	2807	2835	2863	2892	2920	2948	2977	3005	3033	3062	3090	3118	3147
7	3175	3203	3232	3260	3289	3317	3345	3374	3402	3430	3459	3487	3515	3544	3572	3600
8	3629	3657	3685	3714	3742	3770	3799	3827	3856	3884	3912	3941	3969	3997	4026	4054
9	4082	4111	4139	4167	4196	4224	4252	4281	4309	4337	4366	4394	4423	4451	4479	4508
10	4536	4564	4593	4621	4649	4678	4706	4734	4763	4791	4819	4848	4876	4904	4933	4961
11	4990	5018	5046	5075	5103	5131	5160	5188	5216	5245	5273	5301	5330	5358	5386	5415
12	5443	5471	5500	5528	5557	5585	5613	5642	5670	5698	5727	5755	5783	5812	5840	5868
13	5897	5925	5953	5982	6010	6038	6067	6095	6123	6152	6180	6209	6237	6265	6294	6322
14	6350	6379	6407	6435	6464	6492	6520	6549	6577	6605	6634	6662	6690	6719	6747	6776
15	6804	6832	6860	6889	6917	6945	6973	7002	7030	7059	7087	7115	7144	7172	7201	7228
16	7257	7286	7313	7342	7371	7399	7427	7456	7484	7512	7541	7569	7597	7626	7654	7682
17	7711	7739	7768	7796	7824	7853	7881	7909	7938	7966	7994	8023	8051	8079	8108	8136
18	8165	8192	8221	8249	8278	8306	8335	8363	8391	8420	8448	8476	8504	8533	8561	8590
19	8618	8646	8675	8703	8731	8760	8788	8816	8845	8873	8902	8930	8958	8987	9015	9043
20	9072	9100	9128	9157	9185	9213	9242	9270	9298	9327	9355	9383	9412	9440	9469	9497
21	9525	9554	9582	9610	9639	9667	9695	9724	9752	9780	9809	9837	9865	9894	9922	9950
22	9979	10007	10036	10064	10092	10120	10149	10177	10206	10234	10262	10291	10319	10347	10376	10404

APPENDIX C: Spanish Translations of English Phrases*

This appendix includes phrases you might find helpful in working with families during pregnancy, labor, and birth, and after the birth. There are many ways to phrase questions. We have chosen some statements we consider essential and have tried to phrase them in a straightforward way. The phrases are designed to help you in situations in which translation is not possible at the moment.

This list begins with introductory statements, which are presented in a logical conversational flow. The remaining phrases are arranged according to the phases of pregnancy and birth during which they are most applicable.

Essential Introductory Phrases	**Frases Introductoras Esenciales**
Hello	Hola
I am a nurse.	Soy enferera (enfermero).†
I am a student nurse.	Soy estudiante de enfermería.
My name is __________.	Mi nombre es __________. Me llamo __________.
What is your name?	¿Cuál es su nombre? ¿Cómo se llama?
What name should I call you?	¿Cómo quiere que la llamemos? ¿Cómo quiere ser llamada?
Thank you	Gracias
Please	Por favor
Is someone here with you?	¿Hay alquien aquí con usted?
Does he (she) speak English?	¿Habla él (ella) inglés?
Goodbye	Adiós.
Phrases for the Antepartum Period	**Frases para el Periodo Prenatal**
Are you taking any medications now?	¿Está tomando algunas medicinas ahora?
Show me the medicine bottles please.	Por favor, muéstreme los frascos.
Have you ever had trouble with your blood pressure?	¿Ha tenido problemas alguna vez con la presión arterial?
When was the first day of your last period?	¿Cuál fue el primer día de su última regla? ¿Cuál fue el primer día de su última menstruación?
Have you had any spotting or bleeding since your last period?	¿Ha sangrado o ha tenido manchas de sangre desde su última regla?
Have you been on birth control pills?	¿Ha estado tomando píldoras anticonceptivas?
When did you stop taking them?	¿Cuándo dejó de tomarlas?
Do you have an intrauterine device (IUD)?	¿Usa un aparato intrauterino?
How many times have you been pregnant?	¿Cuántas veces ha estado usted embarazada?
Are you having any problems with your pregnancy?	¿Tiene problemas con su embarazo?
Is there anything that is worrying you?	¿Hay algo o alguna cosa que la preocupe?
I would like to take your blood pressure.	Quisiera tomarle la presió arterial.
I would like to take your pulse.	Quisiera tomarle el pulso.
I would like to take your temperature.	Quisiera tomarle la temperatura.
I would like to listen to your heart and lungs.	Quisiera escucharle el corazon y los pulmones.
I would like to check your uterus.	Quisiera examinarle el útero.
Please urinate in this cup and leave it in the bathroom.	Puede orinar en este vaso y dejarlo en el baño.
Please stand up.	Por favor, levántese.
Please sit down.	Por favor, siéntese.
Please lie down.	Por favor, acuéstese.
Phrases Related to Client Safety	**Frases Relacionadas con la Seguridad del Cliente**
I would like to talk to you alone.	Quisiera hablar a solas con usted.

*Prepared by Elizabeth Medina, PhD. Associate Professor of Spanish, Regis University, Denver, Colorado.
†In Spanish, nouns that end in *a* indicate female gender; nouns that end in *o* indicate male gender.

Are you safe at home?	¿Sufre de peligros en casa?
Are you afraid of your partner?	¿Le tiene miedo a su compañero?
During your pregnancy has your partner hit, slapped, kicked, or punched you?	Durante su embarazo, ¿la ha golpeado? ¿la ha abofeteado? ¿la ha pateado? o ¿le ha dado puñetazos?
How many times?	¿Cuántas veces?
Do you have someone for support?	¿Cuénta con alguien que la pueda ayudar?
Questions the Mother or Father May Ask	**Posibles Preguntas que Madres o Padres Hacen**
How big is my baby?	¿De qué tamaño es el (la) bebé?
How much does the baby weigh now?	¿Cuánto pesa el bebé ahora?
When will I feel my baby move?	¿Cuándo lo (la) voy a sentir moverse?
Phrases for the Intrapartum Period	**Frases Durante el Parto**
Note: Review the essential introductory phrases for beginning a conversation.	*Nota:* Repase las frases introductoras para comenzar una conversación.
Are you having labor pains?	¿Tiene dolores de parto?
Are you having contractions?	¿Tiene contracciones?
Are you having pain?	¿Tiene dolores?
Do you need medicine for pain?	¿Necesita medicina para el dolor?
Do you need to urinate?	¿Necesita orinar?
This is a bedpan to urinate in.	Aquí tiene el bacín (la chata) (el pato) para orinar.
Can I help you to the bathroom?	¿La ayudo a ir al baño?
Do you need to have a bowel movement?	¿Necesita mover el vientre (obrar)? Necesita "Hacer caca"—coloquial
Has your bag of water broken?	¿Se le ha roto la bolsa de agua(s)?
Have you had any bright-red bleeding during your pregnancy?	¿Ha tenido algún sangramiento de color rojo durante su embarazo?
How many births have you had?	¿Cuántos niños le han nacido?
I need to do a vaginal examination.	Necesito hacerle un examen vaginal.
I will help you.	La voy a ayudar.
I will stay with you.	Me quedaré con usted.
Please pant. I will show you how.	Por favor, jadee. Le voy a mostrar cómo.
Do not push now.	No puje ahora.
Push now.	Puje ahora.
Stop pushing.	Pare de pujar. No puje más.
The doctor needs to do a cesarean birth.	El doctor le va a hacer una operación cesárea.
This is medicine for your pain. You will feel better soon.	Esta medicina es para el dolor. Va a sentirse mejor pronto.
When is your baby supposed to be born?	¿Cuando está supuesto a nacer el bebé?
January	enero
February	febrero
March	marzo
April	abril
May	mayo
June	junio
July	julio
August	agosto
September	septiembre
October	octubre
November	noviembre
December	diciembre

What is your doctor's name?	¿Cuál es el nombre de su doctor?
What is your midwife's name?	¿Cuál is el nombre de su comadrona (partera)?
Your baby is having some trouble now.	El bebé está pasando por algunos problemas. El bebé está sufriendo algunas dificultades.
I need to put this oxygen mask on you. It will help your baby. It may smell funny, but it is OK.	Le voy a poner esta máscara de oxígeno. Va a ayudar al bebé. Huele extraño, pero no hay problemas.
Please turn on your left side.	Por favor voltéese al lado izquierdo.
Please turn on your right side.	Por favor voltéese al lado derecho.
Your baby is OK.	El bebé está bien.
Phrases for the Postpartum Period and the Newborn Area	**Frases para el Periodo Despues del Parto y el Area del Recien Nacido**
Note: Review the essential introductory phrases for beginning a conversation.	*Nota:* Repase las frases introductoras para comenzar una conversación.
Are you hungry?	¿Tiene hambre?
Are you thirsty?	¿Tiene sed?
Are you cold?	¿Tiene frío?
Are you tired?	¿Está cansada?
I am going to put antibiotic ointment in the baby's eyes.	Le voy a poner al bebé un ungüento antibiótico alrededor de los ojos.
It will help protect your baby from some infections.	Lo (la) va a proteger contra algunos infecciones.
I am going to take some blood from your baby's foot to check the blood sugar and hematocrit.	Le voy a sacar sangre del pie al bebé para determinar el azúcar del la sangre ye el hematocrítico.
If your baby begins to spit up, please turn him (her) on his (her) side.	Si el bebé comienza a vomitar, colóquelo (colóquela) de costado.
It may help to position your baby like this.	Lo (la) ayudará—si lo coloca así. Lo (la) ayudaría—si lo colocara así.
I would like to suggest that you clean your nipples this way before you breastfeed your baby.	Es bueno que se lave los pezones de esta manera antes de darle el pecho al bebé.
It is better that you clean your baby's cord this way.	Es mejor para el bebé que le lave el ombligo de esta manera.
It is better that you bathe your baby this way.	Es mejor que lo (la) bañe de esta manera.
It is better that you clean your baby's penis this way.	Es mejor que le limpie el pene así.
I would like to suggest that you fold the diaper this way.	Le sugiero que doble el pañal así.
I would like to suggest that you fasten the diaper this way.	Le sugiero que asegure el pañal así.
Take the baby's temperature this way.	Tómele la temperature así.
I need to check (your breasts, your uterus, your flow, your stitches, your legs and feet).	Necesito examinarle (los pechos, el útero, el flujo, los puntos, las pierns y los pies).
I need to feel your uterus.	Necesito examinarle el útero.
I need to massage your uterus.	Necesito darle un masaje en la región del útero.
Place your baby on its side.	Coloque al bebé de costado.
Place the baby's used diapers here.	Coloque aquí los pañales usados.
Please rub your uterus every half hour to keep it firm. I will show you how.	Necesita darse un masaje en la región del útero cada media hora para mantenerlo firme. Le voy a mostrar cómo.
Would you like to see your baby now?	¿Quiere ver a su bebé ahora?
Would you like me to help you feed your baby?	¿Quiere que le ayude a alimentarlo (la)?
Your baby needs a car seat to go home in.	El (la) bebé necesita un asiento para bebé en el automóvil.
Special Neonatal Needs	**Necesidades del Recien Nacido**
We are giving your baby oxygen.	Le vamos a dar oxígeno al (a la) bebé.
Your baby is having problems breathing.	El (la) bebé tiene problemas al respirar.
Your baby needs extra help.	El (la) bebé necesita ayuda especial.
Your baby needs to go to a special care nursery.	El (la) bebé necesita ir a la sala de cuidados especiales para bebés.

APPENDIX D: Guidelines for Working with Deaf Patients and Interpreters

1. First, remember that it requires trust on the part of the patient to allow nonsigning caregivers and an interpreter into her life.
2. It is important to use a registered interpreter. Medical interpreters are registered with the Registry of Interpreters for the Deaf. Although family members and friends may offer to interpret, it is best to use registered medical interpreters because they are required to translate the patients' and nurses' words exactly and accurately without adding in any other opinion.
3. Greet the patient and family with a handshake and body posture that indicates welcome. You may point to your name tag and use the American Sign Language (ASL) alphabet cards to spell out your name. The patient may wish to select cards to indicate her name. It is especially important as you work together to make the effort to provide a greeting as you would with speaking patients; greetings help develop rapport.
4. Once the interpreter is present, continue to look at the patient and speak directly to her. There will be a temptation to look at the interpreter, and it will help to remember that you are speaking to the patient.
5. Avoid phrasing your words as if you are talking to the interpreter (e.g., "Can you tell her . . . ?"). Instead, phrase your questions as you do with speaking patients (e.g., "I'm going to ask you some questions now.").
6. Depend on the deaf patient to ask questions.
7. Look at the patient's face for signs of difficulty in understanding. Deaf patients have a behavior of "gesturing" that involves shaking their heads as if to indicate "yes" even when they do not understand. If the patient is nodding "yes," ask her to repeat the directions you have just given.
8. Be as direct as possible. Keep to what you want to know or what you want to convey. Speak in short sentences, using nontechnical words. Avoid colloquial or slang words. Be sure to explain what you want to do before you do it. For instance, tell her you want to start an IV and explain the equipment. Then, with her permission, start the IV.
9. Be aware that deaf patients may have difficulty understanding when to take medications. It will be helpful to associate taking medications or completing some treatment or activity with meals. (For instance, while showing her the two capsules she is to take when she goes home, tell her to take the two capsules at breakfast and another two capsules at bedtime.) Avoid saying, "Take two capsules at 8:00 a.m., 2:00 p.m., and 12:00 a.m."
10. The difference in interpreting time may also affect obtaining a history. It is best to begin with a specific event in the past and work forward.

What to Do Until the Interpreter Arrives

1. Role-play as much as possible.
2. Demonstrate what you want the patient to do or what you want to do.
3. Be resourceful.
4. Remember that some deaf patients can read lips. Some may read written language, but use care in assuming the patient understands.

What to Do to Prepare for Working with a Deaf Patient

1. Contact local agencies that work with deaf patients to see what resources are available. Ask about classes in ASL. Being able to use some basic signs will be very helpful while waiting for an interpreter to arrive.
2. Read to learn more about the deaf culture. Contact your local agency or the National Information Center on Deafness, Silver Springs, Maryland, to get suggestions on books you might read.
3. Investigate your health facility. What is available to assist you? Look for videos used for teaching in the maternal-child unit and note if they have captions. Remember that many deaf patients do not read written language, so it will be important to review the content of the video with an interpreter present.

Prepared with the kind assistance of Mr. Gerald Dement, Interpreter Coordinator, Pikes Peak Center on Deafness, Colorado Springs, Colorado.

Appendix E: Sign Language for Healthcare Professionals

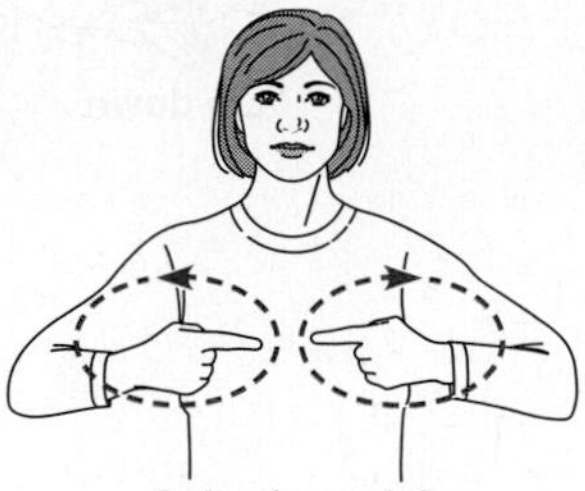

Ache (or pain)

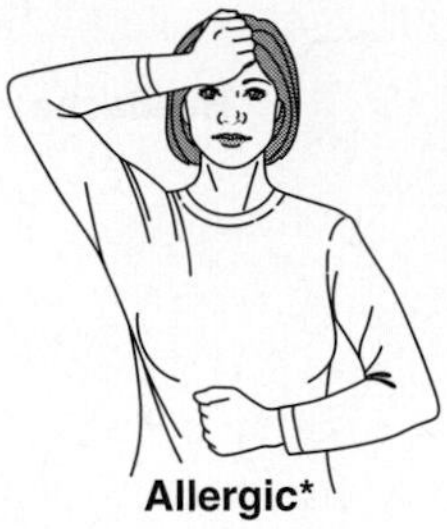

Allergic*

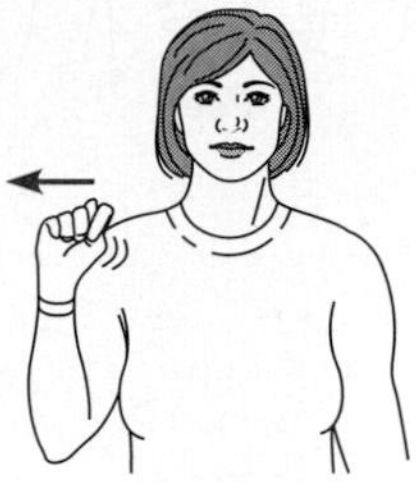

Bathroom

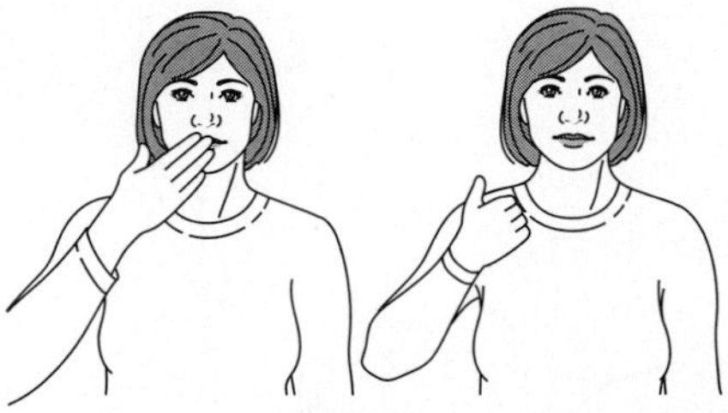

Better

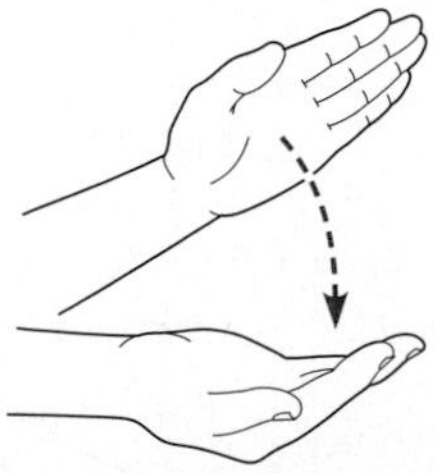

Congratulate (or praise)

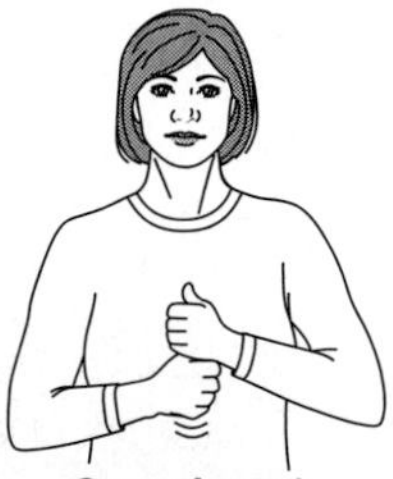

Constipate*

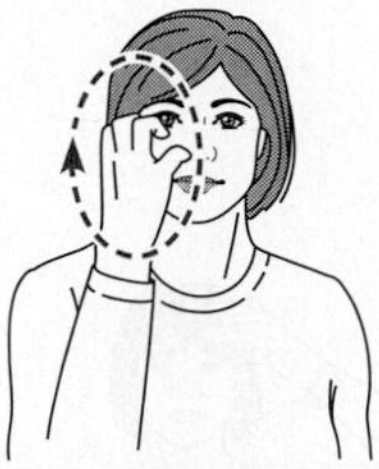

Dizzy

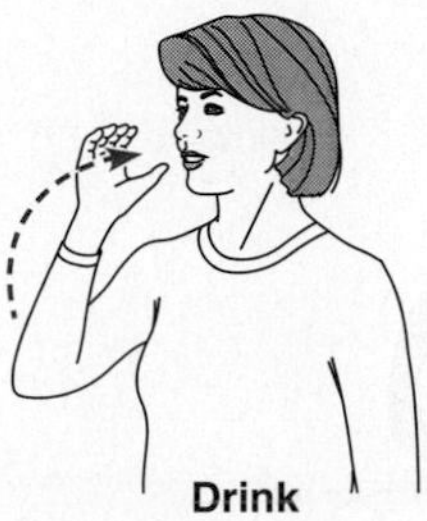

Drink

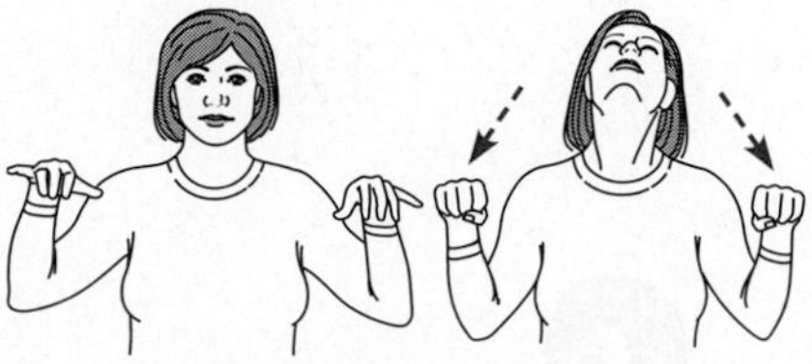

Faint

*Indicates signs that are in manually signed English. Those without an asterisk are in American Sign Language.

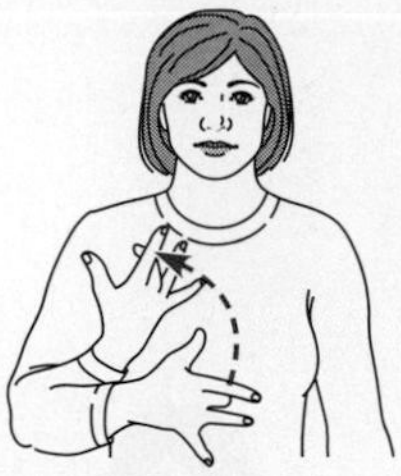

Feel

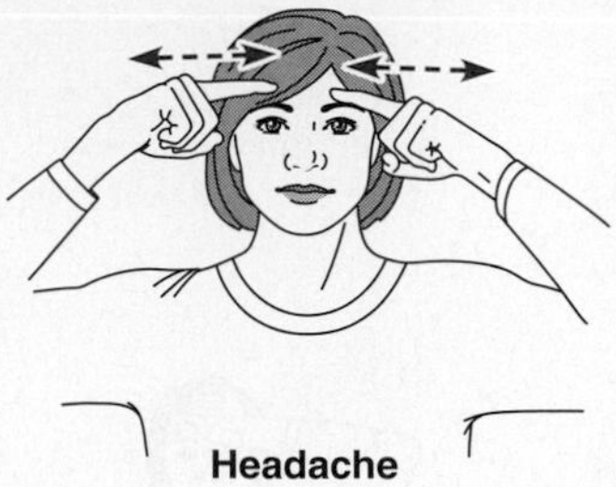

Headache

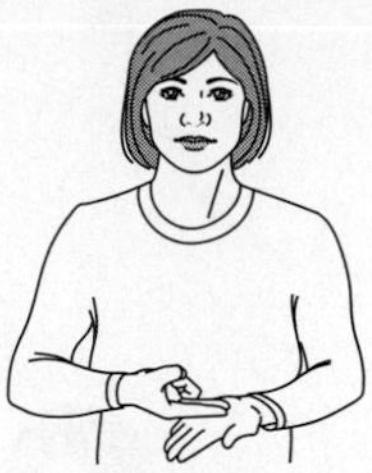

Lie down

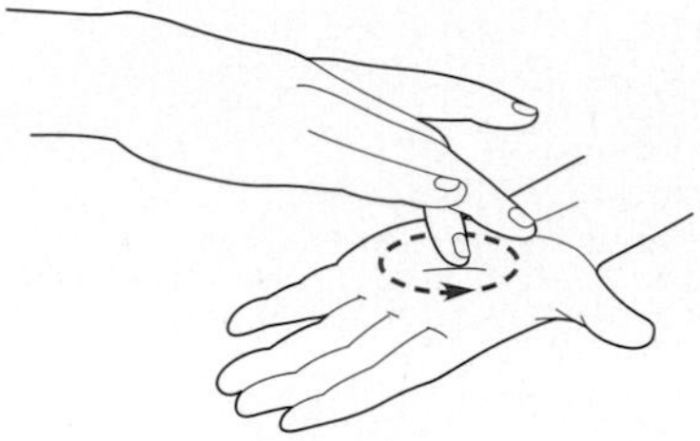

Medicine

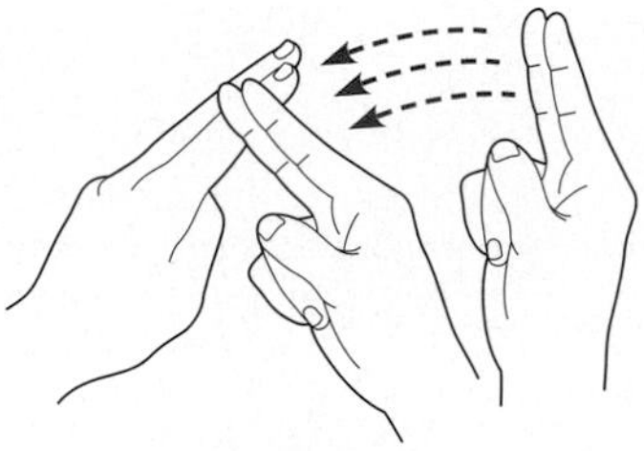

Name

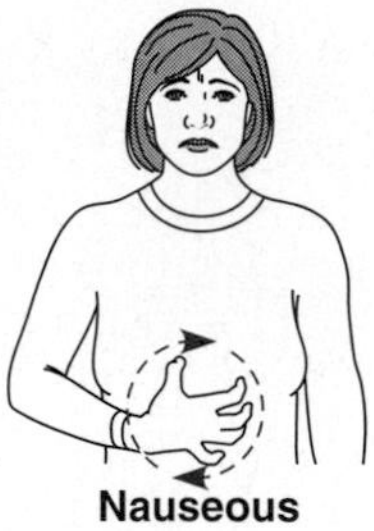

Nauseous

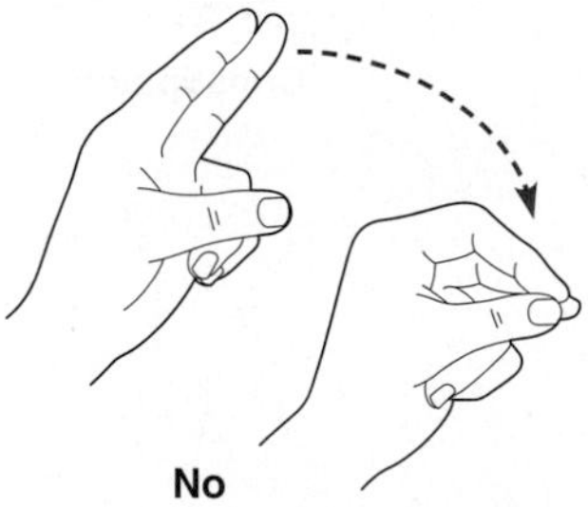

No

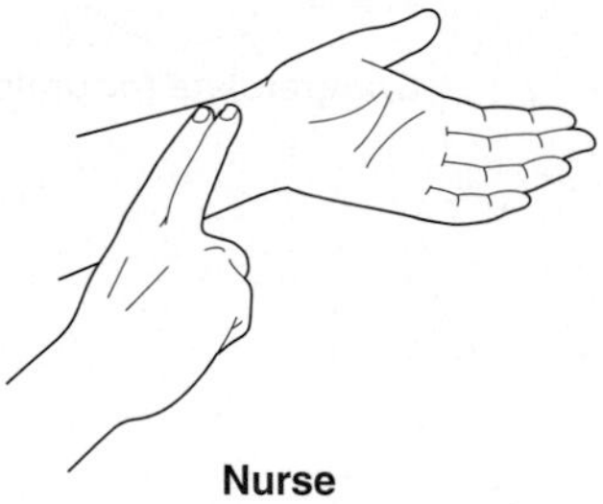

Nurse

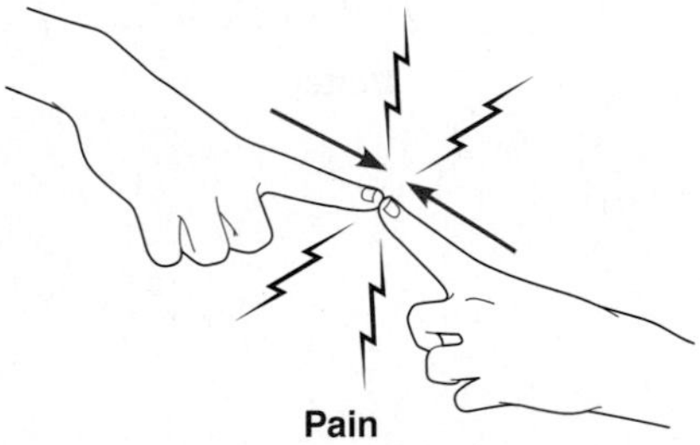

Pain

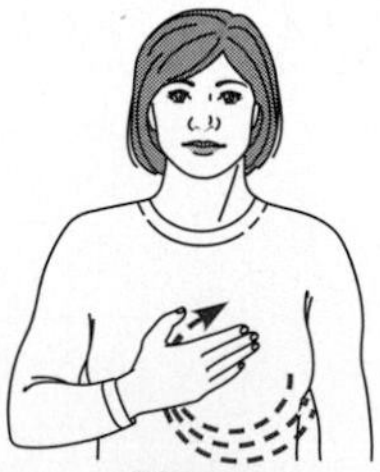

Please

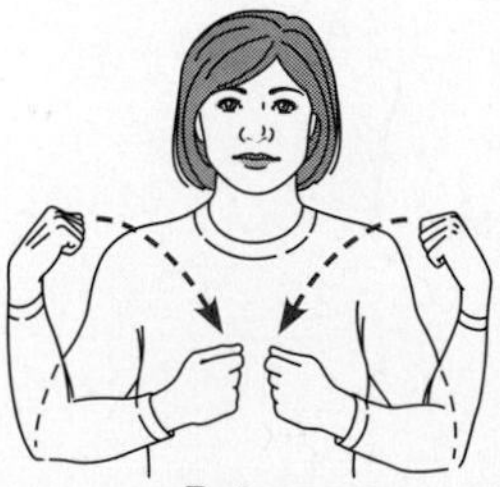

Put on

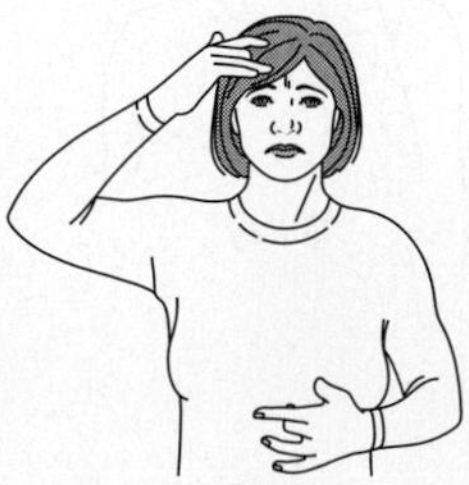

Sick

*Indicates signs that are in manually signed English. Those without an asterisk are in American Sign Language.

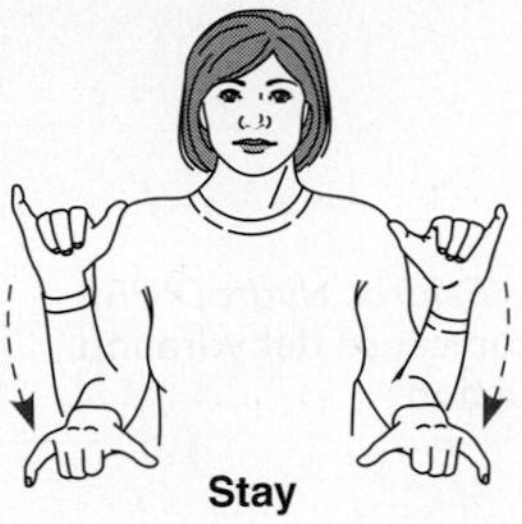

Stay

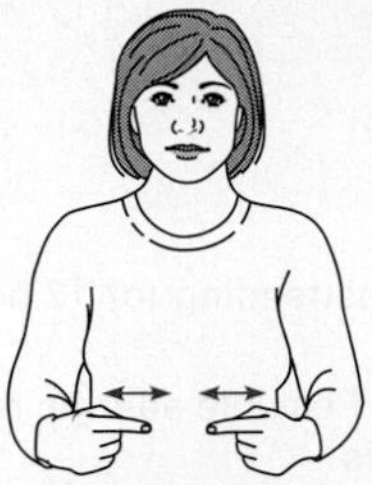

Stomachache*

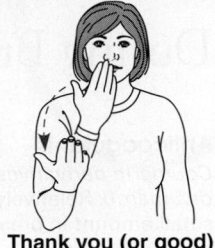

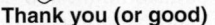

Thank you (or good)

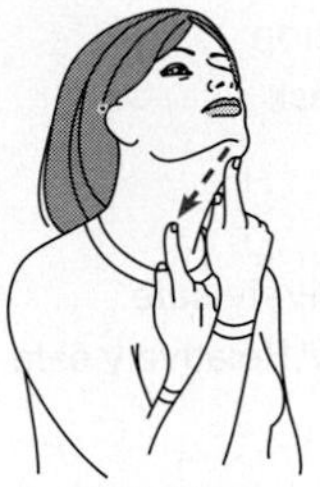

Thirsty

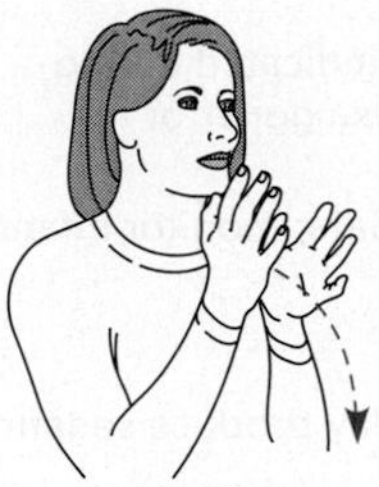

Vomit

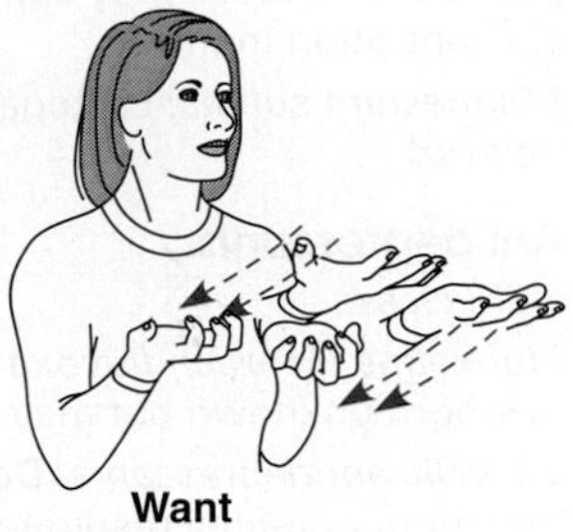

Want

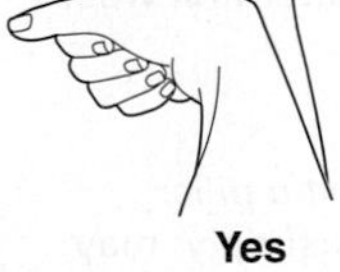

Yes

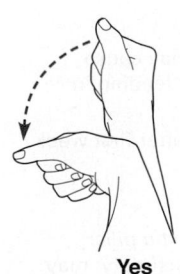

*Indicates signs that are in manually signed English. Those without an asterisk are in American Sign Language.

APPENDIX F: Actions and Effects of Selected Drugs During Breastfeeding*

Anticoagulants

Coumarin derivatives (warfarin, dicumarol): Relatively safe to use; only small amount in breast milk; check PTT

Heparin and derivatives (Lovenox): Does not cross into breast milk; check PTT

Anticonvulsants

Phenytoin (Dilantin), phenobarbital: Generally considered safe; if high doses of phenobarbital are ingested, may cause drowsiness; short-acting phenobarbiturates (secobarbital) preferred, because they appear in lower concentration in milk

Magnesium sulfate: Lactogenesis may be delayed

Antidepressants

SSRI class:

Fluoxetine (Prozac), fluvoxamine: Effect on newborn unknown but may be of concern

Tricyclic antidepressants (Doxepin): Sedation, potential respiratory arrest in infant

Antihistamines

Diphenhydramine (Benadryl), Claritin, Allegra: May cause decreased milk supply; infant may become drowsy or irritable

Clemastine (Tavist): Counterindicated

Antihypertensives

β adrenergic blockers:

Atenolol, acebutolol: Cyanosis, bradycardia, hypotension

Tenormin: Hypotension, bradycardia

Antimetabolites/Antineoplastics

Unknown, probably long-term anti-DNA effect on the infant; potentially very toxic

Antimicrobials

Aminoglycosides: May cause ototoxicity or nephrotoxicity if given for more than 2 weeks

Ampicillin: Skin rash, candidiasis; diarrhea

Azithromycin: No risk to newborn

Chloramphenicol (rarely used): Possible bone marrow suppression; too low a dose for Gray syndrome; refusal of breast

Erythromycin: Accumulates in breast milk, idiopathic hypertrophic pyloric stenosis

Methacycline: Possible inhibition of bone growth; may cause discoloration of the teeth; use should be avoided

Metronidazole (Flagyl): Possible neurologic disorders or blood dyscrasias; delay breastfeeding for 12 hours after dose

Penicillin: Possible allergic response; candidiasis

Quinolones (synthetic antibiotics): Can cause arthropathies

Sulfonamides: May cause hyperbilirubinemia; use contraindicated until infant over 1 week old

Tetracycline: Long-term use and large doses should be avoided; may cause tooth staining or inhibition of bone growth

Antithyroids

Thiouracil: Contraindicated during lactation; may cause goiter or agranulocytosis

Propylthiouracil: Safe; monitor infant thyroid function

Barbiturates

Phenothiazines: May produce sedation

Bronchodilators

Aminophylline: May cause insomnia or irritability in the infant

Leukotriene inhibitors (Zyflo, Accolate): Potential tumorigenicity

Caffeine

Excessive consumption may cause jitteriness or wakefulness

Cardiovascular

Amiodarone: Transient bradycardia, IUGR; contains iodine—potential for thyroid gland problems

Clonidine (Catapres): May reduce milk volume

Methyldopa: May increase milk volume; monitor for hypotension for 48 hours after birth

Propranolol (Inderal): May cause hypoglycemia; possibility of other blocking effects, especially if infant has renal or liver dysfunction

Quinidine: May cause arrhythmias in infant

Reserpine (Serpasil): Nasal stuffiness, lethargy, or diarrhea in infant

Corticosteroids

Adrenal suppression may occur with long-term administration of doses greater than 20 mg/day

Diuretics

Furosemide (Lasix): Not excreted in breast milk

Thiazide diuretics (Esidrix, HydroDIURIL Oretic): Safe but can cause dehydration, reduce milk production

Heavy Metals

Gold: Potentially toxic; gold salts—compatible with breastfeeding

Lead: Excreted in breast milk; high maternal levels can affect neuropsychologic development

Mercury: Excreted in the milk and hazardous to infant

Hormones

Androgens: Suppress lactation

Thyroid hormones: May mask hypothyroidism

Laxatives

Peri-Colace, Dulcolax: Relatively safe

Milk of magnesia, Metamucil: Relatively safe

Narcotic Analgesics

Codeine: Accumulation may lead to neonatal depression

Meperidine: Avoid use. May lead to neonatal depression

Morphine: Long-term use may cause newborn addiction

Nonnarcotic Analgesics, NSAIDS

Acetaminophen (Tylenol): Relatively safe for short-term analgesia

Ibuprofen (Motrin): Safe

Propoxyphene (Darvon): May cause sleepiness and poor breastfeeding in infant

Salicylates (aspirin): Safe after first week of life; monitor PTT

Oral Contraceptives

Combined estrogen/progestin pills: Significantly decrease milk supply; may alter milk composition; may cause gynecomastia in male infants

Progestin only (DMPA, Norplant): Safe if started after lactation is established

Radioactive Materials for Testing

Gallium citrate (67G): Insignificant amount excreted in breast milk; no breastfeeding for 2 weeks

Iodine: Contraindicated; may affect infant's thyroid gland

^{125}I: Discontinue breastfeeding for 24 hours

^{131}I: Breastfeeding should be discontinued until excretion is no longer significant; may be resumed after 10 days

*Based on data from Riordan, J., & Auerbach, K. J. (2010). *Breastfeeding and human lactation* (4th ed., pp. 147–196). Boston: Jones & Bartlett; Briggs, G. G., Freeman, R. K., & Yaffe, S. J. (2008). *Drugs in pregnancy and lactation* (8th ed.). Baltimore: Williams & Wilkins; Hale, T. (2010). *Medications and mothers' milk* (14th ed.). Amarillo, TX: Pharmasoft Publishing; Committee on Drugs, American Academy of Pediatrics. (2001). The transfer of drugs and other chemicals into human milk. *Pediatrics, 108*(3), 776.

Technetium-99m: Discontinue breastfeeding for 24 hours (half-life = 6 hours)

Sedatives/Tranquilizers

Diazepam (Valium): May accumulate to high levels; may increase neonatal jaundice; may cause lethargy, weight loss, and poor suck

Lithium: Contraindicated; may cause neonatal flaccidity, hypotonia, affect thyroid and cardiac arrhythmia

Smoking Cessation

Nicotine patch (Nicoderm, Nicotrol): Irritability, abnormal sleep patterns, poor feeding

Bupropion (Zyban, Wellbutrin): No effect on breastfeeding

Substance Abuse

Alcohol: Potential motor developmental delay; mild sedative effect

Amphetamines: Controversial; may cause irritability, poor sleeping pattern

Cocaine, crack: Extreme irritability, tachycardia, vomiting, apnea

Marijuana: Drowsiness

Heroin: Tremors, restlessness, vomiting, poor feeding

Nicotine (smoking): Shock, vomiting, diarrhea, decreased milk production

GLOSSARY

Abdominal effleurage Gentle stroking used in massage.

Abortion Loss of pregnancy before the fetus is viable outside the uterus; miscarriage.

Abruptio placentae (ab-rŭp'shē-ō pla-sen'tē) Partial or total premature separation of a normally implanted placenta.

Abstinence Refraining voluntarily, especially from indulgence in food, alcoholic beverages, or sexual intercourse.

Acceleration Periodic increase in the baseline fetal heart rate.

Acculturation The process by which people adapt to a new cultural norm.

Acme Peak or highest point; time of greatest intensity (of a uterine contraction).

Acquaintance and date rape Rape in which the assailant is someone with whom the victim has had previous nonviolent interaction (acquaintance rape) or which occurs between a dating couple. Date rape is a form of acquaintance rape.

Acquired immunodeficiency syndrome (AIDS) An immunologic disorder caused by infection with the human immunodeficiency virus (HIV) and characterized by increasing susceptibility to opportunistic infections and rare cancers.

Acrocyanosis Cyanosis of the extremities.

Acrosomal reaction Breakdown of the hyaluronic acid in the corona radiata by enzymes from the heads of sperm; allows one spermatozoon to penetrate the ovum zona pellucida.

Active acquired immunity Formation of antibodies by the pregnant woman in response to illness or immunization.

Active alert state Alert state marked by an increase in facial and body movement, with periods of fussiness occurring. The infant in this state has increased sensitivity to disturbing stimuli. Also called *active awake.*

Active management of labor (AMOL) Medical protocol for augmentation of labor that includes (1) a strict criterion for labor admission, (2) early amniotomy, (3) high-dose oxytocin infusion for inefficient labor contractions, and (4) a commitment to provision of continuous nursing care.

Acupressure Therapy using pressure from the fingers and thumbs to stimulate pressure points.

Acupuncture Therapy using very fine (hairlike) stainless steel needles to stimulate specific acupuncture points depending on the client's medical assessment and condition.

Acute bilirubin encephalopathy (ABE) See *Kernicterus.*

Adequate intake (AI) A value cited for a nutrient when there are not sufficient data to calculate an estimated average requirement.

Adjustment reaction with depressed mood A maternal adjustment reaction occurring in the first few postpartum days, characterized by mild depression, tearfulness, anxiety, headache, and irritability. Also called *postpartum blues.*

Adnexa Adjoining or accessory parts of a structure, such as the uterine adnexa: the ovaries and fallopian tubes.

Adolescence Period of human development initiated by puberty and ending with the attainment of young adulthood.

Afterpains Cramplike pains due to contractions of the uterus that occur after childbirth. They are more common in multiparas, tend to be most severe during breastfeeding, and last 2 to 3 days.

Alpha-fetoprotein (AFP) A fetal protein produced in the yolk sac for the first 6 weeks of gestation and then by the fetal liver.

Alternative therapy Any procedure or approach that is used in place of conventional medicine.

Alveolar surface tension The contracting force between alveoli.

Alveoli Small units of the breast tissue in which milk is synthesized by the alveolar secretory epithelium.

Amenorrhea Suppression or absence of menstruation.

Amniocentesis Removal of amniotic fluid by insertion of a needle into the amniotic sac; amniotic fluid is used to assess fetal health or maturity.

Amnioinfusion (AI) Procedure used to infuse a sterile fluid (such as normal saline) through an intrauterine catheter into the uterus in an attempt to increase the fluid around the umbilical cord to decrease or prevent cord compression during labor contractions; also used to dilute thick meconium-stained amniotic fluid.

Amnion The inner of the two membranes that form the sac containing the fetus and the amniotic fluid.

Amniotic fluid The liquid surrounding the fetus in utero. It absorbs shocks, permits fetal movement, and prevents heat loss.

Amniotic fluid embolism An obstetric emergency that occurs when a bolus of amniotic fluid, fetal cells, hair, or other debris enters the maternal circulation and then the maternal lungs; the cause is unknown but has a 60% to 80% mortality rate.

Amniotic fluid index (AFI) A method of reporting fluid volume. The AFI is calculated by dividing the maternal abdomen into four quadrants with the umbilicus as the reference point. Then the deepest vertical pocket is measured. These measurements are summed to calculate the AFI.

Amniotomy (am-nē-ot'ō-mē) The artificial rupturing of the amniotic membrane.

Ampulla The outer two-thirds of the fallopian tube; fertilization of the ovum by a spermatozoon usually occurs here.

Anaphylactoid syndrome of pregnancy See *Amniotic fluid embolism.*

Androgen Substance producing male characteristics, such as the male hormone testosterone.

Android pelvis Male-type pelvis.

Antepartum Time between conception and the onset of labor; usually used to describe the period during which a woman is pregnant.

Anterior fontanelle Diamond-shaped area between the two frontal and two parietal bones just above the newborn's forehead.

Anthropoid pelvis Pelvis in which the anteroposterior diameter is equal to or greater than the transverse diameter.

Apgar score A scoring system used to evaluate newborns at 1 minute and 5 minutes after birth. The total score is achieved by assessing five signs: heart rate, respiratory effort, muscle tone, reflex irritability, and color. Each of the signs is assigned a score of 0, 1, or 2. The highest possible score is 10.

Apnea A condition that occurs when respirations cease for more than 20 seconds, with generalized cyanosis.

Areola Pigmented ring surrounding the nipple of the breast.

Aromatherapy The use of certain essential oils, derived from plants, whose odor or aroma is believed to have a therapeutic effect.

Artificial rupture of membranes (AROM) Use of a device such as an amnihook or allis forceps to rupture the amniotic membranes.

Assimilation Phenomenon in which a minority group completely changes its cultural identity to become part of the majority culture.

Assisted reproductive technology (ART) Term used to describe the highly technologic approaches used to produce pregnancy.

Attachment Enduring bonds or relationship of affection between persons.

Attachment theory A framework for understanding perinatal loss that begins with the basic premise that human beings are biologically predisposed to bond with emotionally significant persons in their lives.

Autosome A chromosome that is not a sex chromosome.

Ayurveda The classical system of Hindu medicine. The term *ayurveda* means the knowledge of how to live a vital, healthful life.

Babinski reflex Reflex found normally in infants under 6 months of age in which the great toe dorsiflexes when the sole of the foot is stimulated.

Bacterial vaginosis (BV) A bacterial infection of the vagina, formerly called *Gardnerella vaginalis* or *Hemophilus vaginalis,* characterized by a foul-smelling, grayish vaginal discharge that exhibits a characteristic fishy odor when 10% potassium hydroxide (KOH) is added. Microscopic examination of a vaginal wet prep reveals the presence of "clue cells" (vaginal epithelial cells coated with gram-negative organisms).

Bag of waters (BOW) The membrane containing the amniotic fluid and the fetus.

Ballottement (bal-ot-maw') A technique of palpation to detect or examine a floating object in the body. In obstetrics, the fetus, when pushed, floats away and then returns to touch the examiner's fingers.

Barlow maneuver A test designed to detect subluxation or dislocation of the hip. A dysplastic joint will be felt to be dislocated as the femur leaves the acetabulum.

Barr body Deeply staining chromatin mass located against the inner surface of the cell nucleus. It is found only in normal females. Also called *sex chromatin.*

Basal body temperature (BBT) The lowest waking temperature.

Baseline fetal heart rate (BL FHR) The average fetal heart rate observed during a 10-minute period of monitoring.

Baseline variability (BL VAR) Changes in the fetal heart rate that result from the interplay between the sympathetic and the parasympathetic nervous systems.

Battledore placenta Placenta in which the umbilical cord is inserted on the periphery rather than centrally.

Becoming a mother (BAM) See *Maternal role attainment.*

Bed sharing An infant sleeping in close social and/or physical contact with a committed caregiver (usually the mother). Also called *cosleeping.*

Bereavement To have suffered the *event* of loss.

Beta human chorionic gonadotropin (beta hCG) A product of the trophoblast or placenta that is detected through serum testing and is a very accurate marker of the presence of pregnancy and placental health.

Bilirubin encephalopathy See *Kernicterus.*

Biofeedback The use of monitoring devices to help individuals learn to control their autonomic responses.

Biophysical profile (BPP) Assessment of five variables in the fetus that help to evaluate fetal risk: breathing movement, body movement, tone, amniotic fluid volume, and fetal heart rate reactivity.

Birth center A setting for labor and birth that emphasizes a family-centered approach rather than obstetric technology and treatment.

Birth defects Structural abnormalities present at birth.

Birth plan A written document prepared by the expectant parents that is used to identify available options in the birth setting and aspects of the childbearing experience that are most important to them.

Birthing room A room for labor and birth with a relaxed atmosphere.

Birth rate Number of live births per 1000 population.

Bishop score A prelabor scoring system to assist in predicting whether an induction of labor may be successful. The total score is achieved by assessing five components: cervical dilatation, cervical effacement, cervical consistency, cervical position, and fetal station. Each of the components is assigned a score of 0 to 3, and the highest possible score is 13.

Blastocyst The inner solid mass of cells within the morula.

Bloody show Pink-tinged mucus secretions resulting from rupture of small capillaries as the cervix effaces and dilates.

Body stalk Future umbilical cord; structure that attaches the embryo to the yolk sac and contains blood vessels that extend into the chorionic villi.

Bogginess The softening of the uterus due to inadequate contraction of the muscle tissue.

Boggy uterus (uterine atony) A term used to describe the uterine fundus when it is not firmly contracted after the birth of the baby and in the early postpartum period; excessive bleeding occurs from the placental site, and maternal hemorrhage may occur.

Bonding Process of parent-infant attachment occurring at or soon after birth.

Brachial palsy Partial or complete paralysis of portions of the arm resulting from trauma to the brachial plexus during a difficult birth.

Brachial plexus injury Injury due to improper or excessive traction applied to the fetal head during birth that results in damage to the network of nerves that send signals from the spine to the shoulder, arm, and hand.

Braxton Hicks contractions Intermittent painless contractions of the uterus that may occur every 10 to 20 minutes. They occur more frequently toward the end of pregnancy and are sometimes mistaken for true labor signs.

Brazelton's neonatal behavioral assessment A brief examination used to identify the infant's behavioral states and responses.

Breasts Mammary glands.

Breast self-examination (BSE) A manual examination conducted monthly by a woman to evaluate her own breasts for signs of masses, changes, nipple discharge, or evidence of abnormalities.

Breech presentation A birth in which the buttocks and/or feet are presented instead of the head.

Broad ligament The ligament extending from the lateral margins of the uterus to the pelvic wall; keeps the uterus centrally placed and provides stability within the pelvic cavity.

Bronchopulmonary dysplasia (BPD)/chronic lung disease (CLD) of prematurity Chronic pulmonary disease of multifactorial etiology characterized initially by alveolar and bronchial necrosis, which results in bronchial metaplasia and interstitial fibrosis. Appears in x-ray films as generalized small, radiolucent cysts within the lungs.

Brown adipose tissue (BAT) Fat deposits in newborns that provide greater heat-generating activity than ordinary fat. Found around the kidneys, adrenals, and neck; between the scapulas; and behind the sternum. Also called *brown fat.*

Calorie (cal) Amount of heat required to raise the temperature of 1 kg of water 1 degree centigrade.

Capacitation Removal of the plasma membrane overlying the spermatozoa's acrosomal area with the loss of seminal plasma proteins and the glycoprotein coat. If the glycoprotein coat is not removed, the sperm will not be able to penetrate the ovum.

Caput succedaneum (kap'ut suk-s''ĕ-dáne-um) Swelling or edema occurring in or under the fetal scalp during labor.

Cardinal ligaments The chief uterine supports, suspending the uterus from the side walls of the true pelvis.

Cardinal movements The positional changes of the fetus as it moves through the birth canal during labor and birth. The positional changes are descent, flexion, internal rotation, extension, restitution, and external rotation. Also called *mechanisms of labor.*

Cardiopulmonary adaptation Adaptation of the newborn's cardiovascular and respiratory systems to life outside the womb.

Caring theory Consists of five attributes of the caregiver: (1) knowing, (2) being with, (3) doing for, (4) enabling, and (5) maintaining belief.

Centering Group prenatal care.

Cephalhematoma (sef′ăl-hé-mă-tōmă) Subcutaneous swelling containing blood found on the head of an infant several days after birth; it usually disappears within a few weeks to 2 months.

Cephalic presentation Birth in which the fetal head is presenting against the cervix.

Cephalopelvic disproportion (CPD) A condition in which the fetal head is of such a shape or size, or in such a position, that it cannot pass through the maternal pelvis.

Cerclage Surgical procedure in which a stitch is placed in the cervix to prevent a spontaneous abortion or premature birth.

Certified nurse-midwife (CNM) An RN who has received special training and education in the care of the family during childbearing and the prenatal, labor and birth, and postpartal periods. After a period of formal education, the nurse-midwife takes a certification test to become a CNM.

Certified registered nurse (RNC) A registered nurse who has shown expertise in a specific field by passing a national certification examination.

Cervical dilatation Process in which the cervical os and the cervical canal widen from less than 1 cm to approximately 10 cm, allowing birth of the fetus.

Cervical funneling A cone-shaped indentation in the cervical os which is common in cases of cervical incompetence.

Cervical insufficiency Painless dilatation of the cervix without contractions because of a structural or functional defect of the cervix. Also called *incompetent cervix.*

Cervical ripening Softening of the cervix; occurs normally as a physiologic process before labor or is stimulated to occur through the process of induction of labor.

Cervix The "neck" between the external os and the body of the uterus. The lower end of the cervix extends into the vagina.

Cesarean birth Birth of fetus accomplished by performing a surgical incision through the maternal abdomen and uterus.

Chadwick's sign Violet bluish color of the vaginal mucous membrane caused by increased vascularity; visible from about the fourth week of pregnancy.

Chemical conjunctivitis Irritation of the mucous membrane lining of the eyelid; may be due to instillation of silver nitrate ophthalmic drops.

Child abuse Nonaccidental physical or threatened harm, including mental or emotional injury, sexual abuse, and sexual exploitation.

Child neglect Failure by parents or other custodians to meet the medical, emotional, physical, or supervisory needs of a child.

Childbearing decisions The decisions parents face about their childbirth preferences and experiences.

Chiropractic The third largest independent health profession found in the United States. Uses spinal manipulation to address abnormal nerve transmission (subluxation) caused by misalignment of the spine.

Chlamydial infection Caused by *Chlamydia trachomatis,* this infection is the most common bacterial sexually transmitted infection in the United States.

Chloasma (klō-az′mă) **(melasma gravidarum)** Brownish pigmentation over the bridge of the nose and the cheeks during pregnancy and in some women who are taking oral contraceptives. Also called *mask of pregnancy.*

Chorioamnionitis (kō′rē-ō-am′nē-ō-nī′tis) An inflammation of the amniotic membranes stimulated by organisms in the amniotic fluid, which then becomes infiltrated with polymorphonuclear leukocytes.

Chorion The fetal membrane closest to the intrauterine wall that gives rise to the placenta and continues as the outer membrane surrounding the amnion.

Chorionic villus sampling (CVS) Procedure in which a specimen of the chorionic villi is obtained from the edge of the developing placenta at about 8 weeks' gestation. The sample can be used for chromosomal, enzyme, and DNA tests.

Chromosomes The threadlike structures within the nucleus of a cell that carry the genes.

Circumcision Surgical removal of the prepuce (foreskin) of the penis.

Circumvallate (ser-kŭm-val′āt) **placenta** A placenta with a thick, white fibrous ring around the edge.

Civil unions Legally recognized partnerships that involve rights and responsibilities comparable with those enjoyed by married couples. Often used by same-sex couples.

Cleavage Rapid mitotic division of the zygote; cells produced are called *blastomeres.*

Climacteric The period of time that marks the cessation of a woman's reproductive function; the "change of life," or menopause.

Clinical nurse specialist (CNS) A nurse possessing a master's degree and specialized knowledge and competence in a specific clinical area.

Clitoris Female organ homologous to the male penis; a small oval body of erectile tissue situated at the anterior junction of the vulva.

Coitus interruptus Method of contraception in which the male withdraws his penis from the vagina before ejaculation.

Cold stress Excessive heat loss resulting in compensatory mechanisms (increased respirations and nonshivering thermogenesis) to maintain core body temperature.

Colostrum (kō-los′trŭm) Secretion from the breast before the onset of true lactation; contains mainly serum and white blood corpuscles. It has a high protein content, provides some immune properties, and cleanses the newborn's intestinal tract of mucus and meconium.

Colposcopy The use of an instrument inserted into the vagina to examine the cervical and vaginal tissues by means of a magnifying lens.

Combined oral contraceptives (COCs) Commonly called birth control pills or "the pill," COCs are a form of contraception that uses a combination of a synthetic estrogen and a progestin.

Comparable worth The standard that the same wages should be paid for different types of work that require comparable skills, responsibility, education, and experience.

Complementary and alternative medicine (CAM) A group of diverse medical and healthcare systems, practices, and products that are not generally considered part of conventional medicine.

Complementary therapy Any procedure or product that is used together with conventional medical treatment.

Conception Union of male sperm and female ovum; fertilization.

Condoms Rubber sheaths that cover men's penises to prevent conception or disease.

Conduction Loss of heat to a cooler surface by direct skin contact.

Condylomata acuminata Known also as genital or venereal warts, they are a common sexually transmitted infection caused by the human papilloma virus (HPV).

Condylomata lata Wartlike growth of skin, usually seen on the external genitals or anus. There are two types, a pointed variety and a broad, flat form usually found with syphilis.

Conjugate Important diameter of the pelvis, measured from the center of the promontory of the sacrum to the back of the symphysis pubis. The diagonal conjugate is measured and the true conjugate is estimated.

Conjugate vera The true conjugate, which extends from the middle of the sacral promontory to the middle of the pubic crest.

Contraception The prevention of conception or impregnation.

Contraction Tightening and shortening of the uterine muscles during labor, causing effacement and dilatation of the cervix; contributes to the downward and outward descent of the fetus.

Contraction stress test (CST) A method of assessing the reaction of the fetus to the stress of uterine contractions. This test may be utilized when contractions are occurring spontaneously or when contractions are artificially induced by oxytocin challenge test (OCT) or breast self-stimulation test (BSST).

Convection Loss of heat from the warm body surface to cooler air currents.

Coombs' (kōōmz) **test** A test for antiglobulins in the red cells. The indirect test determines the presence of Rh-positive antibodies in maternal blood; the direct test determines the presence of maternal Rh-positive antibodies in fetal cord blood.

Cordocentesis Also called percutaneous umbilical blood sampling (PUBS), a technique used to obtain pure fetal blood from the umbilical cord while the fetus is in utero, which is used for diagnosis of hemophilias, hemoglobinopathies, fetal infections, chromosome abnormalities, nonimmune hydrops, and isoimmune hemolytic disorders, as well as assessment of fetal hemoglobin and hematocrit for calculation of transfusion requirements in the second and third trimesters.

Cornua The elongated portions of the uterus where the fallopian tubes open.

Corpus The upper two thirds of the uterus.

Corpus luteum A small yellow body that develops within a ruptured ovarian follicle; it secretes progesterone in the second half of the menstrual cycle and atrophies about 3 days before the beginning of menstrual flow. If pregnancy occurs, the corpus luteum continues to produce progesterone until the placenta takes over this function.

Cosleeping An infant sleeping in close social and/or physical contact with a committed caregiver (usually the mother).

Cotyledon (kot-i-lē′don) One of the rounded portions into which the placenta's uterine surface is divided, consisting of a mass of villi, fetal vessels, and an intervillous space.

Couplet care A family-centered approach for maternal-child nursing where both the mother and her baby are cared for by the same nurse, with the baby remaining at the mother's bedside. Also called mother-baby care.

Couvade (kū-vahd′) In some cultures, the male's observance of certain rituals and taboos to signify the transition to fatherhood.

Crack A form of freebase cocaine that is smoked.

Crisis intervention Actions taken by the nurse to help the client deal with an impending, potentially overwhelming crisis; regain his or her equilibrium; grow from the experience; and improve coping skills.

Critical thinking Intellectual processes that include separating fact from opinion, identifying prejudices and stereotypes that may influence interpretation of information, exploring differing ideas and views, and arriving at conclusions or insights.

Crowning Appearance of the presenting fetal part at the vaginal orifice during labor.

Crying state A state in the infant sleep-awake cycle in which the infant exhibits increased motor activity, grimaces, eyes that are tightly closed or open, and extreme responsiveness to stimuli.

Cultural beliefs Those beliefs that reflect the predominating values, attitudes, and practices accepted by a population, community, or ethnic group.

Cultural competency Referring to the skills and knowledge necessary to appreciate, understand, and work with individuals from different cultures.

Culture The beliefs, values, attitudes, and practices that are accepted by a population, community, or an individual.

Cycle of violence A theory that postulates that battering takes place in a cyclic fashion through three phases: the tension-building phase, the acute battering incident, and the tranquil phase (honeymoon period).

Cystocele The downward displacement of the bladder, which appears as a bulge in the anterior vaginal wall.

Deceleration Periodic decrease in the baseline fetal heart rate.

Decidua (dē-sid′yū-ă) Endometrium or mucous membrane lining of the uterus in pregnancy that is shed after childbirth.

Decidua basalis The part of the decidua that unites with the chorion to form the placenta. It is shed in lochial discharge after childbirth.

Decidua capsularis The part of the decidua surrounding the chorionic sac.

Decidua vera (parietalis) Nonplacental decidua lining the uterus.

Decrement Decrease or stage of decline, as of a contraction.

Deep sleep State of sleep in which the infant will be nearly still except for occasional startles, twitches, and sucking.

Depo-Provera A long-acting, injectable progestin contraceptive.

Descriptive statistics Statistics that describe or summarize a set of data.

Diagonal conjugate Distance from the lower posterior border of the symphysis pubis to the sacral promontory; may be obtained by manual measurement.

Diaphragm A flexible disk that covers the cervix to prevent pregnancy.

Diastasis (dī-as′tă-sis) **recti** (rek′ti) **abdominis** Separation of the recti abdominis muscles along the median line. In women, it is seen with repeated childbirths or multiple gestations. In the newborn, it is usually caused by incomplete development.

Dietary reference intakes (DRIs) Specific allowances for pregnant and lactating women, DRIs are subdivided into the recommended dietary allowance (RDA) and adequate intake (AI).

Dilation and curettage (D&C) Stretching of the cervical canal to permit passage of a curette, which is used to scrape the endometrium to empty the uterine contents or to obtain tissue for examination.

Dilatation of the cervix Expansion of the external os from an opening a few millimeters in size to an opening large enough to allow the passage of the infant.

Diploid number of chromosomes Containing a set of maternal and a set of paternal chromosomes; in humans, the diploid number of chromosomes is 46.

Disability Impairment in one or more of five function categories: cognition, communication, motor abilities, social abilities, or patterns of interactions.

Disassociation relaxation A pattern of active relaxation in which the woman learns to tighten one area of the body and then relax other areas simultaneously. This relaxation pattern is very effective for some women during labor.

Disenfranchised grief Grief that is not supported by the usual societal customs.

Domestic partnership A mechanism by which public and private employers can provide insurance coverage and pension-rights benefits to the partners of gay and lesbian employees.

Domestic violence Defined as the collective methods used to exert power and control by one individual over another in an adult intimate relationship. Forms of abuse typically fall into three categories: psychologic abuse, physical abuse, and sexual abuse.

Doula A supportive companion who accompanies a laboring woman to provide emotional, physical, and informational support and acts as an advocate for the woman and her family.

Down syndrome An abnormality resulting from the presence of an extra chromosome number 21 (trisomy 21); characteristics include mental retardation and altered physical appearance. Formerly called ***mongolism.***

Drowsy awake state A state in the infant sleep-wake cycle that occurs between light sleep and the quiet alert state. It is marked by infants opening and closing their eyes, but the eyes appear glazed and the face is often still. They may return to sleep or awaken further in response to stimuli.

Drug-exposed infant The newborn of an alcoholic or drug-addicted woman.

Dual process model A view of grief encompassing two competing facets: loss and restoration. The loss orientation is concerned with the individual's need to confront the reality of the loss, and the restoration orientation seeks to regain balance and temper the pain of grief.

Dubowitz tool A clinical gestational age assessment tool.

Ductus arteriosus A communication channel between the main pulmonary artery and the aorta of the fetus. It is obliterated after birth by rising PO_2 and changes in intravascular pressure in the presence of normal pulmonary functioning. It normally becomes a ligament after birth but sometimes remains patent (patent ductus arteriosus, a treatable condition).

Ductus venosus A fetal blood vessel that carries oxygenated blood between the umbilical vein and the inferior vena cava, bypassing the liver; it becomes a ligament after birth.

Duncan's mechanism Occurs when the maternal surface of the placenta rather than the shiny fetal surface presents upon birth.

Duration The time length of each contraction, measured from the beginning of the increment to the completion of the decrement.

Dysfunctional uterine bleeding (DUB) A condition characterized by anovulatory cycles with abnormal uterine bleeding that does not have a demonstrable organic cause.

Dysmenorrhea Painful menstruation.

Dyspareunia Painful intercourse.

Dystocia (dis-tō′sē-ă) Difficult labor due to mechanical factors produced by the fetus or the maternal pelvis or due to inadequate uterine or other muscular activity.

Early adolescence A term referring to adolescents who are age 14 and under.

Early decelerations Periodic change in fetal heart rate pattern caused by head compression; deceleration has a uniform appearance and early onset in relation to maternal contraction.

Early (primary) postpartum hemorrhage See *Postpartum hemorrhage.*

Eclampsia (ek-lamp′sē-ă) A major complication of pregnancy. Its cause is unknown; it occurs more often in the primigravida and is accompanied by elevated blood pressure, albuminuria, oliguria, tonic and clonic convulsions, and coma. It may occur during pregnancy (usually after the 20th week of gestation) or within 48 hours after childbirth.

Ectoderm Outer layer of cells in the developing embryo that gives rise to the skin, nails, and hair.

Ectopic pregnancy Implantation of the fertilized ovum outside the uterine cavity; common sites are the abdomen, fallopian tubes, and ovaries. Also called *oocyesis.*

Effacement Thinning and shortening of the cervix that occurs late in pregnancy or during labor.

Effleurage (e-fler-ahz′) A light stroking movement of the fingertips over the abdominal area during labor; used to provide distraction during labor contractions.

Ejaculation Expulsion of the seminal fluids from the penis.

Elder abuse Any deliberate action or lack of action that causes harm to an elderly person.

Electronic fetal monitoring (EFM) A method of placing a fetal monitor on the fetus in order to obtain a continuous tracing of the FHR, which allows many characteristics of the fetal heart rate to be observed and evaluated.

Emancipated minors Minors who are legally considered to have assumed the rights of an adult. An adolescent may be considered emancipated if he or she is self-supporting and living away from home, married, pregnant, a parent, or in the military.

Embryo The early stage of development of the young of any organism. In humans the embryonic period is from about 2 to 8 weeks' gestation and is characterized by cellular differentiation and predominantly hyperplastic growth.

Embryonic membranes The amnion and chorion.

Endoderm The inner layer of cells in the developing embryo that give rise to internal organs such as the intestines.

Endometrial biopsy (EMB) Procedure providing information about the effects of progesterone produced by the corpus luteum after ovulation and endometrial receptivity.

Endometriosis Ectopic endometrium located outside the uterus in the pelvic cavity. Symptoms may include pelvic pain or pressure, dysmenorrhea, dispareunia, abnormal bleeding from the uterus or rectum, and sterility.

Endometritis (metritis) Infection of the endometrium.

Endometrium (en′dō-mē′trē-ŭm) The mucous membrane that lines the inner surface of the uterus.

En face An assumed position in which one person looks at another and maintains his or her face in the same vertical plane as that of the other.

Engagement The entrance of the fetal presenting part into the superior pelvic strait and the beginning of the descent through the pelvic canal.

Engorgement Vascular congestion or distention. In obstetrics, the swelling of breast tissue brought about by an increase in blood and lymph supply to the breast, preceding true lactation.

Engrossment Characteristic sense of absorption, preoccupation, and interest in the infant demonstrated by fathers during early contact with their infants.

Environmental toxins Chemical compounds found in air, food, and water, whose bioaccumulation can lead to adverse health effects.

Epidural block Regional anesthesia effective through the first and second stages of labor.

Episiotomy (ĕ-piz-ē-ot′o-mē) Incision of the perineum to facilitate birth and to avoid laceration of the perineum.

Epstein's (ep′stīnz) **pearls** Small, white blebs found along the gum margins and at the junction of the hard and soft palates; commonly seen in the newborn as a normal manifestation.

Erb-Duchenne paralysis (Erb's palsy) Paralysis of the arm and chest wall as a result of a birth injury to the brachial plexus or a subsequent injury to the fifth and sixth cervical nerves.

Erythema toxicum Innocuous pink papular rash of unknown cause with superimposed vesicles; it appears within 24 to 48 hours after birth and resolves spontaneously within a few days.

Erythroblastosis fetalis Hemolytic disease of the newborn characterized by anemia, jaundice, enlargement of the liver and spleen, and generalized edema. Caused by isoimmunization due to Rh incompatibility or ABO incompatibility.

Essure Method of permanent sterilization that requires no surgical incision. Under hysteroscopy, a stainless steel micro-insert is placed into each proximal section of the fallopian tube.

Estimated date of birth (EDB) During a pregnancy, the approximate date when childbirth will occur; the "due date."

Estrogens The hormones estradiol and estrone, produced by the ovary.

Ethnicity A social identity that is associated with shared beliefs, behaviors, and patterns.

Ethnocentrism An individual's belief that the values and practices of his or her own culture are the best ones.

Euphemism A substituted word or expression with a more pleasant association than the one which, although more direct, is considered to be harsher.

Evaporation Loss of heat incurred when water on the skin surface is converted to a vapor.

Evidence-based practice An approach to problem solving and decision making based on the consideration of data from research, statistical analysis, quality measures, risk management measurements, and other sources of reliable information.

Exchange transfusion The replacement of 70% to 80% of circulating blood by withdrawing the recipient's blood and injecting a donor's blood in equal amounts, for the purpose of preventing the accumulation of bilirubin or other by-products of hemolysis in the blood.

External cephalic version (ECV) Procedure involving external manipulation of the maternal abdomen to change the presentation of the fetus from breech to cephalic.

External os The opening between the cervix and the vagina.

Fallopian tubes Tubes that extend from the lateral angle of the uterus and terminate near the ovary; they serve as a passageway for the ovum from the ovary to the uterus and for the spermatozoa from the uterus toward the ovary. Also called *oviducts* and *uterine tubes*.

False labor Contractions of the uterus, regular or irregular, that may be strong enough to be interpreted as true labor but that do not dilate the cervix.

False pelvis The portion of the pelvis above the linea terminalis; its primary function is to support the weight of the enlarged pregnant uterus.

Family Two or more persons who are joined together by bonds of sharing and emotional closeness and who identify themselves as being part of a family.

Family assessment The process by which a nurse collects data regarding a family's current level of functioning, support systems, sociocultural influences, home and work environment, type of family, family structure, and needs.

Family-centered care An approach to health care based on the concept that a hospital can provide professional services to mothers, fathers, and infants in a homelike environment that would enhance the integrity of the family unit.

Family development The changes that families experience over time, including changes in relationships, communication patterns, roles, and interactions.

Family planning Actions an individual or a couple take to avoid a pregnancy, to space future pregnancies for a specific reason, or to gain control over the number of children conceived.

Family power The individual who has either the potential or actual ability to change the behavior of other family members.

Family roles The specific roles of individuals within a family unit. Examples of roles include breadwinner, homemaker, mother, father, social planner, and family peacemaker.

Family values A system of ideas, attitudes, and beliefs about the worth of an entity or a concept that consciously or unconsciously bind together the members of the family in a common culture.

Fecundability The ability to become pregnant.

Female condom A thin, disposable polyurethane sheath with a flexible ring at each end that is placed inside the vagina and serves to prevent sperm from entering the cervix, thus preventing conception.

Female genital mutilation (FGM) Also known as *female genital cutting, female circumcision,* and *genital circumcision,* the practice of removing all or parts of a girl's or woman's genitalia for cultural reasons.

Female reproductive cycle (FRC) The monthly rhythmic changes in sexually mature women.

Feminization of later life Worldwide trend for women to comprise a majority of the elderly population.

Feminization of poverty Term used to describe the fact that, in the United States, women comprise a majority of the adult poor.

Ferning capacity Formation of a palm-leaf pattern by the crystallization of cervical mucus as it dries at mid-menstrual cycle. The formation can be helpful in determining time of ovulation. Observed via microscopic examination of a thin layer of cervical mucus on a glass slide. This pattern is also observed when amniotic fluid is allowed to air dry on a slide and is a useful and quick test to determine whether amniotic membranes have ruptured.

Fertility awareness-based (FAB) methods Also known as natural family planning, fertility awareness-based methods are founded on an understanding of the changes that occur throughout a woman's ovulatory cycle. All these methods require periods of abstinence and recording of certain events throughout the cycle; cooperation of the partner is important.

Fertilization Impregnation of an ovum by a spermatozoon; conception.

Fetal acoustic stimulation test (FAST) A fetal assessment test that uses sound from a speaker, bell, or artificial larynx to stimulate acceleration of the fetal heart; may be used in conjunction with the nonstress test.

Fetal alcohol spectrum disorder (FASD) An umbrella term that includes all categories of prenatal alcohol exposure, including fetal alcohol syndrome (FAS); it is not meant to be used as a clinical diagnosis.

Fetal alcohol syndrome (FAS) Syndrome caused by maternal alcohol ingestion and characterized by microcephaly, intrauterine growth restriction, short palpebral fissures, and maxillary hypoplasia.

Fetal attitude Relationship of the fetal parts to one another. Normal fetal attitude is one of moderate flexion of the arms onto the chest and flexion of the legs onto the abdomen.

Fetal blood sampling Blood sample drawn from the fetal scalp (or from the fetus in breech position) to evaluate the acid–base status of the fetus.

Fetal bradycardia A fetal heart rate less than 120 beats per minute during a 10-minute period of continuous monitoring.

Fetal breathing movements (FBM) Intrauterine practice respiratory movements that begin around the 17th to 20th week of gestation.

Fetal death Death of the developing fetus after 20 weeks' gestation. Also called *fetal demise*.

Fetal fibronectin (fFN) A glycoprotein that is produced by the trophoblast and fetal tissues whose presence between 20 and 34 weeks' gestation is a strong predictor of preterm birth associated with preterm spontaneous rupture of membranes.

Fetal heart rate (FHR) The number of times the fetal heart beats per minute; normal range is 120 to 160.

Fetal lie Relationship of the cephalocaudal axis (spinal column) of the fetus to the cephalocaudal axis (spinal column) of the woman. The fetus may be in a longitudinal or transverse lie.

Fetal movement record (FMR) A method for tracking fetal activity taught to pregnant women.

Fetal position Relationship of the landmark on the presenting fetal part to the front, sides, or back of the maternal pelvis.

Fetal presentation The fetal body part that enters the maternal pelvis first. The three possible presentations are cephalic, shoulder, and breech.

Fetal tachycardia A fetal heart rate of 160 beats per minute or more during a 10-minute period of continuous monitoring.

Fetoscope An adaptation of a stethoscope that facilitates auscultation of the fetal heart rate.

Fetus The child in utero from about the seventh to ninth week of gestation until birth.

Fibrocystic breast changes Benign breast changes characterized by bilateral, cyclic breast pain and breast nodularities that may be unilateral or bilateral, and often in the upper outer quadrants of the breasts.

Fibrocystic breast disease Benign breast disorder characterized by a thickening of normal breast tissue and the formation of cysts.

Fimbria Any structure resembling a fringe; the fringelike extremity of the fallopian tubes.

Folic acid An important vitamin directly related to the outcome of pregnancy and to maternal and fetal health.

Follicle-stimulating hormone (FSH) Hormone produced by the anterior pituitary during the first half of the menstrual cycle, stimulating development of the graafian follicle.

Fontanelle (fon′tă-nel′) In the fetus, an unossified space, or soft spot, consisting of a strong band of connective tissue lying between the cranial bones of the skull.

Foramen ovale Special opening between the atria of the fetal heart. Normally, the opening closes shortly after birth; if it remains open, it can be repaired surgically.

Forceps Obstetric instrument occasionally used to aid in childbirth.

Forceps-assisted birth A birth in which a set of instruments, known as forceps, are applied to the presenting part of the fetus to provide traction or to enable the fetal head to be rotated to an occiput-anterior position. Forceps-assisted birth is also known as *instrumental delivery, operative delivery,* or *operative vaginal delivery.*

Forceps marks Reddened areas over the cheeks and jaws caused by the application of forceps. The red areas usually disappear within 1 to 2 days.

Foremilk Breast milk obtained at the beginning of the breastfeeding episode.

Frequency The time between the beginning of one contraction and the beginning of the next contraction.

Functional residual capacity (FRC) The amount of air remaining in the lungs at the end of a normal expiration.

Fundus The upper portion of the uterus between the fallopian tubes.

Galactorrhea Nipple discharge.

Gamete (gam′ēt) Female or male germ cell; contains a haploid number of chromosomes.

Gamete intrafallopian transfer (GIFT) Retrieval of oocytes by laparoscopy; immediately combining oocytes with washed, motile sperm in a catheter; and placement of the gametes into the fimbriated end of the fallopian tube.

Gametogenesis The process by which germ cells are produced.

General anesthesia A state of induced unconsciousness that may be achieved through intravenous injection, inhalation of anesthetic agents, or a combination of both methods.

Genotype The genetic composition of an individual.

Gestation (jes-tā′shŭn) Period of intrauterine development from conception through birth; pregnancy.

Gestational age The number of complete weeks of fetal development, calculated from the first day of the last normal menstrual cycle.

Gestational age assessment tools Systems used to evaluate the newborn's external physical characteristics and neurologic and/or neuromuscular development to accurately determine gestational age. These replace or supplement the traditional calculation from the woman's last menstrual period.

Gestational diabetes mellitus (GDM) A form of diabetes of variable severity with onset or first recognition during pregnancy.

Gestational trophoblastic disease (GTD) Disorder classified into two types: benign (hydatidiform mole) and malignant.

Gonadotropin-releasing hormone (GnRH) A hormone secreted by the hypothalamus that stimulates the anterior pituitary to secrete FSH and LH.

Gonadotropins Hormones that stimulate the gonads (ovaries in women or testes in men).

Gonorrhea A sexually transmitted infection caused by the bacterium *Neisseria gonorrhoeae.*

Goodell's sign Softening of the cervix that occurs during the second month of pregnancy.

Graafian follicle The ovarian cyst containing the ripe ovum; it secretes estrogens.

Grasping reflex Normal newborn reflex elicited by stimulating the palm with a finger or object, resulting in newborn firmly holding on to the finger or object.

Gravida (grav′i-dă) A pregnant woman.

Grief An individual's *reaction* to loss, including physical symptoms, thoughts, feelings, functional limitations, and spiritual responses.

Grief work The inner process of working through or managing the bereavement.

Guided imagery A state of intense, focused concentration used to create compelling mental images. It is sometimes considered a form of hypnosis.

Gynecoid pelvis Typical female pelvis in which the inlet is round instead of oval.

Habituation (ha-bit-chū-ā′shŭn) Infant's ability to diminish innate responses to specific repeated stimuli.

Haploid number of chromosomes Half the diploid number of chromosomes. In humans there are 23 chromosomes, the haploid number, in each germ cell.

Harlequin sign A rare color change that occurs between the longitudinal halves of the newborn's body, such that the dependent half is noticeably pinker than the superior half when the newborn is placed on one side; it is of no pathologic significance.

Hatha yoga The physical branch of yoga; in the United States, it is commonly practiced for wellness, illness prevention, and healing.

Hegar's sign A softening of the lower uterine segment found upon palpation in the second or third month of pregnancy.

HELLP syndrome A cluster of changes including ***h***emolysis, ***e***levated ***l***iver enzymes, and ***l***ow ***p***latelet count; sometimes associated with severe preeclampsia.

Hemolytic disease of the newborn *Hyperbilirubinemia* secondary to Rh incompatibility.

Herpes genitalis A lifelong, recurrent sexually transmitted infection caused by the herpes simplex virus (HSV).

Heterozygous A genotypic situation in which two different alleles occur at a given locus on a pair of homologous chromosomes.

Hindmilk Breast milk released after initial let-down reflex; high in fat content.

Homeopathy Term derived from the Greek word *homos,* meaning "the same," and describing a healing system that uses as remedies minute dilutions of substances that, if ingested in larger amounts, would produce effects *similar* to the symptoms of the disorder being treated.

Homozygous A genotypic situation in which two similar genes occur at a given locus on homologous chromosomes.

Hormone therapy (HT) Administration of hormones, usually estrogen and a progestin, to alleviate the symptoms of menopause.

Hospital disposition The incineration at regular intervals of a dead fetus or infant's body, usually with other body parts.

Human chorionic gonadotropin (hCG) A hormone produced by the chorionic villi and found in the urine of pregnant women. Also called *prolan.*

Human immunodeficiency virus (HIV) A virus that causes a progressive disease that ultimately results in the development of *acquired immunodeficiency syndrome (AIDS).*

Human placental lactogen (hPL) A hormone synthesized by the syncytiotrophoblast that functions as an insulin antagonist and promotes lipolysis to increase the amounts of circulating free fatty acids available for maternal metabolic use.

Hydatidiform (hī-da-tid′i-form) **mole** Degenerative process in chorionic villi, giving rise to multiple cysts and rapid growth of the uterus, with hemorrhage.

Hydramnios (hī-dram′nē-os) An excess of amniotic fluid, leading to overdistention of the uterus. Frequently seen in diabetic pregnant women, even if there is no coexisting fetal anomaly. Also called *polyhydramnios.*

Hydrops fetalis See *Erythroblastosis fetalis.*

Hydrotherapy Type of therapy that makes use of hot or cold moisture in any form. Hydrotherapy is used to relax muscles, promote rest, decrease pain, reduce swelling, promote healing, cleanse wounds and burns, reduce fever, lessen cramps, and improve well-being.

Hyperbilirubinemia (hī-per-bil′i-rū-bi-nē′mē-ă) Excessive amount of bilirubin in the blood; indicative of hemolytic processes due to blood incompatibility, intrauterine infection, septicemia, neonatal renal infection, and other disorders.

Hyperemesis gravidarum Excessive vomiting during pregnancy, leading to dehydration and starvation.

Hyperventilation Rapid breathing that occurs over a prolonged period of time resulting in an imbalance of oxygen and carbon dioxide that can result in tingling or numbness in the tip of nose, lips, fingers, or toes; dizziness; spots before the eyes; or spasms of the hands or feet (carpal-pedal spasms).

Hypnosis Whether guided by a trained hypnotherapist or self-induced, a state of great mental and physical relaxation during which a person is very open to suggestions.

Hypoglycemia Abnormally low level of sugar in the blood.

Hysterectomy Surgical removal of the uterus.

Hysterosalpingography (HSG) Testing by instillation of radiopaque substance into the uterine cavity to visualize the uterus and fallopian tubes.

Hysteroscopy Use of a special endoscope to examine the uterus.

Implanon (subdermal implant) A single-capsule implant inserted subdermally in the woman's upper underarm; it is impregnated with etonogestrel, a progestin, which prevents ovulation, and is effective as a contraceptive method for 3 years.

Inborn error of metabolism A hereditary deficiency of a specific enzyme needed for normal metabolism of specific chemicals.

Incompetent cervix See *Cervical insufficiency.*

Increment Increase or addition; to build up, as of a contraction.

Induction of labor The process of causing or initiating labor by use of medication or surgical rupture of membranes.

Infant A child under 1 year of age.

Infant mortality rate Number of deaths of infants under 1 year of age per 1000 live births in a given population per year.

Infant of diabetic mother (IDM) At-risk infant born to a woman previously diagnosed as diabetic or who develops symptoms of diabetes during pregnancy.

Infant of substance-abusing mother (ISAM) Formerly called infant of an addicted mother, an infant born to a mother who abuses or is addicted to drugs or alcohol.

Inferential statistics Statistics that allow an investigator to draw conclusions about what is happening between two or more variables in a population and to suggest or refute causal relationships between them.

Infertility Diminished ability to conceive.

Informed consent A legal concept that protects a person's rights to autonomy and self-determination by specifying that no action may be taken without that person's prior understanding and freely given consent.

Infundibulopelvic ligament Ligament that suspends and supports the ovaries.

Instrumental style of coping A style of coping by which persons generally use more cognitive skills to navigate loss and value care that includes an emphasis on problem solving.

Integrative medicine An approach that combines mainstream medical therapies with complementary therapies for which there is some high-quality scientific evidence of safety and effectiveness.

Intellectual disability The most common type of developmental disability; formerly called *mental retardation.*

Intensity The strength of a uterine contraction during acme.

Internal os An inside mouth or opening; the opening between the cervix and the uterus.

Internal version Procedure used for the vaginal birth of a second twin. The obstetrician inserts a hand into the uterus, grasps the feet of the fetus, and changes the fetus from a transverse to a breech presentation. Also called *podalic version.*

Intrapartum The time from the onset of true labor until the birth of the infant and expulsion of the placenta.

Intrauterine device (IUD) Small metal or plastic form that is placed in the uterus to prevent implantation of a fertilized ovum.

Intrauterine fetal surgery Surgery performed on a fetus to correct anatomic lesions that are not compatible with life if left untreated.

Intrauterine growth restriction (IUGR) Fetal undergrowth due to any etiology, such as intrauterine infection, deficient nutrient supply, or congenital malformation. A term used to describe fetuses falling below the 10th percentile in ultrasonic estimation of weight at a given gestational age.

Intrauterine pressure catheter (IUPC) A catheter that can be placed through the cervix into the uterus to measure uterine pressure during labor. Some types of catheters may be inserted for the purpose of infusing warmed saline to add additional intrauterine fluid when oligohydramnios is present.

Introitus Opening or entrance into a cavity or canal such as the vagina.

Intuitive style of coping A style of coping by which persons generally feel their way through loss and prefer care with an emphasis on emotional and psychosocial support.

In vitro fertilization (IVF) Procedure during which oocytes are removed from the ovary, mixed with spermatozoa, fertilized, and incubated in a glass petri dish; then up to four viable embryos are placed in the woman's uterus.

Involution Rolling or turning inward; the reduction in size of the uterus following childbirth.

Ischial spines Prominences that arise near the junction of the ilium and ischium and jut into the pelvic cavity; used as a reference point during labor to evaluate the descent of the fetal head into the birth canal.

Isthmus The straight, narrow part of the fallopian tube with a thick muscular wall and an opening (lumen) 2 to 3 mm in diameter; the site of tubal ligation. Also, a constriction in the uterus that is located above the cervix and below the corpus.

Jaundice Yellow pigmentation of body tissues caused by the presence of bile pigments. See also *Physiologic jaundice.*

Karyotype The set of chromosomes arranged in a standard order.

Kegel exercises Perineal muscle tightening that strengthens the pubococcygeus muscle and increases its tone.

Kernicterus (ker-nik′ter-ŭs) An encephalopathy caused by deposition of unconjugated bilirubin in brain cells; may result in impaired brain function or death.

Kilocalorie (kcal) Equivalent to 1000 calories, it is the unit used to express the energy value of food.

Klinefelter syndrome A chromosomal abnormality caused by the presence of an extra X chromosome in the male. Characteristics include tall stature; sparse pubic and facial hair; gynecomastia; small, firm testes; and absence of spermatogenesis.

Labor The process by which the fetus is expelled from the maternal uterus. Also called *childbirth, confinement,* or *parturition.*

Labor augmentation The stimulation of uterine contractions when spontaneous contractions have failed to result in progressive cervical dilation or descent of the fetus.

Labor induction The stimulation of uterine contractions before the spontaneous onset of labor, with or without ruptured fetal membranes, for the purpose of accomplishing birth.

Labor support The emotional, physical, and informational support of the woman during childbirth.

Lactase deficiency (lactose intolerance) A condition characterized by difficulty digesting milk and dairy products. Results from an inadequate amount of the enzyme lactase, which breaks down the milk sugar lactose into smaller digestible substances.

Lactation The process of producing and supplying breast milk.

Lacto-ovovegetarians Vegetarians who include milk, dairy products, and eggs in their diets and occasionally fish, poultry, and liver.

Lactose intolerance A condition in which an individual has difficulty digesting milk and milk products.

Lactovegetarians Vegetarians who include dairy products but no eggs in their diets.

La Leche League International (LLLI) Organization that provides information on and assistance with breastfeeding.

Lamaze method A method of childbirth preparation.

Lanugo (lă-nū'gō) Fine, downy hair found on all body parts of the fetus, with the exception of the palms of the hands and the soles of the feet, after 20 weeks' gestation.

Laparoscopy Procedure that enables direct visualization of pelvic organs.

Large for gestational age (LGA) Excessive growth of a fetus in relation to the gestational time period.

Last menstrual period (LMP) The last normal menstrual period experienced by the woman before pregnancy; sometimes used to calculate the infant's gestational age.

Late adolescence A term referring to adolescents who are ages 18 to 19 years.

Late decelerations Symmetrical decrease in fetal heart rate beginning at or after the peak of the contraction and returning to baseline only after the contraction has ended, indicating possible uteroplacental insufficiency and potential that the fetus is not receiving adequate oxygenation.

Late preterm infant An infant born between 34 and 37 weeks of gestation.

Late (secondary) postpartum hemorrhage See *Postpartum hemorrhage.*

Lecithin/sphingomyelin (les'i-thin sfing'gō-mī'ĕ-lin) **(L/S) ratio** Lecithin and sphingomyelin are phospholipid components of surfactant; their ratio changes during gestation. When the L/S ratio reaches 2:1, the fetal lungs are thought to be mature and the fetus will have a low risk of respiratory distress syndrome (RDS) if born at that time.

Leiomyoma A benign tumor of the uterus, composed primarily of smooth muscle and connective tissue. Also referred to as a *myoma* or a *fibroid.*

Leopold's maneuvers A series of four maneuvers designed to provide a systematic approach whereby the examiner may determine fetal presentation and position.

Let-down reflex Pattern of stimulation, hormone release, and resulting muscle contraction that forces milk into the lactiferous ducts, making it available to the infant. Also called *milk ejection reflex.*

Leukorrhea Mucous discharge from the vagina or cervical canal that may be normal or pathologic, as in the presence of infection.

Lightening Moving of the fetus and uterus downward into the pelvic cavity.

Light sleep State that makes up the highest proportion of newborn sleep and precedes awakening; characterized by some body movements, rapid eye movements (REM), and brief fussing or crying.

Linea nigra (lin'ē-ă ni'gră) The line of darker pigmentation extending from the umbilicus to the pubis noted in some women during the later months of pregnancy.

Local anesthesia Injection of an anesthetic agent into the subcutaneous tissue in a fanlike pattern.

Lochia (lō'kē-ă) Maternal discharge of blood, mucus, and tissue from the uterus; may last for several weeks after birth.

Lochia alba White vaginal discharge that follows lochia serosa and that lasts from about the 10th to the 21st day after birth.

Lochia rubra Red, blood-tinged vaginal discharge that occurs following birth and lasts 2 to 4 days.

Lochia serosa Pink, serous, and blood-tinged vaginal discharge that follows lochia rubra and lasts until the 7th to 10th day after birth.

Lung compliance The ease with which the lung is able to fill with air.

Luteinizing hormone (LH) Anterior pituitary hormone responsible for stimulating ovulation and for development of the corpus luteum.

Maceration The process of tissue breakdown that begins from the moment of death.

Macrosomia (mak-rō-sō'mē-ă) A condition seen in newborns of large body size and high birth weight (more than 4000 to 4500 g [8 lb, 13 oz to 9 lb, 14 oz]), such as those born of prediabetic and diabetic mothers.

Malposition An abnormal position of the fetus in the birth canal.

Malpresentation A presentation of the fetus into the birth canal that is not "normal"—that is, brow, face, shoulder, or breech presentation.

Mammogram A soft-tissue radiograph of the breast without the injection of a contrast medium.

Massage therapy Manipulation of the soft tissues of the body to reduce stress and tension, increase circulation, diminish pain, and promote a sense of well-being.

Mastitis Inflammation of the breast.

Maternal mortality rate The number of maternal deaths from any cause during the pregnancy cycle per 100,000 live births.

Maternal role attainment (MRA) Process by which a woman learns mothering behaviors and becomes comfortable with her identity as a mother.

Maternal serum alpha-fetoprotein (MSAFP) Screening test performed between 16 and 22 gestational weeks that utilizes the multiple markers (the "triple screen") of alpha-fetoprotein (AFP), human chorionic growth hormone (hCG), and urine estriol (uE3) to screen pregnancies for neural tube defect, Down syndrome, and trisomy 18.

Mature milk Breast milk that contains 10% solids for energy and growth.

McDonald's sign A probable sign of pregnancy characterized by an ease in flexing the body of the uterus against the cervix.

Meaning reconstruction A framework for understanding perinatal loss that focuses on redefining ourselves and how we interact with the world after a significant loss. The goal of recovery, as related to meaning reconstruction, is a positive change in self-identity by assigning the loss a meaning, thereby allowing the individual to assimilate the loss into her or his world.

Meconium Dark green or black material present in the large intestine of a full-term infant; the first stools passed by the newborn.

Meconium aspiration syndrome (MAS) Respiratory disease of term, postterm, and SGA newborns caused by inhalation of meconium or meconium-stained amniotic fluid into the lungs; characterized by mild to severe respiratory distress, hyperexpansion of the chest, hyperinflated alveoli, and secondary atelectasis.

Meiosis The process of cell division that occurs in the maturation of sperm and ova that decreases their number of chromosomes by one half.

Melasma gravidarum See *Chloasma.*

Menarche (me-nar'kē) Beginning of menstrual and reproductive function in the female.

Mendelian inheritance A major category of inheritance whereby a trait is determined by a pair of genes on homologous chromosomes. Also called *single gene inheritance.*

Menopause The permanent cessation of menses.

Menorrhagia Excessive or profuse menstrual flow.

Menstrual cycle Cyclic buildup of the uterine lining, ovulation, and sloughing of the lining occurring approximately every 28 days in nonpregnant females.

Mentum The chin.

Mesoderm The intermediate layer of germ cells in the embryo that gives rise to connective tissue, bone marrow, muscles, blood, lymphoid tissue, and epithelial tissue.

Metrorrhagia Abnormal uterine bleeding occurring at irregular intervals.

Middle adolescence A term referring to adolescents who are ages 15 to 17 years.

Milia (mil'ē-ă) Tiny white papules appearing on the face of a newborn as a result of unopened sebaceous glands; they disappear spontaneously within a few weeks.

Milk/plasma ratio The comparison of the concentration of substances in the breast milk and the maternal blood serum.

Miscarriage See *Spontaneous abortion.*

Mitosis Process of cell division whereby both daughter cells have the same number and pattern of chromosomes as the original cell.

Molding Shaping of the fetal head by overlapping of the cranial bones to facilitate movement through the birth canal during labor.

Mongolian blue spots Macular areas of bluish black or gray-blue pigmentation found on the dorsal area and the buttocks of newborns.

Moniliasis Yeastlike fungal infection caused by *Candida albicans.*

Monosomies A genetic condition that occurs when a normal gamete unites with a gamete that is missing a chromosome.

Mons pubis (monz pu'bis) Mound of subcutaneous fatty tissue covering the anterior portion of the symphysis pubis.

Morning sickness A term that refers to the nausea and vomiting that a woman may experience in early pregnancy. This lay term is sometimes used because these symptoms frequently occur in the early part of the day and disappear within a few hours.

Moro reflex Flexion of the newborn's thighs and knees accompanied by fingers that fan, then clench, as the arms are simultaneously thrown out and then brought together, as though embracing something. This reflex can be elicited by startling the newborn with a sudden noise or movement. Also called the *startle reflex.*

Morula Developmental stage of the fertilized ovum in which there is a solid mass of cells.

Mosaicism Condition of an individual who has at least two cell lines with differing karyotypes.

Mother-baby care Also called *couplet care,* a family-centered care approach in which the infant remains at the mother's bedside and both are cared for by the same nurse.

Mottling (mot'ling) Discoloration of the skin in irregular areas; may be seen with chilling, poor perfusion, or hypoxia.

Mourning The process by which individuals incorporate the loss experience into their lives, it is influenced by many factors including personality, gender, family dynamics, and social, religious, and cultural norms.

Mucous plug A collection of thick mucus that blocks the cervical canal during pregnancy. Also called *operculum.*

Multigravida (mŭl-tē-grav'i-dă) Woman who has been pregnant more than once.

Multipara (mŭl-tip'ă-ră) Woman who has had more than one pregnancy in which the fetus was viable.

Multiple gestation More than one fetus in the uterus at the same time.

Music therapy Form of sound therapy using one or more musical instruments and improvisations or musical compositions. *Sound therapy* is based on the premise that when the body is exposed to the correct sound frequency (including some very low and very high frequencies that humans cannot normally hear) the body restores itself.

Myometrium Uterine muscular structure.

Nägele's rule A method of determining the estimated date of birth (EDB): after obtaining the first day of the last menstrual period, subtract 3 months and add 7 days.

Naturopathy A healing system that employs various natural means of preventing and treating human disease, such as foods, herbs, rest, etc. Also called *natural medicine.*

Neonatal morbidity The number of potential cases per year of a disease, illness, or complication occurring in the neonatal period.

Neonatal mortality risk The chance of death within the newborn period.

Neonatal transition The first few hours of life, in which the newborn stabilizes his or her respiratory and circulatory functions.

Neonatology The specialty that focuses on the management of at-risk conditions of the newborn.

Neutral thermal environment (NTE) An environment that provides for minimal heat loss or expenditure.

Nevus (nē'vŭs) **flammeus** (flaem'iŭs) Large port-wine stain.

Nevus vasculosus "Strawberry mark": raised, clearly delineated, dark-red, rough-surfaced birthmark commonly found in the head region.

New Ballard score (NBS) A postnatal gestational age assessment tool, it is a refinement of a previous Ballard score tool with added criteria for more accurate assessment of the gestational age of newborns between 20 and 28 weeks' gestation and less than 1500 g.

Newborn Infant from birth through the first 28 days of life.

Newborn screening tests Tests that detect inborn errors of metabolism that, if left untreated, cause mental retardation and physical handicaps.

Newborns' and Mothers' Health Protection Act (NMHPA) Legislation which states that women who have given birth vaginally cannot be forcibly discharged from the hospital within 48 hours of the time of birth for insurance reasons. Cesarean birth mothers are covered by their insurance for 96 hours following the time of birth.

Nidation Implantation of a fertilized ovum in the endometrium.

Nipple A protrusion about 0.5 to 1.3 cm in diameter in the center of each mature breast.

Nonmendelian (multifactorial) inheritance The occurrence of congenital disorders that result from an interaction of multiple genetic and environmental factors.

Nonstress test (NST) An assessment method by which the reaction (or response) of the fetal heart rate to fetal movement is evaluated.

Nuchal cord Term used to describe the umbilical cord when it is wrapped around the neck of the fetus.

Nuchal folds The accumulation of fluid between the posterior cervical spine and the overlying skin in the fetal neck identified during an ultrasound examination.

Nuchal translucency testing A combination of an ultrasound and maternal serum test that is used to screen fetuses between 11 weeks and 1 day and 13 weeks and 6 days to determine if a fetus is at risk for a chromosomal disorder, such as Down syndrome (trisomy 21) and trisomy 18.

Nulligravida (nŭl-i-grav'i-dă) A woman who has never been pregnant.

Nullipara A woman who has not given birth to a viable fetus.

Nurse practitioner A professional nurse who has received specialized education in either a master's degree program or a continuing education program and thus can function in an expanded role.

Nurse researcher A professional nurse who has an advanced doctoral degree, typically a Doctor of Philosophy (PhD), and assumes a leadership role in generating new research.

Nursing advocacy An approach to patient care in which the nurse educates and supports the patient and protects his or her rights.

Obstetric conjugate Distance from the middle of the sacral promontory to an area approximately 1 cm below the pubic crest.

Oligohydramnios (ol'i-gō-hi-dram'nē-os) Decreased amount of amniotic fluid, which may indicate a fetal urinary tract defect.

Oocyte Early primitive ovum before it has completely developed.

Oogenesis Process during fetal life whereby the ovary produces oogonia, cells that become primitive ovarian eggs.

Ophthalmia (of-thal'mē-ă) **neonatorum** Purulent infection of the eyes or conjunctiva of the newborn, usually caused by gonococci.

Oral contraceptives Birth control pills that work by inhibiting the release of an ovum and by maintaining a type of mucus that is hostile to sperm.

Orientation Infant's ability to respond to auditory and visual stimuli in the environment.

Ortolani maneuver A manual procedure performed to rule out the possibility of developmental dysplastic hip.

Osteoporosis A condition most common in postmenopausal women that is characterized by decreased bone strength related to diminished bone density and bone quality. It is thought to be associated with lowered estrogen and androgen levels. Osteoporosis puts an individual at increased risk for fractures of the hip, forearm, and vertebrae.

Ovarian ligaments Ligaments that anchor the lower pole of the ovary to the cornua of the uterus.

Ovary Female sex gland in which the ova are formed and in which estrogen and progesterone are produced. Normally there are two ovaries, located in the lower abdomen on each side of the uterus.

Ovulation Normal process of discharging a mature ovum from an ovary approximately 14 days before the onset of menses.

Oxytocin Hormone normally produced by the posterior pituitary, responsible for stimulation of uterine contractions and the release of milk into the lactiferous ducts.

Oxytocin challenge test (OCT) See *Contraction stress test*.

Palpation The technique of assessing a uterine contraction by touch.

Pap smear Procedure to detect the presence of cancer of the uterus by microscopic examination of cells gently scraped from the cervix.

Para (par'ă) A woman who has borne offspring who reached the age of viability.

Parametritis Inflammation of the parametrial layer of the uterus.

Parent-newborn attachment Close affectional ties that develop between parent and child. See *Attachment*.

Passive acquired immunity Transfer of antibodies (IgG) from the mother to the fetus in utero.

Patient-controlled analgesia (PCA) A method of pain control where anesthesia, usually morphine or meperidine, is initially administered by the anesthesiologist and subsequent doses are self-administered by pushing a button controlled by a special IV pump system.

Pedigree Graphic representation of a family tree.

Pelvic cavity Bony portion of the birth passages; a curved canal with a longer posterior than anterior wall.

Pelvic cellulitis (parametritis) Infection involving the connective tissue of the broad ligament or, in severe cases, the connective tissue of all the pelvic structures.

Pelvic diaphragm Part of the pelvic floor composed of deep fascia and the levator ani and the coccygeal muscles.

Pelvic floor Muscles and tissue that act as a buttress to the pelvic outlet.

Pelvic inflammatory disease (PID) An infection of the fallopian tubes that may or may not be accompanied by a pelvic abscess; may cause infertility secondary to tubal damage.

Pelvic inlet Upper border of the true pelvis.

Pelvic outlet Lower border of the true pelvis.

Pelvic tilt Exercise designed to reduce back strain and strengthen abdominal muscle tone. Also called *pelvic rocking*.

Penis The male organ of copulation and reproduction.

Percutaneous umbilical blood sampling (PUBS) See *Cordocentesis*.

Perimenopause A term referring to the period of time before menopause during which the woman moves from normal ovulatory cycles to cessation of menses.

Perimetrium The outermost layer of the corpus of the uterus. Also known as the *serosal layer*.

Perinatal hospice A compassionate, structured program that provides a context in which parents can find meaning in the intimate experience of the life and death of their child.

Perinatal loss Death of a fetus or infant from the time of conception through the end of the newborn period 28 days after birth.

Perinatal mortality rate The number of neonatal and fetal deaths per 1000 live births.

Perineal (per'i-nē-ăl) **body** Wedge-shaped mass of fibromuscular tissue found between the lower part of the vagina and the anal canal.

Perineal prep An aseptic cleansing of the woman's vulvar and perineal area before she gives birth.

Perineum (per'i-nē'ŭm) The area of tissue between the anus and scrotum in a man or between the anus and vagina in a woman.

Periodic breathing Sporadic episodes of apnea, not associated with cyanosis, that last for about 10 seconds and commonly occur in preterm infants.

Periods of reactivity Predictable patterns of newborn behavior during the first several hours after birth.

Peritonitis Infection involving the peritoneal cavity.

Persistent occiput posterior (OP) position Malposition of the fetus in which the fetal occiput is posterior in the maternal pelvis.

Persistent pulmonary hypertension of the newborn (PPHN) Respiratory disease resulting from right-to-left shunting of blood away from the lungs and through the ductus arteriosus and patent foramen ovale.

Phenotype The whole physical, biochemical, and physiologic makeup of an individual as determined both genetically and environmentally.

Phenylketonuria (PKU) (fen'il-kē'tō-nū'rē-ă) A common metabolic disease caused by an inborn error in the metabolism of the amino acid phenylalanine.

Phosphatidylglycerol (PG) (fos-fă-tī'dĭl-glis'er-ol) A phospholipid present in fetal surfactant after about 35 weeks' gestation.

Phototherapy The treatment of jaundice by exposure to light.

Physiologic anemia of infancy A harmless condition in which the hemoglobin level drops in the first 6 to 12 weeks after birth, then reverts to normal levels.

Physiologic anemia of pregnancy Apparent anemia that results because during pregnancy the plasma volume increases more than the erythrocytes increase.

Physiologic jaundice A harmless condition caused by the normal reduction of red blood cells, occurring 48 or more hours after birth, peaking at the 5th to 7th days, and disappearing between the 7th and 10th days.

Pica The eating of substances not ordinarily considered edible or to have nutritive value.

Placenta (plă-sen'tă) Specialized disk-shaped organ that connects the fetus to the uterine wall for gas and nutrient exchange. Also called *afterbirth*.

Placenta accreta Partial or complete absence of the decidua basalis and abnormal adherence of the placenta to the uterine wall.

Placenta increta A high-risk condition that occurs when the placenta attaches to the uterine wall and invades or attaches itself within the myometrium.

Placenta percreta A high-risk condition that occurs when the placenta penetrates the myometrium, sometimes attaching to peritoneal structures within the abdominal cavity, where the removal of the uterus (hysterectomy) is sometimes necessary.

Placenta previa Abnormal implantation of the placenta in the lower uterine segment. Classification of type is based on proximity to the cervical os: *total*—completely covers the os; *partial*—covers a portion of the os; *marginal*—is in close proximity to the os.

Placental delivery Placenta and membranes expelled after the birth of the infant, during the third stage of labor.

Platypelloid pelvis An unusually wide pelvis, having a flattened oval transverse shape and a shortened anteroposterior diameter.

Podalic version Type of version used to turn a second twin during a vaginal birth. See *Internal version.*

Polar body A small cell resulting from the meiotic division of the mature oocyte.

Polycystic ovarian syndrome (PCOS) The most common endocrine disorder affecting women of reproductive age, marked by menstrual dysfunction, androgen excess, obesity, hyperinsulinemia, and infertility.

Polycythemia An abnormal increase in the number of total red blood cells in the body's circulation.

Polydactyly (pol-ē-dak'ti-lē) A developmental anomaly characterized by more than five digits on the hands or feet.

Polypharmacy The act of taking multiple drugs to treat symptoms, when the etiology of the symptoms is actually a side effect from one or more prescribed medications.

Positive signs of pregnancy Indications that confirm the presence of pregnancy.

Postcoital emergency contraception (EC) A form of combined hormonal contraception that is used when a woman is worried about pregnancy because of unprotected intercourse, rape, or possible contraceptive failure (e.g., broken condom, slipped diaphragm, missed oral contraceptives, or too long a time between Depo-Provera injections).

Postcoital test (PCT) An examination that evaluates the cervical mucus, sperm motility, sperm-mucus interaction, and the sperm's ability to negotiate the cervical mucus barrier. Also called *Sims-Huhner test.*

Postconception age periods Period of time in embryonic/fetal development calculated from the time of fertilization of the ovum (about 266 days [38 weeks] or 9 1/2 calendar months). Also called *fertilization age.*

Postmature newborn See *Postterm newborn.*

Postmaturity See *Postterm newborn.*

Postpartum After childbirth.

Postpartum blues See *Adjustment reaction with depressed mood.*

Postpartum depression Severe depression that occurs within the first year after giving birth with increased incidence at about the fourth week postpartum, just before resumption of menses, and upon weaning.

Postpartum endometritis (metritis) A reproductive tract infection limited to the uterus and associated with childbirth that occurs at any time up to 6 weeks postpartum.

Postpartum hemorrhage A loss of blood of greater than 500 ml following birth. The hemorrhage is classified as *early* if it occurs within the first 24 hours and *late* if it occurs after the first 24 hours.

Postpartum home care Home visits for postpartum families occurring in the home setting. This provides opportunities for expanding information and reinforcing self- and infant care techniques initially presented in the birth setting.

Postpartum major mood disorder See *Postpartum depression.*

Postpartum psychosis Psychosis occurring within the first 3 months after birth.

Postterm labor Labor that occurs after 42 weeks' gestation.

Postterm newborn Any infant born after 42 weeks' gestation.

Postterm pregnancy Pregnancy that lasts beyond 42 weeks' gestation.

Post-traumatic stress disorder (PTSD) Intense psychologic distress resulting from a traumatic event and evidenced by recurrent, intrusive thoughts; flashbacks, persistent avoidance of stimuli associated with the trauma; a generalized feeling of "numbness"; and persistent signs of arousal.

Post-traumatic stress syndrome (PTSS) See *Post-traumatic stress disorder (PTSD).*

Precipitous birth (1) Unduly rapid progression of labor. (2) A birth in which no physician is in attendance.

Precipitous labor Labor lasting less than 3 hours.

Preeclampsia (prē-ē-klamp'sē-ă) Toxemia of pregnancy, characterized by hypertension, albuminuria, and edema. See also *Eclampsia.*

Premature infant See *Preterm infant.*

Premature rupture of membranes (PROM) See *Rupture of membranes (ROM).*

Premenstrual dysphoric disorder (PMDD) A disorder associated with the luteal phase of the menstrual cycle (2 weeks before onset of menses) in which a woman experiences five or more affective (emotional) or somatic (physical) symptoms, which are relieved with menstruation and have occurred during most cycles during the previous year.

Premenstrual syndrome (PMS) Cluster of symptoms experienced by some women, typically occurring from a few days up to 2 weeks before the onset of menses.

Prenatal education Programs offered to expectant families, adolescents, women, or partners to provide education regarding the pregnancy, labor, and birth experience.

Presentation The fetal body part that enters the maternal pelvis first. The three possible presentations are cephalic, shoulder, and breech.

Presenting part The fetal part present in or on the cervical os.

Presumptive signs of pregnancy Symptoms that suggest but do not confirm pregnancy, such as cessation of menses, quickening, Chadwick's sign, and morning sickness.

Preterm infant Any infant born before 38 weeks' gestation.

Preterm labor Labor occurring between 20 and 38 weeks of pregnancy. Also called *premature labor.*

Primigravida (prî-mi-grav'i-dă) A woman who is pregnant for the first time.

Primipara (prî-mip'ă-ră) A woman who has given birth to her first child (past the point of viability), whether or not that child is living or was alive at birth.

Probable signs of pregnancy Manifestations that strongly suggest the likelihood of pregnancy, such as a positive pregnancy test, enlarging abdomen, and positive Goodell's, Hegar's, and Braxton Hicks signs.

Professional nurse A person who has graduated from an accredited basic program in nursing, has successfully completed the nursing licensure examination (NCLEX), and is currently licensed as a registered nurse (RN).

Progesterone A hormone produced by the corpus luteum, adrenal cortex, and placenta whose function is to stimulate proliferation of the endometrium to facilitate growth of the embryo.

Progressive relaxation A relaxation technique that involves relaxing first one portion of the body and then another portion, until total body relaxation is achieved; may be used during labor.

Prolactin A hormone secreted by the anterior pituitary that stimulates and sustains lactation in mammals.

Prolapsed umbilical cord Umbilical cord that becomes trapped in the vagina before the fetus is born.

Prolonged decelerations Decelerations in which the FHR decreases from the baseline for 2 to 10 minutes.

Prolonged labor Labor lasting more than 24 hours.

Prostaglandins (PGs) Complex lipid compounds synthesized by many cells in the body.

Pseudomenstruation Blood-tinged mucus from the vagina in the newborn female infant; caused by withdrawal of maternal hormones that were present during pregnancy.

Psychologic disorders Abnormal mental or emotional conditions characterized by alterations in thinking, mood, or behavior.

Ptyalism Excessive salivation.

Puberty The developmental period between childhood and the attainment of adult sexual characteristics and functioning.

Pubic Pertaining to the pubes or pubis.

Pubis Pertaining to the pubes or pubic area.

Pudendal (pyū-den′dăl) **block** Injection of an anesthetizing agent at the pudendal nerve to produce numbness of the external genitals and the lower one third of the vagina to facilitate childbirth and permit episiotomy if necessary.

Puerperal infection Infection of the reproductive tract associated with childbirth and occurring any time up to 6 weeks postpartum.

Puerperal morbidity A maternal temperature of 38°C (100.4°F) or higher on any 2 of the first 10 postpartal days, excluding the first 24 hours. The temperature is to be taken by mouth at least four times per day.

Puerperium (pyū-er-pēr′ē-ŭm) The period after completion of the third stage of labor until involution of the uterus is complete, usually 6 weeks.

Quickening The first fetal movements felt by the pregnant woman, usually between 16 and 18 weeks' gestation.

Quiet alert state Alert state characterized by a brightening of the eyes and face. Infants are most attentive to their environment in this state and provide positive feedback to caregivers. Also called *wide awake state*.

Radiation Heat loss incurred when heat transfers to cooler surfaces and objects not in direct contact with the body.

Rape Sexual activity, often intercourse, against the will of the victim.

Rape trauma syndrome A term that refers to a variety of symptoms, clustered in phases, that a rape survivor experiences following an assault.

Reciprocity An interactional cycle that occurs simultaneously between mother and infant. It involves mutual cuing behaviors, expectancy, rhythmicity, and synchrony.

Recommended dietary allowances (RDA) Government recommended allowances of various vitamins, minerals, and other nutrients.

Recurrent pregnancy loss (RPL) Three or more consecutive pregnancy losses before 24 weeks gestation.

Reflexology Form of massage involving the application of pressure to designated points or reflexes on the client's feet, hands, or ears using the thumb and fingers.

Regional analgesia The temporary and reversible loss of sensation produced by injecting an anesthetic agent (called a local anesthetic) into an area that will bring the agent into direct contact with nervous tissue.

Regional anesthesia Injection of local anesthetic agents so that they come into direct contact with nervous tissue.

Reiki Tibetan-Japanese hand-mediated therapy designed to promote healing, reduce stress, and encourage relaxation. During Reiki sessions, practitioners place their hands on or above specific problem areas and transfer energy from themselves to their clients in order to restore the balance of the client's energy fields.

Relaxin A water-soluble protein secreted by the corpus luteum that causes relaxation of the symphysis and cervical dilatation.

Religion An institutionalized system that shares a common set of beliefs and practices.

Relinquishing mothers Those mothers who choose to give their infants up for adoption.

Respiratory distress syndrome (RDS) Respiratory disease of the newborn characterized by interference with ventilation at the alveolar level, thought to be caused by the presence of fibrinoid deposits lining the alveolar ducts. Formerly called *hyaline membrane disease*.

Responding model A set of guidelines for successful interactions with grieving families.

Retained placenta Retention of the placenta beyond 30 minutes after birth.

Retinopathy (ret-i-nop′ă-thē) **of prematurity (ROP)** Formation of fibrotic tissue behind the lens; associated with retinal detachment and arrested eye growth, seen with hypoxemia in preterm infants.

Rh factor Antigens present on the surface of blood cells that make the blood cell incompatible with blood cells that do not have the antigen.

Rh immune globulin An anti-Rh *(D)* gamma globulin given after birth to an Rh-negative mother of an Rh-positive fetus or child. Prevents the development of permanent active immunity to the Rh antigen.

Rhythm method The timing of sexual intercourse to avoid the fertile time associated with ovulation.

Risk factors Any findings that suggest the pregnancy may have a negative outcome, for either the woman or her unborn child.

Roles Patterns of behavior normatively defined and expected of an occupant of a given social position.

Room sharing An arrangement in whichthe infant sleeps in the same room in close proximity to the parents, but in his or her own bed.

Rooting reflex An infant's tendency to turn the head and open the lips to suck when one side of the mouth or cheek is touched.

Round ligaments Ligaments that arise from the side of the uterus near the fallopian tube insertion to help the broad ligament keep the uterus in place.

Rugae (rū′gē) Transverse ridges of mucous membranes lining the vagina that allow the vagina to stretch during the descent of the fetal head.

Rupture of membranes (ROM) Rupture may be PROM (premature), SROM (spontaneous), or AROM (artificial). Some clinicians may use the abbreviation RBOW (rupture of bag of waters).

Sacral promontory A projection into the pelvic cavity on the anterior upper portion of the sacrum; serves as an obstetric guide in determining pelvic measurements.

Salpingitis Infection of the fallopian tubes.

Scalp stimulation A test used during labor to assess fetal well-being by pressing a fingertip on the fetal scalp. A fetus not under excessive stress will respond to the digital stimulation with heart rate accelerations.

Scarf sign The position of the elbow when the hand of a supine infant is drawn across to the other shoulder until it meets resistance.

Schultze's mechanism Expulsion of the placenta with the shiny, or fetal, surface presenting first.

Secondary infertility Condition in which couples are unable to conceive after one or more successful pregnancies.

Self-quieting ability Infant's ability to use personal resources to quiet and console himself or herself.

Semen Thick whitish fluid ejaculated by the male during orgasm and containing the spermatozoa and their nutrients.

Sepsis neonatorum Infections experienced by a newborn during the first month of life.

Sex chromosomes The X and Y chromosomes, which are responsible for sex determination.

Sexual assault A broad term that refers to a variety of types of unwanted sexual touching or penetration without consent, from unwanted sexual contact or touching of an intimate part of another person to forced anal, oral, or genital penetration.

Sexually transmitted infection (STI) Refers to infections ordinarily transmitted by direct sexual contact with an infected individual. Also called *sexually transmitted disease*.

Shaken baby syndrome (SBS) A traumatic brain injury that results from violent shaking, with or without contact between the infant's head and an exterior surface.

Simian line A single palmar crease frequently found in children with Down syndrome.

Sims-Huhner test See *Postcoital test (PCT).*

Situational contraceptives Contraceptive methods that involve no prior preparation (e.g., abstinence or coitus interruptus).

Skin turgor Elasticity of skin; provides information on hydration status.

Skin-to-skin contact Physical contact between the mother and baby whereby the naked baby is placed prone on the mother's chest during the first 24 hours.

Small for gestational age (SGA) Inadequate weight or growth for gestational age; birth weight below the 10th percentile.

Spermatogenesis The process by which mature spermatozoa are formed, during which the number of chromosomes is halved.

Spermatozoa Mature sperm cells of the male animal, produced by the testes.

Spermicides A variety of creams, foams, jellies, and suppositories that, when inserted into the vagina before intercourse, destroy sperm or neutralize any vaginal secretions and thereby immobilize sperm.

Spinal block Injection of a local anesthetic agent directly into the spinal fluid in the spinal canal to provide anesthesia for vaginal and cesarean births.

Spinnbarkheit The elasticity of the cervical mucus that is present at ovulation.

Spirituality A belief in a transcendent power pertaining to the spirit or soul.

Spontaneous abortion Abortion that occurs naturally. Also called *miscarriage.*

Spontaneous rupture of membranes (SROM) The breaking of the "water" or membranes marked by the expulsion of amniotic fluid from the vagina.

Station Relationship of the presenting fetal part to an imaginary line drawn between the pelvic ischial spines.

Sterilization An inclusive term that refers to surgical procedures that permanently prevent pregnancy. In the male, sterilization is achieved through a procedure called a vasectomy. In the female, sterilization is done by tubal ligation.

Stillbirth The birth of a dead infant.

Striae (strī'ă) Stretch marks; shiny purplish lines that appear on the abdomen, breasts, thighs, and buttocks of pregnant women as a result of stretching the skin.

Subconjunctival hemorrhage (sŭb'kon-jŭnk-tī'văl hem'ŏ-rij) Hemorrhage on the sclera of a newborn's eye, usually caused by changes in vascular tension during birth.

Subfertility A couple who has difficulty conceiving because both partners have reduced fertility.

Subinvolution (sŭb-in-vō-lū'shŭn) Failure of a part to return to its normal size after functional enlargement, such as failure of the uterus to return to normal size after pregnancy.

Sucking reflex Normal newborn reflex elicited by inserting a finger or nipple in the newborn's mouth, resulting in forceful, rhythmic sucking.

Sudden infant death syndrome (SIDS) The sudden death of an infant; the primary cause of infant death beyond the neonatal period in the United States.

Supine hypotensive syndrome (vena caval syndrome, aortocaval compression) A condition that can develop during pregnancy when the enlarging uterus puts pressure on the vena cava when the woman is supine. This pressure interferes with returning blood flow and produces a marked decrease in blood pressure with accompanying dizziness, pallor, and clamminess, which can be corrected by having the woman lie on her left side.

Surfactant (ser-fak'tănt) A substance composed of phospholipid, which stabilizes and lowers the surface tension of the alveoli during extrauterine respiratory exhalation, allowing a certain amount of air to remain in the alveoli during expiration.

Suture Fibrous connection of opposed joint surfaces, as in the skull.

Symphysis pubis Fibrocartilaginous joint between the pelvic bones in the midline.

Syndactyly (sin-dak'ti-lē) Malformation of the fingers or toes in which there may be webbing or complete fusion of two or more digits.

Syphilis A chronic, sexually transmitted infection caused by the spirochete *Treponema pallidum.*

Taboos Behaviors or objects that are avoided by individuals or groups.

Telangiectatic nevi (tel-an'jē-ek-tat'ik nē'vī) **(stork bites)** Small clusters of pink-red spots appearing on the nape of the neck and around the eyes of infants; localized areas of capillary dilatation.

Teratogens Nongenetic factors that can produce malformations of the fetus.

Term The normal duration of pregnancy.

Testes The male gonads, in which sperm and testosterone are produced.

Testosterone The male hormone; responsible for the development of secondary male characteristics.

Therapeutic abortion Medically induced termination of pregnancy when a malformed fetus is suspected or when the woman's health is in jeopardy.

Therapeutic insemination Procedure to produce a pregnancy in which sperm obtained from a woman's husband or from a donor is deposited in the woman's vagina.

Therapeutic touch Complementary therapy grounded in the belief that people are a system of energy with a self-healing potential. The therapeutic touch practitioner, often a nurse, unites his or her energy field with that of the client, directing it in a specific way to promote well-being and healing.

Thermogenesis The newborn's physiologic mechanisms that increase heat production.

Thrombophlebitis Inflammation of a vein wall, resulting in thrombus.

Thrush A fungal infection of the oral mucous membranes caused by *Candida albicans.* Most often seen in infants; characterized by white plaques in the mouth.

Tocolysis Use of medications to arrest preterm labor.

Tonic neck reflex Postural reflex seen in the newborn. When the supine infant's head is turned to one side, the arm and leg on that side extend while the extremities on the opposite side flex. Also called the *fencing position.*

TORCH An acronym used to describe a group of infections that represent potentially severe problems during pregnancy. *TO,* toxoplasmosis; *R,* rubella; *C,* cytomegalovirus; *H,* herpesvirus.

Total serum bilirubin Sum of conjugated (direct) and unconjugated (indirect) bilirubin.

Touch relaxation A relaxation technique that involves relaxing an area of one's body as another person provides a "touch" cue to that specific area. Touch relaxation is very effective during labor contractions.

Toxic shock syndrome (TSS) Infection caused by *Staphylococcus aureus,* found primarily in women of reproductive age.

Traditional Chinese medicine (TCM) System of medicine developed more than 3000 years ago in China that seeks to ensure the balance of energy, which is called *chi* or *qi* (pronounced "chee").

Chi is thought to maintain health and vitality and enable the body to carry out its physiologic functions.

Transitional milk Breast milk produced from the end of colostrum production until about 2 weeks postpartum.

Transvaginal ultrasound A follicular monitoring test that is used in women undergoing induction cycles, for timing ovulation for insemination and intercourse, for retrieving oocytes for in vitro fertilization, and for monitoring early pregnancy.

Transverse diameter The largest diameter of the pelvic inlet; helps determine the shape of the inlet.

Transverse lie A lie in which the fetus is positioned crosswise in the uterus.

Trichomonas vaginalis A parasitic protozoan that may cause inflammation of the vagina, characterized by itching and burning of vulvar tissue and by white, frothy discharge.

Trichomoniasis A sexually transmitted infection caused by *Trichomonas vaginalis,* a microscopic motile protozoan that thrives in an alkaline environment.

Trimester Three months, or one third of the gestational time for pregnancy.

Trisomy The presence of three homologous chromosomes rather than the normal two.

Trophoblast The outer layer of the blastoderm that will eventually establish the nutrient relationship with the uterine endometrium.

True pelvis The portion that lies below the linea terminalis, made up of the inlet, cavity, and outlet.

Trunk incurvation (Galant reflex) Reflex resulting from the stroking of the spine that causes the pelvis to turn to the stimulated side.

Tubal embryo transfer (TET) Procedure in which eggs are retrieved and incubated with the man's sperm then transferred back into the women's body at the embryo stage.

Tubal ligation Sterilization of a woman accomplished by transecting or occluding the fallopian tubes.

Turner syndrome A number of anomalies that occur when a woman has only one X chromosome. Characteristics include short stature; little sexual differentiation; webbing of the neck, with a low posterior hairline; and congenital cardiac anomalies.

Ultrasound High-frequency sound waves that may be directed, through the use of a transducer, into the maternal abdomen. The ultrasonic sound waves reflected by the underlying structures of varying densities allow identification of various maternal and fetal tissues, bones, and fluids.

Umbilical cord (ŭm-bil'i-kăl kōrd) The structure connecting the placenta to the umbilicus of the fetus and through which nutrients from the woman are exchanged for wastes from the fetus.

Urinary tract infection (UTI) Significant *bacteriuria* in the presence of symptoms.

Uterine atony Relaxation of uterine muscle tone following birth.

Uterine inversion Prolapse of the uterine fundus through the cervix into the vagina; may occur just before or during expulsion of the placenta; associated with massive hemorrhage, requiring emergency treatment.

Uterine rupture A nonsurgical disruption of the uterine cavity.

Uterosacral ligaments Ligaments that provide support for the uterus and cervix at the level of the ischial spines.

Uterus The hollow muscular organ in which the fertilized ovum is implanted and in which the developing fetus is nourished until birth.

Vacuum extraction An obstetric procedure used to assist in the birth of a fetus by applying suction to the fetal head with a soft suction cup attached to a suction bottle (pump) by tubing and placing the device against the occiput of the fetal head.

Vagina The musculomembranous tube or passageway located between the external genitals and the uterus of a woman.

Vaginal birth after cesarean (VBAC) Practice of permitting a trial of labor and possible vaginal birth for women following a previous cesarean birth for nonrecurring causes such as fetal distress or placenta previa.

Variability Baseline fluctuations of two cycles per minute or greater in the FHR and classified by the visually quantified amplitude of peak-to-trough in beats per minute.

Variable deceleration Periodic change in fetal heart rate caused by umbilical cord compression; decelerations vary in onset, occurrence, and waveform.

Vasa previa Condition occurring when the fetal vessels course through membranes and are present at the cervical os. Although this is a rare cause of antepartum bleeding, it has a high rate of fetal death.

Vasectomy Surgical removal of a portion of the vas deferens (ductus deferens) to produce infertility.

Vegan A "pure" vegetarian; one who consumes no food from animal sources.

Vena caval syndrome Symptoms of dizziness, pallor, and clamminess that result from lowered blood pressure when a pregnant woman lies supine and the enlarged uterus presses on the vena cava. Also known as supine hypotensive syndrome.

Vernix caseosa (ver'niks kā'sē-ō-să) A protective, cheeselike, whitish substance made up of sebum and desquamated epithelial cells that is present on the fetal skin.

Version Turning of the fetus in utero.

Vertex The top or crown of the head.

Viability The potential for the pregnancy to result in a live birth.

Vibroacoustic stimulation (VAS) Application of device delivering 90 dB of sound and vibration for 1 to 3 seconds to the mother's abdomen to stimulate movement in the fetus, thereby accelerating the fetal heart rate. (Also called *FAST* for *fetal acoustic stimulation test* or *VST* for *vibroacoustic stimulation test.*)

Vicarious trauma A condition that can occur as a result of working with people who are trauma victims. Also called *secondary trauma effect.*

Visualization Complementary therapy in which a person goes into a relaxed state and focuses on or "visualizes" soothing or positive scenes such as a beach or a mountain glade. Visualization helps reduce stress and encourage relaxation.

Vulva The external structure of the female genitals, lying below the mons veneris.

Vulvovaginal candidiasis (VVC) A genital infection most often caused by *Candida albicans.* Also called *moniliasis* or *yeast infection.*

Weaning The process of discontinuing breastfeeding and accustoming an infant to another feeding method.

Wharton's (hwar'tunz) **jelly** Yellow-white gelatinous material surrounding the vessels of the umbilical cord.

Zona pellucida Transparent inner layer surrounding an ovum.

Zygote A fertilized egg.

Zygote intrafallopian transfer (ZIFT) Retrieval of oocytes under ultrasound guidance, followed by in vitro fertilization and laparoscopic replacement of fertilized eggs into the fimbriated end of the fallopian tube.

INDEX

Page numbers followed by f indicate figures and those followed by t indicate tables or special features. The titles of special features (e.g., Focus Your Study, Critical Thinking in Action, Research Evidence in Practice, Developing Cultural Competence) are also capitalized.

A

B

C

D

E

F

H

I

J

N

P

Q

R

S

T

V

W

X

Y

Z

TEACHING NEWBORN BATHING

Bath Supplies

Basin for water ♦ Washcloths, towels ♦ Receiving blankets (to rest baby on and dry baby off with) ♦ Hair brush ♦ Mild, unperfumed soap ♦ Diaper ♦ Cotton balls (optional) ♦ Ointment ♦ Alcohol pads/rubbing alcohol (controversial) ♦ Warm water supply

Bathing the Baby

Start at the baby's head while baby is still clothed ♦ Using a wet washcloth (no soap), wipe one eyelid from inner to outer corner ♦ Change the spot on the washcloth to clean the other eye ♦ Wash external ears using index finger in washcloth ♦ Wash rest of face and, using soap now, progress to neck creases ♦ Dry off each area after washing it to decrease heat loss ♦ Remove baby's shirt and wash chest, arms, and hands (use soapy hands instead of washcloth if desired) ♦ Wash trunk and back (hold baby off table, supporting baby while doing the back) ♦ Keep a circumcised baby off his abdomen if possible and wash with warm water only ♦ Keep baby's upper body warm by wrapping in towel or blanket before washing legs and feet ♦ Wash genitalia (wash girls front to back; do not retract foreskin of uncircumcised boys) ♦ Wash hair: put a little water and shampoo on hair; use

(continued)

TEACHING SIGNS OF POSSIBLE ILLNESS DURING NEWBORN PERIOD

Possible Warning Signs

Temperature above 38C (100.4F) axillary and below 36.6C (97.8F) axillary ♦ Continued rise in temperature ♦ More than one episode of forceful vomiting or frequent vomiting (over a 6 hour period) ♦ Refusal of two feedings in a row ♦ Lethargy (listlessness), difficulty in waking ♦ Inconsolable infant (quieting techniques are not effective) or continuous high-pitched cry ♦ Cyanosis (bluish discoloration of skin) with or without a feeding ♦ Absence of breathing longer than 20 seconds ♦ Reddened umbilical cord ♦ Abdominal distention, crying when trying to pass stools, or absence of stools after stool pattern is established ♦ Two consecutive green watery or black, loose stools or increased frequency of stooling ♦ No wet diapers for 18–24 hours or less than 6 wet diapers per day after 4 days of age ♦ Increasing jaundice of the skin and jaundice over abdomen and extremities ♦ Pustules, rashes, or blisters other than normal newborn rashes ♦ Development of eye drainage

If a Warning Sign Develops

Call caregiver ♦ Be prepared to tell caregiver length of time since onset, related activities or problems, specific characteristics of problem, and baby's temperature

(continued)

TEACHING POSTPARTUM COMFORT MEASURES

Relief of Breast Discomfort

Wear supportive, well-fitting bra ♦ Apply ice packs for 20 minutes, 4 times a day ♦ If not breastfeeding avoid breast stimulation

Relief of Uterine Cramping (Afterpains)

Lie on abdomen, with a small pillow placed under it to apply pressure ♦ Apply heat ♦ Walk (obtain assistance for first ambulation) ♦ Take analgesic medication (if breastfeeding, take mild analgesic about 1 hour before breastfeeding)

Relief of Episiotomy Discomfort

Apply ice packs to the perineum during the first few hours after birth ♦ Take 20-minute sitz baths 3–4 times a day ♦ Use perineal analgesic/anesthetics sprays ♦ Keep perineum clean and free from dried discharge ♦ Use gentle spray of warm water on perineum after voiding to provide cleansing; then pat dry, front to back ♦ Take analgesic medication

(continued)

POSTPARTUM DISCHARGE TEACHING

Review Important Self-Care Measures

Care of breasts ♦ Expected positional changes in the uterus, and continued comfort measures for uterine cramping (afterpains) ♦ Care of the episiotomy and hemorrhoids if present ♦ Expected changes in lochia ♦ Need for adequate nutrition and fluid intake ♦ Measures to promote bowel elimination ♦ Strategies to promote rest and relaxation ♦ Postpartum exercises ♦ Resumption of sexual activity ♦ Warning signs of possible problems

Review Important Infant Care Measures

Information and support regarding feeding techniques ♦ Bathing and diaper changes ♦ Umbilical cord care ♦ Care of the uncircumcised and circumcised penis ♦ Recognizing normal characteristics of the newborn ♦ Maintaining safety ♦ Soothing techniques ♦ Recognizing illness or problems in the newborn

How to Obtain Baby's Temperature

Properly place thermometer to ensure greatest accuracy ♦ Never leave baby unattended, no matter which method is used ♦ After taking baby's temperature, find and note the temperature ♦ *Rectal temperatures are not recommended*

Taking Axillary Temperature

Place tip of the thermometer underneath baby's armpit ♦ Hold outer aspect of baby's arm next to his or her body ♦ Hold thermometer securely in place for 3–4 minutes

Helpful temperature ranges (Centigrade and Fahrenheit values)

Temperatures: 36.5C (97.7F), 37.0C (98.6F), 37.8C (100.0F), 38.3C (101.0F), 38.9C (102.0F), 39.4C (103.0F), or 40.0C (104.0F)

hairbrush to work it in; rinse, dry, and brush hair ♦ Brush during shampooing once a week and brush dry hair daily to help prevent cradle cap

General Considerations

Bathe baby in warm, draft-free room ♦ Collect all supplies before starting the bath so baby is never left unattended ♦ Use only tepid water (warm to inner wrists) ♦ Test water each time before putting baby in ♦ Bathe baby every day in warm, humid weather; give full body bath twice a week in dry weather ♦ Keep one hand on baby at all times during bath, cradling baby's head and back with arm while securely holding on to thigh ♦ Ointments are better than lotions for dry, cracked hands and feet ♦ Lotion or talc-free powder may be used, but controversy exists over their use (do not let baby inhale powder) ♦ Do not immerse baby in bath water until umbilical cord falls off ♦ Choose a convenient bath time that allows parents and baby to enjoy the experience ♦ Baths may be useful in soothing a fussy baby

Copyright © by Prentice Hall Nursing

Copyright © by Prentice Hall Nursing

Relief of Hemorrhoidal Discomfort

Take 20-minute sitz baths 3–4 times a day ♦ Apply anesthetic ointments or witch hazel pads ♦ Maintain side-lying or prone position when in bed ♦ Avoid prolonged sitting ♦ Maintain adequate fluid intake ♦ Take stool softener if needed to avoid constipation

Copyright © by Prentice Hall Nursing

place pillow under right hip to displace uterus and avoid venal caval syndrome ♦ Encourage sexual activities enjoyed by both partners as long as they are generally not contraindicated medically ♦ To avoid introducing *Escherichia coli* into the vagina, the couple should *not* go from anal to vaginal penetration without thoroughly washing the penis ♦ Encourage the exploration of other methods of expressing affection such as hugging, cuddling, and stroking each other to increase feelings of closeness ♦ Suggest masturbation, either privately or as a shared experience, to provide release ♦ Woman's orgasmic contractions from masturbation may be unusually intense in later pregnancy ♦ Encourage openly expressing feelings, preferences, and concerns to partner

Contraindications to Sexual Intercourse

Ruptured membranes ♦ Presence of bleeding ♦ Woman with history of preterm labor due to release of oxytocin with orgasm (breast stimulation also triggers the release of oxytocin and should therefore be avoided)

Combined Oral Contraceptives and Other Methods

Combination birth control pills (8% failure) have rare but serious medical complications and may have annoying side effects ♦ Spermicides such as jellies, creams, foam, film, and vaginal suppositories (29% failure) minimally effective if used alone ♦ Operative sterilization (vasectomy [0.15% failure] and tubal ligation [0.5% failure]) theoretically reversible, but 30%–85% reversible in men and 40%–75% reversible in women

Correct Procedure for Using Method

Identify supplies or equipment needed ♦ Provide details of how method is used ♦ Discuss what to do if unusual circumstances arise (missed pill, missed AM temperature, second episode of intercourse with diaphragm)

Warning Signs Requiring Immediate Action

For combined oral contraceptive pill users: shortness of breath or chest pain; severe headaches; severe abdominal pain; visual disturbances such as double vision, reduced visual fields, blindness; severe leg pain or swelling ♦ For IUD users: severe or persistent abdominal pain, late or missed periods, fever, chills, noticeable or foul discharge, spotting, bleeding, heavy periods, clots
Note: Failure rates are percentages of women experiencing an unintended pregnancy with first year of typical use. Failure rates are much lower for perfect use of a method.

Source: Hatcher, R. A., et al. (2004). *Contraceptive technology* (18th ed.). New York: Ardent Media.

If a Warning Sign Develops

Call caregiver immediately ♦ Note any specific information about the sign: how long it has been present, any related signs or symptoms, any other important information

1 c green leafy vegetables) ♦ **Meat, poultry, fish, dry beans, eggs, nuts** normally 2–3 servings daily; increase to 3–4 servings during pregnancy (1 serving = 2 oz cooked lean meat, poultry, or fish; 2 eggs; 1/2 c cottage cheese; 1 c cooked legumes [kidney, lima, garbanzo, or soy beans, or split peas]; 6 oz tofu; 2 oz nuts or seeds; 4 tablespoons peanut butter)

Additional Considerations

Consider calories in making choices (not all nutritionally equivalent foods have same number of calories) ♦ Eat foods with low nutrient value (sometimes called empty calories) sparingly (cakes, doughnuts, potato chips, butter, mayonnaise) ♦ Combine foods to enhance nutrition (eg, 1 c spaghetti with a 2-oz meatball and 1/4 c tomato sauce = 1 serving of meat, 1 1/3 servings of grain, and 1/2 serving of vegetable) ♦ Drink adequate amount of fluids daily, preferably 8–10 8-oz glasses of water or other fluid ♦ Do not eat swordfish, shark, tilefish, or king mackeral because these fish contain high levels of mercury, which may be toxic to the fetal brain ♦ Eat up to 12 oz/week of other fish and shellfish (canned light tuna, shrimp, salmon, catfish, pollock ♦ Avoid soft cheeses such as feta, brick and blue-veined cheeses unless label states they were made with pasteurized milk.

TEACHING ABOUT METHODS OF CONTRACEPTION

Factors to Consider in Choosing a Method of Contraception

Effectiveness ♦ Safety ♦ Age and future childbearing plans ♦ Contraindications in health history ♦ Religious or moral factors ♦ Personal preferences, biases ♦ Lifestyle: frequency of intercourse, number of partners, cost factors, access to medical care ♦ Partner's support and willingness to participate. If no method used, 85% chance of pregnancy

Fertility Awareness or Natural Family-Planning Methods

Include basal body temperature (BBT), calendar (rhythm), cervical mucus (ovulation or Billings), and symptothermal methods ♦ Require periodic abstinence ♦ Generally require no artificial devices or substances ♦ Readily reversible ♦ 25% failure rate

Mechanical Contraceptives

Include male condom (15% typical use failure rate), female condom (21% failure), diaphragm (16% failure), cervical cap (nulliparous → 16% failure), intrauterine device (IUD) (less than 2% failure) ♦ Condoms available over the counter ♦ All barrier methods readily reversible and generally free of side effects in appropriate clients ♦ Women who have had a child may accept an IUD more easily but women who have never given birth are candidates if their uterus is deep enough

(continued)

TEACHING ABOUT SEXUAL ACTIVITY DURING PREGNANCY

During Pregnancy the Woman May Experience

Sexual desire may change or may remain unchanged ♦ *First trimester*: possible decreased sexual desire due to discomforts such as breast tenderness, nausea, fatigue ♦ *Second trimester*: woman tends to feel at her best; sexual desire may increase ♦ *Third trimester*: possible decreased sexual desire due to discomfort and fatigue ♦ More intense orgasms followed by cramping possible in last weeks of pregnancy

During Pregnancy the Partner May Experience

Sexual desire may change or may remain unchanged ♦ Possible changed desire due to feelings about partner's changing appearance, beliefs about sexual activity with a pregnant woman, concern about hurting the woman or fetus, personal view of pregnancy as erotic or not, response to the notion of partner as a mother

Sexual Activities

Suggest positions such as side lying, female superior, or vaginal rear entry for more comfortable intercourse in later pregnancy ♦ If male superior position is used, woman should

(continued)

TEACHING DIETARY CHANGES RECOMMENDED DURING PREGNANCY

General Information

Desired weight gain during pregnancy for woman of normal prepregnant weight is 25–35 pounds (not really "eating for two") ♦ Increased caloric intake of 300 kcal/day sufficient during pregnancy (usually includes 1–2 additional servings of milk and 1 additional serving of meat or a protein alternative) ♦ MyPyramid may be used for planning a nutritionally balanced diet.

Specifics

Dairy normally 2–3 servings daily; increase to 4 servings during pregnancy (1 serving = 1 cup [c] milk or yogurt, 1.5 ounces [oz] hard cheese, 2 c cottage cheese, 1 c pudding made from milk) ♦ **Bread, cereal, rice, & pasta group** 6–11 servings daily (1 serving = 1 slice of bread, 1/2 hamburger roll, 1 oz dry cereal, 1 tortilla, 1/2 c pasta, rice, or grits) ♦ **Fruits** 2–4 servings including at least 1 good source of vitamin C (1 serving = 1 medium size piece of fruit or 1/2 cup juice) ♦ **Vegetables** 3–5 servings vegetables such as tomatoes may also serve as a good source of vitamin C (1 serving = 1/2 cup cooked vegetables, 1 c raw vegetables,

(continued)

TEACHING WARNING SIGNS DURING PREGNANCY

Warning Signs: *Possible Causes*

Sudden gush of fluid from vagina: possible premature rupture of membranes (PROM) ♦ *Vaginal bleeding:* placenta previa or abruptio placentae, cervical lesion, bloody show ♦ *Abdominal pain:* PROM, abruptio placentae, preeclampsia ♦ *Fever at least 101F (38.3C):* infection ♦ *Dizziness, blurred vision, double vision, spots before eyes:* high blood pressure, preeclampsia ♦ *Persistent vomiting:* hyperemesis gravidarum ♦ *Severe headache:* hypertension, preeclampsia ♦ *Edema of hands, face, legs, feet:* preeclampsia ♦ *Muscular irritability, convulsions:* preeclampsia, eclampsia ♦ *Epigastric pain:* preeclampsia, ischemia in major abdominal vessels ♦ *Oliguria* (decreased urination): renal impairment, decreased fluid intake ♦ *Dysuria* (painful urination): urinary tract infection ♦ *Decrease or absence of fetal movement:* maternal medication, obesity, fetal death

(continued)

While Being Monitored

If the woman remains in bed, it is best if she lies on her left side ♦ The right side may also be used ♦ Monitoring can be done while the woman is sitting up in a chair or rocker ♦ Monitoring may continue while the woman ambulates if a telemetry unit is used

Normal Findings with Electric Fetal Monitoring

Normal fetal heart rate baseline between 110 and 160 beats per minute ♦ Variability is present, and average ♦ Accelerations of FHR occur with fetal movement ♦ Early decelerations may be present (indicate pressure of fetal head on the cervix) ♦ Absence of late and/or variable decelerations

Indications of Possible Nonreassuring Fetal Stress

Sustained fetal heart rate baseline below 110 beats/min (bradycardia) or above 160 beats/min (tachycardia) ♦ Decreased variability ♦ Development of periodic decelerations (late or variable) ♦ Meconium-stained amniotic fluid ♦ Signs of nonreassuring fetal status not always clear

Interventions That May Be Used When There Is Possible Nonreassuring Fetal Status

As a result of changes in the FHR pattern, the maternal position may be changed from one side to the other, oxygen administered by face mask ♦ An IV may be started, or, if one is in place, the rate may be increased ♦ Blood pressure is checked more frequently to identify hypotension pitocin should be discontinued.

AWHONN standards) during labor (monitor the woman's vital signs, the uterine contraction pattern, and the fetal heart rate) ♦ Explain assessments and the results (prior to vaginal examinations, explain what will be done and validate the woman's discomfort during the examination) ♦ Assist the woman in pushing when the first stage is completed and the woman has a natural urge to push

Essential Points

Remember that the woman (couple) has the right to determine what happens, and the nurse acts as an advocate when needed ♦ The nurse should be prepared to act as an advocate for analgesia and anesthesia if the woman requests it, regardless of her social status ♦ The nurse should be available to the couple during labor and birth and supportive ♦ Request privacy during the labor and birth if desired

before and cool down after exercising ♦ Wear supportive shoes and supportive bra ♦ Stop exercising if the following signs and symptoms develop: extreme fatigue, dizziness or faintness, sudden sharp pain, difficulty in breathing, nausea and vomiting, pain, vaginal bleeding, excessive muscle soreness; contact caregiver if symptoms persist

Basic Body Conditioning Exercises

Pelvic tilt to reduce back strain and strengthen abdominal muscles (may be done standing, on hands and knees, or lying down) ♦ Exercises to strengthen abdominal tone: abdominal muscle tightening, partial sit-ups (knees must be flexed and feet flat on the floor) ♦ Kegel exercises to improve perineal muscle tone ♦ Tailor sitting to prepare inner thigh muscles for birth

Teaching in the Home

The home provides an excellent setting because the family members are in their own territory and may feel more in control of the visit; the nurse is a visitor ♦ During the introduction, observe family relationships and communication style. Who is the greeter? Who makes the decisions? Who asks the questions and how is information shared? Who is the primary caretaker of the infant? How are siblings incorporated into care of the new baby? ♦ During the assessment of the mother and newborn, continue to provide information regarding findings of each assessment and encourage mother to ask questions ♦ Ask for return demonstrations when appropriate and maintain a supportive environment in which they may occur ♦ Make referrals to appropriate healthcare professionals or agencies as needed ♦ Carry a listing of resources in your community so information can be easily shared ♦ Assist the family in problem solving and locating special resources or in meeting healthcare needs ♦ Act as an advocate for healthcare that meets the needs of the mother, child, and new family

TEACHING NURSING CARE DURING LABOR

During Admission the Birthing Room Nurse Will

Welcome the laboring woman and her partner/support person(s) ♦ Obtain a brief history: include questions regarding woman's physical and psychologic safety and history of domestic violence; provide privacy (just the woman and the nurse for this section of the history) ♦ Assess maternal vital signs, contraction status, membrane status, and fetal heart rate ♦ Perform a vaginal examination if no bleeding is present (provides information about cervical dilatation and effacement; status of amniotic membranes; fetal position, presentation, and station) ♦ Explain findings and answer questions ♦ Orient woman to environment ♦ Establish rapport

During Ongoing Care the Birthing Room Nurse Will

Stay with the woman to provide comfort and reassurance ♦ Be available to assist the woman (couple) with breathing techniques and relaxation ♦ Provide comfort measures such as backrubs, lotion rubs, effleurage, distraction, visualization, music, use of focal point, Therapeutic Touch, coaching, encouragement, perineal care, showers, whirlpool tubs, ambulation, positioning ♦ Provide encouragement and support for the partner/support person ♦ Assess the woman and her fetus on an ongoing basis (according to

(continued)

TEACHING ABOUT FETAL HEART RATE MONITORING

Purpose of Fetal Monitor During Labor and Birth

Provides a useful continuous assessment of numerous characteristics of the fetal heart rate ♦ May indicate the development of nonreassuring fetal status

Types of Fetal Heart Rate Monitoring

Auscultation using special equipment such as a fetoscope (performed intermittently) ♦ Intermittent monitoring by a handheld Doppler ultrasound device ♦ Continuous monitoring by electronic fetal monitor (EFM); the EFM may also be used intermittently, either externally or internally

What to Expect from the Electronic Fetal Monitor

The uterine contraction pattern and the fetal heart rate will be recorded continuously on special graph paper ♦ The nurse and physician or certified nurse-midwife will evaluate the tracing periodically ♦ A light on the front of the monitor will blink with each beat of the fetal heart ♦ A sound dial can be adjusted so that a beep is heard with each fetal heartbeat ♦ The actual count of the fetal heart rate at each moment is displayed on a digital screen ♦ At any moment, the fetal heartbeat is recorded on the graph paper, is heard as a beep, and is seen as a blink of light and on the digital display

(continued)

TEACHING HOME CARE OF THE POSTPARTAL FAMILY

When possible the nurse prepares for the home visit by establishing contact and a beginning relationship with the family while they are still in the birthing center or hospital setting ♦ Purposes of the home visit are to assess maternal, neonatal, and family status, to provide teaching, and to make referrals as needed

Fostering a Caring Relationship with the Family

Introduce yourself to the family ♦ Address family members by their surnames until invited to use the given name ♦ Ask to be introduced to other family members ♦ Ask for permission before sitting ♦ Be genuine; make sure your verbal and nonverbal messages are congruent; do not make assumptions; demonstrate caring behaviors; answer questions honestly and thoroughly; provide opportunity for family members to ask further questions for clarification; provide opportunity for return demonstration if needed ♦ Demonstrate empathy; listen to the family without judgment; be attentive; listen to the family's perspective ♦ Establish trust; do what you say you will do; be on time; be prepared for the visit; provide any follow-up as needed; provide information about community resources

(continued)

TEACHING ABOUT EXERCISE DURING PREGNANCY

Value of Regular Exercise During Pregnancy

Improves maternal fitness and muscle tone ♦ Relieves stress, improves sleep ♦ Helps control weight gain ♦ Promotes more rapid recovery following birth ♦ Promotes sense of well-being ♦ May help prevent certain complications

Choosing the Best Exercise

In general, continue any exercise at which woman is proficient ♦ Avoid learning new, strenuous sports ♦ Avoid high-risk activities or sports that require good balance and coordination ♦ Walking is excellent exercise choice. Non-weight-bearing activities (swimming, cycling) may be more comfortable as pregnancy progresses ♦ When in doubt, contact caregiver

Basic Guidelines for Exercise During Pregnancy

Exercise regularly, most days of the week if possible ♦ Avoid exercising while lying supine ♦ Decrease intensity of exercise as pregnancy progresses and stop when fatigued ♦ Avoid high-risk activities or activities that require good balance and coordination ♦ Avoid prolonged overheating ♦ If woman is unable to talk or feels unable to breathe, exercise is too intense ♦ Warm up

(continued)

TEACHING ABOUT COMMON DISCOMFORTS OF PREGNANCY

General Information about Common Discomforts

Caused by hormonal changes, especially elevated levels of human chorionic gonadotropin (hCG), estrogen, and progesterone, and/or anatomic changes such as enlarged uterus or engorged breasts ♦ Not all discomforts experienced by all women ♦ Generally not health threatening

Self-Care Measures for Relief of Common Discomforts

Nausea and vomiting: eat crackers or dry toast before arising; avoid causative foods and odors; eat small, frequent meals and dry foods with fluids between meals; avoid greasy or highly seasoned foods ♦ *Urinary frequency:* void when urge experienced; increase fluid intake during day ♦ *Breast tenderness:* wear well-fitting, supportive bra ♦ *Increased vaginal discharge:* bathe regularly; avoid douching, nylon underpants, and panty hose; wear cotton underwear; use powder to maintain dryness (light layer; avoid caking) ♦ *Nasal stuffiness and epistaxis* (nosebleed): avoid use of medicated nasal sprays and decongestants; use cool-air vaporizer (may be unresponsive to treatment) or normal saline sprays ♦ *Ptyalism*

(continued)

TEACHING SAFETY CONSIDERATIONS DURING HOME VISITS

Currently, communities are quite complex, and the safety of the nurse may be a concern

Follow Basic Safety Rules

Be aware of your personal body carriage; carry yourself with a sense of determination that demonstrates that you know where you are going and are in charge of yourself (stand straight, shoulders square; appear sure of yourself; look forward); have a determined, steady stance and gait; avoid appearing hesitant, confused, or lost ♦ Establish contact with the family prior to the visit; clearly identify the address and specific characteristics and identifying factors that will enable you to find the family's home ♦ Ask the family for directions ♦ Carry a map and trace out the route on the map prior to the visit ♦ Be sure to take the map along and leave it out of sight from passing cars; if you need to look at the map, do so unobtrusively to avoid drawing attention to yourself (remember, you want to appear as if you are in charge) ♦ Prior to your visit, notify someone of where you are going and when you expect to return ♦ Prior to your visit, remove personal items from the interior of your car and lock them in your trunk ♦ Carry a fully charged cell phone ♦ Wear a name

(continued)

TEACHING BREATHING TECHNIQUES FOR LABOR

Essentials of the Lamaze Method

Involves three patterns of chest breathing ♦ One pattern is maintained until no longer effective, then woman moves to the next pattern ♦ Breathing with each contraction begins and ends with a cleansing breath (inhale through nose and exhale through pursed lips)

First Pattern

Begin with a cleansing breath ♦ Inhale slowly through nose, lift chest up and out during inhalation ♦ Exhale through pursed lips ♦ Maintain breathing rate of 6–9 breaths per minute (2 breaths every 15 seconds) ♦ End with a cleansing breath

Second Pattern

Begin with a cleansing breath, then push out a short breath at the end of this inhalation ♦ Inhale and exhale through mouth at a rate of about 4 breaths every 5 seconds ♦ Keep jaw relaxed and mouth slightly open ♦ End with a cleansing breath

(continued)

CERVICAL DILATATION ASSESSMENT GUIDE

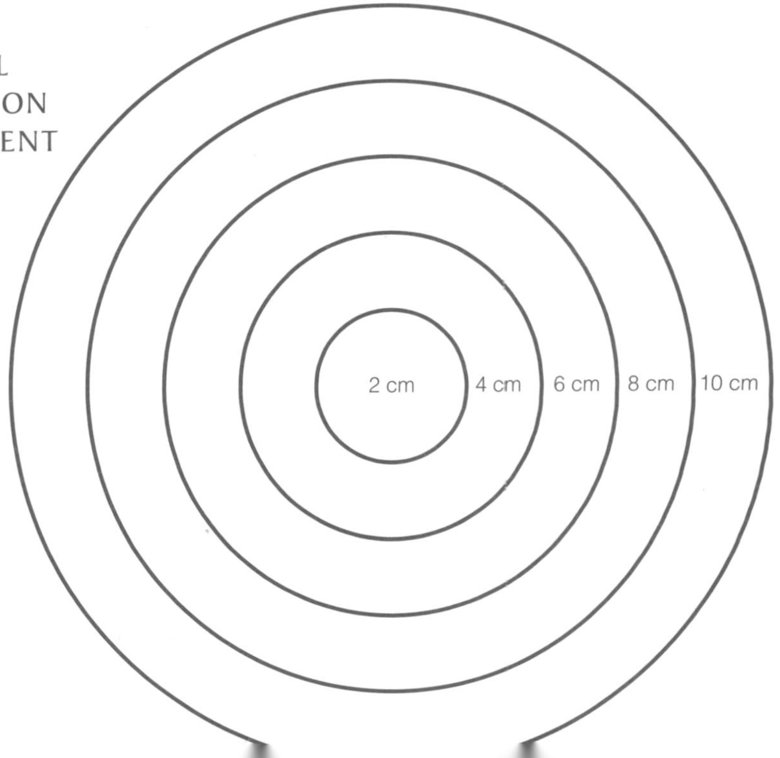

tag that identifies you as a professional nurse ♦ Do not wear expensive jewelry ♦ Always carry enough change so that you can make a phone call from a pay phone if necessary or phone card ♦ Carry needed phone numbers with you in an easily accessible place ♦ If you are very uncomfortable with the location of the home or have concerns for your safety, pay attention to your feelings and leave; contact the family immediately and arrange another appointment at a time when another nurse can accompany you ♦ It is important to follow your intuition

(excessive salivation): use astringent mouthwash; suck on hard candy ♦ *Heartburn:* eat small, more frequent meals; take low-sodium antacids; avoid overeating, fatty and fried foods, lying down after eating, and sodium bicarbonate ♦ *Ankle edema:* elevate legs frequently; dorsiflex feet when standing; avoid tight garters or constricting bands ♦ *Varicose veins:* elevate legs; wear support hose; do not cross legs, wear tight garters, or stand for long periods ♦ *Hemorrhoids:* gently reinsert into rectum as necessary; avoid constipation; use ice packs, topical ointments, anesthetic agents, warm soaks, or sitz baths ♦ *Constipation:* increase fluid intake; eat high-fiber diet; get regular exercise; develop regular bowel habits; use stool softeners as recommended by caregiver ♦ *Backache:* perform good body mechanics; do pelvic-tilt exercise; avoid uncomfortable working heights, high-heel shoes, heavy lifting, and fatigue ♦ *Leg cramps:* dorsiflex foot to stretch affected muscle; apply heat to affected muscle; evaluate diet ♦ *Faintness:* arise slowly from resting position; avoid prolonged standing in warm or stuffy environments ♦ *Dyspnea* (shortness of breath): maintain proper posture when sitting and standing; sleep propped up on pillows if dyspnea occurs at night ♦ *Flatulence:* avoid gas-forming foods; chew food thoroughly; get regular daily exercise; maintain normal bowel habits ♦ *Carpal tunnel syndrome:* avoid aggravating hand movements; use splint as prescribed; elevate affected arm

Third Pattern

Breathe rapidly and shallowly with periodic forced exhalations ♦ Draw lips back to the teeth and make a "Hee" sound during exhalation ♦ Then purse lips and exhale, making a "Hoo" sound ♦ Begin with a pattern of 4 breaths (Hee, Hee, Hee, Hoo) and, as contractions become more intense, change pattern to 3 breaths (Hee, Hee, Hoo), then 2 breaths (Hee, Hoo)

Pushing Breaths

Begin with a cleansing breath ♦ Breathe in 2 additional breaths and, holding them, push down on the perineum ♦ Visualize pushing down through the vagina ♦ Exhale during the pushing effort or hold breath, whichever is more comfortable

TEACHING INITIAL POSTPARTUM CARE

Checking the Uterine Fundus

Determine location of the fundus (normally at umbilicus or one finger breadth above within hours of birth; descends at rate of about one finger breadth per day for first 10–14 days) ♦ Assess position and consistency (affected by distention of bladder, presence of infection, breastfeeding, ambulation, and retention of products of conception) ♦ Gently massage the fundus to alleviate atonic (boggy) uterus ♦ Report recurrence of bogginess to the caregiver immediately

How to Apply Perineal Pads

Apply from front to back ♦ Change after voiding or whenever they are soiled

Caring for the Perineum

Use perineal spray, rinse bottle, or cleansing pads and pat dry with toilet paper ♦ Always clean from front (at the symphysis pubis) to back (around the anus) ♦ May apply witch hazel pads or analgesia sprays

(continued)

TEACHING RESUMPTION OF SEXUAL ACTIVITY AFTER BIRTH

When to Resume Sexual Activity

Couples advised to abstain from intercourse until the episiotomy is healed and the lochial flow has stopped (usually by end of 3rd week). Many practitions advise women to wait for 6 weeks.

The Woman May Experience

Some vaginal dryness for the first few weeks ♦ Difficulty feeling excitement because of fatigue associated with newborn care (moreover, her partner may be unaware of the extreme fatigue she may be experiencing because of the demands of newborn care and her recovery from childbirth) ♦ Awkwardness if there is a leakage of breast milk during sexual activity ♦ Vaginal tenderness ♦ Fear of pain during intercourse ♦ Fear of another pregnancy

(continued)

TEACHING POSTPARTUM WARNING SIGNS

Warning Signs: Possible Causes

Alterations in pattern of lochia (increased amount, change from lochia alba to serosa or from lochia serosa to rubra, and/or presence of clots): possible uterine infection or uterine relaxation ♦ *Development of foul-smelling lochia:* uterine infection ♦ *Maternal temperature elevation above 38C (100.4F):* infection ♦ *Constant uterine tenderness:* infection ♦ *Failure of fundus to descend as expected:* uterine infection or subinvolution ♦ *Continued or increased discomfort in the episiotomy site* (separation of the suture line, development of swelling, increased tenderness, or presence of whitish or gray-green discharge at the site of episiotomy): infection or incomplete approximation of sutures ♦ *Tenderness, swelling, and warmth in any area of the legs:* thrombophlebitis ♦ *Swelling, warmth, and tenderness in any area of the breast:* clogged milk ducts or mastitis

If a Warning Sign Develops

Call caregiver immediately ♦ Note specific information about the sign: length of time it has been present, related problems, or activities, and specific characteristics of the problem

TEACHING BREASTFEEDING

Basics of Milk Production

Milk produced according to demand ♦ Milk stored in ducts under areola ♦ Adequate maternal fluid intake required ♦ Milk supply established by frequent breastfeeding (every 1 1/2 to 3 hours) ♦ Let-down reflex: flow of milk initiated by newborn's sucking, presence, or cry; by mother's thoughts; or during maternal orgasm

Positioning Baby at the Breast

Turn baby's entire body toward mother, with mouth adjacent to nipple and the ear; shoulder and hip are in direct alignment ♦ Mother should assume a comfortable position with arms supported ♦ Direct nipple straight into baby's mouth so that during sucking, jaw compresses ducts directly beneath areola ♦ Lightly brush infant's mouth with breast to stimulate rooting reflex (but avoid touching both cheeks)

(continued)

Beginning Ambulation

Call for assistance the first time ♦ Anticipate some dizziness

Changes in the Lochia

Lochia dark red (lochia rubra) for first 1–3 days (similar to menstrual flow) ♦ Lochia pinkish brown or serous (lochia serosa) after 2–3 days ♦ Moderate flow (use of 4–8 perineal pads per day) and small clots normal ♦ *Signs of possible problems:* increase in amount, change from serosa back to rubra, presence of larger clots, change in odor

Procedure for Feeding

Avoid arbitrary time limits (since let-down reflex may take up to 3 minutes) ♦ Allow baby to suckle at first breast until breast is emptied ♦ Insert finger in baby's mouth near nipple to break suction ♦ Burp baby before changing breast ♦ Burp baby again at completion of feeding ♦ To prevent skin breakdown wash nipple with warm water and dry thoroughly

Helpful Hints

Be certain baby is well awake before attempting feeding ♦ Alternate breast at which baby begins feeding (use safety pin as reminder) ♦ Lift breast slightly or press lightly on breast above nares if mother's large breast occludes infant's nares ♦ Rotate baby's position at breast to avoid undue trauma to nipples and improve emptying of ducts ♦ Avoid supplementary formula feedings until lactation is established ♦ Check with caregiver before taking any medication while breastfeeding (because medications may cross into breast milk)

The Partner May Experience

Fear of the postpartum partner being uncomfortable during sexual activity, particularly intercourse ♦ Disruption of the sexual pattern the couple had established ♦ Fear of partner becoming pregnant again ♦ Reduced interest in sex because of fatigue associated with newborn care

Contraceptive Considerations

Determine the couple's desires regarding contraceptive information ♦ If needed and desired, present factual information regarding different types of contraceptives ♦ Inform couple that 40% of *nonlactating* mothers resume menstruation by the 6th week after birth, and 45% of *lactating* mothers resume menstruation by the 12th week after birth ♦ Breastfeeding does not provide adequate protection against pregnancy because milk is superheated and plastic bottle bags may burst; use "defrost" setting on microwave oven and carefully check temperature of formula before feeding

Positioning the Baby for Feeding

Hold baby close, establishing eye contact as in breastfeeding ♦ Hold baby's bottom or foot firmly, keeping his or her back straight to aid digestion and provide a sense of security ♦ Quiet baby before feeding ♦ Alternate the side baby is fed from to give baby two-sided stimulation ♦ Avoid feeding while baby is on his or her back ♦ Do not prop the bottle

Procedure for Feeding

Nipple hole should allow only drops of milk to flow ♦ Keep nipple full with milk to decrease air ingestion

How to Burp a Baby

Position baby so his or her head rests on mother's shoulder or face down on lap, or sit baby on lap with baby's chin and chest supported ♦ Gently pat or stroke baby's back ♦ Burp baby halfway through feeding and at end of feeding ♦ Learn baby's preferred burping position and whether baby is a slow or quick burper ♦ Regurgitation of small amounts of formula is common ♦ Have burp cloth available

of greenish-yellow material, or reddened areas ♦ Expect tenderness around the cord and darkening and shriveling of cord ♦ A small drop of blood may be present when cord falls off ♦ Never pull on cord or attempt to loosen it ♦ If cultural custom demands binding of the abdomen, a sanitary method such as the use of a clean piece of gauze can be recommended.

Circumcision Care

Squeeze warm water over circumcision with each diaper change ♦ Rinse area off with warm water and pat dry ♦ Apply small amount of petroleum ointment (unless a Plastibell is in place) with each diaper change ♦ Fasten diaper loosely over penis ♦ Since the glans is sensitive, avoid placing baby on his stomach ♦ Check for any foul-smelling drainage, bleeding, swelling or cessation of urination at least once a day ♦ Let Plastibell fall off by itself (about 8 days after circumcision); ♦ Plastibell should not be pulled off, after 8 days have parents consult their health care provider. Light, sticky, yellow film or granulation tissue (part of healing process) may form over head of penis

Uncircumcision Care

Clean uncircumcised penis with water during diaper changes and with bath ♦ Do not force foreskin back over the penis; foreskin will retract normally over time (may take 3–5 years)

How many births have you had?	¿Cuantos niños le han nacido?
I will help you.	La voy a ayudar.
I need to examine your [breasts, uterus, flow, stitches, legs, feet, baby].	Necesito examinarle [los pechos, el útero, el flujo, los puntos, las piernas, los pies, su bebé].
I would like to take your [blood pressure, pulse, temperature].	Quisiera tomarle [la presió arterial, el pulso, la temperatura].
Are you taking any medications now?	¿Está tomando algunas medicinas ahora?
Please pant. I will show you how.	Por favor, jade. Le voy a mostrar cómo.
Do not push now.	No puje ahora.
Push now.	Puje ahora.
Stop pushing.	Pare de pujar.
	No puje mád.
Please turn on your left side.	Por favor voltéese al lado izquierdo.
Your baby is OK.	El bebé está bien.

Techniques for Quieting Baby

Check for soiled diaper ♦ Swaddle or bundle baby (bring arms and legs into midline, which increases sense of security) ♦ Hold swaddled baby upright against mid-chest supporting the buttock and the back of baby's head. ♦ Use slow, calming movements with baby ♦ Softly talk, sing, or hum to baby ♦ Baby can hear heartbeat, feel warmth, and hear parent's softly spoken words or calming sounds.

TEACHING INFANT DISCHARGE CARE

Immediate Safety Measures for the Newborn

Watch for excessive mucus: use bulb syringe to remove secretions ♦ Keep newborn on his or her back in crib or in someone's arms ♦ Avoid leaving newborn unattended in parent's room ♦ Always check that ID bands or sensor is in place when transporting newborn.

Voiding and Stool Characteristics and Patterns

At least 6–10 wet diapers per day after first few days of life ♦ Urine straw to amber color without foul smell ♦ Normal progression of stool changes: (1) meconium (thick, tarry, dark green); (2) transitional stools (thin, brown to green); (3a) breastfed infant: yellow gold, soft or mushy stools; (3b) formula-fed infant: pale yellow, formed and pasty stools ♦ Only 1–2 stools a day for formula-fed baby ♦ 6–10 small, loose yellow stools per day or only one stool every few days after breastfeeding is well established (after about 1 month)

Umbilical Cord Care

Clean cord and skin around base with a cotton swab or cotton ball ♦ Clean 2–3 times a day or with each diaper change ♦ Do not give tub baths until cord falls off in 7–14 days ♦ Fold diaper below umbilical cord to let the cord air-dry ♦ Check each day for any odor, oozing

(continued)

TEACHING NEWBORN FORMULA-FEEDING

Types of Formula

Ready-to-feed: use directly from the can ♦ Concentrate: dilute with water before feeding ♦ Powder: add water and mix well for proper concentration

Amount of Formula

Start with 3 oz in each bottle (since a newborn usually takes 1–3 oz every 2 1/2 to 4 hours) ♦ Expect increases in baby's appetite with demand feeding (as baby needs more he or she will start finishing each bottle) ♦ Do not feed the baby a partially used bottle after 1 hour at room temperature ♦ Prepare a fresh bottle for each feeding: do not add new formula to old ♦ Refrigerate bottles made in advance ♦ Do not feed the baby an opened, refrigerated can of concentrated or ready-to-feed formula after 48 hours ♦ Travel with water and formula separated—carry the premeasured water bottles and bottles with premeasured amounts of powdered formula, or carry premeasured commercially prepared formula packets

Temperature of Formula

Mother can try a bottle directly from the refrigerator, but most babies prefer warm formula, close in temperature to breast milk ♦ Warm bottle under hot tap water, in bottle warmer, or in pan of heated water ♦ Always test temperature of formula by sprinkling a few drops on wrist ♦ BE VERY CAREFUL if using a microwave oven to warm formula,

(continued)

TEACHING TECHNIQUES FOR WAKING AND QUIETING NEWBORNS

Using Waking Techniques

When getting ready for feeding ♦ During feeding if baby is sleepy or goes to sleep ♦ To alter baby's feeding schedule

Techniques for Waking Baby

Loosen clothing, change diaper ♦ Hand express milk onto baby's lips ♦ Talk with baby while making eye contact ♦ Hold baby in upright position (sitting or standing) ♦ Have baby do sit-ups (gently and rhythmically bend baby back and forth while grasping baby under his or her knees and supporting baby's head and back with your other hand) ♦ Play patty-cake with baby ♦ Stimulate rooting reflex (brush one cheek with hand or nipple) ♦ Increase skin contact (gently rub hands and feet)

Use Quieting Techniques

In first months after birth ♦ With a baby who is easily stimulated and excited ♦ To calm an excited baby before feeding ♦ With an overly hungry or overeager baby

(continued)

COMMUNICATING WITH A CLIENT WHO SPEAKS SPANISH

Tips

♦ In Spanish, nouns and adjectives that end in *a* indicate female gender, whereas nouns and adjectives that end in *o* indicate male gender ♦ Most often, the stress in Spanish words is placed on the second-to-last syllable

♦ *ay* is pronounced like the word *eye* ♦ *ll* is pronounced *y* ♦ *cu* is pronounced *qu* ♦ *qu* is pronounced *k* ♦ *h* is silent ♦ *v* is pronounced *b* ♦ *j* is pronounced *h* ♦ *z* is pronounced *s*

Helpful Words and Phrases

Hello	Hola
I am a student nurse.	Soy estudiante de enfermería.
My name is _____ .	Mi nombre es _____ .
What is your name?	¿Cómo se llama?
Please	Por favor
Thank you	Gracias
Is there anything worrying you?	¿Hay algo o alguna cosa que la preocupe?
Are you having pain?	¿Tiene dolores?

(continued)